International Handbook of
Traumatic
Stress Syndromes

The Plenum Series on Stress and Coping

Series Editor:

Donald Meichenbaum, *University of Waterloo, Waterloo, Ontario, Canada*

Editorial Board: Bruce P. Dohrenwend, *Columbia University*
Marianne Frankenhaeuser, *University of Stockholm*
Norman Garmezy, *University of Minnesota*
Mardi J. Horowitz, *University of California Medical School,*
San Francisco
Richard S. Lazarus, *University of California, Berkeley*
Michael Rutter, *University of London*
Dennis C. Turk, *University of Pittsburgh*
John P. Wilson, *Cleveland State University*
Camille Wortman, *University of Michigan*

Current Volumes in the Series:

A CLINICAL GUIDE TO THE TREATMENT OF THE
HUMAN STRESS RESPONSE
George S. Everly, Jr.

COMBAT STRESS REACTION
The Enduring Toll of War
Zahava Solomon

COPING WITH NEGATIVE LIFE EVENTS
Clinical and Social Psychological Perspectives
Edited by C. R. Snyder and Carol E. Ford

DYNAMICS OF STRESS
Physiological, Psychological, and Social Perspectives
Edited by Mortimer H. Appley and Richard Trumbull

HUMAN ADAPTATION TO EXTREME STRESS
From the Holocaust to Vietnam
Edited by John P. Wilson, Zev Harel, and Boaz Kahana

INFERTILITY
Perspectives from Stress and Coping Research
Edited by Annette L. Stanton and Christine Dunkel-Schetter

INTERNATIONAL HANDBOOK OF TRAUMATIC STRESS SYNDROMES
Edited by John P. Wilson and Beverley Raphael

POST-TRAUMATIC STRESS DISORDER
A Clinician's Guide
Kirtland C. Peterson, Maurice F. Prout, and Robert A. Schwarz

THE SOCIAL CONTEXT OF COPING
Edited by John Eckenrode

STRESS BETWEEN WORK AND FAMILY
Edited by John Eckenrode and Susan Gore

THE UNNOTICED MAJORITY IN INPATIENT PSYCHIATRIC CARE
Charles A. Kiesler and Celeste G. Simpkins

WOMEN, WORK, AND HEALTH
Stress and Opportunities
Edited by Marianne Frankenhaeuser, Ulf Lundberg, and Margaret Chesney

A Continuation Order Plan is available for this series. A continuation order will bring delivery of each new volume immediately upon publication. Volumes are billed only upon actual shipment. For further information please contact the publisher.

International Handbook of
Traumatic Stress
Syndromes

Edited by

John P. Wilson
Cleveland State University
Cleveland, Ohio

and

Beverley Raphael
University of Queensland
Herston, Australia

Plenum Press • New York and London

Library of Congress Cataloging-in-Publication Data

International handbook of traumatic stress syndromes / edited by John
P. Wilson and Beverley Raphael.
     p.   cm. -- (The Plenum series on stress and coping)
   Includes bibliographical references and index.
   ISBN 0-306-43795-3
   1. Post-traumatic stress disorder.   I. Wilson, John P. (John
Preston) II. Raphael, Beverley. III. Series.
   [DNLM: 1. Stress Disorders, Post-Traumatic.   WM 172 I6053]
RC552.P67I58 1993
616.85'21--dc20
DNLM/DLC
for Library of Congress   92-49117
                                                               CIP

ISBN 0-306-43795-3

© 1993 Plenum Press, New York
A Division of Plenum Publishing Corporation
233 Spring Street, New York, N.Y. 10013

Printed in the United States of America

To our families

Cassie Rickarby

Matthew Wilson
Michael Wilson

Andrew Colwell
Rachel Colwell

And to the children of the future

Contributors

Inger Agger
Department of Social Studies and
    Organization
Aalborg University
DK-9220 Aalborg, Denmark

David Alan Alexander
Department of Mental Health
University of Aberdeen Medical School,
    Foresterhill
Aberdeen AB 2ZD, Scotland

Ofra Ayalon
School of Education
University of Haifa
Haifa 31999, Israel

Jorge Barros-Beck
Centre Hospitalier Spécialisé
Rouffach 68250, France

Andrew Baum
Department of Psychology
Uniformed Services University of the Health
    Sciences
Bethesda, Maryland 20814

P. Bell
Mater Infirmorum Hospital
Crumlin Road
Belfast BT 14 6 AB, Northern Ireland

Leonard Bickman
Department of Psychology and Human
    Development
George Peabody College of Vanderbilt
    University
Nashville, Tennessee 37203

Dora Black
Department of Child and Adolescent
    Psychiatry
Royal Free Hospital
Pond Street
London NW3, England

Richard Douglas Blackwell
Medical Foundation for the Care of Victims
    of Torture
96–98 Grafton Road
London NW5 3EJ, England

Edward Blanchard
Department of Psychology
State University of New York at Albany
Albany, New York 12222

Arthur S. Blank, Jr.
Readjustment Counseling Service (10B/RC)
Department of Veterans Affairs
Washington, DC 20420

Bennett G. Braun
Center on Psychiatric Trauma and
    Dissociation
Rush Institute of Mental Well-Being
Rush-Presbyterian-St. Luke's Medical
    Center
Chicago, Illinois 60612

Joel Osler Brende
Martin Army Community Hospital
Fort Benning, Georgia 31905;
Adult Outpatient Services
The Bradley Center, Inc.
Columbus, Georgia 31907; and
Department of Psychiatry
Mercer School of Medicine
Macon, Georgia 31206

Elizabeth A. Brett
Department of Psychiatry
Yale University
New Haven, Connecticut 06511

William Buckingham
Office of Psychiatric Services
Health Department
Melbourne, Victoria 3000, Australia

Renate Grønvold Bugge
Vest-Agder Sentralsykehus
4600 Kristiansand South, Norway

Ann W. Burgess
Department of Psychiatric Mental Health
    Nursing
University of Pennsylvania School of
    Nursing
Philadelphia, Pennsylvania 19104

Philip Burgess
Psychiatric Epidemiology and Services
    Evaluation Unit
Health Department Victoria
Parkville, Victoria 3052, Australia

Ed Cairns
Department of Psychology and Centre for
    the Study of Conflict
University of Ulster
Coleraine, Londonderry BT52 1SA,
    Northern Ireland

Stephen R. Couch
Department of Sociology
Pennsylvania State University
Schuylkill Haven, Pennsylvania 17972-2208

Mark Creamer
Health Department Victoria, and
    Department of Psychology
University of Melbourne
Parkville, Victoria 3052, Australia

Marc-Antoine Crocq
Centre Hospitalier Spécialisé
Rouffach 68250, France

Margaret Cunningham
Service for the Treatment and Rehabilitation
    of Torture and Trauma Survivors
28 Nelson Street
Fairfield, New South Wales 2165, Australia

Peter S. Curran
Mater Infirmorum Hospital
Crumlin Road
Belfast BT 14 6 AB, Northern Ireland

Yael Danieli
Group Project for Holocaust Survivors and
    Their Children
345 East 80th Street, Apt. 31-J
New York, New York 10021

Giovanni de Girolamo
Division of Mental Health
World Health Organization
1211 Geneva 27, Switzerland

Jan H. M. de Groen
Department of Clinical Neurophysiology
University of Limburg School of Medicine
6200 MD Maastricht, Netherlands

Owen Dent
Department of Sociology
Australian National University
Acton 2601, Australia

Fabrice Duval
Centre Hospitalier Spécialisé
Rouffach 68250, France

Atle Dyregrov
Center for Crisis Psychology
Fabrikkgt 5
5037 Solheimsvik, Norway

Leo Eitinger
Ö Ullern Terr. 67
0380 Oslo 3, Norway

Liisa Eränen
Department of Social Psychology
University of Helsinki
SF-00100 Helsinki, Finland

George S. Everly, Jr.
Health Psychology Laboratory, Loyola
    College
Baltimore, Maryland, and
Psychological Services and Behavioral
    Medicine
Homewood Hospital Center, The Johns
    Hopkins Health System
204 Glenmore Avenue
Catonsville, Maryland 21228

Paul R. J. Falger
Department of Medical Psychology
University of Limburg School of Medicine
6200 MD Maastricht, Netherlands

Anthony Feinstein
Institute of Neurology and National
    Hospital for Nervous Diseases
Queen Square
London WC1N 3BG, England

Matthew J. Friedman
National Center for PTSD
Veterans Administration Medical and
    Regional Office Center
White River Junction, Vermont 05009, and
Department of Psychiatry and
    Pharmacology
Dartmouth Medical School
Hanover, New Hampshire 03755

Rob Gordon
Department of Psychology
Royal Children's Hospital
Melbourne, Parkville, Victoria 3052,
    Australia

Caroline Gorst-Unsworth
The Medical Foundation for the Care of
    Victims of Torture
96–98 Grafton Road
London NW5 3EJ, England

Kerry Goulston
Repatriation Hospital
Concord 2139, Australia

Mary C. Grace
Traumatic Stress Study Center
Department of Psychiatry
University of Cincinnati College of Medicine
Cincinnati, Ohio 45267-0539

Arthur Green
Department of Psychiatry
Columbia-Presbyterian Hospital
New York, New York 10032

Bonnie L. Green
Department of Psychiatry
Georgetown University Hospital
Washington, DC 20007

Zev Harel
Department of Social Work and Center on
    Applied Gerontological Research
Cleveland State University
Cleveland, Ohio 44115

Laurie Leydic Harkness
Yale University
Community Support Program and
    Psychiatric Rehabilitation Program
Veterans Administration Medical Center
West Haven, Connecticut 06516

Carol R. Hartman
Department of Psychiatric Mental Health
    Nursing
Boston College School of Nursing
Chestnut Hill, Massachusetts 02167

Jean Harris Hendriks
Department of Child and Adolescent
    Psychiatry
Royal Free Hospital
Pond Street
London NW3, England

Judith Lewis Herman
61 Roseland Street
Somerville, Massachusetts 02143

Arc Holen
Department of Psychiatry
University of Oslo
P.O. Box 85
Vinderen N-0319, Oslo 3, Norway

David J de L Horne
Department of Psychiatry, Clinical Sciences
    Block
University of Melbourne
Victoria 3050, Australia

Mardi J. Horowitz
Department of Psychiatry
University of California
San Francisco, California 94143

Alexandra Hough
St. Thomas' Hospital, London, and
The Medical Foundation for the Care of
    Victims of Torture
96–98 Grafton Road
London NW5 3EJ, England

Johan E. Hovens
Department of Psychiatry
Saint Lucas Hospital
1061 AE Amsterdam, Netherlands

Cao Hua
Department of Psychiatry
Flinders University of South Australia
Bedford Park
South Australia 5042, Australia

Edna J. Hunter
3280 Trumbull Street
San Diego, California 92106

Arthur Hyatt-Williams
Scientific Research and Development
    Branch, Home Office, Research and
    Planning Unit
Queen Anne's Gate
London SW1H 9AT, England

Toshiharu Iwadate
Department of Psychiatry
School of Medicine, Tohoku University
Aoba-ku, Sendai 980, Japan

Tony Jaffa
The Medical Foundation for the Care of
    Victims of Torture, London, and
The Adolescent Community Team
32b York Road
Battersea, London SW11, England

Søren Buus Jensen
Center for Psychosocial and Traumatic
    Stress
Aalborg Psychiatric Hospital
Mølleparkvej 10, Aalborg, Denmark

S. Janet Johnston
Dover Counselling Centre
9 Cambridge Terrace
Dover CT16 1YZ, England

Marianne Juhler
Rehabilitation and Research Center for
    Torture Victims
Juliane Mariesvej 34
2100 Copenhagen 0, Denmark

Boaz Kahana
Department of Psychology and Center on
    Applied Gerontological Research
Cleveland State University
Cleveland, Ohio 44115

Eva Kahana
Department of Sociology and Elderly Care
    Research Center
Case Western Reserve University
Cleveland, Ohio 44106

Tony Kaplan
Department of Child and Adolescent
    Psychiatry
Royal Free Hospital
Pond Street
London NW3, England

Terence M. Keane
Department of Veterans Affairs Medical
    Center
Boston, Massachusetts 02130

Brian Kelly
Department of Psychiatry
Royal Brisbane Hospital
University of Queensland
Herston 4029, Australia

J. David Kinzie
Department of Psychiatry
Oregon Health Sciences University
Portland, Oregon 97201-3098

J. Stephen Kroll-Smith
Department of Sociology
University of New Orleans
New Orleans, Louisiana 70148

Henry Krystal
Michigan Psychoanalytic Institute
26011 Evergreen Road, Suite 206
Southfield, Michigan 48076

Richard A. Kulka
National Opinion Research Center
1155 East 60th Street
Chicago, Illinois 60637

Rima E. Laibow
TREAT
13 Summit Terrace
Dobbs Ferry, New York 10522

Louise J. Lasschuit
Department of Psychiatry
Saint Lucas Hospital
1061 AE Amsterdam, Netherlands

C. Shaffia Laue
346 Maine
Lawrence, Kansas 66044

Robert Laufer
Late Professor of Sociology
Brooklyn College of the City University of
    New York
Brooklyn, New York 11210

Anthony C. Leonard
Traumatic Stress Study Center
Department of Psychiatry
University of Cincinnati College of Medicine
Cincinnati, Ohio 45267-0539

Patti Levin
Trauma Clinic
Massachusetts General Hospital, and
Harvard Medical School
Boston, Massachusetts 02114

Karmela Liebkind
Department of Social Psychology
University of Helsinki
SF-00100 Helsinki, Finland

Robert Jay Lifton
Center on Violence
John Jay College of Criminal Justice
City University of New York
New York, New York 10019

Jacob D. Lindy
Department of Psychiatry and Traumatic
    Stress Study Center
University of Cincinnati Medical School
Cincinnati, Ohio 45267-0539

G. C. Loughrey
Mater Infirmorum Hospital
Crumlin Road
Belfast BT 14 6 AB, Northern Ireland

Tom Lundin
Department of Psychiatry
University Hospital
S-58185 Linköping, Sweden

Jean-Paul Macher
Centre Hospitalier Spécialisé
Rouffach 68250, France

Mona S. Macksoud
Project on Children and War
Center for the Study of Human Rights
Columbia University
New York, New York 10027

Mary Bernadette Manolias
Scientific Research and Development
   Branch, Home Office, Research and
   Planning Unit
Queen Anne's Gate
London SW1H 9AT, England

Bertil Mårdberg
Department of Psychiatry
University Hospital
S-58185 Linköping, Sweden

Alexander Cowell McFarlane
Department of Psychiatry
University of Adelaide
Gilles Plains, South Australia 5086,
   Australia

Noach Milgram
Department of Psychology
Tel-Aviv University
Ramat-Aviv 69978, Israel

Jeffrey T. Mitchell
Emergency Health Services Department
University of Maryland, Baltimore County
   Campus
Catonsville, Maryland 21228

Kathi Nader
Program in Trauma, Violence, and Sudden
   Bereavement
University of California, Los Angeles, and
Neuropsychiatric Institute and Hospital
Center for the Health Sciences
Los Angeles, California 90024

Bahman Najarian
Department of Psychology
University of Shahid Chamran
Ahwaz, Iran

Fran Norris
Department of Psychology
Georgia State University
Atlanta, Georgia 30303

Carol S. North
Department of Psychiatry
Washington University School of Medicine
St. Louis, Missouri 63110

Frank M. Ochberg
Department of Psychiatry
Michigan State University
East Lansing, Michigan 48824

Tsunemoto Ōdaira
Department of Psychiatry
School of Medicine, Tohoku University
Aoba-ku, Sendai 980, Japan

Wybrand Op den Velde
Department of Psychiatry
Saint Lucas Hospital
1061 AE Amsterdam, Netherlands

Roderick Jan Ørner
North Lincolnshire Health Authority
Baverstock House, County Hospital
St. Anne's Road
Lincoln LN4 2HN, England

Ulf Otto
Department of Psychiatry
University Hospital
S-58185 Linköping, Sweden

Erwin Randolph Parson
P.O. Box 62
Perry Point, Maryland 21902–0062

Philippa Pattison
Department of Psychology
University of Melbourne
Parkville, Victoria 3052, Australia

Robert S. Pynoos
Program in Trauma, Violence, and Sudden
   Bereavement
University of California, Los Angeles, and
Neuropsychiatric Institute and Hospital
Center for the Health Sciences
Los Angeles, California 90024

Beverley Raphael
Department of Psychiatry
Royal Brisbane Hospital
University of Queensland
Herston 4029, Australia

Magne Raundalen
Asligrenda 8
5095 Ulset, Norway

John Reid
Oregon Social Learning Center
207 East 5th Avenue
Eugene, Oregon 97401

Robert F. Rich
Institute of Government and Public Affairs
University of Illinois
Urbana, Illinois 61801

Derek Roger
Department of Psychology
University of York, Heslington
York 5DD, England

Stewart J. Rosenberg
Centre Hospitalier Spécialisé
Rouffach 68250, France

Rachel M. Rosser
Department of Psychiatry
University College and Middlesex School of
    Medicine
Wolfson Building, Middlesex Hospital
London W1N 8AA, England

Susan E. Salasin
Center for Mental Health Services
Department of Health and Human Services
5600 Fishers Lane
Rockville, Maryland 20857

Jose Saporta
Trauma Clinic, Massachusetts Mental
    Health Center, and
Harvard Medical School
Boston, Massachusetts 02115

William E. Schlenger
Mental and Behavioral Health Research
    Program
Research Triangle Institute
P.O. Box 12194
Research Triangle Park, North Carolina
    27709

Erik G. W. Schouten
Department of Medical Psychology
University of Limburg School of Medicine
6200 MD Maastricht, Netherlands

Robert Schweitzer
Department of Psychology
University of Queensland
St. Lucia, Brisbane, Queensland 4067,
    Australia

Raymond Monsour Scurfield
Pacific Center for PTSD and Other War-
    Related Disorders
U.S. Department of Veterans Affairs
P.O. Box 50188
Honolulu, Hawaii 96850

Derrick Silove
Academic Mental Health Unit
University of New South Wales
Liverpool Hospital
New South Wales 2170, Australia

Michael A. Simpson
Intermedica
P.O. Box 51
Pretoria, South Africa

Elizabeth M. Smith
Department of Psychiatry
Washington University School of Medicine
St. Louis, Missouri 63110

Susan D. Solomon
Disaster Research Program
National Institute of Mental Health
Rockville, Maryland 20857

Zahava Solomon
Research Branch
Department of Mental Health
Medical Corps
Israel Defence Forces
Military P.O. Box 02149, Israel

Daya J. Somasundaram
Department of Psychiatry
University of Jaffna
Jaffna, Sri Lanka

Peter Steinglass
Department of Psychiatry
George Washington University
Washington, DC 20052

Linda Ann Stevenson
104 Moore Road
Mapperley, Nottingham NG3 6EJ, England

Christopher Charles Tennant
Department of Psychiatry
University of Sydney
Sydney, Australia, and
Royal North Shore Hospital
Saint Leonards 2065, Australia

James Thompson
Department of Psychiatry
University College and Middlesex School of
   Medicine, Wolfson Building
Middlesex Hospital
London W1N 8AA, England

Stuart W. Turner
Department of Psychiatry
University College and Middlesex School of
   Medicine, Wolfson Building
Middlesex Hospital
London W1N 8AA, England

Robert J. Ursano
Department of Psychiatry
F. Edward Hebert School of Medicine
Uniformed Services University of the Health
   Sciences
Bethesda, Maryland 20814

Bessel A. van der Kolk
Trauma Clinic, Massachusetts Mental
   Health Center, and
Harvard Medical School
Boston, Massachusetts 02115

Guus van der Veer
Social Psychiatric Centre for Refugees
Cornelis Schuystraat 17
1071 JD Amsterdam, Netherlands

Hans Van Duijn
Department of Neurophysiology
Saint Lucas Hospital
1061 AE Amsterdam, Netherlands

Abdul Wali H. Wardak
Department of Psychology
University of Hull
Cottingham Road
Hull HU6 7RX, England

Lars Weisæth
Division of Disaster Psychiatry
Department of Psychiatry
University of Oslo
Oslo 3, Norway

Daniel S. Weiss
Department of Psychiatry
University of California
San Francisco, California 94143

Tom Williams
Post Trauma Treatment Center
31933 Miwok Trail
Evergreen, Colorado 80439

John P. Wilson
Department of Psychology
Cleveland State University
Cleveland, Ohio 44115

Ronnie Wilson
Department of Psychology and Centre for
   the Study of Conflict
University of Ulster
Coleraine, Londonderry BT52 1SA,
   Northern Ireland

Jessica Wolfe
Department of Veterans Affairs
   Medical Center
Boston, Massachusetts 02130

Ruth Wraith
Department of Child Psychotherapy
Royal Children's Hospital
Melbourne, Parkville, Victoria 3052,
   Australia

Akbar Zargar
Department of Architecture
University of Shahid Beheshti
Tehran, Iran

Foreword

The history of the field of traumatic stress, or what is now called "traumatology," begins with the ancient Egyptian physician's reports of hysterical reactions. These reports, which were published in 1900 B.C. in *Kunyus Papyrus*, became one of the first medical textbooks (Veith, 1965). Thus, this *Handbook*, a remarkable single-volume collection of 84 chapters, represents one of the latest achievements in this long history.

Traumatology is the *investigation and application of knowledge about the immediate and long-term psychosocial consequences of highly stressful events and the factors which affect those consequences.* This discipline emerged only within the last decade, partly because of the coalescence of numerous divergent fields of scholarly investigation and therapeutic treatment. These areas included, but were not limited to, such fields of study and treatment as the Holocaust, family abuse (e.g., family violence, incest), rape and sexual abuse, crime victimization studies and victimology, war trauma, and, in general, stress and coping.

These areas are built upon the cumulative scholarly and clinical literature that began to emerge extensively in the nineteenth century. A number of historians have traced the various major developments in this field (Absem, 1984; Ellenberger, 1970; Trimble, 1981, 1985; Veith, 1965). To appreciate fully this massive work, it is important to consider this nearly 4,000-year history. I will briefly review only the highlights and mention some important references.

In an analysis of the history of hysteria, Veith (1965) suggested that emotional reactions to highly stressful events are found in every century that has records of human behavior. Theories and explanations of these behaviors have varied. The symptoms of flashbacks, dissociation, and startle response were variously viewed as works of God, the gods, the devil, and various types of spirits (Ellenberger, 1970). Thanks to Franz Anton Mesmer, an eighteenth-century physician and inventor of hypnotism, scientific concepts began to replace religious ones, and this led eventually to the analysis of psychological possession and multiple personality (Azam, 1887; Flournoy, 1900; Hodgson, 1891; Veith, 1965).

Hurst (1940) and others (see Trimble, 1981) noted the important contributions of the innovative work being done at La Salpêtrière Hospital in Paris (Briquet, 1959). Jean-Martin Charcot, its most distinguished physician, was the first to demonstrate that hysteria had psychic origins (Charcot, 1889). His work subsequently had considerable influence on such traumatologists as Pierre Janet, Sigmund Freud, John Eric Erichsen, and Helmut Oppenheim.

Pierre Janet is credited as the first psychologist to study and treat traumatic stress, including hysterical and dissociative symptoms (van der Hart, Brown, & van der Kolk,

1989). His work began in the early 1880s (Janet, 1886). Through his numerous publications, spanning over 50 years, Janet made some of the most important contributions to traumatology. Among his contributions are (1) the recognition of the inability to integrate traumatic memories as the core issue in posttraumatic syndromes (van der Hart *et al.*, 1989), (2) the discovery of the importance of the fundamental biphasic nature of traumatic stress (van der Kolk, Brown, & van der Hart, 1989), (3) the articulation of all the symptoms of PTSD that are cited in contemporary diagnostic criteria in the DSM-III (van der Kolk *et al.*, 1989), and other vital research.

Building on Janet and abandoning hypnosis because of its unreliability, Sigmund Freud experimented with direct suggestion, transference, and became involved in the emergence of persuasive therapy (Absem, 1984). Freud's contribution to traumatology (1895, 1914, 1920) is well documented. Less known, however, is the fact that Oppenheim (1911) is credited with coining the term "traumatic neurosis," although Joseph Breuer and Freud (1895/1955) were viewed as the primary contributors. The concept of posttraumatic neurosis emerged with the growing recognition of the emotional impact of highly stressful events.

At that time, there were many examples of human reactions to highly stressful events that resulted in the symptoms of posttraumatic neurosis, or posttraumatic stress disorder (PTSD) in today's parlance. Homer's epic poem, "The Odyssey," describes the psychological travails of Odysseus—a recent veteran of the Trojan Wars who was returning home to Ithaca—that include flashbacks and survivor's guilt. Trimble (1985) illustrated many examples of trauma in literature: for example, Shakespeare's *King Henry IV*, "Why does thou bend thine eyes upon the earth. . . . Why hast thou lost the fresh blood in thy cheeks . . . [have] thick-eyed musing and cursed melancholy?" Charles Dickens's nonfictional account of surviving a major train accident and his "two or three hours work . . . amongst the dead and dying surrounded by terrific sights." His traumatizing experience led to his statement: "I am curiously weak—weak as if I were recovering from a long illness" (Foster, 1969).

Train wrecks were the principal means for the writing of another important chapter in the history of traumatology. Trimble (1981) carefully documented the development of what was called "railway spine" and later "Erichsen's disease," named for its inventor. In 1882, John Eric Erichsen had written a book containing his thesis that the "concussion of the spine" due to "violent shock of railway collision" could account for what would later be described as the symptoms of PTSD. His thesis was confirmed and extended by Clevenger (1889). Both books were used by litigant survivors of various railway accidents to secure a settlement for their ailments that could not be detected physically.

However, Herbert Page (1885), a surgeon working for the London and North West Railway, refuted the spine concussion thesis with his own book. Among other things, Page suggested that survivors of railway accidents who complain of various symptoms, such as sleep disturbances, startle responses, and numbing of various body parts without any organic explanation, are suffering from "nervous shock." He was one of the first writers to suggest a psychosocial origin for this heretofore mysterious disease.

War-related traumatic stress became the context for a continuing tradition of important research and conceptualization. Beginning with the clinical observations in early wars (Hammond, 1883) was the notion of *melancholia*, which was seen in combat veterans of the American Civil War. *Shell shock* emerged during World War I (Glass, 1954) to account for the PTSD-like symptoms observed in many returning war veterans. It was believed to be caused by the air blasts of explosives that left soldiers dazed and confused. Although this term was replaced with "war neurosis" or "traumatic neurosis" (Grinker & Spiegel, 1945), there was still a reluctance to ascribe its cause to exposure to and coping with frightening stressors. The consensus was that a predisposing character or personality defect accounted for why some individuals developed combat-related PTSD and others did not when exposed to the same type of stressor (Figley, 1978). This position generally prevailed until the Vietnam War but did not officially change until 1980 with the publication of the DSM-III (American Psychiatric Association, 1980), which now incorporated the term *PTSD*.

However, the areas of stress and coping seemed to evolve separately from that of traumatic stress with the focus by Claude Bernard (see Selye, 1956) on the *milieu intérieur* (internal environment) of a living organism, the importance of which remains fairly constant irrespective of its external environment. Cannon (1929) built on this concept of "homeostasis," the ability of the body to remain in a constant state, thus providing staying power, which is roughly equivalent to a building's heating system regulated partly by a thermostat.

Hans Selye is widely credited with developing the study of stress. He defined stress as "the state manifested by a specific syndrome which consists of all the non-specifically-induced changes within a biologic system" (Selye, 1956, p. 64). Much later, he defined stress more simply: "The nonspecific response of the body to any demand made upon it" (Selye, 1974, p. 14). Equally important, he was the first researcher to suggest that stress is not simply nervous tension or even exclusively distressing, that stress is something to be avoided, but that complete freedom from stress is death. Even more helpful was Selye's discovery of the biological stress syndrome, which was known more widely as the general adaptation syndrome (Selye, 1974), that describes the body's general method of coping with any type of stressor (Figley, 1989).

Although traumatology has long historical roots, it was in the 1980s that it achieved accelerated growth with important and useful innovations coming to fruition. Among them was the publication of the DSM-III in 1980, the birth of the Society for Traumatic Stress Studies in 1985, and the *Journal of Traumatic Stress*. Today, traumatology is recognized as a separate field of study (Figley, 1988) with thousands of professionals specializing in it worldwide.

The publication of this *Handbook* is one more important development in this growing field of study. The editors, who are internationally recognized scholars, have done a remarkable job of soliciting, organizing, and editing these chapters into a cohesive collection. When a definitive history of traumatology emerges, I am certain that this work will be a prominent feature.

CHARLES R. FIGLEY
Florida State University
Tallahassee, Florida

References

Absem, D. W. (1984). Brief historical overview of the concept of war neurosis and of associated treatment methods. In H. J. Schwartz (Ed.), *Psychotherapy of the combat veterans* (pp. 1–22). New York: Spectrum.

American Psychiatric Association. (1980). *Diagnostic and statistical manual of mental disorders* (3rd ed.). Washington, DC: Author.

Azam, E. E. (1887). *Hypnotisme, double conscience et altération de la personalité.* Paris: Ballière.

Breuer, J., & Freud, S. (1955). *Studies of hysteria.* In J. Strachey (Ed. and Trans.), *The standard edition of the complete psychological works of Sigmund Freud* (Vol. 2). London: Hogarth Press. (Original work published in 1895)

Briquet, P. (1959). *Traité clinique et thérapeutique de l'hystérie.* Paris: Ballière.

Cannon, W. B. (1929). *Bodily changes in pain, hunger, fear, and rage.* New York: Appleton.

Charcot, J. (1889). *Clinical lectures of the disease of the nervous system.* London: New Syndenham Society.

Clevenger, S. V. (1889). *Spinal concussion.* London: F. A. Davies.

Ellenberger, H. F. (1970). *The discovery of the unconscious: The history and evolution of dynamic psychiatry.* New York: Basic Books.

Erichsen, J. E. (1882). *On concussion of the spine: Nervous shock and other obscure injuries of the nervous system in their clinical and medico-legal aspects.* London: Longman, Green.

Figley, C. R. (1978). Introduction. In *Stress disorders among Vietnam veterans: Theory, research, and treatment.* New York: Brunner/Mazel.

Figley, C. R. (1988). Toward a field of traumatic stress. *Journal of Traumatic Stress, 1*(1), 3–16.

Figley, C. R. (1989). *Helping traumatized families*. San Francisco: Jossey-Bass.

Flournoy, T. (1900). *A study of a case of glossolalia*. New York: Harper.

Foster, J. (1969). *The life of Charles Dickens* (Vol. 2). London: J. M. Dent.

Freud, S. (1914). *Psychopathology of everyday life* (A. A. Brill, Trans.). London: T. Fisher Unwin.

Freud, S. (1920). *Selected papers on hysteria: Nervous and mental diseases monograph series*, No. 4.

Glass, A. J. (1954). Psychotherapy in the combat zone. *American Journal of Psychiatry, 110*, 725–731.

Grinker, R., & Spiegel, J. P. (1945). *Men under stress*. Philadelphia: Blakiston.

Hammond, W. A. (1883). *A treatise on insanity in its medical relations*. London: H. K. Lewis.

Hodgson, R. (1891). A cs [case] of double consciousness. In *Proceedings of the Society of Psychical Research*. London: Edward Arnold.

Hurst, A. (1940). *Medical diseases of war*. London: Edward Arnold.

Janet, P. (1886). Les actes inconscients et le dédoublement de la personalité. *Revues Philosophiques, 22*(2), 212–223.

Oppenheim, H. (1911). *Textbook of nervous diseases for physicians and students* (A. T. Bruce, Trans.). London: Foulis.

Page, H. (1885). *Injuries of the spine and spinal cord without apparent mechanical lesion*. London: J. and A. Churchill.

Selye, H. (1956). *The stress of life*. New York: McGraw-Hill.

Selye, H. (1974). *Stress without distress*. Philadelphia: Lippincott.

Trimble, M. R. (1981). *Post-traumatic neurosis*. Chichester, England: Wiley.

Trimble, M. R. (1985). Post-traumatic stress disorder: History of a concept. In C. R. Figley (Ed.), *Trauma and its wake: The study and treatment of post-traumatic stress disorder* (Vol. 1, pp. 5–14). New York: Brunner/Mazel.

van der Hart, O., Brown, P., & van der Kolk, B. A. (1989). Pierre Janet's treatment of post-traumatic stress. *Journal of Traumatic Stress, 2*(4), 379–396.

van der Kolk, B. A., Brown, P., & van der Hart, O. (1989). Pierre Janet's post-traumatic stress. *Journal of Traumatic Stress, 2*(4), 365–378.

Veith, I. (1965). *Hysteria: The history of a disease*. Chicago: University of Chicago Press.

Preface

The field of traumatic stress studies has seen remarkable growth during the last decade since the advent of posttraumatic stress disorder (PTSD) as a diagnostic category in the third edition of the *Diagnostic and Statistical Manual of Mental Disorders*, published by the American Psychiatric Association in 1980. The exponential expansion of the field has moved the study and treatment into the mainstream of modern psychiatry, psychology, the neurosciences, as well as the social and behavioral sciences. To establish some perspective on the rate of growth of the field, one only has to recognize that a decade ago there were no reference books on traumatic stress syndromes, few standardized psychological measures of the disorder, little knowledge about the biological basis of behaviors associated with PTSD, and a limited understanding of effective therapeutic approaches. Today, in contrast, there are over 40 books on trauma and victimization, a *Journal of Traumatic Stress*, and hundreds of scientific articles in the major professional journals. Furthermore, in the United States, there is now the National Center for Post-Traumatic Stress Disorder, which has five specialized divisions at different Veterans Administration hospital locations. It is clear from these and other indicators that the field has come a long way in a short amount of time and will continue to grow rapidly across national boundaries.

The development of the *International Handbook of Traumatic Stress Syndromes* grew out of the recognition that a standard reference volume was needed to organize the subareas of study in the field. The editors undertook an intensive effort to locate important research by some of the leading investigators throughout the world and integrate it within a structured organizational framework. The result of this process of international collaboration is an eight-part *Handbook* containing 84 chapters. These contributions span the breadth and depth of the field at this time concerning theory, research methodology, and treatment considerations across a number of survivor and victim populations. While every effort was made to be as inclusive as possible, some readers will no doubt find omissions or imbalances in areas that they regard as important to the field. In some cases, too, political pressure and the suppression of scientific data by governments prevented the opportunity for some investigators to have their research published, especially in Middle Eastern countries which have been affected by war and civil violence in the last 20 years. Most of this scholarly material pertained to the effects of war trauma and the use of torture in these countries. Despite whatever limitations may exist, it is our hope that this *Handbook* will stimulate additional research, encourage the discovery of new techniques of treatment, and ultimately help to alleviate the pain and suffering of traumatized persons, their families, and their loved ones.

In the broader social sense, the development of the field of traumatic stress studies must symbolize the evolution of a humane concern for the consequences of violence and destruction, and, as such, must surely speak hopefully for the human race. If, at last, compassion for those who are inevitably wounded and hurt can override the aggressive and destructive themes so congruent in many of our cultures, then we may become ready for peaceful, nonviolent, just, and considerate human relationships amongst those who inhabit this small planet. In many respects, this book speaks clearly to the resiliency of human behavior and to the importance of hope in overcoming adversity, pain, suffering, and various forms of evil, cruelty, and unfairness that intrude into the lives of ordinary people throughout the world.

Acknowledgments

The completion of the massive project which became this *Handbook* could not have been accomplished without the assistance and support of many organizations and individuals. First, the College of Arts and Sciences at Cleveland State University in the United States made it possible in 1989 for me (JPW) to have a six-month hiatus from my university teaching schedule in order to work in Australia with Dr. Beverley Raphael at the Royal Brisbane Hospital of the University of Queensland. Appreciation is extended to Dr. Steve Slane, Chairperson of the Department of Psychology, and to Dr. Georgia Lesh-Laurie, former Dean of the College at Cleveland State University, for their efforts on my behalf. I also offer special thanks to Dr. Harry Andrist, Dean of the College of Graduate Studies at Cleveland State University, whose financial support was appreciated.

A special thank-you is extended to the University of Queensland, Herston, Australia, which generously provided a travel grant in order for me to fly from the United States to Australia in June, 1989. Further, the faculty and staff in the Department of Psychiatry at Royal Brisbane Hospital were not only accommodating but also stimulating to work with during the colloquium and other special events. A special debt of gratitude is extended to Jan Parker, administrative assistant to Professor Raphael, who typed and retyped the original manuscripts received in Australia as well as overseeing the entire editing process on a daily basis. On numerous occasions, Ms. Parker worked well beyond her normal responsibilities to insure the proper preparation of the chapters. Thanks are also extended to all of the other secretarial staff who worked with her to complete this task.

During my stay in Australia, the Department of Veterans' Affairs and the Vietnam Veterans' Counselling Service (VVCS) arranged for me to visit every repatriation general hospital (RGH) and VVCS center. This opportunity not only allowed me to travel throughout Australia and Tasmania, but also enabled me to get to know the staff of the service as well. My appreciation and thanks are extended to Trevor Fear, my host on the tour and a good friend, and to Ric Marshall, who was then director of the VVCS.

At Cleveland State University, many individuals labored to see that this *Handbook* was completed in a thorough fashion. First and foremost, we wish to thank Lynn Viola, Secretary in the Department of Psychology, who assumed the responsibility of overseeing the production of 84 chapters on a daily basis. This enormous task was always carried out with a positive attitude and a recognition of the need to produce a reference volume to aid persons suffering the adverse emotional effects of trauma and victimization. Ms. Viola's sincerity and dedication were transmitted to students in the department who likewise worked beyond the call of duty to see that all of the work was correct and properly organized. Expressing our appreciation here does not serve justice to their input and effort, but it is important to single out Sue Roberts, my graduate assistant, without whose dedication to the field of traumatic stress and expertise with computers the *Handbook* would not have become a reality. Thanks are also extended to Steve Mindlin, Brenda Kozie, Adrienne Fitzpatrick, Karen Groth, Dan Ileana, Lisa Weston, Dawn Miller, Nicole Zirzow, Rachel Boyd, Jim Mullin, and David Fleck for their many hours of dedicated work.

We would also like to acknowledge the efforts of the contributors who shared in our vision of creating a state-of-the-art international reference volume on trauma and post-traumatic stress disorder (PTSD) which could be used by practitioners, researchers, scholars, educators, social policymakers, and others concerned with understanding and healing the painful and prolonged effects of traumatization.

Finally, a special thank-you to Dad and Mom, Bernard and Louise Armstrong of Oakey, Queensland, Australia, who graciously provided a wonderful place for the senior editor to live and write with his wife and children. The bucolic splendor of Brookvale Farm made the tasks of editing and writing a labor of love.

JOHN P. WILSON
BEVERLEY RAPHAEL

Contents

III. WAR TRAUMA AND CIVIL VIOLENCE

Theoretical and Conceptual Foundations of Traumatic Stress Syndromes

Throughout the history of mankind, traumatic events of natural and human origin have occurred that have left psychic scars on the inner selves of the victims and the survivors. Our knowledge of how traumatic events have affected the psychological functioning and adaptation of victims has developed gradually until the middle of the twentieth century when global warfare and massive social upheaval throughout the world caused an acceleration in understanding the impact of trauma to individuals and to entire cultures. The need to care for those afflicted by catastrophic events led to more sophisticated medical, epidemiological, and psychiatric studies which began to document and conceptualize the nature of stress-response syndromes. By 1980, with the advent of posttraumatic stress disorder (PTSD) as a category of the mental disorders listed in the third edition of the *Diagnostic and Statistical Manual of Mental Disorders* (DSM-III) of the American Psychiatric Association, scientific interest in traumatic stress syndromes led to a new level of integration of the literature and generated many empirical studies which sought answers regarding the nature and dynamics of the phenomenon. As a part of this process, challenges were posed to theoretical and conceptual explanations of PTSD and allied conditions that were known previously as traumatic neurosis, shell shock, railroad spine, combat fatigue, operational exhaustion, K-Z syndromes, or other names.

Furthermore, as evidence of the rapid progression of the field of traumatic stress studies, both theoretical and clinical insights were integrated in the revised edition of 1987, the DSM-III-R. These diagnostic advances are presented in Table I.1.

At present time, the DSM-IV criteria are being prepared and will reflect only minor changes which incorporate more recently accumulated clinical and empirical studies of stress-response syndromes. Among the major issues yet to be resolved is the classification of PTSD as a disorder. Although debates continue, many researchers and clinicians believe that stress-response syndromes should be a distinct diagnostic category of their own, with distinct subtypes of PTSD.

Despite the extraordinary growth of the field of traumatic stress studies, there is

Table I.1. Diagnostic Criteria for 309.89
Posttraumatic Stress Disorder

A. The person has experienced an event that is outside the range of usual human experience and that would be markedly distressing to almost anyone, e.g., serious threat to one's life or physical integrity; serious threat of harm to one's children, spouse, or other close relatives and friends; sudden destruction of one's home or community; or seeing another person who has recently been, or is being, seriously injured or killed as the result of an accident or physical violence.

B. The traumatic event is persistently reexperienced in at least one of the following ways:
   (1) Recurrent and intrusive distressing recollections of the event (in young children, repetitive play in which themes or aspects of the trauma are expressed)
   (2) Recurrent distressing dreams of the event
   (3) Sudden acting or feeling as if the traumatic event were recurring (includes a sense of reliving the experience, illusions, hallucinations, and dissociative [flashback] episodes, even those that occur upon awakening or when intoxicated)
   (4) Intense psychological distress at exposure to events that symbolize or resemble an aspect of the traumatic event, including anniversaries of the trauma

C. Persistent avoidance of stimuli associated with the trauma or numbing of general responsiveness (not present before the trauma), as indicated by at least three of the following:
   (1) Efforts to avoid thoughts or feelings associated with the trauma
   (2) Efforts to avoid activities or situations that arouse recollections of the trauma
   (3) Inability to recall an important aspect of the trauma (psychogenic amnesia)
   (4) Markedly diminished interest in significant activities (in young children, loss of recently acquired developmental skills, such as toilet training or language skills)
   (5) Feeling of detachment or estrangement from others
   (6) Restricted range of affect, e.g., unable to have loving feelings
   (7) Sense of a foreshortened future, e.g., does not expect to have a career, marriage, or children, or a long life

D. Persistent symptoms of increased arousal (not present before the trauma), as indicated by at least two of the following:
   (1) Difficulty falling or staying asleep
   (2) Irritability or outbursts of anger
   (3) Difficulty concentrating
   (4) Hypervigilance
   (5) Exaggerated startle response
   (6) Physiologic reactivity upon exposure to events that symbolize or resemble an aspect of the traumatic event (e.g., a woman who was raped in an elevator breaks out in a sweat when entering any elevator)

Note: From the *Diagnostic and Statistical Manual of Mental Disorders*, Third Edition—Revised, p. 250. Washington, DC: American Psychiatric Association. Copyright 1987 by the American Psychiatric Association. Reprinted by permission.

still a lack of knowledge about and theoretical understanding of the complex forms of interactions between (1) the nature of the stressor event, (2) the personality attributes and coping processes of the person, (3) the psychobiological mechanisms affected by trauma, and (4) the cultural responses to those who are victimized.

Furthermore, there is presently a lack of consensus on how best to conceptualize stress-response syndromes. For example, in Chapter 4, Mardi J. Horowitz proposes a phase or stage model of PTSD. Yet other theorists and researchers have proposed alternative formulations, such as biphasic models, unconscious motivational process concerning affect regulation, psychobiological models of disordered arousal, and psychoformative processes that shift the emphasis onto the construction of meaning and the reformulation of the trauma's impact to the self-structure. Clearly, future research will be necessary to construct an integrative theoretical model which incorporates these disparate views.

The nine chapters in Part I of this volume address the major theoretical and conceptual issues in the field at the present time. In the contributions are represented a multidisciplinary cross-section of researchers who examine theoretical conceptualizations of stress-response syndromes from various perspectives and orientations, including psychohistorical approaches, biological changes in nervous system functioning, psychoanalytical models, sociological analysis of toxic biospheric contamination, cross-disaster comparisons of response to trauma, the similarity of PTSD to complex dissociative processes, and the nature of anomalous traumatic experiences.

In Chapter 1, Robert Jay Lifton, a pioneer in the field, summarizes the corpus of his research on such groups as survivors of the atomic bomb at Hiroshima, Vietnam veterans, and the Nazi doctors who were involved in medical genocide in the death camps during the Third Reich of Adolf Hitler. Lifton's 10 principles of psychoformative processes are presented in the context of the life/death paradigm indigenous to many traumatic events. Psychoformative theory is distinct because of Lifton's view on how the self-structure is affected by trauma. Injury to the self may lead to profound psychic numbing, survivor guilt, forms of splitting, dissociation, and doubling as psychological processes which attempt to adapt to the nature of the overwhelming and often terrorizing experience. Psychoformative theory also indicates that all survivors face the task of transforming the traumatic episode, and Lifton describes the protean task by which the self can be reintegrated in new forms that are associated with animation, transcendence, and enhanced ego vitality. Through the evolution of Lifton's work, the conceptual framework of PTSD can be readily discerned through his groundbreaking research during the last 30 years.

In Chapter 2, the biological response to trauma is examined. Clearly, traumatic events are experiences which affect organismic functioning directly on four interrelated levels: biological, psychological, social-interpersonal, and cultural. From a holistic perspective, the immediate and long-term effects of trauma may impact on one level more severely than on another (e.g., a disabling physical injury). Nevertheless, they are, in fact, interrelated processes which reciprocally influence each other in direct and subtle ways that define the nature of the mind–body relationship. Although it is now recognized that PTSD can negatively affect each of these four interrelated domains of human adaptive behavior, the most basic impairment to the organism seems to be to the brain and central nervous system, which contain the neurophysiological mechanism that governs memory, affect, thought, and sociability.

In Chapter 2, Bessel A. van der Kolk and Jose Saporta present a detailed analysis of the rapidly growing literature on the psychobiology of PTSD. As they note in their chapter, "the human response to trauma is so constant across traumatic stimuli that it is safe to say that the central nervous system (CNS) seems to react to any overwhelming, threatening and uncontrollable experience in quite a consistent pattern."

Beginning with the early work of Pierre Janet, a contemporary of Sigmund Freud, van der Kolk and Saporta review the attempts to understand a trauma's impact on neurological functioning. As early as 1889, Janet observed that the hyperarousal inherent in posttraumatic behavior interfered with information-processing, verbal memory, and the various functions of consciousness, and resulted in somatic encoding of the residue of the trauma. Furthermore, by means of a comparative analysis and historical review, the authors have discerned common psychobiological mechanisms in response to trauma as noted by Freud, Abraham Kardiner, Grinker and Spiegel, Pavlov, and many other early investigators who studied the relationship between traumatization, learning, and neurophysiological changes which affect overt behavior and cognitive processes.

At the heart of understanding the biological response to psychic trauma is the concept of hyperarousal and overdriven neurophysiological processes. As traditionally conceived, a trauma disrupts the normal steady state (stasis) of the organism and leads to disequilibrium. Disequilibrium occurs, of course, at both the psychological level (i.e., emotional distress and cognitive reliving/reexperiencing) and the physical level. Thus, the psychobiology of PTSD seeks to understand how changes in the CNS and autonomic nervous system (ANS) occur and the intricate neural mechanisms which control symptom expression and behavior. There are many approaches that researchers have employed to understand hyperarousability, disequilibrium, and the overt manifestations of CNS and ANS function. Van der Kolk and Saporta start by examining the core symptomatology of PTSD and then summarize the literature on the neural structures (e.g., limbic system, locus coeruleus) which play specific and general roles in the production of symptom manifestation. Thus, the following neural subsystems and behavioral phenomena are analyzed and then placed into a comprehensive and integrated summary: (1) autonomic hyperreactivity and intrusive reexperiencing, (2) numbing of responsiveness, (3) developmental levels and the effects of trauma, (4) the limbic system, (5) noradrenergic and serotonergic pathways, (6) endogenous opioid system, and (7) the role of the locus coeruleus and related structures. In conclusion, the authors state that

> The rapidly expanding knowledge of the effects of traumatization on the central nervous system, the dawning awareness that nervous functions are at the core of the psychological disruptions in PTSD, combined with the availability of animal models for PTSD, makes the psychobiology of trauma on of the most promising areas in psychiatry.

In Chapter 3, attention is focused on the relationship between dissociative disorders and posttraumatic stress disorder. In particular, Bennett Braun highlights the parallels between multiple personality disorder (MPD) and PTSD. As van der Kolk noted in Chapter 2, in 1889, Janet began to lay out the framework of understanding trauma and the phenomenon of dissociation. In a similar way, Braun notes that

> multiple personality disorder (MPD) and posttraumatic stress disorder (PTSD) were formulated in medical consciousness at about the same time that modern psychiatry was being molded by its Age of Giants. During this period of 1880 to 1920, MPD was pulled from its millennia-old identification with demonology and possession into the rational spheres of psychology. . . . The "cowardice" of warriors who relived scenes of terror in sweating nightmares acquired a new etiology in the trenches of World War I, namely, "shell shock," later to become the "combat fatigue" of World War II, and the PTSD of today.

Since the end of World War II, our clinical and scientific knowledge of both MPD and PTSD has advanced rapidly, and it is not surprising that common psychobiological processes underlie both phenomena; hence there is the beginning of a convergence in the knowledge base for both disorders. To this end, Braun explicates the areas of convergence and divergence in MPD and PTSD and notes that psychological trauma is common to both. Although the responses to trauma vary among individuals, when the event is severe enough or prolonged and repeated, the long-term psychiatric consequences are likely to be pronounced and follow as predictable sequelae. In the way of an example, Braun notes in the child-abuse diathesis of MPD three necessary and sufficient elements that could result in MPD and in PTSD, or either disorder independently. Factor 1 concerns predisposing factors that include a psychobiological capacity to dissociate and repeated exposure to an inconsistently stressful environment. Factor 2 involves the experience of "a specific, overwhelmingly traumatic event which may be present to which the young victim responds by dissociating—that is, dissociating behavior, affect, sensation and knowledge from the main stream of consciousness." Factor 3 identifies the nature of the abusive environment as containing the potential of perpetuating episodes of trauma that would lead to further dissociative responses which might eventuate in distinct personality states or unique identities. Thus, it is clear that dissociation as a mental process plays a central role in the development of both PTSD and MPD. But, as Braun notes, a continuum of dissociation illustrates a natural adaptive mechanism becoming increasingly maladaptive and pathologic dissociation is seen to be at the furthest distance from "full" awareness—farther away than suppression, denial, and repression. This . . . illustrates the definition of dissociation as the separation of an idea or thought process from the main stream of consciousness. Also implied is that dissociation has a significantly greater physiologic component than is found in Freud's concept.

Building on his early model of dissociation (i.e., BASK = behavior, affect, sensation, knowledge), Braun develops a BASK model of PTSD in which the role of dissociation in response to trauma is explored. However, among the hallmark features of PTSD is intrusive recollections of the trauma which appear on the surface to be just the opposite of dissociation. Braun notes that

Intrusive symptoms are seen as breakdowns of the protective mechanisms of denial and amnesia. Both intrusion and denial symptoms are seen as disturbances of the ongoing flow of mental processes. . . . In PTSD as well as in other dissociative disorders, there is a need to dissociate behavior, affect, sensation, and knowledge (BASK) from the integrated flow of mental activity. This dis-integration is a characteristic of dissociative symptomatology.

Throughout his chapter, Braun systematically differentiates how the BASK model of PTSD and MPD overlap in their psychological mechanisms, thus advancing clinical inquiry and the ability to more effectively intervene with treatment strategies. He concludes: "The understanding of PTSD and MPD begins with an awareness that severe psychological trauma is the underlying etiology, and that maladaptive use of dissociation is the underlying pathology."

In Chapter 4, Mardi J. Horowitz presents a synopsis of his research program on posttraumatic stress syndromes. Throughout the years of his multifaceted research programs, Horowitz has attempted to define the nature and process of stress-response syndromes. As an outcome of his many seminal projects with his associates, Horowitz has successfully integrated the principles of psychodynamic functioning with modern information-processing theory. As a result, two parallel sets of stress-response syndromes have been elucidated. The first configuration and sequence recognizes (similar to Lifton) that there is an expectable and predictable sequence of symptoms following an abnormally stressful life event. This sequence of symptom clusters includes phases of outcry (initial distress and psychic overload), denial and avoidance, intrusion of trauma-related imagery and affect, and a phase of "working-through" the continuing affective and psychic problems resulting from the traumatic event until completion is achieved. It is noteworthy that these phases of response to a trauma are regarded as the normal sequence of the stress recovery process. Thus, given sufficient severity in a stressful life event, one would expect such a phasic sequence of stress recovery to occur. However, not all victims are able to enact a healthy stress recovery process and many become pathologically fixated at one of the phases in the recovery. When this occurs, they may enter into states of denial, depression, emotional constriction, avoidance, or, alternatively, experience *flooded states* of affect and imagery (intrusion). Although it is the case that some individuals progress sequentially from denial to intrusion, others experience cyclical swings or alterations between states of avoidance and intrusive (unbidden and involuntary) episodes of reliving what happened in the traumatic event. Horowitz notes, for example:

Such unbidden images tend to occur most frequently when the person is relaxed—for example, when lying down to sleep or closing the eyes to rest. Vivid sensory images occurring during periods of rest or relaxation constitute a *hypnogogic* phenomenon. A similar occurrence on awakening is called *hypnopompic* phenomenon. The stressed person may become anxious that these frightening experiences will recur or may interpret them as a sign of . . . "going crazy."

Because PTSD overlaps with both normal and pathological grief, Horowitz discusses the differences between traumatic bereavement and PTSD. Included here is an examination of how personality and premorbid processes relate to PTSD and bereavement. Finally, his chapter includes an important section on treatment implications and techniques based on the nature and dynamic of a phasic model of stress-response syndromes.

Chapter 5 presents an overview of psychoanalytic contributions to a theory of traumatic stress. Understanding the psychoanalytic perspective of response to trauma is especially important because the earlier frameworks of Sigmund Freud and others were very influential in shaping psychiatric thinking about PTSD. In this chapter, Elizabeth A. Brett reviews the three fundamental psychoanalytic models of trauma.

It was Freud's view that a traumatic event overpowered normal, healthy ego defenses and broke through what he termed the "stimulus barrier" and thus rendered the ego incapable, at least temporarily, of proper reality testing and secondary process thinking. Once overwhelmed, the ego contracted from reality-oriented thinking because attention was directed inwardly to affect and imagery associated with the trauma. A traumatic neurosis was thus characterized by anxiety, nightmares, depression, and persistent concerns about what happened in the trauma itself. However, in Freud's view, the failure to recover from a trauma was not due to the *magnitude* of the stressor events *per se*, but rather to repressed instinctual conflicts that were "unleashed" or activated into awareness upon the breach to the stimulus barrier. Thus, the traditional Freudian view saw the persistence of symptoms as manifestations of premorbid character flaws of innate weaknesses in the ego apparatus. As a consequence, the failure to recover from a trauma or the development of chronic PTSD is attributed to premorbid personality functioning and not to the exposure to extremely stressful life events. As noted by Brett, the full explication of Freud's model of traumatic neurosis included conceptions of (1) early infantile conflict, (2) the breach of the stimulus barrier, and (3) repetition compulsion as coping attempts to master the original trauma.

Post-Freudian psychoanalytic perspectives have attempted to modify the early paradigm which was predicated on a biologically driven instinct model of human psychic functioning. Brett devotes the balance of her chapter to an analysis of the theories of Horowitz (information-processing and psychodynamic control principles); Kardiner and Spiegel's ego contraction and restitutive efforts in defensive functioning; and Krystal's model which developed out of work with Holocaust survivors (cataleptic passivity, constriction, numbing, and primary adaptive failure). She concludes her chapter by reorganizing the models into Type A and Type B phenomena depending on the structural implications of the theory. In Type A models, a trauma leads to distress and the development of defenses against the distress. In Type B models, the trauma causes regression and an inability to modulate affective expression. Although theoretically different, it is possible to integrate the Type A and B paradigms into a more comprehensive framework. Nevertheless, Brett's chapter is quite heuristic in forcing conceptual classification as to the nature of the psychodynamic models and the relatively greater emphasis on intrapsychic processes to event-determined adaptational dilemmas.

In Chapter 6, Lars Weisaeth and Leo Eitinger examine the concept of trauma by elucidating common themes from studies in Norway on World War II refugees, victims of a large industrial accident, victims of an oil rig disaster in the North Sea, and terrorist action in 1984 against a Norwegian merchant ship captured in Libya for 67 days. The authors address many questions germane to theoretical perspectives of trauma, including: (1) Why does the human organism react with similar symptomatology to quite different stressor events? (2) What are the similarities and dissimilarities in symptomatology? (3) What is the most successful form of posttraumatic therapy and when should it be initiated and concluded?

Weisaeth and Eitinger note that the general uniformity inherent in the response to trauma reflects the effects of the stressors to the most basic core psychobiological processes, a fact fully explicated by van der Kolk and Saporta in Chapter 2. However, these authors note, as have many other researchers in the field of traumatic stress studies, that there are at least three central psychological principles inherent in different traumas which concern (1) the degree of threat and danger, (2) the degree of loss (i.e., death) or the witnessing of death, and (3) the degree of actual or perceived responsibility for failure to help in a prosocial manner. This third dimension is similar to what Lifton discusses as a failed enactment or survivor guilt in Chapter 1.

In their comparative analysis of PTSD reactions among the different groups studied who were exposed to extreme stress, Weisaeth and Eitinger note that relatively high rates of PTSD, depression, and associated symptoms were common. Second, although the role of premorbid risk factors could be identified in some of the studies, a more integrative approach identified three dimensions of risk process to PTSD (1) high-risk *situations* which lead to high prevalence rates of PTSD, (2) high-risk *persons* who are vulnerable to developing PTSD at different threshold levels, and (3) high-risk *reactions* and initial coping mechanisms that are associated with the later onset of PTSD. Thus, based on the effective ability to identify the levels of risk proneness an individual exhibits in response to a particular trauma, a variety of therapeutic approaches to treatment are implicated, including critical stress incident debriefing, pretrauma stress inoculation counseling, and posttraumatic intervention by qualified specialists in posttraumatic therapy. Chapter 6 is unique because it is able to formulate *conceptual paradigms* of trauma on the basis of careful empirical and epidemiological studies of trauma which forced health care specialists to identify helpful procedures of intervention for the victims.

In Chapter 7, J. Stephen Kroll-Smith and Stephen R. Couch expand the analysis of theoretical models of traumatic stress syndromes in their sociological examination of technological hazards in which social responses become traumatic stressors. To begin, the authors note that biospheric contamination is emerging as a worldwide crisis. As such, toxic biospheric contaminants are not discrete single-stressor experiences that occur to an individual. Rather, their effects on the biosphere fundamentally disrupt and alter the relation of humankind to the environment and raise the specter that the air, soil, and water may not be safe and hence are potential sources of threat to existence and well-being. As the authors state:

> Contrary to the role of natural disaster response strategies in mitigating the potential psychosocial harm caused by the aversive agent, it is our opinion that socially contested responses to the threat of biospheric contamination are likely to become *stressors* in their own right, producing psychosocial sequelae in conjunction with the physical impact of the aversive agent.

What makes biospheric contamination a potential source of traumatic stress? Among the various principles reviewed in Chapter 7, the concept of pervasive psychological permeation with uncertainty is an important notion since those who are exposed to toxic agents cannot know for certain many important elements of information by which to construct coping and adaptive strategies. For example, what was the dose level exposure and what are the immediate and long-term effects on health and well-being? Are there known risk factors associated with exposure and its aftermath? Can the deleterious effects be treated or reversed? These and many more related questions begin to point to the depth of *adaptational dilemmas* faced by extreme biospheric contamination. And yet the social awareness of environmental contamination

> sets in motion a pattern of claims and counterclaims as groups and organizations assert, sponsor, and attempt to impose on others their definition of the scope and severity of the problem, while challenging, rejecting, and subverting the definitions of others. Somewhat ironically, it is the trauma that ensues from the claims and counterclaims that a hazard or disaster exists that permits us to label toxic exposure a disaster using Barton's definition of the term as a collective stress experience.

Building upon the structural analysis of biospheric contaminations as precipitating traumatic stress via profound psychosocial uncertainty as to the aversive effects and the social controversies which arise out of competing claims, Kroll-Smith and Couch then proceed to explain how the *appraisal* processes of the events are affected at both the individual and collective levels. Of necessity, the appraisal processes include threats to basic belief systems and the generation of psychic distress and social alienation. For example, the authors note that

> interpreting the deleterious effects of these claims about danger in the individual begins with the idea that, "in toxic contamination causes subjective evaluations are closely tied to the development of physical and mental health problems" (Baum, 1987, p. 46). Subjectivity is related to uncertainty. People facing the threat of chemical contamination or asbestos poisoning live in a chronic state of contingent loss. The greater the degree of contingency or uncertainty, the greater the need to construct symbolic claims of the scope and seriousness of the threat.

Chapter 7 concludes with a series of observations and directions for future research in which disruption of man's most basic relation to his environment by biospheric contamination leads to traumatic stress syndromes at both the individual and collective levels which are inextricably linked. Given the specter of increasing global biospheric contamination, this chapter breaks new ground in theoretical approaches to trauma in a manner quite similar to Lifton's pioneering work on the psychic consequence of the atomic bomb at Hiroshima and the advent of the nuclear age.

In Chapter 8, Rima E. Laibow and C. Shaffia Laue discuss PTSD which results from anomalous traumatic experiences. Anomalous traumatic experiences are different from others primarily in that the DSM-III-R PTSD diagnostic Criterion A is problematic, as anomalous stressor phenomena do not conform to discernable "events outside the range of usual human experience that would be markedly distressing to almost anyone." In anomalous trauma, the stressor event or experience is typically hidden, hard to detect, ephemeral, ineffable, and not easily verifiable by conventional scientific methods of assessment, measurement, or quantification. Furthermore, although most victims of trauma are reticent to talk about what happened during the event because it is so painful, distressing, and emotionally overwhelming, the anomalous trauma is even more complicated because the event or experience is uncommon, deviant from the common order, or incongruous as compared to readily verifiable objective stressors. For example, as Laibow and Laue document, until the 1960s, it was not widely believed that childhood sexual abuse actually occurred. Children, and later, adults who reported such experiences were thought to be engaging in fantasies rather than reporting what happened to them. Similarly, as noted by the authors of Chapter 7, toxic biospheric contamination generates traumatic stress precisely because of the uncertainty of its effects and the concomitant tendency for others to disavow the nature or possibility of aversive psychological consequences. Thus, the victims of anomalous traumatic experiences, which include such phenomena as childhood sexual abuse, torture, satanic cult ritualistic abuse, and reported UFO abductions by aliens, pose special challenges to mental health specialists who work with them.

The authors take a cautious and conservative approach to therapeutic intervention and clinical conceptualization of experienced anomalous trauma. First, they note that in many cases there is physical evidence or clues that a hidden traumatic event has occurred, such as scarlike marks, unexplained cervical bleeding, puncture-like wounds, and soft neurological signs, such as dizziness, impaired concentration, and headaches. Second, many individuals report and exhibit the classic symptoms of PTSD without being able to report with clarity the nature of the traumatic event they have experienced. Third, feelings of stigmatization, alienation, and self-consciousness are common in experienced anomalous trauma (a finding reported in Chapter 7 on biospheric contamination as well). Fourth, psychological testing frequently shows that such persons are not overtly psychotic, suffering from a personality disorder, or having a significant premorbid history. Finally, the authors suggest that the proper use of hypnosis is especially valuable in uncovering the previously "hidden" traumatic event and upon successful appraisal, the PTSD symptoms often dissipate spontaneously and with excellent recovery to normal functioning.

Part I concludes with Chapter 9 by Beverley Raphael and John P. Wilson, which looks at theoretical and intervention considerations in working with victims of disaster. The authors begin by noting that there are common themes among victims of personal trauma and those involved in disasters:

> The commonalities between community and personal disaster and across a range of different catastrophes experiences allow a further definition of the principal themes: the various traumatic elements; their interaction with personal factors in the individual; their interrelationship with the sociocultural milieu; the processes of adaptation to the traumatic experience; and the ultimate outcome. . . . The correlates of morbidity, and the factors influencing vulnerability and resilience are now being identified across major and personal disasters, both "natural" and "man-made." Such understandings provide the conceptual rationale on the basis of which intervention may be developed.

Thus, when a disaster strikes, its impact affects both the individual and the community as a system and as such has widespread systematic effects at multiple sociocultural levels (e.g., loss of materials and resources; loss of lives, families, and relatives; loss of economic and social support systems; loss or destruction of institutions and patterns of living). The authors note:

> This concept of threat and damage to the community system as a whole is important in terms of possible consequences for that community and its individual members, and because interventions may be essential at this system level. Thus, understandings and interventions are linked at all system levels, ranging from individual to group systems, organizational systems, community systems, and to society systems.

Starting with a delineation of disaster impacts on the system level, Raphael and Wilson explore next the theoretical considerations of trauma to the individual. Included here is a detailed examination of (1) the nature and dimensions of the traumatic experience, (2) the importance of personal background factors, (3) the influence of the interpersonal and social milieu postdisaster in the recovery environment, and (4) factors affecting the processing of the trauma and long-term considerations in terms of mental health and social policy. With these theoretical and structural analyses in place, the authors have set the stage for discussing the principles of intervention for victims of disaster.

There are many levels of intervention following a disaster in order to help the survivors restore a sense of psychic equilibrium and socioeconomic stability. Raphael and Wilson state that

> Any proposed interventions should have well-defined goals, be targeted to those most in need, be flexible and adaptive to the realities of the disaster and postdisaster community; reflect compassion, warmth, and empathy toward those who have been affected. Clear intake criteria and assessments should be defined, plus proposed therapeutic or preventive measures and their rationale; the outcomes sought and how and when they will be measured; and how the program will be evaluated. There is a dearth of systematic documentation, and studies in the field of postdisaster social and psychological intervention reveal a great need for documentation, further data gathering, and systematic research.

Throughout the balance of this chapter, the authors attempt to systematically explicate each of the various levels of necessary intervention postdisaster and the critical issues that arise during the process. As such, this chapter constitutes a compact guide to understanding disaster and its aftermath for the mental health professional. It specifies most of the major parameters that define the social, psychological, and cultural impact of a disaster while, at the same time, providing specific directions for aiding specialists and others who become responsible for restoring order and well-being out of chaos.

CHAPTER 1

From Hiroshima to the Nazi Doctors

The Evolution of Psychoformative Approaches to Understanding Traumatic Stress Syndromes

Robert Jay Lifton

Introduction

When we gather as an intellectual and moral community in connection with our concern about traumatic events and posttraumatic responses, we seek to have good emerge from the bad. Although I feel this is especially true in my work, which involves so many destructive, indeed evil, events, I think it is also true for all of us. The logical aspect of that paradox for us is that, as we pursue our work, we seek the moment when our work is less necessary. We seek and work toward the cessation of destructive events on a massive scale, such as the Holocaust, the Vietnam War, or Hiroshima. As a result, we must keep a watchful eye on perpetrators, even as we pursue our work to help victims and survivors. At the same time, we have to keep a sharp moral and psychological distinction between victimizers and victims. In that regard, I refer to my own study of Vietnam veterans, *Home from the War* that I subtitled *Vietnam Veterans: Neither Victims nor Executioners* (Lifton, 1973/1992). This title reflects my understanding, as I began to work with Vietnam veterans, that they had been cast into the two roles that Albert Camus warned us never to assume. Those with whom I worked subsequently struggled

courageously to extricate themselves from the roles of executioner and of victim. One does not want to be a victim any more than one wants to be a victimizer.

My purpose in this chapter is to present an overview of my work with victims of trauma from the atomic bomb at Hiroshima to the recent study of Nazi doctors who oversaw massive killing in concentration camps in World War II.

In retrospect, as I consider my earlier work involving victims of Chinese thought reform and survivors of the nuclear attack on Hiroshima (Lifton, 1976/1991), I have come to realize, especially through my more recent work with Nazi doctors, that if we want to understand what has happened to victims and cope with posttraumatic stress reactions, we must understand more about the deed of the victimizers. Moreover, that understanding must include some of the psychology of victimizers, even as we seek to understand the victims. In this sense, we not only seek to help people but also to do things that take a stand against the victimizing process.

The Evolution of Ten Principles of Psychoformative Theory and Traumatic Stress Syndromes

1. *Life/death paradigm and symbolization of the self.* From my own work, as well as from that of others, I have derived 10 fundamental principles that can inform us in our research and treatment of posttraumatic stress disorder (PTSD) (Lifton, 1976b). First is the principle of

Robert Jay Lifton • Center on Violence, John Jay College of Criminal Justice, City University of New York, New York, New York 10019.

International Handbook of Traumatic Stress Syndromes, edited by John P. Wilson and Beverley Raphael. Plenum Press, New York, 1993.

the life/death basis and the recognition that, in the most artificial and harmful way, the issue of death traditionally has been omitted from posttraumatic stress. Although people acknowledge death as an issue, conceptual resistance to death is coupled with a general cultural resistance to the idea of death. In my research on Nazi doctors, I have recognized that victimizers as well as victims experience death immersion. In the case of the Nazi doctors (especially in the death camps) some of their behavior was a means of warding off their own *death anxiety*. Certainly, the issue of death is central conceptually and in every other way, and our task is to confront death personally and conceptually. The more that we do this, the more effective our work will be.

2. *The concept of being a survivor*. The second principle, which is a direct corollary to the first, is the concept of the survivor, and, again, death is a key. The clear point is that survival is an achievement. Moreover, survival has a dialectical nature. The survivor has different alternatives. He or she can remain locked in numbing, or can use that survival as a source of insight and growth. We all seek the second choice in our work. The principle of survival keeps us on a normative level because we know that if one survives something, this is *not* of itself pathological.

3. *The human connectedness of survivors*. Third is what I refer to as the ultimate dimension (Lifton, 1976b). We know that trauma involves very immediate and painful nitty-gritty experiences and we know some of the symptoms as posttraumatic stress disorder (American Psychiatric Association, 1987, DSM-III-R; in press, DSM-IV). But there is also a dimension in posttraumatic stress disorder that involves larger human connectedness. If we review some of our experience with Vietnam War veterans and other groups who have undergone severe trauma (e.g., Holocaust survivors) we find in each case a struggle to reinstate a larger human connectedness or a sense of being "on the great chain of being." This is one of the most poignant and difficult struggles that accompanies the recovery process. We symbolize immortality—our historical and biological connectedness to those who have gone before and those we assume will follow. We do this through our limited life span, whether through children, our works, our influences, or through nature, or through some spiritual principle, or even through experiences of transcendence.

When we experience radical discontinuity in an immediate way, in the intrapsychic self, the self is dislodged from its forms. In the nineteenth century, Pierre Janet (cited in van der Kolk & van der Hart, 1989) described this and Freud later addressed it within the context of depth psychology (see Chapter 5, in this volume, for a review). The vulnerability to dissociation and splitting in this acute or radical discontinuity at the immediate level renders the self susceptible to doubling.

3a. *Vulnerability to stress and dissociation*. Although prior characteristics of the self are of enormous importance in the outcome of any kind of posttraumatic stress reaction, the experience and our knowledge of radical discontinuity teach us that dissociation can be created in anybody. Moreover, severe stress can make contact with some prior vulnerability to dissociation, to splitting, to discontinuity, which exists to some degree in everyone. Although the degree of vulnerability to discontinuity and dissociation may vary in each of us, some such vulnerability is part of the human condition.

4. *Posttraumatic stress disorder as a normal reaction to extreme stress*. Fourth is the normative principle. The posttraumatic stress disorder is a normal adaptive process of reaction to an abnormal situation. Understanding this leads to a greater acceptance, on the part of the therapist and of the person who has undergone that posttraumatic stress reaction, of his or her situation and symptoms.

5. *Survivor guilt and self-condemnation*. Fifth is the issue of self-condemnation. Self-condemnation is the source of what we call *psychological guilt*, which occurs in people who experience extreme trauma and in posttraumatic stress disorders or survivor reactions. I refer to this as a paradoxical form of guilt because, sometimes, one can condemn the self more as a survivor or victim than as the victimizer because the victimizer may numb himself or herself.

5a. *Failed enactment during trauma and self-image*. This self-condemnation is associated with a combined extreme sense of helplessness at the time of the trauma and what I call *failed enactment*. At the time of the trauma, there is a quick and immediate sense that one should respond according to one's ordinary standards, in certain constructive ways, by halting the path of the trauma or evil, or by helping other people in a constructive way. Neither of these may be possible during extreme trauma. At the very most, the response that is possible is less than the ideal expectation.

I speak of this as failed enactment because some beginning, abortive image forms toward that enactment in a more positive way that is never possible to achieve. One can then describe the idea of an image as a schema for enactment that is never completed. The response to this incomplete enactment can be perpetual self-condemnation.

When we say that a survivor or somebody who has undergone stress some time ago is "down" on himself or herself, we may be referring not to a sense of guilt but rather to self-condemnation that is related to that lingering failed enactment and to a residual, traumatized "self" that is still to some degree in that state of helplessness. In other words, the entire functional self is still in that state of helplessness and failed enactment, and the self in that state brings about self-condemnation. The recovery process involves transcending that traumatized self.

6. *Emotional vitality and fragmentation in the self*. The sixth principle is that of feeling versus not feeling. I suggest that the standard psychoanalytic defense mechanisms are less discrete than we claim; they overlap to a great extent and relate to feeling and not feeling. This whole issue of dissociation originally described by Pierre Janet (cited in van der Kolk & van der Hart, 1989) is central to posttraumatic stress reaction and survivor experience.

7. *Psychic numbing: Discontinuity in the self*. This central concern in our work now takes us to a seventh principle, namely psychic numbing. Psychic numbing stops the symbolizing or formative process. The mind needs the nourishment provided by the continuous process of creating images and forms in order to function well. In extreme forms of psychic numbing, such as dis-

sociation, the symbolizing process is interrupted and distorted. In that way, psychic numbing becomes a key, or at least a lever, to looking at this cessation or interruption of the psychic process, the radical discontinuity, that so characterizes PTSD. Analyzing this formative process and applying it to posttraumatic stress disorder is a very hopeful dimension because it is perpetual. If one sees that continuous process, then one can move beyond the traumatized self and radical discontinuity.

8. *The search for meaning: Paradigmatic forms of self-experience.* This brings us to the eighth principle—the principle of meaning. Although psychiatrists and psychologists have sometimes declined to use the term *meaning* on the grounds that it cannot be defined scientifically, we must find a rigorous way of analyzing it because, without addressing this idea of meaning or inner form, we cannot understand posttraumatic stress disorder. Again, meaning must take place at two paradigmatic levels—the proximate level in which one is struggling with issues of connection and separation, of movement and stasis, and of integration versus disintegration, or integrity versus disintegration; and the aforementioned ultimate level at which one is struggling with issues of larger human connectedness. We have witnessed a person coming out of severe stress reexamine his or her sense of meaning about such phenomena as the goodness or badness of human beings, about whether human beings are really tied to each other, and whether we can trust any connections that we have in our lives. This supports my assertion that we cannot really address the issue without those questioned meanings.

9. *The moral dilemmas of trauma.* The ninth principle is the *moral dimension.* War neurosis has been defined by some as a refusal to die coupled with a refusal to kill. That double refusal was the beginning of wisdom for many Vietnam War veterans and points to the importance of the moral context in which behavior occurs. Did the man who refused to fire at My Lai, who kept his gun faced to the ground, very visibly demonstrating that he refused to fire, commit abnormal behavior? Was he a victim of combat neurosis? Or did be exhibit an admirable form of restraint that took unusual personal courage? I believe it was the second. In that sense, the moral context played a fundamental role.

Having addressed these symptoms, I now assert that part of our function is to legitimize the right to have some of these symptoms within the context of trauma. We fulfill that function by accepting and helping people with these symptoms.

At the same time, I think we need to render illegitimate some of the destructive or traumatic situations that create the symptoms. In our discourse, in our relationship to patients, and in our public positions on relevant issues, our moral stance toward destructive behavior is bound up with the effectiveness and the humanity of our work with victims and survivors.

Although this is much more valid in massive, destructive, evil forms of trauma, as opposed to the kind of trauma that occurs in the natural history of human experience, such as the loss of a parent or another loved one, we nevertheless must legitimize the symptoms and the reaction in this case without necessarily trying to de-

legitimize the trauma itself, as we would do in other forms of massive traumata.

10. *Transformation of the self.* Finally, in looking at all these issues, I return to a psychology of the self. I refer not specifically to Heinz Kohut but rather to the overall sense of self, which has constituted an increasing emphasis in the last 10 or 15 years on psychoanalytic psychiatry and psychology and has enabled us to unite these various dimensions. This unification is essential in order for us to see the dialectical nature of the survivor and the capacity for staying numbed, as opposed to a capacity not only for insight, but even special forms of illumination, which a survivor can have as perhaps no one else can.

Any claim to psychological insight must be tested against disorder. I believe that psychoformative theory, the principles around death and continuity, can contribute to an understanding of the major psychiatric syndromes. Yet at the clinical and conceptual heart of psychiatry, death-related issues have been most neglected and here, too, overall symbolizing principles are required most.

There are certain advantages in formulating a consideration of the traumatic syndrome. Over time, I have developed several strong convictions about this general psychological area: direct, intense psychological trauma—perhaps even adult trauma in general—is a kind of stepchild in psychiatry. An exploration of the psychology of the survivor is crucial to understanding such trauma (Lifton, 1976/1991). The study of adult trauma and survival has direct bearing on issues around death and death imagery in ways that shed much light on psychiatric disturbance and on our contemporary historical condition.

Psychoanalytic Contributions to Understanding Posttraumatic Stress Syndromes

We have learned to find models in early childhood experience for later adult behavior. But there is a beginning sense in psychiatry that a reverse process may be just as useful. Intense adult trauma can provide a model (at least in terms of understanding) for the more obscure and less articulated traumata of early childhood. This reversal was not unknown to Freud (1920/1955). And it is the basis for the image model of the human being as a perpetual survivor—first of birth itself and then of "holocausts" large and small, personal and collective, that define much of existence—a survivor capable of growth and change, especially when able to confront and transcend those "holocausts" or their imprints (Lifton, 1976b).

War Neurosis as a Paradigm of Adult Traumatic Stress Reaction

The adult traumatic experience, in the form of war neuroses, played a very special part for Freud in his conceptual development in general and in his ideas about death in particular. Freud gave special attention to war neurosis and the concept of trauma in connection with his elaboration of the death instinct in *Beyond the Pleasure Principle* (1920/1955). That book is a crucial one in Freud's opus. James Strachey, for instance, tells us (in his editor's note for the Standard Edition) that "in the series of Freud's metapsychological writings, *Beyond the Pleasure Principle* may be regarded as introducing the final phase of his views" (Jones, 1953). Robert Waelder, a distinguished second-generation Viennese disciple of Freud, has noted that: "It is probably not accidental that this short work was written soon after World War I . . . [when] Europe was full of shell-shocked soldiers; one could see them shaking in the streets" (Waelder, 1967, p. 222).[1]

Yet the impact of the traumata of World War I on Freud and his movement has hardly been recorded. World War I (as well as his personal affliction with cancer) had considerable bearing on Freud's elaboration of the death instinct and his preoccupation with it in his later, speculative books, and Europe's grotesque death immersion had an equally significant impact on Freud's attitudes toward his own life and toward his struggling psychoanalytic movement. He cared more about the movement than he did about his individual existence. The war's traumata to the movement (personal and professional deprivations, various forms of separation and isolation, as well as the deaths of friends and family members) must have been perceived as a struggle for survival. And although Freud had relatively (for him) unproductive periods during the war, he also had bouts of extraordinary creativity. There can be little doubt that he and many of his followers were energized in some degree by their survival, though it is difficult to say at what cost. It is quite likely that the war's many levels of destruction accelerated the spread of psychoanalytic influence throughout the world. Few other groups could offer as compelling an explanation for the mass killing and the psychological consequences of war. More fundamentally, massive trauma subverts existing systems of symbolization and tends to bring about in its victims a hunger for explanation or formulation, though it also stimulates (perhaps more frequently) an opposite tendency toward a covering-over that requires static closure. Freud's movement undoubtedly encountered both kinds of war-linked responses, but it was the receptivity that was new and especially important. There is also the possibility that this psychoanalytic survival of World War I reactivated earlier death anxieties in the movement and contributed to its fearful sectarianism and antagonism to heretics. (We can take it to be more than coincidence that, in an important letter written by Freud to Ernest Jones in February, 1919, an interesting

discussion of the nature of traumatic neurosis was followed directly by the sentence: "Your intention to purge the London Society of the Jungish members is excellent" (Jones, 1953, pp. 253–254).

The Problem of Adult Traumatic Reactions to Freud's Instinct Theory of Behavior

Clearly, the war experience raised important theoretical questions for sensitive theorists like Freud. These had to do not only with the nature of homicidal destruction but also with the trauma and neuroses that could be observed in its wake. The problem for Freud was to assimilate these experiences into his already well-developed theoretical system, which meant assimilating them to instinct theory in general and to the libido concept and the sexual origin of the neuroses in particular (Freud, 1919/1964).

To be sure, Freud could point out with some pride that earlier psychoanalytic emphases on psychogenic origins of the symptoms of any neurosis, the importance of unconscious impulses, and the part played by psychic gain through or "flight into" illness had been vindicated by widespread observations on the war neuroses. But, at the same time, he was clearly troubled by the fact that those observations had done nothing to confirm psychoanalytic theory to the effect that "the motive forces which are expressed in the formation of symptoms are sexual and that neuroses arise from a conflict between the ego and the sexual instincts which it repudiates" (Freud, 1919/1964). Freud's response to the challenge was ingenious if a bit convoluted and characteristically illuminating beyond its conceptual claim. In two of his writings devoted to the question of war neuroses and in a few letters written at the end of World War I, one to Jones in particular, Freud acknowledged the importance of the external trauma but, at the same time, associated war neurosis with "internal narcissistic conflict" (Jones, 1953). By invoking his newly evolved theory of narcissism, of libido directed not at another person but at one's own self, Freud could at least place this form of traumatic neurosis within the general realm of libido theory. Although Freud was not always entirely clear on the subject, the essence of his argument was that traumatic neuroses of peacetime (railway accidents and other injuries in which there remains considerable neurotic overlay) can be explained by means of sexual energy or libido becoming fastened to the particular organ or to the body or ego in general, whereas traumatic neuroses of war included that narcissistic process along with an added dimension of "the conflict . . . [which] becomes acute as soon as the peace-ego realizes what danger it runs of losing its life owing to the rashness of its newly formed, parasitic double" (Freud, 1919/1964).

That argument carries Freud beyond mere libido theory toward a concept of meaning. The conflict within the self has to do with what one is willing or not willing to die for, and one's "fixation to the trauma" includes a "compulsion to repeat" elements associated with it as a form of mastery or integration. It was, in fact, precisely this compulsion to repeat that Freud described as violating the "pleasure principle" (according to which the quest for pleasure is always a central motivation) and

---

[1]Waelder goes on to explain: "Some of them had merely been exposed to the 'ordinary' experience of trench warfare; others had been subjected to more particular experiences of concentrated shock, such as, for example, being suddenly covered by a load of earth in an explosion—they had barely escaped being buried alive" (p. 222). By then a number of psychoanalysts had worked professionally with such people. The Fifth International Psycho-Analytic Congress, held in Budapest in late September, 1918, had, in fact, included a symposium, *The Psycho-Analysis of War Neuroses*, from which a small book eventually emerged.

carrying the organism "beyond the pleasure principle" (see Chapter 5, in this volume, for further elaboration).

The Stimulus Barrier as a "Protective Shield" for the Ego

Moreover, it was in discussing these questions that Freud emphasized a principle of a "protective shield" by which he meant a kind of psychic skin necessary for the important everyday function of keeping out external stimuli that might otherwise overwhelm the self or ego. Hence "protection against stimuli is an almost more important function for the living organism than reception of stimuli" (Freud, 1919/1964). He could then define as "traumatic" any excitations from outside which are powerful enough to break through the protective shield. And traumatic neurosis became "a consequence of an extensive breach being made in the protective shield against stimuli" (Freud, 1919/1955). Freud could then see in traumatic neurosis something close to a retrospective model for neurosis in general and even for individual acts of repression that may or may not contribute to neurosis.

Not only did Freud make traumatic neurosis a retrospective model for neurosis in general but he did so around a concept of blockage of stimuli or what could be called *diminished feeling* or *psychic numbing*. The protective shield carried out that function toward outside stimuli but, for stimuli arising from within (instinctual impulses or primary process), there had to be an analogous pattern (what Freud called the "binding" of excitations). And "a failure to effect this binding would provoke a disturbance analogous to a traumatic neurosis" (reference unavailable). That failure, incidentally, makes necessary the compulsion to repeat and the operation of the psyche outside or beyond the pleasure principle. Freud is saying the same thing when he concludes his essay on war neuroses with the observation that "we have a perfect right to describe repression, which lies at the basis of every neurosis, as a reaction to trauma—as an elementary traumatic neurosis." Here Freud associates neurosis with a feeling disorder arising out of the organism's attempt to block excitations caused or released by trauma. This stress on the struggle against feeling reverberates throughout his work. Although Freud did not speak of what we have been calling *death imagery*, he did associate this struggle around excitation and feeling (as encountered in traumatic neurosis) with his argument for a death instinct. Traumatic neurosis became a cornerstone for neurosis on the one hand, and Freud's death-related conceptualizations on the other. In this juxtaposition, Freud came closest to creating a death-oriented psychology.

But, at that point, Freud called forth his own protective shield in order to place the traumatic neuroses within libido theory. To do so, he had to ward off the potentially transforming influence of death on theory, on our understanding of human experience. Freud's conceptual shield was his invocation of the concept of narcissism. That concept approaches conflicts within the self in terms of libido or sexual energy "lodged in the ego." Freud could claim that such "ego libido" was released by trauma and could no longer be adequately "bound" or

constructively contained. Similarly, he invoked the concept of narcissism to explain psychological patterns in schizophrenia and, to a lesser extent, those in severe depression or melancholia. In all three conditions, Freud used the idea of narcissism or intense, unmanageable self-directed sexual energies to explain actual processes of disintegration and related death equivalents. In that way, Freud could not only reaffirm libido theory but collapse his own observations on meaning (in traumatic neurosis, conflicts over what one will die for) and impaired feeling (the protective shield and related internal blockage or "binding") into a mechanistic-quantifiable energic principle. Yet the beginnings he made in sorting out these death-related struggles around meaning and feeling have by no means been lost.

Kardiner's Conception of Traumatic Neuroses: Ego Contraction and Symptom Formation

Abraham Kardiner (1959), for instance, who has distilled much of psychiatric thought on the traumatic syndrome emerging from World War II, began with Freud's explorations of trauma (see Chapter 2, in this volume). But by emphasizing his own and Rado's view of "neurosis as a form of adaption," he was able to stress the need "to unravel the sense behind the symptomatology" as well as issues around feeling and numbing. Concerning the letter, he spoke of a "shrinking" of the ego, of the organism's "shrunken inner resources," and above all of "ego contraction" that interferes with virtually all areas of behavior. Kardiner combined this stress on "ego contraction" with the equally important emphasis on "disorganization rather than regression." Contraction and disorganization—what we would call numbing and disintegration—lead readily to the symptom complex, acute or chronic, that just about everyone has observed: fatigue and listlessness, depression, startle reactions, recurrent nightmares, phobias and fears involving situations associated with the trauma (what Rado calls "traumatophobia"), mixtures of impulsive behavior and unsteadiness in human relationships, and projects of all kinds (including work or study) that may take the form of distrust, suspiciousness, and outbursts of violence.[2]

---

[2]Like Freud, Kardiner is struck by resemblances between extreme forms of the traumatic syndrome and schizophrenia but in terms of these principles of contraction and disorganization rather than narcissism and libido theory. Kardiner's thinking closely approximates our own: "Traumatic neurosis is a disease very closely related to schizophrenia, both from the point of view of central psychodynamics and from the ultimate withdrawal from the world which it set in motion. The deteriorations undergone in both conditions have a striking resemblance to each other. In a manner of speaking, the traumatic neurosis is a kind of persecutory delusion. The persecutor is, however, the outer world. The entire syndrome is produced by what appears to be a prominent device in the establishment of schizophrenia, namely, ego curtailment. This 'ego curtailment' or contraction is associated with what other observers have called 'a chronic state of over-vigilance . . . which seriously affects [many combat veterans'] lives' (1959, p. 247).

A convergence of observations suggests that severe threats to the organism produce patterns of structure that have relevance for a wide variety of psychiatric impairments.

What Kardiner neglected, however, is the place of death and death anxiety in the traumatic syndrome (see Lifton, 1976b). His advances depended upon bypassing instinctualism. But, as in the case of much revisionist work, rejecting the death instinct became associated with neglect of death. The neglect is striking in traumatic neuroses, where death is so close. An evolving view puts the death back onto traumatic neurosis. As early as 1953, Joseph D. Teicher entitled a paper on the subject, "'Combat Fatigue' or 'Death Anxiety Neurosis,'" advocating the latter. Teicher (1953) associated his advocacy of "death anxiety neurosis" with classical emphasis on the importance of guilt toward the dead, as intensified by prior guilt from "fantasied murder" (feelings toward one's father, for instance in association with the Oedipus complex). But when he goes on to say that "in the neurotic form of fear of death, the sufferers are afraid to die and afraid to kill; in their illness they avoid death and murder," we find ourselves at first nodding in agreement but quickly sensing that there is something wrong in the way he is putting things. What is right about the approach is its direct stress on dying and killing, its relationship, that is, to death. What is dubious about the statement is its equation of fear of dying and killing as a neurotic state. What Teicher means, of course, is that these fears become incapacitating and therefore associated with "death anxiety neurosis." But the reader's impulse is to say, "Well, if that is the case, the world could use a good bit more of such a neurosis, or a modicum of its symptoms; if not fear, at least reluctance, to die or kill in military combat." The problem here is the reference point of disturbance or neurosis, a matter that turns out to have considerable importance. Both Kardiner and Teicher wrote from the vantage point of World War II, sometimes referred to as "America's last good war." It was, of course, a dreadful war: Its "goodness" lay in the American combination of decisive success and equally deserved moral clarity. So evil was the enemy—at least the Nazi enemy—that to annihilate him could only be perceived as virtuous. Consequently, those soldiers who broke down, who were "afraid to die and afraid to kill" on behalf of this crusade, could be quite comfortably viewed as neurotic.

Not so in the case of the Vietnam War two or three decades later (see Lifton, 1973/1992). That war, for American participants, was ambiguous in the extreme. Its combination of doubtful justification, absence of structure (as a counterinsurgency action in which the enemy was nowhere and everywhere), and consequent frequency of killing or even massacre of civilians all contributed to various forms of confusion and reluctance to fight. Under those conditions, moral revulsion and psychological conflict became virtually inseparable, sometimes in the form of delayed reactions.

Months or even years after their return to this country, many Vietnam veterans combined features of the traumatic syndrome with preoccupation with questions of meaning—concerning the war and, ultimately, all other areas of living (Archibald, Long, Miller, & Tud-

denham, 1962).[3] Most of these men were not incapacitated by their symptoms and could not be called "neurotic" (Sajer, 1971). Indeed, their anxiety, guilt, and anger could serve animating functions in terms of both introspective and "extrospective" (outward-looking or social) exploration. They seemed to need those emotions for their assimilation of the pain and confusion they had experienced. The traumatic experience, or at least elements of it, had a constructive function for them. And, in many of these cases, both the syndrome (or some of its components) and the doubts about the war began with a confrontation that broke through existing patterns of numbing and evoked images of dying or killing in Vietnam. An approach to traumatic syndrome should focus on death and related questions of meaning, rather than requiring us to invoke the idea of "neurosis." This death-centered approach suggests a moral dimension in all conflict and neurosis.

The Death Imprint and the Psychology of the Survivor

The psychology of the survivor helps us greatly here. The survivor is one who has come into contact with death in some bodily or psychic fashion and has remained alive. There are five characteristic themes in the survivor: the death imprint, death guilt, psychic numbing, conflicts around nurturing and contagion, and struggles with meaning or formulation. Each of these has a special relevance for traumatic syndrome, and, in combination, they affect survivors at both proximate and ultimate levels of experience.

Core Themes of Survivors and Victims: The Death Imprint and Its Impact on the Self-Structure

The death imprint consists of the radical intrusion of an image feeling of threat or end to life. That intrusion may be sudden, as in war experience and various forms of accidents, or it may take shape more gradually over time. Of great importance is the degree of unacceptability of death contained in the image—of prematurity, grotesqueness, and absurdity. To be experienced, the death imprint must call forth prior imagery either of actual death or of *death equivalents*. In that sense, every death encounter is itself a reactivation of earlier "survivals." The degree of anxiety associated with the death imprint has to do with the impossibility of assimilating the death imprint—because of its suddenness, its extreme or protracted nature, or its association with the terror of premature, unacceptable dying. Also of considerable importance is one's vulnerability to death imagery—not only to direct life threat but also to separa-

---

[3]The official incidence of traumatic neuroses has been observed to be lower in Vietnam than in World War II. But, as a number of observers have pointed out, these statistics are misleading because they neglect the delayed reactions and nonclinical manifestations of pain and resistance (Lifton, 1973/1992).

tion, stasis, and disintegration—on the basis of prior conflictual experience. But predisposition is only a matter of degree: If the threat or trauma is sufficiently great, it can produce a traumatic syndrome in everyone, as was largely the case in the man-made flood disaster at Buffalo Creek, West Virginia, in 1972 (Lifton & Olson, 1976).[4]

The survivor retains an indelible image, a tendency to cling to the death imprint—not because of release of narcissistic libido, as Freud claimed, but because of continuing struggles to master and assimilate the threat (as Freud also observed) and around larger questions of personal meaning. The death encounter reopens questions about prior experiences of separation, breakdown, and stasis as well as countervailing struggles toward vitality; it reopens questions, in fact, around all of life's beginnings and endings. So bound to the image can the survivor be that one can speak of a thralldom to death or a "death spell."

The death imprint is likely to be associated not only with pain but also with value—with a special form of knowledge and potential inner growth associated with the sense of having "been there and returned." The death encounter undermines our magical sense of invulnerability by means of its terrible inner lesson that death is real, that one will eventually die—and this vies with our relief at no longer having to maintain that illusion. The result can be something resembling illumination.

Death Guilt, Loss, Bereavement, and Grief

Affecting the outcome and the degree of anxiety is the extent of the sense of grief and loss. In severe traumatic experience, grief and loss tend to be too overwhelming in their suddenness and relationship to unacceptable death and death equivalents for them to be resolved. And many of the symptoms in the traumatic syndrome have precisely to do with impaired mourning. What is involved in our terms is the inability to reconstruct shattered personal forms in ways that reassert vitality and integrity.

Thus, the death imprint in the traumatic syndrome simultaneously includes actual death anxiety (the fear of dying) and anxiety associated with death equivalents (especially having to do with disintegration of the self). This powerful coming together of these two levels of threat may well be the most central feature of image response in the traumatic syndrome (Lifton, 1976b).

The extraordinary power of this imagery—its indelible quality—has to do not only with death but with guilt. What is extremely important, in addition to ultimate threat, is the limited capacity to respond to the threat and the self-blame for that inadequate response.

[4]The flood resulted from corporate negligence in the form of dumping coal waste in a mountain stream in a manner that created an artificial dam, which eventually gave way, killing 125 people and leaving 5,000 homeless. I consulted with two law firms concerning questions of psychic damage (or "psychic impairment") and, together with Eric Olson, conducted extensive interviews with Buffalo Creek survivors and found that virtually all of those we examined showed significant traumatic effects.

We have stressed the importance of the image for motivation, its anticipatory quality in the sense of providing a "plan" or "schema" for enactment. But, in the face of severe trauma, precisely that process is radically interrupted. The soldier whose buddy is suddenly killed or blown up right next to him, for instance, experiences an image that contains feelings not only of horror and pity but an immediate inner plan for action—for helping his comrade, keeping him alive, relieving his pain, perhaps getting back at the enemy—or at least a psychic equivalent of any of these forms of action. But under the circumstances—and all the more so in a massive immersion in death (as in Hiroshima and in the Nazi death camps)—both physical and psychic action are virtually impossible. One can neither physically help victims nor resist victimizers; one cannot even psychically afford experiencing equivalent feelings of compassion or rage. Freud raised this kind of issue in trauma when we drew an example from children's play in which he emphasized that "children repeat unpleasurable experiences . . . [so] that they can master a powerful impression far more thoroughly by being active than they could by merely experiencing it passively." And Erikson has similarly stressed the severe psychic consequences of inactivation as opposed to the capacity for activity in any threatening situation. The inactivation of which we speak is within the image itself and therefore a violation of the kind of psychic flow one can ordinarily depend upon. One feels responsible for what one has not done, for what one has not felt, and above all for the gap between that psychical and psychic inactivation and what one felt called upon (by the beginning image formation) to do and feel.

Intrusive Imagery and Memories of Trauma

The image keeps recurring, in dreams and waking life, precisely because it has never been adequately enacted. And there is likely to be, in that repetition, an attempt to replay the situation, to rewrite the scenario retrospectively in a way that permits more acceptable enactment of the image—whether by preventing others from dying, taking bolder action of any kind, experiencing strong compassion and pity, or perhaps suffering or dying in place of the other or others. In that way, the hope is to be relieved of the burden or self-blame. But whatever actual recovery and relief from guilt one achieves depends much more on the capacity to grasp and accept the nature of one's inactivation under such circumstances.

From this standpoint, we can take another look at survivor or death guilt. We have mentioned the survivor's fundamental inner question: "Why did I survive while letting him, her, or them die?" It is a relatively simple step to feel that by having so failed in one's image actions at the time, "I killed him," or that "if I had died instead, he, she, or they would have lived." This last feeling may in part reflect the psychic death one did actually undergo—the extreme stasis or numbing accompanying one's inactivation in the face of death and threat—and the related sense that subsequent resumption of vitality in the absence of true enactment (mostly in the form of preventing the dead from dying) is wrong. Death guilt ultimately stems from a sense that until some such enactment is achieved, one has no right to be alive.

One could define the traumatic syndrome as the state of being haunted by images that can neither be enacted nor cast aside. Suffering is associated with being "stuck" or "trapped in the trauma" (Wilson, 1989). Hence the indelible image is always associated with guilt, and, in its most intense form, it takes the shape of an image of ultimate horror: a single image (often containing brutalized children or dying people whom the survivor loved) that condenses the totality of the destruction and trauma and evokes particularly intense feelings of pity and self-condemnation in the survivor. To the extent that one remains stuck in such images, guilt is static, there is a degree of continuing psychological incapacity, and traumatic syndrome can turn into traumatic neurosis. But there is also the possibility of finding something like alternative enactment for the image that haunts one, of undergoing personal transformation around that image. In that sense, the very association of guilt with the traumatic syndrome makes possible a transforming relationship to its indelible imagery. And here are the beginnings of a psychological explanation for religious visions of realization and moral growth through suffering.

Only part of oneself feels discomfort at having survived—the experience is also associated with relief, even joy or exhilaration. These feelings can, in turn, contribute to additional guilt. The joy at having survived remains tainted by its relationship to that gap between image and enactment, between the excruciating, demanding picture one had constructed and the muted, devitalized, limited actions and feelings one could muster.

Self-Condemnation as Survivor Guilt

In all this, self-condemnation strikes us as quite unfair. The traumatized person seems to have to endure the additional internal trauma of self-blame. This is why there is a "paradoxical guilt" experienced by victimized survivors. This guilt seems to subsume the individual victim–survivor rather harshly to the evolutionary function of guilt in rendering us accountable for our relationship to others' physical and psychological existences. This experience of guilt around one's own trauma suggests the moral dimension inherent in all conflict and suffering. We have no choice but to make judgments about trauma and our relationship to it. Just as there is an inseparability between psychological and moral dimensions of guilt, we may say the same about all psychological disturbance. Psychological pain always includes a moral judgment; moral judgments express psychological conflict and realization.

In that sense there is no such thing as a value-free mechanism in either traumatic syndrome or any form of neurosis or psychosis. If we can speak of evolutionary purpose, we may say that the capacity for guilt was given us so that we might imbue all behavior, per-

haps especially pain, with an ethical dimension. There is no denying the enormity of the cost, of the secondary pain via the guilt itself. That cost is starkly visible in the "paradoxical guilt" of the traumatic syndrome, which, in turn, has bearing on equally "unfair" forms of guilt in many different neurotic and psychotic conditions. In such states, we observe the destructive manifestations of an emotion necessary to humanity, of the emotion concerned with critical self-judgment. And we come to suspect that beyond guilt itself, neurotic and psychotic versions of it are also integral to the human condition.

The Continuum of Psychic Numbing

At the heart of the traumatic syndrome—and of the overall human struggle with pain—is the diminished capacity to feel or *psychic numbing*. There is a close relationship between psychic numbing (including its acute form, "psychic closing-off") and death-linked images of denial ("If I feel nothing, then death is not taking place") and interruption of identification ("I see you dying, but I am not related to you or to your death"). The survivor undergoes a radical but temporary diminution in his or her sense of actuality in order to avoid losing this sense completely and permanently; he or she undergoes a reversible form of symbolic death in order to avoid a permanent physical or psychic death. From the standpoint of formative process, those patterns can be understood as expressions of an internal decision of the organism concerning investment and, therefore, an experience of feeling. When made under conditions of acute trauma, that "decision" is neither voluntary nor conscious.

Freud was acutely aware of such issues. This awareness is reflected in a passage from *Civilization and Its Discontents*:

> No matter how much we may shrink with horror from certain situations—of a galley slave in antiquity, of a peasant during the Thirty Years' War, of a victim of the Holy Inquisition, of a Jew awaiting a pogrom—it is nevertheless impossible for us to feel our way into such people, to divine the changes which original obtuseness of mind, a gradual stupefying process, the cessation of expectations and cruder or more refined methods of narcotization have produced upon their receptivity to sensations of pleasure and unpleasure. Moreover, in the case of the most extreme possibility of suffering, special mental protective devices are brought into operation. (Freud, 1961, pp. 55–56)

Freud (1919) is referring to acute and chronic forms of psychic numbing, in response to the most extreme kinds of trauma. Because he abruptly terminates these observations ("It seems to me unprofitable to pursue this aspect of the problem any further"), I had previously thought that Freud was making a special case of these extraordinary situations of what have been subsequently called "massive psychic trauma" and contrasting them with ordinary existence. But more careful study of the context suggests that Freud is actually making a relativistic statement. The preceding sentence, in fact, reads, "Happiness . . . is something essentially subjective," and Freud was cautioning against making too many assumptions concerning the effects of what we would consider the most extreme forms of trauma on people whose situation was quite removed from our own. He was suggesting that a process of "narcotization" or numbing might well prevent these people from experiencing anything like the degree of pain we might think we would experience. This reading suggests that Freud had a sensitive awareness of the adaptive nature of psychic numbing and of its importance for the whole gamut of human experience. There is perhaps implicit here also an important distinction between this kind of "gradual stupefying process" and more sudden kinds of traumata for which the organism is totally unprepared.

This passage was surely consistent with Freud's earlier observations about the "protective shield" and the extent to which the sense organs not only receive stimuli but "include special arrangements for further protection against excessive amounts of stimulation and for excluding unsuitable kinds of stimuli. To place all this within his instinctual cosmology, however, Freud (in a passage with which we are already familiar) subsumed this narcotization or numbing to the operation of the death instinct in maintaining the "Nirvana principle":

> The dominating tendency of mental life, and perhaps of nervous life in general, is the effort to reduce, to keep constant or to remove internal tension due to stimuli. [Freud went on to say that] our recognition of that fact is one of our strongest reasons for believing in the existence of death instincts. (Freud, 1920/1955)

And he saw this as an alliance between the pleasure principle, operating to reduce the internal tension caused by stimuli of various kinds, and the death instinct. Where this reduction of stimuli could not be considered exactly pleasurable, it was the latter, the death instinct, that took precedence in guiding the organism toward its own demise, in being "concerned with the most universal endeavor of all living substance—mainly to return to the quiescence of the inorganic world." Via instinctual theory, Freud is doing something interesting here. He is suggesting that a struggle with, or primarily against, feeling is the most fundamental characteristic of the human mind. In one place he suggests that in traumatic neuroses the compulsion to repeat derives from the earlier inability to experience feeling appropriate to the trauma—so that repetitive dreams about the traumatic experience "are endeavoring to master the stimulus retrospectively, by developing the anxiety whose omission was the cause of the traumatic neurosis" (Freud, 1920/1955). This is close to what we call *failed enactment*, here a matter of feelings that should have been but were not experienced. But where Freud goes on to see this compulsion to repeat as itself we would emphasize the struggle to assimilate the destructive or annihilating force into prior, or else altered, mental structures.

The numbing in severe versions of the traumatic syndrome consists of the mind being severed from its own psychic forms. To explain this process let us consider two quotations:

> The whole situation around me was very special . . . and my mental condition was very special too. . . . About life and death . . . I just couldn't have

any reaction . . . I don't think I felt either joy or sadness. . . . My feelings about human death weren't really normal. . . . You might say I became insensitive to . . . death. (Lifton, 1976/1991)

> We were all too exhausted to react, and almost nothing stirred our emotions. We had all seen too much. In my sick and aching brain, life had lost its importance and meaning, and seemed of no more consequence than the power of motion one lends to a marionette, so that it can agitate for a few seconds. Of course, there was friendship . . . but immediately behind them (two close friends) there was the hole full of guts, red, yellow, and foul smelling; piles of guts almost as large as the earth itself. Life could be snuffed out like that, in an instant, but the guts remained for a long time, stamped on the memory. (Sajer, 1971)

The first quotation is from a Hiroshima survivor, the second from a former soldier in the German infantry during World War II. In the case of the Hiroshima survivor, the overwhelming trauma was the experience of the bomb and its immediate aftermath of grotesque death immersion. The German soldier had experienced years of perpetual death-linked trauma. Their tone is strikingly similar in its combined suggestion of desensitization toward death and the annihilation of physical and psychic life. In order to dissociate itself from grotesque death, the mind must itself cease to live, become itself deadened. The dissociation becomes intrapsychic in the sense that feeling is severed from knowledge or awareness of what is happening. To say that emotion is lost, whereas cognition is retained is more or less true but does not really capture what the mind is experiencing. What is more basic is the self's being severed from its own history, from its grounding in such psychic forms as compassion for others, communal involvement, and other ultimate values. That is what is meant by the mind's being severed from its own forms. And that severance, in turn, results in the failed enactment and guilt we spoke of previously. This kind of process was described even before Freud by Pierre Janet (cited in van der Kolk & van der Hart, 1989) under the concept of *dissociation*. It includes not only stasis in the sense of inactivation but also disintegration in the sense of a coming apart of crucial components of the self. To be sure, that disintegration, like the stasis, is partial and, to a considerable degree, temporary—in fact, it is in the service of preventing more total and lasting forms of disintegration. But we can say that this dissociative disintegration characterizes the psychic numbing of the traumatic syndrome and is at the heart of that experience.

There is a close relationship between the phrase used by a Hiroshima survivor, "a feeling of paralysis of my mind," and a Buffalo Creek survivor's sense, in explaining his isolation from people around him, "Now . . . it's like everything is destroyed." Those two comments refer, respectively, to patterns of stasis and disintegration and suggest important elements of separation as well. For all three death equivalents are important in the dissociative disintegration of the traumatic syndrome. As a consequence, psychic action, the essence of the formative-symbolizing process, is virtually suspended, and the organism is in a state of severe de-symbolization. In that sense, psychic numbing undermines the most fundamental psychic processes. That is why we can speak of it as the essential mechanism of mental disorder.

The Problems of Intimacy, Nurturance, and Suspicion of the Counterfeit

These manifestations of psychic numbing are directly responsible for the two additional survivor struggles we have not yet discussed: those around suspicion of the counterfeit and quest for meaning. The survivor struggles toward—and in a way, against—reexperiencing himself or herself as a vital human being. Conflicts over nurturing and contagion have to do with the human relationships he or she requires for that revitalization, and with their impaired state. The survivor experiences feelings of weakness and special need, along with resentment of help offered as a reminder of weakness. Any such help is likely to be perceived as counterfeit. This is not only because of its association with weakness but because prior forms of dependency in human relationships have proven themselves unreliable; one's human web has been all too readily shattered, and in rearranging one's image feelings, one is on guard against false promises of protection, vitality, or even modest assistance. One fends off not only new threats of annihilation but gestures of love or help. Part of this resistance to human relationships has to do with a sense of being tainted by death, of carrying what might be called the psychic stigma of the annihilated. This stigma, which victims have always experienced, is usually explained around the idea of *self-concept*: If one is treated so cruelly, one tends to internalize that sense of being worthless. To modify and add to that principle, we could say: Having been annihilated and "killed," one feels oneself to have become part of the entire constellation of annihilation and destruction, to be identified with (live in the realm of) death and breakdown. The whole process, of course, is intensified by others' fear of the survivor's death taint. He or she becomes associated in their minds with a constellation of killing and dying that, should one let him or her get too close, endangers "ordinary healthy people." Consequently, associations to his or her experience can activate latent anxieties in others concerning death and death equivalents.

The struggles around nurturing and contagion are directly related to an insufficiently appreciated survivor emotion, that of *perpetual anger* and *frequent rage*. We discussed various kinds of survivor anger, rage, and violence, as directly related to a sense of inner death and a desperate effort at vitality. The survivor seems, in fact, to require his or her anger and rage—and all too often, violence—as an alternative to living in the realm of the annihilated. Many have noted that anger is relatively more comfortable than guilt or other forms of severe anxiety; it can also be a way of holding onto a psychic lifeline when surrounded by images of death.

The Task of Reformulation: Transformation and Reanimation

Maybe that is something of the way we live all the time, but, in the case of severe trauma, we can say there has been an important break in the lifeline that can leave one permanently engaged in either repair or the acquisition of new twine. And here we come to the survivor's overall task, that of *formulation*, evolving new inner forms that include the traumatic event, which, in turn, requires that one find meaning or significance in it so that the rest of one's life need not be devoid of meaning or significance. Formulation means establishing the lifeline on a new basis. That basis includes proximate and ultimate involvements. The survivor seeks vitality both in immediate relationships and in ultimate meaning, the one impossible without the other. Some Hiroshima survivors, for instance, could reanimate their lives around peace movement activities, which offered a sense of immediate activity in like-minded groups and ultimate significance within which their otherwise unassimilable experience could be understood. If the world could receive a valuable message from Hiroshima, that is, and they could be the agents and disseminators of that message, then what happened to them could be said to have a large purpose. The same principle applies to Nazi death-camp survivors in their struggle to establish and participate in the State of Israel. More typical is the quest for vitality around direct biological continuity—the tendency of many survivors to reassert family ties and reproduce and thereby assert biological and biosocial modes of symbolic immortality. In any case, the ultimate dimension, the struggle for resurgent modes of symbolic immortality, is crucial to the survivor, though rarely recognized as such.

Without this kind of formulation, the survivor remains plagued by unresolved conflicts in the other areas mentioned—by death anxiety, death guilt, psychic numbing, and immobilizing anger and suspicion of the counterfeit. Numbing (in particular, the desymbolizing center of the traumatic syndrome) is likely to persist. For to overcome that numbing, new psychic formations that assert vitality and one's right to it must evolve.

Beyond the Death Encounter: Confrontation, Reordering, and Renewal

A student of people with grief reactions around survival once spoke of their need for "emancipation from bondage to the deceased" (Lindemann, 1944). Even where deaths have not occurred, the survivor of a traumatic situation requires parallel emancipation from the bondage from his or her own inner deadness. In neither case does emancipation mean total severance but rather the creation of imagery that maintains fidelity to the end or to one's experience of inner deadness, fidelity in the sense of remembering what the experience entailed and including its excruciating truths in the self that is being recreated. What one does with feelings of self-condemnation or guilt is crucial to the outcome. There is a three-stage process available to the survivor of actual or symbolic death encounter, consisting of confrontation, reordering, and renewal (Lifton, 1973/1992). The second of these stages, *reordering*, is likely to be dominated by struggles with guilt and especially with converting static to animating forms of guilt. *Confrontation*, in the sense of recognizing the threat to existing forms and allowing for a certain amount of necessary dissolution of them, must precede those struggles. And for them to bear fruit they must be followed by renewal at both proximate and ultimate levels, and, equally important, in centering arrangements that integrate these levels. But without guilt-associated struggles around fidelity to the dead and the experience of deadness and to oneself as a witness, no such renewal or formulation is feasible.

A major difficulty here is the literalism the survivors impose upon themselves in viewing their death encounter. So terrifying and awesome do they find it, so demanding are their requirements of fidelity to it, that they may bind themselves to what they take to be its absolutely unaltered reality and permit themselves no psychic movement from that perceived reality. But where that is the case, the "reality" they lock themselves into is a false one because perception of any experience is achieved only by inner recreation of it. And the literalism they impose upon themselves turns out to be a form of numbing in the area of image formation, a suppression of psychic action. To be literally bound to a traumatic experience is to permit oneself no psychic vitality in relationship to the experience itself and to limit vitality in other areas of life as well. This near sanctification of the literal details of the death immersion was a considerable barrier to writers and artists attempting to give form to Hiroshima. The same issue affects every survivor within the confines of his own psyche. Here we may speak of a vicious circle in which death guilt and death anxiety reinforce numbing, which, in turn, holds one to suspicion of the counterfeit and to a relationship to the death immersion that is literalized and unformulated, which, again in turn, leaves one naked to death anxiety and death guilt.

To break out of this vicious circle in the direction of formulation, survivors must find a balance between appropriate blaming (which may indeed include considerable anger toward those who bear some responsibility for the traumatic events) and scapegoating (total concentration on the target for anger in a way that continues to literalize and inhibits assimilation of the experience). They must look backward in time as well as forward. Their tendency to claim a personal "golden age" prior to the death encounter can, it is true, distort, but may also serve as a source of life-sustaining imagery now so desperately required. To be forward-looking, to be receptive to experience that propels one toward the future, one must assemble those image feelings available to one that can assert, however tenuously, the continuity of life.

The Nazi Doctors: The Concept of Doubling in Response to Extreme Stress

I turn now to the subject of perpetrators and, more specifically, to my work with Nazi physicians (Lifton, 1986). The doctors with whom I worked were involved not only in experiments but also in direct supervision of killing at Auschwitz and other camps. They did selections; they went to the gas chamber; they supervised the insertion of the gas; they were responsible for declaring people dead and for having the gas chambers opened. They also did selections in camp; they did selections on medical blocks, reversing healing and killing in an al-

most literal way. They were part of a vast project—which was put forward in theory, a kind of biomedical theory that was central to Nazi belief—of killing in the name of healing. One cannot kill that many millions of people without a claim to virtue, a healing vision. This is the ultimate paradox of the Nazi movement—the combination of terror and brutality on the one hand and visionary idealism on the other. We must understand this combination in order to comprehend the Nazi movement itself. The fact that physicians were at the center of this paradox points to the biologized nature of the regime. As one doctor told me: "I joined the Nazi party the day after I heard Rudolph Hess declare that National Socialism was nothing but applied biology." The movement saw itself as healing the Nordic race, in a biological way, and doctors were crucial to the process, both in direct, personal ways and in sterilization and so-called euthanasia, or the killing of mental patients. Moreover, they were symbolic figures, biological activists, carrying out this biomedical vision.

The Psychological Functions of Doubling: Intrapsychic Dissociation

1. Interviews with both Nazi doctors and many observant and sensitive survivors of Auschwitz have led me to observe very different patterns of what I call *doubling* in the two groups. This includes the formation of a part self, which ultimately becomes an entire and considerably autonomous self. Although the two selves are interacting parts of a holistic self, a dialectic exists between their connectedness and the considerable autonomy of the second self.

2. Second, there is the holistic principle. The second self functions fully as a whole self; for this reason, it is so adaptable and so dangerous. It enables a relatively ordinary person to commit evil. It has a life/death dimension, in which the perpetrator overcomes his or her own death anxiety by involvement in the killing of others.

3. Another function of this doubling is the avoidance of guilt, or in the case of perpetrators, the transfer of conscience. The conscience becomes associated with the group, with the sense of duty, and with an adaptation to the Auschwitz milieu, so that the self can protect itself from the feelings of conscience over what it should feel guilty about, namely, its involvement in killing other people.

4. Doubling represents a way of adapting to evil. Indeed, it is part of the genius of adaptation of our species, which has carried over into adapting to evil. By doubling, one can sufficiently overcome conflicts in order to commit acts of evil. In the case of the Nazi doctors, once one made a decision to stay in Auschwitz, then one had to double if one were to adapt to that environment.

Situational Context and Determinants of Doubling

We can view Auschwitz as an institution that operated on doubling. Moreover, the institution needed and was provided with a certain degree of ideology, including degrees of anti-Semitism. This belief system, accompanied by extreme numbing and various mixtures of omnipotence and impotence, led to the creation of what can be called an "Auschwitz self," while maintaining a sense of professional identity as physicians. Thus, the doctors conducted experiments in an effort to remain doctors, when in reality they were killing. Sometimes they supported medical work carried out by prisoner–physicians. They saw themselves as physicians who were performing very technical tasks; in so doing, they developed tunnel vision regarding their actions.

Auschwitz prisoners also underwent doubling. Many Auschwitz inmates whom I interviewed said such things as "I was a different person in Auschwitz. I really was. I was a completely different person." They were suggesting different self-formation, this time in the name of the preservation of life. Although the purpose and moral judgment differ drastically, the process has some parallels.

Looking back at some of my own and others' work with Vietnam War veterans, we might recall the words of Philip Kingrey, who wrote in his book, *The Labyrinth of Fear*, that "threat made me threatening. I was two of myself, one human and the other inhuman. I delighted in destruction, and yet was a healer." He struggled with two sides of himself, the way in which any person put into an atrocity-producing situation might struggle in trying to heal. In the early 1970s, a Vietnam War veteran told of a dream in which "I was arguing with myself. There were two separate selves, and one of them finally shot the other, so that I shot myself." Here, a tremendous and painful kind of doubling process occurred, in which the dream was expressing a powerful impulse to end the doubling in some way but was unable to do so in a constructive manner. Instead, the dream served as an opportunity to look at the violence and to move toward a more nonviolent resolution, albeit through a violent act in the dream itself.

The Protean Principle

In conclusion, the experience of an extreme situation really is an assault on and a threat to the entire self. This is the wisdom of theory focused on the self, as articulated by Kohut and Erikson, as well as by Harry Stack Sullivan and, much earlier, Otto Rank. To this we must add a formative principle, as I have previously described—one of continuous psychic action. Furthermore, we must add what I call the *Protean principle*, after the Greek god Proteus. This Protean principle involves something that is historically influenced and has to do with the multifaceted nature of our lives, the way in which we can move from involvement to involvement or have multiple images that are sometimes contradictory, simultaneously in our heads, because of various historical forces to which we are exposed. Such forces include the breakdown of the kinds of classical symbols that held us to a more narrow life pattern in the past, as well as the influence of the mass media (which can be considerable) in making contact with areas of the self that need not only be superficial.

The Transformation of the Self

Given the formative principle and the Protean principle in connection with a focus on self, we can look at posttraumatic disorders, struggles, and survivor reactions in terms of a self-process that is very specific to that traumatic situation. We then are better equipped to look at the process in which people can move in and out of the traumatized self or in and out of symptoms, feelings, or positions with respect to the trauma. As I have stated, moving out of that traumatized self into some reintegration of the self constitutes the recovery process.

The posttraumatic stress reaction can be understood as an effort to restore or create anew the reintegration of the self. The residual symptoms are, on one hand, adaptive; their presence implies their necessity. We struggle with the ambivalence toward the extent to which we want to eliminate these symptoms, because, although they are a problem, they also represent adaptation. Again the symptoms include evidence of residual doubling, which is a continuing adaptation. Indeed, perhaps one never loses a sense of that traumatized self fully but masters it and integrates it into a larger sense of self. Overcoming that doubling is very much the reintegrative and therapeutic process.

Often the unfinished psychological work has to do with not only a new enactment to compensate for that failed enactment at the time of the trauma, in order to eliminate self-condemnation, but also moving out of that entire holistic double self toward a more integrated self. In contrast, for example, the "Rambo" phenomenon is a superficial and malignant mass media effort to chart a false direction of integration, where integration is not present. It is a reintegrative process through violence along with a replay of failed enactment that is absolutely made literal. In the Rambo film, we see the replay of the Vietnam War, and as the film says, "this time, we win." It is very externalized, harmful, and ultimately a false claim to reintegration.

Finally, we can say that the same phenomenon of the formation of a second self can contribute to mass murder in ways that I have described previously. At the same time, it can, in a different guise and in a different moral context, contribute to survival and to the enhancement of life. But doubling and the conditions for doubling are our adversary in our work. Moreover, within the moral context of the work that we do, we are confronting the adversary all the time in our efforts to bring about reintegration. Indeed, our efforts toward that goal, toward contributing to reintegration of the self, require that we grasp the nature of the adversarial forces of disintegration and take our stand against them.

References

American Psychiatric Association. (1987). *Diagnostic and statistical manual of mental disorders* (3rd ed., rev.). Washington, DC: Author.

American Psychiatric Association. (in press). *Diagnostic and statistical manual of mental disorders* (4th ed.). Washington, DC: Author.

Archibald, H. C., Long, D. M., Miller, C., & Tuddenham, R. D. (1962). Gross stress reaction in combat: A 15-year follow-up. *American Journal of Psychiatry*, 119, 317–322.

Freud, S. (1919). *Zur Psychoanalyse der Kriegsneurosen*. Leipzig: Internationaler Psychoanalytischer Verlag.

Freud, S. (1955). Beyond the pleasure principle. In J. Strachey (Ed. and Trans.), *The standard edition of the complete psychological works of Sigmund Freud* (Vol. 18, pp. 7–64). London: Hogarth Press. (Original work published 1920)

Freud, S. (1961). *Civilization and its discontents*. New York: W. W. Norton.

Freud, S. (1964). Introduction to psychoanalysis and the war neuroses, including appendix, "Memorandum on the electrical treatment of war neurotics." In J. Strachey (Ed. and Trans.), *The standard edition of the complete psychological works of Sigmund Freud* (Vol. 17, pp. 205–215). London: Hogarth Press. (Original work published 1919)

Jones, E. (1953). *The life and work of Sigmund Freud* (Vol. 2, pp. 253–254). New York: Basic Books.

Kardiner, A. (1959). Traumatic neuroses of war. In S. Ariete (Ed.), *American handbook of psychiatry* (Vol. 1, p. 256). New York: Basic Books.

Lifton, R. J. (1976). *The life of the self*. New York: Simon & Schuster.

Lifton, R. J. (1986). *The Nazi doctors*. New York: Basic Books.

Lifton, R. J. (1991). *Death in life: Survivors of Hiroshima*. Chapel Hill and London: University of North Carolina Press. (Original work published 1967).

Lifton, R. J. (1992). *Home from the war: Vietnam veterans: Neither victims nor executioners*. (2nd ed.). Boston: Beacon Press. (Original work published 1973).

Lifton, R. J., & Olson, E. (1976). The human meaning of total disaster: The Buffalo Creek experience. *Psychiatry*, 39, 1–17.

Lindemann, E. (1944). Symptomatology and management of acute grief. *American Journal of Psychiatry*, 101, 141–148.

Sajer, G. (1971). *The forgotten soldier*. New York: Harper & Row.

Teicher, J. D. (1953). "Combat fatigue" or "death anxiety neurosis." *Journal of Nervous and Mental Disease*, 117, 232–242.

van der Kolk, B., & van der Hart, O. (1989, December). Pierre Janet and the breakdown of adaptation in psychological trauma. *American Journal of Psychiatry*, 146(12), 1530–1540.

Waelder, R. (1967). Trauma and the variety of extraordinary challenges. In S. S. Furst (Ed.), *Psychic trauma* (pp. 221–234). New York: Basic Books.

Wilson, J. P. (1989). *Trauma, transformation and healing: An integrative approach to theory, research and post-traumatic therapy*. New York: Brunner/Mazel.

CHAPTER 2

Biological Response to Psychic Trauma

Bessel A. van der Kolk and Jose Saporta

They will fail to cope psychologically with their problems until they have a sense of security in their bodies. In losing control over their bodily functions they are not the competent people they were before. (Kolb & Multipassi, 1982)

Background

The recognition that psychological trauma results in enduring biological changes goes back to the very earliest descriptions of the human trauma response. A century ago, Pierre Janet (1889) taught that when people react to experiences with "vehement emotions," this interferes with proper information processing and appropriate action. He held that hyperarousal was responsible for the memory disturbances that accompany traumatization: Interfering with information processing on a verbal, symbolic level, hyperarousal causes memories to be split off from consciousness and to be stored only somatically. Fragments of these "visceral" memories return later as physiological reactions, emotional states, visual images, or behavioral reenactments (van der Kolk & van der Hart, 1989).

Janet thought that the physiological response to trauma accounted for the continued emergency responses to subsequent stresses. He claimed that fear needs to be tamed for proper cognitive appraisal and for appropriate action: Experiences which overwhelm people's coping mechanisms set the stage (or to use Pavlov's later concept "condition" them) to react automatically with excessive emotional reactions to subsequent stressors. These are accompanied by inordinate physical responses, usually without conscious awareness that these extreme reactions to current experiences are rooted in the past.

Freud also suggested that the fixation on the trauma is biologically based: "After severe shock . . . the dream life continually takes the patient back to the situation of his disaster from which he awakens with renewed terror . . . the patient has undergone a physical fixation to the trauma" (Freud, 1919/1954). The feature of hyperreactivity to external stimuli was described by Freud in the clearest neuropsychiatric terms that he knew:

I think that one may venture . . . the traumatic neurosis as the result of an extensive rupture in the barrier against stimuli . . . we seek to understand the effect of the shock by considering the breaking through of the barrier with which the psychic organ is provided.

Pavlov's investigations continued the tradition of explaining the trauma response as the result of lasting physiological alterations (Pavlov, 1927). He, and others employing his paradigm, coined the term *defensive reaction* for a cluster of innate reflexive responses to environmental threat. Many studies have shown how the response to potent environmental stimuli (unconditional stimuli—US) becomes a conditioned reaction. After repeated aversive stimulation, intrinsically nonthreatening cues associated with the trauma (conditional stimuli—CS) become capable of eliciting the defensive reaction by themselves (conditional response—CR). A rape victim may respond to conditioned stimuli, such as

Bessel A. van der Kolk and Jose Saporta • Trauma Clinic, Massachusetts Mental Health Center, and Harvard Medical School, Boston, Massachusetts 02115.

International Handbook of Traumatic Stress Syndromes, edited by John P. Wilson and Beverley Raphael. Plenum Press, New York, 1993.

the approach by an unknown man, as if she were about to be raped again, and experience panic. Pavlov also pointed out that "constitutional factors," that is, individual differences in temperament, accounted for the variability in the human response to traumatic stimuli.

Abraham Kardiner (1941), who first systematically defined posttraumatic stress for American audiences, noted that sufferers from posttraumatic stress disorder (PTSD) continue to live in the emotional environment of the traumatic event, with enduring vigilance for and sensitivity to environmental threat. He described the five principal features of PTSD as (1) persistence of startle response and irritability, (2) proclivity to explosive outbursts of aggression, (3) fixation on the trauma, (4) constriction of the general level of personality functioning, and (5) atypical dream life. He suggested that the startle reaction probably was a conditioned reflex and considered it the central element of the posttraumatic stress reaction, relating it to the development of irritability and psychosomatic symptoms in these patients.

In war stress and neurotic illness, Kardiner and Spiegel (1945) stated that a traumatic neurosis is a physical one, and that the physical sensation endures:

> The nucleus of the neurosis is a physioneurosis. This is present on the battlefield and during the entire process of organization; it outlives every intermediary accommodative device, and persists in the chronic forms. The traumatic syndrome is ever present and unchanged.

In Men under Stress, Grinker and Spiegel (1945) described physical symptoms in the acute posttraumatic state that seem to reflect neurochemical changes of the catecholamine system: They described flexor changes in posture, hyperkinesis, "violently propulsive gait," tremor at rest, masklike faces, absence of associated movement while walking, cogwheel rigidity, gastric distress, urinary incontinence, mutism, and a violent startle reflex. Grinker and Spiegel noted the similarity of many of these symptoms and those of diseases of the extrapyramidal motor system. They seem to depict extraordinary stimulation of certain biological systems and implicate ascending amine projections in particular. Contemporary studies, generally unaware of this earlier research, have continued to scientifically test these conceptions and confirm that the stress hormones of people with PTSD continue to react to minor stimuli as emergencies.

Symptomatology of Posttraumatic Stress Disorder

The phasic posttraumatic symptoms of hyperalertness, hyperreactivity to stimuli, and traumatic reexperiencing have been documented in a vast literature on combat trauma, crimes such as rape (e.g., Burgess & Holstrom, 1974; Kilpatrick, Veronen, & Best, 1985), kidnapping (Terr, 1983), natural disasters (e.g., Shore, Tatum, & Vollmer, 1986), accidents (e.g., Wilkinson, 1983), and imprisonment (Krystal, 1978). The human response to trauma is so constant across traumatic stimuli that it is safe to say that the central nervous system (CNS) seems to react to any overwhelming, threatening, and uncon-

trollable experience in quite a consistent pattern. Regardless of the circumstances, traumatized people are prone to have intrusive memories of elements of the trauma, to have a poor tolerance for arousal, to respond to stress in an all-or-nothing way, and to feel emotionally numb. All these psychological phenomena must have a basis in biological functioning, and some of these relationships between biological abnormalities and psychological states are now ready to be explored. PTSD, as defined in the DSM-III-R (American Psychiatric Association, 1987) highlights those posttraumatic symptoms that are most clearly biologically based; the secondary posttraumatic changes in self-identity and interpersonal relations are slated to be classified in the separate category of Disorders of Extreme Stress Not Otherwise Specified (DESNOS) in the DSM-IV (American Psychiatric Association, in press). As there are good reasons to assume that the current PTSD categories A (intrusive recollections) and C (hyperarousal) are, biologically speaking, intimately related, we will discuss them jointly throughout this chapter.

Autonomic Hyperreactivity and Intrusive Reexperiencing

Kardiner (1941) coined the term physioneurosis to describe posttraumatic stress. He pointed out that while people with PTSD tend to deal with their environment by emotional constriction, their bodies continue to react to certain physical and emotional stimuli as if there were a continuing threat of annihilation. Starting with studies by Dobbs and Wilson (1960), conditioned autonomic arousal to combat stimuli has repeatedly been documented in veterans with PTSD. Using a variety of different techniques, Malloy, Fairbank, and Keane (1983), Kolb and Multipassi (1982), Blanchard et al. (1986), and Pitman et al. (1987) all have found significant conditioned reactions in response to stimuli reminiscent of the original trauma, as measured by heart rate, blood pressure and electromyogram. The relationship between autonomic arousal and intrusive recollections was illustrated by the study of Rainey et al. (1987), which showed that lactate administration elicited PTSD-like flashbacks in 7 out of 7 subjects and panic attacks in 6 in 7 patients with PTSD, 6 of whom also met panic disorder criteria. These findings further support the notion of common biological underpinnings for the flashbacks and panic attacks in PTSD.

The reliability and specificity of the studies of physiological reactions to traumatic stimuli are beginning to raise the possibility that in the future a pychophysiologically based diagnostic test for PTSD will be available to help in making the diagnosis. However, it still is unclear how specific the hyperarousal is as a conditioned response to traumatic stimuli alone. Clinical experience suggests that the increased autonomic arousal can be rather nonspecific, and may occur in response to a variety of stimuli. In fact, some research suggests that habituation may follow repeated exposure to the traumatic stimulus itself, but associated events continue to elicit hyperreactivity (Strian & Klicpera, 1978). These findings can be used therapeutically in implosion therapy (Keane et al., 1989).

The loss of neuromodulation that is at the core of PTSD leads to intensification of emotional reactivity in general: Traumatized people go immediately from stimulus to response without being able to make the intervening psychological assessment of the cause of their arousal, which causes them to overreact and intimidate others. Nonspecific noises played into the rooms of sleeping people with posttraumatic stress may precipitate nightmares in which old traumatic occurrences are recreated in exact detail (Kramer, Schoen, & Kinney, 1984). Hyperarousal also interferes with psychotherapy, in preventing remembering and working through painful memories.

Numbing

Numbing of responsiveness, which may be registered as depression, as anhedonia and amotivational states, as psychosomatic reactions, or as dissociative states, are all associated symptoms of PTSD. In contrast with the intrusive PTSD symptoms, numbing is tonic and part of patients' baseline functioning. It interferes with the ability to explore, remember and integrate memories, and undermines the capacity to fantasize and symbolize, all of which are essential for finding new meaning. Throughout the literature, numbing is all too unquestioningly described as a psychological defense against remembering painful affects. We will argue that numbing is a core, biologically based symptom of PTSD.

Effects of Developmental Level on Psychobiological Effects of Trauma

Although most studies on PTSD have been done on adults, particularly on war veterans, in recent years a small prospective literature has emerged which calls attention to the differential effects of trauma at various age levels. Anxiety disorders, chronic hyperarousal, and reenactments have now been described with some regularity in acutely traumatized children (Bowlby, 1973; Ornitz & Pynoos, 1989; Pynoos & Eth, 1985; Stoddard *et al.*, 1985; Terr, 1988). In addition to reactions to discrete traumatic incidents, chronic intrafamilial abuse must certainly be included among the most severe traumas encountered by human beings. This recognition opens up the boundaries between the current concept of PTSD and what we have called the *trauma spectrum* (van der Kolk, 1988): other posttraumatic disorders ranging from those that result from brief traumatic exposure at an early age, such as phobias and panic, to Borderline Personality Disorder and Multiple Personality Disorder, which are usually associated with chronic intrafamilial abuse (Herman, Perry, & van der Kolk, 1989). Specific neurobiological abnormalities are beginning to be identified along this spectrum: Prospective studies by Putnam *et al.* show neuroendocrine disturbances in sexually abused girls compared with normals while Gilette *et al.* have demonstrated abnormalities of the hypothalamic-pituitary-thyroid axis in adult female psychiatric patients with childhood histories of incest (Gilette *et al.*, 1989). Nonbrain-damaged adult patients who mutilate themselves invariably seem to have a history of severe childhood trauma, and their behavior has been associated with abnormalities of the endogenous opioid and catecholamine systems (Bach-y-Rita, 1974; Pattison & Kahan, 1983; van der Kolk, Greenberg, *et al.*, 1989). Research in the last decade has shown that many children who have been victims of intrafamilial abuse have chronic problems with hyperarousal and aggression against others and themselves (Cicchetti & Rosen, 1984; Green, 1980; van der Kolk, Herman, & Perry, 1989b).

The biological effects of developmental trauma have best been studied in young nonhuman primates, who, in many ways, resemble young human beings. Primate research for forty years has firmly established the fact that early disruption of the social attachment bond reduces the long-term capacity to cope with subsequent social disruptions and to modulate physiological arousal. These studies have demonstrated that trauma early in the life cycle has long-term effects on the neurochemical response to stress, including the magnitude of the catecholamine response, the duration and extent of the cortisol response, as well as a number of other biological systems, such as the serotonin and endogenous opioid system (Kraemer *et al.*, 1984; Reite & Fields, 1985).

Trauma and the Limbic System

The limbic system plays an important role in guiding the emotions that stimulate the behavior necessary for self-preservation and survival of the species. It is responsible for such complex behaviors as feeding, fighting, fleeing, and reproduction, and it also assigns free-floating feelings of significance, truth, and meaning to experience (MacLean, 1985). Destruction of parts of the limbic system abolishes social behavior, including play, cooperation, mating, and care of the young. The apparent similarities between some aspects of temporal lobe epilepsy (TLE), PTSD, and some long-term sequelae of childhood trauma continue to challenge us to further explore the effects of trauma on the limbic system. During this past decade, the relationships between environmental trauma and the organization and function of the limbic system are slowly beginning to be understood, partly because of the pioneering work of such primatologists as Kling and Steklis, whose studies of nonhuman primates have conclusively shown that disruption of early attachment directly affects the maturation of the limbic system (Kling & Steklis, 1976).

The limbic system is also the primary area of the CNS where memories are processed, and is the most likely location to find an explanation for the memory disturbances which follow trauma. The hippocampus, which records in memory the spatial and temporal dimensions of experiences, does not fully mature until the third or fourth year of life. However, the system that subserves memories related to the quality (feel and sound) of things (which is mainly located in the amygdala) matures much earlier (O'Keefe & Nadel, 1978). Thus, in the first few years of life, only the quality of events but not their context can be remembered. Even after that, the hippocampal localization system remains vulnerable to disruption: Severe or prolonged stress can suppress hipppocampal functioning (Squire, 1987), creating context-free fearful associations which are hard to locate in space and time. This results in amnesia for the specifics of traumatic experiences, but not the feelings associated with them (Sapolsky, Krey, & McEwen, 1984). These experiences may then be encoded on a sensorimotor level without proper localization in space and time. They therefore cannot be easily translated into the symbolic language necessary for linguistic retrieval.

A third trauma-related function of the limbic system involves the issue of *kindling*. Intermittent stimulation of the limbic system with an electrical current that was initially too small to produce overt behavioral effects can eventually sensitize limbic neuronal circuits and lower firing neuronal-firing thresholds: Repeated stimulation of the amygdala causes long-term alterations in neuronal excitability (Post, Pickar, Ballenger, Naber, & Rubinow, 1984). It is possible that similar kindling phenomena occur when people are repeatedly traumatized, or when one traumatic event is followed by intrusive reexperiences. Thus, trauma may lead to lasting neurobiological and behavioral (characterological) changes mediated by alterations in the temporal lobe. Kindling may also account for the frequency of neurological abnormalities in trauma victims, especially child victims of physical or sexual abuse (van der Kolk, 1987). Open studies claim that carbamezapine is an effective treatment for the intrusive symptoms of PTSD (Lipper *et al.*, 1986) which lends some support for a role of the limbic system in codifying posttraumatic reactions.

Neuromodulation of Arousal: Noradrenergic versus Serotonergic Pathways

The locus coeruleus (LC) is at the anatomical core of the physiological arousal mechanism. Although the LC contains corticotropin releasing factor (CRF) and opioid neurons, both of which play a role in the biology of PTSD, the LC is also the principal source of noradrenaline (NE) in the CNS, the neurotransmitter responsible for delivering messages to the rest of the brain about the need to prepare for emergencies. The arousal system consists of two groups of NE fibers which emanate from the LC, the dorsal and ventral bundles. Both ventral and dorsal bundles increase the readiness of the hypothalamic mechanisms controlling defensive reactions so that these can be set into action rapidly and vigorously when required. The dorsal noradrenergic bundle connects the LC with the septohippocampal system, the part of the limbic system involved in the evaluation of incoming stimuli. Gray (1982) has proposed that the dorsal bundle to the hippocampal system is the most important projection from the LC; it does not carry specific information, only the general message: This is important (Gray, 1982). Impulses reaching the septohippocampal system from the dorsal noradrenergic bundle influence the way in which this system processes information. Naturally occurring opiates modify the firing of the LC (Bird & Kuhar, 1977), while such pharmacological agents as clonidine and the beta-adrenergic blockers act

by a different molecular mechanism but produce the same final effect: reduced activity in the LC neurons. Antianxiety drugs are thought to interfere with LC activity by increasing the action of gamma-aminobutyric acid (GABA-ergic) inhibition on the cell bodies of the LC.

The function of the septohippocampal system is to evaluate in which way incoming stimuli are important, and whether they are associated with reward, punishment, novelty, or nonreward. Thus, the hippocampus is thought to be the evaluative center involved in behavioral inhibition, obsessional thinking, inhibition of exploratory behavior, scanning, and construction of a spatial map (O'Keefe & Nadel, 1978), and fulfills the crucial function of storing and categorizing information. When categorization is complete, the hippocampus disengages from active control of behavior. External stress increases corticosterone production, which decreases the firing rates of the hippocampus (Pfaff, Silva, & Weiss, 1971). Lesions of the hippocampus lead to paralysis because of excessive susceptibility to interference from competing responses.

The signal that punishment is imminent activates two related mechanisms, one of which inhibits ongoing behavior, while the other increases the level of arousal. The behavioral facilitating system (BFS), mediated by NE fibers emanating from the LC, activates the diencephalic and hypothalamic structures necessary for emergency responses. The BFS is activated when specific goal-oriented aggressive attack patterns require motivated motor support (Dupue & Spoont, 1989). The opposing process, the behavioral inhibition system (BIS), is mediated by the septohippocampal system, primed by ascending serotonergic and cholinergic mechanisms. The crucial role of the septohippocampal system is to activate a descending inhibitory pathway which prevents initiation of emergency responses until it is clear that they will be of use. Numerous studies have shown that serotonergic antagonists reduce the suppression of behavior by punishment. Serotonergic antagonists also cause increased aggression in response to stress, and hyperreactivity to stimuli (Sheard & Davis, 1976). The suppression of behavior by punishment is reversed by serotonin receptor blockers (e.g., Cook & Sepinwall, 1975). Serotonergic pathways play an important role in the control of anxiety-related behavior associated with suppression by punishment. The ascending serotonergic pathways are thought to provide the missing signal the septohippocampus needs if it is to distinguish punishment from reward. The introduction of the serotonin reuptake blockers fluvoxamine, fluoxetine, and gepirone demonstrated how these agents reversed the continued emergency responses and repetitive behaviors following stress in animals, allowing a better understanding about the degree to which decreased serotonin seems to play a role in these behaviors. Current clinical trials of these drugs in people with PTSD suggest that they are by far the most effective biological treatments of PTSD currently available. This makes us believe that in traumatized individuals decreased serotonin decreases the influence of the BIS, thereby disposing the septohippocampal system to interpret noradrenergic signals originating in the LC in response to stress as recurrences of traumatic experiences. Thus, we postulate that lowered serotonin activity in PTSD is at the core of a diminished efficacy of the BIS which, in turn, is responsible for the continuation of emergency responses to minor stresses long after the actual trauma has ceased.

Stress Response and the Psychobiology of PTSD

Arousal

The body responds to increased physical or psychological demands by releasing norepinephrine from the LC and adrenocorticotropin (ACTH) from the anterior pituitary. The precise interactions between the various stress hormones is extremely complex and is still poorly understood, but both norepinephrine and epinephrine play a role in stimulating the release of CRF. The hypothalamus regulates ACTH release by the secretion of CRF. The hypothalamus also secretes thyroxin releasing hormone (TRH), which activates the secretion of thyroid stimulating hormone (TSH) from the pituitary. CRF, as well as vasopressin, activates the release of ACTH and beta-endorphin and stimulates adenylate cyclase activity and the formation of cyclic adenosine monophosphate (cyclic AMP). Peripherally, the body's stress response consists of the secretion of norepinephrine by the sympathetic nerves and of epinephrine by the adrenal medulla, whereas, stimulated by ACTH, the adrenal cortex secretes glucocorticoids. These hormones help the body mobilize the energy necessary to deal with stressors, ranging from increased glucose release to enhanced immune function. In a well-functioning organism, stress produces rapid and pronounced hormonal responses. However, chronic persistent stress blunts this effective stress response and induces desensitization: After prolonged stress, CRF secretion produces less cyclic AMP formation and ACTH release because of down-regulation of CRF receptors. Thus, the release of the stress hormone ACTH is controlled by complex regulatory mechanisms. Multiple factors such as CRF, vasopressin, catecholamines, and other hormones stimulate ACTH release by acting on the anterior pituitary.

It therefore is not surprising that, in the study of the psychobiology of PTSD, stress hormones have figured most prominently, and that abnormalities of these systems are often found in patients with PTSD. Kosten *et al.* (1987) found increased 24-hour norepinephrine and epinephrine secretion in veterans with PTSD compared to patients with other psychiatric diagnoses. Mason *et al.* (1986) found low 24-hour urinary cortisol levels in Vietnam veterans with PTSD. In a different study, PTSD subjects showed blunted ACTH response to CRH stimulation: Smith *et al.* (1989) found that the severity of PTSD was directly related to baseline plasma cortisol. This finding supports the notion that there are chronically increased levels of cortisol in patients with PTSD.

However, Smith and colleagues also suggested the alternative explanation of decreased pituitary function secondary to persistent elevations of endogenous CRH due to chronic hypothalamic-pituitary-adrenal (HPA) axis activity at the level of the hypothalamus.

Changes in receptor activity have been found in PTSD which are consistent with down-regulation secondary to chronic exposure to elevated levels of circulating catecholamines: Perry, Giller, and Southwick (1987) have demonstrated a 40% decrease in the number of platelet alpha-2-adrenergic receptors in 25 patients with PTSD. Lerer *et al.* (1987) reported evidence of desensitization of adenylate cyclase-coupled adrenergic receptors on lymphocytes and platelets in PTSD.

However, persistent activation of stress response is not only a function of the stress hormones themselves, but also of the capacity of the organism to modulate arousal. We discussed before how serotonergic input into the septal hippocampus decreases the relative strength of the noradrenergic input, allowing modulation of emergency responses. The serotonin reuptake blockers fluvoxamine, fluoxetine, and gepirone seem to have a dramatic beneficial effect on the capacity to modulate arousal and decrease posttraumatic repetitions of images, behaviors, or somatic states. The clinical trials with these drugs suggest that they are by far the most effective biological treatments of PTSD currently available.

Numbing

Although the numbing in responsiveness in PTSD has generally been conceptualized only in psychological terms, as a defense against reliving memories of the trauma, our recent research may shed some light on the biological components of this aspect of PTSD. Stress-induced analgesia (SIA) has been described in experimental animals following a variety of inescapable stressors such as electric shock, fighting, starvation, and cold water swim (Akil *et al.*, 1984; Kelly, 1982; Lewis, Cannon, & Liebeskind, 1980). In these severely stressed animals, opiate withdrawal symptoms can be produced equally by termination of the stressful stimulus or by naloxone injections. Thus, severe, chronic stress in animals results in a physiological state which resembles dependence on high levels of exogenous opioids (Terman, Shavit, Lewis, Cannon, & Liebeskind, 1984).

Stimulated by the finding that fear activates the secretion of endogenous opioid peptides (Bolles & Fanselow, 1980) and that SIA can become conditioned to subsequent stressors, and to previously neutral events associated with the noxious stimulus, we tested the hypothesis that in people with PTSD, reexposure to a stimulus resembling the original trauma will cause an endogenous opioid response that can be indirectly measured as naloxone reversible analgesia (Pitman *et al.*, 1990; van der Kolk *et al.*, 1989). We found that two decades after the original trauma, people with PTSD developed opioid-mediated analgesia in response to a stimulus resembling the traumatic stressor, which we correlated with a secretion of endogenous opioids equivalent to 8 mg of morphine. This change in pain response was the most significant factor differentiating the PTSD from the control groups' response to a traumatic stimulus. Self-reports of emotional responses to the combat videotape in the placebo condition indicated a relative blunting of emotional response to the traumatic stimulus, and we interpreted this finding to indicate that opioid-mediated SIA may be involved in psychic numbing. Survivors of severe trauma have repeatedly been described to experience a triad of physical analgesia, psychic numbing, and depersonalization. Our finding of SIA in PTSD may also be relevant to the phenomenon of self-mutilation.

Patients who engage in such self-destructive behavior almost invariably have a history of severe childhood trauma and, in response to even relatively minor emotional stressors, they may experience physical analgesia, dissociative reactions and emotional numbing, which can be abolished by (1) an act of self-mutilation or (2) the administration of naloxone (Richardson & Zaleski, 1983; Sandman, Barron, Crinella, & Donnelly, 1987). Whether the analgesia, dissociative reactions, and emotional numbing reported in these patients are all functions of a conditioned endogenous opioid response to a traumatic stressor remains a subject for further investigation.

Memory Disturbances in PTSD

One of the hallmarks of PTSD is the intrusive reexperiencing of elements of the trauma in nightmares, flashbacks, or somatic reactions. These traumatic memories seem to be triggered by autonomic arousal (Rainey *et al.*, 1987) and are thought to be due to hyperpotentiation of memory pathways and mediated by noradrenergic pathways originating in the LC (van der Kolk, Greenberg, Boyd, & Krystal, 1985). The innervation of the structures of the brain subserving memory functions originates in the LC from which noradrenergic projections go to the limbic system, cerebral cortex, and, to a lesser degree, the hypothalamus (Grant & Redmond, 1981). The LC also facilitates memory retrieval by means of the noradrenergic tracts to the hippocampus and amygdala (Delaney, Tussi, & Gold, 1983). We (van der Kolk *et al.*, 1985) and Pitman (1989) have hypothesized that a long-term augmentation of the LC pathways following trauma underlies the repetitive intrusive reliving of the trauma, particularly after renewed stress. Because autonomic arousal is mediated by the LC, it is plausible that not only flashbacks but also traumatic nightmares occur following autonomic nervous system activation, mediated by the potentiated pathways from the LC to the hippocampus and amygdala. This also could account for the eidetic (picturelike), rather than the oneiric (dreamlike) quality of traumatic nightmares (van der Kolk *et al.*, 1984).

Sleep Studies

Patients with PTSD have been found to have chronically disturbed sleep which appears to be related to chronic physiological hyperarousal. Both Kaminer and Lavie (1988) and van Kammen, Christiansen, van Kammen, and Reynolds (1990) found increased sleep latency, more awakenings, less total sleep time, and less rapid eye movement (REM) time. Kinney and Kramer (1985) found PTSD patients to be exquisitely sensitive to nonspecific auditory stimuli, which provoked autonomic arousal, accompanied by nightmares about traumatic experiences. We (van der Kolk *et al.*, 1984) found that post-

traumatic nightmares may occur during any stage of the sleep cycle; that most occur between 2 and 3 A.M. during Stage II or III sleep, possibly during a transition to REM sleep. When they occur during Stage II or III, patients report exact living experiences of traumatic material, while, during REM, they are more typical anxiety dreams.

Psychosomatic Reactions

Numerous studies for the past one hundred years have established a causal relation between the inhibition of expression of traumatic experience and psychophysiological impairment. These studies have demonstrated a marked increase in symptoms of the respiratory, digestive, cardiovascular, and endocrine systems in people with PTSD (Janet, 1889; Krystal, 1978). Recent studies have indicated that learning to expresss the memories and feelings related to the traumatic event can restore some of the psychophysiological and immunological competence in people with traumatic histories (Pennebaker & Susman, 1988).

Implications for the Psychopharmacological Treatment of PTSD

While giving voice to both the traumatic events and the affects related to them is generally considered the most effective treatment of PTSD, verbal therapies cannot proceed as long as the patient is unable to tolerate the feelings associated with the trauma and continues to experience subsequent emotionally stimulating events as an unmodified recurrence of the trauma. It often is necessary to supplement psychotherapy with medications which decrease autonomic arousal or increase neuromodulation. Clinical studies of war veterans have shown that the autonomic nervous system is centrally involved in many of the symptoms of PTSD, including startle reactions, irritability, nightmares and flashbacks, and explosive outbursts of aggression. It is therefore predictable that those medications which affect autonomic arousal would prove helpful in treating the symptoms of PTSD. Autonomic arousal can be reduced at different levels in the central nervous system: through inhibition of noradrenergic activity (clonidine and the beta-adrenergic blockers), by increasing the inhibitory effect of the GABA-ergic system with GABA-ergic agonists (the benzodiazepines) and through enhancing the serotonergic inhibition system with such agents as lithium carbonate and the serotonin reuptake blockers. Even though positive results have been claimed for any of these medications, at the present time there are no data about which patient, or even what symptom of PTSD will predictably respond to any of these medications. Clinical reports have claimed success for every class of psychoactive medication for the treatment of certain features of PTSD. These have included benzodiazepines (van der Kolk, 1983), tricyclic antidepressants (Burstein, 1984; Reist, Kaufmann, & Haier, 1989), serotonin reuptake blockers (van der Kolk, 1983), mono-amine oxidase (MAO) inhibitors (Frank, Kosten, Giller, & Dan, 1988; Hogben & Cornfeld, 1981; Shetatsky, Greenberg, & Lerer, 1988), lithium carbonate (van der Kolk, 1983), beta-adrenergic blockers and clonidine (Kolb, Burris, & Griffiths, 1984), carbamezapine (Lipper et al., 1986) and antipsychotic agents. However, no carefully controlled studies documenting the differential effects of various psychotropic medications on the symptoms of PTSD exist at this time. The only psycho-tropic medications whose efficacy in PTSD symp-tomatology have been evaluated in double-blind studies are tricyclic antidepressants and MAO-inhibitors (Birk-heimer et al., 1985; Bleich et al., 1987; Davidson et al., 1990; Frank et al., 1988; Shetatsky et al., 1988). One study showed that amitriptyline is an effective antidepressant in patients with PTSD but does little for core PTSD symptomatology, including psychological numbing. Tri-cyclic antidepressants generally are thought to be most effective in treating nightmares, depression, sleep disor-ders, and startle reactions, but were less able to relieve numbing. Hogben and Cornfield (1981) found MAO-inhibitors effective in the treatment of PTSD; that anec-dotal study was contradicted by Shetatsky et al. (1988), but to some degree supported by Frank et al. (1988).

Conclusions

The rapidly expanding knowledge of the effects of traumatization on the central nervous system, the dawn-ing awareness that memory (mal)functions are at the core of the psychological disruptions in PTSD, combined with the availability of animal models for PTSD make the psychobiology of trauma one of the most promising areas in psychiatry. This developing understanding of the neurobiological correlates of traumatization is al-ready providing further clues about effective therapy for PTSD. The implications of these findings are not only relevant to better pharmacological management, but also for psychodynamic, cognitive-behavioral, and activity therapies. A variety of psychopharmacological agents that affect the physiological arousal system, including clonidine, benzodiazepines, MAO inhibitors, and tri-cyclic antidepressants, decrease the long-term effects of inescapable shock in animals and seem to have some use in the pharmacotherapy of PTSD. The recent discovery that serotonin reuptake inhibitors seem to act by quite a different mechanism and may be extremely effective in reducing the intrusive and the numbing symptoms of PTSD needs to be carefully documented and under-stood. Further exploration during the coming decades of how trauma affects neuroendocrine emergency systems, neuromodulation, and memory should provide us with a much greater understanding about the interplay be-tween soma and psyche in coping with potentially over-whelming experiences.

References

American Psychiatric Association. (1987). *Diagnostic and statisti-cal manual of mental disorders* (3rd ed., rev.). Washington, DC: Author.

American Psychiatric Association. (in press). *Diagnostic and sta-tistical manual of mental disorders* (4th ed.). Washington, DC: Author.

Akil, H., Watson, S. J., Young, E., Lewis, M. E., Khachaturian, H., & Walker, J. M. (1984). Endogenous opioids: Biology and function. *Annual Review of Neuroscience, 7,* 223–255.

Bach-y-Rita, P. (1974). Habitual violence and self-mutilation. *American Journal of Psychiatry, 131,* 1018–1020.

Bird, S. J., & Kuhar, M. J. (1977). Iontophoretic application of opiates to the locus coeruleus. *Brain Research, 122,* 523–533.

Blanchard B. E., Kolb, L. C., Gerardi, R. J., Ryan, P., & Pal-lmeyer, T. P. (1986). Cardiac response to relevant stimuli as an adjunctive tool for diagnosing posttraumatic stress disorder in Vietnam veterans. *Behavior Therapy, 17,* 592–606.

Bleich, A., Siegel, B., Garb, B., Kottler, A., & Lerer, B. (1987). PTSD following combat exposure: Clinical features and phar-macological management. *British Journal of Psychiatry, 149,* 365–369.

Bolles, R. C., & Fanselow, M. S. (1980). A perceptual defensive recuperative model of fear and pain. *Behavior and Brain Sci-ences, 3,* 291–323.

Bowlby, J. (1969). *Attachment and loss* (Vol 1: Attachment). New York: Basic Books.

Bowlby, J. (1973). *Attachment and loss* (Vol 2: Separation). New York: Basic Books.

Burchfield, S. R. (1979). The stress response: A new perspec-tive. *Psychosomatic Medicine, 41,* 661–672.

Burgess, A. W., & Holstrom, L. (1974). Rape trauma syndrome. *American Journal of Psychiatry, 131,* 981–986.

Burstein, A. (1984). Treatment of posttraumatic stress disorder with imipramine. *Psychosomatics, 25,* 681–686.

Cicchetti, D., & Rosen, K. S. (1984). Theoretical and empirical considerations in the investigation of the relationship be-tween affect and cognition in an atypical population of in-fants. In C. Izard, J. Kagan, & R. Zajanc (Eds.), *Emotions, cognition and behavior.* New York: Cambridge University Press.

Cook L., & Sepinwall, J. (1975). Behavioral analysis of the effect and mechanism of action of the benzodiazepines. In E. Costa & P. Greengard (Eds.), *Mechanisms of action of the ben-zodiazepines* (pp. 1–28). New York: Raven.

Davidson, J. R. T., Kudler, H. S., Smith, R. D., Mahorney, S. L., & Lipper, S. L. (1990). Amitriptyline and placebo in the treat-ment of posttraumatic stress disorder. *Archives of General Psy-chiatry, 47,* 259–266.

Davidson, J. R. T., & Nemeroff, C. B. (1989). Pharmacotherapy in PTSD: Historical and clinical considerations and future di-rections. *Psychopharmacology Bulletin, 25,* 422–425.

Davis, N. M., & Gray, J. A. (1983). Brain 5-hydroxytryptamine and learned resistance to punishment. *Behavioral Brain Re-search, 8,* 129–137.

Delaney, R., Tussi, D., & Gold, P. E. (1983). Long-term potentia-tion as a neurophysiological analog of memory. *Pharmacology, Biochemistry, & Behavior, 18,* 137–139.

Dobbs, D., & Wilson, W. P. (1960). Observations on the per-sistence of traumatic war neurosis. *Journal of Nervous & Mental Disease, 21,* 40–46.

Dupue, R. A., & Spoont, M. R. (1987). Conceptualizing a sero-tonin trait: A behavioral model of constraint. *Annals of the New York Academy of Science, 187,* 47–62.

Frank, J. B., Kosten T. R., Giller, E. L., & Dan, E. (1988). A randomized clinical trial of phenelzine and imipramine in PTSD. *American Journal of Psychiatry, 145,* 1289–1291.

Freud S. (1954). Introduction to psychoanalysis and the war neuroses. In J. Strachey (Ed. and Trans.), *The standard edition of the complete psychological works of Sigmund Freud* (Vol. 17, pp. 207–210). London: Hogarth Press. (Original work published 1919)

Gold, P. E., & Zornetzer, S. F. (1983). The mnemon and its juices: Neuromodulation of memory processes. *Behavioral and Neural Biology, 38,* 151–189.

Grant, S. J., & Redmond, D. E., Jr. (1981). The neuroanatomy and pharmacology of the nucleus locus coeruleus. In H. Lal & S. Fielding (Eds.), *Pharmacology of clonidine.* New York: Liss.

Gray J. (1982). *The neuropsychology of anxiety: An inquiry into the functions of the septohippocampal system.* New York: Oxford University Press.

Gray J. (1988). *The psychology of fear and stress* (2nd ed.). Cambridge, England: Cambridge University Press.

Green, A. H. (1980). *Child maltreatment.* New York: Jason Aronson.

Grinker, R. R., & Spiegel, J. J. (1945). *Men under stress.* New York: McGraw-Hill.

Herman, J. L., Perry, J. C., & van der Kolk, B. A. (1989). Childhood trauma in borderline personality disorder. *American Journal of Psychiatry, 146,* 390–395.

Hogben, G. L., & Cornfeld, R. B. (1981). Treatment of traumatic war neurosis with phenelzine. *Archives of General Psychiatry, 38,* 440–445.

Jacobs, W. J., & Nadel, L. (1985). Stress-induced recovery of fears and phobias. *Psychological Review, 92,* 512–531.

Janet, P. (1889). *L'Automatisme psychologique: Essai de psychologie expérimentale sur les formes inférieures de l'activité humaine.* Paris: Félix Alcan.

Kagan, J., Reznick, S., & Snidman, N. (1987). The physiology and psychology of behavioral inhibition in children. *Child Development, 58,* 1459–1473.

Kaminer, H., & Lavie, P. (1988). Dreaming and long-term adjustment to severe trauma. *Sleep Research, 18,* 146.

Kardiner A. (1941). *The traumatic neurosis of war.* New York: Paul B. Hoeber.

Keane, T. M., Fairbank, J. A., Caddell, J. M., *et al.* (1989). Implosive (flooding) therapy reduces symptoms of PTSD in Vietnam combat veterans. *Behavior Therapy, 20,* 245–260.

Kelly, D. D. (1982). The role of endorphins in stress-induced analgesia. *Annals of the New York Academy of Science, 398,* 260–271.

Kilpatrick, D. G., Veronen, L. J., & Best, C. L. (1985). Factors predicting psychological distress in rape victims. In C. Figley (Ed.), *Trauma and its wake* (pp. 113–141). New York: Brunner/Mazel.

Kling, A., & Steklis, H. D. (1976). A neural substrate for affiliative behavior in nonhuman primates. *Brain Behavior Evolution, 13,* 216–238.

Kolb, L. C., Burris, B. C., & Griffiths, S. (1984). Propranolol and clonidine in the treatment of posttraumatic stress disorders of war. In B. A. van der Kolk (Ed.), *Posttraumatic stress disorder: Psychological and biological sequelae.* Washington, DC: American Psychiatric Press.

Kolb, L. C., & Multipassi. L. R. (1982). The conditioned emotional response: A subclass of chronic and delayed posttraumatic stress disorder. *Psychiatric Annals, 12,* 979–987.

Kosten, T. R., Mason, J. W., Giller, E. L., Ostroff, R. B., & Harkness, L. (1987). Sustained urinary norepinephrine and epinephrine elevation in PTSD. *Psychoneuroendocrinology, 12,* 13–20.

Kraemer, G. W., Ebert, M. H., Lake, C. R., *et al.* (1984). Cerebrospinal fluid measures of neurotransmitter changes associated with pharmacological alteration of the despair re-

sponse to social separation in rhesus monkeys. *Psychiatry Research, 11,* 303–315.

Kramer, M., Schoen, L. S., & Kinney, L. (1984). The dream experience in dream disturbed Vietnam veterans. In B. A. van der Kolk (Ed), *Posttraumatic stress disorder: Psychological and biological sequelae.* Washington, DC: American Psychiatric Press.

Krystal, H. (1968). *Massive psychic trauma.* New York: International Universities Press.

Krystal, H. (1978). Trauma and affects. *Psychoanalytic Study of Children, 33,* 81–116.

Krystal H. (1979). Alexithymia and psychotherapy. *American Journal of Psychotherapy, 33,* 17–31.

Krystal, J. H., Kosten, T. R., Southwick, S., Mason, J. W., Perry, B. D., & Giller, E. L. (1989). Neurobiological aspects of PTSD: Review of clinical and preclinical studies. *Behavior Therapy, 20,* 177–198.

Lerer, B., Ebstein, R. P., Shetatsky, M., Shemesh, Z., & Greenberg, D. (1987). Cyclic AMP signal transduction in posttraumatic stress disorder. *American Journal of Psychiatry, 144,* 1324–1327.

Lewis, J. W., Cannon, J. T., & Liebeskind, J. C. (1980). Opioid and nonopioid mechanisms of stress analgesia. *Science, 208,* 623–625.

Lipper, S., Davidson, J. R. T., Grady, T. A., *et al.* (1986). Preliminary study of carbamezapine in posttraumatic stress disorder. *Psychosomatics, 27,* 849–854.

MacLean, P. D. (1985). Brain evolution relating to family, play, and the separation call. *Archives of General Psychiatry, 42,* 505–517.

Maier, S. F., & Seligman, M. E. P. (1976). Learned helplessness: Theory and evidence. *Journal of Experimental Psychiatry General, 105,* 3–46.

Malloy, P. F., Fairbank, J. A., & Keane, T. M. (1983). Validation of a multimethod assessment of posttraumatic stress disorders in Vietnam veterans. *Journal of Consulting & Clinical Psychology, 51,* 4–21.

Mason, J. W., Giller, E. L., Kosten, T. R., Ostroff, R. B., & Podd, L. (1986). Urinary free cortisol levels in posttraumatic stress disorder. *Journal of Nervous & Mental Disease, 174,* 145–149.

Mason, J. W., Giller, E. L., Kosten, T. R., *et al.* (1988). Elevated norepinephrine/cortisol ratio in PTSD. *Journal of Mental & Nervous Disease, 176,* 498–502.

O'Keefe, J., & Nadel, L. (1978). *The hippocampus as a cognitive map.* Oxford, England: Clarendon Press.

Ornitz, E. M., & Pynoos, R. S. (1989). Startle modulation in children with posttraumatic stress disorder. *American Journal of Psychiatry, 146,* 866–870.

Pattison, E. M., & Kahan, J. (1983). The deliberate self-harm syndrome. *American Journal of Psychiatry, 140,* 867–872.

Pavlov, I. P. (1927). *Conditioned reflexes: An investigation of the physiological activity of the cerebral cortex* (G. V. Anrep, Ed. and Trans.). New York: Dover.

Pennebaker, J. W., & Susman, J. R. (1988). Disclosure of traumas and psychosomatic processes. *Social Science Medicine, 26,* 327–332.

Perry, B. D., Giller, E. L., & Southwick, S. M. (1987). Altered plasma alpha-2 adrenergic receptor affinity states in PTSD. *American Journal of Psychiatry, 144,* 1511–1512.

Pfaff, D. W., Silva, M. T., & Weiss, J. M. (1971). Telemetered recording of hormone effects on hippocampal neurons. *Science, 172,* 394–395.

Pitman, R. K. (1989). Posttraumatic stress disorder, hormones, and memory. *Biological Psychiatry, 26,* 221–223.

Pitman, R. K., Orr, S., Laforgue, D., *et al.* (1987). Psychophysiology of PTSD imagery in Vietnam combat veterans. *Archives of General Psychiatry, 44,* 970–976.

Pitman, R. K., van der Kolk, B. A., Orr, S. P., & Greenberg, M. S. (1990, June). Naloxone reversible stress-induced analgesia in posttraumatic stress disorder. *Archives of General Psychiatry, 47*(6), 541–544.

Post, R. M., Pickar, D., Ballenger, J. C., Naber, D., & Rubinow, D. R. (1984). Endogenous opioids in cerebrospinal fluid: Relationship to mood and anxiety. In R. M. Post & J. C. Ballenger (Eds.), *Neurobiology of mood disorders* (pp. 356–368). Baltimore: Williams & Wilkins.

Putnam, F. W. (1984). The psychophysiological investigation of multiple personality disorder: A review. *Psychiatric Clinics of North America, 7,* 31–41.

Pynoos, R. S., & Eth, S. (1985). Developmental perspective on psychic trauma in childhood. In C. R. Figley (Ed.), *Trauma and its wake* (pp. 36–52). New York: Brunner/Mazel.

Rainey, J. M., Aleem, A., Ortiz, A., et al. (1987). Laboratory procedure for the inducement of flashbacks. *American Journal of Psychiatry, 144,* 1317–1319.

Reist, C., Kaufmann, C. D., & Haier, R. J. (1989). A controlled trial of desipramine in 18 men with PTSD. *American Journal of Psychiatry, 146,* 513–516.

Reite, M., & Fields, F. (Eds.). (1985). *The psychobiology of attachment and separation.* Orlando: Academic Press.

Richardson, J. S., & Zaleski, W. A. (1983). Naloxone and self-mutilation. *Biological Psychiatry, 18,* 99–101.

Sandman, C. A., Barron, J. L., Crinella, F. M., & Donnelly, J. F. (1987). Influence of naloxone on brain and behavior of a self-injurious woman. *Biological Psychiatry, 22,* 899–906.

Sapolsky, R., Krey, L., & McEwen, B. S. (1984). Stress down-regulates corticosterone receptors in a site specific manner in the brain. *Endocrinology, 114,* 287–292.

Sheard, M. H., & Davis, M. (1976). Shock elicited fighting in rats: Importance of intershock interval upon effect of PCPA. *Brain Research, 111,* 433–437.

Shetatsky, M., Greenberg, D., & Lerer, B. (1988). A controlled trial of phenelzine in posttraumatic stress disorder. *Psychiatry Research, 24,* 149–155.

Shore, J. H., Tatum, E. L., & Vollmer, W. M. (1986). Psychiatric reactions to disaster: The Mount St. Helens experience. *American Journal of Psychiatry, 143,* 590–595.

Smith, M. A., Davidson, J., Ritchie, J. C., Kudler, H., Lipper, S., Chappell, P., & Nemeroff, C. B. (1989). The corticotropin releasing hormone test in patients with posttraumatic stress disorder. *Biological Psychiatry, 26,* 349–355.

Squire, L. R. (1987). *Memory and the brain.* New York: Oxford University Press.

Stoddard F. (1985). *Stress disorders in burned children and adolescents.* Paper presented at the Annual Meeting of the American Psychiatric Association, Dallas, TX.

Strian, F., & Klicpera, C. (1978). Die Bedeuting psycho-autonomische Reaktionen im Entstehung und Persistenz von Angstzustanden. *Nervenartzt, 49,* 576–583.

Terman, G. W., Shavit, Y., Lewis, J. W., Cannon, J. T., & Liebeskind, J. C. (1984). Intrinsic mechanisms of pain inhibition: Activation by stress. *Science, 26,* 1270–1277.

Terr, L. (1983). Chowchilla revisited: The effects of psychic trauma four years after a school bus kidnapping. *American Journal of Psychiatry, 140,* 1543–1550.

Terr, L. (1988). What happens to early memories of trauma? *Journal of the American Academy of Child & Adolescent Psychiatry, 1,* 96–104.

van der Kolk, B. A. (1983). Psychopharmacological issues in posttraumatic stress disorder. *Hospital & Community Psychiatry, 34,* 683–691.

van der Kolk, B. A. (1987). *Psychological trauma.* Washington, DC: American Psychiatric Press.

van der Kolk, B. A. (1988). The trauma spectrum: The interaction of biological and social events in the genesis of the trauma response. *Journal of Traumatic Stress, 1,* 273–290.

van der Kolk, B. A., Blitz, R., Burr, W., et al. (1984). Nightmares and trauma. *American Journal of Psychiatry, 141,* 187–190.

van der Kolk, B. A., Greenberg, M. S., Boyd, H., & Krystal, J. H. (1985). Inescapable shock, neurotransmitters and addiction to trauma: Towards a psychobiology of posttraumatic stress. *Biological Psychiatry, 20,* 314–325.

van der Kolk, B. A., Greenberg, M. S., Orr, S. P., & Pitman, R. K. (1989). Endogenous opioids and stress-induced analgesia in posttraumatic stress disorder. *Psychopharmacology Bulletin, 25,* 417–421.

van der Kolk, B. A., Herman, J. L., & Perry, J. C. (1989). *Childhood trauma and self-destructive behavior.* Paper presented at the 146th annual meeting of the American Psychiatric Association, San Francisco.

van der Kolk, B. A., & van der Hart, O. (1989). Pierre Janet and the breakdown of adaptation in psychological trauma. *American Journal of Psychiatry, 146,* 1530–1540.

van Kammen, W. B., Christiansen, C., van Kammen, D. P., & Reynolds. (1990). Sleep and the POW experience: Forty years later. In E. L. Giller (Ed.), *Biological assessment and treatment of PTSD.* Washington DC: American Psychiatric Press.

Wilkinson, C. B. (1983). Aftermath of disaster: Collapse of Hyatt Regency Hotel Skywalks. *American Journal of Psychiatry, 140,* 1134–1139.

CHAPTER 3

Multiple Personality Disorder and Posttraumatic Stress Disorder

Similarities and Differences

Bennett G. Braun

Introduction

Multiple personality disorder (MPD) and posttraumatic stress disorder (PTSD) were formulated in medical consciousness at about the same time that modern psychiatry was being molded by its Age of Giants. During this period of 1880 to 1920, MPD was pulled from its millennia-old identification with demonology and possession into the rational spheres of psychology (Ellenberger, 1970). The "cowardice" of warriors who relived scenes of terror in sweating nightmares acquired a new etiology in the trenches of World War I, namely, "shell shock," later to become the "combat fatigue" of World War II, and the PTSD of today. All too often throughout history the MPD and PTSD patient shared similar fates: isolation or death for the "possessed," rejection or execution for the craven. Until recently, however, it was not realized that MPD and PTSD had two similarities in etiology and phemonenology: origin in exposure of the victim to shattering psychological trauma—in childhood in the instance of MPD, in later life in PTSD—and the subsequent need for the person to dissociate as a coping mechanism.

The similarities in etiology and phenomenology are not fully appreciated unless one examines them through the lens of dissociation (Braun, 1986a; Braun & Sachs, 1985; Frankel, unpublished manuscript; Putnam, 1985; Spiegel, 1984). The history of revival of interest in dis-

sociation is a fascinating journey through the history of modern psychiatry, but not one that will be pursued here (Braun, 1986a; Decker, 1986; Ellenberger, 1970). Dissociation is, however, the unifying concept that will be used to link etiology and phenomenology to diagnosis and treatment (Braun, 1988a,b) of both MPD and PTSD. The linkage may be strong enough to suggest that both are psychopathologic stress syndromes and dissociative disorders—disorders of arousal.

Commonality of Trauma to Dissociation and Forms of MPD and PTSD

The psychopathological trauma that lies somewhere in the history of all MPD and PTSD patients is the "traumatic event" defined in DSM-III-R (American Psychiatric Association, 1987): "an event that is outside the range of usual human experience and that would be markedly distressing to almost anyone" (p. 250).

Response to trauma is quite varied. Different people who seem to have experienced similar trauma, such as father–daughter incest (Herman, 1981), or exposure to war as a soldier or civilian victim (Horowitz, 1983; Walker & Cavenar, 1982) have been shown to have a varying intensity of response.

Variable responses to trauma may be due in some degree to characteristics of the event (Eth & Pynoos, 1985; Herman, 1981; Oswald & Bitner, 1968; Wilson, Smith, & Johnson, 1985):

1. The degree of life threat, for example, witnessing violence versus subjection to violence
2. Speed of onset, for example, the sudden, unexpected attack versus prolonged anticipation and fear prior to the traumatic event(s)

Bennett G. Braun • Center on Psychiatric Trauma and Dissociation, Rush Institute of Mental Well-Being, Rush-Presbyterian-St. Luke's Medical Center, Chicago, Illinois 60612.

International Handbook of Traumatic Stress Syndromes, edited by John P. Wilson and Beverley Raphael. Plenum Press, New York, 1993.

3. Duration of trauma, for example, a mugging or hit-and-run rape versus prolonged sexual assault and ritual torture
4. Potential for recurrence
5. Proportion of a group or community affected

Writing about PTSD in United States veterans of the Vietnam conflict, Wilson (1988) and Walker and Cavenar (1982) cited factors that may influence degree of response, including degree of aloneness in the experience, sociocultural opposition to the event, the type of transition period after the trauma, and the lack or presence of early intervention.

A number of authors have pointed out the probability of different responses to naturally occurring violence, such as tornadoes and earthquakes, and violence inflicted by another person (Eth & Pynoos, 1985; Herman, 1981; Oswald & Bitner, 1968). The single, apparently random natural disaster is a different order of experience from deliberately inflicted injury. Rose (1986) said in a discussion of rape victims that it is easier for a victim to psychologically reorganize against a random act of nature than to do so for personal violence, especially when the injury is an act of premeditated violence inflicted by another human being.

In particular, premeditated violence may undermine the victim's basic assumptions about his or her own invulnerability and the fundamental nature of man (Janoff-Bulman, 1985). Thus, the personal beliefs of the victim may mediate response to psychic trauma.

Terr (1988) suggested that there are two types of trauma: (1) Type I follows from single, unanticipated traumatic events that penetrate coping and defensive mechanisms by sheer force and surprise. (2) Type II follows from long-standing or repeated exposures to extreme traumatic events. She also noted four characteristics that are common to all severe traumatic stress disorders: (1) visualization—the ability to revisualize a terrible event or series of events, (2) reenactment, (3) fear, and (4) a sense of futurelessness.

When response to trauma cannot be worked through, for whatever reason, the victim becomes "stuck" (Horowitz, 1983). Moreover, if exposure to severe trauma occurs in late adolescence or adulthood, the response usually is concordant with a diagnosis of PTSD as opposed to MPD (Putnam, 1985). Although PTSD is probably a dissociative reaction if the trauma occurs in adulthood, it is not usually associated with the development of alternate personality states (Braun, 1988a; Putnam, 1985; Spiegel, 1984).

Almost all authors who have treated or studied MPD patients agree that its development is linked to trauma in childhood—more often than not inside the immediate family—that interrupts normal personality development. The victim dissociates as a coping mechanism, then becomes trapped in a dissociative pattern of giving pain, hate, outcry, and emotional numbing to one or more "others" to handle (Braun & Sachs, 1985).

Braun (1984c), Braun and Sachs (1985), and Kluft (1984b) independently proposed similar models that focus on the child-abuse diathesis of MPD. The 3-P model of Braun and Sachs (Figure 3.1) conceptualizes three necessary, and together sufficient, elements in the development of multiple personality disorder: predisposing, precipitating, and perpetuating factors.

Predisposing Factors

An inborn biopsychological capacity to dissociate is usually identifiable by a high responsiveness to hypnosis.

There is also repeated exposure to an inconsistently stressful environment—for example, an abusive family where the child may receive irregularly administered physical, sexual, and/or psychological abuse from parents, uncles, aunts, or other "loving" caregivers. Irregularity may be in both timing and reasons for abuse (affection at one time and abuse at another for the same act).

Precipitating Event

A specific, overwhelmingly traumatic event may be present to which the young victim responds by dissociating, that is, dissociating behavior, affect, sensation, and knowledge from the main stream of consciousness (see Figure 3.4). If the event is isolated or far separated in time from similar events, the result may be a single dissociative episode.

Perpetuating Factors

Repetition of interactive behaviors between abuser and victim create the psychic environment for repeated dissociations by the victim, linked by a common affective theme. After continuous exposure, the victim has files of affectively chained memories and associated response patterns separated by amnestic barriers. The psychic stage is thus set for development of different personality states, each with its own adaptive functioning.

A number of investigators have concluded, on the basis of studies with a combined sample of more than 1,000 patients, that MPD is one of the major sequelae of child abuse (Braun, 1984b; Braun & Gray, 1986; Putnam, Guroff, Silberman, Barban, & Post, 1986; Putnam, Post, Guroff, Silberman, & Barban, 1983; Schultz, Braun, & Kluft, 1989). In these studies child abuse was identified as an etiologic factor ranging from 95.2% (Braun & Gray, 1986) to 98% (Schultz et al., 1989) of patients.

Childhood trauma reported retrospectively by 100 patients in a National Institutes of Mental Health survey included sexual abuse by nearly 83%, repeated physical abuse in 75%, combined physical and sexual abuse in 68%, followed in descending order by extreme neglect, witness to violent death, other abuses, and extreme poverty (Putnam et al., 1986). Reports of abuse from MPD patients are often startling, frightening, and even difficult to believe. Putnam (1989b) observed that the abuse associated with MPD is usually far more sadistic, ritualistic, and bizarre than that suffered by most child victims of abuse.

Braun (1985a) was among the first to suggest a "transgenerational" aspect to MPD, that is, that MPD and abusive behaviors may be found in successive generations of families at a rate of occurrence beyond the

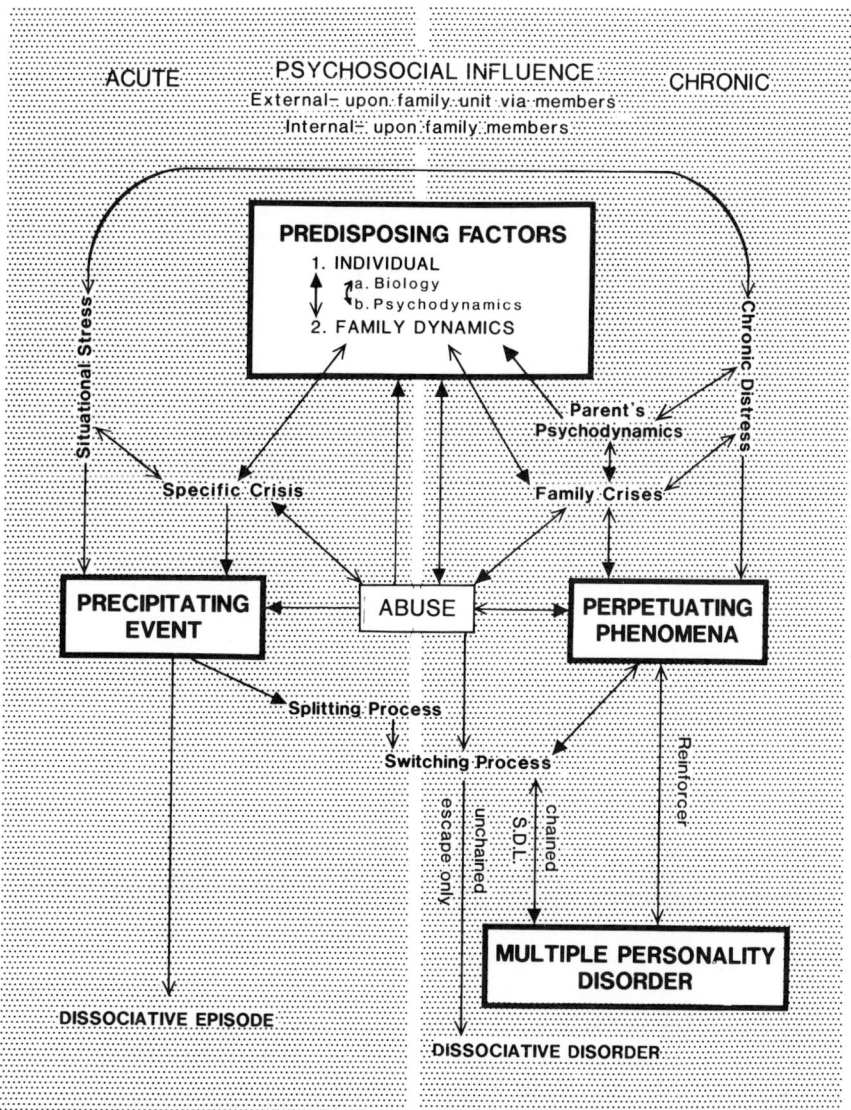

Figure 3.1. A model of dissociative phenomena in multiple personality disorder. From "The Development of Multiple Personality Disorder: Predisposing, Precipitating, and Perpetuating Factors," by B. G. Braun and R. G. Sachs, in R. Kluft (Ed.), *Childhood Antecedents of Multiple Personality*, p. 53. Copyright 1985 by the American Psychiatric Association. Reprinted by permission.

probability of chance. The suggestion has continued to be intriguing (Putnam, 1989b), but no firm data yet support the hypothesis. Widom (1989) criticized suggestions of intergenerational transmission of child abuse on grounds that many studies are methodologically weak because of overdependence on self-report and retrospective data, inadequate documentation of childhood abuse and neglect, and infrequent use of baseline data from control groups.

The World Health Organization (Carballo, 1985) reported that child abuse occurs at rates of 13 to 21 per thousand population in industrialized nations. Rates in developing nations are not known because data are lack-

ing. A fundamental constraint to data gathering internationally is the variation in definitions between countries. Carballo (1985) noted that lack of uniformity in definitions of child abuse also reflects differences in technical approaches and terminology of physicians, psychologists, sociologists, forensic experts, and others concerned with these problems.

The three extracts that follow contain terminology adopted for the WHO report on child abuse (Carballo, 1985):

Child abuse refers only to parental acts that constitute a misuse or exploitation of the rights of parents and guardians with regard to the control and disciplining of children under their care. According to this usage, child abuse occurs when a parent or guardian knowingly misuses his privileged position to commit acts that transgress social norms and damage the child's development. (pp. 31–32)

Child neglect, or passive child abuse, refers to the failure by parents or guardians to perform duties and obligations that are basic to the child's well being, including nurture, protection, supervision, and the provision of food, clothing, medical care and education. (p. 32)

Child exploitation refers to forms of child abuse from which the perpetrator gains economic benefits. (pp. 32–34)

Widom (1989) and Putnam (1989b) confirmed the judgment of a number of investigators that debate regarding the definition of child abuse; uncertainty about its prevalence and ultimate effects are methodological problems that only well-constructed research studies will resolve.

Issues and Implications

Phenomenology of MPD and PTSD as Dissociative Disorders

Lowenstein (1988) proposed that MPD and PTSD be viewed as paradigmatic stress syndromes that could take their place in modern psychopathology along with, but different from, the organic, affective, and schizophrenic disorders. Both MPD and PTSD may occur at about a 1% rate in the general population according to Lowenstein. The lowest incidence reported is 0.17% in a study by Worrall (1987).

Considered as dissociative disorders, both disorders manifest a need to cope with the psychic sequelae of overwhelming trauma by dissociating information from its integration with mental activities. Yet the use of dissociation as a coping or adaptive mechanism implies (1) a biopsychological ability to dissociate and (2) a need to use the ability (Braun & Sachs, 1985). Using a Dissociative Experiences Scale (DES) to survey various groups, Bernstein and Putnam (1986) showed that patients with MPD and PTSD had the highest mean scores of all patient groups. The self-administered questionnaire requires respondents to indicate the frequency with which they experience specific dissociative or depersonalization experiences.

Dissociation is a normal process, exhibited by many persons in everyday life for such activities as daydreaming. Used as a coping mechanism to deal with traumatic experience, it may evolve into a maladapted, patholog-

ical activity. On a continuum of awareness (Figure 3.2), dissociation is seen to be at the furthest distance from "full" awareness—farther away than suppression, denial, and repression. This graph illustrates the definition of dissociation as the separation of an idea or thought process from the main stream of consciousness. Also implied is that dissociation has a significantly greater physiologic component than is found in Freud's concept.

Braun (1988a,b) and Putnam (1989a) pointed out the nature of dissociation as a continuum. A continuum of dissociation (Figure 3.3) (Braun, 1984b, 1988a) illustrates a natural adaptive mechanism becoming increasingly maladaptive and pathologic. The "normal" dissociation of daydreaming and hypnosis do not usually represent any significant disruption in identity or behavior; "normal" life probably has many small dissociational experiences which occur "if we look for them" (E. R. Hilgard, 1977, 1984).

Many writers (Putnam, 1989a) have identified the high incidence of dissociation in persons who experience severe psychic trauma and/or threat to life. Braun (1985b, 1986a, 1988a,b) mapped the dissociation experience onto a model representing the psychophysiological processes of behavior, affect, sensation (including perception), and knowledge in temporal motion. This BASK model (Figure 3.4) can be adapted to illustrate that dissociation can occur in any one or more of the processes: (1) in behavior (automatism), (2) in affect and sensation (hypnotic anesthesia) (see Figure 3.5), and (3) in behavior-affect-sensation-knowledge (psychogenic amnesia) (see Figure 3.6).

The BASK model illustrates the maladaptive dissociational psychopathology of PTSD and MPD. Mental health is defined in the BASK model as the congruence of the levels of BASK and their confluence over time.

Posttraumatic Stress Disorder

Horowitz (1976) authoritatively discussed stress response syndromes, including the phenomenology of PTSD.

Freud postulated effects of trauma on the individual that closely parallel the "intrusion" and "denial" symptoms of PTSD: (1) fixations to the trauma, or attempts to repeat the trauma and (2) defensive reactions directed toward assuring that the trauma will be neither repeated nor remembered.

Figure 3.7 shows the intrusion and denial symptoms of PTSD. On the BASK model, they are seen as dissociation of behavior, affect, sensation, and knowledge from the stream of ongoing mental processes. The model is an outline of the phenomenology of PTSD.

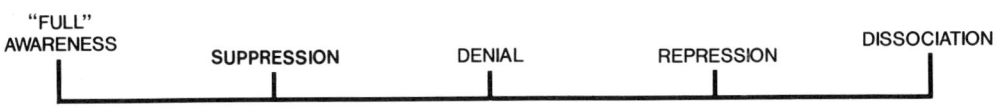

Figure 3.2. Levels on a continuum of awareness in PTSD and MPD.

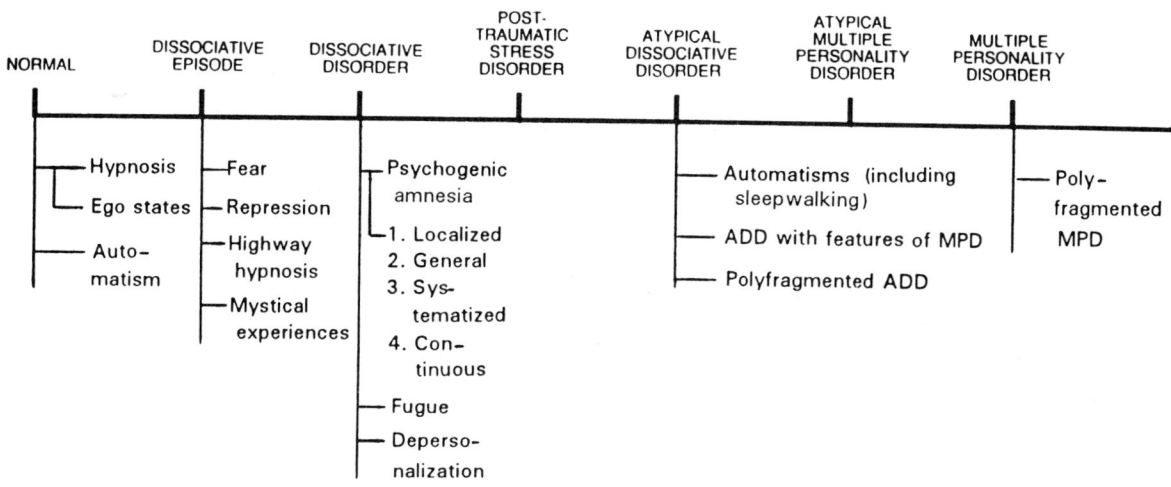

Figure 3.3. Levels on a continuum of dissociation in PTSD and MPD.

Figure 3.4. The BASK paradigm for PTSD and MPD. (The arrows signify the passage of time.)

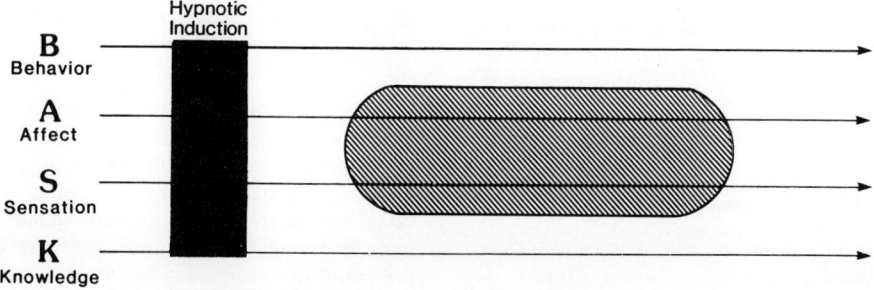

Figure 3.5. BASK model of hypnotic anesthesia.

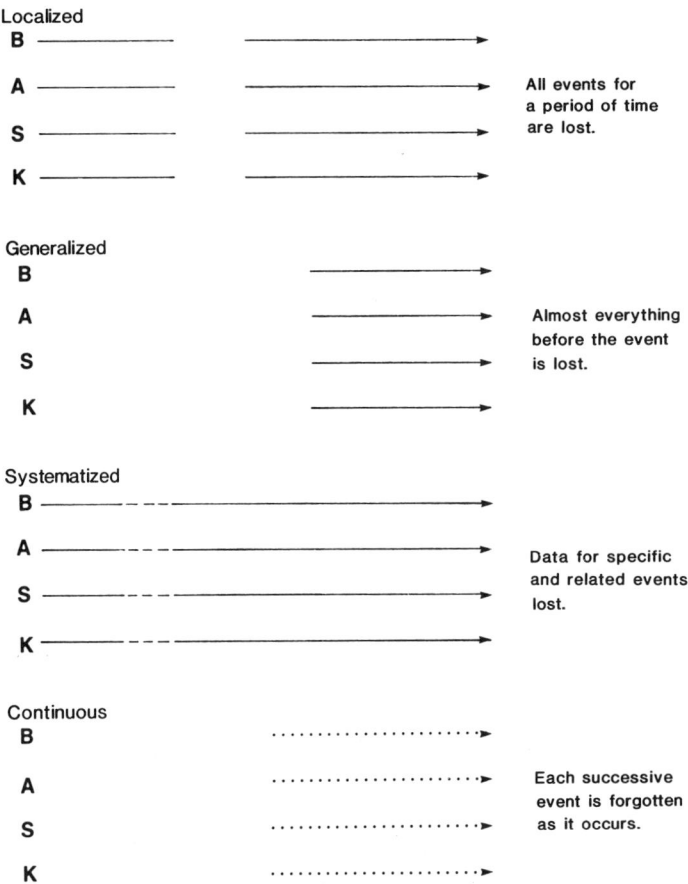

Figure 3.6. BASK model of amnesia.

The BASK Model of PTSD: A Comparative Analogue to MPD

Intrusive Symptoms

1. Recurrent, intrusive, distressing recollections of the event(s)
2. Recurrent distressing dreams of the event(s)
3. Sudden acting or feeling as if the event was recurring
4. Hypervigilance, difficulty falling asleep
5. Irritability, pangs of strong emotion
6. Exaggerated startle response
7. Intense psychological distress at exposure to events that symbolize or resemble an aspect of the traumatic event, including an anniversary of the trauma.

Denial Symptoms

1. Efforts to avoid thoughts or feelings associated with the trauma
2. Psychogenic amnesia: inability to recall important aspects of the trauma (see Figure 3.6)

3. Markedly diminished interest in significant activities
4. Feelings of detachment from others
5. Restricted range of affect
6. Sense of a foreshortened future.

A case report illustrates these dissociative aspects of PTSD:

H. H., a 46-year-old white male, suffered from PTSD since return from his second military tour of duty in Vietnam. He claimed to have reenlisted for a second tour in hopes of being killed as retribution for atrocities he had committed. Just before his return from the second tour of duty his best friend, who had been involved in some of the atrocities, stood up in the middle of a fire fight and was mortally wounded, dying in the patient's arms.

After discharge, H. H. developed classic PTSD signs: (1) intrusive memories so powerful that he sometimes felt that he was back in Vietnam; (2) flashbacks triggered by certain loud noises that would cause him to drop to the ground and hide under bushes; (3) fear of things that would remind him of Vietnam, for example, news programs or movies; and (4) futurelessness expressed in fear that he would harm his wife or children in the same way he had killed Vietnamese, and as he had been harmed as a child.

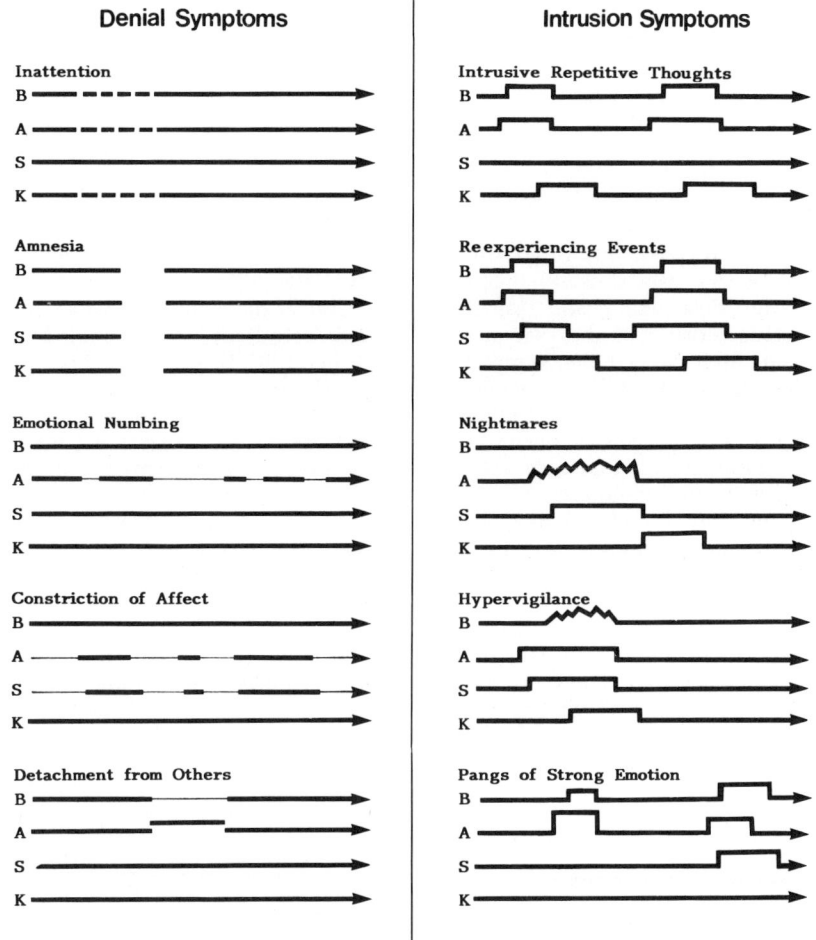

Figure 3.7. PTSD symptoms classified by the BASK paradigm.

The patient was reared in an extremely abusive home (predisposing factor for PTSD). His father regularly had vaginal and anal intercourse with the patient's sister, while H. H. was forced to watch. He was sodomized by his father and forced to perform fellatio. If he attempted to protect his sister or himself, he was severely beaten and threatened with castration. His mother also beat him frequently, with a broom or any object at hand.

In Vietnam, H. H. reenacted his abusive childhood in the role of the father. He cut off prisoners' genitalia, and discharged his M-16 weapon into the vaginas and anuses of Vietnamese women and men. In the role of his mother, he clubbed a Vietnamese woman to death.

The signs and symptoms manifested by H. H. are congruent with Terr's Type II PTSD, following from long exposure to extremely traumatic events.

Even though PTSD has been considered an anxiety disorder in the DSM-III-R (American Psychiatric Association, 1987), its symptoms are more understandable as manifestations of a dissociative disorder. The essential feature of an anxiety disorder is the existence of anxiety and the numerous intrapsychic, cognitive, behavioral, and interpersonal strategies for its avoidance. The essential feature of a dissociative disorder is disturbance or alteration in the normally integrative functions of identi-

ty and memory. It can be seen as an insertion or withdrawal from the ongoing flow of consciousness. Although anxiety and avoidance are prominent in PTSD and in dissociative disorders, the major and essential features are dissociative symptoms.

The intrusion symptoms of PTSD (intrusive thoughts, nightmares, hypervigilance, episodes of strong emotion) and denial symptoms (inattention, amnesia, constriction of thought processes, emotional numbing) can be conceptualized as opposite sides of dissociation: Intrusive symptoms are seen as breakdowns of the protective mechanisms of denial and amnesia. Both intrusion and denial symptoms are seen as disturbances of the ongoing flow of mental processes.

In PTSD as well as in other dissociative disorders, there is a need to dissociate behavior, affect, sensation, and knowledge (BASK) from the integrated flow of mental activity. This dis-integration is a characteristic of dissociative symptomatology. If one identifies PTSD as a dissociative disorder, it may be appropriate to begin to think of MPD as a special case of PTSD, as first proposed by Spiegel (1984) and Braun (1988a).

The parallels between MPD and PTSD are profound in clinical experience. When a clinician works with MPD patients, the diagnostic features of PTSD are nearly always encountered. In both instances, the patients have been traumatized by events far out of the normal range of human experience. MPD patients may, during phases of their illness and during treatment, be troubled by recurrent and intrusive recollections of the traumatic events, have nightmares in which the events are experienced as if they were being relived, and have the feeling that the events are recurring. These recollections may have a significant physiologic dimension.

Like PTSD sufferers, MPD patients often try to avoid thoughts and experiences associated with the trauma. Amnesia, withdrawal, detachment, and restricted ranges of affect are characteristics of the personality types frequently encountered in MPD. Other symptoms that MPD patients often share with PTSD patients include sleep disturbances, affective outbursts, trouble in concentrating, abrupt startle responses, hypersensitivity, and, in some cases, irrational guilt, for example, guilt at being the "cause" of their own trauma, and guilt at having survived. Many feel they should have died. Most have a foreshortened sense of the future.

The link between dissociative disorders and trauma seems an increasingly firm relationship. Dissociative disorders, in particular those that are more severe, have a high correlation with trauma as noted in the MPD/trauma retrospective studies cited earlier. The trauma link together with the dissociative nature of symptoms are strong arguments for conceptualizing MPD and PTSD as dissociative disorders.

Multiple Personality Disorder

Although MPD and PTSD share much dissociative phenomenology, there are distinct differences in epidemiology and demographics of the two disorders, as well as in the difficulty of establishing a diagnosis.

MPD occurs most often in women, if currently recorded cases are a true indication of incidence in the population (Putnam, 1989b; Putnam et al., 1986). Female-to-male ratios run from 9-to-1 to 2-to-1 (Horevitz & Braun, 1984). The reasons remain speculative and include (1) sex-linked genetic characteristics, (2) cultural determinants, (3) higher incidence of severe sexual and physical abuse among female children, (4) greater expectation by therapists in finding MPD in women than in men, and (5) women MPD patients finding their way into the mental health system, whereas men, more likely to express violent behavior, are more often sent to prisons (Putnam, 1984; Putnam, Loewenstein, Silberman, & Post, 1984; Wilbur, 1985).

Age at diagnosis is most likely to be in the third or fourth decade of life, although MPD has its genesis in childhood. Kluft (1984b) suggested that MPD symptoms become most "florid" at this time. However, the average patient may have been in the mental health system about seven years (Braun & Gray, 1986; Putnam, 1985; Putnam et al., 1984). This is the length of time that has often been required before an MPD patient is correctly diagnosed, generally because of a lack of an index of suspicion.

Figure 3.8 characterizes the phenomenology of MPD on the BASK model. A major difference between MPD and PTSD phenomenology is immediately apparent. In PTSD (Figure 3.7) the same "person" is seen dealing with the B-A-S-K components of PTSD symptoms. In MPD (Figure 3.8), two or more "persons" have been created to deal with problems of fear, rage, and the like.

The presence of two or more "persons" in a single body presents the therapist with the typical MPD phenomenology (Braun, 1984b, 1986b, 1988a):

1. Domination of the patient by one of two or more personalities occurs at any one time (occasionally with one personality being in executive control and another in an observer or advisory role).

2. Each personality presents a full or nearly full range of different, frequently opposite, mental characteristics.

3. Transitions between personalities may be abrupt or may be gradual. A patient adept at "covering up" the presence of MPD may be able to accomplish covert switching of personalities in the presence of the therapist.

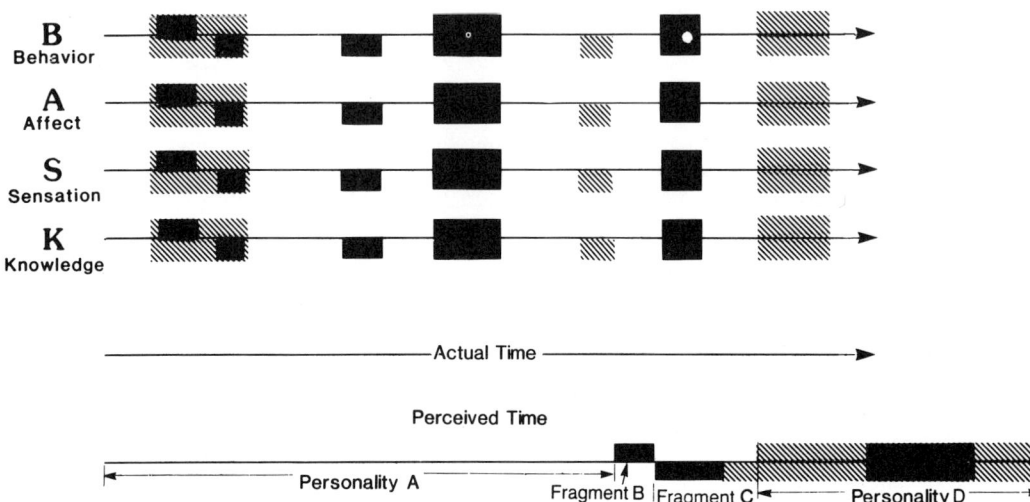

Figure 3.8. Multiple personality classified by the BASK paradigm.

4. Amnestic barriers are present between personalities (two-way amnesia), but some may be aware of others' existence (one-way amnesia), and two or more may share information on a limited basis.

5. Any one personality will have "lost time" that represents periods when other personalities were in executive control; however, the sum of all personalities' memories may appear to represent more time than actually passed in any given period (see Figure 3.8).

6. The patient may manifest a broad spectrum of physical and mental complaints, for example, gastrointestinal problems, weight control, depression, anxiety, difficulties with thoughts or attempts, fugues, substance abuse, and headache among others (Bliss, 1980; Coons & Milstein, 1986; Kluft, 1984a; Putnam, 1985).

7. Because of the sometimes astounding range of symptoms, and because of the tendency for patients to "cover up" their "crazy" thought processes, the adult patient often has a long history of varied and failed diagnoses (Kluft, 1985).

PTSD/MPD Similarities and Differences: Implications for Diagnosis and Treatment

In both MPD and PTSD, a variety of medical problems as well as mental disorders may obscure a diagnosis. Rage, fear, depression, and anxiety may appear in their own guises, or as physical "conversion" or dissociative manifestations of psychopathophysiology.

Coons, Bowman, Pellow, and Schneider (1989) investigated the occurrence of posttraumatic stress and dissociation in women who had suffered sexual abuse and incest in childhood or young adulthood. Using the DES, the study confirmed previous (Bernstein & Putnam, 1986) work indicating high Dissociative Experience Scale (DES) scores in patients with PTSD and MPD. Patients with eating disorders—bulimia and anorexia nervosa—had low DES scores. Dissociation appeared to be a discriminating factor in the young women studied, many of whom had common presenting symptoms of depression, anxiety, and physical complaints.

The link between trauma and dissociation is the defensive mobilization of dissociation to contain and distribute the psychic residue of trauma (Spiegel, 1986). The price paid for this defense is often subsequent psychic fragmentation manifested as dissociative symptoms. The labile behavior, memory, and affect of PTSD may be understood as a dissociative phenomenology akin to the multiple "memory receptacles" of MPD.

Spiegel, Hunt, and Dondershine (1988) reported further studies with the hypnotizability of PTSD patients and control groups, concluding that spontaneous dissociation, imagery, and hypnotizability are important components of PTSD symptoms. Hypnotizability scores were higher for PTSD patients than for controls or for patients with schizophrenia, major depression, bipolar disorder, and generalized anxiety disorder.

There appears to be a relationship between dissociability and hypnotizability (Bliss, 1980, 1984; Braun, 1980). There also appears to be a relationship between hypnotizability and child abuse. J. R. Hilgard (1970), Nash, Lynn, and Givens (1984), Nash and Lynn (1986), and Frischholz, Lipman, and Braun (1984) showed increased hypnotizability in MPD patients.

The DES supplements and complements previous data showing that MPD patients in general display the highest dissociation and hypnotizability scores of all categories of patients (Bernstein & Putnam, 1986; Braun, 1983, 1984a; Lipman, Braun, & Frischholz, 1984; Spiegel, 1986). The 3-P Model of Braun and Sachs (1985) characterizes the central role that dissociation plays in the genesis of MPD.

High hypnotizability also contributes to professional skepticism about MPD and fears of iatrogenically inducing MPD. Beginning with Braun's 1979 presentation and papers by Kluft (1982) and Braun (1984a) addressing the myth of iatrogenically induced MPD, professional fears on this point appear to be declining (Putnam, 1989b).

Skepticism regarding the very existence of MPD as a clinical entity may still exist and contributes to the chances that an MPD patient will encounter an abusive and harrassing therapist (Dell, 1988). Braun (1985a) has pointed out that skepticism about factitious MPD is warranted until a discretely separate personality has been seen in several therapeutic encounters and confirmed as a stable true personality state. Braun (1982) and Putnam (1988) also noted that clinicians usually identify alternate personalities first by observing psychophysiological changes in the patient, for example, changes in voice, facial musculature, eye gaze, and right/left handedness. These should not be taken as prima facie evidence of MPD but should be seen consistently and repeatedly over time.

Issues of Differential Diagnosis

Concern that MPD could be confused with transient ego-state phenomena may be allayed by the appropriate uses of hypnosis and tests for hypnotizability. Ego states may only reach consciousness and be communicated within formal hypnotic trance (J. Watkins & H. Watkins, 1980).

Horevitz and Braun (1984) observed that as many as 70% of MPD patients may also meet DSM-III-R criteria for borderline personality disorder. This observation was independently confirmed by Schultz, Braun, and Kluft (1986). MPD can be distinguished from borderline personality disorder in that (1) there is a reliable pattern of intrapersonality consistency in MPD patients not seen in borderline patients, and (2) symptoms of other disorders are also present in MPD patients (Braun & Kluft, unpublished manuscript). On the DES, non-MPD borderline patients do not score as high as MPD and PTSD patients (borderline or not), a fact which may be used cautiously in differential diagnosis.

Schizophrenia offers one of the most difficult problems in differential diagnosis of MPD (Kluft, 1987). MPD patients may display from one to eight of Schneider's 11 first-rank symptoms at initial assessment. The presence of these symptoms should not exclude a diagnosis of MPD, but rather should encourage the therapist to consider MPD. Subtle clues to one diagnosis or the other may be overlooked; for example, the "voices" heard by a schizophrenic patient are usually perceived as coming from outside the head, whereas MPD patients usually hear the voices coming from inside, as when alters are heard arguing.

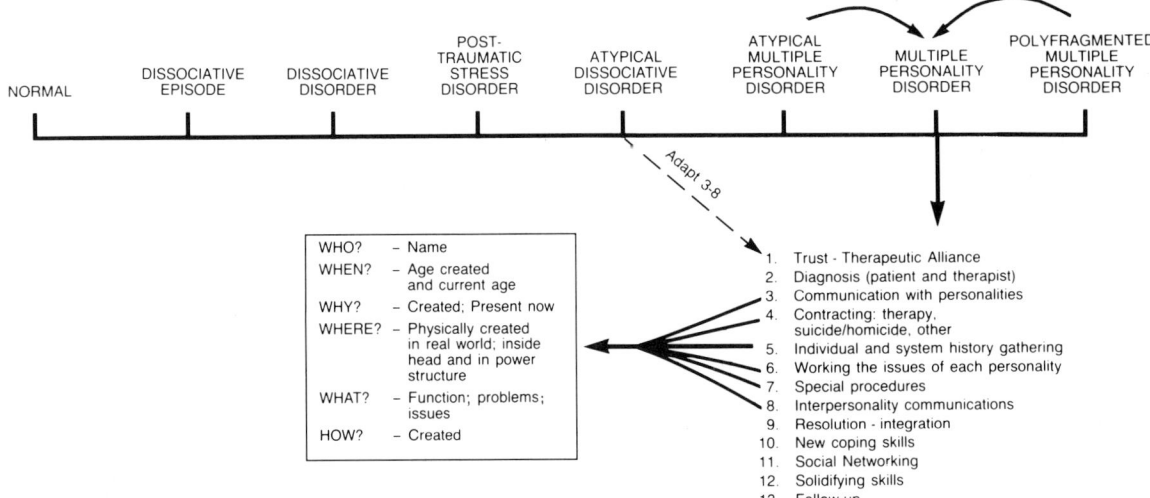

Figure 3.9. Treatment considerations in PTSD and in MPD.

Because trauma and its accompanying fear and rage are the specific underlying causes of PTSD and MPD, the specific and essential commencement of treatment is the establishment of trust. A firm therapeutic alliance is the key to successful therapy (Braun, 1986b).

In Figure 3.9, Braun (1986b) adapted the dissociation model to outlining the issues that must be addressed in treatment of the dissociative psychopathology of the traumatic stress syndromes. Although Issues 3 through 8 are specifically directed toward treatment of MPD, the same rationale is also adaptable to PTSD: (3) opening communication; (4) contracting to further therapy and prevent suicide; (5) history gathering; (6) working the issues, including gaining mastery; (7) use of special procedures, such as sand tray therapy (Sachs & Braun, 1986), abreactive therapy (Young, 1986; Sachs, Braun, & Shepp, 1988), and group psychotherapy (Ochberg, 1989); (8) about Issue 9, reaching a resolution of the problems that sustain the behaviors.

MPD is markedly different from PTSD in the central role that secrecy plays in the lives of so many patients (Braun, 1986a,b; Braun & Sachs, 1985; Goodwin, 1985; Kluft, 1985). Secrecy is imposed upon the physically/sexually abused child in an abusive family to maintain the facade of "normalcy" to the outside world and, in a threatening manner, to assure that the child will not "tell." The mandate for secrecy is reinforced in later life when the patient is compelled to camouflage the odd behavior of presenting different personalities to the world. MPD patients will characteristically resist attempts to gain their trust and will test the trustworthiness of a therapist at many points in the therapeutic process. This pattern is also seen during the treatment of many PTSD patients.

The therapist must be consistent in all dealings with these patients as they are exquisitely suspicious of inconsistent authority figures. Patients will attempt to manipulate therapists throughout the course of treatment, trying to "set the therapist up" to be proven inconsistent and untrustworthy (Braun, 1986b).

In both MPD and PTSD, the therapist may experience significant problems of countertransference (Danieli, 1982). Victims of rape, abuse, torture, and other personal violence can raise troublesome issues for the therapist. These issues can be potentiated when the patient is manipulative, deceitful, insulting, or threatening. Exposure of horrible acts in a patient's personal history, accompanied by violent abreaction, can create over time a "secondary" PTSD in a therapist, or in therapists who consistently encounter stressful events in group therapy.

Psychopharmacology in MPD and PTSD

Pharmacotherapy, especially in MPD patients, requires careful approach and close monitoring (see Chapter 66, in this volume). Response of MPD patients to any drug may be variable and can be unpleasantly surprising. MPD patients do not respond to drugs in a consistent and predictable manner (Barkin, Braun, & Kluft, 1986). MPD is associated with significant differences and changes across personalities that may be psychological, psychophysiological, or neurophysiological, depending upon which personality has executive control of the body at the time of drug administration.

Misdiagnosis may lead to an MPD patient's receiving inappropriate psychoactive drugs (Putnam, 1989b). A drug prescribed for a misdiagnosed schizophrenia may actually reinforce pathologic dissociation. For example antidepressants, anxiolytics, and sedatives may all have a useful role at one time or another in treatment of MPD symptoms, but no pharmacotherapy should be undertaken without a thorough review of the literature and, if possible, the collaboration of an MPD therapist experienced in the use of medication.

Drugs that may be particularly useful in PTSD and highly fragmented MPD are the central adrenergic "blockers." Kolb, Barris, and Griffiths (1984) suggested that PTSD involves an abnormal arousal of the central adrenergic system that can be blocked, thereby lessening explosiveness, nightmares, intrusive thoughts, startle responses, and hyperalertness. Extremes of anxiety and hyperactivity are sometimes controlled in MPD patients by the administration of beta-adrenergic blockers (propranolol) and an alpha-adrenergic agonist (clonidine). Both drugs decrease adrenergic activity, albeit by different mechanisms.

I have applied Kolb *et al.*'s (1984) ideas to MPD, exceeding 160 mg/day, the maximum dose of propranolol prescribed in their study, carefully increasing it to 1600+ mg/day in many patients. High dose treatment has proven successful in more than 150 patients on high doses (500 mg/day or more) of propranolol, with few side effects. I have treated several cases with doses of clonidine, 1.6 to 4.0 mg/day, mainly patients diagnosed with MPD, but also many cases of PTSD. The use of medications to lower noradrenergic activity in MPD and PTSD must still be regarded as unusual and should not be pursued without thorough investigation and safeguards including consultation when necessary (Braun, 1990).

Discussion and Summary

Conceptualizing multiple personality disorder (MPD) as a special case of posttraumatic stress disorder (PTSD), and both as disorders with dissociative components, brings dissociation into focus as a major mechanism for responding to psychological trauma. Dissociation is a unifying concept that permits the linkage of etiology and phenomenology to diagnosis and treatment.

The etiology of PTSD is trauma as defined in the DSM-III-R: "an event that is outside the range of usual human experience and that would be markedly distressing to almost anyone" (p. 250). This is also true of MPD.

Occurring in adult life, under such conditions as war, natural disaster, rape, or other personal violence, the dissociative response may develop into PTSD. If it is not readily resolved to a dissociative episode, the dissociated event(s) are ruminated upon and "develop a life of their own," being reactivated by various stimuli. The stimuli are mainly external but may be internal as well. Through association, the flashbacks and/or other symptoms are released, and if they remain without resolution are self-reinforcing (Braun, 1984b, 1986a, 1989; van der Kolk, 1987; Wolf & Mosnaim, 1990). The negative effects appear to be greater when the trauma is organized and carried out by human beings (war, personal violence, or child abuse as opposed to random natural disaster) and encountered more than once (military combat and child abuse).

Dissociative responses to repetitive trauma that occur in childhood, in the setting of an abusive family, may become "chained" by common affective themes. Over time, separate files of affectively chained memories and associated response patterns may develop, separated by amnestic barriers. Thus, the stage is set for dissociating rage and emotionally numbing fear into the files of alter personalities or personality fragments.

The experience of severe trauma leaves the child and the adult victim with a sense that the world has become unpredictable and dangerous. The victim's sense of invulnerability is destroyed; he or she is left with death anxiety, a loss of ability to feel and be involved with the world, and impaired human relationships accompanied by cynicism, irritability, and rage (Lifton, 1968, 1973, 1979; Lifton & Olson, 1976).

In those children and adults who have a high biopsychological capacity to dissociate, the normal process of dissociation becomes a coping mechanism to deal with the psychological sequelae of severe physical or psychological trauma. The dissociative process that manifests itself in everyday life as daydreaming or highway hypnosis may evolve into a maladaptive, pathological activity. Ideas and thought processes that are unacceptable sequelae of trauma are dissociated from the mainstream of consciousness, creating the dissociative phenomenology of PTSD and MPD that will manifest itself often at inopportune times.

The understanding of PTSD and MPD begins with an awareness that severe psychological trauma is the underlying etiology, and that maladaptive use of dissociation is the underlying pathology. This understanding is facilitated by the cross-pollination of ideas from both fields. The approach to treatment flows from the same understanding. This must be interpreted by the therapist as a mandate to found the therapeutic alliance upon the establishment of trust—bringing trust and mastery into the life of a person whose belief in the world, in humanity, and in him- or herself has been shattered.

References

American Psychiatric Association. (1987). *Diagnostic and statistical manual of mental disorders* (3rd ed., rev.). Washington, DC: Author.

Barkin, R., Braun, B. G., & Kluft, R. P. (1986). The dilemma of drug therapy for multiple personality disorder. In B. G. Braun (Ed.), *Treatment of multiple personality disorder* (pp. 107–132). Washington, DC: American Psychiatric Press.

Bernstein, E. M., & Putnam, F. W. (1986). The development, reliability and validity of a dissociation scale. *Journal of Nervous and Mental Disease, 174*, 727–734.

Bliss, E. L. (1980). Multiple personalities: A report of 14 cases with implications for schizophrenia and hysteria. *Archives of General Psychiatry, 37*, 1388–1397.

Bliss, E. L. (1984). Spontaneous self-hypnosis in multiple personality disorder. In B. G. Braun (Ed.), Symposium on multiple personality. *Psychiatric Clinics of North America, 7*, 135–148.

Braun, B. G. (1979, October). *Hypnosis creates multiple personality: Myth or reality?* Paper presented at the 31st Annual Meeting of the Society for Clinical and Experimental Hypnosis, Denver.

Braun, B. G. (1980). Hypnosis for multiple personality. In H. J. Wain (Ed.), *Clinical hypnosis in medicine* (pp. 209–218). Chicago: Yearbook Medical Publishers.

Braun, B. G. (1982). Multiple personality: Form, function and phenomena. Privately printed and distributed (1992 version available free from author).

Braun, B. G. (1983). Psychophysiologic phenomena in multiple personality and hypnosis. *American Journal of Clinical Hypnosis, 16*, 124–137.

Braun, B. G. (1984a). Hypnosis creates multiple personality:

Myth or reality? *International Journal of Clinical and Experimental Hypnosis, 32*, 191–197.

Braun, B. G. (1984b). Towards a theory of multiple personality and other dissociative phenomena. In B. G. Braun (Ed.), Symposium on multiple personality. *Psychiatric Clinics of North America, 7*, 171–194.

Braun, B. G. (1984c). *International Journal of Family Psychiatry, 5*(4), 303–313.

Braun, B. G. (1985a). The transgenerational incidence of dissociation and multiple personality disorder. In R. P. Kluft (Ed.), *Childhood antecedents of multiple personality* (pp. 127–150). Washington, DC: American Psychiatric Press.

Braun, B. G. (1985b). Dissociation: Behavior, affect, sensation, knowledge. In B. G. Braun (Ed.), *Dissociative disorders 1985: Proceedings of the Second International Conference on Multiple Personality/Dissociative States* (p. 6). Chicago: Rush-St. Luke's-Presbyterian Medical Center.

Braun, B. G. (1986a). *Dissociation: An overview*. Annual Meeting of the American Psychiatric Association, Washington, DC.

Braun, B. G. (1986b). Issues in the psychotherapy of multiple personality disorder. In B. G. Braun (Ed.), *Treatment of multiple personality disorder* (pp. 1–28). Washington, DC: American Psychiatric Press.

Braun, B. G. (1988a). The BASK (behavior, affect, sensation, knowledge) model of dissociation. *Dissociation, 1*(1), 4–23.

Braun, B. G. (1988b). The BASK model of dissociation: Treatment. *Dissociation, 1*(2), 16–23.

Braun, B. G. (1989). Dissociation as a sequela to incest. In R. P. Kluft (Ed.), Symposium on psychotherapy of the survivor of incest with a dissociative disorder. *Psychiatric Clinics of North America, 12*, 307–324.

Braun, B. G. (1990). Unusual medication regimens in the treatment of dissociative disorder patients: Part I. Noradrenergic agents. Dissociation, 3(3), 144–150.

Braun, B. G., & Gray, G. T. (1986). Report on the 1985 questionnaire on multiple personality disorder. In B. G. Braun (Ed.), *Dissociative disorders 1986: Proceedings of the Third International Conference on Multiple Personality/Dissociative States* (p. 111). Chicago: Rush-St. Luke's-Presbyterian Medical Center.

Braun, B. G. & Sachs, R. G. (1985). The development of multiple personality disorder. In R. P. Kluft (Ed.), *Childhood antecedents of multiple personality* (pp. 37–64). Washington, DC: American Psychiatric Press.

Carballo, M. (1985). Introduction. In Z. Benkowski & M. Carballo (Eds.), *Battered children and child abuse* (pp. 1–45). Bern, Switzerland: World Health Organization.

Coons, P. M., Bowman, E. S., Pellow, T. A., & Schneider, P. (1989). Posttraumatic aspects of the treatment of victims of sexual abuse and incest. *Psychiatric Clinics of North America, 12*, 325–335.

Coons, P. M., & Milstein, V. (1986). Psychosexual disturbances in multiple personality: Characteristics, etiology and treatment. *Journal of Clinical Psychiatry, 47*, 106–110.

Danieli, Y. (1982). Families of survivors of the Nazi Holocaust: Some short- and long-term effects. In C. D. Speilberger, I. G. Sarason, & N. A. Milgram (Eds.), *Stress and anxiety* (Vol. 8). New York: Hemisphere Publishing.

Decker, H. S. (1986). The lure of non-materialism in materialist Europe: Investigations of dissociative phenomena, 1880–1915. In J. Quen (Ed.), *Split minds/split brains* (pp. 31–62). New York: New York University Press.

Dell, P. F. (1988). Professional skepticism about multiple personality. *Journal of Nervous and Mental Disease, 176*, 528–531.

Ellenberger, H. F. (1970). *The discovery of the unconscious: The history and evolution of dynamic psychiatry*. New York: Basic Books.

Eth, S., & Pynoos, R. S. (1985). Developmental perspective on psychic trauma in childhood. In C. R. Figley (Ed.), *Trauma and its wake: The study and treatment of post-traumatic stress disorders* (pp. 36–52). New York: Brunner/Mazel.

Frankel, F. H. (in preparation). *Dissociation as a coping mechanism*. Unpublished manuscript.

Frischholz, E. J., Lipman, E. S., & Braun, B. G. (1984). Hypnosis in multiple personality disorder: Part II, special hypnotic phenomena. In B. G. Braun (Ed.), *Dissociative disorders 1984: Proceedings of the First International Conference on Multiple Personality/Dissociative States* (p. 101). Chicago: Rush-St. Luke's-Presbyterian Medical Center.

Goodwin, J. (1985). Credibility problems in multiple personality disorder patients and abused children. In R. P. Kluft (Ed.), *Childhood antecedents of multiple personality* (pp. 1–20). Washington, DC: American Psychiatric Press.

Herman, J. (1981). *Father-daughter incest*. Cambridge: Harvard University Press.

Hilgard, J. R. (1970). *Personality and hypnosis*. Chicago: University of Chicago Press.

Hilgard, E. R. (1977). *Divided consciousness: Multiple controls in human thought and action*. New York: Wiley.

Hilgard, E. R. (1984). The hidden observer and multiple personality. *International Journal of Clinical and Experimental Hypnosis, 32*, 248–253.

Horevitz, R. P., & Braun, B. G. (1984). Are multiple personalities borderline? In B. G. Braun (Ed.), Symposium on multiple personality. *Psychiatric Clinics of North America, 7*, 69–88.

Horowitz, M. J. (1976). *Stress response syndromes*. Northvale, NJ: Jason Aronson.

Horowitz, M. J. (1983). Post-traumatic stress disorders. *Behavioral Sciences and the Law, 1*(3), 9–23.

Janoff-Bulman, R. (1985). The aftermath of victimization: Rebuilding shattered assumptions. In C. R. Figley (Ed.), *Trauma and its wake: The study and treatment of post-traumatic stress disorders* (pp. 15–35). New York: Brunner/Mazel.

Kluft, R. P. (1982). Varieties of hypnosis intervention in the therapy of multiple personality. *International Journal of Clinical and Experimental Hypnosis, 24*, 230–240.

Kluft, R. P. (1984a). An introduction to multiple personality disorder. *Psychiatric Annals, 14*, 19–24.

Kluft, R. P. (1984b). Treatment of multiple personality disorder: A study of 33 cases. In B. G. Braun (Ed.), Symposium on multiple personality. *Psychiatric Clinics of North America, 7*, 9–29.

Kluft, R. P. (1985). The natural history of multiple personality disorder. In R. P. Kluft (Ed.), *Childhood antecedents of multiple personality* (pp. 197–238). Washington, DC: American Psychiatric Press.

Kluft, R. P. (1987). First-rank symptoms as a diagnostic clue to multiple personality disorder. *American Journal of Psychiatry, 144*, 293–298.

Kolb, L. C., Barris, B. C., & Griffiths, S. (1984). Propranolol and clonidine in treatment of the chronic post-traumatic stress disorders of war. In B. van der Kolk (Ed.), *Post-traumatic stress disorder: Psychological and biological sequelae* (pp. 97–107). Washington, DC: American Psychiatric Press.

Lifton, R. J. (1968). *Death in life*. New York: Random House.

Lifton, R. J. (1973). *Home from the war: Vietnam veterans: Neither victims nor executioners*. New York: Simon & Schuster.

Lifton, R. J. (1979). *The broken connection*. New York: Simon & Schuster.

Lifton, R. J., & Olson, E. (1976). The human meaning of total disaster: The Buffalo Creek experience. *Psychiatry, 39*, 1–18.

Lipman, L. S., Braun, B. G., & Frischholz, E. J. (1984). Hypnotizability and multiple personality disorder: Part I, overall hypnotic responsivity. In B. G. Braun (Ed.), *Dissociative disorders 1984: Proceedings of the First International Conference on Multiple Personality/Dissociative States* (p. 100). Chicago: Rush-St. Luke's-Presbyterian Medical Center.

Lowenstein, R. J. (1988). The spectrum of phenomenology in multiple personality disorder: Implications for diagnosis and treatment. In B. G. Braun (Ed.), *Proceedings of the Fifth International Conference on Multiple Personality/Dissociative States* (p. 7). Chicago: Rush-St. Luke's-Presbyterian Medical Center.

Nash, M. R., & Lynn, S. J. (1986). Child abuse and hypnotic ability. *Imagination, Cognition and Personality, 5*, 211–218.

Nash, M. R., Lynn, S. J., & Givens, D. L. (1984). Adult hypnotic susceptibility, childhood punishment and child abuse: A brief communication. *International Journal of Clinical and Experimental Hypnosis, 32*, 6–11.

Ochberg, F. M. (1989). Traumatic therapy and victims of violence. In F. M. Ochberg (Ed.), *Posttraumatic therapy and victims of violence* (pp. 3–23). New York: Brunner/Mazel.

Oswald, R., & Bitner, E. (1968). Life adjustment after severe persecution. *American Journal of Psychiatry, 124*, 1393–1400.

Putnam, F. W. (1984). The psychophysiologic investigation of multiple personality disorder. In B. G. Braun (Ed.), *Symposium on multiple personality. Psychiatric Clinics of North America, 7*, 31–40.

Putnam, F. W. (1985). Dissociation as a response to extreme trauma. In R. P. Kluft (Ed.), *Childhood antecedents of multiple personality* (pp. 65–98). Washington, DC: American Psychiatric Press.

Putnam, F. W. (1988). The switch process in multiple personality disorder. *Dissociation, 1*(1), 24–32.

Putnam, F. W. (1989a). Dissociation. In F. W. Putnam, *Diagnosis and treatment of multiple personality disorder* (pp. 1–25). New York: Guilford Press.

Putnam, F. W. (1989b). Etiology, epidemiology, and phenomenology. In F. W. Putnam (Ed.), *Diagnosis and treatment of multiple personality disorder* (pp. 45–70). New York: Guilford Press.

Putnam, F. W., Guroff, J. J., Silberman, E. K., Barban, L., & Post, R. M. (1986). The clinical phenomenology of multiple personality disorder: A review of 100 recent cases. *Journal of Clinical Psychiatry, 47*, 285–293.

Putnam, F. W., Loewenstein, R. J., Silberman, E. K., & Post, R. M. (1984). Multiple personality in a hospital setting. *Journal of Child Psychiatry, 45*, 172–175.

Putnam, F. W., Post, R. M., Guroff, J. J., Silberman, E. K., & Barban, L. (1983). One hundred cases of multiple personality disorder. *New Research Abstract No. 77*. American Psychiatric Association annual meeting, New York.

Rose, D. S. (1986). "Worse than death": Psychodynamics of rape victims and the need for psychotherapy. *American Journal of Psychiatry, 143*(7), 817–824.

Sachs, R. G., & Braun, B. G. (1986). The use of sand trays with the MPD patient. In B. G. Braun (Ed.), *Dissociative disorders 1986: Proceedings of the Third International Conference on Multiple Personality/Dissociative States* (p. 61). Chicago: Rush-Presbyterian-St. Luke's Medical Center.

Sachs, R. G.., Braun, B. G., & Shepp, E. (1988). Technique for planned abreactions with MPD patients. In B. G. Braun (Ed.), *Dissociative disorders 1988: Proceedings of the Fifth International Conference on Multiple Personality/Dissociative States* (p. 85). Chicago: Rush-Presbyterian-St. Luke's Medical Center.

Schultz, R., Braun, B. G., & Kluft, R. P. (1986). The interface between multiple personality disorder. In B. G. Braun (Ed.), *Dissociative disorders 1986: Proceedings of the Third International Conference on Multiple Personality/Dissociative States* (p. 111). Chicago: Rush-Presbyterian-St. Luke's Medical Center.

Schultz, R. G., Braun, B. G., & Kluft, R. P. (1989). Multiple personality disorder: Phenomenology of selected variables in comparison to major depression. *Dissociation, 2*, 45–51.

Spiegel, D. (1984). Multiple personality as a post-traumatic stress disorder. In B. G. Braun (Ed.), *Symposium on multiple personality. Psychiatric Clinics of North America, 7*, 101–110.

Spiegel, D. (1986). Dissociating damage. *American Journal of Clinical Hypnosis, 29*, 123–131.

Spiegel, D., Hunt, T., & Dondershine, H. E. (1988). Dissociation and hypnotizability in posttraumatic stress disorder. *American Journal of Psychiatry, 145*, 301–305.

Terr, L. C. (1988). An overview of psychic trauma in children. In B. G. Braun (Ed.), *Dissociative disorders 1988: Proceedings of the Fifth International Conference on Multiple Personality/Dissociative States* (p. 173). Chicago: Rush-St. Luke's Medical Center.

van der Kolk, B. (1987). *Psychological trauma*. Washington, DC: American Psychiatric Press.

Walker, J. I., & Cavenar, J. O. (1982). Forgotten warriors: Continuing problems of Vietnam veterans. In J. O. Cavenar & H. Brodic (Eds.), *Critical problems in psychiatry*. Philadelphia: J. B. Lippincott.

Watkins, J., & Watkins, H. (1980). Ego-states and hidden observers. *Journal of Altered States of Consciousness, 5*, 3–18.

Widom, C. S. (1989). The cycle of violence. *Science, 244*, 160–166.

Wilbur, C. B. (1985). The effect of child abuse on the psyche. In R. P. Kluft (Ed.), *Childhood antecedents of multiple personality* (pp. 21–36). Washington, DC: American Psychiatric Press.

Wilson, J. P. (1988). Understanding the Vietnam veteran. In F. Ochberg (Ed.), *Post-traumatic therapy and victims of violence*. New York: Brunner/Mazel.

Wilson, J. P., Smith, W. R., & Johnson, S. (1985). A comparative analysis of PTSD among various survivor groups. In C. R. Figley (Ed.), *Trauma and its wake: The study and treatment of posttraumatic stress disorder* (pp. 142–172). New York: Brunner/Mazel.

Wolf, M. E., & Mosnaim, A. D., (1990). *Posttraumatic stress disorder: Etiology, phenomenology and treatment*. Washington, DC: American Psychiatric Press.

Worrall, W. A. (1987). Multiple personality in Alaska. In B. G. Braun (Ed.), *Dissociative disorders 1987: Proceedings of the Fourth International Conference on Multiple Personality/Dissociative States* (p. 60). Chicago: Rush-St. Luke's-Presbyterian Medical Center.

Young, W. C. (1986). Restraints in the treatment of a patient with multiple personality. *American Journal of Psychotherapy, 40*, 601–606.

CHAPTER 4

Stress-Response Syndromes

A Review of Posttraumatic Stress and Adjustment Disorders

Mardi J. Horowitz

Introduction

The signs and symptoms of response to a stressful life event are expressed in two predominant phases: the *intrusive state*, characterized by unbidden ideas and feelings and even compulsive actions, and the *denial state*, characterized by emotional numbing and constriction of ideation. In this review of stress-response syndromes, I will outline those phases, discuss the DSM-III (American Psychiatric Association, 1980) diagnoses for stress-response disorders, and consider the mutual etiologic effects of stressful life events, psychiatric disorders, and preexisting conflicts or functional deficits. Guidelines for brief dynamic psychotherapy for patients who need more than transient support are presented.

Stress-response syndromes are composites of signs and symptoms that occur after serious life events or threatening life circumstances. In clinical practice, the experiences most frequently observed as precipitants of stress disorders are injury, assault, or loss of a loved one.

The clinician evaluating a person with a stress-response syndrome must appraise the degree of external stress imposed and the degree of stress experienced. An evaluation must be made as to how they interact with the person's preexisting personality characteristics as well as how the response compares with typical responses in a representative population. For these tasks, it is essential that the clinician understand the processes underlying normal as well as abnormal psychological responses.

Therefore, in this review of stress-response syndromes, I will first discuss general signs and symptoms of psychological responses to traumatic life events. Then I will consider how these elements are combined in the formal diagnostic nomenclature and will discuss various etiological considerations and treatment.

Historical Background

In the late nineteenth century, the prevailing European view was that someone who developed symptoms after a stressful life event was predisposed to them by hereditary weakness of the nervous system (Trimble, 1981). Breuer and Freud (1893–1895/1955) rejected this theory, proposing instead a theory that unconscious psychological processes contributed to stress responses, and that traumatization contributed to the formation of neurotic symptoms.

Studies in the twentieth century indicated that while patients with posttraumatic neuroses sometimes were malingerers, malingering was not a major factor in posttraumatic neuroses (Trimble, 1981). As yet, hereditary predisposition to stress-response syndromes has not been clearly demonstrated. However, preexisting personality features have been found to be a factor in individual responses to serious life events (Horowitz, 1986). In addition, earlier studies of larger populations exposed to disaster or combat indicated that as the severity of the life event increased, so did the proportion of the exposed population manifesting disorders (Grinker

Parts of this chapter first appeared in *Psychiatry* (Vol. 1), edited by Robert Michels, 1985, Philadelphia: J. B. Lippincott. Copyright 1985 by M. J. Horowitz. Adapted by permission.

Mardi J. Horowitz • Department of Psychiatry, University of California, San Francisco, California 94143.

International Handbook of Traumatic Stress Syndromes, edited by John P. Wilson and Beverley Raphael. Plenum Press, New York, 1993.

& Spiegel, 1945). In some cases, personality factors predisposed the individual to greater resilience, and in others to greater vulnerability. It became clear that some mental disorders followed traumatic life events and that psychological factors played an important role.

States and State Transition: A Theory of Phases of Response

States of mind theory has been developed in order to amplify observations that the constellation of ideational, emotional, defensive, coping, and interactional responses of an individual are not consistent across time even after a singularly traumatic life event. The person does exhibit patterned behavior, in that certain characteristics of expression and experience tend to occur in the same mood. But mood and state, very similar concepts, vary in a way that can lead to observation of relatively distinct phases of response. The formal properties, as distinguished from the contents of thinking and communication, can identify these phases in a way that allows a generalization across different types of stressful or traumatic life events, and even to a large extent across different types of people, and different cultures. Naturally, personality typology, culture, and other factors that affect style, habit, and schematization will also affect how the person experiences and expresses ideas and emotions in response to stressful events.

Figure 4.1 summarizes the prototypical set of phases that may follow a traumatic life event. This prototype is a generalization from clinical observation and field studies of many different types of individuals. No single individual will necessarily fit the prototype, nor is there any sharply defined transition point between one phase and another. The working-through phase, for example, often combines somewhat attenuated features of both the intrusive and denial states, as will be described below.

Outcry Phase

The immediate response to a serious life event is often alarm, accompanied by strong emotion, most often fear. This initial appraisal leads to a short period of emotional outcry: The person quickly processes the crude implications of the event, has an alarm reaction that interrupts ordinary activities, and expresses warning signals (Lazarus, 1966). The person may call out a warning, such as "Watch out!" or may scream for rescue, as "God!" or "Mama!" or may sob or grimace in anguish. In a precursor of what will occur more prominently in the denial phase, the person may exclaim passionately, "Oh, no! It can't be true!" Outcry may also consist of only a stunned stare and the feeling of inability to comprehend the trauma.

An outcry phase does not invariably take place. Some people confronted by severely stressful events continue to demonstrate effective, well-modulated behavior, with emotional expressivity. However, once their immediate coping efforts are no longer required, an inward or outward "crying out" may occur. Later, when such persons are alone and begin to relax and lower their defensive barriers, phases of denial and intrusion may ensue.

Such outcry phenomena are normal responses to shocking news. Abnormal outcry phenomena include panic, misdirected enraged destructiveness, sudden episodes of giving up, or other instances in which the person is so swept away by emotional responses that possible adaptive actions are neglected.

Denial and Intrusion Phases

Some signs and symptoms of stress-response syndromes tend to occur together in coherent, empirically demonstrated clusters (Lazarus, 1966; Zilberg, Weiss, & Horowitz, 1982). They are manifested in two predominant states of mind, which may succeed each other: the intrusive state, characterized by unbidden ideas, sudden rushes of feeling, and even compulsive actions, and the denial state, in which the individual ignores implications of threats or losses, forgets important problems, and experiences emotional numbing, withdrawal of interest in life, and behavioral constriction.

Symptoms that may emerge during the denial and the intrusive phases of stress-response syndromes are listed in Tables 4.1 and 4.2. The most important denial experiences may include such patterns as staring blankly into space, even avoiding the faces of others who can provide emotional support. The individual may experience a narrowing of focus and may fail to react appropriately to new stimuli, sometimes stubbornly adhering to tasks and stimuli considered important before the new and drastic changes in the life situation occurred. For example, after a nearby plane crash, the person might compulsively clean house.

Another important experience during the denial phase is an inner sense of clouding of perception, with a feeling that the world has become grayer than before. The individual may experience a diminished awareness of bodily sensations, even a feeling of being "dead in life" (Lifton & Olson, 1976). It is important for the clinician to ask after these and other signs and symptoms listed in Table 4.1, as most patients do not have adequate descriptive language for mental experiences to report them spontaneously.

Many of these denial signs and symptoms are normal ways of modulating emotional responses to serious events into tolerable, time-spaced doses. Abnormal denial is characterized by such extreme avoidance that the person does not cope with stressors and may resort to extreme countermeasures, such as excessive drug use or thrill-seeking events.

In contrast, intrusive phases are characterized by hypervigilance (excessive alertness to threatening stimuli), often evidenced by the subjects constantly scanning the environment for threatening cues (Janis, 1958). This hypervigilance can prompt startle reactions to relatively innocuous stimuli, especially if loud noises or shocking visual stimuli were part of the traumatic event. The startle reactions may range from clenching a single muscle group to suddenly assuming a globally protective position. The individual's readiness to interpret a new stim-

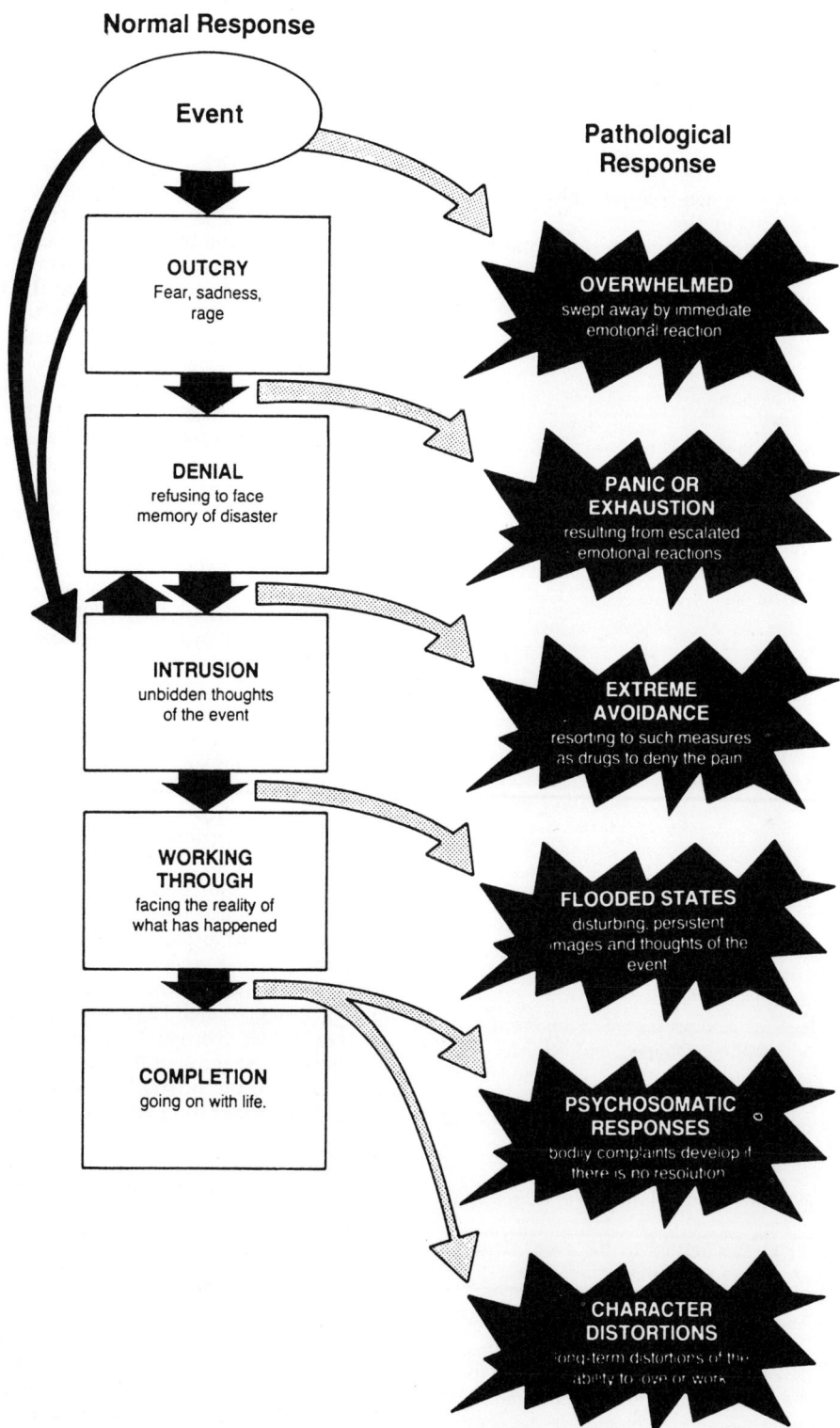

Figure 4.1. Normal and pathological phases of poststress response. From Horowitz, M. J., *Stress-Response Syndromes*, 2nd ed. Northvale, NJ: Jason Aronson, 1986.

Table 4.1. Common Symptoms or Signs during Denial Phases of Stress-Response Syndromes

Perception and attention
  Daze
  Selective inattention
  Inability to appreciate significance of stimuli
  Sleep disturbances (e.g., too little or too much)
Consciousness of ideas and feelings related to the event
  Amnesia (complete or partial)
  Nonexperience of themes that are consequences of the event
Conceptual attributes
  Disavowal of meanings of current stimuli in some way associated with the event
  Loss of a realistic sense of appropriate connection with the ongoing world
  Constriction of range of thought
  Inflexibility of purpose
  Major use of fantasies to counteract real conditions
Emotional attributes
  Numbness
Somatic attributes
  Tension-inhibition responses of the autonomic nervous system, with sensations such as bowel symptoms, fatigue, headache, and muscle pain
Activity patterns
  Frantic overactivity
  Withdrawal
  Failure to decide how to respond to consequences of the event

Table 4.2. Common Symptoms or Signs during Intrusive Phases of Stress-Response Syndromes

Perception and attention
  Hypervigilance, startle reactions
  Sleep and dream disturbances
Consciousness of ideas and feelings related to the event
  Intrusive-repetitive thoughts, emotions, and behaviors (illusions, pseudohallucinations, nightmares, unbidden images, and ruminations)
  Feelings of being pressured, confused, or disorganized when thinking about themes related to the event
Conceptual attributes
  Overgeneralization of stimuli so that they seem related to the event
  Preoccupation with themes related to the event, with inability to concentrate on other topics
Emotional attributes
  Emotional "attacks" or "pangs" of affect related to the event
Somatic attributes
  Sensations or symptoms of flight or fight-readiness (or of exhaustion from chronic arousal), including tremor, diarrhea, and sweating (adrenergic, noradrenergic, or histaminic arousals) with sensations such as pounding heart, nausea, lump in throat, and weak legs
Activity patterns
  Compulsive repetitions of actions associated with the event or of searching for lost persons or situations

ulus as a repetition of traumatic life events may, in turn, lead to illusions.

During the intrusive state, mental misperceptions through any of the senses, including sight, hearing, and smell, may appear. In a hallucinatory experience, the person interprets inner sensations that have no external basis as real. In a pseudohallucination, the person understands that vivid, subjective images are not true signals of external reality but nonetheless responds emotionally as if they were real. Such unbidden images, whether of hallucinatory, pseudohallucinatory, illusory, or mnemonic quality, include "sensing" the presences of others who may have died during the traumatic event (Horowitz, 1983). They may be the sources of paranormal phenomena, such as seeing or hearing ghosts of the deceased.

Such unbidden images tend to occur most frequently when the person is relaxed—for example, when lying down to sleep or closing the eyes to rest. Vivid sensory images occurring during periods of rest or relaxation constitute a *hypnogogic* phenomenon. A similar occurrence on awakening is called a *hypnopompic* phenomenon. The stressed person may become anxious that these frightening experiences will recur or may interpret them as a sign of losing control or "going crazy."

Patients can immediately be reassured that hypnogogic phenomena and other unbidden perceptual experiences are not serious portents of psychosis but are common after a traumatic event. Reassurance is especially useful if denial states have created a latency period of weeks before the phenomena occur. In such instances, intrusive experiences come as a major surprise if the person believes he or she has mastered the stressful life event.

During the intrusive phase the stressed person often ruminates unproductively about themes related to the serious life event. Themes that predated or occurred after the traumatic circumstance may also be incorporated; that is, the broader themes are contaminated by reactions to the trauma, a process called *overgeneralization*. If the individual then reacts normally, such wide-ranging associational linkages diminish in a process called *extinction*. If a denial phase is entered, the person disavows the meaning of the event, a development often complemented by constriction of associations about any theme. Sometimes the stressed person maintains a contrived continuation of "life as usual," which contains an altered subjective quality; the person feels like an automaton, carrying out habitual patterns in an unspontaneous, devitalized manner.

This brings us to two important emotional phenomena: the sense of *numbness* that may be present during the denial phase and its opposite, the *pangs of strong emotion* that may characterize an intrusive phase. Numbness is not simply an absence of emotions; it is a sense of being "benumbed." The individual may actually feel surrounded by a layer of insulation. Emotional blunting may alter patterns of interaction with people in support systems, affecting family life, friendships, and work relations. Members of the support network may be offended by the change in the relationship and withdraw, reducing support just when it is most needed.

The opposite experience, that of emotional pangs, eventually becomes familiar during the intrusive phase to the person under stress. Emotion occurs in intense waves that seem almost unbearable at their peak. The subject comes to know that these peaks will be followed by a reduction in intensity, making it possible to "live through them."

Intrusive phases sometimes contain reenactments of traumatic life events and fantasized responses. These compulsive repetitions may be a reliving of the event or a symbolic mastery of the event with the self now placed in an active rather than in a passive role. During denial states, activity may increase, but it takes a different form. It may include excessive engagement in sports, work, or sexual activities as an attempt to jam channels of thinking and feeling so that ideas and emotions related to the stressful event are stifled.

A phase of working through is characterized by progress on thinking and feeling, communicating and relating to others, that is, on the themes that have been so distressful during the intrusive phase. This includes forming new schemas or revising schemas to accommodate internal information structures to the news to the self embodied not only in the traumatic life event, but also in everything that has been serially affected by it. There are both omissions and preoccupations, returns of denial and intrusive-type signs and symptoms during the working-through phase. The edge is taken off either extreme, helping to promote the gradual restoration of equilibrium that will be marked at the end of this phase by movement into a state of relative completion of processing the meaning to the self of the traumatic event.

During the working-through phase, there may also be periods of relaxation in which neither defensive avoidances nor flooding with emotion is observed to be prominent.

There is considerable schematic and information-processing work, as well as frequent social interaction changes during the working-through process. In terms of bereavement, this has been called "the work of grief." During this process, the stressful life events, and events subsequently associated with them, are all reviewed according to different working models, and different schematic models, of the self and the articulation of the self to others and to the nonhuman environment. As each individual may have multiple self schemas, there may be a working through of the event in relationship to each of the important constellations of self-organization. In this process, there may be activation of weak, dependent, or childlike self schemas, or of grandiose, domineering, and aggressive ones. Thus, the meaning of the stress event is assessed not only by the most realistic self schemas but also by extremes that may also infuse the event with meaning.

The working-through phase involves some kind of decision about what it all means for the overall self-organization. The process is thus an evolutionary, survival-of-the-species function, preparing the person to make new commitments after a loss or injury, and to accept the self and the world for the true view of what the new and present situation now consists of. Before this adaptive end of the stress review process, there is not adequate differentiation of fantasy from reality. In the working-through phase, fantasy is differentiated from reality. What was real, but seems unreal, comes to feel more real. What was fantastically elaborated from the event, and seemed to be a real implication of it, is now recognized as an exaggeration or imagination.

Because of this review process, there may be gains in conflict resolution or growth of self-organization beyond the level achieved by the person before the stressful life event. Thus, there may be some "silver lining," as the person learns greater resiliency, sagacity, and capacity, in spite of the inevitable and enduring losses of any traumatic life event.

Preexisting neurotic character structure will make ambivalence, and hence conflict, more likely during the stress review process of the working-through phase. Abnormal schemas of self and other, and tendencies to image-distorting or information-distorting control processes in order to avoid emotional pain, may also impair the individual's ability to reschematize the self and the world in the most adaptive way. Reactive decompensation where character limitations exist may result.

Although listed as such in Figure 4.1, completion is not so much a phase as it is a milestone. It marks the relative end of the most active phases of processing these serious life events in question. Completion is always "relative" because memories and schemas related to the traumatic event will tend to persist throughout the lifetime. I do list this as a phase because it contains a sense that the person has of being complete, of having restored self-coherence, and of being ready now for new relationships and activities of the self.

Normal and Pathological Grief

Thus far, the discussion has focused on reactions to personal traumatic assaults and injuries. Bereavement reactions follow many of the same forms and have a prototypical course of resolution.

In differentiating normal from pathological grief, Abraham (1927) and Freud (1917/1957) characterized normal grief as feelings of painful dejection, with loss of interest in life functions and inhibition of activities. Pathological grief reactions, they believed, were marked by additional features, such as panic, hostility toward the self, regression to narcissistic forms of self-preoccupation, and other signs of deflated self-esteem. They explained these additional features by a theory of pathological mourning, postulating that the subject had a preexisting ambivalent relationship with the deceased. After the death, this complex of ideas and feeling led to self-hatred, to internalization of attributes of the lost object, and to direction of aggressive drives toward the self.

Subsequent field studies of bereavement and continued clinical investigations indicate that hostility toward oneself, characterized as pathogenic by Abraham and Freud, is not an uncommon grief reaction in persons who do not otherwise warrant diagnosis as mentally disordered (Parkes, 1972; Raphael, 1983). Self-blame, hatred, and disgust may normally occur. States of mind characterized by inertia, hypochondriasis, numbness, irritability, feelings of worthlessness, and apathy are also noted in normal grief reactions (Bibring, 1982; E. Jacobson, 1946; J. Jacobson, 1971).

These feelings are usually transient, however. Gen-

Table 4.3. Common Experiences during Grief and Their Pathological Intensifications[a]

Phase	Normal response	Pathological intensifications
Dying	Emotional expression and immediate coping with the dying process	Avoidant; overwhelmed, dazed, confused, self-punitive; inappropriately hostile
Death and outcry	Outcry of emotions with news of the death and turning for help to others or isolating self with self-succoring	Panic; dissociative reactions; reactive psychoses
Denial	Avoidance of reminders, social withdrawal, focusing elsewhere, emotional numbing, not thinking of implications to self of certain themes	Maladaptive avoidances of confronting the implications of the death. Drug or alcohol abuse, counterphobic frenzy, promiscuity, fugue states, phobic avoidance, feeling dead or unreal
Intrusion	Intrusive experiences including recollections of negative relationship experiences with the deceased, bad dreams, reduced concentration, compulsive enactments	Flooding with negative images and emotions, uncontrolled ideation, self-impairing compulsive reenactments, night terrors, recurrent nightmares, distraught from intrusion of anger, anxiety, despair, shame or guilt themes, physiological exhaustion from hyperarousal
Working through	Recollections of the deceased and contemplations of self with reduced intrusiveness of memories and fantasies, increased rational acceptance, reduced numbness and avoidance, more "dosing" of recollections and a sense of working it through	Sense that one cannot integrate the death with a sense of self and continued life. Persistent warded off themes may manifest as anxious, depressed, enraged, shame-filled, or guilty moods, and psychophysiological syndromes
Completion	Reduction in emotional swings with a sense of self-coherence and readiness for new relationships. Able to experience positive states of mind	Failure to complete mourning may be associated with inability to work, create, to feel emotion or positive states of mind

[a]From Horowitz, 1990.

erally the bereaved person progressively develops a sense of mastery, which reduces secondary anxiety about being overwhelmed. When painful subjective experiences are overwhelming or remarkably persistent, interfering with love and work, the reaction may be regarded as pathological (Horowitz, Wilner, Marmar, & Krupnick, 1980). Table 4.3 summarizes some of the differences between normal and pathological in terms of the varied states theory of the general phases of stress response syndromes.

Formal Diagnoses

Under the *Diagnostic and Statistical Manual of Mental Disorders*, third edition (DSM-III) (American Psychiatric Association, 1980), the diagnoses made most frequently for patients with pathologically intense reactions to stressful life experiences are posttraumatic stress disorder, adjustment disorder, and brief reactive psychosis.

Posttraumatic Stress Disorder

A posttraumatic stress disorder (PTSD) characteristically includes experiences that in some way repeat the traumatic event, often as intrusive ideas accompanied by unbidden feelings. This compulsive repetition may be associated with the other main set of symptoms, those of denial states, for instance, numbness or unresponsiveness to, or reduced involvement with, the external world.

The stressor event that produced the syndrome is usually one that would evoke significant symptoms in most people and that lies outside the range of such common experiences as simple bereavement, chronic illness, business loss, or marital conflicts. Rapes, muggings, assaults, military combat, torture, natural disasters, traumatically frightening or painful medical experiences, deaths of loved ones, and accidents, such as airplane and car crashes, can all evoke the reactions that characterize posttraumatic stress disorders. The most prominent features of such events are the sudden helplessness and shocking perceptions they provoke.

Intrusive experiences and psychic numbing (emotional anesthesia) are two major symptoms that lead to the diagnosis of posttraumatic stress disorder. Unbidden images, dreams, and nightmares frequently occur. In rare instances, the patient may experience dissociative states that last for hours or days; during these states he or she may compulsively relive the event. Recurrent or prolonged episodes of depression, anxiety, guilt, shame, and rage are also common. Minor stimuli may trigger explosive, hostile behavior. In addition, the disorder may include components of sympathetic nervous system hyperarousal, such as difficulty relaxing or falling asleep, with persisting tachycardia, sweating, and pupillary dilation.

A latency period of months or even years may intervene between the stressful event and the maximum symptomatic response. According to DSM-III, when the symptoms begin within 6 months of the traumatic event, the disorder is acute. In such cases the prognosis for remission is good. If more than 6 months have elapsed between the event and the emergence of symptoms, the reaction is considered delayed, and if the symptoms have lasted 6 months or more, the disorder is considered chronic. Delayed or chronic subtypes are usually more difficult to treat.

In making comprehensive diagnoses, it is important to consider the possibility of concussion in acute physical traumas or malnutrition in prolonged stress responses. Very mild concussions may leave no immediate apparent neurological signs but may have residual long-term effects on mood and concentration (Trimble, 1981). Malnutrition during extended stressful periods may also lead to organic brain syndromes. Furthermore, persons with posttraumatic stress disorders commonly cope in ways that may lead to other disorders; for example, they may commence excessive use of alcohol, narcotics, sedatives, or food.

If the life event is not severe enough to meet the criteria for posttraumatic stress disorder, the diagnosis of adjustment disorder may be made. These stress-response syndromes may also have signs and symptoms of the intrusive and denial phases.

Adjustment Disorder

Adjustment disorders are defined by DSM-III as maladaptive reactions to identifiable psychosocial pressures, with the reactions emerging within 3 months after the onset of the stressor. Signs and symptoms, not as specifically defined as those for posttraumatic stress disorder, include a wide variety of disturbances in interpersonal and work functioning as well as maladaptive extremes of anxiety, depression, rage, shame, and guilt. According to DSM-III, if these signs and symptoms meet the criteria for another Axis I mental disorder, such as anxiety disorder or depressive disorder, then the diagnosis of adjustment disorder should not be made.

The identifiable psychosocial pressures that may precipitate adjustment disorders include such changed life circumstances as divorce, difficulties with child-rearing, illness or disability, financial difficulties, a new form of work, graduation, moving, retirement, and cultural upheaval.

DSM-III lists categories of adjustment disorders that are classified by the patient's predominant complaints. They include depressed or anxious mood, combined out-of-control emotional states, disturbance of social conduct, work or academic inhibition, and withdrawal from others. Thus, adjustment disorder is a very open diagnostic entity, and in each case it is important to reach a specific individualized formulation.

Neither posttraumatic stress disorder nor adjustment disorder should be regarded as a minor mental disorder. In either instance, suicidal ideation may be high, and severe dysfunction may be found in such areas as work, social life, and parenting. Both disorders may cause high levels of personal distress. The prognosis for full recovery, however, is usually excellent.

Brief Reactive Psychosis

Brief reactive psychosis has a sudden onset immediately following exposure to a stressful event and may last from a few hours to no more than 2 weeks. The clinical picture includes emotional turmoil and at least one gross psychotic symptom, a criterion that primarily differentiates this condition from posttraumatic stress disorder and adjustment disorder. A paranoid delusion would be one such symptom.

Epidemiological studies suggest that brief reactive psychoses are less common than posttraumatic stress disorders. The studies are limited, however, by the fact that they are almost invariably retrospective. The absence of prospective studies means a lack of knowledge about preexisting pathology of characteristics that might predispose individuals to brief reactive psychosis (Rabkin, 1982).

Suggestions for the Revision of Psychiatric Diagnosis

At the present time, posttraumatic stress disorder is found within the anxiety disorders. Pathological grief reactions are difficult to diagnose because of a clause that is variously interpreted about the required nature of the event for PTSD as "beyond the usual range of experience" (American Psychiatric Association, 1980). Of course, the death of a loved one, especially a shocking or unexpected death, is well beyond the ordinary range of experience for that individual! But because all persons experience the death of loved ones, usually at first in the form of the death of their parents, there is a tendency for some clinicians to regard a bereavement as "an ordinary life experience." It really depends on whether one is taking an epidemiological or an individual perspective. Taking an individual perspective, which is appropriate to psychiatry, means that a bereavement reaction can become a posttraumatic stress disorder when the person has an abnormal response that fits the sign- and symptom-defined criterion of PTSD.

There is no particular reason why PTSD should be grouped with the anxiety disorders. It is true that increasing levels of anxiety are present, if for no other reason than that the person is having increasing levels of intrusion. But they are also present as a primary fear response, because of the injury or loss sustained by the self in any stressful or traumatic experience. It seems wise, therefore, to take PTSD diagnosis out of the anxiety disorders and list it under a separate category.

This reclassification would be a real advantage to the future level of diagnosis: With the stress-response syndromes, we have the first categories for which we can understand etiology and can, therefore, offer some explanations of why the signs and symptoms develop. We have a clear anchor in knowledge of the external events. And eventually, in the future, we will be able to understand much more about relationships among information structure, mental symptoms, brain structure, and any physiological changes. Thus, with the stress-response syndromes, we have a sort of leading edge toward diagnosis, for which we may eventually have an etiologically or causatively based nomenclature rather than one that is simply descriptive.

Although there are a variety of syndromes, such as PTSD, pathological grief, and reactive psychosis which may be traced and related to the interaction of persons, environment, and the occasion of serious life events, the life event structure of individuals will also affect their rate of succumbing to other types of disorder, both physical and mental.

The Role of Trauma in Mental Illness

About 60% of persons diagnosed as having a mental disorder have experienced a severely stressful life event in the 2 weeks preceding the onset of that disorder. In contrast, about 20% of comparison groups not diagnosed as having a mental disorder have experienced a stressful event in the previous 2 weeks (Brown & Harris, 1978). Paykel (1978) summarized such studies as indicating that in the months following a traumatic life event, there is a sixfold greater risk of suicide, a twofold greater risk of depressive disorders, and a slight increase in the risk of developing a schizophrenic syndrome.

Besides leading to posttraumatic and adjustment disorder, stressful experiences can lead to concomitant physiological disturbances and can contribute to other anxiety disorders. Preexisting episodes of separation trauma have been suggested as a predisposition to panic disorders (Klein, 1981). In addition, serious or threatening life events have been implicated in the onset of phobic disorders. For example, Weekes (1978) found that the majority of 528 agoraphobic men and women reported that either sudden or prolonged stress created by difficult life situations was an antecedent to the development of their anxious states of mind; only 5% could offer no cause. Of course, these are impressionistic, retrospective data.

Sim and Houghton (1966), who developed a list of ten types of stressful factors, found that the most common precipitants of phobic disorder in their sample of 191 patients with agoraphobia and other phobias were bereavement and "sudden shock." As Rabkin (1982) pointed out, however, the absence of control groups and a lack of precision in defining stressors and diagnosis render those findings questionable.

Such data on the relation of stress to anxiety, depressive, and schizophrenic disorders do not indicate whether a patient's incipient mental disorder may have contributed to the life events in question. It is probably best to view causation as interactional, with environmental, biological, and psychological causes and predispositions. After all, many serious losses, injuries, and disasters do not lead to psychiatric disorders (Hamburg & Adams, 1967).

Most studies show marked individual differences among stress-response subjects; the person who seemed most disturbed before an event is not always the one who develops a disorder afterward. Nonetheless, it does seem to hold true that the more previous trauma a person experiences, the more likely he or she is to develop symptoms after a stressful life event. Experimentally, persons with more previous trauma found vicarious stress more disturbing (Horowitz, 1975).

When stressors become extreme, as in extended combat or in concentration camps, the rate of morbidity increases. Chapman (1962), for example, reported that a postdisaster psychiatric syndrome may be found in from 0% to 30% of victims, depending on the severity of the stressor.

An up-to-date and fully comprehensive set of studies evaluated victims of the 1972 Buffalo Creek flood in West Virginia, which wreaked sudden, unexpected devastation with considerable loss of life (Erikson, 1976; Gleser, Green, & Winget, 1978; Lifton & Olson, 1976; Titchener & Kapp, 1976). Up to 2 years after the flood, survivors showed symptoms of intrusive recollection, reactive anxiety, depression, and social dysfunction comparable to levels of distress found in patients treated in mental health clinics for anxiety and depressive disorders. Workers exposed to dead and dismembered bodies after a disaster may themselves suffer posttraumatic stress disorders (Raphael, 1983). For children exposed to disasters or trauma, there may be a long latency period followed by manifestation of altered social function (Newman, 1976; Terr, 1981).

Perhaps the most studied personal disaster is the death of a loved one. Reports of increased morbidity of surviving spouses have been questioned, but clearly the death of a loved one may lead to suicidal ideation and to increased use of potential toxins, such as cigarettes, alcohol, and mood-altering drugs. A comparison of reactions by two groups of persons whose parent had died—those who sought brief therapy for symptomatic grief reactions after the death and those who did not—was reported by Horowitz and colleagues (Horowitz, Krupnick, Kaltreider, Wilner, Leong, & Marmar, 1981); a summary of the levels of distress in both groups is shown in Table 4.4. High levels of distress on stress-specific self-report measures, such as the Impact of Event Scale (IES) (Horowitz, Wilner, & Alvarez, 1979), were noted by some subjects in both groups, but a significantly greater proportion of the patient group had high levels of signs or symptoms.

Table 4.4. Distress Levels of Patients Who Sought Brief Psychotherapy after the Death of a Parent and Persons Who Did Not (by Percentage of Persons)[a]

Distress variable[b]	Patients seeking brief therapy			Persons not seeking therapy			X^2	$p <$
	Low	Medium	High	Low	Medium	High		
Self-rating Intrusion (IES)	3	36	61	28	39	33	8.98	.01
Avoidance (IES)	10	32	58	61	17	22	19.02	.001
Depression (SCL-90)	7	32	61	46	31	23	15.23	.001
Anxiety (SCL-90)	23	26	51	65	6	29	13.32	.001
Total symptoms (SCL-90)	23	23	54	66	17	17	13.68	.001
Clinician's rating Intrusion (SRRS)	17	40	43	67	19	14	16.91	.001
Total neurotic symptoms (BPRS)	3	52	45	42	47	11	17.56	.001

[a]From Horowitz, M., Krupnick, H. J., Kaltreider, N., Wilner, N., Leong, A., & Marmar, C. (1981). Initial psychological response to parental death. *Archives of General Psychiatry, 38,* 316–323.
[b]IES indicates rating on the Impact of Event Scale; SCL-90, the Symptom Checklist-90; SRRS, the Stress Response Rating Scale; and BPRS, the Brief Psychiatric Rating Scale.

Individuals whose spouse or parent dies appear more likely to experience pathological grief reactions if the preexisting relationship was characterized by guilt and anger as well as by strong attachment (Horowitz, 1990). Deaths that are unexpected, complicated, or experienced in some way as "unfair" are also harder to assimilate in mourning. Escalating consequences, such as economic difficulties, social disengagement, and disruption of place of residence, can increase the risk of pathological response, and feelings of hopelessness and helplessness will increase the likelihood of depressive reactions. In general, human contact provides major sustenance in grief. The lack of such contact may make mourning difficult and lead to increased likelihood of psychological morbidity (Clayton, 1975).

Preexisting Conflicts or Functional Deficits

In some instances, pretrauma neuroses may make a person unusually resilient. Someone accustomed to anxious or sad states of mind will not be as surprised or frightened by them as will a person who has no experience of distress. Generally, however, preexisting neurotic conflicts may be impediments to processing stressful life events.

Among the neurotic impediments to an adaptive response to stressful life events are the following:

1. Irrational but enduring attitudes that "Bad thoughts cause real harm," "Wishing makes it so," or "One must always be loved or protected by another in order to survive."
2. Active, incompatible, and so conflicted sets of wishes and values whose content is associatively similar to traumatic events. Contradictory person schemas, leading to emotional ambivalence and containing previous ambivalent attitudes, also may dispose to pathological responses.
3. Habitual use of information-distorting control processes that lead to pathological defenses, such as externalization, projection, devaluation, dissociation, extreme repression, and global disavowal or splitting. Habitual overcontrol may also block adaptation and lead to pathological prolongations of denial and intrusive phases of response.
4. Excessive preoccupation with fantasy-based reparations of deficits, involving fantasies related associatively to what was threatened by or lost in the stressful life event.
5. Self-concepts, role-relationship models, scripts, and other person schemas that organize stressful information by the view that the self is bad, damaged, worthless, or incompetent. Deficits in development may also lead to impoverished self schemas and a pathological sense of being unable to cope with stressors.

Processing of Stressor Events

Responses to traumatic events are often discussed in terms of processing new information that is incongruent with preexisting inner schematizations or mental models—our cognitive maps of how the self articulates with the world. Serious life events are those that will eventually change cognitive maps.

It is essential that persons who experience stressful life events have time to review the implications of the news inherent in those events. The mind continues to process the new information until reality and inner models are brought into accord, in what can be called a "completion tendency."

Until memories of traumatic life events can become integrated with mental schematizations, they are stored in an especially active form of coding. These "memory contents" tend toward repeated mental representation; that is, they tend to be repeatedly examined. Each repeated representation once again sets in motion information processing that may eventually revise cognitive schematizations. As new schematic structures are established, the news about the individual's revised circumstances becomes part of long-term memory, and the codifications in active memory decay.

Codification in active memory tends to decay anyway, as is shown by experiments on short-term memory. Following a traumatic event, however, the news is so important that the active memory of the stressors is not, like ordinary short-term memories, automatically erased or replaced by other sets of information. Indeed, this process of decay may not occur at all.

The first processing of the news of a stressful life event entails a rapid appraisal of how best to cope with it (Lazarus, 1966). A low level of inhibitory regulation leads to excitation of emotional systems and to the behaviors associated with emotional outcry (Horowitz, 1991). The amount of information required to change cognitive schematic models is usually so great that complete processing and integration are impossible in a short time. The emotional implications are too overwhelming. Inhibiting regulatory efforts are initiated so that the stressful information can be gradually assimilated, dose by dose.

Excessively high inhibitory controls may interrupt the assimilation and accommodation process. A high level of control leads to the denial and numbing phase of stress-response syndromes. Failures of control lead either to a continuation of outcry, as in prolonged panic-stricken states, or to an intrusive state. Optimally, adaptive controls reduce ideational and emotional processing to tolerable levels. Under such circumstances, the person can gradually make new decisions and record new intentions and beliefs as plans and schematizations. By mental processing of memories and fantasies in such working states of mind the person can gradually complete his or her adaptation to the stressful life event.

Biological as well as psychological factors are involved in these sequences. One theory, as yet inadequately tested experimentally or empirically, is that the processing of psychological meanings of traumatic perceptions activates certain neural or neurohormonal networks in unusual ways (Kandel, 1983; Redmond, 1981). For example, the continued strain of processing might exhaust certain neurotransmitter systems, disposing the person to depressive states. Conversely, excessive arousal of certain neurotransmitter systems, such as the noradrenergic systems, could perpetuate anxious states of mind, leading to more active information transfer at synapses along alarm-system neural pathways. Once certain biological systems are hyperaroused, depleted, or deregulated, other metabolic functions aimed at reestablishing equilibrium may be set in motion.

During this course toward equilibrium, it may be difficult to process psychological meanings in a way that leads toward adaptation to stress.

Treatment

Early intervention has distinct advantages. Immediate distress is reduced, chronic or delayed responses may be prevented, and pathological responses may not be fixed, making for a briefer intervention (Caplan, 1964; Lindemann, 1944). In crisis work of this type, human relationship support through communication and ministration to physical and emotional needs is a powerful method of reducing distress and should be used as the first form of intervention.

If the patient has insomnia, which may produce fatigue and lowered coping capacity, sedation with one of the antianxiety agents may be used on a single night or night-by-night basis. Smaller daytime doses of the same agent may be prescribed, again on a dose-by-dose basis. The patient, and persons close to him, should be cautioned against continued use of these agents or use of multiple mood-control agents, especially against combining alcohol with prescribed medications. Antidepressive agents should not be prescribed to relieve sadness and despondency as immediate responses to loss. Patients in the acute phase of response to a traumatic event should be advised to avoid driving, operating machinery, or engaging in other tasks that require alertness; they may suffer lapses of attention, concentration, and sequential planning or have startle reactions that disrupt motor control.

Transient support may be all that is required. However, if the patient fails to progress well through the adaptive phases of a stress response within a few weeks, further intervention is needed. A formal course of brief dynamic psychotherapy is one appropriate modality.

Elsewhere my colleagues and I have presented detailed expositions of brief dynamic therapy for stress disorders (Horowitz, 1986, 1987; Horowitz & Kaltreider, 1979). In that literature, we advocate brief psychotherapy for recent stressful events both as an immediate treatment procedure and as a way of preventing chronic disorders. We are most experienced in conducting these brief therapies in once-a-week hourly sessions for 12 visits. Several principles are summarized here and in Table 4.5.

When a person seeks help, the therapist establishes an alliance that allows helping the patient work through any reactions. In addition, the therapist may seek to modify preexisting conflicts, developmental difficulties, and defensive styles that rendered the patient unusually vulnerable to traumatization by this particular experience.

Therapy begins with the establishment of a safe and communicative relationship that, together with specific interventions, alters the status of the patient's controls. The patient can then proceed to reappraise the stressful life event, and the meanings associated with it, and make the necessary revisions of inner models of self and of the world. As the patient reappraises and revises, new decisions are made and adaptive actions are engaged. Desired behavioral patterns can be practiced until they gradually become automatic.

As the patient achieves new levels of awareness, this process is repeated and deepened; there is more trust in the therapist, and the patient is able to modify controls further and assimilate more thoughts about the current stress that had previously been warded off.

Table 4.5. An Outline of Brief Dynamic Therapy for Stress Disorders

Session	Relationship issue	Patient activity	Therapist activity
1	Initial positive feeling for helper	Patient tells story of stress event	Preliminary focus is discussed
2	Lull as sense of pressure is reduced	Event is related to previous life of patient	Takes psychiatric history. Give patient realistic appraisal of syndrome
3	Patient testing therapist for various relationship possibilities	Patient adds associations to indicate expanded meaning of events	Focus is realigned; resistances to contemplating stress-related themes are interpreted
4	Therapeutic alliance deepened	Implications of events in the present are contemplated	Defenses and warded-off contents are interpreted, linking of latter to stress event and responses
5	—	Themes that were avoided are worked on	Active confrontation with feared topics and re-engagement in feared activities are encouraged
6	—	Future is contemplated	Time of termination is discussed
7 to 11	Transference reactions interpreted and linked to other configurations; acknowledgment of pending separation	Working through of central conflicts and issues of termination, as related to the life event and reactions to it, is continued	Central conflicts, termination, unfinished issues, and recommendations are clarified and interpreted
12	Saying goodbye	Work to be continued by patient alone and plans for future are discussed	Real gains and summary of future work for patient to do alone are acknowledged

Note: From *Stress-Response Syndromes* (2nd ed.) by M. Horowitz, 1986, New York: Jason Aronson. Copyright 1986 by Jason Aronson. Reprinted by permission.

When, several sessions before the final one, the therapist introduces a plan for the termination of therapy, the patient reexperiences loss, often with a return of symptoms. This time, however, the loss can be faced gradually, actively rather than passively, and in the context of a communicative and helping relationship. The final hours of therapy should center on the specific interpretations of the link between the termination experience and the stressful event. Case histories, provided elsewhere, are of course necessary to more fully convey the nature of such therapeutic approaches (Horowitz, 1986; Horowitz, Marmar, Krupnick, *et al.*, 1984).

ACKNOWLEDGMENT

Research and preparation of this chapter was supported by the John D. and Catherine T. MacArthur Foundation.

References

Abraham, K. (1927). A short study of the development of the libido. In *Selected papers of Karl Abraham, M.D.* New York: Basic Books.

American Psychiatric Association. (1980). *Diagnostic and statistical manual of mental disorders* (3rd ed.). Washington, DC: APA Press.

Bibring, E. (1982). The mechanism of depression. In P. Greenacre (Ed.), *Affective disorders*. New York: International Universities Press.

Breuer, J., & Freud, S. (1955). Studies on hysteria. In J. Strachey (Ed. and Trans.), *The standard edition of the complete psychological works of Sigmund Freud* (Vol. 2, pp. 1–307). London: Hogarth Press. (Original works published 1893–1895)

Brown, G., & Harris, T. (1978). *Social origins of depression: The study of psychiatric disorder in women*. London: Tavistock.

Caplan, G. (1964). *Principles of preventive psychiatry*. New York: Basic Books.

Chapman, D. (1962). A brief introduction to contemporary disaster research. In G. Baker & D. Chapman (Eds.), *Man and society in disaster*. New York: Basic Books.

Clayton, P. (1975). The effects of living alone on bereavement symptoms. *American Journal of Psychiatry, 132*, 133–137.

Erikson, K. (1976). *Everything in its path: Destruction of communality in the Buffalo Creek flood*. New York: Simon & Schuster.

Freud, S. (1957). Mourning and melancholia. In J. Strachey (Ed. and Trans.), *The standard edition of the complete psychological works of Sigmund Freud* (Vol. 14, pp. 243–258). London: Hogarth. (Original work published 1917)

Gleser, G., Green, B., & Winget, C. (1978). Quantifying interview data on disaster survivors. *Journal of Nervous and Mental Disease, 166,* 209–216.

Grinker, R., & Spiegel, J. (1945). *Men under stress.* Philadelphia: Blakiston.

Hamburg D., & Adams, J. (1967). A perspective on coping behavior: Seeking and utilizing information in major transitions. *Archives of General Psychiatry, 17,* 277–284.

Horowitz, M. J. (1975). Intrusive and repetitive thoughts after experimental stress: A summary. *Archives of General Psychiatry, 32,* 1457–1463.

Horowitz, M. J. (1983). *Image formation and psychotherapy.* New York: Jason Aronson.

Horowitz, M. J. (1986). *Stress-response syndromes* (2nd ed.). New York: Jason Aronson.

Horowitz, M. J. (1987). *States of mind: Configurational analysis of individual psychology* (2nd ed.). New York: Plenum Press.

Horowitz, M. J. (1990). A model of mourning: Change in schemas of self and other. *Journal of the American Psychoanalytic Association, 38,* 297–324.

Horowitz, M. J. (1991). Person schemas. In M. J. Horowitz (Ed.), *Person schemas and maladaptive interpersonal patterns* (pp. 13–31). Chicago: University of Chicago Press.

Horowitz, M. J., & Kaltreider, N. (1979). Brief therapy of the stress-response syndrome. *Psychiatric Clinics of North America, 2,* 365–377.

Horowitz, M. J., Krupnick, J., Kaltreider, N., Wilner, N., Leong, A., & Marmar, C. (1981). Initial psychological response to parental death. *Archives of General Psychiatry, 38,* 316–323.

Horowitz, M. J., Marmar, C., Krupnick, J., Wilner, N., Kaltreider, N., & Wallerstein, R. (1984). *Personality styles and brief psychotherapy.* New York: Basic Books.

Horowitz, M. J., Wilner, N., & Alvarez, W. (1979). The Impact of Event Scale: A measure of subjective stress. *Psychosomatic Medicine, 41,* 209–218.

Horowitz, M. J., Wilner, N., Marmar, C., & Krupnick, J. (1980). Pathological grief and the activation of latent self images. *American Journal of Psychiatry, 137,* 1157–1162.

Jacobson, E. (1946). The effects of disappointment on ego and superego formation in normal and depressive development. *Psychoanalytic Review, 33,* 129–147.

Jacobson, J. (1971). *Depression.* New York: International Universities Press.

Janis, I. (1958). *Psychological stress.* New York: Wiley.

Kandel, E. (1983). From metapsychology to molecular biology: Explorations into the nature of anxiety. *American Journal of Psychiatry, 140,* 1277–1293.

Klein, D. (1981). Anxiety reconceptualized. In D. Klein & J. Rabkin (Eds.), *Anxiety: New research and changing concepts.* New York: Raven Press.

Lazarus, R. (1966). *Psychological stress and the coping process.* New York: McGraw-Hill.

Lifton, R. J., & Olson, E. (1976). The human meaning of total disaster: The Buffalo Creek experience. *Psychiatry, 39,* 1–18.

Lindemann, E. (1944). Symptomatology and management of acute grief. *American Journal of Psychiatry, 101,* 141–148.

Newman, C. (1976). Children of disaster: Clinical observations at Buffalo Creek. *American Journal of Psychiatry, 133,* 306–312.

Parkes, C. (1972). *Bereavement: Studies of grief in adult life.* London: Tavistock.

Paykel, E. (1978). Contribution of life events to causation of psychiatric illness. *Psychological Medicine, 8,* 245–254.

Rabkin, J. (1982). Stress and psychiatric disorders. In L. Goldberger & S. Breznitz (Eds.), *Handbook of stress: Theoretical and clinical aspects.* New York: Free Press.

Raphael, B. (1983). *The anatomy of bereavement.* New York: Basic Books.

Redmond, R. M. (1981). *Maternal deprivation reassessed.* Harmondsworth, England: Penguin Books.

Sim, M., & Houghton, H. (1966). Phobic anxiety and its treatment. *Journal of Nervous and Mental Disease, 143,* 484–491.

Terr, L. (1981). Psychic trauma in children: Observations following the Chowchilla schoolbus kidnapping. *American Journal of Psychiatry, 138,* 14–19.

Titchener, J., & Kapp, F. (1976). *Family and character change at Buffalo Creek.* New York: Simon & Schuster.

Trimble, M. (1981). *Post-traumatic neurosis.* New York: Wiley.

Weekes, C. (1978). Simple, effective treatment for agoraphobia. *American Journal of Psychotherapy, 32,* 357–369.

Zilberg, N., Weiss, D., & Horowitz, M. J. (1982). Impact of Event Scale: A cross-validation study and some empirical evidence. *Journal of Consulting and Clinical Psychology, 50,* 407–414.

CHAPTER 5

Psychoanalytic Contributions to a Theory of Traumatic Stress

Elizabeth A. Brett

Introduction

In the last several decades, a new field has emerged focusing on the impact of stressors of unusual severity. Based on investigations of soldiers, Holocaust survivors, and victims of nuclear war, natural, and manmade disasters, this field has variously been called the study of *extreme environmental stress* (Hocking, 1970), *traumatic stress* (Figley, 1986), and *catastrophic trauma* (Krystal, 1978). Psychoanalysts share with the investigators in this new field a fundamental concern with the impact of trauma on an individual's psychic life. However, psychoanalysts or those psychodynamically oriented toward the understanding of intrapsychic processes have traditionally been interested in stressors of a different type, stressors which symbolically represent aspects of infantile conflict. The similarity between the two fields has meant that psychoanalytic formulations of trauma have been useful in the development of models of traumatic stress. The differences between the two fields has meant that traditional psychoanalytic formulations need to be revised and amended when applied to the new field of traumatic stress.

Three Fundamental Psychoanalytic Models of Trauma

There are three fundamental conceptualizations of trauma which still have wide currency within psychoanalysis and which also have influenced the field of traumatic stress. They are the traditional psychoanalytic

Elizabeth A. Brett • Department of Psychiatry, Yale University, New Haven, Connecticut 06511.

International Handbook of Traumatic Stress Syndromes, edited by John P. Wilson and Beverley Raphael. Plenum Press, New York, 1993.

model of symptom formation (Fenichel, 1945), Freud's stimulus-barrier definition of trauma (Freud, 1920/1953), and his repetition and defense model of trauma based on the operation of the repetition compulsion (Freud, 1939/1953). This chapter will examine the ways in which this legacy of interest in trauma has been responded to and revised by psychoanalytic investigations of traumatic stress.

The Question of Etiology

These traditional models of trauma leave three critical problems with which new psychoanalytic investigators of traumatic stress have had to grapple. The first is an etiological issue: How does one conceptualize the relative importance as pathogenic factors of the individual's history as opposed to the nature of the traumatic stressor? This is sometimes referred to as the problem of premorbidity (see Chapter 1, in this volume). The second problem area is the definition of the traumatic state itself: How does one conceptualize trauma as an adult phenomenon, and what distinguishes catastrophic trauma from the traditional psychoanalytic view of infantile trauma? The third issue is the conceptualization of the posttraumatic state: Is the posttraumatic state an identifiable syndrome in which distinctive mechanisms account for symptom formation?

After reviewing the traditional psychoanalytic formulations of trauma, I will examine the ways in which investigators of traumatic stress have addressed these questions.

Traditional Psychoanalytic Formulations of Trauma

In order to place recent contributions in perspective, I will begin with a more detailed examination of the traditional psychoanalytic formulations of trauma. The first is the traditional model of symptom formation outlined by Fenichel (1945) in his classic work, *The Psychoanalytic Theory of Neurosis*. As reviewed by Fenichel, symptoms form when current frustrations revive infantile conflict. Under the impact of the later frustration, a regression occurs to the point of fixation of the original conflict. In this manner, the current symptoms come to reflect ways of feeling and defending that were operative at much earlier times. The conflict, if experienced consciously by the child, would have proven traumatic, that is, overwhelmingly dangerous or extremely anxiety provoking. Hence defenses are used to encapsulate the conflictual material, and a fixation occurs preventing normal development of the impulses involved in the conflict. This impact of the fixation on the form of the symptoms is used by the clinician to locate the point of the original developmental arrest (Fenichel, 1945). In order for symptoms to form, the combined intensity of the current frustration and the infantile conflicts must be sufficiently great. The severity of the current frustration and infantile conflicts form a "complemental series": If one of the two sources of pathogenesis is high, the other one need only be low (Freud, 1917/1953). This view allows for the situation in which a sufficiently intense current frustration is the primary determinant of pathology. However, for the most part in psychoanalytic theories of neurosis and treatment, the infantile conflict is the principal pathogenic factor.

There are several problems with this model for the field of catastrophic trauma: (1) there is minimal focus on the nature or severity of the stressor except as a stimulant to the revival of early conflict, (2) pathogenesis is accounted for by early infantile conflict, and (3) the regression following the current stress is understood as important for the information it conveys about the nature of the early fixation.

The second psychoanalytic formulation of trauma is found in one of Freud's most widely cited definitions of trauma. He states that a trauma occurs when the intensity of stimuli became so great that the stimulus barrier is overwhelmed. The organism is then flooded with unmanageable impulses and its functioning is disrupted (Freud, 1920). This definition is useful because it emphasizes the intensity of a stressor, the importance of modulating stimuli, and the disorganization secondary to a failure of modulation. This definition does not address the question of whether there are differences between an infantile and adult trauma nor does it answer the question about whether there are any differences between the experience of a trauma that occurs as a result of infantile conflict or as a result of a catastrophic stressor.

The third psychoanalytic formulation of trauma is Freud's repetition and defense model based on the operation of the principle of *repetition compulsion*. Freud developed this model specifically to account for the repetitive return of traumatic material in the nightmares of soldiers who fought in World War I. Because his theory could not account for this distinctive posttraumatic symptom, he extended his stimulus-barrier formulation. Following the overwhelming assault on the stimulus barrier, a regression occurs, leading to the use of an early and primitive defense, the repetition compulsion. This

defense consists in repeating a disturbing event in an effort to master it. By actively recreating the event, rather than passively experiencing it as in the original situation, the individual is given an opportunity to reexperience it with a higher degree of preparedness and efficacy in preventing the ego from being overwhelmed. Freud stated that the aftermath of trauma in this model consists of the repeated return of traumatic material propelled by the repetition compulsion alternating with defenses against remembering or repeating the trauma (Freud, 1939/1953). The significance of this model is that it identifies a distinctive symptom of posttraumatic states and includes new explanatory mechanisms in order to account for it. This leaves the question of whether there are other identifiable unique characteristics or dynamics in posttraumatic states.

Traumatogenesis

One of the areas specifically addressed by the recent analytic investigators of catastrophic trauma is how to conceptualize most usefully the etiology of trauma. As many authors have noted, there is a tendency to focus on either of two possibilities: (1) the factors related to the individual are decisive in traumatogenesis, or (2) the factors related to the stressor are decisive in the development of trauma (Figley, 1978; Green, Lindy, & Grace, 1985; Hendin & Hass, 1984; Hocking, 1970). Alternatively, however, Wilson (1989) and Wilson, Smith, and Johnson (1985) have proposed interactional models which simultaneously include both sets of variables.

One extreme position is represented by the use of the traditional psychoanalytic theory of symptom formation as a model for understanding trauma. In that view, the factors related to the individual are responsible for the pathogenesis. Infantile conflict is the source of the pathology and later symptoms are understood primarily as reflections of the early conflicts and defenses. Later symptomatology has no particular distinctive form of its own.

In reaction against the classical model of symptom formation, Kardiner took up the other extreme position (Kardiner & Spiegel, 1947). His view that pathogenesis arises from the nature of the traumatic event led him to dismiss the etiologic significance of all individual factors. For Kardiner, the decisive factor in the genesis of trauma is the individual's inability to adapt effectively to the traumatic event. Further understandings of the unique personal meaning of or fears about the traumatic event are not relevant. This is in contrast to the typical neurosis, in which a further understanding of fears and meanings uncovers the unconscious conflict which is responsible for the pathology. Kardiner conceded that an old conflict may be symbolically revived by a traumatic event, but this occurs as an independent accompaniment to the trauma; it is not what causes the event to be traumatic. In sharp contrast to the traditional view, Kardiner believed that the psychic meaning of the trauma is organized after the event. It is only when the individual tries to defend against the damage done to his functioning by the trauma, after it has occurred, that meanings symbolic of old conflicts are attributed to it. In addition to this alternative to conceptualizing the relationship of individual factors and the stressor, Kardiner went on to describe a characteristic posttraumatic syndrome, making the point that stress pathology is distinctive and nonreducible to early forerunners.

Several recent theorists have disagreed with Kardiner's views and taken a position intermediary between the two extreme etiologic positions. Hendin and Hass (1984) believed that pretraumatic personality factors are involved in determining what events become traumatic. They pointed out that similar events have different meanings to different individuals and that it is the meanings of events which determine whether they become overwhelming and hence traumatic. Furthermore, a person's prior life experience is an important contributor not only to trauma development but also to the nature of the ensuing stress symptoms. Hendin and Hass stated that the two extreme positions, the one that attributes pathology to earlier conflicts and the one that attributes pathogenesis to intrinsic qualities of the stressor, are both inaccurate. It is the integration of the individual's unique response and the nature of the stressful event which is crucial. They clarified that their focus on characteristics of the individual does not mean that individual characteristics are necessarily pathological or in a general way a predisposion to trauma.

Similar to Hendin and Hass, Krystal (1978, 1985) believed that it is the meaning of an event which determines whether it becomes traumatic. He began with Freud's statement that trauma is caused by the subjective experience of helplessness. This position includes taking into account those individual factors which contribute to the individual's judgment that he or she is helpless. Although he does not clearly address the etiological question in terms of the relative contributions of the individual or stressor factors, he would agree with Hendin and Hass's critiques of the two extreme positions which have been taken in the controversy over etiology.

How adequate are these current psychoanalytic responses to the question of etiology and what is their significance for the evolution of a model of catastrophic trauma? It is important that Hendin and Hass and Krystal have brought back the emphasis on the unique, individual nature of the reaction to an event as a factor in its appraisal as overwhelming. However, for this view not to be misinterpreted as a reversion to an infantile conflict model, it must be emphasized that the primary pathogenic force comes from the nature of the traumatic event. Hocking (1970) and Green et al. (1985), in considering the etiologic controversies while reviewing the empirical research on catastrophic stress, proposed models of catastrophic trauma in which the nature and intensity of the stressor are the primary but not sole etiological ingredients. A variety of individual and societal factors affect whether the response to a stressor persists and becomes a disorder. Such a model is able to accommodate two findings from the growing body of research on catastrophic stress. The first finding is that as exposure to stress increases, so does the number of individuals who develop stress disorders (Egendorf, Kadushin, Laufer, Rothbart, & Sloan, 1981; Green et al., 1985; Hocking, 1970). The second finding is that particular types of events are more associated with the development of stress disorders than others (Gleser, Green, &

Winget, 1981; Jones, 1985; Laufer, Brett, & Gallops, 1985; Lund, Foy, Sipprelle, & Strachan, 1984; Sales, Baum, & Shore, 1984; Wilson, Smith, & Johnson, 1985). The recent revision of the DSM-III criteria for posttraumatic stress disorder (PTSD) is the first formal diagnostic attempt to spell out the nature of those events which are likely to produce stress disorders (American Psychiatric Association, 1980, 1987). They include the threat of injury or loss of life to one's self or loved ones, destruction of one's community, hearing about the kidnap or torture of loved ones, and witnessing mutilation or violent death. In summary, it is important to embrace a model of catastrophic trauma in which the pathogenic force is seen as originating primarily from the exposure to the traumatic event. It is important to do this without renouncing the complexity involved in the individual's subjective experience of the event as well as the complexity involved in the position that a continuum would exist along which predisposition factors are increasingly important as contributors to susceptibility to traumatic stress.

Definition of Trauma

As mentioned above, one of Freud's definitions of trauma is based on the notion that the organism's protective barrier which modulates incoming stimuli is overwhelmed by the intensity of the organism's reaction to the stressor. Although a number of authors continue to use this essential notion (Hendin & Hass, 1984; Schwartz, 1984), alternative definitions of trauma are proposed by Krystal (1985), Emery and Emery (in press), and Parson (1984).

Krystal, also mentioned above, approached the definition of trauma by examining the individual's subjective experience. He was in agreement with Freud's view that trauma involves the subjective experience of helplessness. In this light, he was critical of Freud's primarily economic stimulus-barrier definition of trauma. Both the notions of the stimulus barrier and the intensity of stimuli which overwhelm it focus on quantity. They do not explain how individuals determine that they are helpless nor how they experience this helplessness. This leads Krystal to distinguish two types of trauma: infantile and adult.

Infantile trauma occurs when an infant is overwhelmed by excessively intense affect. In this situation, levels of affect will continue to escalate because the child is unable to manage an undifferentiated, massive psychosomatic reaction to an event. In order to understand the adult's response to potentially overwhelmingly intense affect, Krystal takes pains to examine affective development. He describes a developmental process in which affects are increasingly desomatized, differentiated, and verbalized, making them available for use as signals of potential danger. The child experiences affect as an undifferentiated psychosomatic state which cannot be articulated or sampled in small bits for use as a signal. Thus, the child is unable to anticipate and prevent the possibility of being overwhelmed. The adult, however, can differentiate nuances of feeling, increasingly separate feelings from purely somatic sensations, and anticipate danger. For the adult in a danger situation, levels of affect increase initially as they do for the child. However, at the point when the danger is judged to be unavoidable, the adult using affects as signals is able to anticipate and prevent the state of being overwhelmed by intolerable levels of emotion by blocking affects. According to Krystal, the adult trauma occurs, then, when the individual surrenders to the sense of helplessness and blocks the affect. The inhibition and constriction of affect progress to include all cognitive functioning. Following Stern (1968), Krystal called this a *catatonoid reaction*; continued unabated, it can inhibit life-preserving action and all adaptive functioning, resulting in psychogenic death. Seligman (1975) described a similar syndrome of surrender in animals faced with unavoidable danger. This learned helplessness has been widely used in attempts to understand depression. There are two reasons Krystal believed the catatonoid reaction a particularly useful one for describing adult trauma: It conforms to the subjective experience of the traumatized individual, and it takes into account the impairment of affective and cognitive functioning so often seen following a trauma.

There are a number of ways in which Krystal's contribution is crucial for the development of a model of catastrophic stress. First, he clearly distinguished what is commonly understood as trauma in the psychoanalytic literature from catastrophic trauma. The term *trauma* is used so loosely in psychoanalytic writings that it has lost a great deal of its utility (Furst, 1967). Krystal pointed out that what is meant by trauma in the traditional model of symptom formation is actually the threat of trauma which is warded off by defensive maneuvers and symptom formation. He reserved the term *catastrophic trauma* to refer to his models of adult and infantile surrender to helplessness. Second, Krystal gave a clear clinical description of the traumatic state. The use of the theoretical stimulus-barrier definition, without an accompanying clinical description, left an important gap in the phenomenology of traumatic stress. Third, Krystal distinguished between infantile and adult trauma. His definition of infantile trauma is essentially the same as Freud's. What is new is Krystal's definition of adult trauma. His definition of trauma based on the catatonoid reaction is different in its description of the clinical experience of trauma as well as in its theoretical formulation of the traumatic state. Although Freud as well as other writers have noted the stunned responses following a trauma, Krystal carefully attended to the significance of these symptoms and accorded them critical roles in the traumatic state itself.

Emery and Emery (in press) have proposed a psychoanalytic model of traumatic stress based on the importance of aggression and repetition phenomena. They believe that traditional psychoanalysis has focused on libidinal conflicts, without adequately recognizing the independent and primary role of aggression in development. In the Emery and Emery view, trauma occurs when an individual acts on an intention to harm someone, creating a conflict between the wish to destroy and the desire to maintain object relations. At the traumatic moment, a *split in the ego* occurs, reflecting a double identification with the aggressor and the victim in the traumatic situation. The two identifications condense,

forming a *pathological ego structure*, which is then regulated by the repetition compulsion. It is not clear what Emery and Emery mean by the pathological ego structure. It is clear, however, that the identifications forming this structure are repeated both in relation to external objects or situations and internally, with different portions of the psyche taking the victim and aggressor stances. Thus, a traumatized person might reenact a victim or aggressor role with others. A person might, for example, reenact the two identifications internally by feeling helpless against hallucinations that command him or her to kill. Emery and Emery state that the identifications with the victim and aggressor account for the *generic meaning* common to all traumatic events. Individual meanings based on personal histories color the generic meaning but are not responsible for the pathogenesis of PTSD.

Emery and Emery attempt to bring aggression into focus. They state that traumatic stress may be caused by a rise in aggression, a conflict over aggression, and later manifested by the identifications with the two roles involved in the aggressive act. This view emphasizes that the stressed individual perceives the stressor—person or event—as aggressive and also feels a rise in aggression as the threatening situation is confronted. One difficulty with the Emery and Emery model is that it is narrow, for example, in contrast with Krystal's position, in which helplessness and surrender can occur in reaction to a variety of affects, such as fear or grief as well as aggression.

Another new definition of trauma is offered by Parson (1988). A full consideration of his proposal necessitates a more detailed explanation of his view of the sequelae to trauma so this will be discussed in the succeeding section.

The Posttraumatic State

The third problem area for a psychoanalytic model of catastrophic trauma is how to conceptualize the posttraumatic state. There are two models for understanding the sequelae to trauma which have influenced formulations of catastrophic posttraumatic states: the traditional model of symptom formation and the *repetition-compulsion* model of trauma. In order to examine the utility of these models and evaluate the current responses to them, I will discuss each model on the basis of the symptoms it accounts for, the mechanism it uses to explain the process by which stress leads to symptoms, and the nature of posttraumatic regression.

The classical model of symptom formation is used to account for neurotic symptoms, that is, symptoms which are conceptualized as compromise formations between infantile impulses and the defenses against those impulses. Aside from this stipulation, the form of the symptoms is not restricted, and a wide variety of symptoms can be understood using this model. The symptoms are formed when the impact of the current frustration leads to regression to the etiologically significant fixation (Fenichel, 1945). Freud's repetition and defense model of trauma was in part a reaction to the inadequacy of this model and represented a significant departure from it in each of the three areas chosen for discussion. First, Freud was trying to account for specific posttraumatic symptoms, principally for the symptoms involving traumatic repetitions; to a lesser extent, he was interested in the defenses against the traumatic repetitions. Second, Freud introduced a new mechanism, the repetition compulsion, to explain the return of traumatic material. Third, regression does not lead to the emergence of the pathogenic conflict as in a fixation. The regression is simply an impoverishment in functioning: a reversion to an old and primitive defense. In summary, Freud moved toward a model focused on accounting for unique posttraumatic symptoms formed by the operation of a new pathological mechanism in which regression was not a pathway to the primary etiological factor.

A number of authors have presented alternatives and supplements to these traditional models. Brende and McCann (1984) have focused explicitly on the regression involved in war experiences. In their model, they described aspects of character pathology, particularly diffusion, rigidity, and disintegration of ego boundaries. They explained that these symptoms occurred originally in response to the regression fostered by military training, in which dependency on leaders and comrades is encouraged, and in response to the phylogenic regression to a primitive survival mentality which occurs during combat. These regressive behaviors recur after the war experience is over. They made the points that (1) regressive behaviors are necessary to adapt to a war situation, and (2) that this regression may persist and account for later symptoms. These particular war-related contributors to vulnerability to trauma have also been discussed by Grinker and Spiegel (1945), Shatan (1977), and Wilson (1980). This mode does not address the question of differences between regression secondary to situations fostering a generalized regressive response and discrete events precipitating an abrupt and extreme regressive reaction. This model is useful in contributing to understanding the strain of warfare, but it does not account for the communality of symptoms across traumatically stressed populations.

Hendin and Hass (1984), in trying to explain the symptoms of PTSD catalogued in DSM-III as well as chronic personality adaptations based on guilt, paranoia, and depression, contended that the form of these stress symptoms is determined by the meaning of the trauma to the individual. They used the etiological contributions of the individual's precombat history to explain the nature of the stress symptoms. However, they referred primarily to the content and meaning of the symptoms, for example, whether one's dreams or intrusive memories are dominated by paranoia or depression. Their work did not address the question of why nightmares or intrusive memories are typical posttraumatic symptoms and they did not develop mechanisms to explain this aspect of symptom formation.

DeFazio (1984) cited Fairbairn's model of war trauma. In the selection cited, Fairbairn attempted to account for both a global contraction of ego functioning and for the specific symptomatic belief that the world is a dangerous and malevolent place. Fairbairn understood these symptoms as consequences of a regression to the earliest ego processes involving splitting, introjection, and projection. For example, the stressed individual's sense of the world as terrifying is attributed to a regression to the time when the child is unable to keep internalized bad objects repressed and thus experiences internally disturbing events as external. This notion of regression is similar in certain respects to the one used in the traditional model of symptom formation. The focus of attention shifts from the stressor to early intrapsychic conflict. The experience of actual danger to the adult is understood by appeal to intrapsychic danger in the infant. The fact that the adult's experience of a traumatic stressor is described by mechanisms used to account for the child's early ego development means that the distinctive features of traumatic stress go unnoticed and unexplained.

Parson (1988) proposed a two-part model of response to traumatic stress. First, PTSD develops in response to a traumatic stressor. Second, a posttraumatic self disorder (PTsfD) may develop in response to *sanctuarial stress*, that is, the failure of the environment to empathically respond to the stressed individual. The symptoms of the self disorder include a variety of symptoms of narcissistic rage and vulnerability including low self-esteem, alienation, paranoid ideation, fantasies of retaliation and revenge, and sensitivity to slights, phoniness, and failures to care for and attend to the stressed individual. Parson developed this conceptualization for several reasons: (1) the pervasiveness of narcissistic phenomena in Vietnam veterans, (2) the relative neglect of these symptoms in the literature, and (3) his belief that the posttraumatic self disorder is more severe than the stress disorder since it affects the self as a whole. Parson effectively brought these symptoms to our attention by providing excellent clinical descriptions. The other theorists who have been as impressed as Parson with the pervasiveness of the damage to the psyche and the consequent passivity and constriction are Kardiner and Krystal, who understand these sequelae as continuations of the adaptive failure at the traumatic moment. Parson's self-psychology perspective enabled him to describe in more detail narcissistic features of these symptoms. The danger, as in Fairbairn's case, of borrowing models developed for clinical groups with early developmental disorders is that the unique characteristics of posttraumatic pathology may be overlooked or that the power of situational stressor attributes may be minimized.

Kardiner pointed to five cardinal features of stress disorders (see Chapter 1, in this volume, for a review of this position): (1) traumatic nightmares, (2) fixation on the trauma, (3) startle response, (4) aggressive reaction, and (5) generalized contraction of functioning (Kardiner & Spiegel, 1947). He posited two mechanisms which account for symptoms. The first is the destruction of adaptive functioning, which is the immediate response to the traumatic event. This adaptive failure consists of a massive psychological and physiological constriction and withdrawal of those adaptive systems responsible for the maintenance of contact and interaction with the environment. The second mechanism in his model is a restitutive one. In the second stage of traumatic neurosis, the personality reorganizes in an attempt to compensate for its impoverished adaptive capability. The difference between Kardiner's and Fairbairn's views is that Kardiner would not look to earlier explanations for the fact or form of the regressed functioning. His explanation of the fear of the return of the trauma is that it is a manifestation of the impaired adaptive functioning, that is, the organism's inability to modulate its memory of the trauma. He would not consider this a regression to a specific early level of functioning which accounts for the fearfulness. Rather he would understand this regression to be more in the nature of an impoverishment or disorganization of functioning at the time of the trauma.

Like Kardiner, Krystal was most impressed by the cognitive and affective constriction observed in posttraumatic states. He posited a progressive catatonoid process to account for this disruption in functioning. Although a result of the trauma is an impairment of affect tolerance and a regression along developmental lines to earlier modes of managing affect, the catatonoid reaction is a successful defense against a regression to the earliest modes of experiencing overwhelming affect, that is, to the infantile traumatic state. Krystal emphasized that the adult cannot experience affects as the child does. Symptoms are therefore determined by the adult's developed defensive capabilities as well as by regressive forces.

Krystal's model is a bold and innovative development in psychoanalytic contributions to the study of catastrophic stress. The most important aspect of this contribution is that it is a model which is trying to account for the unique and particular symptoms and pathological mechanisms of catastrophic trauma, not trying to understand these features in terms of theories developed for other clinical groups. A second advantage of Krystal's approach is that he examines the impact of an event on the adult, developed psychic apparatus; he does not immediately reduce symptomatology to manifestation of early ego processes. These are extremely important advances in legitimizing a model which is not a subtly revised version of the usual psychoanalytic model of symptom formation.

In contrast to Kardiner's and Krystal's interest in numbing and constriction, Emery and Emery embrace a psychoanalytic model of traumatic stress which focusses much more narrowly on the reexperiencing dimension of the disorder. The primary identifications with the victim and aggressor which occur at the traumatic moment are repeated endlessly in the posttraumatic state. Emery and Emery use this conceptualization to account not only for the traditionally acknowledged reexperiencing symptoms, such as nightmares and intrusive images, but also for the variety of aggressive, rageful responses on the one hand and the helpless and withdrawn behaviors on the other hand which are understood as direct continuations of the identifications with the aggressor and victim internalized at the traumatic moment. This understanding of the nature of repetition, that is, that elements of a situation are repeated both internally and in relation to external objects, does not differ from the usual psychoanalytic use of the term. What is different is the statement that the identifications with the victim and aggressor are central. However, a weakness in this formulation is that it ignores reenact-ments that involve emotions and imagery unrelated to aggression.

Conclusion

There are several reasons why it has been important to examine these psychoanalytic models and weigh their utility. The first is that in this chapter I have argued that traditional psychoanalytic ideas have contributed to, but also have impeded, the development of models of traumatic stress. Unless the contributions and impediments can be clearly distinguished, we are in danger of throwing out the contributions along with the impediments or we are in danger of unwittingly allowing the impediments to reenter our theories in new guises. With respect to this later danger, the chief problems left by traditional psychoanalytic theory have had to do with conceptualizing etiology and with the analogy with disorders of the early ego. A clear appreciation of the problems this legacy has caused for the development of models of traumatic stress would prevent an uncritical acceptance of comparisons between traumatic stress and forms of early ego pathology. A satisfactory model of traumatic stress must have the following characteristics: a view of etiology in which the primary etiological factor is exposure to a traumatic stressor and a recognition of the distinctive nature of the major symptoms of traumatic stress accompanied by a detailed explanation of the unique aspects of stress symptom formation. The second reason why it has been useful to examine the different models is that each concentrates on different aspects of the response to traumatic stress. They illuminate and help us to penetrate the clinical material in new ways. We see and attend to constellations of symptoms or relationships between elements of the disorder that we had not appreciated before, as with Krystal's elaboration of the catatonoid response. The third reason for a careful scrutiny of these models is that they have significant and differing implications for treatment. A particular behavior or symptom would be understood, and consequently responded to, differently in each model. For example, helplessness might be understood by Krystal as a consequence of the severe constriction of functioning resulting from the catatonoid response, by Parson as narcissistic vulnerability secondary to sanctuarial stress, or by Emery and Emery as a repetition of the sense of victimization at the traumatic moment. The manner in which the meanings of symptoms are unraveled and related to the traumatic event differs. Thus, these models lead to varied treatment strategies whose utility will have to be compared and assessed.

Where do these contributions leave us as far as the evolution of a psychoanalytic model of catastrophic trauma is concerned? Advances in psychoanalytic formulations of trauma have been made in developing a more complex view of etiology, a more precise definition of trauma, and more developed concepts about the distinctive nature of posttraumatic symptoms and the mechanisms responsible for their operation. What work remains to be done? In a review of theories of trauma, Ostroff and I (1985) noted that there are at least two

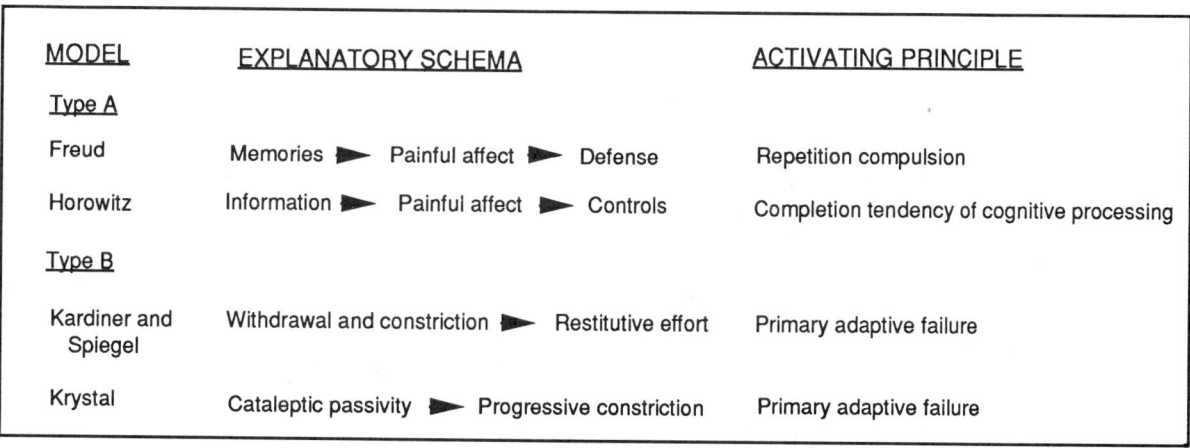

Figure 5.1. Models of stress disorder.

types of models of trauma. In Type A models, exemplified by Freud's repetition-compulsion notion, trauma is followed by two tendencies: (1) to repeat the trauma and (2) to defend against these repetitions. Horowitz (1986) has taken this fundamental idea, translated it into information-processing language, and proposed the most developed model of this type. In his theory, states of "intrusion," that is, *repetition*, and "denial," that is, *defense*, oscillate until the cognitive processing of the trauma can be completed. In Type A models, then, the skeletal framework of the model is that trauma-linked imagery and thoughts lead to painful affect, which leads to defenses. Each theorist posits a mechanism which governs this process, the repetition compulsion in the case of Freud. Figure 5.1, which is a modification of one used in my original review, illustrates this framework.

Type B models are based on the progressive unfolding of one process rather than on the alternation of two states. Kardiner and Spiegel's and Krystal's models are of this type. The trauma directly initiates a massive adaptive failure. In Kardiner and Spiegel's model, this leads to progressive withdrawal and constriction followed by reorganization in an attempt to cope with its diminished capacities (the restitutive phase). In Krystal's model, the catatonoid reaction leads to severe disturbances in affect and can continue to the point of psychogenic death. Both Kardiner and Spiegel, and Krystal, consider reexperiencing important but they view it as a secondary phenomenon, as a result of the organism's disrupted functioning. Because adaptive functioning has been so crippled, the person cannot modulate and defend against memories of the trauma. Although both models, in a broad sense, view reexperiencing as a result of the inability of the organism to adapt to the trauma, the emphasis in each model is different. In Type A models, the need to repeat is an immediate result of the trauma and regressive defensive functioning, such as numbing, is seen as a response to the reexperiencing phenomenon. In Type B models, the trauma leads directly to a massive regression in defensive functioning which, in turn, leads to the inability to modulate memories of the trauma.

Thus, there are two principal differences between these models: (1) the contrast between a model embracing two states (*reexperiencing* and *defensive functioning*) versus a model describing one state (*massive adaptive failure*); and (2) the contrast between a reexperiencing phenomenon viewed as primary and leading to defensive functioning, and a reexperiencing phenomenon viewed as secondary, that is, caused by the breakdown in defensive functioning. In the discussion of these two models, I speculated that the differences might be due to the severity of the disorders. Freud did not have extensive experience with victims of catastrophic trauma, and Horowitz's work is based on stressors of peacetime, such as accidents, illnesses, and bereavement, whereas Kardiner and Krystal worked with severely traumatized combat veterans and Holocaust survivors. In the most severe cases of traumatic stress, it may be that the reexperiencing dimension is less prominent. The differences between the two models raise a host of questions: Is reexperiencing a primary effect of trauma? To what extent is the defensive dimension of the disorder a response to the reexperiencing phenomenon and to what extent a direct manifestation of adaptive failure? Do reexperiencing and defensive functioning vary along a continuum of severity of stress? Perhaps the two most important implications of these questions are that (1) we need a more elaborate description of the reexperiencing dimension of the disorder comparable to Krystal's discussion of the defensive dimension and (2) we need more complex perspectives on the relationship of the two dimensions to each other.

In summary, Krystal and Hendin and Hass proposed models of traumatic stress in which the pathogenic force originates from the traumatic event while taking into account the person's subjective experience and past history. Kardiner, Krystal, and Parson contributed to further development of our understanding of the defensive dimension. Emery and Emery provide a narrowed, aggression-based conceptualization of the reexperiencing dimension. A comprehensive model of traumatic stress must be able to describe the unique features of both dimensions, explain their relationship to each other, and understand their relative prominence in the variety of symptom pictures.

References

American Psychiatric Association. (1980). *Diagnostic and statistical manual* (3rd ed.). Washington, DC: Author.

American Psychiatric Association. (1987). *Diagnostic and statistical manual* (3rd ed., rev.). Washington, DC: Author.

Brende, J. O., & McCann, I. L. (1984). Regressive experiences in Vietnam veterans: Their relationship to war, post-traumatic symptoms and recovery. *Journal of Contemporary Psychotherapy, 14,* 57–75.

Brett, E., & Ostroff, R. (1985). Imagery and post-traumatic stress disorder: An overview. *American Journal of Psychiatry, 142,* 417–424.

DeFazio, V. J. (1984). Psychoanalytic therapy and the Vietnam veteran. In H. J. Schwartz (Ed.), *Psychotherapy of the combat veteran* (pp. 23–46). New York: Spectrum Publications.

Egendorf, A., Kadushin, D., Laufer, R. S., Rothbart, G., & Sloan, L. (1981). *Legacies of Vietnam: Comparative adjustment of veterans and their peers.* Washington, DC: U.S. Government Printing Office.

Emery, P. E., & Emery, O. B. (in press). Psychoanalytic considerations on post-traumatic stress disorder. *Journal of Contemporary Psychotherapy.*

Fenichel, O. (1945). *The psychoanalytic theory of neurosis.* New York: W. W. Norton.

Figley, C. R. (Ed.). (1978). *Stress disorders among Vietnam veterans.* New York: Brunner/Mazel.

Figley, C. R. (Ed.). (1986). *Traumatic stress points: News from the Society for Traumatic Stress Studies* (Vol 1[2]). Dayton, OH: Society for Traumatic Stress Studies.

Freud, S. (1953). Introductory lectures on psycho-analysis. In J. Strachey (Ed. and Trans.), *The standard edition of the complete psychological works of Sigmund Freud* (Vol. 16, pp. 243–463). London: Hogarth Press. (Original work published 1917)

Freud, S. (1953). Beyond the pleasure principle. In J. Strachey (Ed. and Trans.), *The standard edition of the complete psychological works of Sigmund Freud* (Vol. 18, pp. 7–64). London: Hogarth Press. (Original work published 1920)

Freud, S. (1953). Moses and monotheism. In J. Strachey (Ed. and Trans.), *The standard edition of the complete psychological works of Sigmund Freud* (Vol. 23, pp. 7–56). London: Hogarth Press. (Original work published 1939)

Furst, S. S. (Ed.). (1967). *Psychic trauma.* New York: Basic Books.

Gleser, G. C., Green, B. L., & Winget, C. N. (1981). *Prolonged psychosocial effects of disaster: A study of Buffalo Creek.* New York: Academic Press.

Green, B. L., Lindy, J. D., & Grace, M. C. (1985). Post-traumatic stress disorder: Toward DSM-IV. *Journal of Nervous and Mental Disease, 173,* 406–411.

Grinker, R., & Spiegel, J. (1945). *Men under stress.* Philadelphia: Blakiston.

Hendin, H., & Hass, A. P. (1984). *Wounds of war: The psychological aftermath of combat in Vietnam.* New York: Basic Books.

Hocking, F. (1970). Psychiatric aspects of extreme environmental stress. *Diseases of the Nervous System, 31,* 542–545.

Horowitz, M. (1986). *Stress response syndromes* (2nd ed.). New York: Jason Aronson.

Jones, D. R. (1985). Secondary disaster victims: The emotional effects of recovering and identifying human remains. *American Journal of Psychiatry, 142,* 303–307.

Kardiner, A., & Spiegel, H. (1947). *War stress and neurotic illness.* New York: Paul B. Hoeber.

Krystal, H. (1978). Trauma and affects. *Psychoanalytic Study of the Child, 33,* 81–116.

Krystal H. (1985). Trauma and the stimulus barrier. *Psychoanalytic Inquiry, 5,* 131–161.

Laufer, R. S., Brett, E., & Gallops, M. S. (1985). Dimensions of post-traumatic stress disorder among Vietnam veterans. *Journal of Nervous and Mental Disease, 173,* 538–545.

Lund, M., Foy, D., Sipprelle, C., & Strachan, A. (1984). The Combat Exposure Scale: A systematic assessment of trauma in the Vietnam war. *Journal of Clinical Psychology, 40,* 1323–1328.

Parson, E. R. (1984). The reparation of the self: Clinical and theoretical dimensions in the treatment of Vietnam combat veterans. *Journal of Contemporary Psychotherapy, 4,* 4–56.

Parson, E. R. (1988). Post-traumatic Self-Disorder (PTsfD): Theoretical and practical considerations in psychotherapy of Vietnam veterans. In J. P. Wilson, Z. Harel, & B. Kahana (Eds.), *Human adaptation to extreme stress: From the Holocaust to Vietnam* (pp. 245–279). New York: Plenum Press.

Sales, E., Baum, M., & Shore, B. (1984). Victim readjustment following assault. *Journal of Social Issues, 40,* 117–136.

Schwartz, H. J. (1984). *Psychotherapy of the combat veteran.* New York: Spectrum Publications.

Seligman, M. E. P. (1975). *Helplessness.* San Francisco: W. W. Freeman.

Shatan, C. (1977). Bogus manhood, bogus honor: Surrender and transfiguration in the United States Marine Corps. *Psychoanalytic Review, 64,* 585–610.

Stern, M. M. (1968). Fear of death and neurosis. *Journal of the American Psychoanalytic Association, 16,* 3–31.

Wilson, J. P. (1980). Conflict, stress, and growth: Effects of war on psychosocial development. In C. R. Figley and S. Leventman (Eds.), *Strangers at home: The Vietnam veteran since the war* (pp. 123–165). New York: Praeger.

Wilson, J. P. (1989). *Trauma, transformation, and healing: An integrative approach to theory, research, and post-traumatic therapy.* New York: Brunner/Mazel.

Wilson, J. P., Smith, W. K., & Johnson, S. (1985). A comparative analysis of PTSD among various survivor groups. In C. R. Figley (Ed.), *Trauma and its wake: The study and treatment of post-traumatic stress disorder* (Vol. 1, pp. 142–172). New York: Brunner/Mazel.

CHAPTER 6

Posttraumatic Stress Phenomena

Common Themes across Wars, Disasters, and Traumatic Events

Lars Weisæth and Leo Eitinger

Introduction

Over a period of many years, results from studies on psychological traumatizations were described with more or less typical symptomatology until the American Psychiatric Association in 1980 suggested the diagnosis of posttraumatic stress disorders (PTSD). This fascinating diagnosis (1987), however, introduces several riddles: Why does the human organism react with similar symptomatology to quite different experiences, such as torture, rape, natural disaster, and the like? What are the similarities and dissimilarities in symptomatology? What is the most appropriate form of posttraumatic therapy and when and how should it be initiated and concluded? Considering the enormous variety of traumata and stressors inherent in disaster, war, and other traumatic situations, it is even more astonishing that the human response is so similar across social, demographic, and other variables.

This uniformity of response probably reflects the common basic traumata emanating from these events, of which the most important are: (1) the psychological effects of the physical suffering and of the *danger trauma*, that is, the overwhelming *threat to life*; (2) the *loss trauma*, that is, the death of close ones, often witnessed by the helpless victim; and (3) what we have called the *responsibility trauma*, that is, the attack on one's psychological self. To illustrate a combined and severe trauma, torture may serve as an example.

The evil instincts of torturers throughout the ages and, even worse, the training of modern torturers, have exploited human vulnerability in these three areas. Modern torture includes the worst possible infliction of physical suffering with repeated threats of death (see Part IV, in this volume). The torture victim is forced to experience fear of death a thousand times in fantasy. Particularly vicious torture also inflicts threat of loss trauma or actual loss trauma by threatening to kill or actually killing the victim's child, spouse, or parent in the presence of the victim. This creates the loss trauma, as well as the responsibility trauma, the insoluble conflict between sacrificing one's loved ones or betraying the cause. One of the central aims of torture is to destroy the personality of the victim. However, it is a common effect of intentional trauma that not only is a person's body attacked, but also his or her psychological sense of self. After the torture, many victims are forced into exile and their fate as refugees adds to their helplessness and deprivation.

It is more commonly assumed that the degree of responsibility trauma seems to vary with the agent causing the trauma, the most severe being deliberate, humanly instigated violence, the second worst being an accidental man-made trauma, such as a technological disaster (see Chapter 7, in this volume), and the third level represented by any trauma caused by nature (Raphael, 1986). Although the three traumata described above account for many of the similarities in posttraumatic stress phenomena, the degree of exposure to the responsibility trauma seems to be related to the degree of violence inflicted on the victim.

The striking *common thread* in posttraumatic stress phenomena may also reflect the limited avenues of human responses to such basic traumata. Why is there not more divergence and variability in response to trauma? Stereotyped responses may indicate that it is a basic psy-

Lars Weisæth • Division of Disaster Psychiatry, Department of Psychiatry, University of Oslo, Oslo 3, Norway. **Leo Eitinger** • Ö Ullern Terr. 67, 0380 Oslo 3, Norway.
International Handbook of Traumatic Stress Syndromes, edited by John P. Wilson and Beverley Raphael. Plenum Press, New York, 1993.

chobiologically founded reaction pattern which has psychological adaptation and survival value.

Considering the great diversity of human nature and the fact that stress research in general has shown quite clearly the overriding importance of the individual's interpretation and experience of the stressful situation, the uniformity of the response is all the more important in understanding posttraumatic adaptations.

Comparison of PTSD Reactions among Different Groups Exposed to Extreme Stress

This chapter concerns investigations by Norwegians on posttraumatic responses to (1) human violence against groups of the civilian population during World War II (resistance underground fighters, refugees, concentration camp survivors, and war sailors), (2) accidental humanly caused traumata (technological disasters), (3) personal events connected with extreme violence (terror, rape, bank robberies), and (4) military and paramilitary accidents (ship's crews under bombardment, avalanche disasters). It will focus on the similarities of the responses, but we also raise the question of whether there are not important differences regarding time of onset, course, and some symptoms that may have consequences for the diagnosis and treatment of posttraumatic stress reactions and PTSD.

Space does not allow us to give a detailed picture of all the investigations or results, but we shall discuss the control issues for future research.

Before World War II

Before the introduction of PTSD diagnosis in 1980, posttraumatic psychopathology was labeled either (1) *after the event* thought to be of etiological importance, such as the war-sailor syndrome or the concentration-camp syndrome; or (2) *after the response*, such as the posttraumatic neurosis. The third possibility was an ordinary psychiatric diagnosis (see Chapter 1, in this volume).

There have been many negative consequences of this lack of some unifying clinical or diagnostic concept bridging similar conditions. For example, it has hindered public and professional understanding and has greatly hampered clinical practice and research. Similarly, Norway had no legislation regarding compensation for war victims. New laws had to be promulgated and amendments added several times as a result of the medical and psychiatric findings in the postwar period in order to adequately care for war victims.

The lack of a specific diagnosis may have been particularly unfortunate for those poor victims who were given a general psychiatric diagnosis instead (e.g., schizophrenia). The reluctance to accept posttraumatic psychopathology in some countries, such as post-World War II Germany, and the similarity of some of its symptoms to certain other psychiatric conditions, such as the autistic symptoms of schizophrenia, resulted in the frequent use of this diagnosis as well as anxiety neurosis,

depressions, and alcohol abuse. A similar situation existed in the United States and elsewhere following World War II and other wars (Wilson, Harel, & Kahana, 1988).

The posttraumatic stress syndrome was well described at an early stage (Trimble, 1981). However, during the last century, the changing views of the medical profession on the nature of posttraumatic psychopathological states, whether of an organic, psychological, or social nature, have offered a rare case of the extent to which economic, sociological, military, and political interests and stakes in the medical field have clearly influenced the clinical practitioners and researchers at various times. Thus, the history of traumatic neurosis offers interesting reading (Fischer-Homberger, 1975; Weisæth & Eitinger, 1991).

Early on in his practice, Freud experienced the traumatic neurosis patient, following accidents, and was of course decisively influenced by the power of psychogenetic factors through his work with Jean-Martin Charcot. When Freud had separated the anxiety neurosis from the other neurotic states, and subsequently had the opportunity to study and treat the many psychological casualties in the First World War, one would have expected that he would have succeeded in finding a distinct diagnosis for the posttraumatic stress cases. However, he struggled for the rest of his life with the question of whether or in what ways posttraumatic neurosis was different, and he left the question of etiology open (see Chapter 5, in this volume, for a discussion).

Among the first researchers who systematically studied civilian populations exposed to one and the same trauma was Edward Stierlin (1909) from Zurich. In 1906, he investigated 21 survivors of an accidental manmade disaster (mining catastrophe) and 135 persons 2 months after a natural disaster, the earthquake in Messina in Sicily in 1908. Stierlin singled out the cases of traumatic neurosis, as well as subjects who developed Freudian *Angstneurosen*. He described latency periods among the psychic cases in contrast to the cerebral-organic cases, the resilience of children, the vulnerability of elderly people, and the rarity of classical hysteria, but also the triggering effect as well as the shock-curative effect of trauma upon hysteria, the absence of compensation issues, the frequent physiological disturbances, and the posttraumatic sleep disorder. Stierlin emphasized the etiological role of fright, both for *Schreck-psychosen* (fright psychosis) and *Erdbebenneurosen* (earthquake neurosis)—in the first, creating hallucinations; in the latter, compulsive images of extraordinary intensity.

The change in symptomatology concerning posttraumatic phenomena may have added to the complexity and complicated the task of reaching a diagnosis with a satisfactory face and descriptive validity. The changing pattern has been most clearly seen in combat reactions of soldiers as described during the last hundred years or so as exemplified by the high frequency of conversion reactions during World War I, as compared to the high frequency of open-anxiety reactions during World War II and later wars. The fact that the German armed forces in World War I and World War II did not allow the diagnosis of anxiety states must have had an influence on the symptomatology of the soldiers. On the other hand we know that the number of anxiety and other psychogenic reactions increased substantially among Finnish soldiers during World War II, immediately after they had crossed the original prewar border of their country, that is, moving from a defensive to an offensive type of warfare.

The educational level of the soldiers and the understanding of stressors and acceptance of stress reactions by the military organization and society go a long way toward explaining such changes. Cultural factors also play a role as evidenced in cross-cultural studies of stress reactions in soldiers. We found, for example, that the attitude toward death among United Nations (UN) soldiers from various continents on difficult peacekeeping assignments was influenced by their religious convictions; if they believed in reincarnation after a glorious death in battle, or in predetermination of their fate, this was likely to reduce their fear (Weisæth & Sund, 1982).

After World War II

Refugees in Norway

A case control study was carried out comprising all the postwar refugees who came to Norway and had been in contact with psychiatric institutions during the first 10 years after their arrival. They have been followed up personally by Eitinger (1958, 1960; Eitinger & Grunfeld, 1966).

The frequency of psychosis for the total refugee population when compared with the Norwegian population was 5 to 10 times higher. Each of the refugee patients was matched with a Norwegian patient for control. Among the refugee patients, *paranoid persecutory* reactions were statistically significantly higher than among the Norwegian patients. Jealousy reactions, another expression of feelings of insecurity, were present in one out of six psychotic refugee cases as compared to none in the control cases. The refugees were either married or engaged to a Norwegian partner, whose families would not accept them, and were exposed to many humiliations, forced feelings of inadequacy, and insecurity about their own worth. Psychosomatic and somatic reactions were found more frequently among refugees than among the controls.

The refugees' psychogenic traumatization consisted mainly of isolation and insecurity which resulted not only in delusions of persecution but also in jealousy, and, last but not least, various somatic reactions.

These findings reflect the sum total of the traumatizing war experiences and the accumulated effects of stress, loss, and deprivation. Both depressions and paranoid psychotic reactions were prevalent among the refugees and masked frequently the basic posttraumatic symptoms which were present in all cases. This raises the question of the role of depression in the differential diagnosis of PTSD.

Norwegian Concentration Camp Survivors

The largest group investigated after World War II were the Norwegian concentration camp (NCC) survivors. The initiative to start systematic medical studies in postwar Norway came from some elite units of the Norwegian resistance fighters and combat soldiers who had noticed that some of the rigorously selected, healthy, and well-trained men who had coped successfully with the stress of war, started to deteriorate physically and mentally. Similar observations were made among the concentration camp survivors. "The Board of Norwegian Doctors of 1957" carried out an exceptionally thorough and comprehensive study of persons who had been exposed to severe and long-lasting stress. More than 6,000 were deported, and about 1,500 died, among them 30 children under the age of 10 years (Eitinger & Strøm, 1973; Strøm, 1968). The mortality of all the ex-concentration camp prisoners has been controlled and compared with the mortality of the total Norwegian population. From 1945 to 1976, that is, during a period lasting up to over 30 years after the liberation, the diagnosed mortality was higher for the ex-prisoners than for the average population.

Owing to the cooperation of the compulsory National Health Insurance system in Norway, it is possible to follow a person's health record even if he or she is moving from place to place throughout the country. A representative sample of 500 ex-prisoners was controlled and matched with nonprisoners of the same sex, the same age group, members of the same branch of an insurance organization, of the same socioeconomic status, and the same occupational category as the ex-prisoners. In this way, the possibility of errors because of, for instance, varying sick-leaves, which may be especially prominent in the different occupational categories, was eliminated.

Health is not merely the absence of disease, and we were therefore also interested in the general adjustment of ex-prisoners in the postwar period. As an index of adaptation we have used the number of professions, the number of residences, the changes of occupational status, and the stability of work.

We found that ex-concentration camp prisoners were forced to change their professions more often than the controls. The stability of the Norwegian population is demonstrated by the fact that nearly 98% of the controls had one residence only, whereas the ex-prisoners moved much more, either because of their difficulty in settling down or in order to find new jobs. The ex-prisoners were also less successful in their professional life. One out of four could be characterized by an obvious professional decline, whereas this could be seen in only 1 out of 25 controls. The ex-prisoners were less capable of sticking to their professions and jobs. One out of three had to find four or more jobs during the observation period in order to remain in some sort of occupation.

To demonstrate the morbidity, we registered every sick period for each person and each diagnosis, and how many days of the period were spent in a hospital. The number of sick periods and diagnoses in the two groups were on a statistically significant level, higher among the ex-prisoners than among the controls; this was not linked to any special diagnosis. Only about 5% of the controls as compared to 20% of the ex-concentration camp prisoners had more than 10 sick periods.

When the days spent in hospital are considered, there are statistically highly significant differences between the two groups. As expected the ex-prisoners are more severely and frequently ill, and they had to spend

Table 6.1. Hospitalization of Ex-Concentration Camp
Prisoners ($n = 498$)

Number and length of hospitalization periods	Ex-prisoners (%)	Controls (%)	
0–5 periods	94	99.1	($p < .001$)
6 or more	6	0.9	
Hospitalized	40.3	60.8	
Less than 30 days	25.9	25.8	($p < .001$)
31 or more days	33.8	13.4	

longer periods being treated for their disease in hospital than the controls did, 33% being hospitalized for more than 30 days as compared to 13% of the controls. The differences are marked in all diagnoses, somatic or psychiatric. The issue of premorbidity prior to trauma seems to be of little importance in this group and the increased morbidity influences almost all their psychic and somatic functions. Even small additional life-stress situations can upset the labile equilibrium and result in a manifest illness. In a more recent study, Eitinger and Strøm (1981) demonstrated that the frequency of the so-called endogenous psychosis was not higher in NCC survivors than in the average Norwegian control groups, whereas the frequency of organically caused psychosis and reactive psychosis (i.e., psychosis provoked by situational stress) was substantially higher.

Latency and Delayed Onset of PTSD

For years, the prevailing international opinion was that since the ex-prisoners had recovered soon after the war and had been at work often for several years without symptoms, the later appearance of an illness could not be referred to events which had happened during the war. However, the existence of a latency period was recognized. The medical community had also been reluctant to accept that nonorganic chronic mental illnesses could develop in persons who had had a harmonious childhood. This fact, however, was established. On the one hand, the finding of chronic psychiatric disorders challenged the traditional views of psychodynamic psychiatry, with its emphasis on individual predisposition as a necessary condition for psychiatric disorders to develop; on the other hand, it supported one of the less understood basics of dynamic psychiatry, that several years may pass before the effects of a traumatic experience, such as the pathogenic factors of childhood, become manifest. Usually an extreme, long-lasting stress situation involves both psychological and physical stressors. However, the stress on the allied merchant seamen during World War II was purely psychological in those who were not torpedoed.

Norwegian Merchant Marine Sailors

One third of the Norwegian sailors who survived their service in the Merchant Marine during World War II were disabled (Askevold, 1976/1977) and nearly all were

marked by their war experience. The stress the sailors were exposed to during the five war years was characterized by a constant threat to their lives, and frequent or even continuous interruption of sleep. The foremost dangers were represented by enemy submarines and attacking airplanes. The freight was based on highly explosive gasoline, explosive materials, and ammunition. During 1942–1943, on average, one Norwegian ship was torpedoed every third day. Out of 1,000 ships, 500 were lost. In contrast to the concentration camp prisoners, the sailors experienced only psychological stress. That stress, however, was constant and consisted of a long-lasting confrontation with dangers since they had no possibility to fight back or escape from it—a particularly vicious kind of helplessness. In addition to the physical threat, the sailors were separated from their families for several years and many of them lost brothers, a father, or close friends on ships in the same convoy without having any chance to make rescue efforts.

These findings help to establish that PTSD can be evoked by long-lasting psychological stress only and that physical traumatization is not a necessary prerequisite. Initially, this fact was not understood or recognized, the view being that the war sailors had often suffered from no direct life threat, only exposure to the chance of being torpedoed.

The lack of knowledge about the "war-sailor syndrome" may have contributed to too much weight being put on the causal effect of more recent physical trauma, like explosion, in Leopold and Dillon's study (1963). The war-sailor syndrome demonstrates that chronic stress is conducive to a general lowering of the powers of resistance of the total organism, as proved among concentration camp survivors and prisoners of war (POW) in Japan (see Chapter 19, in this volume).

Case control studies, such as were examined, can establish the threshold of human endurance to extreme stressors, provide knowledge about the coping factors that may make a difference even in such situations, establish prevalence estimates of various types of psychopathology in differentiated risk groups, clarify the nature and symptomatology of various posttraumatic syndromes, and give much information regarding the possibilities and limitations of therapy and tertiary prevention (Wilson et al., 1988).

Research Perspectives

Based on the Norwegian experiences, some of the topics which necessitated further research are: (1) the role of individual predisposition; (2) the subjective experience during the trauma; (3) the early risk reactions; (4) the primary and secondary prevention; (5) the effect of therapy on the course of illness; (6) the question of the mechanisms of pathogenesis, latency period, and bridge symptoms; and (7) the associated features.

We had to acknowledge the need for controlled prospective studies of trauma-exposed populations which could be followed closely over a sufficient time period using clinical methods. There was also a lack of knowledge about the effects of less extreme trauma of briefer duration occurring under peacetime circumstances. We were able to conduct such studies, which will be treated next. However, a research problem which has only been partially solved has been the question of providing reliable baseline (pretraumatic) data on previous health and other individual risk factors, such as vulnerable personality traits, specific coping skills, and the like.

Industrial Disaster in Norway

A major disaster occurred in Norway's largest paint production plant. As a result of an accidental explosion, the entire factory was destroyed. Thirty thousand square meters of the building were consumed by fire, which, at its height, reached 1,200 feet. The fire was brought under control after 36 hours. Remarkably, there were only six fatalities. Two of the 125 survivors suffered severe injuries and another 21 had minor injuries. Psychiatric assistance was made available to all workers immediately after the explosion and constituted the start of the research project (Weisæth, 1984, 1985, 1989).

In order to measure the intensity of the primary disaster stress, the 125 survivors were divided into 2 groups according to the distance from the explosion center and then compared with a control group consisting of workers from the same factory, but not at work at the time of the explosion, though most of them (65%) had witnessed the extremely visual disaster from some distance, and 12% of this control group had been active in the rescue operations. The three groups were comparable (with a few small differences) before the disaster. Their health was generally good, both in terms of physical, psychosomatic, and mental health, as could be expected in a cohort of fully employed persons, many managing shift work as well.

Data were collected from each person at 3 different points in time: the acute period, after 7 months, and after 4 years. A more therapeutically oriented intervention was used toward the persons who were considered as risk cases—judged according to the symptomatology. A 100% completion rate was achieved for practical purposes.

As far as the symptomatology is concerned, the following posttraumatic stress reactions were present in the 3 groups with clearly varying frequency: startle responses, 86% in Group A, 80% in Group B, and 34% in Group C; sleep disturbance, 83%, 76%, and 36%, respectively, in the 3 groups; repetitive anxiety, 82%, 71%, and 19%, respectively; fear of the destroyed area, 79%, 69%,

and 19%, respectively; and traumatic nightmares, 61%, 41%, and 14%, respectively.

These five symptoms can be considered as an immediate reaction to an extremely frightening experience, constituting a tightly knit posttraumatic anxiety syndrome. Of the other symptoms of the posttraumatic stress syndrome, that is, tremor, social withdrawal (avoidance behavior), guilt, shame, depressive mood, and irritability were found in 15–40% only, but always together with the 5 above-mentioned anxiety symptoms.

The differences were even more marked when severity of the symptoms was judged, and when the time factor was considered. Moderate up to severe reactions were found 1 week after the explosion in 43% in Group A, 22% in Group B, and 10% in Group C. After 7 months, there was a decline in the point prevalence of PTSD to 36%, 17%, and 4%, respectively, in the 3 groups. After 4 years, when 238 out of 246 were still alive, the percentages were 19, 1.8, and 2.6, respectively, in the 3 groups.

All symptoms except irritability decreased in frequency as well as in intensity with time. The moderate symptoms had a higher tendency to improve than the severe ones.

There was a strong correlation between the development of the PTSD and some background variables, such as adaptational problems in childhood and adult life, previous psychiatric impairment, high psychosomatic reactivity, character disorders, current life stressors, but most important of all was the intensity of disaster stress. (No correlation was found with age, civil status, education, secondary disaster stressors, and independent life events after the disaster.) We must therefore conclude that the actual trauma is a necessary and pathogenetic cause of the manifestation of PTSD. Furthermore, 10 of the survivors of the explosion were considered as chronically incapacitated: 9 of them belonged to Group A.

One of the variables which turned out to be of statistical importance was prior experience and training in coping with disaster or other danger situations. There was an unusually high frequency of *disaster-competent* employees in all three groups owing to their maritime background and partly to their participation in the Norwegian Merchant Marine during World War II. Many of them had experienced, for brief periods, accidental threats to their lives. The majority of the latter displayed optimal or suboptimal disaster behavior. Nobody with little or no disaster training responded optimally to the

Table 6.2. Percentages of Posttraumatic Stress Reactions during Early Acute Phase after an Industrial Disaster

	Group A (high stress) $n = 66$	Group B (medium stress) $n = 59$	Group C (low stress) $n = 121$
Anxiety	82	71	19
Sleep disturbances	83	76	36
Traumatic nightmares	61	41	14
Startle response	86	80	34
Fear of destroyed areas	79	69	19
Irritability	24	2	4
Social withdrawal	38	9	2

Table 6.3. Prognosis and Course of Posttraumatic Stress Disorders in Subjects of Industrial Disaster

PTSD	1 week	7 months	2 years[a]	3 years[a]	4 years[b]
			Group A (%)		
Severe	29	11	9	8	
Marked	8	20	9	5	
Moderate	6	6	9	9	
Total	43	37	27	22	19
			Group B (%)		
Severe	7	2	2	2	
Marked	7	10	2	0	
Moderate	9	5	9	2	
Total	23	17	13	4	2
			Group C (%)		
Severe	3	0			
Marked	3	1			
Moderate	4	3			
Total	10	4			3

[a]Minimum numbers based on examination of risk group only.
[b]Numbers based on questionnaire study.

disaster and one half of this unprepared group reacted inadequately. More important to our discussion is the fact that there was a negative association between adequacy of disaster behavior and the likelihood of PTSD. Those who behaved well during the emergency were less likely to suffer posttraumatic shock and PTSD. This is an interesting finding, since it implies that we can reduce the frequency of PTSD by adequate training or stress-inoculation techniques.

It is worth mentioning that during the follow-up period, there was hardly any other psychiatric morbidity except what could be associated with the disaster. The only exceptions were a case of cerebral tumor and one of manic-depressive psychosis. This suggests that the PTSD has a tendency toward recovery and will usually not be replaced by other pathological reactions.

We have not observed any cases of long latency, which might be construed to the effect that acute frightening stress experiences of brief duration give immediate reactions, in contrast to the long-lasting stress experiences where delayed reactions had been observed.

Risk-Proneness to PTSD: Situations, Persons, and Reactions

Based on our observations, it has been possible to identify risk cases as far as the development of PTSD is concerned by defining:

1. High-risk *situations*, the presence of particularly severe trauma dimensions
2. High-risk *persons*, the presence of high-risk factors (vulnerability) in exposed persons
3. High-risk *reactions*, the presence of early response variables that predict later illness

This categorization has been the foundation of primary and secondary prevention in our intervention work. The number of disaster-affected persons may be large, whereas the interventive resources may be limited, as is the time available to prevent psychiatric cases from developing.

Disaster in the North Sea

Another industrial disaster, the capsizing of an oil-drilling rig in the North Sea, happened on March 27, 1980. Of the 212 on board, 123 (58%) were killed. The study of the survivors confirmed the findings referred to above on PTSD and are described in detail by Holen (1990). However, for our present discussion, we only wish to mention that practically all the survivors had an acute form of the PTSD syndrome, 40% developed psychiatric problems, and only one tenth had delayed onset.

In addition to the survivors, the rescuers were investigated after 9 months (Ersland, Weisæth, & Sund, 1989). Their symptoms were similar to those of the survivors, though somewhat milder and less frequent, suggesting a disaster-related etiology. The percentage of rescuers suffering from posttraumatic stress lies at a level between the above-mentioned Groups B and C (i.e., about 25%). One third of the rescuers had experienced serious life danger, 50% had had close relationships to those who were killed, and many saw them die. Seventy-five percent had to make difficult decisions about priorities during the rescue of victims. The main stressor was the fact that they were "helpless helpers." Between 47% and 65% of the rescuers experienced some kind of stress reactions during the rescue activities and in a little less than 20% this factor reduced the functional capacity of the rescuers.

As in the study of the disaster behavior of the survivors of the industrial disaster described first, these problems were mainly seen in rescuers with little disaster education and training.

Terror against a Civilian Ship's Crew in Libya

During the summer of 1984, 14 seamen, the entire crew of a Norwegian ship, were seized upon arrival in Libya. They were kept under arrest for 67 days and subjected to *psychological* and *physical torture* because they were suspected of being enemies of the Libyan state. Within the first few days of imprisonment, one seaman had been murdered, another had been abducted and was believed to be dead, and a third had been severely physically maltreated (Weisæth, 1989). The immediate reactions to the extreme stress were fear, depression, and rage. Not a single seaman capitulated during the torture.

Shortly after their release, all the seamen underwent thorough medical examinations. Six of them suffered from clear-cut posttraumatic stress disorder and one seaman developed the disorder 2 months later. In spite of comprehensive treatment, the same 7 sailors, or 54% of the crew, still suffered from PTSD 6 months after their release. Three and a half years later, 5 of the 6 seamen, and 1 previously unaffected, were still suffering from serious posttraumatic stress symptoms.

Compared with the industrial disaster that was described, the torture experience seems to have produced a greater number of severe health failures. Both groups consisted of healthy and well-functioning, fully employed individuals before the exposure, and both were offered comprehensive preventive and therapeutic programs immediately afterward. The difference in resulting psychopathology must be ascribed to differences in the intensity, duration, and kind of traumatic exposure.

Although the industrial explosion was unprecedented and unexpected, and caused typical stunned shock reactions, the event was easy to comprehend since it was well within the borders of the victims' conceptual frame of reference. On the other hand, the regular merchant sailors, who were suddenly treated as dangerous enemy agents, naturally found their imprisonment and torture completely meaningless and difficult to comprehend.

Neither the disaster training as seamen nor the immediate therapeutic intervention was sufficient to overcome the impact of the severe and incomprehensible traumatization. Although the figures are small, they demonstrate very clearly that the intensity of the stress exposure is closely related to the manifestation of PTSD; two were exposed to extreme stress and both had PTSD. Seven were exposed to severe stress, four of them had PTSD, and three none. Four had moderate stress, one had PTSD, the other three none (see Table 6.4).

Compared to the traumatic reactions in the survivors of the technological industrial disaster, two striking differences appeared in the contents of the clinical symptoms of the posttorture PTSD victims. First, it was always one or more actors who made up the threatening element in the recurring experiences of the threat. This seemed to reflect the constant threat of death created by the captors and interrogators, in contrast to the material/technological dangers that dominated the PTSD symptoms after the industrial disaster. Second, the aggression in the seamen was a direct reaction to the violence they had suffered. In the technological disaster, on the other hand, angry feelings only developed after some time and then as a neurasthenic irritability secondary to long-standing anxiety and long-lasting sleep deprivation. This difference in development and content of aggression symptoms may be a distinguishing clinical feature between man-made and accidental causation of PTSD.

Table 6.4. Distribution of Posttraumatic Stress Disorder at 6-Month Follow-Up

Intensity of stress exposure	Seamen (N)	PTSD
Extreme	2	2
Severe	7	4
Moderate	4	1
Total ($p = 0.22$)	13	7

The meaninglessness is enhanced by a lack of a cause, contrary to what soldiers experience during wartime. The same lack of motivation can be found in victims of terror and must be considered as one of the causes of the so-called Stockholm Syndrome. It seems that individuals exposed to human violence develop paranoid ideations and fear of human beings which are more disturbing than fear located to a limited disaster area or phobic situation.

Rape

In Norway, the findings on rape problems were very strongly supported in the research of S. Dahl, while she was affiliated with our institute. She found the same posttraumatic stress symptoms in the large majority of rape victims, along with psychophysiological symptoms that were of somewhat different character. These symptoms reflected disgust against the rape and the rapist as well as against the somatic part of the traumatization. Rape victims suffered much more from feelings of shame and depression (see Chapter 44, in this volume, for a discussion). Very often these feelings seemed to be induced (subconsciously) by prevalent social attitudes expressed through educational forms, history, and, mainly, by sensation-hungry mass media, toward the hero, the conqueror, the strong man—the victimizer, the torturer, and the rapist—on the one hand, and the weak, the conquered, the victim—the raped—on the other. The general attitude is to admire the strong and despise the weak. Thus, victims felt "duty bound" by the general attitude of society to feel shame at being a victim; this sense of obligation produced guilt feelings about having been debased, tortured, or raped, yet having survived the ordeal. If a victim had not survived, the sympathy of the press and society would have been overwhelming. Survivors, however, demonstrate that the strong, admired hero has done something wrong, something unacceptable; this outcome provokes feelings of unease and confusion in the public. It is this discrepant public opinion which projects and forces on the victims the feelings of shame and guilt which have become an accepted symptom of PTSD (Dahl, 1989).

We have found a hierarchy of feelings of shame—and guilt—among PTSD patients. Victims of bank robberies who are not actively involved in handing over the stolen money would become angry with the robbers and thus conform to the views of our society. They are perhaps a little ashamed in addition to their anger, but they would not have guilt feelings. Victims of natural disasters may not have guilt feelings either, but victims of man-made disasters, of torture, and especially of rape feel both debased and shameful.

Military and War-Related Disasters

The following two groups of traumatization which are connected with military service/actions are currently being studied longitudinally at our institute. The final results, however, are not available at the time of writing and this presentation must therefore be considered a preliminary one (Herlofsen, 1989).

A platoon of 46 men was hit by an avalanche about midday on March 5, 1988. Thirty-one men sent directly into the valley were struck by the avalanche and were completely or partly buried. Sixteen soldiers died, while 15 survived, some of whom had various degrees of physical injuries. None of these injuries were serious, but three soldiers were kept in the hospital for 2 weeks.

The other 15 men in the platoon were ordered to stay outside the valley, and so were not involved in the disaster, or in the rescue operation. They were thus "natural experimental control subjects." Unexpectedly, several of the posttraumatic stress symptoms were more marked in this latter group than among the involved survivors. The most probable explanation is that the enforced passivity provided no possibility for abreacting the stress experience. Another possible explanation is uncertainty and fantasies about the dimensions of the disaster.

The same observation was made in the study previously mentioned, namely, the merchant marine gas and oil tankers that sailed in the Persian Gulf during the Iran/Iraq war in the 1980s (Weisæth & Lie, 1990). The sailors had no chance of fighting back or escaping and were forced into passivity while repressing any aggression. However, those who were actively engaged in fire extinguishing had obviously less posttraumatic stress symptoms. Similar results have been found in the UN peace-keeping forces in Lebanon (Weisæth & Sund, 1982).

The other most intriguing finding in the avalanche-exposed group was a complete absence of PTSD. The reason might be that they all had been exposed to immediate emotional first aid and crisis intervention and were taking part in a comprehensive psychiatric prevention program. Also, the bereaved families, the comrades of the deceased, and the rescuers were studied and treated intensively and simultaneously in the prevention program.

Malt (1991) has carried out several longitudinal studies on various kinds of accidental physical injuries (traffic accidents and the like). The main findings were rather frequent psychiatric complications, whereas PTSD was infrequent. His explanation is that these traumata are of very short duration, not completely unexpected, and most lack the terror of impending death. However, some serious injuries, such as extensive burns, will usually prompt psychological reactions, not only because of their social implications but mainly because of the horrifying experience of being on fire (Malt, 1988; Malt, Blikra, & Høivik, 1989; Malt, Myhre, Blikra, & Høivik, 1987).

Looking back at the result of the studies as far as the therapeutic consequences to the victims are concerned, concentration camp survivors and war sailors could receive only financial and social help. Thus, the symptoms became chronic and were practically inaccessible to other therapeutic intervention (Malt, 1980).

The industrial disaster led to a systematic intervention for the individual survivors, and the outcome of the PTSD symptoms was positively influenced by this intervention. This finding is based on clinical experiences even if we, for obvious ethical reasons, do not have control groups.

Conclusion

Based on our experiences, a comprehensive intervention program has gradually evolved that provides (1) group debriefing; (2) anticipatory guidance concerning posttraumatic stress symptoms; and (3) information about what the victims themselves can do, what others can do, and when to seek guidance and help from specialists. Such intervention increases a sense of control, reduces uncertainty and helplessness, and contributes to making the victim master of his or her fate. Most often, the psychiatrist works through cooperation with others, mainly professionals who are outside the medical field and primary health care services. This comprehensive intervention program has been practiced and has proven its importance and effectiveness in both the above-mentioned avalanche disaster and in a long series of minor catastrophic events that occurred in Norway and that did not result in any serious posttraumatic stress complications.

References

American Psychiatric Association. (1987). *Diagnostic and statistical manual of mental disorders* (3rd ed., rev.). Washington, DC: Author.

Askevold, F. (1976/1977). The war sailor syndrome. *Psychotherapy and Psychosomatics, 77*(27), 133–138.

Dahl, S. (1989). Acute response to rape—A PTSD variant. *Acta Psychiatrica Scandinavica, 80*(Suppl. 355), 56–62.

Eitinger, L. (1958). *Psykiatriske undersøkelser blant flyktninger i Norge* [Psychiatric investigations of refugees in Norway]. Oslo: Universitetsforlaget.

Eitinger, L. (1960). The symptomatology of mental disease among refugees in Norway. *Journal of Mental Science, 106,* 947–966.

Eitinger, L., & Grünfeld, B. (1966). Psychoses among refugees in Norway. *Acta Psychiatrica Scandinavica, 42,* 315–326.

Eitinger, L., & Strøm, A. (1973). Mortality and morbidity after excessive stress. Oslo: University Press.

Eitinger, L., & Strøm, A. (1981). New investigations on the mortality and morbidity of Norwegian ex-concentration camp prisoners. *Israel Journal of Psychiatry and Related Sciences, 18,* 173–195.

Ersland, S., Weisæth, L., & Sund, A. (1989). The stress upon rescuers involved in an oil rig disaster. *Acta Psychiatrica Scandinavica, 80*(Suppl. 355), 38–49.

Fischer-Homberger, E. (1975). *Die traumatische Neurose: Vom somatischen zum sozialen Leiden* [Traumatic neurosis: From somatic to social suffering]. Bern, Switzerland: H. Huber.

Herlofsen, P. (1992). Individual and group reactions to an avalanche trauma. In Ursano, R. J., McCaugley, B., & Fullerton, C. S. (Eds.), *The Structure of human chaos: Individual and community responses to trauma and disaster.* New York: Cambridge University Press.

Holen, A. (1990). *A long-term outcome study of survivors from a disaster.* Oslo: University of Oslo.

Leopold, R. L., & Dillon, H. (1963). Psycho-anatomy of a disaster: A long-term study of post-traumatic neuroses in survivors of a marine explosion. *American Journal of Psychiatry, 119,* 913–921.

Malt, U. F. (1980). Long-term psychosocial follow-up studies of burn injuries: A review. *Journal of Burns, 6,* 190–197.

Malt, U. F. (1988). The long-term consequences of accidental injury. *British Journal of Psychiatry*, 810–818.

Malt, U. F. (1991). Psychiatric aspects of accidents and traumatic injuries. In Seva, A. (Ed.), *The European handbook of psychiatry and mental health* (pp. 1349–1361). Barcelona: Editorial Anthropos.

Malt, U. F., Blikra, G., & Høivik, B. (1989). The 3-year biopsychosocial outcome of 551 hospitalized accidentally injured adults. *Acta Psychiatrica Scandinavica*, *80*(Suppl. 355), 84–93.

Malt, U. F., Myhre, T., Blikra, G., & Høivik, B. (1987). Psychopathology and accidental injury. *Acta Psychiatrica Scandinavica*, *76*, 261–271.

Raphael, B. (1986). *When disaster strikes*. New York: Basic Books.

Stierlin, E. (1909). Über psycho-neuropathische Folgezustände bei den Überlebenden der Katastrophe von Courrieres am 10. März 1906. Unpublished doctoral dissertation. Zürich, Switzerland.

Strøm. A. (Ed.) (1968). *Norwegian concentration camp survivors.* Oslo: University Press.

Trimble, M. R. (1981). *Post-traumatic neurosis.* Chichester: Wiley.

Weisæth, L. (1984). *Stress reactions to an industrial disaster: An investigation of disaster behaviour and acute post-traumatic stress reactions, and a prospective, controlled, clinical and interventive study of subacute and long-term post-traumatic stress reactions.* Unpublished doctoral thesis, University of Oslo, Oslo, Norway.

Weisæth, L. (1985). Post-traumatic stress disorder after an industrial disaster. In Pichot, P. *et al.* (Eds.), *Psychiatry—The state of the art* (pp. 299–307). New York: Plenum Press.

Weisæth, L. (1989). The stressors and the post-traumatic stress syndrome after an industrial disaster. *Acta Psychiatrica Scandinavica*, *80* (Supp. 355), 25–37.

Weisæth, L. (1989). Torture of a Norwegian ship's crew. *Acta Psychiatrica Scandinavica*, *80*(Suppl. 355), 63–72.

Weisæth, L., & Eitinger, L. (1991). Research on PTSD and other post-traumatic reactions: European literature. *PTSD Research Quarterly*, *2*(2), 1–2.

Weisæth, L., & Sund, A. (1982). Psychiatric problems in UNIFIL and the UN-soldiers' stress syndrome. *Review of International Service Santé*, *44*, 109–116.

Wilson, J. P., Harel, Z., & Kahana, B. (Eds.). (1988). *Human adaptation to extreme stress: From the Holocaust to Vietnam.* New York: Plenum Press.

CHAPTER 7

Technological Hazards

Social Responses as Traumatic Stressors

J. Stephen Kroll-Smith and Stephen R. Couch

Introduction

Natural disasters in industrially developed countries are frequently experienced as emotional shocks but only rarely do they result in long-term psychosocial impairment (Mileti, Drabek, & Haas, 1975, p. 103; Schorr, Goldsteen, & Cortes, 1982; Smith, North, & Price, 1986, p. 60). The trauma of technological hazards that disrupt the relationship between people and the biosphere, however, frequently last for years, impeding the psychosocial development of victims (Baum, 1987; Erikson, 1976; Gleser, Green, & Winget, 1981). Chronic psychosocial impairment does not fit the common core of expected posthazard responses and must give us pause to consider the unique problems posed by willful or negligent contamination of the environment. Kasperson and Pijawka observed that the "major burden of hazard management in developed societies has shifted from risks associated with natural processes to those arising from technological development and application" (1985, p. 17).

Rates of natural disaster occurrence have varied little through the years. There are roughly as many hurricanes and tornadoes now as there were one hundred years ago. What has changed is our ability to adapt to these natural phenomena. Early warning detection devices and pre- and postdisaster emergency response policies have greatly reduced the number of fatalities and the amount of property damage while increasing the chances that survivors will successfully recover and re-

vitalize their communities (Wijkman & Timberlake, 1984, pp. 11–17; Kroll-Smith, Couch, & Levine, in press). These pre- and postimpact response capacities prompted one expert to write that only rarely do natural disasters "result in significant long-term economic, social and political change" (Kreps, 1980, p. 38; Fritz, 1961). It is reasonable to assume that the comparatively low rate of long-term psychosocial sequelae following a natural disaster is related to advanced warning technology and the prompt and effective recovery and rehabilitation efforts that follow impact.

Biospheric Contamination: Emerging Crisis Worldwide

Human contamination of the biosphere, however, is a comparatively new crisis. It is not a natural act, or an act of God. Because corporate actions, government initiatives, and political alignments result in pollution, contaminating the environment is more than an ecological emergency, it is also a social and political crisis (Shrivastava, 1987). Complicating the picture is the bewildering uncertainty of environmental contamination itself. Vyner (1988) argued that it is both phenomenologically and medically invisible. Dioxin and ionizing radiation, for example, are not present in forms that allow people to see, hear, smell, taste, or touch them. "It is quite impossible," he observed, "for humans to determine if and when they are being exposed" (p. 13). It is also true that most contaminants are "invisible to physicians evaluating and treating" exposed patients (p. 13). Finally, because the United States National Disaster Relief Act (1974) does not cover biospheric contamination, whatever official authority exists to respond to it is diffuse and often lodged within a variety of agencies operating at different levels of government (LaPlante & Kroll-Smith, 1989; Zimmerman, 1985).

J. Stephen Kroll-Smith • Department of Sociology, University of New Orleans, New Orleans, Louisiana 70148. **Stephen R. Couch** • Department of Sociology, Pennsylvania State University, Schuylkill Haven, Pennsylvania 17972–2208.

International Handbook of Traumatic Stress Syndromes, edited by John P. Wilson and Beverley Raphael. Plenum Press, New York, 1993.

Contrary to the role of natural disaster response strategies in mitigating the potential psychosocial harm caused by the aversive agent, it is our opinion that socially contested responses to the threat of biospheric contamination are likely to become *stressors* in their own right, producing psychosocial sequelae in conjunction with the physical impact of the aversive agent.

This chapter develops a conceptual basis for interpreting the social stressors that accompany toxic hazards. It is a search for the social sources of psychopathology in chemical contamination crises.

Our primary assumption is that natural disasters have much more direct and nonsymbolic effects on human lives and social processes than technological disasters whose invisibility and uncertainty create a comparatively larger arena for the interplay of symbol, social structure, and event. The basic "facts" of contamination, for example, are not known by the interested parties. Characterizing these crises is a pervasive uncertainty regarding such issues as the scope and the severity of the contamination, exposure, liability, and responsibility for clean-up and community rehabilitation. If tangible objective signs are not available to reduce the stress of uncertain threat, then we are apt to seek something representational or symbolic to reduce it.[1]

From a symbolic perspective, the terms *hazard* and *disaster* are not objective conditions characterized by concrete markers; rather, they are linguistic devices employed by individuals and groups to assert grievances and claims with respect to some alleged changes in their environment. To assert the existence of a hazard or a disaster is to make a moral claim on society to mobilize whatever resources are necessary to relieve the affected parties of the danger and to compensate them for their losses. Claim-makers do not simply say, "Hey, look, our backyards are oozing black oily slime that ignites when we throw a match on it!" They say, "It's not right that this should be happening! This is wrong and unjust! It's dangerous and threatens my family! It violates our basic constitutional rights!"

The extreme uncertainty of biospheric contamination, however, insures that counterclaims are likely to emerge. One source of these claims—potentially liable corporations or responsible government agencies—frequently responds by cautioning against a worst-case interpretation until the knowable laws of physical nature are applied to the threat and measurable aspects of its presence are calculated. "Perhaps the slime is dangerous, perhaps it's not. Let's not panic until we know what the 'facts' are." An institutional counterresponse issued from potentially responsible parties should not surprise us. Counterclaims, however, are also likely to issue from neighbors who do not live near the alleged contamination or do not "see" the environmental changes that others claim exist.

Biospheric contamination sets in motion a pattern of claims and counterclaims as groups and organizations assert, sponsor, and attempt to impose on others their definition of the scope and severity of the problem, while challenging, rejecting, and subverting the definitions of others. Somewhat ironically, it is the trauma that ensues from the claims and counterclaims that a hazard or disaster exists that permits us to label toxic exposure a disaster using Barton's definition of the term as a collective stress experience in which "many members of a social system fail to receive expected conditions of life from the system" (1969, p. 38). "Adapting to an invisible exposure," Vyner suggested, "is a toxic process" (1988, p. 195).

The following two sections create a conceptual framework for interpreting human responses to environmental contamination as the activities of groups and organizations making assertions and counterassertions regarding alleged changes in the biosphere. We begin by developing a particular perspective on an individual's subjective apprehension of such risks and conclude with a revision of the traditional disaster stage model as a moral vocabulary that is employed by various groups to stake claims regarding the "real" degree of danger.

A Question of Perception: Biosphere Contamination as Threat

Why do technological disasters diminish the long-term psychosocial health of victims to a greater extent than natural disasters? Perhaps it is because toxic spills, asbestos decay, or core meltdowns "contaminate rather than merely damage . . . they pollute, befoul, taint, rather than just create wreckage and they scare human beings in new and special ways" (Erikson, 1991, p. 15). The primordial antipathy to the thought of being poisoned requires little commentary. Surely here is the essential reason for the prolonged impact of environmental contamination. Indeed, if more complex forms of human development are contingent on gratification of the need for physical safety (see Maslow, 1970), the perception of one's house, backyard, or neighborhood park as poisoned would interfere with such growth. But we will complicate the picture considerably if we ask an additional question: Where does the *perception* of contamination come from?

There are two quite different answers to this question. If people behave as engineers, as some have argued (see Starr, 1969), then they will seek all the facts and deduce from them the degree of threat posed by the contaminant. The image is of an objective world to be known and a rational knower sorting and assessing the facts. Assumed here, however, is that all the facts are known and are communicated in a manner that makes them knowable to the nonscientist; also assumed is that people act as isolated individuals and that behavior naturally follows the rational accumulation of facts. A major criticism of the rational actor answer, however, is that the scientific formulation of reality does not exhaust the possible range of human actions, most of which are based on nontheoretical or commonsense assumptions about the world (see Berger & Luckmann, 1966, p. 15). Indeed, the postmodern view of science itself now as-

---

[1]Such a search necessitates the addition of a new approach to the field of disaster-impact studies. We are accustomed to examining disaster effects through clinical-descriptive, epidemiological, or quasi-experimental designs (see Baum, 1987). Although all of these approaches are useful, they are not designed to identify the *sociocultural* sources of stress.

sumes the subjective biases of scientists as critical in understanding how "rational" inquiry is accomplished (see Kuhn, 1962).

If ordinary people do not engage solely in logico-deductive reasoning to make sense out of their world, what else do they do? Another answer suggests that they construct reality in concert with others. "Humans experience their environment," Douglas wrote, "mediated by conceptual categories fabricated in social interaction" (1985, p. 34). Assumed here is that "safe" and "hazardous" are socially constructed categories of meaning. The sense people make out of their world, in other words, is shaped more by the activities of others than by "objective facts."

Between events and behavior formed in response to those events, there is a social process of definition (see Blumer, 1969, p. 687). Persons experiencing a flood or hurricane are not just responding to the physical events themselves, but to what those events mean and represent to them as socially constructed crises. Between the physical environment and the human response is a social process that constructs the meaning of a situation or event as dangerous, hazardous, challenging, or benign. A social constructionist view of the perception of risks and threats suggests that although psychosocial distress is experienced by concrete individuals, it arises from and is resolved or intensified in a social context. A comprehensive interpretation of disaster trauma, in other words, will include an account of the sociocultural processes that shape the experience of distress. We "are disturbed," wrote Epictetus, "not by things, but by the views which [we] take of things" (Lazarus & Folkman, 1984, p. 19).[2]

To this view of the person as appraising and fashioning a world in concert with others we modify the traditional disaster stage model to fit the case of biospheric contamination and add the complementary notion that it is more than an objective sequence of event-bounded steps; it is also a moral vocabulary encouraging, discouraging, and justifying responses to the event.

A New Look at an Old Model: The Disaster Stage Paradigm

We can advance our understanding of the social bases of psychosocial trauma in toxic exposure situations by recasting the traditional academic view of the disaster stage model. The stage model was originally developed to identify the sequence of social and cultural responses to natural disasters that take place before, during, and after impact (for extended discussions of the model, see Wallace, 1956, pp. 1–19; and Baker & Chapman, 1962).

[2]Perhaps a caveat is in order here. It is not our intention to deny the importance of physical or nonsocial factors in understanding human response to natural and technological crises. We agree with Dunlap and Catton who claimed that "sometimes the physical environment has direct, unmediated impacts upon humans" (1983, p. 126). People may actually be contaminated by PCBs; or their houses may be destroyed by hurricanes. Our contention, however, is that people do not experience these traumas in isolation from society.

This linear model presupposes a period of stasis interrupted by *warnings* or apprehension that a calamity may occur and moves through the *threat* and *impact* stages, to the *inventory, rescue,* and *remedy* stages, and finally, to the *recovery* and *rehabilitation* stages.

The purpose of this stage model is to assist disaster planners and emergency response personnel in anticipating the typical sequence of events that move a community from order, to chaos, to the reconstitution of order. From structure to the terror, ambiguity, and confusion of impact, to the remaking of structure, settlements move through a cycle to bring closure to a catastrophic moment. With the reconstitution of order, the disaster enters the collective memory, recalled on those occasions deemed appropriate to remember a shared experience of horror. The stages were originally conceived as objective markers of the original flow of events in natural disasters. Assumed is the existence of an objective division of activities and events carrying victims, emergency response teams, social service agencies, and others from one temporal period to another.

There are some obvious problems with the model if we attempt to use it wholesale in making sense out of human responses to environmental contamination. First, the presence or perceived presence of environmental toxins tends to trap portions of a population in the warning, threat, or impact stages, freezing them in extended moments of apprehension, dread, or horror of contamination. Radiation spreading silently through the food chain or the foundations of houses, polychlorinated biphenyls (PCB) carried unseen throughout the workplace, toxic chemicals leaching quietly throughout underground swales, these do not strike swiftly, leave visible devastation, and disappear. They do, at times, present various signals that danger is near, but the signals are frequently vague and open to dispute. Technological hazards that disrupt the relationships between communities and their biophysical environments, in other words, do not create a moment betwixt and between points of stability. Rather, they create fixed, seemingly permanent periods of unstructure—times within which conventional patterns of meanings, organization, and behavior no longer seem to work. This coincidence of a depreciating fund of practical knowledge and an amplified awareness of the need to respond means that people are experiencing the contamination of water, soil, and air in a highly charged context of uncertainty. Essential questions remain unanswered: "Are we in an environment in which invisible contamination is present? Is this contaminant actually being absorbed by body tissue? Is the absorbed dose dangerous?" (Vyner, 1988, p. 14).

Moreover, exposure is rarely uniform. Some neighborhoods or workplaces are more at risk than others. Variations in the perceived threat of exposure are likely to lead to varying or conflicting accounts of the danger. Long-term exposure to warning and threat, particularly when it is unevenly distributed throughout the population, places severe demands on the coping resources of a person or group.

The extreme uncertainty characterizing this type of crisis suggests the utility of rethinking the traditional approach to the disaster stage model. First, sufficient evidence to reach consensus on the question of what stage a community or neighborhood is experiencing is not available. Thus, government officials, corporations, the media, citizen's groups, and individuals more often than not move through the disaster cycle at different rates. Assume, for example, that as a government agency assesses the evidence of contamination and concludes that there is sufficient cause to declare a public warning, a citizen's group is already convinced that they are being poisoned. From their perspective a simple warning is hardly adequate. Each side will develop its claim roughly within the boundaries of either the warning, the threat or the impact stage, with one party trying to convince the other that there is no reason to panic or that there is every reason to take immediate corrective action. The issue here is that both parties want something from the other and perceive the other as able but unwilling to comply.

Second, when the question of what stage a community is experiencing is a contested issue, organizations and groups are likely to transform the stages into a moral vocabulary used to justify a line of conduct. Morals or "values are invoked to justify claims or demands, to express dissatisfaction, indignation, or outrage" with someone who is viewed as able but unwilling to act on our behalf (Spector & Kitsuse, 1977, pp. 93, 95). "The language of morality," Gouldner writes, "arises in the social world in situations where what men want, the gratifications they seek, are precarious and uncertain" (1970, p. 266). It is not that the words *warning* or *impact* are necessarily themselves invoked by a group or organization; rather, if members of a citizen's group, for example, perceive themselves to be absorbing dangerous doses of radiation, they are likely to construct their interpretation of the situation as one of impact and identify others who *should* be as frightened as they are and others who *ought* to assume responsibility for the contamination and relocate and recompense them.

In other words, perceived threats or impacts are transformed into moral claims pressed against parties who are identified as being obligated to respond. In a complementary fashion, however, government engineers, geologists, or corporate public relations experts who perceive the situation as less critical, perhaps at the warning stage, admonish "hyperactive" citizens and a "sensationalist" press to act in a more "responsible" and "rational" manner toward what might very well prove to be no threat at all. In these examples, the affected parties treat one another as able but unwilling to respond to their claims for action based on what they "know" to be the "correct" interpretation of the problem.

Appraisal Process in Technological Disasters

Thus far, we have developed a perspective on the person as a symbol user, appraising, defining, and constructing a world in collusion with others. The natural disaster stage model was reworked to account for the quite different way in which a community moves through a human-induced environmental crisis. A case was made that the stages themselves are experienced as moral imperatives by groups and organizations who

launch claims and counterclaims on the ethical obligations of others who are seen as able but unwilling to respond appropriately to their demands. The collective stress generated in this contested milieu of uncertainty creates doubt and despair as families and friendship networks, communities, and institutions are reappraised as no longer able to provide the conditions of life that are expected from these important human resources. Technological hazards that disrupt the relationship between communities and the biosphere are preeminently social disasters that tear at the roots of civil order.

Attempted here is a sociocultural formulation of a clinical problem. "Although physical and psychological distress is experienced individually," Boehnlein noted, "it often arises from, and is resolved [or intensified] in, a social context" (1987, p. 520). Between the individual and the hazard, in other words, is a social process set in motion by the particular attributes of the aversive agent itself and the symbolic capacities of human agents. In the second half of this chapter, we pull together a wealth of primary and secondary data to document the deleterious consequences of claims and counterclaims on the victims of toxic poisoning.

Toxic Exposure and the Reappraisal of Self

The idea of the self is derived from our imagined appearance to other people, our imagined judgment of that appearance, and a subsequent self-appraisal that we are worthy or unworthy, deserving of respect or disreputable, and so on (Cooley, 1922, p. 183). The social basis of self-esteem and self-worth signal the importance each of us has for one another in creating and maintaining a healthy self-image. We look to one another to confirm our value and social worth. If social support systems are critical for positive evaluations of self and emotional health, then any interference with these systems is likely to prove detrimental to affected individuals. At the moment, there are little more than impressionistic data on the relationship of toxic exposure to the self. What we do have, however, suggests that it is the first casualty of chemical contamination.

With few exceptions, the warning signs of most natural disasters are officially communicated to potentially affected populations through radio, television, and local authorities. The flow of warning notices is usually from the top down. On the other hand, the signs of toxic poisoning, are usually first noticed and brought to the attention of the community by the potential victims themselves.[3]

Someone notices that the water has a foul smell. While tending his garden, a man sees oil-stained soil at the south end of the plot. A mother witnesses changes in the health of her children. A former resident of a highly contaminated neighborhood, the Love Canal, recalls:

> My son had to come home for lunch, and I had to go pick him up and take him back because by the time he'd get to

[3]The fact that affected residents are the first to claim a danger exists should not be confused with the fact that in some cases authorities may already know of the hazardous conditions but do not make this knowledge public (see Finsterbusch, 1987).

school he'd have an asthma attack. And I used to think it was pollen. (Edelstein, 1988, p. 51)

For some residents, the warning signs point to the real possibility that their bodies are ingesting poison. Purity of the body and the freedom to exercise control over it are values with deep roots in Western secular humanism (Erikson, 1991; Vidich, 1980). With the exception of intentional ingestion, the cultural meaning of the word *poison* violates both of these values. To "be poisoned," that is, not to poison one's self, expresses the loss of hegemonic control over one's body. An agency outside the person willfully or negligently exposed his or her body to a foreign, impure substance. It is reasonable to assume that people who begin to perceive themselves and their families as poisoned are experiencing a profound life change event. Janoff-Bulman and Frieze (1983) argued that exposure to toxins is likely to result in changing several of the basic assumptions the individual has about the world, including a positive belief in the self (see also Gibbs, 1986).

A negative reappraisal of the self, however, is related to more than the experience of exposure. It is also related to the response that others make to victims' claims that the environment is now a hazard and that they are being poisoned. Situated between the experience of contamination and self-reappraisal, in other words, is a social process. The role of informal support networks, friends, relatives, work associates, in dampening or ameliorating the stress of crises events is well documented (Dohrenwend, 1978; Kaplan, Cassel, & Gore, 1977; Litwak & Messeri, 1989). In periods of personal turmoil, these groups are critical in offering assistance, assurances, and affirmation that, in spite of the difficulty, the person is still worthy of respect and part of a wider, caring community. People who define themselves as victims of invisible contamination are likely to believe that their supportive others are able and willing to respond empathetically to this particular trauma, as they have responded to other traumas in the past.

How do these informal support systems respond to the claims made by fellow members that their houses and bodies are contaminated? "Outside the immediate family," Edelstein observed, "toxic victims frequently find that exposure changes their relationships with friends, relatives, co-workers, and others" (1988, p. 110). It would appear that the more the claims are believed by members of the support network, the more likely those members are to modify their behavior toward the claimmakers. Victims of asbestos contamination in a mobile-home park report that friends

act as if we're going to spread some disease or something. I was at a Christmas party where the couple got themselves a new sofa, and you know, the woman asked me—just me—if I'd mind sitting on a newspaper while I was there, as if I was carrying in something dirty on my clothes. (Cuthbertson, 1987, p. 68)

A former resident of a town ravaged by an underground mine fire remembers listening to the parents of her child's best friend explain that with the threat of gases it would be impossible for the children to play together until the doctor says it is safe. "It made me feel horrible, like I was the mother of dirty children," she

recalled (Kroll-Smith, 1983). A man whose well water is contaminated reports:

Only my mother will come here. It's like we have the plague the way they avoid Legler. They feel that they don't want to expose themselves to our house. My wife's parents don't even want to know about it. (Edelstein, 1988, p. 111)

An asbestos victim recalls:

We soon found that we victims were being persecuted, harassed, ridiculed, and threatened by strangers, friends, and family. (Cuthbertson, 1987, p. 67)

When friends and family begin to act like uncaring and hostile strangers, the traditional support network is no longer available as a source of self-worth and self-esteem. People who claim to be contaminated are likely to be treated as contagious and routinely placed outside the boundaries of their emotional community. A Love Canal resident describes going to a local bar for her "usual 'pick me up,' no matter what end of the bar I stand at," she muses, "the rest of the people stand bunched at the other end" (Kroll-Smith, Couch, & Levine, in press).

It is reasonable to assume that the negative self-appraisal resulting from the dreadful apprehension that one's body is being poisoned could be muted and softened by a therapeutic response on the part of a support network. The emergence of "altruistic communities" following a natural disaster is now a commonplace observation and their role in mitigating the immediate after-effects of impact is well understood (Drabek & Key, 1984; Moore, 1958). Intensifying the shock of exposure, however, is a quite different process: It is the realization that victims are no longer members of a traditional community of people who depend on one another for sympathy and support. The rituals of avoidance and shame enacted by neighbors, friends, and relatives serve notice on the exposed that they are outside the boundaries of "pure" or "safe" society. To be associated with them is to risk impurity or danger. "Our lives mean nothing to our neighbors," concluded a victim of the Centralia mine fire (Kroll-Smith, 1983, unpublished manuscript).

Not only is the support of friends and neighbors lacking in technological hazard situations, but so is effective help from large-scale institutions. An industrial corporation is often seen as the culprit responsible for the contamination in the first place, and local, state, and federal governmental agencies are blamed for a lack of regulatory effectiveness prior to the contamination and for inadequate response measures once the problem occurred. Victims experience a loss of trust in the ability of our economic and social institutions to help them in time of need.

Psychological Alienation and Distress

This breakdown of a person's social support system at all levels can result in what has been termed *alienation*. This concept has been given a number of different meanings over the years, but most mean by it a sense of disaffection from the social world or various parts of it (e.g., from one's job, or one's family, or one's community). By and large, scholars believe that alienation is composed of a number of related parts, including social isolation (i.e., lack of meaningful contact with others), powerlessness (lack of ability to control life's events), and normlessness (a belief that socially approved behaviors are not adequate to achieve one's ends).

In general, the link between high levels of alienation and psychological distress is well established (Mirowsky & Ross, 1986). For example, powerlessness (or very similiar concepts) has been linked to demoralization (Wheaton, 1980), lack of coping ability (Wheaton, 1983), stress (Pearlin, Lieberman, Menaghan, & Mullan, 1981), depression (Garber, Miller, & Seaman, 1979), problem drinking (M. Seeman, A. Z. Seeman, & Budros, 1988), and emotional distress following a natural disaster (Lima *et al.*, 1989). And normlessness has been found to be correlated with such problems as mistrust, paranoia, brooding, and worrying (Mirowsky & Ross, 1983). Summarizing their extensive primary and secondary work on the social causes of psychological distress, Mirowsky and Ross concluded that alienation is one of the most important causes of psychological distress. They stated: "Of all the things that might explain the social patterns of distress, one stands out as central, the sense of control over one's own life" (1989, p. 167).

Technological hazard situations shatter that sense of control. Victims feel powerless to summon the resources to adequately protect their families and themselves. The commonly accepted norms of social behavior are inadequate for solving the problem at hand. One's friends, neighbors, and government will not help and cannot be trusted. People feel at the mercy of forces beyond their control and comprehension, threatened by a physical world which used to provide security and alienated from the social world which once gave them comfort, solace, and meaning.

Theoretically, then, alienation provides an interesting link between a type of environmental event and the social breakdown it sets in motion, and individual patterns of psychological distress. Empirically, recent preliminary evidence supports this link. A number of standard alienation measures were administered to residents of two communities which were contaminated by toxic wastes, and to a control group from a nearby community. Results show that alienation levels were significantly higher among residents of the contaminated communities than among members of the control group (Couch & Kroll-Smith, 1990).

Threat Beliefs and Trauma

In addition to psychological distress caused by the experience of contamination, by stigma, and by alienation, people must also cope with difficulties presented by the socially constructed claims of danger. Although these claims are a way of making sense out of an uncertain situation, they may also set in motion social processes which are more detrimental to adjustment than they are helpful.

Interpreting the deleterious effects of these claims about danger in the individual begins with the idea that

in toxic contamination cases, "subjective evaluations are closely tied to the development of physical and mental health problems" (Baum, 1987, p. 46). Subjectivity is related to uncertainty. People facing the threat of chemical contamination or asbestos poisoning live in a chronic state of contingent loss. The greater the degree of contingency or uncertainty, the greater the need to construct symbolic claims of the scope and seriousness of the threat. "In situations . . . involving exposure to invisible contaminants . . . one finds that invisible health threats are met by the development of nonempirical belief systems about the nature of the threats" (Vyner, 1988, p. 21; cf. Kroll-Smith & Couch, 1987). Several studies suggest that these symbolic claims "may be more important in determining chronic stress and mental health effects than is the actual threat or danger posed" (Baum, 1987, p. 45; Baum, Singer, & Baum, 1981; Fowlkes & Miller, 1982; Kroll-Smith & Couch, 1990; Vyner, 1988). Thus, a key question in the study of the social sources of trauma concerns the meaning of beliefs in victim's emotional and behavioral response to threat or to loss.

In an earlier article we called nonempirical or symbolic constructions of danger *threat belief systems* and distinguished them from risk perceptions (Kroll-Smith & Couch, 1987; see also Kroll-Smith, Couch, & Levine, in press). Most studies of risk rely on the concept of "perception" to convey the link between the hazard and the person's appraisal of danger. Even though we have learned a great deal about the individual's potential response to risk situations through the study of perception, the ego orientation of the concept has tended to narrow interpretations to the psychological makeup of the perceiver. Beliefs, we suggest, more profoundly influence the believer than perceptions influence the perceiver. To perceive is to become aware of something directly through the senses; to believe, on the other hand, is to commit with conviction to a publicly ratified view of some aspect of the world. Beliefs are internalized; they are located deeper in the psyche than perceptions and are far less easily modified.[4]

The tenacity of beliefs is explained in part by the fact that they are social phenomena. Although perceptions issue from sensory stimuli, beliefs are constructed in conversation among people who agree that the world or a portion of it is sacred, safe, dangerous, worthy of trust or distrust, and so on (see Borhek & Curtis, 1975; Parsons, 1951, Chap. 8; the classic statement on the sociology of belief remains Durkheim, 1915). Collective agreement strengthens the hold beliefs have on believers. Perceptions are more private matters, easier to revise; to violate a belief, however, is to risk censure and disapproval. Thus, embedded in beliefs is a moral claim on believers who are required to emote and behave in ways consistent with the social reality symbolized by the beliefs.

---

[4]Mileti, Drabek, and Hass (1975) noted that the concept of risk perception "has not been particularly fruitful as a predictor of . . . socially important behaviors, e.g., adoption or not of lifesaving adjustments. It appears that hazard perception studies are not likely to get very far until the social constraints within which perception-behavior links are occurring are explicitly incorporated into theory and research design" (1975, pp. 33–34).

As previously discussed, toxic contamination situations result in the estrangement of victims from their normal community support networks. The more the claims of contamination are believed in by members of the support network, the more likely they are to avoid and withdraw from claims-makers. Victims tend to respond to this avoidance by forming groups of their own. The core members of these new support networks are usually other people who claim to be poisoned or who fear the threat of contamination. Together, they frequently affirm each other's fears, developing a set of cognitive and emotive assumptions about danger that places them farther outside the boundaries of ordinary community life.

The first and most important grassroots group to emerge at Love Canal was organized on the basis of a shared belief system regarding the amount and kind of danger it was facing and what its members were entitled to as taxpaying citizens (Levine, 1982, pp. 167–177). Similarly, Love Canal residents talked about chemical migration and risk using "the conditional language of belief" (Fowlkes & Miller, 1982, p. 47). Residents of Centralia, Pennsylvania, responded to the risks of an underground mine fire with a "shared set of linked ideas concerning the amount and kinds of dangers facing their families" (Kroll-Smith & Couch, 1987, p. 264; Kroll-Smith & Couch, 1990, Chap. 5). Similarly, people residing near the Three Mile Island (TMI) nuclear facility developed coherent beliefs about safety and trust in government after the TMI accident (Vyner, 1984). Several families in a trailer park contaminated with asbestos "developed new linguistic/emotional definitions of the situation" and "a new basis from which to view and respond to their environment" (Cuthbertson, 1987, p. 61).

Threat belief systems do vary according to the specific type of environmental contamination, and the social, historical, and cultural differences between communities. However, there is a thematic continuity across the four systems we examined.[5] These common themes include (1) the certainty that the environment, or a portion of it, is now dangerous and to be avoided; (2) the certainty that the bodies of believers and the bodies of their children are being poisoned; (3) the conclusion that victims can expect little empathy or assistance from neighbors or government (Note: This theme is not represented in the Three Mile Island threat belief system, but we would be surprised if it were not a constituent part of the system that was simply not written up.); (4) the conclusion that escape or relocation is the only reasonable way to avoid further damage.

Beliefs confer certainty on reality. They reduce the hazard that accompanies the acute experience of uncertainty. Technical experts may disagree over the presence of PCBs or dioxin in people's backyards, but believers are certain the chemicals are there. Certainty is also extended to the ambiguous events and incidents coincident with technological hazards. For believers, the meanings of a power surge in a gas monitor, a neighbor diagnosed with cancer, or an agency official who cites evidence that the risks are not as severe as first indi-

cated, does not reside in the events themselves but in the logic of the belief system. Believers can stop asking questions about the scope and degree of danger. Certain of the "true" extent of the danger, they require little supporting information to confirm their threat beliefs and an extraordinary amount of contrary evidence to disconfirm them. A heavy cigarette smoker in Centralia scoffed at the idea that his two-pack-a-day habit might be the source of a chronic, productive cough. "I've been smoking all my life," he reasoned, "but it's only been since this mine fire that I started to cough" (Kroll-Smith, 1983).

The certainty with which believers believe in the reality of loss and threat appears to be independent of the statistical frequency of the losses or threats themselves. Interviews with Centralia residents who constructed a threat belief system discovered that not every believer could recount personal experiences to confirm the reality of the threat of poisonous gases and substances, and the personal encounters some people did have with the fire varied in number and intensity. Although personal experiences were not available to all believers, two sources of accredited public information were: the worst case situations of seven families who experienced persistently high gas readings in their homes, and the three crisis events that occurred in the vicinity of the fire. These atypical cases were frequently talked about as if they were the typical experiences—as if the most extreme was also the most representative. Claims of damage and loss were based on the relatively few catastrophic events and clearly dangerous situations in the history of the blaze, not the long and tedious chronology of events that might have encouraged a less dreadful apprehension of the situation (Kroll-Smith & Couch, 1990).

There is, of course, a sound *ecological* basis for this apprehension. Extreme cases may be statistically unrepresentative of people's experiences at the moment, but there is no way of providing unqualified assurances that, the next day or the day after, new victims will not be discovered. Seemingly simple questions defy empirical answers: How much, if any, of the toxic substances are present? What is a dangerous dose? Am I absorbing any? Probabilities and professional opinions are the best the scientific community can provide. Beliefs, however, are definitive.

Complementing the ecological basis of hyperalterness is a social process that results in the intensification of threat beliefs. It stems from victims' experiences of social isolation following toxic exposure. Already discussed is the tendency of traditional support networks to abandon members who claim they are contaminated. Believers in a threat belief system quickly find that they are no longer welcome among nonbelievers. Placed outside the boundaries of their support groups and local communities, believers are likely to see themselves as a separate group and begin to rely on one another for support (Stone & Levine, 1985). With a high amount of *intragroup* activity among believers and a low number of *intergroup* exchanges, few believers will have a chance to survey the range of interpretations and responses others hold about the crisis. Nor are they encouraged to seek new information relevant to further evaluations of alternatives. As believers avoid and are avoided by non-

[5]We culled beliefs from the following four contamination crises: Love Canal, Three Mile Island, Centralia, and Globe, Arizona. Globe is a lesser known incident of asbestos poisoning.

believers, social isolation works to intensify their fears.

In summary, threat beliefs are intensely held claims about danger and loss of communal support. These highly charged verities are also greedy, tending to demand almost all the attention of the believers. The behavior of believers is characterized by hyperalertness to any sign of possible danger, a strong motivation to avoid people who disagree with the beliefs, obsessional concern with any detail related to the problem, a tendency to reduce the complexity of the world into the radically simplified idea that everything is threatening and few options exist for reducing the danger, and a readiness to identify others who are able but unwilling to assist in overcoming the crisis. It is reasonable to assume that the steady state of hypervigilance required by such intense claims might cause enough chronic apprehension to be productive of further anxiety in its own right (Boehnlein, 1987; Kroll-Smith & Couch, 1990; Vyner, 1988). Chronic preoccupation with danger accompanied by the idea that there is little anyone can or will do about it is a source of traumatic stress in people's lives arguably as significant as the physical danger of the hazard itself.

Contested Claims, Social Hatred, and the Expanding Scope of Victimization

Loss of solidary group support, negative reappraisal of self, alienation, and chronic apprehension encoded in a threat belief system are several of the social sources of traumatic stress accompanying environmental contamination. An additional stressor that further intensifies the trauma of the original victims and expands the scope of victimization is the frequently bitter, vitriolic conflict that ensues when someone claims that the biosphere is no longer safe. The hostility generated by environmental contamination frequently evolves into a form of social hatred as individuals and groups perceive each other as threats to their essential ideas of well-being (Cuthbertson, 1987; Cuthbertson & Nigg, 1987; Kaperson & Pijawka, 1985; Kroll-Smith & Couch, 1990).

Claims-making, a form of moral discourse, charges that some person or group is able but unwilling to act in a responsible and just manner toward a problem. The emotional intensity of claims that the environment is contaminated and the local community is now a dangerous place to live rarely go uncontested. Counterclaims are likely to emerge from neighbors and others charging the believers with hyperbole and incendiary actions. Claims-making insures that technical controversies are transformed into moral controversies. Claims-makers are likely to find allies among various stakeholders in the crisis. Professional voluntary associations, the press, politicians, and lawyers, among others, provide public ratification that the world is as the claims-makers portray it. Armed with a casuistic logic, each group and organization competes for public ratification of its particular version of the crisis. Human agents, social organizations, and economic policies are responsible for creating technological hazards, and claims-making controversies are a principal means by which these hazards become traumatic stressors, insuring that more than just the immediate victims of contamination will be adversely af-

fected. The questions addressed in this section are "How do these claims-making conflicts emerge?" and "How do they become traumatic stressors adversely affecting the psychosocial stability of most community residents?"

Sources of Controversy: Invisible Contamination and Threat to Beliefs

The sources of controversy in biospheric contamination crises originate in the geographic particularism of the largely invisible contamination plume and the formation of a threat belief system that places believers in the impact stage, while the rest of the community experiences the problem as manageable and questions the histrionic displays of the believers. Most studies of air, water, and soil contamination report the uneven, erratic course of the contaminants (Brown, 1991; Couch & Kroll-Smith, 1985; Levine, 1982). Not everyone is immediately affected. In this type of crisis different sectors and subsystems of a community can be expected to be experiencing divergent levels of environmental disruption and stress. Underground swales, wind currents, streams, and past engineering practices are among the variables that result in the absence of a uniform dispersion of pollutants. "Well in our area there was none [chemicals]," remembers a Love Canal resident, "We never even thought of it. It's probably at the south end but we're at the north end" (Fowlkes & Miller, 1982, p. 42). "I was born and raised in Globe [Arizona]," observes one man, "I've had sulfur smoke on one side and the asbestos mill on the other, and I'm as healthy as a new horse" (Cuthbertson, 1987, p. 37). Consider the case of the Centralia mine fire:

> Burning eyes, the taste of sulfur, and an acrid odor accompanied by headaches, lassitude, and respiratory troubles were unequivocal evidence for residents on the "hot side," . . . that the gases caused by the fire were circulating in the borough. For residents on the north end ("cold") side of town, however, gas was not "in the air." (Kroll-Smith & Couch, 1990, pp. 44–45)

For some residents the threat of contamination is remote or simply nonexistent. For others, however, contamination is not a remote possibility but an immediate reality. For believers it is no longer a matter of paying attention to warning cues, to signals of danger, for they are already in the impact stage. In a water-pollution case, a woman recalls listening to a "sixteen-year-old girl tell . . . of her fears that the creek's contaminants would affect her ability to have children. I was standing over at the door, crying with her, and I thought then, Lord Jesus, this can't go on!" (Cable & Walsh, 1990). For other residents, however, the problem is not as immediate, perhaps not as severe, and calls for a less volatile and drastic response. A resident of Love Canal recalls spending "a lot of time down in the creek [purportedly contaminated] and I never got any skin rash. . . . We've had so much wildlife . . . schools of fish, rabbits" (Fowlkes & Miller, 1982, p. 48). Biospheric contamination creates a crisis requiring a choice as to which of several competing experiences of the same world, each of which tacitly claims to have faithfully reflected that world, will be credentialed as *the* version of the world.

Thus, a segment of a neighborhood or a community is now experiencing its environment as the source of disease, adverse generational effects, and human loss; their homes are viewed as dangerous and certain areas in their neighborhoods are redefined as life threatening and to be avoided. Groups emerging around a threat belief system move quickly to the impact stage and talk about the possibility of "suffering," "fear," and "death." With a firm belief in their status as victims of contamination, believers are likely to use the emotionally charged vocabulary of impact to place moral demands on neighbors, friends, and others to accept their claims that adverse effects are now occurring and that immediate action is necessary. People who define the problem as at worst a warning, or perhaps as no problem at all, are likely to begin viewing believers and their emergent groups as threats to property values and valued lifestyles, perhaps as threats to the very continuance of the neighborhood or town itself (Cuthbertson & Nigg, 1987; Fowlkes & Miller, 1982; Kroll-Smith & Couch, 1990). Those who do not find in the environmental cues a warrant for extreme concern are likely to see themselves as victims of a fictive, or at best exaggerated, crisis.

Controversies as Traumatic Stressors

Claims-making controversies over the question of biospheric contamination create two sources of stress: *cultural* and *structural* (Kasperson & Pijawka, 1985). The primary cultural stressor originates with the disruption of a shared assumption that is basic to inhabitants of a geographic area. While neighbors frequently disagree over politics, a barking dog, or matters of taste, they continue to live and invest in their houses because they mutually trust that the air, water, and soil about them is safe and able to nurture life. But technological hazards sever their trust in that environment and place them in immediate conflict with others who do not "see" the threats and impacts which they claim exist.

A challenge to a community's primitive belief in a safe environment (perhaps best pictured as the bottom block in Abraham Maslow's hierarchy of needs) tears at the seams of a cultural theme basic to social survival. If the water or soil *is* contaminated, there is little reason for me to continue investing in my community. However, the evidence of contamination is likely to be less than certain. Perhaps my experience of the local biosphere does not lead to the conclusion that an immediate threat exists. In that case, continued investment in my community makes sense, and challenges to that investment are likely to be interpreted as threats to my civil rights. Both interpretations are likely to evolve into competing belief systems, with believers in one interpretation disliking other believers the more intensely they are felt to threaten their view of the world (Fowlkes & Miller, 1982, p. 95; Kroll-Smith & Couch, 1990). Biospheric contamination more often than not creates situations where no one interpretation of the crises can monopolize the public imagination and competing interpretations evolve into competing belief systems. What emerges are

competing views of the same local world: It is dangerous and uninhabitable; you should be concerned. No, the environment is safe and habitable; you should get control of yourself.

Phenomenologists refer to this type of cognitive conflict as a "reality disjuncture" and suggest that it can be the source of considerable psychosocial stress (Coulter, 1975; Eglin, 1979). Disputants in a reality disjuncture look at what they perceive to be the same world and experience it in contrary ways. The social validation necessary to affirm the individual's trust that the world is as he or she sees it is transformed into a source of social conflict. The very nature of claims-making activity insures that the conflict is not waged over whatever verifiable information is available about the hazard. Rather, the dispute is between people who perceive their antagonists as able but unwilling to cooperate in a "realistic" and "justifiable" definition of the threat. Thus, disputants are defined as persons with special motives to make false claims. Fear, hysteria, and greed are among the several labels antagonists apply to each other to explain away opposing claims (see Cuthbertson, 1987; Fowlkes & Miller, 1982; Kroll-Smith & Couch, 1990). Negative labeling heightens the emotional intensity of the conflict, exacting a toll on the psychosocial stability of disputants.

Toxic chemicals leaching through underground swales or asbestos fibers floating through the air do not destroy buildings or level houses, but they do damage the moral rules for local community life. When the presence of contamination is defined by a segment of a neighborhood as "impact," the high degree of uncertainty accompanying this type of hazard insures that competing definitions will emerge, creating a marked crisis in the local culture. Insofar as each of the disputants in this crisis maintains his or her own experiences as the ineradicable grounds for further action, dispute resolution is all but impossible as potentially endless cycles of reciprocal blaming, censure and condemnation ensue. "The fire has split us up," observed a mine fire victim, "it has torn us apart, you know—divided us. We're divided this and that way. We're worse than a pie cut into eight pieces" (Kroll-Smith & Couch, 1990, p. 6). The intensity of this cultural crisis and the psychosocial stress that it creates increases dramatically as emergent groups alter the local social structure.

The second stressor related to the intramural conflict over competing claims that the environment is habitable or uninhabitable is structural change in the routine organizational life of the community or settlement. Local social structures operate in routine, nonemergency contexts and are usually ill-prepared for the type of innovative action necessary to address the demands of biospheric contamination (Kroll-Smith & Couch, in press; Wolensky & Miller, 1981). The milieu of extreme uncertainty characterizing environmental contamination episodes initiates against the effective functioning of organizations designed to operate in noncrisis situations.

Social organizations can respond to threat in one of two fashions: *anticipation* and *resilience* (Kroll-Smith & Couch, 1990). Local community organizations can reduce threat by anticipating it only when it is possible to know with a high degree of certainty what to expect and how to prevent it. Life in "Tornado Alley," for example, is organized around early warning detection technologies, designated shelters, and postimpact procedures. Organizational resiliency, on the other hand, is the ability of the local community to bounce back from insult, to cope with unanticipated dangers after they have become manifest. By its ability to accommodate variability and the unexpected, resilience is an important resource in the social response to extreme uncertainty. The technological nature of community social organizations, however, their manifest design and purpose, and their customary and methodical arrangements are more suited to anticipation than to resilience. The amount of organizational stress varies inversely with the predictability of the aversive agent. The less predictable and controllable the hazard, the more likely customary organizations are perceived as inadequate to respond to the threat.

If routine social arrangements could accommodate the acrimonious claims-making, the level of hostility would be contained by the organizational history of the club or association and the institutionalized means of problem definition and resolution. If the Chamber of Commerce, for example, could incorporate a particular claim, the chamber's traditional civic organization would refashion it to fit its mandate and goals. People who adopt a threat belief system, however, are not likely to find the Chamber of Commerce or other civic organizations amenable to their volatile claims of danger.

The apparent discrepancy between the demands of biospheric contamination and the inherit limitations of nonemergency social systems insures that routine social arrangements will not give people access to roles consistent with their particular appraisals of danger. In this case, the emergence of competing beliefs usually leads to the emergence of competing groups. Three distinct grassroots groups emerged at the Love Canal, each organized around a different perception of the amount and kind of danger posed by the chemicals (Levine, 1982). Similarly, seven local protest groups emerged in the wake of the accident at Three Mile Island (Walsh, 1981). The Centralia mine fire resulted in the formation of seven citizen's groups in a town of fewer than a thousand people (Kroll-Smith & Couch, 1990). Asbestos contamination of a trailer park in Globe, Arizona, was the cause of two emergent groups, each with quite different beliefs about the "real" dangers (Cuthbertson & Nigg, 1987).

It would appear that establishing protocols of survival in conditions of extreme uncertainty demands mitigative adjustments that are likely to be inconsistent with routine social arrangements. Evident throughout the literature on psychosocial stress and contamination is the idea that social responses to environmental crises restructure communities by creating subcultures of hostility that frequently prove as debilitating as the environmental problem itself.

A team of community psychologists explains its problems with effective intervention at the Love Canal:

> Our frustrating and saddening experience in consulting with United Way agencies . . . was that the murkiness and pessimism of the situation resulted in divisions among victims . . . effective community organization was nearly impossible in an atmosphere of hopelessness

and misplaced conflict. (J. Kliman, Kern, & A. Kliman, 1982, p. 267)

In cases of asbestos and pesticide contamination, competing "victim clusters" emerged, which "attempted to demonstrate the correctness of their own interpretations of the . . . risk level of the disaster agent. . . . [The] emotional climate that emerged was one of anger, frustration [and] bitterness" (Cuthbertson & Nigg, 1987, p. 480).

Characterizing the dilemma of the Centralia mine fire were

> two irreconcilable goals: the preservation of health and safety, and the preservation of Centralia. For most residents . . . achievement of one goal meant sacrificing the other. Since the stakes were high, the dissension left little room for compromise, and since the evidence was equivocal . . . and vague, even contradictory interpretations were officially and experientially confirmed. (Kroll-Smith & Couch, 1990, p. 52)

In a self-reporting stress study in Centralia, over two thirds of the respondents identified the community conflict caused by the fire as more of a stressor in their lives than the fire itself (Kroll-Smith & Couch, 1990).

Under some circumstances, conflict can serve to solidify a group or community. In the recovery and rehabilitation stages of a natural disaster, for example, conflict facilitates the restructuring of neighborhoods, civic associations, and so on, by helping to realign group interests and reestablish the competitive milieu necessary for an exchange-based social order (Turner, 1976). The sociocultural conflict that emerges in cases of biospheric contamination, however, does not strengthen the consensual bases of community life; it puts the basic consensus itself in question. Groups emerging in response to technological hazards do not resolve their differences on the basis of an underlying unity; quite the contrary, they splinter on the basis of their differences. Erikson argued that people experience the conflicts that destroy the consensual basis of their social life as collective traumas:

> By collective trauma, I mean a blow to the tissues of social life that [is experienced as a] form of shock—a gradual realization that the community no longer exists as a source of nurturance and that a part of the self has disappeared. (1976, p. 302)

Summary and Implications

This chapter began with the assumption that the extreme uncertainty accompanying many technological disasters forces victims to fashion their own appraisals of danger. It is not spontaneous reactions to threat that mark human responses to biospheric contamination, but a kind of forensic analysis as people sift and sort the ambiguous and uncertain evidence to construct conclusions regarding the "real" degree of danger. Also assumed in this chapter is the idea that the uneven distribution of biospheric contamination frequently results in various neighborhoods, indeed neighbors themselves, moving through the disaster stage model at quite different rates. For some families, their backyards and basements are already poisoned. For others, the signs of enviromental damage are too vague and indeterminate to define themselves or their neighbors as threatened.

With these two assumptions we have attempted to show that the reality of toxic contamination differs considerably from the reality of natural disasters. Indeed, it make more sense to speak of the "realities" of a human-caused contamination of the environment, because the ambiguity of the situation sets in motion social processes that virtually insure the creation of differing versions of the degree and scope of danger. People who define themselves as victims of contamination are also likely to be defined by others as people to be avoided. Friendships begin to subside and once sociable neighbors no longer seem to have anything to say. Intensifying the experience of environmental pollution is the social trauma of being acted toward as a polluted person, someone to be avoided.

Threat belief systems are likely to emerge, responding to the vacuum of reliable and objective assessments of the degree of danger. Ironically, however, although these beliefs are constructed to reduce the uncertainty of threat, they are likely to encourage a belief in danger while offering little hope for escape. Threat beliefs are also likely to mobilize residents into citizens' groups that call for immediate action to address contamination. To the degree that these groups challenge the "normal" order of a neighborhood or community, they are likely to cause the emergence of competing groups who view the "real" crisis as their "hysterical" neighbors. The result is community polarization and destructive conflict. Whatever the real threat of toxic poisoning might be, a no less traumatic experience for many victims is their inability to keep the social and emotional consequences of the problem within manageable bounds.

This analysis has some disturbing implications for professionals who wish to help victims cope with technological hazards (Kroll-Smith & Couch, in press). For one thing, the belief that more accurate risk communication will solve these problems appears to be false. For many technological risks, the degrees of danger can only be guessed at, and the uneven pace of scientific advancement, along with the constant creation of new hazards, insures that ambiguities about risks will remain. Moreover, even in cases where scientific knowledge offers assurances, the quick formation of groups dominated by threat beliefs makes it unlikely that reassuring information will be easily assimilated.

Other apparently obvious strategies also dissolve in the face of this analysis. Ordinarily, emergency and technical response personnel work through local governments to gain the cooperation of the community in abating the hazard and protecting families. All too often, however, local governing bodies are perceived by organized opposition in a town or neighborhood as partisan and unwilling to represent their needs. More often than not, attempts to work through these bodies increase the anxiety of residents. Or what of the support engendered by an activist group? While providing emotional support to its members, activity in such a group will also solidify ingroup/outgroup boundaries and will make community-wide consensus building difficult. What of

individual counseling to help victims adjust to reality? Which, or whose, reality is the "correct" one?

Perhaps the best approach to technological hazards would be to shift the focus of discussion. The problem is usually considered to be technical and medical. Budgeting money to clean up the contamination and conduct epidemiological research is the routine official response to this type of disaster. With a few exceptions, money cannot at present buy a clean-up; the technology is simply not adequate to the task. Moreover, epidemiological studies are almost always open to considerable debate and are likely to become themselves sources of stress. Simply put, if the goal is to reduce the trauma of the victims, intervention strategies based solely on technical and medical approaches will fail.

In our opinion, an additional intervention strategy is necessary, one that complements the issue of contamination by concentrating on reducing the bewildering array of emotive and behavioral responses to it. If the social responses to contamination are themselves sources of trauma, effective intervention will depend, in part, on developing strategies for mitigating these responses. The key to this type of intervention is to arrest the social dynamics producing the stress. A framework for thinking about these strategies is found in the literature on dispute resolution (see, e.g., Coleman, 1957; Deutsch, 1973). A key distinction in this literature is the difference between *competitive* processes and *cooperative* processes. Transposed to the contaminated community, the primary task is to shift residents from a destructive model of disaster response to a constructive model, one that encourages people to view their predicament as a common problem in which the conflicting parties have a joint stake in resolving.

Left unfettered, human responses to toxic contamination are likely to create communication styles that enhance distortion and encourage the emergence of hostile groups commited to nonnegotiable outcomes. Communication between people who are organized around contrasting appraisals of danger is likely to be interpreted as unreliable. People report little confidence in the information they obtain directly from competing others. A zero-sum logic emerges as people struggle to enhance their own power while minimizing the power of others. The struggle to maintain a favorable power position shifts the focus of attention from the toxins to imposing one's definition of the threat on the other person. Suspicion and hostility between victims enhance sensitivity to differences and threats while minimizing the awareness of similarities.

Arresting this destructive process and creating the conditions for cooperative problem-solving requires the active intervention of people who are trained in the arts of conflict resolution and consensus building. We have identified the following tasks as necessary, though hardly sufficient, for successful intervention to occur:

1. Create a communicative context that encourages residents to view the diversity of opinions on the amounts and kinds of danger caused by exposure as a predictable pattern in this type of crisis. The reality is that people are affected in different ways. The task is to create a forum for the exchange of conflicting definitions that encourages people to be tolerant of the differences,

and, perhaps, to benefit from being made aware of them. The problem here is how to get people to agree to disagree.

2. Defuse the highly charged emotive setting by creating public contexts that encourage people to keep their emotional responses within manageable bounds. Do not ask people to deny the powerful feelings that follow the experience of exposure or the threat of losing one's home, but balance the expression of these fears with concrete activities that serve to remind them that they are still in charge of their lives. The problem here is how to legitimate people's fear without letting it dominate their lives.

3. Environmental contamination requires a considerable amount of local political activity to insure a just and equitable response by culpable and responsible parties. This activity can help people shift their anger from neighbors and friends to groups and agencies outside the boundaries of the community. The problem here is how to encourage people with widely different views of the crisis to recognize the legitimacy of the other's interests and identify their struggle as a common one.

If these few suggestions fall far short of a comprehensive intervention strategy, they nonetheless hint at what a successful mitigation approach might look like. What is clear is the role of sociocultural factors in intensifying the trauma of environmental contamination and the attendant need to rethink our routine disaster-management procedures.

References

Baker, G. W., & Chapman, D. W., (Eds.). (1962). *Man and society in disaster*. New York: Basic Books.

Barton, A. H. (1969). *Communities in disaster: A sociological analysis of collective stress situations*. Garden City, NY: Doubleday.

Baum, A. (1987). Toxins, technology and natural disasters. In G. Van Den Bos & B. Bryant (Eds.), *Cataclysms, crises and catastrophes* (pp.5–54). New York: Brunner/Mazel.

Baum, A., Singer, J., & Baum, C. (1981). Stress and the environment. *Journal of Social Issues, 37*, 4–35.

Berger, P., & Luckmann, T. (1966). *The social construction of reality*. New York: Doubleday.

Blumer, H. (1969). *Symbolic interaction*. Englewood Cliffs, NJ: Prentice-Hall.

Boehnlein, J. K. (1987). Culture and society in post-traumatic stress disorder: Implications for psychotherapy. *American Journal of Psychotherapy, 41*, 519–530.

Borhek, J. T., & Curtis, R. F. (1975). *A sociology of belief*. New York: Wiley.

Brown, P. (1991). The popular epidemiology approach to toxic waste contamination. In S. R. Couch & J. S. Kroll-Smith (Eds.), *Communities at risk: Collective responses to technological hazards* (pp. 133–156). New York: Peter Lang.

Cable, S., & Walsh, E. (1991). The emergence of organized protest in chronic technical emergencies. In S. R. Couch & J. S. Kroll-Smith (Eds.), *Communities at risk: Collective responses to technological hazards* (pp. 113–132). New York: Peter Lang.

Coleman, J. (1957). *Community conflict*. Glencoe, IL: Free Press.

Couch, S. R., & Kroll-Smith, J. S. (1985). The chronic technical disaster: Toward a social scientific perspective. *Social Science Quarterly, 66*, 564–575.

Couch, S. R., & Kroll-Smith, J. S. (1989). *Toxic exposure and social alienation: Two case studies*. Paper presented at the Fourth National Environmental Health Conference, San Antonio, TX.

Cooley, C. H. (1922). *Human nature and the social order*. New York: Scribner's.

Coulter, I. (1975). Perceptual accounts and interpretive asymmetries. *Sociology, 9*, 385–396.

Cuthbertson, B. H. (1987). *Emotion and technological disaster: An integrative analysis*. Unpublished doctoral dissertation, Arizona State University, Tempe, AZ.

Cuthbertson, B. H., & Nigg, J. M. (1987). Technological disaster and the nontherapeutic community: A question of true victimization. *Environment and Behavior, 19*, 462–483.

Deutsch, M. (1973). *The resolution of conflict*. New Haven: Yale University Press.

Dohrenwend, B. S. (1978). Social stress and community psychology. *American Journal of Community Psychology, 6*, 1–14.

Douglas, M. (1985). *Risk acceptability according to the social sciences*. New York: Russell Sage Foundation.

Drabek, T. E., & Key W. H. (1984). *Conquering disaster: Family recovery and long-term consequences*. New York: Irvington.

Dunlap, R. E., & Catton, W. R. (1983). What environmental sociologists have in common. *Sociological Inquiry, 53*, 113–135.

Durkheim, E. (1915). *The elementary forms of the religious life*. New York: Macmillan.

Edelstein, M. (1988). *Contaminated communities: The social and psychological impacts of residential toxic exposure*. Boulder, CO: Westview Press.

Eglin, P. (1979). Resolving reality disjunctures on Telegraph Avenue: A study of practical reasoning. *Canadian Journal of Sociology, 4*, 359–377.

Erikson, K. T. (1976). Loss of communality at Buffalo Creek. *American Journal of Psychiatry, 133*, 302–305.

Erikson, K. T. (1991). A new species of trouble. In S. R. Couch & J. S. Kroll-Smith (Eds.), *Communities at risk: Collective responses to technological hazards* (pp. 11–30). New York: Peter Lang.

Finsterbusch, K. (1987, July). Typical scenarios in twenty-four toxic waste contamination episodes. Paper presented at the Annual Meeting of the International Association of Impact Assessment, Barbados, British West Indies.

Fowlkes, M. R., & Miller, P. Y. (1982). *Love Canal: The social construction of disaster*. Washington, DC: FEMA.

Fritz, C. E. (1961). Disaster. In R. K. Merton & R. A. Nisbet (Eds.), *Contemporary social problems* (pp. 651–694). New York: Harcourt, Brace, Jovanovich.

Garber, J., Miller, W. R., & Seaman, S. F. (1979). Learning helplessness, stress, and the depressive disorders. In R. A. Depue (Ed.), *The psychobiology of the depressive: Implications for the effects of stress* (pp. 335–363). New York: Academic Press.

Gibbs, M. S. (1986). Psychopathological consequences of exposure to toxins in the water supply. In A. H. Levovits, A. Baum, & J. E. Singer (Eds.), *Advances in environmental psychology: Vol. 6. Exposure to hazardous substances* (pp. 47–70). Hillsdale, NJ: Lawrence Erlbaum.

Gleser, G. C., Green, B. L., & Winget, C. N. (1981). *Prolonged effects of disasters: A study of Buffalo Creek*. New York: Academic Press.

Gouldner, A. (1970). *The coming crisis of western sociology*. New York: Basic Books.

Janoff-Bulman, R., & Frieze, I. H. (1983). A theoretical perspective for understanding reactions to victimization. *Journal of Social Issues, 39*, 1–17.

Kaplan, B. H., Cassel, J. C., & Gore, S. (1977). Social support and health. *Medical Care, 15*, 47–58.

Kasperson, R. E., & Pijawka, D. (1985). Societal response to hazards and major hazard events: Comparing natural and technological hazards. *Public Administration Review, 45*, 7–18.

Kliman, J., Kern, R., & Kliman, A. (1982). Natural and human-made disasters: Some therapeutic and epidemological implications for crisis intervention. In U. Rueveni, R. V. Speck, & J. L. Speck (Eds.), *Therapeutic intervention: Healing strategies for crisis intervention* (pp. 253–280). New York: Human Sciences Press.

Kreps, G. (1980). Research needs and policy issues on mass media. In *Disasters and the mass media: Proceedings of the committee on disasters and the mass media workshop, February, 1979, Committee on Disasters and the Mass Media* (pp. 37–74). Washington, DC: National Academy of Sciences.

Kroll-Smith, J. S. (1983). *Interviews with residents of Centralia, Pennsylvania.* Unpublished manuscript.

Kroll-Smith, J. S., & Couch, S. R. (1987). A chronic technical disaster and the irrelevance of religious meaning: The case of Centralia, Pennsylvania. *Journal for the Scientific Study of Religion, 26*, 25–37.

Kroll-Smith, J. S., & Couch, S. R. (1990). *The real disaster is above ground: A mine fire and social conflict.* Lexington, KY: University Press of Kentucky.

Kroll-Smith, J. S., & Couch, S. R. (1991). Technological hazards, adaptation and social change. In S. R. Couch & J. S. Kroll-Smith (Eds.), *Communities at risk: Collective responses to technological hazards* (pp. 193–320). New York: Peter Lang.

Kroll-Smith, J. S., Couch, S. R., & Levine, A. G. (in press). Technological hazards and disasters. In R. A. Dunlap & W. Michelson (Eds.), *Handbook on environmental sociology.* Wesport, CT: Greenwood Press.

Kuhn, T. S. (1962). *The structure of scientific revolutions.* Chicago: University of Chicago Press.

LaPlante, J. M., & Kroll-Smith, J. S. (1989). Coordinated emergency management: The challenge of the chronic technological disaster. *International Journal of Mass Emergencies and Disasters, 7*, 134–150.

Lazarus, R. S., & Folkman, S. (1984). *Stress, appraisal, and coping.* New York: Springer.

Levine, A. G. (1982). *Love Canal: Science, politics, and people.* Lexington, MA: Lexington Books.

Lima, B. R., Chavez, H., Samaniego, N., Pompei, M. S., Pal, S., Santacruz, H., & Lozano, J. (1989). Disaster severity and emotional disturbance: Implications for primary mental health care in developing countries. *Acta Psychiatrica Scandinavica, 79*, 74–82.

Litwak, E., & Messeri, P. (1988). Organizational theory, social supports and mortality rates: A theoretical convergence. *American Sociology Review, 54*, 49–66.

Maslow, A. H. (1970). *Motivation and personality.* New York: Harper & Row.

Mileti, D. S., Drabek, T. E., & Haas, J. H. (1975). *Human systems in extreme environments: A sociological perspective.* Boulder, CO: Institute of Behavioral Science.

Mirowsky, J., & Ross, C. E. (1983). Paranoia and the structure of powerlessness. *American Sociological Review, 48*, 228–239.

Mirowsky, J., & Ross C. E. (1986). Social patterns of distress. In A. Inkeles (Ed.), *Annual review of sociology* (pp. 23–45). Palo Alto, CA: Annual Reviews.

Mirowsky, J., & Ross, C. E. (1989). *Social causes of psychological distress.* New York: Aldine de Gruyter.

Moore, H. E. (1958). *Tornadoes over Texas.* Austin: University of Texas Press.

Parsons, T. (1951). *The social system.* New York: The Free Press.

Pearlin, L. I., Lieberman, M. A., Menaghan, E. G., & Mullan, J. T. (1981). The stress process. *Journal of Health and Social Behavior, 22*, 337–356.

Seeman, M., Seeman, A. Z., & Budros, A. (1988). Powerlessness, work, and community: A longitudinal study of alienation and alcohol use. *Journal of Health and Social Behavior, 29*, 185–198.

Schorr, J. K., Goldsteen, R., & Cortes, C. H. (1982). *The long-term impact of a man-made disaster: A sociological examination of a small town in the aftermath of the Three Mile Island nuclear reactor accident.* Paper presented at the Tenth World Congress of Sociology, Mexico City, Mexico.

Shrivastava, P. 1987. *Bhopal: Anatomy of a crisis.* Cambridge, MA: Ballinger Press.

Smith, E., North, C. S., & Price, P. C. (1986). Response to technological accidents. In M. Lystad (Ed.), *Mental health response to mass emergencies* (pp. 52–95). New York: Brunner/Mazel.

Smith, E. M., Robins, L. N., Przybeck, T. R., Godring, E., & Solomon, S. D. (1986). Psychosocial consequences of a disaster. In J. H. Shore (Ed.), *Disaster stress studies: New methods and findings* (pp. 50–76). Washington, DC: American Psychiatric Press.

Spector, M., & Kitsuse, J. I. (1977). *Constructing social problems.* Menlo Park, CA: Cummings Press.

Starr, C. (1969). Social benefit versus technological risk. *Science, 165*, 1232–1238.

Stone, R. A., & Levine, A. G. (1985). Reactions to collective stress: Correlates of active citizen participation at Love Canal. *Prevention in Human Services, 4*, 153–177.

Turner, R. H. (1976). Types of solidarity in the reconstitution of groups. *Pacific Sociological Review, 10*, 60–68.

Vidich, A. J. (1980, May/June). The theodicy of man-made hazards. *ARC Newsletter*, p. 3.

Vyner, H. M. (1984). *The psychosocial effects of invisible environmental contaminants.* Paper presented to the Three Mile Island Public Health Fund's Workshop on the Psychosocial Effects of Invisible Environmental Contaminants.

Vyner, H. M. (1988). *Invisible trauma.* Lexington, MA: Lexington Books.

Wallace, A. F. C. (1956). Tornado in Worcester. *National Academy of Sciences/National Research Council Disaster Study #3.* Washington, DC: National Academy of Sciences.

Walsh, E. (1981). Resource mobilization and citizen protest in communities around Three Mile Island. *Social Problems, 29*, 1–21.

Wheaton, B. (1980). The sociogenesis of psychological disorder. *Journal of Health and Social Behavior, 21*, 100–124.

Wheaton, B. (1983). Stress, personal coping resources, and psychiatric symptoms. *Journal of Health and Social Behavior, 24*, 208–229.

Wijkman, A., & Timberlake, L. (1984). *Natural disasters: Acts of God or acts of man?* Washington, DC: International Institute for Environment and Development.

Wolensky, R. P., & Miller, E. J. (1981). The everyday versus the disaster role of local officials—citizen and official definitions. *Urban Affairs Quarterly, 16*, 483–504.

Zimmerman, R. (1985). The relationship of emergency management to governmental policies on man-made technological disasters. *Public Administration Review, 45*, 29–39.

CHAPTER 8

Posttraumatic Stress Disorder in Experienced Anomalous Trauma

Rima E. Laibow and C. Shaffia Laue

Introduction

Experienced anomalous trauma (EAT) is seen in patients exhibiting signs of stress-response traumata in the absence of a readily identifiable traumatic event despite careful investigation. Posttraumatic stress disorder (PTSD) is frequent in these patients. Such persons are generally free of major psychopathology and may show physical and emotional traumatic sequelae. Prior to treatment, memorylike traces may or may not be present for scenarios which correlate with the psychological and physical stigmata of the stressful event. As will be discussed in this chapter, EAT may be seen in patients in any ethnic and/or demographic cohort. As noted elsewhere in this volume, PTSD was first described adequately in the context of battle fatigue (Kardiner, 1941), although it may present in a wide variety of clinical guises (van der Kolk, 1987).

Traumatic versus Anomalous Stressor Events

Our current understanding of PTSD has evolved from the careful examination of patients whose lives have been significantly disrupted by traumatic events which cannot readily be identified and fixed in time and place. Although recall may be impeded by such defenses as repression, the notion of posttraumatic stress presupposes a clearly identifiable traumatic stressor with a

knowable, or implied, set of reality parameters which define both the stress and the circumstances surrounding it. We usually have no difficulty understanding why the stressor perpetuates itself in the experiential reality of the patient. We can begin to propose biochemical and neurological models for the encoding, and for the unlearning, of the effects of real-life tragic and traumatic events (see Chapters 2 and 66, in this volume, for a review). Deficits of memory may be (at least hypothetically) reversed and worked-through via the process of retrieval of information and affect associated with the traumatic stress itself. The response, meaning, and emotional "envelope" of the stress may also be anticipated, at least on a hypothetical basis, for most types of traumatic events. The field of traumatic stress studies is, in fact, devoted to the development of increasing sophistication and clarity in identifying, retrieving, treating, and healing the psychological wounds of those exposed to overwhelming stressors. Numerous modalities have been attempted and evaluated in studies designed to assess the treatment and outcome of trauma (Wilson, 1989; see also Chapter 70, in this volume).

Stressful life events can precipitate the anguish of posttraumatic functional impairment long after they have ceased to be represented in the physical world of the patient. It is clear that there has been an event which has occurred in society and can be recognized by its members. Although we may deplore the exploitative or tragic nature of the events which have impacted upon the patient, we are able to comprehend without significant challenge to our prevailing paradigms of reality that there has, in fact, been a traumatic event.

In dramatic contrast, patients who report anomalous trauma events in the absence of psychopathology severe enough to account for the production of such material often show the clinical picture associated with PTSD. This is remarkable when one considers that it is possible that no traumatic event occurred except that which may be rooted in fantasy. These "traumata" are,

Rima E. Laibow • TREAT, 13 Summit Terrace, Dobbs Ferry, New York 10522. **C. Shaffia Laue** • 346 Maine, Lawrence, Kansas 66044.

International Handbook of Traumatic Stress Syndromes, edited by John P. Wilson and Beverley Raphael. Plenum Press, New York, 1993.

in large measure, split off, denied, and repressed as they are in other occurrences of PTSD.

Culturally Bound Definitions of Trauma and Awareness of Stressor Experiences

It is well to remember that our commonly shared, culturally bound perception of the real, possible, comprehensible, and knowable is neither fixed nor immutable. Only a few decades ago, the notion that children, from their earliest days, and in horrifyingly large numbers at that, were being sexually and physically abused by the adults entrusted with their care was utterly repugnant, unthinkable, and unacceptable even to professionals who saw the evidence with their own skilled eyes. Westrum (1982) offered a model by which events become "hidden" and therefore remain anomalous to the perception of society in a circular process: The hidden event is disbelieved and its disbelief helps to keep it hidden. Long after ample documentation by radiologists and pediatricians (Astley, 1953; Bakwin, 1956; Caffey, 1946, 1957; Silverman, 1972; Wooley & Evans, 1955) was available, battered children and their battering parents remained hidden because of social and emotional factors in the observers who could not see the data despite their clarity. In fact, it was not until Frederic N. Silverman elected to preside over a session of the American Academy of Pediatrics devoted to the "Battered Child Syndrome" in October of 1961 that the problem was officially recognized by the medical community. Furthermore, not until the ground-breaking national survey of hospitals and district attorneys by Kempe, Silverman, Steele, Droegemueller, and Silver, published in 1962, was significant public and professional reaction stirred so that at last, decades after it was first reported, it became possible for the collective cultural reality to admit the unthinkable: Some parents could, and did, severely damage and even kill their own children. Within just a few years of this seminal survey, which found 749 cases, legal action had been taken making the battered child syndrome reportable in every state in the United States (McCoid, 1965). By 1977, this hidden event had become visible and the number of reported cases had surpassed 500,000 (Sheils, Afrest, Maier, & Sethi, 1977).

On the Nature of Hidden Events

Speaking of hidden events in general, Westrum (1982) stated:

> An event is hidden if its occurrence is so implausible that those who observe it hesitate to report it because they do not expect to be believed. The implausibility may cause the observer to doubt his own perceptions, leading to the event's denial or misidentification. Should the observer nonetheless make a report, he/she can expect to be treated with incredulity or even ridicule. Since the existence of a hidden event is contrary to what science, society, and perhaps even the observer believes, the event re-

mains hidden because of strong social forces which interfere with reporting. The actual degree of underreporting is sometimes difficult to believe, a skepticism which itself acts as a deterrent to taking seriously those reports which do surface.

Therapists do not entertain a diagnosis of posttraumatic stress in the absence of known or surmised stress, yet in patients suffering from experienced anomalous trauma, this is often the clinical reality. Although the posttraumatic state of the patient experiencing EAT may be clear, what is a great deal less clear is the traumatic event which has presumably produced it. These patients may exhibit acute, chronic, delayed, or immediate PTSD or some combination of these clinical pictures.

Physical Symptoms (Clues) to Hidden Traumatic Events

Frequently reported *physical symptomatology* may include burn or scarlike marks (which may appear old but which are reported as previously absent); red, watery, painful eyes, optic swelling, swollen or crusted lids, blurred vision; headaches; scaling, dry, patchy, or irritated skin, especially on exposed surfaces; scooplike or other defects in striated muscle under apparently unbroken skin which suddenly appear; sudden and unexpected lactation in nonlactating females; unexplained cervical or uterine bleeding; rashes; copious nocturnal nasal hemorrhages; puncturelike wounds on any body surface; genital irritations and disruptions of reproductive functions of a variety of types, sometimes including reported loss of a pregnancy (up to and including late first trimester) without the passage of any fetal or material tissue; bruises (which may be symmetrically placed); incisions which are generally painless (and which sometimes show accelerated or other aberrant wound healing); percutaneous punctures and wheals, often in a symmetrical pattern; genital mutilations; alleged implants both subcutaneously and at deeper levels. It should be noted that medical documentation supports the sudden and anomalous appearance of many of these reported signs while others await definitive clarification.

Common Psychological Symptoms of Anomalous Trauma

Psychological and psychophysiological manifestations include sleep disturbances, phobic or anxiety-ridden states, intrusive images (identical with the flashback states previously described in PTSD), decreased libido, anhedonia, memory lapses, "lucid dreaming," distractibility, loss of interest in previous pursuits, preoccupation with new and inexplicable subjects and interests, "spiritual awakening or crisis," religiosity, depression, headaches, and somatic complaints.

EAT patients often experience abrupt changes in their coping ability and suddenly increased anxiety or phobic concerns. However, they may report that these facets of their lives have remained constant over a span of years, often since childhood. Such symptoms may have resisted previous therapeutic intervention. But in all these cases there is a conspicuous lack of known, easily understood trauma and the presence of a post-traumatic-like state which, despite careful investigation, has no known, easily discernible antecedents. There may be recurring dreamlike memory fragments, either "lucid dreams" or less vivid ones, which seem to hold special significance for the patient, even though it is sometimes hard for him or her to articulate the precise nature of this special significance. There may be frightening and perplexing "index events" which seem to the patient as if they, too, hold great significance but which may be vague and indistinct. These index events may be dreamlike and are hard to credit as an event-level reality for most of us sharing the common reality of our times and our culture, including the therapist and the patient. A typical index event of this type might be a "bedroom visitation" or an interruption of a car trip followed by capture and levitation on board an unidentified flying object (UFO), a medical examination-like procedure, apocalyptic or other kinds of *visual* experiences, and a return or a frightening visitation by spirits; an experience of astral projection or the apparition of deceased relatives. Upon return to ordinary awareness, the patient may report a significant dislocation in one or more aspects of reality, such as time, location, or state of awareness. These experiences commonly alarm and greatly distress the witness although recall may range from fragmentary and partial to complete. The patient often attempts a "prosaicization" of events which make little rational sense as recounted but which can be intellectualized to some degree if certain highly improbable assumptions are allowed into the scenario.

For example, Errol is a 32-year-old man who has been married for 5 years and is actively parenting his 10-year-old stepson. Errol displays an 11.5 cm ruler-straight, deeply scarred incisionlike old wound precisely parallel to the long axis of the leg on the posterior surface of the left calf muscle over the area of greatest circumference. This scar shows 1.25 cm striations of even length and regular placement perpendicular to the long axis of the scar every 2.5 cm. Despite the strikingly regular appearance of this scar, which Mike reports he has had since age 10, he accounts for it by saying, "I fell about 10 feet from a tree onto a barbed wire fence on a farm where I lived with my foster parents." Pressed for details, he reports that although he does not recall any such event, he does recall standing dazed and confused next to the fence after watching a "bright light" recede in the afternoon sky. When he returned home, his foster parents had already initiated a police search since he had been missing for several hours although he felt he had been gone for no more than 20 minutes. No other possibility suggested itself at the time to account for the large, fresh, painless wound on his calf and, since the barbed wire was nearby, he invoked this improbable source of injury, despite the lack of any memory of being impaled on it (and in spite of the straight-line nature of the wound) to "prosaicize" or normalize the occurrence.

This desperate attempt to make ordinary what nonetheless feels quite extraordinary to the patient is a common feature of these memorylike traces in EAT. Such memories are frequently laden with fear and distress for pa-

tients who find their strangeness and the memory itself dystonic. These absurd prozaicizations only partly bind the anxiety which these episodes contain. The patients anxiously return to these events over and over in their own minds (often telling no one of their concerns).

Whether through the intervention of a therapist or by spontaneous processing, there may be a dramatic unfolding of additional memorylike material. When this occurs, there is frequently a rapid and spontaneous working-through and resolution of previously troublesome symptoms and a dramatic return to the premorbid level of functioning or a significant increase in functional capacity. During this process, however, the anxiety level of the patient may become disorganizing and require support and sensitivity from those who are providing assistance. Despite the sudden, sometimes incapacitating, level of anxiety and panic which may accompany this process in some patients, there may be a significant and rapid lessening of the anxiety, panic, sleep disorder, and so forth, once this process is well underway or has reached completion.

Spontaneous Recovery Following Successful Appraisal

The rapid improvements following successful appraisal are generally robust and long-lasting, unlike "flights into health," "transference cures," Pentecostal or charismatic cures, and similar phenomena. This is in sharp distinction to the result of ordinary fantasies that reach conscious awareness. Although such fantasies may aid in the process of working-through and conflict resolution, their production, in itself, is not known to result in the long-term resolution of severe and pervasive, possibly life-long, symptomatology upon simply being made available for conscious recall and/or processing.

Physical Event Reality or Intrapsychic Process: A Challenge to the DSM PTSD Stressor Criterion "A"

EAT presents a series of challenges to our understanding of both trauma and its sequelae. Similarly, the customary assignment of reality value to events customarily held to be outside the realm of physical events may be challenged as well. If, on the one hand, it is possible for fantasies originating solely on an intrapsychic basis to produce both PTSD and physical stigmata (wounds, burns, corneal swelling, radiation-like effects, loss of late first trimester pregnancies without passage of tissue, etc.) of the profound sort seen in these cases, it is of great importance for the behavioral sciences to expend significant effort in attempting to understand the mechanisms, susceptible population, frequency, and nature of these events. Our understanding of the capacities of the intrapsychic world could well be expanded and revised by what is learned from this investigation. On the other hand, if, in fact, there is trauma occurring at event-level reality, or something similar enough to it to account for these effects, then our commonly held view of reality is open for some serious revision as it becomes necessary to admit significant new possibilities to that construct. In either event, there is good reason to explore the class of posttraumatic states represented by patients demonstrating EAT.

Current research suggests that as many as one person in five may report paranormal experiences (Kramer, 1989; Targ & Hastings, 1987). No one knows how frequently such anomalous experiences are accompanied by painful affect. No data exist to indicate how frequently the reported experience of anxiety-laden contact with UFOs occurs although both of these occurrences appear to be far from rare (Sprinkle, 1990). It is not known what proportion of these experiences are accompanied by, or followed by, PTSD-like sequelae and how many are integrated into the affective and experiential state of the individual without the traumatic sequelae which are the focus of this chapter.

Stigmatization, Alienation, and Self-Consciousness in Anomalous Trauma

More information regarding the differences in individual experience would be very helpful in identifying effective coping mechanisms and vulnerable segments of the population. Nonetheless, it is clear that there are many individuals who are burdened by these events yet whose reality testing is fully intact contemporaneously with these experiences. One aspect of this excellent reality testing is evident when we realize that many patients screen this material intentionally: Knowing that disbelief and ridicule await those presenting a scenario or "memory" widely disparate from ordinarily accepted reality, these patients withhold this information from the helping professionals with whom they come in contact and, indeed, often from everyone around them. Showing an excellent assessment of the social realities which surround them, they fear that sharing these memorylike data will result in labeling and penalization by professionals and nonprofessionals alike. They bear a heavy burden in suffering discomforts which have no cause they can believingly identify, fearing the loss of their psychological equilibrium and sanity, fearing that if they share their dreadful suspicions or secret fears they will be separated from the good opinion of those they interact with, being seen as "crazy" and knowing that what they feel is neither safe, "normal," nor tolerable by the society at large. They are the guilty victims of some terrible secret which even they do not clearly know. Thus, they are burdened not only with the effects of the traumatic state which is thoroughly anomalous (because there is no known trauma to be seen which will account for their suffering), they are also heavily burdened with a secret and, often, with shame over having the secret.

In fact, they are quite correct in their assessment of the response which generally awaits them. During the process of active retrieval of memorylike material referred to above, Errol experienced overwhelming anxiety and depression. He became suicidal and attempted to kill himself. In the subsequent hospitalization, Errol debated whether to tell his attending psychiatrist whether he believed that he had been abducted and scarred by UFO (extraterrestrial) aliens many times in his life or to sequester this information. He reasoned that although he now partly believed this to be the case, sharing such information would result in hospitalization for a presumed psychotic state while his psychiatric assessment without this information would not. As he predicted, although he was referred for psychiatric treatment for his depression and anxiety, no psychotic features were present and he was released from hospital since he did not share this material with the examining or treating staff. It is likely that he was accurate in his assessment of the result sharing this material would have had on his opportunity to leave the hospital once the short-term effects of his suicide attempt had been counteracted. It is noteworthy that extensive psychometric and psychiatric evaluation at that time did not disclose any evidence of impaired reality testing and found that although he was quite clearly depressed, his emotional state seemed related to overwhelming but unidentified stress rather than underlying psychopathology (Vassos, personal communication, 1990).

Paradigms and Models of Anomalous Traumatic Events

Although parapsychological models suggest themselves, the paradigmatic example of EAT is contained in the example of the UFO abduction scenario. Typically able to present only partial recall to the clinician, the abductee may recall events which, if they *were* factual recounts of event-level reality, would certainly qualify as obvious precursors to PTSD states. Physical stigmata may remain after the experience, and fuller recall can often be potentiated by the same procedures which can be expected to yield similar results in trauma of a more prosaic sort. Yet clarity on the externally mediated reality state of these events is elusive. Significantly, sufficient psychopathology to account for either psychotic decompensation and delusion or self-mutilation is generally absent in these individuals. Thus, the prejudice of the listener may impose psychopathology on the patient even where it is not present. If an anxious and phobic patient were, for example, to confide to a therapist that he had been abducted by aliens who took him aboard a UFO and performed a series of medical procedures and examinations on him, that report alone might precipitate a diagnosis of psychosis in the absence of any other support for that assessment.

The material presented commonly lies so far outside the confines of personal and cultural belief systems that it would seem intolerably anomalous to most of us. We would probably dismiss or repudiate it using a few comfortable and familiar assumptions which hold so much obvious wisdom that they do not seem to require specific examination. Our index of suspicion for it would be so low that the diagnosis of PTSD very likely would not be considered even if the patient were showing classical signs of this disorder. Instead, the manifest content of the scenario alone might well precipitate a pathological assessment of the patient to be made in the absence of significant psychopathology. Following a diagnosis of major psychopathology, treatment would be instituted for the diagnosis, not for the patient's symptomatology.

In order to protect our reigning paradigms of reality, we make a rapid and comfortable series of determinations which dismiss the unacceptable and anomalous from our purview. This effectively precludes the open evaluation of the anomaly. Westrum identified several fallacies which hinder the open evaluation of anomalous events. The first is the self-reinforcing system of perception which holds that "It can't be; therefore, it isn't," the second is the belief that "if anomalous events are observed, they will usually be reported," and the third is that, once reported, the "relevant 'experts' will be aware of the reports." However, the self-protective nature of paradigm-based screening precludes the serious consideration of the anomalous event by experts whose expertise is built on a worldview which excludes the possibility of the anomaly's occurring. Hence the "expectable" response of most clinicians and laymen alike upon hearing of a UFO abduction account or other example of EAT would be an immediate dismissal of even the possibility that such an episode might occur rather than a rational, nonprejudicial, and therapeutically focused series of evaluations and interventions.

In the service of this paradigm protection, a variety of mechanisms may be brought to bear. First and foremost is the pathologization of the clinician's view of the individual who reports the paradigm-violating material as mentioned above. Treatment may then follow, including involuntary hospitalization (or incarceration), medication against the wishes of the patient (who may be deemed incompetent solely because of the content of the report), and potential violation of the civil liberties of the patient.

Clinicians frequently invoke a variety of "explanations" to further protect their own state of comfort. Dream states, suggestibility, poor reality testing, screen memories, outright dissembling, borderline psychopathology, or frank psychosis are customarily offered and accepted as evident and reasonable organizing models by which the presentation of this unacceptable anomalous material may be dismissed. These facile explanations, however, frequently fail to account for the often total lack of supporting evidence for these diagnoses present in the psychological state of the individual who reports the anomalous material. Further, they fail to account completely for either the posttraumatic status of the individual or the anomalous physical evidence which may be present. These are typical maneuvers by which the presentation of information which challenges paradigmatic assumptions is dismissed or screened out before the assumptions can be adequately tested for predictive value, reliability, and possible accuracy.

Historical Analogues of Anomalous Scientific Phenomena

Recounting the controversy surrounding the reality of meteorites, Ernst Friedrich Flourens Chladni wrote of

the time when, before the incontrovertible evidence of the fall of meteorites at l'Aigle in 1803, the European scientific community stridently agreed that no such thing as meteorites either existed or could exist. They validated those beliefs by denying (and even destroying) information to the contrary. He observed that there had been a time, "when people thought it necessary to throw away or explain as error everything that did not conform to a self-constructed model" (Clark & Westrum, 1987). Confirming this observation in 1759, James Pringle, a preeminent man of science, member of the Royal Society, and eventually its president, wrote of the impossibility of meteors: "And here I venture to affirm that, after perusing all the accounts I could find of these *phenomena*, I have met with no well-vouched instance of such an event; nor is it to be imagined, but that, if these meteors had really fallen, there must have been long ago so strong evidence of the fact, as to leave no room to doubt of it at present" (Pringle, 1759).

Our confident reality testing on behalf of our own paradigms and the well-being of our patients can, like that of Pringle, fail to take into account the nature of hidden information and the fact that the reporting of anomalous material does not, in itself, preclude truthful reporting based on the nonpathological reality of the patient. Good reality testing, including an open and fair assessment of the *actual*, not the *presumed*, emotional and psychopathological state of the individual, is highly desirable because it offers us the opportunity to apply the scientific method to our current level of theoretical sophistication and thereby refine our understanding of reality further still. Of course, this process is severely impeded when the new data are excluded from consideration strictly because they are too anomalous for assessment.

Paradigm of the UFO Abduction Scenario as Anomalous Trauma

In the increasingly frequently reported UFO abduction scenario, the patient (who may be a young child or an elderly patient, of any ethnic or national group, well or poorly educated, or otherwise demographically varied) typically reports some version of a scenario in which alien creatures, usually hominoid, short in stature, with large, dark, almond-shaped eyes, seemingly quite emotionless, compel his or her participation in an abduction. The abduction typically is composed of episodes which follow each other in predictable, but not inevitable, sequence. The segments generally include capture, medical examination, theophany, communication, and return (Bullard & Haines, Treat II). These events occur in strikingly uniform order, rarely include extraneous events, and are quite robust in their orderliness. Although not every segment is present in every scenario, there are some which are invariably present. Those present follow each other in rigidly predictable order although there is no intrinsic logic as to why, for example, theophany should follow examination rather than preceed it. Nonetheless, when theophany is present, it is present in its proper place.

Folklorist T. Edward Bullard examined 312 cases of UFO abduction reports going back as far as 1878. A facile dismissal asserts that all such stories represent variations on the widely publicized Betty and Barny Hill abduction story of 1962, first made widely public in 1966 (Fuller, 1966), is belied by the fact that similar stories describing similar creatures have been reported from around the world long before this particular case compelled worldwide attention.

Using "story-type" analysis familiar to folklore studies, Bullard (1987) found that

> Abduction stories follow a consistent pattern. A complex sequence of episodes orders the abduction story and a complex sequence of events orders several episodes. Reports stick to this order with remarkable fidelity. The events themselves are reasonable, but the most noteworthy thing about this persistent order is that the sequence is not inevitable. Interchanges of episodes and events could happen without disrupting the meaning of the story. No necessary logic holds the parts in place, yet even little-published elements stay in the same location time after time. In [nonabduction] stories from oral tradition the flexible parts flex and the result is swarms of variants all with twists of their own, alike in general themes but not fine details. Faithfulness to one pattern seems too much to expect of subjective experiences spread among many independent people, but an assumption of real experience easily accounts for the consistent order.

Furthermore, although about 75% of the UFO abduction scenarios available to us in English are in part or entirely the result of hypnotic regression techniques, the 25% which emerge without any hypnosis conform with the same exactitude to the story type and episode order as those which have emerged with the aid of hypnosis (Bullard, 1989).

Further still, Bullard stated that the easy "out" of a scenario offered and accepted consciously or unconsciously to the hypnotized, hypersuggestible patient by a believing hypnotist is equally unsupported by the available data because the same scenario, true to story type, emerged during sessions conducted by both UFO abduction-believing and -disbelieving hypnotists, knowledgeable hypnotists, and those totally ignorant of the topic.

Thus, careful examination of this anomalous material suggests that it cannot be dismissed out-of-hand solely as the product of disordered minds or of zealous believer-hypnotists. Looking closely at the population reporting this material, we find other features which are themselves a violation of commonly held assumptions about people reporting anomalous events, especially about those reporting UFO abduction as well. It is widely believed that this population must be a highly disordered one. Surprisingly, however, there is a remarkable lack of measurable psychopathology within this group. Although the assessment of this population remains preliminary, the indications contained in the the work which has been done strongly suggest that the population of those reporting this anomalous experience is primarily within normal limits for psychological integration and functional state. It is not our purpose here to attempt to ascribe relative reality value to the experience of abduction reported by these patients. Rather, precisely because it lies outside the realm of clinical expertise to assess *with absolute certainty* whether these events have actually occurred or if they represent a special type of fantasy state uniquely capable of precipitating a posttraumatic state, it is mandatory for the clinician to examine the impact upon the patient of these experiences, *whatever their source*. This must be done in a clear-sighted and open-minded fashion so that the impact of the experiences may be dealt with therapeutically rather than made into hidden events.

Absence of Gross Psychopathology

Intuitive assessment of the likely state of reality testing among the population reporting abduction experiences might suggest that psychotic-level distortions or other serious psychopathology would be found as a general rule. But it would also follow that one would expect these individuals to show other aspects of their affective, interpersonal, and adaptive realms to be impaired in significant ways as well. If such a level of distortion and delusion were present, a patient could be expected to demonstrate other evidence of significant reality disruption. Psychopathology of such magnitude would not be predicted to be present in a well-integrated, mature, and nonpsychotic individual. Instead, one would expect clinical and psychometric tools to reveal serious problems in numerous areas of adaptive functioning. It would be highly anomalous if otherwise well-functioning persons were to demonstrate a single area of floridly psychotic distortion leaving work, love, and play untouched. Indeed, if this single *idée fixe* were totally circumscribed, noninvasive, and discrete, that in itself would be highly anomalous. Furthermore, a coherent, shared system of delusion found principally in otherwise high-functioning individuals at all points on the developmental spectrum where speech is present which matches to a remarkable degree the similar circumscribed delusional systems of other equally high-functioning individuals strains credulity far more seriously than the notion that perhaps there is some kernel of experiential reality (of whatever type) which would account for these anomalous reports and traumata. Well-developed, fixed, delusional states with numerous elaborated and sequential components, physical, psychophysiological, and emotional, are not seen in otherwise healthy individuals, to say nothing of closely parallel and shared delusional systems among persons who are widely psychologically and demographically divergent.

The clinical picture presented by those claiming UFO abduction experiences, however, is a surprising one because, contrary to intuitive expectations, these persons are often basically well-functioning individuals attempting to cope with overwhelming stressors. There is a conspicuous absence of psychopathology of the magnitude necessary to account for the production of floridly delusional and presumably psychotic material. Although large-scale studies, long-term follow-up, and better sampling techniques are needed, preliminary clinical and psychometric results suggest, instead, a noteworthy absence of dissociative states, delusions, borderline symptomatology, hysteria, and conversion symptoms (Rodeghiler, personal communication, 1990).

Psychological Assessment of Anomalous Trauma: Preliminary Findings

In order to evaluate the psychometric status of a small number of UFO abductees, people who believed that they had, once or more in their lives, been subjected to UFO abductions ($n = 9$, 5 male, 4 female) were asked to participate in a psychological and psychometric evaluation. Elizabeth Slater, an experienced licensed clinical psychologist, carried out an investigation using interviews, projective tests (Rorschach, TAT, Draw a Person, and the MMPI), and the Wechsler Adult Intelligence Scale, but she did so under a false premise. Slater was told "the subjects were being evaluated to determine similarities and differences in personality structure, as well as psychological strengths and weaknesses." She was led to believe that the focus of the study was an interest in determining which psychological factors might account for creativity or its absence. The subjects withheld information pertaining to UFO abductions or UFO-related events but were instructed not to withhold other information. Although she understood her task to be that of identifying similarities and differences within these subjects, Slater (1990) was not able to determine a significant commonality in the psychometric evaluation of these people. She wrote:

while the subjects are quite heterogeneous in their personality styles, there is a modicum of homogeneity in several respects: (1) relatively high intelligence with concomitant richness of inner life; (2) relative weakness in the sense of identity, especially sexual identity; (3) concomitant vulnerability in the interpersonal realm; (4) a certain orientation towards alertness which is manifest alternately in a certain perceptual sophistication and awareness or in interpersonal hypervigilance and caution. . . . Perhaps the most obvious and prominent impression left by the nine subjects is the range of personality styles they present. . . . There is little to unite them as a group from the standpoint of the overt manifestations of their personalities. . . . They [are] very distinctive, unusual and interesting subjects. [But] along with above average intelligence, richness in mental life, and indications of narcissistic identity disturbance, the nine subjects also share some degree of impairment in personal relationships. For [some] subjects, problems in intimacy are manifest more in great sensitivity to injury and loss than in lack of intimacy and relatedness.

. . . The last salient dimension of impairment in the interpersonal realm relates to a certain mildly paranoid and disturbing streak in many of the subjects, which renders them very wary and cautious about involving themselves with others. It is significant that all but one of the subjects had modest elevations on the MMPI paranoia scale relative to their other scores. Such modest elevations mean that we are not dealing with blatant paranoid symptomatology but rather oversensitivity defensiveness, and fear of criticism and susceptibility to feeling pressured. To summarize, while this is a heterogeneous group in terms of overt personality style, it can be said that most of its members share being rather unusual and very interesting. They also share brighter than average intelligence and a certain richness of inner life that can operate favorably in terms of creativity or disad-

vantageously to the extent that it can be overwhelming. Shared underlying emotional factors include a degree of identity disturbance, some deficits in the interpersonal sphere, and generally mild paranoia phenomena (hypersensitivity, wariness, etc.). (p. 10)

Instead of a seriously disordered population with paranoid, delusional, hallucinatory, or other symptomatology, Slater found a group of people creatively enhanced, slightly impaired in the capacity for intimate trust, rather sensitive, and well within the range of normal functioning.

When she was informed of the true reason for the selection of the subjects for this evaluation (i.e., their shared belief that they had been abducted by aliens), Slater (1988) wrote an addendum to the original report. The addendum consists of a reevaluation of the data in light of the new information with which she was provided. In it she states:

The first and most critical question is whether our subjects' reported experiences could be accounted for strictly on the basis of psychopathology, i.e., mental disorder. The answer is a firm no. In broad terms, if the reported abductions were confabulated fantasy productions, based on what we know about psychological disorders, they could only have come from pathological liars, paranoid schizophrenics, and severely disturbed and extraordinarily rare hysteroid characters subject to fugue states and/or multiple personality shifts. . . . It is important to note that not one of the subjects, based on test data, falls into any of these categories. Therefore, while the testing can do nothing to prove the veracity of the UFO abduction reports, one can conclude that the test findings are not inconsistent with the possibility that reported UFO abductions have, in fact, occurred. In other words, there is no apparent psychological explanation for their reports. (p. 12)

Premorbid Disposition: Anomalous Trauma versus Prior Vulnerability

Preliminary assessment of the abduction population does suggest an important link with early childhood abuse. The relationship, however, is not a simple one. Although early traumatization (including birth trauma) (Lawson & McCall, 1985) has been advanced as the causative factor in the production of these scenarios, the personality sequelae of early abuse (sexual or nonsexual) and/or trauma do not seem to correlate to this material's presentation either. It has been noted that reports of early abuse are frequent in this population, but the significance of this remains unclear (Laibow, 1989; Ring, 1990). Wider and more carefully controlled studies are necessary to assess what, if any, link does exist between child abuse and later UFO-abduction scenario production (see Wilson, 1988, 1989, for a discussion of stress vulnerability and predisposition).

Demographic Variables

Equally intriguing is the demographic variability of those who give us these reports. Even though the reporters range from people as diverse as a mestizo Brazilian farmer (Creighton, 1969), an American corporate lawyer, a writer of horror and fantasy novels, and a black Midwestern minister, there is an intriguing and puzzling concordance of elements in these reports. Particular details of the scenarios repeat themselves with disturbing regularity no matter what the educational, national, social, experiential, or other demographic characteristics of the reporter. Young children, grandfathers, mothers, English speakers, and descendants of the Incas living in the high Andes, the rich, the poor, the literate, and the illiterate, the urban and the agrarian, in short, anyone emerging from any cultural matrix may tell basically the same tale.

High Degrees of Concordance in Individual Reports

In the abduction scenarios, both specific details and themes repeat themselves with great regularity. In general, the appearance and *modus operandi* of the aliens, their affect and procedures, their tools and interests, their crafts and physical features, all tally from report to report with a high rate of concordance (see e.g., Fuller, 1966; Fowler, 1979; Hopkins, 1981; Streiber, 1988). This intriguing fact seems impervious to the socioeconomic, educational, national, or cultural background of the abductee. Some writers argue that no one is free of the pervasive impact of science fiction and aliens which bombard us and point to the similarity of themes which might pertain to the scenarios (Kottmeyer, 1989; Laibow, 1989). Careful examination of these themes shows them to be quite divergent and rather remote from stories of UFO abduction. As previously mentioned, Bullard documents that the same stories were being reported over 100 years ago, rendering this notion a weak one. Furthermore, young children in remote parts of the globe probably are not reading science fiction in English or watching old movies on TV in villages in which there is no electricity. We are perhaps at a point in our cultural evolution which is the last at which it will be possible to find large numbers of truly naive subjects in this area in the global community. Thus, the need for good investigation is timely as well as intellectually and clinically relevant. Similarly, whether the individual has had previous contact with the literature of abduction or not seems to make little difference in this vein since the reports of individuals who can be shown to have had no exposure to abduction literature also contain these common features (Bullard, 1987).

Over and over again, when working with abductees who reported spectacular and mysterious events, skilled clinicians and investigators have reported that they are convinced that their subjects were being wholly truthful in their reports. Lie detectors, hypnosis, personality evaluations, and expert testimony have been employed in making these determinations. In general, in addition to concordant bits of data which puzzle the clinician, there is also a strong concordance of high anxiety and a PTSD-like response to the stress level of these experiences presented as part of the clinical picture which may be disorganizing for the individual. This PTSD-like response may be delayed in onset owing to the emergence of the stress-laden material long after its purported occurrence. Alternatively, it may be acute and chronic, either with or without recognition of the abduction-related material at a conscious level of awareness. Symptomatic relief is often rapid when exploration of this material takes place (Laibow, 1990a,b).

Thus, an intriguing adherence to type in terms of content, form, and the concordance of both content and event in these reports makes them unlike other fantasy-generated material. So striking is this adherence to type that certain frequently reported aspects of the abduction scenarios have been withheld by researchers in order to provide a "check" on the material being presented to them by individuals who may have had access to the relevant literature. But these details are routinely included in the patient's recall of scenarios despite the fact that they have never been made available to the general public. Reasoning that abductees may have been influenced at either the conscious or the unconscious level by material which they do not recall having encountered before, these sequestered details are important in the determination of reporter reliability. They are similarly important to the patient whose working through frequently includes a process of coming to terms with a level of reality which he or she can reasonably ascribe to these experiences. Interestingly, in cases in which the patient has read some of the abductee literature, the previously withheld material (of which the abductee is unaware) is often offered to the therapist with a sense of personal invalidation, apology, and embarrassment. The abductee may express concern that this information is less likely to be believed than the other material with which he or she is already familiar.

Hypnosis and the Memory of Trauma

It is useful for the clinician to bear in mind that most of what is known about reliability of memory under hypnosis has emerged from studies which either focus on simulated trauma or in nontraumatic recall. The memory traces and mode of storage of traumatic memory may not be similar to those of nontraumatic recall. It should also be noted that the clinical picture of the traumatized patient retrieving repressed material pertinent to the trauma is one in which, at least in our experience, suggestibility plays little or no part. Patients who are recounting traumatic experiences while in trance will verbally struggle and protest strongly if the therapist attempts to change the scenario as they have recounted it, in clear distinction to the hypersuggestibility of patients who recount material not traumatically weighted. In fact, clinicians investigating traumatic incidents (including abduction scenarios) have learned to make use of leading questions on a routine basis. When a patient supposedly recounting a traumatic episode allows the accretion of material into the scenario, it is a good indication that the recall being tapped is at least partly due to factors other than direct and traumatic experience (see Sollod, 1990). This is consistent with current thinking on state-dependent learning.

Alternatively, patients may also recall the events

leading to the traumatic episode but have an amnesia-like blank for the episode itself. This is true in UFO-abduction cases as it is in other types of trauma. Interestingly, the sighting of a UFO may be remembered but the events following may be absent from memory. For some individuals, the UFO sighting may include one or more humanoid forms. When considering the memory which does not seem to be available in spite of a concerted (often years-long) attempt to retrieve it, the patient may show either a nagging and anxious quality to this absence of recall or a bland indifference. Both the anxiety and the bland response tend to be replaced by more appropriate affect when this amnesia-like state is pierced. Patients may report a gap in time recall quite unlike a fugue state. This gap may range from a few minutes to a few hours. There may simply be only a perceived gap in remembered activities to suggest any anomalous occurrence to the patient, yet this gap is returned to over and over again in the patient's own mind. When asked "What is the strangest thing that ever happened to you," this episode, or the circumstances around it, may be produced as the response to this question even decades later. In many cases other witnesses experienced some aspect of this episode. It is frequent that they have, by mutual (but usually unspoken) agreement, come to terms with at least part of the anomaly by never referring to it either to each other or to "outsiders" then later. When this agreement is "renegotiated," corroboration is often forthcoming which assists the patient in clarifying aspects of this episode. The treating therapist may find him- or herself also treating an unexpected partner to the episode as the recall efforts of the identified patient leads to an upwelling of material in a co-experiencer.

Examination of the transcripts of hypnotic sessions which yield abduction material reveals that although subjects are sufficiently suggestible to enter the trance state as directed by the therapist, they resist having material "injected" into their account. They customarily refuse to be "led" or distracted by the therapist's attempts to change either the focus or content of their report. The subject characteristically insists upon correcting errors or distortions suggested or implied by the hypnotist during the session. Hence it is difficult to account for the similarities and concordances of these scenarios through the mechanism of suggestibility when these subjects so steadfastly refuse to be led by hypnotists.

In fact, it is even more striking that while these patients feel data which they are producing both in and out of hypnosis as experientially "real," nonetheless, they frequently seek to discount or explain away this bizarre and frightening material. This behavior occurs even though sharing the story regularly results in a significant remission of anxiety-related symptoms and discomfort. These abduction scenarios may be so ego-dystonic that the patients have frequently not shared the material with anyone at all or with only a small and highly select group of trusted intimates. Contrary to the common perception of publicity-seeking behavior, in the vast preponderance of cases, patients are reluctant to allow themselves to be publicly identified as having had these experiences. They perceive that the abduction scenario is so highly anomalous that they expect to experience ridicule and repudiation if they become associated with it publicly. It therefore functions like a guilty secret in the way that rape, incest, and other abuses have in the past.

Developmental Viscissitudes in Children Reporting Anomalous Trauma

It is helpful to look at Lenore Terr's case study of early memories of trauma (Terr, 1985) since even very young children have reported EAT. In her sample of 25 severely traumatized children, 18 showed consistent and prevalent behavioral memories in the form of (1) posttraumatic play, (2) personality changes related to frequent reenactments or to long-standing grief and/or rage, and (3) trauma-specific fears. She also noted a consistency of these behavioral memories with outside documentation of the trauma which often included parts, *but not the totality*, of the experience. These children were 2½ to 3 years of age at the time of the trauma. One girl who was 34 months at the time of the trauma was still having dreams which could be directly linked to the trauma at age 15 years. This symptom could be related to the fact that she had not received any psychotherapeutic treatment.

It is important to note that as children get older, they can give contemporary addenda and additions to verbal traumatic memories as well as reappraisal through new cognitive advances. Hence, a female abduction victim's referral to a perpetrator as "the devil" might well change over time as she becomes developmentally able to reconsider her old memories using new knowledge and cognitive skills. Just as a 4-year-old girl might remember an experience with male genitalia 30 months earlier as being "scared by a finger part," her explanation of "the devil" is commensurate with her emotional, social, and verbal development and may change with continued development.

Persons reporting the symptoms of PTSD secondary to EAT may show physical marks or various disruptions of development related to reproductive functions. In a non-EAT case, a child of 2 years was observed placing his penis in his 6-month-old sister's mouth in an effort to gain control over his own experienced abuse. There was no doubt that he had been taught the behavior. Any child who has experienced this type of invasive and inappropriate touching, no matter what the source, and who has received no treatment is at risk for infecting his or her peer group. Terr has documented cases of secondary symptoms, such as a young girl showing symptoms of PTSD after several months of playing a particularly frightening playground game ("wolf and rabbit") at recess. The game had been invented by a classmate who, it was later discovered, had been molested. The wolf-and-rabbit game was her attempt to master the position of the helpless victim which she has been forced to experience. Unfortunately, the trauma, instead of being mastered, was communicated to her peers, and it was there that the symptomatology of PTSD was first recognized and treated.

Without treatment, the risk of contagion between those who have experienced trauma (anomalous or not) and their peers (especially including family members) is high.

The abductions experience, whatever its origin, has been repeatedly observed to cluster in families. Thus, it is not surprising that both primary and secondary PTSD would be especially likely in families in which one member has had an anomalous trauma.

Just as there is a risk of underdiagnosis and mismanagement of the presenting symptoms, there is also the risk of a variation of the disorder which appears to be related to the Münchausen syndrome. In this condition, also called *chronic factitious disorder with physical symptoms*, individuals present their medical history with dramatic flair, but are extremely vague and inconsistent when questioned in detail. At times, parents with this disorder may present their children with reported fictitious ailments and watch as their children are subjected to various medical procedures for conditions which they know do not exist.

Conclusion

As can be seen from clinical vignettes and material presented in this chapter, the possibility of anomalous trauma presenting as, for example, alien abduction carries with it a wide spectrum of possible presentations. Even though it is not possible to evaluate with certainty the ultimate locus of reality of these experiential events, we can be sure that they provide an important and challenging source of trauma and its expectable sequelae. Clinicians and researchers would do well to devise research schemata to delineate more clearly the objective and the subjective components of reality which confound the topic of improbable, but not impossible, sources of trauma and their uniquely interesting sequelae.

But, even before closure can be achieved on the issue of the locus of these events, it is of crucial importance to treat the patient as he or she presents, not as we clinicians expect patients to present in the light of the data which we expect (and therefore allow ourselves) to see. Thus, the patient reporting (or suggesting) UFO abduction-related material, or other EAT, should be further assessed because that individual may or may not be a repository of ill health mentally or emotionally. Underlying pathology must, of course, be addressed, but so must underlying good health. If accurate assessment points out a healthy personality burdened by a traumatic load, then it is the responsibility of the clinician to treat the burden while respecting the strength in the personality. Pathologizing beyond the data simply because that is what we believe we *should* see is as unwarranted as ignoring the anomalous trauma because confronting it makes us uncomfortable. We cannot afford to take the tack of some clinicians of the recent past who just could not allow themselves to believe that parental abuse could happen, so they left the abusive sequelae untreated. Thus, the understanding of anomalous trauma serves to further refine our collective knowledge of traumatic stress syndromes.

References

Astley, R. (1953). Multiple metaphyseal fractures in small children. *British Journal of Radiology, 26,* 577–583.

Bakwin, H. (1956). Multiple skeletal lesion in young children due to trauma. *Journal of Pedicatrics, 49,* 7–15.

Bullard, T. E. (1987a). *UFO abductions: The measure of a mystery.* Washington, DC: The Fund for UFO Research.

Bullard, T. E. (1987b). *On stolen time: A summary of a comparative study of the UFO abduction mystery.* Washington, DC: The Fund for UFO Research.

Bullard, T. E. (1989). *Hypnosis and UFO abductions: A troubled relationship.* Washington, DC: The Fund for UFO Research.

Bullard & Haines, Treat II need ref & date; cited p.

Caffey, J. (1946). Multiple fractures in the long bones of infants suffering from chronic subdural hematoma. *American Journal of Roentgenology, Radium Therapy and Nuclear Medicine, 56,* 163–173.

Caffey, J. (1957). Some traumatic lesions in growing bones other than fractures and dislocations: Clinical and radiological features. *British Journal of Radiology, 30,* 225–238.

Clark, T., & Westrum, R. (1987). Paradigms and ferrets. *Social Studies of Science, 17,* 3–33.

Creighton, J. (1969). The amazing case of Antonio Villas Boaz. In C. Bowen (Ed.), *The humanoids* (pp. 200–238). Chicago: Contemporary Books.

Fowler, R. (1979). *The Andreasson affair.* New York: Bantam Books.

Fuller, J. G. (1966, October). Aboard a flying saucer. *Life.*

Hopkins, B. (1981). *Missing time: A documented study of UFO abductions.* New York: Ballantine Books.

Kardiner, A. (1941). *The traumatic neuroses of war.* New York: Paul B. Hoeber.

Kempe, C. J., Silverman, F. N., Steele, B. B., Droegemueller, W., & Silver, H. K. (1962). The battered child syndrome. *Journal of the American Medical Association, 181,* 17–24.

Kottmeyer, M. M., & Laibow, R. (1989). Dual victims: The abused and the abducted. *IUR,* pp. 3–9.

Kramer, W. H. (1989). *Recent experiences with PSI-counseling in Holland.* Paper presented at the 38th International Conference of the Parapsychology Foundation, London, England.

Laibow, R. (1989).

Laibow, R. (1990a). Some clinical considerations on patients regarding UFO abductions. In I. von Ludwinger (Ed.), *CES* Vol. XI.

Laibow, R. (1990b). Psychodynamic and psychophysiological . . . (TREAT II proceedings).

Lawson & McCall. (1985).

McCoid, A. H. (1965). The battered child and other assaults on the family: Part one. *Minnesota Law Review, 50,* 1–58.

Pringle, J. (1759).

Ring, K. (1990). *UFO and NDE self reporters: Results from the Omega project.* TREAT II proceedings.

Rodeghiler, M. (1990). Personal conversation with the author.

Sheils, M., Afrest, S., Maier, F., & Sethi, P. J. (1977, October 10). The battered children. *Newsweek,* pp. 112–116.

Silverman, F. N. (1972). Unrecognized trauma in infants, the battered child syndrome, and the syndrome of Ambroise Tardieu. *Radiology, 104,* 337–353.

Slater, E. (1988). *Results of 9 psychologicals.* Washington, DC: The Fund for UFO Research.

Slater, E. (1989). Results of MMPI testing on persons reporting UFO abductions. Personal communication with the author.

Slater, E. (1990).

Sollod, R. (1990). *An integrated psychotherapeutic approach to anomalous experiences.* Paper delivered at the Second Conference on Experienced Anomalous Trauma.

Sprinkle, L. (1988). The changing message of UFO activity: From empirical science to experimental science. In M. L. Ab-

103

selson, D. Ward, & K. P. Freeman (Eds.), *Paranormal research.* Fort Collins: Colorado State University.

Streiber, W. (1988). *Communion.* New York: Avon Books.

Targ, R., & Hastings, A. (1987). Psychological impact of psychic abilities. *Psychological Perspectives, 18,* 45.

Terr, L. (1985). Remembered images and trauma. *Psychoanalytic Study of the Child, 40,* 493–533.

van der Kolk, B. A. (1987). *Psychological trauma.* Washington, DC: American Psychiatric Press.

Vassos, L. (1990). Person communication with the author.

Westrum, R. (1982). Social intelligence about hidden events. *Knowledge: Creation, Diffusion, Utilization, 3*(3).

Wilson, J. P. (1988).

Wilson, J. P. (1989). *Trauma, transformation, and healing: An integrative approach to theory, research, and post-traumatic therapy.* New York: Brunner/Mazel.

Wooley, P. V., & Evans, W. A. (1955). Significance of skeletal lesions in infants remembling those of traumatic origin. *Journal of the American Medical Association, 158,* 539–543.

CHAPTER 9

Theoretical and Intervention Considerations in Working with Victims of Disaster

Beverley Raphael and John P. Wilson

Introduction

Compassionate and humanitarian concerns have dictated the intense response that occurs following most major disasters throughout the world. Such catastrophes are evocative, fill the onlookers with vicarious dread, and, at the same time, provide a focus for the altruism and good will that will strengthen and sustain those affected throughout the crisis period. Although the shock, horror, and grief that may follow have long been recognized, the more profound psychological consequences that will affect significant numbers of people are only now being systematically and consistently quantified (Raphael, 1986).

The commonalities between community and personal disaster and across a range of different catastrophic experiences allow a further definition of the principal themes: the various traumatic elements; their interaction with personal factors in the individual; their interrelationship with the sociocultural milieu; the processes of adaptation to the traumatic experience; and the ultimate outcome (Wilson, 1989). The correlates of morbidity, and the factors influencing vulnerability and resilience are now being identified across major and personal disasters, both "natural" and "man-made." Such understandings provide the conceptual rationale on the basis of which interventions may be developed (e.g., Lystàd, 1988).

Beverley Raphael • Department of Psychiatry, Royal Brisbane Hospital, University of Queensland, Herston 4029, Australia. John P. Wilson • Department of Psychology, Cleveland State University, Cleveland, Ohio 44115.
International Handbook of Traumatic Stress Syndromes, edited by John P. Wilson and Beverley Raphael. Plenum Press, New York, 1993.

However, the systematic implementation of preventive and treatment programs is still in its infancy. There is also a need for controlled trials with a range of goal-oriented programs, to evaluate the most effective interventions for communities, individuals, and groups and the most cost-effective ways of achieving optimal outcomes.

Trauma of Disaster

By definition, disasters overwhelm, at least temporarily, the coping resources of the community and of individuals. They do so by the threat inherent in them: the threat of death, loss, and destruction to the community or the individual. The system at macro- or micro-level must respond to this threat, deal with the trauma and its consequences, if it is to survive. Such overwhelming trauma will always be remembered, must be made meaning of, will be reworked and adapted to, in a variety of ways. The consequences of damage, loss, and altered functioning will be mitigated by the response of the organism or the system itself in its interaction with and support from wider systems. The ultimate consequences are never unitary but include an incorporation of the event into a view of the world, an incorporation of the trauma and confrontation with it into identity and perceptions of strength and vulnerability, and residua of pain and power, hurt and survival.

Trauma and the Community: Theoretical Considerations

When the community is struck by catastrophe, it faces threat, perhaps with little warning beforehand,

and cannot escape. There is the threat of death and destruction to its integrity as a whole, as well as to its members. It is likely to suffer losses, including both material losses and the sense of invulnerability. At least temporarily, its usual systems of functioning are overwhelmed, so that response systems come into play to deal with the trauma. Response to the trauma occurs in patterns which may facilitate or hamper survival and adaptation. Rescue, recovery, and restitution begin as damage and losses are counted, cared for, mended, and mourned. Meaning is made of what has happened and why. The events are reviewed, incorporated, and moved on from as part of the experience of ongoing existence. Rituals, memories, and memorials may give testimony to its occurrence and to mastery. Or painful scars, wounds, and disintegration may be present, reflecting what has unalterably occurred.

This concept of threat and damage to the whole community system implies potentially important consequences, and may govern intervention strategy and its impact at all system levels—individual, group, organization, community, and society—because these levels are interlinked. These parameters of emergency and disaster response have been well described by sociological researchers such as Quarantelli (1978, 1982, 1984) and especially Drabek (1986). How and to what degree these different systems are affected depends on the severity, extent, and focus of a disaster, and whether key systems are affected or destroyed (e.g., communication centers, hospitals). In the 1989 earthquake in Newcastle, Australia, damage to telephone exchanges, a major hospital, and city core buildings added to response difficulties.

The nature of the community, its organizational systems, its leadership, its networks and communication will influence its capacity to perceive and respond to the threat of disaster, and its preparation and training for this or other emergencies. The community's background level of integration, its strength as a unit, and its disintegration, deprivation, or impaired functioning will influence its capacity to respond to the trauma and may influence adaptation and outcome afterward. In the period of impact, responses may be adaptive or nonadaptive. The levels of death and destruction that follow may be such as to impair the very fabric and nature of the community. Emergency organizational systems that arise to respond may succeed or fail. The recovery organizational system that subsequently evolves may reflect active mastery and strength of the community or may function poorly if it is dominated by personal or political motives, scapegoating, splitting, inflexible bureaucratic responses, and aggrieved bitterness and entitlement.

If destruction of buildings and property has been great, evacuation and dislocation of families may alter permanently the human nature of the community. Key elements of functioning include: (1) patterns of communication and information; (2) resources and their sharing and distribution; (3) leadership, both regular and the spontaneous natural leadership that may arise; (4) social networks and their support of their members and others; (5) sociocultural prescriptions which define the nature of catastrophe in general and this catastrophe in particular, acknowledging both suffering and strength; (6) the roles of "victims," "helpers," and others; and (7) the recovery pathways.

Such systems may be highly functional, providing excellent two-way communication with the rapid availability of and access to accurate information (e.g., what to do, where to go, extent of death, damage, and loss, how to get help); adequate resources and access to them, with power over and equity in their distribution; strong leadership oriented to survival in the emergency, comfort and care in the recovery, and promoting hope, mastery, and active involvement in the restitution of the community; strong, supportive, communicating, caring, and flexible social networks; sociocultural prescriptions which recognize strength, are compassionate to suffering, and do not marginalize, blame, or scapegoat but rather empower.

Negative parameters in these dimensions are likely to threaten adaptation of the community as well as its individual members.

The time course of adaptation to trauma is often usefully considered in terms of phases, although these may not be simple, clear-cut, or occur in a fixed time frame. Initially, there is the period of euphoria, altruism, intense affiliation, and supportive interaction in the immediate postemergency phase. This is the "honeymoon" or "therapeutic community" phase, lasting through the early days or weeks, when good feelings and hopefulness predominate. Gradually, this gives way to the "phase of disillusionment," during which the realities of loss and damage are faced, when promised support and restitution fall short, and bitterness, grief, frustration, conflict, and deprivation come to the fore. Progressively there is a return to equilibrium—which may be at a new and more positive level as a result of the successful mastery of the challenge and trauma; or a level much as was present before, but inevitably different because of what has happened; or to ongoing disillusionment, despair, and perhaps disintegration in the "second disaster" as it may be called.

Thus, the ultimate adaptations for the community and society systems and subsystems will reflect the response to and mastery of these challenges and the incorporation of them into the community's identity and functioning. The disaster is often named for the community (e.g., the San Francisco earthquake) and this may mean significant issues for the community's view of itself, how it is viewed by the wider society, and important aspects of its future successful functioning.

Trauma and the Individual: Theoretical Considerations

When extreme events outside ordinary experience occur, whether they occur as a major disaster affecting the community as a whole or to individual members in their personal disasters, there are a number of important dimensions which will influence reactions to them and the pattern of outcomes that may be a consequence. The theoretical and conceptual basis of response is usefully considered in terms of the model of Green, Wilson, and Lindy (1985) and more recently of Wilson (1989). Such models take into account: features of the traumatic event and experience; personal and background factors of the individual; the sociocultural milieu of the recovery environment; the processing of the experience by the indi-

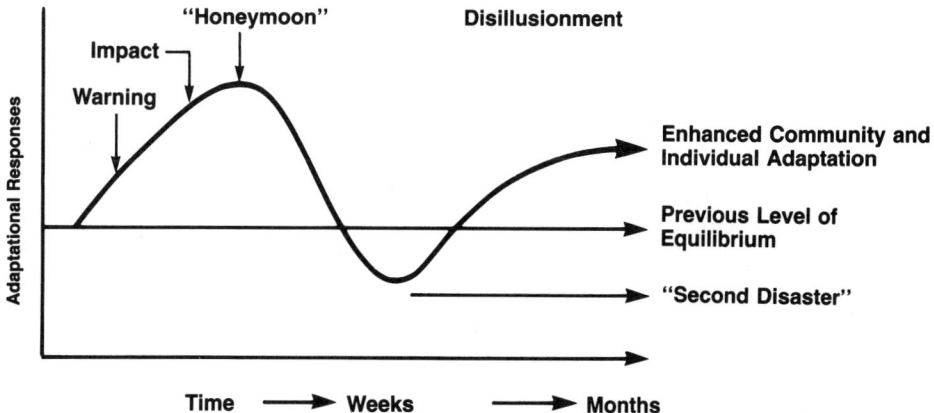

Figure 9.1. Phases of response to disaster.

vidual; and the spectrum of altered states and outcome both cross-sectionally and longitudinally.

This overview, of course, makes the assumption of defining those affected by the experience: a difficult task in community disasters, as indicated by Green (1982), because effects may depend on presence, propinquity to the event, perceptions of it as a threat or challenge, and direct and indirect experience of it. "Victims" have been variously defined as primary, secondary, and so forth. The near-miss may become a victim in the psychological sense, similar to the distant bereaved, neither of whom may have personally experienced the episode. Nevertheless, and bearing these issues in mind, the elements that follow have been shown to be of significance.

The Traumatic Experience

While early disaster and traumatic stress research tended to present a unitary view of the trauma, there is increasing recognition of the multiple stressor dimensions and the fact that they may each be identified by more quantitative parameters, such as severity, duration, potential for recurrence, and so forth. The principal dimensions of trauma have been identified by Raphael (1976), Horowitz (1976), Parker (1977), Western and Doube (1979), Weisæth (1977–1983), Holen, Sund, and Weisæth (1979), Wilson, Smith, and Johnson (1985), Wilson (1989) and more recently reviewed (Raphael, 1986; see also Chapter 49, in this volume). They encompass as primary traumata (1) *encounter with death and destruction,* either the personal threat to life or the massive, shocking, mutilating, and gruesome deaths of others; (2) *loss of person, property,* or other such variables as home, community, social network, workplace, and the like.

Other traumatic dimensions arise in association with these and include (1) *dislocation* following evacuation and loss of community, home, or family; (2) *moral conflict* and *responsibility* trauma in relation to roles of the individual in the event; (3) receipt of *intentional* harm or injury; (4) *causing* death or severe harm to another; (5) exposure to *subtle threat* of life and health as in toxic or noxious exposure; and (6) loss of sense of *personal invulnerability.*

Perceived exposure, severity, and duration operate with each of these traumata, as do degree of expectation, anticipation, warning, and preparation. All parameters influence consequences.

Finally, the *causative influence* of the trauma may be significant, whether an "act of God" or man, or an interaction of these two. An individual may be the victim of fate, of unfortunate accident, neglect, or negligence, or of the action of human beings with innocent or malevolent and violent intent. Particular trauma may reside with this latter aspect, particularly breach of trust, fearfulness, anger, and problems of acceptance and resolution.

Personal Background Factors

A number of research studies have attempted to identify the parameters of vulnerability and resilience in individuals, and how the traumatic experience is responded to in terms of these. Although early studies saw individual vulnerability (with the inference of inadequacy) as the chief cause of morbid outcome (see Chapter 5, in this volume for detailed consideration of the role of revived early conflict and other psychoanalytic formulations), more recent research and clinical experience emphasizes the critical importance of the traumatic event.

The most recent research findings and clinical accounts of major community and personal disasters point to the *interaction* of certain personality constellations and previous experiences with the traumatic experience and its processing. These factors range from possible psychiatric vulnerability as indicated by past and/or family psychiatric history, issues of past experience, to training which may influence the person's reaction to and way of dealing with the trauma. "Neuroticism" has been identified as correlating with vulnerability (see Chapter 34, in this volume) and may indicate certain temperamental and personality constellations that respond to stress by heightened arousal and greater risk for development of disorder. Clearly there may be other variables as yet unidentified by research, and the findings with regard to past psychological problems are by no means clear-cut.

Sociodemographic factors may also indicate groups at heightened risk, for example those with lower education, socioeconomic deprivation, and marginal ethnic or racial status. Some studies have suggested women to be more at risk, at least for the development of PTSD, but others have emphasized their resilience in the face of adversity (Gibbs, 1989). Such variables are not themselves readily amenable to intervention at the time of disaster but may help to target programs to those in greatest need.

There is much evidence to suggest that previous *training and preparation* will be helpful. The mechanisms may be through increasing the sense of personal mastery at the time of the trauma, thereby lessening the feelings of helplessness: knowing "what to expect," "what to do," may enhance cognitive as well as practical mastery and may thus decrease "shock," lessen terror, and prevent dissociation.

Vulnerability issues related to behavior and experiences during the period of occurrence of the trauma may also be important. It is increasingly obvious that *dissociation* during this time of the acute episode of threat correlates with the subsequent development of morbidity for many people (see Chapter 39, in this volume). Disorganized and other nonadaptive behaviors during the episode are similarly associated with unfavorable outcome (Weisæth, 1983). Distortion of cognitive process including time perception, the inability to save another's life in the process of fighting for one's own survival, or other behaviors evoking terror, shame, guilt, or negative affects may further complicate the capacity to process and integrate the experience subsequently.

Coping styles reflecting individual personality in interaction with the environment may influence perception of the trauma, response to it, and adaptation afterwards. Problem-solving active styles may be more significant in the emergency; other styles, such as expression of feelings, may prove more adaptive subsequently. Gibbs (1989) reviewed many of these factors and found that there is evidence that more active, approach coping styles, rather than avoidance/denial may be more effective, and there is considerable support for the value of active coping. Higher internal locus-of-control scores have been associated with better outcome in some studies, but these may really represent an active coping process.

Past experience of trauma might create further vulnerability, especially if it remains unresolved. Balanced against this risk is the concept of "stress inoculation," which may be theorized as helping to prevent extreme reactions and enhancing the capacity to cope with stress. Certainly, clinical experience suggests that some individuals may be more vulnerable because of previous traumatization and loss, with recent trauma opening into these earlier issues. For example, one older woman who suffered in the Newcastle earthquake had suffered in concentration camps during the war. She had also experienced several serious earthquakes in her European country of origin and multiple bereavements. She had moved to Newcastle because there were "no earthquakes there." She had managed her earlier traumatic experiences, but this was the final trauma which brought past unresolved trauma and grief to be dealt with. Yet protective influences may exist from experience with, survival through, and mastery of stressful events. Research is needed to clarify the contribution of such experiences and the differential effects they may have on outcome.

Many workers highlight the *meaning* made of the traumatic event, which may link to *perceptions*, past experience, and many of the variables above. The delineation of all these factors, their interrelationship to each other and to the past experience and personality of the individual, and how they affect outcome are very complex and need much further research to identify their significance and contribution.

Interpersonal and Social Milieu: Recovery Postdisaster

How the society defines the event, influences and prescribes a response, and facilitates recovery will influence ultimate outcome. The *meaning* made of the event by the society may influence all other parameters.

Sociocultural prescriptions may be critical, regarding what is acknowledged as legitimate "suffering" and who are legitimate "victims"; what is appropriate "care," who is eligible for it, and who can provide it; and what are the sanctioned pathways to recovery. Victims may be seen as passive and helpless and may be expected to stay that way if they are to be helped by powerful helpers. The more powerful role of survivor may be readily acquired in the transition from victim state, or it may not be accessible. Restitution, retribution, and compensation may be expected and available or may become, through societal influences, complex and further stressors. Justice and its meaning and actuality in the society may strongly influence processing of the trauma and outcome.

Specific *cultural norms* regarding response to trauma and its healing may be influential: For instance, some societies may favor avoidance, denial, and privacy, whereas others may prefer ritual, expression of feelings, and working through. Some cultures make specific provision (e.g., American Indian healing rituals; see Wilson, 1989).

A very specific area of difficulty may relate to the *talking cure* of psychotherapy. Although adaptations have been made to enhance the telling of the trauma story in situations as widely different as South African township youth in the Sanctuary Project described by Straker (personal communication, 1988), to the Cambodian refugees cared for by Kinzie (see Chapter 26, in this volume), this westernized approach may not sit comfortably with an ethos of privacy and control of feelings that is part of many other cultures. Similarly, in the personal disaster of bereavement, traditional Australian Aboriginal culture affirms powerful ceremonial rituals expressing the affects of grief and promoting mastery (Reid, 1979), while traditional Anglo-Saxon culture has deritualized and curtailed these.

Social networks with social support are crucial variables in the recovery process in both personal and community disasters. This has been well documented in bereavements (Raphael, 1983) and in other traumatic situations of personal and community disaster (Solomon, 1986). Supportive interactions may occur between the traumatized individual and his *primary confidant* and/or *family group*. Or they may arise from networks of *workplace and neighborhood* or social and leisure situations. The natural groups that arise postdisaster, particularly those groups that have shared a specific experience, are likely to be valuable in helping with talking-through, cathar- sis, and making personal and shared meaning of what has happened. These intense attachments of the "thera- peutic community effect" may be extremely helpful and may merge into organizations to facilitate recovery, as, for instance, in self-help and recovery groups which are likely to promote active mastery.

Perceptions of social support have been identified in many personal traumatic situations and in the face of adversity as being influential in outcome. Those who perceive their social networks as inadequate, or unhelp- ful, or who lack a personal confidant, may be the more vulnerable.

The *basic resources of the community*, the degree to which these are damaged or lost, particularly in terms of the extent of destruction, will be powerfully influential in the capacity of the social environment to support the individual's recovery process. Most of the world's disas- ters occur in countries where economic and other re- sources are at a low level, impacting on the possibility of preparing for, responding to, and recovering from disas- ter. This degree of deprivation will override all others and the struggle is one of survival.

Processing of the Trauma

Horowitz (1976, 1986) provided the most widely adapted model of processing the traumatic experience. His model of *cognitive processing* with alternating intru- sive reexperiencing and avoidant numbing, leading to a gradual working-through of the overwhelming experi- ence, is now widely accepted (see Chapter 4, in this volume). It is likely that these phenomena, as well as the accompanying arousal, occur frequently as part of the early reactive processes after an overwhelming experi- ence, and that they are extremely common. For most people, they settle and do not continue into further dis- tress, vulnerability, or to the development of disorder (see Chapter 34, in this volume).

An important issue which has not been widely rec- ognized is the different processing, that is, *grieving and mourning*, involved in adapting to loss. This issue is par- ticularly complicated because many of the losses which have been studied have been those occurring in disasters (e.g., Lindemann, 1944), or other very traumatic circum- stances of loss, and the reactions described are often more related to the traumatic encounter with death (i.e., the *circumstances* of the loss) than the processes of grief and bereavement to resolve it. Preoccupations of the be- reaved are with the circumstances of the trauma, often including traumatic images of the dead person, rather than grieving and mourning with yearning, sadness, and the sorting through of many different memories of the person in the past.

Earlier research (Raphael & Maddison, 1976) identi- fied these separate processing aspects. Work carried out by Lindy, Green, Grace, and Titchener (1983) also de- fined the separateness of these processes and the need to deal with the trauma-processing aspect in psycho- therapy before the loss-processing aspect could be worked with in their group of disaster victims. The Pynoos studies with children clearly identify, with sepa- rate research instruments, the differential effects of grief and encounter with death (Pynoos, 1989). Similarly, re-

search currently in progress (Middleton & Raphael, 1987–1990) is defining these processes and phenomena further.

To summarize, *processing the traumatic encounter with death* will bring heightened arousal, alternating reex- periencing with affect, and avoidance and numbing of affect. There may be different patterns of predominance of these components and their related phenomena. The affects are usually those of fear and terror. For most, this process settles within days or weeks of the event, unless maintained or locked into high levels of response be- cause traumatization was so great, or because of interac- tion with the elements of vulnerability outlined above, or because of the failure of facilitating processes to help deal with the trauma, or because of inhibitory processes which prevent successful working-through. This latter might include ongoing or new stresses, such as those related to the battle for survival.

After the initial shock, the processes of *grieving and mourning* for people, structures, and things that have been destroyed bring heightened arousal and anxiety associated with loss: The survivor searches and scans the environment, seeking familiar persons and aroused for their return. The perceptual set of the bereaved antic- ipates the lost objects, whose images are constantly in mind. This grief-related anxiety is, therefore, separation anxiety (which would be assuaged by return of the de- ceased), not the anxiety of expectation of continued life threat, as in trauma processing.

When a lost person fails to "return" and the pangs of grief with yearning and longing for him or her are not requited, they gradually attenuate. There may be efforts to mitigate or shut out pain associated with the remind- ers of the loss, but the memories of the person are nei- ther images of horror nor intrusions in the sense noted above (unless there are traumatic phenomena associated with the death). Mourning processes involve review of the memories, both positive and negative, with sadness, and sometimes further anger at the loss, guilt on some occasions, fear about managing without the deceased, or any of the wide-ranging feelings relevant to the com- plexity of all human relations. Emotions of sadness may overlap with and be difficult to distinguish from depres- sion.

Here, too, there is an intense early phase in the initial weeks of mourning, but for most people this phase gradually attenuates, leaving some residual phe- nomena of memories and affect. Such normal phenome- na may lead into one of the forms of pathological grief, to depression, or to some other morbid outcome specific or nonspecific to loss, depending on the severity of the loss, the presence of concomitant traumatic stressors, and other vulnerabilities extant at the time of bereave- ment or occurring subsequently (Raphael, 1983).

It is useful to consider these as normal reactions to abnormal experiences and to recognize that, for the most part, there will be intense early response and subse- quent adaptation and resolution. Some individuals will go on to suffer disorders specifically reflecting the pro- cessing phenomena (e.g., PTSD, pathological grief); others will demonstrate nonspecific morbid patterns. Time courses vary enormously and there are no clear and exact endpoints to the processing of these two pri- mary experiences (i.e., encounter with death and loss) as they merge into the ongoing realities of human life and existence.

Outcomes

From the range of phenomena described in PTSD, outcomes may vary from co-morbidity, such as depressive disorders, anxiety, substance abuse, through to character pathology, physical health problems, pathological bereavement syndromes, and impacts on social behavior, personal relationships, work, personal functioning, and enjoyment of life. These outcomes have been summarized elsewhere (Raphael, 1986). As noted, there may be a complex spectrum of positive and negative adaptations which need to be understood. Much of the determination of outcome will depend on the multiple variables described above as stressor dimensions of the traumatic event and processing issues, the interactions of these variables with the societal systems as a whole, the time frames that are current, what has passed, and the distance to which the individual has progressed on the pathway to integrating the experience. If he or she is still locked into reliving it, preoccupied months and years later, it is likely that other negative outcomes will result as well, and the moving-on process may only be facilitated by the full assessment of and intervention with each one of these factors.

Interventions for Victims of Disaster

Interventions may be developed before disaster and trauma occur or be provided during and afterward. Goals may include *prevention* of negative outcomes and the facilitation of positive ones in individuals (through normal reactive processes and their support) or *treatment and management* of persons already suffering distress and impairment as a consequence of experienced disaster.

Planning and development of such interventions require not only a thorough understanding of the issues outlined above, but also sanctions for such interventions, including access and consultancy to the organizational systems involved in disaster response and management (Raphael, 1986).

Any proposed interventions should have well-defined goals, be targeted to those most in need, be flexible and adaptive to the realities of the disaster and postdisaster community, and reflect compassion, warmth, and empathy toward those who have been affected. Clear intake criteria and assessments should be defined, as should proposed therapeutic or preventive measures and their rationale, outcomes sought and how and when they will be measured, and how the program will be evaluated. There is a dearth of systematic documentation and studies in the field of postdisaster social and psychological intervention; documentation, further data gathering, and systematic research are greatly needed. Such programs provide an ideal opportunity for evaluation, although the emergency ethos favors a rapid and sometimes emotional response and a tendency to bypass these formal requirements. This is well attested to by the scientific literature of disaster studies, which reports only a few attempts to investigate the effectiveness of interventions (Lindy *et al.*, 1983; Singh & Raphael, 1981) either in a preventive framework (as to workers in critical incident stress debriefing) or in treatment of posttraumatic stress disorder in direct victims of disaster.

There are, however, theoretical and empirical evidence as well as some research findings which can provide a framework for interventions, utilizing what is known and has been briefly outlined above. Interventions will be considered in three major frameworks: social system interventions, personal interventions dealing with death encounter, and personal interventions dealing with loss.

Social System Interventions

These interventions are those initiated by the mental health consultant to prevent or deal with those negative aspects of social system response either before, during, or after the disaster. As indicated previously, the consultant can only provide such interventions if he or she has sanctions to do so. The military ethos of many counterdisaster organizations, a community ethos of "it can't happen here," the life-threatening, overwhelming, and practical problems confronted in the crisis, have all, in the past, led to mental health issues taking second place. However, most systems now recognize, acknowledge, and utilize some consultancy of this kind, especially in the United States.

This involvement may encompass ideally pre- and postdisaster programs and should aim to (1) promote *predisaster* awareness and knowledge and skills about common psychological reaction patterns to disaster threat, impact, and aftermath and the most adaptive responses and behavior. There is ample evidence that this will enhance resilience and provide some protective effect against the traumata of disaster. Exercises and training further familiarize people with adaptive responses, thereby lessening anxiety and helplessness at the time of catastrophe (and probably increasing survival). Information and education are extremely valuable, as are the enhancement of networks of communication and support.

(2) *Acute phase* consultancy can provide interventions ranging from support for disaster leaders and opportunities for them to debrief; to guidance for emergency and rescue workers, both professional and volunteer; to triage and emergency management of victims whose behavior is disorganized, nonadaptive, or showing the "disaster syndrome" or who are psychiatrically decompensated. Guidance can be given regarding the importance of keeping families together and preventing further traumatic effects of separation by retaining social networks as far as possible when evacuation is essential; maintaining early, rapid, accurate, effective communication of information to all those affected and involved, including families and workers; having body identification procedures and providing those bereaved in a disaster the opportunity to see and say their good-byes to the deceased (Singh & Raphael, 1981). It is vital to educate media and publication systems employees who record and publicly present the catastrophe, to limit tours of

duty and the amount of traumatic exposure of disaster workers, and to ensure subsequent debriefing for these persons (see Chapter 76, in this volume). Of interest in this latter context is the brief report of Tyrer (1989) following the Lockerbie disaster, where with support, shorter tours of duty, rotation and relief, he appears to have mitigated against posttraumatic effects for those involved in body handling.

Although there is considerable empirical support for such *debriefing* to deal with the stresses experienced by all those who respond to the emergency, there is still a need for systematic controlled trials to establish the effectiveness of such interventions (Raphael, 1990).

(3) Assessment should be made of the need and planning for mental health systems response in the *postdisaster* phase. The mental health consultancy may need to negotiate for a place in the postdisaster recovery organizational systems, to ensure that adequate resources, access, and expertise are available to deal with the likely mental health problems that will arise. *Estimates* will relate to the numbers in identified risk categories (e.g., the bereaved, those exposed to life threat and the deaths of others, the dislocated, the separated, the injured, and children). Mental health expertise will be required to carry on consultancy efforts during the recovery phase (in schools, local government, and community organizations) as well as to provide specific personal interventions for those at risk or affected.

At a systems level, there is a need for *generic educational programs* to provide information about normal responses, sources of help, and preventive and helpful measures. Such education is necessary for the public, including helpers involved in the recovery phase, such as welfare, housing, volunteer, and all health and relief workers. Programs should deal with the normality of responses, the patterns for different groups (e.g., children), the likely positive outcomes and how to facilitate them, as well as how to assist or refer those in need of counseling or psychiatric help. The importance of such *information* cannot be underestimated but must be appropriately presented.

Organizational interventions may range from the identification of organizational stressors, to analysis of and intervention with organizational difficulties which arise after the disaster. These range from inadequacy to splitting, to over-response, to successful management. The critical importance of the affected community's involvement in and decision-making about its own recovery process may need to be reinforced through interventions (as, e.g., to promote the development of self-help organizations with goals for recovery and renewal). Special assistance may be needed to promote recognition of, and management for, the stresses carried by workers through formal organizational interventions sanctioning debriefing, counseling and support services, or other work and roles. Scapegoating, splitting, blame, and political manipulations are particularly destructive and interventions may need to assist organizations to recognize or prevent and deal with these themes.

Interventions may also be aimed at *mobilizing and strengthening social networks* (Solomon, 1986). This may mean promoting access to kinship networks which are most often those involved, and helping to develop extra assistance through other systems, such as friends,

neighbors, informal care-givers, and community gate-keepers. Media education, network development, utilization of indigent-support persons, and self-help systems may all be useful. These networks are important sources of information, comfort, advice, and practical assistance. Policies postdisaster should take each of them into account and promote, utilize, and develop them as far as possible.

Guidance to and debriefing for *community leaders* may be valuable but needs to be provided sensitively. They are likely to take on very heavy responsibilities, and often become overinvolved and unable to utilize the skills of others, or subsequently to hand over control so that the community can provide its own response and organizations. This may reflect a "counterdisaster syndrome"; assistance with this may facilitate a more consultative and effective recovery process involving other community leaders and representatives.

Defining phases and promoting community recovery processes of *grieving*, *thanksgiving*, memorialization, and celebration of survival through testimony in commemorative theatre, art, and writing may help the community gradually and progressively, as its own time frames permit, move on from the trauma and loss to the phase of renewal and recovery, in which the disaster is integrated into its ongoing existence and is seen as a symbol in the past, not only of the hurt and loss, but also of community strengths.

Personal Interventions Dealing with Death Encounter and Its Consequences

With personal interventions, clinicians aim to deal with the traumatically stressful reactions of individuals who have either experienced threat to their own lives, or witnessed, seen, or been associated with the deaths of others under violent, shocking, or horrific circumstances. Important elements include the severity of the perceived threat, elements of helplessness and terror, inescapable horror, or massive gruesome, mutilating, or otherwise horrific violent deaths of others, especially children. Assault or horrific threat to self or others may also create a similar trauma. Those likely to be so exposed are those close to the center of violent natural (cyclone, tornado) or man-made (crash) catastrophes, where they might have died themselves, have seen others do so, or were severely injured and threatened with death. Elements of fear, terror, and helplessness, gruesome images (e.g., decapitation) are prominent, or there may have been dissociation and isolation of affect. The person may or may not have responded appropriately to the threat with resultant feelings of either pride and mastery, or shame, conflict, guilt, and regret. The remembered images or specific screenlike images and their associated feeling states are likely to constitute the form of intrusive and reexperiencing components of the reaction; the shutting out, deadening, and numbing of these, comprise the avoidant responses. Arousal, a mechanism initially appropriate in response to a threat, is maintained or returns, inappropriately for the reality now that the danger has gone.

Prevention approaches may be directed toward those

who are seen as vulnerable through exposure to such experiences, including those severely exposed (e.g., survivors of an air crash) and others who perceive threat as significant in association with such circumstances, or those who might be considered vulnerable for other reasons (concurrent injury or loss). A group for whom such approaches have been used includes such emergency workers as fire service, police, ambulance, paramedic, medical and nursing, body handling, and victim identification personnel.

Traumatic or critical incident *stress debriefing* has been a format applied since the late 1970s in an attempt to assist with worker stress and centers on early intervention in groups for emergency workers. The processes include review of the experience, expression of feelings, provision of information on responses and their normality, and advice to help adaptive coping. Although early work (see Chapter 76, in this volume) emphasized intervention in the first 24 to 48 hours, most workers now find the first few days and even the first week appropriate. Follow-up contact or debriefing, and supportive counseling programs complement this model, which promotes confrontation with the experience, expression of feeling about it, and active cognitive and practical mastery. Similar methods are used to assist individuals who have been through traumatic experiences, including such personal disasters as armed hold-ups, assault, rape, violent attack, or witnessing death. Empirically, there is need to support this approach, but its scientific basis and optimal format are yet to be established in controlled trials.

General evidence to support the value of *personal preventive interventions* involving catharsis, discussion, and sharing what has happened comes from a number of sources. Military psychiatrists demonstrated the effectiveness of the "forward psychiatry" treatment concept of immediacy, proximity, and expectancy in a rapid return of the soldier to function with his combat unit. That this may only be effective in the short term is clearly indicated by Zahava Solomon's work with Israeli army combat stress sufferers who were, despite such treatment, clearly very vulnerable to subsequent reactions with the development of PTSD (see Chapter 27, in this volume). Mitchell's reports are anecdotal, but his very considerable experience supports the view that debriefing for emergency workers, which involves catharsis, talking-through, and making meaning of the experience, is perceived as helpful by these workers and may indeed be so. Rosser reported that in her group studies of those who were affected by the King's Cross rail disaster in London, there were positive associations between better mental health and having been able to talk-through the experience, although these results are preliminary (see Chapter 37, in this volume). Studies by Pennebaker, Kiecolt-Glaser, and Glaser (1988) in less acute situations support the benefit of describing on paper life experiences of the trauma. There is a need to establish scientifically relationships between talking-through what has happened, affective expression and release, and outcome; optimal methods of facilitating such processes must be determined if evaluation shows that they prevent the development of disorder.

Where a preventive approach merges into *treatment*, where reactive process moves into severe reaction and disorder, is often difficult to say. In such instances, intervention would involve the treatment of either early or established phenomenology in the PTSD spectrum. Here, too, we find goals of helping the individual to confront what has happened, to express feelings associated with the event, and to construct meaning and gain mastery of the experience. Whether advocating a behavioral or psychodynamic approach, the same principles apply; they are core aspects of treatment even when pharmacotherapy is utilized. How much, how soon, what aspects of the trauma, at what rate it should be dealt with, and at what level of affect expression are all areas of importance not yet clearly identified in systematic research. Clinical work, however, places great importance on helping this confrontation to occur at a rate and degree that can be managed by the individual, with a progressive and appropriate "dosing" of affect expression.

Any such therapies rest on the basis of *trust* in the therapeutic relationship. The patient or client may feel secure to progress to dealing with his trauma only when confident that the therapist is not only genuine, empathic, and warm, but also capable of understanding the significance of the trauma, bearing to hear of it, and able to helping the traumatized person manage the affect it evokes. All therapeutic modalities must rest on this basis. The same applies even if a decision is made for group or family therapy as major or adjunctive methods.

Behavioral and cognitive conceptualization of PTSD and its management in those frameworks have been reviewed by Foa, Steketee, and Rothbaum (1989) and Keane, Fairbank, Caddell, Zimering, and Bender (1985). Behavioral methods range from trauma desensitization to implosive (flooding) therapy. Foa suggested that many behavioral treatments may be specific for the fear, avoidance, and phobic components of PTSD, which in established cases are often difficult to resolve, but there are, as yet, inadequate data from controlled trials to refine recommendations in this sphere (Keane, 1989). *Trauma desensitization* has been investigated in comparison with hypnotherapy and psychodynamic therapy with a wait-listed control group (Brom, Kleber, & Defares, 1989). These therapists utilized this approach by training the patient in relaxation techniques and then encouraging him or her to reexperience, in imagination, a hierarchy of situations of the traumatic event. The patient was encouraged to confront the previously avoided traumatic stimuli and gain a sense of mastery and control. This therapy had significant benefits (as did the other modalities), compared to a wait-list group of controls, even for established disorder. Effects on intrusion phenomena were greatest, with far less on the avoidant ones, in contradiction to predicted benefits noted above (i.e., on avoidant phenomena). This may relate to the consideration by Foa *et al.* as to the need to take into account the meaning made of the experience and the fact that a perceived threat is a stronger predictor of PTSD than an actual threat. These matters remain to be elucidated.

Hypnotherapy is also described as one of the successful entities in the Brom *et al.* study. In this research, the hypnotherapy had a behavioral orientation aiming to help the patient confront the trauma and to decrease his conditioned responses triggered by it. There has recently been other work suggesting hypnotherapy to treat rape victims (Ebert, 1988) and war-related trauma (Kingsbury, 1988). Here the goals are confronting the trauma and assisting mastery, control, and empowerment. Brom's studies indicated positive benefits, although, as with the other therapies, they were limited in extent.

Psychodynamic Therapies. Lindy (1986) described a psychoanalytic psychotherapy for PTSD which involved an opening phase, a working-through phase, and termination. However, evaluation of this type of therapy and its contribution to posttrauma phenomena and PTSD is still in its infancy.

Theoretical frameworks for such approaches link to the Horowitz model of cognitive processing, in which intrusive and avoidant processes alternate, each with its associated affect, as the individual attempts to integrate the death encounter experience (Horowitz, 1986). This conceptualization suggests that therapeutic approaches will vary according to the predominence of intrusion/painful reexperiencing and avoidant phenomena. When the former are most profound and distressing, the goals are control, lessening of affect, and diminution of these phenomena, possibly assisted by pharmacotherapy. When avoidance predominates, catharsis, abreactive, and expressive measures are utilized. Although Horowitz's group reported on the benefits of some brief therapy in traumatic situations, their studies are principally oriented to bereavement and will be discussed below (Krupnick & Horowitz, 1985). Psychodynamic approaches may also utilize concepts related to the breaching of ego boundaries by the traumatic stimulus and methods of assisting in restitution. Lindy's group described their attempts at psychotherapeutic outreach to the victims of the Beverly Hills nightclub fire. Their approach was helpful, but only small numbers of survivors could be involved. They demonstrated that the experience of the therapist was one of the factors in successful outcome, such therapists being more likely to engage the patient and keep him or her in therapy until some successful outcome was reached (Lindy *et al.*, 1983).

Brom's group also reported on the effectiveness of psychotherapeutic treatments in their comparative trial; as with behavioral treatments, not everyone benefited. The behavioral approach aimed at breaking through the process of avoidance; psychodynamic therapy was oriented more to exploration of and dealing with the mechanisms relating to the need to avoid. Horowitz supervised this therapy. As with the behavioral and hypnotherapy treatments, sessions ranged from 14 to more than 18 in number, with 60% of subjects in all treatment groups showing improvement compared to 26% of the wait-list control group. Psychodynamic therapy was more effective than the other therapies with avoidant processes. This finding is important in view of the resistance of this area of phenomenology, the treatment generally, and the profound impairment of personal functioning that may be associated with avoidance/numbing. One difficulty with this study is that almost three fourths of the subjects were bereaved, so that while they were all diagnosed as suffering from PTSD and showed substantial change on scores on the IES (Horowitz, Wilner, & Alvarez, 1979), it is not clear to what degree effects of trauma and loss are distinguished

and how specifically death issues were dealt with in therapy.

These findings are useful because they all emphasize common themes, but still leave many unanswered questions. For instance, how much confrontation with the traumatic event/stimulus is appropriate? How much may be potentially damaging by again overwhelming the ego, retraumatizing, or rendering the individual once more powerless and out of control? This opens into the concept of "dosing" of affect, which Lindy's group postulated as important with their experience of disaster survivors and a suggestion which fits well with clinical experience. So much affect may be manageable, may be able to be expressed, confronted, and worked-through at a particular time. More may be "too much" or "too soon." Individual vulnerabilities, coping styles, and personalities will clearly contribute, but how and to what extent they do, and how this may affect clinical practice is not well established.

The "trauma membrane" may form to protect the traumatized person and his network against reexperiencing or talking of the trauma with others; it is one form of defense. Many other defenses may exist, ranging from dissociation, denial, and repression to overinvolvement in distracting, busy activities or the care of other traumatized people.

These defenses may exist for good reasons in terms of the dynamics of the individual who may be vulnerable to posttraumatic or other damage, or who may be struggling with many survival issues. Thus, any process that helps to confront the traumatic experience should involve assessment of defensive and coping styles and analysis of the functions they may be serving, so that therapeutic approaches of whatever orientation take these into account.

McFarlane (1989) reported on his treatment of 56 patients with PTSD, of whom 46 were victims of a natural disaster—the Ash Wednesday bushfires in Australia. He emphasized the establishment of the therapeutic alliance, specific (e.g., arousal) and nonspecific components, treatment of PTSD and associated disorders, the context of illness, perpetuating factors, and the traumatic event itself, highlighting difficulties and the need for further research.

Pharmacotherapy for the symptoms, in particular for disordered arousal, plays a role in the management of established PTSD, but little is known about whether its effect could be used preventively for early and intense reactive phenomena. Friedman (1988) described the biological profile of PTSD in terms of alterations of sympathetic arousal, neuroendocrine systems, and the sleep/dream cycle. He suggested here and later (see Chapter 66, in this volume) that medication, particularly antidepressants, may be helpful in dampening hyperarousal because of their panic-reducing effects. Benzodiazapines have been used and may be helpful in dealing with excessive anxiety, but the dangers of dependence, especially in PTSD groups, warrant a cautious approach. Clonidine has also been reported as useful for some patients, but again there is a need for controlled trials. All the workers in this field highlighted the need for an eclectic approach, and as Friedman suggested, drug treatment alone is never sufficient to alleviate the suffering in PTSD. Pharmacotherapy is primarily useful as an adjunct to psychological (psychotherapeutic and/or behavioral) treatment of PTSD. As he went on to say, pharmacological treatments facilitate therapeutic work to deal with the various painful conflicts, traumata, and affects involved in PTSD.

The *encounter with death* is the key theme that must be dealt with throughout this spectrum; it is not easy for the victim or for those who care for him. Going back to face the experience of death again; the terror, and the reality one could have died; the joy and shame that one did not and others did; the horror of gruesome and violent death; the unforgettable smell, coldness, and sight of death; the helplessness and the fact that death cannot be controlled are all painful and fearful. They are painful and fearful for client and therapist alike and both may wish to avoid touching upon or reworking the experience. Sensitivity, but at the same time a belief in the value of confronting the trauma and the capacity to survive with strength as these experiences are dealt with, is part of the therapeutic work. In retrospect, each element of mastery in dealing with the affect will revitalize the victim and bring feelings of trust and joy in the ongoing nature of life and survival. The therapist needs to be very aware of countertransference issues, his or her own perceptions and fantasies of death and destruction, and be able to recognize how these may influence interactions with, understandings of, and responses to those who have been traumatized in this way. Clearly, these issues can be confronted, but the work is difficult and often avoided; the therapist may require extra support and supervision. Countertransference may be reflected across the spectrum from enmeshment and overinvolvement to detachment and avoidance (Wilson, 1989). Nevertheless, if both client and therapist can endure, a successful outcome is likely.

Personal Interventions in Dealing with Loss

Personal interventions also aim to deal with the various losses the individual may have experienced through personal or community disaster, including the loss of a loved one, home, or valued property, community, or place of work. It may be that the loss by death has been associated with very traumatic circumstances so that reactions overlie and intertwine with one another (i.e., reactions to the trauma of a death encounter and the loss). Important elements in outcome will be the severity of the perceived loss, the presence or absence of such traumatic circumstances of death, factors in the individual, factors in the social milieu, especially perceptions of inadequate support, the grieving or processing of the experience, and other stressors that occur at the same time or arise subsequently (Raphael, 1983).

Here, the early reactive processes here may also be intense and may gradually attenuate or go on to pathology. *Prevention* approaches are aimed at facilitating normal adaptations. They might range from interventions regarding policy, such as seeing the body of the deceased, funeral ceremonies, and inquiries, to public recognition and support for those grieving in a disaster. Here, too, education is important in helping those who

are distressed and others near them to be aware of and facilitate normal processes. In recent years, social prescriptions have clearly improved in this way with heightened awareness.

Prevention directed toward the individual is aimed at helping him or her to grieve normally and involves approaches such as those adopted and reported by Lindemann (1944) in the bereaved victims of the Coconut Grove night club fire. He reported changing patterns of grieving to "normal" over several therapeutic sessions which were aimed at promoting the grief work.

Systematic evaluation of preventive interventions with high-risk bereaved individuals (widows) has been carried out in a randomized controlled trial (Raphael, 1977). Here the aims were to (1) facilitate the expression of grief, (2) review the lost relationship in its positive and negative aspects, (3) promote social network support, and (4) deal with any specifically relevant risk variables, such as preexisting difficulties in the relationship between the bereaved and the dead person, or concurrent traumatic stress or other stress issues. This study established the effectiveness of preventive intervention with such high-risk bereaved widows. Other studies subsequently have extended this work—for instance, Parkes (1979)—and are reviewed elsewhere (Raphael & Nunn, 1989).

Treatment Intervention

As with the experience of reaction to threat and encounter with death, reactions to loss may be intense and may become prolonged or pathological, merging into disorder. It is difficult to draw the boundary between distress and disorder, especially as there are not as yet diagnostic criteria for pathological grief. Treatment interventions for pathological grief (Raphael, 1983) include specific exploration of the lost relationship and review of its ambivalent and dependent aspects; helping the bereaved to confront and deal with anxiety, anger, and guilt over abandonment, death wishes, and neediness; promoting and facilitating supportive interactions with family and social network; dealing with shock, rage, and resentment over the act of fate/God/man in such unanticipated and traumatic loss. The bereaved tends to become "locked" into the tragedy and unable to move on from the death and dead person, who may become an idealized focus and preoccupation, sometimes to the exclusion and destruction of other relationships and functioning. Moving on to life without the deceased may be difficult and more complicated if there is an unconscious need to atone and suffer for the death; or if the body has not been found and the farewell finalized; or if justice, compensation, and/or revenge dominate.

Most approaches to the management of pathological forms of grief have taken a *psychotherapeutic* approach, relying on actively confronting and dealing with the loss, encouraging the expression of grief and catharsis, and reviewing and processing the memories of the lost person in the process of undoing, bit by bit, the bonds of the relationship. This is likely to be most effective where grief has taken pathological forms of delay or inhibition. Where there is extreme, continuing, external expression, as in chronic grief, this is more difficult.

Here, psychotherapeutic approaches may aim to explore underlying dynamics of the role of this grief in holding onto the lost person, punishing the bereaved and others, and in gaining care. In each instance, the dynamics of the defenses need to be understood and taken into account. There may also be questions of what aspects can be fact, to what degree and when there has been enough or too much expression of grief, and when the time has come to allow or help the bereaved person to draw his or her mourning to a close. It is clear that some grief, remembrance, and sadness may continue for a long time, but in normal circumstances, this does not dominate the life of the bereaved or interfere with his or her relationships and personal functioning.

Behavioral approaches have been used but, on the whole, represent similar themes of helping the bereaved to confront and deal with the realities of the loss gradually, and express the affect that is associated with it. This approach may be helpful with chronic grief or where there are phobic components (e.g., about visiting the grave), but on the whole this form of grief (chronic) is difficult to treat by any modality.

Other disorders that arise in association with trauma and stress (e.g., depression, anxiety disorders, or substance abuse) can be treated in their own right, alongside work of a psychotherapeutic kind to deal with the grief and trauma issues.

Family interventions are often very helpful in view of the fact that family members are at the same time comforters and bereaved. Different rates and patterns of grieving, individual relationships to the lost person, and differing roles and responsibility as well as family dynamics may all interfere with the working-through of the loss.

Traumatic bereavements, such as occur in personal or community disasters (Lundin, 1984), are always particularly stressful and frequently difficult to resolve. They affect the young, the innocent, and cut violently across the fabric of everyday life. For these reasons, special sensitivity and care are required in dealing with them.

Pharmacotherapy has rarely been seen as a major factor in bereavement counseling or management, as there appears to be a longer established tradition of successfully working-through and dealing with these issues without drug treatment, unless other pathology has supervened.

Specific evaluation of a bereavement outreach program after a major Australian disaster (Singh & Raphael, 1981) has shown some effectiveness but also highlighted the extra difficulties of such traumatic bereavements, the problems of providing services for the people, and the great reluctance or unwillingness that many have about utilizing counseling services.

Here, too, the *therapeutic relationship* is of primary importance, and *trust* is a key issue. The therapist may find it personally stressful to deal with losses which could have affected him or her, too, and where it is painful to stay with the bereaved through their anger, grief, despair, and deprivation. Transference may be difficult, particularly if the counselor is regarded as some sort of replacement figure and where dependency issues have been prominent.

Nevertheless, there is increasing recognition of the value of bereavement counseling by bereaved people and their families, and evidence of its effectiveness from scientific studies (Raphael & Nunn, 1989). It is a useful modality of personal intervention, both preventive and therapeutic, for the care of disaster victims.

Other Themes and Stresses

Clearly, *many other stressors* and reactions to them may complicate the experience and adaptation of those who have been through community and personal disasters. Interventions need to be focused (as defined above) but they may also need to address supplementary factors, such as guilt and conflict, practical problems of disaster recovery, subsequent stressors, and the multiple complications of long-standing personal or family difficulties, or ongoing psychological problems, psychiatric disorder, or character pathology. Separate contracts in other care, or care alongside the trauma focus, may be necessary to deal with these issues.

Practical problems requiring assistance from the earliest postdisaster period may lead to the need for consultation work with other professionals and community agencies. The practical assistance that can be offered will provide a useful therapeutic opportunity for counseling alongside such issues; these approaches have been shown to be particularly valued by those affected (e.g., Singh & Raphael, 1981). The dynamics of this situation are important and it may take great therapeutic skill to avoid the practical problems' becoming a defensive avoidance of real emotional and psychological stresses that must be dealt with.

Outreach programs are often advocated and implemented because of the difficulties victims may have in seeking help. They, too, bring special opportunities for therapy, but also dynamics of the helper relationships which are quite different from traditional settings. These need to be recognized and taken into account.

Finally, disasters occur to *families* and the primary group will inevitably be stressed far beyond its usual capacity. Reactions to death and loss may reverberate throughout the family system. It is often useful to intervene with family members to facilitate interaction, sharing of the experience, mutual understanding, comforting and support, catharsis, cognitive mastery, and eventual integration of the disaster and what it has meant to this family as a unit, as well as to its individual members. This is appropriate and especially important where children are involved.

Conclusion

There is a greatly enhanced understanding of the response to community and to personal disaster, from both theoretical and research points of view. At systems and personal levels, traumatization can occur and reactive processes can be set in motion. Ample evidence demonstrates that interventions at system and personal levels to deal with death encounter and losses will be effective in promoting adaptation and in lessening the likelihood of morbid outcomes. Such interventions need to be further developed, utilized, and researched to enhance our knowledge of stress, response, and disease processes, particularly in relation to catastrophe. Much that is good can occur despite the pain, horror, and loss, not the least of which is the altruism, care, and compassion shown by human beings to each other as a consequence.

References

Brom, D., Kleber, R. J., & Defares, P. B. (1989). Brief psychotherapy for post-traumatic stress disorders. *Journal of Consulting and Clinical Psychology, 57*(5), 607–612.

Drabek, T. E. (1986). *Human system responses to disaster: An inventory of sociological findings.* New York: Springer-Verlag.

Ebert, B. W. (1988). Hypnosis and rape victims. *American Journal of Clinical Hypnosis, 31*(1), 50–56.

Foa, E. B., Steketee, G., & Rothbaum, B. O. (1989). Behavioral cognitive conceptualizations of post-traumatic stress disorder. *Behavior Therapy, 20*, 155–176.

Friedman, M. J. (1988). Toward rational pharmacotherapy for post-traumatic stress disorder: An interim report. *American Journal of Psychiatry, 145*(3), 281–285.

Gibbs, M. (1989). Factors in the the victim that mediate between disaster and psychopathology: A review. *Journal of Traumatic Stress, 2*(4), 489–514.

Green, B. L. (1982). Assessing levels of psychological impairment following disaster. *Journal of Nervous and Mental Diseases, 170*(9), 544–552.

Green, B. L., Wilson, J. P., & Lindy, J. D. (1985). Conceptualizing post-traumatic stress disorder: A psychosocial framework. In C. R. Figley (Ed.), *Trauma and its wake: The study and treatment of post-traumatic stress disorder* (pp. 53–69). New York: Brunner/Mazel.

Holen, A., Sund, A., & Weisæth, L. (1979). *Predictors of disaster morbidity.* Paper presented at the Symposium on Disaster Psychiatry, Stavanger, Norway.

Horowitz, M. J. (1976). *Stress response syndromes.* New York: Jason Aronson.

Horowitz, M. J. (1986). *Stress response syndromes* (2nd ed.). New York: Jason Aronson.

Horowitz, M. J., Wilner, N., & Alvarez, W. (1979). Impact of Events Scale: A measure of psychosomatic stress. *Psychosomatic Medicine, 41*, 209–218.

Keane, T. M. (1989). Post-traumatic stress disorder: Current status and future directions. *Behavior Therapy, 20*(2), 149–153.

Keane, T. M., Fairbank, J. A., Caddell, R. M., Zimering, R. T., & Bender, M. E. (1985). A behavioral approach to assessing and treating post-traumatic stress disorder in Vietnam veterans. In C. R. Figley (Ed.), *Trauma and its wake: The study and treatment of post-traumatic stress disorder* (pp. 257–294). New York: Brunner/Mazel.

Kingsbury, S. J. (1988). Hypnosis in the treatment of post-traumatic stress disorder: An isomorphic intervention. *American Journal of Clinical Hypnosis, 31*(2), 81–90.

Krupnick, J., & Horowitz, M. J. (1985). Brief pysychotherapy with vulnerable patients: An outcome assessment. *Psychiatry, 48*, 223–233.

Lindemann, H. (1944). Symptomatology and management of acute grief. *American Journal of Psychiatry, 101*, 141–148.

Lindy, J. D. (1986). An outline for the psychoanalytic psychotherapy of post-traumatic stress disorder. In C. R. Figley (Ed.), *Trauma and its wake: Traumatic stress theory, research, and intervention* (Vol. 2, pp. 195–212). New York: Brunner/Mazel.

Lindy, J. D., Green, B. L., Grace, M., & Titchener, J. (1983). Psychotherapy with survivors of the Beverly Hills Supper Club fire. *American Journal of Psychotherapy, 37*, 593–610.

Lundin, T. (1984). Morbidity following sudden and unexpected bereavement. *British Journal of Psychiatry, 144*, 84–88.

Lystad, M. (Ed.). (1988). *Mental health response to mass emergencies: Theory and practice.* New York: Brunner/Mazel.

McFarlane, A. C. (1989). The treatment of post-traumatic stress disorder. *British Journal of Medical Psychology, 62*, 81–90.

Middleton, W., & Raphael, B. R. (1987–1990). *Study of bereavement reaction following death of a primary family member.* Research in progress, University of Queensland, Australia.

Parker, G. (1977). Cyclone Tracy and Darwin evacuees: On the restoration of the species. *British Journal of Psychiatry, 130*, 547–555.

Parkes, C. M. (1979). Evaluation of a bereavement service. In A. Devries & I. Carmi (Eds.), *The dying human* (pp. 389–402). Ramat Gan, Israel: Turtledove.

Pennebaker, J. W., Kiecolt-Glaser, J. K., & Glaser, R. (1988). Confronting traumatic experience and immunocompetence: A reply to Neale, Cox, Valdimarsdottir, and Stone. *Journal of Consulting and Clinical Psychology, 56*(4), 638–639.

Pynoos, R. (1989, May). Paper presented at Bereavement Conference, Seattle, WA.

Quarantelli, E. L. (1978). *Disasters: Theory and research.* London: Sage.

Quarantelli, E. L. (1982). *Inventory of disaster field studies in the social and behavioral sciences: 1919–1979.* Columbus, OH: Disaster Research Center, Ohio State University.

Quarantelli, E. L. (1984). *Organizational behavior in disasters and implications for disaster planning.* Emmitsburg, MD: National Emergency Training Center, Federal Emergency Management Agency.

Raphael, B. (1977). Bereavement and prevention. *New Doctor, 4*, 41–45.

Raphael, B. (1983). *Anatomy of bereavement.* New York: Basic Books.

Raphael, B. (1986). *When disaster strikes.* New York: Basic Books.

Raphael, B. (1990). *Prospective study of primary prevention in groups at high risk of post-traumatic stress disorder.* Research in progress, University of Queensland, Australia.

Raphael, B., & Maddison, D. C. (1976). Care of bereaved adults: Modern trends. In O. W. Hill (Ed.), *Psychosomatic medicine–3* (pp. 491–506). London: Butterworth.

Raphael, B., & Nunn, K. (1989). Counselling the bereaved. *Journal of Social Issues, 44*(3), 191–206.

Reid, J. (1979). A time to live, a time to grieve: Patterns and processes of mourning among the Yolngu of Australia. *Cultural Medical Psychiatry, 3*(4), 319–346.

Singh, B., & Raphael, B. (1981). Postdisaster morbidity of the bereaved: A possible role for preventive psychiatry. *Journal of Nervous and Mental Disease, 169*(4), 203–212.

Solomon, S. D. (1986). Mobilizing social support networks in times of disaster. In C. R. Figley (Ed.), *Trauma and its wake: Traumatic stress theory, research, and intervention* (Vol. 2, pp. 232–263). New York: Brunner/Mazel.

Straker, J. (1988). Personal communication with the author.

Tyrer, M. (1989). Lockerbie air disaster. *Journal of the Royal Army Medical Corps, 135*(2), 93–94.

Weisæth, L. (1983). *The study of a factory fire.* Unpublished doctoral dissertation, University of Oslo, Norway.

Western, J. S., & Doube, L. (1979). Stress and Cyclone Tracy. In G. Pickup (Ed.), *Natural hazards management in North Australia.* Canberra: Australian National University.

Wilson, J. P. (1989). *Trauma, transformation and healing*. New York: Brunner/Mazel.

Wilson, J. P., Smith, W. K., & Johnson, S. K. (1985). A comparative analysis of PTSD among various survivor groups. In C. R. Figley (Ed.), *Trauma and its wake: Traumatic stress theory, research, and intervention* (pp. 142–172). New York: Brunner/Mazel.

Assessment, Methodology, and Research Strategies

As the field of traumatic stress studies has evolved, diversified, and increased in complexity, the development of an armamentarium of objective and projective psychometric techniques of assessing stress-response syndromes has shown a correspondence to theoretical and conceptual advances in our knowledge base. Similarly, the rapid accumulation of empirical studies of PTSD and associated characteristics has led to the development of more adequate and sophisticated research methodologies by which to test hypotheses and theoretical constructs. Part II of this volume contains eight chapters which specifically address the issues of assessment of PTSD by different research strategies, including epidemiological studies, objective and projective psychometric procedures, structured clinical interview techniques, and prospective and retrospective studies of traumatic events.

In Chapter 10, Andrew Baum, Susan D. Solomon, Robert J. Ursano, and their colleagues present a concise review of critical issues in the field of disaster research and the study of psychic trauma. They begin by noting that investigators face a number of practical issues in the early stages of research. These critical issues include a proper and timely assessment of the population, a realistic estimate of the costs and time frame required to carry out the project, securing access to the victim population within legal and ethical limits, and conceptualizing the structure and dimensions of the trauma itself. Careful planning around these practical aspects of the research protocol can help to avoid mistakes that could result in an incomplete or inadequate data set.

In the second half of this densely packed chapter, the authors review a number of methodological issues that have grown out of the empirical literature on disasters and trauma. This is an especially valuable task because it summarizes "lessons learned" and therefore aids in designing more rigorous scientific research designs in the future. Included in their analysis are such considerations as retrospective versus prospective design problems; the nature and adequacy of outcome measures; the types of psychological scales of measurement (e.g., diagnostic instruments, biological markers, behavioral measures, etc.); stressor measures; appropriate cohort and control groups; sampling designs and pitfalls; and statistical analyses.

In Chapter 11, Bonnie L. Green, one of the principal investigators of the Buffalo Creek dam disaster, addresses the question of identifying survivors at risk, especially in regard to the nature of the trauma and the specific stressors to which they were exposed. In this regard, she states:

the most fruitful approach to examining aspects of events at this point in time, then, appears to be looking within a particular event, for individual differences in how the event unfolded and attempting to specify generic dimensions that might apply to a variety of events.

But what is a traumatic event? It is clear that disasters and traumas often contain multiple stressors and are rarely unidimensional. Furthermore, although some stressors are objective and readily verifiable, others are not easily *quantified*, and there are large individual differences in subjective reactions to trauma which are *qualitative* in nature. The issue of stress vulnerability and *threshold effects* at which a person develops PTSD is a very important one. There is also the related question of chronic or ongoing stressors as well as the *interaction* between the original, primary stressors and a host of secondary stressors. All these considerations have, of course, direct implications for the proper measurement of stressors in order that their relationship to identifying individuals at risk can be assessed. Green concludes her lucid analysis by identifying five areas of investigation that would help to advance the field in terms of conceptualizing and differentiating the acute, chronic, and life-course impact of stressors on the onset of psychopathology and psychosocial adaptation.

In the medical sciences, epidemiological studies are critical to understanding the prevalence and nature of disease processes. In Chapter 12, Richard A. Kulka and William E. Schlenger present a comprehensive analysis of survey research and field designs for the study of PTSD. In particular, they "focus on four specific problems that are common in such studies: (1) identification of target populations and selection of representative samples, (2) identification of relevant comparison groups, (3) case identification, and (4) collection of comprehensive data." Because the authors were part of a team that conducted the landmark National Vietnam Veteran Readjustment Study (NVVRS), one of the most heralded epidemiological studies ever undertaken, they bring a wealth of experience and knowledge regarding the potential limits to survey research in the study of stress-response syndromes. In addition, they are able to use the NVVRS study as illustrative of how to design and carry out such an epidemiological study. This is quite important heuristically because the kinds of difficulties and successes they experienced can be of enormous value to other investigators throughout the world who would wish to study other disaster and trauma victims to identify the prevalence, severity, and comorbidity of PTSD and allied symptoms. In terms of the NVVRS study, the authors state, relative to their objectives, that

> of particular interest were its antecedents, its course, its consequences, and its relationship to other physical and emotional disorders. Relationships between PTSD and other postwar psychological problems, on the one hand, and physical disabilities, substance abuse, minority group membership, and criminal justice involvement, on the other, were also to be examined, as was the impact of postwar psychological problems on veterans' families and on their use of VA [medical] facilities. In short, nothing less was required than perhaps the most far-reaching and ambitious national mental health epidemiological study ever attempted on any population.

In their chapter, Kulka and Schlenger review the development of the NVVRS study, its design, choice of measures, procedures, and problems of method. This process is most informative because it details the logic and rationale, step by step, for every major set of decisions made in the study. The result is a wealth of information and a ground plan of the necessary measures that researchers must follow to insure the reliability and validity of their findings, especially in terms of case identification (caseness). This remarkable chapter breaks new ground in the study of PTSD and demonstrates that scientific creativity is necessary to advance methods by which to obtain information that becomes the springboard for new directions of inquiry in the acquisition of knowledge.

Although it is the case that epidemiological surveys study persons who have already experienced a traumatic event, there are few *prospective* studies that follow the progression and sequelae of a trauma from its beginning to a given point in time posttrauma. In Chapter 13, Anthony Feinstein presents research data in one of the first prospective studies of victims of physical trauma. In this regard, the prospective study method allows us to see the natural history of a disorder, such as PTSD, in a longitudinal way.

Feinstein's study was conducted at Whittington Hospital in London, England. All the patients had been victims of physical injuries which resulted from motorbike accidents, motorcar collisions, sports injury, assault, domestic violence, falls, and pedestrian accidents, and had suffered fractures of the femur, tibia, or fibula without a loss of limb. The *criteria* also included being between 15 and 60 years of age, being admitted to an orthopedic ward for surgical correction, showing no evidence of head trauma, witnessing no fatalities in the accident, or self-inflicted injuries.

The patients were initially assessed in the hospital orthopedic ward by standard medical procedures as well as objective measures of their injuries on two rating scales. The psychological measures included the General Health Questionnaire, the Clinical Interview Schedule, the Impact of Events Scale, and the Standardized Assessment of Personality instrument. The patients were followed-up 6 weeks and 6 months after accidental injury. PTSD symptoms were assessed using the DSM-III-R criteria by an experienced clinician familiar with the disorder and its diagnosis.

Among the important results of this prospective study is that upon initial assessment in the hospital, about two thirds (67%) had symptoms sufficient to be classified as psychiatric cases. Among the "case"-identified individuals, 25% were suffering from PTSD as well as anxiety and depressive symptoms. Dissociative reactions were relatively rare, and the general pattern of recovery indicated a reduction of symptoms over time. As Feinstein stated:

> A consistent decline in all measures of symptoms was observed over time. At the group level, the maximum symptomatology was reported in the first week following the trauma when almost two thirds of the victims were classified as psychiatric cases. This had fallen to about 25% by 6 weeks and 6 months. . . . The fact that there was no significant change in the number of cases from 6 weeks to 6 months is not indicative of a stable situation having been reached by 6 weeks, since 5 patients deteriorated in their condition while a similar number had improved.

Thus, among the many important findings reported in this study is the fact that for some patients, PTSD symptoms were immediately present whereas for others there was a delayed onset. Given the current DSM-III-R criteria for classifying PTSD after one month's duration, these results suggest that it may be necessary to reevaluate the idea of when to diagnose, a factor currently under consideration in DSM-IV. Finally, Feinstein's study illustrates the need for more prospective studies of different victim populations so that comparative analyses between populations can be made in order to deepen our knowledge of the natural history of PTSD (i.e., the posttraumatic sequelae) in order to discern common pathways as well as areas of deviation specific to exposure to stressor events.

As the quality of theoretical and conceptual paradigms of PTSD have become better defined in terms of psychobiological processes, the ability to develop and validate psychometric measures of the syndrome has increased accordingly. It is a truism that, to a large degree, the quality of psychometric assessment techniques is determined by the *quality* of the theoretical constructs which define stress-response syndromes. In Chapter 14, Jessica Wolfe and Terence M. Keane review the evolution of the assessment of PTSD, especially as it pertains to war stressors and combat exposure. They note that

> The publication in 1980 of the DSM-III, in conjunction with clinicians' growing awareness of the span of environmentally based trauma, thus provided an important catalyst for the development of assessment procedures specific to PTSD. The existence of a classification schema

encouraged the development and application of psychological assessment tools in two specific ways: First, it provided preliminary scientific credibility for the disorder, stimulating the need to attempt further validation of the diagnostic category itself. Second, by proposing particular symptom patterns, the categorization stirred an interest in examining and detailing the various components of PTSD. From this point on, several new questions became pivotal in the assessment of PTSD.

In their chapter, Wolfe and Keane review, largely in a historical chronology, various psychological scales which have been used to measure PTSD. These instruments include the MMPI, the Impact of Events Scale, the Vietnam Era Stress Inventory, the Mississippi Scale, structured clinical interview procedures such as the SCID (which is discussed fully in Chapter 15), psychophysiological measures, and measures of personality and psychopathology. Each instrument is considered in terms of its psychometric qualities (e.g., reliability, validity, internal consistency, etc.) along with a discussion of the respective strengths and weaknesses of the scales. The result of this process is the identification of measures that can be of use to researchers in the field. In their conclusion, the authors state that "further research is needed to assess the effects of different typologies of stressors as well as their variations in frequency and duration on the development of PTSD." Clearly, this position is congruent with that of Green in Chapter 11 and points to the convergence in our understanding of where systematic research and programmatic efforts need to be made to discover new information about the interaction between the person, the trauma, and the specific stressors which impact on the self-structure and personality processes of the victim.

In the psychometric tradition of objective personality assessment, the individual responds to a set of items structured by the questionnaire which are then scored, tabulated, and interpreted accordingly. Although this is a time-honored and tested procedure, it has its inherent limitations, as discussed by Wolfe and Keane. However, in recent years, efforts have been made to develop structured clinical interview techniques to diagnose all the DSM-III-R mental disorders on Axis I and Axis II. In Chapter 15, Daniel S. Weiss discusses the SCID module for the diagnosis and assessment of PTSD.

Weiss begins his chapter by placing the assessment of psychological distress into a historical context and states that

> The recognition of the basic uniformity of psychological and biological reactions following exposure to the range of traumatic stressors has been aided by the formalization of diagnostic criteria. The social . . . consequence of displaying a near universal pattern of reactions subsequent to surviving exposure to a traumatic stressor are weighty and need social attention.

Thus, the specialist or researcher who seeks to make a differential diagnosis can benefit from the utilization of a standardized protocol which constitutes an algorithm for scientific decision-making. The advantages of such a protocol are numerous, of course, but perhaps the primary factor is that once the user is proficient with the procedure, it eliminates errors that are due to rater bias, lack of experience with the disorder, and inefficient or improper history taking. Thus, the SCID PTSD module can be considered a "yardstick" by which to validly measure the symptoms which make up the A, B, C, and D criteria of PTSD in DSM-III-R, both in the present and during the lifetime.

In his chapter, Weiss explains the logic and rationale for the questions which make up the SCID module for PTSD. Furthermore, examples are given for each of the DSM-III-R criteria, a strategy which results in "walking" the reader through the use of the protocol. In his conclusion, Weiss states that

> The roles of structured clinical interviews and the data made available by their use are crucial to the ongoing evolution of diagnostic criteria for PTSD or response to traumatic stress. What other psychological and/or physiological phenomena co-occur after exposure to traumatic stress continues to be an evolving and growing area of attention. For this reason alone, ignor-

ing the increase in precision and the possibility for comparability of results, the regular use of standard structured clinical interviews ought to be a regular activity for those who work with survivors of trauma.

The development of objective psychometric measures of PTSD has clearly demonstrated the need for assessment procedures that are sensitive to the dimensions of the disorder. As noted by van der Kolk and Saporta in Chapter 2, PTSD is a disorder of arousal in which the ability to modulate affect is adversely altered. The disruption of the steady state (stasis) causes a disequilibrium in the psyche which has, of course, manifestations in affect, cognition, and behavior.

In Chapter 16, Patti Levin presents an analysis of PTSD by the Rorschach projective technique. The Rorschach is a simple test in which an individual is asked to view 10 inkblot cards, five of which contain color, and explain the nature of his or her perceptions of the parts of the inkblots. Developed in 1921 by Hermann Rorschach, the test was further codified as a clinical assessment tool by psychologists in the United States—Beck, Klopfer, Piatrowski, and Rappaport among them—who created complex and detailed scoring systems. In 1974, John E. Exner further modified the Rorschach into the Comprehensive Scoring System, an objective procedure which generated norms for pathological and normal subjects.

Levin summarizes the results of her study of 27 adults who had a positive PTSD diagnosis. The subjects all had experienced trauma in adulthood (e.g., rape, major accidents) and none of them had a premorbid history on Axis I or Axis II diagnosis. The individuals were each administered the Rorschach and their results were compared to Exner's normative data. Over 200 variables were compared to the normative national sample, and about one half were found to be significantly different for the PTSD sample. In her chapter, Levin discusses her six major hypotheses, all of which were supported by the data which reveal a detailed portrait of PTSD symptoms that are operating on an unconscious level. As predicted, the PTSD sample showed high degrees of unmodulated affect, impaired reality testing, interpersonal detachment, emotional constriction, and hypervigilance. In her conclusion, Levin notes that

> the Rorschach was able to tap unconscious mental processes in a manner which highlighted and underscored reports of PTSD throughout the literature. Yet the Rorschach was able to go beyond the "ballpark" snapshots of other psychometric instruments, which may be less sensitive to the specific process of PTSD. Rather, the Rorschach demonstrated a finely tuned calibration of the discrete and subtle levels of the syndrome, suggesting its applicability as a sensitive and exquisite measure of PTSD.

This finding appears to be a very important one because the procedure is a projective one in which the person generates his or her own percepts onto the stimulus field. Without prompting by a cue contained in an item on an objective measure of PTSD, the individual's pathology is expressed quite readily without conscious awareness. Thus, Levin's work appears to have identified a *PTSD profile* (Rorschach codes using the Exner system) which is sensitive to all the major DSM-III-R dimensions of the disorder. Clearly, this discovery adds yet another assessment technique to the domain of reliable measures of PTSD and will stimulate many further studies to discern commonalities and differences among objective and projective techniques of personality assessment.

In Chapter 17, Mark Creamer and his colleagues present a *retrospective* study of a multiple shooting which took place in Melbourne, Australia, in December, 1987. Nine people were killed and five were wounded by a berserk gunman who wielded a semiautomatic rifle and fired randomly at employees on two floors of an 18-story office building. In addition to the individuals who directly witnessed the shootings on the 5th and 12th floors, many others in the building were aware that a serious crisis was at hand.

To study the effects of the shooting on the workers in the building, Creamer and his colleagues mailed surveys to all people employed in the building with data collection occurring at 4, 8, and 14 months. The researchers found a contrast (control) group of nontraumatized office workers in a similar-sized office building in downtown Melbourne. The subjects were administered the Impact of Event Scale, the SCL-90-R, and the General Health Questionnaire. Sociodemographic and social support network data were also obtained from the participants. The response rate to the survey groups was relatively high (55%) and consistent across the time intervals sampled.

The result produced a rich set of findings concerning psychological symptoms after the shooting. As expected, the traumatized groups had PTSD symptoms and more depression, anxiety, poor concentration, and relationship problems than did the contrast group. The general level of psychological distress experienced by the traumatized group diminished very little between the 4- and 14-months posttrauma follow-up, a finding that is in accord with Feinstein's *prospective* study of victims of physical injury reported in Chapter 13. Perhaps among the most important aspect of Creamer's study is the quality of the research design as a retrospective study of trauma. As the authors state:

> The current study also has implications for future research in the area. In particular, the results highlight the importance of utilizing a longitudinal methodology to adequately chart the course of posttrauma reactions. With the current subject group, there is also a need for longer term follow-up, given the relatively high level of psychological problems reported at 14-months posttrauma.

CHAPTER 10

Emergency/Disaster Studies

Practical, Conceptual, and Methodological Issues

Andrew Baum, Susan D. Solomon, and Robert J. Ursano
with (alphabetically) Leonard Bickman,
Edward Blanchard, Bonnie L. Green, Terence M. Keane,
Robert Laufer, Fran Norris, John Reid,
Elizabeth M. Smith, and Peter Steinglass

Introduction

During the fall of 1987, a group of behavioral scientists involved in the study of disaster effects and traumatic stress met to discuss a range of issues related to research in these areas. This chapter, which summarizes these discussions, is intended to identify the central issues and obstacles to the development of research on traumatic stress.

The difficulties in studying trauma are abundant and include the necessity of doing naturalistic field studies, the problems of trying to apply experimental control to settings that resist this application, and the nascent quality of underlying conceptual frameworks. In this chapter, we address each of these issues in our discussion, which is divided into three sections. The first deals with practical problems associated with the nature of the phenomenon under investigation. The second considers conceptual issues associated with defining and classifying disasters along meaningful dimensions. Finally, the third section discusses methodological issues, particularly in relation to measurement and sampling.

Andrew Baum • Department of Psychology, Uniformed Services University of the Health Sciences, Bethesda, Maryland 20814. Susan D. Solomon • Disaster Research Program, National Institute of Mental Health, Rockville, Maryland 20857. Robert J. Ursano • Department of Psychiatry, F. Edward Hebert School of Medicine, Uniformed Services University of the Health Sciences, Bethesda, Maryland 20814. Leonard Bickman • Department of Psychology and Human Development, George Peabody College of Vanderbilt University, Nashville, Tennessee 37203. Edward Blanchard • Department of Psychology, State University of New York at Albany, Albany, New York 12222. Bonnie L. Green • Department of Psychiatry, Georgetown University Hospital, Washington, DC 20007. Terence M. Keane • Department of Veterans Affairs Medical Center, Boston, Massachusetts 02130. Robert Laufer • Late Professor of Sociology, Brooklyn College of the City University of New York, Brooklyn, New York 11210. Fran Norris • Department of Psychology, Georgia State University, Atlanta, GA 30303. John Reid • Oregon Social Learning Center, 207 East 5th Avenue, Eugene, Oregon 97401. Elizabeth M. Smith • Department of Psychiatry, Washington University School of Medicine, St. Louis, Missouri 63110. Peter Steinglass • Department of Psychiatry, George Washington University, Washington, DC 20052.

This chapter is based on the *Proceedings of the Workshop on Research Issues: Emergency, Disaster, and Post-Traumatic Stress* (September, 1987), Uniformed Services, University of the Health Sciences (USUHS), Military Stress Studies Center, Bethesda, MD. This work was supported by a grant from the National Institute of Mental Health (NIMH) (MH-40106). The opinions or assertions contained herein are the private ones of the authors and are not to be considered as official or reflect the views of the Department of Defense, USUHS, or NIMH.

International Handbook of Traumatic Stress Syndromes, edited by John P. Wilson and Beverley Raphael. Plenum Press, New York, 1993.

Practical Problems

Because research on traumatic stress is not readily adaptable to a laboratory setting, it must generally be conducted in the field. The practical problems that characterize this kind of field research are myriad. Laboratory settings, however, simply cannot replicate the real-life traumatic situation with its actual threat. Some traumatic events are so extremely stressful that there is no way to come close to an analogue. Furthermore, although treatment-seeking populations have much to teach us about responses to catastrophe, many important questions in this area are related to the impact of a range of stressor experiences on a range of individuals, *most* of whom never seek treatment. Thus, the *population* under study as well as the *phenomena* under study are widely dispersed and must be sought out rather than screened at a treatment facility.

Timely Assessment

Clearly, the sources of most of the difficulties in doing this research is the nature of the phenomena under study. Because traumatic events are not predictable, it is usually difficult, if not impossible, to get predisaster baseline data. In most cases, the disaster simply occurs, and the researcher must then design a study as rapidly as possible in order to ensure timely data collection. Because many traumatic events strike quickly and without warning, the researcher may have little time even to get to a geographical area much less prepare for a full-blown research effort. Timing is often critical in studying these events, and logistical concerns never imagined by the laboratory researcher can become predominant in a quick, field-based study of a disaster or trauma.

In some cases, advance preparation can be made possible through advance funding. In the United States, the National Institute of Mental Health (NIMH) regards funding in advance of a disaster to be an appropriate and feasible research strategy for studies which have as their focus a particular mental health research question rather than a particular emergency event, and require immediate postimpact assessment as an essential element in the study design. This process acknowledges that although the exact location and timing of a particular disaster cannot be predicted, the overall occurrence of emergency events is regular and frequent. Funding *prior to* the event allows investigators the opportunity to prepare in advance for such events by developing relevant instruments, devising sampling plans, training interviewers, and pilot testing the instruments in areas of high risk.

Estimating Costs and Time Frame

Even with advance funding, however, these studies are likely to face other practical problems. Particularly problematic for studies which obtain advance funding is that it is extremely difficult to estimate the costs of conducting such a study and the time frame that will be necessary to complete it. Depending on the area of the country in which one is conducting research, cultural differences may play an important role in access to subjects (e.g., no telephones in motels, subjects will not be interviewed on Sundays, etc.). The ability of subjects to understand the goals of the research may vary with education, and, in some rural areas, subjects may be suspicious of researchers from the "big city," or may not take seriously the scheduling of specific appointment times. Because these problems are often difficult to anticipate, budgets are likely to underestimate the true costs of research.

Furthermore, managing travel arrangements and interviewing in the field over time is extremely complicated. The researcher must to some extent be flexible and adaptable to the subjects, the locale, and the situation. An administrative person who interacts with the university system (travel authorizations, budgets, expense reporting) and plans the practical aspects of the work (car rental, airline reservations, room rental, expense tracking) is nearly always needed. The large amount of time (and funding) it takes to conduct such a study with its unique logistical requirements can only be appreciated by actual hands-on experience.

Gaining Access to Victims

Obtaining access to victims may be the most difficult problem for any study of disaster. In some cases, it may be necessary to elicit the cooperation of several government agencies in order to obtain objective information about affected areas. Many agencies may be unwilling to provide names of victims because of confidentiality. Also, potential subjects may be reluctant to participate in interviews because they are involved in legal litigation.

It should be noted that subject recruitment must be approached with great sensitivity, because some proportion of subjects will have had very traumatizing experiences, and the researcher must not increase this distress. Subjects may be reluctant to share their experience because it is painful, a fact which increases recruitment difficulties. Thus, clinical input into the subject recruitment process, as well as the interview process, is useful. Also, since the investigator is on the subject's turf in a field study, she or he must gain an appreciation of local norms and customs and incorporate these into the research design.

Conceptual Issues

Research designed to study the effects of disasters has the potential for adding to our understanding of a broad range of issues of critical importance to mental health and prevention (e.g., stress response, family disruption, social and economic factors). However, the degree to which this potential is realized may depend on the extent to which study goals are grounded in relevant theory. Many disaster studies focus on the *disaster event itself* rather than on the theoretical underpinnings of the research or broader links to other areas of mental health or psychosocial outcomes. Integrating the methods and theories of other fields within the study of these events may serve to broaden a particular study's significance. There is, therefore, a need for greater emphasis on the underlying issue being studied. For example, if variables thought to differentiate response to different disasters are psychological processes, such as appraisal of stressors, uncertainty, loss, or fear, these processes should be most prominent. This emphasis increases the significance of a study by adding or highlighting information about basic processes that may be applicable to other areas.

Theory-driven research, or research which attempts to identify mechanisms, predictors, and mediators or response to trauma, is stronger and more likely to yield interesting or useful findings than is research which is purely descriptive. Not only does theory allow one to focus and refine measurement of the phenomenon of interest, it also guides design decisions about subject sampling, selection of control or comparison groups, and other procedural problems. However, neither the literature on disasters nor the smaller but growing literature on traumatic stress syndromes provides easily derivable or testable conceptual frameworks. This section addresses some of the conceptual issues that have emerged from previous studies of traumatic stress.

Utility of Identifying the Dimensions of Disaster

An important aspect of research in the area of traumatic stress is designing and delineating the salient dimensions of the event, or events, to which the subjects/survivors are responding (see Chapter 9, in this volume, and Wilson, Smith, & Johnson, 1985). The *meaning* to a subject of a particular event may influence the nature and extent of the response. However, it is also the case that certain types or aspects of events are associated with higher levels of symptoms and rates of disorders than other types of events, regardless of individual meaning, suggesting differential pathogenicity of experiences.

Learning which types of experiences are most likely to lead to problems in which groups or subgroups of victims is important for several reasons. First, some experiences may be preventable. For example, if specific aspects of body handling after air crashes are shown to have negative long-term effects, then clean-up activities following mass casualties might be planned with this in mind (perhaps using trained individuals rather than civilian volunteers for these duties). Also, if we can identify which experiences are most likely to lead to later problems, populations of exposed individuals most in need can be targeted for outreach/intervention, and public education efforts can be aimed at helping people assess their own risk and understand any symptoms that may develop.

In addition, there are implications for treatment. If certain aspects of experiences are associated with more psychological distress, and those who are more distressed are most likely to seek treatment, it is probable that those individuals who show up for treatment have had some of these experiences. Such information would be helpful to therapists in terms of knowing what to look for in patients' experience and what experiences are going to need addressing in the treatment setting.

Finally, the identification of psychologically relevant aspects of disaster or trauma will guide measurement and hypotheses testing. The impact of a given disaster may be viewed as the impact of various parts of the event or consequences of it: terror, loss, inconvenience, bereavement, and helplessness are all parts of victimization, and some aspects may be more or less salient in different events. Study of targeted aspects as well as the overall impact may help to refine our knowledge of the pathological aspects of these events.

For all these reasons, studies that investigate links between aspects of stressor experiences and later psychological functioning are extremely important. In terms of psychiatric nosology as well, experiences which are more likely to be followed by symptoms can and should be delineated empirically. Such empirical data would serve to advance treatment beyond accumulated clinical reports and shared stereotypic knowledge of posttraumatic adaptation.

Conceptualizing the Trauma's Structure

Researchers in this area often deal with catastrophic trauma as if it were undifferentiated. For example, we talk about earthquakes, floods, fires, or war as if they represent equivalent events; in point of fact, they are rarely undifferentiated events. Even the most basic term *disaster* has not been adequately defined. One of the most immediate problems associated with the conduct of disaster research in general is the lack of agreement about what constitutes a disaster. A number of typologies and classification systems have been proposed, but further work is needed in conceptualizing and classifying disasters (Raphael, 1986; Wilson, 1989).

In order for knowledge regarding the effects of a disaster to become cumulative it must be possible to compare results from various studies. Wide variation in the types of disasters studied and lack of systematic classification of factors of various components of disaster has made cross-study comparisons difficult. For example, Bromet and Schulberg (1986) noted that part of the reason for the extreme difficulty in identifying consistent predictors of mental health impairment following disasters is the fact that the various studies have focused on disasters which are quite different in nature and severity. The problem of comparability is compounded by the diverse methodologies used in these investigations.

Furthermore, the *Diagnostic and Statistical Manual of Mental Disorders* (DSM-III-R) (American Psychiatric Association, 1987) makes a formal distinction between an *enduring circumstance* (repeated traumatization within the same setting, as in war or a concentration camp) and an *acute, discrete event* with clearly defined beginning and ending points. However, in deciding whether the trauma is an acute event or an enduring process, the DSM-

III-R is less helpful. Insofar as natural disasters are concerned, some may be very short term and can be categorized as acute events, but many, such as a succession of earthquakes or the leakage of deadly gas from a lake, may occur over a period of days or even weeks and thus become enduring processes. The same, of course, is true of human-made disasters, such as Three Mile Island or Chernobyl. The precise point at which the event/process ends and the posttrauma process begins is often less than obvious. This is a crucial methodological issue which requires considerable attention prior to attempting to investigate how catastrophic trauma is related to posttrauma adaptation.

Even in most acute events, it is often the case that one can and should distinguish both the nature of individual traumata and the differences between them. In the literature on the effects of war, it has now become commonplace to talk about war-stress as a concept which encompasses particular types of trauma, such as combat, the loss of a buddy, medical personnel stress, and the witnessing of and participation in atrocities. Originally, however, the war experience was thought by some to encompass only combat experience. The change occurred as a function of researchers' discovering that there were distinct dimensions to the war experience which were differentially related to postwar outcomes (Wilson & Krauss, 1985).

Methodological Issues

Although studies of disasters and other traumatic events share the basic methodological concerns common to other field studies, they also must overcome problems unique to this topic. There is a need for well-designed studies which use standardized instruments and data collection techniques, careful selection and description of victim and comparison groups, and repeated assessment over time. Studies such as these would permit cross-study comparison, replication, and generalization of findings. At present, it is difficult to draw valid conclusions regarding the extent of impairment resulting from different kinds of disaster experiences.

Many methodological problems arise when conducting field studies of disaster. First, most traumatic stress studies are post hoc, that is, subjects were not studied *before* they were traumatized. A few investigators have been able to acquire pre- and/or posttrauma data when a catastrophe occurs in an area where a study is already underway. Sometimes it is also possible to access existing records on victims (e.g., physician, school, hospital), and categorize these data into "before" and "after" measures. For the most part, however, researchers must rely on subjects' retrospective reports of functioning over time. Of course, the subject's account of what happened to him or her with regard to the actual traumatic experience is very important. It may also be possible to supplement this material with corroborating information, for example, by showing that the stressor measures relate to other more objectively determined indices such as the relative destruction of various parts of a town. Nevertheless, studies which focus on individual differences require knowledge of what happened to

a particular subject, and group measures may be of limited interest in studies of this kind.

Other goals, such as maintaining experimenters "blind" with regard to where subjects live or whether they are in the traumatized or control group is usually not possible, since subjects in a comparison group are likely to live in another area. Comparison groups from the same area are likely to contain secondary victims, who will show effects of their own. In addition, diagnostic assessments of posttraumatic stress disorder (PTSD) require knowledge of such experiences as trauma. In studies examining individual experiences, subjects are likely to volunteer information about what happened to them, thus potentially affecting interviewer assessment. For these cases, we recommend including stressor measures that are as objective as possible, and psychological status measures that have well-defined criteria so that interviewers do not have to make many judgments. Stressor measures should focus on what actually happened to the person rather than on the subject's feelings about what happened, unless emotions are designated as a particular interest (as in some events, such as toxic or nuclear leaks, where objective harm cannot be assessed).

In the following section, we will discuss each of the above issues in greater depth. Beginning with a focus on measurement, we will examine strategies for defining the measure of both outcomes and stressors, as well as considerations involved in scheduling the timing of the assessment. We will then focus the discussion on a range of sampling issues, including defining the victim and comparison groups, designing a sampling strategy, and managing attrition.

Measurement Issues

What data to collect and how to collect them are, of course, critical for the development and growth of this research field. The use of unstandardized and investigator-developed unique measures, although necessary in some cases, can contribute to low statistical power, wasted study resources, and an inability to compare findings across studies. However, it must also be stressed that uniformity can lead to rigidity and the possible misapplication of standardized instruments. The art of assessment therefore reflects a balance between these two forces. There is no single set of valid measures that are always appropriate; the application of multilevel assessment of variables for which standardized measures are not available can strengthen a research design.

Outcome Measures

One problem fundamental to disaster research involves defining relevant outcomes. Some researchers in the field maintain that it is necessary to establish the presence of diagnosable psychopathology or "caseness," in order for disaster to be considered etiologically significant. Others hold that research needs merely to demonstrate that disasters bring about an increase in the prevalence or persistence of symptoms that are, to a greater or lesser degree, present within the normal population. Recommendations about the most appropriate ways of measuring symptomatic outcomes would seem to rest on the resolution of this issue. However, it should be noted that evidence for severe psychopathology has been found to be fairly limited. Recently, a great deal of attention has been focused on PTSD as an outcome measure. The comorbidity of other disorders with this diagnosis (in particular, alcoholism and depression) mandates thoughtful consideration in research designs (see Rundell, Ursano, Holloway, & Silberman, 1989).

The use of "homemade" scales should be abandoned in favor of standardized outcome measures. In the past, selection of measurement instruments for disaster studies was problematic, since most of the previous disaster investigators had devised a new questionnaire for each study. Panel members emphasized the importance of using standardized instruments when conducting disaster research, for purposes of cross-study comparability.

To date, few measures have been validated for use in the systematic assessment of psychological trauma. Researchers seeking to assess the aftermath of exposure to highly stressful events have relied upon a wide range of measures to assess psychological functioning. Typically these measures have been psychiatric symptom-oriented, although some researchers have attempted to evaluate social functioning, marital functioning, vocational functioning, changes in attitudes, and biological correlates of exposure. The work of several of the panel members supports the use of a multimethod approach to the assessment of adjustment: behavioral, psychophysiological, and subjective stress measures. Subjective measures have clearly been given precedence in the research conducted to date. However, recent studies have demonstrated the value of complementing subjective indices with measures from the biological and behavioral spheres (Baum, Grunberg, & Singer, 1982). These studies have used multimethod assessment in the field and in the laboratory, thus demonstrating the broad-based applicability and feasibility of this approach for the assessment of traumatic response.

To facilitate consistency in the measures used to assess traumatic outcomes, the panel assembled the types of instruments that have been successfully used by researchers in the field. Although it is difficult to recommend the use of any specific battery of measures for a given study, the following instruments are worthy of serious consideration when designing a study of the effects of disaster or other traumatic events:

1. *Subjective measures of psychological symptoms*
   (a) Minnesota Multiphasic Personality Inventory (MMPI) and the use of its PTSD subscale (Keane, Malloy, & Fairbank, 1984; Wilson, 1989)
   (b) Symptom Checklist-90 (Derogatis, 1977)
   (c) Beck Depression Inventory (Beck, 1967)
   (d) Center for Epidemiologic Studies Depression Scale (CES-D) (Radloff, 1977)
   (e) Spielberger State-Trait Anxiety Inventory (Spielberger, Gorsuch, & Lushene, 1970)
   (f) Impact of Events Scale (Horowitz, Wilner, & Alvarez, 1979)
   (g) Mississippi Scale for Combat-related PTSD (Keane, Caddell, & Taylor, 1988)
   (h) Zung Depression Scale (Zung, 1965)
   (i) Vietnam Era Stress Inventory (Wilson & Krauss, 1989)
2. *Diagnostic instruments*
   (a) Structured Clinical Interview for DSM-III-R (SCID) (Spitzer & Williams, 1985)
   (b) Diagnostic Interview Schedule/Disaster Supplement (DIS/DS) (Robins & Smith, 1983)
3. *Family functioning*
   Family Environment Scale (R. H. Moos & B. S. Moos, 1986)
4. *Biological measures or psychophysiological measures*
   (a) Physiological reactivity to cues reminiscent of the traumatic event (heartrate, blood pressure, skin conductance, finger temperature) (Blanchard, Kolb, Pallmeyer, & Gerardi, 1982; Malloy, Fairbank, & Keane, 1983)
   (b) Basal levels of corticosteroids and catecholamines (epinephrine and norepinephrine) (e.g., Baum, Gatchel, & Schaeffer, 1983)
   (c) Ratio of cortisol to norepinephrine (e.g., Mason, Giller, Kosten, & Harkness, in press)
   (d) Basal systolic and diastolic blood pressure (Blanchard et al., 1982)
5. *Behavioral measures*
   (a) Continuous performance tests, tests of attention (Asarnow & MacCrimmin, 1978; Rosvold, Mirsky, Sarason, Bransome, & Beck, 1956)
   (b) Information-processing assessments (Rey, 1964; Stroop, 1935)

The above instruments are not intended to be exhaustive of all potentially useful outcome measures. However, the listing contains measures that have been successfully used in past traumatic stress research and are generally viewed favorably in the clinical research literature. Acceptable levels of reliability and validity have been demonstrated for many of these measures, a factor that should enhance their acceptance in the mental health research field. Inclusion of these measures in a research protocol would not necessarily preclude the use of other favored or theoretically derived assessment measures selected by the scientist.

In fact, there may be some areas where the field could advance by developing new measures. There are reasons to believe that symptomatic reactions to disasters may vary over time and across situations. Although the cyclical nature of symptoms may be captured via repeated measurements, their situation-specific (or situationally enhanced) nature is not captured well by most standardized scales. For example, Endler and Magnusson (1976) argued that individuals differ in their proneness to anxiety in different situations. Some may become anxious in interpersonal situations; others, when confronted by physical danger. They suggested that trait anxiety scales primarily tap the anxiety that arises in interpersonal situations and are less likely to tap anxieties that arise in novel or physically dangerous situations. Certain situations could reasonably be expected to be more difficult for victims than other situations, and, as a result, disaster effects may be underestimated by current methods.

Furthermore, in postdisaster study designs it may be difficult to disentangle true increases in psychopathology from apparent increases that result from a tendency of those exposed to blame the disaster for difficulties that may actually have predated it. However, studies using the DIS, for example, have shown that this reversal of the sequence of events can be minimized if, rather than relying on global health assessments, the investigator inquires about specific symptoms and behaviors and also makes the effort to carefully date the onset of specific symptoms. Specific questions set in a life-history context reduce the halo effect that may arise from the respondents' feelings that the disaster should have caused particular effects.

Stressor Measures

Quantifying dimensions of catastrophic experiences is a difficult task for several reasons. First, because each traumatic event differs from other events in important ways, no existing instrument covers all potential aspects. Investigators may have to invent questions to fit the situation. Second, some events are extremely difficult to quantify because the harm done during the event is not immediately evident. As a result, although the damage resulting from an earthquake may be obvious (e.g., loss of a family member, loss of a house, exposure to dead bodies), the damage done by a toxic or nuclear accident (e.g., Times Beach, Three Mile Island) may not manifest itself for years. In the latter case, beliefs and perceptions of harm become crucial, making stressor measures, such as proximity to the site, imperfect. Third, some aspects of events are more difficult to quantify than others because of their subjective quality or complexity. For example, threat to life is, to some extent, a judgment based on degree of warning, potential avenues of escape, closeness to the death agent, predictability, and so forth. Consistent with the portrayal by Lazarus (1966) of stress and coping as a dynamic cognitive and behavioral process, appraisal of an event may vary with the individual, yielding a range of effects from the same experience.

In spite of these problems, traumatic events can indeed be described and classified along dimensions (see Wilson *et al.*, 1985). Investigators are beginning to identify aspects of events that are associated with later symptoms and are attempting to look for generic aspects that transcend different types of events. Several suggestions derive from this approach. First, rather than starting from scratch, the researcher should look for elements that other investigators have explored in other events. It is important that the explored dimensions include those that are highly salient in the particular event under study. Unless these aspects are already known, open-ended interviews to determine them are warranted. Measurement of stressors should be as objective and as close to the experience as possible. Research has shown that recall of factual information (e.g., such and such happened) can be quite good over long periods of time, while frequency is less well recalled, and reliability for aspects requiring judgment is fairly poor.

Measurement of both the intensity and the distinguishing qualitative features of a trauma are necessary to achieve a full understanding of the impact of the trauma on subsequent adjustment; that is, it is necessary to distinguish between the relative effects of differences in degree of traumatization and differences in kind of traumatization. This suggests that interval scales and qualitative or categorical measures are both necessary, since no single measure will suffice to capture the complexity of trauma. In most studies of war, for example, respondents are asked to indicate whether they have been exposed to any of a range of identified experiences and, if so, their degree of exposure to each of the specified events (Wilson & Krauss, 1985). The individual items are usually part of a checklist, and the frequency of exposure multipliers consists of a series of five-point Likert-style scales ranging from "Never" to "Often."

Frequency multipliers are often highly redundant with event components of a scale. A scale which captures a reasonable number of the events within a dimension may actually provide a latent measure of the frequency of exposure to the range of events. With regard to war experience, for example, a respondent who indicates exposure to a broad range of combat experiences is much more likely to have been routinely exposed to these events than a respondent who indicates exposure to only one or two events. It is also possible to identify those experiences which are most traumatic within a dimension and then weight those events so that not all events have an equal impact on the scale. Here again, the most traumatic events are generally associated with exposure to a greater range of events.

In most cases, interval measures of particular dimensions are likely to provide better estimates of the relation between trauma (and adaptation to the trauma) than either nominal or ordinal measures. However, there are some instances in which quantifying an experience does not significantly contribute to a better understanding of the relation between trauma and response. Using the war literature as an example, the loss of a close buddy *appears* to be an event whose identifiable pathogenic impact is not enhanced by measuring the number of times the event occurs. Yet this is still open to empirical analysis.

The above approach may also be used to explore dose-response issues, such as the following: Is there a minimum dose? How large a dose of a particular component of the trauma is required before we see evidence of a pathogenic response to the trauma? At what level do most humans show some evidence of a pathogenic effect of the trauma? At what point is there no additional incremental effect on the pathogenic response to the trauma? And, most intriguingly, what is the dose-response pattern over the range of the trauma, that is, the threshold effect for individual differences in stress response? Addressing these issues requires the construction of interval scales suitable for use in analytic models which may contain both linear and nonlinear terms. (For an example of dose-response disaster research, see Shore, Tatum, & Vollmer, 1986.)

Scheduling Assessments

Longitudinal studies using repeated measurements are valuable, if not essential, in the study of disaster effects. To date, little is known about the natural course of psychological reactions. Thus, many crucial questions remain: Do mental health effects occur immediately after exposure or are they delayed? How long do these mental health changes persist? Are they constant or do they fluctuate in a cyclical pattern? Whether or not long-term effects are observed may depend on the severity of the disaster, length of the follow-up interval, and the timing of the follow-up interview. If data are collected only once, the nature of the findings will depend on *when* the interview takes place.

It is difficult to develop generally applicable recommendations about the most appropriate length for a follow-up interval; the ideal timing probably varies across settings and across physical agents. For example, in settings where there is a recurring threat of disaster (a tornado or flood season) it seems advisable to conduct interviews in the midst of that season and during other times of the year. In other situations, anniversary dates could be important, although depending on the purpose of the study, such dates may be inappropriate for measurement. The ability to identify a return to baseline or presumed pretrauma levels of functioning can compensate somewhat for the lack of pretrauma measures and can provide important information about the effects of trauma.

Sampling Issues

In this section, we discuss a range of methodological issues related to locating a study sample, including defining exposure and identifying victims, selecting a valid comparison group, designing a sampling strategy, and dealing with attrition.

Defining Victims and Comparison Groups

The definition of exposure can be a problem for an otherwise well-designed study, as was found in a study of the mental health effects of various environmental hazards (Smith, Robins, Pryzbeck, Goldring, & Solomon, 1986). Although the tornadoes and floods that struck the study area seemed self-evident, difficulties arose when respondents reported they were out of town when the event occurred or their business was flooded but not their residence. A new category (*not at home*) was subsequently added for those who were away during the disaster or whose primary residence was unaffected.

Toxic disasters present problems in identifying victims that are not usually found in studies of natural disasters. Flood damage can be seen, but toxic hazards such as dioxin, methane gas, hydrogen sulfide, and many others often provide little visual evidence of damage. Victims themselves may be unaware of exposure until they are notified by officials. One solution in these cases is to add a new category: *self-perceived exposure*. Of course, this strategy gives rise to additional research questions, such as assessing differences between the objective-exposure and the perceived-exposure groups. However, these questions can be important ones, particularly if the differences between such groups are small.

Most studies of disaster define the victim sample in terms of the extent to which given individuals personally experience injury or property damage. Many definitions of victimization, however, recognize the broader, collective context of disaster. Bolin (1985) observed that there are two broad categories of victims. *Primary victims* are those who directly experience physical, material, or personal losses. *Secondary victims* are those who live in the affected area but have no personal injuries or damages. Nonetheless, they may have witnessed destruction, been subjected to postdisaster economic problems, or been inconvenienced by washed-out roads and bridges. This two-category definition of victimization recognizes that a disaster is more than an individual's life event; it is a community event with the potential to precipitate change and stress among persons suffering no direct damage. Of course, there may be other victims as well (e.g., relief workers, relatives or friends of primary victims) but most research in this area concentrates on these two classes.

In many studies, "nonvictim" controls would be better described as secondary victims. Until more is known about the consequences of secondary or indirect exposure across various types of incidents, the inclusion of indirect or secondary victim groups as well as nonvictim groups is recommended. Thus, control groups may reflect "less affected" rather than unaffected populations.

This approach to defining victims has disadvantages, however. It will increase difficulties in establishing the equivalence of the comparison groups in ways other than exposure to disaster. For example, if Cincinnati were to be hit by a tornado, and if residents not personally experiencing property damage were considered as secondary victims, who would be an appropriate nonvictim group? The nearby residents of Dayton, Ohio? At Three Mile Island (nuclear accident), researchers were forced to go beyond nearby communities using areas of 80 to 100 or more miles away as comparison sites (e.g., Baum *et al.*, 1983; Bromet, 1980). Behavioral scientists, in particular, may find that they need to increase their knowledge of other disciplines, such as demography or economics, to make such decisions. It may be that more than one nonvictim site is needed, particularly when predisaster conditions are not known and cannot be controlled for in the analysis. Thus, for example, in studies at Three Mile Island a variety of control groups have been used, including people living near undamaged reactors, near traditional plants, or near no power plants, allowing for control of a number of variables.

Since few investigators are in the position of having predisaster information on victims, several comparison groups may be needed. Identifying an appropriate control group can be fraught with difficulties. In trying to choose controls as similar as possible to disaster victims in all respects except for the experience of the disaster, individuals from the same area with minimal or indirect exposure to the disaster may be included in the control group. However, individuals indirectly exposed to disasters (e.g., only vicariously via experiences of relatives or close friends) may exhibit adverse psychological experiences not shared by those never exposed and may, therefore, not be a suitable comparison group. Also, it can be argued that the effects of technological disasters may be widespread with respect to confidence and perceived control.

Even though those indirectly exposed may be more

similar to the disaster victims, individuals without any exposure may differ in ways which are related to their mental health status but are independent of their disaster experience. Exposure to disaster is not an entirely random occurrence, and disaster victims may start out with a higher risk of developing mental problems. Population and economic pressures may cause people to live in marginal or vulnerable areas, predisposing them to victimization.

Designing a Sampling Plan

The use of traditional sampling techniques may not be possible in disaster studies and, in fact, may not be necessary if the investigator is not attempting population estimates. Because the prevalence of many mental health disorders may be low in untreated populations, sampling from high-risk groups actually enhances the investigator's ability to detect significant disaster-related effects. However, it must be recognized that compiling a proper sampling frame and obtaining the cooperation of participants in high-risk cohorts can be more difficult than in general population surveys.

Because of the difficulties (and costs) involved in obtaining suitable comparison groups, investigators should consider other sources of data as well. One source is the Epidemiologic Catchment Area (ECA) project funded by NIMH which provides longitudinal data on the incidence and prevalence of psychiatric disorders in five sites across the country (Eaton & Kessler, 1985). These data are now available for public use. Investigators using the DIS or DIS/DS on a sample exposed to disaster in a demographically similar community could use ECA data in lieu of collecting longitudinal data on a "no exposure" control group.

Attrition

Longitudinal studies inevitably bring attrition, the loss of subjects owing to respondent death, disinterest, illness, physical incapacity, or migration. There is mounting evidence (e.g., Norris, 1987) that attrition is generally overrated as a threat to the validity of panel studies. However, attrition may be critical in instances when it occurs as a result of the event under study. For example, in most epidemiological studies, death is not a source of bias since the panel continues to be representative of the surviving cohort. However, if that death is linked to the disaster, either directly or indirectly, it is a cause for concern. Even in this case, deaths would have to occur with considerable frequency to produce a sizable bias. Migration is more problematic because it is not presently known whether those who leave a disaster-stricken area are the "best-off," that is, those with the assets that allow them to leave, or the "worst-off," those who perceive themselves as least able to cope. The solution here may be to study migration as an important outcome of disaster in its own right.

Of course, investigators should assess who drops out (and why) in any study involving multiple waves of data collection and, when necessary, should use that information to qualify their findings. They must also devise procedures to minimize attrition. Expectations should be realistic, however. The only way to avoid attrition is not to do longitudinal studies, or to begin with a sample of volunteers who are selected because they will agree, in advance, to participate in a given number of interviews. The latter approach is obviously unsound, since self-selection on this criterion may introduce a different and undetectable kind of bias.

Conclusions

In this chapter, we have highlighted some important practical, conceptual, and methodological considerations in the design of studies of disaster and traumatic stress. Although interest in the effects of trauma has been longstanding (e.g., Trimble, 1981) the scientific study of traumatic stress is relatively recent. The field needs to develop, not so much in terms of devising a new set of methods and theories, but rather in terms of adapting those from other areas of research to the specific needs of traumatic stress studies.

The phenomenon of traumatic stress is both important and complex. Each research question may be investigated in many different ways, and the optimal strategy will depend on the host of factors unique to each situation. Although the panel members have used many different approaches to the study of traumatic stress, all agreed on the need for increased codification and standardization of the field. This was seen as best accomplished by enhanced communication among researchers, with one important goal being the development of both common-focus research and multisite studies. Investigators were also encouraged to adopt standardized assessment batteries and instruments, and to place greater emphasis on conceptual development. It is only by these means that the field of traumatic stress research, which is still in its infancy, will develop into a rich resource for assisting victims of disaster.

References

American Psychiatric Association. (1987). *Diagnostic and statistical manual of mental disorders* (3rd ed., rev.). Washington, DC: Author.

Asarnow, R. F., & MacCrimmin, D. J. (1978). Residual performance deficit in clinically remitted schizophrenics: A marker of schizophrenia. *Journal of Abnormal Psychology, 87*, 597–608.

Baum, A., Gatchel, R. J., & Schaeffer, M. A. (1983). Emotional, behavioral and physiological effects of chronic stress at Three Mile Island. *Journal of Consulting and Clinical Psychology, 51*, 565–572.

Baum, A., Grunberg, N. E., & Singer, J. E. (1982). The use of psychological and neuroendrocrinological measurements in the study of stress. *Health Psychology, 1*(3), 217–236.

Beck, A. T. (1967). *Depression: Clinical, experimental, and theoretical aspects.* New York: Paul B. Hoeber.

Blanchard, E. B., Kolb, L. C., Pallmeyer, T. P., & Gerardi, R. J. (1982). The development of a psychophysiological assessment procedure for post-traumatic stress disorder in Vietnam veterans. *Psychiatric Quarterly, 54*, 220–229.

Bolin, R. (1985). Disaster characteristics and psychosocial impacts. In B. J. Sowder (Ed.), *Disasters and mental health: Selected* contemporary perspectives (pp. 3–28). Rockville, MD: U. S. Department of Health and Human Services.

Bromet, E. (1980). Three Mile Island: Mental health findings. Pittsburgh: Western Psychiatric Institute and Clinic and the University of Pittsburgh.

Bromet, E. J., & Schulberg, H. C. (1986). The TMI disaster: A search for high risk groups. In J. H. Shore (Ed.), Disaster stress studies: New methods and findings. Washington, DC: American Psychiatric Press.

Derogatis, L. R. (1977). The SCL-90 Manual 1. Scoring, administration and procedures for the SCL-90. Baltimore: Johns Hopkins University School of Medicine, Clinical Psychometrics Unit.

Eaton, W. W., & Kessler, L. G. (Eds.). (1985). Epidemiologic field methods in psychiatry: The NIMH epidemiologic catchment area program. Orlando: Academic Press.

Endler, N. S., & Magnusson, D. (1976). Toward an interactional psychology of personality. Psychological Bulletin, 83(5), 956–974.

Horowitz, M. J., Wilner, N., & Alvarez, W. (1979). Impact of events scale. A measure of psychosomatic stress. Psychosomatic Medicine, 41, 209–218.

Keane, T. M., Caddell, J. M., & Taylor, K. L. (1988). Mississippi scale for combat-related posttraumatic stress disorder: Three studies in reliability and validity. Journal of Consulting and Clinical Psychology, 56, 85–90.

Keane, T. M., & Fairbank, J. A. (1983). Survey analysis of combat related stress disorders in Vietnam veterans. American Journal of Psychiatry, 140, 345–350.

Keane, T. M., Malloy, P. F., & Fairbank, J. A. (1984). Empirical development of an MMPI subscale for the assessment of combat-related posttraumatic stress disorder. Journal of Consulting and Clinical Psychology, 52, 888–891.

Lazarus, R. S. (1966). Psychological stress and the coping process. New York: McGraw-Hill.

Malloy, P. F., Fairbank, J. A., & Keane, T. M. (1983). Validation of a multimethod assessment of post-traumatic stress disorders in Vietnam veterans. Journal of Consulting and Clinical Psychology, 51, 488–494.

Mason, J. W., Giller, E. L., Kosten, T. R., & Harkness, L. (in press). Elevation of urinary norepinephrine/cortisol ratio in post-traumatic stress disorder. Journal of Nervous and Mental Disorders.

Moos, R. H., & Moos, B. S. (1986). Family Environment scale manual (2nd ed.). Palo Alto: Consulting Psychologists Press.

Norris, F. H. (1987). Effects of attrition on relationships between variables in surveys of older adults. Journal of Gerontology, 42(6), 597–605.

Radloff, L. S. (1977). The CES-D scale: A self-report depression scale for research in the general population. Applied Psychological Measurement, 1(3), 385–401.

Raphael, B. (1986). When disaster strikes: How individuals and communities cope with catastrophe. New York: Basic Books.

Rey, A. (1964). L'examen clinique en psychologie. Paris: Presses Universitaires de France.

Robins, L. N., & Smith, E. M. (1983). Diagnostic Interview Schedule/Disaster Supplement. St. Louis: Washington University School of Medicine, Department of Psychiatry.

Rosvold, H. E., Mirsky, A. F., Sarason, I., Bransome, E. D., & Beck, L. H. (1956). A continuous performance test of brain damage. Journal of Consulting Psychology, 20, 343–350.

Rundell, J. R., Ursano, R. J., Holloway, H. C., & Silberman, E. K. (1989). Psychiatric responses to trauma. Hospital and Community Psychiatry, 40(1), 68–74.

Shore, J. H., Tatum, E. L., & Vollmer, W. M. (1986). Evaluation of mental effects of disaster: Mt. St. Helen's eruption. American Journal of Public Health, 76 (Suppl.), 76–83.

Smith, E. M., Robins, L. N., Pryzbeck, T. R., Goldring, E., & Solomon, S. D. (1986). Psychosocial consequences of disaster. In J. Shore (Ed.), Disaster stress studies: New methods and findings. Washington DC: American Psychiatric Press.

Spielberger, C. D., Gorsuch, R. L., & Lushene, R. E. (1970). Manual for the State-Trait Anxiety Inventory (self-evaluating questionnaire). Palo Alto: Consulting Psychologists Press.

Spitzer, R. L., & Williams, J. B. (1985). Structured clinical interview for DSM-III-R, patient version. New York: Biometrics Research Department, New York State Psychiatric Institute.

Stroop, J. R. (1935). Studies of interference in serial verbal reactions. Journal of Experimental Psychology, 18, 643–662.

Trimble, M. (1981). Post-traumatic neurosis. New York: Wiley.

Wilson, J. P. (1989). Trauma, transformation and healing. New York: Brunner/Mazel.

Wilson, J. P. & Krauss, G. E. (1985). Predicting post-traumatic stress disorder among Vietnam veterans. In W. Kelly (Ed.), Posttraumatic stress disorder and the war veteran patient (pp. 102–147). New York: Brunner/Mazel.

Wilson, J. P., Smith, W. K., & Johnson, G. (1985). A comparative analysis of various survivor groups. In C. R. Figley (Ed.), Trauma and its wake: The study and treatment of post-traumatic stress disorder (pp. 142–172). New York: Brunner/Mazel.

Zung, W. (1965). A self-rating depression scale. Archives of General Psychiatry, 12, 63–70.

CHAPTER 11

Identifying Survivors at Risk

Trauma and Stressors across Events

Bonnie L. Green

Introduction

A great deal of interest has been recently paid to symptoms and diagnoses that follow exposure to events that are outside of the normal range. In particular, post-traumatic stress disorder (PTSD) entered the psychiatric nomenclature in 1980 (American Psychiatric Association [APA], 1980) and was somewhat modified with the revision of the third edition of the *Diagnostic and Statistical Manual of Mental Disorders* (DSM-III) in 1987 (DSM-III-R, APA, 1987). However, the earlier versions of the DSM also contained diagnoses related to stress, and such symptoms and diagnoses have long been acknowledged, particularly in association with wartime experience (Trimble, 1981). Recent work by Horowitz and his colleagues (Horowitz, 1986; Horowitz, Weiss, & Marmar, 1987) has suggested a generic category of "stress-response syndromes" that may arise following a variety of individual and collective events including bereavement.

Most of the literature on traumatic stress has focused on describing either the specific symptoms that are associated with exposure to such events or the dynamic or associational processes which connect the event with the symptomatic outcome. The event itself, and/or particular aspects of the event, have received little attention. Recent research on Vietnam War veterans has begun to address empirically which aspects of the war experience are most associated with prolonged symptoms. Although few authors in other areas of traumatic stress have focused on the nature of the experience as a predictor of who is more or less *at risk* following a traumatic event, in the process of doing empirical research, any number of investigators have examined particular aspects of events and attempted to link them to the symptoms studied.

In this chapter, I will focus on the events and dimensions of events that set in motion the symptoms and syndromes that are of interest to clinicians and researchers working in the area of traumatic stress. Before explaining specifically what will be covered in the chapter, however, a general framework for the focus on stressor events needs to be addressed. A number of years ago, two colleagues and I presented a general model of the factors that are important in understanding the development of a particular outcome in the processing of a traumatic event. In that model (Green, Wilson, & Lindy, 1985), we proposed that three types of factors are important in such a process. The first category of factors covers the *traumatic event* itself or what objectively occurred to the person in terms of life threat, loss, and so forth, and what role the person played in the event. Two additional types of factors were also seen to contribute to the processing of the particular experience(s). *Individual factors*, primarily those which precede the event, include the person's characteristic defense mechanisms and coping styles along with his or her history of psychiatric illness, the specific meaning of the event to the person based on past experience, and other innate characteristics of the individual, such as intelligence and temperament. Also in this category would be coping efforts the person brought to bear in the particular case of coping with the event, which is actually an interaction of the person's style with the nature of the event.

A second group of factors contributing to adaptation to an event were those factors in the *recovery environment* that generally follow the event. These include the availability and use of social supports and networks, the meaning of the event to society at large, and, thus, how society regards the person who went through the event

Bonnie L. Green • Department of Psychiatry, Georgetown University Hospital, Washington, DC 20007.

International Handbook of Traumatic Stress Syndromes, edited by John P. Wilson and Beverley Raphael. Plenum Press, New York, 1993.

as well as subsequent events that either result from or follow the original trauma.

Within this schema, the traumatic event(s) themselves set the processing into motion. As noted, the adaptation may be more or less difficult depending on the nature or intensity of the event itself and the impact of personal strengths/deficits and social/environmental forces on its processing. Although all these factors are important, I will deal with the first category, the event itself, conceptually and as it implicated in outcome.

This chapter consists of five sections. In the first section, some *background/historical information* will be given with regard to early studies of stress, early conceptual schemes about stressors, and shifts in the types of events that have been studied. The second section covers current conceptualizations of stressors and trauma, including the DSM-III-R, types of events that are considered to constitute trauma, and conceptual problems with multiple and/or chronic traumatic exposure. The third section will suggest some *generic dimensions* of trauma and will review empirical findings from a variety of events that support these dimensions. *Measurement problems* in stressor research will be addressed in the fourth section. The final section will suggest *future directions* that might be fruitful to pursue with regard to questions about stressors.

Background

The earliest investigations of traumatic events tended to be those dealing with situations of extreme stress, such as war and concentration camp internment. In those contexts, it probably seemed as if people's experiences were so stressful as to be impossible to differentiate at an individual level, so little attention was paid to differences in specific aspects of the overall experience. This approach is not helpful, however, when it comes to describing less extreme events where experiences may vary widely. This is particularly important to understand with collectively based traumatic events. One may experience a tornado by having one's mailbox knocked down, or by having one's child killed by flying debris. In both instances, a tornado is being experienced, but the psychological responses might be expected to be quite different. Even in extreme individual situations, such as rape, studies have shown that knowing specific aspects of the event increases the prediction of psychological outcomes.

In the disaster literature, there has been some attempt to delineate dimensions of disastrous events in order that categories of events could be created. For example, Barton (1969) suggested that the scope of the impact, the speed of onset, the duration, and the social preparedness of the community are all likely to affect responses. Berren, Beigel, and Ghertner (1980) suggested five dimensions that distinguish events: type (man-made vs. natural), duration, degree of personal impact, potential for recurrence, and control over future impact. Although such distinctions seem potentially important, for the most part there has been no attempt to link these types of dimensions with outcome. The primary reason for this is probably that investigations tend

to study only one event at a time, so there is no variability on the above-stated dimensions of that particular event. In order to link such dimensions to psychological outcome, a number of events would need to be studied in the same time frame with the same instruments. A number of investigators are beginning to do exactly that (Baum, personal communication [study in progress]; Steinglass & Gerrity, 1990), but results are just beginning to be available (see Chapter 10, in this volume, for an analysis). The most fruitful current approach to examining aspects of events, then, appears to be looking within a particular event for individual differences in how the event unfolded and attempting to specify generic dimensions that might apply to a variety of events.

Another approach is to compare a group exposed to a particular stressor to a group without this experience. This is an approach that characterized much of the research in the 1970s; for example, families that experienced a flood were compared to those who did not (Bennett, 1970; Melick, 1978). However, this approach will produce information about specific aspects of events only if experimental and control groups vary on one dimension only. If they vary on several dimensions, it will be more difficult to pinpoint specific effects.

It appears that, over the years, there has been a shift from studying "natural" phenomena to studying those events and incidents of human origin. The exception to this is war, a person-induced event with potentially devastating human consequences which has been studied on and off for decades. Those investigators studying disaster have turned more and more to "technological" events (Baum, Fleming, & Davidson, 1983) as a subject of study. In these events, control that should be maintained over technology is lost (Baum, Fleming, & Davidson, 1983) as opposed to natural events, where there was never control in the first place. Although this distinction is a potentially important one, oftentimes the "causation" is a mixture of human and natural so that a clear distinction cannot be drawn (Bolin, 1988; Smith, North, & Price, 1988; see also Chapter 33, in this volume). Also receiving more attention in the 1980s and 1990s is the deliberate, human-perpetrated traumatic event, such as rape, assault, and politically motivated torture. In the stress/trauma literature, the victims of such events have been subjects of investigation.

These distinctions thus lead to a conceptualization of types of events that fall along a *continuum of deliberateness* or *causality*. At one end are those events which are completely natural, over which persons have no control (e.g., a tornado). In the middle of the continuum would be those events that would be categorized as resulting from "error," or "mishap" (e.g., a toxic waste spill). The upper end of the continuum would include events that were deliberately perpetrated with an intent to harm (e.g., assault, rape).

New types of catastrophes challenge our capacity to classify them. These new types of events, which are increasingly the subject of study, are those in which the impact is "invisible," at least initially. Examples of this type of event are the Three Mile Island radiation leak, the Times Beach toxic spill, and contraction of the human immunodeficiency virus (HIV), leading to acquired immune deficiency syndrome (AIDS). Initially, the only indication of these events is the receipt of the information that they have occurred. One could even conceptualize the information as the stressor. Even though contraction of HIV is considered to be ultimately fatal, toxic and nuclear leaks have no clear-cut, definite effects for an individual, making this type of stressor a difficult one to conceptualize. Later in this chapter, I will propose that such stressors require a category of their own.

This section has not provided an exhaustive historical perspective. Rather, the intention has been to sample how stressors have tended to be conceptualized and delineated (or not) as well as to indicate a trend toward a broader definition of potentially traumatic events, including, more recently, technological and health-related events. This expanded definition encompasses more survivors who can be understood within the traumatic stress framework and who are potentially in need of clinical services.

Current Conceptualizations of Stressors and Trauma

Conceptualizations of trauma, or of what constitutes a "stressor" worthy of our interest and empirical investigation, are nearly as varied as the scientists who write about them. Historically, a number of schemes were reviewed for differentiating events. In the next section, I will focus on particular aspects of events where some generic dimensions of traumatic events will be suggested. Here, I will focus on a broader look at what constitutes trauma as currently defined.

Most easily at hand is the definition of stressor events that may set in motion the syndrome of post-traumatic stress disorder, found in recent editions of the *Diagnostic and Statistical Manual* (DSM) of the APA (1980, 1987). Posttraumatic stress disorder (PTSD) is a combination of intrusive, avoidant/numbing, and physiological arousal symptoms that are seen to arise following extremely stressful events. The criteria for defining such events have changed somewhat from the initial definition in DSM-III (APA, 1980) to the present definition in DSM-III-R (APA, 1987). This definition is currently under review for potential modification in the forthcoming DSM-IV (Davidson & Foa, 1991), so that even pinning down the "official" mental health definition of a stressor is like shooting at a moving target.

Brett, Spitzer, and Williams (1988) described the changes from the early DSMs, where the focus was on characteristics of the environment, to the more recent ones (DSM-III and DSM-III-R) where more emphasis has been placed on the individual's contact with a particular type of situation. Unfortunately, some of the language in the present nosology is circular (Green, 1990), for example, a stressor for the purpose of assessing PTSD is an event that would "be markedly distressing to almost anyone" (APA, 1987, p. 250). DSM-III-R continues to emphasize the rare occurrence of the stressor and its capacity to cause symptoms. However, it suggests some general dimensions that are applicable to the person's experience (Brett *et al.*, 1988). This list includes threat of injury to one's self or loved one(s), sudden destruction of one's home or community, and witnessing mutilation or violent death. Thus, the etiology of PTSD is seen to be

personal exposure to particular aspects of events that would in some universal way be considered extraordinary or extreme with a negative valence. Although not specifically stated, with one exception (community destruction) these aspects all involve exposure to death or injury, or threat of death or severe injury, suggesting a latent dimension that might help organize our thinking about what is potentially traumatic.

Other sources have been less subtle about this organizing principle and have placed specific emphasis on the importance of the theme of death in traumatic response. Lifton (1988) specifically mentioned the "death imprint" as an important aspect of the survivor syndrome. This imprint makes it impossible for the survivor to deny the reality of death and brings him or her face-to-face with feelings of personal vulnerability and consequent anxiety. This confrontation would be the cause of the symptoms in the syndrome and would require the survivor to grapple with the formulation of a rationale for his or her continued existence. It has yet to be determined empirically whether this "death encounter," actual or symbolic, is a necessary condition for producing PTSD symptoms.

Breslau and Davis (1987b) raised questions about the DSM-III conceptualization with regard to whether the stressor in PTSD is unique because of its magnitude (quantitative aspects) or because of its nature (qualitative aspects). They suggested that the DSM-III definition moves toward defining the uniqueness of the stressor in terms of its magnitude rather than in terms of a qualitative difference. Such a conceptualization makes it difficult to define a cutoff between ordinary and extraordinary events wherein extraordinary events produce one type of specific pathology and where ordinary events (i.e., those that would be addressed in adjustment disorder and that have been studied in life-events research) produce a different type. This issue has also been raised by Solomon and Canino (1990). Their research on two different types of disasters using the same methodology suggested that PTSD symptoms also result from more "ordinary" stressors. These two points of view (Lifton, on the one hand, arguing for the death imprint, and Breslau and Davis, and Solomon and Canino the other, arguing that PTSD and non-PTSD stressors may not be discontinuous) are both currently represented in the field. Between DSM-III and DSM-III-R, as noted, more emphasis was placed on specific qualitative events that put individuals at higher risk for PTSD. However, the magnitude/quality of the event issue remains with regard to the conceptualization of traumatic events. There is disagreement about what constitutes a traumatic event and whether several more ordinary events (or even one) might "add-up," psychologically, to a traumatic event. More empirical data are needed to address this question adequately.

One potential "solution" to the issue of specifying traumatic events is to incorporate the person's own evaluation of the event into the definition, which, in fact, is being considered for the DSM-IV. Although it is clear that the person's subjective appraisal of the event is quite important—critical to know, clinically—and is likely to increase the prediction of who develops stress reactions, incorporation of it into stressor definitions is not recommended. This is because confounding objective and subjective descriptions of events may prevent us from doing research which might help answer the questions raised above more definitely (Green, 1986).

Staying within a general conceptualization of trauma, as related to extreme or extraordinary events, and what is considered to constitute a "trauma" are becoming more varied; many different types of events are seen as potentially "traumatic." From wars and natural disasters, the original traumatic events most discussed and studied, we have shifted to interest in technological events and deliberate episodes of violence toward fellow human beings. Refugees fleeing repressive governments where they are threatened with injury, death, or torture, and police and emergency medical personnel who come in constant contact with either the threat of death and injury or death and dying are seen as individuals at risk for stress disorders. Chronic stress symptoms have been identified among people who have been exposed to radiation or toxic contamination and who fear early death or debilitation or the passing on of defective genes to their offspring. Individuals infected with HIV or with AIDS, who know they will die but not how long it will take or how agonizing it will be, are also among those currently conceptualized as experiencing extreme stressors that are expected to produce at least some symptoms of a stress response (see Chapter 45, in this volume, for a discussion). This identification of such groups for targeted study attests to the change in mental health professionals' view of disorder and a focus on external events as at least providing the trigger for psychological reactions.

An issue that complicates the conceptualization of stressors is that of repeated or multiple traumatization or of chronic, ongoing exposure to stressors. Ongoing stressor experiences, such as war, incest, and spouse battery, do not lend themselves to easy classification or measurement. Laufer (1988) wrote in great detail about war as "routinized traumatization." In this conceptualization, ongoing events like war are seen as processes rather than as catastrophic events. The process is ongoing and contains within it a number of discrete events. Because war in contemporary society is out of the range of usual human experience, at least in some countries, its ongoing nature would be expected to be more disruptive and discontinuous of normal developmental processes than would a single discrete event, no matter how severe. This conceptualization could also apply to such other chronic stressors as incest and battery.

DSM-III-R acknowledged the difference between single and multiple or chronic events with its recent revisions of the criteria for Axis IV-severity of psychosocial stressors. Events are seen as predominantly acute (i.e., duration less than 6 months) or predominantly enduring circumstances (duration greater than 6 months). Inspection of the examples indicates that acute events are those that tend to happen once, although they clearly may have enduring sequelae that produce ongoing stress (divorce, rape, death of spouse), while enduring circumstances include situations of repeated trauma, such as war or captivity. Although this distinction is a welcome one, multiple or prolonged traumatic experiences still pose particularly difficult conceptual and measurement problems, because they may contain a number of different stressor experiences or experiences that have happened more than one time. Such experiences might be quantitatively and qualitatively different than more acute events, making comparisons extremely difficult.

Generic Dimensions of Trauma

I recently suggested some generic dimensions of stressor experiences that could be used to define a variety of traumatic events (Green, 1990). I would like to present those here and review the literature that supports the association of these particular dimensions with PTSD or other stress-response symptoms. At present, investigations of events may be characterized in a variety of ways. There may be some variability within events along certain dimensions, whereas other circumstances may have less variability. There may be overlap in the dimensions. However, some agreement about dimensions would allow systematic research to be done to assess which aspects of events put people most at risk for short- or long-term psychological problems or symptoms. Such information would allow for more precise education around psychological effects of events and should be relevant to assessing who would be in potential need of psychotherapeutic services. Also, if specific dimensions can be identified across events, it should be possible to do more precise research about the role of nonstressor factors in the processing of traumatic events.

The proposed dimensions are focused at an *individual level*, that is, at what happened to the particular person, rather than at a group or community level. This approach assumes that even within a collective event, experiences vary widely and that the individual's experience will play an important role in how the event is processed. This is somewhat obvious for events that occur individually (e.g., rape), but may be unclear for disasters and other group events, where the overall impact on the group is likely to mediate the response as well.

Dimension I: Threat to Life and Limb

The first dimension is probably one of the most obvious and most studied of the dimensions of trauma. It involves an encounter with the environment in which the person may not know for certain whether he or she will survive and is often thought of as a "brush with death." Evidence for the association of this dimension

Table 11.1. Generic Dimensions of Trauma

Dimension	Experienced trauma
I	Threat to life and limb
II	Severe physical harm or injury
III	Receipt of intentional injury/harm
IV	Exposure to the grotesque
V	Violent/sudden loss of a loved one
VI	Witnessing or learning of violence to a loved one
VII	Learning of exposure to a noxious agent
VIII	Causing death or severe harm to another

with stress symptoms is fairly extensive. Threat to life has been shown to significantly predict long-term outcome in the Buffalo Creek dam collapse of 1972 (Gleser, Green, & Winget, 1981; Green *et al.*, 1990). The Beverly Hills and Baldwin Hills fires (Green, Grace, & Gleser, 1985; Maida, Gordon, Steinberg, & Gordon, 1989) also showed this relationship of life threat with stress symptoms. Life threat related to combat exposure for Vietnam veterans has been documented as a risk factor for PTSD symptoms in a number of studies (e.g., Foy & Card, 1987; Green, Lindy, Grace, & Gleser, 1989; Kulka *et al.*, 1990; Laufer, Gallops, & Frey-Wouters, 1984), as it has in World War II and in Korean war veterans (Elder & Clipp, 1988). Crime victim samples have also shown this relationship (Kilpatrick *et al.*, 1989).

Dimension II: Severe Physical Harm or Injury

The fact of actual injury to the person is a dimension, related to life threat, which is not usually examined separately in research on traumatic events, except those falling into Dimension III (below). A disaster study examining this dimension after the Beverly Hills fire showed that injury predicted symptoms of affective distress and hostility up to 2 years following the event (Green, Grace, & Gleser, 1985).

Dimension III: Receipt of Intentional Injury/Harm

Injury has been more often examined within intentionally perpetrated traumatic events. These events *per se* have been shown to be associated with PTSD or other types of stress symptoms when people who have experienced them are compared with people who have not. Rape (Kilpatrick *et al.*, 1989; Steketee & Foa, 1987), family abuse (McCormack, Burgess, & Hartman, 1988), battery violence (Shields & Hanneke, 1983), incest (Donaldson & Gardner, 1985), and torture (Goldfeld, Mollica, Pasavento, & Faraone, 1988; Kinzie, 1988) have all been shown empirically to be associated with increased symptoms of anxiety, depression, and PTSD. This stressor dimension may be similar physically to Dimension II, however, the injury is a result of human malfeasance and should probably be separately categorized. Such incidents of interpersonal violence may be qualitatively different in a psychological sense than threat or injury arising from nature or mishap, since betrayal by other human beings must be dealt with in addition to the vulnerability and helplessness caused by the sudden threat.

Even within these types of events, the extent of the injury has some predictive power in terms of outcome, further supporting Dimension II as a generic dimension of trauma. Specifically, the extent of injury was shown to be related to outcome within groups of treatment-seeking Vietnam veterans (Lund, Foy, Sipprelle, & Strachan, 1984), rape victims (McCahill, Meyer, & Fischman, 1979; Sales, Baum, & Shore, 1984), and victims of crime (Kilpatrick *et al.*, 1989).

Dimension IV: Exposure to the Grotesque

This category is meant to cover experiences wherein the individual is exposed to the death (or near death) of another (during or after the fact) and where the death is particularly disfiguring, mutilating, or otherwise grotesque (e.g., burned, mangled, swollen, or otherwise disfigured bodies). This aspect of a traumatic event has been shown to be highly disturbing in a number of technological catastrophes, such as air crashes (Taylor & Frazer, 1982), a supper club fire (Green, Grace, & Gleser, 1985), and Vietnam combat (witnessing mutilation of enemy soldiers or working "graves and registration"; Green *et al.*, 1989). The latter two studies particularly point to the long-lasting consequences of this particular type of exposure.

Dimension V: Violent/Sudden Loss of a Loved One

Loss of a loved one is sometimes thought of as a normal, expectable experience that happens to most people over their lifetime. However, loss through traumatic or catastrophic events is likely to be sudden and violent and thus conceptually shares a great deal with sudden life threat or injury experiences. Even if one is not present at the time of the death, there is likely to be vicarious perception of the event and the potential for intrusive imagery associated with the individual's reconstruction of the death. This aspect of traumatic events has been well studied in the disaster/trauma literature and has been shown to be predictive of stress or PTSD symptoms across a wide variety of events. These include such natural disasters as the Australian bushfires (McFarlane, 1986) and volcanic eruptions (Murphy, 1984), and such technological events as dam collapses (Gleser *et al.*, 1981), structure fires (Green, Grace, & Gleser, 1985), and bus accidents (Milgram, Toubiana, Klingman, Raviv, & Goldstein, 1988). Loss in the context of combat has been shown to predict PTSD symptoms (Breslau & Davis, 1987a; Green *et al.*, 1989) as has experiencing the murder of a loved one (Amick-McMullan, Kilpatrick, Veronen, & Smith, 1989).

Dimension VI: Witnessing or Learning of Violence to a Loved One

At present, although this dimension is mentioned in the DSM-III-R as a possible precipitant for PTSD, little research has been done to document this relationship. One presentation was located which indicated that some PTSD symptoms were present in a majority of partners of rape victims, and a few met full criteria for diagnosis (Resnick, Veronen, & Saunders, 1988). As would be the case for Dimension V, violent or sudden loss, the violence against the loved one, if not witnessed directly, is likely to be experienced vicariously based on reports of what happened. In addition to the example given above (one's partner being raped), other types that would fall into this category would include having one's child severely injured, kidnapped, or abused and having one's partner mugged or tortured.

Dimension VII: Learning of Exposure to a Noxious Agent

This aspect was discussed earlier with regard to its relatively recent appearance in the disaster/trauma literature as a type of event that may cause symptoms of stress. As noted, the stressor may be the information that one has been exposed to a substance which may prove fatal or harmful in the long run. In order for this information to be stressful, the individual would have to believe that death/illness was possible. In some cases, such fears may be well grounded (e.g., HIV infection); in other cases, the threat may be more vague (e.g., exposure to toxic waste) and experts may not know the actual risk of harm. There is evidence that exposure to toxic waste at Times Beach (Smith, Robins, Przybeck, Goldring, & Solomon, 1986) and to a radiation leak at Three Mile Island (Baum, Gatchel, & Schaeffer, 1983; Dew, Bromet, Schulberg, Dunn, & Parkinson, 1987) were associated with higher risk for PTSD symptoms and other psychological and physical symptoms of stress. Learning that one has been infected with the human immunodeficiency virus has also been shown to increase risk for stress reactions (Atkinson *et al.*, 1988). These experiences are also likely to involve blaming someone else for the exposure, perhaps overlapping with Dimension III, and undoubtedly complicating the psychological processing of the event.

Dimension VIII: Causing Death or Severe Harm to Another

This final category involves the individual as a perpetrator and thus makes her or him the agent of the stressor experience. The focus of this category is on individuals who commit such acts because their particular role requires them to, or their role puts them in situations where there is strong pressure to commit such acts. I am not addressing perpetration of crimes, such as murder, burglary, and rape in a civilian setting because these are seen to fall outside the range of traumatic stress studies, although examination of such individuals for a history of trauma certainly seems a potentially worthwhile pursuit.

These experiences are likely to occur to people who are on duty in military or paramilitary roles, such as soldiers and police (see Chapter 32, in this volume). It is assumed that in a case where the dead or injured person is an innocent bystander, the impact would be more pronounced. This variable has been examined somewhat carefully in studies of surviving Vietnam combat veterans and indeed has been shown to be associated with higher levels of PTSD symptoms (Breslau & Davis, 1987a; Laufer, Gallops, & Frey-Wouters, 1984; Lund *et al.*, 1984). Few studies have dealt with causing death in the line of duty in civilian settings; more systematic study in this area is beginning to occur. For example, shooting incidents have been shown to predict symptoms of PTSD in police officers (Solomon & Horn, 1986).

Our research group at the Traumatic Stress Study Center of the University of Cincinnati recently completed a study which combined data sets from three traumatic events: (1) the Buffalo Creek dam collapse and flood of 1972 (2 and 14 years posttrauma), (2) the Beverly Hills Supper Club fire of 1977 (1 year), and (3) military service in the Vietnam War (12 to 15 years). The study was primarily focused upon creating profiles of symptoms for different groups in order to see whether type or recency of trauma, or demographic or cultural characteristics influenced the shape of the profiles. In conjunction with this study, we created several stressor categories that cut across and applied to the various events: life threat, bereavement/loss, and exposure to the grotesque, three of the dimensions proposed above (I, IV, V). Although these were originally defined somewhat differently in each event, comparable categories were created and subjects were designated as having significant experiences in these areas on a dichotomous basis. Further, we had a variable of causing death or harm to others for the Vietnam sample. Outcome measures included a diagnosis of PTSD, Intrusion and Avoidance subscales of the Impact of Event Scale (IES) (Zilberg, Weiss, & Horowitz, 1982), and a symptom checklist for stress symptoms, the Cincinnati Stress Response Schedule (CSRS), derived, in part, from Symptom Checklist-90 (SCL-90) items (Derogatis, 1983). PTSD diagnosis and IES symptoms were available only for the Buffalo Creek follow-up sample and the Vietnam veterans. The CSRS and SCL-90 were available on all groups. Each of the three dimensions of trauma (threat, loss, grotesque) significantly predicted a diagnosis of PTSD, with life threat being the strongest predictor ($r = .32$). Similarly, life threat was the strongest predictor of Intrusion and Avoidance (IES) scores ($r = .36$) and of the total score on the stress-related self-report items from the SCL-90 ($r = .32$). Exposure to the grotesque also significantly predicted each of the three sets of scores. The relationships with loss were somewhat weaker. Although this variable significantly predicted the CSRS total and IES Avoidance, the correlations were relatively low (.15 and .12, respectively) and intrusion symptoms on the IES were not predicted. The total stress score (a summary of the three dimensions just described) significantly predicted IES, PTSD, and CSRS items ($r = .31$ to .37) indicating a clear-cut "dose-response" relationship between stressors and outcome across samples. Even though stressors do not account for all the variance in outcome, they clearly play an important role. For the Vietnam sample, perpetration of atrocities against Vietnamese (abusive violence), as expected, predicted PTSD, IES, and self-report (CSRS) stress at moderate levels ($r = .32$ to .44).

These findings, together with the review of the association between generic stressor dimensions and stress reactions, provide strong evidence that specific aspects of stressors are important risk factors for psychological problems, particularly PTSD and similar symptoms, following a traumatic event. Similar results were reported by Wilson, Smith, and Johnson (1985). These stressors set into motion appraisal of the events and subsequent cognitive processing to incorporate them psychologically (Horowitz, 1986). As mentioned earlier, other factors are seen to affect the processing and the individual's ultimate adaptation (Green, Wilson, & Lindy, 1985; Green, Grace, Lindy, Gleser, & Leonard, 1990) but the nature and intensity of the experience itself clearly play a role.

141

As noted earlier, multiple and chronic events do not fit as neatly into a stressor conceptualization as more acute events, and there has been no work trying to compare more chronic events. Baum and his colleagues are presently gathering data to address this issue. Most research in the area of traumatic stress tends to be on specific survivor groups who have experienced either acute or chronic trauma. Examples of more chronic, prolonged events include war (combat and other war stressors), incest, battery, torture, and life-threat stressors associated with duty as police or other emergency personnel. Indirectly, based on the descriptive accounts, one could hypothesize that prolonged or multiple trauma would result in more complicated and/or more severe pathology than acute events.

This area is only beginning to be explored and the work on this to date has involved the examination of acute versus chronic sexual assault. A recent study by Kramer (1989) examined directly the role of multiple versus single trauma with regard to sexual assault. In that study, chronic (multiple assault) victims were more likely to be diagnosed with PTSD than victims of acute (single) assault. Chronic victims were not more likely to meet criteria for borderline personality disorder; however, there was an age effect, with more women assaulted before the age of twelve being more likely to meet criteria for borderline personality. Chronic victims had similar MMPI profiles as acute victims with significantly higher pathology on Scales 1 (Hypochondriasis), 3 (Hysteria), and 8 (Schizophrenia). This work indicates that acute and chronic or repeated victimization are related, but effects may be somewhat different, with potentially more severe effects from multiple traumatic experiences. It also suggests that age at the time of the event(s) is an important factor to consider in assessing the long-term impact of traumatic events.

Measurement Problems in Stressor Research

It has been clearly demonstrated that the objective nature of the stressor is associated with symptomatic outcome in the short and in the long term. March (1990) likewise concluded that the evidence for a dose-response relationship of objective stressor to PTSD and related symptoms was quite strong. Thus, it seems fairly evident that continued attention to the area of stressors in future research is not only worthwhile but strongly indicated.

Although there is a clear role for stressor experiences in our model of which factors influence post-trauma adaptation, the conceptualization and measurement of these experiences raise a number of sticky problems for research. A few of these will be briefly addressed in this section.

One of the major questions has to do with how stressors are measured and the extent to which victim self-report is the best source of accurate information for this variable. On the one hand, subjects are the best source of information about what happened to them because they were there when it happened. On the other hand, it is certainly possible that the subject's present adjustment to the traumatic event colors his or her recall about the detail of what happened. In our Buffalo Creek follow-up, we were able to address to some extent the reliability of recall of stressor experiences between 1974 (2 years postflood) and 1986 (14 years postflood) (Green & Grace, 1988). For the initial ratings, we had diagnostic reports that varied with regard to how much specific information was collected about life threat, loss of friends and family, and exposure to grotesque death. In 1986, we asked specific questions to obtain more complete data in these areas. Loss and life threat were constructed as dimensions varying from "none" to "severe" with specific anchors for each scale point (Gleser et al., 1981). Reliability for loss was quite good ($r = .58$) for a 12-year period, and contrasting losses of friends with losses of family members, the same level of loss was reported at both time periods.

Recall of life threat was less reliable, with an association of only .36. Furthermore, the amount of life threat during the flood reported by the subjects at the two time points decreased significantly over the 12-year period. There are several explanations for these findings: (1) the problem is "within time" rater reliability, that is, raters must make more subjective judgments about life threat than about bereavement; (2) recall decays over time, so that details of the threat remembered after 14 years are fewer than those remembered after 2 years; (3) the source of the data changed from a family narrative, where the family constructed the story together, to a gathering of individual data, where only one person reported the event; and (4) there is a systematic element to recall that involves people with less symptomatology recalling less severe threat as they retrospectively remember the traumatic event. Unfortunately, our data were not gathered with a reliability study in mind and are only suggestive that later recall does not show a one-to-one correspondence with earlier recall of the same event. We had no way of addressing the issue of accuracy of recall (see Erdelyi & Kleinbard, 1978, and McCloskey, Wible, & Cohen, 1988, for overviews on recall and hypermnesia).

These problems and issues suggest several points that need to be addressed with regard to measuring stressors. The first has to do with exploring the possibility of a third-party account of the events that happened. In studies of military veterans, there may be some "objective" indices available for validating the information given by the subject. However, this validation is likely to apply only with regard to gross factors: Was the veteran in combat in Vietnam? Was his unit overrun? For specific aspects of experiences, it is highly unlikely that neutral sources exist. For example, one exception might be a robbery that is on videotape. Relying on others who were present at the event, who are likely to be victims themselves and/or relatives of the traumatized subject, does not help much. Thus, the reality is that we must rely on subjects' self-reports for our information. If this is the case, we need to maximize the accuracy of the accounts.

Clearly, one way of doing this is to get details about what happened as early as possible from the subject so that the information is less subject to memory decay and less confounded with the subject's adjustment to the event.

A second strategy is to make the measure of stressors as objective and detailed as possible and to ask about each aspect separately. Our original Buffalo Creek scales were aggregated into dimensions. For example, loss included home, pets, family, friends, and household members, placed on an ordinal scale. However, constructing the ordinal scale required some assumptions (e.g., that losing a member of one's lateral extended family is more extreme than losing a friend) that may not actually apply. Loss is a dimension in the sense mentioned earlier (ranging from no losses to loss of important people in one's life). However, it may make more sense for scaling purposes to inquire about each type of loss separately. These separate questions can then be summarized into a dimension after the fact. With regard to accuracy, *a priori* scales are extremely important as well as scales that do not require inference on the part of the subject. For example, having the subject self-rate extent of life threat on a subjective scale is likely to be more confounded with psychological states than asking specific questions (obviously dependent upon the event being studied) about amount of warning, contact with noxious agent (e.g., flood waters, fire/smoke) amount of struggle to escape, threats of violence, and presence of a weapon. A study by Robins *et al.* (1985) showed that correspondence between sibling reports of aspects of early home environment was quite good if the presence or absence of an event was the unit of measurement (71% agreement). They also found that people agreed well with themselves over time. However, correspondence between sibling reports (which would be a gross measure of the validity/accuracy of the account) decreased notably when the frequency of the event was reported and notably again (to the point of very low correspondence), when inferential data were reported.

The only caveat about using *a priori* objective scales is in the case where the investigator is less than intimately familiar with all possible aspects of the stressor experience. Important aspects may be missed unless pilot work allows for open-ended reporting of the event and/or open-ended or "other" categories are included for aspects the investigators may have missed.

Of course measuring the subjective aspects of the stressor is completely legitimate as an additional source of information that is likely to be quite predictive of outcome (e.g., Green, Grace, & Gleser, 1985; Kemp, Rawlings, & Green, 1991). However, the two should be measured separately so that they are as unconfounded with outcome as possible (Breslau & Davis, 1987b; Green, 1986).

A further measurement problem is related to the linking of the stressor experience with the psychological sequelae and whether that link needs to be made by subjects. Specifically, this issue has been raised in regard to the Diagnostic Interview Schedule (Robins, Helzer, Croughan, & Ratcliff, 1981) in which PTSD questions are asked in the format "Did you ever see something so horrifying or frightening or have something so horrible happen to you that you kept having symptom X?" It has been shown that this format *underestimates PTSD symptoms* reported in other contexts (Solomon & Canino, 1990) and that it underestimates the prevalence of the disorder itself (Kulka *et al.*, 1991). However, more cogent to the present discussion is that it evidently also underestimates the prevalence/occurrence of *traumatic events* which can only be reported in the context of a symptom that subjects themselves link to the event (Hough, 1988; Kilpatrick & Resnick, in press). Thus, asking about stressors and symptoms simultaneously, particularly in a format where subjects are required to make dynamic links between the two, is likely to yield ungeneralizable data.

Future Directions

A number of suggestions have already been made or implied throughout the body of this chapter. They will be briefly reviewed and summarized below, and several additional points will be made. This area of research is relatively new and good information about the specific links between stressors and psychological symptoms is just beginning to be recognized as an important area of investigation.

1. Consider using the generic dimensions described above as a framework for constructing questions about traumatic experiences. Even though each dimension will clearly not apply to each study, separately covering those areas that do apply will allow convergent data from divergent studies to inform us about stressor dimensions.

2. Use detailed questions about aspects of the subject's stressor experience that are as objective and specific as possible, remembering that the most valid data are likely to be gathered in this manner.

3. In research in which several trauma populations are potentially included in the sample, take a careful history of traumatic events that is conducted completely independently of symptoms that are assessed. Avoid instruments where stressors and symptoms are gathered simultaneously in the same questions and particularly those that require the subject to make a causal link between stressors and symptoms.

4. Include in the history of stressful events more "ordinary" events and examine the extent to which they predict stress symptoms and PTSD symptoms.

5. More broadly, stressors should be conceptualized as independent and dependent variables in research studies on traumatic events. When they are the independent variables, we can investigate which specific symptoms and syndromes are associated with particular types of events. This approach allows us to expand our thinking beyond the DSM definition of "stress disorders" to determine empirically which aspects of events are associated with which psychological sequelae. Such information will help us do a better job of diagnosis in the future.

Conversely, as noted above, we need to measure the symptoms of certain diagnoses like PTSD that are delineated in the nosology and to determine empirically just which dimensions of events are most highly associated with these various diagnoses. In this type of research, stressors are the dependent variables. Both types of research will help us to understand which human experiences are most pathogenic and to better delineate the symptoms, syndromes, and conditions that arise from various types of events.

References

American Psychiatric Association. (1980). *Diagnostic and statistical manual of mental disorders* (3rd ed.). Washington, DC: Author.

American Psychiatric Association. (1987). *Diagnostic and statistical manual of mental disorders* (3rd ed., rev.). Washington, DC: Author.

Amick-McMullan, A., Kilpatrick, D. G., Veronen, L. J., & Smith, S. (1989). Family survivors of homicide victims: Theoretical perspectives and an exploratory study. *Journal of Traumatic Stress, 2,* 21–35.

Atkinson, J. H., Grant, I., Kennedy, C. J., Richman, D. D. Spector, S. A., & McCutcheon, J. A. (1988). Prevalence of psychiatric disorders among men infected with human immunodeficiency virus. *Archives of General Psychiatry, 45,* 859–864.

Barton, A. H. (1969). *Communities in Disaster: A sociological analysis of collective stress situations.* Garden City, NY: Doubleday.

Baum, A., Fleming, R., & Davidson, L. M. (1983). Natural disaster and technological catastrophe. *Environment and Behavior, 15,* 333–354.

Baum, A., Gatchel, R. J., & Schaeffer, M. A. (1983). Emotional, behavioral, and physiological effects of chronic stress at Three Mile Island. *Journal of Consulting and Clinical Psychology, 51,* 565–572.

Bennett, G. (1970). British floods 1968. Controlled survey of effects on health of local community disaster. *British Medical Journal, 3,* 454–458.

Berren, M. R., Beigel, A., & Ghertner, S. (1980). A typology for the classification of disasters. *Community Mental Health Journal, 16,* 103–111.

Bolin, R. (1988). Response to natural disasters. In M. L. Lystad (Ed.), *Mental health response to mass emergencies: Theory and practice* (pp. 22–51). New York: Brunner/Mazel.

Breslau, N., & Davis, G. C. (1987a). Post-traumatic stress disorder: The etiologic specificity of wartime stressors. *American Journal of Psychiatry, 144,* 578–583.

Breslau, N., & Davis, G. C. (1987b). Post-traumatic stress disorder: The stressor criterion. *Journal of Nervous and Mental Disease, 175,* 255–264.

Brett, E. A., Spitzer, R. L., & Williams, J. B. (1988). DSM-III criteria for post-traumatic stress disorder. *American Journal of Psychiatry, 145,* 1232–1236.

Davidson, J. R. T., & Foa, E. B. (1991). Diagnostic issues in posttraumatic stress disorder: Considerations for the DSM-IV. *Journal of Abnormal Psychology, 100,* 346–355.

Derogatis, L. R. (1983). *SCL-90-R version: Manual I.* Baltimore, MD. Johns Hopkins University.

Dew, M. A., Bromet, E. J., Schulberg, H. C., Dunn, L. O., & Parkinson, D. K. (1987). Mental health effects of the Three Mile Island nuclear reactor restart. *American Journal of Psychiatry, 144,* 1074–1077.

Donaldson, M., & Gardner, R. (1985). Diagnosis and treatment of traumatic stress among women after childhood incest. In C. R. Figley (Ed.), *Trauma and its wake: The study and treatment of post-traumatic stress disorder* (pp. 356–377). New York: Brunner/Mazel.

Elder, G. H., Jr., & Clipp, E. C. (1988). Combat experience, comradeship, and psychological health. In J. P. Wilson, Z. Harel, & B. Kahana (Eds.), *Human adaptation to extreme stress: From the Holocaust to Vietnam* (pp. 131–156). New York: Plenum Press.

Erdelyi, M. H., & Kleinbard, J. (1978). Has Ebbinghaus decayed with time?: The growth of recall (hypermnesia) over days. *Journal of Experimental Psychology: Human Learning and Memory, 4,* 275–289.

Foy, D. W., & Card, J. J. (1987). Combat-related post-traumatic stress disorder etiology: Replicated findings in a national sample of Vietnam-era men. *Journal of Clinical Psychology, 43,* 28–31.

Gleser, G., Green, B. L., & Winget, C. (1981). *Prolonged psychosocial effects of disaster: A study of Buffalo Creek.* New York: Academic Press.

Goldfield, A. E., Mollica, R. F., Pesavento, B. H., & Faraone, S. V. (1988). The physical and psychological sequelae of torture: Symptomatology and diagnosis. *Journal of the American Medical Association, 259,* 2725–2729.

Green, B. L. (1986). On the confounding of "Hassles," stress, and outcome (Comment on R. S. Lazarus *et al.*, & B. P. Dohrenwend *et al.*, articles). *American Psychologist, 41,* 714–715.

Green, B. L. (1990). Defining trauma: Terminology and generic stressor dimensions. *Journal of Applied Social Psychology, 20(2),* 1632–1641.

Green, B. L., & Grace, M. C. (1988). Conceptual issues in research with survivors and illustrations from a follow-up study. In J. P. Wilson, Z. Harel, & B. Kahana (Eds.), *Human adaptation to extreme stress: From the Holocaust to Vietnam* (pp. 105–124). New York: Plenum Press.

Green, B. L., Grace, M. C., & Gleser, G. C. (1985). Identifying survivors at risk: Long-term impairment following the Beverly Hills Supper Club fire. *Journal of Consulting and Clinical Psychology, 53,* 672–678.

Green, B. L., Grace, M. C., Lindy, J. D., Gleser, G. C., & Leonard, A. (1990). Risk factors for PTSD and other diagnoses in a general sample of Vietnam veterans. *American Journal of Psychiatry, 147,* 729–733.

Green, B. L., Lindy, J. D., Grace, M. C., & Gleser, G. C. (1989). Multiple diagnosis in post-traumatic stress disorder: The role of war stressors. *Journal of Nervous and Mental Disease, 177,* 329–335.

Green, B. L., Lindy, J. D., Grace, M. C., Gleser, G. C., Leonard, A. C., Korol, M., & Winget, C. (1990). Buffalo Creek survivors in the second decade: Stability of stress symptoms. *American Journal of Orthopsychiatry, 60,* 43–54.

Green, B. L., Wilson, J. P., & Lindy, J. D. (1985). Conceptualizing PTSD: A psychosocial framework. In C. R. Figley (Ed.), *Trauma and its wake: The study and treatment of post-traumatic stress disorder* (pp. 53–69). New York: Brunner/Mazel.

Horowitz, M. J. (1986). *Stress response syndromes* (2nd ed.). Northvale, NJ: Jason Aronson.

Horowitz, M. J., Weiss, D., & Marmar, C. (1987). Commentary: Diagnosis of post-traumatic stress disorder. *Journal of Nervous and Mental Disease, 175(5),* 267–268.

Hough, R. (1988, October). *PTSD: How do we find it, where do we look?* Panel presented at the annual meeting of the Society for Traumatic Stress Studies, Dallas, TX.

Kemp, A., Rawlings, E. I., & Green, B. L. (1991). Post-traumatic stress disorder (PTSD) in battered women: A shelter sample. *Journal of Traumatic Stress, 4,* 137–148.

Kilpatrick, D. G., & Resnick, H. S. (in press). *PTSD associated with exposure to criminal victimization in clinical and community populations.* In J. R. T. Davidson & E. B. Foa (Eds.), *Posttraumatic stress disorder in review: Recent research and future directions.* Washington, DC: American Psychiatric Press.

Kilpatrick, D. G., Saunders, B. E., Amick-McMullan, A., Best, C. L., Veronen, L. J., & Resnick, H. S. (1989). Victim and crime factors associated with the development of crime-related post-traumatic stress disorder. *Behavior Therapy, 20,* 199–214.

Kinzie, J. D. (1988). The psychiatric effects of massive trauma on Cambodian refugees. In J. P. Wilson, Z. Harel, & B. Kahana (Eds.), *Human adaptation to extreme stress: From the Holocaust to Vietnam* (pp. 305–317). New York: Plenum Press.

Kramer. T. L. (1989). *Post-traumatic stress disorder and borderline personality disorder in victims of single vs. multiple sexual assaults.* Unpublished doctoral dissertation, University of Cincinnati, Cincinnati, OH.

Kulka, R. A., Schlenger, W. E., Fairbank, J. A., Hough, R. L., Jordan, B. K., Marmar, C. R., & Weiss, D. S. (1990). *Trauma and the Vietnam War generation.* New York: Brunner/Mazel.

Kulka, R. A., Schlenger, W. E., Fairbank, J. A., Jordan, K., Hough, R. L., Marmar, C. R., & Weiss, D. S. (1991). Assessment of PTSD in the community: Prospects and pitfalls from recent studies of Vietnam veterans. *Psychological Assessment: A Journal of Consulting and Clinical Psychology, 3,* 547–560.

Laufer, R. S. (1988). The serial self: War trauma, identity, and adult development. In J. P. Wilson, Z. Harel, & B. Kahana (Eds.), *Human adaptation to extreme stress: From the Holocaust to Vietnam* (pp. 33–53). New York: Plenum Press.

Laufer, R. S., Gallops, M., & Frey-Wouters, E. (1984). War stress and trauma: The Vietnam veteran experience. *Journal of Health and Social Behavior, 25,* 65–85.

Lifton, R. J. (1988). Understanding the traumatized self: Imagery, symbolization, and transformation. In J. P. Wilson, Z. Harel, & B. Kahana (Eds.), *Human adaptation to extreme stress: From the Holocaust to Vietnam* (pp. 7–31). New York: Plenum Press.

Lund, M., Foy, D., Sipprelle, C., & Strachan, A. (1984). The combat exposure scale: A systematic assessment of trauma in the Vietnam war. *Journal of Clinical Psychology, 40,* 1323–1328.

Maida, C. A., Gordon, N. S., Steinberg, A., & Gordon, G. (1989). Psychosocial impact of disasters: Victims of the Baldwin Hills fire. *Journal of Traumatic Stress, 1,* 37–48.

March, J. S. (1990). The nosology of post-traumatic stress disorder. *Journal of Anxiety Disorders, 4,* 61–82.

McCahill, T. W., Meyer, L. E., & Fischman, A. M. (1979). *The aftermath of rape.* Lexington, MA: D. C. Heath.

McCloskey, M., Wible, C. G., & Cohen, N. J. (1988). Is there a special flashbulb-memory mechanism? *Journal of Experimental Psychology: General, 117,* 171–181.

McCormack. A., Burgess, A. W., & Hartman, C. (1988). Familial abuse and post-traumatic stress disorder. *Journal of Traumatic Stress, 1,* 231–242.

McFarlane, A. C. Post-traumatic morbidity of a disaster: A study of cases presenting for psychiatric treatment. *Journal of Nervous and Mental Disease, 174,* 4–13.

Melick, M. (1978). Life changes and illness: Illness behaviors of males in the recovery period of a natural disaster. *Journal of Health and Social Behavior, 19,* 335–342.

Milgram, N. A., Toubiana, Y. H., Klingman, A., Raviv, A., & Goldstein, I. (1988). Situational exposure and personal loss in children's acute and chronic stress reactions to a school bus disaster. *Journal of Traumatic Stress, 1,* 339–352.

Murphy, S. A. (1984). Stress levels and health status of victims of a natural disaster. *Research in Nursing and Health, 7,* 205–215.

Resnick, H. S., Veronen, L. J., & Saunders, B. E. (1988, October). Symptoms of PTSD in rape victims and their partners: A behavioral formulation. In H. Resnick (Chair), *The impact of rape on family functioning: Empirical findings and treatment implications.* Panel conducted at the meeting of the Society for Traumatic Stress Studies, Dallas, TX.

Robins, L. N., Helzer, J. E., Croughan, J., & Ratcliff, K. S. (1981). The NIMH Diagnostic Interview Schedule: Its history, characteristics, and validity. *Archives of General Psychiatry, 38,* 1381–1389.

Robins, L. N., Schoenberg, S., Holmes, S., Ratcliff, K., Benham, A., & Works, J. (1985). Early home environment and retrospective recall: A test for concordance between siblings with and without psychiatric disorders. *American Journal of Orthopsychiatry, 55,* 27–41.

Sales, E., Baum, M., & Shore, B. (1984). Victim readjustment following assault. *Journal of Social Issues, 40,* 117–136.

Shields, N. M., & Hanneke, C. R. (1983). Battered wives' reactions to marital rape. In D. Finkelhor (Ed.), *The dark side of families: Current family violence research* (pp. 131–148). Beverly Hills, CA: Sage Publications.

Smith, E. M., North, C. S., & Price, P. C. (1988). Response to technological accidents. In M. L. Lystad (Ed.), *Mental health response to mass emergencies: Theory and practice* (pp. 52–95). New York: Brunner/Mazel.

Smith, E. M., Robins, L. N., Przybeck, T. R., Goldring, E. S., & Solomon, S. D. (1986). Psychosocial consequences of a disaster. In J. H. Shore (Ed.), *Disaster stress studies: New methods and findings* (pp. 50–76). Washington, DC: American Psychiatric Press.

Solomon, R. M., & Horn, J. M. (1986). Postshooting traumatic reactions: A pilot study. In J. T. Reese & H. H. Goldstein (Eds.), *Psychological services for law enforcement* (Publication No. 85–600538, pp. 383–393). Washington, DC: U. S. Government Printing Office.

Solomon, S. D., & Canino, G. J. (1990). Appropriateness of DSM-III criteria for post-traumatic stress disorder. *Comprehensive Psychiatry, 31,* 1–11.

Steinglass, P., & Gerrity, E. (1990). Natural disasters and post-traumatic stress disorder: Short-term vs. long-term recovery in two disaster-affected communities. *Journal of Applied Social Psychology, 20*(1), 1746–1765.

Steketee, G., & Foa, E. B. (1987). Rape victims: Post-traumatic stress responses and their treatment: A review of the literature. *Journal of Anxiety Disorders, 1,* 69–86.

Taylor, A. J. W., & Frazer, A. G. (1982). The stress of post-disaster body handling and victim identification work. *Journal of Human Stress, 8,* 4–12.

Trimble, M. (1981). *Post-traumatic neurosis.* New York: Wiley.

Wilson, J., Smith, W. K., & Johnson, S. K. (1985). A comparative analysis of PTSD among various survivor groups. In C. R. Figley (Ed.), *Trauma and its wake: The study and treatment of post-traumatic stress disorder* (pp. 142–172). New York: Brunner/Mazel.

Zilberg, N. J., Weiss, D. S., & Horowitz, M. J. (1982). Impact of Event Scale: A cross-validation study and some empirical evidence supporting a conceptual model of stress response syndromes. *Journal of Consulting and Clinical Psychology, 50,* 407–414.

CHAPTER 12

Survey Research and Field Designs for the Study of Posttraumatic Stress Disorder

Richard A. Kulka and William E. Schlenger

Introduction

The purpose of this chapter is to elucidate some of the scientific and practical challenges involved in studying posttraumatic stress disorder (PTSD) in the community. By "in the community," we mean that we will focus not on studies of people who come to a clinic, hospital, or other treatment provider seeking treatment for PTSD (i.e., not on clinical studies), but rather on studies of people who have PTSD regardless of whether they have sought treatment or have otherwise come to the attention of mental health professionals. Such community studies are conducted to provide estimates of the *prevalence* of PTSD among specific population groups (e.g., Vietnam veterans, crime victims, persons exposed to a natural disaster), and to identify *risk factors* for the development of PTSD, and represent the only means of formulating unbiased estimates of these parameters (cf. Weissman, Myers, & Ross, 1986).

The design and conduct of epidemiologic studies in the community present a wide variety of challenges to the researcher. In this chapter, we will focus on four specific problems that are common in such studies: (1) identification of target populations and selection of representative samples, (2) identification of relevant comparison groups, (3) case identification, and (4) collection of comprehensive data.

As noted by Tom Wolfe in *The Right Stuff* (1979)—his documentary of life among the inner circle of test pilots who became America's early astronauts—one of the central themes or phrases running through conversations of these test pilots, whose achievements dominated the flying fraternity in the late 1950s, was "pushing the outside of the envelope":

> The "envelope" was a flight-test term referring to the limits of a particular aircraft's performance, how tight a turn it could make at such-and-such a speed, and so on. "Pushing the outside," probing the outer limits, of the envelope seemed to be the great challenge and satisfaction of flight test. (p. 12)

In many respects, as eloquently documented by Jean Converse in her recent book, *Survey Research in the United States* (1987), the history of survey and public opinion research has also been characterized by a continuing series of efforts to "push the outside," to test repeatedly the outer limits of this versatile research methodology, often in the face of vocal and influential doubters regarding its capacity to meet these challenges. The most obvious of these challenges have related to subject matter, what she (1987) refers to as "the luxuriant fields of self-report":

> Survey professionals had to feel their way and learn what things people were willing to discuss and what they were not.
>
> In the course of the 1935–60 years, investigators pushed at the borders of inquiry, and they learned that most people were willing to discuss almost anything. For good or ill, people were in general willing to express

Richard A. Kulka • National Opinion Research Center, 1155 East 60th Street, Chicago, Illinois 60637. William E. Schlenger • Mental and Behavioral Health Research Program, Research Triangle Institute, P. O. Box 12194, Research Triangle Park, North Carolina 27709.

International Handbook of Traumatic Stress Syndromes, edited by John P. Wilson and Beverley Raphael. Plenum Press, New York, 1993.

opinions and attitudes not only on innumerable imper- sonal topics but also on subjects very close to the bone of personal revelation, emotion, and intimacy. Whether they did so with candor and completeness was an ongo- ing question, but survey research did indeed expand the realms of inquiry. (pp. 403–404)

Such expansion, epitomized by the so-called Kinsey Reports that documented American sexual practices—as well as by surveys of drug and alcohol use, delinquent and criminal behavior, psychological distress, and the like—has also extended to the more "mechanical" as- pects of the survey method, including the diversity and complexity of measurement methods employed (e.g., use of psychological and IQ tests, physiological assess- ments, environmental monitors, diary keeping), the de- gree of burden these may entail, and the basic modes of data collection. For example, less than a decade ago, it was still relatively easy to locate texts and articles assert- ing with "absolute authority" that it was not possible to obtain valid data and/or adequate response rates with mail or telephone surveys, and/or that telephone inter- views must by necessity be restricted in length to 15 minutes or less. "Flight-tests" reported by Dillman (1978) and others have clearly "expanded the envelope" in this regard, and ongoing research continues to test and extend these limits.

In short, although the survey research enterprise has become broadly institutionalized and—to a great extent—"standardized," the challenges posed for it by an increasingly complex society require the continual development of innovative survey designs that entail considerable "risks of failure." Such innovations are risky in the sense that numerous colleagues both within and without the profession are quite willing to conjec- ture that the study in question "can't be done," at least not in accord with "acceptable" current standards.

One such "impossible" survey was a recent study conducted by Rossi, Fisher, and Willis (1986) on "The Condition of the Homeless in Chicago," a survey that required (among other things) the screening and inter- viewing of persons who occupied randomly selected blocks throughout the city in the dead of night (i.e., between the hours of 1:00 to 6:00 A.M.). Similarly, while this chapter was being written, preliminary work was underway to design a National Household Seropreva- lence Survey to obtain accurate estimates of current lev- els of human immunodeficiency virus (HIV) infection in the general population. This survey will require the col- lection of blood samples and descriptions of sensitive risk behavior from over 50,000 men and women nation- wide, and will require extremely high levels of participa- tion.

Another such study was the National Vietnam Vet- erans Readjustment Study (NVVRS), an ambitious na- tionwide epidemiologic study of Vietnam veterans that incorporated several features which, in combination, tested some of our preconceptions regarding the poten- tial limits of survey research (Kulka et al., 1990). Because of our involvement in the design and conduct of the NVVRS, we will use our experiences in that study to illustrate some of the major problems that must be ad- dressed in carrying out field studies of PTSD.

National Vietnam Veterans Readjustment Study

As part of the Veterans Health Care Amendments of 1983 (Public Law 98-160), the U. S. Congress directed that the Veterans Administration (VA; now the Depart- ment of Veterans Affairs) conduct a systematic and com- prehensive "study of the prevalence and incidence of posttraumatic stress disorder and other psychological problems in readjusting to civilian life" among Vietnam veterans. This study was to be of sufficient size, scope, complexity, and design that it would provide national estimates of the extent of the mental health and other health needs of Vietnam veterans and also permit so- phisticated analyses of the nature, scope, covariation, and etiology of their readjustment difficulties.

As specified by the Congress—and evolved by the VA, its consultants, and the NVVRS research team—the NVVRS had three broad goals. The first major goal was to provide information about the incidence, prevalence, and effects of posttraumatic stress disorder and related postwar psychological problems among Vietnam vet- erans. A second major goal of the study was to provide a comprehensive description of the *total* life adjustment of Vietnam theater veterans and to compare their adjust- ment to that of Vietnam era veterans (i.e., persons who served in the Armed Forces during the Vietnam era but did not serve in the Vietnam theater) and of *civilian coun- terparts* (i.e., persons who did not serve in the military during the Vietnam era). Third, the study was to provide detailed scientific information about one specific type of postwar psychological problem: PTSD. Of particular in- terest were its antecedents, its course, its consequences, and its relationship to other physical and emotional dis- orders. Relationships between PTSD and other postwar psychological problems, on the one hand, and physical disabilities, substance abuse, minority group member- ship, and criminal justice involvement, on the other hand, were also to be examined, as was the impact of postwar psychological problems on veterans' families and on their use of VA facilities. In short, nothing less was required than perhaps the most far-reaching and ambitious national mental health epidemiologic study ever attempted on *any population*.

Clearly, achieving these broad objectives required a large-scale, complex study with careful attention to re- search design, sampling and location procedures, in- strument development and validation, data collection, and numerous other special methodological issues. In addition, the controversial nature of some of the study's subject matter (e.g., PTSD), the intense interest in the study on the part of groups across the political spec- trum, and the programmatic implications of the study's findings all acted to underscore the importance of the design to the ultimate utility of the study's findings. If the findings were to be useful to policymakers, they had to be credible to the scientific community, to the various political interest groups, and ultimately to Congress. As with all research projects, the credibility of the findings from the NVVRS was predicated on the defensibility of its research design.

To meet the Readjustment Study's ambitious informational and methodological objectives, we developed a design with multiple components (full details of the design of the NVVRS can be found in Kulka *et al.*, 1990). The component that was designed to meet the study's major informational objectives was the National Survey of the Vietnam Generation (NSVG). The NSVG research design involved in-depth face-to-face interviews averaging 3 to 5 hours in length with samples drawn to represent the study's three major groups. These were: (1) Vietnam *theater* veterans—persons who served on active duty in the U. S. Armed Forces during the Vietnam era (August 5, 1964 through May 7, 1975) and who served in the Republic of Vietnam or its surrounding waters or airspace; (2) Vietnam *era* veterans—persons who served on active duty in the U. S. Armed Forces during the Vietnam era but who did *not* serve in the Vietnam theater; and (3) civilian counterparts—persons who did not serve in the military during the Vietnam era, matched on age and sex, and race/ethnicity (for men only) or occupation (for women only) to the theater veterans. In order to assure that critical statistical comparisons could be made reliably, certain subgroups were oversampled. These included blacks, Hispanics, women, and veterans with service-connected disabilities.

The content of the survey interview was designed to cover the broad spectrum of adjustment. Components covering such topics as marriage and family, education, occupation, military service and Vietnam experience, stressful and traumatic life experiences, mental and physical health status, use of health and mental health services, and social support were included in the survey interview.

Two additional components of the Readjustment Study that are closely related to the NSVG are worth mentioning. These are the Clinical Examination Component and the Spouse/Partner Interview Component. For the Clinical Examination Component, 440 veterans underwent a follow-up assessment by a mental health professional. The assessment included a semistructured diagnostic interview, using the Structured Clinical Interview for DSM-III-R (SCID) (Spitzer, Williams, & Gibbon, 1987) and a variety of psychometric instruments. The purpose of the assessment was to provide additional information about the presence or absence of a variety of psychiatric disorders, particularly PTSD. Clinical assessments were conducted by mental health professionals located in 28 of the largest Standard Metropolitan Statistical Areas (SMSAs) around the country who were experienced in working with stress disorders. The Clinical Examination sample was drawn from among veterans in the NSVG survey interview sample who lived within "reasonable commuting distance" of these 28 areas, and included all those who appeared on the basis of their survey interview to be PTSD positive and a sample of those who appeared to be PTSD negative.

The Spouse/Partner Component involved interviews with the spouse or "significant other" of 450 theater veterans. The purpose of these interviews was to collect information about the veteran from a collateral, and to assess the impact of postwar psychological problems on persons who share the lives of those with such problems. The Spouse/Partner subsample was selected to include adequate numbers of both spouses of veterans whose survey interviews suggested substantial levels of postwar psychological problems and spouses of those without such problems.

Target Populations and Representative Samples: Who Are We Studying?

An important first step in conducting community epidemiologic studies, particularly studies of the prevalence of PTSD, is the specification of an operational definition of the target population group(s) of interest. Although on the surface this may seem a simple, or even trivial, exercise, it can have important implications for the design of the study. For instance, consider something as apparently simple as defining the term *Vietnam veteran*. For example, should veterans with limited active duty during the Vietnam era or in the Vietnam theater be excluded, or those older veterans who had also participated in the Korean Conflict and/or in previous wars? What about those currently in the Reserves or National Guard or those still on active military duty (noting that the latter technically are not "veterans")?

Our ultimate choice in the NVVRS was to include in the study virtually all "official" Vietnam veterans, defining the veteran respondent universe as

> all persons who served on active duty [180 days or more] in the military forces of the United States during the Vietnam era (August 5, 1964 through May 7, 1975), except those who are currently [at the time the sample was drawn] on active duty. (Kulka *et al.*, 1990, p. 11)

This definition included men and women of all ages, from all branches of the service, draftees, career retirees, enlistment terminations, and persons who served on active duty during the Vietnam era who were currently reservists or National Guard personnel. Under this definition, the study population contained an estimated 93% to 94% of the total number of persons who served on active duty during the Vietnam era, which represented the most comprehensive sample coverage of the Vietnam veteran population of any study conducted to date. As a result, however, rates of PTSD and other postwar psychological problems estimated from the NVVRS sample may differ substantially from those reported in prior research or from those that would have been obtained if the Readjustment Study had excluded some of the subpopulations noted above, or had included those "veterans" still on active duty.

Second, the basic epidemiologic objectives of the NVVRS dictated that a national probability sample be drawn of *all* veterans of the Vietnam era, excluding only those currently on active duty. As noted above, this would include men and women of all ages, from all branches of the service, draftees, career retirees, enlistment terminations, and persons who served on active duty during the Vietnam era who are currently reservists or National Guard personnel. Because no comprehensive list of this population existed, one had to be created. The most common means for doing this in past studies was to screen households either by telephone or in-person to identify Vietnam era veterans. However, this approach necessarily relies on self or proxy reports to identify veterans, and the screening rates obtained by the two most rigorous surveys employing this method (Fischer, Boyle, Bucuvalas, & Schulman, 1980; Rothbart, Fine, & Sudman, 1982) suggest significant underreporting of Vietnam era veteran status, resulting in undercoverage rates on the order of 32% to 38% relative to 1980 Census data.

As a result, we decided to draw the NVVRS samples of veterans directly from military personnel records. Rather than screening households, then, this option involved the screening and abstraction of information from literally tens of thousands of military records to obtain the desired sample.

Although identification of the veteran samples from military records provided the advantage of a more representative sample than could have been achieved through identification via household screening, it had two important practical disadvantages. First, doing so required us to create a frame from which the veteran samples could be drawn. In other words, we first had to create a virtually complete list of the more than 8 million veterans who served in the military during the Vietnam era, so that each veteran selected into the sample would have a known probability of selection. Creation of this list, or sampling frame, required us to obtain military records from the many places where they are stored to assure completeness.

The second disadvantage of opting for military records-based samples of veterans, rather than relying on household screening techniques, is that it required that we track down all sampled veterans wherever they were currently living so that we could interview them. Samples that result from household screening can take advantage of geographic clustering techniques, so that the persons selected in the sample are located in a relatively small number of geographic areas. The records-based sample, by contrast, was scattered literally throughout the world, and tracing information available from the military records consisted largely of "home of record" and next of kin addresses that were often up to 20 years old. However, because these veterans were judged to have been exposed to an "occupational health risk" as a result of their military service, it was possible, through an interagency agreement with the National Institute of Occupational Safety and Health (NIOSH), to obtain current addresses for most veterans from the Internal Revenue Service (IRS). Those for whom the IRS could not supply an accurate current address were located by means of specialized tracing procedures, including contacts with relatives, credit bureau and state motor vehicle record checks, and, ultimately, "on the street" field investigations. Through the use of these various sources it was possible to locate successfully over 95% of the sampled veterans (over 96% of the theater and 93% of the era veterans).

Even when located, however, the sample was *very* widely scattered, and interviews were conducted in virtually every corner of the 50 states and Puerto Rico, ranging from two cases in South Dakota to over 400 in California (who, in turn, were scattered throughout virtually every county in the state). As a result, the average interviewer travel mileage required to conduct an interview with a Vietnam theater veteran was almost 200

miles, with an average travel time of over 7 hours. For interviews with Vietnam era veterans, these averages were 160 to 170 miles and over 6 hours, respectively, and those for interviews with nonveterans only slightly lower. Thus, a substantial price was paid, in terms of the effort (and, ultimately, the cost) required to complete an interview, for the increased population coverage (and therefore representativeness) that resulted from drawing the study's veteran samples from military records.

Specification of Comparison Groups: Compared to What?

A fundamental design problem that must be addressed in virtually any community study of PTSD involves the specification of comparison groups. Comparison groups are important as a means of examining and ruling out alternative hypotheses about a study's findings. For example, having comparison groups allows one to examine the hypothesis that the PTSD prevalence observed in the target group is due primarily to the assessment method or to the base rate in the population. In the context of the NVVRS, it was important not only to determine the prevalence of PTSD among Vietnam theater veterans, but also to determine whether the prevalence among theater veterans was significantly different from (higher than) the prevalence among Vietnam era veterans and civilian counterparts. Establishing that PTSD prevalence differs between the target group and one or more comparison groups helps to increase confidence that the prevalence rate observed in the target group is not merely a function of the particular assessment method or of the population base rate.

A second need for comparison groups arises from the fact that exposure to traumatic stress, a necessary condition for the development of PTSD, is never applied at random. Rather, exposure to events that can precipitate PTSD may be related to a wide variety of background and other "predisposing" characteristics, and observed differences in PTSD prevalence between groups might be due to differences in such characteristics. In the example of the NVVRS, persons were not assigned at random to service in the military, and within the military, to service in Vietnam. As a result, differences that we observe today in the current prevalence of PTSD between theater veterans and the comparison groups may be attributable to differences in the basic experiences of the groups (e.g., service in Vietnam), but they may also result from differences in the characteristics or experiences that Vietnam theater veterans brought with them to their military service.

The Congressional mandate for the NVVRS called for a study of the prevalence of postwar psychological problems among Vietnam theater veterans. In principle, such a mandate could have been fulfilled simply by studying theater veterans. However, it was quite clear that any information about the current adjustment of Vietnam veterans would be much more meaningful when viewed in the context of the adjustment of other comparable groups. Consequently, it was decided that comparison groups were a necessary aspect of the research design.

That decision led, in turn, to an important question: What was/were the most appropriate comparison group(s)? One obvious choice was Vietnam *era* veterans—that is, those who were in the military at the same time but did not serve in the war—and era veterans were indeed included in the NVVRS design as a comparison group. If theater veterans are found to have more adjustment problems than era veterans, one possible explanation is that the excess is due to their Vietnam experience. However, it is also possible that such differences are due to differences in characteristics between the two groups, especially given the fact that soldiers were not assigned to Vietnam duty at random. Therefore, the Vietnam era veteran sample was drawn in such a way as to be capable of producing reliable estimates for the population of era veterans *and* for era veterans matched on age and race with theater veterans. If the prevalence of postwar psychological problems among theater veterans was found to be higher than among era veterans with similar age-race characteristics, then the hypothesis that the differences are due to Vietnam experience becomes more credible. Other competing hypotheses (e.g., that any observed differences are due to differences between the groups in childhood experiences) could be assessed by controlling statistically for a variety of risk factors and other characteristics in making the prevalence rate comparisons.

An additional consideration with regard to comparison groups addresses the hypothesis that part or all of the prevalence of adjustment problems among veterans—theater or era—is attributable to their having been in the armed forces *per se*. As was the case with decisions within the military about which troops went to Vietnam, the process by which people were inducted into the armed forces was also not random (though it may have seemed so to some at the time). Consequently, those who served in the armed forces may be different from those who did not on characteristics that are related to their current adjustment levels. The hypothesis that current adjustment problems of veterans are due to military experience *per se* could be evaluated in part by comparing the adjustment of veterans to their civilian counterparts—that is, persons who did not serve in the military. Therefore, a civilian counterpart group was also included in the Readjustment Study design. This group was selected to match the age-race distribution of theater veterans, allowing for comparisons of prevalence rates for theater veteran, era veteran, and civilian counterpart groups with similar age-race characteristics. Again, other competing hypotheses could be assessed by controlling statistically for a variety of other risk factors in making these comparisons.

A special problem in specifying appropriate comparison groups for female theater veterans resulted from the fact that the vast majority of them—about 85%—were nurses. To control for the effects of this occupational (and, therefore, educational and socioeconomic status) homogeneity, the female era veteran and civilian counterpart samples in the NVVRS included oversamples of nurses so that they could be matched by occupation to the theater veteran sample.

One additional comparison group issue arose as a consequence of the broad definition of *Vietnam veteran* adapted for the NVVRS. Obviously, not everyone who

serves in a war effort is exposed to combat. In fact, the conventional wisdom in military circles is that about four support troops are required for each combat soldier in the field. Because exposure to combat and other stressors of service in a war zone were hypothesized as the "active ingredient" that would produce differences in PTSD prevalence between Vietnam theater veterans and the comparison groups, the inclusion of many support troops in the theater veteran group might serve to reduce the prevalence difference between the study groups and thus mask a true difference.

To guard against this possibility, we needed a way of assessing war zone stress exposure in the theater veteran group, such that we could subdivide theater veterans into *high* and *low* exposure groups. The prevalence of PTSD among high war zone stress exposure theater veterans could then be compared to the prevalence in the comparison groups as a more powerful test of the hypothesis that the prevalence of PTSD would be elevated in a group of "war veterans."

A basic premise underlying our effort to develop a comprehensive assessment of exposure to war zone stress, based on the prior research literature in this area (e.g., Egendorf, Kadushin, Laufer, Rothbart, & Sloan, 1981; Laufer, Gallops, & Frey-Wouters, 1984), was that the phenomenon of war trauma is multidimensional. Moreover, with few exceptions, the basic concepts and measures required to conduct a multidimensional assessment of combat and war zone stress exposure were already represented in the research literature and were adapted for use in the NVVRS. We began by compiling measures within eight broad areas suggested by recent research: (1) general indicators of degree of involvement in combat; (2) exposure to stresses of serving in Vietnam other than combat; (3) number, nature, and duration of service in principal combat roles; (4) specific dimensions of combat exposure or involvement, including extent, type, and frequency of exposure to enemy fire, degree of involvement in engaging the enemy, and degree of exposure to injury and death of American soldiers; (5) exposure to and participation in injury or death of Vietnamese civilians or abusive violence; (6) degree of perceived risk, threat, or danger to life and limb; (7) extent and nature of positive war zone experiences; and (8) aspects of war stress of particular relevance to nurses, medics, and others assigned to work with the dead and dying. It was assumed that a comprehensive assessment of Vietnam war stress must assess each of these broad dimensions to at least some degree, either as empirically distinct in their own right *or* as aspects included in a broader, more general measure to describe adequately the war experiences of *all* participants.

In our overall assessment of war zone stress exposure, almost 100 items representing these broad domains were subjected to principal components analyses to identify ways of combining specific experiences such that the important underlying dimensions of war zone stress were appropriately represented. These analyses, conducted separately for male and female veterans who served in the Vietnam theater, resulted in the identification of four basic clusters of items for males and six for females. In addition to the retention of an individual item indicating experience as a prisoner of war, the items retained for men (94 of 97) clustered along four basic dimensions: (1) exposure to combat, (2) exposure to abusive violence and related conflicts, (3) deprivation, and (4) loss of meaning and control. For women, in addition to the POW item and another indicating receipt of a combat medal, the items retained (87 of 97) represented six basic dimensions: (1) exposure to wounded and dead, (2) exposure to enemy fire, (3) direct combat involvement, (4) exposure to abusive violence, (5) deprivation, and (6) loss of meaning and control. Indices were created for each of these clusters, with internal consistency reliabilities (coefficient alpha) ranging from .704 to .937 (median .873). In spite of the orthogonal rotation algorithm used to derive these clusters, correlations among these indices were moderate to high, suggesting some degree of potential redundancy or overlap, and each was at least moderately correlated with one of our PTSD measures—the Mississippi Scale for Combat-Related PTSD (Keane, Caddell, & Taylor, 1988).

In further analyses designed to explore the possibility of deriving a single overall summary measure of war zone stress exposure, one of these indicators (loss of meaning and control) was dropped because of possible confounding of exposure and reactions to stress, and those remaining were subjected to *second-order* principal components analyses. These analyses indicated a single component for males and two for females (with the second being substantially weaker than the first in the latter case), thereby allowing in each case for the creation of a *general* index representing "overall war zone stress" as a weighted linear combination (factor score) of the individual indices. Correlations of these overall indices with PTSD symptomatology (assessed by the Mississippi scale) were .575 and .516 for males and females, respectively.

Although this war zone stress index—a continuous measure—is suitable for correlation and regression analyses, there is good reason to believe that the relationship between war zone stress and PTSD, for example, may not be strictly linear, that is, there may well be a "threshold effect." For this reason, as well as for ease of presentation, it was desirable to identify groups of Vietnam theater veterans who are relatively *high* on this measure, versus those who are relatively *low*. Rather than making this dichotomization decision arbitrarily, a series of analyses was conducted to examine the extent to which different "cutoff" scores on the war zone stress index were able to distinguish those relatively low from those relatively high on the *component* war zone stress indices from which the factor scores were derived. These analyses suggested a cutoff score in the 75% low/25% high range for men and the 60/40 range for women.

Since this derived measure of war zone stress exposure was based solely on self-report measures, it was important to examine it in relation to somewhat more *objective* indicators to independently establish its validity. Thus, the relationship between this measure and several indicators abstracted from military records was examined (Kulka *et al.*, 1990). Fortunately, we found good correspondence between the self-report measure and information contained in respondents' military records (e.g., receipt of combat medals, combat military occupational specialty). For example, 70% of the men who received Purple Hearts were classified as having been exposed to high stress, versus 22% of those who did not

receive a Purple Heart. Also, 49% of the men who served in the Marine Corps and 31% of those who served in the Army were classified as high-stress exposure, versus 10% of those who served in either the Navy or Air Force. Such findings increased our confidence in the self-report measure.

Thus, the NVVRS design included theater veteran subgroups defined by their level of exposure to war zone stress, and nationally representative samples of Vietnam era veterans and civilian counterparts as comparison groups. An example of the importance of these comparison groups in evaluating competing hypotheses can be found in the NVVRS examination of the issue of "predisposition." To examine the role of "predisposing factors," or characteristics that theater veterans brought with them to the war, we selected over 80 characteristics and experiences that predated military or Vietnam experience and that might conceivably have accounted for differences in current PTSD prevalence rates between the study groups. The impact of these factors was assessed via a series of multiple regression analyses that provided estimates of the differences in current prevalence for each of the study group contrasts with the effects of the predisposing factors controlled (Kulka *et al.*, 1990).

Findings of the regression analyses indicated that the adjustment for predisposing factors decreased the current PTSD prevalence differences between theater veterans and the comparison groups. This suggests that there is a role for personal characteristics in the prevalence of PTSD. However, the PTSD prevalence differences between theater veterans and the comparison groups remained large and statistically significant even after adjustment for predisposing factors, indicating that predisposing factors alone do not account for these differences. Additional analyses conducted within the theater veteran group indicated a strong role for exposure to war zone stress in the prevalence of PTSD. In combination, these analyses provide strong evidence that the hypothesis that the current adjustment problems of Vietnam veterans result from their personal characteristics does not adequately explain the findings. Rather, the NVVRS findings are consistent with a model of PTSD that posits a role for individual vulnerability and a role for exposure to environmental factors in determining which war participants develop PTSD.

Case Identification

One of the most important scientific challenges facing community epidemiologic studies is the issue of case identification: How does one determine who is a case and who is not? In clinical studies, people who come seeking treatment present with certain problems, or symptoms, and a "story" to tell (e.g., "I'm here because . . ."). Diagnostic interviews in clinical settings, therefore, often begin with such questions as: "Tell me why you are here. How I can help you?" In community studies, however, the respondent has not come to the interviewer with a story to tell. On the contrary, the interviewer has come to the respondent in an attempt to learn his or her story, but does not have a "presenting problem" as a starting point for the assessment process.

Reflecting the emphasis on PTSD in the Congressional mandate, the NVVRS research team wanted to create a research design for the NVVRS that would maximize the accuracy of the study's estimate of the prevalence of PTSD among Vietnam theater veterans. This concern was expressed through two important features of the NVVRS design. First, when the NVVRS was being planned, the American Psychiatric Association (APA) was in the process of revising the third edition of its *Diagnostic and Statistical Manual of Mental Disorders* (DSM-III) (APA, 1980), the document that provides the "official" definition of psychiatric disorders in the United States. To assure that the NVVRS assessment of PTSD was consistent with the official definition of PTSD that would be in place when the NVVRS findings became available, the research team coordinated its efforts with the group working on revising the psychiatric taxonomy, the APA's Work Group to Revise DSM-III. Research Triangle Institute co-sponsored the meeting of the Ad Hoc Panel on the Definition and Measurement of PTSD, whose recommendations for revising the diagnostic criteria for PTSD were incorporated into the revised PTSD definition. As a result of this coordination, the NVVRS clinical estimates of PTSD prevalence are estimates of the prevalence of the disorder *as defined in the current official taxonomy* (DSM-III-R) (APA, 1987).

Second, the bedrock of the accuracy of any diagnostic procedure is its *validity*—that is, the extent to which the procedure classifies individuals in whom the disorder is truly present as "cases," and those in whom the disorder is truly absent as "noncases." To achieve the objective of diagnostic accuracy, we developed a "double validation" design that involved first conducting a preliminary validation study and then conducting a second validation study to run concurrently with the national survey.

The need to conduct a preliminary validation study prior to launching the national survey component of the NVVRS arose out of the fact that *no published information* existed concerning the validity of *any* of the existing survey instruments used to identify PTSD in earlier research. Therefore, the NVVRS design called for a preliminary study to examine the ability of several candidate survey measures to discriminate *true cases* of PTSD from *true noncases*. This validation study involved administering a package of candidate PTSD instruments to a group of subjects whose diagnostic status was known. The diagnostic status of subjects, who were mostly veterans undergoing psychiatric treatment, was "known" because their chart diagnosis *and* the diagnosis made by an expert clinician *agreed* on the presence or absence of PTSD. The expert clinician's diagnosis was made on the basis of an independent diagnostic interview conducted blind to the chart diagnosis. Results of the preliminary validation study (Schlenger & Kulka, 1987) indicated that several instruments in the package could classify people as cases or noncases of PTSD with acceptable accuracy. These findings served as the basis for decisions about the package of instruments to be included in the NSVG.

Although the preliminary validation study provided important information about the ability of certain instruments to identify PTSD among people who were undergoing psychiatric treatment, it did not (and we did not

intend it to) provide *complete* information about every aspect of the validity of the study's PTSD measures. Because the national survey component of the NVVRS involved a community sample, rather than a treatment-seeking sample, the relationship between the diagnostic measures and "true" diagnosis (i.e., the validity of those measures) could be expected to be at least somewhat attenuated from the estimate made on the basis of a treatment-seeking population.

For this reason the NVVRS design contained a Clinical Examination Component. The primary purpose of the clinical examination was to provide additional information about the correspondence between PTSD measures included in the survey interview and "true" PTSD. The Clinical Examination Component was designed as a multimethod validity study, in which multiple PTSD measures, including a semistructured interview conducted by an experienced mental health professional, could be brought to bear on the diagnostic decision. Thus, we planned a "triangulation" method for PTSD case identification, in which the diagnostic decision process would take into account information collected through a variety of methods and from a variety of sources.

The Clinical Examination Component represented the second stage in a two-stage case determination procedure (Dohrenwend, Levav, & Shrout, 1986) that is common in community epidemiologic studies. At the first stage, the study cohorts were screened during the NSVG interview with the Mississippi Scale for Combat-Related PTSD (Keane *et al.*, 1988), a brief, self-report instrument whose ability to identify cases of PTSD had been independently demonstrated. At the second stage, a subsample stratified on the basis of screening results was selected to undergo a detailed diagnostic assessment in the Clinical Examination Component. Diagnostic findings from the clinical examination were then projected statistically to make national prevalence estimates for the study cohorts.

Each clinical examination participant underwent a semistructured clinical interview that resulted in a diagnostic decision about PTSD. In addition, the clinician who conducted the interview completed several clinical scales describing his or her clinical impression of the participant, and the participant completed several self-report PTSD scales. In addition, the spouse/partner of each clinical examination participant was also interviewed, if there was one. As a result, the research team had at its disposal five self-report scales directly related to PTSD (plus a number of other psychiatric symptom scales related to PTSD but less directly so), and four clinical judgment scales, for clinical subsample respondents. The specific measures included in the assessment are described in Table 12.1.

The case determination process for clinical examination participants was based on analysis of a set of five primary indicators of current PTSD. The diagnostic decision for each subject was made on the basis of the weight of the evidence: At least three of the five indicators had to be positive before a clinical examination subject could be considered to be a current case. In fact, for 87% of the subjects at least four out of the five primary indicators agreed on the diagnosis, and for the remaining 13% three out of five agreed. The diagnosis based on

Table 12.1. Posttraumatic Stress Disorder Indicators Available for National Vietnam Veterans Readjustment Study Clinical Examination Participants

Name	Description	Type	Source
M-PTSD	Mississippi Combat-Related PTSD Scale	Self-report	Survey interview
MMPI-PTSD	MMPI PTSD Scale (Fairbank–Keane Scale)	Self-report	Clinical interview
SCIDX	PTSD diagnosis from the SCID interview	Clinician judgment based on self-report	Clinical interview
SXCTCURR	Number of PTSD symptoms reported as having occurred within the past 6 months	Interview self-report	Survey interview
SRRS_INT	Intrusion subscale; of the Stress Response Rating Scale—assesses the presence of signs/symptoms of intrusive thoughts	Clinical judgment based on observation	Clinical interview
SRRS_AVD	Avoidance subscale of the Stress Response Rating Scale—assesses the presence of signs/symptoms of avoidance	Clinical judgment based on observation	Clinical interview
SRRS_REA	Reactivity subscale of the Stress Response Rating Scale—assesses the presence of signs/symptoms of psychological reactivity	Clinican judgment based on observation	Clinical interview
IES_INT	Intrusion subscale of the Impact of Event Scale—assesses the presence of signs/symptoms of intrusive imagery during R's self-selected worst period	Booklet self-report	Clinical interview
IES_AVD	Avoidance subscale of the Impact of Event Scale—assesses the presence of signs/symptoms of avoidance during R's self-reported worst period	Booklet self-report	Clinical interview
ASSES_SC	Global Assessment Scale—assesses overall level of psychosocial functioning	Clinician judgment based on observation	Clinical interview

information from multiple indicators is called the *composite diagnosis*.

The first three primary indicators were: (1) the clinical interviewer's determination of the presence or absence of PTSD, made on the basis of the SCID interview; (2) the person's score on the Mississippi Scale for Combat-Related PTSD; and (3) the person's score on the PTSD subscale of the MMPI. These indicators were included separately because of the strong prior evidence of their reliability and validity in making the diagnosis of PTSD (Keane *et al.*, 1988; Keane, Malloy, & Fairbank, 1984; Schlenger & Kulka, 1987).

In addition, we created two other primary indicators by statistically combining information from the study's other independent measures of PTSD. The statistical combinations were developed on the basis of analysis of data from the subset of participants for whom there was no discrepancy among the first three diagnostic indicators. Analyses showed that information from the Stress Response Rating Scale (Weiss, Horowitz, & Wilner, 1984), the Impact of Event Scale (Horowitz, Wilner, & Alvarez, 1979), and the Global Assessment

Scale (Endicott, Spitzer, Fleiss, & Cohen, 1976) could be combined into two indicators whose diagnosis agreed with the diagnosis of the three independently validated assessments for more than 97% of the agreed-upon cases (Kulka *et al.*, 1990).

Clinical examination diagnostic findings were extended to the full survey sample via logistic regression, using as predictors only variables from the survey interview (prediction model $R_2 = .737$). Comparison of the prevalence rates that resulted from the composite diagnosis procedure with those that resulted from a variety of alternative case determination algorithms, including reliance solely on the clinical interviewer's diagnosis, suggested that alternate algorithms produced prevalence estimates that fell in a relatively narrow band, and those produced by the composite diagnosis procedure fell in the middle of that band.

NVVRS findings indicate that an estimated 15.2% of male and 8.5% of female Vietnam theater veterans are current PTSD cases (Kulka *et al.*, 1990). This represents about 480,000 of the nearly 3.2 million veterans who served in the Vietnam theater. Among both male and female theater veterans, the current prevalence of PTSD was found to be significantly higher ($p < .0001$) for those exposed to high levels of war zone stress than for those with low/moderate stress exposure (a fourfold difference for men and sevenfold for women). Also for both sexes, current PTSD prevalence rates for theater veterans are consistently higher than rates for comparable era veterans (males 2.5%, $p < .0001$; females 1.1%, $p < .0001$) or civilian counterparts (males 1.2%, $p < .0001$; females 0.3%, $p < .0001$).

Among male Vietnam theater veterans, 27.9% of Hispanics are estimated to be current cases of PTSD, as are 20.6% of blacks and 13.7% of white/others (each subgroup is significantly different from each other subgroup, all $p < .0001$). Moreover, the current prevalence rate differences between theater veterans, era veterans, and civilian counterparts were found to hold within all three race/ethnicity subgroups: Theater veteran rates are consistently higher than rates for era veterans and civilians (all $p < .0001$).

Collection of Comprehensive Data

Community epidemiologic studies typically have both descriptive and analytic objectives. The basic descriptive objective involves formulating estimates of the prevalence of the disorder being studied in various population groups or subgroups. The analytic objective, however, involves the investigation of risk factors and other etiologic issues.

Scientifically, a comprehensive study should address descriptive and analytic objectives. Pragmatically, however, examination of risk factors requires the collection of much more information than is needed for the estimation of prevalence. Taken together, the amount of information required to address the important descriptive and analytic objectives can be quite substantial, raising two pragmatic questions: (1) Can the amount of data required be collected without unduly burdening or stressing respondents, and if so, (2) are the resources available to support the substantial cost of collecting large volumes of data? With respect to the second of these, it is important to note that the marginal cost of collecting the information needed to examine risk factors is relatively small, given that one is committed to addressing the prevalence objective (i.e., if one has committed the resources necessary to select samples and collect data to formulate prevalence estimates, the marginal cost of collecting additional data concerning risk factors is relatively small). Because of its Congressional mandate, the NVVRS represented a rare instance in which the substantial resources required could be made available.

The Congressional mandate for the NVVRS suggested the need for a comprehensive study. Reflecting the very comprehensive description of veterans requested by Congress and the Veterans Administration, the content of the survey interview was designed to cover the broad spectrum of adjustment, including such topics as marriage and family, education and occupation, military service and Vietnam experience, stressful and traumatic events, substance use, psychiatric disorder, physical health, social support, and the use of health and mental health services. This provision for comprehensiveness resulted in a survey interview *averaging* 5 hours in length for Vietnam theater veterans, and 4 and 3 hours for Vietnam era veterans and nonveterans, respectively. Moreover, over 80% of these interviews were conducted in a single session. In addition to their *length*, these interviews were quite sensitive for many respondents, dealing as they did with exposure to war and other trauma, invoking painful memories of experiences one might prefer to forget.

To address the possible problems that might occur as a result of the potentially sensitive material covered in the interview, an elaborate training and support system was devised for interviewers. NSVG interviews were conducted by experienced survey research interviewers, trained in administering the NSVG interview in a 10-day training session. In addition to covering the mechanics of the interview process, the training also focused on issues of interviewer sensitivity. During this stage of training, the trainers helped interviewers identify the parts of the interview that were most likely to evoke emotional responses from respondents, recognize the behavioral cues indicating emotional reactivity, and manage emotionality should it occur. This portion of the training was provided by a team of recognized expert clinicians experienced in diagnosing and treating stress disorders, particularly among combat veterans.

In addition to this training, we established support networks for both respondents and interviewers. Interviewers carried with them to each interview a list of local mental health treatment resources (e.g., Veterans Centers and mental health centers) in the event that the respondent requested referral information. In addition, we instructed interviewers to report to the clinical training team anything "unusual" that occurred in their contacts with respondents. The clinician would then review the facts of the case with the interviewer, and they would together decide on a course of action (e.g., the clinician might call the respondent to check up on him or her, or to make a treatment referral). Finally, each respondent was recontacted by telephone a week or so after the interview and asked specifically about the interview and its impact. During this telephone call, we offered referral assistance to those who requested it.

The number of interviews in which respondents were distressed was quite small, and no reactions were severe. About one in every hundred NSVG interviews resulted in either the respondent or the interviewer invoking the support network. These few cases were resolved by applying the above procedures in a manner that addressed the individual needs and specific circumstances of the respondent. Interviewers had both professional and peer supports to help them. In addition to their special training, interviewers had access to clinical backup (for advice, support, and other needs) at all times. In addition, we scheduled conference calls for small groups of interviewers with members of the training team to provide peer support and to allow interviewers to benefit from the experiences of their colleagues.

Another factor that contributed to the complexity of this interview was the inclusion as a major questionnaire component of the NIMH Diagnostic Interview Schedule (DIS), an instrument developed by Robins and her colleagues (cf. Helzer & Robins, 1988) to permit the generation of psychiatric diagnoses from interviews conducted by specially trained lay (survey) interviewers, rather than by mental health professionals. Although a series of large-scale surveys using this instrument has been conducted at five specific sites as part of the NIMH Epidemiologic Catchment Area (ECA) Program (Regier *et al.*, 1984), this instrument had not previously been used in a *national* epidemiologic survey conducted by interviewers scattered throughout the United States. Reflecting the level of training, practice, and supervision required to conduct this interview properly, interviewer training for the NVVRS required *10 full days*, and a special "certification" interview was required of each interviewer to demonstrate proficiency in using the DIS. Over 140 interviewers were ultimately trained for the study, about 20% of whom were unable or unwilling to achieve this certification.

In spite of the many unique and formidable challenges just noted, the national survey component of the NVVRS was able to achieve virtually all of the performance standards set for it. The 3,016 total interviews conducted exceeded the targeted number of 2,980. For Vietnam theater veterans, over 83% of those sampled and eligible were interviewed, with subgroup response rates ranging from 81% among Hispanic male theater veterans to 86% for female theater veterans. Those not located (cited previously) were included among the nonrespondents for these response rate calculations; in fact, almost 87% of those located and eligible were interviewed, and the only veterans excluded as ineligible were those determined to be still on active duty and those residing outside of the 50 states and Puerto Rico during the entire field period. Response rates for Vietnam era veterans and nonveterans were 76% and 70%, respectively, reflecting in part the lower salience of the survey to these groups in relation to the level of burden required for their participation.

These results were not achieved without extraordinary effort, however. Interviewing was conducted with three random replicates of the total sample over a 15-month period, involving the use of over 100 interviewers. Respondent incentives (mandated by federal legislation) of $25, $20, and $15 were paid to Vietnam theater, era, or nonveterans, respectively, and these were increased to as high as $50 toward the end of the field period to maximize response rates. In addition, as the remaining sample cases became more scattered and difficult to interview, *interviewer* bonuses ranging from $25 to $75 per case were also instituted, and the most successful interviewers traveled throughout the country to contact the most difficult cases.

The two other survey components of the NVVRS, both of which involved follow-up interviews triggered by responses to the initial interview, also posed some significant new challenges, especially the clinical interview component. The clinical examination sample was drawn from among both theater and era veteran respondents to the survey interview who lived within "reasonable commuting distance" of 28 population centers (SMSAs) around the country. Mental health professionals in these areas who were experienced in working with

stress disorders were recruited and specially trained to use the nonpatient version of the SCID, a semistructured diagnostic interview adapted specifically for the study (SCID-NP-V). The sample included all those who appeared on the basis of the survey interview to be PTSD positive, and a sample of those who appeared to be negative, with the latter also selected so as to oversample those at highest risk of being "false negatives." Veterans selected for this component were asked to schedule an appointment and travel to the clinician's office for an additional 3-hour clinical assessment.

The required travel distances were often quite substantial, and most of these veterans had never before been to a psychiatrist or clinical psychologist. Although a $20 incentive (later raised to $50) and travel expenses were paid, the follow-up interview clearly represented a substantial additional burden and commitment on the part of these veterans. In fact, at one point it appeared that no better than a 65% to 70% response rate would be obtained for this component. At that time, a plan by which some of the clinicians agreed to travel to veterans' homes to conduct these interviews was initiated where necessary. A total of 440 veterans selected from among survey interview participants underwent the clinical assessment, yielding a clinical examination response rate of over 85%. Since, to our knowledge, the use of follow-up clinical assessments conducted by mental health professionals across the nation is unprecedented in the United States, the feasibility of this component was somewhat in doubt at the outset.

By contrast, the spouse/partner component, involving 1-hour follow-up survey interviews with co-resident spouses or partners of veterans, selected from the *entire* theater veteran sample (i.e., not restricted to 28 SMSAs) using the same criteria as the clinical follow-up, was decidedly "conventional" and presented no particular challenges at all! (We thought that the staff was entitled to at least one fairly conventional survey component!) Of the 557 theater veterans selected for this family interview follow-up, for whom there was an eligible family member (co-resident spouse or partner), 474 resulted in a family interview. This translates into an 85% spouse/partner interview response rate, with subgroup rates ranging from 83% for the spouse/partners of black and Hispanic males to 91% for the spouse/partners of female theater veterans.

In short, although several features of the comprehensive survey design for this project were regarded as at least "iffy" at the outset by some of our colleagues in the industry (and, candidly, at least partially by ourselves), in most respects we have been quite gratified (though not entirely satisfied) by these results. In spite of legitimate concerns regarding the feasibility of this study, it was possible to successfully achieve virtually all the performance objectives established for this landmark survey, while also learning a great deal in the process about how it might have been done even better. This represents the very essence of the concept of "pushing the outside of the envelope" as applied to any field of endeavor, and we are pleased to have had the opportunity to add this modest "flight-test" to the distinguished tradition in survey research of continually testing and expanding the limits of the method and its legitimate realms of inquiry.

Conclusion

In this chapter, we have identified several of the major problems that face the researcher attempting to conduct a field study of PTSD. We have used our experiences in conducting the National Vietnam Veterans Readjustment Study to provide examples of both the problems and some possible solutions. We hope that our experiences have "expanded the envelope," and that others will make use of these experiences to generate further expansions.

References

American Psychiatric Association. (1980). *Diagnostic and statistical manual of mental disorders* (3rd ed.). Washington, DC: Author.

American Psychiatric Association. (1987). *Diagnostic and statistical manual of mental disorders* (3rd ed., rev.). Washington, DC: Author.

Converse, J. M. (1987). *Survey research in the United States: Roots and emergence 1890–1960*. Berkeley, CA: University of California Press.

Dillman, D. A. (1978). *Mail and telephone surveys: The total design method*. New York: Wiley-Interscience.

Dohrenwend, B. P., Levav, I., & Shrout, P. E. (1986). Screening scales from the Psychiatric Epidemiology Research Interview (PERI). In M. M. Weissman, J. K. Myers, & C. E. Ross (Eds.), *Community surveys of psychiatric disorders*. New Brunswick, NJ: Rutgers University Press.

Egendorf, A., Kadushin, C., Laufer, R. S., Rothbart, G., & Sloan, L. (1981). *Legacies of Vietnam: Comparative adjustment of veterans and their peers*. Washington, DC: U. S. Government Printing Office.

Endicott, J., Spitzer. R., Fleiss, J., & Cohen, J. (1976). The Global Assessment Scale: A procedure for measuring overall severity of psychiatric disturbance. *Archives of General Psychiatry*, *33*, 766–771.

Fischer, V., Boyle, J. M., Bucuvalas, M., & Schulman, M. A. (1980). *Myths and realities: A study of attitudes toward Vietnam era veterans*. Washington, DC: U. S. Government Printing Office.

Helzer, J. E., & Robins, L. N. (1988). The Diagnostic Interview Schedule: Its development, evolution, and use. *Social Psychiatry and Psychiatric Epidemiology*, *23*(1), 6–16.

Horowitz, M. J., Wilner, N., & Alvarez, W. (1979). Impact of Event Scale: A measure of subjective stress. *Psychosomatic Medicine*, *41*, 209–218.

Keane, T. M., Caddell, J. M., & Taylor, K. L. (1988). Mississippi scale for combat-related post-traumatic stress disorder: Three studies of reliability and validity. *Journal of Consulting and Clinical Psychology*, *56*, 85–90.

Keane, T. M., Malloy, P. F., & Fairbank, J. A. (1984). Empirical development of an MMPI subscale for the assessment of combat-related post-traumatic stress disorder. *Journal of Consulting and Clinical Psychology*, *52*, 888–891.

Kulka, R., Schlenger, W. E., Fairbank, J. A., Hough, R. L., Jordan, B. K., Marmar, C. R., & Weiss, D. S. (1990). *Trauma and the Vietnam war generation*. New York: Brunner/Mazel.

Laufer, R. S., Gallops, M. S., & Frey-Wouters, E. (1984). War stress and trauma: The Vietnam veteran experience. *Journal of Health & Social Behavior*, *25*, 65–85.

Regier, D. A., Myers, J. K., Kramer, M., Robins, L. N., Blazer, D. G., Hough, R. L., Eaton, W. W., & Locke, B. Z. (1984). The NIMH Epidemiologic Catchment Area Program: Historical context, major objectives, and study population characteristics. *Archives of General Psychiatry*, *41*, 934–941.

Rossi, P. H., Fisher, G. A., & Willis, G. (1986). *The condition of the homeless in Chicago: A report based on surveys conducted in 1985 and 1986*. Amherst, MA: Social and Demographic Research Institute, University of Massachusetts.

Rothbart, G. S., Fine, M., & Sudman, S. (1982). On finding and interviewing the needles in the haystack: The uses of multiplicity sampling. *Public Opinion Quarterly*, *46*(3), 408–421.

Schlenger, W., & Kulka, R. (1987, August 28). *Performance of the Fairbank-Keane MMPI scale and other self-report measures in identifying post-traumatic stress disorder*. Paper presented at the 95th annual meeting of the American Psychological Association, New York.

Spitzer, R., Williams, J., & Gibbon, M. (1987). *Structured Clinical Interview for DSM-III-R, Version NP-V*. New York: New York State Psychiatric Institute, Biometrics Research Department.

Weiss, D., Horowitz, M., & Wilner, N. (1984). The Stress Response Rating Scale: A clinician's measure for rating the response to serious life events. *British Journal of Clinical Psychology*, *23*, 202–215.

Weissman, M. M., Myers, J. K., & Ross, C. E. (Eds.). (1986). *Community surveys of psychiatric disorders*. New Brunswick, NJ: Rutgers University Press.

Wolfe, T. (1979). *The right stuff*. New York: Farrar Straus Giroux.

CHAPTER 13

A Prospective Study of Victims of Physical Trauma

Anthony Feinstein

Introduction

Almost a decade has passed since the diagnostic category of posttraumatic stress disorder (PTSD) first appeared in the third edition of the *Diagnostic and Statistical Manual of Mental Disorders* (DSM-III) of the American Psychiatric Association (APA) (1980). Despite the subsequent appearance of a large literature devoted to the subject, the disorder continues to remain controversial and to promote intense debate among researchers and clinicians. Those in agreement with Breslau and Davis (1987) have voiced misgivings of the entire concept, whereas advocates of the disorder feel they are being asked to attain a strength of validity for PTSD beyond that of most other psychiatric disorders (Horowitz, Weiss, & Marmar, 1987).

A source of this controversy can be traced to the problem of establishing the significance of the "stressor." This has had the effect of continuing the long standing *stress-vulnerability* debate in psychiatric research (see Chapter 11, in this volume, for a discussion). The majority of research studies on PTSD have been retrospective in nature, often identifying cohorts of subjects or patients months or years after the traumatic event. These studies have performed the useful task of supplying phenomenological and empirical data, but the methodological weaknesses apparent in such designs have precluded the prospective study of issues such as stressor events themselves. In addition, they have been unable to address questions concerning the *natural history of the disorder* and which factors exert a modifying influence. Thus, there is a need for prospective, longitudinal studies to rectify the situation. In the process, the nosological status of PTSD could be clarified, for even though the disorder currently has a place among the anxiety disorders, concomitant depressive and dissociative symptomatology have frequently been recorded (Wilson, 1988a, 1989).

Although medical and public attention is naturally drawn to such major disasters as the Lockerbie aircrash, less dramatic but potentially serious and disabling events take place on a daily basis, causing physical and emotional suffering to a large group of individuals. This group includes victims of assault and motor vehicle (see Chapter 43, in this volume, for a review) and industrial accidents. Emotional traumata in these contexts may be frequently overlooked or dismissed for no better reason than they constitute relatively commonplace events and in terms of magnitude are dwarfed by the drama of major disasters. However, PTSD and its debilitating effects are to be found among victims of these individual disasters with different stressor dimensions (Wilson, Smith, & Johnson, 1985).

The aim of this chapter was to address a deficiency in current PTSD literature; to undertake a prospective, longitudinal study documenting posttraumatic psychological sequelae in a sample of patients injured in motor vehicle accidents and similar events.

The following criteria had to be met by participants before they were included in the study:

1. *Age.* All subjects had to be between 15 and 60 years of age.
2. *Trauma.* Subjects had to have suffered a fracture of the femur, tibia, or fibula without a loss of limb.
3. *Site.* Subjects required admission to an orthopedic ward for surgical correction of the fracture and were discharged from the hospital by the time the first follow-up assessment was completed (6 weeks).
4. Subjects had no evidence of a head injury or any

Anthony Feinstein • Institute of Neurology and National Hospital for Nervous Diseases, Queen Square, London WC1N 3BG, England.

International Handbook of Traumatic Stress Syndromes, edited by John P. Wilson and Beverley Raphael. Plenum Press, New York, 1993.

other physical trauma and had good recall of events surrounding the accident.

5. No fatalities must have occurred in the accident.
6. Patients with self-induced injuries, that is suicide attempts, were excluded.

Although the victims may all have experienced injuries of similar severity, the nature of the trauma differed from person to person.

Initial Assessment: Location and Procedures

Patients were initially assessed on the orthopedic wards of the Whittington Hospital, London, England. The extent of physical injury was documented using the Abbreviated Injury Scale (AIS) and Injury Severity Score (ISS) (Greenspan, McLellan, & Greig, 1985).

All patients were initially assessed within 4 to 7 days of admission. The rationale for allowing a minimum duration of 4 days to elapse prior to the first assessment was the fact that all patients would have had some surgical intervention necessitating an anesthetic and a period of recovery from this seemed advisable. Demographic data were collected on all patients, including age, sex, marital status, nature of employment, social class, and past psychiatric history and treatment. Furthermore, whether or not the person had been drinking prior to the accident and the number of units of alcohol consumed per week were evaluated.

The nature of the stressor experienced was ascertained from the type of injury. Information was obtained on whether the victims had been either active or passive participants in the traumatic event. The patients were also asked to assess their responsibility for the event on a three-point scale: (1) fully responsible, (2) partially responsible, or (3) not at all responsible. They were also asked to rate their opinion as to the stressfulness of the event on a four-point scale: (1) life threatening, (2) moderate threat, (3) little threat, and (4) no threat.

Psychological Measures

Measures used included the 28-item General Health Questionnaire (GHQ) (Goldberg & Hillier, 1979), which was scored in the traditional manner (0-0-1-1) and using the Likert method (0-1-2-3), and the Clinical Interview Schedule) (CIS) (Goldberg, Cooper, Eastwood, Kedward, & Shepherd, 1970). Although both the CIS and the GHQ are designed to detect neurotic symptomatology, the CIS contains items dealing with dissociation and phobic avoidance behavior. It is also possible to rate psychotic symptoms with the CIS should the need arise. A score of 14 or higher on the CIS was taken as an indication of psychiatric caseness. Other measures were the Impact of Event Scale (IES) (Horowitz, Wilner, & Alvarez, 1979) and the Standardized Assessment of Personality (SAP) (Mann, Jenkins, Cutting, & Cowen, 1981). The SAP was administered by interviewing an

informant—a person close to the patient who had known him or her for a period exceeding 5 years.

Follow-Up Assessments

The patients were subsequently followed up at two points: 6 weeks and 6 months after the accidental injury. At the 6-week follow-up, the length of each patient's stay in the hospital was recorded. At 6 months, the presence of litigation was noted. The above rating scales, with the obvious exception of the SAP, were repeated.

Patients were assessed for PTSD using a self-report symptom checklist derived from the DSM-III-R (APA, 1987) criteria for PTSD. Responses were either Yes or No to symptoms that had been present during the previous week. In addition, the patients completed the Beck Depression Inventory (BDI) (Beck, Ward, Mendelson, Mock, & Erbaugh, 1961) and the Spielberger State-Trait Anxiety Scale (STAI) (Spielberger, Gorsuch, & Lushene, 1970). According to Beck's criteria, patients scoring greater than 17 or 26 on the BDI were judged to have depression of moderate or severe intensity, respectively. The follow-up PTSD questionnaire, GHQ, IES, BDI, and Spielberger scales were completed by postal return; the CIS was completed when patients returned to the orthopedic outpatient clinic or by visiting patients at home.

Results

Population

Forty-eight cases seen over a 6-month period met the criteria for inclusion. In terms of severity of injury, all patients rated as either 4 or 9 on the Abbreviated Injury Scale (AIS), which is well below the LD_{50} and indicative of mild to moderately severe injury.

Of those selected, 34 were male and 14 female. The mean age of the sample was 30.5 years ($SD = 11.7$ years) with a range from 16 to 60 years. Marital status revealed 33 single patients (68.8%), 11 married (22.9%), 3 divorced (6.3%), and 1 widowed (2.1%). The distribution of the subjects by social class I to V was 4.2%, 14.6%, 39.6%, 25%, and 16.7%, respectively. Thirty-six (75%) of the patients were employed and 12 (25%) were unemployed.

Four patients had a past history of psychiatric disorder. The mean alcohol consumption of the sample was 11.8 units/week ($SD = 13.3$ units/week) with a range of 0 to 48 units (median = 5.5 units/week). Twelve patients (25%) admitted to drinking prior to their accident. Details of their blood alcohol levels were not known. One female victim and 10 male victims could be classed as problem drinkers (in excess of 14 or 21 units of alcohol per week, respectively). The mean length of stay in the hospital was 11.5 days ($SD = 6.9$ days) with a range of 5 to 35 days. Ten patients (20.8%) were involved with some form of medicolegal action.

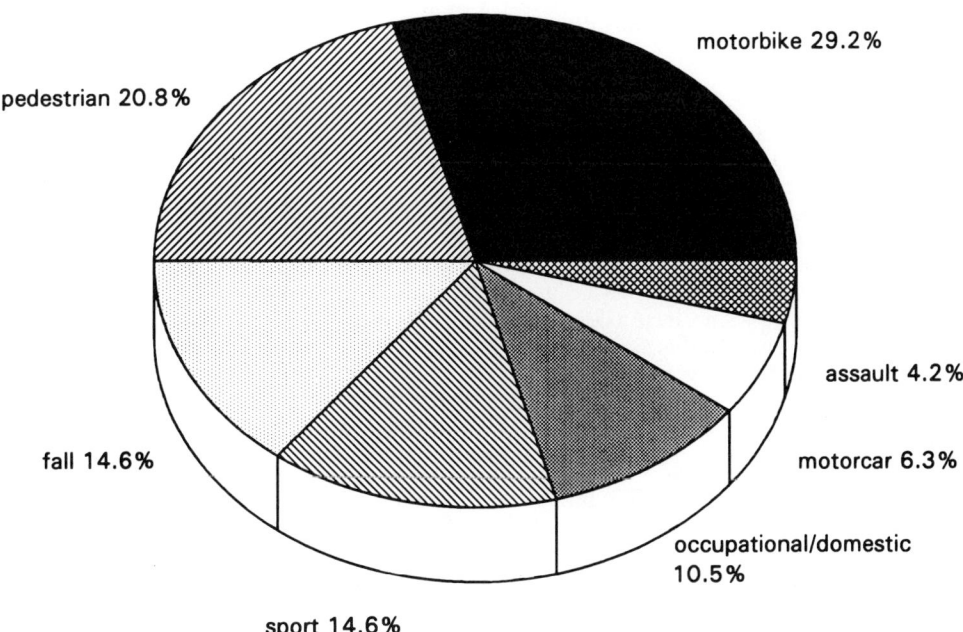

Figure 13.1. Nature of the traumatic accident.

Stressor Events

A breakdown of the nature of the trauma involved is shown in Figure 13.1. Motorbike accidents accounted for almost a third of all the stressors (29.2%). Fifteen patients felt entirely responsible for the trauma that befell them; 16 patients partially responsible, and 17 patients not responsible at all. Thirty-three patients had been actively involved in the traumatic event, whereas 15 had been passive participants. The majority of the victims (58.3%) rated their accidents as life-threatening; 12.5% as little threat; and the remainder as moderate but not life-threatening.

Initial Assessment

The results of the initial assessment done while the patients were still hospitalized are shown in Table 13.1. On the basis of scores of 14 or greater on the Clinical Interview Schedule, 30 (62.5%) patients were rated as psychiatric cases at initial interview.

Dissociative phenomena (assessed from the CIS) were endorsed by 40 patients at the initial assessment, of which 20 patients reported that they had only experienced the phenomenon once.

Fourteen patients had dreams related to the traumatic event. A breakdown of the personality traits obtained from the Standard Assessment of Personality revealed that in 52% no traits were discernible. Of 21 patients in whom personality traits were recordable, only 4 were severe enough to warrant the classification of a personality disorder. Compulsive traits were noted in 6 (12.5%); antisocial in 5 (10.4%); and borderline in 3 (6.3%), with single patients in most of the remaining DSM-III-R categories.

Those meeting the criteria of psychiatric caseness were more likely to have been female ($p < .02$) and had "life-threatening" accidents ($p < .05$). All 4 patients with a previous psychiatric history were cases, and there was a trend for cases to report their role in the traumatic event as "not at all responsible" ($p < .07$). Those who met caseness criteria had higher scores than noncases on all questionnaires administered ($p < .001$ for all) the exception being the social dysfunction scale of the GHQ.

Assessment at the 6-Week Follow-Up

Four patients were lost to follow-up. Although all 4 were traceable, they refused further participation in the study citing their reluctance to have a psychiatrist ask any further questions. The results of the 6-week assessment are shown in Table 13.2.

The number of psychiatric cases (as defined by a CIS score of 14 or higher) was 12 (27.3%). Sixteen patients reported dissociative phenomena 6 weeks posttrauma, of which 5 cases reported the experience more than once within the past week. Seven patients reported dreams related to the traumatic event within the previous week. Of these, 5 had experienced the dream more than once.

On the basis of scores from the Beck depression scale, 4 male and 2 female patients were rated as moderately or severely depressed. Combined scores for both sexes showed that the state anxiety score was significantly higher than the trait anxiety score ($p < .0001$).

Twelve victims (25%) were classified as suffering from PTSD. Patients who were classified as meeting psychiatric caseness were more likely to be suffering from PTSD than those who were not cases ($p < .03$) and to have a past psychiatric history ($p < .02$). Furthermore,

Table 13.1. Results of the Initial Assessment ($N = 48$)

	Mean	SD	Minimum	Maximum
Clinical Interview Schedule	17.21	9.02	3	40
Impact of Event Scale	24.36	12.53	2	51
Intrusion subscale	14.87	7.71	1	31
Avoidance subscale	9.56	6.65	0	25
General Health Questionnaire (traditional)	11.62	5.03	1	26
General Health Questionnaire (Likert)	34.75	10.93	15	63
General Health Questionnaire (Somatic)	9.00	3.54	2	16
General Health Questionnaire (Anxiety/Insomnia)	10.40	4.55	0	19
General Health Questionnaire (Social Dysfunction)	13.71	1.82	8	16
General Health Questionnaire (Depression)	2.27	3.91	0	15

they had significantly higher scores on the IES, Intrusion and Avoidance subscales, the BDI, and the Spielberger State and Trait scores ($p < .001$ or $p < .0001$ for all the above). In addition, all the GHQ subscales were elevated (e.g., somatic complaints [$p < .04$] and depression [$p < .0001$].

Comparisons between Initial (Week 1) and 6-Week Assessments

The decline in the number of individuals classified as psychiatric cases over 6 weeks (30 to 12) was significant ($p < .0007$; McNemar test). Ten patients had remained classified cases, 2 new cases had developed, 15 patients had remained noncases, and 17 had improved to noncase status. The differences between case and noncase status noted on initial assessment regarding sex, nature of the trauma, and responsibility for the trauma were no longer apparent.

When the mean scores obtained at 6 weeks for each individual rating scale were compared with those obtained at the initial interview, all had decreased over time at a statistically significant level. Thus, significant *decreases* in scores over time were noted for the CIS ($p < .0001$), IES total ($p < .005$), IES Intrusion subscale ($p < .001$), GHQ ($p < .008$), Somatic subscale ($p < .007$), Social Disability subscale ($p < .0001$), and the Depression subscale ($p < .05$). However, no significant differences were found between the initial and follow-up Avoidance subscales from the IES and Anxiety subscales from the GHQ.

Seven patients were still experiencing dreams related to the trauma as compared to 14 at the first assessment. Dissociative phenomena were reported by 16 subjects, a substantial decrease from the 40 subjects in the first assessment.

Assessment at 6 Months

Five additional patients had dropped out of the sample at the 6-month assessment. The percentage of patients who completed the full assessment was 81.25%. The results of the rating scales and repeat CIS assessment are shown in Table 13.3.

Table 13.2. Results of the 6-Week Follow-Up ($N = 44$)

	Mean	SD	Minimum	Maximum
Clinical Interview Schedule	12.35	10.05	0	43
Impact of Event Scale	18.45	15.59	0	57
Intrusion subscale	10.32	8.63	0	29
Avoidance subscale	8.14	8.49	0	36
General Health Questionnaire (traditional)	9.86	5.01	1	25
General Health Questionnaire (Likert)	30.59	10.93	13	62
General Health Questionnaire (Somatic)	7.41	4.41	1	19
General Health Questionnaire (Anxiety/Insomnia)	9.48	4.85	0	19
General Health Questionnaire (Social Dysfunction)	12.07	2.00	8	16
General Health Questionnaire (Depression)	1.64	3.08	0	14
Beck Depression Inventory	9.07	7.43	0	32
Spielberger State scores	39.42	13.13	20	71
Males	38.12	13.17	20	64
Females	43.00	12.87	20	71
Spielberger Trait scores	32.80	11.67	20	67
Males	32.30	12.40	20	50
Females	34.16	9.56	20	67

Table 13.3. Results of the 6-Month Follow-Up ($N = 39$)

	Mean	SD	Minimum	Maximum
Clinical Interview Schedule	6.92	7.50	0	27
Impact of Event Scale	15.89	15.17	0	51
Intrusion subscale	7.64	7.83	0	30
Avoidance subscale	8.24	9.04	0	31
General Health Questionnaire (traditional)	6.21	6.89	0	23
General Health Questionnaire (Likert)	22.62	14.54	5	58
General Health Questionnaire (Somatic)	5.76	4.38	0	16
General Health Questionnaire (Anxiety/Insomnia)	5.71	5.28	0	19
General Health Questionnaire (Social Dysfunction)	8.97	3.32	1	17
General Health Questionnaire (Depression)	2.45	3.64	0	13
Beck Depression Inventory	7.41	7.83	0	34
Spielberger State scores	36.64	12.56	20	65
Males	34.60	11.60	20	65
Females	41.20	13.98	20	48
Spielberger Trait scores	35.15	12.59	20	69
Males	32.70	11.60	20	44
Females	40.60	13.60	24	69

The number of persons classified as psychiatric cases was down to 10. Of the 7 (14.6%) victims who were suffering from PTSD at 6 months, 6 were psychiatric cases. Of these, 5 individuals had experienced dissociative phenomena within the previous week. In one of these cases, the experiences had occurred more than once. Nine subjects experienced dreams related to the trauma within the previous week; of these, 4 had had them more than once.

Three patients had moderately severe depression and two had severe depression classified by the BDI. Combining the male and female scores showed that the 6-months state anxiety score was not significantly higher than the trait anxiety score ($p < .09$).

Of all the discrete variables documented at the initial interview, the only distinguishing feature between case and noncase status was whether or not the victim had been drinking before the accident, with those who had more likely to be grouped as psychiatric cases ($p < .06$). In addition, those victims who had been drinking *before* the accident had a significantly higher weekly alcohol consumption than those who had not ($p < .001$; Mann-Whitney test). Although they drank more per week, this group was not more likely to be classed as problem drinkers (as defined by 21 units or more of alcohol per week) compared to those who had not been drinking before the accident. The above figures refer to drinking habits before the accidental injury. Similar information was not obtained postaccident.

Individuals who met psychiatric case status had significantly higher scores on all 4 subscales from the GHQ, the IES, Intrusion and Avoidance subscales ($p < .001$), BDI, and Spielberger State-Trait Anxiety scores ($p < .001$ or less for comparisons).

Comparisons between 6-Week and 6-Month Assessments

The decrease in the number of psychiatric cases from 12 to 10 was not statistically significant. Twenty-four patients had remained as noncases; 5 had remained as cases, 5 had improved to noncaseness, and 5 new patients met caseness at 6 weeks posttrauma. The number of individuals with PTSD had decreased from 12 to 7. Of the original 12 victims with PTSD, 2 had dropped out of the study by the time the 6-month assessment was carried out. This change in the number of victims with PTSD over time was not significant.

A comparison between the mean scores for individual rating scales obtained at 6 months and those obtained at 6 weeks revealed that significant decreases over time had occurred with respect to the GHQ ($p < .0005$) on the subscales of Social Disability ($p < .0001$), Somatic Complaints ($p < .02$), and Anxiety/Insomnia ($p < .0001$). A nonsignificant change over time was noted ($p = .2$; Wilcoxon signed-ranks test) with respect to the BDI. The Impact of Event Scale and its subscales did not show any statistically significant change over time. Similarly, there was no significant difference between the Spielberger state anxiety scores at 6 weeks and at 6 months.

However, the Spielberger trait anxiety score reported at 6 months was significantly higher than the 6-weeks score ($p < .04$), indicating that the cohort's general level of arousal had significantly increased since the accident. This is further confirmed by the fact that although at 6 weeks there was a significant difference between the state and trait anxiety scores, this was no longer apparent at 6 months. As noted above, the state anxiety scores had not significantly changed from 6 weeks to 6 months, so the narrowing of the gap between state and trait anxiety scores was due to an *increase* in the trait scores over time. Finally, the number of victims experiencing dreams related to the trauma had increased from 7 to 9. Only 5 patients reported dissociative phenomena compared with 16 at the 6-week assessment.

Predictive Factors of Poor Outcome

The victims who were of most interest to this study were those who remained as psychiatric cases at 6 months. These were the cases who were assigned to the poor-outcome category. In order to predict which individual victims would end up with a poor outcome, a discriminant analysis was performed on all the variables available at the first assessment. The initial Impact of Event score, which assesses symptoms of PTSD, was the most powerful predictor of poor outcome at 6 months. On the basis of this variable alone, we could predict psychiatric caseness at 6 months with a 82.05% accuracy.

Discussion

At the initial interview, almost two thirds ($N = 32$) of the patients reported sufficient symptoms to be labeled as psychiatric cases. Without any therapeutic intervention the natural history of these sequelae revealed that the majority improved with time. Comparing psychiatric cases with noncases at 6 months revealed that case-identified patients drank more alcohol per week and had higher scores when it came to subjectively rating their response to the trauma on the Impact of Event Scale.

It is difficult to place these data in perspective because there is a paucity of information with which to compare them. Whereas numerous studies have documented symptoms of posttraumatic stress reactions at varying times ranging from weeks to years following a traumatic insult, few studies have documented symptoms within a uniform time period soon after such an event and then performed follow-up analyses. With the exception of a Norwegian study (Malt, 1988), no prospective, longitudinal studies examining the natural history of the symptomatology have been undertaken. The fact that all patients in this study were selected on the basis of injuries of similar severity controls for yet another variable that has made the interpretation of numerous other researchers' results problematic. In sum, a combination of the above criteria sets this study apart from others and answers some of the criticisms leveled at methodological weaknesses in previous research on traumatic stress reactions.

Clinical Assessment versus Diagnosis

In assessing these patients, the purpose was to document their symptomatology with no attempt to formulate formal clinical diagnoses. The design of the study, with the emphasis on self-report questionnaires, was not considered a valid means of arriving at a diagnosis, the exception being the case of PTSD where a comprehensive symptom checklist derived from the DSM-III-R was used. Psychiatric caseness as defined by scores on the CIS, rather than the diagnosis of PTSD, was taken as the index of psychological distress. Psychiatric caseness implies a broader definition of pathology than PTSD, encompassing most cases of PTSD in addition to other psychological difficulties that may have arisen following the injury. Psychiatric caseness was not synonymous with PTSD although the two were highly correlated.

Demographic Characteristics

The sample was heavily biased toward younger male patients with only 9 patients older than 40 years and approximately 60% under 30 years of age. This probably reflects the nature of the trauma, of which almost a third were due to motorbike injuries. This bias toward younger male patients is consistent with previous findings from the accident literature, particularly among victims of traffic accidents (Maguire, 1976; Shaffer, Schmidt, & Zlotowitz, 1977).

The high unemployment rate and preponderance of patients with social class III, IV, and V is indicative of the catchment area served by the Whittington Hospital and probably accurately reflects the situation in a deprived inner London borough.

Natural History of Postaccident Psychological Sequelae

A consistent decline in all measures of symptoms was observed over time. At the group level, the maximum symptomatology was reported in the first week following the trauma when almost two thirds of the victims were classified as psychiatric cases. This had fallen to about 25% by 6 weeks and 6 months. The percentage of victims who were classified as psychiatric cases by the CIS at the follow-up periods is higher than figures derived from community samples (Andrews, Schonell, & Tennent, 1977), but slightly lower than those seen by general practitioners (Goldberg & Blackwell, 1970). The fact that there was no significant change in the number of cases from 6 weeks to 6 months is not indicative of a stable situation having been reached by 6 weeks: Five patients deteriorated in their condition while a similar number had improved. (An analogous situation exists with respect to PTSD.) Thus, the natural history of these posttraumatic reactions following accidental injury would seem to be that in the majority of cases the victims improve spontaneously and consistently over time, but in one small subgroup, the sequelae run a fluctuating course; in another, their onset is delayed. DSM-III-R allows for a delayed onset of symptoms stipulating at least 6 months to have passed before this criterion is met but does not address the issue of symptom fluctuation over time. Horowitz (1976) has incorporated into his model of traumatic stress reactions a pattern of oscillation between the denial and intrusion stages of symptom expression. The results from a small subgroup of patients within the present study seem to confirm the concept.

The results of this study support the DSM-III-R criteria for PTSD (namely, the minimum duration of one month's symptomatology before a diagnosis can be reached), because by 6 weeks the number of psychiatric cases had fallen considerably as had the scores on all other rating scales. The high percentage of psychiatric cases found at initial assessment could be explained by the distress experienced by the victims as a consequence of the trauma.

The percentage of patients with PTSD and the scores on the IES reported in this study were significantly higher than the results from the Norwegian longitudinal study of accidents (Malt, 1988), despite the fact that the extent of injuries suffered by victims in both studies were similar. The Norwegians reported only a single case of PTSD at 6 months and none at 2 years after the accident. The reason for the discrepancy seems unclear. One could argue that the more rigid assessment of patients in the Norwegian study (extensive clinical interviews as opposed to self-report symptom checklists in the present study) may have reduced the number of PTSD false positives, but this would not explain the discrepancy with respect to scores on the Impact of Event Scale. The fact that almost 60% of the present sample rated their accident as life threatening may account for their high IES, and it is conceivable that the Norwegian group's self-assessment of their trauma may not have been as severe; information on this was not available. It is also possible that by 2-year follow-up the results of the present study may more closely approximate those of Malt and his colleagues. However, the results do suggest that 6 months following accidental injury the diagnosis of PTSD and intrusive and avoidant characteristics are part of the psychological sequelae.

Factors Influencing Development of Psychopathology

At the initial assessment, more severe trauma (e.g., motor vehicle accidents) and more extreme subjective ratings of severity of trauma (e.g., "life threatening"), were more prevalent among psychiatric cases as opposed to noncases. By the 6-week and 6-month follow-up, this distinction had disappeared. These two variables may therefore be regarded as influencing the degree of postaccident distress experienced but not in terms of exerting any lasting influence on the development of psychopathology. What is more influential in this regard are scores on the initial Impact of Event Scale, which was found to be the single most important predictor of psychiatric morbidity at 6 months. The fact that this score correlated highly with scores from the two follow-up scales suggests that when it comes to accidental injury, the DSM-III-R concept of the stressor is important but not totally determinant. Rather, it is the way the individual cognitively assimilates and copes with the traumatic event that ultimately has the most influence in determining outcome. These findings are in broad agreement with those of McFarlane (1988) who found psychiatric impairment after a natural disaster (as measured by the GHQ-12) to be more closely related to levels of distress following the disaster (as measured by the IES) than to the victim's severity of exposure or loss.

Employment status appeared transiently as a variable discriminating case status from noncase status at the 6-week follow-up. Most patients were back at work by 6 weeks, suggesting that a return to work soon after the accident may have a beneficial effect. Employment status was not controlled for during the follow-up period, and it is conceivable that some unemployed patients found work, which may account for the disappearance of employment status as a predictor variable of morbidity at 6 months. The alternative view is that employment status is not a robust discriminator of psychiatric morbidity following traumatic injury.

The fact that female patients endorsed more symptoms than their male counterparts confirms the findings of researchers into gender differences in the reporting of neurotic and affective symptomatology in general (Jenkins, 1985).

Phenomenology of Posttraumatic Stress Reactions

By examining the symptomatology recorded, observations could be made concerning the nature of the stress reactions. On the GHQ, scores on the Anxiety subscale were appreciably higher than the depressive ones for all 3 stages of assessment. Of all 4 subscale scores on the GHQ, Depression scores were the lowest. However, the GHQ items for depression are directed toward the more severe end of the spectrum, and it is conceivable that more moderate forms of depressive reactions could be overlooked. Examination of the Beck depression scores tends to confirm this. Thus, of the 12 individuals designated as psychiatric cases at the 6-week follow-up and on the basis of cut-off points derived from the Beck scale, half were either moderately or severely depressed. This finding of depression was found at the 6-month follow-up as well. These figures replicate the findings of Malt (1988), who found 9 out of 18 patients with posttraumatic psychiatric sequelae to be suffering from depression of varying degrees of severity.

The results of the Spielberger State-Trait Anxiety scores tended to support the finding of raised scores on the anxiety component of the GHQ. Of note was the fact that although the state scores decreased over time, the trait scores at 6 months were significantly higher than the 6-week scores, which suggests that the victims were functioning at a higher general state of arousal 6 months after the trauma. This was mainly applicable to the female patients.

The results of this study do not support the concept of PTSD as being primarily a dissociative disorder. Although a high percentage of patients initially reported dissociative phenomena within the first week following accidental injury, in half of these subjects dissociation had only occurred once. These numbers had substantially fallen by 6 weeks and 6 months and if present were only endorsed as a single, brief episode in the majority of patients. In addition, psychiatric case status and persons with PTSD were not more likely to have experienced the phenomenon when compared to noncase status, or those without PTSD. It would therefore appear that in regard to postaccident psychological traumata following motorbike and sports injuries, dissociative phenomena are brief and transitory experiences and do not correlate with levels of psychological distress.

Thus, these results highlight the fact that posttraumatic psychological sequelae following accidental injury have both an anxiety and a depressive component. Since caseness in this study correlated highly with the diagnosis of posttraumatic stress disorder, one may assume that despite its nosological status as an anxiety disorder, PTSD either has a depressive component or else frequently coexists alongside other Axis I diagnoses of depression of various grades. This is in accord with the results of certain retrospective studies (Sierles, Chen, McFarland, & Taylor, 1983).

Methodological Considerations

Certain methodological problems must be borne in mind when interpreting the results of this study. The sample size was small and was further reduced when 9 individuals dropped out during the follow-up period. Nevertheless, the 80% response rate by 6 months is relatively strong for purposes of statistical analysis. The sample was also skewed by having more males than females. In addition, the follow-up period of 6 months is probably too short a time by which to draw any conclusions concerning the final long-term sequelae.

It can also be argued that the stressor in this case points out the difficulty with the DSM-III-R requirements for PTSD, namely an "event outside the range of usual human experience." However, a traumatic fracture of either femur or tibula/fibula requiring admission via an accident and emergency department and necessitating surgery within a few days was considered sufficiently severe to fulfil this DSM-III-R A criterion. Although all patients had injuries of similar severity, the different ways in which they acquired them added another potentially confounding variable to the analysis. Ideally, it would have been desirable to have included only a single type of traumatic event (e.g., motorbike injury), but such a step added to the list of other inclusion/exclusion criteria would have made the collection of such a sample too lengthy for this present study.

Since this study was predominantly a descriptive one, no attempts were made to control for a host of other variables that may have influenced the development of psychopathology during the follow-up period, such as subsequent life events and extent of social support. As their role in this study is uncertain, caution has to be exercised in drawing too many conclusions from the present findings.

Conclusion

The results of this prospective, longitudinal study can only be regarded as applicable to the types of accidental injuries of moderate severity that we studied. Nevertheless, they do give some tentative pointers as to the natural history of posttraumatic stress reactions, the phenomenology and nosological status of the condition, and factors that determine prognosis. Future research requires prospective studies of which this model is but one approach.

References

American Psychiatric Association. (1980). *Diagnostic and statistical manual of mental disorders* (3rd ed.). Washington, DC: Author.

American Psychiatric Association. (1987). *Diagnostic and statistical manual of mental disorders* (3rd ed., rev.). Washington, DC: Author.

Andrews, G., Schonell, M., & Tennent, C. (1977). The relationship between physical, psychological and social morbidity in a suburban community. *American Journal of Epidemiology, 105,* 324–329.

Beck, A. T., Ward, C. H., Mendelson, M., Mock, J., & Erbaugh, J. (1961). An inventory for measuring depression. *Archives of General Psychiatry, 4,* 53–63.

Breslau, N., & Davis, G. C. (1987). Post-traumatic stress disorder: The stressor criterion. *Journal of Nervous and Mental Disease, 175,* 255–264.

Goldberg, D. P., & Blackwell, B. B. (1970). Psychiatric illness in general practice. A detailed study using a new method of case identification. *British Medical Journal, 11,* 439–443.

Goldberg, D. P., Cooper, B., Eastwood, M. R., Kedward, H. B., & Shepherd, M. (1970). A standardized psychiatric interview for use in community surveys. *British Journal of Preventive Social Medicine, 24,* 18–23.

Goldberg, D. P., & Hillier, V. F. (1979). A scaled version of the General Health Questionnaire. *Psychological Medicine, 9,* 39–145.

Greenspan, L., McLellan, B. A., & Greig, H. (1985). Abbreviated injury scale and injury severity score: A scoring chart. *Journal of Trauma, 25,* 60–64.

Horowitz, M. J. (1976). *Stress response syndromes.* New York: Jason Aronson.

Horowitz, M. J., Weiss, D. S., & Marmar, C. (1987). Diagnosis of post-traumatic stress disorder. *Journal of Nervous and Mental Disease, 175,* 267–268.

Horowitz, M. J., Wilner, N., & Alvarez, W. (1979). Impact of Event Scale: A measure of subjective stress. *Psychosomatic Medicine, 41,* 209–218.

Jenkins, R. (1985). Sex differences in minor psychiatric morbidity. *Psychological Medicine, Monograph Supplement 7.* New York: Cambridge University Press.

Malt, U. (1988). The long-term psychiatric consequences of accidental injury: A longitudinal study of 107 adults. *British Journal of Psychiatry, 153,* 810–818.

Mann, A. H., Jenkins, R., Cutting, J. C., & Cowen, P. J. (1981). The development and use of a standardized assessment of abnormal personality. *Psychological Medicine, 11,* 839–847.

McFarlane, A. C. (1988). Relationship between psychiatric impairment and a natural disaster: The role of distress. *Psychological Medicine, 18,* 129–139.

MacGuire, F. L. (1976). Personality factors in highway accidents. *Human Factors, 18,* 433–442.

Shaffer, J. W., Schmidt, C. W., & Zlotowitz, H. I. (1977). Social adjustment profiles of female drivers involved in fatal and nonfatal accidents. *American Journal of Psychiatry, 134,* 801–804.

Sierles, F. S., Chen, J. J., McFarland, R. E., & Taylor, M. A. (1983). Post-traumatic stress disorder and concurrent psychiatric illness: A preliminary report. *American Journal of Psychiatry, 140,* 1177–1179.

Spielberger, C. D., Gorsuch, R. L., & Lushene, R. E. (1970). *Manual of the State-Trait Anxiety Inventory.* Palo Alto: Consulting Psychologists Press.

CHAPTER 14

New Perspectives in the Assessment and Diagnosis of Combat-Related Posttraumatic Stress Disorder

Jessica Wolfe and Terence M. Keane

Introduction

Evolution of Assessment

Although the psychological consequences of exposure to severe life stressors such as war have been observed for centuries, the technical classification of posttraumatic stress disorder (PTSD) has been documented in the psychiatric nomenclature only since 1980 (*Diagnostic and Statistical Manual of Mental Disorders*, 3rd ed. [DSM-III], American Psychiatric Association [APA], 1980). As a result, the development of criteria-based, formal evaluation procedures has been relatively recent. Nonetheless, a review of the literature on combat-related disorders shows that a number of researchers made significant early contributions in the definition of features now known to accompany PTSD.

In 1945, Grinker and Spiegel employed psychiatric terminology to describe symptoms consistent with combat-related PTSD. The symptoms they observed in a World War II sample of combatants are the clear forerunners of current diagnostic criteria for PTSD (*Diagnostic and Statistical Manual of Mental Disorders*, 3rd ed., rev., [DSM-III-R], APA, 1987), specifically, anxiety, depression, rage reactions, sleep disturbance, and guilt. The label *gross stress reactions*, a diagnosis included in the DSM-I, was, in fact, frequently applied to survivors of

combat and other extreme stressors. However, the publication of the DSM-II in 1968 omitted this diagnosis, preferring to classify reactions during combat under the rubric of adjustment disorders. As a consequence, minimal scientific interest was directed at the investigation of trauma syndromes, and essentially no systematic evaluation of combat (or civilian) PTSD took place until considerably later.

In 1960, Dobbs and Wilson provided some of the first evaluation-based data on combat stress when they empirically demonstrated psychophysiological reactivity to combat stimuli in a group of World War II patients apparently suffering from PTSD. Later, Merbaum (1977), using a psychometric approach, was able to show a distinctively elevated symptom profile on the Minnesota Multiphasic Personality Inventory (MMPI) (Hathaway & McKinley, 1967) performance of combat veterans serving in various wartime conflicts. All these data were among the first to highlight some of the distinguishing phenomenologic aspects of PTSD (cf. Fairbank, Keane, & Malloy, 1983; Malloy, Fairbank, & Keane, 1983). Yet the information was not incorporated into broader diagnostic schema for PTSD until the publication of the DSM-III in 1980. In the interim, assessment approaches for trauma (combat or otherwise) remained limited to more traditional diagnostic approaches; these involved the gathering of diagnostic data through semi- or unstructured interview procedures. Two factors affected the overall adequacy of this approach: First, since explicit diagnostic criteria for PTSD had not yet been established, few clinicians inquired in detail about the nature and extent of various traumatizing life experiences. Second, since there were no standardized psychiatric interviews for traumatic disorders available before at least the late

Jessica Wolfe and Terence M. Keane • Department of Veterans Affairs Medical Center, Boston, Massachusetts 02130.

International Handbook of Traumatic Stress Syndromes, edited by John P. Wilson and Beverley Raphael. Plenum Press, New York, 1993.

1970s, any inquiry into traumatic exposure was more likely to be guided by the interviewer's own orientation and training in psychopathology than adherence to any overarching or comprehensive diagnostic schema. Hence there was little serious investigation of presumed life stressors or their pathological sequelae in any uniform, widespread, or objective fashion.

The publication in 1980 of the DSM-III, in conjunction with clinicians' growing awareness of the span of environmentally based trauma, thus provided an important catalyst for the development of assessment procedures specific to PTSD. The existence of a classification schema encouraged the development and application of psychological assessment tools in two specific ways: First, it provided preliminary scientific credibility for the disorder, stimulating the need to attempt further validation of the diagnostic category itself. Second, by proposing particular symptom patterns, the categorization stirred an interest in examining and detailing the various components of PTSD. From this point on, several new questions became pivotal in the assessment of PTSD, particularly as viewed through the topic of combat-related PTSD. These included: the ability of the evaluation procedure to identify the disorder as distinct from other syndromes (cf. Andreasen, 1982); the capacity of the approaches to evaluate the nature of the stressor phenomenon and the accompanying symptom criteria (cf. DSM-III-R; APA, 1987); and the scientific adequacy of the assessment instruments themselves (cf. Hyer *et al.*, 1986). The evolution of assessment efforts in PTSD from the late 1970s until the late 1980s will be considered in terms of these issues.

Conceptual Models

Multidimensional Approaches

Overall, the most recent approaches to the assessment of combat-related PTSD have advocated an orientation which is multidimensional in scope and multimodal in application (Keane, Wolfe, & Taylor, 1987; Wolfe, Keane, Lyons, & Gerardi, 1987). *Multidimensional* implies the need to assess the patient across a wide (and critical) range of psychological functions, including developmental, social, familial, educational, vocational, medical, cognitive, interpersonal, behavioral, and emotional spheres. Because PTSD is considered to have long-term pervasive effects, particularly if undetected over periods of time, information in all the preceding spheres is obtained in detail for the pre-, para-, and postmilitary periods. This material is crucial in determining to what degree, if any, pre- and postmilitary experiences may have contributed to adjustment following exposure to military trauma. In addition to diagnosis, these data have obvious implications for treatment planning as well. Multimodal assessment refers to an assessment approach that incorporates structured clinical interviews, psychometric measures, behavioral observation, and psychophysiological evaluation.

Early Phases of Assessment Procedures

Measurement of Symptomatology

Descriptive Studies

Early assessment procedures in combat-related PTSD were strongly concerned with the validation of this disorder. The majority of efforts were therefore designed to provide accurate phenomenologic descriptions of combatants suffering from PTSD versus combatants who were unaffected, and develop instruments which were valid and reliable in detecting precise patterns of symptomatology. Before the development of instruments specific to PTSD, evaluation procedures focused exclusively on self-report measures in which subjects reported on a range of symptoms. Using this approach, authors such as Figley (1978), Wilson (1978a,b; 1980), and Silver and Iacono (1984) successfully showed that subsets of combatants from Vietnam, in fact, shared the PTSD symptom picture described some 40 years before in work by Grinker and Spiegel (1945). In one of the first major *epidemiological* surveys of the psychological aftermath of the Vietnam War, Egendorf, Kadushin, Laufer, Rothbart, and Sloan (1981) confirmed this symptom picture using a much broader sample. Hence early assessment efforts, relying primarily on self-report measures and interview formats, were able to discriminate distinct and pronounced symptoms of reexperiencing, interpersonal difficulties, affective numbing, guilt, nightmares, depression, and anxiety in a range of combat-exposed male veterans.

Vietnam Era Stress Inventory (VESI). In 1981, Wilson and Krauss developed the Vietnam Era Stress Inventory which was one of the first comprehensive assessment tools for PTSD based in large part on the DSM-III. This questionnaire used a self-report format to cover biographical information and assess functioning in terms of combat participation, PTSD symptomatology, and current adjustment. One application supporting the utility of the VESI was a study of PTSD in women veterans from the Vietnam War (Schnaier, 1986). In that study, analyses of VESI scales yielded Cronbach alphas ranging from 0.87 to 0.98. Additionally, the VESI was used in another study to compare PTSD symptoms across nine stressor events (Wilson, Smith, & Johnson, 1985).

Psychometrics

Minnesota Multiphasic Personality Inventory (MMPI). In the early 1980s, Penk *et al.* (1981) and Roberts *et al.* (1982) pioneered some of the first applications of traditional psychological test measures in the assessment of combat-related disorders. In a study by Penk *et al.* (1981), the MMPI was administered to a series of combat and noncombat Vietnam veterans specifically seeking treatment for substance abuse. By using the MMPI findings in conjunction with other measures, the investigators found that the degree of combat exposure (i.e., heavy combat) was a significant predictor of greater psychological disturbance. In a subsequent MMPI investigation, Roberts *et al.* (1982) divided a similar sample into high and low/no PTSD groups using the existing DSM-III criteria for the disorder. The authors found that the MMPI profiles of the PTSD "positive" group were significantly different from their nonaffected cohorts, showing, in particular, elevations on scales tapping psychopathy, paranoia, and social introversion. These studies were the first to distinguish high- and low-combat exposed subjects using psychometric evaluation. However, the studies were limited by the fact that they included veterans seeking treatment for substance abuse and PTSD status was not confirmed through an independent clinical interview. Nonetheless, the value of using psychometrics in the assessment of trauma was empirically demonstrated.

Shortly after, two other studies further supported the utility of the MMPI in the assessment of combat-related PTSD. Using more carefully selected samples than earlier studies, Fairbank *et al.* (1983) compared three well-matched groups, including Vietnam veterans with PTSD, Vietnam era veterans with other psychological disturbances, and positively adjusted combat controls, on the MMPI and several other psychological symptom measures. Through statistical analyses, the authors determined that PTSD combat veterans could, in fact, be differentiated on the basis of their MMPI performance as found in a distinctive 8–2 clinical scale elevation. This pattern was similar to that of Merbaum (1977) who had previously used the MMPI to investigate the dysfunction of combatants from other wars. Furthermore, when use of the MMPI was combined with a series of psychological measures tapping a range of functions, for example, the Spielberger State-Trait Anxiety Inventory (Spielberger, Gorsuch, & Lushene, 1970), the Beck Depression Inventory (Beck, Mendelson, Mock, & Erbaug, 1961), and the Zung Depression Scale (Zung, 1965), diagnostic classification rates for PTSD reached 83%.

Foy, Sipprelle, Rueger, and Carroll (1984) also provided information on the usefulness of the MMPI as an assessment instrument for adjustment in combatants. Using a discriminant function analysis on the clinical scale scores, these authors obtained an 82% correct classification rate based on the use of the MMPI in Vietnam combatants. In this study, the authors grouped their sample along a continuum of PTSD symptoms, a procedure that precluded clinical adjudication of the PTSD diagnosis. In addition, the responses of PTSD patients to individual MMPI items were not analyzed, so it was unclear which specific items differentiated the two groups.

Keane, Malloy, and Fairbank (1984) employed a substantially larger sample to attempt further validation of the PTSD diagnosis through use of the MMPI. These authors conducted comprehensive *a priori* assessments in order to assign patients to PTSD or non-PTSD diagnostic groupings. Using an empirically derived decision rule for the clinical scales, they were able to classify 74% of the patients among the two groups. More importantly, statistical analyses yielded a unique set of 49 MMPI items which correctly classified 82% of the 200 subjects. The validity of this PTSD subscale was additionally strengthened when Fairbank, McCaffrey, and Keane (1985) investigated the ability of a variety of subjects to feign PTSD on the basis of their MMPI performance. In this study, the authors succeeded in using the PTSD and *F* scales of the MMPI to differentiate at the 90% level between veterans with PTSD and two groups consisting of mental health professionals and well-adjusted combatants, both instructed to feign the disorder's symptomatology. Wilson (1989) has reviewed the literature on the MMPF and MMPI subscales for PTSD.

Mississippi Scale. The Mississippi Scale for Combat-Related PTSD (Keane, Caddell, & Taylor, 1988) represents one of the first validated self-report measures of PTSD symptomatology. Particular strengths of the instrument are its basis in DSM-III criteria for the disorder and the fact that it provides a continuous measure of PTSD symptomatology. Unlike other psychometric instruments which may have a special use in PTSD but were derived for use with other disorders (e.g., the Beck Depression Inventory), the Mississippi explicitly addresses the primary and secondary symptomatology associated with PTSD as defined in the DSM. Consequently, it provides a common frame of reference for clinicians who hope to adapt uniform approaches to assessment. Recent findings on the reliability and validity associated with this instrument are discussed in Current Status (see below).

Other Symptom Scales. The Impact of Event Scale (IES), developed by Horowitz, Wilner, and Alvarez (1979), is a 15-item, self-report instrument designed to assess the impact of extreme life stressors on psychological functioning. The IES, developed before the first formal DSM conceptualization of PTSD (i.e., the DSM-III), yields scores along two important PTSD components—intrusion and avoidance—thus providing quantification of these dimensions. The instrument is based in one of the earliest conceptual models of traumatic stress syndromes (Horowitz, 1976) which specifically predicts alternation (i.e., phaseology) between these constructs. Hence a special use of the IES in assessment has been its ability to help define changes along these parameters over time as well as at any given point. As Schwarzwald, Solomon, Weisenberg, and Mikulincer (1987) noted, until recently, findings from the IES were largely based on assessment of small civilian samples who had been exposed to stressors involving personal injury or bereavement. The instrument thus lacked validation with larger PTSD populations and with combat-exposed veterans in particular.

Interviews

Structured PTSD Interviews. The concept of a multi-modal orientation in assessing PTSD implies that various typologies of measurement instruments should be used, including, for example, interview formats, psychometrics, and laboratory procedures. Within these, both clinician-administered and self-report formats are helpful. Several structured interviews have existed for use in combat-related PTSD, including, for example, the Jackson Structured Interview for Combat-related PTSD (Keane, Fairbank, Caddell, Zimering, & Bender, 1985) and the Brecksville Interview for PTSD (Smith, 1985). Both of these interviews emphasize the need for structured questioning of a combatant's lifetime experiences in a systematic fashion, including the reported period of combat traumatization (cf. Scurfield, Corker, Gongla, & Hough, 1984). In addition, most authors note that, unless directly addressed, many PTSD sufferers will not spontaneously offer information to support a diagnosis of that disorder. This appears to hold true for victims across a variety of trauma categories (see, for example, Wolfe, 1987, on response modes in victims of childhood abuse). One particular factor contributing to the reticence in veterans may be the extraordinary lag time between the period of initial traumatization and the time when the individual first feels able to come for assessment. This suggests that the mode of interpersonal interaction is especially critical with this population and requires particular attention by clinicians.

Generic Interviews. The Structured Clinical Interview for DSM-III/III-R (SCID) (Spitzer & Williams, 1985) and the Diagnostic Interview Schedule (DIS) (Robins, Helzer, Croughan, Williams, & Spitzer, 1981) have served as the two primary generic interviews employed in the overall assessment of PTSD (see Chapter 15, in this volume, for a review). Their primary contribution stems from their ability to provide other Axis I diagnoses, an important factor considering the high rates of co-morbidity now being established in combat-related PTSD (Keane, Gerardi, Lyons, & Wolfe, 1988; Keane & Wolfe, 1990). Generally speaking, interviews of this type should be used in conjunction with a range of other assessment devices according to the multimodal model offered above; other instruments would preferably include a series of psychometrics validated for use with PTSD and a structured PTSD interview. The combined use of such instruments has helped ensure delineation of the exact traumatizing circumstances in addition to the presence of symptom criteria.

Laboratory Procedures

Psychophysiological Assessment. Over the past 7 years, psychophysiologic assessment procedures have come to play an important role in combat-related PTSD. Based in part on the work of Lang (1977), a multimethod assessment of anxiety was devised which included measures of overt behavior, subjective distress, and psychophysiological arousal (e.g., heartrate and galvanic skin response) in combat veterans. Two sets of investigators, Blanchard, Kolb, Pallmeyer, and Gerardi (1982) and Malloy *et al.* (1983), developed laboratory paradigms for the assessment of PTSD in Vietnam veterans using graduated exposure to mild combat stimuli. Both groups were able to demonstrate specific patterns of increased psychophysiological arousal across a number of major measurement channels (e.g., heartrate, skin conductance response (SCR), electromyograph (EMG), and blood pressure) in combat veterans diagnosed with PTSD. Furthermore, these changes seemingly occurred directly in response to the explicit presentation of combat stimuli. Subsequent studies by Knight, Keane, Fairbank, Caddell, and Zimering (1984), Blanchard, Kolb, Gerardi,

Ryan, and Pallmeyer (1986), and Pallmeyer, Blanchard, and Kolb (1986) confirmed the utility of this assessment approach when they conducted similar laboratory procedures which included critical comparison groups of non-PTSD combat veterans carrying a range of psychiatric diagnoses. Pallmeyer *et al.* (1986) in particular was able to demonstrate empirically that psychophysiological measures in their sample were actually more accurate than psychological tests in discriminating PTSD combat veterans from diagnostically heterogeneous groups of veterans. Taken collectively, these studies provided convincing proof of the importance of psychophysiological reactivity as a central component of PTSD, and led the way for consideration of potential markers in this disorder.

Other Considerations

Family and Premorbidity Studies. Few systematic assessment procedures originally existed for the study of either preexisting or familially associated psychological disturbance in PTSD. Early evaluation efforts were limited by both a lack of appropriate instrumentation and sampling biases, although Davidson, Swartz, Storck, Krishnan, and Hammett (1985) found greater rates of family morbidity among PTSD veterans. In addition, analyses of combat veterans' views of their backgrounds some 10 to 40 years past the reported traumatizing event are undoubtedly affected by reporting distortion secondary to the effects of chronic PTSD (cf. Green, Wilson, & Lindy, 1985, for effects on civilians).

Other studies have examined the issue of predisposition more directly. Generally, early assessment efforts did not confirm the presence of preexisting individual or familial psychopathology as predictive of subsequent combat-related PTSD (Card, 1983; Foy *et al.*, 1984; Helzer, Robins, Wish, & Hesselbrock, 1979). In one of the most convincing studies in this area, Card (1983) used archival data to compare the behavioral and academic performance of Vietnam veterans with PTSD, those without PTSD, and nonveteran controls. Findings from her study indicated that few premorbid conditions or factors predicted the ultimate development of PTSD. Similarly, research into the nature, availability, and use of social support networks by combatants (Keane, Scott, Chavoya, Lamparski, & Fairbank, 1985) found that these types of factors failed to differentiate veterans with PTSD from other veteran control groups during the pre-Vietnam period. However, immediately following wartime exposure, PTSD veterans reported significantly greater levels of impairment in social support systems.

Measuring Stressor Dimensions

Exposure Scales

Combat Exposure Scales

A second aspect in the use of scales for diagnosing PTSD relates to assessment of the stressor criterion. Since 1980, diagnostic criteria for PTSD have included the requirement of exposure to a life-threatening event which is outside the realm of usual human experience.

As attention grew toward the measurement of behavioral and emotional symptoms associated with PTSD, some interest was expressed in the need to address aspects or parameters of the stressor experience itself. Although many researchers would consider exposure to combat sufficient to meet the criterion described above, from a scientific point of view it became necessary to consider improved definitions of situational stressors capable of evoking PTSD. Presumably, this type of understanding would enhance sophistication about the psychological consequences of exposure to extreme stressors.

Before 1987, there were several combat exposure scales available that attempted to delineate the nature of the combat experience. These scales took two forms: checklists which dichotomously reflected the presence or absence of exposure to various combat-related events (Gallops, Laufer, & Yager, 1981) and instruments comprised of self-ratings by the subject (typically 5-point) providing a range of exposure to combat phenomena (Figley & Stretch, 1980; Wilson & Krauss, 1981). In both formats, certain items connoting greater traumatization (e.g., being wounded) were often weighted more heavily to reflect presumed differential contributions to the development of combat PTSD (Wilson & Krauss, 1985). A third type of exposure scale was developed by Lund, Foy, Sipprelle, and Strachan (1984). These investigators ranked a series of war stressors ordinally from more common to rarest, assuming that combatants who had been exposed to rarer stressors would have also encountered more common battlefield occurrences. Accordingly, scoring on this Gutman scale was accomplished through summing all of the events endorsed. Foy et al. (1984), investigating this scale further, found a high correlation between combatants' scores on that scale and the one previously described by Gallops et al. (1981), thus suggesting some degree of construct validity.

Current Status of Assessment

Measurement of Symptomatology

Descriptive Studies

The VESI. A modified version of the VESI was partially validated in a pair of studies (Wilson, 1989) which compared it to the Beck Depression Inventory (Beck et al., 1961), the Sensation Seeking Scale (Zuckerman & Linn, 1968), the Impact of Event Scale (Horowitz et al., 1979), and the MMPI PTSD subscale (Keane et al., 1984). Results of these studies have shown that the VESI is strongly associated with the other measures and that it appears to tap components of PTSD similar to those found by the MMPI PTSD subscale. These components include survivor guilt and depression, intrusive imagery, fear of loss of control, hyperarousal and sleep disturbance, numbing and alienation, memory loss and problems of concentration, and demoralization.

Psychometrics

The MMPI. Recently, several studies have reviewed the ability of the MMPI to diagnose combat-related PTSD (see Gerardi, Keane, & Penk, 1989, for a review). Some of these studies have raised important questions about the use of this instrument and its existing decision rules for PTSD. Vanderploeg, Sison, and Hickling (1987) examined four distinct diagnostic groups (PTSD, psychotic, depressed, and chronic pain) to assess the utility of previously established decision rules for diagnosing combat veterans (Keane et al., 1984). Their study revealed that these empirically derived rules (scales F, 8, 2) were only slightly better than chance (57%) in accurately classifying veterans with PTSD. However, marked variability in symptom presentation within the PTSD group appears to have accounted for some of this discrepancy as does the restricted range of assessment procedures used for original subject classification (e.g., chart review or clinician judgment, exclusively). Nonetheless, future research on the MMPI clearly must provide further documentation on the effectiveness of the decision rules on the clinical scales.

McCaffrey and Bellamy-Campbell (1989) reexamined the findings of Fairbank et al. (1985) which demonstrated the usefulness of the F scale and the PTSD subscale for detecting feigning of PTSD symptomatology. These investigators advanced the methodology of the earlier study by including a group of Vietnam veteran mental health professionals who were specifically instructed to feign the symptoms of this disorder in completing the MMPI. In their study, none of those professionals were misclassified as having PTSD when the F and PTSD subscale criteria were used as group predictors. Hence the high sensitivity and specificity of these predictors was supported.

Cannon, Bell, Andrews, and Finkelstein (1987) have raised other current questions in the use of the MMPI for diagnosing combat-related PTSD. In this study, the investigators found that application of the clinical decision rules for the MMPI as reported by Keane et al. (1984) resulted in a high false-positive rate for PTSD diagnosis within their population. However, as these authors pointed out, this limitation may have stemmed from the particular composition of their sample which included a broad-based psychiatric patient population and a significantly lower base rate of PTSD than the sample originally employed by Keane and colleagues. An additional factor in rates of diagnostic accuracy may have been due to differences between the two studies in their reliability for determining a PTSD diagnosis: By their own report, the Cannon study used a less comprehensive basis for establishing the initial diagnosis, thus increasing the likelihood that some subjects were included in the PTSD group who did not actually warrant this diagnosis. As the authors correctly noted, any of these factors would be likely to affect the basis for comparison of sensitivity and specificity rates for the MMPI when compared to their original derivation (i.e., Keane et al., 1984). In summary, all these issues point to the need for evaluation-based studies to consider such factors as the reliability of the *a priori* methods used for determining group inclusion and the importance of determining base rates of PTSD in the populations under study before attempting to make reliability comparisons within (or across) diagnostic instruments.

Hyer, Woods, Harrison, Boudewyns, and O'Leary (1989) assessed the tendency of Vietnam veterans to overreport symptoms and examined to what degree this overreporting influenced the eventual diagnosis of PTSD. Using the MMPI *F-K* index as a widely accepted measure for the identification of dissimulation or over-reporting of symptoms (cf. Grow, McVaugh, & Eno, 1980; Webb, McNamara, & Rodgers, 1981), the authors examined a large series of Vietnam incountry and era patients. Their findings confirmed previous work indicating that a high percentage of all Vietnam veterans show overreporting patterns on the MMPI. This tendency was most pronounced with increasing PTSD subscale scores. The authors interpreted these findings in two ways: that many veterans from that war continue to seek validation of their wartime experiences, and that individuals continuing to struggle with symptoms of PTSD may exhibit patterns of symptom overreporting as a component of the disorder (i.e., as a cry for help).

Last, two studies have provided novel information on the use of the MMPI in assessing noncombat-related PTSD. Koretzky and Peck (1990) found that a noncombat PTSD group scored significantly higher on the MMPI compared to a group of non-PTSD psychiatric controls; furthermore, the 8–2 clinical profile was once again observed in the PTSD patients. However, a PTSD subscale score of 19 most efficiently separated the two groups in this study compared to the previous cutoff of 30 usually obtained in veteran samples with this disorder. In another study, McCaffrey, Hickling, and Marrazo (1989) found that the 8–2 scale elevations obtained with PTSD veterans successfully characterized civilians with PTSD in their study sample. However, no statistically significant difference was found between mean scores on the PTSD subscale for the PTSD and non-PTSD civilian groups. This led the authors to conclude that certain diagnostic decision rules developed in combat PTSD populations may be limited in their generalizability to civilian populations with this disorder. However, this conclusion may reflect a tautological dilemma in the diagnosis of PTSD. This relates to the fact that criteria for group inclusion are generally based on a single, non-standardized clinical interview designed to assess DSM-III or DSM-III-R criteria for PTSD. As many investigators in combat-related PTSD have now pointed out, the disorder is sufficiently complex to warrant a comprehensive, multimodal evaluation which uses a variety of diagnostic instruments to collectively increase diagnostic accuracy. Until more of these are developed and employed in civilian populations being studied for PTSD, it will remain difficult to determine definitively the value of a single instrument for assessing PTSD in nonveteran populations.

Recently, a new standardization of the MMPI, the MMPI—2 (Butcher, Dahlstrom, Graham, & Tellegen, 1989), has become available. This version provides new normative performance data; it also contains long-awaited revisions of 82 (or 14%) of the original test items. These changes were carefully directed at eliminating such features as obsolete or idiomatic language, awkward and ambiguous wording, and statements reflecting sexist or cultural bias. In addition, the revision contains items aimed at addressing new (and critical) problem areas of functioning, for example, family difficulties and personality problems. A major change in the MMPI—2 is that it provides a unique set of content scales which augment the existing clinical scales. These content scales reflect the use of an empirical approach to psychometric measurement. In terms of PTSD, the 15 content scales permit assessment of such factors as treatment outcome and interpersonal behavior, variables of extreme importance in the evaluation of PTSD and ones not directly addressed by the original MMPI. Importantly, the 49-item PTSD subscale has remained relatively unchanged in the MMPI—2 with the exception that three repeat items have been omitted. Overall then, the MMPI—2 constitutes a distinct improvement over its predecessor in a number of areas related to the assessment of PTSD. The availability of content scales, along with clinical profiles, should provide important diagnostic information as well as a comparative basis for the psychological functioning of trauma victims in veteran and in nonveteran PTSD populations. It will also serve as a superior measure for studies of treatment outcome.

Mississippi Scale. Keane, Caddell, and Taylor (1988) have conducted three studies on the reliability and validity associated with the Mississippi Scale. These studies successfully identify the psychometric properties of the scale, specifically its internal consistency (alpha = .94) and factorial structure, its test-retest reliability over a 1-week period ($r = .97$), and the instrument's sensitivity (.93), specificity (.89), and overall diagnostic hit rate (.90). Despite the adequacy of these psychometric properties, Keane and colleagues emphasize that the use of multiple-assessment procedures (i.e., comprehensive interviews, various psychometric instruments, psychophysiological evaluation, chart review, and collateral reports) remains essential for arriving at the PTSD diagnosis. However, when multiple instruments are used, diagnostic discrepancies among them must be resolved. These discrepancies do not necessarily indicate an inability to confer the diagnosis; rather, they may suggest a number of other factors, including, for example variability in presentation of the disorder, construct or psychometric limitations of the assessment instrument, variability in base rates in the sample under study (cf. Shrout, Dohrenwend, & Levav, 1986), and unknown estimates of the prevalence of the disorder (cf. Kulka *et al.*, 1988). Any or all of these factors can influence the findings yielded by a single diagnostic instrument. In these instances, clinical adjudication is the recommended approach to resolution.

Impact of Event Scale. Several investigations have now explored the use of the IES (Horowitz *et al.*, 1979) with combat veterans. In one study, Schwarzwald *et al.* (1987) examined the ability of the IES to distinguish between two groups of Israeli veteran subjects who had been diagnosed with or without combat-related PTSD on the basis of the DSM criteria. Their results indicated that the IES was, in fact, sensitive to between group differences in this population; in addition, the validity of the scale's two major factors (Intrusion and Avoidance) was confirmed. In a second study, Weisenberg, Solomon, Schwarzwald, and Mikulincer (1987) assessed the interrelationship between the DSM-III PTSD criteria and responses on the IES in Israeli combatants. The authors specifically considered whether different diagnostic contributions were made by evaluation procedures utilizing dichotomous (i.e., DSM-based) versus continuous (IES) measures. Results indicated that subjects diagnosed with PTSD based on the DSM criteria had significantly higher scores on both factors of the IES than subjects without the disorder. Furthermore, even though both IES factors correlated significantly with each of the three DSM-III diagnostic criteria, the Intrusion factor was most strongly associated with the PTSD diagnosis. The authors emphasized that, despite empirical support for the use of the IES, the instrument remains limited in its ability to assess PTSD symptomatology comprehensively. This is due to the fact that the measure assesses primarily the dimensions of intrusion and avoidance and does not yield a broader appraisal of other PTSD symptomatology (e.g., arousal factors). Nonetheless, performance of the IES in the National Vietnam Veterans Readjustment Study (NVVRS) (Kulka *et al.*, 1988) provides further support for the scale's usefulness in assessing combat-related PTSD.

New Symptom Scales. One pressing question in the assessment of PTSD continues to be the quantification of the disorder's symptomatology. Instruments like the Mississippi Scale and the PTSD subscale of the MMPI aid in the determination of the PTSD diagnosis and contribute to an understanding of the severity of the disorder. Although the development of such scales often conceptually reflects the DSM criteria for PTSD, no scales exist which were directly and comprehensively formulated for the assessment of these criteria. The Clinician Administered PTSD Scale (CAPS) (Blake, Weathers, Kaloupek, Klauminzer, & Keane, 1989) is one of the first instruments to measure the frequency and severity of the DSM-III-R criteria for PTSD. The scale consists of 17 examiner-administered questions which explicitly inquire about the presence, intensity, and frequency of each of the DSM criteria. Responses to these items are scored in a way to permit determination of the PTSD diagnosis. In addition, eight other questions address a series of secondary symptom dimensions frequently associated with the disorder, including depression, anxiety, guilt, homicidality, and suicidality. Hence a quantifiable estimate of numerous dimensions of PTSD can be readily obtained. Finally, the CAPS provides for inquiry and rating about the degree of impairment in social and occupational functioning for each of the symptoms. Consequently, both qualitative and quantitative indices of impairment across a range of important functions are available. The CAPS can be administered using nearly any specified time period (e.g., daily, weekly, lifetime) as a point of reference. Hence change scores over time and as a measure of the effectiveness of pre- and posttreatment interventions will be possible as a component of PTSD assessment.

Interviews

Structured Interviews. The use of structured clinical interviews for PTSD has recently been expanded considerably. Rosenheck and Fontana (1989) developed an instrument called the War Stress Inventory (WSI). The interview is composed of questions which systematically assess the veteran's functioning over many areas. Al-though most questions are based in a self-report format, the WSI also requires clinician-based confidence ratings to help assess the reliability of the subject's report. In addition, the WSI contains portions or, in some cases, validated subsets of preexisting assessment instruments, including, for example, the Addiction Severity Index (McLellan *et al.*, 1985), the Symptom Checklist-90 (Derogatis, Lipman, & Covi, 1973), and the Mississippi Scale for Combat-related PTSD (Keane, Caddell, & Taylor, 1988). The assessment of behavior critically linked to combat-related PTSD, for example, the witnessing of or participation in atrocities, is also directly addressed through inclusion of the Laufer-Parson Guilt Scale (Laufer & Frey-Wouters, 1988).

The advantage of this approach overall is that it combines interview-based inquiries with psychometric assessment. In addition, the WSI is one of the first formats in which various existing methods of PTSD assessment can be systematically combined. The WSI also contains items aimed at examining the veteran's use of treatment resources as well as provision for follow-up assessment at a series of prescribed intervals. Information from the WSI will yield some of the first program evaluation data detailing the use of PTSD treatment resources by Vietnam veterans in conjunction with evaluation of their functional status. Since the WSI is being used by 23 PTSD Clinical Treatment teams distributed nationally within the VA system of the United States, this evaluation system will provide a large-scale data base. It will also have the capacity to examine the contribution of such factors as geographic locale in the presentation of veterans seeking PTSD assessment and treatment.

Generic Interviews. A host of recent studies (cf. Centers for Disease Control, 1988; Escobar *et al.*, 1983; Keane, Gerardi, Lyons, & Wolfe, 1988; Helzer, Robins, & McEvoy, 1987; Kulka *et al.*, 1988; Sierles, Chen, McFarland, & Taylor, 1983; Sierles, Chen, Messing, Besyner, & Taylor, 1986) have shown that PTSD is associated with the co-occurrence of certain major psychological disorders, for example, substance abuse or dependence, major depression, and anxiety-based disturbances, such as panic disorder. This appears to be the case regardless of the interview format employed for diagnosis (e.g., the SCID or the DIS), the background qualifications of the interviewer (lay vs. professional), or the presence of specific demographic characteristics (patient vs. nonpatient; veteran vs. civilian) (Keane & Wolfe, 1990). Hence the importance of using comprehensive diagnostic interviews to review the full range of diagnostic possibilities in PTSD is clear. Despite this benefit, careful review of the available psychiatric interview procedures shows considerable variation in the degree and accuracy with which PTSD is likely to be assessed (cf. Keane & Wolfe, 1990). This variability relates in part to structural characteristics of the interviews themselves. For example, the strict standardization of the DIS negates the need for clinical adjudication of diagnoses by experienced clinicians; thus, use of the instrument by lay interviewers in some surveys may have contributed to a degree of inaccuracy in several areas including PTSD diagnoses, comorbidity estimates, and also information on the nature of the collateral disturbance (Keane & Wolfe, 1990). The combination of intrinsic methodologic limitations of any one diagnostic instrument plus the tendency toward polythetic presentation by these patients therefore argues strongly for the use of multidimensional and multimodal assessment procedures when assessing PTSD.

Personality Assessment. Although PTSD is classified along the DSM's Axis I, there has been considerable interest in whether individual personality disorders contribute to (or are influenced by) the presence of this disorder. Although earlier work did not substantiate the presence of any definitive premorbid personality factors in the development of PTSD (Wilson & Krauss, 1985), studies of this type have been unavoidably limited by retrospective and self-report methodologies. In addition, because the diagnostic validity of the disorder was a primary concern (Breslau & Davis, 1987; Wolfe & Keane, 1990), earlier studies often focused intensively on efforts to identify the disorder's overt symptom profile which seemed more readily measurable. As the diagnostic picture has become clearer, interest has extended to the range of Axis II disorders potentially accompanying PTSD. In combat veterans, several studies have provided evidence for the coexistence of certain personality disorders with PTSD, primarily antisocial. Generally, these investigations indicate rates of a co-diagnosis of antisocial personality disorder ranging from 26% to 64% of sample participants (cf. Keane & Wolfe, 1990; Sierles *et al.*, 1986). The recently completed NVVRS (Kulka *et al.*, 1988) found that 31% of their sample evidenced lifetime diagnoses for antisocial disturbance. The generalizability of these findings to noncombat-related PTSD, however, remains to be investigated.

In addition to the antisocial personality diagnosis, borderline personality disturbance is frequently considered in conjunction with PTSD. Essentially, no systematic study of the incidence of this disorder in PTSD veterans has yet been conducted. A recent finding by Herman, Perry, and van der Kolk (1989) has shown that an inordinately high percentage (exceeding 80%) of patients with a diagnosis of borderline personality disorder showed, in fact, clear evidence of early histories of traumatization, specifically sexual or physical abuse. This raises the question as to what degree early traumatizing experiences (or disorders) may have gone undetected in the evaluation efforts of borderline patients. This issue will require further research consideration in veteran and in civilian populations, and highlights the degree to which diagnosis can be directly affected by the parameters included in an assessment.

The Millon Clinical Multiaxial Inventory (MCMI) (Millon, 1983) has recently been applied in the assessment of personality disorders and PTSD. The MCMI is composed of 11 personality scales which correspond more directly than the MMPI with the DSM Axis II diagnostic categories. Hyer, Woods, Boudewyns, Bruno, and O'Leary (1988) employed the MCMI with a sample of Vietnam veterans hospitalized for treatment of PTSD. The authors found that passive-aggressive and avoidant personality patterns were characteristic of this group and that borderline and schizoid features were common accompaniments. As the authors noted, their findings are limited in part by the lack of a control group and the fact that the observed profiles have typified some other psychiatric samples in states of extreme distress (cf. Millon, 1983). In summary, although the scientific assessment of personality disorders is a technology that is still in its infancy, the data collected to date on the high rates of personality disorder associated with PTSD indicate the importance that must be placed on enhancing the sophistication of these assessment methods.

Laboratory Procedures

Psychophysiological Assessment. Assessment of combat-related PTSD in the laboratory has generally relied on the presentation of auditory and visual combat stimuli. Recently, several investigators (cf. Pitman, Orr, Forgue, de Jong, & Claiborn, 1987; Pitman, Altman, & Macklin, 1989) have explored the use of neutral, positive, and trauma-derived autobiographical scripts for determining patterns of psychophysiological responsivity in Vietnam veterans. The use of individually derived images and scripts is based on earlier work by Lang (1977), who successfully demonstrated patterns of heightened physiologic reactivity in subjects presented with affectively and semantically meaningful cues. The application of affectively intense, individualized stimulus cues now appears to be useful in examining the physiological reactivity associated with combat PTSD. However, comparisons across types of laboratory methodologies (e.g., autobiographical vs. generic stimuli; heartrate vs. skin conductance) are still needed to assess the psychophysiological approach's unique contribution to evaluation and diagnosis.

New Approaches

Neuropsychology and Cognition. Several authors have recognized the limits of an overreliance on phenomenologic and psychosocial approaches to the conceptualization and assessment of PTSD. These investigators have stressed the need for increasing attention to the biochemical and neuropsychiatric components of this disorder (cf. van der Kolk, Greenberg, Boyd, & Krystal, 1985; Watson, Hoffman, & Wilson, 1988). Mason, Giller, Kosten, Ostroff, and Podd (1986) and other investigators have offered preliminary findings on proposed hormonal and neurotransmitter alterations in PTSD; however, this avenue of diagnostic assessment is just emerging and is beyond the scope of this chapter.

Kolb (1987) offered a neuropsychological theory of PTSD in which he posited the existence of certain cortical neuronal changes leading to the loss of inhibitory lower brainstem functions. The PTSD symptoms of intrusion and hyperarousal are conjectured to be a result of this inhibitory failure. At the present time, no firm empirical evidence exists to support this particular model. Moreover, there are no comprehensive or well-controlled studies to date investigating neuropsychological dysfunction in veterans with PTSD; the few reports of this type are clinically based and reveal no clear-cut or distinguishing pattern of cognitive deficits (Krystal, Kosten, Perry, & Southwick, 1989). Future studies involving response parameters (e.g., evoked brainstem potentials) and information processing patterns (e.g., attentional processes) in combat-related PTSD should provide new opportunities for evaluating cognitive changes associated with this disturbance. Until paradigms are developed demonstrating their specificity for PTSD, however, these procedures are likely to remain outside of the mainstream of routine assessment methods.

Measuring Stressor Dimensions

A major issue in the assessment of PTSD relates to the current diagnostic schema for this disorder. This schema specifically requires delineation of exposure to an unusual and severely stressful life event as one component for the determination of the disorder (Breslau & Davis, 1987). In this respect, PTSD is distinct from all other syndromes which do not explicity consider exposure to externally generated events as "etiologic" in their diagnostic criteria. The inclusion of external traumatization as a diagnostic criterion, rather than as a predictor, has seriously influenced the development of formal assessment procedures in this disorder. Specifically, it has raised important issues relating to the best approach to measurement of the occurrence and effect of these events (see Chapter 11, in this volume, for a review). Recent developments in terms of exposure scales demonstrate the growth in this area while simultaneously highlighting some of the remaining problems.

Exposure Scales

Combat Exposure Scales

Over the past few years, there has been further development in the assessment of external combat stressors. Wilson and Krauss (1985) found through factor analysis that combat exposure scales were predictive of different dimensions of PTSD. In 1987, Solomon, Mikulincer, and Hobfoll reported on an objective military stress scale which they had devised in their work with Israeli combatants. The scale contains four dichotomous items relating to past military preparedness, experiences near the front line, engagement in battle, and exposure to the evacuation of bodies. Watson, Kucala, Manifold, Vassar, and Juba (1988) developed a Military Stress Scale which combines the use of both dichotomous and Likert (i.e., scaled) ratings. This scale covers a range of combat events including involvement in atrocities. According to the scale's authors, events deemed to be of greater severity (i.e., on a conceptual basis) were weighted differentially.

Keane *et al.* (1989) presented three studies demonstrating the psychometric properties of a self-report combat exposure scale which they developed. Their instrument is comprised of seven Likert-scaled items: three from the earlier scale by Figley and Stretch (1980) and an additional four statements developed consensually by clinicians highly familiar with the assessment of PTSD. In this scale, the authors also weighted items differentially according to the presumed severity of the event. Studies of the scale's psychometric properties involving internal consistency and factor structure, test-retest reliability, and group comparisons among comba-

tants with and without the PTSD diagnosis showed that the instrument was psychometrically sound. In particular, the authors noted the importance of structuring retrospective report in as scientific (e.g., quantitative) a fashion as possible. Nonetheless, they recognized that current adjustment might still influence subject ratings on such measures.

Watson, Juba, and Anderson (1989) recently compared the properties of five previously described exposure scales. Using information from the military record to ascertain the likelihood of prior trauma exposure (e.g., medals awarded and military occupational specialty), the authors derived a trauma measure for each participant. They then conducted correlational analyses between this information and the various combat scales as well as among the combat scales themselves. According to their findings, the scales by Gallops *et al.* (1981) and Watson *et al.* (1988) were the most directly related to combat history and the least confounded by the diagnosis of PTSD. Unfortunately, the Keane scale (Keane *et al.*, 1989) was not included in this study. Also, as Watson and colleagues noted, military records may be unreliable in their ability to reflect actual combat history, a notion supported by those authors' failure to obtain significant correlations among their independent trauma history variables.

In summary, some methodologic questions remain about the most valid format for assessing actual combat exposure. To date, all methods have focused upon self-report of combat experiences. This approach has obvious inherent limitations. Furthermore, although higher degrees of combat exposure have been shown to be strongly associated with the development of wartime PTSD (Foy *et al.*, 1984; Friedman, Schneiderman, West, & Corson, 1986; Kulka *et al.*, 1988), the majority of combatants do not eventually develop this disorder. Hence the issue of how exposure interacts with individual vulnerability and posttraumatic environments remains a large area for future scientific inquiry.

Women's Military Exposure Scale

Considerable historical and autobiographical information has suggested that women veterans have been subjected to a variety of severe or traumatizing events during wartime (cf. Walker, 1986). For the most part, there has been a dramatic failure to recognize or identify these events in any systematic fashion (Quester, 1982). Despite this, the results of the recent NVVRS (Kulka *et al.*, 1988) clearly indicate that wartime exposure for in-country women exists and in fact has contributed to a current PTSD incidence of nearly 9% in female Vietnam veterans and a lifetime rate approaching 28%.

The assessment of PTSD in women to date has been seriously limited by the use of evaluative procedures developed primarily for male combatants. As such, use of these procedures with women veterans may contribute to diagnostic inaccuracies. Wolfe, Furey, and Sandecki (1989) have recently developed the first of a series of instruments designed to address empirically the psychological adjustment of women veterans exposed to war. The Women's Military Exposure Scale, modeled after the Combat Exposure Scale by Keane *et al.*

(1989), contains a range of statements which highlight the exposure of women to potentially traumatizing wartime events. These include events in the professional, environmental, and psychosocial spheres. Two sample statements are presented in the Appendix. When this scale is empirically validated, information will be be available about the instrument's psychometric properties and its overall utility for comprehensive PTSD assessment.

Conclusion

As the assessment of combat-related PTSD becomes increasingly refined, stringent new questions are being asked of evaluative procedures. One question is the degree to which assessment techniques should be challenged to seek correlations among symptom categories rather than provide documentation of a symptom's presence. For example, should evaluative procedures attempt to relate hyperarousal to symptoms of reexperiencing or avoidance? A second issue is whether assessment procedures should begin to consider findings supporting the PTSD diagnosis in terms of Axis II findings (cf. Brett, Spitzer, & Williams, 1988; Ramchandani, 1989). For example, to what degree do findings of Axis II disturbance bear on the diagnosis of PTSD? Although these questions are raised in terms of assessment procedures, they relate to the larger issue of a field in search of an integrated model for the disorder.

Other future trends in assessment deal with the notion of an interaction between person and environmental factors in the determination of PTSD. It is increasingly clear that measurement of "newer" variables, for example, guilt (cf. Opp & Samson, 1989), attributional style (Peterson *et al.*, 1982), and coping resources (Green, Lindy, & Grace, 1988) will prove to be important based in their apparent influence on the expression of the disorder. To the degree that motivation is a factor in adjustment, the ability of diagnostic instruments to assess feigning or factitious PTSD will also remain an important consideration. This is particularly true in veteran populations and cases involving litigation where compensation benefits are often inextricably linked with both diagnosis and help-seeking.

Last, further research is needed to assess the effects of different typologies of stressors as well as their variations in frequency and duration on the development of PTSD. Accompanying this is a growing need to consider the extent to which methodologies developed for the assessment of combat-related PTSD are generalizable to civilian populations. Because of the progress made in the study of combat-related PTSD, evaluation models from this area can serve as a critical basis for the establishment of systematic assessment procedures in nonveterans. We believe that this approach would significantly advance the conceptual and empirical bases of comprehensive diagnostic procedures and, in addition, would dramatically enhance our understanding of PTSD as a whole.

Appendix

Sample questions from the Women's Military Exposure Scale:

1. How many times did you have to decide who would receive lifesaving medical care?

   0 = never, 1 = 1–2 times, 2 = 3–12 times, 3 = 13–50 times, 4 = more than 50 times

2. What percentage of the time did you encounter verbal or physical sexual harassment?

   0 = never, 1 = between 1% and 25%, 2 = between 26% and 50%, 3 = between 51% and 75%, 4 = more than 75%

ACKNOWLEDGMENTS

This work was conducted at the National Center for PTSD, Behavioral Science Division. The research was supported by Merit Review Awards to each author individually from Medical Research of the Department of Veterans Affairs and also by a grant from the National Institute of Mental Health (MH5–21424). Deborah Polk and Timothy Carey assisted in the preparation of this chapter.

References

American Psychiatric Association. (1980). *Diagnostic and statistical manual of mental disorders* (3rd ed.). Washington DC: Author.

American Psychiatric Association. (1987). *The diagnostic and statistical manual of mental disorders* (3rd ed., rev.). Washington DC: Author.

Andreasen, N. C. (1982). The diagnosis and classification of affective disorders. In J. M. Davis & J. W. Maas (Eds.), *The affective disorders* (pp. 135–149). Washington, DC: American Psychiatric Press.

Beck, A. T., Mendelson, M., Mock, J., & Erbaug, J. (1961). An inventory for measuring depression. *Archives of General Psychiatry, 12*, 63–70.

Blake, D. D., Weathers, F., Kaloupek, D., Klauminzer, G. W., & Keane, T. M. (1989, November). *Clinician Administered PTSD Scale (CAPS)*. (Available from Dudley Blake, National Center for PTSD [116B], Boston VA Medical Center, 150 S. Huntington Ave., Boston, MA 02130)

Blanchard, E. B., Kolb, L. C., Gerardi, R. J., Ryan, P., & Pallmeyer, T. P. (1986). Cardiac response to relevant stimuli as an adjunctive tool for diagnosing posttraumatic stress disorder in Vietnam veterans. *Behavior Therapy, 17*, 592–606.

Blanchard, E. B., Kolb, L. C., Pallmeyer, T. B., & Gerardi, R. J. (1982). The development of a psychophysiological assessment procedure for posttraumatic stress disorder in Vietnam veterans. *Psychiatric Quarterly, 54*, 220–229.

Breslau, N., & Davis, G. C. (1987). Posttraumatic stress disorder: The stressor criterion. *Journal of Nervous and Mental Disease, 175*, 255–264.

Brett, E. A., Spitzer, R. L., & Williams, J. B. (1988). DSM-III-R criteria for post-traumatic stress disorder. *American Journal of Psychiatry, 145*, 1232–1236.

Butcher, J. N., Dahlstrom, W. G., Graham, J. R., & Tellegen, A.

(1989). *Minnesota Multiphasic Personality Inventory—2*. Minneapolis: University of Minnesota Press.

Card, J. J. (1983). *Lives after Vietnam: The personal impact of military service*. Lexington: D. C. Heath.

Cannon, D. S., Bell, W. E., Andrews, R. H., & Finkelstein, A. S. (1987). Correspondence between MMPI, PTSD measures and clinical diagnosis. *Journal of Personality Assessment, 51*, 517–521.

Centers for Disease Control. (1988). Health status of Vietnam veterans. *Journal of the American Medical Association, 259*, 2715–2719.

Davidson, J., Swartz, M., Storck, M., Krishnan, R. R., & Hammett, E. (1985). A diagnostic and family study of posttraumatic stress disorder. *American Journal of Psychiatry, 142*, 90–93.

Derogatis, L. R., Lipman, R. S., & Covi, L. (1973). SCL-90: An outpatient psychiatric rating scale—Preliminary report. *Psychopharmacology Bulletin, 9*, 13–25.

Dobbs, D., & Wilson, W. P. (1960). Observations on the persistence of traumatic war neurosis. *Journal of Nervous and Mental Disease, 21*, 40–46.

Egendorf, A., Kadushin, C., Laufer, R. S., Rothbart, G., & Sloan, L. (Eds.) (1981). *Legacies of Vietnam: Comparative adjustment of veterans and their peers*. New York: Center for Policy Research.

Escobar, J. I., Randolph, E. T., Puente, G., Spiwak, F., Asamen, J. K., Hill, M., & Hough, R. L. (1983). Posttraumatic stress disorder in Hispanic Vietnam veterans: Clinical phenomenology and sociocultural characteristics. *Journal of Nervous and Mental Disease, 171*, 585–596.

Fairbank, J. A., Keane, T. M., & Malloy, P. F. (1983). Some preliminary data on the psychological characteristics of Vietnam veterans with posttraumatic stress disorder. *Journal of Consulting and Clinical Psychology, 51*, 912–919.

Fairbank, J. A., McCaffrey, R. J., & Keane, T. M. (1985). Psychometric detection of fabricated symptoms of posttraumatic stress disorder. *American Journal of Psychiatry, 142*, 501–503.

Figley, C. R. (1978). Symptoms of delayed combat-stress among a college sample of Vietnam veterans. *Military Medicine, 143*, 107–110.

Figley, C. R., & Stretch, R. H. (1980). Vietnam veterans questionnaire combat exposure scale. In *Vietnam veterans questionnaire: Instrument development. Final report*. West Lafayette, IN: Purdue University.

Foy, D., Sipprelle, R. C., Rueger, D. B., & Carroll, E. (1984). Etiology of posttraumatic stress disorder in Vietnam veterans: Analysis of premilitary, military, and combat exposure influences. *Journal of Consulting and Clinical Psychology, 52*, 79–87.

Friedman, M. J., Schneiderman, M. A., West, A. N., & Corson, J. A. (1986). Measurement of combat exposure, posttraumatic stress disorder, and life stress among Vietnam combat veterans. *American Journal of Psychiatry, 143*, 537–539.

Gallops, M., Laufer, R. S., & Yager, T. (1981). Revised combat scale. In R. S. Laufer & T. Yager (Eds.), *Legacies of Vietnam: Comparative adjustments of veterans and their peers* (Vol. 3, p. 125). Washington, DC: U. S. Government Printing Office.

Gerardi, R. J., Keane, T. M., & Penk, W. (1989). Utility: Sensitivity and specificity in developing diagnostic tests of combat-related post-traumatic stress disorder (PTSD). *Journal of Clinical Psychology, 45*, 691–703.

Green, B. L., Lindy, J. D., & Grace, M. C. (1988). Long-term coping with combat stress. *Journal of Traumatic Stress, 1*, 399–412.

Green, B. L., Wilson, J. P., & Lindy, J. D. (1985). Conceptualizing post-traumatic stress disorder: A psychosocial framework. In C. R. Figley (Ed.), *Trauma and its wake: The study and treatment of post-traumatic stress disorder* (pp. 53–69). New York: Brunner/Mazel.

Grinker, R., & Spiegel, J. P. (1945). *Men under stress*. Philadelphia: Blakiston.

Grow, R., McVaugh, W., & Eno, T. (1980). Faking and the MMPI. *Journal of Clinical Psychology, 36*, 910–917.

Hathaway, S. R., & McKinley, J. C. (1967). *Minnesota Multiphasic Personality Inventory: Manual for administration and scoring*. New York: Psychological Corporation.

Helzer, J., Robins, L. N., Wish, E., & Hesselbrock, M. (1979). Depression in Vietnam veterans and civilian controls. *American Journal of Psychiatry, 136*, 526–529.

Helzer, J. E., Robins, L. N., & McEvoy, L. (1987). Post-traumatic stress disorder in the general population: Findings of the Epidemiological Catchment Survey. *New England Journal of Medicine, 317*, 1630–1634.

Herman, J. L., Perry, J. C., & van der Kolk, B. A. (1989). Childhood trauma in borderline personality disorder. *American Journal of Psychiatry, 146*, 490–495.

Horowitz, M. J. (1976). *Stress response syndromes*. New York: Jason Aronson.

Horowitz, M. J., Weiss, D. S., & Marmar, C. (1987). Diagnosis of post-traumatic stress disorder—Commentary. *Journal of Nervous and Mental Disease, 175*, 267–268.

Horowitz, M. J., Wilner, N., & Alvarez, W. (1979). Impact of Event Scale: A measure of subjective stress. *Psychosomatic Medicine, 41*, 209–218.

Hyer, L., O'Leary, W., Saucer, R., Blount, J., Harrison, W., & Boudewyns, P. (1986). Inpatient diagnosis of the post-traumatic stress disorder. *Journal of Consulting and Clinical Psychology, 54*, 698–702.

Hyer, L., Woods, M., Harrison, W. R., Boudewyns, P., & O'Leary, W. C. (1989). MMPI F-K index among hospitalized Vietnam veterans. *Journal of Clinical Psychology, 45*, 250–254.

Hyer, L., Woods, M. G., Boudewyns, P. A., Bruno, R., & O'Leary, W. C. (1988). Concurrent validation of the Millon Clinical Multiaxial Inventory among Vietnam veterans with post-traumatic stress disorder. *Psychological Reports, 63*, 271–278.

Keane, T. M., Caddell, J. M., & Taylor, K. L. (1988). Mississippi scale for combat-related post-traumatic stress disorder: Three studies in reliability and validity. *Journal of Consulting and Clinical Psychology, 56*, 85–90.

Keane, T. M., Fairbank, J. A., Caddell, J. M., Zimering, R. T., & Bender, M. E. (1985). A behavioral approach to assessing and treating posttraumatic stress disorder in Vietnam veterans. In C. R. Figley (Ed.), *Trauma and its wake: The study and treatment of post-traumatic stress disorder* (pp. 257–294). New York: Brunner/Mazel.

Keane, T. M., Fairbank, J. A., Caddell, J. M., Zimering, R. T., Taylor, K. L., & Mora, C. A. (1989). Clinical evaluation of a measure to assess combat exposure. *Psychological Assessment: A Journal of Consulting and Clinical Psychology, 1*, 53–55.

Keane, T. M., Gerardi, R. J., Lyons, J. A., & Wolfe, J. (1988). The interrelationship of substance abuse and posttraumatic stress disorder. In M. Galanter (Ed.), *Recent developments in alcoholism* (Vol. 6, pp. 27–48). New York: Plenum Press.

Keane, T. M., Malloy, P. F., & Fairbank, J. A. (1984). Empirical development of an MMPI subscale for the assessment of combat-related post-traumatic stress disorder. *Journal of Consulting and Clinical Psychology, 52*, 888–891.

Keane, T. M., Scott, W. O., Chavoya, G. A., Lamparski, D. M., & Fairbank, J. A. (1985). Social support in Vietnam veterans with posttraumatic stress disorder. *Journal of Consulting and Clinical Psychology, 53,* 95–102.

Keane, T. M., & Wolfe, J. (1990). Comorbidity in post-traumatic stress disorder: An analysis of community and clinical studies. *Journal of Applied Social Psychology, 20,* 1776–1788.

Keane, T. M., Wolfe, J., & Taylor, K. L. (1987). Post-traumatic stress disorder: Evidence for diagnostic validity and methods of psychological assessment. *Journal of Clinical Psychology, 43,* 32–43.

Knight, J., Keane, T. M., Fairbank, J. A., Caddell, J. M., & Zimering, R. T. (1984). *Empirical validation of DSM-III criteria for PTSD.* Paper presented at the annual meeting of the Association for Advancement of Behavior Therapy, Philadelphia, PA.

Kolb, L. C. (1987). A neuropsychological hypothesis explaining post-traumatic stress disorder. *American Journal of Psychiatry, 144,* 989–995.

Koretzky, M. B., & Peck, A. (1990). Validation and cross-validation of the PTSD subscale of the MMPI with civilian trauma victims. *Journal of Clinical Psychology, 46,* 296–300.

Krystal, J. H., Kosten, T. R., Perry, B. D., & Southwick, S. (1989). Neurobiological aspects of PTSD: Review of clinical and preclinical studies. *Behavior Therapy, 20,* 177–198.

Kulka, R. A., Schlenger, W. E., Fairbank, J. A., Hough, R. L., Jordan, B. K., Marmar, C. R., & Weiss, D. S. (1988). *National Vietnam veterans readjustment study (NVVRS).* Research Triangle Park, NC: Research Triangle Institute.

Lang, P. J. (1977). The psychophysiology of anxiety. In H. Akiskal (Ed.), *Psychiatric diagnosis: Exploration of biological criteria.* New York: Spectrum Publications.

Laufer, R., & Frey-Wouters, E. (1988). *War trauma and the role of guilt in post-war adjustment.* Paper presented at the annual meeting of the Society for Traumatic Stress Studies, Dallas, TX.

Lund, M., Foy, D., Sipprelle, C., & Strachan, A. (1984). The combat exposure scale: A systematic assessment of trauma in the Vietnam war. *Journal of Clinical Psychology, 40,* 1323–1328.

Malloy, P. F., Fairbank, J. A., & Keane, T. M. (1983). Validation of a multimethod assessment of post-traumatic stress disorders in Vietnam veterans. *Journal of Consulting and Clinical Psychology, 51,* 488–494.

Mason, J. W., Giller, E. L., Kosten, T. R., Ostroff, R. B., & Podd, L. (1986). Urinary free-cortisol levels in post-traumatic stress disorder patients. *Journal of Nervous and Mental Disease, 174,* 145–149.

McCaffrey, R. J., & Bellamy-Campbell, R. (1989). Psychometric detection of fabricated symptoms of combat-related post-traumatic stress disorder: A systematic replication. *Journal of Clinical Psychology, 45,* 76–79.

McCaffrey, R. J., Hickling, E. J., & Marrazo, M. J. (1989). Civilian-related post-traumatic stress disorder: Assessment-related issues. *Journal of Clinical Psychology, 45,* 72–76.

McLellan, A. T., Luborsky, L., Cacciola, J., Griffith, J., Evans, F., Barr, H. L., & O'Brien, C. P. (1985). New data from the Addiction Severity Index: Reliability and validity in three centers. *Journal of Nervous and Mental Diseases, 173,* 412–423.

Merbaum, M. (1977). Some personality characteristics of soldiers exposed to extreme war stress: A follow-up study of post hospital adjustment. *Journal of Clinical Psychology, 33,* 558–562.

Millon, T. (1983). *Millon Clinical Multiaxial Inventory manual.* Minneapolis: National Computer Systems.

Opp, R. E., & Samson, A. Y. (1989). Taxonomy of guilt for combat veterans. *Professional Psychology: Research and Practice, 20,* 159–165.

Pallmeyer, T. P., Blanchard, E. B., & Kolb, L. C. (1986). The psychophysiology of combat-induced post-traumatic stress disorder in Vietnam veterans. *Behavioral Research and Therapy, 24,* 645–652.

Penk, W. E., Rabinowitz, R., Roberts, W. R., Patterson, E. T., Dolan, M. P. & Athers, H. G. (1981). Adjustment differences among male substance abusers varying in degree of combat experience in Vietnam. *Journal of Consulting and Clinical Psychology, 49,* 426–437.

Peterson, C., Semmel, A., von Baeyer, C., Abramson, L. Y., Metalsky, G. I., & Seligman, M. E. P. (1982). The attributional style questionnaire. *Cognitive Therapy and Research, 6,* 287–300.

Pitman, R. K., Altman, B., & Macklin, M. L. (1989). Prevalence of post-traumatic stress disorder in wounded Vietnam veterans. *American Journal of Psychiatry, 146,* 667–669.

Pitman, R. K., Orr, S. P., Forgue, D. F., de Jong, J. B., & Claiborn, J. M. (1987). Psychophysiological assessment of post-traumatic stress disorder imagery in Vietnam combat veterans. *Archives of General Psychiatry, 44,* 970–975.

Quester, G. H. (1982). The problem. In N. L. Goldman (Ed.), *Female soldiers—Combatants or noncombatants? Historical and contemporary perspectives* (pp. 217–235). Westport, CT: Greenwood Press.

Ramchandani, D. (1989). Diagnosis of post-traumatic stress disorder. *American Journal of Psychiatry, 146,* 684–685.

Roberts, W. R., Penk, W. E., Gearing, R., Rabinowitz, R., Dolan, M. P., & Patterson, E. T. (1982). Interpersonal problems of Vietnam combat veterans with symptoms of PTSD. *Journal of Abnormal Psychology, 91,* 444–450.

Robins, L. N., Helzer, J. E., Croughan, J. L., Williams, J. B. W., & Spitzer, R. L. (1981). *NIMH diagnostic interview schedule, Version III.* Rockville, MD: NIMH, Public Health Service (Publication No. ADM-T-42–3 [5–81]).

Rosenheck, R., & Fontana, A. (1989). *The war stress inventory.* Available from the Veterans Administration Northeast Program Evaluation Center, West Haven, CT.

Schnaier, J. A. (1986). A study of women Vietnam veterans and their mental health adjustment. In C. R. Figley (Ed.), *Trauma and its wake: Vol. II. Traumatic stress theory, research, and intervention.* New York: Brunner/Mazel.

Schwarzwald, J., Solomon, Z., Weisenberg, M., & Mikulincer, M. (1987). Validation of the Impact of Event Scale for psychological sequelae of combat. *Journal of Consulting and Clinical Psychology, 55,* 251–256.

Scurfield, R. M., Corker, T. M., Gongla, P. A., & Hough, R. L. (1984). Three post-Vietnam "rap/therapy" groups: An analysis. *Group, 8,* 3–21.

Shrout, P. E., Dohrenwend, B. P., & Levav, I. (1986). A discriminant rule for screening cases of diverse diagnostic types: Preliminary results. *Journal of Consulting and Clinical Psychology, 54,* 314–319.

Sierles, F. S., Chen, J., McFarland, R. E., & Taylor, M. A. (1983). Post-traumatic stress disorder and concurrent psychiatric illness. *American Journal of Psychiatry, 140,* 1177–1179.

Sierles, F. S., Chen, J., Messing, M. L., Besyner, J. K., & Taylor, M. A. (1986). Concurrent psychiatric illness in non-Hispanic outpatients diagnosed as having post-traumatic stress disorder. *Journal of Nervous and Mental Disease, 174,* 171–173.

Silver, S. M., & Iacono, C. U. (1984). Factor-analytic support for DSM-III's post-traumatic stress disorder for Vietnam veterans. *Journal of Clinical Psychology, 40,* 5–14.

Smith, J. R. (1985). *Brecksville psychological assessment manual*. Brecksville, OH: Veterans Administration Medical Center.

Solomon, Z., Mikulincer, M., & Hobfoll, S. E. (1987). Objective versus subjective measurement of stress and social support: Combat-related reactions. *Journal of Consulting and Clinical Psychology, 55*, 577–583.

Spielberger, C. D., Gorsuch, R. L., & Lushene, R. E. (1970). *Manual for the State-Trait Inventory (self-evaluation questionnaire)*. Palo Alto: Consulting Psychologists Press.

Spitzer, R. L., & Williams, J. B. (1985). *Structured clinical interview for DSM-III (SCID)*. New York: Biometrics Research Department of NYSPI.

van der Kolk, B. A., Greenberg, M., Boyd, H., & Krystal, J. (1985). Inescapable shock, neurotransmitters, and addiction to trauma: Towards a psychobiology of post-traumatic stress. *Biological Psychiatry, 20*, 314–325.

Vanderploeg, R. D., Sison, G. F. P., Jr., & Hickling, E. J. (1987). A reevaluation of the use of the MMPI in the assessment of combat-related posttraumatic stress disorder. *Journal of Personality Assessment, 51*, 140–150.

Walker, K. (1986). *A piece of my heart: Stories of 26 American women who served in Vietnam*. Novato, CA: Presidio Press.

Watson, C. G., Juba, M. P., & Anderson, P. E. D. (1989). Validities of five combat scales. *Psychological Assessment: A Journal of Consulting and Clinical Psychology, 1*, 98–102.

Watson, C. G., Kucala, T., Manifold, V., Vassar, P., & Juba, M. (1988). Differences between post-traumatic stress disorder patients with delayed and undelayed onsets. *Journal of Nervous and Mental Disease, 176*, 568–572.

Watson, I. P. B., Hoffman, L., & Wilson, G. V. (1988). The neuropsychiatry of post-traumatic stress disorder. *British Journal of Psychiatry, 152*, 164–173.

Webb, J., McNamara, K., & Rodgers, D. (1981). *Configural interpretation of the MMPI and CPI*. Columbus, OH: Psychiatric Publications.

Weisenberg, M., Solomon, Z., Schwarzwald, J., & Mikulincer, M. (1987). Assessing the severity of post-traumatic stress disorder: Relation between dichotomous and continuous measures. *Journal of Consulting and Clinical Psychology, 55*, 432–434.

Wilson, J. P. (1978a). *Forgotten Warrior Project*. Cincinnati: Disabled American Veterans.

Wilson, J. P. (1978b). *Identity, ideology and crisis: The Vietnam veteran in transition* (Vol. 2). Washington, DC: Disabled American Veterans.

Wilson, J. P. (1980). Conflict, stress and growth: Effects of war on psycho-social development among Vietnam veterans. In C. Figley & S. Leventman (Eds.), *Strangers at home: Vietnam veterans since the war* (pp. 123–165). New York: Praeger.

Wilson, J. P. (1989). *Trauma, transformation, and healing*. New York: Brunner/Mazel.

Wilson, J. P., & Krauss, G. E. (1981). *The Vietnam Stress Inventory. A scale to assess war stress and post-traumatic stress disorder among Vietnam veterans*. Cleveland, OH: Cleveland State University.

Wilson, J. P., & Krauss, G. E. (1985). Predicting post-traumatic stress disorders among Vietnam veterans. In W. E. Kelly (Ed.), *Posttraumatic stress disorder and the war veteran patient* (pp. 102–147). New York: Brunner/Mazel.

Wilson, J. P., Smith, W. K., & Johnson, S. K. (1985). A comprehensive analysis of PTSD among various survivor groups. In C. R. Figley (Ed.), *Trauma and its wake: The study and treatment of post-traumatic stress disorder* (pp. 142–172). New York: Brunner/Mazel.

Wolfe, D. (1987). *Child abuse. Implications for child development and psychopathology* (Vol. 10). Newbury Park, CA: Sage Publications.

Wolfe, J., Furey, J., & Sandecki, R. (1989). *Women's Military Exposure Scale*. (Available from Jessica Wolfe, National Center for PTSD [116B], Boston VA Medical Center, 150 S. Huntington Ave., Boston, MA 02130.)

Wolfe, J., & Keane, T. M. (1990). The diagnostic validity of posttraumatic stress disorder. In M. E. Wolf & A. P. Mosnain (Eds.), *Post-traumatic stress disorder: Biological mechanisms and clinical aspects* (pp. 48–63). Washington, DC: American Psychiatric Press.

Wolfe, J., Keane, T. M., Lyons, J. A., & Gerardi, R. J. (1987). Current trends and issues in the assessment of combat-related post-traumatic stress disorder. *Behavior Therapist, 10*, 27–32.

Zuckerman, M., & Linn, K. (1968). Construct validity of the sensation seeking scale. *Journal of Consulting and Clinical Psychology, 32*, 420–426.

Zung, W. (1965). A self-rating depression scale. *Archives of General Psychiatry, 12*, 63–70.

CHAPTER 15

Structured Clinical Interview Techniques

Daniel S. Weiss

Introduction

Historical Context

The assessment of the depth and degree of impairment or distress following exposure to traumatic stress has long been an activity of the clinician who has endeavored to assist those who are suffering from traumatic stress syndromes. The issue of whether or not a psychiatric diagnosis such as posttraumatic stress disorder (PTSD) (in the DSM-III-R; American Psychiatric Association, 1987) or prolonged posttraumatic stress disorder (in the ICD-9-CM) best characterizes the psychological processes following exposure to traumatic stressors depends on a variety of factors, not all of which are scientific. Nonetheless, the recognition of the basic uniformity of psychological and biological reactions following exposure to the range of traumatic stressors has been aided by the formalization of diagnostic criteria. The social implications of carrying a psychiatric diagnosis as a consequence of displaying a near universal pattern of reactions subsequent to surviving exposure to a traumatic stressor are weighty and need social attention. But the continuing understanding of the features and phenomena of traumatic stress has been considerably advanced by the appearance and use of structured diagnostic interview techniques.

The use of such interview techniques has not been confined to the diagnosis of the PTSD; in fact, specific structured techniques solely for PTSD followed the development and initial use of such techniques with other psychiatric disorders. The promulgation of the Research

Diagnostic Criteria (e.g., Williams & Spitzer, 1982) and the push for standard instrumentation in research on psychopathological conditions (e.g., Endicott & Spitzer, 1978; Wing, Cooper, & Sartorius, 1974) were key forces in spurring the development and use in empirical research of structured clinical interviews. Inevitably, this Zeitgeist spread to research activities with individuals suffering from PTSD.

This chapter will examine several of the structured clinical interview techniques that have been offered. In the process, some general considerations will be discussed, details of the individual techniques will be presented, a presentation of some of the published research evidence for reliability, validity, utility, and comprehensiveness will be conducted, and a series of concluding recommendations for future work in the area will be offered.

Defining the Domain

The definition of structured clinical interview techniques will be broadened somewhat in this chapter to include information about methods that might not universally be agreed upon as structured clinical interview techniques. Generally, a structured clinical interview technique is understood to be a formalized interview process or procedure that has internally logical or consistent rules that govern the content of questions asked of an interviewee, the order in which topics are covered, and the specific kind of information sought. Generally, rules are also provided that govern the making of diagnostic decisions. Additionally, structured clinical interview techniques are designed to be administered by individuals with clinical training and experience—hence they are differentiated from other diagnostic interview schedules which do not require that the interviewer have clinical training. A related and key feature of this distinction is the format in which questions are posed and asked. In structured clinical interviews, the questions posed are

Daniel S. Weiss • Department of Psychiatry, University of California, San Francisco, California 94143.

International Handbook of Traumatic Stress Syndromes, edited by John P. Wilson and Beverley Raphael. Plenum Press, New York, 1993.

adds important clinical information to any study, whether the techniques are used to their fullest to make diagnostic decisions or whether they are simply used to guide the interview itself.

Structured Clinical Interview for DSM-III-R

Introduction

The most widely used, and probably the most thoroughly researched structured clinical interview is the Structured Clinical Interview for DSM-III-R (SCID) (Spitzer, Williams, & Gibbon, 1987). Unlike the other structured interviews designed for use by clinicians discussed in this chapter, the SCID covers more than just PTSD and more than just the anxiety disorders. This feature may be more or less desirable, depending upon the purposes that suggested the use of a structured interview. All other things being equal, which they sometimes are not, the recommendation would be to use a comprehensive structured diagnostic interview like the SCID in order to collect information about co-morbidity and to have the option to discover other co-occurring symptoms following exposure to traumatic stress that are not currently included in the diagnostic criteria for PTSD.

The SCID has been under continual development and refinement by Spitzer's group at the New York State Psychiatric Institute. First being keyed to the DSM-III criteria, the current version of the SCID is keyed to the DSM-III-R criteria. More likely than not, when the DSM-IV appears, a version of the SCID keyed to DSM-IV will not be far behind. For Axis I disorders, there are currently three versions of the SCID: the SCID-P (patient version), which is designed for use with those groups in which differential diagnosis with psychotic disorders is likely; the SCID-OP (outpatient version), which is designed for use with those groups in which disorders are likely but psychotic disorders are not; and the SCID-NP (nonpatient version), which is designed for use with groups in which interviewees are not necessarily identified as psychiatric patients. The SCID has an accompanying manual of instructions with do's and don'ts; its review and study are essential for proper use of the instrument.

The SCID comprises modules for each disorder assessed. These are presented after an initial open-ended narrative that includes identifying information and a history of the present illness in the patient versions or a history of the periods of most emotional distress in the SCID-NP. This feature of the SCID is crucial. Its proper and sensitive use is often the difference between an interview process that seems smooth, empathic, and concerned, versus one that is choppy, insensitive, and treats the interviewee as an object of study. The introductory section also sets the tone for the respondent to understand that inquiry will be directed at current status as well as lifetime status. For the PTSD module, which will generally be the main focus of attention for those who have suffered traumatic stress, an additional introductory narrative may be used, especially when the subject population is known to have been exposed, or the stressor that subjects might share is common.

To illustrate this point, our use of the SCID in the National Vietnam Veterans Readjustment Study (NVVRS) (Kulka *et al.*, 1990) included such an open-ended narrative by respondents in which they could tell their stories about the trauma experiences (mostly, but not exclusively, combat-related) as an initial starting point for more specific and detailed exploration following the SCID protocol for the PTSD module. The use of the SCID PTSD module in the NVVRS also deviated from usual practice in that all items were administered to all respondents, even if, in the judgment of the interviewer, the traumatic event did not clearly qualify for Criterion A. The purpose of this strategy was to be able to investigate symptom patterns, over and above the goal of making reliable and valid diagnoses. Currently, the PTSD module is a special addition to the SCID.

The PTSD Module and Interview Criteria

The SCID provides the clinician the opportunity to assess the presence or absence of each of the DSM-III-R criteria for occurrence currently, as well as over the course of the respondent's lifetime. As a consequence, meeting the criteria for PTSD can be assessed for current status as well as lifetime. In assessing the presence or absence of any sign or symptom, the SCID instruction manual notes that the SCID allows the clinician to indicate that the presentation of the criterion item is subthreshold, that is, "the threshold for the criterion is almost met." Such a provision is also provided for the diagnosis of the disorder itself: "The full criteria are not quite met but clinically the disorder seems likely." This may be especially true with PTSD where three avoidance symptoms are required to meet the diagnosis, and survivors may clearly manifest only two or one. To the degree that it is possible, clarifying what goes into the decision-making process about the presence or absence of a criterion symptom should be done beforehand. A thorough presentation of this issue, which is, in fact, the key issue in cross-method studies of reliability and validity, is presented for the SCID PTSD module. Similar materials, however, should be developed for any structured interview technique.

The NVVRS clinical research team prepared materials for its clinical interviewers illustrating what clinical phenomena were appropriately coded for each item. This section is based on those materials, and attempts to show what counts as a "present" instance for each of the SCID items linked to the DSM-III-R criteria, as well as examples of clinical phenomena that do not meet the criteria.

1. *Recurrent and Intrusive Distressing Recollections of the Event*

In order to be coded present, the recollections must be recurrent, intrusive, and distressing. These recollections are typically characterized as spontaneous and uncontrollable, and seem to have "a life of their own." They are unbidden, unwelcome, and unable to be stopped once started. Examples that meet this criterion would include a veteran driving along in a car, not focusing on any particular thoughts, who has a sudden and distressing memory of placing mutilated corpses in body bags after a rocket attack (referring to a specific wartime experience). Another example would be a victim of a mudslide who is reading a novel and suddenly has the interfering thought, "If only I had checked the foundation of the house and had it reinforced—I could have prevented the damage" during which the memory of the house inspection is recalled.

Clinical phenomena that do not meet the criterion for intrusive recollections include the repeated ruminative thoughts of the severely depressed individual who thinks "I am worthless" outside of the context of a traumatic event; the ruminative and obsessive thoughts of the individual who feels "I am sinful," or the intrusive thoughts of an individual with social fears who thinks "I will make a fool of myself in front of all these people." These are three examples of intrusive thoughts that do not relate to traumatic life events but are specific for other disorders. Another example of phenomena that do not meet this criteria is the combat veteran who frequently thinks of his Vietnam experiences, and may be saddened by the memories, but does so volitionally, without a sense of intrusion to the memories.

2. *Recurrent and Distressing Dreams of the Event*

Dreams must be recurrent and distressing. Night terrors should be scored as present, and the content of the dream should align with the traumatic exposure. The content of trauma-related nightmares may consist of relatively straightforward dreams of aspects of the event(s) (e.g., repetitive dreams of specific firefights for a veteran) or symbolic representations with some form of trauma-relevant combat theme (e.g., running in terror through a jungle with one's spouse and children while trying to escape an unseen assailant).

Clinical phenomena that do not meet the criterion include dreams or recurrent nightmares of falling off a cliff that are of a fantasy nature and not linked to traumatic experiences, dreams of monsters or other threatening fantasy figures, or anxiety dreams related to conflicts or fears involving daily living rather than traumatic exposure.

3. *Sudden Acting or Feeling as if the Traumatic Event Were Recurring*

This phenomenon includes a sense of reliving the experience, illusions, hallucinations, and dissociative (flashback) episodes, even those that occur upon awakening or when intoxicated. The important distinction is between an intrusive memory—in which the person perceives him or herself to be remembering the event—and a feeling as if the event were happening again, during which the individual loses the ability to distinguish the past from the present. Behavior during reliving experiences is dissociative-like, and sometimes is unknown to the subject until described by another person who has observed the behavior (often a spouse or close friend). Phenomena that qualify for this item include the case of a war veteran who hears a car backfire, hits the dirt, and sees a battle scene pass before his eyes with the dissociative quality of reliving the experience. Reliving experiences are often set off by the sight of blood, or a dead, mutilated animal at the side of the road, or any stimulus reminiscent of the trauma. Another example would be someone who experienced severe shaking in an earthquake, and, when a truck passes by and shakes the building, relives the earthquake experience, including the sense of distorted time and terror about safety.

4. *Intense Psychological Distress at Exposure to Events*

The focus is on psychological distress—fear, anxiety, anger, sense of impending doom—in the face of a representation that symbolizes or resembles an aspect of the traumatic event (including anniversaries of the event). A classic example of this phenomenon is the assault victim who becomes fearful and anxious whenever approaching the scene of the attack, or a survivor of torture with electrodes who needs to have an electrocardiogram. Being unable to face certain situations or continue on with the ordinary course of daily activities because of the possibility of reminders or reexposure is the feature. The survivor of a tornado is unable to step inside a mobile home, because it was inside such a structure that she witnessed her child being killed.

Phenomena that do not meet criterion for distress upon reexposure are the sad feelings experienced at anniversaries of a trauma, but ones that do not impede ongoing functioning.

5. *Deliberate Efforts to Avoid Thoughts or Feelings Associated with the Event*

Intentional efforts to avoid thoughts or feelings or deliberate efforts to avoid activities or situations that arouse recollections of the event must have been made, but need not have been successful. However, in instances where avoidance has been attempted but not succeeded, there must be evidence that distress occurred. Avoidance strategies may vary on several dimensions. They may be obvious or subtle, relatively adaptive or clearly maladaptive. Obvious forms of avoidance include the refusal to discuss or talk about the trauma, the use of alcohol or drugs to cloud memories, and the avoidance of places and things that are a reminder of the trauma. Overworking is also a strategy used to avoid thoughts and feelings about trauma. Sometimes the interviewee is self-aware of these strategies; other times, the phenomena are clinically more subtle.

Phenomena that do not meet the criterion for avoidance include the inability to remember aspects of the event; avoidance of social situations that provoke anxiety unrelated to a traumatic event (declining to give sales presentations), and depressive social withdrawal and overall loss of interest in things.

6. *Inability to Recall an Important Aspect of the Event (Psychogenic Amnesia)*

The clinical phenomenon here is not simply that the person could not keep track of everything that happened, but rather that the individual is aware of important details that cannot be remembered—that is, there are gaps and holes in the story as it is told. Psychogenic amnesia may be either partial or complete. High levels of distress often accompany descriptions of events in which the respondent is unable to recall important details.

Examples that are instances of the phenomenon include the combat veteran who cannot remember an episode in which a buddy was killed or how he survived;

another is the automobile accident victim whose wife was killed and who cannot remember being told that his spouse died. Phenomena that do not meet the criterion for psychogenic amnesia include forgetting minor details or a victim with head injury, alcohol-induced "blackouts," or other neurologic memory failures.

7. *Markedly Diminished Interest in Significant Activities*

The essential feature here is a change in level of interest subsequent to the trauma or the onset of symptoms. Activities in which interest is lost must have been meaningful to the respondent prior to the trauma, as evidenced by continued interest or focus on the activity. Developmental changes must be ruled out in assessing this item.

Examples that fit this phenomenon include the athletically active woman who gives up all physical fitness after a scarring automobile accident; the witness to a shooting who abandons a lifelong passion of hunting; or the volunteer paramedic who no longer teaches CPR after having failed to revive a clearly moribund victim after a disaster. Examples that do not meet the criterion are changes in activity because of physical limitations and the severe anhedonia of someone with major depression. Thus, if both PTSD and major depression are present, a clinical determination must be made of whether the loss of interest is clearly tied to the response to trauma.

8. *Feeling of Detachment or Estrangement from Others*

Here, too, the essential aspect is change after the trauma. The phenomenon is common in psychological disturbance, but the key feature is a marked increase in feelings of distance and detachment. An example is a parent, an active churchgoer, whose child is abducted: The parent continues to participate in the church, but feels alone and alienated, receives no comfort, and feels that faith has betrayed him or her. An example that is not scored as present would be the emergency/disaster worker who feels that civilians cannot appreciate what he has been through but does not feel socially isolated from others who have not had similar experiences.

9. *Restricted Range of Affect*

The restriction of affect or "numbing" is relative to the range available prior to the trauma. The phenomenon is often recognized by people who are unable to have loving feelings; they are numb, and do not have feelings they think they should. An example would be an earthquake survivor whose co-worker was killed and who does not feel choked up, or moved, or sad about the lost co-worker and continues to function in a mechanical, lifeless, business-only manner.

10. *Sense of Foreshortened Future*

Examples that fit this phenomenon would be a child who does not expect to have a career, a marriage, children, or a long life. Other examples include the hurricane survivor who does nothing to prepare for future emergencies because he "won't be around, anyway" and the combat veteran who drifts in and out of employment, because he does not have a sense of a job history or the implications of this for any future opportunities.

This symptom is to be distinguished from a chronic lack of regard for future consequences from someone with antisocial personality disorder, for example.

11. *Difficulty Falling or Staying Asleep*

This item requires no further elaboration.

12. *Irritability or Outbursts of Anger*

This phenomenon is often observed by the interviewee with some chagrin and apology. There is a sense of loss of control, sometimes coupled with a fear of even greater expression of anger or hostility. Examples include the supervisor at work, having been robbed at gunpoint, who angrily explodes at a subordinate for having thoughtlessly told a joke about mugging. This item needs to be scored in relation to pretrauma anger expression.

13. *Difficulty Concentrating*

Trauma survivors very frequently report difficulties concentrating, in both the acute and chronic phases of response. For example, a combat veteran might report that he or she found it extremely difficult to concentrate on classroom lectures and assigned reading materials, whereas a sexual assault victim may find that he or she is no longer able to concentrate on the computational and accounting tasks of employment. The report of difficulty concentrating is to some extent a function of intrusive images and thoughts that may interfere with cognitive tasks that allow attention to wander, such as reading or mental arithmetic.

14. *Hypervigilance*

This phenomenon represents excessive attention to external stimuli beyond that called for given a realistic appraisal of the level of external threat. This symptom can often be observed during the interview, especially if the interview situation may have reminders of the trauma (e.g., a victim of falling books and furniture during an earthquake will not sit near the clinician's books). This item is to be differentiated from the generalized suspiciousness in a person with longstanding paranoid trends or paranoid personality disorder. Another example would be of the assault victim who continually looks over her shoulder when walking down streets and in stairwells.

15. *Exaggerated Startle Response*

This must not predate the trauma and can sometimes be witnessed during the interview, if some unusual noise or sound occurs.

16. *Physiological Reactivity to Events That Symbolize or Resemble an Aspect of the Event*

The clinical phenomenon here includes reactivity expressed in a variety of ways: heavy or irregular breathing, lightheadedness, tingling in the extremities, tightness in the chest, knot in the stomach, damp or cold palms or feet, and other indicators of arousal. Frequently occurring in conjunction with attempts at avoidance of stimuli reminiscent of the traumatic event (e.g., a woman who was raped in an elevator breaks out in a sweat when entering an elevator), these episodes can be extremely distressing and approach a level of arousal that is exhausting.

NVVRS Research with the Instrument

The NVVRS used the SCID in two ways. The first was a prevalidation study aimed at selecting measures of PTSD to be used in the household survey. The set of survey-based measures was administered to 243 Vietnam theater veterans in treatment for PTSD or other psychiatric disorders at VA Medical Centers or Veterans Centers in addition to veterans without psychiatric disorder. Eight sites across the country were employed, and subjects' diagnoses had to be double-determined to be used in this phase; that is, the chart diagnosis had to agree with the diagnosis made by an independent expert clinician who had administered the SCID and was blind to the chart diagnosis.

The results of that study suggested that a survey interview measure that was similar to the DIS and the Mississippi Scale for Combat-Related PTSD (Keane et al., 1988) were the best candidates, yielding kappa coefficients of .714 and .753, respectively, when scored as scales with a cutoff. The DIS-type diagnostic measure yielded a coefficient of .639 when scored using DSM-III-R algorithm rules. In this study the SCID was used as one part of a "gold standard."

The second study utilized the Clinical Interview component of the NVVRS. It provided a second validity check on the household survey measures of PTSD. Over 300 theater and 100 era veterans were selected to undergo a follow-up clinical interview with one of 29 expert mental health clinicians using the SCID. Participants were selected to include all those who appeared on the basis of the NSVG survey data to be current cases, and a sample of those whose results indicated they were not cases. A second constraint on participants was that they lived within 28 standard metropolitan statistical areas. The response rates were 85% for theater veterans and 83% for era veterans for a total of 440 interviews.

All 440 SCID PTSD modules were reviewed (with audiotape) for accuracy, completeness, and clinical veracity by one of five study expert clinicians. Additional scrutiny was given to those cases in which a subthreshold diagnostic decision was made or in which the review indicated an additional opinion was needed for a two-clinician review of any change. The quality review of the 440 cases resulted in major changes in the initial interviewer's diagnosis of either or both lifetime or current PTSD in only 11 cases. For current PTSD, three were changed from negative to subthreshold or partial, two were changed from negative to positive, two were changed from positive to subthreshold or partial, and four were changed from positive to negative. For the lifetime SCID PTSD diagnosis, one case was changed from negative to subthreshold or partial, five cases from negative to positive, one case from positive to partial, and one case from positive to negative.

A blind interrater reliability study on 15 randomly selected PTSD definite cases and 15 randomly selected PTSD subthreshold or absent cases was conducted, with each of the three clinical co-principal investigators re-

viewing 10 of the cases subject only to the constraint that the case was not reviewed in the prior quality review procedure. Kappa coefficients (Cohen, 1960) were computed between the blind reviewer's diagnosis and the initial interviewer's diagnosis before quality review for both lifetime and current PTSD in the sample of 30 cases. The coefficient for lifetime PTSD was .94 and for current was .87. Although this study cannot be considered a full-scale reliability study, the results do suggest that the SCID can produce reliable diagnoses of both lifetime and current PTSD.

Other Structured Interviews

Anxiety Disorders Interview Schedule—Revised

The group at the State University of New York at Albany has developed the Anxiety Disorders Interview Schedule (ADIS) (DiNardo, O'Brien, Barlow, Waddell, & Blanchard, 1983) and the Anxiety Disorders Interview Schedule—Revised (ADIS—R) (DiNardo & Barlow, 1985). The goal of this interview schedule was to be able to go into greater detail regarding the anxiety disorders. The items were developed by the group at Albany as well as being borrowed from other previously developed interview schedules.

The ADIS—R also attempts to avoid the problem of hierarchical diagnostic decisions and skip outs, so as to minimize the possibility of overlooking valuable information. Initial results using the ADIS were promising for all the anxiety disorders studied (Barlow, 1988). Unfortunately, this group of anxiety disorders did not include PTSD.

The only published study located from this group that examined PTSD was conducted by Blanchard; it employed the ADIS rather than the ADIS—R (Blanchard, Gerardi, Kolb, & Barlow, 1986). The ADIS allows diagnoses for past or current conditions, and as presented in the published paper, skips out if a traumatic event is not presented. Using 43 male Vietnam combat veterans, the ADIS was administered by Gerardi who was blind to the criterion diagnosis. In this study, the criterion diagnosis was a clinical diagnosis made by another physician. The criterion diagnosis indicated 28 with PTSD, 11 without PTSD, and 4 with PTSD in remission. There was agreement in 40 of the 43 cases, and the kappa coefficient was .86. Although these results by themselves are encouraging, given that all the interviewees appeared to be VA patients, it is not clear how well the ADIS or ADIS-R would do in a sample in which the base rate of PTSD was lower. Also missing are interrater reliability data for PTSD where both raters use the ADIS—R for making the diagnosis.

Nonetheless, the ADIS—R may be a useful alternative structured clinical interview where anxiety disorders are the major focus. The data for anxiety disorders other than PTSD are quite encouraging. It is the relative underemphasis of PTSD and attention to PTSD using this technique that might suggest caution if PTSD is the major area of interest.

Structured Interview for PTSD

The Structured Interview for PTSD (SI-PTSD) (Davidson, Smith, & Kudler, 1989) is a relatively recent addition to the structured interview techniques available to diagnose PTSD. The SI-PTSD is the only interview schedule discussed in this chapter that focuses only on PTSD. Whether this is a strength or limitation partially depends upon the purpose for which a structured interview technique is being employed.

The SI-PTSD is designed to elicit information not only about the presence or absence of symptoms, but also attempts to scale the severity of the experience of these symptoms, from both a current and lifetime perspective. The published study using the SI-PTSD was made using DSM-III rather than DSM-III-R diagnostic criteria. The interview schedule itself, however, includes items allowing for diagnoses using either set of criteria.

The data presented included 116 veterans of the Vietnam, Korean, and Second World Wars, all of whom were in treatment. In a subsample of 41 patients, the SCID for DSM-III was administered by a separate interviewer. Thirty-seven of 41 diagnoses were in agreement. The kappa coefficient for these data was .786.

A second goal of the SI-PTSD appears to be to combine the dimensional and the categorical approaches to PTSD. The diagnostic decisions are made based on the interviewer assessing symptom severity to be at least moderate (e.g., 2 on a 0 to 4 scale). The items comprising the syndrome can then be summed and used as a continuous variable measuring the severity of symptoms. Analyses are presented of this score with other measures and some cutoffs are tentatively offered. It seems that from the initial sample, promising results have been generated.

The authors noted, however, that their measure has so far been confined only to study with combat veterans. For the dimensional claims of the SI-PTSD, the burden of using other groups is heavier than it is solely for the issue of diagnosis.

Diagnostic Interview Schedule

The background, history, and findings of the NIMH Diagnostic Interview Schedule (DIS) have been chronicled extensively and in many different places (e.g., Regier et al., 1988; Robins, Helzer, Croughan, & Ratcliff, 1981; Robins, Helzer, Croughan, Williams, & Spitzer, 1981). The logic and background of the DIS and the goals and objectives of its use and relationship to operationalizing the diagnostic criteria formulated in various nomenclatures are very thoroughly and compellingly presented by Robins (1989). Despite its development and use in epidemiological contexts, much of the reliability/validity studies of the DIS have included use of other structured clinical interviews. Hence it seems important to present some information about this instrument.

Despite early positive reports about the validity of DIS computer-generated diagnoses, Anthony et al. (1985) reported results that were not encouraging. Kappa coefficients ranged from −.02 to .35 for a variety of disorders, none of them PTSD. In this study, a clinical reappraisal of all DIS positives and a sample of DIS negatives from the Baltimore Epidemiologic Catchment Area (see Regier et al., 1988) site was conducted using an interview instrument based on the Present State Examination (Wing et al., 1974) but modified to obtain DSM-III diagnoses. After examining the bulk of the reports, Burke (1986) concluded that the DIS works reasonably well for alcohol abuse and major depression, but that it may have significant difficulty assessing the presence of panic disorder. Robins (1985, 1989) suggested that, for many reasons, the research published to date does not begin to resolve the question of the validity of the DIS.

With respect to PTSD, initially the DIS did not contain a module for PTSD. The NVVRS utilized a form of the DIS that had included items relevant for the diagnosis of PTSD, and, subsequently, other data about PTSD have been reported (CDC, 1988; Helzer, Robins, & McEvoy, 1987). Nonetheless, the NVVRS data probably provide the best estimate of the validity of the diagnosis of PTSD.

A comparison of the diagnostic decisions based on the DIS survey data with those from the clinician's SCID diagnosis indicated that though the DIS had performed acceptably in the Preliminary Validation Component with treatment-seeking veterans, in the full community sample it could not be used to make a current diagnosis of PTSD. For the 440 cases, using the SCID diagnosis of PTSD as the standard, the DIS PTSD module achieved a sensitivity of only 21.5, a specificity of 97.9, and a kappa coefficient of .256. Thus, some disquieting questions remain about the use of the DIS with lay interviewers in a community sample for the diagnosis of PTSD.

Composite International Diagnostic Interview

A new entry into the arena of structured interviews is the Composite International Diagnostic Interview (CIDI) (Robins et al., 1988). A combination of elements of the DIS and the Present State Examination, it is fully structured to allow administration by lay interviewers and scoring by computer, and is designed for international use with a variety of different nomenclatures. Sponsored in part by the World Health Organization and the Alcohol, Drug Abuse, and Mental Health Administration, the CIDI includes in its original version a module for PTSD. Because of the scope and international significance of the enterprise, it seemed important to note its place in the sphere of structured interviews.

Currently, the CIDI is undergoing international field testing. One potential advantage of the CIDI for future work is that items are being modified to use in different cultures. Presumably, questions about exposure to trauma will be appropriately calibrated to the cultural arena. If the results are promising, it may be that the PTSD module of the CIDI can serve useful purposes in the epidemiologic realm. Whether such a structured interview can be used in clinical situations will remain to be evaluated.

Summary

This chapter has described a variety of structured interviews, some more "clinical" than others. An attempt was made to differentiate between those interviews with broader or narrower coverage, those designed to be administered by nonclinicians and those requiring a clinician for administration, those that produce diagnoses, and those that produce diagnoses and summary scores of severity. It is clear that the whole issue of diagnosis of PTSD as response to traumatic stress is one that transcends the technical issues of measurement validity and reliability. A case was made to the added benefits that might be derived clinically in using a structured interview, even if the focus of attention is not research.

Using the SCID, issues regarding lifetime and current diagnosis, presence, absence, and subthreshold status of symptoms was discussed. Information about the status of the ADIS—R, the SI-PTSD, and the DIS was offered. The CIDI was introduced and its international character was noted.

The role of structured clinical interviews and the data made available by their use are crucial to the ongoing evolution of diagnostic criteria for PTSD or response to traumatic stress. What other psychological and/or physiological phenomena co-occur after exposure to traumatic stress continues to be an evolving and growing area of attention. For this reason alone, ignoring the increase in precision and the possibility for comparability of results, the regular use of standard structured clinical interviews ought to be a regular activity for those who work with survivors of trauma. The choice of technique will vary with preference, time, training, and the desire for comparison with other work. As more investigations are conducted with the instruments discussed in this chapter, it may become clearer that some have features that make them more or less preferable. At this point, it is fair to say that this aspect of measurement is still in its youth.

References

American Psychiatric Association. (1987). *Diagnostic and statistical manual of mental disorders* (3rd ed., rev.). Washington, DC: Author.

Anthony, J. C., Folstein, M., Romanoski, A. J., Vonkorff, M. R., Nestadt, G. R., Chahal, R., Merchant, A., Brown, C. H., Shapiro, S., Kramer, M., & Gruenberg, E. M. (1985). Comparison of lay Diagnostic Interview Schedule and a standardized psychiatric diagnosis. *Archives of General Psychiatry, 42,* 667–676.

Barlow, D. H. (1988). *Anxiety and its disorders.* New York: Guilford Press.

Blanchard, E. B., Gerardi, R. J., Kolb, L. C., & Barlow, D. H. (1986). The utility of the Anxiety Disorders Interview Schedule (ADIS) in the diagnosis of post-traumatic stress disorder (PTSD) in Vietnam veterans. *Behavioral Research and Therapy, 24,* 557–580.

Burke, J. (1986). Diagnostic categorization by the Diagnostic Interview Schedule (DIS): A comparison with other measures of assessment. In J. E. Barrett & R. M. Rose (Eds.), *Mental disorder in the community: Progress and challenge.* New York: Guilford Press.

Centers for Disease Control, Vietnam Experience Study (CDC). (1988). Health status of Vietnam veterans I: Psychosocial characteristics. *Journal of the American Medical Association, 259,* 2701–2707.

Cohen, J. (1960). A coefficient of agreement for nominal scales. *Educational and Psychological Measurement, 20,* 37–46.

Davidson, J., Smith, R., & Kudler, H. (1989). Validity and reliability of the DSM-III criteria for posttraumatic stress disorder: Experience with a structured interview. *Journal of Nervous and Mental Disease, 177,* 336–341.

DiNardo, P. A., Barlow, D. H. (1985). *Anxiety Disorders Interview Schedule—Revised (ADIS—R).* Albany, NY: Phobia and Anxiety Disorders Clinic, State University of New York at Albany.

DiNardo, P. A., O'Brien, G. T., Barlow, D. H., Waddell M. T., & Blanchard, E. B. (1983). Reliability of DSM-III anxiety disorder categories using a new structured interview. *Archives of General Psychiatry, 40,* 1070–1074.

Endicott, J., & Spitzer, R. L. (1978). A diagnostic interview: A schedule for affective disorder and schizophrenia. *Archives of General Psychiatry, 35,* 837–844.

Endicott J., Spitzer, R. L., Fleiss, J., & Cohen, J. (1976). The Global Assessment Scale: A procedure for measuring overall severity of psychiatric disturbance. *Archives of General Psychiatry, 33,* 766–771.

Helzer, J. E., Robins, L. N., & McEvoy, L. (1987). Post-traumatic stress disorder in the general population. *New England Journal of Medicine, 317,* 1630–1634.

Horowitz, M. J., Wilner, N., & Alvarez, W. (1979). The Impact of Event Scale: A measure of subjective stress. *Psychosomatic Medicine, 41,* 209–218.

Keane, T. M., Caddell, J. M., & Taylor, K. L. (1988). Mississippi scale for combat-related posttraumatic stress disorder: Three studies in reliability and validity. *Journal of Consulting and Clinical Psychology, 56,* 85–90.

Kendell, R. E. (1988). What is a case? Food for thought for epidemiologists. *Archives of General Psychiatry, 45,* 374–376.

Kulka, R. A., Schlenger, W. E., Fairbank, J. A., Hough, R. L., Jordan, B. K., Marmar, C. R., & Weiss, D. S. (1990). *Trauma of the Vietnam generation: Report of the findings from the National Vietnam Veterans Readjustment Study* (Vol. 1). New York: Brunner/Mazel.

Regier, D. A., Boyd, J. H., Burke, J. D., Rae, D. S., Myers, J. K., Kramer, M., Robins, L. N., George, L. K., Karno, M., & Locke, B. Z. (1988). One-month prevalence of mental disorders in the United States. *Archives of General Psychiatry, 45,* 977–986.

Robins, L. N. (1985). Epidemiology: Reflections on testing the validity of psychiatric interviews. *Archives of General Psychiatry, 42,* 918–924.

Robins, L. N. (1989). Diagnostic grammar and assessment: Translating criteria into questions. *Psychological Medicine, 19,* 57–68.

Robins, L. N., Helzer, J. E., Croughan, J., & Ratcliff, K. S. (1981). National Institute of Mental Health Diagnostic Interview Schedule: Its history, characteristics, and validity. *Archives of General Psychiatry, 38,* 318–389.

Robins, L. N., Helzer, J. E., Croughan, J., Williams, J. B. W., & Spitzer, R. L. (1981). *NIMH Diagnostic Interview Schedule: Version III-A* (May, 1981). Rockville, MD: National Institute of Mental Health.

Robins, L. N., Wing, J., Witchen, H. U., Helzer, J. E., Babor, T. F., Burke, J. D., Farmer, A., Jablenski, A., Pickens, R.,

Regier, D. A., Sartorius, N., & Towle, L. H. (1988). The Composite International Diagnostic Interview (CIDI): An epidemiologic instrument suitable for use in conjunction with different diagnostic systems and in different cultures. *Archives of General Psychiatry*, 45, 1069–1077.

Spitzer, R. L., Williams, J. B. W., & Gibbon, M. (1987). *Structured Clinical Interview for DSM-III, Version NP-V*. New York: New York State Psychiatric Institute, Biometrics Research Department.

Weiss, D. S., Horowitz, M. J., & Wilner, N. A. (1984). The Stress Response Rating Scale: A clinician's measure for rating the response to serious life events. *British Journal of Clinical Psychology*, 23, 202–215.

Williams, J. B. W., & Spitzer, R. L. (1982). Research diagnostic criteria and the DSM-III: An annotated comparison. *Archives of General Psychiatry*, 39, 1283–1289.

Wing, J. K., Cooper, J. E., & Sartorius, N. (1974). The description and classification of psychiatric symptoms: An instruction manual for the PSE and CATEGO systems. London: Cambridge University Press.

Zilberg, N. J., Weiss, D. S., & Horowitz, M. J. (1982). Impact of Event Scale: A cross-validation study and some empirical evidence supporting a conceptual model of stress response syndromes. *Journal of Consulting and Clinical Psychology*, 50, 407–414.

CHAPTER 16

Assessing Posttraumatic Stress Disorder with the Rorschach Projective Technique

Patti Levin

Introduction

The literature on the theory and clinical implications of posttraumatic stress disorder (PTSD) has grown enormously over the past 10 years, yet clearly in striking contrast to the relative paucity of literature regarding psychometric assessment. There are few psychological instruments in use which have adequate norms for the evaluation of PTSD, particularly for nonmilitary traumatic events. Currently, there is much evidence that many kinds of "civilian" disasters (e.g., rape, violent assault, natural disasters, hostage situations, etc.) can produce a stress response (Green, Lindy, & Grace, 1985; Horowitz, 1976, 1985; Krystal & Niederland, 1968; Sales, Baum, & Shore, 1984).

At this time, such measures include a PTSD subscale for the Minnesota Multiphasic Personality Inventory (MMPI) (Burke & Mayer, 1985; Keane, Malloy, & Fairbank, 1984; Wilson, 1989), the Impact of Events Scale (Horowitz, Wilner, & Alvarez, 1979; Zilberg, Weiss, & Horowitz, 1982), and the Diagnostic Interview Schedule (Robins, Helzer, Croughan, & Ratcliff, 1981), all essentially self-report instruments. An inherent problem with such tests is the reliability of retrospective, subjective narrative (Green & Grace, 1988).

The Rorschach Test and Assessing PTSD

Projective testing has been shown to have numerous advantages over self-reports, including the ability to

Patti Levin • Trauma Clinic, Massachusetts General Hospital, and Harvard Medical School, Boston, Massachusetts 02114.

International Handbook of Traumatic Stress Syndromes, edited by John P. Wilson and Beverley Raphael. Plenum Press, New York, 1993.

tap unconscious thoughts and feelings (Thorndike & Hagen, 1969). The Rorschach is ideally suited for assessment of PTSD in that it is believed to bypass conscious cognitive and affective experience, or resistance, and can tap unconscious mental processes. Therefore, it can provide valuable information even with clients who present with completely dissociated, denied, or walled-off traumatic stressors. "Emotional constriction may well be the most common expression of PTSD, and the diagnosis is likely to be missed during this phase" (van der Kolk & Ducey, 1989). In addition, patients often present with symptoms which are not consciously linked to the traumatic event either by the patient or the therapist (Green *et al.*, 1985; Horowitz, 1976; Scurfield, 1985). Most victims are ambivalent about discussing their traumata in their attempts to avoid the painful recollections. Such avoidance or denial and the complex nature of the symptomatology can complicate diagnosis and subsequent appropriate treatment (Lindy, Green, Grace, & Titchener, 1983). In addition, the Rorschach has been shown to have discriminant validity in effectively differentiating conscious attempts at faking psychopathology (Seamons, Howell, Carlisle, & Roe, 1981). The Rorschach was advocated in workers' compensation cases, as early as 1951, to distinguish malingering from PTSD (Trimble, 1981).

Previous studies of the Rorschach with Vietnam veterans have indicated that the neutral stimulus of the Rorschach provoked "uncontrolled and apparently trauma-related responses" (Souffront, 1987; van der Kolk & Ducey, 1989) particularly from the five chromatic cards (II, III, VIII, IX, X)—"even in subjects who denied preoccupation with the trauma in their daily lives" (van der Kolk & Ducey, 1989).

The Rorschach is a diagnostic tool which provides an ideal instrument in bypassing conscious mental processes, understanding coping strategies, and delineating cognitive and affective states and traits. It can facilitate differential diagnosis, aid in treatment planning, and possibly serve to speed up therapist/client understanding in linking trauma to symptomatology.

Brief Overview of the Rorschach

In 1921, a Swiss psychiatrist, Hermann Rorschach, introduced the Rorschach Inkblot Test. It was brought to the United States in 1925 and systematized by five psychologists: Beck, Klopfer, Piotrowski, Hertz, and Rappaport (with Shafer, Gill, and Holt), each of whom developed separate systems for scoring and interpretation. From the 1920s through the 1970s all five systems were used, "despite the absence of standardized data for (these) measures" (St. Pierre, 1988). Each systematizer brought his or her own theoretical orientation to the administration, scoring, and interpretation.

There was much criticism of the Rorschach owing to the lack of consensus among systematizers, as well as lack of objective criteria for scoring (Parker, 1983). In 1974, Exner created the first standardized system for administration, scoring, and interpretation in the Comprehensive System. Exner spoke with the four systematizers still living and asked what revisions they would make if they could revamp their systems. He conducted three surveys of over 1,000 clinical psychologists regarding issues of design and analysis, training and administration, and practices and opinions. Exner subjected all existing studies (more than 4,000 articles and 30 books) of the five systems to analysis, evaluation, and replication, in an attempt to consolidate the most valid and reliable parts of each system into one common, standardized language. Exner's system is data-based: it is atheoretical and closely linked to replicated and validated studies. In addition, the Rorschach Workshops under Exner's supervision, continually update the Comprehensive System through ongoing research (Exner, 1974, 1986, 1990). Perhaps the most important aspect of the Comprehensive System was the creation of normative samples for nonpatients (both adults and children), as well as certain adult psychiatric populations.

The structural features of the system are based on all the scores, including the determinants. These features are used to ascertain the psychological operations employed by the subject in responding to the inkblots. Each response is coded systematically, which generates an understanding of the subject's unconscious experience and dealings with self and world. The determinants are used in a number of ratios and percentages in the Structural Summary, which provides information on cognitive, ideational, and affective processes, coping styles, relationship between available resources and stimulus demands, self-image and interpersonal attitudes, and specific psychopathology. Interpretations are tied closely to data, with an emphasis on quantitative and structural variables, including the importance of the total configuration of results rather than a focus on any single score. Results are compared to nonpatient and psychiatric patient sample norms and standard deviations.

The earliest reported study of the use of the Rorschach in assessing the effect of environmental stressors was done in 1965 (Shalit, 1965). The Rorschach was administered to 20 servicemen in the Israeli Navy during a severe storm at sea, when the storm was 10 hours old, and compared to Rorschachs previously administered in the routine selection process. It had been hypothesized that the human movement response (M) would remain consistent as a representation of a basic personality trait, but that inanimate movement (m) would increase owing to the state reaction of a subjective experience of helplessness in the face of intense situational stress. Results confirmed the hypotheses.[1]

In 40 subjects demonstrating a postaccident anxiety syndrome, total responses to the 10 Rorschach cards averaged between 8 and 9 (Modlin, 1967). Although Exner (1986) considered records of 10 or fewer answers to be invalid, Modlin related the findings (with no mention of Rorschach results other than number of responses) to the premorbid characteristics of a particularly homogeneous sample: "simple, literal, unimaginative . . . stoic . . . conventional," with limited and constricted capacity for emotional expression (Modlin, 1967). The Rorschach results were viewed as evidence of vulnerability to the syndrome, as opposed to an indication of the effects of the traumatic events.

In contrast, the van der Kolk and Ducey study (van der Kolk, 1984; van der Kolk & Ducey, 1989) interpreted the four severely constricted records as evidence of psychic numbing, and subsequent inability to use fantasy or "thought as experimental action." Eight subjects with markedly extratensive (Experience Balance [EB]) styles demonstrated "extensive use of unstructured color (CF and pure C), and diminished ego functions" represented by few human movement (M) determinants. This study seemed to show a particular bias in the authors' considering introversive EB styles as evidence of "higher cognitive processes." The authors modified the standard EB ratio ($M:WsumC$) by weighing ideation against both ideation and affect ($M:M + WsumC$). However, Rorschach's formulation of the EB did not imply a value judgement; rather, both introversive and extratensive EB styles are simply preferred coping styles, and are equally effective. The "markedly" extratensive protocols were seen as an example of the intrusive phase of PTSD. However, the extratensive style is not, in itself, indicative of unmodulated affect. Rather, it is the extensive use of unstructured color ($FC:CF + C$) that could be a symbolic equivalent of the intrusive phase.

In addition, the authors found an unusually high number of (m) responses (mean of 3.64), indicating a subjective sense of helplessness and "the perception of threatening forces beyond one's control" (van der Kolk & Ducey, 1989). There was extensive use of concrete, uncensored references to traumatic war events, including numerous blood and anatomy contents.

A study of two Vietnam veterans with PTSD "beautifully illustrated how the Rorschach may act as a releaser of highly charged fantasies" (Bersoff, 1970). Both subjects' responses were replete with direct and symbolic trauma content "to the almost exclusion of pre-

---

[1]All responses on the Rorschach are coded by a letter and/or numerical index.

vious, more time-spanning, characterological concerns" (Bersoff, 1970).

Salley and Teiling (1984) wrote an article on the Rorschach responses of a Vietnam veteran who had dissociated rage attacks. They noted the plethora of divider themes in the content, which were interpreted as the patient's need to wall off certain aspects of his inner experience. Percepts included subground explosions and a preoccupation with morbid subjects in a concrete, trauma-related fashion, such as wounded people, body parts, and blood, particularly on the chromatic cards. There was extensive use of shading determinants, indicating intensely painful affect and helplessness. No psychotic thought process was apparent. Fortunately, the authors did not make any other formulations based on the structural aspects of this case, as a review of their scoring found a number of errors. Of note were the missed inanimate movement scores which would have significantly distinguished the mean m from Exner's norms, found to be meaningful in other studies (Shalit, 1965; Souffront, 1987; Swanson, Blount, & Bruno, 1990; van der Kolk & Ducey, 1989).

Carr responded to the content interpretation of Salley and Teiling's study and made mention of the similarity to several of his own patients' Rorschach responses. Examples of specific trauma-related percepts corroborated the "essence of PTSD . . . the concretization of very specific stimuli that have served to precipitate anxiety around a trauma not yet appropriately integrated" (Carr, 1984).

Kowitt (1985) replied to Carr by suggesting that "unconscious fantasies and conflicts may be concealed within the traumatic imagery" and can be overlooked because of the compelling nature of the trauma itself. Carr (1985) answered Kowitt (a former student) by succinctly stating that what one does with insight, regarding concrete trauma responses in the Rorschach, is dependent upon one's own theoretical and treatment biases.

Souffront (1987) used the Rorschach in the differential assessment of 60 Vietnam veterans with and without PTSD. Results indicated two predictors that were significant discriminants: an elevation in (m) and the FC:CF + C ratio weighted in the direction of unstructured color. Souffront considered the results of her discriminant analysis predicting PTSD group membership as consistent with the DSM-III diagnosis. Statistically significant Rorschach variables indicated an inability to integrate intrusive recollections, psychic numbing as the result of severe situational stress, and an inability to modulate affect.

In a study of stressful life events and Rorschach content, Aron examined 56 undergraduate students who were chosen on the basis of extreme scores (both high and low) on the College Schedule of Recent Experience (CSRE), a self-report checklist (Marx, Garrity, & Bowers, 1975, cited in Aron, 1982). Subjects "who have experienced real-life, unhappy, stressful events" had significantly more anxious content on the Rorschach.

Lewis and Arsenian (1982) observed the phasic PTSD qualities of intrusion and suppression, or expression and denial, in a case example of a murderer's Rorschach, administered 10 years after the crime. Following percepts of trauma images, the patient would respond to the inkblot with a "vigilant warding off of

associated images" in an "attempt to undo by wish fulfillment the associated train of responses set off in his mind" (Lewis & Arsenian, 1982).

The Rorschach test was advocated in the differential diagnosis of elderly patients (Nichols & Czirr, 1986). The aged often present with depressive symptomatology, physical complaints, and even occasionally psychotic conditions. The authors found that "while PTSD patients often show depressive indications and color stress (on the Rorschach), form level is generally good and bizarre responses tend to be related to actual experiences, such as body parts, or explosions" (Nichols & Czirr, 1986). Hartman et al. (1990) presented Rorschach data from 41 Vietnam veterans who were being treated on an inpatient PTSD unit. Results suggested that reality-testing was impaired (mean $X + \% = .56$ and $F + \% = .50$). Subjects utilized ineffective coping strategies (18 were ambitensive). The authors suggested that PTSD subjects were similar to Exner's (1986) character disorder norms. It is interesting to note that the authors were inconclusive regarding Rorschach correlates in their study of the phenomenon of emotional numbing, only suggesting the high lambda (mean 1.06) as attempts to avoid or distance from emotions. However, the mean Affective Ratio (Afr) in their study was .45, which is significantly lower than normal, and reflects attempts at avoiding affect.

In contrast, Swanson et al. (1990) found low Afr's (mean .49) among their 50 Vietnam combat veteran subjects with PTSD, and linked this result with the tendency to "avoid emotionally laden situations." Other results indicated impaired reality testing ($X + \% = .46$, $F + \% = .48$, $X - \% = .29$); low stress tolerance (D Score = -1.82); situational anxiety ($m = 2.84$); and unmodulated affect ($FC:CF + C = .86:2.16$). Subjects engaged in passive ideation ($Mp > Ma$) and experienced painful, negative introspection ($V = 1.46$).

The literature review of the Rorschach and trauma reveals general agreement regarding *unmodulated affect*, as indicated by the use of unstructured color, and an ongoing experience of tension, helplessness, and discomfort, as indicated by a significant amount of inanimate movement and shading scores. In addition, many of the studies reviewed found Rorschach protocols to contain concrete, trauma-related percepts.

Methods

This study compared the Rorschach protocols of adults diagnosed with PTSD with Exner's nonpatient norms (Exner, 1990). Based on a review of the literature, the following hypotheses have been tested:

1. That the sample population will demonstrate a disorder of thinking, involving imagination, reasoning, and active ideation, as an example of trauma's disorganizing effect on cognitive processing. It is hypothesized that human movement (M) will be affected in one, or both, of two ways: poor form quality (M-) as evidence of difficulty with interpersonal relationships (Exner, 1986); and low numbers of M responses indicating inability to use ideation in translating, or responding to the stimulus field.

2. That the sample population will demonstrate a disorder of affect. It is hypothesized that the *FC:CF + C* ratio will be either significantly weighted toward the use of unstructured color, or severely constricted.

3. That there will be a disordered Affective ratio (*Afr*) indicating either over- or underresponsiveness to one's emotional environment.

4. That there will be an elevation of *m* and *Y* responses owing to subjective feelings of helplessness and the perception of being out of control of one's environment.

5. That there will be evidence of hypervigilance as indicated by a positive finding on the Hypervigilance Index (HVI).

6. That concrete trauma-related material will appear as an example of unintegrated reliving of traumatic events. Criteria for concrete content will be specific aspects of individual traumatic events that have been described and reported by the clinician as part of the diagnosis of PTSD.

Subjects

The volunteer subjects of this study were 27 adults who had no Axis I or Axis II diagnosis prior to a trauma that met the DSM-III-R criteria, whose pretrauma level of functioning was within normal limits, and who, at the time of testing, carried a diagnosis of PTSD confirmed by two clinicians. Eleven of the subjects were women; 16 were men. They ranged in age from 19 years to 60 years (mean: 36 years). Twenty-five were white, one was black, and one was Hispanic. On average, they had 13 years of education but ranged from completing the 9th grade to postdoctorate education. Forty-five percent were married, 26% single, 19% separated or divorced, and 7% living with a significant other. Traumata included rapes, violent assaults, electrical and chemical accidents, bombing, fires, and other major accidents. Traumata occurred from age 18 to age 59, and from 6 months to 10 years (mean: 3 years) prior to the date of testing.

Procedure

The Rorschach protocols were administered by me or other qualified testers using the Exner method of administration and scoring. All Rorschach protocols were checked for scoring accuracy by either myself or by other testers in the case of protocols administered by myself.

Data Analysis

The data were analyzed using *t*-tests for determining whether statistically significant differences existed between the sample and Exner's (1990) normative populations. Hypothesis 6 resulted in descriptive information only, as normative data do not currently exist for comparison.

Results

All tested hypotheses proved significant to <.001 on two-tailed *t*-tests (*df* = 26) (see Table 16.1). In addition, the statistical analyses yielded significant differences between the sample and Exner's norms on almost half of the 205 variables. (Hypothesis 6 will be discussed in a later section.)

Discussion

The PTSD sample appears significantly different from Exner's normal population, not only on the 5 hypothesized variables tested, but also on 44 other means and 32 miscellaneous frequency variables. However, I will also discuss the significance of the *lack* of difference in a number of theoretically important variables.

The inferences drawn from the statistical analyses must be considered tentative or exploratory in light of the sample size of 27. To be assured that outcome data are representative of all similar adults with PTSD would require a larger sample.

Further, Exner's nonpatient normative data were randomly selected, beginning in 1978. The diagnostic category of PTSD did not appear in the psychiatric nomenclature until 1980. It is therefore possible that some of Exner's subjects had PTSD. Recent epidemiological surveys not yet published appear to indicate that for Vietnam combat veterans, the lifetime incidence of PTSD is approximately 80% (Keane, personal communication, 1989). It is not unreasonable to assume that PTSD from nonmilitary stressors might also be more prevalent than previously acknowledged.

Finally, a satisfactory interpretation of the Rorschach requires more than an analysis of the structural data. To do full justice to the Rorschach, one must also analyze and integrate both the sequence of scores and the verbalizations. A full integration necessitates attention to the quantitative and the qualitative material to flesh out, or humanize, the nomothetic skeleton. Unfortunately, it is beyond the scope of this chapter to do more than a relatively blind interpretation of the structural data, which is a beginning, not an end.

Hypothesis 1

The sample demonstrated peculiarities in ideation, as reflected in the significant finding of poor quality human movement (*M*-) scores. Thinking activity among the subjects reflects deviations from consensually based reality. The literature on PTSD found numerous indications that the trauma imprint is experienced in a chronically intrusive form; such fixation disrupts ideation when event-related thoughts impinge (Freud, 1920/1954; Horowitz, 1985; Kardiner, 1941; van der Kolk & van der Hart, 1989; Wilson, 1989).

A similar finding, the occurrence of human movement scores without form usage (*M* none), further signifies marked problems in thinking. *M* none responses represent attempts at detaching from or disregarding the

Table 16.1. Significant Variables in Rorschach Study of PTSD

Variable	Exner (N = 700) Mean	SD	Sample (N = 27) Mean	SD	t-score (two-tailed)
D	12.89	3.54	11.15	7.34	2.56**
FQX+	0.90	0.92	0.04	0.19	4.78****
FQXo	16.99	3.34	18.60	4.63	5.30****
FQXu	3.25	1.77	6.07	5.15	8.29****
FQX−	1.44	1.04	3.48	2.08	10.20****
Mo	3.52	1.89	2.04	1.53	4.11****
Mu	0.20	0.45	1.04	1.02	9.33****
m	1.12	0.85	3.70	2.69	16.13****
FC	4.09	1.88	1.30	1.27	7.75****
FC + CF + C + Cn	6.54	2.52	4.63	2.92	3.98****
es	8.21	3.00	13.07	4.67	8.38****
D Score	0.04	1.09	−1.48	1.76	7.24****
p (passive)	2.69	1.52	4.41	2.65	5.93****
Intellect Index	1.56	1.29	0.12	0.10	5.76****
Zf	11.81	2.59	13.48	5.87	3.34***
Zd	0.72	3.06	−0.89	5.67	2.73**
Afr	0.69	0.16	0.48	0.25	7.00****
X + %	0.79	0.08	0.60	0.09	9.50****
F + %	0.71	0.17	0.64	0.24	2.33*
X − %	0.07	0.05	0.15	0.08	8.00****
Xu%	0.14	0.07	0.23	0.10	9.00****
Isolation Index	0.20	0.09	0.13	0.09	3.50***
H	3.39	1.80	2.26	1.29	3.23***
Hd	0.69	0.89	2.59	2.48	11.18****
(Hd)	0.14	0.35	0.70	1.03	8.00****
A	8.16	2.04	7.22	2.62	2.41*
Bt	2.48	1.29	1.04	1.48	5.76****
Cg	1.29	0.93	1.96	1.99	3.72****
Sum6 Sp Sc	1.59	1.25	0.81	0.96	3.25***
COP	2.07	1.52	0.73	1.14	4.62****

Proportional variables

Variable	Exner (N = 700) n	%	Sample (N = 27) n	%	t-score (two-tailed)
Dd	452	65%	24	89%	2.67**
FQXnone	58	8%	6	22%	2.80***
Mu	123	18%	17	63%	9.33****
M−	20	03%	11	41%	12.67****
M none	8	1%	4	15%	7.00****
C	51	7%	13	48%	8.20****
Sum T	620	89%	11	41%	8.00****
Sum V	137	20%	12	44%	3.00***
Sum Y	274	39%	25	93%	6.00****
Fr + rF	47	6%	5	19%	2.40*
FD	553	79%	16	59%	2.50**
Col/Shad Blend	252	36%	17	63%	3.00***
Hx	8	1%	5	19%	9.00****
(A)	88	13%	10	37%	4.00****
An	244	35%	16	59%	2.67**
Bl	96	14%	14	52%	5.43****
Sx	30	4%	10	37%	8.25****
DV	373	53%	4	15%	3.80****

continued

Table 16.1. (Continued)

Proportional variables

Variable	Exner (N = 700) n	%	Sample (N = 27) n	%	t-score (two-tailed)
INCOM	323	46%	6	22%	2.40*
FABCOM2	12	2%	3	11%	3.00***
Sum6 Sp Sc2	23	3%	4	15%	4.00****
AB	98	14%	10	37%	3.29***
PSV	34	5%	8	30%	6.25****
Ambient EB	143	20%	13	48%	3.50***
D Score = 0	455	65%	8	30%	3.89****
D Score < 0	89	13%	16	59%	7.67****
D Score < −1	30	4%	13	48%	11.00****
Adj D = 0	428	61%	11	41%	2.22*
Adj D < 0	66	9%	10	37%	4.67****
Zd < −3.0	37	5%	9	33%	7.00****
X + % < .70	71	10%	21	78%	11.33****
X + % < .61	12	2%	15	56%	18.00****
F + % < .70	313	45%	18	67%	2.20*
Xu% > .20	109	16%	16	59%	6.14****
X − % > .15	24	3%	12	44%	13.67****
X − % > .20	9	1%	7	26%	4.17****
X − % > .30	2	03%	1	4%	3.70****
SCZI = 4	2	03%	2	4%	3.70****
DEPI = 6	3	04%	1	4%	3.60***
CDI = 5	3	04%	3	11%	10.60****
CDI = 4	18	3%	6	22%	6.33****
Dd > 3	33	5%	13	48%	10.75****
Sum T = 0	80	11%	16	59%	8.00****
Sum T > 1	75	11%	9	33%	3.67***
Fr + rF > 0	47	7%	6	22%	3.00***
Afr < .40	11	2%	13	48%	15.33****
Afr < .50	50	7%	18	67%	12.00****
COP = 0	145	21%	15	56%	4.38****
COP > 2	271	39%	2	7%	3.56**
MOR > 2	22	3%	9	33%	10.00****
Level 2 SpSc > 2	03	3%	4	15%	4.00****
Sum 6 SpSc > 6	1	01%	8	30%	49.83****
Pure H < 2	69	10%	8	30%	3.33***
p > a + 1	6	1%	7	26%	12.50****
Mp > Ma	72	10%	8	30%	3.33***

*p < .05; **p < .02; ***p < .01; ****p < .001.

stimulus field, similar to a delusion or a hallucinatory operation. None of the Rorschach studies reviewed in the literature showed evidence of a formal psychotic thought process. Yet the literature on PTSD had many references to the nature of traumatic imagery, to the extent that mental representations can mimic psychosis, specifically thought disorders (Brett & Ostroff, 1985; Horowitz, 1985; van der Kolk & Ducey, 1989). This disordered thinking can appear in the form of illusions or pseudohallucinations.

Nevertheless, the sample showed no significant evidence of psychosis, as corroborated by normal outcomes on the Schizophrenia Index (*SCZI*). The only evidence of cognitive slippage was represented by the significant elevation of Level 2 Fabulized Combinations (*FABCOM2*).

Examples were "two people with their hearts outside of themselves" and "clouds with an Oreo cookie in the middle." As FABCOMs are construed as very loose associations which posit implausible relationships between two or more objects, their elevation might be interpreted as an obvious and visible metaphor: The traumas experienced by the subjects in this sample were themselves implausible events. Who would have expected such painful and distressing traumatic events to have occurred to them? The stressor events were unforeseen and radically different from the ordinary, predictable occurrences of everyday life. Trauma victims unanimously wonder "why me?" It is almost predictable that of all the special scores representative of cognitive slippage, FABCOMs are the specific primary process example manifested in PTSD.

An alternate hypothesis regarding ideation was the expectation that the total occurrence of human movement (M) would be lower than normal. This hypothesis was not confirmed. As M responses are a form of delayed action, a deliberate use of ideation in mediating the stimulus field, the sample suggests that the capacity to reason, fantasize, conceptualize, and harness ego resources is not completely extinguished. This outcome contradicts data found in the van der Kolk and Ducey (1989) study, but confirms an earlier study by Shalit (1965).

Hypothesis 2

Disordered affect, as represented by the FC:CF + C ratio weighted in the direction of unstructured color, was highly significant. The overwhelming affective states reported throughout the literature on PTSD is reflected by the sample's inability to modulate feelings. Affect is discharged with little or no control; the cognitive mechanisms that normally modulate emotional display are severely impaired. It is possible to speculate that feelings reach levels of intensity that intrude upon, or even usurp, cognitive processing. The issue of capacity for affective control is related to the D and adjusted D scores, which will be discussed elsewhere. The disordered FC:CF + C ratio is more representative of a failure to use available resources in a manner which can invoke emotional modulation. Pure C responses signify emotions essentially void of control and are an indication of failure in modulating impulses.

The literature on PTSD is replete with examples of trauma's disorganizing impact on emotion. PTSD is synonymous with feeling overwhelmed, fearing a loss of emotional control, having marked difficulty controlling emotions, and fearing affect overload (Durham, McCammon, Allison, & Williamson, 1987; Lindy, 1985; Newman, 1987; Souffront, 1987; Titchener & Kapp, 1976; van der Kolk & Ducey, 1989; Wilson, 1989). Such affective states are more representative of the experience of the trauma itself, and perhaps represent memory encoded on the most primitive level. The Rorschach taps unconscious, primary process material. It may be that the neutral stimulus of the inkblot captured the hallmark of PTSD: the diminished capacity to exert control over one's level of arousal.

The alternate hypothesis, that access to affect would be severely constricted, was partially confirmed. Only one subject had no color responses. The primary difference between the sample and control group indicated less access to affect, as opposed to total constriction (less total use of color: FC + CF + C + Cn). Moreover, the sample differed from the normals to the extent that, where color was used, it was disproportionately unstructured. The interpretation from the van der Kolk and Ducey study (1989) that such affective constriction was an example of psychic numbing appears in this study to be more connected to the hypothesis regarding Afr.

Hypothesis 3

Although two subjects had Afr's one standard deviation above the mean, the overwhelming majority were one or more standard deviations below the mean. The mean Afr was significantly reduced. The sample was clearly underresponsive to the emotional environment and avoidant in their attempts to circumvent emotional overload. This finding may be seen as a strength when considered together with the amount of unmodulated affect predominating.

Exner found a bimodal distribution of Afr among the EB styles, with ambitents falling in the middle range (1986). Introversives and extratensives were significantly different from each other, with extratensives becoming more involved with affect in their coping operations. In fact, while introversives had a wider range of Afr, not one extratensive had an Afr below the normal range. This study found just as many extratensives with significantly lower Afr's. Therefore, even among those subjects whose coping styles include a psychological receptiveness to affect, considerable effort is exercised to avoid overloading resources, and to use constraint against affective responsivity. It appears that despite the predominant coping style, trauma produces a tendency to back away from affect as a coping mechanism. This reaction is echoed throughout the literature.

Krystal noted the defensive strategy of affective blocking in PTSD (1988). Defenses against the full impact of emotional sequelae to trauma are universal (Lifton & Olson, 1976). Trauma victims ward off affect, feel incapable of confronting emotional experience, and develop overcontrolled states of mind (Horowitz, 1985; Lifton, 1976; Wilson, 1989). Denial and avoidance of affective experience to counteract states of overwhelmed intrusive reliving is a prime example of the biphasic response pattern in PTSD (van der Kolk & Ducey, 1989).

St. Pierre (1988) found low Afr's in her sample of sexually abused children and adolescents. Her interpretation of the finding was related to the use of avoidance and denial, not only during the abuse (invalidation of reality common among family members and/or significant others), but also as a mechanism of defense and coping in abuse sequelae. A similar factor among trauma survivors is not only their own need to avoid thinking about or emotionally reliving the events, but also the common response pattern of significant others' requiring that victims "get on with life . . . forget what happened."

Hypothesis 4

Almost every study on the use of the Rorschach with trauma found significant elevations in inanimate movement responses (m) (Exner, 1986; Hartman et al., 1990; Shalit, 1965; Souffront, 1987; van der Kolk & Ducey, 1989). This study corroborated previous research and showed markedly significant elevations in both m and Y (diffuse shading responses). Salley and Teiling's (1984) Rorschach study also showed an elevation in shading responses among trauma survivors.

The literature on PTSD is full of references to emotional states of helplessness, persistent irritability, chronic tension and anxiety, and loss of control (Davidson & Jackson, 1985; Durham et al., 1987; Hartman & Burgess, 1988; Janoff-Bulman, 1985; Kardiner, 1941; Niederland, 1964; van der Kolk, 1987; Wilson, Smith, & Johnson, 1985; Wilson, Harel, & Kahana, 1988). Y and m responses indicate feelings of helplessness produced by feeling out of control. Indeed, the traumatic event is one in which the "rug" gets pulled out from under one's feet—it is a state beyond one's control—someone or something else controls a life or death decision. Clinicians concur that no matter how effectively victims responded during the traumatic event, they continue to struggle with "if only" scenarios in attempts to master such feelings as powerlessness.

Inanimate movement is seen by some researchers as related to dissociation. Schachtel (1966) characterized the (m) response as "the attitude of the impotent spectator." This expression describes unintegrated thoughts during extreme threat in which an individual's helplessness precludes other active defensive operations. The Salley and Teiling (1984) study of a Vietnam veteran with dissociated rage attacks similarly emphasized inanimate movement elevations as suggestive of dissociation. Clinical reports of victims' descriptions of trauma stories are remarkably consistent in the use of dissociation employed as a coping strategy during the traumatic event. Similarly, Exner (1986) conceptualized an elevation of inanimate movement scores as "thoughts or drives that are not well integrated into the cognitive framework." The inability to integrate traumatic material is ubiquitous throughout the literature on PTSD. Unprocessed stressor events are the basis of being "trapped in the trauma" (Wilson & Zigelbaum, 1986).

Hypothesis 5

The Hypervigilance Index (HVI) was found to be positive with statistical significance. HVI describes a style that is similar to paranoia, but without pejorative implications regarding health of ego functioning. It is a tendency to be overly alert to the possibility of threat. A positive HVI suggests a tendency to avoid or mistrust close interpersonal relationships, to be more concerned with issues of personal space, and to be overly alert in daily routines. Hypervigilant people tend to be pessimistic in the anticipation of negative outcomes, or expect that others will take advantage of them. Hypervigilance requires the maintenance of an energy system that functions even without environmental clues or stimuli.

This description characterizes the portrait of PTSD drawn throughout the literature. The Hypervigilance Index is an example of the type of disordered relationships suggested by the elevation in (M-) responses in Hypothesis 1.

Horowitz (1985) conceptualized hypervigilance as evidence of the intrusive phase of PTSD. Van der Kolk (1987) found a pervasive expectation of doom and consequent hypervigilance among subjects with PTSD, regardless of type of stressor. Rape victims experience profound mistrust and become obsessively vigilant to their environment (Burgess & Holmstrom, 1974; Rose, 1986). Mugging victims assume newly vigilant attitudes, with the impact of human cruelty profoundly disrupting interpersonal relationships (Lejeune, 1973; Ochberg, 1988). There is a tendency to withdraw from and avoid others, as well as a loss of the capacity to use common supports (Krystal, 1984; Niederland, 1964). Clinicians echo the literature in noting that survivors believe that if it happened once, it can happen again. Therefore hypervigilance is a defensive strategy used to protect oneself from further feared invasions of self (Bard & Sangrey, 1986; Titchener & Kapp, 1976).

Hypothesis 6

The diagnosis of PTSD reflects the period of time in a trauma survivor's life before he or she has successfully integrated the traumatic event. It is the period before the "torturing presence" of the trauma is transformed into a "poignant memory" (Lifton, 1988). Concrete trauma-related percepts represent the undigested reliving of the traumatic experience, similar but not identical to a flashback. This study showed trauma percepts in 19 of the subjects' protocols, particularly in response to the chromatic cards (II, III, VIII, IX, X). This finding is believed to corroborate the literature in that such responses are indicative of fixation on the trauma and evidence of the enduring, unintegrated aspects of traumatic experience. Specific examples follow.

A man who survived the bombing of a building resulting in massive deaths and injuries saw "two people getting blown up and the back of their heads getting blown up and hearts being pulled out" (Card III), and "explosion . . . rocket coming in being blown up. Smoke and fire coming up. This is blood. When the rocket came down there were people there who were dead" (Card IX).

A man who was run over by a car while on his bicycle said in response to Card VIII, "I see some death. This mask looks like death because when I was almost killed I saw these two colors." A woman who was violently attacked by a masked man saw masks with piercing, frightening eyes in two responses to Card I. A man who witnessed his girlfriend being raped saw "a woman's vagina bleeding" on Card II. Two different women who were each raped by two masked men saw masked men repetitively throughout their protocols.

Three emergency medical workers saw numerous bloody anatomy percepts: "A heart with blood coming out. You can see the valves in the heart" on Card II; "massive traumatic amputation, legs missing, blood" on

Card II; "looks like anatomy structures. Ribs out in front, breaking open to cause a flailed chest" on Card III. Two fire-fighters saw "the head of a dragon with fire and smoke" on Card IX. In fire-fighting, "the head of the dragon" is the term used to describe the critical moment during a fire when there is a sudden, massive explosion of flames. A man whose thumbs were violently disjointed during an accident saw thumbs numerous times in responses. An artist who lost most of the use of his preferential hand after being attacked by a Doberman pinscher saw dogs, specifically Dobermans, in two responses.

In his original formulation of the test, Rorschach believed that responses were related to psychological and behavioral characteristics, and he avoided or minimized content. Later revisionists applied Freudian and Jungian psychoanalytic theory to content interpretation and idiographic analysis. Exner (1986) stated that it is essential to review the free associations "to capture the rich idiography" that might be found in projected material. State or trait influences, particularly the intense psychological states seen in PTSD, appear to direct the quality and quantity of projected material.

This study found corroboration for the plethora of trauma-related state influences emphasized in the literature (Carr, 1984; Lewis & Arsenian, 1982; Salley & Teiling, 1984; van der Kolk & Ducey, 1989). PTSD sufferers have been described as fixated in, trapped by, and attached to the trauma (Freud, 1920/1954; Kardiner, 1941; van der Kolk, 1984, 1987, 1989; Wilson & Zigelbaum, 1986).

Profile of PTSD

The Rorschach captures the process of perception and describes the subject's basic psychological organization in terms of behavioral functioning. Other significant findings can be heuristically clustered as follows.

Reality Testing

Reality testing among the sample was impaired, as measured by poor form quality ($X + \%$, $X - \%$, $F + \%$). There was significant perceptual-mediational distortion. The inclusion of good form in a response is considered to be an ego operation. Clearly, failures in modulating affect throughout the sample subjects' responses were the major contributing factor in the diminishment of appropriate reality testing. Additionally, there was an overcommitment to individuality, as measured by the elevation in unusual form quality ($Xu\%$), which also had an impact on consensual reality perception. However, the sample indicated an ability or willingness to see the more commonplace features of the cards, represented by the lack of significant difference in Popular responses.

Problems in emotional control, as well as preoccupation, appear to have had a disorganizing effect on subjects' cognitive processing. As the discussion of Hypothesis 1 suggested, intrusive thoughts and feelings can create disorganization, confusion, and other symptoms of mental impairment.

The combination of poor reality testing ($X + \%$, $X - \%$, $F + \%$), a normal amount of Popular responses, and significantly lower D scores because of intense situational distress suggests that PTSD sufferers may be aware of conventional reality, but simply unable to modulate their emotions in a way that would allow them to utilize more adaptive forms of behavior.

Thinking

Other significant variables support Hypothesis 1, which showed how trauma impairs ideational operations. The sample used considerable effort and cognitive sophistication in organizing or synthesizing their responses in a meaningful way (Zf). Such activity can be seen as an analogue for the constant need among trauma survivors to make meaning out of their experience: to make sense of what happened to them. This process is described throughout the literature as necessary to the transformation and recovery from PTSD (Bard, Arnone, & Nemiroff, 1986; Horowitz, 1976; Krystal, 1988; Lifton, 1976, 1988; van der Kolk, 1984; Wilson, 1989).

Although the sample organized more than normals, they were less efficient in their attempts to process information. It appears that being affectively overwhelmed, along with attempting to avoid emotionally provocative stimuli, may have created hasty decision-making and negligence in information processing. This impulsive approach to problem-solving was seen in the significantly lower Zd (Organizational Efficiency). Wilson (personal communication, 1990) suggested that the trauma imprint creates the tendency for premature closure of the stimulus field.

Underlying cognitive schema prepare or even buffer people in their capacity for adaptation. The unusual significance of Ambitensive EB styles suggests that the majority of sample subjects do not have a preferential style with which they can more efficiently accommodate and assimilate the traumatic events and sequelae. The Hartman *et al.* (1990) study also found an unusually large proportion of Vietnam veterans with PTSD to have ambitent EB styles. Ambitents take more time to achieve solutions, and are therefore more stress-vulnerable. It is possible to speculate that the lack of stable response style might create more difficulty in successfully coping with and integrating the trauma. In this study, neither the preference for using one's inner life to exert control over feelings during ideational operations (introversive), nor the routine propensity toward manifesting affect in an interchange with the environment (extratensive) were effective in the face of such overwhelming events.

The sample showed significant rigidity in thinking (either side of the a:p ratio being three times higher), which indicates a narrowness or inflexibility in thought processes. This lack of ability to try a wide range of thinking operations may be an inherent psychological style, or may be the result of emotional numbing. Clearly, it is possible to speculate that the presence of cognitive or ideational rigidity diminishes the ability to accommodate and assimilate new material, and may be the "pivotal hook" upon which the syndrome continues to swing, rather than an enablement to recovery.

Another indication of rigid thinking is the significant elevation in Perseveration responses (*PSV*) which shows either difficulty in switching sets, or some kind of psychological preoccupation. This finding is analogous to emphasis in the literature on the universal fixation on the trauma, and the resulting psychological paralysis (Freud, 1920/1954; Horowitz, 1985; van der Kolk, 1987; van der Kolk & Ducey, 1989). The significant amount of behavioral passivity (*p > a*) and passive-dependency (*Mp > Ma*) seen in the sample can be interpreted in the framework of learned helplessness, discussed in the literature as a common reaction to trauma (Lifton & Olson, 1976; Peterson & Seligman, 1983; Titchener & Kapp, 1976; van der Kolk, 1987). Subjects appear to use passive forms of fantasy in a defensive maneuver. This passive-dependent style has implications on the interpersonal level, and will be elaborated further in a later section.

Where the van der Kolk and Ducey study (1989) found a lack of capacity to use thought as a delaying or perspective-taking tactic, this study found a significantly lower use of intellectualization as a similar defensive strategy. Perhaps the profound nature of trauma and its disruptive effect on thinking diminishes the ability to cope through intellectualization. Only one dependent variable of the Intellectualization Index, *AB* (abstract, symbolic reference), was elevated. This finding may indicate that, while attempts are made to ward off threats to the self, intellectualization remains an unsuccessful defensive tactic.

Affect and Control

The sample showed evidence of unmodulated affect, constricted access to affect, and avoidance of affectively provocative stimuli. In addition to the intensely distressing affect found in the elevation in diffuse shading responses (*Y*), the sample had an elevation in Vista responses (*V*), which represent the most painful affective states. Certainly, trauma residue includes intensely painful feelings of terror, disgust, rage, anxiety, irritation, and apprehensiveness.

Although depression is viewed in the literature by some authors as the final common pathway of unresolved PTSD, this study found only slight indications of depressive features—two subjects scored positive on the Depression Index (DEPI). It is possible to speculate that this finding may be related to length of time since the stressor which in this study was an average of 3 years, but not more than 10 years. It is important to remember, however, that Exner (1986) suggests a rule-in, rather than rule-out, approach. Therefore, depression cannot be ruled-out as a corollary of PTSD.

The capability for control is related to capacity for stress tolerance. The sample was markedly overloaded by stimulus demands (minus *D* Scores), even though subjects had a normatively average amount of available resources (Experience Actual [EA]). The elevations in (*m*) and (*Y*) accounted for most of the stimulus overload. Therefore, under ordinary conditions (one might postulate, pretrauma conditions) it is reasonable to infer that subjects had sufficient ego resources with which to tolerate stress. There was no difference in EA between the

sample and normal populations. EA is an index of the availability of ego resources. This outcome bolsters the conclusion that resources are organized in such a manner that make them potentially available for use under ordinary circumstances. Because trauma is defined by the DSM-III-R (American Psychiatric Association, 1987) as a stressor "outside the range of usual human experience" (p. 250), it seems obvious that such situational demands would impair available resources.

There was significant lack of normal censoring, which is another indication of diminished controls. Sex (*Sx*) and Blood (*Bl*) responses were markedly elevated, indicating a reduced ability to suppress impulses, owing to a tenuous hold on affect. Clearly, despite attempts to avoid or deny affectively provocative stimuli, unmodulated affect was in excess of the capacity to control.

In addition, elevations in the use of Space responses (*S*) suggest the existence of anger or hostility, particularly when autonomy is threatened. As Freud (1920/1954) and Lindy (1985) suggested, trauma creates a breach of the stimulus barrier. The normal "membrane" becomes easily perforated from within, yet as a later section on interpersonal issues will discuss, the membrane is less permeable to the outside world.

Sample subjects, however, do use some defensive mechanisms to counteract losing control. Along with attempts to avoid affective stimulation (low *Afr*), subjects tend to narrow the field. They create a more limited environment, which may seem easier to manage. The emphasis on uncommon detail responses (*Dd*) is a way of selectively attending to specific portions of the inkblot and thereby delimiting the fuller picture.

Relationship to Self and Others

One of the most compelling results of the statistical analyses was the bimodal distribution of texture responses (*T*). For the most part, subjects had *T*-less protocols, but when texture did occur, it occurred with unusual frequency. An elevation in texture is usually the product of some recent, significant emotional loss. Along with the loss of the belief in a just or ordered world, the trauma survivors in this study lost the illusion of invulnerability. Moreover, some lost functioning body parts, some lost loved ones and were bereaved, and some lost the ability to function independently in the world. It is not surprising that for some victims, the loss-stress relationship created stronger needs for affective closeness.

However, most of the subjects appear to have stopped reaching out to others. The criteria for subjects included normal functioning pretrauma, and it is assumed, therefore, that most subjects would have fallen within the normal range of affective reaching out, rather than assuming they did not know how to reach out in the first place. As a whole, the sample can be characterized as distant, or interpersonally guarded. They are more concerned about issues of personal space, as corroborated by the Hypervigilance Index (HVI). Further, the elevation in Clothing contents (*Cg*) underscores subjects' need to maintain a guarded, self-protective position. This guarded stance is reminiscent of a hardened "outer shell," or body armor: the creation of a trauma membrane to protect oneself from further feared threats (Lindy, 1985).

The elevation in human detail responses (*Hd* and [*Hd*]) suggests that subjects are overly suspicious of others. There is a distorted view of people, who are seen as unreal, or unavailable. Indeed, people are viewed more as unreal fragments than whole human beings. It is not surprising that victims do not look to other people for help, or yearn for closeness. Relationships are impaired, as previously suggested by *M*- responses in Hypothesis 1. Trauma is often synonymous with betrayal. Trust is shattered. How can relationships not be affected?

It seems contradictory that the sample was significantly passive-dependent, in light of their guardedness and lack of reaching out, and this finding is probably indicative of an area of internal conflict. For some victims, human relationships may be impaired by the conflict over need and nurturing versus a decreased sense of trust.

In the PTSD sample, thinking is marked by pessimism, which is pervasive in relationships. The elevation in Morbid responses (*MOR*) also relates to a damaged self-image. The self is perceived quite negatively, with considerable, painful focus on liabilities and defects (Vista responses). There is significant bodily concern, as indicated by the elevation in Anatomy contents (*An*).

Although the sample spends an average amount of time in self-focusing activity (normal $3r + (2)/R$), subjects avoid the kind of introspection most related to insight or self-awareness (low *FD*). Considering the amount of damage to self-image, it is not surprising that victims appear unable to look inward without loathing. Clearly, trauma creates considerable changes in self-perception.

Conclusions and Recommendations

The Rorschach was able to tap unconscious mental processes in a manner which highlighted and underscored reports of PTSD throughout the literature. Yet the Rorschach was able to go beyond the "ballpark" snapshots of other psychometric instruments, which may be less sensitive to the specific process of PTSD. Rather, the Rorschach demonstrated a finely tuned calibration of the discrete and subtle levels of the syndrome, suggesting its applicability as a sensitive and exquisite measure of PTSD.

Furthermore, this study suggests a need for amplification and clarification of the DSM-III-R categories. Specifically, Category B3 regarding flashback-type phenomena appears to be a "garbage-pail" category. Data from this study imply the need to differentiate such dissociative phenomena more discretely. The neutral stimulus of the Rorschach was able to trigger intense psychological distress, which suggests that there may be emotional overload without ideation—without an obvious trigger as delineated in Category B4. Similarly, no other reexperiencing (*B*) category actually deals with affect overload (see Wilson, 1989, for a discussion).

Rorschach and PTSD

Based on the current study and those reviewed, Table 16.2 supplies the Rorschach variables that correspond to DSM-III-R categories.

The avoidance symptoms described in Category C were all corroborated by Rorschach data. However, this study underscores the combination of avoidant features

Table 16.2. Comparison of DSM-III-R Categories and Rorschach Variables

DSM-III-R category	Rorschach variables
B: Reexperiencing symptoms	
1. Intrusions	$M-$; $CF + C > FC$; m & Y; HVI; PSV; Sx & Bl
2. Dreams	Indices not found
3. Dissociative symptoms: Flashbacks and reliving illusions and hallucinations	Pure C; concrete trauma-related responses; m & Y; $M-$; M no form; $FAB2$; $X + \%$; $X - \%$; AB
4. Distress at triggers	m & Y; $CF + C > FC$; D score; $?V$
C: Avoidance symptoms	
1. Avoid thoughts or feelings	Afr; AB
2. Avoid situations	Afr; HVI; Zd; $Hd > H$
3. Amnesia	Indices not found
4. Diminished interest	Afr; brief records
5. Detachment	M no form; Afr; $M-$; HVI; no T; FD; Pure $H < 2$
6. Restricted range of affect	Afr; $FC + CF + C + Cn$
7. Sense of doom	HVI; ?Morbid responses
D: Arousal symptoms	
1. Difficulty with sleep	Indices not found
2. Irritability	m & Y; $AdjD$ score
3. Difficulty concentrating	?Pure C; Zd
4. Hypervigilance	HVI
5. Startle	?Pure C
6. Physiologic reactivity	?Afr & $CF + C > FC$; ?Pure C; ?concrete trauma-related response

and intrusive symptomatology rather than the common misperception that the biphasic process is one reaction alternating with the other. Although the behavior of patients with PTSD may suggest more pure phasic responses, this study suggests that PTSD sufferers undergo dualistic and complex unconscious cognitive and affective processes. They use many conscious and unconscious avoidance operations including narrowing the stimulus field, selective attention, and avoidance of emotionally provocative stimuli as defensive strategies to counteract unmodulated emotion, intensely distressing affects, and diminished ability to harness ego resources in the service of controlling impulses.

This finding has particular relevance for clinical practice. Clinicians must understand PTSD as having a volatile and dynamic relationship between avoidance and reexperiencing: it is a tension state in which both aspects exist concurrently. Therefore, the first goal of treatment must be the creation of a positive, empathic alliance in which the therapist is seen as a "safe other." Respect for the patient's need to feel a sense of control in the treatment process must be paramount. The therapist and patient can form a temporary unit in which both can tolerate and digest affect-laden material. In such a way, the therapist temporarily replaces the impaired cognitive mechanisms which normally modulate intense affects, by linking feelings or fragments of sensations to real events, and by validating and normalizing that such responses are normal reactions to abnormal events. This prerequisite necessitates a delicate balance between allowing the patient to set the pace of unfolding the trauma story, and helping the patient titrate the amount of affect-laden memories until self-regulation and equilibrium are achieved.

Finally, the Rorschach can be utilized as a sensitive measure of recovery. As such, the Rorschach can provide an objective, data-based outcome of therapeutic intervention. Clearly, a goal of treatment is for the patient to escape the "tentacles" of the trauma, to "spring" the trauma trap, and thus, to be able to live more fully in the present.

References

American Psychiatric Association. (1980). *Diagnostic and statistical manual of mental disorders* (3rd ed.). Washington, DC: Author.

American Psychiatric Association. (1987). *Diagnostic and statistical manual of mental disorders* (3rd ed., rev.). Washington, DC: Author.

Aron, L. (1982). Stressful life events and Rorschach content. *Journal of Personality Assessment, 46*(6), 582–585.

Bard, M., Arnone, H., & Nemiroff, D. (1986). Contextual influences on the post-traumatic stress adaptation of homicide survivor-victims. In C. R. Figley (Ed.), *Trauma and its wake: Vol. II. Traumatic stress theory, research, and intervention.* New York: Brunner/Mazel.

Bard, M., & Sangrey, D. (1986). *The crime victim's book* (2nd ed.). New York: Brunner/Mazel.

Bersoff, S. (1970). Rorschach correlates of traumatic neurosis of war. *Journal of Projective Techniques and Personality Assessment, 34*(3), 194–200.

Brett, E., & Ostroff, R. (1985). Imagery and post-traumatic stress disorder: An overview. *American Journal of Psychiatry, 142*(4), 417–424.

Burgess, A., & Holmstrom, R. (1974). Rape trauma syndrome. *American Journal of Psychiatry, 131,* 981–985.

Burke, H., & Mayer, S. (1985). The MMPI and the post-traumatic stress syndrome in Vietnam era veterans. *Journal of Clinical Psychology, 41*(2), 152–156.

Carr, A. (1984). Content interpretation re: Salley and Teiling's "Dissociated rage attacks in a Vietnam veteran: A Rorschach study." *Journal of Personality Assessment, 48*(4), 420–421.

Carr, A. (1985). Rorschach content interpretation in post-traumatic stress disorders: A reply to Kowitt. *Journal of Personality Assessment, 49*(1), 25.

Davidson, P., & Jackson, C. (1985). The nurse as a survivor: Delayed post-traumatic stress reaction and cumulative trauma in nursing. *International Journal of Nursing Studies, 22*(1), 1–13.

Durham, T., McCammon, S., Allison, Y., & Williamson, J. (1987). *Psychological adjustment of rescue workers following two disasters.* Paper presented at the national meeting of the Academy of Criminal Justice Sciences, St. Louis, MO.

Exner, J. (1974). *The Rorschach: A comprehensive system.* New York: Wiley.

Exner, J. (1985). *A Rorschach workbook for the comprehensive system* (2nd ed.). New York: Rorschach Workshops.

Exner, J. (1986). *The Rorschach: A comprehensive system: Vol. I. Basic foundations* (2nd ed.). New York: Wiley.

Exner, J. (1990). *A Rorschach workbook for the comprehensive system* (3rd ed.). , North Carolina: Rorschach Workshops.

Freud, S. (1954). Beyond the pleasure principle. In J. Strachey (Ed. and Trans.), *The standard edition of the complete psychological works of Sigmund Freud* (Vol. 3). London: Hogarth Press, 1954. (Original work published 1920)

Green, B. L., & Grace, M. (1988). Conceptual issues in research. In J. Wilson, Z. Harel, & B. Kahana (Eds.), *Human adaptation to extreme stress: From the holocaust to Vietnam.* New York: Plenum Press.

Green, B. L., Lindy, J., & Grace, M. (1985). Post-traumatic stress disorder: Toward DSM-IV. *Journal of Nervous and Mental Disease, 173*(7), 406–411.

Hartman, C., & Burgess, A. (1988). Rape trauma and the treatment of women. In F. Ochberg (Ed.), *Post-traumatic therapy and victims of violence.* New York: Brunner/Mazel.

Hartman, W., Clark, M., Morgan, M., Dunn, V., Fine, A., Perry, G., & Winsch, D. (1990). Rorschach structure of a hospitalized sample of Vietnam veterans with PTSD. *Journal of Personality Assessment, 54*(1 & 2), 149–159.

Horowitz, M. (1976). *Stress response syndromes.* New York: Jason Aronson.

Horowitz, M. (1985). Disasters and psychological responses to stress. *Psychiatric Annals, 15*(3), 161–167.

Horowitz, M., Wilner, N., & Alvarez, W. (1979). Impact of event scale: A measure of subjective stress. *Psychosomatic Medicine, 41*(3), 209–218.

Janoff-Bulman, R. (1985). The aftermath of victimization: Rebuilding shattered assumptions. In C. R. Figley (Ed.), *Trauma and its wake: The study and treatment of post-traumatic stress disorder* (pp. 15–35). New York: Brunner/Mazel.

Kardiner, A. (1941). *The traumatic neuroses of war.* New York: Paul B. Hoeber.

Keane, T. (1989). Personal communication with the author.

Keane, T., Malloy, P., & Fairbank, J. (1984). Empirical development of an MMPI subscale for the assessment of combat-related posttraumatic stress disorder. *Journal of Consulting and Clinical Psychology, 52*(5), 888–891.

Kowitt, M. (1985). Rorschach content interpretation in posttraumatic stress disorders: A reply to Carr. *Journal of Personality Assessment, 49*(1), 21–24.

Krystal, H. (1984). Psychoanalytic views of human emotional damages. In B. van der Kolk (Ed.), *Post-traumatic stress disorder: Psychological and biological sequelae* Washington, DC: American Psychiatric Press.

Krystal, H. (1988). *Integration and self healing: Affect, trauma, alexithymia.* New York: Analytic Press.

Krystal, H., & Niederland, W. (1968). Clinical observations on the survivor syndrome. In H. Krystal (Ed.), *Massive psychic trauma* New York: International University Press.

Lejeune, A. (1973, October). On being mugged. *Urban Life and Culture,* 254–287.

Lewis, C., & Arsenian, J. (1982). Psychological resolution of homicide after ten years. *Journal of Personality Assessment, 46*(6), 647–657.

Lifton, R. J. (1976). *The life of the self.* New York: Simon & Schuster.

Lifton, R. J. (1988). Understanding the traumatized self: Imagery, symbolization, and transformation. In J. P. Wilson, Z. Harel, & B. Kahana (Eds.), *Human adaptation to extreme stress: From the Holocaust to Vietnam* (pp. 7–31). New York: Plenum Press.

Lifton, R. J., & Olson, E. (1976). The human meaning of total disaster: The Buffalo Creek experience. *Psychiatry, 39,* 1–18.

Lindy, J. (1985). The trauma membrane and other clinical concepts derived from psychotherapeutic work with survivors of natural disasters. *Psychiatric Annals, 15*(3), 153–160.

Lindy, J. D., Green, B. L., Grace, M., & Titchener, J. (1983). Psychotherapy with survivors of the Beverly Hills Supper Club fire. *American Journal of Psychotherapy, 37,* 593–610.

Modlin, H. (1967). A post accident anxiety syndrome: Psychosocial aspects. *American Journal of Psychiatry, 123*(8), 1008–1012.

Newman, J. (1987). Differential diagnosis in post-traumatic stress disorder: Implications for treatment. In T. Williams (Ed.), *Post-traumatic stress disorder: A handbook for clinicians* Cincinnati, OH: Disabled American Veterans.

Nichols, B., & Czirr, R. (1986). Post-traumatic stress disorder: Hidden syndrome in elders. *Clinical Gerontologist, 5*(3 & 4), 417–433.

Niederland, W. (1964). Psychiatric disorders among persecution victims: A contribution to the understanding of concentration camp pathology and its after-effects. *Journal of Nervous and Mental Diseases, 139,* 458–474.

Ochberg, F. (1988). Post-traumatic therapy and victims of violence. In F. Ochberg (Ed.), *Post-traumatic therapy and victims of violence.* New York: Brunner/Mazel.

Parker, K. (1983). A meta-analysis of the reliability and validity of the Rorschach. *Journal of Personality Assessment, 47*(3), 227–231.

Peterson, C., & Seligman, M. (1983). Learned helplessness and victimization. *Journal of Social Issues, 2,* 103–116.

Robins, L. N., Helzer, J. E., Croughan, J., & Ratcliff, K. S. (1981). The NIMH Diagnostic Interview Schedule: Its history, characteristics, and validity. *Archives of General Psychiatry, 38,* 1381–1389.

Rose, D. (1986). "Worse than death": Psychodynamics of rape victims and the need for psychotherapy. *American Journal of Psychiatry, 143*(7), 817–824.

Sales, E., Baum, M., & Shore, R. (1984). Victim readjustment following assault. *Journal of Social Issues, 40*(1), 117–136.

Salley, R., & Teiling, P. (1984). Dissociated rage attacks in a Vietnam veteran: A Rorschach study. *Journal of Personality Assessment, 48*(1), 98–104.

Schachtel. (1966). *Experimental foundations of Rorschach's test.* New York: Basic Books, p. 186.

Scurfield, R. (1985). Post-traumatic stress assessment and treatment: Overview and formulations. In C. Figley (Ed.), *Trauma and its wake: The study and treament of post-traumatic stress disorder* (pp. 219–256). New York: Brunner/Mazel.

Seamons, D., Howell, R., Carlisle, A., & Roe, A. (1981). Rorschach simulation of mental illness and normality by psychotic and non-psychotic legal offenders. *Journal of Personality Assessment, 4*(2), 130–135.

Shalit, B. (1965). Effects of environmental stimulation on the M, FM and m responses in the Rorschach. *Journal of Projective Techniques and Personality Assessment, 29,* 228–231.

Souffront, E. (1987). The use of the Rorschach in the assessment of post-traumatic stress disorder among Vietnam combat veterans. (Doctoral dissertation, Temple University, 1987.) *Dissertation Abstracts International, 48,* 04B.

St. Pierre, J. (1988). *Rorschach responses of sexually abused children.* Unpublished doctoral dissertation, Massachusetts School of Professional Psychology, MA.

Swanson, G., Blount, J., & Bruno, R. (1990). Comprehensive system Rorschach data on Vietnam combat veterans. *Journal of Personality Assessment, 54*(1 & 2), 160–169.

Thorndike, R., & Hagen, E. (1969). *Measurement and evaluation in psychology and education.* New York: Wiley.

Titchener, J., & Kapp, F. (1976). Family and character change at Buffalo Creek. *American Journal of Psychiatry, 133*(3), 295–299.

Trimble, M. (1981). *Post-traumatic neurosis: From railway spine to whiplash.* New York: Wiley.

van der Kolk, B. (1984). *Adult psychic trauma: Psychological and biological sequelae.* Washington, DC: American Psychiatric Press.

van der Kolk, B. (1987). The psychological consequences of overwhelming life experiences. In B. van der Kolk (Ed.), *Psychological trauma* (pp. 1–30). Washington, DC: American Psychiatric Press.

van der Kolk, B., & Ducey, C. (1989). The psychological processing of traumatic experience: Rorschach patterns in post-traumatic stress disorder. *Journal of Traumatic Stress, 2*(3), 259–274.

van der Kolk, B., & van der Hart, O. (1989). Pierre Janet and the rediscovery of psychological trauma. *American Journal of Psychiatry, 146*(12), 1530–1540.

Wilson, J. (1989). *Trauma, transformation, and healing: An integrative approach to theory, research and post-traumatic therapy.* New York: Brunner/Mazel.

Wilson, J. P. (1990). Personal communication with the author.

Wilson, J., Harel, Z., & Kahana, B. (Eds.). (1988). *Human adaptation to extreme stress: From the Holocaust to Vietnam.* New York: Plenum Press.

Wilson, J., Smith, W. K., & Johnson, S. (1985). A comparative analysis of PTSD among various survivor groups. In C. R. Figley (Ed.), *Trauma and its wake: The study and treatment of post-traumatic stress disorder* (pp. 142–172). New York: Brunner/Mazel.

Wilson, J., & Zigelbaum, S. D. (1986). Post-traumatic stress disorder and the disposition to criminal behavior. In C. R. Figley (Ed.), *Trauma and its wake: Vol. II. Traumatic stress theory, research and intervention* (pp. 305–321). New York: Brunner/Mazel.

Zilberg, N., Weiss, D., & Horowitz, M. (1982). Impact of Event Scale: A cross-validation study and some empirical evidence supporting a conceptual model of stress response syndromes. *Journal of Consulting and Clinical Psychology, 30,* 407–414.

CHAPTER 17

Posttrauma Reactions Following a Multiple Shooting

A Retrospective Study and Methodological Inquiry

**Mark Creamer, Philip Burgess, William Buckingham,
and Philippa Pattison**

Introduction

This chapter describes an investigation of psychological reactions among the survivors of a multiple shooting that occurred in a Melbourne city office block on December 8, 1987. Nine people died and a further five were injured in an incident that has become known as the Queen Street Shootings. The research was undertaken to examine levels of posttrauma reactions over time and to identify those factors that may affect reaction to, and recovery from, trauma.

Reaction to trauma has been defined as "an emotional state of discomfort and stress resulting from memories of an extraordinary, catastrophic experience which shattered the survivor's sense of invulnerability to harm" (Figley, 1985b, p. xviii). Such posttrauma reactions have been the focus of considerable interest over the last few years, particularly since the recognition of Posttraumatic Stress Disorder (PTSD) as a separate diagnos-

tic entity in the third edition of the *Diagnostic and Statistical Manual of Mental Disorders* (DSM-III) (American Psychiatric Association [APA], 1980). The last decade has seen a substantial amount of research in the area, much of which has addressed the psychological sequelae of combat or natural disasters. Rates of morbidity vary according to the criteria used and the extent and nature of the trauma. It appears, however, that the presence of psychological symptoms following exposure to a traumatic incident is the norm rather than the exception, particularly in the period immediately posttrauma (Quarantelli, 1985; Wilson, Smith, & Johnson, 1985). Unfortunately, however, longitudinal studies are rare and few attempts have been made to chart the course of posttrauma reactions over time.

Studies investigating reactions to disasters of human origin are less common. Such research is of great importance, however, especially given the increasing interest in cognitive processing models of posttrauma reactions (Foa, Steketee, & Rothbaum, 1989; Green, Wilson, & Lindy, 1985). Those traumata resulting from pure human malevolence may be expected to shatter more basic assumptions (Janoff-Bulman, 1985) and be harder for victims to understand and cognitively process (Figley, 1985a) than those resulting from combat experiences or natural disasters. In addition, traumata of human origin are thought to result in more severe psychological reactions than natural disasters (APA, 1980). Such incidents constitute a challenge for the helping professions in their efforts to assist survivors in processing and integrating the trauma.

The current research sought to investigate the psychological effects of a multiple shooting, as well as iden-

Mark Creamer • Health Department Victoria, and Department of Psychology, University of Melbourne, Parkville, Victoria 3052, Australia. **Philip Burgess** • Psychiatric Epidemiology and Services Evaluation Unit, Health Department Victoria, Parkville, Victoria 3052, Australia. **William Buckingham** • Office of Psychiatric Services, Health Department, Melbourne, Victoria 3000, Australia. **Philippa Pattison** • Department of Psychology, University of Melbourne, Parkville, Victoria 3052, Australia.

International Handbook of Traumatic Stress Syndromes, edited by John P. Wilson and Beverley Raphael. Plenum Press, New York, 1993.

tifying those factors that may predispose an individual to the development of posttrauma reactions. A three-stage, prospective research design was utilized. This chapter is based on findings from a more detailed report of the research (Creamer, Burgess, Buckingham, & Pattison, 1989)

The Incident

The shootings occurred in an 18-story office building located in the center of Melbourne, a city of approximately three million people. A gunman entered the building late on a Tuesday afternoon and proceeded to the fifth floor where he asked to see a particular staff member. (It emerged during the coronial inquest that the gunman had known this person at school and had developed an intense and irrational hatred of him in the intervening years.) When the staff member appeared, the gunman produced a sawed-off, semiautomatic rifle. As people ran for cover, he pursued them, firing a number of shots and killing a 19-year-old female staff member.

Unable to catch his intended victim, he proceeded to the 12th floor although it is unclear why he chose this level. He entered the work area and fired repeatedly at people hiding under desks and behind partitions. He killed three people on this floor and severely injured one other. He then left this work area and proceeded down the stairs to the 11th floor. In a similar fashion, he paced up and down between the desks, firing frequently at individuals where they were hiding. He killed four people on this floor and injured another four. He reportedly spoke often throughout the incident, saying such things as "You're all scum; well, who's laughing now? I'm going to take you all with me." Individual killings were prolonged and sadistic in nature, with the gunman tormenting and mocking his victims. Eventually he was tackled from behind and a brief struggle ensued, during which the gun was taken from him. He managed to break free and clambered through a broken window. Despite attempts by staff to hold on to him, he finally kicked loose and fell to his death on the pavement below.

It should be noted that the gun was not functioning properly throughout the incident. A total of 41 shots were fired, but a further 184 unspent cartridges were ejected from the rifle during the incident as the gunman repeatedly tried to make it operate. Thus, a number of people had the gun pointed at them and the trigger pulled, with the weapon failing to discharge. There is no doubt that the carnage would have been considerably worse had the gun been functioning properly.

At the time of the shootings, approximately 850 people were employed in the building, although many had left to go home by the time the incident occurred. Those who were still there experienced a range of exposure to trauma: As well as those who received physical injuries, some saw their colleagues being shot, some had the gun pointed at them with the rifle failing to discharge, and some attempted to assist their dead and injured workmates before the emergency services arrived. Many people in the building were in fear for their lives: Even those on the floors not directly affected knew that a shooting was taking place and barricaded themselves into their work areas; they did not know that they were safe until the police came through the building some time later. Staff not in the building at the time were obviously affected also, as were the families of those involved.

It is clear that the shootings constituted a severe trauma for the subjects of this research. The incident was characterized by a number of features normally associated with severe posttrauma reactions, such as significant threat to life, bereavement, unpredictability, exposure to grotesque sights, and sudden onset (Green, 1982).

An extensive mental health recovery program was mounted in the building following the shootings and was retained throughout the first year posttrauma. The program was integrated into the affected community and was coordinated by the senior author. As well as a range of community-based strategies, individual and group treatment was made readily accessible. Unfortunately, a controlled empirical evaluation of this program was neither ethically nor practically possible. Thus, the extent to which these interventions affected recovery from the trauma remains purely speculative.

Research Design

The research utilized a repeated measures survey methodology, with data collection at 4-, 8-, and 14-months posttrauma. Timing of data collection was dictated by the practicalities of the research: As well as ensuring appropriate measurement intervals, other events that may have affected levels of distress (such as the coronial inquest and the anniversary) had to be taken into account. The method of data collection (self-report) was chosen for practical reasons, given the large subject group, as well as to provide comparability with earlier research. Consideration was given to the possibility of obtaining a formal diagnosis, particularly with reference to PTSD. Unfortunately, this would have been possible only by means of a structured clinical interview and was considered to be beyond the scope of the current study.

Research Subjects

All people employed in the building at the time of the shootings were utilized as a potential subject pool; thus, individuals did not have to actively volunteer to receive a copy of the survey. Nevertheless, this group remains a volunteer population in that participation in the research was not compulsory. This group of subjects is referred to in this chapter as the *trauma group*.

Because the study was concerned with adaptation as a function of trauma, a *contrast group* was used to enable results to be compared with a nontraumatized sample. A group of office workers from a similarly sized office building in the Melbourne city area was selected. The organization employing these subjects was a public sector corporation similar to that of the trauma group.

Thus, although such a group does not constitute a matched control, it does provide a very appropriate comparison. Despite differing from the trauma group on some sociodemographic variables (see below), the contrast group is a closer match than, for example, the groups cited for the published normative data on tests used in the research.

The Survey

In the process of survey development, the authors attempted to operationalize psychosocial factors that have been speculated to affect recovery from trauma (see, for example, Raphael, 1986). Previous posttrauma research and an earlier version of guidelines recommended by Raphael and her colleagues (Raphael, Lundin, & Weisaeth, 1989) were also considered. A major consideration was also the time required to complete the survey; it was felt that a more lengthy survey would jeopardize a reasonable response rate. Full details of the survey have been provided elsewhere (Creamer et al., 1989); only a brief summary will be provided here. The survey included three well-established scales and covered a number of other relevant areas, as follows:

1. *Impact of Events Scale (IES)* (Horowitz, Wilner, & Alvarez, 1979): This 15-item scale is widely used in posttrauma research and taps the two most commonly reported experiences in response to stressful events (intrusive thoughts and avoidance). The IES has good psychometric properties (Zilberg, Weiss, & Horowitz, 1982) and its use has been recommended by Raphael and her colleagues (1989).

2. *The Symptom Checklist 90 Revised (SCL-90-R)* (Derogatis, 1977): This scale was included to provide a broad, objective measure of symptomatology. It provides information on nine specific symptom subscales as well as overall indices of symptom severity. The Global Severity Index (GSI), an overall measure of the number and severity of problems, represents the most useful single indicator of current distress and is used for most of the analyses reported in this chapter. The SCL-90-R has been widely used in previous studies of posttrauma reactions (Davidson & Baum, 1986; Woolfolk & Grady, 1988).

3. *General Health Questionnaire (GHQ)* (Goldberg, 1972): The 12-item version of the GHQ was included primarily to provide comparisons with previous studies in Australia. The GHQ is a well respected and widely used instrument for the detection of psychiatric morbidity in posttrauma research (McFarlane, 1988; Parker, 1977) and its use has again been recommended by Raphael et al. (1989).

4. *Sociodemographic Information*: This category was included both to provide descriptive data on subjects and to identify any high-risk categories in terms of symptom development.

5. *Social Support Networks*: Social support has been widely considered to be an important factor in recovery from trauma (Cohen & Willis, 1985; Solomon, 1986). In the absence of a well-validated social support scale for use in posttrauma research, these questions were developed specifically for the current study. This approach is in common with many previous studies (Green & Berlin, 1987; Green, Grace, & Gleser, 1985).

The social support scale comprised seven questions. Principle components analysis revealed two factors. Factor 1 (Need) comprised three questions and covered need for, availability of, and use of social support networks. The second factor (Help), comprising four questions, covered the degree of perceived helpfulness of social support networks. Responses were aggregated to arrive at values for Need (with high scores indicating a high degree of need for, availability of, and use of social support networks) and Help (with high scores indicating a high degree of perceived helpfulness of social support networks). Alpha coefficients for Need (3 items) ranged from .52 to .73 and for Help (4 items) from .68 to .74. Given the low number of questions in each scale, these figures suggest reasonable levels of internal consistency.

6. *Treatment*: A detailed description of treatment received following the shootings was beyond the scope of the current survey. Nevertheless, subjects were asked whether they had received medication or counseling during each stage of the research.

7. *Stressful Life Events*: A seven-item list of stressful life events was derived from consideration of the relevant research (Zimmerman, 1983), because existing life events scales were considered to be too lengthy for inclusion in the current survey. Much previous posttrauma research has used similar short lists (McFarlane, 1987) or has simply asked respondents to report any stressful life events occurring during the period of the research (Green, Grace, & Gleser, 1985). Subjects were asked if they had experienced any of these events in either the year before or the period since the shootings. The number of events reported was summed to give a total score (SLE), possible scores ranging from 0 to 7.

Although it would have been desirable to obtain some indication of the way in which the individual coped with these events, there appeared to be no efficient measurement strategy. However, subjects were asked if they had received individual counseling for a psychological problem in the 5 years preceding the shootings. This question was used as a crude indicator of the presence of previous psychological problems. It is recognized that this is an assumption; people may receive treatment for a variety of reasons, ranging from relatively minor situational disturbances through to severe psychiatric disorders. There would have been some difficulty, however, in accessing more detailed information about previous psychological functioning.

8. *Avoidance*: As well as the Avoidance subscale of the IES, subjects were asked the extent to which they had avoided going to the floors on which the shootings took place. Respondents answered on a nine-point scale ranging from "I have not avoided it" to "I always avoid it."

9. *Exposure to Trauma*: A series of questions was designed to measure the subjects' experience of the shootings. On the basis of a brief pilot study, a hierarchical four-point measure of objective exposure to trauma was developed. The criteria comprised being in the building at the time of the shootings, being on one of the floors on which the shootings occurred, and being on an affected floor *and* on the side of the floor on which the shootings took place (i.e., the east side of the building). A single objective index was calculated by summing

these exposure indicators to give a total possible score of 3. Those individuals not in the building at the time scored 0 on the exposure index.

More complex indices of exposure to trauma were investigated, including sighting the gunman and dead or injured co-workers, but these were rejected because they contributed little to the analyses. In addition, such indices were less objective and considered to be of lower validity; for example, more people reported seeing the gunman than could possibly have been the case. It is thought that this confusion arose from the fact that many people saw a reflection of the gunman in the windows of the building opposite when he flung himself out of the window and jumped to his death.

Three subjective questions of experience of the trauma were included and were scored by subjects on nine-point scales. The first of these covered the degree of fear experienced at the time, while the remaining two inquired about the extent to which subjects felt guilty about the way they had behaved during the incident. Responses to the two latter questions were highly correlated (.54, $p < .001$) and were therefore summed for future analyses to give a single "guilt" score.

Although the above questions attempted to assess experience of the trauma, subjects were also asked on which floor they normally worked, regardless of whether they were present at the time of the shootings.

The questionnaire for the contrast group was similar to that described above; a few questions were modified or omitted if they would have made no sense to contrast subjects. Since the research utilized a repeated measures design, questionnaires for Stages 2 and 3 were essentially the same as that for Stage 1. Questions inquiring about information that could not have changed over the intervening period (such as some of the sociodemographic questions) were omitted. The Exposure to Trauma section was omitted in its entirety, since this information had been obtained in Stage 1.

A new section was included at Stages 2 and 3. Developed specifically for the research, it comprised two scales, *Understanding* and *Sense of Security*. The Understanding scale comprised seven questions based on the work of Figley (1985a), and covered the subjects' understanding of what had happened, why it had happened, why it had happened to them, and why they had acted and felt as they did during and since the trauma. The second scale comprised a further four questions inquiring about feelings of insecurity and vulnerability.

Procedure

All staff employed in the building at the time of the shootings were surveyed at 4-months posttrauma, with responders being followed up at 8 and 14 months. Each questionnaire was numbered to allow follow-up data to be compared. All subjects received the survey in a personally addressed envelope delivered to their workplace. It was accompanied by a letter outlining the rationale for the research, the arrangements for ensuring confidentiality and assurances that participation in the study was entirely voluntary. Subjects were asked to return the questionnaire to the senior investigator, regardless of whether it had been completed.

Results

Response Rates

A total of 838 surveys were distributed to the trauma group and 338 to the contrast group at 4-months posttrauma. Of these, 447 trauma and 192 contrast surveys were returned completed, giving response rates of 53% and 57%, respectively. These rates are higher than expected for an unsolicited survey methodology, especially given the nature of the research. Certainly, the response rates for the current research are higher than those for many comparable studies (e.g., Green, Grace, & Gleser, 1985; McFarlane, 1987). In addition, while it remains a volunteer group, it does not suffer from the biases in subject selection (such as restricting the study to those who have presented for treatment) that have characterized much previous research.

At 8-months posttrauma, all those who had responded to Study 1 were resurveyed with the full instrument described above. Response rates of 78% (trauma) and 67% (contrast) were obtained. Those who responded at 8 months were resurveyed at 14 months, with response rates of 76% (trauma) and 68% (contrast).

Comparison of Participants and Nonparticipants

As noted above, 391 of the possible 838 trauma group respondents chose not to participate in the research. This raises questions about the degree to which the trauma group in the research adequately represents the total possible sample. It was therefore decided to survey those individuals who had chosen not to participate in the research with a very brief, anonymous questionnaire. The content and results of this survey have been reported in detail elsewhere (Creamer *et al.*, 1989) and therefore will not be repeated here. Nevertheless, it was clear that nonparticipation was largely a result of practical concerns. The most frequently cited reasons for not responding to the survey included "It was too long," "I was too busy," and "It didn't seem to apply to me." It was also clear that the group who chose not to participate did not differ from the research sample in the terms of degree of exposure to trauma.

More detailed analyses were possible with those subjects who discontinued the research at Stages 2 or 3, since data collected at 4-months posttrauma were available for this group. Information obtained at Stage 1 was categorized into five groups: sociodemographic data; stressful life events; exposure to trauma indices; recovery factors (e.g., social support and avoidance); and symptom levels. For the trauma group, there was no difference on any of these variables between those subjects participating in Stage 2 and those who discontinued the research. The only difference apparent at Stage 3 was country of birth, with those subjects not born in Australia more likely not to continue. This may have been a result of language or cultural factors. In the contrast group, those people on lower salaries were more likely to discontinue the research at Stage 2, whereas younger subjects were more likely to discontinue at Stage 3. It is therefore reassuring to note that those subjects who discontinued the research at Stages 2 or 3 differed little from those who continued to participate.

Description of the Subject Groups

1. *Sociodemographic Data*: The trauma group comprised slightly more males (58%) than females; this compares favourably with the gender breakdown in the total possible sample, which contained 56% males. The trauma group ranged in age from 17 to 64 years, with a mean of 34.9 years ($SD = 9.8$). The majority (60%) were married or in de facto marital relationships, and 40% had at least one child. The average salary was in the A$20,000 to A$25,000 range; 94% had received at least four years of secondary school education and 73% had completed secondary school.

The contrast group did not differ from the trauma group in terms of gender, marital status, children, or educational background. The contrast group, however, were younger (mean = 31.4, $SD = 10.7$, $t[635] = 4.04$, $p < .001$) and, perhaps as a function of this age difference, earned a slightly lower annual salary ($t[624] = 4.74$, $p < .001$). Respondents in the contrast group were more likely than those in the trauma group to have been born in Australia ($X^2[1] = 6.84$, $p < .01$).

2. *Stressful Life Events*: A difference was apparent between the groups in terms of the reporting of stressful life events, with 62% of the trauma group and 52% of the contrast group reporting a major stressful life event in the 12-months pretrauma ($X^2[1] = 5.94$, $p < .01$). Although this may be a reflection of reality, it may also be a "reporting bias." In other words, those people who have recently been through a trauma may be more likely to remember (and report) unpleasant events occurring in their lives. The trauma group continued to report a higher number of stressful life events at all three stages of the research (Stage 1: $X^2[1] = 9.4$, $p < .01$; Stage 2: $X^2[1] = 17.2$, $p < .001$; Stage 3: $X^2[1] = 10.4$, $p < .01$).

3. *Exposure to Trauma*: Approximately two thirds of the trauma group were in the building at the time of the shootings and about 13% were on the floors on which the shootings occurred. The range of scores on the exposure index is inevitably skewed, with large numbers of respondents scoring low on the scale and few scoring highly. This is to be expected given the nature of the trauma and the time at which it occurred; a significant proportion of people had already left to go home and those in the building were distributed across all 18 floors. In fact, the number of respondents on the three affected floors is higher than would be predicted if the population had been distributed equally throughout the building.

4. *Treatment*: Nearly 15% of the trauma group received individual counseling during the first 4-months posttrauma; this figure dropped to 9% and 10%, respectively, at Stages 2 and 3. This compares with 1% or less for the contrast group at each stage. Although the trauma group reported increased use of medication following the shootings, there was no difference between the groups at any stage of the research in the number of subjects taking prescribed medication.

Table 17.1. Alpha Coefficients of, and Pearson Correlation Coefficients between, IES, GSI, and GHQ at 4-, 8-, and 14-Months Posttrauma

	Stage 1			Stage 2			Stage 3		
	IES	GSI	GHQ	IES	GSI	GHQ	IES	GSI	GHQ
IES	.92	.58	.46	.93	.64	.51	.92	.64	.52
GSI		.98	.72		.98	.74		.98	.76
GHQ			.93			.93			.91

Note. Alpha coefficients are shown on the diagonals. All correlations are significant at the .001 level.

Symptom Levels

In order to allow for comparisons across time, only data collected from those subjects who responded to all three surveys will be reported in this section. As noted above, there was no difference in symptom levels for either the trauma or contrast groups between those subjects who participated in all three stages and those who discontinued the research at Stages 2 or 3. The trauma group for these analyses comprised 251 subjects and the contrast group, 84. For analyses involving the SCL-90-R, the Global Severity Index (GSI) is quoted.

As shown in Table 17.1, the three primary symptom measures (IES, GSI, and GHQ) are highly correlated with each other at all three stages of the research. The GSI and GHQ, being general measures of psychological problems, are more closely related with each other than with the trauma-specific measure, the IES. The diagonals in Table 17.1 show the alpha coefficients of each scale.

Although the two subscales of the IES are sensitive to different symptom groups, previous research has shown a strong relationship between them, with interscale correlations ranging from .42 (Horowitz *et al.*, 1979) to .78 (Zilberg *et al.*, 1982). In the current study there was a high correlation between the Intrusion and Avoidance subscales at all three stages (Stage 1: .75, Stage 2: .77, and Stage 3: .76; all these correlations are significant at the .001 level).

Table 17.2 shows the raw scores on the SCL-90-R, IES, and GHQ for the trauma and contrast groups at the three stages of the research. In addition, the table shows an "effect size" of the differences between the groups, calculated by subtracting the contrast group mean from the trauma group mean and dividing by the standard deviation of the contrast group. GHQ scores are commonly interpreted by the use of cut-off points with scores of two or more classified as "cases." Table 17.2 also shows the percentage of respondents in each group scoring 2 or more.

Of interest are the effect sizes for the subscales of the SCL-90-R. The greatest variation between the groups consistently occurred on the Depression (DEP) and Anxiety (ANX) subscales, with effect sizes of at least 1.00 at each stage of the research. The two other scales consistently showing the largest effect sizes between the groups were Lack of Concentration (OCD) and Interpersonal Sensitivity (INT). These four groups of psychologi-

Table 17.2. Trauma and Contrast Group Scores on SCL-90-R, IES, and GHQ at 4-, 8-, and 14-Months Posttrauma

	Stage 1					Stage 2					Stage 3				
	Trauma		Contrast		Effect size	Trauma		Contrast		Effect size	Trauma		Contrast		Effect size
	Mean	SD	Mean	SD		Mean	SD	Mean	SD		Mean	SD	Mean	SD	
SCL-90-R															
SOM	.46	.55	.27	.34	.56	.49	.59	.32	.42	.40	.51	.65	.27	.40	.60
OCD	.72	.78	.35	.42	.88	.71	.75	.38	.44	.75	.71	.81	.30	.44	.93
INT	.64	.74	.31	.38	.87	.67	.78	.37	.41	.73	.65	.81	.31	.40	.85
DEP	.70	.74	.23	.30	1.57	.73	.78	.32	.41	1.00	.69	.80	.26	.31	1.39
ANX	.57	.69	.18	.28	1.39	.54	.67	.20	.28	1.21	.54	.72	.19	.34	1.03
HOS	.55	.69	.27	.37	.82	.60	.76	.29	.44	.70	.55	.72	.29	.48	.54
PHO	.31	.54	.09	.27	.81	.24	.48	.07	.24	.71	.29	.56	.09	.29	.69
PAR	.56	.69	.29	.36	.75	.60	.78	.34	.47	.55	.55	.76	.28	.43	.63
PSY	.34	.54	.15	.28	.69	.32	.49	.17	.35	.43	.34	.57	.14	.33	.61
GSI	.56	.59	.25	.27	1.29	.57	.59	.28	.33	.88	.56	.64	.25	.32	.97
IES															
Intrusion	11.5	8.4	2.1	3.5	2.68	9.6	8.4	1.4	3.1	2.65	9.0	7.8	1.5	2.9	2.59
Avoidance	11.4	9.0	2.5	4.7	1.89	10.4	9.1	1.7	3.6	2.42	9.8	9.1	2.0	4.0	1.95
Total	22.9	16.0	4.6	7.6	2.41	20.0	16.0	3.2	6.1	2.75	18.8	15.6	3.4	6.4	2.41
GHQ score	2.9	3.7	0.8	2.1	1.00	3.3	4.0	1.5	2.6	0.69	2.8	3.6	1.3	2.5	0.60
Proportion scoring > 1	47.6%		16.8%			48.6%		30.2%			46.3%		26.2%		

cal problems correspond closely with the diagnostic criteria for PTSD, which include a number of symptoms normally associated with depression, anxiety, impaired concentration, and problems with interpersonal relationships.

Although not a significant effect, observation of mean scores on the GHQ indicates a small fluctuation over time, with both groups scoring more highly at Stage 2. A possible explanation for this finding lies in the timing of the study: Stage 2 was distributed in August—the middle of the Melbourne winter when colds, influenza, and other minor ailments are rife. This finding suggests that the 12-item version of the GHQ may be sensitive to relatively minor changes in mood and physical health. This instability over time is also apparent when the cut-off scores are examined; the percentage of contrast group subjects scoring 2 or above increases from 17% to 30% in 4 months (i.e., Stage 1 to Stage 2), before dropping back to 26% at Stage 3. This lack of stability suggests that there may be some problems associated with using the 12-item GHQ as a stable and reliable indicator of psychological distress. In addition, the fact that it is not a truly dimensional measure (such as the SCL-90-R), renders it less appropriate for the regression analyses reported below.

Repeated measures multiple analyses of variance (MANOVA) were conducted separately on the SCL-90-R, IES, and GHQ data. Significant group effects were found for all three measures (SCL-90-R: $F[9,318] = 4.47$, $p < .001$; IES: $F[92,324] = 52.86$, $p < .001$; GHQ: $F[1,327] = 23.65$, $p < .001$). Subsequent univariate tests indicated that differences between the groups were significant at the .001 level on all subscales of both the IES and the SCL-90-R. Thus, averaged over time, the trauma group

obtained higher mean scores on the SCL-90-R, IES, and GHQ than the contrast group.

No significant effects were found for time on the SCL-90-R ($F[18,309] = 1.60$, $p > .05$) or the GHQ ($F[2,326] = 2.61$, $p > .05$). There was, however, a significant time effect on the IES ($F[4,322] = 6.20$, $p < .001$). Comparisons between Stage 1 and Stage 2 revealed a significant difference for both the Intrusion ($t[326] = -3.34$, $p < .001$) and Avoidance ($t[326] = -2.27$, $p < .05$) subscales. Comparisons between the mean of Stages 1 and 2, and Stage 3 showed similar effects (Intrusion: $t[326] = -3.67$, $p < .001$; Avoidance: $t[326] = -2.21$, $p < .05$). Thus, there is no evidence to suggest that scores on the SCL-90-R or GHQ reduced over the three stages of the research. Scores on the IES, however, did show a decrease over time, particularly on the intrusion subscale.

There was no significant interaction between group and time effects on any of the three scales. This suggests that differences between the groups on the SCL-90-R, IES, and GHQ were constant over the three stages of the research.

Factors Predicting Symptom Levels

Those variables that may have influenced the development and course of psychological symptoms following the trauma were divided into two groups, namely, *vulnerability factors* and *recovery factors*. Vulnerability factors comprised sociodemographic characteristics, prior psychological treatment, other stressful life events, and experience of the shootings. It is argued that these variables may predispose an individual to the development

Table 17.3. Abbreviated Variable Names and Descriptions

Name	Description
SEX	Female = 2; male = 1
MARR	Marital status; 1 = married or de facto; 2 = not married
SAL	Salary, coded into nine levels per original survey
PRIOR	Counseling for a psychological problem in the 5 years prior to the shootings; 1 = yes; 2 = no
GUIL	Feelings of guilt associated with the shootings (low scores indicate strong feelings)
FEAR	Feelings of fear at the time of the shootings
FLR	Floor on which the individual normally worked, coded by floors where the shooting occurred: 5, 11, 12 = 1; other floors = 0
SLE1	Number of stressful life events in the first 4-months posttrauma
SLE2	Number of stressful life events in the second 4-months posttrauma
SLE3	Number of stressful life events in the third period of the research
NEED1	Need for, availability of, and use of social support networks in the first 4-months posttrauma
NEED2	As for NEED1, in the second 4-months posttrauma
NEED3	As for NEED1, in the third period of the research
HELP1	Perceived helpfulness of social support networks in the first 4-months posttrauma
AVO1	Avoidance of the affected floors during the first 4-months posttrauma
AVO3	As for AVO1, in the third period of the research
REC1	Received individual counseling in the first 4-months posttrauma
REC3	As for REC1, in the third period of the research
MED3	Took prescribed medication in the third period of the research
UND2	Understanding about the incident and personal reactions to trauma in the second 4-months posttrauma
UND3	As for UND2, in the third period of the research
SEC2	Sense of security in the second 4-months posttrauma
SEC3	As for SEC2, in the third period of the research

Table 17.4. Regression Coefficients for Significant Vulnerability Factors and Recovery Factors on the GSI and IES at 4-Months Posttrauma

	Vulnerability factors alone		Vulnerability and Stage 1 recovery factors	
	S1GSI	S1IES	S1GSI	S1IES
SEX	.16**	.14*		
MARR		−.12*		−.11*
SAL		−.15*		−.16*
PRIOR	.18**		−.15**	
GUIL	−.18***	−.17***	−.18***	−.17***
FEAR	.15**	.31***		.19***
FLR			.12*	.18**
SLE1	.22***	.13*	.17**	
NEED1			.20**	.16**
HELP1			−.13*	
REC1			−.11*	
AVO1			.21***	.34***
Variance	33%	37%	42%	50%

* = $p < .05$; ** = $p < .01$; *** = $p < .001$.

4-months posttrauma. Only those variables showing significant regression coefficients are presented.

Thus, vulnerability factors alone accounted for 33% of the variance on GSI scores and 37% on IES scores at 4-months posttrauma, with gender, subjective experience of the trauma, and stressful life events all showing significant regression coefficients on both symptom measures. The addition of recovery variables increased the variance accounted for on the IES and GSI by 13% and 9%, respectively. Perceived need for social support and avoidance of the affected floors were both powerful predictors of symptom levels. In addition, the floor on which the individual normally worked became a signifi-

Table 17.5. Regression Coefficients for Significant Vulnerability Factors and Recovery Factors on the GSI and IES at 8-Months Posttrauma

	Vulnerability factors alone		Vulnerability and Stage 1 and 2 recovery factors	
	S2GSI	S2IES	S2GSI	S2IES
PRIOR	−.14*			
SEX	.17*	.16*		
MARR		−.17*		−.17*
GUIL	−.15*	−.14*	−.15*	−.14*
FEAR	.16*	.30***		.18**
FLR			.15*	.18**
SLE1	.17*		.15*	
SLE2	.19**			
NEED2			.16*	.14*
Variance	35%	39%	46%	51%

* = $p < .05$; ** = $p < .01$; *** = $p < .001$.

of posttrauma reactions. Recovery factors comprised those variables occurring after the trauma that may have influenced recovery, including social support and avoidance of the affected floors. In order to facilitate the reporting of data in this chapter, abbreviated variable names have been used in subsequent tables; Table 17.3 describes these abbreviations.

Symptom levels (i.e., IES and GSI scores) at 4-months posttrauma were predicted from the independent variables by means of a multiple regression analysis. Vulnerability factors were entered first, followed by recovery factors. These analyses were carried out only with the trauma group. Table 17.4 shows the regression coefficients for the vulnerability and recovery factors at cant predictor when recovery factors were added to the equation.

A similar procedure was followed for the prediction of symptom levels at 8-months posttrauma. Table 17.5 shows the significant regression coefficients for variables predicting symptom levels at that stage of the research. Again, vulnerability factors were entered first, followed by recovery factors from both 4- and 8-months posttrauma.

Vulnerability factors again accounted for more than one third of the variance on the symptom measures. Recovery factors added relatively little at this stage, with perceived need for social support being the only variable from this group to demonstrate a significant effect.

Symptom levels at 14-months posttrauma were predicted from both vulnerability factors and recovery factors occurring throughout the period of the research. Table 17.6 shows the regression coefficients from this analysis; again, vulnerability factors were entered prior to recovery factors, and only those variables demonstrating significant regression coefficients are reported.

Tables 4, 5, and 6 provide an indication of those factors that predict outcome in the absence of any knowledge regarding earlier symptom levels. Sociodemographic variables, experience of the trauma, and other stressful life events together accounted for between 30% and 43% of the variance on the outcome measures. The addition of the recovery variables increased this figure by between 11% and 14%. The only sociodemographic characteristic to independently predict symptom levels at all three stages of the research was gender (with females scoring more highly than males). Gender ceased to be significant, however, when recovery factors were also considered, suggesting a possible interaction effect with either social support or avoidance behavior. Both marital status and salary predicted functioning over the first 4 to 8 months, with married subjects and those on lower salaries scoring higher on the IES. Interestingly, the objective measure of exposure to trauma was not a predictor of large symp-

Table 17.7. Regression Coefficients for Significant Variables on the GSI and IES at 14-Months Posttrauma When Earlier Symptom Measure Scores Are Included

	S3GSI	S3IES
GUILT	.12**	
SLE3	.09*	
NEED1	−.25***	
NEED2	−.12*	−.15*
NEED3	.28***	.17*
UND2	−.19**	
SEC2	.21**	
SEC3	−.25**	
REC3	.13*	
S1GSI	.43***	—
S2GSI	.56***	—
S1IES	—	.27***
S2IES	—	.51***
Variance	86%	80%

* = $p < .05$; ** = $p < .01$; *** = $p < .001$.

tom levels when subjective indices (notably fear during the incident) were also included.

Finally, scores on the outcome measures from earlier stages were entered in the equation to determine whether symptom levels at 4 and 8 months following the shootings could predict scores at 14 months. The results of this analysis are shown in Table 17.7; again, only those variables demonstrating significant regression coefficients are shown.

It is clear that symptom levels at Stage 1, and particularly Stage 2, are strong predictors of symptom levels at Stage 3. If an individual was reporting a high level of psychological problems 4 months after a trauma, he or she was still likely to be experiencing those problems 10 months later. The inclusion of these earlier symptom measures in the equation increased the total variance to 86% for the GSI and 80% for the IES. The regression coefficients of the other variables are particularly important, however, because they provide information about those individuals who do not conform to that pattern. It appears that the utilization of social support networks, acknowledgment of guilt feelings in the first few months following the trauma, and an understanding about both the event and personal reactions to the trauma were all associated with improved functioning at 14-months posttrauma.

It is also important to note that many variables investigated in the current research did not prove to be significant in the prediction of later symptom development. For example, age, education, country of birth, living situation, number of children, stressful life events in the year pretrauma, and objective indices of exposure to trauma all failed to show a significant effect.

Table 17.6. Regression Coefficients for Significant Vulnerability Factors and Recovery Factors on the GSI and IES at 14-Months Posttrauma

	Vulnerability factors alone		Vulnerability and Stage 1, 2, and 3 recovery factors	
	S3GSI	S3IES	S3GSI	S3IES
SEX	.17*	.16*		
GUIL	−.19**	−.17*		
FEAR	.18*	.27***		.18*
FLR		.20*		.22**
SLE1			.17*	
SLE3	.23**		.23**	
MED3			−.18*	
AVO3			.31**	.23*
Variance	30%	43%	44%	54%

* = $p < .05$; ** = $p < .01$; *** = $p < .001$.

Discussion

Although posttrauma reactions typically comprise a number of core symptoms, the disorder is characterized by a variety of associated problems and a general impairment in functioning. This was reflected in the range of problems reported by the trauma group. In the absence of any pretrauma measures, it is difficult to be certain that such symptoms were not present before the shootings. However, comparisons with the contrast group, as well as the nature of the symptoms reported, render this possibility unlikely. It is reasonable, therefore, to assume that the psychological problems reported by the trauma group were largely a result of exposure to a traumatic incident. Other factors, of course, may have exacerbated these problems in an already vulnerable population.

One of the clearest findings in terms of symptom levels was noted on the trauma specific measure, the IES. Subjects in the trauma group reported frequent thoughts and memories of the incident, including dreams and vivid images. In an attempt to cope with these intrusive memories and thoughts, survivors of the shootings were likely to attempt to avoid reminders of the incident and to avoid thoughts and feelings associated with it whenever possible. These attempts to avoid sometimes resulted in social withdrawal, isolation, and feeling numb or emotionally flat.

The SCL-90-R covered a large range of psychological symptoms, and subjects in the trauma group reported a higher level of all of these problems than the contrast group. This highlights the pervasive and broad nature of posttrauma reactions. In particular, symptoms associated with depression and anxiety were reported to a much greater extent in the trauma group, as well as problems associated with concentration and relationships with other people. These symptoms are typical of posttrauma reactions and correspond closely with the diagnostic criteria for PTSD.

The GHQ confirmed the findings of the SCL-90-R in terms of the global measure of psychological well-being. The trauma group reported a lower level of psychological well-being than the contrast group on this measure at all three stages of the research.

Thus, those people employed in the affected building, regardless of whether they were present at the time of the shootings, were more likely than those in the contrast group to report a range of psychological, physical, and behavioral symptoms following the trauma. The question then arises as to the course of these symptoms over time. The IES demonstrated a reduction in trauma-specific symptom levels (i.e., intrusive thoughts and avoidance) over the period of the research. Most of the other measures, however, remained relatively stable between 4- and 14-months posttrauma. This suggests that, while memories of the incident and attempts to avoid reminders of the trauma reduced in severity over time, subjects in the trauma group were left with a range of psychological symptoms that affected their quality of life. These tended to be more general symptoms such as depression, anxiety, concentration difficulties, and problems with interpersonal relationships. At 14-months posttrauma, subjects in the trauma group were significantly more distressed than those in the comparable contrast group. It may be that such reactions are part of the normal recovery process following trauma. In addition, no information is available on the course of psychological symptoms between the trauma itself (December 8th) and Stage 1 of the research (April 8th). It is probable

that a good deal of recovery took place during this period.

It is also clear that a number of factors affected the development and course of these symptoms. Those variables were divided into two groups, *vulnerability factors* and *recovery factors*, and each group will be discussed separately. The first group comprised sociodemographic information, experience of the shootings, and other stressful life events. It is argued that these factors may predispose an individual to the development of posttrauma reactions.

Of the sociodemographic factors, gender was consistently a predictor of psychological distress, with females reporting a higher level than males. This may reflect a reluctance on the part of males to acknowledge psychological problems; in other words, males may perceive such reactions as a sign of weakness. Another possible explanation lies in the broader issue of the role of women in society. Females are, in reality, more often the target of physical assault than males. It is therefore understandable that they are at higher risk of developing psychological problems following a trauma such as the Queen Street shootings that involved a violent assault. It is possible, of course, that gender would not be a predictive variable following other kinds of traumatic incidents such as natural disasters.

There was some evidence that those people with a prior history of psychological problems were more vulnerable to the development of general symptoms, as measured by the SCL-90-R. This, however, only applied in the acute, or early, stages of recovery, up to 8 months following the shootings; at 14 months this variable no longer predicted symptom levels. Although it may be that those people were more sensitive to (and therefore more likely to report) psychological symptoms in the early stages of the research, it is also possible that they were, in reality, more vulnerable to acute reactions to severe stressors.

Interestingly, salary was a predictor of symptom levels on the IES at 4-months posttrauma. That is, those people on higher salaries were less likely to complain of intrusive memories or of attempts to avoid reminders of the incident. Again, this was only in the acute stages of recovery; this effect was no longer evident at 8- or 14-months posttrauma. Although a number of explanations for this finding are possible, the effect was relatively small and any interpretation remains largely speculative.

Marital status also seems to have affected scores on the IES, with those people who were married reporting an increased occurrence of intrusive memories and tendencies to avoid trauma-related situations, thoughts and feelings. Again, this effect was no longer important at 14 months following the shootings. The finding is surprising, however, since it may be argued that those people in stable relationships would have better social support networks available to them. It may be that the closeness of a marital or de facto relationship results in added strain, as the victim struggles to come to terms with the trauma while, at the same time, trying to maintain the relationship. Spouses may be unable to understand the changes in their partners following the trauma and may feel rejected as the victims withdraw and refuse to talk about the incident or their reactions. Spouses may also feel inadequate in their ability to help, resulting in further tension and increased symptoms. An alternative explanation is that spouses may encourage more discussion of the trauma and their partner's responses. This may serve to sensitize the survivor to psychological reactions and perhaps reduce any tendency to deny symptoms.

One of the clearest findings in terms of vulnerability factors concerned the role of subjective experience of the trauma; that is, those people who were most frightened and those who felt most guilty about their behavior during the incident were at high risk of developing more severe posttrauma reactions. Although a high level of fear during the incident continued to be predictive of high symptom levels throughout the period of the research, feelings of guilt in the first few months were predictive of improved functioning by 14 months following the shootings. This suggests that such feelings, as well as being a normal reaction to trauma, may be adaptive in terms of assisting the individual to process and come to terms with the incident. Of interest is the fact that the objective degree of exposure to trauma did not have predictive value when these subjective indices were also considered. However, this should not be taken to mean that the actual experiences of the individual were not important; they, of course, determined to a large extent the degrees of fear and guilt. Nevertheless, it does appear that the objective danger that an individual faced during the shootings was of less significance in the development of subsequent symptoms than the perceived threat. It has long been accepted that the severity of the threat is an important predictor of posttrauma reactions. Green and her colleagues (Green, Lindy, & Grace, 1985) argued that the primary determinant of outcome in posttrauma reactions is the nature and intensity of the external threat. As the degree of threat becomes more severe, an increasing proportion of individuals will develop subsequent psychological problems. The finding in the current research that the perceived threat is more important than the actual threat in predicting posttrauma reactions adds an extra dimension to these hypotheses.

A predictor related to experience of the trauma is the floor on which individuals normally worked. Although this, of course, was related closely to actual experience of the trauma, the fact that approximately one third of the research sample were not in the building at the time renders this variable important in its own right. As with the indices of exposure to trauma discussed above, this variable predicted scores on the outcome measures at all three stages of the research. Those people who normally worked on the floors where the shootings took place, regardless of whether they were present at the time of the shootings, reported higher symptom levels. A number of explanations for this finding are possible. First, people not in the building at the time may be thought of as secondary victims, vulnerable to the realization that if they had not left early or taken the day off, they too could have been killed. Second, they were more likely than others in the building to be repeatedly exposed to vivid accounts of what had happened during the incident. Third, since they worked with those who died, grief and bereavement may have complicated their recovery to a greater extent than people on other

floors. Finally, it was in these areas that the most disruption to work practices was experienced following the shootings and considerable pressure was experienced for some months as the sections involved were relocated and a large backlog of work developed. This, of course, constitutes an additional stressor in the period following the shootings.

The existence of other stressful life events in the period following the shootings was also a predictor of high symptom levels, particularly on the global measure of psychological distress, the SCL-90-R. (Interestingly, the trauma-specific measure, the IES, was relatively unaffected by these events.) In other words, such stressors as a death or illness in the family, relationships breaking up, or work and financial problems seem to have resulted in increased vulnerability to psychological distress. Generally speaking, adverse life events affected scores only during the period in which they occurred and had no effect on later measures. There is some evidence, however, that those occurring during the first 4 months following the shootings had longer term effects; that is, they continued to affect scores on the SCL-90-R up to 14 months later. It is likely that such events had a greater and longer lasting impact if they occurred when people were still struggling with the immediate aftermath of the shootings and were at their most vulnerable. It should also be recognized, of course, that these events alone are likely to result in psychological distress. Increased scores on a measure such as the SCL-90-R would be expected following such stressors, irrespective of the shootings. Nevertheless, the fact that they were most powerful in the first few months following the shootings suggests an interaction effect; adverse life events in the period immediately following a disaster may interact with the effects of the trauma to impede recovery.

As well as vulnerability factors, or those characteristics that may predispose an individual to the development of posttrauma reactions, the research also attempted to identify those factors that occurred following the shootings that may have assisted or impaired the individual's recovery from the trauma. There were, however, certain limitations on the extent to which this was possible. The community based recovery program referred to earlier, for example, is likely to have had some effect on the development and course of symptoms. In addition, there may have been other variables operating in the recovery process of which the research team were unaware; indeed, it is to be expected that each individual will be exposed to a number of idiosyncratic influences that may affect recovery from trauma. The findings of the current research in terms of recovery variables are therefore limited, although a number of factors emerged as being significant.

An attempt was made to determine the extent to which effective social support networks may have facilitated recovery from the trauma. It should be noted that the social support scale may have had less relevance to respondents in this research than it would have had in other posttrauma studies. This is because subjects in the current research spent considerable time at work, where naturally occurring support networks existed, and thus the impact of external social supports may have been reduced. Nevertheless, the social support scale had some predictive value. The main effects were from the first factor, which covered need for, use of, and availability of social support networks. This variable acted more as an indication of vulnerability than as a recovery variable for the time at which it was measured; in other words, those people in most distress were likely to seek out and use their support networks. On the other hand, it was also a predictor of later symptom levels, with those people who needed and used their support networks in the early stages of the research reporting a lower level of psychological problems at 14-months posttrauma. In addition, those people who perceived such support as being helpful were likely to report fewer symptoms. This suggests that effective social support may have been an important factor in recovery.

Avoidance of the floors on which the shootings took place was also a powerful predictor of later symptom development. Avoidance is, of course, a common feature of posttrauma reactions. The fact that it is associated with high symptom levels is in line with many theories of posttrauma reactions which suggest that such avoidance impairs an individual's ability to process the trauma (Foa *et al.*, 1989). If survivors continue to avoid situations that remind them of the trauma, they will not be in a position to confront, and come to terms with, what has happened to them.

The Understanding scale was included in an attempt to assess the degree to which the individual had processed or integrated the trauma. It was hypothesized that successful cognitive processing of the event would be evidenced by an understanding of the incident and personal reactions to the trauma and would be associated with reduced symptom levels. Although not reported in this chapter, questions on this scale, and particularly those regarding personal reactions to trauma, were highly correlated with symptom levels; that is, those people who felt that they understood their reactions were likely to be reporting lower symptom levels. In addition, there was evidence of a delayed effect; those people who demonstrated a high level of understanding at Stage 2 of the research showed reduced symptom levels at Stage 3. The Sense of Security scale was a stronger predictor of symptom levels; not surprisingly, feelings of insecurity and vulnerability were associated with more global psychological problems.

Summary and Conclusions

Methodological Implications for Future Research

Although a number of limitations were inherent in the current research, some general conclusions are possible. First, it is clear that subjects in the trauma group reported a range of psychological problems in the 14 months following the shootings. These included intrusive thoughts and memories of the trauma; cognitive, behavioral, and affective avoidance; and general psychological distress, including symptoms of depression, anxiety, poor concentration, and relationship problems. There is little evidence to suggest that the severity of these problems diminished between 4- and 14-months posttrauma.

Second, a number of factors rendered subjects more susceptible to the development of posttrauma reactions at all three stages of the research. These included experience of the shootings, particularly the relative amount of fear that an individual felt during the incident; working on a floor on which the shootings occurred, regardless of whether they were present at the time; the occurrence of other stressful events in a person's life during the first 4 months following the trauma; and gender, with females being more vulnerable than males. Both salary and marital status rendered individuals more susceptible to short-term problems, with those on lower salaries and those people who were married or in de facto marital situations being at higher risk.

Third, a number of factors occurring after the shootings appeared to promote recovery from the trauma, including the availability and use of effective social support networks; reduced avoidance of thoughts and situations associated with the trauma; and a good understanding of both the event and the personal reactions to the trauma (i.e., why they had been feeling as they had since the shootings).

The current study also has implications for future research in the area. In particular, the results highlight the importance of utilizing a longitudinal methodology to adequately chart the course of posttrauma reactions. With the current subject group, there is also a need for longer-term follow-up, given the relatively high level of psychological problems reported at 14-months posttrauma. It is important to determine whether these levels are maintained over a number of years, or whether they reflect specific difficulties inherent in the first year following a disaster.

It is hoped that future research will continue to address the issue of cognitive processing of the traumatic event. The Understanding scale, which was shown to predict symptom levels in the current study, represents an initial attempt to operationalize this processing. The findings, although tentative at this stage, highlight the importance of effectively educating survivors about the psychological sequelae of trauma, to assist them toward a greater understanding of their own personal reactions. Future research in the area of cognitive processing following trauma will have major implications for the prevention and treatment of posttrauma reactions.

ACKNOWLEDGMENT

This research was funded in part by the Victorian Health Promotion Foundation and supported by the Office of Psychiatric Services, Health Department, Victoria, Australia.

References

American Psychiatric Association. (1987). *Diagnostic and statistical manual of mental disorders* (3rd ed., revised). Washington DC: Author.

Cohen, S., & Willis, T. A. (1985). Stress, social support and the buffering hypothesis. *Psychological Bulletin, 98*, 310–357.

Creamer, M., Burgess, P., Buckingham, W., & Pattison, P. (1989). *The psychological aftermath of the Queen Street shootings.*

Parkville, Victoria, Australia: Department of Psychology, University of Melbourne.

Davidson, L. M., & Baum, A. (1986). Chronic stress and post-traumatic stress disorders. *Journal of Consulting and Clinical Psychology, 54*, 303–308.

Derogatis, L. (1977). *SCL-90-R Version: Manual-I* Baltimore, MD: Johns Hopkins University Press.

Figley, C. (1985a). From victim to survivor: Social responsibility in the wake of catastrophe. In C. Figley (Ed.), *Trauma and its wake: The study and treatment of post-traumatic stress disorder* (pp. 398–415). New York: Brunner/Mazel.

Figley, C. (Ed.). (1985b). *Trauma and its wake: The study and treatment of post-traumatic stress disorder*. New York: Brunner/Mazel.

Foa, E. B., Steketee, G., & Rothbaum, B. O. (1989). Behavioral-cognitive conceptualizations of post-traumatic stress disorder. *Behavior Therapy, 20*, 155–176.

Goldberg, D. P. (1972). *The detection of psychiatric illness by questionnaire*. London: Oxford University Press.

Green, B. L. (1982). Assessing levels of psychological impairment following disaster: Consideration of actual and methodological dimensions. *Journal of Nervous and Mental Disease, 170*, 544–552.

Green, B. L., Grace, M. C., & Gleser, G. C. (1985). Identifying survivors at risk: Long-term impairment following the Beverly Hills supper club fire. *Journal of Consulting and Clinical Psychology, 53*, 672–678.

Green, B. L., Lindy, J. D., & Grace, M. C. (1985). Post-traumatic stress disorder: Toward DSM IV. *Journal of Nervous and Mental Disease, 173*, 406–411.

Green, B. L., Wilson, J. P., & Lindy, J. D. (1985). Conceptualizing post-traumatic stress disorder: A psychological framework. In C. Figley (Ed.), *Trauma and its wake: The study and treatment of post-traumatic stress disorder* (pp. 53–69). New York: Brunner/Mazel.

Green, M. A., & Berlin, M. A. (1987). Five psychosocial variables related to the existence of post-traumatic stress disorder symptoms. *Journal of Clinical Psychology, 43*, 643–649.

Horowitz, M. J., Wilner, N., & Alvarez, W. (1979). The Impact of Events Scale: A measure of subjective stress. *Psychosomatic Medicine, 41*, 209–218.

Janoff-Bulman, R. (1985). The aftermath of victimization: Rebuilding shattered assumptions. In C. Figley (Ed.), *Trauma and its wake: The study and treatment of post-traumatic stress disorder* (pp. 15–35). New York: Brunner/Mazel.

McFarlane, A. C. (1987). Life events and psychiatric disorder: The role of a natural disaster. *British Journal of Psychiatry, 151*, 362–367.

McFarlane, A. C. (1988). The etiology of post-traumatic stress disorders following a natural disaster. *British Journal of Psychiatry, 152*, 116–121.

Parker, G. (1977). Cyclone Tracy and Darwin evacuees: On the restoration of the species. *British Journal of Psychiatry, 130*, 548–555.

Quarantelli, E. L. (1985). An assessment of conflicting views on mental health: The consequences of traumatic events. In C. Figley (Ed.), *Trauma and its wake: The study and treatment of post-traumatic stress disorder* (pp. 173–215). New York: Brunner/Mazel.

Raphael, B. (1986). *When disaster strikes*. London: Century Hutchinson.

Raphael, B., Lundin, T., & Weisaeth, L. (1989). A research method for the study of psychological and psychiatric aspects of disaster. *Acta Psychiatrica Scandinavica, 80*, Suppl. 353 (pp. 1–75).

Solomon, S. D. (1986). Mobilizing social support networks in times of disaster. In C. Figley (Ed.), *Trauma and its wake: Vol. II. Traumatic stress theory, research, and intervention* (pp. 232–263). New York: Brunner/Mazel.

Wilson, J. P., Smith, W. K., & Johnson, S. K. (1985). A comparative analysis of PTSD among various survivor groups. In C. Figley (Ed.), *Trauma and its wake: The study and treatment of post-traumatic stress disorder* (pp. 142–172). New York: Brunner/Mazel.

Woolfolk, R. L., & Grady, D. A. (1988). Combat related post-traumatic stress disorder. *Journal of Nervous and Mental Disease, 176*, 107–111.

Zilberg, N. J., Weiss, D. S., & Horowitz, M. J. (1982). The Impact of Events Scale: A cross validation study and some empirical evidence supporting a conceptual model of stress response syndromes. *Journal of Consulting and Clinical Psychology, 50*, 407–414.

Zimmerman, M. (1983). Methodological issues in the assessment of life events: A review of issues and research. *Clinical Psychology Review, 3*, 339–370.

PART III

War Trauma and Civil Violence

Section A: Trauma and the Aging Process: Studies Related to World War II

During the twentieth century, two great wars and many others throughout the world have taken a toll of over 50 million lives and created conditions of social chaos and economic ruin. These different wars have always left a psychic legacy in the lives of the survivors. Part III, Section A comprises five chapters which examine the long-term effects of trauma experienced in World War II on the aging process and on psychosocial adaptation. Included in these studies are the following groups:

1. Dutch Resistance fighters who fought against the Nazi occupation of Holland
2. Australian ex-service personnel who were held as prisoners of war by the Japanese
3. Victims of the Nazi Holocaust
4. French civilians living in the region of Alsace-Lorraine who were conscripted into the German army and later were captured by the Russian army and interned, mistakenly, as German prisoners of war, despite their French heritage
5. Former United States servicemen who were stationed in Hawaii at Pearl Harbor on December 7, 1941, when the Japanese attacked the naval base there and launched the United States into World War II.

These chapters share a common feature of prolonged psychological effects of exposure to war trauma which persists in an active form today. In some instances (e.g., the Dutch Resistance fighters and the Alsace-Lorraine POWs), the severity of their current symptoms meets the diagnostic criteria for chronic PTSD. However, whether or not an individual or the cohort group meets the standard for psychiatric "caseness," the results are unequivocal in showing that in memory, dreams, and daily activity the effects of the events experienced during the war are very much alive and, for many survivors, emotionally troublesome. Table III.1 presents a summary overview of these chapters.

In Chapter 18, Wybrand Op den Velde and his colleagues report on the Dutch Resistance fighters who carried out a variety of tasks against the Nazi occupation of Holland which began on May 10, 1940. The role of the Resistance fighter was an extremely dangerous one since discovery by the German Army could result in execu-

Table III.1. A Summary Overview

Chapter/study and authors	Population studied	Median age and related features	Measures used and time period assessed	Symptoms evident	Major findings
18 Dutch Resistance fighters Op den Velde *et al.*	N = 813 World War II Dutch Resistance fighters	64.1 years 93% married 50 imprisoned	21-item self-rating scale Maastricht Questionnaire SCID-R PTSD DSM-III-R N = 147 completed questionnaires	Recurrent dreams Detachment Sleep disturbance Guilt Memory impairment Constricted affect Depression Alienation	84% PTSD rate Vital exhaustion common in PTSD Marital conflicts High divorce rate
19 Australian POWs of Japanese Tennant *et al.*	N = 170 POWs N = 172 matched (controls)	65.0 years (POWs) 66.5 years (controls)	Zung Depression Scale State-Trait Anxiety Eysenck Personality Questionnaire Jackson Hostility Scale Structured interviews	POWs had more Alcohol abuse Anxiety Depression Symptoms of PTSD	POWs had more Medical problems Depression Multiple episodes of psychiatric problems Anxiety
20 Nazi Holocaust survivors Harel *et al.*	N = 168 Holocaust N = 180 Israeli Holocaust N = 155 immigrants (controls)	62.6 years 65.1 years (Israel) 63.0 years (controls)	Philadelphia Geriatric Center Morale Scale Social network Self-disclosure Social support Social affiliations	PTSD symptoms related to Holocaust Symptoms of aging (e.g., depression)	Survivors with social support had better mental health Self-disclosure to significant others associated with mental health Reconstructing social networks associated with mental health
21 French POWs of Russians Crocq *et al.*	N = 1400 former POWs surveyed N = 525 completed questionnaires	66.7 years 1 year in POW camp 4 years military duty as German conscripts	DSM-III PTSD DSM-III-R PTSD SCFD-R PTSD	Intrusive recollections Depression Anxiety Alienation Sleep disturbance Anomie Nightmares	89% nightmares 82% intrusive imagery 39% survivor guilt 73% active avoidance 71% foreshortened future 76% sleep disturbance 75% startle response
22 Pearl Harbor survivors Harel *et al.*	N = 350 former servicemen at Pearl Harbor	65 years Members of Pearl Harbor Survivors Association	DSM-III-R PTSD Affect balance Locus of control Altruism Generic PTSD	Intrusive recollections Group pride Survivor identity	89% nightmares/dreams 87% intrusive imagery 42% survivor guilt 17% active avoidance 24% startle response

tion. Although the roles of the Resistance fighters were varied, they included (1) aid to persons in hiding, primarily Jews; (2) reporting the news of the war since the Nazis had censored the press and radio; (3) providing aid to Allied pilots who had been shot down over Holland; (4) espionage activity; and (5) active armed resistance against German soldiers. Clearly, there were many stressors experienced in the role of a Resistance fighter, and those who survived faced a difficult postwar recovery environment as well because there was no formal recognition of their sacrifices in the climate of national reconstruction and preoccupation with establishing economic sovereignty. As a consequence, many Resistance fighters became isolated, embittered, and alienated from those who did not resist occupation and who did not wish to be reminded of their passivity in the face of Nazi occupation and aggression.

Op den Velde and his colleagues surveyed all male Dutch Resistance fighters who were still living in 1984. From this available pool ($n = 813$) 147 eventually completed a set of questionnaires designed to study a broad range of psychological reactions and psychiatric symptoms. In terms of the prevalence of PTSD as assessed by the SCID technique, 55.8% met the diagnostic criteria and another 27.9% had PTSD in remission. Only 16.3% never met the criteria. Thus, nearly 84% of the sample suffered from PTSD at some time since the end of World War II. Moreover, careful analysis of separate PTSD symptoms indicated that there were very high levels of all of the B, C, and D, DSM-III-R PTSD criteria whether or not the individual had a current diagnosis of PTSD. Op den Velde and his associates provide a detailed discussion of their findings and their interpretation and suggest that "the subjects with war trauma-related PTSD suffered from vital exhaustion to a significantly larger degree than male cardiac patients. . . . It may be thought that *vital exhaustion* might be clearing the way to the onset or the recurrence of PTSD symptoms in subjects with traumatic antecedents in their life history."

In Chapter 19, Christopher Charles Tennant and his colleagues report on former Australian servicemen who were captured and interned as POWs by the Japanese, initially in the Malay Peninsula of Southeast Asia, and later in other locations as well. In the study, Tennant and his colleagues compare a random sample of Australian POWs to a cohort group of former combatants who were not POWs. After a careful selection procedure to ensure the representativeness of the sample, 170 POWs and 172 controls were selected and given medical and psychiatric evaluations as well as psychological testing. The test battery included measures of depression, anxiety, hostility, and neuroticism.

The results produced a number of significant differences between the two groups. As expected, the POWs had more medical problems (e.g., dysentery, malaria, beriberi) during the war than the combatants. Second, the risk of developing clinical psychiatric disorders was also higher for the POWs in terms of anxiety, depression, and alcohol dependence. Third, in terms of the frequency of multiple episodes of psychiatric disorder, the POWs had more recurrences from 1943 to 1984. Although there were no specific measures of PTSD in this study, the obtained pattern of results is quite similar to that found by Op den Velde in the preceding chapter. Thus, given the extreme severity of the stressors experienced by the former POWs, it would be surprising if their rate of chronic PTSD was not similar to the Dutch Resistance fighters, especially those who were placed in concentration camps by the German Army. Clearly, future research may allow such comparisons to be made, using the more recently standardized measures of PTSD reported in Part II of this volume.

In Chapter 20, Zev Harel and Boaz and Eva Kahana present another in a series of analyses of their large-scale research project on aging Holocaust survivors who are living in the United States and in Israel. In this study, attention is focused on social resources and mental health. In a simplified way, the central question being addressed is the determination of the factors that allow for positive mental health and coping in this aging population of former internees in Nazi death and concentration camps. Based on the extant gerontology literature, the authors argue that integration into and utilization of social networks has a salutary effect on mental health. By being integrated into a social network, the aging survivor has sources of social, psychological, and economic support that permit a meaningful connection to a community of peers and relations. Furthermore, these social bonds facilitate having a sense of self-esteem and integrity as well as the opportunity to self-disclose important personal concerns.

The sample consisted of 168 survivors of the Holocaust who came to the United States between the end of World War II and 1975 and a control cohort of 155 European immigrants who arrived in the United States prior to the war.

The central findings of this study were impressive: Aging survivors who utilized social support from their primary group and friends had far better mental health than individuals who were more isolated and disconnected from potential sources of support in a meaningful network. Particularly noteworthy was the finding that on a number of social resource variables, the survivors actually had higher indices of integration and well-being. Although there are many alterative interpretations of these data, it appears that where the survivors have successfully *reconstructed* social networks and communities that were destroyed by the Holocaust and World War II, they were able to make a recovery environment that was in itself a therapeutic milieu. What contributed to this healing psychological community was the opportunity to disclose important personal concerns in the context of a shared historical identity that gave rise to patterns of social interaction that ultimately led to positive mental health during the aging process.

Considered from another perspective, the recovery from war trauma, internment, and extreme stress was not in the psychoanalyst's office but among family and friends in a psychologically meaningful community of supportive others who, perhaps, tacitly knew the nature of private suffering and prolonged stress effects. This does not mean, of course, that the survivors were without symptoms of anxiety, depression, or PTSD. Rather, while previous research has shown these symptoms to exist, their deleterious effects appear to have been attenuated by the degree to which they were able to stay tightly involved in social networks that facilitated personal self-esteem with a meaningful community.

Chapter 21 presents a detailed analysis of PTSD in World War II POWs from Alsace-Lorraine who were conscripted into the German Army and then held in captivity in the Soviet Union. This study by Marc-Antoine Crocq and his colleagues is especially interesting because of the cultural dimension of the conscripts. The Alsace-Lorraine region borders Germany and France and throughout its history has alternately belonged either to Germany or France. The people in the region are bilingual and have cultural roots in both heritages.

During the battle of Krusk in July and August of 1943, men from Alsace-Lorraine were captured in large number by the German army and were forced into military duty, some against the advancing Russian forces. Upon capture by the Russian army, the French citizens were mistaken as Germans and subsequently treated brutally by their captors as POWs.

In 1988, the authors surveyed the former POWs, who now belonged to a survivors organization in France. Among the 1,400 completed surveys, a random sample of 525 questionnaires was analyzed. Similar to the study by Op den Velde in Chapter 18, the investigators used the SCID and DSM-III and DSM-III-R diagnostic criteria for PTSD.

The results were remarkably similar to those obtained for the Dutch Resistance fighters. For example, 82% still experience intrusive recollections and nightmares of their wartime captivity; 73% actively attempt to avoid thoughts or feelings associated with the trauma; 71% report a foreshortened sense of the future; and over 70% still have sleep disturbance and startle reactions as a manifestation of physiological hyperarousal. Additionally, nearly 40% report survivor guilt. These major findings are only part of a larger set of results that suggest that there were enduring personality changes in the survivors who, like the Dutch Resistance fighters, returned to their home culture uncelebrated, embittered, and psychologically isolated, because others in the region were less affected by the war and did not have the difficult task of recovering from being mistakenly treated as German soldiers by the Russian captors who failed to recognize their French heritage and nationality. As such they were caught in a web of ambiguity both during the war itself and upon return to the recovery environment in which the French had surrendered early in the war to Nazi occupation. Thus, the social forces were in place to create anomie, alienation, isolation, and prolonged stress effects of chronic PTSD.

The final chapter examines the long-term effects on the survivors of the Japanese attack at Pearl Harbor. During the 45th reunion of the Pearl Harbor Survivors Association in Honolulu, Hawaii, in 1986, the opportunity arose to survey the 800 members in attendance at the meeting. In Chapter 22, Zev Harel, Boaz Kahana, and John P. Wilson report on the results of this survey. The first wave of respondents ($N = 350$) completed questionnaires which were then subjected to statistical analysis.

The authors utilized the DSM-III-R criteria in the questionnaire as well as measures of locus of control, self-disclosure, affect balance, and adjustment to aging. The results obtained were nearly identical to those reported by Crocq in Chapter 21. Eighty-seven percent of the men still experience intrusive recollections of the attack on Pearl Harbor; 29% report nightmares about their experiences on the "day of infamy"; and over 25% report sleep disturbance, startle reactions, and symptoms of physiological hyperactivity. Quite similar to Crocq's data, 42% still report survivor guilt.

The multiple regressive analyses performed indicated that locus of control, self-disclosure, and altruism were important variables in current mental health and positive affect, a finding which parallels the results for aging Holocaust survivors reported by Harel and his co-workers in Chapter 20. Particularly noteworthy here is the fact that the Pearl Harbor survivors and the Holocaust survivors are of a similar age range and both groups maintain strong supportive social networks. Thus, the replication of results in two diverse populations of survivors suggests that although PTSD symptoms may persist in memory, affect, and behavior, they are attenuated to a significant degree by membership in a highly cohesive group that ensures positive ego identity and continuity in the context of a psychologically meaningful environment. Finally, Harel coded the open-ended data from the survey questionnaire and found that the memories of the attack were clear, detailed, and readily retrievable with powerful affect. All the available information suggested that this monumental historical event that propelled the United States into World War II was an important part of the identity and an active influence on the course of the aging process itself.

CHAPTER 18

Posttraumatic Stress Disorder in Dutch Resistance Veterans from World War II

Wybrand Op den Velde, Paul R. J. Falger,
Johan E. Hovens, Jan H. M. de Groen, Louise J. Lasschuit,
Hans Van Duijn, and Erik G. W. Schouten

Introduction

At present it is generally accepted that extensive war traumata can cause permanent damage to a person's mental and physical health. However, the precise nature of the associations between traumatic war experiences and subsequent disorders remains uncertain.

In the Netherlands, the largest group of patients with chronic posttraumatic stress pathology consists of middle-aged and elderly victims of World War II. There is evidence that more than 182,000 adults (over 1% of the entire Dutch population) may be categorized as such (Department of Welfare, Health and Cultural Affairs,

Wybrand Op den Velde • Department of Psychiatry, Saint Lucas Hospital, 1061 AE Amsterdam, Netherlands. **Paul R. J. Falger** • Department of Medical Psychology, University of Limburg School of Medicine, 6200 MD Maastricht, Netherlands. **Johan E. Hovens** • Department of Psychiatry, Saint Lucas Hospital, 1061 AE Amsterdam, Netherlands. **Jan H. M. de Groen** • Department of Clinical Neurophysiology, University of Limburg School of Medicine, 6200 MD Maastricht, Netherlands. **Louise J. Lasschuit** • Department of Psychiatry, Saint Lucas Hospital, 1061 AE Amsterdam, Netherlands. **Hans Van Duijn** • Department of Neurophysiology, Saint Lucas Hospital, 1061 AE Amsterdam, Netherlands. **Erik G. W. Schouten** • Department of Medical Psychology, University of Limburg School of Medicine, 6200 MD Maastricht, Netherlands.

International Handbook of Traumatic Stress Syndromes, edited by John P. Wilson and Beverley Raphael. Plenum Press, New York, 1993.

1987). Former members of the Resistance movement comprise a relatively large group of the war victims in the Netherlands. In 1985, 43,000 Resistance participants were still alive. Also, in 1985, an investigation into the current complaints and states of health of Dutch Resistance veterans who had been subjected to episodes of prolonged stress during World War II was developed. For this purpose the cooperation of Stichting 1940–1945, a foundation that actively promotes the interests of Resistance veterans (the only one of its kind in the Netherlands), was obtained.

Studies of Nazi concentration camp survivors showed strongly reduced involvement in their surroundings, loss of interest in everyday activities, apathy, pessimism, premature aging, and impaired sexual needs (Abalan, 1987). This complex of symptoms originally became known as *post-concentration camp syndrome* or *KZ-syndrome* (Schmolling, 1984; Thygesen, 1980). Interestingly, it was found that people who had not been imprisoned but who had been exposed to gross wartime stress might also develop a mental disorder with characteristics strikingly similar to those of post-concentration camp syndrome (Häfner, 1968; Venzlaff, 1964).

It is now generally recognized that an acute reaction to extreme war stress can be followed by a period in which the victim does not appear to have any complaints or show obvious signs of having problems with coming to terms with prior traumatic experiences (Bastiaans, 1957; Bieder, 1984; Christensen, Walker, Ross, & Maltbie, 1981; Dimsdale, 1974; Lorenzer, 1968; Luchterland, 1970). Yet, frequently after a period of many years, a delayed form of post-concentration camp syndrome may develop.

Scientific Studies of Resistance Veterans

In the immediate postwar period, attention was directed mainly to the somatic sequelae of the surviving victims. Many camp inmates suffered from malnutrition, deficiencies, injuries, and infectious diseases. Treatment was based on the combination of rest and good nutrition. Apparent psychological reactions to war stress were seen as a temporary burden, which would disappear spontaneously. In the Netherlands, physicians and psychologists persuaded patients "to work hard and to forget." Lasting psychological troubles were interpreted as a manifestation of preexisting personality disturbances (see Chapter 5, in this volume, for a discussion of premorbid biases).

Studies of Nonimprisoned Veterans

In 1951, Rümke described a 44-year-old Dutch Resistance veteran, who had developed headaches, memory impairment, restlessness, and insomnia 4 years after the liberation. Contrary to the then prevailing professional opinion that delayed traumatic reactions were nonexistent, Rümke attributed these complaints to the man's horrible war experiences, after a careful analysis of the content of his intrusive thoughts. Truly, in 1951, this appeared to be a revolutionary idea.

Ten years later, Wibaut (1961) examined a group of Dutch Resistance veterans, who had applied for a special war pension (Registers), and a group who after a period of Resistance work had been subsequently arrested and imprisoned in a concentration camp (Internees). His findings are summarized in Table 18.1.

Wibaut (1961) observed a quite unexpected fact for which he could not provide an explanation: namely, that the disability rates were higher with respect to participation in the Resistance itself than with respect to subsequent imprisonment. He further concluded that the duration of imprisonment was not linked to the development of "neuropsychic" diseases. A positive relationship between the degree of maltreatment (torture) and neuropsychic disorders was established. Late onset of neuropsychic disorder was found in 37% of the 464 subjects, in 11.5% of which the disorder became apparent more than 2 years after the liberation of Europe in 1945. Wibaut attempted to establish the possible effects of a death sentence which had been pronounced but not executed, a method of torture often employed by the

Table 18.1. Percentage of Disability in Former Dutch Resistance Fighters

Disability	Registers (N = 161)	Internees (N = 303)
Somatic disease	19	13
Neuropsychic disease	56	32
Somatic and neuropsychic disease	20	55

Note. From *Diseases and Disorders Resulting from Resistance Work and Imprisonment* by F. Wibaut, 1961. The Hague, Netherlands: World Veterans Federation. Copyright 1961–1962 by the World Veterans Federation. Reprinted by permission.

Nazis. His figures indicated a delayed influence of a death sentence on subsequent mental disorders.

Flaten and Aasen (1976) studied Norwegian Resistance fighters who had not been taken prisoner. The local health insurance offices provided information about the morbidity of the veterans in the period 1945–1970. Control norms were obtained from the files in these offices. In the health insurance files, Flaten and Aasen found no signs of late sequelae, such as concentration camp syndrome. The Resistance fighters even showed significantly less somatic morbidity than normal, in terms of the lengths of sick leaves and hospital stays. However, these veterans were neither interviewed nor examined with the aim to identify war-related pathology.

Studies of Imprisoned Resistance Veterans

Important follow-up studies of Resistance fighters who had survived the German concentration camps were carried out in Denmark and Norway. At that time, the living conditions and the nature of the Resistance work in the occupied Scandinavian countries were very similar to those in the Netherlands. Thygesen *et al.* (1970) and Strøm (1968) studied imprisoned Resistance veterans with employment and adaptation problems; their findings are summarized in Table 18.2. These Scandinavian investigators also reported the onset of symptoms after many years, in particular among young individuals. Once established, the post-concentration camp syndrome might remain stationary, but often the condition gradually worsened.

Nielsen (1983) examined all Danish Resistance veterans who had survived the Porta-Stutthof concentration camp. In 1980, 187 ex-prisoners were still alive, and 69% of this group suffered from post-concentration camp syndrome.

In a long-term follow-up study (1945–1970) of nearly all Norwegian concentration camp survivors, of which the majority appeared to have been Resistance veterans,

Table 18.2. Percentage of Symptoms in Scandinavian Resistance Veterans with Mental Problems

Symptoms	Norway[a] (N = 191)	Denmark[b] (N = 321)
Fatigue	84	92
Memory impairment	87	87
Affective instability	85	85
Insomnia	65	64
Depressive mood	32	59
Concentration difficulties		56
Headaches	60	51
Nightmares	52	49
Premature aging		48
Anxiety symptoms	58	35
Alcohol abuse	13	12
Suicide attempts		4
Psychotic disorder		7

[a]From Strøm, 1968.
[b]From Thygesen *et al.*, 1970.

a much higher mortality, longer sick leaves, and longer hospitalization periods were found than in the persons of the control group (Eitinger & Strøm, 1973).

From a clinical perspective, Bastiaans (1974), who had treated several hundred Dutch Resistance veterans who had survived the concentration camps, observed that post-concentration camp syndrome consisted of three phases, which were based on Selye's General Adaptation Syndrome.

Bastiaans' Modification of Selye's Model of Stress

Phase 1: "Alarm." This phase, which may last from months to years, is the expression of psychosomatic distress, failing self-defense, ego weakness, in fact, a state of intense arousal. This phase is marked by unspecific nervous behavior, neurasthenia, insomnia, nightmares, chronic weariness, and vague complaints stemming from dysharmonic functioning of the different organ systems.

Phase 2: "Adaptation." This phase is characterized by pathological adaptation to so-called normality and intense repression of traumatic war experiences. In this phase, which may last for many years, neurotic overactivity combined with tenseness and irritability may develop. In other veterans, chronic asthenic–depressive reactions are seen. This phase is often marked by the *Targowla syndrome* (i.e., paroxysms of sudden reexperiencing of what happened in the concentration camp). Psychosomatic syndromes, such as hypertension, myocardial infarction, asthma, and gastric ulcers are likely. These symptoms constitute a group in between the fight reactions (overactivity) and the flight reactions (asthenia and depression).

Phase 3: "Exhaustion." Following a latency period of what may often be many years (Phase 2), there is a sudden uncontrolled return of the repressed mental contents. Afflicted individuals again start dreaming, having nightmares, and feeling depressed and ill-treated. The break-through of the *repression barrier* is promoted by new threats that are formed by daily television programs and newspapers.

Stress as a Consequence of Participation in the Dutch Resistance

In order to understand the specific problems faced by the aging Resistance veterans, it is a prerequisite to study their war experiences.

The Psychological Climate during World War II

On May 10, 1940, the Netherlands was invaded by Hitler's army. The badly equipped Dutch army offered stubborn resistance but was forced to capitulate 5 days later. This defeat occurred after the heavy bombing of Rotterdam, the second largest city in the Netherlands, when the threat to annihilate more towns was imminent.

At the beginning of the military occupation, the Nazis allowed daily life to continue normally. After a short period of time, most of the imprisoned Dutch soldiers were released. In the course of the year of 1940, however, the persecution and deportation of the sizable Jewish community began. The Dutch population reacted with growing horror. In February 1941, in reaction to this persecution, a general strike was called in Amsterdam, where most Jews were living. This strike, the only one of its kind in Europe during the Nazi rule, was bloodily repressed (Warmbrunn, 1963).

A pro-Nazi political party already existed in the Netherlands before the German occupation. It was supported by roughly 4% of the population (then about 8.5 million people) and became very influential during the occupation. Many members of this party were appointed to important positions during the war and acted as informers to the German secret police (*Sicherheitsdienst*) (Warmbrunn, 1963).

Development of the Resistance Movement

The gradually developing resistance to the Nazi occupation in the Netherlands took a variety of forms, with the most characteristic and important being the following:

1. *Aid to persons in hiding*. The aid was primarily for Jews, but also for adolescent and young adult males who refused to do forced labor in Germany and for Resistance fighters who were wanted. This aid consisted primarily of finding both temporary shelters and more permanent hiding places in the towns and countryside, helping wanted individuals reach these places, providing them with food, supplying false identity cards, and the like.

2. *News reporting*. The Germans who occupied the Netherlands heavily censored the press and radio. Numerous illegal newspapers and bulletins were printed and distributed in which news items that were broadcast by British radio stations were reported and in which the Dutch people were urged to get involved in the Resistance.

3. *Aid to Allied pilots*. Members of the Allied air forces who had crashed over occupied territory were offered shelter and transport to Great Britain, usually via secret routes through Belgium, France, Spain, and Portugal.

The following types of Resistance work were carried out on a more modest scale:

1. *Espionage*. A number of espionage groups were set up to gather both military and economic information. Their reports were sent to Great Britain by courier or through secret radio transmissions.

2. *Armed resistance*. Even at that time, the Netherlands was a densely populated country where real guerrilla warfare was not feasible. The armed Resistance fighters usually lived at home and were only called to action in small groups for special offensives. Armed aggression against the occupiers was carried out on a small

scale. The Nazis reacted to armed attacks on German soldiers with severe reprisals in the form of executions of innocent people.

Acts of armed resistance included the "liquidation" of dangerous collaborators, raids on distribution offices, destruction of population registers, and attacks on prisons in order to free imprisoned Resistance fighters. Sabotage, such as blowing up railway tracks, was committed to hinder transportation.

In top secrecy, an army was put together and trained to assist during the advance of the Allied forces. This underground army—"the Forces of the Interior" (*Binnenlandse Strijdkrachten*)—was supplied with weapons which were dropped by planes of the Allied forces.

The Resistance Participants

The Resistance movement was comprised of very heterogeneous groups acting together to achieve a common goal and thus subjecting themselves to the same perils. Men and women, young and old, participated in the Resistance. Not only healthy individuals, but also the weak and the infirm did their bit. All classes of Dutch prewar society were represented in the Resistance although, in fact, only approximately 4% of the entire population either supported the movement or actually took part in Resistance work. It was not until the end of 1943 that the Resistance became a larger, relatively well-organized movement with its own general command structure and well-defined communication lines. In general, most Resistance fighters were poorly prepared and badly equipped for the extraordinary work they were to perform. Only a few individuals had had previous formal military training. Numerous partisans were arrested because of carelessness or betrayal. Many of them did not survive. They were cruelly interrogated and subsequently executed or put into concentration camps where a large proportion of them died.

Psychological Consequences and Stressors in Resistance Work

The various traumatic experiences that Resistance veterans had to cope with may be categorized as follows:

1. *Tension of the Resistance work itself.* There was no escaping the knowledge that one would have to kill when necessary and that one's life and the lives of one's family were constantly endangered. Not only were the Resistance fighters preoccupied with the fate of their families, but they were forced to conceal all knowledge of underground activities from the ones closest to them. In addition to all this was the perpetual fear of betrayal.

Individuals belonging to orthodox Christian denominations faced especially troubling conflicts of conscience by joining the Resistance, for they were often compelled to commit extreme acts of violence that clashed fundamentally with their religious upbringings (Van Scheyen, 1982).

The above-mentioned continual fear and stress to which Resistance fighters were exposed have been extensively reported by the historian De Jong. We quote from his research on the German occupation (De Jong,

1976, Volume 7, p. 1030; translation provided by the authors):

> This tension resulted from a situation in which one had consciously put oneself or in which one had drifted almost without noticing. Not one single Resistance fighter did not know what the consequences would be of being caught: cruel interrogation, imprisonment in jail or a concentration camp, possibly execution. The enemy was ever-present and on the lurk. Dutch, and sometimes German, policemen patrolled on the trains with a list of wanted persons. The same policemen, often in plainclothes, waited at station exits or patrolled on bicycles and demanded of any passers-by they fancied that they identify themselves. However good the forged identity card one possessed was, it could not pass a scrutinizing control. Moreover, one had really put one's fate in other people's hands: those of the people one collaborated with on underground matters. We do not think the importance of this dependency can be stressed heavily enough. In their normal ways of life, most people do not, and certainly not for any length of time, find themselves in a situation in which they realize that their lives depend directly on the behavior of their fellow men. In time of war, this could be the case for members of military units, they each know that whether they survive or not is determined by the adequate reaction of their comrades. However, actual combat situations as such do not occur that frequently as a rule. The Resistance work, however, meant being in permanent danger. . . . Many a Resistance fighter felt that he was imperiled every hour of the day and night. This was in fact the case. His life was perpetually threatened by the activities of the "Sicherheitsdienst," a formidable enemy whose tentacles had penetrated to every corner of the country.

2. *Time spent in prison, a correctional institution, or a concentration camp.* Besides referring to the torture that an individual was subjected to, it also includes the stress brought on by fear of "spilling the beans," the time spent on death row, and the accompanying tormenting feelings of submissiveness and uncertainty (Wibaut, 1961).

In several studies of the Nazi concentration camps, the mortality rate has been used as a measure for the hardship of the regime. However, mortality is only a very rough indicator of the conditions in a particular camp during a circumscribed period. Leliefeld and Van Staden ten Brink (1982) studied the Dutch prisoners of the concentration camp at Dachau, the majority of whom were Resistance workers. Of the 1,366 male Dutch prisoners, 697 perished before the end of World War II. The highest mortality numbers were found for the period until December 1942. Further, mortality was strongly correlated to the age of the prisoners, as shown in Table 18.3.

Adaptation to Life in the Concentration Camp

Hers (1988), himself a physician, a Resistance fighter, and a concentration camp survivor, described the three general phases of adaptation to life in the con-

Table 18.3. Mortality of Dutch Male Prisoners at Dachau

Year of birth	Mortality (%)
1871–1884	100
1885–1889	69
1890–1894	75
1895–1899	64
1900–1904	48
1905–1909	48
1910–1914	27
1915–1919	22
1920–1924	21
1925–1929	18

Note. From *Dutch Prisoners of the Concentration Camp Dachau 1941–1979: A Study of Mortality and Causes of Death* by H. Leliefeld and A. Van Staden ten Brink, 1982. Leiden: Samson/Sijthoff. Reprinted by permission.

centration camp: (1) the acute or alarm phase, lasting 2 weeks; (2) the adaptation phase, with an average duration of 6 weeks; and (3) the apathy phase, of 3 to 5 months. Hers also described a fourth phase, the "low-level subsistence phase." The transition from apathy to low-level subsistence was characterized by the disappearance of hunger edema, despite an unchanged and insufficient diet. The prisoner, aroused from his apathy and lethargy, became clear-headed and the prevailing indifference toward his fellow prisoners or death gradually was replaced by comradely assistance and gallows humor. This phase could last for years. Usually, death, in this phase, resulted from concomitant infections or serious injuries.

Also, many individuals suffered greatly from the absolute feeling of *powerlessness* that they experienced during their stay in captivity, a feeling caused by seeing fellow prisoners, Russian prisoners of war, Poles, and Jews being hung or beaten to death before their eyes.

The Postwar Psychological Climate

In the immediate postwar years, the population hardly gave themselves time to reflect on the previous period or to deal with their emotions. The disorganized and plundered country immediately claimed all its energy for recovery and reconstruction. Collectively and individually, people tried to forget the five frightening years of occupation.

Although many Resistance veterans found their families safe and sound after rejoining them at the end of the war, many were still suffering from "survival guilt." This was the result of having lost comrades in the Resistance, people to whom they had come to feel so close.

The soldiers and the war sailors, returning home after the defeat of the Nazis, were welcomed as the liberators and heroes. Generally, they readjusted easily to society. The position of the Resistance veterans, however, was more complex. The vast majority of the population had strongly disapproved the behavior of the German occupiers, but only a few really offered active

Resistance. Most people did not have the courage to risk their lives for such ideals as freedom and justice. Thus, the social position of the Resistance veterans was beset with ambivalent reactions and feelings. Most people do not appreciate being reminded of their own cowardice. The result was that the Resistance veterans were ignored as a special group of people. This attitude of hidden neglect was present in "the man in the street," as well as in the highest levels of the government. As a consequence, most Resistance veterans learned to keep quiet about their wartime experiences. Only in the presence of fellow Resisters and in friendly gatherings did they feel safe enough to express their deeper emotions. This restraint resulted in feelings of isolation and rejection by society in general. A kind of "conspiracy of silence" emerged.

In the postwar years, many Resistance veterans left their native country and settled in nations such as Australia, New Zealand, Canada, and the United States. Generally, nowadays, the neighbors of a Resistance veteran are not even aware of the fact that he or she played a heroic role during the occupation. This lack of awareness could have contributed to the chronic feelings of bitterness and mistrust, which are so characteristic of many elderly Dutch Resistance veterans. When they express what they feel, the comments are always that "Nobody has learned any lessons from the Second World War," that "Nothing has changed," and that "Nobody can understand what I feel." Even today, this ambivalence plays an important role in Dutch society. In 1985, the current administration proposed to stop celebrating officially the liberation of 1945 annually, and celebrate it once every 5 years instead. In 1988, the termination of the special war pension laws was advocated, with the argument that there was now good social security for everyone in the Netherlands and that there was no longer any need for special compensation for disabled war veterans (Op den Velde, 1988).

Hence it may be said that the position of the Dutch Resistance veterans was quite different from the position of the Allied World War II combat veterans in a social and historical sense. Their position was also entirely different from that of returning Vietnam veterans in the United States in the 1960s and 1970s. First, Vietnam veterans operated in a well-organized military hierarchical structure. They received orders from their superiors instead of taking their own decisions day after day, as Resistance veterans had to do. Furthermore, the Vietnam veteran returned to a society where the social ambivalence about his role was openly present and expressed (Wilson, 1988a,b; Wilson & Krauss, 1985; Wilson, Smith, & Johnson, 1985). The Vietnam veteran was seen both as the brave man who had performed his duty for his nation and as a potential war criminal. The Dutch Resistance veterans, on the other hand, had kept silent for the most part and were ignored. They could not even blame their country or the Dutch government for the hardships and misery that they had endured, but only their own "stupidity." These peculiar negative social reactions toward the Resistance veterans may have exerted a negative influence on their coping with past traumatic experiences. It also might have blocked a thorough working-through of and a giving of sense to their still recent war experiences, which might have contributed to the fixation of traumatic reactions and traumatic personality changes.

From the perspective of the psychotherapist, it may be thought that the special position of the Resistance veterans resembles that of incest victims, who are also subject to social ignorance and disbelief. We have seen many psychiatric files and hospital records of incest victims as well as Resistance veterans, and found that in many cases their traumatic antecedents were not even mentioned (Op den Velde, 1985). This social tendency to ignore may explain why scientific studies of Dutch Resistance veterans are so scarce and, when published, hardly attract any attention.

The Study

The Subjects

In this study, 147 Dutch male former Resistance fighters participated. They were all born between January 1, 1920, and January 1, 1926. Thus, during World War II, they were between 15 and 25 years old, whereas, at the time of this study, they were between 60 and 65 years old. These veterans had all been granted a special government pension that was based on established war-related disabilities, either mental or physical, partial or complete. Most of these veterans had been exposed to severe and prolonged periods of war stress. Their traumatic war experiences (e.g., the actual duration of their participation in the Resistance and, for some, the time spent in German prisons and in concentration camps) were documented objectively by several independent witnesses' reports as an essential part of their application for this particular war veterans pension (Op den Velde *et al.*, 1990).

Sampling Procedure

All Dutch male Resistance veterans, who satisfied the age and pension criteria and who were living in the Netherlands ($N = 813$) received a letter from Stichting 1940–1945 in 1983 with a request to participate in the study. Subsequently, 619 veterans (76%) gave a positive reply and completed a 21-item self-rating questionnaire (the Maastricht Questionnaire) for the assessment of vital exhaustion (Appels, Höppener, & Mulder, 1987). Because of more than 5 missing items in the completed questionnaire, 32 subjects had to be omitted. From the remaining 582 eligible subjects, a sample of 182 was drawn for further examination. In the course of the study, a complete set of data was obtained from 147 subjects.

Results

Some of the general findings are presented here. Pertinent sociodemographic characteristics of this group are given in Table 18.4. These data show that the Resistance veterans who were studied have a relatively high level of education. The war experiences of the 147

Table 18.4. Sociodemographic Characteristics of Male Dutch Resistance Veterans

	Percentage	N = 147
Mean age 64.1 years		
Highest completed level of education		
Primary school	36.7	54
Vocational training	27.2	40
High school	30.0	44
University	6.1	9
Current employment status		
Partially employed	4.1	6
(Partially) unemployed	1.4	2
(Partial) disability pension	94.5	139
Marital status		
Married	93.9	137
Married more than once	29.1	43
Never married	2.1	3
Widowed	1.4	2
Widowed and remarried	9.5	14
Divorced	2.7	4
Divorced and remarried	19.6	29

Resistance veterans of this study are summarized in Table 18.5.

Posttraumatic Symptomatology

The prevalence of current posttraumatic stress disorder as currently defined in the *Diagnostic and statistical manual of mental disorders* (3rd ed., revised [DSM-III-R], American Psychiatric Association [APA], 1987), was assessed by means of the SCID-R-PTSD module and is given in Table 18.6.

The diagnosis of PTSD in remission was often a difficult one. This diagnosis, which was made in retrospect, was based on the personal statements made by

Table 18.5. War Experiences of the Subjects Studied

	Percentage	N
Resistance participation		
0–6 months	9.4	14
7–12 months	14.0	21
13–24 months	27.2	40
25–36 months	15.6	23
37–48 months	10.3	15
49–60 months	23.5	34
Concentration camp imprisonment following Resistance participation		
No imprisonment	49.1	72
0–6 months	12.3	18
7–12 months	15.7	23
13–24 months	9.6	14
25–36 months	8.2	12
37–48 months	4.8	7

Table 18.6. Prevalence of Posttraumatic Stress Disorder

	Percentage	N
Current PTSD	55.8	82
PTSD in remission	27.9	41
Never had PTSD	16.3	24
Total	100.0	147

the subjects so that the percentage given for PTSD in remission is an estimate.

The PTSD symptoms in the group of subjects who currently fulfilled the diagnostic criteria of the stress disorder were compared with subjects who did not meet these diagnostic criteria (Table 18.7).

Many Resistance veterans suffering from chronic PTSD, who sought medical treatment, primarily present rather unspecific complaints like unusual tiredness, diminished effort tolerance, lack of initiative, and fatigue (Op den Velde, 1985). In order to get more insight into the role of these complaints, a questionnaire measuring "vital exhaustion" was administered. *Vital exhaustion* is a complex of signs of unusual tiredness and general malaise. So far, vital exhaustion has been studied primarily in middle-aged males who were suffering from various forms of coronary heart disease (Appels & Mulder, 1988). Several current studies indicate that middle-aged males with fatal or nonfatal myocardial infarction tend to have suffered from vital exhaustion prior to the coronary event to a significantly larger extent than age-matched reference groups (Appels *et al.*, 1987; Falger, Schouten, Appels, & DeVos, 1988). The scores on the Maastricht Questionnaire, indicating the degree of vital exhaustion of the Resistance veterans are given in Table 18.8.

Table 18.7. Percentage of Clinical Ratings of DSM-III-R Symptoms of Current PTSD

Symptoms	Current PTSD	No current PTSD	p
Number of subjects	82	65	
Intrusive recollections	90.2	21.9	<.000
Recurrent dreams	65.9	22.2	<.000
Sudden acting or feeling as if the traumatic events reoccurred	59.8	10.9	<.000
Diminished interest	48.8	6.3	<.000
Feelings of detachment	56.8	10.9	<.000
Constricted affect	63.0	12.7	<.000
Hyperalertness	72.8	37.5	<.000
Sleep disturbances	86.6	43.8	<.000
Feelings of guilt	63.0	27.0	<.000
Memory impairment	66.7	30.2	<.000
Avoidance of signals that resemble the trauma	66.7	40.6	<.002
Intensification of emotions at exposure to events that resemble the trauma	90.1	54.8	<.000

Table 18.8. Measuring the Occurrence of Vital Exhaustion as Measured with the Maastricht Questionnaire

	N	Mean score[a]	SD
Resistance veterans with current PTSD	82	30.09	9.96
Resistance veterans without PTSD	65	15.48	10.91

[a]Score range: 0–42.

The Lifetime Course of PTSD

In the literature, relatively little information on the lifetime developmental course of PTSD is available; therefore, special attention was given to the occurrence of the first symptoms of the disorder (Table 18.9).

Many Resistance veterans reported considerable fluctuations over the years of their PTSD-related symptoms. Several types of life-span developmental courses were found that might be conducive to current PTSD (see Table 18.10):

1. A (sub)acute PTSD which gradually developed into a chronic condition
2. A delayed form of PTSD, in which the first symptoms developed between 5 and 35 years after the end of World War II
3. A mixed condition with PTSD complaints for a period of approximately 5 years immediately after the war, followed by symptom-free intervals of 15 to 30 years, after which manifestations of PTSD began to reoccur.

The Significance of the Type of War Trauma

The group of war victims who were studied was, in fact, composed of two groups. The first group participated actively in acts of resistance and, as a result, lived a life of uninterrupted emotional tension, perpetual anxiety, and hypervigilance for sustained periods of time.

Table 18.9. First Occurrence of Symptoms Suggestive of PTSD in 147 Resistance Veterans[a]

First symptoms	Percentage	N
1945–1950	31.7	39
1951–1955	4.1	5
1956–1960	5.7	7
1961–1965	8.1	10
1966–1970	16.3	20
1971–1975	13.0	16
1976–1980	15.3	19
1981–1985	5.7	7
Total		123

[a]Numbers based on the personal statements of the subjects.

Table 18.10. PTSD in Resistance Veterans

Types and course	Percentage	N
(Sub)acute onset (between 1944 and 1950) chronic progressive course	9.7	12
Delayed onset (between 1951 and 1985) chronic progressive course	12.2	15
(Sub)acute onset (between 1944 and 1950) duration of symptoms less than 5 years	8.1	10
Delayed onset (between 1951 and 1985) duration of symptoms less than 5 years	20.3	25
(Sub)acute onset (between 1944 and 1950) remissions and exacerbations	13.8	17
Delayed onset (between 1951 and 1985) remissions and exacerbations	35.8	44

The other group was also exposed to anxiety and hyper-vigilance but, in addition, were arrested, interrogated, and imprisoned in a concentration camp. It is generally acknowledged that staying in a Nazi concentration camp was an extremely horrible and traumatic experience. Only one in three concentration camp inmates survived. These survivors had been through countless events which, under more normal circumstances, would have been, when taken separately, sufficiently severe and outside the normal range of usual human experience to cause acute PTSD as defined in the DSM-III-R. In addition to all this, the concentration camp inmates underwent extreme physical hazards, resulting from malnutrition, injuries that were afflicted by frequent beatings, and exhaustion that was caused by hard labor as well as

the hardships of exposure to cold winters without sufficient shelter and clothing, and infectious diseases. It can be considered a miracle that so many survivors recovered with time, and that some of them never even developed any clear signs of PTSD or any other mental disorder. (In a forthcoming paper we will describe the characteristics of the small group of concentration camp survivors without PTSD.)

In order to study whether the various types of war traumata had any effect on the actual symptom patterns, those veterans who participated only in Resistance work were compared with those who were arrested and imprisoned subsequently in concentration camps (Table 18.11).

Table 18.11 clearly shows that the symptom profiles of PTSD between the two groups were not significantly different. In particular, it had been expected that more signs of numbing of responsiveness would be present in the PTSD symptom profiles of concentration camp survivors, this did not appear to be the case.

Life History Interview

In a semistructured life history interview, information was obtained on several prewar and postwar factors that might have influenced the vulnerability to PTSD. Separate data are given for the veterans with and without current PTSD (see Table 18.12).

Discussion

The Symptoms of Chronic PTSD

There were considerable differences in the symptom profiles between the Resistance veterans with cur-

Table 18.11. Prevalence of DSM-III-R Symptoms
of Current Posttraumatic Stress Disorder[a]

Symptoms	Only Resistance	Resistance and concentration camp	p
Number of subjects	72	74	
Prevalence of current PTSD	54.9	53.8	
Intrusive recollections	66.1	59.5	<.838
Recurrent dreams	50.7	43.2	<.368
Sudden acting or feeling as if the traumatic events reoccurred	36.1	40.5	<.582
Diminished interest	33.8	26.4	<.333
Feelings of detachment	35.2	37.8	<.742
Constricted affect	40.3	41.7	<.865
Hyperalertness	54.2	60.3	<.457
Sleep disturbance	68.1	67.6	<.949
Guilt feelings	48.6	45.8	<.738
Memory impairment	53.5	47.9	<.503
Avoidance of signals that resemble the trauma	57.7	52.7	<.541
Intensification of emotions at exposure to events that resemble trauma	73.2	76.4	<.664

[a]The presence or absence of the symptoms was scored. The presence is given in percentages.

Table 18.12. Life-History Data of the Resistance Veterans

Life history	No current PTSD	Current PTSD	p
Prewar period			
No chronic illness of a parent	47	53	
Chronic illness of a parent	17	29	<.255
No conflicts in the family	55	57	
Conflicts in the family	10	23	<.056
No unemployment of father	58	63	
Unemployment of father	7	16	<.122
No financial problems	54	51	
Financial problems	11	31	<.005
Postwar period			
No marital problems	52	43	
Marital problems	13	36	<.001
No divorce	52	63	
At least one divorce	13	16	<.970
No death of wife	57	73	
Death of wife	8	6	<.342
No problems with colleagues	55	66	
Problems with colleagues	10	20	<.155
No problems with own children	53	48	
Problems with own children	10	27	<.008

rent PTSD and those without PTSD, or with PTSD in partial or complete remission (see Table 18.7). Those veterans who did not meet the SCID-R criteria for PTSD exhibited relatively few symptoms of numbing of responsiveness and of reexperience, but often signs of physiological hyperarousal were present. In particular, insomnia and intensification of their symptoms at exposure to events that resembled the trauma were frequently reported. This finding is a warning that if the symptoms of PTSD fade, one cannot simply conclude that the patient is truly cured. Residual symptoms, in particular those belonging to the DSM-III-R Criterion D (Physiological Arousal) can be more permanent.

The subjects with war trauma-related PTSD suffered from vital exhaustion to a significantly larger degree than male cardiac patients in the period preceding their first myocardial infarction (see Table 18.8; see also Falger & Op den Velde, 1991). It may be thought that vital exhaustion might be clearing the way to the onset or the recurrence of PTSD symptoms in subjects with traumatic antecedents in their life history, which is in accordance with the clinical observations of concentration camp survivors done by Bastiaans (1974) (cited in the literature review).

DSM-III-R PTSD is characterized by symptoms around three dimensions of stress response: reexperiencing, avoidance and numbing, and physiological arousal (Brett, Spitzer, & Williams, 1988). The fact that vital exhaustion, or a similar concept, has not been included in the DSM-III-R PTSD seems to be the consequence of defining posttraumatic disturbances proceeding from the study of the acute reactions, rather than the chronic sequelae. Vital exhaustion might be considered a fourth dimension of chronic PTSD, in addition to the dimensions of reexperience, avoidance and numbing, and physiological hyperarousal.

The Etiology of PTSD

At the beginning of this study, we expected that a high prevalence of mental as well as physical problems would be found in particular within the group of concentration camp survivors. For the mental symptoms this expectation was not corroborated (Table 18.11). A similar finding has been reported previously by Wibaut (1961) (see Table 18.1). The comparisons between the Resistance veterans with and without concentration camp imprisonment (see Table 18.11) lead to the assumption that exposure to a high level of anxiety and hypervigilance as such might be considered to be the primary cause of the mental as well as the physical complaints that are present after more than 40 years. It may also be concluded that the many physical traumata are of lesser importance. Thus, a period of several years with uninterrupted, enhanced vigilance and fear may be considered as an extremely virulent psychotrauma.

In this respect, the war situation of the Dutch Resistance fighters differed from those of World War II military combat veterans. Military combat during World War II was generally characterized by the alternation of periods of fighting and danger with periods of rest and the absence of imminent threat. However, the sailors of the Allied merchant marines were in a situation that could be said to resemble that of the Resistance fighters. For long periods at sea, on vulnerable ships in enemy-controlled waters, there was the ever-present danger of a sudden attack by German submarines or aircraft, thus prolonging a constant fear of death.

Askevold (1980) studied a group of Norwegian war sailors, and compared them to Norwegian concentration camp survivors. Of the 35,000 Norwegian sailors in the merchant navy who sailed for the Allied forces, 6,000 were killed at sea. He recognized in both groups an almost similar symptom complex, with fatigue, irritability, lack of initiative, emotional incontinence, disturbed sleep, and recurrent dreams. For the sailors, these dreams were typically filled with alarm bells, torpedo hits, explosions, and burning ships. Eitinger and Askevold (1968) interpreted the frequent "neurasthenic symptoms" and memory impairment in concentration camp prisoners as signs of organic brain damage, resulting from malnutrition, physical damage, and emaciation by infection. The similar neurasthenic symptoms in the war sailors were, in Askevold's opinion, also an indication of organic brain damage. He concludes: "Our findings make it probable that brain damage may arise from non-physical violence via mechanisms which are quite unknown" (Askevold, 1980). In a critical review of the Scandinavian studies of war sailors, Sjaastad (1986) concluded that there was insufficient neurological proof for organic brain damage in the sailors. The description of the aging Norwegian war sailors is strikingly similar to our observations in the Dutch Resistance veterans. However, Askevold did not use the DSM-III PTSD concept. What he described, however, is a combination of signs of PTSD and what in the present study has been called "vital exhaustion." From a clinical point of view, PTSD in older subjects indeed has several aspects often observed in patients with organic brain damage, and the symptomatology of chronic PTSD might be said to be isomorphic to organic brain syndromes. In fact, such symptoms are not necessarily the result of anatomical brain damage, but they can be summoned by exposure to a long-lasting period of extreme emotional strain and uninterrupted fear of death. This might be relevant for a comparison of World War II military veterans with soldiers who have been involved in guerrilla warfare. In guerrilla warfare, imminent danger is hardly foreseeable, and, in fact, is never absent, whereas in more "classical" combat the dangers are limited to more or less restricted periods of attack or defense, with subsequent possibility for some relaxation and recuperation.

The Course of PTSD

This study, done on a group of subjects who are presently approaching old age, all of whom have been exposed to very severe and prolonged war stress, showed that PTSD often may take a chronic course and can have severe and debilitating effects. More than 40 years after the end of World War II, a considerable number of Resistance veterans still suffered from full-blown PTSD. In the majority of the cases, PTSD occurred for the first time after a symptom-free period of highly variable duration (see Table 18.9).

Although it used to be assumed that PTSD characterized by symptoms which first occur many years after the traumatic experiences was not plausible (e.g., Kluznik, Speed, Van Valkenburg, & Magraw, 1986; Scrignar, 1984), the present empirical findings (Table 18.9) do not support this assumption. The first appearance of war trauma-related PTSD symptoms, even after more than 35 years, was observed in several cases. This finding might be relevant for the interpretation of follow-up studies of trauma victims. In most recent studies of PTSD, the prevalence of trauma-related sequelae is studied in a relatively short period following the exposure to a serious stressful event. This might lead to a far too optimistic picture with regard to the long-term effects. It can be tentatively supposed that traumatic experiences can be warded off for a long time, but in many instances this will be at the cost of much invisible effort, which can progress into a condition characterized by chronic vital exhaustion. In the state of exhaustion, the subject is no longer capable of suppressing traumatic memories, and intrusive recollections as well as signs of numbing of responsiveness begin to appear. This might happen to persons who in the postwar years have gone through a period with PTSD-related phenomena, but also in subjects who never had any complaints before.

No differences were observed between the courses of the PTSD in veterans with and without subsequent concentration camp imprisonment. In a study of Holocaust survivors living in Israel, no significant differences were found between concentration camp survivors and those who had lived in hiding (Shanan & Shahar, 1983; see also Kahana, Kahana, & Harel, 1988, and Chapter 20, in this volume).

Both the Resistance veterans with and those without the concentration camp incarceration can be characterized by significantly more physical complaints than the control group of the same age taken from the general Dutch population. However, we did not find any intergroup differences. This is in accordance with the findings in the study of the Norwegian concentration camp prisoners (Eitinger & Strøm, 1973), and of Holocaust survivors living in Montreal (Eaton, Sigal, & Weinfeld, 1982). These observations underscore the remarkable adaptive and reintegrative capacities of the human body after exposure to extreme physical hardships and injuries. The results also underscore the narrow relationship between psychological stress and somatic dysfunctions.

Life History Characteristics

A matter of continuing controversy is whether the vulnerability to PTSD is influenced by early experiences and personality development. In a retrospective study of elderly people, it is impossible to identify relevant premorbid personality disturbances. However, some aspects of prewar life might be indicative of developmental problems. Chronic illness of one of the parents, conflicts in the family, and unemployment of the father were not clearly related to current PTSD. The influence of these kinds of factors on vulnerability toward PTSD is complex. Problems at a young age may exert a negative effect, but a kind of "hardening" can be positive. We observed that financial problems during childhood were positively related to current PTSD (Table 18.12, $p < .005$). An explanation for this finding remains a matter of speculation.

The general impression of the life-history interviews of the Resistance veterans warrant the conclusion that severe traumatization and subsequent PTSD symptoms do not preclude good or even excellent social and professional functioning for considerable periods of time. However, most of the subjects retired or were granted a disability pension at the age of 50 to 55 years. (At the time of the study only 6 of the 147 subjects were still partially employed. The mean year of retirement was 1975; $SD = 7.33$.) Problems and conflicts with colleagues at work often played a role and promoted early retirement.

It was often observed that the symptoms of PTSD not only continued but sometimes became worse after retirement, especially if compensation had been granted. Most Resistance veterans stated that the loss of work was a burden which exerted an unexpected negative effect on their coping with their traumatic past. A similar pattern was observed in the Scandinavian war sailors (Hartvig, 1977). Several Resistance veterans reported the onset of PTSD in relation to the loss of their jobs because of unemployment or the abolishment of their companies.

Marital problems were often reported (Table 18.12). The divorce rate in the group of 147 Resistance veterans was much in excess of that of the general population of comparable age and social background. In the group with current PTSD, marital conflicts were much more frequent than compared to the group without current PTSD ($p < .001$, Table 18.12). On the other hand, the divorce rates did not differ between the two groups ($p < .970$). It remains obscure whether the high frequency of marital problems is the result of traumatic experiences or can be seen in relation to the personality characteristics which also influenced the decision to join the Resistance. Furthermore, Table 18.12 shows that current PTSD goes together with problems with the partner as well as with educational problems with the children.

Concluding Remarks

A group of 147 Dutch male World War II Resistance veterans was studied. Some of the findings are remarkable, such as the high prevalence of current PTSD more than 40 years after the end of the war, the often extensive delay between the war trauma and the first onset of symptoms, and the role played by vital exhaustion. An important question that has to be answered, however, is whether these findings can be extrapolated to other groups of trauma victims.

First of all, the group that was studied here is not representative of the general Dutch population. Most of these veterans belonged to the "hard core" of the Resistance movement, and should be considered as true heros. They represent the rather small minority of the population that made the decision to actively resist the Nazi occupiers, and they deliberately took an enormous risk, while they could not possibly foresee all consequences. Certain personality characteristics might have influenced their attitude and decision to participate. In the interviews, most of the veterans struck the interviewers as modest and shy, and shameful rather than proud. They all stated to always having had a strongly developed sense of justice. With respect to Friedman's and Rosenman's typology, most of them could be called Type A personalities (Falger & Op den Velde, 1991). Furthermore, without exception, they all were exposed to very severe war traumata, although of differing natures during the war, generally for a period of several years. At the time of the actual Resistance participation they were young, between 15 and 25 years of age.

Dutch people generally do not give way to their feelings. In the postwar years the subjects under study hardly gave themselves time to reflect on the previous period or to deal with their emotions. The five frightening years of occupation became an unfinished chapter in their pasts. Social acceptance of the veterans was hindered by a peculiar ambivalent attitude among the vast majority of the population. When symptoms of PTSD emerged, these were often not recognized as being related to their war experiences, neither by the veterans themselves, nor by their family members, nor by their physicians. Only a few of them received anything which resembled what would now be generally accepted as a proper treatment for posttraumatic disorders. This general lack of treatment might have contributed to the fixation of their symptoms, suffering, bitterness, and feelings of estrangement.

The debt was able to remain silent for a long time, but often the bill was presented quite unexpectedly many years later. The heroic resistance to the Nazi occupiers was full of risks. Many Resistance fighters paid the price with their lives. The survivors are still paying the price now with exhaustion, insomnia, anxiety, depression, and nightmares.

ACKNOWLEDGMENTS

This study was made possible through grants from Stichting Dienstverlening Verzetsdeelnemers and Stichting 1940–1945 (Grant No. 1984.012).

References

Abalan, F. (1987). Les conséquences neuropsychiques de la déportation dans les camps de concentration Nazis de la seconde guerre mondiale chez les adultes. Doctoral dissertation, University of Bordeaux.

American Psychiatric Association. (1980). *Diagnostic and statistical manual of mental disorders* (3rd ed.). Washington, DC: Author.

American Psychiatric Association. (1987). *Diagnostic and statistical manual of mental disorders* (3rd ed., rev.). Washington, DC: Author.

Appels, A., Höppener, P., & Mulder, P. (1987). A questionnaire to assess premonitory symptoms of myocardial infarction. *International Journal of Cardiology, 17,* 15–24.

Appels, A., & Mulder, P. (1988). Excess fatigue as a precursor of myocardial infarction. *European Heart Journal, 9,* 758–764.

Askevold, F. (1980). The war sailor syndrome. *Danish Medical Bulletin, 27,* 220–224.

Bastiaans, J. (1957). *Psychosomatische gevolgen van onderdrukking en verzet* [Psychosomatic sequelae of persecution and resistance]. Doctoral dissertation, University of Amsterdam.

Bastiaans, J. (1974). The KZ-syndrome: A thirty year study of the effects on victims of Nazi concentration camps. *Revue de Medecine et Chirurgie, 78,* 573–580.

Bieder, J. (1984). Séquelles tardives et retardées de la catastrophe concentrationnaire. *Annales Médico-Psychologique, 142,* 277–283.

Brett, E. A., Spitzer, R. L., & Williams, J. B. W. (1988). DSM-III-R criteria for posttraumatic stress disorder. *American Journal of Psychiatry, 145,* 1232–1236.

Christensen, R. M., Walker, J. I., Ross, D. R., & Maltbie, A. A. (1981). Reactivation of traumatic conflicts. *American Journal of Psychiatry, 138*, 984–985.

De Jong, L. (1976). *Het Koninkrijk der Nederlanden in de tweede wereldoorlog* [The Netherlands during the Second World War] (Vol. 7, pp. 1029–1052). The Hague: Staatsuitgeverij.

Department of Welfare, Health and Cultural Affairs. (1987). *Rapport van de Commissie voor de Vereenvouding en Coördinatie van de Wetten voor Oorlogsgetroffenen* [Report of the Commission for the Adjustment of the Laws for War Victims]. Rijswijk.

Dimsdale, J. E. (1974). The coping behavior of the Nazi concentration camp survivors. *American Journal of Psychiatry, 131*, 792–797.

Eaton, W. W., Sigal, J. J., & Weinfeld, M. (1982). Impairment in Holocaust survivors after 33 years: Data from an unbiased community sample. *American Journal of Psychiatry, 139*, 773–777.

Eitinger, L., & Askevold, F. (1968). Psychiatric aspects. In A. Strøm (Ed.), *Norwegian concentration camp survivors* (pp. 45–84). Oslo: Universitetsforlaget.

Eitinger, L., & Strøm, A. (1973). *Mortality and morbidity after excessive stress.* Oslo: Universitetsforlaget.

Falger, P. R. J., & Op den Velde, W., (1991). Long-term health consequences of being a World War II Resistance veteran: Post-traumatic stress disorder and cardiovascular disease. *Psychosomatic Medicine, 53*, 226.

Falger, P. R. J., Schouten, E. G. W., Appels, A., & De Vos, Y. C. M. (1988). Sleep complaints, behavioral characteristics and vital exhaustion in myocardial infarction cases. *Psychology and Health, 2*, 231–238.

Flaten, O., & Aasen, B. M. (1976). Morbidity in two groups of resistance fighters from World War II. Prag: VI. Int. Med. Kongress der FIR, 1–2.

Häfner, H. (1968). Psychological disturbances following prolonged persecution. *Social Psychiatry, 3*, 79–88.

Hartvig, P. (1977). Krigsseilersyndromet [The war sailor syndrome]. *Nordisk Psykiatrisk Tidsskrift, 29*, 302–312.

Hers, J. F. P. (1988). The pathophysiology of imprisonment, deportation and resistance. In J. F. P. Hers & J. L. Terpstra (Eds.), *Stress: Medical and legal analysis of World War II suffering in the Netherlands* (pp. 77–84). Leiden: Samson/Sijthoff.

Kahana, B., Kahana, E., & Harel, Z. (1988). Study of 180 Holocaust survivors. *Journal of Traumatic Stress, 1*, 413–429.

Kluznik, J. C., Speed, N., Van Valkenburg, C., & Magraw, R. (1986). Forty-year follow-up study of United States prisoners of war. *American Journal of Psychiatry, 143*, 1443–1446.

Leliefeld, H., & Van Staden ten Brink, A. (1982). *Nederlandse gevangenenvan het concentratiekamp Dachau 1941–1979, onderzoek naar mortaliteit en doodsoorzaken* [Dutch prisoners of the concentration camp Dachau 1941–1979: A study of mortality and causes of death] (Part 2). Leiden: Samson/Sijthoff.

Lorenzer, A. (1968). Some observations on the latency of symptoms in patients suffering from persecution sequelae. *International Journal of Psycho-Analysis, 49*, 316–318.

Luchterland, E, (1970). Early and late effects of imprisonment in Nazi concentration camps. *Social Psychiatry, 5*, 102–110.

Nielsen, H. (1983). Invaliditeten og dens forløb 1946–79 blandt svaert deportationsbelastede KZ-fanger [Disability and its course during the period 1946–79 among severely strained concentration camp prisoners]. *Ugeskr Laeger, 145*, 935–940.

Op den Velde, W. (1985). Posttraumatisch stress-syndroom als laat gevolg van verzetsdeelname [Posttraumatic stress syndrome as a late sequel of Resistance participation]. *Nederlands Tijdschrift Geneesk, 129*, 834–838.

Op den Velde, W. (1988). Specific psychiatric disorders. In J. F. P. Hers & J. L. Terpstra (Eds.), *Stress: Medical and legal analysis of World War II suffering in the Netherlands* (pp. 121–128) Leiden: Samson/Sijthoff.

Op den Velde, W., Falger, P. R. J., De Groen, J. H. M., Van Duijn, H., Hovens, J. E., Meijer, P., Soons, M. & Schouten, E. G. W. (1990). Current psychiatric complaints of Dutch Resistance veterans: A feasibility study. *Journal of Traumatic Stress, 3*, 351–358.

Rümke, H. C. (1951). Late werkingen van psychotraumata [Delayed effects of psychotraumata]. *Nederlands Tijdschrift Geneesk, 95*, 2928–2937.

Schmolling, P. (1984). Human reactions to the Nazi concentration camps: A summing up. *Journal of Human Stress, 10*, 108–120.

Scrignar, C. B. (1984). *Posttraumatic stress disorder: Diagnosis, treatment and legal issues.* New York: Praeger.

Shanan, J., & Shahar, O. (1983). Cognitive and personality functioning of Jewish Holocaust survivors during their midlife transition (46–65) in Israel. *Archiv für Psychologie, 135*, 275–294.

Sjaastad, O. (1986). The war sailor and KZ syndrome. *Functional Neurology, 1*, 5–19.

Strøm, A. (Ed.). (1968). *Norwegian concentration camp survivors.* Oslo: University Press.

Thygesen, P. (1980). The concentration camp syndrome. *Danish Medical Bulletin, 27*, 224–228.

Thygesen, P., Hermann, K., & Willanger, R. (1970). Concentration camp survivors in Denmark. Persecution, disease, disability, compensation. A 23 year follow-up. *Danish Medical Bulletin, 17*, 65–108.

Van Scheyen, J. D. (1982). Over verzetsmentaliteit en het "Verzetssyndroom" [On Resistance mentality and the "Resistance syndrome"]. *Zeeuws Tijdschrift, 2*, 49–54.

Venzlaff, H. (1964). Mental disorders resulting from racial persecution outside concentration camps. *International Journal of Social Psychiatry, 4*, 177–185.

Warmbrunn, W. (1963). *The Dutch under German occupation, 1940–1945.* Stanford, CA: Stanford University Press.

Wibaut, F. (1961, November/1962). *Diseases and disorders resulting from resistance work and imprisonment* (pp. 126–145). The Hague, Netherlands: World Veterans Federation: International Conference on the Effects of Imprisonment and Deportation.

Wilson, J. P. (1988a). Treating the Vietnam veteran. In F. Ochberg (Ed.), *Posttraumatic therapy and victims of violence* (pp. 255–278). New York: Brunner/Mazel.

Wilson, J. P. (1988b). Understanding the Vietnam veteran. In F. Ochberg (Ed.), *Posttraumatic therapy and victims of violence* (pp. 225–254). New York: Brunner/Mazel.

Wilson, J. P., & Krauss, G. E. (1985). Predicting posttraumatic stress disorders among Vietnam veterans. In W. E. Kelly (Ed.), *Posttraumatic stress disorder and the war veteran* (pp. 102–147). New York: Brunner/Mazel.

Wilson, J. P., Smith, W. K., & Johnson, S. K. (1985). A comparative analysis of PTSD among various survivor groups. In C. R. Figley (Ed.), *Trauma and its wake: The study and treatment of posttraumatic stress disorder* (pp. 142–172). New York: Brunner/Mazel.

CHAPTER 19

Medical and Psychiatric Consequences of Being a Prisoner of War of the Japanese

An Australian Follow-Up Study

Christopher Charles Tennant, Kerry Goulston, and Owen Dent

Introduction

During World War II, Singapore was the strategic British base defending India and Australasia from Japanese attack. Despite adequate warning of the impending Japanese invasion of the Malay Peninsula, and adequate time to prepare a strategic withdrawal, the British command blundered and the island of Singapore fell to the Japanese with many thousands of British, Australian, and Canadian troops falling captive. For the next three and a half years, these troops were subject to gross privations. Initially, this large labor force was put to work in and around Singapore, and then subsequently large work parties were sent out to other areas to support the Japanese war effort. Some worked in coal mines in Japan and others were sent to the most notorious location of all—the Burma/Thailand railway. These captives were separated from loved ones without any contact or communication throughout that period and most believed they would never return to their homes. All troops, particularly those working on the railway, suffered a wide range of ongoing adverse stressors, including starvation, malnutrition, multiple infectious diseases, inadequate shelter and clothing, enforced prolonged marches, physical labor to the point of exhaustion, severe and often random physical violence, and punishments that were both brutal and unpredictable, and ultimately, because of these abuses, a high probability of dying. Some 30% overall died in captivity. Apart from findings from this present study (Dent et al., 1987; Goulston, Dent, & Chapuis, 1985; Tennant, Goulston, & Dent, 1986a,b), there have been no Australian empirical research studies of Japanese prisoners of war (POWs) although some descriptive research has been published (Hinden, 1981).

In contrast, there have been a number of morbidity studies of North American survivors of Japanese POW experience who have been followed-up for a period of some 20 years postwar (Beebe, 1975; Richardson, 1965). These North American studies have documented medical and psychiatric complications postwar in American and Canadian servicemen captured in the Pacific by the Japanese (Beebe, 1975; Richardson, 1965). Most of their data are based on subjects admitted to hospital over a 20-year period and are confounded by issues of "utilization of service" or "illness behavior." Thus, these morbidity estimates are distorted by such selection biases. In the first of these studies, POWs of the Japanese were compared with veterans of the Pacific campaign who had not been captured (Beebe, 1975). The former group had significantly more admissions over the 20-year period for 28 of 34 medical conditions. Despite issues of service utilization, nonetheless, these findings provide significant evidence of greater medical morbidity in the POW sam-

Christopher Charles Tennant • Department of Psychiatry, University of Sydney, Sydney, Australia, and Royal North Shore Hospital, Saint Leonards 2065, Australia. Kerry Goulston • Repatriation Hospital, Concord 2139, Australia. Owen Dent • Department of Sociology, Australian National University, Acton 2601, Australia.

International Handbook of Traumatic Stress Syndromes, edited by John P. Wilson and Beverley Raphael. Plenum Press, New York, 1993.

ple. Furthermore 8 of the 28 conditions identified were *psychiatric disorders* (Beebe, 1975). A subsample of these subjects was interviewed using the Cornell Medical Index and the POWs reported significantly more psychological symptoms than did the control group (Beebe, 1975). In contrast, the present study is that of a random sample of Australian POWs of the Japanese comparing their medical and psychiatric histories and examination with that of a combatant control group.

Methods

Sampling Frame

The Central Army Records Office keeps records of all persons who have ever served in the Australian Army. However, it was impossible to use these records as a sole basis for sampling, because of the very large numbers of files involved and because these files are indexed neither according to the areas in which the veterans served nor according to whether or not a veteran had been a prisoner of war. An alternative method was to attempt to obtain complete lists of veterans who had returned alive to Australia at the end of the war after imprisonment or after serving elsewhere in Southeast Asia or in the Southwest Pacific area.

The first step was to identify POWs from the Eighth Division who survived the war. All official records of the division were destroyed before the surrender, but during imprisonment, nominal rolls of troops in some units were recompiled and maintained throughout to the conclusion of the war. Some of these rolls were made available to us by veterans who had kept them since the war, and these formed the basis of the sampling frame. These nominal rolls were matched against honor rolls available from the Australian War Memorial to ensure that the names of soldiers who had died in action or during imprisonment were deleted. From these sources, it was possible to compile apparently complete lists of 4,008 names of returned members of six units of the Eighth Division. Obtaining a suitable comparison group was difficult. There was an insufficient number of Eighth Division members who were not captured to form a control group. In the absence of a suitable sampling list, it was not practical to match POWs with civilians who were in the same age group during the war. Because of different conditions of service, it was inappropriate to compare the POWs with all World War II veterans, of whom some had served only in Europe and some had never left Australia.

Ultimately, members of the Sixth, Seventh, and Ninth Divisions were selected as controls. These veterans had served in Southeast Asia or in the Southwest Pacific area during the period in which Eighth Division members were captives of the Japanese. The health status of these veterans at the time of enlistment, their age structure, the method of selection for service, and the conditions under which they served were similar to those of the Eighth Division. Unfortunately, official rolls for these divisions were destroyed after the war, but we were able to obtain apparently complete lists of 6,900 members of certain units where unit associations or individuals had maintained membership rolls over the

years. The units from which samples were drawn and the numbers of members in each of these units are listed as follows:

1. *POW group*:
   2/18th Battalion (8th Division) (770)
   2/19th Battalion (8th Division) (1,072)
   2/20th Battalion (8th Division) (736)
   2/30th Battalion (8th Division) (724)
   2/15th Field Regiment (8th Division) (421)
   8th Division Signals (283)
   Total = 4,008
2. *Non-POW group*:
   2/4th Battalion (6th Division) (1,959)
   2/23rd Battalion (7th Division) (1,615)
   6th Division Cavalry Commandos (803)
   2/2nd Machine Gun Battalion (9th Division) (803)
   2/3rd Anti-Tank Regiment (9th Division) (1,719)
   Total = 6,900

Sample Selection

It was intended to select at random 170 veterans from each group to attend the Repatriation General Hospital, Concord, Sydney for medical and psychiatric assessment. To avoid inconvenience to veterans and contain costs, only those living within the Sydney metropolitan area were included.

Each list of names was numbered consecutively, and a table of random numbers was used to select a sample from each group. If a number was repeated, a replacement random number was drawn. As the selected names were traced in the Department of Veterans Affairs in the Unit Associations and in other records, many were excluded from the study for a variety of reasons. In some cases, no records could be found: some veterans had not served in Southeast Asia or the Southwest Pacific; many had died since the war; many were not currently living in the Sydney metropolitan area; and a small number of those who were supposedly living in Sydney could not be located by letter or by telephone (see Table 19.1). Sampling continued until the required numbers of participants had been obtained. Ultimately, of 193 Eighth Division veterans who met the requirements of entry into the study and who were located and asked to participate, 170 (88%) agreed. Of 201 veterans from other divisions, 172 (86%) agreed to participate in the study. When a veteran agreed to take part in the study, an appointment was made, transport was arranged, and a further explanatory letter was sent to him. Containers for the purpose of collecting stool specimens were sent with this letter.

Accuracy of the Sample

The cost of bringing veterans to Concord Hospital, and the costs of medical examinations and nursing and administrative support, were major constraints on sample size. On the one hand, we needed to contain these costs as far as possible, while on the other hand, we had to draw a sample large enough to make sound estimates of the prevalence of various conditions and to detect differences of clinical importance in the population of all

Table 19.1. Demographic Details

	POWs	Non-POWs	Significance (p)
Australian born	92.4%	95.3%	—
Mean age (years)	66.5	65.0	.004
Mean age on leaving school (years)	14.9	14.7	.25
Occupational prestige (ANU 2)	530.0	526.0	.72
AIF recruits	88.8%	87.2%	.66
Army service to the end of World War II (months)	64.5	58.8	.0001
Private or corporal	79.4%	74.6%	.29
Retired	80.0%	73.3%	.18
Married	82.4%	82.6%	.96
Height (cm)	171.5	172.7	.1
Weight (kg)			
On enlistment	69.4	68.0	.18
On release from captivity	44.6		
On discharge from the Army	63.4	69.1	.0001
Current	74.7	77.3	.07

veterans from the Southeast Asian and Southwest Pacific theaters of World War II.

Since the study was aimed at extending knowledge rather than making a specific practical decision, the consequences of a Type I error were not serious, and a significance level of .05 was acceptable for statistical tests. With an alpha of .05, by convention beta (the probability of a Type II error) was set at four times alpha, giving power of 1 minus .02 = .8. Thus, given our sample of 170 POWs and 172 other veterans, we can determine the minimum true difference in the rate of occurrence of a disease between the two groups in the population that would be detected for a significance level of .05 and a power of .8. This difference is approximately 15%; that is, if the true difference in the case rate for a given disease is less than 15% in the population, it will probably not be detected by this sample.

Assessment Procedure

Assessment of subjects was carried out on an outpatient basis and comprised self-administered questionnaires, clinical interviews, and physical examinations carried out by specialist physicians and surgeons. A wide variety of laboratory investigations and a flexible sigmoidoscopy were carried out. The whole assessment took half a day.

Clinical Assessment

Psychological assessment comprised the following self-administered instruments: a depression inventory (Zung, 1965), the State-Trait Anxiety Scale (Spielberger, Eursuch, & Lushenere, 1970), the Eysenck Personality Questionnaire (H. Eysenck & S. B. Eysenck, 1975), and a hostility questionnaire (Jackson, 1967). Findings relating to these instruments have been published elsewhere (Tennant *et al.*, 1986). A semistructured clinical psychiatric interview was also administered to elicit psychiatric morbidity and alcohol history. The interview, an abbreviated derivation of the Diagnostic Interview Schedule, administered by a psychiatrist (C.T.), focused on affective and alcohol-related disorders using DSM-III criteria (American Psychiatric Association, 1980).

Anxiety disorders assessed were generalized anxiety, panic disorders, obsessive–compulsive neurosis, agoraphobia, social phobias, and posttraumatic stress disorder, while alcohol-related disorders comprised alcohol abuse and dependence. Affective disorders were classified as being either major affective disorder or "other depression." The diagnosis of major affective disorders did not seem too difficult, but diagnosis of other affective conditions was more polemical. For example, it was often difficult to know whether an identified episode (not qualifying as a major affective episode) had been preceded by a stressor (in order to diagnose an adjustment disorder), whether those disorders of at least two years' duration were so consistently chronic as to be called *dysthymic disorder* or, alternatively, whether they were more appropriately diagnosed as *atypical affective illness* (of the type where remissions lasted for more than a few months). In most analyses, these primary affective disorders (other than those meeting criteria for major affective illness) are collapsed and designated as "other affective disorders."

For all diagnostic groups, two further clinical judgments were made. First, a clinical judgment of severity was made for each diagnosed episode (clinically present, moderate, or severe). (This was in addition to any assessment of symptom severity already embraced by DSM criteria.) This judgment was necessarily clinical and was based on a global judgment of all symptoms and thus possibly lacks sensitivity. Second, a judgment was made about duration of episodes. A single episode was one which was clinically discrete and lasted for less than 2 years (but was usually briefer); subjects could have experienced more than one such episode. A chronic episode was one lasting for more than 2 years with symptoms largely remitting, while episodic disorder lasted for at least 2 years but symptoms showed considerable fluctuation.

Given the possibility that organic factors might have contributed to disorders, particularly affective illness, this possibility was excluded in the following ways. First, psychiatric and medical histories and examinations (the former by a psychiatrist, the latter by specialist physicians) were carried out. Second, routine screening investigations were performed; these were selected on the basis of presumed differences between POWs and controls based on war-related experiences. All subjects had full biochemical profile, full blood count and erythrocyte sedimentation rate (ESR), serum folate, serum B-12 assay, serum iron and iron binding, VDRL (test for syphilis), hepatitis antibodies, and liver function tests, including gamma glutamic transaminase. Where indicated, other tests could be ordered. Apart from a single case of alcohol-related dementia with depression, no organic factors could be clearly implicated in the affective disorders. Where alcohol abuse/dependence occurred in conjunction with depressive illness, an attempt was made to distinguish them on the basis of the temporal relationship of alcohol consumption and depressive symptoms.

Analysis of these data utilized the Statistical Package for the Social Sciences (SPSS Inc., 1983) and the analyses reported here comprise primarily 2 times 2 analyses of cross-tabulated data.

Results

The demographic details of the POWs and the non-POW controls are set out in Table 19.1. The significant findings are that the POWs from the Eighth Division were marginally older, having enlisted somewhat earlier than the divisions and they were more malnourished upon their discharge from the army.

Medical Morbidity

Table 19.2 sets out the rate of occurrence of specific illnesses in World War II as recalled by POWs and non-POWs. It is clear the POWs suffered excessive physical illnesses during their war service.

The detailed findings of the medical history and examinations have been published elsewhere (Goulston *et al.*, 1985). Only one postwar medical condition of the many assessed by medical history, namely, peptic ulcer, was recorded more by 24% of POWs compared with 10.5% of non-POWs ($p < .001$). The comprehensive clinical examination by specialist physicians showed no significant differences in the groups. Of importance perhaps, from a psychiatric point of view, was the similarity in POWs and non-POWs of the stigmata of liver disease, diseases such as gynecomastia (4.5% and 3.5%, respectively), spider nevi (2.9% and 2.3%), palmar erythema (10.6% and 9.9%), Dupuytren's contractures (9.4% and 12.2%), and parotidomegaly (4.1% and 5.3%). The wide range of clinical investigations (including FBC and ESR, biochemical profile, serum B-12 and folate, serum iron, iron binding capacity, liver function tests, hepatitis antibodies, and VDRL) revealed no significant difference between the groups; however, microbiology revealed *Strongyloides stercoralis* were positive in six POWs but only in one of the non-POWs. In essence, with one exception, the physical health of the two groups was remarkably similar.

Initial appraisal of the postwar mortality, however, seems to show many more deaths in the POW group (404 deaths) than in the non-POW group (222 deaths). This is an artifact that is due to an age difference in the two samples. Although the two groups were not significantly different in their age distribution, the comparison sample overall tended to be a few years younger than the POW groups. Given the current age of the sample, deaths are now occurring frequently. When two samples are adjusted for age, there is not a significant difference in overall death rates, illness-specific death rates, or timing of deaths over the postwar years. Most deaths have been in more recent years, as the sample has aged.

Table 19.2. Mean Rate of Occurrence of Specific Illness during World War II

Illness	Percentage POWs ($N = 170$)		Percentage non-POWs ($N = 172$)		Significance (p)
Dysentery	90.8	(2.3)	71.5	(3.4)	.0001
Malaria	85.3	(1.7)	66.3	(2.6)	.0001
Cholera	7.1	(2.0)	0.0	—	—
Hookworm	35.3	(3.6)	7.0	(1.9)	.0001
Jaundice	18.2	(3.6)	12.8	(2.5)	.16
Skin rashes	85.9	(2.7)	59.9	(3.7)	.0001
Leg ulcers	60.6	(3.7)	12.8	(2.5)	.0001
Tuberculosis	1.2	—	1.7	—	.66
Beriberi	82.9	(2.9)	1.2	—	.0001
Peptic ulcers	11.8	(2.5)	2.3	—	.0006
Mount ulcers	38.8	(3.7)	8.7	(2.1)	.0001
"Happy feet"	48.8	(3.8)	4.1	(1.5)	.0001
Nervous illness	27.5	(3.5)	23.5	(3.3)	.39

Table 19.3. Risk of Postwar Clinical Psychiatric Disorders

	Percentage			
	POWs (n = 170)	Non-POWs (n = 172)	χ^2	p
Any diagnoses	71	46	21.4	<.0001
Anxiety disorders	45	27	11.3	<.001
Major depression	6	3	1.2	>.05
Other depression	41	20	15.6	<.001
Alcohol abuse and dependence	16	15	0.2	>.05

Psychiatric Morbidity

In terms of *clinical psychiatric status*, Japanese POWs had greater risk of having a postwar clinical psychiatric disorder (71%) than did the comparison group (46%) (X^2 = 21.4, p < .0001). Table 19.3 sets out the proportion of POWs and non-POWs having specific postwar diagnoses of anxiety disorders, major depression, "other depression" and alcohol abuse or dependence. A greater proportion of POWs had anxiety disorder, "other depression" and major depression, but in the latter case the difference just failed to reach statistical significance. The two groups had similar risks of alcohol abuse or dependence.

As discussed earlier, disorders were defined as being either a single episode, episodic, or chronic and it was conceivable that for any single disorder, any subject could have had a single episode (with remission) followed later, for example, by chronic disorder. In order to assess individuals according to the chronicity of their disorder (rather than examining episodes of disorder *per se*), we designated individuals as having (1) chronic disorder (even if they had experienced earlier single episodes or had had episodic disorder) and (2) episodic disorder (even though they may have had an earlier single episode), whereas those who had only single episodes were designated as single episodes. In essence, this was a hierarchy, giving preference (in terms of defining the individual subject) to chronic over episodic and in turn over single episode(s) (see Table 19.4). There

were no significant differences in chronicity of disorder between POWs and non-POWs for alcohol abuse/dependence, or for major depression. In the case of both "other depression" and anxiety, the proportion of POWs having chronic or episodic disorders was virtually double that of the non-POWs, and these differences were statistically significant (Table 19.4). When only those having a specific disorder were assessed however, the difference in the distribution of POWs and non-POWs according to "chronicity" did not reach statistical significance, largely owing to the reduction of statistical power by the removal of the unaffected subjects. When subjects were assessed as to whether their disorders were still present at the time of interview (current impairment), in all cases but two, the subjects were designated as having either chronic or episodic impairment. The two exceptions were both subjects with major affective disorder with onset within the 2 years before the interview.

When the frequencies of single episodes alone were assessed for specific disorders in POWs and non-POWs, there was no significant difference between the groups. However, when single episodes, episodic disorder, and chronic disorder were each treated as an "episode," significantly more POWs had multiple "episodes" for certain disorders than non-POWs (Table 19.5). More POWs had multiple episodes of anxiety disorders and "other depression" than non-POWs. However, when those without disorder were removed from the analyses, there was no significant difference for these disorders between the groups. Finally, there were no significant differences between the groups for major depression or for alcohol abuse/dependence.

Table 19.6 shows the distribution of all "episodes" of individual disorders (as defined above) by year of onset for POWs and non-POWs. There was no significant difference between the two groups in time of onset for any disorder. Table 19.7 shows the distribution of "episodes" by clinical severity in POWs and non-POWs. There was no significant difference in the distribution according to clinical severity (i.e., global symptom intensity). There was no significant difference between the groups on the current use of psychotropic drugs. The proportions of POW and non-POWs, respectively, currently taking the following drugs were: hypnotics, 20% and 18%; minor tranquillizers, 18% and 15%; and other psychotropic drugs, 4% and 3%.

Table 19.4. Risk of Postwar Clinical Psychiatric Disorder

Disorder	Subjects	Percentage				χ^2 (df = 3)
		Chronic	No disorder	Single episode	Episodic	
Anxiety disorders	POWs (n = 170)	55	6	26	13	14.3
	Non-POWs (n = 172)	73	5	17	5	
Major depression	POWs (n = 170)	94	4	2	0	4.9
	Non-POWs (n = 172)	97	2	0	1	
Other depression	POWs (n = 170)	60	6	32	2	16.6
	Non-POWs (n = 172)	80	3	16	1	
Alcohol abuse and dependence	POWs (n = 170)	84	4	2	10	1.1
	Non-POWs (n = 172)	86	2	2	10	

Table 19.5. Risk of Postwar Clinical Psychiatric Disorder

Disorder	Subjects	None	One	Two	Three	χ^2	p
Anxiety disorders	POWs ($n = 170$)	94	73	3	0	13.8	<.01
	Non-POWs ($n = 172$)	162	44	1	1	($df = 3$)	
Major depression	POWs ($n = 170$)	160	7	1	2	2.9	
	Non-POWs ($n = 172$)	167	4	1	0	($df = 3$)	
Other depression	POWs ($n = 170$)	101	65	4	—	16.9	>.05
	Non-POWs ($n = 172$)	137	34	1	—	($df = 2$)	
Alcohol abuse and dependence	POWs ($n = 170$)	142	28	—	—	.12	>.05
	Non-POWs ($n = 172$)	147	25	—	—	($df = 1$)	

Table 19.6. Distribution of "Episodes" of Disorder by Years of Onset

Disorder[a]	Subjects	1943–1953[b]	1954–1963	1964–1973	1974–1983	Total
All disorders	POWs	130	11	26	31	198
	Non-POWs	73	10	123	20	116
Anxiety disorders	POWs	60	3	9	7	79
	Non-POWs	36	3	4	6	49
Major depression	POWs	5	3	0	7	15
	Non-POWs	0	1	4	1	6
Other depression	POWs	40	5	14	14	73
	Non-POWs	18	3	3	12	36
Alcohol abuse and dependence	POWs	22	0	3	3	28
	Non-POWs	19	3	2	1	25

[a]These are episodes, not subjects (one subject may have had more than one "episode" of a disorder).
[b]One phobic disorder, one obsessional neurosis, one schizophrenic illness (all in POWs) occurred in 1943–1953. No significant difference in the distribution of onset of any disorder in POWs and non-POWs.

Table 19.7. Distribution of "Episodes" of Disorder by Clinical Severity

Disorder[a]	Subjects	Present	Moderate	Severe	Total
All disorders	POWs	46	44	108	198
	Non-POWs	27	29	60	116
Anxiety disorders	POWs	12	22	45	79
	Non-POWs	12	8	29	49
Major depression	POWs	11	0	4	15
	Non-POWs	5	1	0	6
Other depression	POWs	14	4	55	73
	Non-POWs	6	2	28	36
Alcohol abuse and dependence	POWs	7	17	4	28
	Non-POWs	4	18	3	25

[a]These are episodes of subjects (one subject may have had more than one "episode" of a disorder). No significant difference in the distribution of clinical severity of any disorder in POWs and non-POWs.

**Table 19.8. Number of Hospital Admissions since World War II
for POWs and Mean Controls**

Disorder	1943–1953	1954–1963	1964–1973	1974–1983	χ^{2b}	p
Neuroses	32	14	30	9	15.1	<.01
Other psychiatric disorder	3(1)[a]	6(2)[a]	10(5)[a]	15(9)[a]	9.6	<.05
Medical illness	156	120	224	375	174.2	<.001

[a]Alcohol-related disorders principally.
[b]Chi-square calculations compare observed frequencies with expected frequencies of an even distribution of admission over time ($df = 3$).

Hospital Psychiatric Admissions

Of the combined sample of 342 subjects, more than a quarter (27%) had been admitted to hospital in the postwar years for a psychiatric illness. These admissions included a small number to hospitals apart from the Repatriation General Hospital, Concord. The primary diagnoses for these admissions were neuroses (70%), alcohol dependence (14%), psychosomatic conditions (6%), psychoses (6%), personality disorders (3%), and stress or adjustment reactions (2%). The distribution of the different diagnostic groups in POWs and controls was not significantly different.

When admission rates were examined over time for the combined sample, different patterns were suggested for neuroses and other psychiatric conditions (see Table 19.8). Neurotic admissions were greatest in the earliest postwar years and least common in the most recent period. Admission for "other disorders" increased over time and was largely accounted for by alcohol-related psychiatric conditions, but age-related conditions (a few cases of endogenous type depression) may also have made a minor contribution.

A comparison of psychiatric admissions among POWs and the control groups revealed a few statistically significant differences. For POWs, 30% had at least one psychiatric admission, compared with 23% of non-POWs ($p > .05$). The median number of psychiatric admissions was 0.21 and 0.15 ($p > .05$), respectively. No significant differences emerged when neurotic admissions or admissions from "all other conditions" were separately assessed. When only those subjects having at least one psychiatric admission were compared, POWs had significantly fewer admissions (median = 1.05) than non-POWs (median = 1.27, $p < .05$). In contrast, medical admissions (usually occurring in the early postwar years) were more likely in POWs (92%) than controls (83%) ($p > .05$); indeed, the POWs were virtually routinely admitted to hospitals immediately on their return to Australia for thorough medical assessment and treatment. There was, however, no significant association between frequency of medical and psychiatric admissions ($R = -.01$).

Discussion

At the outset, it is worthwhile commenting on the limitations of the data. First, the reliability of diagnoses of individual episodes of disorder is more unreliable, the more distant in time was the episode from the time of interview. For this reason, we believe that our diagnoses of single episodes of disorder are likely to *under-represent* the true frequency, owing to problems of recall. Any such underestimate is more likely to affect the group having more frequent postwar episodes. Thus, we believe that POWs are more likely to be so affected and so the observed differences between groups are conservative estimates. For chronic and episodic disorders, recall was less of a problem, since all these subjects had assessable impairment close to (indeed usually at) the time of interview. The problem in this instance was that of accurately dating the time of onset of these disorders; it was, however, a problem affecting POWs and non-POWs equally, since the interviewer was blind as to subject's "war" status at the time of psychiatric interview.

On the other hand, the strengths of the study are, first, that both POWs and non-POWs were randomly selected; they were not selected on the basis of hospital attendance. Second, the comparison group was well matched on prewar variables since, in both groups, individuals were randomly assigned to various battalions formed during the war years. A third strength is that the comparison group is not "normal" in that most men had seen active combat in Pacific campaigns; they, too, were a high-stressed group. To have used a comparison group that did not see service overseas would have been less appropriate however, since most young men of that era volunteered for army service and the majority was sent overseas. It could even be argued that to choose any other group would have introduced bias, since those men who did not join the army (or those who did remain in Australia) could be said to be "different." The use of our "combat" comparison group merely reinforces the conclusions we can draw about the effects of the stress for POWs. The stressful experiences of both groups were substantial, but that of the POWs was almost incomprehensible. They suffered from malnutrition, chronic infection, lack of shelter, enforced work, arbitrary brutality, and possible execution; the Japanese systematically humiliated the POWs because they had surrendered, surrender being something unthinkable to Japanese troops.

Given these experiences, it is not surprising that at the end of the war the 70% of Australian POWs who survived were in abject physical health and resembled survivors of Nazi concentration camps. In the early postwar years, virtually all were admitted to medical wards (often repeatedly) for treatment, usually for their nutrition-related disorders. Thus, it is not surprising that the POWs had significantly more postwar medical admissions that non-POWs. What does seem remarkable is that after 40 years (being at the time of our assessment) their medical health was no worse than that of the comparison group. This was reflected in their medical histories, examinations, and clinical investigations; the only difference was a significant excess of peptic ulcers. The most likely explanation for peptic ulcers in POWs is the chronic and severe psychological stress that they experienced during their captivity and that resulted in postwar depressive and anxiety states with associated autonomic arousal and, consequently, the risk of ulcer disease. Other "physical" explanations for their great risk of peptic ulceration do not seem plausible; the two groups, for example, did not differ in their smoking habits, alcohol consumption, or ingestions of a wide variety of other drugs. The relative similarity of the two groups in the above respects might perhaps be a reflection of the fact that the POWs had 30% mortality during the war years. Those who survived were presumably the fittest and were thus possibly an exceptional group.

Our findings do reveal, however, a significant excess of clinical psychiatric disorders in POWs compared with non-POWs in the postwar period. This morbidity is that of generalized anxiety disorder and "other" depressive disorders. In addition, these disorders are both more frequent and more chronic or episodic in the POWs than in non-POWs. The distributions of time of onset or of clinical severity, however, were not significantly different in the two groups. Although major affective illness was twice as common in POWs, the total number of episodes was relatively small and the differences between groups were not statistically significant. Our clinical psychiatric findings are confirmed in other elements of our data (Tennant *et al.*, 1986). For example, POWs had significantly higher scores on a depression inventory and on a state anxiety scale, although in the latter, statistical significance was not achieved.

The similarity of the groups with respect to clinically diagnosed alcohol abuse and dependence was consistent with their similarity on (1) self-reports of alcohol consumption, (2) the prevalence of liver disease assessed by medical history, (3) the prevalence of liver disease (at specialist medical examination), and (4) the similar rates of abnormal liver function tests which are reported elsewhere (Goulston *et al.*, 1985).

We believe that the etiology of the "affective" disorders (including anxiety) in the POWs can be attributed to the horrendous and prolonged psychological stress to which they were exposed. We have no evidence that organic factors directly account for the differences in rates of psychiatric illness. We argue this since the two groups were no different in terms of (1) postwar history of medical conditions (except for peptic ulcer), (2) postwar age-adjusted mortality, (3) findings from an extensive medical examination, (4) results of clinical investigations, and (5) ingestion of current "medical" drugs which might predispose one to psychiatric illness (including steroids, antihypertensives, nonsteroidal anti-inflammatory drugs, beta blockers, etc.) (see Goulston *et al.*, 1985).

The nature of their psychiatric disorders is also worthy of some comment. Almost all those with anxiety syndromes had generalized anxiety; no case fulfilled all the criteria for posttraumatic stress disorder, although

some specific "posttraumatic" symptoms were observed. Perhaps most frequent were occasional nightmares about war experiences and, for some, avoidance of activities that might arouse recollection of their experiences; but these occurred in a minority of subjects.

Of those with major affective disorder, none had bipolar disorder, none was psychotic, and none had melancholia. Of those with "other depression," those with chronic disorder would be called *dysthymic*, whereas those with episodic depression would be regarded as *atypical depression* of the type where there may have been periods of normal mood lasting for more than a few months (American Psychiatric Association, 1980).

Disorders, furthermore, were often mixed; many subjects, for example, had some features of both anxiety and depression. A clinical judgment was therefore made as to which disorder was most prominent: for example, "other depression" did not necessarily take precedence over generalized anxiety. In these subjects who had posttraumatic symptoms, for example, most had diagnosed depression which was deemed to be more disabling than their posttraumatic symptoms; a depressive diagnosis was thus made. (Had the depressive symptoms not been present, no subjects would have qualified for a diagnosis of posttraumatic stress disorder.)

Despite having more postwar psychiatric morbidity than the comparison group, the POWs did not have significantly more psychiatric admissions. Indeed, they had significantly fewer multiple admissions. It could be argued that perhaps they were more often selectively treated in other settings, either by general practitioners or in psychiatry outpatient departments, but we do not see any reason why this would be so. We could interpret these findings in either of the following ways: First, it may be that those who have had catastrophic stress more often expect to have psychological symptoms (since there is some understandable "cause"); thus, they may not perceive their symptoms as being due to illness and so do not initiate medical contact. A second explanation relates to their use of particular ego defenses. We know, clinically, that POWs use denial and suppression to cope with their unpleasant memories of the war. If similar defenses are used to cope with emotional symptoms, then it may influence their illness behavior: it is our impression that many POWs actively minimize the significance of their symptoms.

When admissions are examined over time, the pattern for the whole group (Table 19.4) was not unusual, in that neurotic admissions were most common in the earliest years postwar, whereas admissions for other psychiatric conditions (largely alcohol-related) increased with the passage of time. Why these admission findings (i.e., less frequent psychiatric admissions in POWs) are so different from those in the United States is, however, hard to explain. Perhaps the "stoicism" alluded to above is greater in Australian than in American POWs, but this must remain speculation.

The nature of clinical morbidity at interview is also of some interest. In general, the morbidity was episodic or chronic depression or anxiety. The depression best fits the description of neurotic depression or dysthymic disorder; the anxiety, that of generalized anxiety syndrome; the reasons why no PTSD diagnoses were made are discussed above.

The greater risk of psychiatric disorder in POWs was also reflected in the rate of Totally and Permanently Incapacitated (TPI) pensions, being 24% in POWs and 8% in non-POWs. We believe that psychiatric morbidity accounted for most of this, since there was little difference in self-report for postwar medical disorders (peptic ulcer being the exception) and there was no significant medical differences between the groups at the time of assessment. Sensitive data on the attribution of pension status, however, were difficult to obtain, as most subjects had multiple disabilities accepted (medical and psychiatric) as being due to war services.

In the general literature on traumatic stress syndrome, there are very few empirical studies of the long-term effects of catastrophic stress. There is a large literature on survivors of the Holocaust, but it is typified by samples that have not been randomly selected. For example, Eitinger (1972) studied those subjects in contact with medical services and had no useful comparison data. Recently, however, there have been two community studies of randomly selected survivors of the Holocaust. Both Levav and Abramson (1984) and Eaton, Segal, and Weinfield (1982) found that concentration camp survivors, compared with community controls, had significantly greater symptomatic morbidity, as assessed by self-completion questionnaires, 25 and 33 years, respectively, after their release. Some of our data (that for the Zung depression scale) (Zung, 1965) show similar results.

Our study, however, goes somewhat further, for we assessed medical and psychiatric morbidity by a comprehensive clinical examination and by laboratory investigations; we examined admissions to hospital and postwar mortality. Medical morbidity and mortality were very similar in POWs and the comparison group. Clinical depression and anxiety at the time of interview was, however, greater in POWs, but this was not reflected in psychiatric admissions where POWs had no more admission than non-POWs. Not surprisingly, catastrophic stress thus continues to have psychological effects over very many years, but in this remarkable group of men, it did not appear to affect significantly their physical health or consumption of drugs or alcohol, nor did it influence illness-related behaviors.

References

American Psychiatric Association. (1980). *Diagnostic and statistical manual of mental disorders* (3rd ed.). Washington, DC: Author.

Beebe, G. W. (1975). Follow-up of studies of World War II and Korean war prisoners: Motility, disability and maladjustments. *American Journal of Epidemiology, 101,* 400–419.

Eaton, W. W., Segal, J. J., & Weinfield, D. M. (1982). Impairment in Holocaust survivors after 33 years: Data review in abused community people. *American Journal of Psychiatry, 139,* 773–777.

Eitinger, L. (1972). *Concentration group survivors in Norway and Israel.* The Hague: Martinus Nighoff.

Eysenck, H., & Eysenck, S. B. (1975). *Eysenck Personality Questionnaire.* London: Hoddeb & Staunton.

Goulston, K., Det, O., & Chapius, P. (1985). Gastrointestinal morbidity among World War II prisoners of war: 40 years on. *Medical Journal of Australia, 143,* 6–10.

Hinden, D. C. (1981). Prisoners of war: Long-term effects. *Medical Journal of Australia, 1,* 565–566.

Jackson, D. N. (1967). *Personality Research Form manual research.* New York: Psychiatrists Press.

Levav, I., & Abramson, J. H. (1984). Treatment distress among concentration camp survivors: A community study in Jerusalem. *Psychological Medicine, 14,* 215–218.

Nie, N. H., Holl, C. H., & Jenkins, J. G. (1970). *Statistical package for the social sciences.* New York: McGraw-Hill.

Richardson, H. J. (1965). *Disabilities and problems of Hong Kong veterans 1964–1965.* Ottawa: Canadian Pensions Commission Department.

Spielberger, C. D., Eursuch, R. L., & Lushenere. (1970). The state-trait anxiety inventory consulting. California: Psychiatrists Press.

Tennant, C., Goulston, K., & Dent, O. (1986a). Clinical psychiatric illness in prisoners of war of the Japanese: Forty years after release. *Psychological Medicine, 16,* 833–839.

Tennant, C., Goulston, K., & Dent, O. (1986b). Australian prisoners of war of the Japanese: Post-war psychiatric hospitalisation and psychological morbidity. *Australian and New Zealand Journal of Psychiatry, 20,* 334–340.

Zung, W. W. (1965). A self-rating depression scale. *Archives of General Psychiatry, 12,* 63–70.

CHAPTER 20

Social Resources and the Mental Health of Aging Nazi Holocaust Survivors and Immigrants

Zev Harel, Boaz Kahana, and Eva Kahana

Holocaust Literature

A review of the literature dealing with the effects of the Nazi Holocaust documents a wide range of physical and psychic impairments suffered by survivors (Chodoff, 1966; Eitinger, 1961). There is a basic agreement among most of the writers that survivors have indeed suffered lasting physical, mental, psychological, and social impairments. As a result, many survivors are characterized as being severely handicapped in a variety of life situations (Chodoff, 1966; Eitinger, 1961; Krystal, 1968). Recent reports within the clinical psychiatric tradition continue to provide evidence of the scarring effects of the Holocaust on survivors (Marcus & Rosenberg, 1989). The literature also suggests that following World War II, the survivors' recovery was made more difficult because the families and communities, through which they might have found comfort and help, no longer existed (Davidson, 1979; Levav & Abramson, 1984).

Similarly, there are assertions that aging survivors of the Holocaust, as they grow older and weaker, are especially vulnerable as they face death, lose loved ones, and spend time in institutions (hospitals or nursing homes). Their physical frailty and psychological vul-

nerability may stimulate memories of traumatic experiences which occurred in camps, in ghettos, or in hiding. These posttraumatic processes cause added burden, along with the challenges of everyday life (Danieli, 1982).

Steinitz (1982) noted that as Holocaust survivors age, the various symptoms of the survivor syndrome, which they had been able to bring under control, come to the surface and assume a dominant role in their lives. The losses and disabilities associated with aging interact with the unhealed psychic wounds and chronic health problems stemming from the events of World War II, thus leaving the aging survivor in a particularly vulnerable position and creating a situation which places strain on family members. As a result, the children of these survivors may begin to enact a pattern of transference and guilt in relation to their parents. They may also begin to experience in a personal way many of the problems of their parents (Steinitz, 1982). The entire family system may be dynamically affected through such reciprocal effects.

In considering the second-generation effects of the Holocaust, it is believed that it was almost impossible for a child living in a "concentration camp family" to grow and mature normally. It has been observed that members of survivor families were more closely enmeshed than those of "American" families, that attachments were stronger, and separations or losses produced greater difficulty. Frequently, children of survivors also described themselves as protective of their parents (Podietz et al., 1984). It has also been suggested that intensive involvement of children through communication with their parents about the Holocaust caused greater disturbances in psychological development of the second generation than for children less actively involved in their parents' traumatic experiences (Robinson & Winnik, 1981).

Zev Harel • Department of Social Work and Center on Applied Gerontological Research, Cleveland State University, Cleveland, Ohio 44115. **Boaz Kahana** • Department of Psychology and Center on Applied Gerontological Research, Cleveland State University, Cleveland, Ohio 44115. **Eva Kahana** • Department of Sociology and Elderly Care Research Center, Case Western Reserve University, Cleveland, Ohio 44106.

International Handbook of Traumatic Stress Syndromes, edited by John P. Wilson and Beverley Raphael. Plenum Press, New York, 1993.

Generalizations based on the medical psychiatric literature underscore the presence of severe pathological consequences of the Holocaust among survivors and their children. As a consequence of these effects, survivors and their children can be viewed as emotionally and socially impaired. On the basis of such conclusions, it may be expected that the social interaction and social relations of Holocaust survivors with their children, family members, and friends tends to be problematic. Conversely, it may be argued that the ability to activate social resources and maintain positive social functioning in the face of extreme trauma represents a hallmark of healing and facilitates mental health among victims of extreme trauma.

However, recent reviews of the clinical literature and cross-sectional studies on the effects of the Holocaust on survivors and children of survivors have raised serious questions about the validity of generalizations based on clinical observations and studies which lack methodological sophistication (Harel, 1983; Solkoff, 1981).

Harel (1983) and Solkoff (1981), following critical evaluations of clinical and experimental studies of Holocaust survivors and their children, questioned the wisdom of basing assertions about the effects of persecution experiences solely upon clinical observations and on poorly designed studies relying primarily on psychoanalytic perspectives of traumatic neurosis. Methodologically, Solkoff (1981) found the studies of Holocaust survivors that he reviewed to be problem-laden, with samples haphazardly selected and control groups nonexistent or poorly described. He concluded that investigators and clinicians often follow personal hunches, looking at survivor populations for evidence to substantiate their personal beliefs. Solkoff (1983) stated that one must guard against vast theoretical leaps from inadequately gathered and reported data, especially from treatment-seeking populations.

More recently, there have been a number of empirical studies specially designed to ascertain the long range effects of the Holocaust on survivors and their children. These studies underscore the remarkable adaptive and reintegrative capacities of Holocaust survivors, their creation of healthy families and social achievements (Anthony & Koupernick, 1973; Bergman & Jucovy, 1982; Davidson, 1981; Klein, 1971; Last & Klein, 1984; Leon, Buthcher, Kleinman, Goldberg, & Almagot, 1981; Pilcz, 1979; Shanan & Shahar, 1983; Weinfeld, Sigal, & Eaton, 1981). Moreover, Davidson (1981) stated that the presence of symptoms of trauma does not preclude good social and family functioning. He advised against generalizations applied to the large heterogeneous population of survivors and their families. Findings from these studies suggest that those writing in the medical psychiatric perspective may have derived their conclusions from observations of biased samples of persons seeking psychiatric help and those applying for restitution from Germany.

There is also a recognition in the professional literature that earlier clinical assumptions based on the medical–psychiatric literature may have been exaggerated. Rustin (1980) warned against the temptation to view all survivors of the Holocaust and their children as one homogeneous group. The particular circumstances of each individual and his or her family must be examined if helpful therapy is to result. Feuerstein (1980) also cautions against the trend, present in the psychological literature on the Holocaust, to view survivors as a homogeneous group. In agreement with this view, Krell (1982) asserts that the successful adaptation of survivor families has not as yet received sufficient attention in the professional literature.

A number of more recent studies have made strides in the direction of addressing adaptation of Holocaust survivors based on broader theoretical perspectives and methods with logically sound approaches. This research indicates that although some Holocaust survivors have been scarred by their experiences, there is also evidence that a large number of survivors are well-adjusted individuals and have made substantial contributions in their new environments. Similarly, while there is evidence indicating that children of survivors sought professional help, there is also considerable evidence which indicates that large numbers of survivors' children have adjusted well personally and enjoy healthy family relationships (Klein-Parker, 1988). Survivors also indicate that their adjustment problems were more difficult because of reactions toward them which included open hostility, indifference, and an attitude of "blaming the victim." Survivors state that the adjustment of stress victims is likely to be aided by more sensitive and more understanding attitudes on the part of the general public and the professional and scientific communities toward their individual and collective concerns. Understanding the role of social resource factors in the reduction or amelioration of long-term stress effects and in aiding the psychological well-being of survivors represents a much needed and potentially useful avenue for developing a more comprehensive understanding of Holocaust survivors and victims of other major trauma.

Social Resources and Mental Health

There has been considerable interest in the gerontological literature concerning the social resources and mental health of the aged. This interest has been stimulated by attempts in gerontological research to identify salient elements of "successful aging" and predictors of well-being, and by efforts to delineate dimensions of frailty and vulnerability among the aged (Federal Council on the Aging, 1978; Harel, Sollod, & Bognar, 1982; E. Kahana, B. Kahana, & Kinney, 1990; Larson, 1978; Palmore, 1979). Cross-sectional studies on the well-being of the aged have shown that mental health is best predicted by health and functional status, socioeconomic status, social resources, and the degree of social integration. There are consistent indications in the literature that psychological well-being in the aged is associated with better health, higher socioeconomic status, and higher economic resources (Larson, 1978). Psychological well-being has also been found to be associated with social interaction, social activity and social support (Harel et al., 1982; Harel & Deimling, 1984).

Although higher social resources are generally found to be associated with better mental health, lower social resources, as well as social losses, have been found to be predictive of poorer mental health (Harel & Deimling, 1984). Older people often experience a decline in social roles, contacts, and relationships (Harel *et al.*, 1982; Larson, 1978), placing them at special risk for negative psychosocial outcomes (E. Kahana *et al.*, 1990).

Research shows that greater support received by the individual in the form of close relationships with family members, friends, acquaintances, co-workers, and the like, *decreases* the likelihood that the individual will experience stress or illness; thus, the level of well-being increases (Dean & Lin, 1977). Mental health may also be enhanced by perceived availability of social resources that are responsive to the needs elicited by stressful life events (Ben-Sira, 1985; Burchfield, Hamilton, & Benks, 1982; Cohen & Wills, 1985; Krause, 1987). There are indications that specific types of social support (e.g., emotional support, integration, tangible help) buffer the impact of specific types of stressors (e.g., death of close family member, crime, and family crises) (Cohen, Teresi, & Holmes, 1986; Krause, 1987). Research also indicates that giving assistance to others (E. Kahana, B. Kahana, Harel, & Rosner, 1988) benefits psychologically in terms of enhanced competence and self-esteem.

There is no clear indication, as yet, as to why and how social support plays a role in preventing stress and illness. House (1981) suggests that social support may act as a buffer between stress and the individual's health. Dean and Lin (1977) conclude that social support may act either as an antecedent factor that reduces the effect of the undesirable experience or as a buffer following the experience.

Social Interactions and Networks

Social interaction (i.e., visiting, phone calls, going places) with family members and friends has also been implicated as playing a role in facilitating mental health and well-being of the elderly, but the exact nature of this role has not been specified. Lemon, Bengtson, and Peterson (1972) suggested that informal activity, which is part of an ongoing relationship, is a strong correlate of life satisfaction because these relationships provide the role supports necessary for maintaining an individual's self-esteem and self-concept. Other studies lend support to their positions, indicating that informal activity with friends sustains morale and life satisfaction (Rosow, 1967).

Evidence continues to accumulate indicating both direct and indirect effects of a social network on illness. Findings indicate that social networks exert a direct effect on reducing physical health symptoms. Social networks also act to reduce symptoms by buffering the effect of increased levels of stress (Cohen & Wills, 1985; Krause, 1987). There is evidence that these effects are not due to the amount of social contact or the quantity of social relationships, but to the extent to which a supportive network reduces feelings of isolation and provides support and help when needed. Accordingly, stress resistant groups were found to have better family support than their counterparts in the distressed group (Dean, 1986; Holahan & Moos, 1985).

There have been few studies which systematically investigated patterns of social interaction and social support and their relative importance for the mental health and/or psychological well-being of extreme stress victims. There is some evidence to indicate that greater social support is associated with better mental health among survivors of extreme stress (Elder & Clipp, 1988; B. Kahana, Harel, & E. Kahana, 1988; Wilson, Harel, & Kahana, 1988).

In summary, it may be concluded that better social resources may be associated with better mental and physical health in the aged. This association is also found in studies with individuals who experienced traumatically stressful events. Social networks generally provide informal support to older individuals and families and, therefore, serve as a buffer between stress and physical and mental impairment. Conversely, losses in resources, and especially losses of irreplaceable social resources, serve as serious stressors in the lives of the aged. It is important to underscore, however, that social networks may also create stresses, and this is especially evidenced in cases of burdens imposed by the care needs of the impaired aged (Noelker & Harel, 1983).

Social Resources and Psychological Well-Being of Holocaust Survivors

With burgeoning evidence in the field of stress research and gerontology illustrating direct, mediating, or moderating effects of support, the benefits of formal and informal aid to the aged who experienced extreme trauma may be very much expected. Yet the potential or actual roles played by social resources in protecting victims of extreme trauma from the long-term impact of stress on psychosocial well-being have seldom been addressed in the literature. Specifically, studies of Holocaust survivors have only recently begun to reflect social science perspectives and move beyond documentation of the adverse consequences of posttraumatic stress syndromes to a much broader view of survivorship and adaptive functioning.

Thus, although there has been an increased interest in the role and importance of social support for persons during their advanced years of life, there have been few attempts to investigate empirically the relative importance of social affiliations, social interaction, social support, and self-disclosure for the psychological well-being of the aged victims of extreme stress. To the extent that extreme stress places individuals at special risks for adverse mental health consequences—there is reason to expect that social resources should be particularly important as predictors of psychological well-being among survivors of traumatic experiences. In order to advance our theoretical formulations in social gerontology, there is a need for more empirical investigations on the importance of social resource variables for the psychological well-being of the aged who have experienced extreme stress.

In our research (B. Kahana *et al.*, 1988) we explored differences in social resources and their relative importance as predictors of psychological well-being among survivors of the Holocaust and comparison groups of European immigrants in the United States and in Israel.

Survivors came to the United States and Israel following World War II, while the comparison groups arrived in the United States and Israel prior to the war. The data presented in this chapter are part of a larger study discussed elsewhere (B. Kahana *et al.*, 1988). One of the primary objectives of this research was to examine differences in social resources and the relative importance of social resource variables for the psychological well-being of aging survivors of the Holocaust and members of the comparison groups.

In our view, it is important to explore not only the pathological consequences and the scars caused by the Holocaust but to also ascertain the factors which are likely to reduce these adverse consequences and aid the psychosocial adjustment of survivors.

Measurement of Social Resources

Measurement of social resources has moved from unidimensional conceptualization to its consideration as a multidimensional construct. Yet there is no agreement as to what salient dimensions of social resources are and how these dimensions may be interrelated. In this chapter, we offer a differentiation of social resource dimensions and theoretical foundations for the importance of the differentiation. Earlier studies of social resources have considered this variable to be a single construct. Recently, however, there have been attempts to differentiate between various indicators of social resources. In research on social resources and mental health (Harel & Deimling, 1984), a factor analysis of the social resource measures included in the OARS instrument yielded a differentiation between social affiliations, social interaction, and social support, and the perceived adequacy of social interaction. Another study which examined the relationship between social resources and mortality differentiated between three components: roles and attachments, social interaction, and social support (Blazer, 1982). These studies, which illustrate the multidimensional nature of the term *social resources*, represent significant conceptual and methodological refinements and should prove useful in stimulating future research in these areas. Therefore, the present study of Holocaust survivors also differentiates between social networks, social interaction, self-disclosure, and social support. One of the central distinctions in the social science literature relates to the conceptualization of social resources and social integration as consisting of two components: an environmental dimension (defined by social network) and a personal dimension (reflections and behaviors) (Cassel, 1976; Rosow, 1967).

Social Networks—Structural Dimensions

Social networks may be seen as structural linkages within which interaction and support occur. *Social resources* may be seen as constituting those interactions and supports which meet psychosocial as well as instrumental needs of the person and may sustain identities of the individual. In the social science literature, *social networks* are viewed as potential sources of support and, as such, these are perceived as resources which are also likely to enhance well-being in the aftermath of stressful life events. Embeddedness in social networks is generally considered in terms of family, friendships, neighbors, and associational or organizational linkages. Although this structural definition of social networks focusing on presence of family ties may be environmentally defined, a closer scrutiny reveals that only family of orientation is truly independent of the actions of a person. Families of procreation, informal friendships, and organizational memberships all reflect on person–environment transactions requiring proactive behaviors to generate them.

In the case of survivors of extreme stress and survivors of the Holocaust, the traumatic experience itself impacted in a major way on the size of the survivors' social networks. The Holocaust resulted in loss of members of the family of origin and the family of procreation. It left survivors bereft of parents, siblings, friends, and neighbors who comprised the essence of their earlier social networks.

In the aftermath of such trauma, major questions arise that relate to desire and ability of such individuals to reconstruct new social networks through marriage, procreation, and affiliation with friends, informal groups, and organizations. Thus, it becomes apparent that social networks are not merely "available" or "given" sources of support in the stress-resources-outcome paradigm as applied to survivors, but these reflect dynamic adaptations resulting from initiatives and activation of resources in the aftermath of traumatic life experiences. Social networks may thus be viewed as the structural framework that is necessary, but perhaps insufficient, to provide the reference groups and the boundaries where interaction and support take place. Our research addresses the question to what extent are there differences in the size of the social networks of survivors and members of the comparison groups. We consider the social network to consist of families of orientation (siblings and other relatives) and families of procreation (spouses and children).

Social Interaction and Social Support— Functional Dimensions

A second aspect of social resources refers to social behaviors or transactions which are likely to activate or reinforce the giving and receipt of support from members of one's social network and which serve to develop and/or sustain these networks. We thus consider under the heading of social resources diverse social behaviors or transactions that have been used as proxies for social resources in the social science and gerontological literature. These include social interactions, self-disclosure, helpfulness to others, and support received.

Social Interactions. This social resource dimension involves visiting, writing, telephoning, and going places with others. Social interactions represent transactions that include personal as well as socioenvironmental initiatives and response patterns. Thus, if victims of extreme trauma are stigmatized by others, they may be less likely to initiate visits, to receive visits or to be invited to go to places with others. At the same time, persons suffering from posttraumatic stress disorder may behave in socially isolated or anxious ways; hence the consequences of their traumatic stress may diminish their degree of involvement with others. Social interactions, in turn, may also be related to support received in times of need, with those more socially interactive or integrated receiving more frequent support. It is important to note, however, that frequency of social interaction should not be equated with closeness or intensity of social ties.

Self-Disclosure. Self-disclosure represents a form of social behavior that is particularly relevant to victims of trauma. Although self-disclosure has been seldom considered to be a specific component of social resources, there is evidence that close and emotionally satisfying relationships comprise important components of social support (Lowenthal & Berkman, 1967). Self-disclosure in social interactions may represent an important prerequisite for forming close social bonds with others and securing confidants. Self-disclosure in social interactions may also be the consequence of the formation of close social bonds. In the aftermath of traumatic life events, the ability to share with others concerns, discomfort, and painful feelings can serve cathartic functions and also activate social supports needed to deal with stress. Recent research (Pennebaker, 1985) suggests that confiding in others in the aftermath of trauma plays a major protective role and reduces the adverse effects of trauma on health. The adaptive functions of self-disclosure in enhancing psychosocial well-being of Holocaust survivors have been demonstrated in our earlier work (B. Kahana et al., 1988). We have noted, however, previously explored differences in self-disclosure between survivors and those who did not endure extreme trauma. Self-disclosure, considered here as a social resource, requires both a personal initiative and a socioenvironmental response.

Social Support Received and Given. Social support is more typically considered in the gerontological literature as assistance received by older persons. In our research, we differentiated between being helpful (giving assistance) to others and receiving assistance. Consideration of social support given to others and being helpful is particularly salient in the framework of the stress research paradigm because it may impact directly on a person's competence and self-esteem, which are likely to be undermined under conditions of traumatic stress (E. Kahana, Midlarsky, & B. Kahana, 1987). Considering social supports in an exchange framework, the provision of support at one point in time may enhance the probability of receiving support at a future time when such supports are needed. Provision of aid to others may be particularly salient to adaptation of Holocaust survivors who found that assisting fellow victims was a major viable form of proactive adaptation during the war (B. Kahana, E. Kahana, Harel, & Segall, 1986).

Such social behaviors as interaction, self-disclosure, and helping comprise important aspects of a multidimensional consideration of social resources. We see these behaviors as proactive rather than environmentally defined, although opportunities and responses of the environment play an important role in their expression. For example, "the conspiracy of silence" concept, which assumed that the Holocaust survivors did not wish to share their traumatic experiences, limited opportunities for self-disclosure among Holocaust survivors.

Support received represents the most extensively studied component of the social resource paradigm. The gerontological literature has focused extensively on instrumental and socioemotional supports received by older persons as major buffers of stress in late life. Instrumental support refers to concrete and tangible services which help persons meet their needs. Instrumental support may be activated at times when individuals have difficulty in coping with certain environmental demands. Instrumental supports, including receiving help with chores, shopping, transportation, or cooking, may have direct effects on well-being and diminish stress in cases of vulnerability. To the extent that survivors have built close family ties with their children, we may expect that the elderly survivors will receive support from their children which, in turn, will enhance their well-being. Socioemotional support helps to maintain a sense of self and facilitates coping (Thoits, 1983). It has been argued that the opportunity for intimacy and fulfillment of expressive needs improves the individual's ability to deal with crises (Dean & Lin, 1977). The value of affective support has been underscored in much of the social support literature as having a stress buffering function. There is evidence that perceived support may be just as important as received support (Wethington & Kessler, 1987) in contributing to the feeling of being valued. In turn, this enhances self-esteem and internal locus of control that subsequently enhance coping with stress.

Meaningful social interactions, self-disclosure, and social support have been found to contribute to the morale of the aged. The research reported here ascertained the extent to which these social resource dimensions are portrayed and the degree to which they facilitated psychological well-being of Holocaust survivors and members of the comparison groups.

Variables and Their Measurement

Four social resource variables were employed in this research, including *social network* (being married, having children, having brothers/sisters, and having relatives), *social interaction* (going places with others, visiting, telephoning, discussing, and confiding), *self-disclosure* (everyday issues, important issues, sex, finances, and the Holocaust), and *social support*. Social support was ascertained both in terms of being helpful (giving assistance) to others and receiving assistance. Both esteem support (concern for well-being, attention to ideas) and instrumental support (transportation, shopping, repairs, cooking, finances, and support at time of illness) were considered in assessing this construct.

Psychological well-being (morale) in this research was measured by 15 items from the Philadelphia Geriatric Center (PGC) Morale Scale (Lawton, 1975). Morale was selected as one of the outcome variables because it is an extensively used measure of psychological well-being in later life. Morale has been shown in prior research to be influenced by stress and to be responsive to situational influences.

Two sets of research questions were explored in this study. The first question relates to the differences in social network, social interaction, self-disclosure, and social support between survivors of the Holocaust and members of the comparison groups who arrived in the United States and Israel from the same countries prior to World War II. It was hypothesized that survivors would have a more restricted social network and more limited social interaction and social support. They were also expected to be less likely to share concerns, ideas, and feelings with others. These expectations were based on observations from the Holocaust literature (Chodoff, 1966) which suggest that the social world of Holocaust survivors is more constricted. The second set of questions addressed the importance of social resource variables in predicting morale in both groups. Based on observations from the Holocaust literature (Danieli, 1982; Steinitz, 1982), it was expected that the social interaction and social support of Holocaust survivors would be more problematic and, consequently, adversely affect their psychological well-being. The gerontological literature, however, suggests that higher levels of social interaction, and especially social support, are associated with better mental health among the aged. Because there have been no previous studies in which the importance of social network, social interaction, self-disclosure, and social support for predicting psychological well-being was systematically ascertained, this research aimed to provide answers to these questions.

Survivors and Controls

Respondents in this research included a survivor group and a comparison group in the United States and two similar groups in Israel. Participants in the United States research included a group of 168 survivors of the Holocaust who immigrated to the United States between the end of World War II and 1965 and a group of 155 immigrants who arrived in the United States prior to World War II. Respondents in both groups were from countries that were under the occupation of Nazi Germany during the Second World War. Respondents ranged in age from 45 to 90, women (55%) outnumbered men slightly, and a somewhat higher percentage of survivors were married compared to controls (82% vs. 69%).

The Israeli sample included a group of 180 survivors of the Holocaust who immigrated to Israel after World War II and 160 persons from similar Eastern European countries who immigrated to Israel prior to the onset of the war and the German occupation of their respective countries. Both respondent groups included individuals 55 years of age and older from European countries. Respondents ranged in age from 55 to 90, with the survivors' average age being somewhat younger than respondents in the comparison group. A slightly higher percentage of respondents in both groups were women, and the overwhelming majority of the respondents were married.

Comparing Survivors and Immigrants on Social Resource Variables

The United States Sample

Details concerning patterns of social affiliation, social interaction, self-disclosure, and social support among survivors and immigrants in the United States are found in Table 20.1. A comparison of United States survivors and immigrants on social network indices reveals that survivors were significantly more likely to be married and had a higher average number of children. There were some differences noted between survivors and immigrants in social interaction. The extent of visiting, telephoning, and discussing issues was somewhat higher among survivors, even though the differences were not statistically significant between the two groups.

Survivors were also more likely than members of the comparison group to portray self-disclosure, sharing everyday concerns with their children, family members, friends, and co-workers and to discuss sex issues and finances. However, only the discussion of finances was significantly different between the two groups.

There were a number of significant differences found between the two groups in giving support to others. Survivors were more likely than members of the immigrant group to give assistance with shopping, repairs, cooking, and finances and more likely to offer assistance in times of illness. It is noteworthy that, although survivors engaged in giving behaviors more often than the comparison group, they did not receive more assistance than the comparison group either in the form of instrumental or socioemotional support.

These findings indicate very clearly that in terms of social network, social interaction, self-disclosure, and social support, aging survivors of the Holocaust in the United States are doing as well and, in some instances, better than members of the comparison group.

The Israeli Sample

Details concerning patterns of social affiliation, social interaction, self-disclosure, and social support among survivors and immigrants in Israel are found in Table 20.2. The comparison of aged survivors and immigrants in Israel on social network reveals that both groups had a similar proportion of respondents who were married. However, survivors had a slightly lower average number of children. Respondents in the immigrant group had somewhat higher number of brothers/sisters and relatives; however, these differences were not significant.

There was little difference noted between survivors and immigrants in social interaction. The extent of going places, visiting, telephoning, discussing issues, and confiding was not at all different for the two groups.

Survivors were more likely than members of the comparison group to share with their children, family members, friends, and co-workers everyday concerns, important concerns, and to discuss sex issues and finances. There were only some slight differences found

Table 20.1. Holocaust Study of United States Social Resources

	Survivors		Immigrants		
	Mean	SD	Mean	SD	F value
Morale	8.17	3.03	10.48	2.40	57.01***
Social affiliation					
Marital status	1.81	.39	1.69	.46	6.49**
Number of children	2.30	1.07	1.92	1.28	8.09**
Brothers/sisters	1.39	1.61	1.08	1.14	3.65
Relatives	3.77	4.55	4.23	4.75	.76
Social interaction					
Going places	7.74	2.75	7.79	2.59	.03
Visiting	9.53	2.82	8.90	2.97	3.58
Phone calls	12.12	2.61	11.83	3.01	.78
Discussion	13.86	3.33	13.47	3.67	.95
Confiding	1.04	.20	1.06	.25	.82
Self-disclosure					
Everyday	13.60	3.91	12.79	3.30	3.46
Important	13.62	4.08	12.90	3.50	2.49
Sex	7.16	2.21	6.92	2.23	.83
Finances	11.69	2.96	10.92	2.67	5.41*
Social support given					
Well-being	12.43	2.03	11.96	2.24	2.87
Ideas	10.53	2.19	10.43	1.92	.13
Transportation	7.79	1.69	7.52	1.48	1.42
Shopping	8.09	1.66	7.47	1.46	8.72**
Repairs	7.31	1.60	6.41	.43	29.41***
Cooking	7.56	1.71	6.98	1.16	8.96**
Finances	8.14	1.85	7.57	1.53	6.40*
Illness	8.43	2.21	7.38	1.75	17.14***
Social support received					
Well-being	11.24	2.31	10.85	2.39	.73
Ideas	10.20	2.11	9.65	1.91	2.07
Transportation	7.82	1.81	7.49	1.53	.91
Shopping	7.65	1.44	7.32	1.07	1.31
Repairs	8.05	1.48	7.51	1.15	5.58*
Cooking	7.58	1.18	7.49	.92	.16
Finances	7.00	.89	6.74	.95	1.49
Illness	8.62	2.05	8.29	2.29	.61

*$p = .05$; **$p = .01$; ***$p = .001$.

between the two groups in offering of assistance. Survivors were slightly but significantly more likely than members of the immigrant group to give assistance in times of illness and assistance with cooking.

Survivors were also slightly more likely to offer assistance with shopping, repairs, and finances, to listen to the ideas of others, and to show more concern for the well-being of their children, family members, and friends. There were also some differences found between the two groups in receiving social support. Survivors were more likely than members of the comparison group to receive assistance with repairs, to get help in times of illness, to have others be concerned about their well-being, and to have their ideas listened to.

Again, these findings indicate very clearly that, in terms of social interaction and social support, aging survivors of the Holocaust both in Israel and in the United

States are doing as well and in some instances better than members of the comparison groups. These results regarding social networks and the extent of social interaction, self-disclosure, and social support are clearly contrary to the expectations based on the Holocaust literature. Survivors developed meaningful social networks and utilized their social networks to engage in social interaction, to share with others their concerns and ideas, and to develop supportive relationships to a somewhat greater extent than members of the immigrant groups. These findings clearly indicate that survivors engaged in deliberate efforts to be involved with others and to regain social contact as much as possible. Contrary to some of the portrayals in the Holocaust literature (Chodoff, 1966; Danieli, 1982; Steinitz, 1982), survivors had to overcome indifference and misunderstanding in their respective social environments to

Table 20.2. Holocaust Study of Israeli Social Resources

	Survivors		Immigrants		
	Mean	SD	Mean	SD	F value
Morale	9.32	3.91	10.99	3.56	17.03***
Social affiliation					
Marital status	1.80	.40	1.76	.60	.42
Number of children	1.73	1.04	2.16	1.01	14.79***
Brothers/sisters	1.62	1.09	1.89	1.46	.59
Relatives	5.08	5.89	6.78	6.60	2.07
Social interaction					
Going places	6.69	3.02	6.57	2.75	.15
Visiting	8.90	2.77	9.14	2.60	.64
Phone calls	11.42	2.69	11.53	2.84	.13
Discussion	13.56	3.90	13.62	3.06	.03
Confiding	1.13	.33	1.18	.38	2.14
Self-disclosure					
Everyday	14.94	4.63	14.87	4.36	.02
Important	14.46	4.58	14.17	4.01	.35
Sex	7.44	2.75	7.36	2.66	.06
Finances	11.20	3.47	10.88	3.33	.70
Holocaust	17.58	6.37	13.09	6.04	36.76***
Social support given					
Well-being	10.04	1.53	9.60	2.34	.61
Ideas	9.64	1.34	8.82	2.04	2.87
Transportation	6.85	.98	7.12	1.94	.49
Shopping	7.89	1.11	7.65	1.44	.36
Repairs	7.02	1.09	6.82	1.45	.26
Cooking	7.68	1.01	6.95	1.41	4.27*
Finances	7.70	1.05	7.27	1.30	1.48
Illness	8.53	1.17	7.46	1.55	7.06**
Social support received					
Well-being	8.69	2.30	8.50	2.39	.49
Ideas	8.98	2.26	8.82	2.27	.34
Transportation	6.72	1.09	6.78	1.08	.22
Shopping	6.84	.97	6.82	1.03	.03
Repairs	7.21	1.27	7.10	1.23	.60
Cooking	6.86	1.05	6.87	1.25	.01
Finances	6.58	.89	6.56	.94	.01
Illness	7.38	1.57	7.25	1.70	.45

*p = .05; **p = .01; ***p = .001.

actively pursue and develop meaningful networks of social support. Survivors' accomplishments in these areas are noteworthy and are indicative of deliberate efforts reflective of other active coping patterns and social achievements despite evidence of their lower morale and higher psychiatric symptomatology (E. Kahana *et al.*, 1988).

Social Resources and Psychological Well-Being

The importance of social affiliation, social interaction, self-disclosure, and social support for the prediction of psychological well-being of survivors and immigrants is summarized in Table 20.3. The analyses of the

importance of social network for psychological well-being reveal that those who are married and who have children and relatives are likely to be generally better off than others. Interestingly, having brothers/sisters has little impact on psychological well-being in either group.

The data on social interaction in our research followed the general patterns found in the gerontological literature, indicating that those who have higher interaction with others have slightly higher psychological well-being (Larson, 1978). Of the social interaction variables, however, only discussion with others was significant for survivors in Israel. Among the Israeli immigrant comparison group, this association also approximated significance.

The review of data on self-disclosure confirmed general findings from the gerontological literature that those who are more likely to share everyday and impor-

Table 20.3. Correlation with Morale

	United States sample		Israeli sample	
	Survivors	Immigrants	Survivors	Immigrants
Social affiliation				
Marital status	.121	.156	.325***	.137
Number of children	.021	.155	.177	.108
Brothers/sisters	−.028	−.050	−.009	.022
Relatives	.093	.109	.015	.083
Social interaction				
Going places	.006	.036	.095	.137
Visiting	−.009	−.084	.060	.107
Phone calls	.084	−.058	.130	.038
Discussion	.041	.116	.228*	.195*
Confiding	.104	.108	.001	.080
Self-disclosure				
Everyday	−.056	.021	.340***	.241**
Important	−.061	.105	.247**	.213*
Sex	.095	.133	.276***	.092
Finances	.114	.002	.114	.164
Holocaust			.106	−.031
Social support given				
Well-being	.020	.067	.032	.112
Ideas	−.046	.015	.118	.116
Transportation	.107	.017	.039	.072
Shopping	.131	−.040	.003	−.026
Repairs	.032	.017	.058	.081
Cooking	.095	−.142	.025	−.058
Finances	.010	.078	−.049	.089
Illness	.264	.131	.072	.010
Social support received				
Well-being	−.099	−.015	.084	.141
Ideas	−.096	−.073	.168	.146
Transportation	−.032	−.110	.000	−.199*
Shopping	.023	−.015	.062	−.009
Repairs	.044	−.102	−.125	−.145
Cooking	.041	−.016	.082	.069
Finances	−.039	−.206*	−.004	−.006
Illness	−.087	−.087	−.001	−.024

*$p = .05$; **$p = .01$; ***$p = .001$.

tant matters as well as those who are more likely to talk with others about sex and finances are likely to have higher morale (Lowenthal & Berkman, 1967).

Indicators of social support revealed, again, what is typically found in the gerontological literature—namely, receiving attention and assistance is associated with lower psychological well-being. Conversely, giving attention and assistance is more likely to be associated with better psychological well-being. However, both giving and receiving of attention and assistance were only minimally associated with psychological well-being in the two groups.

Multiple Regression Analyses

Multiple regression analyses were performed to ascertain the explanatory power of the social resource vari-

ables on psychological well-being; results are shown in Table 20.4. The multiple regression analyses conducted on the data from the survivors in the United States reveal that social resource variables account for a 24% variance in morale. Of the social resource variables, three variables, namely, (1) self-disclosure, talking with others about the Holocaust, (2) giving assistance to others in times of illness, and (3) marital status, accounted for 15% of the total 24% variance accounted for by all social resource variables. Among the immigrants in the United States, a 23% variance was accounted for by all social resource variables. Of these, three variables—marital status, receiving assistance with finances, and offering assistance with cooking—accounted for 11% of the total 23% variance in morale accounted for by all social resource variables.

Data from the multiple regression analyses reveal that social resource variables account for 32% explained variance in the psychological well-being of survivors in

Table 20.4. Multiple Regression Analyses

	United States sample		Israeli sample	
	Survivors	Immigrants	Survivors	Immigrants
All variables				
Multiple r	.49	.48	.56	.46
Multiple R^2	.24	.24	.32	.21
Significant variables				
Multiple r	.39	.33	.49	.35
Multiple R^2	.15	.11	.24	.12
	Beta coefficients			
Social network				
Marital status	.18*	.25**	.24***	
Self-disclosure				
Everyday			.27***	.23**
Assistance given				
Illness	.30***			
Cooking		−.17*		
Assistance received				
Well-being				.15*
Repairs			−.14*	
Finances		−.24**		
Transportation				−.24**

*p = .05; **p = .01; ***p = .001.

Israel. Of the social resource variables, marital status, receiving assistance with repairs and discussing everyday matters with others were significant and accounted for 24% of the total 32% variance accounted for by all social resource variables. Among the immigrants in Israel, 21% of the variance was accounted for by all social resource variables. Of these, three variables—sharing everyday concerns with others, receiving assistance with transportation, and concern of others for one's well-being—accounted for 12% of the total 21% variance in morale accounted for by all social resource variables.

Discussion

Scientific and professional efforts are guided by (1) attitudinal, ethical, and value predispositions; (2) assumptional and knowledge bases; and (3) practice skills. The purpose of this chapter was to address only the second of these three components: namely, to provide a better understanding of the ways in which older survivors of extreme stress cope with their aging experiences, and to derive implications from the data reviewed for aiding future research and clinical practice in the area of social resources and extreme stress. Sensitivity is a prerequisite for work with all groups of elderly and it is equally, if not more important dealing with older persons who are coping with consequences of earlier extreme stress experiences.

Our research data clearly indicate that the availability of social support and of communication with members of one's primary group and friends are indeed important contributors toward higher levels of psychological well-being. The data clearly indicate that survivors have reconstructed social networks to a equal or greater extent than persons of similar sociocultural background who have not experienced the horrors of the Holocaust. Furthermore, survivors are actively engaged in social interactions and social support with their family members and friends and that these relationships and exchanges contribute to their psychological well-being in ways similar to other populations of older persons.

Implications for Mental Health Research

The Holocaust literature reviewed in this chapter has important implications for mental health research and practice. First, victims who seek professional services may have indeed been more seriously affected by their traumatic experiences. Every effort should be made to make available the services which victims need and seek in treatment. At the same time, results of studies conducted exclusively with those seeking mental health services cannot be generalized to the entire survivor population. Such studies have lead to faulty conclusions and misleading generalizations about the entire population of Holocaust survivors.

Data from studies of general groups and samples of Holocaust survivors reviewed in this chapter underscore the necessity for appropriate conceptual and methodological perspectives for theoretical formulations and generalizations about victims and survivors of extreme stress. It is important to employ conceptual approaches that are anchored in the social and behavioral sciences in order to ascertain the range of personal characteristics and resources, as well as the social and environmental factors, which may aid or hinder the adjustment of Holocaust survivors. It is also important that proper methodological procedures be employed in research with survivors of extreme stress not only to assure the validity of findings but also to assure their generalizability. In the absence of conceptual sophistication and methodological rigor, faulty conclusions are derived which serve to further disadvantage victims and survivors of extreme stress.

It is important to underscore, therefore, the following program and practice implications for understanding the needs of older survivors of traumatic stress. There is a clear need for more programs that specifically address conditions within the older family unit and the needs of aging survivors of extreme stress. Programs which will enhance and strengthen the social network and social support of survivors may be as clinically significant as implementing a medical procedure.

It is important for clinical practitioners to recognize that the social life and social resources of extreme stress victims are similar rather than different when compared with persons who are of similar sociocultural background and who relocated to the United States and Israel. Working with survivors of extreme stress is challenging, difficult, and emotionally taxing. Yet it must be kept in perspective that models for the treatment of older survivors of extreme stress are only as useful as they aid the survivors to make an adjustment to current challenges and to consequences of their earlier stressful experiences. There is a potential danger to our clinical efforts if we uncritically accept treatment approaches based on unsubstantiated evidence. Research has begun to show that there are multiple patterns of coping with extreme stress. Aiding the adjustment of survivors will continue to challenge the genius of health and human service professionals.

References

Anthony, E. J., & Koupernick, C. (1973). *The child in his family: The impact of disease and death* (Vol. 2). New York: Wiley.

Ben-Sira, Z. (1985). Potency: A stress-buffering link in the coping stress–disease relationship. *Social Science and Medicine, 21*(4), 397–406.

Bergman, M. S., & Jucovy, M. E. (1982). *Generations of the Holocaust*. New York: Basic Books.

Blazer, D. (1982). Social support and mortality in an elderly community population. *American Journal of Epidemiology, 115,* 684–694

Burchfield, S. R., Hamilton, K. L., & Banks, K. L. (1982). Affiliative needs, interpersonal stress and symptomatology. *Journal of Human Stress, 8*(1), 5–10.

Cassel, J. (1976). The contribution of the social environment to host resistance. *American Journal of Epidemiology, 104,* 107–123.

Chodoff, P. (1966). Effects of extreme coercive and oppressive forces: Brainwashing and concentration camps. In S. Arieti (Ed.), *American handbook of psychiatry, III* (pp. 384–405). New York: Basic Books.

Cohen, C. I., Teresi, J., & Holmes, D. (1986). Assessment of stress-buffering effects of social networks on psychological symptoms in an inner-city elderly population. *American Journal of Community Psychology, 14*(1), 75–91.

Cohen, S., & Wills, T. A. (1985). Stress, social support, and the buffering hypothesis. *Psychological Bulletin, 98*(2), 310–357.

Danieli, Y. (1982). Families of survivors of the Nazi Holocaust: Some short- and long-term effects. In C. D. Spielberger, I. G. Sarason, & N. A. Milgram (Eds.), *Stress and anxiety* (pp. 405–421). Washington, DC: Hemisphere Publishing.

Davidson, S. (1979). Massive psychic traumatization and social support. *Journal of Psychosomatic Research, 23,* 395–402.

Davidson, S. (1981). Clinical and psychotherapeutic experience with survivors and their families. *The Family Physician, 10*(2), 313–321.

Dean, A., & Lin, N. (1977). The stress-buffering role of social support. *Journal of Nervous and Mental Disease, 165,* 403–417.

Dean, K. (1986). Social support and health. *Pathways of Influence Health Promotion, 1*(2), 133–150.

Eitinger, L. (1961). Pathology of the concentration camp syndrome: A.M.A. *Archives of General Psychiatry, 5,* 79–87.

Elder, G., & Clipp, E. (1988). Combat experience, comradeship, and psychological health. In J. P. Wilson, Z. Harel, & B. Kahana (Eds.), *Human adaptation to extreme stress: From the Holocaust to Vietnam*. New York: Plenum Press.

Federal Council on the Aging. (1978). *Public policy and the frail elderly*. Washington, DC: U.S. Government Printing Office.

Feuerstein, C. W. (1980). Working with the Holocaust victims psychologically: Some vital cautions. *Journal of Contemporary Psychotherapy, 11*(1), 70–77.

Harel, Z. (1983). Coping with stress and adaptation: The impact of the Holocaust on survivors. *Society and Welfare, 5,* 221–230.

Harel, Z., & Deimling, G. (1984). Social resources and mental health: An empirical refinement. *Journal of Gerontology, 39,* 747–752.

Harel, Z., Sollod, R., & Bognar, B. (1982). Predictors of mental health among semi-rural aged. *Gerontologist, 22,* 499–504.

Holahan, C. J., & Moos, R. H. (1985). Life stress and health: Personality, coping and family support in stress resistance. *Journal of Personality and Social Psychology, 49*(3), 739–747.

House, J. (1981). *Work stress and social support*. Reading, MA: Addison-Wesley.

Kahana, B., Harel, Z., & Kahana, E. (1988). Predictors of psychological well-being among survivors of the Holocaust. In J. P. Wilson, Z. Harel, & B. Kahana (Eds.), *Human adaptation to extreme stress: From the Holocaust to Vietnam* (pp. 171–192). New York: Plenum Press.

Kahana, B., Kahana, E., Harel, Z., & Segall, M. (1985–1986). Victims as helpers. *Humboldt Journal of Social Relations, 13,* 357–373.

Kahana, E., Kahana B., Harel, Z., & Rosner, T. (1988). Coping with extreme trauma. In J. P. Wilson, Z. Harel, & B. Kahana (Eds.), *Human adaptation to extreme stress: From the Holocaust to Vietnam* (pp. 55–79). New York: Plenum Press.

Kahana, E., Kahana, B., & Kinney, J. (1990). Vulnerability and personal resources. In Z. Harel, P. Ehrlich, & R. Hubbard (Eds.), *Vulnerable aged: People, policies and programs*. New York: Springer.

Kahana, E., Midlarsky, E., & Kahana, B. (1987). Beyond dependency, autonomy and exchange: Prosocial behavior in late life adaptation. *Social Justice Research, 1,* 439–459.

Klein, H. (1971). Families of Holocaust survivors in the Kibbutz: Psychological studies. In H. Krystal & W. Niederland (Eds.), *Psychic traumatization: After-effects in individuals and communities*. Boston: Little, Brown.

Klein-Parker, F. (1988). Dominant attitudes of adult children of Holocaust survivors toward their parents. In J. P. Wilson, Z. Harel, & B. Kahana (Eds.), *Human adaptation to extreme stress: From the Holocaust to Vietnam* (pp. 193–218). New York: Plenum Press.

Krause, N. (1987). Chronic financial strain, social support, and depressive symptoms among older adults. *Psychology and Aging, 2*(2), 185–192.

Krell, R. (1982). Family therapy with children of concentration camp survivors. *American Journal of Psychotherapy, 36,* 513–522.

Krystal, H. (1968). Studies of concentration camp survivors. In H. Krystal (Ed.), *Massive psychic trauma.* New York: International Universities Press.

Larson, R. (1978). Thirty years of research on the subjective well-being of older Americans. *Journal of Gerontology, 33,* 109–129.

Last, U., & Klein, H. (1984). Impact of parental Holocaust traumatization on offsprings' reports of parental child-rearing practices. *Journal of Youth and Adolescence, 13*(4), 267–283.

Lawton, M. P. (1975). The Philadelphia Geriatric Center Morale Scale: A revision. *Journal of Gerontology, 30,* 85–89.

Lemon, B. W., Bengtson, V. L., & Peterson, J. A. (1972). Activity types and life satisfaction in a retirement community. *Journal of Gerontology, 27,* 511–523.

Leon, G., Buthcher, J., Kleinman, M., Goldberg, A., & Almagot, M. (1981). Survivors of the Holocaust and their children: Current status and adjustment. *Journal of Personality and Social Psychology, 41,* 503–516.

Levav, I., & Abramson, J.H. (1984). Emotional distress among concentration camp survivors—A community study in Jerusalem. *Psychological Medicine, 14,* 215–218.

Lowenthal, M. F., & Berkman, P. (1967). *Aging and mental disorders in San Francisco.* San Francisco: Jossey-Bass.

Marcus, P., & Rosenberg, A. (Eds.). (1989). *Healing their wounds: Psychotherapy with Holocaust survivors and their families.* New York: Praeger.

Noelker, L., & Harel, Z. (1983). The integration of environment and network theories in explaining the aged's functioning and well-being. *Interdisciplinary Topics in Gerontology, 17,* 84–95.

Palmore, J. (1979). Predictors of successful aging. *Gerontologist, 19,* 427–431.

Pennebaker, J. (1985). Traumatic experience and psychosomatic disease: Exploring the roles of behavioral inhibition, obsession and confiding. *Canadian Psychology, 26,* 82–95.

Pilcz, M. (1979). Understanding the survivor family: An acknowledgement of the positive dimensions of the Holocaust legacy. In L. Y. Steinitz & D. M. Szonyi (Eds.), *Living after the Holocaust: Reflections by the post-war generation in America* (rev. ed.). New York: Block Publishing.

Podietz, L., Belmont, H., Shapiro, M., Zwerling, I., Ficher, I., Eisenste, T., & Levick, M. (1984). Engagement in families of Holocaust survivors. *Journal of Marital and Family Therapy, 10,* 43–51.

Robinson, S., & Winnik, H. (1981). Second generation of the Holocaust: Holocaust survivors' communication of experience to their children, and its effects. *Israeli Journal of Psychiatry and Related Sciences, 18*(2), 99–107.

Rosow, J. (1967). *Social integration of the aged.* New York: Free Press.

Rustin, S. (1980). The legacy of loss. *Journal of Contemporary Psychotherapy, 11*(1), 32–43.

Shanan, J., & Shahar, O. (1983). Cognitive and personality functioning of Jewish Holocaust survivors during the midlife transition (46–65) in Israel. *Archiv für Psychologie, 135,* 275–294.

Solkoff, N. (1981). Children of survivors of the Nazi Holocaust: A critical review of the literature. *American Journal of Orthopsychiatry, 51*(1), 29–41.

Steinitz, L. Y. (1982). Psycho-social effects of the Holocaust on aging survivors and their families. *Journal of Gerontological Social Work, 4*(3–4), 145–152.

Thoits, P. A. (1983). Multiple identities and psychological well-being: A reformulation and test of the social isolation hypothesis. *American Sociological Review, 48,* 174–187.

Weinfeld, M., Sigal, J., & Eaton, W. (1981). Long-term effects of the Holocaust on selected social attitudes and behaviors of survivors: A cautionary note. *Social Forces, 60*(1), 1–19.

Wethington, E., & Kessler, R. C. (1987). Perceived support, received support and adjustment to stressful life events. *Journal of Health and Social Behavior, 27,* 78–89.

Wilson, J., Harel, Z., & Kahana, B. (Eds.). (1988). *Human adaptation to extreme stress: From the Holocaust to Vietnam.* New York: Plenum Press.

CHAPTER 21

Posttraumatic Stress Disorder in World War II Prisoners of War from Alsace-Lorraine Who Survived Captivity in the USSR

Marc-Antoine Crocq, Jean-Paul Macher, Jorge Barros-Beck, Stewart J. Rosenberg, and Fabrice Duval

Introduction

We studied the prevalence of long-term posttraumatic stress disorder (PTSD) symptoms in a population of men from Alsace-Lorraine who were forcibly drafted into the German armed forces during World War II (WW II), subsequently taken prisoners on the Russian front, and kept in Soviet captivity until repatriation to France several months or years later. They can be considered a homogeneous group with respect to age and their cultural and geographical backgrounds.

Specific posttraumatic symptoms and long-term personality changes after major stress have been described as early as the late nineteenth century (Oppenheim, 1892). More recently, the *Diagnostic and statistical manual of mental disorders* (3rd ed., rev., [DSM-III-R]), (American Psychiatric Association [APA], 1987) proposes a distinct diagnostic category and the latest draft of the ICD-10 (International Classification of Diseases) (World Health Organization, 1989) distinguishes two separate diagnostic categories (viz. posttraumatic stress disorder, F 43.1; and enduring personality changes after catastrophic experience, F 62.0).

Posttraumatic psychiatric symptoms have been recognized in military personnel after combat (Grinker &

Marc-Antoine Crocq, Jean-Paul Macher, Jorge Barros-Beck, Stewart J. Rosenberg, and Fabrice Duval • Centre Hospitalier Spécialisé, Rouffach 68250, France.

International Handbook of Traumatic Stress Syndromes, edited by John P. Wilson and Beverley Raphael. Plenum Press, New York, 1993.

Spiegel, 1945) or following recent captivity (Ahrenfeldt, 1958; Andersen, 1975; Brill, 1946; Corcoran, 1982; Sitter & Katz, 1973; Sledge, 1980; Ursano, Boydstun, & Wheatley, 1981; Wolf & Ripley, 1947). A few studies have also addressed the persistence of symptoms over decades in prisoners of war (POWs) who returned from World War II or Korean War captivity (Beebe, 1975; Goldstein, Van Kammen, Shelley, Miller, & Kammen, 1987; Khan, 1988; Kluznick, Speed, Van Valkenburg, & Magraw, 1986; Speed, Endgahl, Schwartz, & Eberly, 1989; Tennant, 1986; Zeiss & Dickerman, 1989) or in veterans of the French colonial wars in Indochina and Algeria (L. Crocq & M. A. Crocq, 1987).

Historical Background

Alsace-Lorraine comprises Alsace and the northernmost part of Lorraine. It is a borderland between France and Germany. A large part of its population is bilingual, speaking both a German dialect and French. The area has been successively claimed by both countries. It became French in the second half of the seventeenth century, and was German again between 1870 and 1918. After being a part of the French Republic in the two decades preceding World War II, it came under direct German rule during the war and again became a part of France at the war's end.

The shortage of manpower suffered by the German forces on the Russian front led to the introduction of compulsory military service for men in Alsace-Lorraine in August, 1942: those who were born between 1920 and

1924 were drafted into the Wehrmacht. In 1943 and 1944, this practice was extended also to men born between 1906 and 1928. The Nazi government took reprisals against the families of those who attempted to evade the draft. It is noteworthy that some of the recruits previously fought against the German forces in the French army in 1939–1940. Often considered unreliable by the German command, the recruits were dispersed among those from Germany and were kept away from key assignments such as radio communications. The majority served as enlisted men and had to face the fierce fighting between retreating Germans and the advancing Soviet troops.

Men from Alsace-Lorraine were captured in large numbers in July and August, 1943 (the battle for the city of Kursk), June and July, 1944 (the Russian offensive in Byelorussia), and in 1945 (operations that occurred between the Vistula and the Oder rivers), and upon the capitulation of Germany. A substantial number of Alsatians voluntarily surrendered at the Russian lines, mistakenly expecting to be treated as French citizens and turned over to the Western Allies. Whether they had been captured or surrendered voluntarily, POWs were treated with notorious brutality by both sides on the Eastern front. Of more than 100,000 soldiers captured at Stalingrad, only 6,000 returned. The mortality rate for Russian POWs in Germany approached two thirds. Many POWs did not survive the forced marches or the transportation to camp in boxcars. A considerable number reported the summary execution of the wounded and of those who were too exhausted to follow the marches. Most POWs from Alsace-Lorraine were eventually regrouped in a camp near Tambov in central Russia. Once there, they were herded into underground barracks and slept cramped on long plank beds. Captivity in camp was marked by malnourishment. In 1944 and 1945 in Tambov, the rations were meager, typically consisting of bread and thin soup, with an estimated caloric value of 1,340 calories per day. On this insufficient diet, the prisoners were pressed into forced labor in lumbering, mining (coal, peat, asbestos, tungsten), or were forced to work in the fields. Food was further reduced when daily norms of production were not fulfilled. Arbitrary punishments and deadly chores were dealt out by fellow-prisoners turned "kapos," that is, those who collaborated with their captors to enforce a strict camp discipline in return for better treatment. Prisoners invariably developed protein deficiency edemas and were afflicted with dysentery and pneumonia. Hygiene was extremely poor and infestation with lice was constant. The Russian winter also levied a heavy toll in lives. Some POWs suffered a long catastrophic captivity whereas others were captured in 1945 when conditions seemed less harsh than during the earlier war years, or were repatriated relatively early (1,500 POWs were turned over to the British in July, 1944 and sent to French-controlled North Africa). Overall, 130,000 youths from Alsace-Lorraine were forcibly drafted into the Wehrmacht during the war. Of that number, 40,000 disappeared while in Russia on the front or in captivity (ca. 17,000) between 1943 and 1955. It is estimated that 52% of the inmates of the camp at Tambov did not return.

Method

In June, 1988, a 117-item bilingual French-German questionnaire (available upon request) was mailed to about 2,000 POWs from Alsace-Lorraine who survived captivity in the Soviet Union and who were members of the Association of Survivors from Tambov and other Russian POW Camps (*Fédération des Anciens de Tambow et Internés en Russie*). This represents an almost complete survey; only a few members of the association were not able to participate (e.g., because of a severe physical ailment) and did not receive a questionnaire.

The items of the questionnaire surveyed extensively the traumata experienced during combat, capture, and captivity and, among other factors, addressed all the DSM-III (*Diagnostic and statistical manual of mental disorders*, 3rd ed., APA, 1980) and DSM-III-R diagnostic criteria for PTSD (APA, 1987). The Structured Clinical Interview for the DSM-III (SCID) (Spitzer, Williams, & Gibbons, 1987) was used for the phrasing of questions concerning PTSD and anxiety symptoms. The questionnaire had both multiple-choice items and questions to which it was possible to reply in writing.

Valuable additional information was obtained in the numerous personal interviews carried out either in the hospital or in the homes of the subjects. Furthermore, several subjects were regularly followed up in outpatient consultation. We have received responses from approximately 1,000. A sample of 525 completed questionnaires was randomly selected and analyzed to serve as a basis for the statistical results which are presented here.

Analysis of Symptoms

Table 21.1 summarizes the demographic and biographical characteristics of the sample. The age of the subjects was 66.7 years ± 4.3 (SD) (range: 56–80). They had spent 25.6 months ± 6.8 (SD) (range: 3–44) of active service in the Wehrmacht before capture. The duration of captivity in Soviet POW camps was 11.7 months ± 5.8 (SD) (range: 2–78). The estimated weight upon repatriation averaged 48 kilos.

Table 21.2 presents the frequency of symptoms, as reported by the subjects in the questionnaires.

Nightmares

Eighty-four percent of the respondents still reported recurrent distressing dreams or nightmares of wartime and captivity events. The disturbances occurred at a varying frequency: weekly in 13%, monthly in 27%, only a few times a year in 44%. Thus, it may be said that 40% of the sample was still troubled by frequent nightmares. An important feature of these dreams was the concomitant reexperiencing of anxiety, the men often waking with a racing heart and perspiring. It typically took several minutes for the anxiety to subside and for the subjects to be fully awake and aware of their surroundings.

In 31% of the questionnaires, the subjects narrated "repetition" nightmares of factual events which they ex-

Table 21.1. Percentage of Demographic and Biographic Characteristics of POWs (N = 525)

Main age classes	
1919	4.4
1920	8.7
1921	8.9
1922	8.5
1923	11.6
1924	10.8
1925	14.6
1926	7.1
1927	3.3
Year of draft into Wehrmacht	
1942	14.1
1943	65.2
1944	20.3
1945	0.4
Main periods of conscription	
October, 1942	9.1
January, 1943	16.1
May, 1943	13.5
October, 1943	8.7
Rank in German military	
Common soldier	84.6
Private 1st class or NCO	14.5
Cadet or officer	0.5
Military branch	
Infantry	62.8
Tank	8.6
Artillery	5.0
Navy	5.0
Signal corps (Kradmelder)	5.0
Year of capture by Soviet Army	
1943	15.1
1944	42.2
1945 before capitulation	30.5
1945 at capitulation	12.2
Mode of capture	
Crossed the lines to surrender	37.4
Let themselves be captured during retreat	19.6
Captured forcibly	43.0
Camp experiences reported by survivors	
Protein deficiency edemas	
Legs only	43.5
Generalized	29.2
Loss of teeth in camp	40.5
Typhus or typhus-like syndrome	23.8
Night blindness	22.0
Solitary confinement	18.7
Occupation after repatriation	
Industrial	35.0
Business	17.0
Agricultural	16.0
Professional	14.0
Mining	5.0

Table 21.2. Percentage of Ex-POWs Currently Reporting Symptoms (N = 525)

Symptom[a]	Did not answer	No	Yes
Intrusive distressing recollections of wartime or captivity events; B (1)	10.0	8.0	82.0
Recurrent distressing dreams of wartime or captivity events; B (2)	4.6	11.3	84.1
Sudden reliving or reexperiencing of wartime or captivity events; B (3)	12.1	31.7	56.2
Acting suddenly as if the traumatic events were recurring; B (3)	11.8	31.8	56.3
Intense anxiety when exposed to stimuli associated with war or captivity; B (4)	6.0	52.4	41.6
Efforts to avoid thoughts or feelings associated with the traumata; C (1)	6.1	20.9	72.9
Efforts to avoid activities or situations that arouse recollections of the traumata; C (1)	9.6	22.1	68.3
Feeling of being different from others; C (5)	9.2	35.7	55.1
Need to stay away from others	9.2	43.3	47.5
Inability to have loving feelings; C (6)	10.1	61.5	28.4
Increased dependence on love and support from others	6.3	24.6	69.1
Did captivity change the way you see future? C (7)	7.3	21.8	70.9
Sense of a foreshortened future; C (7)	5.9	23.2	70.9
Difficulty falling asleep; D (1)	3.7	20.2	76.0
Frequent outbursts of anger; D (2)	3.7	57.0	39.3
Significant difficulty concentrating; D (3)	3.5	49.1	47.4
Startle reactions when confronted with sudden noise; D (5)	6.5	18.1	75.4
Feeling more anxious than peers	10.2	35.2	54.5
Frequent spontaneous anxiety	4.9	61.0	34.0
Frequent occurrence of panic-like symptoms	7.1	74.6	18.3
Survival guilt (DSM-III)	6.3	54.4	39.3

[a]Letters and digits after the items refer to the DSM-III-R diagnostic criteria for PTSD that are identical or closely corresponding.

perienced during the war or in captivity. Another 25% of the questionnaires contained nightmare narrations with more symbolic themes or general images of war and captivity (44% of the questionnaires contained no narration of nightmares). Symbolic dreams frequently revolved around returning to camp. The subjects were snatched from their homes by the "Russians" or they voluntarily returned to camp after a "furlough." They wandered endlessly from camp to camp, without finding the "right gulag," or woke up in camp and blamed themselves for choosing to return. Other typical scenes included pleading with the captors for mercy, being lost and tongue-tied in a Russian-speaking crowd, or being chased by a pack of wolves and left naked and shivering in the snow. Narrations of repetition nightmares by other subjects typically included: life in camp, "like a movie which cannot be stopped", staying awake all night after capture and interrogation, expecting execution at daybreak, and being eventually spared to see one's companion being hanged; witnessing the suicide of a POW who dived into the camp's well; reliving hand-to-hand combat in the trenches and waking up with a scream when one was about to be bayoneted; hearing the screams of Russian POWs whom they had been ordered to bayonet in "reprisal" for killing a German officer; hearing the "hurrahs" of the attacking Russian infantry; and carting the bodies of the dead and unloading them into the camp's mass grave. Dreams often expressed guilt toward dead friends and conflicts between the wish to remain at home and the duty to rejoin friends in camp.

Many (39%) reported that the recurrence of nightmares was often triggered by a daytime event, such as discussing memories or watching a movie. Only 15% said that their nightmares usually recurred spontaneously. Subjects usually described themselves as active (39%) rather than passive spectators (19.5%) in their dreams. The frequency of nightmares was said to remain constant (39%) or to decrease (30%) rather than to increase (17%) over time (no answer: 14%). The date of onset of nightmares was difficult to record with precision after four decades. However, a delayed onset, more than 6 months after repatriation, was mentioned by 18.5%.

Spouses often reported that the subjects fitfully tossed and turned in bed and screamed during their sleep. This often happened shortly after falling asleep and, therefore, suggested the possibility of night terrors. The frequency of the repetition nightmares fluctuated according to current circumstances. A new physical aggression revived old traumata and survivors reported a sharply increased frequency of captivity nightmares after being assaulted or threatened in the street.

Intrusive Recollections

Distressing daytime recollections were also common. The subjects described them as protracted periods of daydreaming filled with painful images of war and captivity and ruminations about death and violence. Distressing recollections flowed in "cascades" and could not be interrupted voluntarily. Many survivors said that they would then sit alone brooding. They were often deeply absorbed in their memories, partly out of touch with their present environment. Recollections occurred either when the subjects were relaxing or they were triggered by stimuli associated with captivity, such as hearing news about hostages, eating very thin soup, or walking in the forest or in snow. Triggering stimuli may have been specific to a subject and were avoided. One interviewee had to cut down a birch tree in his garden because it reminded him of Russia. Many could not watch a movie about World War II to the end because it made them unbearably anxious. Some described an anticipa-

tory anxiety related to the recurrence of these ungovernable recollections and stayed busy and avoided discussing memories to prevent them. When asked to narrate the content of their intrusive recollections in the questionnaire, the subjects recounted general scenes of war and captivity more often (44%) than the repetition of distinct traumata which they had personally experienced (29%) (no narration: 28%). Intrusive recollections were very often tinged with guilt toward dead friends. One respondent was employed as a grave-digger in camp and reported being haunted by the faces of the friends he buried. Intrusive daytime recollections were significantly associated with repetition nightmares ($X^2 = 14.78$, df: 9, $p < .001$).

Acute Anxiety Symptoms

The frequent occurrence of panic-like symptoms, such as sudden tachycardia resulting in consultation with a cardiologist, was reported by 18% of the sample. However, two thirds of the panic-like attacks were not of a spontaneous origin but were triggered by stimuli associated with war or captivity such as movies about World War II. Spontaneous panic attacks were also observed, and the same patients usually presented both spontaneous and situation- or stimulus-related attacks. The report of panic-like attacks was associated with complaints of nightmares ($X^2 = 6.47$, df: 1, $p = .01$).

Dissociative Phenomena

While we examined them, the men often described reliving or "seeing again" their experiences in camp. At these times, they became noticeably ill at ease and distracted. They appeared conspicuously detached from their surroundings and were anxious and appeared to be dissociating. Moist hands and other symptoms of somatic anxiety were often observed during the interviews. In a few cases, we saw a dramatic emotional catharsis. The reexperiencing of captivity was also provoked by a variety of other recent events, such as a sudden unpleasant confrontation, for example, being harshly rebuked or insulted by a superior or threatened by a mugger. Some events were easily associated with experiences of captivity (an orchestra playing Russian music). Another man described the sudden feeling of being back in a *Kolkhoz* (collective farm) when he entered a crowded city square. Feelings of derealization and depersonalization are often expressed, though they have abated since repatriation.

Enduring Traits

In addition to the preceding discrete symptoms which indicate the recurrent reexperiencing of the traumata, some other chronic features can best be described as enduring characteristics which border on personality changes. Inability to tolerate social contact and social withdrawal were maximal immediately after repatriation. Subjects shunned intimate conversations ("I pretended to be asleep and waited till my girlfriend arose, two hours later if necessary"). They also avoided festive occasions such as dances. Another survivor reported that he could not bear listening to the radio during the first 2 months after his repatriation. This improved with time, and the majority started families and took up jobs.

As residual effects, social phobias have tended to persist, and many spoke of the inability to speak in public. Most subjects still avoided social gatherings and groups. Today, many feel unconcerned, estranged, and out of touch with the world around them. A frequent profile in the interviewed survivors is the paradoxical association of a constantly apprehensive attitude with a careless, apathetic, ambitionless, or "tramp" mentality ("*mentalité de clochard*"). They point to this seeming contradiction: "To be a beggar or a king is of no importance to me, but I worry about the smallest things."

Many subjects developed dependent traits, took few initiatives, and passively expected that such basic needs as clothing and food should be taken care of for them. These dependent traits "reawakened" upon retirement. Many subjects then presented a general lack of interest, became negligent and unkempt, but paradoxically worried about inconsequential things.

Another question was the role of previous personality in survival. Many ex-POWs attributed their survival to the fact that they were strong-willed or had faith. A common comment was that those who gave up hope died quickly.

Associated Features

Guilt about surviving was a diagnostic criterion for PTSD in DSM-III, but was abandoned in DSM-III-R (Brett, Spitzer, & Williams, 1988). However, 40% of our sample reported that they "often" wondered why they survived when their friends had died. Guilt was a prevalent symptom. For instance, this was the case in one interviewee who felt extreme guilt for failing to hear the last words of a dying comrade. He was told one evening in camp that his friend was urgently asking for him; he did not answer that request immediately but deferred his visit to the following day and then discovered the lifeless body of his friend who had died during the night. He tried to make up for what he saw as his failure to assist his friend by visiting his friend's family after repatriation, but obsessive guilt nevertheless persisted.

Interaction with another disorder occurred at times in a striking fashion. One man who survived 18 months of captivity later developed bipolar disorder. He had a regular recurrence of posttraumatic symptoms during the early phases of his manic episodes. He then developed paranoid delusions concerning "Communists" and once spectacularly killed his pet dog in a transient dissociative state.

Role of Duration of Captivity and Other Markers of Severity of Stressors

An association was observed between the reported presence of symptoms and the previous duration of captivity (Table 21.3). Significant symptoms included DSM-III-R PTSD criteria, such as repetitive nightmares, reliving of the traumatic experiences, intense anxiety caused by stimuli associated with war and captivity, feeling of

Table 21.3. Symptoms Significantly Associated with Longer Captivity ($N = 525$)

Symptom[a]	Number of months in captivity (mean + SD)	
	Subjects reporting absence of symptoms	Subjects reporting presence of symptoms
Recurrent distressing dreams of wartime or captivity events; B (2)	10.3 + 5.3	11.9 + 5.8*
Sudden reliving or reexperiencing of wartime or captivity events; B (3)	10.6 + 4.6	12.3 + 6.4**
Intense anxiety when exposed to stimuli associated with war or captivity; B (4)	11.0 + 4.9	12.5 + 6.7**
Feeling of being different from others; C (5)	11.0 + 4.8	12.3 + 6.4*
Increased dependence on love and support from others	10.8 + 5.0	12.1 + 6.1*
Sense of a foreshortened future; C (7)	10.5 + 4.6	12.1 + 6.1†
Frequent outbursts of anger; D (2)	11.2 + 5.0	12.6 + 6.8*
Frequent spontaneous anxiety	11.3 + 4.8	12.7 + 7.3*
Frequent occurrence of panic-like symptoms	11.2 + 4.9	13.5 + 8.3††

[a]Letters and digits after the items refer to the DSM-III-R diagnostic criteria for PTSD that are identical or closely corresponding.
Note. Mean duration of captivity significantly different (Student's t test, two-tailed): *$p < .05$; †$p < .01$; **$p < .005$; ††$p < .001$.

being different from others, sense of a foreshortened future, and outbursts of anger. There were also associations with increased emotional dependence on others, frequent spontaneous anxiety, and panic-like symptoms.

The frequency of repetition nightmares was also associated with the severity of wartime and captivity traumata. Nineteen percent reported having been punished by solitary confinement while in camp. This group also reported a higher incidence of nightmares ($X^2 = 5.21$, df: 1, $p = .02$). Similarly, 93.4% of a group of 30 who survived attempts at their own execution or were submitted to a mock execution after capture, reported repetition nightmares.

Reports of head injury (104 out of 525 respondents) were significantly associated with increased intrusive distressing recollections of wartime or captivity events ($p = .01$), acting suddenly as if the traumatic events were recurring ($p = .01$), intense anxiety when exposed to stimuli associated with war or captivity ($p = .02$), change in the way of seeing the future ($p = .02$), efforts to avoid thoughts or feelings associated with the traumata ($p = .02$), frequent outbursts of anger ($p = .04$), increased dependence on love and support from others ($p = .04$), and a tendency toward more marked inability to have loving feelings ($p = .06$). In all cases, head wounds were more closely associated with PTSD symptoms than other body wounds (187 out of 525 subjects), which were significantly associated only with stimulus-provoked intense anxiety ($p = .04$). It is of course to be expected that those who suffered head injury would have had more stressful combat experiences.

Previous authors (Zeiss & Dickerman, 1989) have reported no association between length of captivity and prevalence of symptoms. However, this might be due to the greater heterogeneity of their study samples in terms of previous traumatic experience. Contrary to other studies, we found no significant association with age or rank at the time of capture. This might be explained by the greater homogeneity of our population with regard to age and rank.

Five Case Histories

The case histories that we offer provide the best perception of the complex interaction of multiple stressors and personal experiences in Alsatian POWs. They illustrate the intricate association of different symptoms.

CASE 1—REPETITION NIGHTMARES

Mr. C. frequently dreams that he is in a railway station with his wife and children. He suddenly turns around and realizes with a fright that the station is empty and that his family has vanished. He has weekly nightmares in which he misses a boat or a train and, waking in a sweat, several minutes pass before his fright dissipates. He relates these dreams to events in which he almost missed his repatriation. He relates an occasion when the guards had announced a surprise for the French on the eve of July 14th, Bastille Day, and had issued them new clothes. On July 14th a train was stationed on the tracks and the POWs firmly believed it meant repatriation. They were disconcerted to discover that it was laden with coal but they unloaded it believing the promise that they would board the train after it had been emptied. In what Mr. C. understands today as a sadistic game of cat and mouse, they were told at the end of the day that their new clothes were now too dirty for them to go home and that they would have to return to camp.

CASE 2—SOCIAL WITHDRAWAL AND PHOBIAS

René H. was born in 1925 in Wissembourg in northern Alsace and was drafted into the Wehrmacht at the beginning of 1943. He spent two years on the frontline in a sanitary company. He started worrying very soon after his father stopped writing and he was not reassured by his mother's explanations that his father could not write because of a hand injury. It was only after returning from captivity that he found out that his father had been deported to a German concentration camp. His most frightening combat experience was being buried alive with ten other soldiers and a sergeant in an underground shelter by heavy shelling of Russian artillery. Some men panicked; others prayed. They survived in total darkness on a few cans of milk. He lost track of time, but the German sappers who dug them out said that they had remained buried for only three days. Back into daylight, he was amazed to see that the hair of

one of his fellow soldiers had turned completely white on one side of his head. They were allowed a short rest in a field dressing station where they were given rice cooked in milk and chocolate.

The patient was first seen in consultation by us in 1988 on the day following the anniversary of his capture by the Russians, on April 16, 1945, near Königsberg in East Prussia. He spent the anniversary of his capture suffering from intrusive recollections of the painful events that occurred on that day. The days following capture were brutal and chaotic. The men were beaten with sabers, whipped, and randomly shot at. Prisoners died everyday during the seven-week transportation to camp in locked freight cars with the limited diet of a bucket of foul potatoes, herrings and very little water. Our patient felt hopeless when he crossed the large width of the Volga with the other prisoners and he felt it to be very unjust that he was treated "as a German" by his captors. Several died very shortly after arriving in the camp having drunk excessive quantitites of water. Fear was constant in camp; he recalls how a prisoner was summarily shot by a sentry when he bent down to pick up his cap that had fallen. They slept on planks, without straw or blankets. He estimates that 20% of the prisoners died during the first nine months in his camp near Sverdlovsk in the Urals; the death rate was extremely high for those over 35. He was put to work in a mine and subsequently at a furnace. Repatriation came unexpectedly as groups of non-German POWs were told to board a train one night. They were delivered to the British seven weeks later.

He was too weak to work for the first year and a half after repatriation. His wife became aware of his nightmares, nightly shouting and bruxism shortly after they were married in the early 1950s. She says that he usually looks defeated and taciturn the next morning. Symptoms abated slightly with time, but worsened again after he turned sixty. There was no period when he did not have nightmares. Nightmares now occur a few times a month. Enemies are chasing him and he has to flee; he is in battle, experiences artillery fire and tanks, shouts and gives orders; "I am in the action, fear only comes later." At times, he wakes up in a sweat with the feeling that someone wants to harm him; he then has to get up and turn the lights on. A television fim about WW II will always trigger nightmares. Intrusive recollections concern very specific events (POW camp, or prisoners shot by the SS). These recollections are unavoidable and pursue him like the devil on his heels ("*comme le diable à mes trousses*"). He does not only remembers events, but reexperiences them. He suffers from constant free-floating anxiety, and is also anxious when confronted with others whom he instinctively perceives as threats or enemies. He cannot be assertive, avoids interaction with people, and does not enjoy having visitors at home. Anxiety is minimal at his home, his "fortress," and anticipatory anxiety builds up whenever he has to leave home. He even has difficulty sleeping when he knows that he will have to baby-sit for his grandchildren the next day. He prefers going out on Monday morning because fewer people are outside. He avoids department stores and cannot drive his car unaccompanied. Similarly, he avoids elevators and small rooms. He had to get rid of his dog because he could not tolerate its barking. He often uses alcohol as an "anesthetic" to bring some peace and tranquility. He has been constantly treated with psychotropic compounds for the last 12 years, and felt that antidepressant compounds (Viloxazine, Fluoxetine) diminished the severity of his nightmares, whereas this was not the case with benzodiazepines. He considers that his personality was altered by the war, and points out that he was a "happy" person before and became withdrawn since the war. Others cannot understand what he feels, and one of the main benefits of our consultations was that he found a person who listened with interest and understanding to his problems.

CASE 3—REPETITION NIGHTMARES AND PANIC ATTACKS

Mr. B. spent 26 months in Russian captivity. He surrendered to Russian troops near Tula in August of 1943 as the front broke and the Germans troops fled. He and an Alsatian friend, M., decided to hide in a bunker and wait for the Russian advance. This was risky. They were aware that a German officer had just shot two German soldiers in an attempt to stop the retreat. When they first encountered Russian troops, they came out of hiding shouting *"kamerad"* and showed a small tricolor which they had sewn on the inside of their lapels to vouch for their French citizenship. They were beaten, and boots, watches, and rings were taken from them. A political commissar appeared storming with rage and Mr. B. was filled with the fear of execution. As he tried to explain his forced incorporation in pidgin Russian—*"nyet germanski, frantsuzski"*—the commissar fired his submachine gun on them. He dived to the ground and pretended to be dead. He remembers that he lost his sense of time and had an image of his family in a dreamlike "movie" in front of his eyes. When the commissar had left, he saw his dead friend lying in a pool of blood. He again nearly lost his life when a Russian soldier took him to the rear where he was beaten by cavalry troops. He reexperiences the execution of his friend very vividly as he retells it. He is still awakened by nightmares in which he sees again and again the same "movie" of his life. His spouse adds that he sometimes screams at night. However, the nightmares are now less frequent. He thinks he survived miraculously because he tried to speak to the Russians, instead of keeping silent like his friend M. He feels guilty for the death of M. because he had persuaded his friend to give himself up for capture. He often ruminates about this event in hour-long daydreams accompanied by a degree of depersonalization. This state can be triggered by the meeting of old friends.

He had a constant anxiety in camp, which he contrasts with the "normal" fear he experienced during combat. Guards would burst into the barracks at night and beat up the prisoners. He suffered dysentery, lost considerable weight, and several of his teeth fell out. He worked at lumbering jobs in the forest. One night when ice had thawed in the spring, he was assigned to empty the morgue where the dead were stored during the winter. He vividly remembers having to break the mountain of frozen bodies with a pick to take them off in sleds to a mass grave. He says that the guards threatened to shoot anyone who related what they saw. It is not surprising that those corpses still appear in his nightmares and daytime recollections. As he recalls, the nightmares started during the captivity and became less frequent over the years. Upon repatriation to France, he discovered that his wife was pregnant by another man and had sold all their belongings.

He experienced a first panic attack in camp. Panic attacks recurred after repatriation as well as some simulated angina pains to the extent that he was admitted to a cardiology unit in 1947. Symptoms of agoraphobia followed and he is still afraid of losing his balance when shopping in department stores. He feels dizzy and has to sit down when visiting the zoo with his grandchildren. He also fears speaking in public. He describes himself as permanently apprehensive and anxious. Once when answering the phone he had the sudden feeling that someone behind him would strangle him and he dropped the receiver. He hates to discuss his captivity and was very reluctant to be interviewed about it.

CASE 4—DEPERSONALIZATION AND GENERALIZED ANXIETY

Mr. N. was a medic on the front near Leningrad where he dispensed medicine and food to his section. He recalls that he himself had no one to turn to for support. He acted out his anxiety on several occasions. The first time was when he rescued a wounded soldier in full view of Soviet tanks. He said a prayer, climbed out of the trench, planted his rifle conspicuously in the snow, and walked to the wounded man without seeking cover. He evacuated the wounded man to the rear, only after arguing with an NCO who wanted the task for himself in order to get away from the danger of the front line. Shortly after this, he returned to the front to discover that his company had been totally annihilated in a tank attack. On another occasion he broke away from his company during a skirmish with the intent of letting himself be captured by the Russians. He heard his company being ambushed and destroyed. He was repeatedly beaten after capture. An officer drew his gun and took aim at him; he screamed pathetically and was unexpectedly spared. After 20 months of captivity, he returned home to a destroyed family. One of his brothers had been deported to a German concentration camp for evading the draft and died shortly after the end of the war. His adoptive father was sentenced to death by the French in 1945 and had to go into hiding in Germany—many years passed before he could make contact again with his adoptive parents. He wept openly when telling the story of his lost family.

Mr. N. frequently experiences depersonalization and derealization. "I often feel that I did not really come back from captivity. I am not really here, only my spirit returned and my body remained there because it is impossible that anyone really survived that. At times, I forget that we are at peace and I am afraid that they'll come back and take me." His professional activity helped him to keep links with others and with his surroundings, but feelings of depersonalization have increased since his retirement. He says that personality changes appeared immediately after repatriation and have persisted ever since. He is constantly apprehensive, as if the world were about to come to a brutal end. He feels very concerned by all news of disasters. He very seldom smiles or laughs and says that hearing his son singing reminds him of "gallows humor." He does not experience panic attacks, but feels extremely uncomfortable when speaking in public and still feels shame for bursting into tears once when he had to speak at a meeting. He regularly consults psychiatrists and is treated with benzodiazepines. He owns a beautiful house but spends most of his time in a more modest lodging to avoid being exposed to the commotion caused by his son's restaurant and children. He feels guilty for not being able to tolerate the noise made by his grandchildren. He is often afraid that his wife might abandon him or cheat him, but says that he is not jealous and acknowledges that his fears are absurd. He is very anxious at nightfall, anxiety with which he associates standing guard on the front in Russia. Nightmares have become very rare with time and he reports only a few symbolic dreams such as "being locked in a pigsty with swine and attempting to break out." His wife reports that he talks and groans in his sleep.

CASE 5—INTRUSIVE RECOLLECTIONS

Mr. M. was an adjutant and fought during the winter of 1943–1944 in what was mostly trench warfare. He had the feeling that the Germans distrusted soldiers from Alsace-Lorraine and Luxembourg, whom they called *"Beute-Deutsche"* ("Germans" taken as spoils of war), and older corporals watched him discreetly despite his higher rank. One night, six men from Lorraine deserted after disabling the machine gun. However, they were wearing German uniforms and the Russians shot them and displayed their bodies on the parapet of the trenches. To give a lesson to others who might be tempted, a Wehrmacht officer ordered 10 men to retrieve the bodies. Mr M. was one of them; they crawled at night between the lines and dragged back three bodies.

He was captured in June, 1944. The POWs were made to run in front of Russian tanks. Some prisoners were run over by tanks while Mr. M. was deafened by cannon fire. It was two weeks before he began to recover some of his hearing. He worked in mines near Stalino and was later transported by freight car to Tambov. The dead were thrown out at every stop of the train. To this day, he remembers very clearly the voice of the nurse who would ask about the daily count of dead—*"skol'ko (how many) kamerad kaputt?"* In camp, he was subjected to "training" sessions conducted by a political commissar, and survived by eating birch leaves and drawing sap from trees.

He was shocked upon returning home to see his brother wearing his best jacket. Mr. M. had been reported dead and the church's bells had tolled for him. His mother had died during his captivity—"out of grief"—and he feels guilty about that. He says that captivity changed his personality from energetic and buoyant to reserved, apathetic and submissive. He had planned before the war to be a forestry engineer but was now content with being an ordinary lumberjack. He was traveling in a train, four years after repatriation when a door squealed . . . he dived to the floor to the astonishment of everyone present and to his embarrassment. Repetition nightmares started after he gained weight and recovered physically, and have persisted ever since.

We made recordings of his sleep in our laboratory. REM sleep latencies were normal over five consecutive nights. However, he woke up three times in the same night with a shout, without remembering the incident on the following morning. The coming of winter always makes him anxious, because he associates it with his captivity. He feels some relief when he sees the carnival on television because it heralds the return of spring. He often has intrusive recollections of war and captivity. He has anticipatory anxiety related to the recurrence of these recollections. He stays busy and avoids discussing his memories, in order to try to avoid recalling them. He never talked about his camp experience with his wife or children and now recounts them with little affect. He testified about his experience after the war but thinks that the committee made fun of him; he got no compensation for his deafness because he could find no witness to prove that it was related to captivity.

Specific Characteristics of Alsatian POWs

The incidence of long-term PTSD symptoms appeared to be high in the present population. This agrees with results from previous studies in other populations (Kluznik *et al.*, 1986; Zeiss & Dickerman, 1989). The large response rate can be ascribed to the fact that the association of ex-POWs was responsible for the diffusion of the questionnaires, and that the completed questionnaires could be returned during the weekly or biweekly get-togethers which the POW association regularly holds in several cities. It is possible that a number of respondents were motivated by hope of better compensation. However, the very specific nightmare contents and other symptoms narrated in the questionnaire support the sincerity of the replies.

In this long-term PTSD, the reexperiencing of the traumatic events (repetitive nightmares, intrusive recollections, emotional reliving of the traumatic events) is a central feature. These symptoms have very specific contents, are true to history, and are triggered by stimuli which clearly recall the wartime and captivity events. This close association between the traumatic event and its reexperiencing confirms the findings of van der Kolk, Blitz, Burr, Sherry, and Hartman (1984).

Other important features, notably the paradoxical association of constant anxious apprehension, avoidance of social events, feelings of detachment, and lack of ambitions would be more aptly described as enduring personality changes rather than distinct DSM-III-R anxiety symptoms. Enduring personality changes are difficult to describe in a systematic way. Nonetheless, they constitute a background of disturbed relationships with others who are perceived as dishonest or potentially harmful. Social interactions generate anxiety and are avoided. These subjects lack confidence in themselves and have difficulties being assertive and facing interpersonal conflict. Perhaps this explains the fact that this group has not formulated a forceful demand for compensation.

Two etiological factors contribute to the severity of symptoms in this population. First, they underwent a succession of multiple extreme stressors, including combat, where sudden destruction was avoided only miraculously, capture and the threat of summary execution, and captivity marked by constant anxiety and the complete loss of any sense of human dignity. It would seem virtually impossible to separate out distinct etiological roles of each stressor.

Second, a very specific characteristic of this group is the ambiguity of its mixed French and Germanic cultural heritage. This ambiguity made it difficult for these subjects to find a meaning for their experience or a country to turn to, and generated feelings of inferiority, guilt, and isolation. They were forced, under the threat of deportation of family members, to serve in an army which most considered foreign, and where they were considered unreliable. They were surprised to be treated as German soldiers when captured by the Soviet army. Likewise, they felt misunderstood by some of their French fellow countrymen who saw their forced incorporation into the German military and tattered Wehrmacht uniforms as treason. Repatriation to a transformed postwar society was abrupt and was not prepared by prolonged hospital observation or welcoming committees. Some subjects had been reported dead and their wives had remarried; others had difficulty obtaining credit for school achievements during the German occupation. A few survivors were even drafted for military service in the French army after repatriation. Post-

261

traumatic stress disorder was not recognized as such in this population, and the sole psychiatric disorder justifying compensation was initially "asthenia." Another debated issue was which government, French or West German, should be responsible for compensation.

Today, many subjects feel that the long-term psychological consequences of captivity have been even a more severe handicap than the physical consequences. They find it impossible to convey this and generally avoid discussing their camp experiences, even with close family members. Interviews with POWs, or groups of POWs, must largely be directed toward alleviating their feelings of inferiority, guilt, isolation, and exclusion from a broader cultural support, their fear of not being believed, and the difficulty they have in discussing their experience and its consequences. No psychological support was organized when these survivors were repatriated. In similar instances today, it would seem useful to organize structured discussion groups with psychological support, immediately upon repatriation, and thereafter on a regular basis. Still, a number of World War II POWs in Alsace-Lorraine may well derive benefit from regular psychological consultation.

ACKNOWLEDGMENTS

We gratefully acknowledge the help of Jean Thuet, President of the Federation ot the Survivors from Tambov and other Russian POW camps (*Fédération des anciens de Tambow et internés en Russie—F-68200 Brunstatt-Mulhouse*), who kindly helped us to obtain access to the population reported in this study.

We acknowledge the valuable comments of Dr. Zack Cernovsky, St. Thomas Psychiatric Hospital, St. Thomas, Ontario, Canada, Dr. John C. Kluznik, Minneapolis, Minnesota, in the United States, Dr. Iain Montgomery, University of Tasmania, Hobart, Australia, and Dr. Charles Van Valkenburg, Carson City, Nevada, United States of America.

We thank Ms. Cornelia Dürrmeier for help in writing the German-language version of the questionnaire.

References

Ahrenfeldt, R. H. (1958). *Psychiatry in the British Army in the second world war* (p. 312). New York: Columbia University Press.

American Psychiatric Association. (1987). *Diagnostic and statistical manual of mental disorders* (3rd Ed., rev.). Washington, DC: Author.

Andersen, R. S. (1975, February). Operation homecoming: Psychological observations of repatriated Vietnam prisoners of war. *Psychiatry, 38,* 65–74.

Beebe, G. W. (1975). Follow-up studies of World War II and Korean war prisoners, II. Morbidity, disability, and maladjustments. *American Journal of Epidemiology, 101,* 400–422.

Brett, E. A., Spitzer, R. L., & Williams, J. B. W. (1988). DSM-III-R criteria for post-traumatic stress disorder. *American Journal of Psychiatry, 145,* 1232–1236.

Brill, N. Q. (1946). Neuropsychiatric examination of military personnel recovered from Japanese prison camps. *Bulletin of the U.S. Army Medical Department, 5,* 249–438.

Corcoran, J. F. T. (1982). The concentration camp syndrome and USAF Vietnam prisoners of war. *Psychiatric Annals, 12*(11), 991–994.

Crocq, L., & Crocq, M. A. (1987). Trauma and personality in the causation of war neuroses. In G. B. Belenky (Ed.), *Contemporary studies in combat psychiatry* (pp. 103–16). New York: Greenwood Press.

Goldstein, G., Van Kammen, W., Shelly, C., et al. (1987). Survivors of imprisonment in the Pacific theater during World War II. *American Journal of Psychiatry, 144,* 1210–1213.

Grinker, R. R., & Spiegel, J. P. (1945). *Men under stress* (p. 484). Philadelphia: Blakiston.

Khan, K. (1988, October). *Long-term psychiatric morbidity amongst ex-POWs and DSM-III.* Paper presented at the World Psychiatric Association Regional Symposium, Washington DC.

Kluznik, J. C., Speed, N., Van valkenburg, C., & Magraw, R. (1986). Forty-year follow-up of United States prisoners of war. *American Journal of Psychiatry, 143,* 1443–1446.

Oppenheim, H. (1892). *Die traumatischen Neurosen* (p. 253). Berlin: Verlag von August Hirschwald.

Sitter, S. C., & Katz, C. J. (1973). American prisoners of war held by the Japanese. In W. S. Mullins & A. J. Glass (Eds.), *Neuropsychiatry in World War II* (Vol. 2, pp. 931–975). Washington DC: Office of the Surgeon General, Department of the Army.

Sledge, W. H. (1980). Self-concept changes related to war captivity. *Archives of General Psychiatry, 37,* 430–443.

Speed, N., Endgahl, B., Schwartz, J., & Eberly, R. (1989). Post-traumatic stress disorder as a consequence of the POW experience. *Journal of Nervous and Mental Disease, 177,* 147–153.

Spitzer, R. L., Williams, J. B. W., & Gibbon, M. (1987). *Structured clinical interview for DSM-III non-patient version* (SCID-NP-V, 2-1-87). New York: New York State Psychiatric Institute, Biometrics Research Department.

Tennant, C. C., Goulston, K. J., & Dent, O. F. (1986). The psychological effects of being a prisoner of war: Forty years after release. *American Journal of Psychiatry, 143,* 618–621.

Ursano, R. J., Boydstun, J. A., & Wheatley, R. D. (1981). Psychiatric illness in U.S. Air Force Vietnam prisoners of war: A five-year follow-up. *American Journal of Psychiatry, 138,* 310–314.

van der Kolk, B., Blitz, R., Burr, W., Sherry, S., & Hartman, E. (1984). Nightmares and trauma: A comparison of nightmares after combat with lifelong nightmares in veterans. *American Journal of Psychiatry, 141,* 187–190.

Wolf, S., & Ripley, H. S. (1947). Reactions among allied prisoners of war subjected to three years of imprisonment and torture by the Japanese. *American Journal of Psychiatry, 104,* 180–193.

World Health Organization. (1989). *International classification of diseases.* Geneva, Switzerland: Author.

Zeiss, R. A., & Dickerman, H. (1989). PTSD 40 years later: Incidence and person-situation correlates in former POWs. *Journal of Clinical Psychology, 45,* 80–87.

CHAPTER 22

War and Remembrance

The Legacy of Pearl Harbor

Zev Harel, Boaz Kahana, and John P. Wilson

Introduction

As the dawn of the twenty-first century begins to rise on the horizon, the generations who were the product of the last five decades will look back on an era of world history characterized by archetypal forces which have counterbalanced the processes of creation and destruction of social systems and civilization. The destructiveness of warfare during the twentieth century has claimed over 40 million human lives, eliminated cultures, and ushered in the specter of the total annihilation of the human race with the advent of the atomic bombing of Hiroshima, Japan, near the end of World War II.

There can be little disagreement that World War II was unique in the annals of world and United States history. The fascist philosophy of Nazi Germany, the intent of Chancellor Hitler and his allies to conquer and subjugate Europe to the vision of Nazi ideology, and the horrendous crimes committed by Hitler's regime were unparalleled in human history. Furthermore, from the perspective of the United States, the Japanese attack at Pearl Harbor initiated a change from a foreign policy of economic and political nonintervention and began America's involvement in the war. For these and other reasons, participation in World War II by members of the U.S. military forces was perceived as highly patriotic and was very much appreciated by the general Ameri-

can public. Today, a half century later, which has included United States involvement in the Korean and Vietnam Wars, the perspective on war and peace has changed drastically throughout the world. The Cold War appears to have ended and many forms of barriers to freedom have literally and symbolically been destroyed.

The events of war are often diverse and traumatic. Human lives are altered by these experiences which seem always to retain a special place in memory even as time heals psychic wounds that once tore the soul. To understand the full meaning of traumatic stress reactions is to address the question of how trauma impacts on memory, identity, consciousness, and adaptation within the life cycle. In this regard, we will focus our attention on the issue of traumatic memories among Pearl Harbor survivors, a unique group of aging U.S. veterans of World War II (Elder & Clipp, 1988).

We begin by asking the question of what it means to be a survivor. Such a seemingly simple question is, in reality, a very complex one when examined in depth. Clearly, survivorship means that the *biological* process of living continues despite the fact that severe trauma may affect many systems of the organism (Rossi, 1986). In an *epigenetic* sense, the life course itself continues to pose challenges, tasks and hardships associated with the various stages of ego development and the aging process. Yet the legacy of trauma, stored in memory and being, may alter the quality and form of existence at any point in the life cycle (Wilson, 1980, 1989; Wilson & Krauss, 1985). And the stages of epigenetic development themselves may function as stressors which can activate latent memories of trauma (Wilson, 1989).

Evidence indicates that the events and traumas of war impact on all levels of organismic functioning and personality; but the exact nature of these effects is not well understood at this time. There are large individual differences in posttraumatic adaptation. However, we

Zev Harel • Department of Social Work and Center on Applied Gerontological Research, Cleveland State University, Cleveland, Ohio 44115. **Boaz Kahana and John P. Wilson** • Department of Psychology, Cleveland State University, Cleveland, Ohio 44115.

International Handbook of Traumatic Stress Syndromes, edited by John P. Wilson and Beverley Raphael. Plenum Press, New York, 1993.

also know that some survivors never fully recover psychological health and well-being after extreme stress and trauma whereas others somehow transform it and emerge more fully human, wise, compassionate, and self-actualizing. These alternative pathways of adaptation to war trauma as well as the later processes of survivorship indicate that it is difficult to establish the boundary between what is a pathological response and what is a normally occurring psychic legacy of the experience (Wilson, 1989). Nowhere is this more evident than when we consider the issue of the memory of trauma, because the psychology of survivorship is inextricably linked to the transformations and vicissitudes of the memories of traumatic events (Kahana *et al.*, Laufer, 1988).

This chapter is concerned with war experience, war effects, and remembrance in Pearl Harbor survivors, former U.S. military servicemen who were stationed at the Pearl Harbor Naval Station on the Hawaiian island of Oahu at the outbreak of World War II in 1941. As such, it constitutes a preliminary attempt to address some of the questions concerning objective and subjectively perceived effects of war stress as well as issues related to adjustment to conventional life in the postwar years. Although empirical research findings will be reported, our purpose is more heuristic in nature; to attempt to show that experiencing phenomena (e.g., "symptoms") associated with war trauma is not pathological in itself. Rather, factors that shape the definition of traumatic stress syndromes being considered pathological are not the symptoms *per se*, but the psychohistorical, social, and cultural context in which they occurred and the subsequent response of society to the victim which, in turn, affects identity development and functioning in survivors. In this regard, the study of Pearl Harbor survivors presented a unique opportunity in which to explore some of the issues regarding the meaning of survivorship and the persistence of symptoms of posttraumatic stress syndromes.

It is important to note that the survivors of the Japanese attack at Pearl Harbor on December 7, 1941, are a unique historical group because the event initiated the United States involvement in World War II. Second, the majority of the survivors of the attack subsequently fought against the Japanese forces in the South Pacific and ultimately emerged victorious. Third, to date there is only one major study of this population of aging war veterans, who are now in their mid- to late 60s (Wilson, Harel, & Kahana, 1989). Fourth, the unique status of Pearl Harbor survivors enables us to explore how a psychohistorical context influences the manner in which the traumatic events are retained in memory and associated with symptom manifestation as well as with individual and group identity. This latter issue is particularly important since the Pearl Harbor Survivors Association (PHSA) is an organization of over 11,000 members which regularly holds local, state, regional and national reunions to affirm, remember, and celebrate their status as survivors. Fifth, in December, 1986, the 45th reunion commemorating the Japanese attack on Pearl Harbor was held by the PHSA in Honolulu, Hawaii, in the United States and created a unique opportunity to carry out a research study. Over 800 members (who refer to each other as "survivors") participated in this historic

reunion. We attended that reunion as well and were granted permission to conduct a study of the membership in attendance. However, prior to the conference, a 16-page Pearl Harbor Research Questionnaire (PHRQ) was developed, which we have described in detail elsewhere (see Wilson *et al.*, 1989).

Sample Characteristics

The initial sample of 250 members that we obtained (Wave I) of the PHSA is unique in several ways and the data reported in this chapter are based on this sample. First, it represents those who volunteered to complete the questionnaire and return it to us. At present, it is not possible to determine whether or not this wave of respondents is representative of the larger membership of the PHSA or of other survivors who do not belong to the organization. Second, this sample represents only those who were healthy enough to attend the 45th reunion in Hawaii. Thus, it is possible that this group of survivors may be different in important ways from other veterans who could not make the long trip to Honolulu to attend this historic meeting. However, within the respondents, the first 50 sets were compared with the next four sets of 50 questionnaires of later respondents, and no significant differences were found on any of the variables, a fact which gives some confidence in the representativeness of the sample in terms of those who attended the reunion. In another data set obtained on 30 survivors who did not attend the reunion and were members of a local chapter located in Ohio, no significant differences were found in the responses, a fact which bolsters the limitations in generalizability of these findings in any attempt to draw conclusions from this study of all survivors of the Pearl Harbor attack.

The mean age of the participants in this research in 1986 was 65, with a range of 62 to 85 years. The average age of the veterans at the time of the attack in 1941 was 19 years. Seventy-two percent of our sample served in the U.S. Navy and 18% were in the Army. The others, representing less than 15% of the sample, were in the Marine and Air Corps. Nearly all the men (93%) enlisted for military service and 71% had graduated from high school or had higher education. In terms of demographic variables, 92% of the men are married and only 17% have been divorced. In terms of religious affiliation, the majority of the veterans (61%) were Protestant and 28% were Catholic.

Retrospective Memories

Witnessing the Attack

This section is based on content analysis of the accounts provided by members of the U.S. Armed Forces, stationed on the island of Oahu, Hawaii, who observed or experienced the Japanese attack on Pearl Harbor on December 7, 1941. Responses in this section include: (1) length and type of service in Hawaii *prior to* the Japanese attack on Pearl Harbor; (2) duty assignment and location of service; (3) observations and experiences on December 7, 1941; and (4) length of service at Hawaii *following* the Japanese attack. (See Wilson, 1989, for a copy of the research questionnaire.)

Assignment and Location

Of the 269 veterans, 240 (89%) answered this question. Of the 240 respondents, 158 (66%) served in the navy and 82 (34%) served in other branches of the U.S. military forces. There were 14 (9%) veterans who served in the navy but were not stationed on a naval ship. Of the 158 that served in the navy, 144 (91%) served on a ship. Of these 144, 127 (88%) specifically named the ship that they served on, while 17 assignments were not specifically mentioned. Nearly all ships stationed at Pearl Harbor were named specifically by the subjects (see Wallin, 1968, for a discussion).

Respondents mentioned a wide range of service duties. Of the 144 respondents who served on ships, 112 (78%) listed their duty or assignment. Some indicated that they were members of a gun crew or division; others were gunners mate, or a pointer and trainer on the ships guns. Some served as engineers, did boiler-room duty, or worked as crew members or deck hands, and electricians. Others functioned as radiomen, strikers or signalmen, damage controllers, performed "watch duty," or were signalmen strikers, and firemen, cooks, maintenance workers, and musicians. Two of the respondents indicated they were deck officers. A few mentioned treating casualties or other such assignments (medical corps duty).

There were 47 (20%) non-U.S. Navy-related responses to this question. The nonnaval military locations listed on the day of the attack included U.S. Army, Marine Corps, and Air Force bases located throughout the geographical areas of the island: (1) Schofield Barracks, (2) Hickam Field, (3) Wheeler Field, (4) Fort Shafter, (5) Fort Weaver, and (6) Ford Island.

Among the 47 nonnaval respondents, there were those who indicated some form of combat duty which included pilot, officer, gun captain, platoon sergeant, antitank leader, field artillery, rifle squad leader, corporal of rifle squad, rifleman, intelligence, artillery, and guard duty. There were others performing some type of service, such as hospital duty, fuel distribution, radio operator, medical aide, band member, operator of corp-fire control equipment, supply-room attendant, telephone operator, fireman, personnel or clerical staff, weather observer, and auto driver. There were those who served as aircraft mechanics, maintenance workers, engineers, radio operators, aerial photographer, and instructor. All in all, the respondents represented a cross-section of those military personnel stationed at Pearl Harbor.

The Japanese Attack

Observations and Actions

Respondents were asked what they remembered from "The day of infamy," as President Franklin D. Roosevelt called it, in 1941. Answers to this question were subdivided into three parts: (1) observational details of the attack (what they experienced and observed), (2) personal reactions (what they did and felt), and (3) observations of the effects of the attack. Of the 269 total respondents, 254 (94%) veterans answered this question. It should be noted that only a small number, 15 (5%) did not answer this question at all.

Details of the Attack—What Was Heard and Observed

Of the 269 respondents, 235 (93%) offered some details about the attack. One half (117) of the veterans stationed at Pearl Harbor said that they saw the Japanese planes in the sky. Some respondents said that they could actually see the pilots' faces, and some recalled seeing the Japanese pilots smiling. Some veterans clearly saw the insignia on the Japanese planes. The Japanese insignias on the planes were referred to as "meatballs," "rising suns," "tomatoes," "red balls," and "orange balls."

There were veterans who heard or observed explosions, the roar of plane engines, or other loud noises. Some men specifically recalled hearing or observing the explosion of bombs and ships, or naval and field targets being hit. Some respondents reported being awakened by explosions, bombs, or other loud noises.

Of the veterans who gave some details about the attack, 75 (32%) saw the Japanese planes dropping bombs on various barracks or ships. There were some whose barracks or ship was strafed directly before their eyes. There were others who either sounded the General Quarters or heard it sound where they were stationed.

Of all the islands and barracks that were mentioned as part of the details of the attack (Ford Island, Wheeler Field, Hickam Field, Schofield Barracks, and the 27th Infantry Division), a small number of respondents mentioned that they saw Ford Island being bombed or under attack. Still others saw Wheeler Field, Hickam Field, Schofield Barracks, and the 27th Infantry under siege.

Of the veterans who said that they saw specific ships being attacked, some saw "battleship row" under attack. There were also those who reported seeing their own ship, barracks, or assigned area being hit by bombs. Of the ships specifically mentioned by respondents to have been seen under attack, the most frequently mentioned was the USS *Arizona*, which many of the respondents witnessed as being under attack and capsizing, as 1,100 U.S. Naval personnel drowned or were entombed on the sunken *Arizona*. Other ships seen under attack were the USS *Oklahoma*, the USS *Utah*, the USS *West Virginia*, the USS *Nevada*, the USS *Raleigh*, the USS *Shaw*, and the USS *California*.

There were those who mentioned seeing blood, and injured or dead people. There were others who saw Japanese planes shot down by antiaircraft fire and oil burning on the water in the harbor.

The overall picture emerging from these accounts is one of being unprepared and surprised by the unexpected attack, witnessing considerable destruction and death inflicted by the Japanese assault, and very minimal response by the U.S. forces stationed at Pearl Harbor.

Personal Reactions

Of the 254 respondents, 222 (87%) reported some kind of personal reaction to the attack. Reactions recalled by the veterans were primarily instrumental in nature, detailing what they did in response immediately or following the attack. Eighty-five (38%) respondents said that they retrieved, loaded, manned, or fired guns at one time or another during the attack. Two stated that they successfully hit one or more Japanese planes while returning fire. Some respondents stated that they reported immediately to their battle stations—as soon as they did when they became aware of being under attack. Some recalled that they ran to a porthole or topside to see what was going on or whether they could help in some way.

Other respondents reported that they helped carry and pick up the dead men, and some respondents looked for fellow comrades in the water. Some men recalled that they fought fires or that they went to another ship to help out. Other survivors indicated that they joined a damage control party or helped repair planes, ships, or other damaged equipment in an effort to assist in postattack measures. Some veterans recalled that they abandoned ship. Some of these were ordered and some did this on their own. Some persons mentioned that they actually swam away, primarily to nearby Ford Island, located in the center of the harbor.

Interestingly, only a small number of veterans mentioned how they felt on that day. Maybe the honor of the occasion, the 45th Anniversary of the Day of Infamy, inspired the giving of testimony in the realm of observations and actions rather than the recall and reporting of feelings that occurred during the attack. Those who reported feelings indicated that they were scared, shocked, terrified, frozen, or physically and emotionally exhausted. And, of course, there were some individuals who were injured during the attack.

Effects of the Attack

Of the 254 respondents who answered this question, about one third (36%) discussed the effects of the attack. The majority of the respondents mentioned specifically the memory of "battleship row" or specific ships being hit. Of these, some vividly recalled that the USS *Arizona* blew up and sank in the shallow waters of the harbor. There were those who saw the USS *Oklahoma* and the USS *Utah* capsize, and others who saw the bombing and sinking of the USS *Nevada*. There were respondents who saw the USS *West Virginia* catch fire, the USS *Raleigh* get bombed, the USS *California* burn, and the USS *Shaw* explode. Some of the respondents mentioned that their own ship began to sink or was bombed by the Japanese attack planes. A significant number of respondents mentioned seeing nearby land bases being bombed, these including Ford Island, Hickam Field, and Wheeler Field. Death, injury, and destruction were other frequent themes. There were respondents who saw crew members, peers, or other servicemen killed. There were others who said that either they or fellow crew members had been injured. Some mentioned that the effects of the attack were devastation and destruction, damage to buildings, and oil and fire

on the water of the harbor. Others mentioned seeing downed Japanese planes or sinking Japanese submarines as part of the effects of the attack. A few men recalled how they observed that units were organizing or preparing to fight; others reported details of fighting against the Japanese, the launching of search parties, and the initiation of repair work. Finally, other veterans recalled the emotional reactions of others, as they struggled to help or save comrades who had been wounded or injured.

Assignments after the Attack

Of the 210 respondents who answered this question, one third remained at Pearl Harbor for less than a month before being assigned to other duty, and 37 (18%) remained at Pearl Harbor between 1 and 3 months. More than one half of the respondents left Pearl Harbor less than 3 months after the attack. A second group of 31 (15%) stayed between 4 and 6 months, and a third group of 23 (11%) remained in Pearl Harbor between 7 and 12 months before being assigned to other duty. Others spent from one to several years before being assigned to other duty. Almost all those who witnessed the day of infamy went on to fight in the Pacific theater and contributed to the United States victory and to the ultimate surrender of the Japanese forces.

Empirical Analyses

Combat Exposure, Recall, and Imagery

Table 22.1 describes the types and degrees of combat exposure. Veterans reported high levels of combat exposure, including firing weapons at the enemy, being subjected to enemy fire, seeing unit members killed and wounded in action, seeing towns destroyed by combat, and experiencing life-and-death situations.

Recall and Intrusive Imagery of War Trauma

Table 22.2 summarizes the results of the descriptive analysis of recall and intrusive imagery reported in 1986 within the context of the Japanese attack at Pearl Harbor. The results are organized according to the diagnostic categories of posttraumatic stress disorder defined in the DSM-III-R manual (American Psychiatric Association, 1987). The table shows the results in terms of a specific psychohistorical context. In 1986, 65% of the veterans reported experiencing some type of intrusive imagery related to the attack in 1941. Recurring thoughts and memories which sometimes "just pop into my mind" were most prevalent (79%). Dreams of the attack were reported by 29% of the veterans. Intrusive symptoms of PTSD were reported four times as often as were symptoms characteristic of avoidance. Yet, 45 years later, one third of the veterans reported difficulty in expressing their feelings about what happened at Pearl Harbor. Thirteen percent indicated that they do not remember much of what happened and 6% found it difficult to be close to people after the attack. On the average, 17% of

Table 22.1. Degree of Combat Exposure

Type of combat exposure in World War II	Percentage of sample ($N = 250$)
Fired a weapon at the enemy	61
Killed someone	46
Under enemy fire	95
Wounded by enemy action	17
Hospitalized because of a wound	8
Received a life-threatening wound	2
Received a wound which left me impaired	6
Received a wound which led to discharge	3
Unit members killed	8
Unit members wounded	7
Unit members killed and wounded	58
Friends, family, or relatives killed	23
Friends, family, or relatives wounded	5
Friends, family, or killed and wounded	36
Saw allies killed	5
Saw allies wounded	8
Saw allies killed and wounded	54
Saw enemy killed	20
Saw enemy wounded	3
Saw enemy killed and wounded	32
Saw allies tortured	3
Saw allies mutilated	2
Saw allies tortured and mutilated	2
Saw enemy tortured	4
Saw and participated in enemy torture	1
Saw towns destroyed by combat	68
Saw civilians killed	2
Saw civilians wounded	4
Saw civilians killed and wounded	20
Under direct attack by enemy	
Once or twice	25
Sometimes	20
Many times	50
Experienced a war incident that was so awful that it changed views on life	23
Experienced a life-or-death situation	66
Experienced unbearable combat fatigue	28

Table 22.2. PTSD Symptoms in 1986

Symptom dimension	Percentage
Intrusion (DSM-III-R-B)	
I have had, at times, recurring thoughts about "the day of infamy" (December 7, 1941) and what happened at Pearl Harbor.	87
I have had, at times, dreams of the attack on Pearl Harbor.	29
Thoughts about the attack at Pearl Harbor sometimes just pop into my mind.	73
I have had, at times, memories of the bombed ships and airfields at Pearl Harbor.	77
I have had, at times, memories of the explosions, screaming, and confusion at Pearl Harbor on the day of infamy.	59
Avoidance (DSM-III-R-C)	
I sometimes find it difficult to express my feelings about what happened at Pearl Harbor.	32
I cannot remember much of what happened at Pearl Harbor.	13
After the attack at Pearl Harbor, I found it difficult to be real close to people.	6
Hyperarousal (DSM-III-R-D)	
When I hear the sounds of certain engine noises, it reminds me of the Pearl Harbor attack.	22
I am easily startled or made "jumpy" by loud or unexpected noises.	24
Survivor guilt	
Sometimes I wonder why I survived the Japanese attack and my buddies died.	42
Associated features	
On December 7, I have special feelings about the attack on Pearl Harbor.	90
I have, at times, bad feelings toward Japanese and avoid them when I can.	36
I have, at times, difficulty going to sleep or staying asleep.	27
Even today, I still have, at times, anger at the Japanese for the attack on Pearl Harbor.	47
Looking back, I believe that the Pearl Harbor experience had a deep influence on the course of my life.	67
I have returned to Hawaii to visit Pearl Harbor.	89

the Pearl Harbor survivors reported avoidance of some or all aspects of the attack at Pearl Harbor. Hyperarousal and startle responses were still present in one quarter of the veterans and survivor guilt was reported by 42% of the veterans. Approximately 42% of the veterans reported having anger or bad feelings toward the Japanese and avoided them whenever possible. Twenty-seven percent reported having difficulty going to sleep or staying asleep. Two thirds of the veterans believed that the Pearl Harbor experience had a deep influence on the course of their lives. Almost all the veterans (90%) had returned to Hawaii to visit Pearl Harbor and reported having special feelings on December 7, the day of the attack.

Posttraumatic Stress Symptoms at Reentry

Table 22.3 presents the percentage of PTSD symptoms reported at reentry and in 1986. As expected, in terms of the *context-specific* hypothesis, symptoms of PTSD were reported less often at these periods than were symptoms reported specific to the attack at Pearl Harbor. Intrusive imagery was the most frequently reported symptom. On the average, 23% of the veterans reported some type of intrusive imagery at reentry which decreased to 12% reported in 1986. One quarter of the veterans reported "nightmares in which I relive my World War II experiences" at reentry. Seven percent reported nightmares in 1986 related to war experiences. On the average, intrusive symptoms decreased by 48% from reentry to 1986. However, "anger at what actually happened during the war" was one of the symptoms most resistant to change. At reentry, 35% of the veterans

Table 22.3. PTSD Symptoms at Reentry and 1986

	Percentage	
Symptom dimension	Reentry	1986
Intrusion (DSM-III-R-B)		
Nightmares in which I relive my World War II experiences	26	7
Recurrent upsetting thoughts about the war	21	10
Felt upset when things reminded me of my World War II experiences	8	5
Felt angry at what actually happened in the war	35	25
Avoidance (DSM-III-R-C)		
Felt depressed	14	11
Felt numb or unable to feel emotions	9	2
Deliberate avoidance of things that remind me of World War II	8	2
Problems remembering what happened during the war	7	9
Felt distant or estranged from people	11	4
Difficulty concentrating	10	9
Hard to express my feelings	22	13
Avoided talking about the war	20	7
Felt isolated	9	5
Hyperarousal (DSM-III-R-D)		
Startled easily	30	12
Difficulty in sleeping	22	16
Felt emotionally overcharged (extremely "hyped up")	13	9
Easily irritated	19	14
Felt nervous or anxious	22	9
Hard to settle down, get "feet on the ground"	20	3
Associated features		
Drinking problem	12	5
Felt guilt about surviving	10	7
Drug addiction	.5	.5
Felt mistrustful of people	10	7
Problems at work	6	2
Marital difficulties	9	7
An urge to catch up on living	28	14

reported anger which decreased to only 29% in 1986. One quarter of the survivors still felt angry at what happened during the war.

On the average, avoidance symptoms were reported half as frequently as intrusive symptoms at reentry and in 1986. About 20% of the veterans report that it was "hard to express my feelings" and "avoided talking about the war" at reentry, and half as many report those symptoms in 1986. On the whole, symptoms of avoidance are the most resistant to change.

Symptoms of hyperarousal were reported at approximately the same frequency as intrusion (21% at reentry and 10.5% in 1986). Thirty percent of the veterans reported that they "startled easily" at reentry. In 1986, this number was reduced to 12% reporting a startle response. "Difficulty in sleeping" continued to be a problem for 16% of the veterans which was only a slight decrease from the 22% reporting sleeping problems at

reentry. One fifth of the veterans reported that at reentry it was "hard to settle down, get their feet on the ground" which decreased by 85% to only 3% reporting feeling this way in 1986. Twenty-eight percent felt "an urge to catch up on living" at reentry as compared to half as many reporting this feeling within the last year.

Overall, there was a 47% decrease in the number of veterans reporting symptoms in 1986 as compared with reentry. However, it is unclear whether the veterans reporting symptoms at reentry are now experiencing fewer symptoms or whether some have improved while others may have developed symptoms more recently. Alternatively, symptoms may have abated after reentry from World War II into civilian life only to reappear after retirement.

Correlates of Posttraumatic Stress Disorder Symptoms

Table 22.4 summarizes the bivariate correlations between select demographic measures, war stress, comradeship, personal attributes, and the three measures of PTSD: (1) at reentry, (2) in 1986, and (3) Pearl Harbor contextual. The results indicate that lower prewar education is positively and significantly correlated with PTSD symptoms at reentry ($r = .21$, $p < .05$). The veteran's use of the GI Bill is also significantly correlated with PTSD symptoms at reentry ($r = .25$, $p < .05$) and PTSD symptoms in 1986 ($r = .1$, $p < .05$).

In terms of war stress, all the measures are significantly correlated with the three measures of PTSD (r's = .18 to .48, $p < .05$). However, the measure of *combat stress* produced the highest correlation with PTSD at reentry ($r = .48$), in 1986 ($r = .38$), and in the context of the Pearl Harbor experience ($r = .49$, $p < .05$).

In terms of postwar evaluation of war experiences, a negative attitude toward military service at discharge and the negative evaluation of military duty are significantly correlated with PTSD symptoms at reentry ($r = .20$, $p < .05$). Further, the negative perception of war's effect on current emotions is significantly correlated with all three measures of PTSD (r's = .38). Membership in veteran's organizations is also significantly correlated with PTSD symptoms reported at reentry ($r = .22$, $p < .05$) and specific to the attack at Pearl Harbor ($r = .18$, $p < .05$). Finally, veterans with an external locus of control reported more symptoms of PTSD at reentry and in 1986 (r's = −.21 and −.32, $p < .05$).

Predictors of Posttraumatic Stress Symptoms

A standard multiple regression was conducted for PTSD symptoms reported at reentry to civilian life. Table 22.5 indicates that there are five variables with significant F-values ($p < .05$): (1) combat stress ($F = 15.55$), (2) postwar evaluation of war's effect on current emotions ($F = 8.12$), (3) external locus of control ($F = 7.00$), (4) use of the GI Bill ($F = 5.90$), and (5) lower prewar education ($F = 4.05$). Forty-one percent of the explained variance in PTSD symptoms at reentry was accounted for by these five variables.

Table 22.6 summarizes the results of the regression analyses for PTSD symptoms in 1986. The variables with

Table 22.4. Correlations between Variables and Measures of PTSD

Variable	PTSD—1946	PTSD—1986	Pearl Harbor Stress 1986
Education			
Prewar education	−.21*	−.17	−.15
Use of GI Bill	.25**	.18*	.14
War stressors			
War stress	.30**	.23*	.36***
Combat stress	.48***	.38***	.44***
Exposure to stress	.22*	.18*	.27**
Receive medical treatment	.33***	.31*	.23*
Postwar evaluation of war experience			
Attitude toward service at discharge	.20*	.17	.06
Evaluation of military experience	.20*	.13	.08
Training helpful later	−.13	−.04	.02
War's effect on aging	.10	−.10	−.07
War's effect on current emotions	.38***	.37***	.38***
Comradeship and veteran's organizations			
Reserve unit membership	.04	.08	.06
Current contact with service buddies	−.02	−.11	.03
Membership in veteran's organizations	.22*	.08	.18*
Personal resources			
Locus of control	−.21*	−.32***	−.08
Altruism	−.01	−.16	−.04
Disclosure	−.02	.06	.07

*$p < .05$; **$p < .01$; ***$p < .001$.

Table 22.5. Correlations between Variables and the Bradburn Affect Balance Scale

Variable	Bradburn Affect Balance Scale	
	Positive affect	Negative affect
Education		
Prewar education	.06	−.04
Use of GI Bill	−.07	.12
War stressors		
War stress	.01	.16
Combat stress	.01	.20*
Exposure to stress	.07	.02
Receive medical treatment	−.07	.28**
Postwar evaluation of war experience		
Attitude toward service at discharge	−.28**	.15
Evaluation of military experience	−.06	.08
Training helpful later	.11	−.13
War's effect on aging	.14	−.10
War's effect on current emotions	−.11	.25**
Comradeship and veteran's organizations		
Reserve unit membership	.01	.02
Current contact with service buddies	.10	−.11
Membership in veteran's organizations	.07	.06
Personal resources		
Locus of control	.20*	−.28**
Altruism	.12	−.08
Disclosure	.16	−.02

*$p < .05$; **$p < .01$.

**Table 22.6. Multiple Regression for PTSD Symptoms
at Reentry—1946**

Variable	B	Beta	F
Education			
Prewar education	−.23	−.11	4.05*
Use of GI Bill	1.14	.14	5.90*
War stressors			
War stress	.45	.09	2.18
Combat stress	.91	.32	15.55*
Exposure to stress	−.77	−.06	.57
Receive medical treatment	.55	.09	2.00
Postwar evaluation of war experience			
Attitude toward service at discharge	.14	.03	.16
Evaluation of military experience	.33	.06	.84
Training helpful later	−.47	−.08	1.88
War's effect on aging	−.19	−.03	.32
War's effect on current emotions	1.06	.18	8.12*
Comradeship and veteran's organizations			
Reserve unit membership	−.44	−.04	.54
Current contact with service buddies	−.64	−.03	.21
Membership in veteran's organizations	.77	.12	3.43
Personal resources			
Locus of control	−.97	−.15	7.00*
Altruism	.62	.07	1.60
Disclosure	−.65	−.08	1.90

*$p < .05$. $R^2 = .41$.

Table 22.7. Multiple Regression for PTSD Symptoms in 1986

Variable	B	Beta	F
Education			
Prewar education	−.10	−.07	1.48
Use of GI Bill	.40	.06	.90
War stressors			
War stress	.11	.05	.71
Combat stress	.47	.24	7.98*
Exposure to stress	−.21	−.02	.08
Receive medical treatment	.67	.15	5.43*
Postwar evaluation of war experience			
Attitude toward service at discharge	.94	.02	.14
Evaluation of military experience	−.38	.00	.00
Training helpful later	.48	.01	.04
War's effect on aging	−.21	−.05	.73
War's effect on current emotions	.69	.17	6.51*
Comradeship and veteran's organizations			
Reserve unit membership	.24	.03	.31
Current contact with service buddies	−.18	−.11	2.99
Membership in veteran's organizations	.13	.03	.18
Personal resources			
Locus of control	−1.10	−.25	16.87*
Altruism	−.12	−.07	1.36
Disclosure	−.40	−.07	1.32

*$p < .05$. $R^2 = .35$.

significant *F*-values included: (1) external locus of control ($F = 16.87$), (2) combat stress ($F = 7.98$), (3) postwar evaluation of war's effect on current emotion ($F = 6.51$), and (4) medical treatment received for a combat-related injury ($F = 5.43$). Thirty-five percent of the explained variance in PTSD symptoms in the last year was predicted by these five variables.

Table 22.7 summarizes the findings for PTSD symptoms in the context of the Pearl Harbor experience reported in 1986. The significant *F*-values are: (1) postwar evaluation of war's effect on current emotion ($F = 12.16$), (2) subjective perception of war stress ($F = 7.49$), and (3) actual combat stress ($F = -6.60$). Thirty-one percent of the explained variance in PTSD symptoms related to the attack on Pearl Harbor was accounted for by the five variables.

Subjective Evaluations of World War II Experiences

Perceived Effects on Postwar Life

In the survey of Pearl Harbor survivors, the veterans were asked to respond to the question: "How did your military service in World War II affect your postwar life? Describe some of the desirable and undesirable aspects of this experience." Content analysis of the answers to this question revealed that 87 (32%) of the responses contained totally positive indications, 36 (13%) were totally negative, and 64 (24%) had both positive and negative aspects. It is important to note that out of the 269 surveyed, 43 (16.2%) elected not to answer this question and another 38 (14%) stated that the war had had no effect or undesirable effects on their lives.

The generally positive nature of answers to this question are also confirmed by responses of these veterans to other questions. Other answers by these men reveal that (1) the majority (65%) perceived military training to have been helpful later in their lives; (2) over two thirds (68%) reported strong positive feelings toward military service after discharge; (3) the majority (51%) perceived that their military experience had strong or very strong influence on their lives; and (4) almost one half (48%) of the veterans who participated in this research perceived their military experiences as "good" or "very good." Interestingly, only 1% perceived their military service as "bad" or "very bad." In the following sections, we describe some of the major themes, positive and negative, reported by the veterans in our research.

Positive Effects of World War II Experiences

Responses of veteran Pearl Harbor Survivors Association members indicative of positive adjustment included: (1) the acquisition of work skills which were helpful in finding employment during the postwar years; (2) planning and leadership skills which were helpful in career advancement; and (3) educational and training opportunities provided for veterans. Additionally, some men stated that their wartime experiences facilitated marital adjustment and family life as well as

the ability to relate to life with a broader perspective. Overall, the themes reflected personal growth, maturity, and a willingness to continue on with adult responsibility in a positive way because of the effects of the war experience.

Negative Effects of World War II Experiences

In terms of negative effects of their war experiences, some of the veterans stated that they had difficulties in various areas of social and psychological adjustment. Overall, the reported negative effects were extremely few. However, they included securing and maintaining employment, establishing interpersonal and intimate relations, and relying excessively on alcohol in order to cope. Related to this, perhaps, was the report of distressing wartime memories. There was also resentment expressed at "losing" precious years of life because of the war.

Intrusive memories and imagery related to Pearl Harbor and World War II remained very much on the minds of many veterans in our study. Here are some examples of what they said: (1) "Bad memories remain"; (2) "Scarred me for the rest of my life"; (3) "Have not been the same and never will because of the war"; (4) "I always think of bad things in life, never think of good things." A few stated that the hardest part of the war was seeing their "best buddies" die and that so many other young men had to lose their lives. Still others said that their experiences were invaluable but that they would not like to go through them again. They also felt that it was what they had to do for their country.

Physical Health

It is evident that the war affected the physical health of some of the veterans. A few also volunteered that they developed excessive reliance on alcohol which persisted for many years. Some of the veterans indicated that their physical injuries had a complicating effect on their ability to secure employment and begin a career.

A review of answers to the question about the effects of the wartime service indicate more positive than negative responses. The major areas mentioned as positive effects were acquired work skills (12%), experiences which helped in obtaining employment (8%), positive outlook on life (14%), educational benefits (8.0%), and relating to others (8.7%). The negative effects included interpersonal problems (7%), the time that the war took away from their families, education, careers, and life in general (8%), and difficulties in getting or keeping a job (4%).

From Pearl Harbor to the Present: Mediating Factors of Adjustment

Social and Environmental Support

Survivors of Pearl Harbor show a strong identification with their military backgrounds. In addition to their involvement with the Pearl Harbor Survivors Association, more than two thirds (68%) are members of such other groups as the Veterans of Foreign Wars, the American Legion, and the Disabled American Veterans.

In addition to formal organizational membership, there are clear indications that affiliations with service buddies has been continuing over the years and that it is a meaningful aspect of the interpersonal world of the Pearl Harbor survivor.

Approximately three quarters of the veterans reported active participation in previous reunions—78% reported exchanging letters, 77% exchanged greeting cards, and 67% had phone contact with their buddies in 1986, the year of the reunion.

Such continuing involvement reflects opportunities for self-disclosure and shared remembrances with others who experienced the trauma as well as the victory of war. At the same time, it contributes to keeping the memories of war alive rather than having them recede into the past.

Regarding the sharing of World War II experiences with significant others, wives of veterans rank highest (76% share "much" or "a lot"), followed by children (57%), close friends (55%), and co-workers (40%). Interestingly, veterans did not seem to share much with their own fathers (25%) or mothers (25%). A rather interesting finding is the fact that the veterans shared their experiences *least* with the clergy (8%) and with counselors (psychiatrists, psychologists, and social workers) (7%).

Pearl Harbor survivors actively remember and keep alive their experiences. Thus, 78% state that they will never forget their combat and military experiences in the war. They go on to state that their experiences constituted one of the most intensive feelings in their lives (70%). The vast majority have revisited the sites of their military service (75%). Thus, the strong social supports which our survivors have developed enable them to actively remember these turbulent times with a feeling of strength behind them.

Perhaps for this reason, the majority stated their military training was helpful later on in their lives (65%), and over two thirds (68%) reported strong positive feelings toward the service after their discharge. These feelings are consistent with the subjective perception of their military experience as good or very good (48%) despite surviving the Pearl Harbor attack and serving four long years. It is noteworthy that only 1% perceived the military experience as bad or very bad. Consistent with the above, the majority (51%) perceived the military influence on their lives as being strong or very strong. This is also reflected in their evaluation of the effects of wartime service on adjustment to aging. Only 9% stated that their military service had a negative effect on their adjustment to aging, whereas as much as 44% went as far as to say it had a positive effect on their adjustment to aging.

In considering social supports of Pearl Harbor survivors, there is a general pattern of cohesiveness with family and friends. Gerontological literature has documented the important role of spouses as sources of both effective and instrumental support in later life. The vast majority of Pearl Harbor survivors (91%) were married at the time of the interview. Only 5% were divorced and only 3% were widowed. Furthermore, 7% were remarried after widowhood and 12% were remarried after di-

vorce. Only 1% of the respondents were never married. In addition to the availability of spouses as potential and actual sources of social support, 88% of respondents also had children. Only 12% of the sample had no children.

Self-disclosure reflects the maintenance of social bonds with others through sharing of experiences. It exemplifies interaction where the veteran may obtain understanding and support for others. Our study also examined the extent to which veterans engage in nurturant interactions and express altruistic attitudes and a desire to be of assistance to others. Pearl Harbor survivors reported strong and consistent evidence of altruistic attitudes. Thus, 97% reported that they enjoy doing things for others, and 96% reported that they help others even when others do not help them. In addition, 89% were willing to risk their lives to help others, thereby reflecting that they preserve, as an enduring value, the serviceman's tradition of self-sacrifice.

Messages for Future Generations

As part of our research with members of the Pearl Harbor Survivors Association, on the occasion of their 45th reunion, veterans were asked to respond to the question: "Considering all of your experiences in World War II and at Pearl Harbor, what would you like to say about this to future generations?" The majority of those answering this question addressed the need for military alertness and strength. The reasons for this assessment may be reflected in the appraisal of one of the veterans in his observations about Pearl Harbor and the war:

The most important part of our nation's history since 1776 is considering the fact that the Pearl Harbor command was not fully informed by our leaders in Washington and with a shortage of patrol planes, we were surprised by the Japanese attack. Our reaction was so quick that we were defending ourselves within minutes; probably this was one of the reasons why they didn't continue the attack. Though Japan claimed victory, it contributed to their own defeat, for they failed to destroy our oil reserves and repair facilities—a major factor in keeping our fleet in the mid-Pacific. Our greatest loss was the young men who gave their lives, not the old battleships which were too slow to keep up with the fast carriers and their escorts. Within weeks we were able to assemble a task force of fast carriers, cruisers, and destroyers, striking back and turning the war in our favor, six months later, in the Battle of Midway. Closing out the war, I was aboard the fast carrier USS *Bennington*, striking back at Japan, fighting off kamikaze attacks, which gave me the satisfaction of being off the coast of Tokyo when the war came to an end. Today, many people debate the atomic bomb and Hiroshima. Although it killed many civilians, Japan agrees it saved millions of lives, Japanese and Americans. The Japanese, young and old, were being trained as human bombs to defend their homeland. Thousands of 14 and 15 year olds were trained as kamikaze pilots to sacrifice their life to destroy enemy naval forces. Admiral Kimmel and General Short were made "scapegoats," their records should be cleared of any fault. General MacArthur, the best informed commander, was surprised in the Philippines, nine hours after Pearl Harbor, losing his bombers and fighter planes on the ground. He was allowed to escape, then promoted and later returned to the Philippines as a hero. We must never forget Pearl Harbor, a very important part of our nation's history. Freedom is precious. A strong military and a united nation will survive.

The first set of responses to this question by veterans included (1) pleas to remember what happened at Pearl Harbor; (2) the need to stay alert and to keep a strong military; (3) the importance for young people to serve their country; and (4) the need for effective communication between the political and military leadership.

Advice for Future Generations

Eighty-nine individuals (33%) offered some type of advice for future generations, based on their experiences in World War II. Here are the suggestions, most of which are indicative of the need to assure the military alertness and strength of the United States:

- Be proud to be an American.
- Never let us become complacent militarily.
- Give something of yourself to your country.
- Never underestimate your enemy.
- Keep abreast of the news and current world events.
- Don't ever allow yourselves to become complacent with freedoms.
- Keep abreast of current changes and positions on foreign policy and American attitudes toward our foreign policy.
- Just as dangerous as annihilation is the danger of erosion from within which could strip us of our liberty and deliver us to a type of government that denies us those freedoms and liberties which we cherish today.
- There is no glamour nor glory in war. It is grotesque and horrible and dehumanizing. There are enough material things and sufficient ideological room for all. We should not have to fight over either. While we stay strong out of necessity, we can and should work toward a peaceful utopia. Learn about the lives, languages, culture, and needs of other social systems. Then we can understand the necessity and logic of tolerance and sharing. And maybe even the compromises necessary to make it work.

Discussion

The results of this study are interesting in several ways despite some limitations of the sample. First, the men in this study, predominantly veterans who served at Pearl Harbor and the South Pacific in the navy during World War II, report moderate to high levels of combat exposure. More than half of the sample report the following types of war stress experiences: firing a weapon at the enemy; being subjected to enemy fire; seeing members of their unit or allies wounded; seeing towns or villages destroyed by combat episodes; being under direct enemy attack on many occasions; and experiencing a life-and-death survival situation. Although these retrospective memories are subject to the problems that are inherent with the passage of time and the cognitive reformulation of these experiences in terms of clarity and meaning, these recollections are nevertheless important. Moreover, in examining the open-response comments about what happened on the day of infamy, the lucidity and detail of recollection in the veterans' memories are highly impressive. This is in contrast to the general view in the psychological literature which suggests that individuals tend to forget unpleasant experiences.

In our view, life crises and momentous events of great historical and personal meaning become stored and embedded in one's memory and are likely to be recalled and/or will intrude periodically in very vivid imagery. And, as noted in the introduction, this raises the fundamental questions of what it means to be a "survivor."

Traumatic Memories versus Posttraumatic Stress Disorder

By what set of criteria do we discern the difference between the memory of trauma and the so-called pathological forms of intrusive imagery that are the *sine qua non* in the diagnosis of posttraumatic stress disorder (PTSD)? Traumatic events, by definition, are painful, difficult, often overwhelming, and full of emotional and moral conflict. They are profoundly distressing experiences which get stored in memory and have attached to them different forms of affect, most of which are negative. Thus, when a survivor remembers what happened during the trauma, is it necessarily to be considered pathological? Moreover, if the recall of trauma is involuntary, unbidden, and intrusive in nature is that sufficient, in itself, to be labeled as a pathological symptom, even if the memory is accompanied by distressing affect, such as sadness, grief, anger, depression, or no affect at all? Similarly, if the survivor wishes to purposely forget or avoid the memory of what happened in the traumatic event, is that necessarily a pathological response or simply a variant on coping in order to attend to present day responsibilities? Clearly, most clinicians would agree that when the symptoms which comprise the definition of PTSD or some other psychiatric diagnosis are severe enough to impair basic personal functioning, such as the ability to work, relate meaningfully to others, and find enjoyment in life, they can be construed as pathological in their effect—that is, they have deleterious consequences on adaptive functioning in the environment.

In attempts to delineate the nature of coping, defense, and adaptation of survivors who are highly functional and well-adjusted to culturally defined patterns of life-course development, it is critical to attempt to understand the subjective perception and importance of the trauma in their lives. Survivors of wartime stress may continue to have memories that are often salient and distressing; nevertheless, these may be very meaningful to them. Furthermore, it is important to underscore the symbolic and collective meaning of the wartime experiences in the lives of veterans. Returning to the sites of the experiences, public recognition, memorials, and commemorations become extremely meaningful and important. The intrusion, recall, and processing of traumatic wartime events need not be considered only in pathological terms. This may be a normally expected process of integrating traumatic memory into individual identity, consciousness, and value system. Alternatively, it must be recognized, too, that when the reactive process leads to disturbance in identity and consciousness, and when physiological functioning becomes impaired because of overwhelmingly stressful experiences, it is appropriate to characterize PTSD behaviors as pathological.

Finally, it is important to underscore the subjectively attributed meaning by the veterans to their wartime experience. This is especially true for veterans of World War II and especially for survivors of the Japanese attack of Pearl Harbor specifically. The majority of these veterans went from being victims of a surprise attack to being conquering heroes—victors of World War II. Upon their return, they were perceived as war heroes and the various social and economic benefits enabled them to acquire education and/or vocational training and to establish themselves as contributors to the postwar industrial and economic development of the United States. These may be among the reasons why these veterans perceived their wartime experiences to have had a positive impact on their postwar vocational and social adjustment, and why so many of them were willing to share the legacy of their experiences.

Beyond all these considerations is the undeniable and deeply ingrained sense of identity in Pearl Harbor veterans who formally refer to each other as fellow "survivors." These are overtly proud, ordinary men whose adult lives were profoundly influenced by momentous historical events that changed the course of history during the middle years of the twentieth century. In the *context* of their experiences and emergence as victors, they began their early adult years with a special sense of achievement and collective involvement. Eventually, those qualities gave birth to an organization (PHSA) to preserve, honor, and bind them together into a *group identity* as survivors that ensured social support and

well-being. As this study has shown, their remembrance of war is vivid, clear, and still very much a part of their lives, despite the inevitable changes that occur in the aging process.

References

American Psychiatric Association. (1987). *Diagnostic and statistical manual of mental disorders* (3rd ed., rev.). Washington, DC: Author.

Elder, G. A., & Clipp, E. C. (1988). Combat experiences, comradeship, and psychological health. In J. P. Wilson, Z. Harel, & B. Kahana (Eds.), *Human adaptation to extreme stress: From the Holocaust to Vietnam* (pp. 131–156). New York: Plenum Press.

Kahana, B., Harel, Z., & Kahana, E. (1988). Predictors of psychological well-being among survivors of the Holocaust. In J. P. Wilson, Z. Harel, & B. Kahana (Eds.), *Human adaptation to extreme stress: From the Holocaust to Vietnam* (pp. 171–192). New York: Plenum Press.

Laufer, R. S., Frey-Wouters, E., & Gallops, M. S. (1985). Traumatic stressors in the Vietnam War and post-traumatic stress disorder. In C. R. Figley (Ed.), *Trauma and its wake: The study and treatment of post-traumatic stress disorder* (pp. 73–89). New York: Brunner/Mazel.

Wilson, J. P. (1980). Conflict, stress and growth: The effects of war on psychosocial development among Vietnam veterans. In C. R. Figley & S. Grentman (Eds.), *Strangers at home: Vietnam veterans since the war*. New York: Praeger.

Wilson, J. P. (1989). *Trauma, transformation and healing*. New York: Brunner/Mazel.

Wilson, J. P., Harel, Z., & Kahana, B. (1989). The day of infamy: The legacy of Pearl Harbor. In J. P. Wilson (Ed.), *Trauma, transformation and healing* (pp. 129–156). New York: Brunner/Mazel.

Wilson, J. P., & Krauss, G. E. (1985). Predicting post-traumatic stress syndromes among Vietnam veterans. In W. Kelly (Ed.), *Post-traumatic stress disorder and the war veteran patient* (pp. 102–147). New York: Brunner/Mazel.

PART III

War Trauma and Civil Violence

Section B: Research from World War II to the Present

Section B of Part III comprises 10 chapters that present an interesting cross-section of research studies which examined the effects of war trauma and civil violence in a diverse sector of survivor populations. These chapters document further the acute and long-term effects of exposure to extremely stressful life events that contribute to psychiatric disorders, and the alteration of the self-structure and life-course trajectories. The groups studied in these chapters include (1) Vietnam veterans and POWs, (2) British Falkland Islands War veterans, (3) Cambodian and Southeast Asian refugees, (4) Israeli combat veterans, (5) survivors of the war in Sri Lanka, (6) victims of civil violence and terrorism in Northern Ireland, (7) victims of the war in Afghanistan, and (8) survivors of civil violence in the United Kingdom. Table III.1 presents a summary of these chapters.

In Chapter 23, Raymond Monsour Scurfield presents an overview of the nature and dynamics of PTSD among Vietnam veterans. His chapter abounds with information which summarizes the evolution of research studies which led to the identification of PTSD as the central psychological difficulty for Vietnam veterans. These studies are reviewed and then connected to the development of the readjustment counseling program of the Veterans Administration in the United States. Furthermore, among the many rich sections of this chapter is a discussion of the central dynamics of PTSD in Vietnam veterans, which include numbing, rage, fear, grief, blame, survivor mode functioning, and complex interactions and combinations of these painful affective reactions. Of special interest in the chapter is the discussion of the unique needs and problems faced by minority veterans, such as women who served in the medical corps, blacks, Hispanics, and Native Americans as well as disabled ex-servicemen. Later on, in Chapter 74, Scurfield will build on all the insights presented in Part III to layout a systematic approach to the treatment of PTSD by specialized inpatient and outpatient programs in PTSD units in hospital settings.

America's longest war, Vietnam, produced 600 prisoners of war who returned home in 1973 under a program known as Operation Homecoming. Edna J. Hunter, author of Chapter 24, directed this California-based project for many years in San Diego. Her research on military families, and especially of the POWs from Vietnam and

275

Table III.1. An Overview of Research on War Trauma and Civil Violence from World War II to the Present

Chapter/study and authors	Population studied	Age and related features	Measures used and time period assessed	Symptoms evident	Major findings
23 Vietnam veterans Raymond Monsour Scurfield	Vietnam veterans	40–50+	Review of literature	PTSD Depression Alcohol Rage Grief Shame	26.7% PTSD rate nationally
24 Vietnam POWs Edna J. Hunter	Vietnam POWs and families	40–50 families N = 651 POWs	1973–present Center for POW Studies in San Diego, CA	PTSD Depression Personality changes Psychic numbing	Issue of control prevalent Families destabilized High divorce rate Overcontrolled states Long-term period of readjustment
25 British Falklands War veterans Roderick Jan Orner	Falklands War veterans	N = 53	DSM-III PTSD General Health Questionnaire (GHQ)	PTSD Anxiety Anger Depression Alienation Numbing Interpersonal conflict	60% PTSD rate War injury correlated with PTSD 68% attribute current problems to the war 54.7% caseness on GHQ
26 Southeast Asian refugees J. David Kinzie	Cambodian refugees and Southeast Asian refugees (Laotian) (Vietnamese) (Mein)	N = 75 adults N = 40 children	DSM-III-R PTSD Clinical interviews Specific stressor endured (e.g., torture)	Depression Nightmares Numbing Startle response Shame Loss of appetite Sleep disturbance Avoidance	85% PTSD rate Lack of ETOH abuse Comorbidity very high Tricyclic antidepressant medication useful Need cross-cultured mental health worker
27 Israeli war veterans Zahava Solomon	Lebanon War	N = 104 male veterans (IDF forces)	1983–1986 Combat stress reaction DSM-III PTSD Clinical interviews SCL-90 Social functioning scale	Psychic numbing Anxiety reactive Guilt Depression Psychosomatic symptoms Hostility	62% PTSD rate at 1-year follow-up Symptoms decreased with time PTSD associated with general psychiatric distress More social dysfunctioning with PTSD Increased alcohol and cigarette use

28 War in Sri Lanka Daya J. Somasundaram	Civilians in Sri Lanka War	Children to elderly Cross-section of persons treated psychiatrically	1983–1988 DSM-III-R ICD-9 Case analysis Screening at psychiatric hospitals	Fatigue Intrusive images Sleep disturbance Poor concentration Anxiety/fear Mistrust Headache	PTSD common Wide range of psychiatric complaints No increase in admission rates Stress reactions the major problem suffered
29 War in Afghanistan Abdul Wali H. Wardak	Afghan refugees and controls	N = 120 Afghan refugees N = 120 controls N = 40 adolescents N = 40 young adults N = Mature adults	State-Trait Anxiety (STAI) Beck Depression (BDI) Crown-Crisp Experimental Inventory (CCEI) GHQ	Anxiety Depression PTSD Alienation	Young adults most severely affected Psychiatric disturbance high for new refugees Anxiety, depression very common PTSD rate appears high Symptoms decrease with time
30 Political violence in Northern Ireland Ed Cairns & Ronnie Wilson	Psychiatric admission in Northern Ireland	Review of literature Children and adults	1968–present	Anxiety Depression General psychiatric complaints	Stress reaction the major problem in adults Children prone to behavioral problems
31 Violence: Northern Ireland Peter S. Curran, G. C. Loughrey, & P. Bell	Civil violence victims	N = 499 persons referred for medical evaluation All over age 16 victims of civil violence seeking compensation 53% women 47% men	DSM-III-R PTSD Clinical interviews ICD-9	Depression Anxiety PTSD symptoms Sleep disturbance Poor concentration Startle response Constricted affect	PTSD rate 23.2% PTSD associated with suicide risk Increased alcohol abuse Marital disharmony Depression associated with PTSD
32 Police using firearms in United Kingdom Mary Manolias & Arthur Hyatt-Williams	Police officers in U.K.	N = 25 male police officers who used weapons	DSM-III PTSD 16-PF Clinical interviews	Depression Anxiety PTSD symptoms Alienation Sleep disturbance Emotional lability Social withdrawal Sweating Problems of concentration	67% PTSD rate 60% perceptual distortions during shooting

their families, has given her a wealth of clinical experience and a set of empirical studies by which to place their problems of readjustment and reunification into a broad but meaningful perspective. This chapter summarizes her insights into the short- and long-term effects of the POW experience.

Hunter begins her chapter by noting that the American POWs in Vietnam were held in captivity longer than in any previous United States wars: an average of 5 years. The captors were brutal, using solitary confinement, brain-washing procedures, and methodical torture as part of their repertoire of social influence techniques. The POWs held captive in North Vietnam were treated more harshly than those interned in the South, below the demilitarized zone (DMZ). Also, prisoners who were taken before 1969 had been treated far more harshly than the captives later on account of the death of Ho Chi Minh in September, 1969, and efforts by the POW families to draw attention to the severe plight of the men who, according to Hunter, at that time "would have resembled the skeletonlike survivors of Bataan of World War II."

In 1971, with the establishment of the Center for Prisoner of War Studies in San Diego, operations and planning began for the eventual release and repatriation of the POWs. Hunter and her colleagues studied extensively over 600 former POWs and their families; the results are reviewed in her chapter. Although these findings are too extensive to summarize adequately here, a few of the major points can be highlighted:

1. Behaviors learned in captivity for survival purposes often made reintegration with families very difficult. Such characteristics as obsessive-compulsiveness, blunted affect, overly controlled emotions, habitual "mental gymnastics," and preference for a rigidly ordered environment often led to interpersonal conflict.

2. Survivors learned to cope with captivity in a much stronger way than they ever thought possible. However, coping patterns were quite varied among the POWs: discovering *what worked* for them was important to survivorship.

3. Similar phenomena and challenges confronted families of the POWs both *during captivity* and upon *repatriation*. Families, too, had to discover what worked for them in terms of coping with the absence of the spouse or father and, later, how to adapt to his return and its effects upon the family system. Not surprisingly, issues of *control* and decision-making were important both to the POW in captivity and to the family system, in which control/decision-making functions may have shifted in the serviceman's absence. Reflected in this changed family system were problems which led to marital dissolutions whose rate was three times higher than carefully matched control groups.

4. Parent–child relationships were altered by the POW experience: the mother's stability and coping style had a large influence on her children's adjustment.

5. Finally, Hunter's analysis makes it clear that the readjustment process following repatriation is not simple, easily dealt with, or to be understood by the initial reactions at homecoming. The longitudinal study of former POWs reveals a picture of human and family struggle to overcome massive life-course disruption to reconnect to sources of social support that offer an enhanced sense of self-esteem and well-being.

It is quite possible to argue that the rather extensive empirical literature on Vietnam veterans not only helped to codify the diagnostic category of PTSD in the DSM-III, but also renewed research efforts with other victim and survivor populations who had endured psychic trauma. As noted by Scurfield in Chapters 23 and 74, the research on the postwar problems of Vietnam veterans generated new questions about the nature and duration of deleterious psychiatric symptoms associated with high levels of combat exposure. Thus, as the clinical and research literature on PTSD spread through professional journals and other periodicals, it is not surprising that mental health professionals in other parts of the world beyond the United States began similar (and often comparative) investigations with veterans and survivors of other wars and areas of civil violence.

In Chapter 25, Roderick Jan Orner examines PTSD among British veterans of the Falklands War, which was fought for about 2 months in 1982. Similar to other surveys reported in Section A of Part III, Orner administered a set of questionnaires to 53 former servicemen who had fought in the Falklands War. These men were about equally representative of the armed services: Navy (26%), Army (30%), Paratroopers (23%), and Royal Marines (21%). The test battery included the DSM-III criteria for PTSD, an adjustment problem checklist, and the General Health Questionnaire (GHQ).

The central findings indicated that 60% of the sample had PTSD, a result consistent with the prevalence rate reported in other chapters in Part III of this volume. Moreover, a factor analysis performed on the adjustment checklist produced orthogonal factors which were labeled general adjustment problems and posttraumatic stress disorder symptoms. The first four factors account for about 64% of the total variance. Additional analyses identified alienation and relationship problems (especially with authority figures) to be significant areas of concern in adjustment. Finally, in examining attribution of their current problems of adjustment, 68% of the sample directly mentioned their involvement in the Falklands War, a result congruent with many studies of Vietnam veterans.

After the United States involvement in Vietnam ended in 1975, another holocaust occurred in Cambodia, a form of *autogenocide* sometimes referred to as "The Killing Fields," which claimed the lives of over two million people under the Marxist Pol Pot regime. At the same time, hundreds of thousands of Southeast Asian refugees were fleeing to Thailand, the United States, Australia, China, and other destinations to find freedom after the Vietnam War.

In Chapter 26, J. David Kinzie reports on PTSD and its treatment among Southeast Asian refugees. This chapter largely reflects the clinical and research efforts of Kinzie and his colleagues at the Indochinese refugee clinic in Portland, Oregon.

To begin, Kinzie makes the point that it is difficult to work with patients from a different culture who present many challenges to assessment, diagnosis, and treatment because of non-Western belief systems, religious orientations, cultural norms and mores, and language barriers which create unique problems in obtaining an adequate history and in discerning the story of the trauma. Suggestions are made in how to manage these problems in order to design effective treatment programs, which in themselves demand innovation, creativity, and flexibility in order to meet the special needs of the refugee patients. A potential problem of significance, if proper steps are not taken to address cross-cultural differences, is the possibility of grossly underestimating (diagnosing) the true prevalence of PTSD, which runs as high as 95% because of multiple stressors endured in Cambodia or in the refugee escape process. For example, among Cambodian concentration camp survivors, 99% experienced forced labor, 79% were separated from their families, 81% were starved, 96% witnessed the death by execution of a family member, and 63% of the children lost a parent. In terms of psychiatric symptom patterns, major depression, dysthymia, and PTSD were present in 75% of all the patients and were chronic in nature.

Given the level of massive traumatization of the Southeast Asian refugees, a number of treatment considerations are reviewed in Kinzie's chapter. Additionally, the potentially valuable role of pharmacological treatment is reviewed, with success found in the proper use of clonidine and imipramine. Finally, at the end of this compassionate, thoughtful, and pragmatic chapter 16 research questions are listed for future psychiatric work with refugee populations of a non-Western origin.

In Chapter 27, Zahava Solomon details the immediate and long-term effects of combat stress among Israeli soldiers who were involved in the Lebanon War of

1982—the seventh and perhaps most controversial of Israel's conflicts since the founding of the nation state.

Solomon begins her chapter by observing that during the war and in its immediate aftermath, there were several hundred psychiatric casualties and that later, this number swelled considerably because of delayed-onset effects. Solomon's chapter is interesting because it reports the major findings of a 7-year research project.

About one year after the Lebanon War ended, 104 male veterans were interviewed in depth. These interviews were then transcribed, coded, and subjected to rigorous statistical methods. Factor analysis of the coded transcripts revealed six major factors with eigenvalues greater than one, including (1) psychic numbing, (2) anxiety reactions, (3) guilt over performance, (4) depressive reactions, (5) psychosomatic reactions, and (6) psychoticlike states. These forms of combat stress reaction (CSR) were considered to be a kind of taxonomy of the typical domain of affective and psychological processes to combat exposure and war trauma.

Using the assessment interview protocol, evaluation of PTSD according to the DSM-III criteria revealed, after one year, 62% suffering from the disorder (a figure identical to that obtained by Orner for the British Falklands War veterans), which diminished to 43% after 3 years.

In addition to analyzing the prevalence of PTSD for the sample, global psychiatric symptoms were measured by the SCL-90 questionnaire. The overall results showed more severe psychopathology at the 1-, 2-, and 3-year intervals postcombat. In particular, there were significant elevations on the scales that measure anxiety, obsessive-compulsive tendencies, and paranoia, a finding parallel to that found in previous research with Vietnam veterans and victims of other forms of trauma (Wilson, 1989).

Among the other fine-grained analyses presented in the chapter, Solomon examined psychosocial functioning and found that the combat stress-reaction casualties presented more problems in social, family, sexual, and occupational functioning than did a control group when assessed at three intervals after the war. Thus, consistent with findings cited in the other chapters in Part III of this volume, prolonged effects of the stressors of combat were not limited to intrusive recollections of the experiences and powerful affective reactions, but began to permeate adaptive behavior at all levels, creating a full range of psychosocial problems of coping in terms of intimacy, the use of leisure time, and the ability to focus on career and family.

A careful reading of all the chapters in Part III begins to reveal a repetitive pattern of themes and common psychiatric sequelae following experience with the multitude of stressors indigenous to combat exposure and war trauma. In Chapter 28, Daya J. Somasundaram details posttraumatic sequelae of the war in Sri Lanka, a conflict which has existed from 1983 to the present between the Tamil militants in the North and the State of Sri Lanka. Consequences of this guerrilla warfare have affected nearly all aspects of Sri Lankan society. Combatants and civilians alike have been both perpetrators and victims of terroristic activity, conventional fighting, torture, interrogation, and other forms of brutality, and have been exposed to the grotesque, death, dying, and social upheaval.

In this chapter, Somasundaram not only documents the range and prevalence of psychiatric reactions to the stressors of this particular war but also presents a series of clinical vignettes which illustrate the diversity of individual reactions to the varied forms of trauma that impact on innocent bystanders or those ideologically committed toward one system of values opposed to another. The result is an enormously elaborate presentation of material that demonstrates the plasticity of human behavior in response to overwhelming events embedded in trauma. Nevertheless, the most consistent theme that emerges from these case analyses is that at their core lie posttraumatic stress reactions which can then be "layered" by many other attempts at coping and adaptation.

In Chapter 29, Abdul Wali H. Wardak examines the effects of the war in Afghanistan on the refugees in the North-west Frontier Province (NWFP) region of Pakistan. Since 1978, the war has continued in Afghanistan:

> Many people have been exposed to horrific events and a terrifying environment. They have witnessed the death of people in combat or bombardment, mutilations, the retrieval of bodies, and the complete devastation of houses, villages, and agricultural land. Some of them have actively participated in the killing of their enemies, in mortar bombing, ambush, hand-to-hand fights, assassinations, and interrogations. Many of them have been through the experience of a prolonged journey through mountains and very rough terrain. In this journey, they experienced fatigue, changes in diet and climate, and travel across time zones coupled with the constant fear of being caught, killed, or imprisoned.

Clearly, these multiple-stressor events have had an impact on individuals, families, and the fabric of the culture itself. In his chapter, Wardak examines the psychiatric and stress-related sequelae of the war stressors on 120 Afghan refugees and 120 matched controls of native Pakistani people from the NWFP region. Furthermore, the refugee sample was stratified into adolescents (13–16 years), young adults (20–30 years), and mature adults (40+ years). Additionally, the sample was classified into two groups (short- versus long-stay) depending on how long they had been in refuge (i.e., less or more than 2 years duration).

All subjects were given a battery of questionnaires which included the State-Trait Anxiety Inventory (STAI), the Beck Depression Inventory, the Crown-Crisp Experiential Inventory (CCEI), and the General Health Questionnaire (GHQ). The results of the statistical analysis confirmed the authors hypotheses and are consistent with those reported in the other chapters in Part III in this volume. First, the refugee group as a whole manifested greater degrees of anxiety, depression, obsessive-ruminative thoughts, somatic anxiety, and psychiatric "caseness" (as discerned by the GHQ). Second, the refugees who had less time in Pakistan (the safe haven) had more severe psychiatric symptoms than did those who had spent over 2 years out of Afghanistan. Third, adolescents exhibited fewer stress-related symptoms than did the mature adults. Finally, the young adults had a higher range of psychological disturbances than did the older adults in the sample.

Wardak's findings parallel those reported by Kinzie in Chapter 26 and show age-related, developmental, and situational effects (time spent in recovery environment). Furthermore, with high levels of exposure to traumatically stressful events, there is an expectable pattern of psychiatric and stress-related reactions; Wardak's data match closely those reported by Somasundaram in Chapter 28. Thus, in four different countries with many subcultures (Cambodia, Vietnam, Sri Lanka, and Afghanistan), the human pattern of adaptation to extreme stress is remarkably uniform in its expression.

In Chapters 30 and 31, the focus of traumatic stress reactions shifts to the effects of *enduring civil violence* in Northern Ireland, where political unrest and dissension have ripped through the Catholic and Protestant communities since 1968. Since that time, over 2,710 individuals have died and over 30,000 have been injured in the political conflict. As with other traumatic events that involve violence, killing, search and detention tactics, interrogations, and torture, there are both individual and sociocultural consequences that affect the adaptive behavior and well-being of the citizens.

In Chapter 30, Ed Cairns and Ronnie Wilson review the literature on the psychiatric sequelae of exposure to enduring civil violence among adults and children. Their review includes an examination of different types of studies which include statistical analysis of psychiatric admission rates and types of diagnoses (e.g., alcohol-related disorders); clinical- and community-based studies in which the General Health Questionnaire (GHQ) has been used to determine psychiatric symptom severity and "caseness." The results of the GHQ survey data show high levels of disturbance in areas of greater violence, a result consistent with that obtained by Wardak for the Afghan refugees reported in Chapter 29. Finally, among the interesting results on studies of children is that those "who had had a relative or friend injured in the troubles, and children who thought that their area was 'not safe to live in,' tended to have higher Rutter scores" [a measure of disturbance]. These findings parallel those reported by Kinzie in Chapter 26 on Cambodian and Southeast Asian refugee children who had witnessed the killing of a relative or parent, or who had suffered the loss of them through violent actions.

In Chapter 31, the issue of PTSD and civil violence is explored by Peter S. Curran, G. C. Loughrey, and P. Bell. The authors carried out a research project on 499 referrals for medicolegal assessment by trained specialists who were knowledgeable about PTSD and differential diagnosis. Additionally, a psychiatric symptom checklist was administered to the patients. The sample consisted of about equal numbers of men and women with the average age being 37.3 years. Only 6.6% had a previous psychiatric history. All subjects had been exposed to incidents of civil violence in Northern Ireland which included (1) assassination attempts (18%), (2) violent personal assault (6.8%), (3) captivity by terrorists (15%), (4) witnessing violent actions against other at personal risk for injury (38.3%), (5) sustained personal injuries (28.3%), (6) witnessing someone being killed (17%), and (7) the loss of a close friend (11.6%). These were among the various stressors experienced by ordinary citizens living in Northern Ireland.

The results, once again, are quite similar to those found among Dutch Resistance fighters, Cambodian refugees, Alsace-Lorraine POWs, and Pearl Harbor survivors. For example, 84.5% had recurrent intrusive recollections; 52.6% reported recurrent dreams of the violence; 66.4% had forms of hyperalertness and manifestations of physiological hyperreactivity; 77.6% had symptom intensification by exposure to events that symbolize or resemble the original trauma; and 96.3% had sleep disturbance. Moreover, increased alcohol abuse, explosive outbursts, depression, and attempted suicide were associated with a diagnosis of PTSD. These findings are also remarkably similar to those found by Somasundaram among persons exposed to civil violence in Sri Lanka; they suggest that while PTSD is a common consequence of traumatic exposure, there is likely to be comorbidity in the form of anxiety reactions, depression, increased alcohol abuse, and behavioral manifestation in attempts at coping and adaptation.

The last chapter in Section B of Part III concerns the traumatic effects of firearms use by police officers in the United Kingdom. In Chapter 32, Mary Bernadette Manolias and Arthur Hyatt-Williams look at the issue of what happens when firearms are used in the course of duty in a country where such an event is a rarity and contrary to normal police activity (i.e., most police officers walk their beat unarmed).

Twenty-five specially trained officers who were permitted to carry firearms were interviewed extensively and were administered a measure of PTSD (the Reaction Index of Frederick) along with the Sixteen Personality Factor Questionnaire. The interesting set of results that were produced parallel those reported by Tom Williams in Chapter 78 for traumata experienced in the workplace:

1. Sixty-one percent of the officers had acute emotional reactions after a shooting, which included sleep disturbances, cold sweats, nightmares, anxiety, depression, and symptoms of gastrointestinal distress.

2. Sixty percent of the officers interviewed reported *perceptual distortions* during the incident, which included tunnel vision, time alterations (e.g., deceleration), and distortions in visual and auditory perceptions (e.g., face enlargement or loss of sound).

3. Postshooting reactions also involved feelings of anomie and alienation from fellow police officers who did not carry firearms.

4. Appearance in court to render testimony increased PTSD symptoms and was a source of anxiety over the event itself.

Among the authors' conclusions are a set of recommendations that include the need for critical incident stress debriefing, supportive counseling and appraisal with regard to legal proceedings, and adequate preparation for testimony.

CHAPTER 23

Posttraumatic Stress Disorder in Vietnam Veterans

Raymond Monsour Scurfield

Introduction

March, 1968. I'm in uniform (2nd Lt., Medical Service Corps, U.S. Army), on a plane ride between Pittsburgh (my hometown) and Philadelphia, flying on my way to the West Coast to depart to Vietnam. The plane filled up, except it seemed for the seat next to me. And then I saw, in the front of the plane, a young, uniformed Army youth being assisted onto the plane. He had no legs, and a patch over one eye, and he was coming down the aisle, very slowly, after everyone else had been seated. I thought, selfishly, "Oh, no, please don't sit down next to me, soldier." And, of course, he did. . . . And, after exchanging a polite hello, I was so very awkward in my silence and caught up in my own thoughts about the "irony" of being on my way to Vietnam and sitting next to a severely disabled vet—promoting my own worst catastrophic fantasies about *my* fate. After we took off, he started talking, obviously wanting to engage with me in conversation. Among other things, I remember him telling me how rough it was the last time he had gone home on leave from his hospital recovery process, especially when one of his high school buddies had told him, "It's such a shame that you lost your legs and eye for nothing." "That really hurt," he said to me. . . . And then, a little later, he turned to me and said, "But you know, sir, I'm the lucky one—no one else in the foxhole survived." (Scurfield, 1988a)

Raymond Monsour Scurfield • Pacific Center for PTSD and Other War-Related Disorders, U.S. Department of Veterans Affairs, P.O. Box 50188, Honolulu, Hawaii 96850 (formerly at Northwest Posttraumatic Stress Treatment Program, American Lake VA Medical Center, Tacoma, Washington). The views expressed in this chapter are solely those of the author and do not necessarily reflect those of the U.S. Department of Veterans Affairs or the Pacific Center for PTSD.

International Handbook of Traumatic Stress Syndromes, edited by John P. Wilson and Beverley Raphael. Plenum Press, New York, 1993.

This chapter discusses various aspects of posttraumatic stress disorder (PTSD) in Vietnam veterans. I will discuss military psychiatry operations in Vietnam through my perspective as an Army social work officer on an Army psychiatric team. There also is an elaboration of the centrality of rage, grief, fear, and blame dynamics in PTSD. Special consideration is given to the role of positive reappraisal of war experiences in the successful stress recovery process.

Prevalence of PTSD among Vietnam War Veterans: Recent Findings

Out of the 3.14 million Vietnam theater veterans who served in the war zone in Southeast Asia between 1964 and 1975, it is estimated that 15.2% currently have complete PTSD classified by the DSM-III-R diagnostic criteria (American Psychiatric Association [APA], 1987). An additional 11.2% currently have "partial PTSD," that is, one or more PTSD symptoms, but do not meet full diagnostic criteria. These findings were reported by the most comprehensive and sophisticated psychiatric epidemiological survey (RTI) ever conducted on veterans of any era of service in the United States (Kulka *et al.*, 1988). Thus, over one fourth of the entire Vietnam veteran population have war-related problems some 17 years since the last American troops were evacuated from Vietnam. In terms of clinical utilization, fully 85% of the veterans with current PTSD reported that they have never seen a mental health professional for their PTSD.

Another recent landmark study reports on the effects of the Vietnam War on PTSD among 2,042 male veteran twin pairs (Goldberg, True, Eisen, & Henderson, 1990). This study dramatically corroborates the prevalence rates reported in the National Vietnam Veterans Readjustment Study (NVVRS), for example, 16.8% of the twins who served in Vietnam had PTSD in contrast to 5% of the co-twins who did not serve in Vietnam. There was a ninefold increase in the prevalence of PTSD among twins who experienced high levels of combat in comparison with their cotwin who did not serve in Vietnam.

The findings cited above are significantly higher than estimates of the PTSD prevalence rate reported in another large-scale study conducted by the Center for Disease Control (CDC) (Houk, 1988). There are impressive research instrumentation and sampling differences between the NVVRS and CDC studies that provide a strong argument for the accuracy of the higher prevalence rate of 15.2% (Kulka et al., 1988) or 16.8% (Goldberg et al., 1990). I am among other researchers who argue that even the 6-month cutoff criterion for PTSD symptoms that was utilized in the RTI study is too narrow and results in an underreporting of the true prevalence rate. However, no matter which set of figures one accepts as reflective of the problems of Vietnam veterans, it is obvious to many observers that remarkable numbers of Vietnam veterans previously and currently have serious readjustment problems. It is the purpose of this chapter to illustrate and discuss the specific nature of these war-related difficulties.

Overview of the Research Literature

In the late 1960s and early 1970s, United States military psychiatry was proudly announcing its success in dramatically reducing the *acute* psychiatric casualty rate in the Vietnam theater of war in contrast to rates for Korea and World War II (Bourne, 1970; Colbach & Parrish, 1970; Borus, 1974). At the same time, however, there was a growing number of clinical descriptive reports about the unique aspects of the Vietnam war experience and the evidence of "readjustment problems" among returning veterans (Solomon, Zarcone, Yoerg, et al., 1971; Strange & Brown, 1970; Fox, 1972; Lifton, 1972, 1973; Van Putten & Emory, 1973; Haley, 1974; Stenger, 1974; DeFazio, 1975; Horowitz & Solomon, 1975; Wilson, 1977, 1978). There were also accounts of the growing Vietnam veteran "self-help" movement, characterized by "rap groups" in community settings where the emphasis was on discussions about war experiences rather than on individual psychopathology (Shatan, 1973, 1974; Egendorf, 1975; Lifton, 1978). In the absence of a PTSD diagnostic category in DSM-II, such terms as *post-Vietnam syndrome* (PVS), *delayed stress syndrome* (DSS), *postcombat syndrome* (PCS), and *combat stress reaction* (CSR) became somewhat popularized among veterans and clinicians working with Vietnam veterans (Wilson, 1978, 1980a).

In more recent years, at least 11 major studies have looked at the etiology, nature, frequency and severity of the readjustment problems of Vietnam veterans (Borus, 1973, 1974; Card, 1983; Egendorf, Kadushin, Laufer, Rothbart, & Sloan, 1981; Goldberg et al., 1990; Harris, 1980; Houk, 1988; Kulka et al., 1988; Laufer, Yager, Frey-Wouters, & Donnellan, 1981; Nace, O'Brien, Mintz, et al., 1978; Robins, Davis, & Goodwin, 1974; Robins, Helzer, & Davis, 1975; Stellman & Stellman, 1988; Wilson, 1977, 1978, 1989; Wilson & Krauss, 1981, 1985). Perhaps the most salient and consistent finding in these studies was a significant association between PTSD (and such other presenting problems as depression, anxiety, and substance abuse) and higher levels of combat exposure versus other predictive factors. Important associations with some *postwar* factors also were reported. Second, there has been the development of a multidimensional approach to the concept of war stress, rather than only the undimensional concept of level of amount of exposure *per se*; for example, the significance of exposure to and/or direct participation in atrocity like behavior (Laufer, 1985; Laufer, Brett, & Gallops, 1985; Laufer, Gallops, & Frey-Wouters, 1984; Wilson, 1989; Wilson & Krauss, 1985). These findings have been presented at local and national conferences of the various professional mental health organizations and in numerous smaller-sized research reports, journal articles, and books, to include several edited works specifically or primarily about Vietnam veterans (Figley, 1978; Figley & Leventman, 1980; Kelly, 1985; Sonnenberg, Blank, & Talbot, 1985a,b; Williams, 1980, 1987). There is also a selected bibliography, updated periodically, with over 1,000 published references about Vietnam and war trauma-related topics (Arnold, 1987) that recently has been incorporated into a much larger bibliographic database by the Department of Veterans Affairs National Center on PTSD.

Department of Veterans Affairs Readjustment Counseling Program

In the late 1970s, the U.S. Department of Veterans Affairs medical care system (its 172 hospitals and clinics make it the largest medical system in the Western world) belatedly began to implement a number of specialized treatment programs for PTSD and associated problems of Vietnam veterans. However, there was and continues to be to some degree considerable resistance to the support of "specialized" PTSD treatment programs. The VA's first specialized treatment program for war-related problems of veterans that was national in scope was the Vet Center Program, now known as the Readjustment Counseling Service. This innovative, community-based, and peer-counseling-oriented program was not instituted until 1979 following congressional-mandated legislation. An earlier similar program was privately established in 1978 by the Disabled American Veterans (DAV) in 80 cities based on the research of the Forgotten Warrior Project (Wilson, 1977, 1978). The VA program has grown from some 90 sites and an initial 3-year delimiting date to over 190 sites (Blank, 1985). Through 1987, Vet Centers were utilized by over 480,000 veterans of whom an estimated 158,000 had PTSD (Gronval, 1988).

In the 1980s, the VA moved to provide a more centralized initiating, coordinating, and facilitative role regarding PTSD research and treatment initiatives (see Chapter 77, in this volume, for a discussion). Several service organizations (such as the Disabled American Veterans, the Paralyzed Veterans of America, the American Legion, and the Vietnam Veterans of America) and the U.S. Senate Committee on Veterans Affairs have been instrumental in an oversight and advocacy role with the VA. Some of the most important PTSD-related initiatives have been (1) a National Advisory Committee (non-VA membership) on the Readjustment of Vietnam-era Veterans; (2) the Chief Medical Director's Special Committee on PTSD; (3) establishment of over 40 specialized PTSD Clinical Teams that have been recently established at various medical centers; (4) a VA National Center for PTSD (NC-PTSD) established in 1989 to promote and coordinate PTSD research, education, training, and information exchange activities throughout the VA system (the NC-PTSD publishes and circulates two newsletters, the *NCP Clinical Newsletter* and the *PTSD Research Quarterly*); and (5) 22 designated specialized inpatient PTSD units that have received special start-up resource allocations from the VA Central Office. I directed one of only four such units west of the Mississippi River in the United States at the American Lake VA Medical Center (Tacoma, Washington). For over four years, this program has had a waiting list of about 200 veterans and up to an 18-month wait to enter the 11-week inpatient phase—the longest such waiting time in the country.

Clearly and unequivocally there has been a growing and impressive evolution of PTSD-related theory, research, and program developments during the past 20 years that have focused primarily on Vietnam veterans. There still is considerable resistance concerning the concept of PTSD, particularly the chronic and delayed subtypes and the extent of the prevalence of PTSD symptoms among Vietnam veterans.

Resistance to Understanding PTSD and Associated Reactions to Trauma

Why is there still such a continuing disbelief and prejudice about the existence of PTSD after all these years and several major world wars and conflicts? It is important to note that the difficulties of veterans following wars has been well documented in the literature on traumatic neurosis (Trimble, 1981). Yet war-related problems persist along with a substantial disbelief about the longer-term impact of both war and civilian trauma, such as rape and industrial accidents (Scurfield, 1992).

Premorbid Bias in Psychoanalytic Thinking

The psychoanalytic school of psychiatry traditionally has placed emphasis on premorbid factors to explain the development of personality (see Chapter 5, in this volume, for a discussion). Psychoanalytic theory did not consider either the environment or adult experiences to be central to personality development in the life span. In terms of adult traumatic reactions, it was presumed that emotional distress would dissipate and hence that postwar psychological sequelae would be transitional in nature. If, however, the symptoms persisted over a longer period of time, the explanation would lie in predisposing personality factors that were triggered by the event. It was also believed that there

was a secondary gain from the continuance of the symptoms. A fixation of symptoms occurred because (1) the person felt justified to receive compensation for the symptoms and/or (2) the symptoms provided some other "gain," such as the receipt of sympathy for being sick, being able to remain dependent on others and stay in a sick role. The bias inherent in the psychoanalytic perspective was that it denied attaching importance to environmental factors and therefore to the traumatic event and hence disavowed the meaningful exploration and consideration of the event itself (for a PTSD-sensitive psychoanalytic perspective, see Lindy, 1988).

It is important to note that the rigorously conducted twin study (Goldberg *et al.*, 1990) dramatically corroborates the importance of war zone exposure (vs. premorbid) factors in the etiology of PTSD. It also controls for premorbid factors in a way that even rigorous retrospective analysis of premorbid self-report histories could not begin to accomplish.

Societal Reactions to the War and the Veterans

It was common for Americans and Australians to confuse their feelings and perceptions about the Vietnam War with their feelings about the warriors who fought in it (Wilson, 1978, 1980a). Instead of directly confronting their own feelings about the American war policy, many ordinary citizens and veterans of earlier wars scapegoated Vietnam veterans. "Baby-killers," "losers," "crybabies," and "walking time bombs" were common pejorative labels and, to some degree, still continue to be. It is interesting to note that Operation Desert Storm resulted in a different kind of confusion about "warriors and the war"—"support for our *troops*" seemed to be considered equivalent to "support for the *war*" (Scurfield, 1992).

Countertransference Reactions among Therapists

Today, mental health clinicians are not exempt from confusing their feelings about the Vietnam War versus those for the warrior (see Brende & Parson, 1985; Scurfield, in press; and Wilson, 1989; on countertransference reactions). A parallel dynamic had occurred between clinicians and survivors of Nazi concentration camps. The countertransference reactions of the clinicians often were complex reactions toward the Holocaust (i.e., the event) and the horrors of the Nazi concentration camps (Danieli, 1984). Therapists' reactions to war, death and dying, violence, and traumatic loss are aroused when working with veterans. If not properly appreciated by the therapist, the reactions can be projected onto the client. As with Nazi concentration camp survivors, there was often a "conspiracy of silence" between the clinicians and Vietnam veterans to *not* discuss war experiences and their implications for personal development.

Psychological Isolation of Vietnam Veterans

Vietnam veterans, especially in the several years immediately following their service in Vietnam, denied and avoided directly talking about their war experiences with most everyone. After all, there was little positive to be gained to identify oneself as a Vietnam veteran, let alone try to talk about troubling war experiences and memories. And, like other trauma survivors, Vietnam veterans with PTSD were either embarrassed, fearful, ashamed, enraged, or ignorant of the link between postwar problems and the war itself. Many men and women withdrew and became psychologically isolated (Wilson & Krauss, 1985).

Department of Defense Resistance

In the U.S. Department of Defense (DOD) and among "prodefense"-oriented individuals there continues to be great difficulty in accepting the concept of prolonged stress reactions. It is acceptable to such individuals that some otherwise healthy and well-adjusted soldiers could have immediate and short-term combat stress reactions to war—but not longer-term problems related to war trauma. It is sometimes believed that soldiers with continuing problems from the war must not have the right moral fiber and character to be good soldiers. There is a second source for such disbelief among prodefense and elements of politically conservative civilian groups that PTSD is inherently an antiwar concept. If the problems that war duty can inflict on veterans for years and even decades following service are emphasized, then this could lead to a serious lessening of the commitment or willingness of young men and women to rush to serve their country when called.

Fear of Self-Disclosure

There are also a number of veterans of World War II, the Korean, and the Vietnam Wars who vigorously deny the validity of PTSD as a valid condition in order not to admit to themselves their own problems that may be at least partly war-related. How can a career military person admit to continuing personal difficulties related to war experiences when the impact on a career is likely to be negative and he or she may experience much loss of self-esteem? Robert J. Lifton (see Chapter 1, in this volume) has indicated that survivors often have a death taint which is aversive to others. It is important to note that the extreme fear and terror that many combat personnel have experienced almost never was disclosed during war duty. Presently, the soldier might be self-condemning for feeling the fear or that others might be cruelly and brutally condemning of the emotional state produced by difficult situations.

False Optimism over Psychiatric Casualty Rates

In contrast to other war veterans, the acute psychiatry casualty rate in Vietnam was significantly less than half that of Korea, which, in turn, was about half that of World War II. This resulted in a number of optimistic medical pronouncements in the late 1960s and early 1970s that "military psychiatry had worked in Vietnam" (Bourne, 1970; Colbach & Parrish, 1970); for example, it had dramatically reduced the *acute* casualty rate. Since the concept of PTSD was not well understood, many persons were labeled as *character disorders* or with inappropriate diagnoses. The dramatic impact that the fixed tour of duty (DEROS) had on suppressing PTSD issues until after the war was only beginning to be realized by the end of the war.

Difficulties for Diagnosis: Symptom Overlap

Another difficulty in working with Vietnam veterans and other trauma survivors is that many PTSD symptoms are not exclusive to PTSD (Scurfield, 1985; Wilson, 1988a,b,c). Few standardized psychological instruments were able to discriminate PTSD until the late 1970s and early 1980s. Moreover, the other adaptive problems related to chronic PTSD, including relationship difficulties, substance abuse, impulse control disorders, and depression, become intertwined or fused with the PTSD. Hence "pure PTSD" is extraordinarily rare among chronic PTSD and adds further difficulty to an accurate diagnostic assessment (Wilson, 1988a,b).

Additionally, there are a number of key symptoms that have not been included in DSM-III-R criteria for PTSD, such as blame and survivor guilt, moral/ethical conflicts, fragmented identity, self-denigration, impulse control problems, phobias related to the trauma, existential malaise, fragmented ego identity, and excessive Type A behaviors which are important to understand.

Treatment in Vietnam for Combat and War Trauma

As noted above, our current understanding of the concept of PTSD did not exist during the war years. In DSM-I, there was a concept of *gross stress reaction* (APA, 1952) that recognized acute reactions. Even this rather rudimentary concept of acute PTSD was removed from the psychiatric nomenclature in 1968 with the publication of DSM-II (APA, 1968). Ironically, 1968 was the height of the troop mobilization in Vietnam and the only acute reaction that could be considered for psychiatric casualties was adult situational reaction.

It also is important to note that neither I (nor practically any other psychiatric personnel) had training in military psychiatry *prior* to arrival in Vietnam. I was assigned to be the executive officer and psychiatric social work officer of one of the two United States Army psychiatric teams in Vietnam. Real training was learned on the job.

Principles of Treatment

The principles of military psychiatry implemented in Vietnam were derived from experiences in World War II and in the Korean War. These are as follows:

1. *Proximity*—Treat as close to the front lines as possible.
2. *Expectancy*—State explicitly to the soldier (and to his unit) that he will be returning to his prepsychiatric state of functioning within a very short period of time.
3. *Immediacy*—Guarantee that the soldier be returned to duty without delay (Grinker & Spiegel, 1945; Goodwin, 1987).
4. *Simplicity*—Explain that the acute psychiatric casualty required only very basic intervention; that is, a relatively safe place for a few days, three meals and a cot, some rest and sleep (induced with medications if necessary), and an opportunity to ventilate and express some of his feelings and reactions.
5. *Centrality*—Be prepared to consolidate medical authority to approve any out-of-country evacuations (Jones & Hales, 1987).

Clearly, the decision-making strategies used in Vietnam reinforced psychiatric thinking employed in previous wars. Thus, the overriding concern was to reduce the chance for secondary gain to occur. The central concern was that the further someone was removed from the front lines and the longer he stayed away, the more difficult it would be to get him to return. A second concern within the psychiatric unit was that a new unit member was potentially dangerous and that a combat unit would much prefer to have an experienced soldier who was "a little crazy" and savvy to the jungle. Operationally, perhaps the major psychiatric indoctrination about secondary gain was the belief that if the veteran were prematurely evacuated out-of-country, there would be a fixation of symptoms, an entrenchment of the psychiatric condition that would become chronic. In effect then, as psychiatric personnel in the war zone, we were responsible for the task of determining if a soldier was "too crazy to be sent back to kill people" or "too sane to be evacuated out of the war zone."

In 1984, I discovered through locating my former commanding officer, a most disturbing fact that no one in our unit had known about in Vietnam except him; his annual efficiency report had been based in part on our unit's having a minimal psychiatric casualty evacuation rate out-of-country. Consequently, he has had considerable guilt about having sent young boys back to the front lines and not knowing how many may have been killed. Sadly, we psychiatric personnel operated in a total vacuum in which we rarely received feedback about the results of our decisions. To my knowledge, the U.S. military does not know today if the treatment and disposi-

tion we performed in Vietnam was effective at all. Other than reducing the acute psychiatric casualty rate, for example, was there a *long-term* difference in psychiatric condition among psychiatric casualties who were evacuated out of the war zone versus those who were returned to duty?

Administrative versus Medical Charges

I would be remiss not to at least mention one additional phenomenon that occurred during the Vietnam War—the unprecedented utilization of administrative channels to discharge soldiers from active duty (Kubey *et al.*, 1985). In other words, the labeling of a soldier as *unfit* or *unsuitable* for military duty (because of disciplinary or other behavioral problems that were judged to be volitional or characterological in nature) resulted in numerous "other than honorable" discharges. In contrast, to consider behaviors to be valid psychiatric cases might result in a discharge through medical channels, which, of course, would not have such a pejorative postactive duty sequelae. Our rudimentary knowledge of PTSD at the time, our ignorance of the profound impact of the nature of the Vietnam War on the morale, willingness, and ability of American soldiers to perform their duties, the absence of a legitimate, acute, gross, stress-reaction, diagnostic label, and the systematic suppression of acute psychiatric casualties all strongly influenced disposition through administrative rather than medical channels. Unfortunately, many Vietnam veterans have been living for decades with the consequences of such practices.

Virtues and Concerns of PTSD Criteria

At this writing, PTSD is an anxiety disorder in the DSM-III-R and includes three major sets of symptoms. The conceptualization of both acute and chronic manifestations is noteworthy—neither of which existed in the DSM-II (1968) during the height of the Vietnam War and when psychiatric casualty rates began to increase dramatically (Colbach & Parrish, 1970).

I have several concerns about the DSM-III-R version of PTSD. These include (1) the removal of survival guilt as a symptom (Scurfield, 1988c); (2) the lack of emphasis on the rage component; (3) the profound impact on poor self-esteem and identity (Scurfield, Kenderdine, & Pollard, 1990); (4) other unlisted features (e.g., self-fragmentation, alienation, moral conflict, etc.); and (5) the fact that PTSD is inappropriately designated as an anxiety disorder and would be more properly defined as a set of *stress response syndromes* with adjustment disorders, brief reactive psychoses, and the like (Marmar & Horowitz, 1988). However, in spite of these concerns, the existence of a trauma-related psychiatric condition with both acute and chronic manifestations is light years ahead of DSM-II (1968) or the DSM-I (1952).

Central Dynamics of PTSD among Vietnam Veterans

It is important to understand the dynamics of the various PTSD symptoms and how they interact with each other since there appear to be two central dynamics.

Many expert clinicians in PTSD will agree that a central dynamic is an *alternation* between reexperiencing symptoms and avoidance symptoms (see Marmar & Horowitz, 1988). I would add that *arousal* symptoms also are exacerbated with the onset of reexperiencing symptoms and abate to some degree with the return of the avoidance mode (see Wilson, 1989, for a discussion).

Interaction of Rage, Terror, Grief, and Blame

In addition to the core dynamics of posttraumatic stress listed in the DSM-III-R, I postulate a second core dynamic: an interaction between rage, grief, and terror. Rage, grief, and terror are intrinsic to, or embedded in, most traumatic experiences. Traumatic events will provoke rage, terror, and grief *if* the survivor allows such affect to be felt and expressed. However, because a conscious acceptance and full expression of these symptoms or emotions during the trauma usually would not be productive to survival (and afterward would tend to elicit painful reexperiencing reactions), the individual typically denies, avoids, or numbs them in order to maintain a homeostasis for physical and mental survival. Subsequently, if the trauma experience is not worked through, there is a perpetuation of numbing, denial, and avoidance of the rage, grief, and/or terror.

Emergency Survival Modes

During and between traumatic events, one or more *survival modes* of functioning will develop. Typical modes in Vietnam included: (1) numbing and detachment, (2) hypervigilance, and (3) aggression and rage. It was not unusual that the survivor would flip back and forth between two or all three of these survivor modes (see Wilson, 1980, 1988c, and Wilson & Zigelbaum, 1986, for a discussion of survivor mode functioning).

Rage, Grief, Terror, and Blame Reactions

The actual sources of posttraumatic symptoms of rage, grief, terror, and blame might derive from pretrauma experiences, trauma itself, and from posttrauma experiences. Pretrauma sources of emotional reactions must be determined through careful assessment; therefore, there may be characterological or other psychiatric problems carried over from preadult life. However, owing to space limitations, I want to focus in this discussion on sources of rage, grief, terror, and blame that derive from the traumatic event.

Rage and grief reactions have at least four combinations of internally and externally directed manifestations (e.g., internal rage–external grief) which create a complex set of reactions that need to be understood. For example, there is rage directed outward toward persons perceived as responsible for the trauma, and grief directed internally for the personal hurt suffered in response to loss of a significant other. Thus, trauma-related sources of rage and grief are inherent aspects of exposure to trauma. Although most concepts of grief do include a rage component, I believe that there are rage dynamics intrinsic to trauma exposure and separate from the grief reaction. It is inherent to experience both rage and grief when the self or significant others are threatened or harmed. Such losses and threats extend to body parts and body functions, belief systems and ideologies, and the affiliative connection to others.

Trauma-related terror derives from several sources which include the emergent risk and consequent lack of control over the initial traumatic situation as well as the seemingly never-ending and frightening reexperiencing phenomena. Trauma also is the source of externally and internally directed blame attributions. Survivors attempt to make some sense out of the event by asking the inevitable question, "Why did this happen?" Affixing attribution for the "cause" of the trauma will naturally occur among victims but becomes manifested in PTSD as a preoccupation with affixing responsibility and blame. If the blame is on the self, there is insufficient consideration allowed for the role of others or of the terrible circumstances of the trauma itself. Arriving at a balanced perspective so that appropriate levels of blame or responsibility are owned oftentimes becomes central to the resolution of PTSD (see Williams, 1987, for a discussion of forms of survivor guilt). Finally, being blamed by others further exacerbates guilt and rage issues.

Maintaining a Survival Mode Following the Trauma

There is a strong tendency for the survivor to maintain, or become fixated at, a numbed survivor mode or to present a combination of numbing and rage, grief, or fear. These maladaptive patterns of numbing or a combination of numbing and a predominant emotional state enable the survivor to attempt to control the varying degrees of unresolved emotional difficulties in their PTSD.

Postwar Coping among Veterans with PTSD

Based upon my clinical experiences with Vietnam War veterans with PTSD these past 24 years, I have observed three primary postwar coping patterns. These are described in the frequency of occurrence among help-seeking veterans. (For a discussion of four patterns of adjustment and personality integration based upon Eriksonian theory and research in the mid-1970s for Vietnam veterans, see Wilson, 1980.)

Pattern I: Numbing Combined with Outer-Directed Rage and Blame

During warfare in Vietnam, the combat soldier typically used numbing or denial by such means as dehumanizing the enemy (i.e., as being only "gooks" or "slopes"), or through repeating the mantra, "Fuck it, it don't mean nothing." Such survival tactics protected the soldier from the horror of what he was experiencing. There was also a tendency to become periodically enraged toward the military command structure. Such patterns helped the soldier to avoid further the horror of killing and maiming and the underlying grief and terror reactions. Such accumulated rage emanated from having one's buddies killed or wounded, the frustrations and horror of fighting a guerrilla war, and perhaps from the frustrations and impotence regarding troubles at home, such as receiving a "Dear John" letter from a lover. In addition, the outward expression of rage facilitated the frontline combat veteran's execution of his mission. Rageful expressions, and perhaps particularly those that were seen by others as somewhat extreme, brought the soldier some self-respect as a man—"Hey, he's one crazy dude, but I want him with me when the going gets rough." On the other hand, acting out through rageful and violent expressions, including during sexual activity, oftentimes became a source of shame, guilt, and self-degradation years later, and a source of preoccupation with fear that one might once again become "evil" or violent as one did during the war. The difficult therapeutic task is to allow sufficient expression of outwardly directed rage and blame by not denying its legitimacy and, at the same time, not allowing the veteran to remain stuck in the rageful blame pattern. Usually, this involves helping the person to let go of the rage and blame to be able to acknowledge other aspects of the trauma. Often, this process is difficult because there is a tendency for survivors to use rage as a means of avoiding grief or their own issues of responsibility. Military basic training also prepped the soldier to channel both grief and terror into outward expressions of anger. It is essential not to consider rage simply as a component of a grief reaction but to realize that rage is an inherent legacy of trauma.

Pattern II: Numbing Combined with Inner-Directed Rage

Soldiers cast in such military roles as medic, nurse, or other medical staff person in a war zone, and persons on bodybag details, in graves registration (who collected, tagged, sorted, and stuffed body parts and bodies into plastic bags), and body escort of corpses back to the United States often used numbing, denial, or cognitive distortion to survive the massive and repeated exposures to death and dying. These were the primary survival modes that allowed for avoidance or denial of painful affect and were conducive to performing these specialty roles. Whatever emotions were not avoided tended to be directed inwardly, since there were few constructive channels of emotive expression other than substance abuse, which are numbing and denial behaviors. These persons face the therapeutic task of moving beyond numbing and internally directed rage and blame to recognition of valid external sources of rage, impacted grief, and profound fear—fear of "going crazy" over a seeming inability to forget the immersion in death trauma.

Pattern III: Numbing Combined with Fear and Anxiety

A number of veterans went through the war experience in a very high state of fear, anxiety, and agitation. In my experience, such persons typically were in combat-support roles, such as field wireman, sentry duty at a base, or involved in ammunition supply. These individuals were often targets for the enemy and could not fight back effectively or prevent harassment fire. In this category were also veterans stationed offshore on ships or other duty which entailed observer experiences of *witnessing trauma* occurring to others (such as a returning fighter plane crash-landing on a carrier deck). Observing such experiences was accompanied by a constant state of fear, seldom or never taking chances, avoiding certain activities, excessive ruminating about one's safety, and "counting down to DEROS" (date of estimated return from overseas) in an obsessive way. Today, such men may present clinically as numb in response to unconscious levels of anxiety reactions and repressed fears, or with more generalized and severe anxiety and panic-like attacks.

Sources of Rage among Vietnam Veterans

This little kid was running down the trail towards us, and the sergeant yelled at me to shoot him. I froze, thinking that "I can't shoot a little kid. My God, he's not trying to hurt any of us." The sergeant quickly pointed his own rifle and shot the kid right in the chest, not 20 yards away. The kid went tumbling through the air, he was so small, and then he literally exploded right in front of me. . . . You see, he had explosives strapped to his body by the VC (Viet Cong). . . . But, even so, I can't get rid of the sight of him running, getting hit and exploding practically in my face. I thought, "What kind of war is this to use little kids to kill, *and* to have to kill them? I had to learn *real* quick to get *real* hard." (Scurfield, 1987)

For Vietnam veterans, there were sources of rage peculiar to the Vietnam War and its aftermath back in the United States. Although it would be beneficial to those reading this chapter to have a detailed description of the various sources of rage among Vietnam veterans, especially those seeking treatment, space limitations preclude such a discussion at this point. Other researchers have written similar accounts (e.g., Kelly, 1985; Brende & Parson, 1985; Scurfield *et al.*, 1984; Wilson, 1978, 1980a,b; Wilson & Krauss, 1985). In an oversimplified listing, I mention briefly only the items that follow:

1. The nature of guerrilla warfare in which there are hit-and-run ambush tactics, the involvement of all segments of the population (i.e., women, children, and elderly), and the promotion of terror
2. The body count as a measure of progress in the war rather than terrain objectives
3. Political versus military decision-making
4. The 1-year tour of duty in a maximally stressful environment
5. The veterans' rejection and betrayal or nonresponse by society upon return to the United States

6. The absence of knowledgeable health care programs for war-related PTSD and other veteran-specific mental health concerns
7. The absence of counseling programs for veterans and their families
8. The abandonment of the Vietnamese people and armies to be overrun by Communist forces
9. The difficulties in securing employment and educational opportunities after the war
10. The uncertainties of herbicidal exposure (e.g., Agent Orange) and denial or minimalization of any responsibility by the government and private industry.

Special Subgroups of Vietnam Veterans

There are special populations of Vietnam War veterans who deserve discussion, including ethnic minorities, the physically disabled, women, and nonmilitary volunteers. It is important to note that within each group (especially among ethnic minorities) there is *considerable* heterogeneity; that is, Hispanics can include Mexican-Americans, Puerto Ricans, Cubans, Central Americans, and South Americans. There are over 200 American Indian tribes in North America with Vietnam veterans. There also is a varying amount of cultural identity present (e.g., traditional Hispanic vs. assimilation into Anglo culture, reservation vs. nonreservation Native Americans, etc.) (Borrego, 1985; Montour, 1985; Egendorf *et al.*, 1981; Kulka *et al.*, 1988; Scurfield & Blank, 1985; Scurfield, in press).

Ethnic Minority Veterans

Blacks, Hispanics, Native Americans, Asian Americans, and Pacific Islanders are perhaps the major ethnic groups represented among United States Vietnam veterans (who are "of color" rather than of Western European background). Unfortunately, ethnic minority veterans rarely have been included in PTSD or veteran studies in numbers sufficient to permit accurate analysis of ethnicity *per se*. Where such an analysis has been possible (for blacks in the *Legacies of Vietnam*, 1981, and blacks and Hispanics in the National Vietnam Veterans Readjustment Study, 1988), the findings were startling in terms of elevated PTSD prevalence rates. Such findings are at least partly attributable to greater exposure to combat. In addition to level of combat exposure, I assume that all minority veterans of color, to varying degrees, have had their prewar, war, and postwar experiences complicated and exacerbated by what has been described as the "triple oppression" of poverty, racism, and cultural oppression that faced Hispanic Vietnam veterans (Borrego, 1985). Complications specific to minority veterans included fighting a "white man's war" against a Third World country, blatantly racist attitudes and behaviors by the military (e.g., basic training conditioning to kill "gooks," "chinks," or "slopes") (Eisenhart, 1975; Parson *et al.*, 1986; Scurfield, in press), racist incidents in country that occurred in rear-echelon areas, and continuing racist issues in the United States.

Physically Disabled Veterans

Particularly problematic to ethnic minorities were the disabled veterans. The legacy of Vietnam includes at least 303,704 wounded American veterans of whom over half required hospitalization, an unprecedented number of seriously disabled (over 75,000), and a *300%* higher rate of amputations or of crippling wounds to the lower extremities than occurred to personnel in World War II. Ironically, the very advances in medical evacuation procedures and superior emergency medical care accessible to the front lines contributed to improved survival rates for substantial numbers of seriously disabled personnel (Tice, 1988). However, the medical evacuation, hospitalization, and rehabilitation process by and large focused on *physical* recovery, and vocational and monetary issues. Denial and numbing of emotions were associated with combat and physical trauma tended to occur during *physical* recovery. There also was profound avoidance by both veteran and provider to attend to the numerous traumatic experiences that were intrinsic to the entire medical evacuation and triage process (Scurfield & Tice, 1992). Also, drugs and alcohol were sanctioned to numb both physical and emotional pain (Tice, 1988). Perhaps the most difficult complication in treating the PTSD aspects of seriously disabled war veterans were two of the primary methods of treating the *physical* trauma: drugs and cognitive "pain-control" techniques. Although, these interventions may be very helpful in terms of dealing with physical pain, they present, at the same time, considerable reinforcement of denial and avoidance symptoms that are central to PTSD. To deal adequately with the psychological pain of the PTSD may well result in an exacerbation of the physical pain because it is almost impossible to relax denial and avoidance defenses to allow adequate processing of psychological pain without, at the same time, removing some of the pain buffers that have been developed (Scurfield, in press). This is a particularly cruel dilemma facing the disabled veteran and the counselor. (For a comprehensive discussion of disabled veteran dynamics, see Tice *et al.*, 1988.)

Female Vietnam Veterans

Estimates of the number of women who served in the Vietnam war zone range from 7,000 to 10,000 (Kubey *et al.*, 1985; Kulka *et al.*, 1988). Although the majority served in medical capacities as nurses, other women did serve in intelligence, security, supply, clerical, and air traffic control (Schnaier, 1985). Some 260,000 women served in the military during the Vietnam era, an untold number in direct medical care in receiving hospitals in Japan and on the West Coast, treating massive numbers of casualties evacuated directly from the war zone or transferred from more acute treatment facilities. Female Vietnam veterans, of course, suffered many stressors experienced by many male Vietnam veterans (exposure to death and dying, threat to personal safety, etc.)—and then some. In my experience in Vietnam at the 8th Field Hospital, where I worked and lived alongside both active duty and nonmilitary women, and in my subsequent clinical and collegial contacts with numerous female veterans since the war, distinctive stressors experienced by women in the war zone included the following: sexual harassment, coercion, and rape; sexual stereotyping and bias against women being in the war zone; false idealization as women on pedestals; role-bound restrictions against emotional expressiveness; and inadequate treatment by VA hospitals (Van Devanter, 1983; Sandecki, 1987; Thompson *et al.*, 1982; Ott, 1985; Scurfield, in press).

Nonmilitary Volunteers

There is a subgroup of women who were in Vietnam who may be the most isolated group to have served in the war zone—the nonmilitary volunteers who were in the Red Cross, in civilian nursing capacities working with the Vietnamese, in the orphanages, and the like. I consider these women to be Vietnam veterans who (like the Vietnam veterans with dishonorable discharges) have not had any Veterans Administration program officially available to them. Just whom could such women possibly talk to who would be knowledgeable and sensitive to their very special status and experiences? They also were probably *least* recognized for their contributions in Vietnam by anyone. (For poignant descriptions of United States women in Vietnam, see Walker, 1985.)

Summary and Conclusions

Unfortunately, the legacy of PTSD from the Vietnam War is impressive in terms of the large number of individuals who present significant PTSD symptomatology today or during the past decades. It is particularly noteworthy that such longstanding war-related symptomatology exists in spite of the psychiatric treatment that occurred in the battlefields of Vietnam. Some of the biases that have minimized or prevented adequate recognition of the phenomenon of PTSD among Vietnam veterans in a timely manner and that have further contributed to a prolonging of the denial of PTSD symptoms have been mentioned in this chapter. It is important to emphasize that such biases have risen out of at least two general sources. One source of bias includes the varying unresolved issues that many Americans, United States institutions, and the country as a whole have about the Vietnam War itself. These biases, in turn, have been projected upon the warriors who fought the war. Indeed, perhaps the most profound discovery that I made during my 1989 return to Vietnam with a therapy group of Vietnam veterans with PTSD was not that these veterans have been relating to a Vietnam that existed over two decades ago, but rather that partly because of our government's isolation policy toward Vietnam, the United States has continued to be "stuck" two decades in the past with practically no realization of the Vietnam of today (Scurfield, 1989). The second source stems from the lack of knowledge of how PTSD impacts in lifecourse adaptation and development and the historic disbelief about the longer-term impact of trauma. Ironically, Vietnam veterans have again had "to walk the point" in terms of being overly criticized *or* credited for the initial emergence of PTSD as an officially recognized psychi-

atric disorder. Then, adding insult to injury, Vietnam veterans have been blamed for being angry, untrusting of, and alienated from our country's institutions.

There is another side to the legacy of the Vietnam War; the incredible strength and conviction and sense of purpose in life that many Vietnam veterans have been able to develop in that too-little-understood-or-talked-about phenomenon of *transforming trauma* (Scurfield, in press; Wilson, 1989). Many survivors know deeply how injurious war is to all living creatures—not least of all the warriors who fight and the nation that supports warfare. It is full acceptance of the shorter- and longer-term wounds of war by all of us, survivor and ordinary citizen alike, that will allow for the possibility of appropriate diagnosis, treatment, and resource allocation for alleviating PTSD among our veterans and others in our country.

References

American Psychiatric Association. (1952). *Diagnostic and statistical manual of mental disorders* (1st ed.). Washington, DC: Author.

American Psychiatric Association. (1968). *Diagnostic and statistical manual of mental disorders* (2nd ed.). Washington, DC: Author.

American Psychiatric Association. (1987). *Diagnostic and statistical manual of mental disorders* (3rd ed. rev.). Washington, DC: Author.

Arnold, A. (1987). Selected bibliography IV: Post-traumatic stress disorder with special attention to Vietnam veterans. Birmingham Southeast Regional Medical Education Center, Department of Veterans Affairs, September. VA monograph.

Blank, A. S. (1985, July). Psychological treatment of war veterans: A challenge for mental health professionals. *Medical Hypnoanalysis*, 6(3), 91–96.

Borrego, R. (1985). Hispanic veterans. In C. Kubey, D. Addlestone, R. O'Dell, K. Snyder, B. Stichman, & Vietnam Veterans of America (Eds.), *The Viet vet survival guide: How to cut through the bureaucracy and get what you need and are entitled to* (pp. 120–121). New York: Ballantine Books.

Borus, J. F. (1973). Reentry II: "Making it" back to the States. *American Journal of Psychiatry, 130*, 850–854.

Borus, J. F. (1974). Incidence of maladjustment in Vietnam returnees. *Archives of General Psychiatry, 30*, 554–557.

Bourne, P. G. (1970). Military psychiatry and the Vietnam experience. *American Journal of Psychiatry, 127*, 481–488.

Brende, J. O., & Parson, E. R. (1985). *Vietnam veterans: The road to recovery.* New York: Plenum Press.

Card, J. (1983). *Lives after Vietnam: The personal impact of military service.* Lexington, MA: Lexington Books.

Colbach, E. M., & Parrish, M. D. (1970). Army mental health activities in Vietnam: 1965–70. *Bulletin of the Menninger Clinic, 34*, 333–342.

Danieli, Y. (1984). Psychotherapists' participation in the conspiracy of silence about the Holocaust. *Psychoanalytic Psychology, 1*(1), 23–42.

DeFazio, V. J. (1975, Winter). The Vietnam era veteran: Psychological problems. *Journal of Contemporary Psychotherapy, 7*(1), 9–15.

Egendorf, A. (1975). Vietnam veteran rap groups and themes of postwar life. *Journal of Social Issues, 31*(4), 111–124.

Egendorf, A., Kadushin, C., Laufer, R., Rothbart, G., & Sloan, L. (1981). *Legacies of Vietnam: Comparative adjustment of veterans and their peers.* A study prepared by the Center for Policy Research for the Veterans Administration. Superintendent of Documents, Government Printing Office, Washington, DC.

Eisenhart, R. (1975). You can't hack it little girl: A discussion of the covert psychological agenda of modern combat training. *Journal of Social Issues, 31*(4), 13–23.

Figley, C. R. (Ed.). (1978). *Stress disorders among Vietnam veterans.* New York: Brunner/Mazel.

Figley, C. R., & Leventman, S. (1980). *Strangers at home: Vietnam veterans since the war.* New York: Brunner/Mazel.

Fox, R. P. (1972). Post-combat adaptational problems. *Comprehensive Psychiatry, 31,* 435–443.

Goldberg, J., True, W. R., Eisen, S. A., & Henderson, W. G. (1990). A twin study of the effects of the Vietnam war on post-traumatic stress disorder, *JAMA, 263*(9), 1227–1232.

Goodwin, J. (1987). The etiology of combat-related posttraumatic stress disorders. In T. Williams (Ed.), *Post-traumatic stress disorders: A handbook for clinicians* (pp. 1–18). Cincinnati, OH: Disabled American Veterans.

Grinker, T., & Spiegel, J. (1945). *Men under stress.* Philadelphia: Blakiston.

Gronval, J. (1988). Statement before the Committee on Veterans' Affairs, U.S. Senate oversight hearing on PTSD and the Veterans Administration. Washington, DC: *Congressional Record.*

Haley, S. A. (1974, February). When the patient reports atrocities: Specific treatment considerations of the Vietnam veteran. *Archives of General Psychiatry, 30*(2), 191–196.

Harris, L. (1980). *Myths and realities: A study of attitudes toward Vietnam era veterans.* Washington, DC: U.S. Government Printing Office.

Horowitz, M. J., & Solomon, G. J. A. (1975). Prediction of delayed stress response syndromes in Vietnam veterans. *Journal of Social issues, 31,* 67–79.

Houk, V. N. (1988). Testimony by the Director, Center for Environmental Health and Injury Control, Centers for Disease Control, before the U.S. Senate Committee on Veterans' Affairs, oversight hearing on PTSD and the Veterans Administration. Washington, DC: *Congressional Record.*

Jones, F. D., & Hales, R. E. (1987). Military combat psychiatry: A historical review. *Psychiatric Annals, 17*(8), 525–527.

Kelly, W. E. (1985). Posttraumatic stress disorder and the war veteran patient. New York: Brunner/Mazel.

Kubey, C., Addlestone, D., O'Dell, R., Snyder, K., Stichman, B., & Vietnam Veterans of America (Eds.). (1985). *The Viet vet survival guide: How to cut through the bureaucracy and get what you need and are entitled to.* New York: Ballantine Books.

Kulka, R., Schlenger, W., Fairbank, J., Hough, R., Jordan, B. K., Marmar, C., & Weiss, D. (1988). *National Vietnam veterans readjustment study (NVVRS): Description, current status and initial PTSD prevalence estimates.* Research Triangle Park, NC: Research Triangle Institute.

Laufer, R. S. (1985). War trauma and human development: Vietnam. In S. Sonnenberg, A. Blank, & J. Talbot (Eds.), *Psychiatric effects of the Vietnam War.* Washington, DC: American Psychiatric Association.

Laufer, R. S., Brett, E., & Gallops, M. S. (1985). Dimensions of posttraumatic stress disorder among Vietnam veterans. *Journal of Nervous and Mental Disease, 173*(9), 538–545.

Laufer, R. S., Gallops, M. S., & Frey-Wouters, E. (1984). The Vietnam experience. *Journal of Health and Social Behavior, 25*(1), 65–85.

Laufer, R. S., Yager, T., Frey-Wouters, E., & Donnellan, J. (1981).

Post-war trauma: Social and psychological problems of Vietnam veterans in the aftermath of the Vietnam War. In A. Egendorf, C. Kadushin, R. S. Laufer, G. Rothbart, & L. Sloan (Eds.), *Legacies of Vietnam* (Vol. 3, pp. 19–44). Washington, DC: U.S. Government Printing Office.

Lifton, R. J. (1972). Home from the war: The psychology of survival. *Atlantic Monthly, 230,* 56–72.

Lifton, R. J. (1973). *Home from the war: Vietnam veterans: Neither victims nor executioners.* New York: Simon & Schuster.

Lifton, R. J. (1978). Advocacy and corruption in the healing profession. In C. Figley (Ed.), *Stress disorders among Vietnam veterans* (pp. 209–230). New York: Brunner/Mazel.

Lindy, J. D. (1988). *Vietnam: A casebook.* New York: Brunner/Mazel.

Marmar, C., & Horowitz, M. (1988). Diagnosis and phase-oriented treatment of PTSD. In J. Wilson, Z. Harel & B. Kahana (Eds.), *Human adaptation to extreme stress: From the Holocaust to Vietnam* (pp. 81–103). New York, New York: Plenum Press.

Montour, F. (1985). Native American veterans. In C. Kubey, D. Addlestone, R. O'Dell, K. Snyder, B. Stichman, & Vietnam Veterans of America (Eds.), *The Viet vet survival guide: How to cut through the bureaucracy and get what you need and are entitled to* (pp. 121–123). New York: Ballantine Books.

Nace, E., O'Brien, C. P., Mintz, J., Ream, N., & Meyers, A. L. (1978). Adjustment among Vietnam drug users two years post-service. In C. R. Figley & S. Levantman (Eds.), *Stress disorders among Vietnam veterans* (pp. 71–128). New York: Brunner/Mazel.

Ott, J. (1985). Women Vietnam veterans. In S. Sonnenberg, A. S. Blank, & J. A. Talbot (Eds.), *The trauma of war: Stress and recovery in Vietnam veterans* (pp. 309–320). Washington, DC: American Psychiatric Press.

Parson, E. R., Doughty, H., Woods, A., Henry, R. H., Porter, L., Johnson, G., Jones, L., & Armstead, R. (1986). The struggle continues. Report of the Working Group on Black Vietnam Veterans. Report submitted to Readjustment Counseling Service, Department of Veterans Affairs, Washington, DC. Unpublished manuscript.

Robins, L. N., Davis, D. H., & Goodwin, D. W. (1974). Drug use by U.S. Army enlisted men in Vietnam: A follow-up on their return home. *American Journal of Epidemiology, 99,* 235–249.

Robins, L. N., Helzer, J. E., & Davis, D. H. (1975). Narcotic use in southeast Asia and afterward. *Archives of General Psychiatry, 32,* 955–961.

Sandecki, R. (1987). Women veterans. In T. Williams (Ed.), *PTSD: A handbook for clinicians* (pp. 159–168). Cincinnati, OH: Disabled American Veterans.

Schnaier, J. (1985). Women veterans. In C. Kubey, D. Addlestone, R. O'Dell, K. Snyder, B. Stichman, & Vietnam Veterans of America (Eds.), *The Viet vet survival guide: How to cut through the bureaucracy and get what you need and are entitled to* (pp. 257–268). New York: Ballantine Books.

Scurfield, R. M. (1985). Post-traumatic stress assessment and treatment: Overview and formulations. In C. R. Figley (Ed.), *Trauma and its wake* (pp. 219–256). New York: Brunner/Mazel.

Scurfield, R. M. (1987). Clinical progress note from group therapy session. American Lake VA Medical Center, Tacoma, WA.

Scurfield, R. M. (1988a). Olin E. Teague award ceremony acceptance speech. Department of Veterans Affairs Central Office, Washington, DC, December 2.

Scurfield, R. M. (1988b). *Post-traumatic stress treatment in the Veterans Administration.* Testimony on VA oversight hearings before the U.S. Senate Committee on Veterans Affairs. Washington, DC: *Congressional Record*.

Scurfield, R. M. (1988c). Counterpoint: Disagreement with the exclusion of survivor guilt from DSM-III-R. *PTSD Quarterly Newsletter, 5*(2), 3 (Center for Stress Recovery, VA Medical Center, Cleveland, OH).

Scurfield, R. M. (1989). *Techniques of peer group therapy for PTSD in Vietnam veterans*. Paper presented at the American Psychiatric Association Annual Meeting, San Francisco, May 8.

Scurfield, R. M. (1992). The collusion of sanitization and silence about war: One aftermath of "Operation Desert Storm." *Journal of Traumatic Stress*, July.

Scurfield, R. M. (in press). Treatment of war-related trauma. In H. B. Williams & J. F. Sommer (Eds.), *The handbook of post-traumatic therapy*. Westport, CT: Greenwood Publishing.

Scurfield, R. M., & Blank, A. S. (1985). A guide to obtaining a military history from Vietnam veterans. In S. Sonnenberg, A. S. Blank, & J. Talbot (Eds.), *The trauma of war: Stress and recovery in Vietnam veterans* (pp. 265–291). Washington, DC: American Psychiatric Press.

Scurfield, R. M., Corker, T. M., Gongla, P. A., and Hough, R. L. (1984). Three post-Vietnam rap/therapy groups: An analysis. *Group, 8*(4), 3–21.

Scurfield, R. M., Kenderdine, S. K., & Pollard, R. J. (1990). Inpatient treatment for war-related post-traumatic stress disorder: Initial findings on a longer-term outcome study. *Journal of Traumatic Studies, 3*(2), 1–37.

Scurfield, R. M., & Tice, S. T. (1992). Interventions with medical and psychiatric evacuees: From Vietnam to the Gulf War. *Military Medicine, 157*(2), 88–97.

Shatan, C. F. (1973). The grief of soldiers: Vietnam combat veterans self-help movement. *American Journal of Orthopsychiatry, 43*(4), 640–653.

Shatan, C. F. (1974). Through the membrane of reality: "Impacted grief" and perceptual dissonance in Vietnam combat veterans. *Psychiatric Opinion, 11*(6), 6–15.

Solomon, G. F., Zarcone, V. P., Yoerg, R., Scott, N. R., & Maurer, R. G. (1971). Three psychiatric casualties from Vietnam. *Archives of General Psychiatry, 25*, 522–524.

Sonnenberg, S., Blank, A., & Talbot, J. (Eds.). (1985a). *Psychiatric effects of the Vietnam War*. Washington, DC: American Psychiatric Association.

Sonnenberg, S., Blank, A., & Talbot, J. (Eds.). (1985b). *The trauma of war: Stress and recovery in Vietnam veterans*. Washington, DC: American Psychiatric Press.

Stenger, G. A. (1974). The Vietnam veteran: Review of several studies on Vietnam veterans. *Psychiatric Opinion, 11*(6), 33–37.

Stellman, J., & Stellman, S.(1988). The American Legion Vietnam Veteran's Study. Washington, DC: *The American Legion Bulletin*, No. 58–88 (19–5).

Strange, R. E., & Brown, D. E. (1970). Home from the war: A study of psychiatric problems in Viet Nam returnees. *American Journal of Psychiatry, 127*, 130–134.

Thompson, J., Sandecki, R., Barajas-Gallegos, L., Alvarez, E., Garcia, C., & Solganick, M. (1982). *Report of a working group on women Vietnam veterans and the operation outreach Vietnam vet center program*. Washington, DC: Readjustment Counseling Service (IOB/RC), VA Central Office. Unpublished manuscript.

Tice, S. (1988). *Physically disabled Vietnam vets: Treatment issues*. Paper presented at conference, Healing from the trauma of Vietnam. University of Oregon, Eugene, OR, April 15.

Tice, S., Hinds, R., Bialobok, E., Carter, H., Cecil, J., Koverman, D., Makowski, N., Pierson, R., & Batres, A. R. (1988). Report of the Working Group on Physically Disabled Vietnam Veterans. Submitted to Readjustment Counseling Service, Department of Veterans Affairs, Washington, DC, April.

Trimble, M. (1981). *Post-traumatic neurosis*. New York: Wiley.

Van Devanter, L. (1983). *Home before morning: The story of an army nurse in Vietnam*. New York: Beaufort.

van Putten, T., & Emory, W. H. (1973). Traumatic neuroses in Vietnam returnees: A forgotten diagnosis? *Archives of General Psychiatry, 29*(5), 695–698.

Walker, K. (1985). *A piece of my heart—The stories of twenty-six American women who served in Vietnam*. New York: Ballantine Books.

Williams, T. (1980). *Post-traumatic stress disorders of the Vietnam veteran*. Cincinnati, OH: Disabled American Veterans.

Williams, T. (Ed.). (1987). *PTSD: A handbook for clinicians*. Cincinnati, OH: Disabled American Veterans.

Wilson, J. P. (1977). *Identity, ideology, and crisis: The Vietnam veteran in transition. Part I, Identity, ideology, and crisis: The Vietnam veteran in transition. Forgotten Warrior Project*. Cleveland, OH: Cleveland State University.

Wilson, J. P. (1978). *Identity, ideology, and crisis: The Vietnam veteran in transition. Part II, Psychosocial attributes of the veteran beyond identity. Patterns of adjustment and future implications. Forgotten Warrior Project*. Cleveland, OH: Cleveland State University.

Wilson, J. P. (1980a). Conflict, stress and growth: Effects of war on psychosocial development. In C. Figley & S. Leventman (Eds.), *Strangers at home* (pp. 123–165). New York: Charles R. Figley.

Wilson, J. P. (1980b, May). *Towards an understanding of post-traumatic stress disorder among Vietnam veterans*. Testimony before the U.S. Senate subcommittee on Veterans Affairs.

Wilson, J. P. (1988a, October 23). *Towards an MMPI Trauma Profile*. Paper presented at the annual meeting of the Society for Traumatic Stress studies, Dallas, TX.

Wilson, J. P. (1988b). Treating the Vietnam veteran. In F. Ochberg (Ed.), *Post-traumatic therapy and victims of violence* (pp. 255–278). New York: Brunner/Mazel.

Wilson, J. P. (1988c). Understanding the Vietnam veteran. In F. Ochberg (Ed.), *Post-traumatic therapy and victims of violence* (pp. 225–254). New York: Brunner/Mazel.

Wilson, J. P. (1989). *Trauma, transformation, and healing: An integrative approach to theory, research, and post-traumatic therapy*. New York: Brunner/Mazel.

Wilson, J. P., & Krauss, G. E. (1981). *The Vietnam Era Stress Inventory*. Cleveland, OH: Cleveland State University.

Wilson, J. P., & Krauss, G. E. (1985). Predicting post-traumatic stress disorders among Vietnam veterans. In W. E. Kelly (Ed.), *Post-traumatic stress disorder and the war veteran patient*. New York: Brunner/Mazel.

Wilson, J. P., & Zigelbaum, S. D. (1986). PTSD and the disposition to criminal behavior. In C. R. Figley (Ed.), *Trauma and its wake: Vol. II. Traumatic stress theory, research, and intervention* (pp. 305–321). New York: Brunner/Mazel.

CHAPTER 24

The Vietnam Prisoner of War Experience

Edna J. Hunter

When they threw me in that room I just couldn't believe that they would put me in a place like that . . . the shock of when they put you in irons . . . then the type of treatment you got there . . . you couldn't see out . . . you couldn't see night or day. . . . You didn't get out of irons . . . no exercise. . . . It was obvious we were going to be solo. I said . . ."We are going to have a tough time in here if we are here for any length of time because the problem is going to be a psychological problem." I was more concerned with the mental problem than I was with the physical problem.

—Personal communication, 1974[1]

United States military prisoners of war (POW) held in Southeast Asia from 1964 through 1973 were held longer than any previous group of American POWs—an average of 5 years, compared to the 3 years for World War II POWs, 2 years for those held in North Korea during the late 1950s, and approximately a year for the Pueblo crew (1960s). Those men held the longest in Southeast Asia were imprisoned there for almost 9 years.

The first American captured in South Vietnam had been held since the spring of 1964. The first pilot shot down over North Vietnam occurred in August of that year. The latter was the *sole* captive of the North Vietnamese for almost 6 months. From February 1965 until November 1968, the prisoner of war population grew steadily, and with the increasing number of men taken,

captor treatment worsened, with most being methodically tortured for varying lengths of time.

Harshness of Captivity in Southeast Asia

Virtually all American POWs held by North Vietnam spent their first days of captivity in solitary confinement. Many spent much longer periods alone. Forty percent spent over 6 months in solitary confinement; 20% from 1 to 2 years; 10% for over 2 years; and 4 POWs spent over 4 years in solitary confinement (Hunter, 1978b). Social isolation *per se* produces stress, without any consideration of the added factors of untreated injuries incurred immediately prior to capture, malnutrition, physical punishment, and techniques used by the captor to induce thought control ("brainwashing") (Hunter, 1976).

Factors Related to Harshness of Captivity

Time of capture and location of capture were both found to be related to the severity of treatment received for Vietnam-era POWs.

---

[1]All personal communications cited are from direct communications with the author or from audiotapes to which the author had access.

Edna J. Hunter • 3280 Trumbull Street, San Diego, California 92106.

International Handbook of Traumatic Stress Syndromes, edited by John P. Wilson and Beverley Raphael. Plenum Press, New York, 1993.

Location as a Predictor of Severity

Prisoners held in the North had a very different experience than those held in South Vietnam. They generally suffered more systematic torture and brutality and more frequent interrogations and "indoctrinations" than those captured in the South. However, the latter suffered an experience marked by severe physical deprivation and had very realistic concerns about basic personal survival. Thus, for POWs held in North Vietnam, the stressors were more *psychological*, whereas they were more likely to be *physical* stressors for those held in South Vietnam, making for very different coping strategies during captivity. Although the men held in the North were subjected to borderline food and living conditions, severe initial physical torture, and intermittent psychological mistreatment for interrogation and propaganda purposes, if they survived the initial capture and torture sessions, chances were good they would survive until formal repatriation. Among those POWs held in the South during the war, fewer returned of the total number missing. The prisoners themselves talked of a "ratio for survival"—the greater the distance from Hanoi where one was captured, the less likely one would survive the POW experience.

Time of Capture as a Predictor

Time of capture (i.e., pre-1969 versus post-1969) was also a factor to consider in understanding the severity of the Vietnam POW experience, and thus the possibility of survival. American military men captured prior to 1969 had a much more stressful experience than those who became POWs subsequent to October, 1969—a point in time when the treatment of the prisoners took a definite turn for the better. The definitive explanation for this change is unknown, but it can probably be attributed to some combination of three factors: (1) the death of Ho Chi Minh in September 1969; (2) statements made about harsh prisoner treatment by two POWs released by their captors in August of 1969; and (3) the efforts on the part of the POW and Missing in Action (MIA) families to bring world attention to the plight of the men who were being threatened with death as "criminals" by their captors at that time (Hunter, 1978b). Had the men been released in 1969 instead of 1973, they would have resembled the skeleton-like survivors of Bataan of World War II. The captor had time to fatten up their "bargaining chips" prior to negotiations for peace.

Research on Vietnam POWs and Their Families

Five hundred sixty-six Americans, including 25 civilians, were repatriated in early spring, 1973 (see Table 24.1). An additional 84 men, held prisoner anywhere from 36 hours to 5.5 years, escaped prior to 1973, and one man (who was later court-martialed by the Marine Corps) did not obtain release from his North Vietnam captors until 1976 (Hunter, 1978b). Compared to the numbers of POWs repatriated following World War I, World War II, and the Korean conflict, the numbers were

Table 24.1. Number of POWs during World War I, World War II, Korean War, and Vietnam[a]

	Captured/ interned	Died in captivity	Returned to United States
World War I	4,120	147	3,973
World War II	130,201	14,702	116,129
Korean War	7,140	2,701	4,418[b]
Vietnam	766	114	651[c]

[a]These statistics were developed in cooperation with the Department of Defense, National Research Council, National Archives, and other sources (Stenger, 1990).
[b]Twenty-one military men refused repatriation at the time of release.
[c]One man still remains in the official POW status.

small indeed, and yet much attention was focused on this group of POWs and their family members. Why so much attention?

Center for Prisoner of War Studies

The Vietnam POW experience offered a unique opportunity to study the effects of prolonged extreme stress that could never have been duplicated in a laboratory. It was also an opportunity to better understand the etiology of the excessively high POW morbidity and mortality rates of POWs of other wars which had been reported in the research literature. For example, ex-POWs of the Japanese after World War II and of the Korean conflict showed a significantly higher mortality rate the first 10 years after their return, compared with those veterans who were not captured (Plag, 1974). However, humanitarian concerns for the eventual welfare of the returning prisoners of war during the late 1960s, as well as concerns for the immediate and long-term welfare of their families and the families of those men declared missing in action were the major motivating factors which led to the establishment of a Center for Prisoner of War Studies (CPWS) in San Diego in late 1971, when it appeared the war was winding down and the men would soon be released (Hunter & Plag, 1973).

Although CPWS was a joint Navy, Army, and Marine Corps effort, ongoing liaison with the U.S. Air Force (AF) personnel who dealt with AF POWs was maintained, and *all* service branches participated in the medical plans for Operation Homecoming. The AF effort differed from the center's plan in two major ways: (1) the AF did not include families in their follow-up, and (2) mental status examinations for each returning AF POW were not carried out "unless clinically indicated."

Current Status of CPWS

Most of the conclusions in this chapter about how American POWs and their families coped with the Vietnam POW experience are based on the 7-year research efforts carried out at the center for 2 years prior to their homecoming, and for 5 years postreturn. Medical, occupational, social, and family adjustments of this group of ex-POWs were monitored. When the center was disbanded rather suddenly in 1978 because of political pressures from senior ranking POWs themselves, no final report on the 7-year project had yet been prepared, and no further funding was provided by the government to prepare such a report.

VA Lessons Learned Conference

Much later, in the mid-1980s, concern that many of the lessons learned from the Vietnam-era POW experience would be lost, prompted an effort by the Veterans Administration (VA) to salvage a portion of the knowledge derived from the Vietnam POW experience. In 1985, the Central Office of the VA called together a group of authorities, many of whom had been involved in Operation Homecoming following the Vietnam conflict, along with others who had been involved in earlier repatriation efforts, for a "Conference on Follow-up Care for Returning POWS." They met to work on a comprehensive lessons learned report, a state-of-the-art of preparing ex-POWs and their families to cope with their captivity experiences, as well as for preparing them for the postreturn period (Veterans Administration, 1985). In the words of the late Ransom J. Arthur, the psychiatrist who made the original proposal to set up the Center for POW Studies at the Naval Health Research Center in 1971 and who also participated in the 1985 VA Conference:

> The basic goal of this conference is to make things better for the present released POWs and for any future captives through the application of accurate and precise knowledge. We are pooling data from a wide variety of sources, many of them first hand. We want to make sure that none of this precious knowledge and wisdom is lost and that enthusiasm for supporting former and future POWs is not extinguished. (Arthur, 1985, p. 25)

Comparison of Vietnam POW Experience with Prior POW Experiences

Although strains of commonality run through all POW experiences, in many respects each captivity situation is quite different from all others. The Vietnam captivity experience was unique in several respects. One difference already mentioned was the length of its duration. In other ways it was quite similar to the earlier harsh prisoner experiences in Korea and those Americans held captive by the Japanese during World War II. Based on earlier research on the long-term effects of incarceration by an Asian captor, in planning for the return of the men from Southeast Asia, the worst was expected. The excellent outward appearance of the Vietnam POWs immediately after release surprised many observers. But we must remember that we got back only the *survivors*. Those men who were not able to cope with the long years of deprivation, torture, and degradation, or who were not given even the opportunity to cope because of captor treatment, had already been plucked from the group.

Survivors

For the most part, those who came back had experienced extended weeks, months, or even years in solitary confinement, harsh treatment, poor nutrition, and minimal medical attention during their captivities. At Operation Homecoming in 1973, instead of discovering the worst possible conditions among these men, we found a group of exceptionally strong individuals. They had to have been strong, or they could never have survived their ordeal.

Coping Strategies and Family Reintegration

Ironically, the very psychological characteristics or adaptive behaviors which made survival possible in captivity tended to make the family reintegration process subsequent to release more difficult; for example, obsessive-compulsiveness, blunted affect/tightly controlled emotions, rigidity/intolerance, extreme patriotism, "gearing down," structured time/time-filling activities, habitual mental gymnastics, concern over physical health almost to the point of hypochrondiasis, ability or preference for solitude, and need for organization or "sameness" (Hunter, 1984).

Comparison of Rehabilitation of Vietnam POWs and Combat Veterans

Perhaps a few words should be said about how being a Vietnam-era POW differed from the postreturn of the ordinary military men who saw combat in Vietnam but who were not taken prisoners. Recall that the Vietnam War was very unpopular with the American public. Because of its unpopularity, American fighting men who saw combat in Vietnam also had to "fight" for recognition upon their return home for what many felt was their "right" or, at the least, their "duty." They were not given a "Hero's Welcome" or a "Job Well Done!" as were the small group of ex-POWs when they were released and came home to grateful adulation.

Vietnam POWs as "Heroes"

In 1973, the POWs were probably the only heroes of that war. The government *made* them heroes. Most of the returning POWs had been committed career military men prior to captivity. As a group, they tended to be older family men, flyers/flight crew members, mainly officers, who were highly intelligent and well educated. Upon release, they were showered with honors, gifts, choice assignments, and medical attention. They had supported one another during their captivity, and they continued close contact with the group with whom they had shared the POW experience in the postrelease years.

Vietnam Combat Veterans as "Baby Killers"

In contrast, many returning Vietnam combat veterans had initially been drafted to serve. They tended to be younger and less experienced militarily, and were not as highly educated or committed to a career in the military. Most had been required to serve a limited 1-year combat duty tour in Vietnam and were then hastily returned Stateside, alone, not with their units. Their comrades were not beside them to talk about what the war experience had meant to them. Upon their return, some veterans were spat on by antiwar civilians. Their enlisted periods ending, disheartened, they disappeared into the civilian crowds, or into the solitude of the dense woods of the Northwest to ruminate for the next decade. After a period of years, many made a trip to "The Wall," followed by an eventual coming to terms with their Vietnam combat experience. Being a former combat veteran in Vietnam was indeed very different from having been a POW during the Vietnam conflict. It would not be unexpected if Vietnam combat veterans, in future years, demonstrate greater long-term effects from their experience than the former POWs who were held by their captors throughout the conflict.

Guilt and the "Hero Role"

Insightful comments were made by one former Vietnam-era POW 4 months after his release:

> We were a national asset for Vietnam. When we came home, we were a national asset in the United States. The public reaction was overwhelming. The response made the POWs have a moral obligation. We had to make public appearances, even if the wives were upset . . . [but] . . . we needed more instruction. The doctors should have limited the number of speeches we could make. We had problems with trying to answer the mail we received. Saying the right thing, smiling all the time. It got to me. We are so devout and righteous we can't stand ourselves. We have so much guilt. POWs were "used" by both North Vietnam and the United States. (It made us) a bit bitter. (personal communication, 1973)

Research on Vietnam-Era POW/MIA Families

Research carried out on Vietnam POWs differed from research efforts on prior captive groups. Although there were definite limitations to the CPWS effort and no final report of the entire 7-year project was ever forthcoming, it was, nonetheless, a noteworthy study. It was the first large-scale, federally funded study which included the *family* of the military man. It was a prospective study, with matched controls. Most earlier studies of POWs were retrospective, did not include family members, and had no comparison groups. Much of what is currently known concerning how families cope with a prolonged, ambiguous, stressful situation, such as a captivity or hostage situation, derive from the CPWS studies.

Generalizing to Other Populations

The "support group" concept, which was found so helpful for POW/MIA families, could also apply to cancer patients, patients with chronic neurological disease, and patients with other long-term care needs. Also, generalizing from the knowledge base derived from studies of family separation and reintegration, knowledge of the captivity experience is transferable to other "victim" experiences: spouse abuse, child abuse, sexual assault, rape, terroristic acts, and indoctrination of young adults into "cults." It even generalizes to our understanding of the effects of certain child-rearing practices (Hunter & Hestand, 1984).

Benefits to Military Families Generally

Other benefits for military families in general have their origin in the CPWS studies. For example, a social work program (active duty and civilian social workers) was proposed and implemented for the Navy in 1973 (Hunter & Plag, 1973). There had been no active duty social workers within that service branch at the time CPWS was founded. Moreover, the recently established Family Service or Support Centers for all service branches throughout the world are a direct result of the early research findings and recommendations emanating from CPWS. The support centers were developed subsequent to suggestions presented at a Conference on Military Family Research: Current Trends and Directions hosted by CPWS in 1977 (Hunter, 1978a). The Department of Defense level triservice Military Family Resource Center in Washington, DC, can also be traced to these early efforts at CPWS. The POW research carried out at the center has provided a better understanding generally of a variety of family dynamics, such as the effects of a missing parent on children and the general usefulness of increasing the skills of a mother who must act as the head of household during her husband's absences. It would appear that it was indeed a cogent decision to study the POW's family along with the POW (Hunter, 1986).

Lessons Learned from Vietnam POW Research

Readers may often wonder how they personally would be able to cope if suddenly they were in a captive or hostage situation. Probably better than expected. Research showed that most of the Vietnam POWs and their family members did. Nonetheless, there is no "one" way to cope with such situations. Captives and their families found they coped in their own somewhat unique manner. Much depends upon the circumstance of the capture and the prisoners or family members own adaptive resources. Many questions must be addressed before one can answer the question about how well a particular individual will cope, such as:

- Were marital relationships satisfactory prior to capture? Was the marriage an established one?
- Were injuries sustained during capture? Was there good basic health prior to captivity?
- Were there supportive friends or family members to lean on when needed?
- Was becoming a captive pure happenstance, or was there strong commitment to a "cause" that placed the captive in jeopardy in the first place? For the spouse left behind, was there commitment to the military spouses' duty?

- What about the captor's culture? Does it place a high value on the individual's life?
- Are the captives or family members left behind very young, not really knowing who they are and what they stand for? Is there a firmly ingrained sense of values?
- Does the POW have a family that waits for his return? Children? Is ongoing communication with them possible during incarceration?
- What about their own family of origin? Did their upbringing give them a good sense of right and wrong? Early religious or moral training? Is there high self-esteem? An internal rather than external locus of control?

Factors such as the above are important in determining how a particular captive copes with captivity, and, in turn, what the long-term effects will be after his return to freedom (Hunter, 1991).

Discovering Effective Coping Methods

Although research shows there are wide differences among individuals with respect to their abilities to withstand pain and suffering, most individuals are much stronger than they thought they were, and can cope with far more stress than they had ever imagined prior to the trauma they faced. Research has taught us that each person must discover his or her best coping techniques, and the same holds true for families who wait in limbo.

Importance of Taking Action

For example, some families of Vietnam POWs found that talking frequently in public, to the press, or visiting foreign embassies to plead for humane treatment for their captives, were excellent coping strategies. They were not merely sitting passively, feeling hopeless and helpless to do anything for their captive loved ones. They were taking *direct action*—doing something. On the other hand, other family members found that talking to the press about their situations was exceedingly stressful, and they avoided it at all costs. Instead, they might have chosen to write letters to Congressmen, foreign embassies, or perhaps sell POW bracelets as their direct action for coping with their own situations.

Issue of Control

In hostage or POW situations, or any stressful ambiguous situation, it is important to feel one still has some degree of control. But how do individuals maintain control over their lives, even when they may in reality find themselves in an almost totally dependent situation? Certainly, the POW cannot lash back and refuse the captor's orders totally. He can, however, tacitly disobey. For example, Vietnam POWs were ordered not to communicate with one another, and yet they clandestinely communicated by tap code through cell walls to fellow prisoners. Thus, the POW maintained a modicum of control, and was not totally helpless and powerless.

Mind and Coping

The body may be in shackles, but prisoners still have their minds. Vietnam POWs found they could visualize past events, practice foreign languages they once knew, compute square roots mentally, recall Bible passages learned as small children but thought they had long forgotten, remember motion pictures in detail which they had once enjoyed, and they could plan for the freedom they hoped for in the future.

Release as a Rebirth

Unlike many of us, former POWs can usually state with confidence, "I now know who I am and what is truly important in life." Many viewed their release as a kind of "rebirth"—a second chance in life. One of the returning POWs offered the following prayer during a church service at Clarke Air Force Base in the Philippine Islands on that first Sunday of freedom in 1973:

> Few men have the opportunity to be born again . . . to be able to stand in freedom again . . . to see the sun shining on the flowers, the trees, and the grass . . . to see clouds rolling past the hills in the distance . . . to hear birds sing . . . and more than that, to be able to share love with our families and friends again. (personal communication, 1973)

The Importance of Family and Friends

POWs came to realize how important their early childhood training had been; how important fellow prisoners were who gave them support and encouragement when sorely needed; and how motivating the thoughts about their beloved wives and children were in giving them that "will to live" without which individuals may curl up in the fetal position and die. Some individuals react in this manner to any extreme stress. Those POWs who do, usually do not live to return home.

Strength from Adversity

It has often been stated that "that which doesn't kill us makes us stronger." Benefits did accrue from the Vietnam POW experience, for former POWs and for their families. Even for families of servicemen missing in action (MIA), who still live each day with some measure of unsolved grief and continuing ambiguity, positive outcomes may be perceived. Over 20 years after the father's disappearance in Vietnam, one child (now an adult) of an MIA stated:

> I *can* say that the pain will lessen, and life is still worth living. It is ironic that the most painful event in my life has also brought about the most changes of a positive nature. I have learned to value and appreciate relationships and life itself, for it can be so very short. I have pondered the existential questions of life at an early age, and [in] so doing, have been enriched with wisdom to help me though life's ups and downs. I have learned the importance of being honest with myself and others, for my life may be short and I may not have a second chance to make things right. . . . It is difficult at times to live

with unanswered questions. Some questions may never be answered. But some may. (personal communication, 1988)

Another MIA adult "child" had not been able to deal with the ambiguous loss of his parent in as positive a manner:

Not knowing what happened, I always wonder what happened to my father. I have difficulty in putting it behind me since it's an open issue. I am resentful of traditional families that have not had to deal with and can't understand the tragedy. Because of that I'm very discreet about my personal life and past and am not able to discuss these things at all. I feel like I'm hiding a deep dark secret that no one could understand. The bitterness and hostility toward the war especially aggravate this. (personal communication, 1988)

Coping with Freedom

After years of learning to cope with captivity, it takes time to learn to cope with freedom. In prison, POWs had "geared down" to cope with the boredom of an unstimulating environment. With freedom, they had to "gear up" again but found they had come to enjoy solitude more than they had previously. Many tended to avoid crowds. In the words of one of the returning Vietnam POWs:

I had a problem adapting to crowds of people. I found myself on several occasions actually becoming claustrophobic in large crowds of people and having to depart the scene. In the hospital it happened to me and a couple of times [later] so I just left. [On another occasion] at a party, the conversation got [to be] just idle prattle, and I suddenly just got fed up with it and the crowd of people who were there and being in the enclosed room, and the whole thing just irritated me. I just got up and walked out and it felt great! (personal communication, 1974)

Keeping their emotions under tight control, a response called psychological numbing, proved to be an effective coping technique while they were prisoners. Back with the family, however, some of them discovered that demonstrating overt affection toward wives and children was extremely difficult. And after all those years, a few still startle when they hear keys jingling. The noise takes them back to Hanoi, where jingling keys meant the guard was coming down the hall and perhaps more torture or interrogations would follow.

Depression was also an issue with which many ex-POWs had to deal. Attaining freedom had been a long-cherished goal. Like Buzz Aldrin, the astronaut who, after returning from the moon, found himself asking, "After such an experience, what now?" It was much the same for some of the ex-POWs, especially for those men who returned to splintered families, deceased parents, decreased physical conditions, acting-out teenagers, or stagnating careers because of the large "black hole" in their lives. Guilt feelings were there; for some, lowered self-esteem. Socially, men who were still bachelors at the time of captivity came home feeling like "35-year-old men in 25-year-old bodies" (Hunter, 1991).

Family Reintegration after Captivity

It takes time for family reintegration after any long separation. Roles within the family must again be reshuffled, as had occurred when the captive was suddenly snatched from its midst. Research on Vietnam POW families showed that it did not really matter whether or not the family structure returned to its original form (usually a traditional father/breadwinner, mother/homemaker), and most did not. What mattered in the area of family readjustment after prolonged captivity was whether or not there was good communication and spousal agreement on the family's structure (e.g., traditional, matriarchal, egalitarian). Wives had learned how to communicate very well with others while their military men were captives, whereas men had learned to remain silent, not to express themselves.

Dependency/Independency Issues

During the Vietnam era, research showed that for the majority of married ex-prisoners, the biggest readjustment they were forced to face upon return was to the vast changes which had occurred both in society and in their wives during their absences. Most wives had become very independent; but of course, they had to in order to survive the practicalities of day-to-day living. They had become mature, competent, coping women. Ironically, one year after the men's return from Southeast Asia, when wives were asked what the "biggest" surprise for them was in regard to their husbands, many stated, "How little he's changed!" They had expected considerable changes to have occurred, but they had not. What changes were observed were in terms of degree of change. Tolerant men tended to become more tolerant subsequent to captivity; rigid men more rigid; patriotic men more patriotic; and the like. In other words, basic personality had not seemed to change as a result of prolonged, harsh captivity. Rather, basic traits seem to have become solidified.

Marital Dissolution

Needless to say, for most families, there was a long period of learning and readjusting to the many changes that had occurred during the separation. By the end of the first year postreturn, although marital dissolution among returning Vietnam POWs was approximately equal to United States population rates in general (approximately 30%), these rates were two and a half to three times the rates (11% to 12%) in a carefully matched comparison group of Vietnam era military families who were not POW families. In firmly established marriages which had good marital relationships prior to captivity, partners usually were able to work out any readjustments which were necessary. These families, for the most part, were still stable families at the end of the fifth year postreturn.

Parent–Child Relations after Captivity

As for children's adjustment, research showed that their mothers were critical factors in the children's adjustment during and after their fathers' absences. If mothers had coped well with the situation, children also appeared to do well. Again, good family communication seemed to be the key to good parent–child relationships, just as it was in predicting good marital relationships.

A Closing Note on Vietnam-Era POWs and Families

To quote one physician who followed the Vietnam ex-POWs closely during the years subsequent to their release from captivity:

It is now apparent that the process of recovery from the stress of shootdown, capture, captivity, and repatriation appears to *require*, among other things, recovery of self-esteem through reintegration with the group: the POW group, the military, the family, and society. . . . To the degree that there is failure, there will be . . . psycho-pathology. We are by nature "being with" creatures. (O'Connell, 1976, pp. 21–22)

In conclusion, research on Vietnam era prisoners of war showed that loved ones around us, self-confidence, the ability to communicate, direct action when threatened, a refusal to ruminate about the hurts of the past, a will to live, service to others, a future orientation, and a firm commitment to a personal "cause" are the key variables in coping with stress, whatever that stress may be. Many of the reactions and behaviors in the years subsequent to a trauma which former POWs or family members may initially have assumed to be abnormal or peculiar, should instead be considered as very normal reactions to an abnormal situation. Finally, those captives and families who were able to view the entire episode retrospectively as a *growth* experience, rather than in completely negative terms, seemed to have been more effective in integrating the experience into their lives and in going forward in the years following release from bondage.

References

Arthur, R. J. (1985). History of research and professional practice in health care of returned POWs: Comments on the utility of theory. In *Proceedings: Conference on follow-up care for returning prisoners of war, March 12–14, 1985, San Diego, California*

(pp. 21–27). Washington, DC: Veterans Administration, Department of Medicine and Surgery.

Hunter, E. J. (1976). The prisoner of war: Coping with the stress of isolation. In R. H. Moos (Ed.), *Human adaptation: Coping with life crises* (pp. 322–331). Lexington, MA: D. C. Heath.

Hunter, E. J. (1978a). First National Conference on Military Family Research. *U.S. Navy Medicine, 69,* 10–13.

Hunter, E. J. (1978b). The Vietnam POW veteran: Immediate and long-term effects of captivity. In C. Figley (Ed.), *Stress disorders among Vietnam veterans: Theory, research, and treatment* (pp. 188–206). New York: Brunner/Mazel.

Hunter, E. J. (1984). Treating the military captive's family. In F. Kaslow & R. Ridenour (Eds.), *Treating the military family: Dynamics and treatment* (pp. 167–196). New York: Guilford Press.

Hunter, E. J. (1986). Families of prisoners of war held in Vietnam: A seven-year study, *Evaluation and program planning (Special Issue).* 243–251.

Hunter, E. J. (1991). Prisoners of war: Readjustment and rehabilitation. In R. Gal & A. D. Mangelsdorff (Eds.), *Handbook of military psychology* (pp. 741–757). Chichester, England: Wiley.

Hunter, E. J., & Hestand, R. (1984). Thought control: From parenting, to behavior mod, to cults, to "brainwashing." In *Proceedings of the Ninth Biennial Psychology in the Department of Defense Symposium* (pp. 20–24). Colorado Springs, CO: U.S. Air Force Academy.

Hunter, E. J., & Plag, J. A. (Eds.). (1973). *An assessment of the needs of POW/MIA wives residing in the San Diego metropolitan area: A proposal for the establishment of family services* (Technical Report No. 73–39). San Diego: Center for POW Studies, Naval Health Research Center.

O'Connell, P. (1976). Trends in psychological adjustment: Observations made during successive psychiatric follow-up interviews of returned Navy, Marine Corps POWs. In R. Spaulding (Ed.), *Proceedings of the Third Annual Joint Medical Meeting Concerning POW/MIA Matters* (pp. 251–255). San Diego, CA: Center for POW Studies, Naval Health Research Center.

Plag, J. A. (1974). *Proposal for the long-term follow-up of returned prisoners of war, their families, and the families of servicemen missing in action: A basis for the delivery of health care services.* San Diego, CA: Center for POW Studies, Naval Health Research Center.

Stenger, C. A. (1990). *American prisoners of war in WWI, WWII, Korea and Vietnam: Statistical data concerning numbers captured, repatriated and still alive as of January 1, 1990.* Washington, DC: VA Advisory Committee on Former POWs.

Veterans Administration. (1985). *Proceedings: Conference on follow-up care for returning prisoners of war, March 12–14, 1985, San Diego, California.* Washington, DC: VA Department of Medicine and Surgery.

CHAPTER 25

Posttraumatic Stress Syndromes among British Veterans of the Falklands War

Roderick Jan Ørner

Background to Military Engagement in the South Atlantic

Great Britain laid claim to the Falkland Islands Group, which includes the Falkland Islands and South Georgia, some 150 years ago. In recent times, the larger islands have been settled by a small number of expatriate United Kingdom citizens renowned for their strong sense of loyalty to the British Crown. The Head of State was represented by a Governor General and a defense force consisting of a Company of Royal Marines garrisoned on 6-month tours of duty. On South Georgia Island, seasonal industrial activity centered on a whaling station at Grytviken. Permanent habitation was established in 1982 by 30 members of the British Antarctic Survey.

Being situated in the South Atlantic more than 18,000 kilometers from the United Kingdom but only 650 kilometers due east of Southern Argentina, the islands have for long been the subject of recurrent controversy not only between the Argentine and British Governments but also the Government of the United States. Argentina's claims to the Falkland Islands are made on the strength of its having controlled the offshore land mass from the time of the breakup of the Spanish Empire in the early nineteenth century. A colony had been established from 1826 to 1831, but the USS *Lexington* destroyed this in a local dispute centered on fishing rights.

British Argentine talks about the islands never progressed significantly toward a negotiated settlement, and it now appears that the ruling junta of General Galtieri started planning an occupation in 1981. A public and diplomatic furor followed a report in March, 1982 that a group of Argentine scrap metal merchants had landed in South Georgia where they set about dismantling the whaling station. Whether this action was a planned pretext for escalation of tension is uncertain, but Argentine forces successfully invaded South Georgia and the Falkland Islands during two days of the first week of April, 1982.

Diplomatic initiatives centered on the United Nations could not resolve conflicts of interest by peaceful means. A Task Force of troops and ships with the Royal Air Force in support had sailed from England by April 9th and reached its destination at San Carlos Water some weeks later. Sea, air, and land engagements occurred during a 74-day period. The land campaign lasted 25 days, culminating in Argentine surrender at Port Stanley on June 16, 1982.

British troops returned to the United Kingdom during the summer months in a phased operation that ensured a time gap of several weeks between military engagement and being reunited with the civilian population at home. Exceptions were made when a prompt return was indicated for medical, logistic, or other pressing reasons. Every returning war veteran able to walk was given a hero's welcome with street parties being held all over the United Kingdom to mark the conclusion of a successful military campaign.

Roderick Jan Ørner • North Lincolnshire Health Authority, Baverstock House, County Hospital, St. Anne's Road, Lincoln LN4 2HN, England.

International Handbook of Traumatic Stress Syndromes, edited by John P. Wilson and Beverley Raphael. Plenum Press, New York, 1993.

Background to Current Survey

The South Atlantic engagement was small in scale and short in duration compared to other recent wars, and achieved its intended objectives for Britain. Casualty statistics bear witness to the costs of modern warfare: 237 British soldiers killed, 777 wounded out of which 446 received significant hospital treatment as a consequence of injuries sustained (Price, 1984). The rate of evacuated psychiatric casualties was 2% of all wounded, being the 16 personnel who received treatment on the hospital ship *Uganda*. Such a low rate of psychiatric morbidity has its parallel in early American studies from the Vietnam War era which suggested psychiatric morbidity in Stateside forces exceeded those reported among troops stationed in Southeast Asia. By the time United States military engagement in Vietnam was finally terminated in March, 1973, the overall psychiatric casualty rate for all branches was reported as 12/1,000 as compared to 37/1,000 in the Korean War and 101/1,000 during World War II (Bourne, 1970).

Throughout the 1970s and 1980s, the limitations inherent in such statistics have become apparent. Increasing numbers of Vietnam War veterans reported distressing psychological reactions and adjustment problems related to their war experiences some time after removal from the combat setting or even after returning to a civilian environment (Figley, 1978). Shatan (1973) described a not untypical scenario of symptom onset occurring between 9 and 30 months after returning to civilian life when the person has to come to terms with the unconsummated grief of soldiers who by their training and war experiences find civilian existence utterly deprived of meaning. Other studies have comprehensively documented the longer-term prevalence of adjustment difficulties among Vietnam War veterans (Kulka *et al.*, 1988). Public and professional recognition of these difficulties was slow in coming with Neff (1975) describing veterans as "invisible patients" in the sense that their presentations involving intense chromic psychological and somatic problems failed to conform to distinct diagnostic categories. From a social adaptation point of view, Yankelovich (1974) found Vietnam veterans to have double the unemployment rate of same-age cohorts. Lower morale, more prevalent pessimism about their future, and feelings of estrangement from society in general were other frequently reported complaints.

Against this background of growing international recognition that the psychological and social consequences of modern warfare are long term and usually not amenable to categorization using conventional psychiatric nomenclature, I was surprised to establish that by 1985 only one paper had been published addressing the psychological and psychiatric morbidity arising from the Falklands War (Price, 1984). This chapter deals exclusively with morbidity during the war itself. Further enquiries consolidated the impression that information pertaining to possible long-term traumatic stress reactions in Falklands War veterans was either not being gathered of kept from public knowledge. Such lack of response and concern from the research and caring professionals was astounding, so a decision was made in the spring of 1986 to carry out a long overdue survey among ex-servicemen who are veterans of the Falklands War.

Review of Literature on PTSD among Falklands War Veterans

In April, 1989, a computer search using posttraumatic stress disorder (PTSD) and Falklands War veterans as keywords identified only two publications concerned with this problem. These are the journal article by Price (1984) on psychiatric casualties during the war plus a speculative and anecdotal report (Jones & Lovett, 1987) of three young men known to staff at a psychiatric outpatient clinic having in common a period of service in the South Atlantic during the Falklands War.

Price (1984) examined factors assumed to account for the low reported rate of psychiatric casualties among British servicemen involved in the recapture of the Falkland Islands. Particular importance was attributed to early psychiatric screening of personnel by trained staff deployed in frontline units. The brief intermittent nature of combat engagements interspersed with more prolonged periods of indirect fire was noted, as was the use of elite units trained for warfare under arctic and subarctic conditions. Price concluded that experiences gained in the South Atlantic offer a unique perspective on how well military personnel can, in fact, function in a combat situation when the total scenario incorporates a constellation of factors known to reduce psychiatric morbidity.

An early indication that delayed traumatic stress reactions were being experienced by Falklands War veterans was suggested in a subsequent paper by Jones and Lovett (1987). Three case studies were presented giving details of their patients' war experiences and subsequent psychological adjustment difficulties. These include excessive drinking, social isolation, panic attacks, intrusive reexperiencing, guilt, depression, marital friction, and deterioration in work performance. No attempt at formal diagnosis of PTSD was made, reference being made instead to "a neurotic disorder with many features in common, coming on six months or more after an unusually severe life threatening stress." Having come upon these three veterans by chance Jones and Lovett speculate about their being "the tip of an iceberg." The authors suggested that veterans' home communities successfully contain traumatized servicemen who consequently do not come to the attention of the National Health Service. It is interesting that in none of the cases reported did the opportunity arise to implement the complete treatment program! Jones and Lovett ended with a plea for the need to establish by comprehensive epidemiological studies the true prevalence of the psychological, social, and adjustment problems experienced by Falklands War veterans. A newspaper article subsequently quoted the estimate of a naval psychiatrist of a one in eight prevalence of PTSD among naval personnel who had returned form the South Atlantic, and Orner (1988) presented a preliminary analysis of the survey data that is the subject of this chapter to the First European Conference on Traumatic Stress.

In 1991, O'Brien and Hughes reported a 5-year follow-up of currently serving paratroopers who fought in the South Atlantic. Twenty-two percent met diagnostic criteria for PTSD: chronic subtype. Only 29% of the whole veteran group reported no symptoms at all. Another interesting aspect of this study is the comparative data obtained from the two paratrooper battalions sent to the Falklands and the battalion stationed in Europe throughout the war.

Survey Methodology

Investigations of PTSD symptomatology within the British Forces is generally considered a matter for sanctioning and implementation by the Ministry of Defense. On the other hand, epidemiological surveys involving ex-servicemen who are veterans of the Falklands War are a prerequisite to making appropriate needs-based services available to the British equivalents of the invisible patients of Neff (1975), and those who would make up the submerged part of Jones and Lovett's (1987) metaphorical iceberg. In recognition of the Ministry of Defense's special public responsibilities to ex-servicemen who served their country so well on or near the Falkland Islands one might have assumed that the importance of fostering of a spirit of open and free cooperation with clinical researchers and service planners would be appreciated. Sadly, this is not so. When I approached the Ministry of Defense with a research protocol requesting help with circulating a questionnaire to Falklands War veterans who were no longer in active military service, I received a reply in July, 1986, to the effect that such help would only be forthcoming subject to an understanding not to publish the survey findings, or inform the media of the project without first consulting with a senior ranking officer at the Ministry and "taking (his) comments into account."

Such infringement of a clinical researcher's freedom to openly investigate and report results of community surveys is not acceptable. Consequently, the epidemiological study was severely compromised by the stance of the Ministry of Defense, as is the potential value of the findings to traumatized servicemen, their families, the helping professions, and our community in general. Rather than circulate questionnaires to ex-servicemen known to the military authorities, the investigation proceeded using a derivative of network sampling as discussed by Sirkin (1979) and later adapted for the Vietnam Era Project by Rothbart, Fine, and Sudman (1982). Media publicity for the project was secured at national and local levels, but unexpectedly large access problems plagued the survey prompting a decision to bring it to a close after 3 years. By that time, the survey sample population consisted of 53 Falklands War veterans who are no longer in military service.

All subjects have completed and returned by post a questionnaire covering basic demographic data, the DSM-III criteria for posttraumatic stress disorder, an adjustment problem checklist adopted from Panzarella, Mantell, and Bridenbaugh (1978), and other questions relating to their origins and subsequent manifestations. The questionnaire set also included the 60-item version of the General Health Questionnaire (GHQ) (Goldberg, 1978), which is a self-administered screening instrument designed for use in general population settings. It identifies two main classes of problems: namely, the inability to carry out normal "healthy" functions and the appearance of new psychological and social symptoms of a distressing nature. Studies of reliability and validity recommend this questionnaire (McDowell & Newell, 1987).

Characteristics of the Population Surveyed

All veterans are self-selected in volunteering to complete the questionnaires. Inclusion criteria are to have served with the British Armed Forces in the engagement zone during the Falklands War and to have subsequently resumed civilian status. This will have occurred by the contracted service period expiring, a serviceman requesting early demobilization, or a formal recommendation from, for example, a senior officer or health personnel that early release form contractual commitments is indicated.

The deployed services are represented by the Navy (26%), Army (30%), Paratroopers (23%), and Royal Marines (21%), of which 9% have officer ranking, 26% are noncommissioned officers, and 65% are of lower rank. The age range at the time of completing the questionnaire spans from 21 years to 46 years, with mean and modal ages being 30 years and 27 years, respectively. At the time of the survey, 45% reported being married, 23% are either separated or divorced, and 32% are single.

Physical injuries had been sustained by 22 (42%) of the population sampled. Physical disability must therefore account in part for the reported prevalence of two in every three of the surveyed group stating that they left the Armed Services because of their war experiences. A total of 13 veterans (25%) gave other war-related considerations as their reason for leaving the services and a further 18 veterans (33%) left for other reasons (e.g., end of service contract). In this connection, it should also be noted that during the time that has lapsed since the Falklands War the year of demobilization is not consistently related to giving the war as the reason for leaving ($p = .67$).

PTSD Symptomatology among Falklands War Veterans

In the obtained sample of 53 veterans, a total of 32 (60%) meet DSM-III criteria for the chronic subtype of posttraumatic stress disorder. This differential diagnosis is significantly associated with having incurred physical injury during the military engagement ($p = .03$). Such other variables as leaving the Armed Services because of war experiences, and period of time lapsed between termination of hostilities and being demobilized show markedly weaker associations ($p = .08$ and $p = .54$). Giving war experiences as the reason for leaving the services does not appear to be a determinant of the time that lapsed between the war and eventual return to civilian life. Neither age ($p = .24$), marital status ($p = .42$), rank ($p = .08$), or unit served with during the war ($p = .15$) carries significant predictive power for PTSD diagnosis.

In the light of the importance American researchers have attributed to the generally unwelcoming reception that awaited Vietnam veterans returning from an unpopular war, it is interesting to reflect on the possible repercussions of the entirely different experience of their British colleagues who returned as heroes of a victorious campaign. To what extent this is, on its own, an important factor for the development and course of chronic or delayed traumatic stress reactions cannot be established by a community survey alone principally because most Falklands War veterans had a staged and protracted period of being "homeward bound." In the observed sample, there is nevertheless an interesting lack of association between meeting criteria for PTSD and veterans' assessment of the amount of support they found within their families at the point of resuming civilian status (p = .13) and at the time of completing the questionnaires (p = .09).

A measure of the degree to which PTSD symptomatology is being experienced in the two subpopulations is provided by calculating the average number of symptoms reported by each veteran. In the traumatized sample, the mean value is 8.7 symptoms out of a maximum total of twelve. Those veterans who do not meet the PTSD criteria experience an average of 5.1 symptoms (p > .05). When symptom occurrence and nonoccurrence is cross-tabulated against PTSD diagnosis, the probability values of all comparisons are statistically significant to the .05 level or less. Most frequently reported symptoms in the index group are: flashbacks and dreams about the war, disturbed sleep, being unable to get close to people, fewer interests, restricted range of feelings, and being easily startled.

Overall, the findings on PTSD symptomatology in this sample reveal professionally trained servicemen exposed to modern warfare in the South Atlantic to be far from immune to developing traumatic stress reactions that run a chronic course. A positive differential diagnosis during the time span of this survey is associated with experiencing a large number of symptoms compared to fellow veterans who do not meet criteria for chronic traumatization. War injury is the single factor investigated to have a significant association to PTSD. The predictive power for diagnostic purposes of having incurred or being free from injury is such that in only 6 out of 10 instances will correct predictions be made. Age, marital status, ranking, units served with, and home support at the time of demobilization and at the time of completing the questionnaire are factors with no statistically significant relationship to PTSD in this sample.

Adjustment Problems

Research reports on traumatic stress following military combat experience do not always make explicit distinctions between PTSD symptomatology and adjustment problems. A tendency has existed to imply the latter to be synonymous with the former (Strayer & Ellenhorn, 1975) but this is at odds with community prevalence surveys (e.g., of Vietnam War veterans) which demonstrate that symptomatology does not of necessity preclude a person from achieving an overall level of life satisfaction in keeping with his own or his family's aspirations (Kulka *et al.*, 1988).

Consequently, the Falklands War Veterans Survey inquired in detail about possible adjustment problems taking these to be independent variables. The checklist used required subjects to indicate on a four-point scale to what extent a particular difficulty is being experienced. The scale ranges from "not at all" through "rarely" to "sometimes" and "often"; each one carrying a numerical weighing from which a total problems score was calculated by simple addition.

A factor analysis of all 53 subjects' responses on the problems checklist was undertaken. This comprised a principal component solution followed by a varimax rotation. The analysis produced eight factors with eigne values of more than one, with Factor 1 being highly significant in accounting for 47.2% of the total variance. All items on the checklist except one ("being worried about members of my family") intercorrelate to a level at or greater than .30. This result confirms the internal consistency of the problem checklist in assessing Factor 1, labeled *General Adjustment Problems*. Correlation in excess of .75 is found for those checklist items that portray the veteran as an alienated and unhappy individual (being discouraged and unhappy, confused, nervous and touchy, lonely and cutoff, unable to get along with family, no sense of purpose in life, feel angry, unable to make decisions, feel helpless, need help, cannot fit in, and having painful memories).

Factors 2, 3, and 4 labeled *PTSD Symptomatology*, *Control*, and *Numbing* together account for a further 16.2% of the total variance. In total, 63.4% are accounted for by Factors 1 through 4.

Subgroup means for the total adjustment problems scores are 99.1 for traumatized veterans and 64.2 for those not so affected. Using the *t*-test generated a probability value less than .0001. The questionnaire may therefore help to distinguish Falklands War veterans categorized by PTSD diagnosis, but a much larger sample has to be surveyed before valid standard error scores can be calculated.

Macroanalyses of 39 adjustment problem variables in a population sample of 53 veterans is contentious, so a plea for a measure of constraint in interpreting these findings is indicated. In recognition of this, a microanalysis was undertaken based on cross-tabulations of adjustment problems checklist scores against diagnostic status for PTSD. This produces four-by-two tables which have several cells with expected frequencies less than five. The risk of obtaining high chi-square values because of a small sample was reduced by also recoding scores into a two-by-two cross-tabulation. Clusters of significant problems could then be identified using both sets of cross-tabulations which identify those configurations of observed frequency distributions that achieve probability values equal to or less than .05.

In those instances where the subpopulations are clearly distinguished by a polarization of problem presence in the PTSD group and problem absence in the nontraumatized group, the adjustment difficulties listed are almost exclusively those that make up DSM-III criteria for PTSD. There are elements of reexperiencing (e.g., having troublesome memories of war experiences), numbing (e.g., feeling bored, wasting time), and arousal (e.g., being nervous and touchy, difficulties sleeping at night, head, back, and stomach aches). In addition, differentiation is achieved by the traumatized group's recognizing a need for change both in themselves and in their current life situation; the latter being strongly linked with a specific problem of "not getting along with family members."

In fact, this particular pattern is achieved by PTSD symptoms that feature in the adjustment problem checklist. Given that the survey sample is subdivided according to these same diagnostic signs, it is not surprising that differences are found, but it is important to note that the degree of polarization on these specific problems is extreme indicating very limited overlap between subgroups.

Also of great interest is the result emerging from a cross-tabulated cluster where the traumatized group record to an equal extent both absence and presence of a given problem, and the nontraumatized subjects consistently report their absence. In other words, differentiation is achieved by the nonoccurrence of a problem in the latter group, rather than by its consistent presence in the former. Linked to a set of relationship problems (e.g., difficult to form deep relationships, unable to trust people, and feeling unattractive to other people) and a residue of PTSD symptoms (having nightmares, poor concentration, and being violently angry), the largest single group of difficulties experienced fall within the category of alienation (e.g., being lonely, cut off from others, discouraged, unhappy, not caring about anything very much, being helpless, no sense of purpose, and distress at how people treat one another). These coexist with some recognition of "a need for help."

Alienation is therefore shown to be experienced to a varied degree within the traumatized group. Those who are not traumatized by their war experiences very rarely report this particular type of problem. This is very much in keeping with early American surveys of Vietnam War veterans (Pollock, White, & Gold, 1975; Wikler, 1974) which concluded that the final "reintegration" or "renewal" phase of the transition back to civilian life for the war veterans as described by Lifton (1973) is for many blocked or obstructed by feelings of alienation among veterans who experienced combat.

Statistically significant cross-tabulations were also achieved by a configuration indicating that certain problems are absent in both groups. An overall low prevalence applies in respect of "being unable to defend myself" and "not fitting into my neighborhood." Other adjustment problems of poor discriminative power are those where cross-tabulations failed to achieve statistical significance at the .05 level. These fall broadly within clusters defined by control issues (daydreaming and fantasizing about doing violence, feeling controlled by others, eating or smoking too much, and sexual frustration) and relationship problems (difficulties with authority figures, feeling of being badly treated by others, and difficulties in getting along with other people). Guilt and self-blame are experienced both by the PTSD and the non-PTSD group.

A noteworthy trend discernible in the data is that in terms of the listed problems, traumatized and nontraumatized Falklands War veterans are most clearly distinguished by personal difficulties included as symptoms in the DSM-III criteria for PTSD. Alienation is prevalent in the index group to a varying degree but is hardly ever reported among their colleagues. To the ex-

tent that adjustment problems arise for traumatized veterans, there is a strong link with PTSD symptomatology and alienation. Guilt, excessive eating, drinking, and relationship problems are found in both groups to an equal extent.

Sixty-eight percent (36) of the sample attribute their current adjustment difficulties to their involvement in the Falklands War. This figure includes eight veterans who do not meet DSM-III criteria for PTSD, reinforcing the impression that it is unhelpful to view diagnosis as the sole criterion for whether or not severe postwar difficulties are being experienced. One in three (17) of these war veterans do not link their current adjustment difficulties to experiences in the war zone. Such attribution is overwhelmingly linked to having fewer problems now compared to other times since the war ($N = 10$), delayed onset of an increasing number of problems ($N = 3$), or a fluctuating but increasing number of problems ($N = 3$). One person attributed current problems to a recent near-fatal accident.

Among the 30 veterans who report having more adjustment problems now, nearly half (14) report fluctuations in intensity over time, 9 (30%) indicate problem prevalence to have increased relentlessly since the war, and a further 7 (20%) report an initial period of well-being to have been followed by steadily increasing difficulties up to the time of the survey. Of the 30 who report more problems now, 73% ($N = 22$) belong to the group of traumatized veterans. This result further cautions against having the PTSD diagnosis the sole criterion for identifying veterans adversely affected by the experience of war.

Reporting, as did 23 veterans, fewer adjustment problems now than at other times since the war is in itself no guarantee that a veteran does not show all the symptoms required for a DSM-III diagnosis. In this group, 10 veterans still meet diagnostic criteria. The first 3 years after the war are most frequently reported to have been the most difficult period for adjustment problems, so here is further indication that the natural course of PTSD symptomatology does not exactly parallel development or resolution of adjustment problems.

General Health

The extent to which traumatizing war experiences in the South Atlantic are associated with long-term poor health is richly illustrated by this survey. Goldberg's (1978) recommendation of a cutoff score of 12 for "caseness" places 54.7% ($N = 29$) of the sample within this category. Cross-tabulated with PTSD a clustering of caseness with positive diagnosis and vice versa is revealed ($p = .0001$). Only seven subjects with a differential diagnosis do not meet the GHQ criteria. Group means of 26.5 and 6.1 for traumatized and nontraumatized veterans are significant to the .0001 level.

Assessing the discriminative power of GHQ caseness to PTSD reveals that seven traumatized veterans achieve scores below the cutoff. Thirty percent of the PTSD group would therefore be missed were such a criterion applied and more than one in eight (13.8%) of those not meeting DSM-III criteria would be wrongly classified. Again, there is support for the conclusion that PTSD symptomatology should be distinguished from other difficulties experienced by war veterans, even when the disorder runs a chronic course.

Correlated with other sample variables, General Health Scores are unrelated to age ($r = +.089$, $p = .53$), but a strong positive association exists with summated scores on the adjustment problems checklist ($r = +.85$, $p = .000$). The impact of reported adjustment problems extends not only into the social and interpersonal facets of life but also compromised the health status of Falklands War veterans.

Concluding Remarks

Until such time as the British Ministry of Defence resolves to match the courage and commitment of its military personnel in the Falklands War with an unqualified acceptance of its public responsibilities to those ex-servicemen who are traumatized by active military service, we shall remain uncertain of the true predicament of our veterans, the continuing impact on their families, their general social adjustment, and their health status (see Chapter 83, in this volume, for a review of these issues). As long as professional journals are in no position to publish the results of comprehensive community surveys, planners cannot make appropriate provisions reflecting demonstrated needs. In spite of methodological limitations, this first survey of the prevalence of chronic traumatic stress syndrome in the lives of Falklands War veterans sets a benchmark against which the results of future studies must be compared. Until access to this much neglected population of war veterans is secured and survey findings can be freely reported, the results of this investigation amount to the sum total of our knowledge. No one can now state that there is no documented evidence that Falklands War veterans have been chronically traumatized by their experiences in the war zone. The proportion of veterans who showed acute traumatic stress reactions will always have to be a matter of conjecture. However, chronic traumatic stress reactions are brought into sharp focus by the results of this survey. Associated with such diagnostic status is a range of adjustment problems, and feelings of alienation in a society that appears and is, mostly, oblivious to the plight of its most recently acquired group of war veterans whose existence is also marred by poor physical health.

References

Bourne, P. G. (1970). Military psychiatry and the Vietnam experience. *American Journal of Psychiatry, 127,* 481–488.

Figley, C. R. (1978). Psychosocial adjustment among Vietnam veterans: An overview of the research. In C. R. Figley (Ed.), *Stress disorders among Vietnam veterans: Theory, research and treatment* (pp. 57–70). New York: Brunner/Mazel.

Goldberg, D. (1978). *Manual of the General Health Questionnaire.* Windsor, England: NFER Publishing.

Jones, G. H., & Lovett, J. W. (1987). Delayed psychiatric sequelae among Falklands War veterans. *Journal of the Royal College of General Practitioners, 37,* 34–35.

Kulka, R. A., Schlenger, W. E., Fairbank, J. A., Hough, R. L., Jordan, B. K., Marmor, C. R., & Weiss, D. S. (1988). *National Vietnam veterans' readjustment study.* North Carolina: Research Triangle Institute.

Lifton, R. J. (1973). *Home from the war.* New York: Simon & Schuster.

McDowell, I., & Newell, C. (1987). *Measuring health: A guide to rating scales and questionnaires.* Oxford, England: Oxford University Press.

Neff, L. (1975, August). *Traumatic neuroses.* Paper presented at the Annual meeting of the American Psychological Association, California.

O'Brien, L. S., & Hughes, S. J. (1991). Symptoms of posttraumatic stress disorder in Falklands War veterans five years after the conflict. *British Journal of Psychiatry, 59,* 135–141.

Ørner, R. J. (1988, August). *P.T.S.D. in Falklands war veterans.* Paper presented at the First European Conference on Traumatic Stress, Lincoln, England.

Panzarella, R. F., Mantell, D. M., & Bridenbaugh, R. H. (1978). Psychiatric syndromes, self concepts and Vietnam veterans. In C. R. Figley (Ed.), *Stress disorders among Vietnam veterans: Theory, research and treatment* (pp. 148–172). New York: Brunner/Mazel.

Pollock, J. C., White, D., & Gold, F. (1975). When soldiers return: Combat and political alienation among white Vietnam veterans. In D. Schwartz & S. Schwartz (Eds.), *New directions in political socialization* (pp. 317–333). New York: Free Press.

Price, H. H. (1984). The Falklands: Rate of British psychiatric combat casualties compared to recent American wars. *Journal of the Royal Army Medical Corps, 130,* 109–113.

Rothbart, G. S., Fine, M., & Sudman, S. (1982). On finding and interviewing the needles in the haystack: The use of multiplicity sampling. *Public Opinion Quarterly, 46,* 408–421.

Shatan, C. F. (1973). The grief of soldiers: Vietnam combat veterans' self-help movement. *American Journal of Orthopsychiatry, 43,* 640–653.

Sirkin, H. (1979). *Network sampling in health surveys.* Paper presented at the Third Biennial Conference on Health Survey Research Method, Virginia.

Strayer, R., & Ellenhorn, L. (1975). Vietnam veterans: A study exploring adjustment patterns and attitudes. *Journal of Social Issues, 31,* 81–94.

Wikler, N. J. (1974, April). *Vietnam and the veterans' consciousness.* Paper presented at the annual meeting of the Pacific Sociological Association, California.

Yankelovich, D. A. (1974). *A study of American youth.* New York: McGraw-Hill.

CHAPTER 26

Posttraumatic Effects and Their Treatment among Southeast Asian Refugees

J. David Kinzie

Introduction

War and conflict with its destruction and violence have been a tragic and common occurrence in the Indochinese area of Asia. Struggles with invaders, colonial powers, internal political factions, and the awesome power of the American military in Vietnam and in Southeast Asia have all led to widespread ruin, injury, and death. Some of the most savage destruction and genocide occurred within the countries of Cambodia, Vietnam, and Laos by their fellow countrymen upon their own people. All these events resulted in various physical and psychological traumata ranging from the known effects of war on civilian populations to the truly massive catastrophic events endured by the Cambodians.

After the United States' withdrawal from Vietnam and the subsequent fall of the existing governments in 1975, millions of Southeast Asians fled their homeland and became refugees. Through 1988, nearly one million have been accepted into the United States. They are a varied group of people with a wide range of socioeconomic status and education, as well as their own ethnic identity. The latter consist of Vietnamese, Chinese-Vietnamese, the Khmer of the Cambodians, Lowland Laotians, and Highland Laotian tribesmen, the Mein and Hmong being the outstanding examples of the latter. Although many refugees made spectacular successes in their new country, studies have documented a high level of psychological distress and the high needs

for psychiatric services (Gong-Guy, 1985; Lin, Tozuma, & Masuda, 1979; Rumbant, 1985).

For 11 years, the Department of Psychiatry of the Oregon Health Sciences University has offered a clinic for Indochinese refugees. This very active program, which currently treats 350 patients, has five transcultural psychiatrists and seven ethnic mental health counselors (Kinzie, 1989). The results of our clinical efforts lead us to identify increasingly the effects of trauma on these refugees. In this chapter, I will describe the known effects of trauma in both clinical and nonclinical populations, the natural course of the stress syndromes, and the treatment approaches. Just as our recognition of posttraumatic stress disorder (PTSD) among Cambodians was slow, we are just now becoming aware of the full extent of PTSD among other Indochinese refugees. Since there is very little literature on the trauma of the refugees of Asian cultures, we first will address the difficulties in diagnosis of PTSD across cultures.

Cross-Cultural Diagnosis of PTSD

The recognition of psychosocial problems and the assessment of psychiatric disorders of patients from different cultures has become more sophisticated, and several excellent references exist (Owen, 1985; Williams & Westermeyer, 1986). Despite this, the recognition of PTSD as an official diagnosis of the American Psychiatric Association since 1980, and the widespread public knowledge of the hardships endured by refugees, most reports on their psychiatric status did not include or simply ignored the diagnosis of PTSD (Gong-Guy, 1985; Kinzie & Manson, 1983; Nguyen, 1982; Westermeyer, 1988). Until there is recognition of the existence of PTSD among refugees and of the diagnostic problems involved

J. David Kinzie • Department of Psychiatry, Oregon Health Sciences University, Portland, Oregon 97201–3098.

International Handbook of Traumatic Stress Syndromes, edited by John P. Wilson and Beverley Raphael. Plenum Press, New York, 1993.

in assessing Asians, we will never know the true prevalence of PTSD and allied forms of psychopathology among Indochinese refugees.

One of the reasons for the unusual avoidance of this diagnosis is the lack of awareness among both public and clinicians. Unlike the concern for Vietnam veterans, POWs, and Nazi Holocaust victims where comparatively more research is available, there is little public information or outcry on the effects of the Indochinese conflicts on the civilian population. Perhaps the marked ambivalence about the Vietnam War in the United States further pushes these tragic consequences for civilians outside of our awareness (see Chapter 57, in this volume, for an alternative cultural perspective).

The Asian patients themselves clearly are different than Americans and the contrast leads to difficulty in diagnosis. Language barriers make interviewing difficult. Interpreters are often poorly trained and unsophisticated about psychiatric diagnoses, leading to further difficulty. The patients' culture often leaves them to assume a shy, unassertive, and unemotional display of their symptoms, especially in the presence of American professionals. Furthermore, there is no economic advantage for them to exaggerate or even accurately describe the traumas since no compensation could be involved. Additionally, the presence of a codiagnosis, usually depression, is so obvious that it may cover the primary symptoms of PTSD. Usually a patient complains of a sleep disorder, poor appetite, lack of interest, and fatigue, but not of the most typical intrusive and avoidance aspects of PTSD. The disorder itself, with its psychic amnesia and numbing, often prevents patients from "remembering" the painful events of the past. For the Cambodians, and probably other Buddhist cultures, the collective sense of shame limits the ability of the patient to acknowledge the problems and traumas endured in their own country by their own countrymen.

However, the largest problem in diagnosis may be the clinician's bias. The most extreme form may be ethnic stereotyping, that is, "death does not matter to Asians," "Asians are stoic and not affected by trauma." This bias often leads to a failure to ask about trauma in a sensitive manner, allowing only a discussion of events in a limited way, and does not expose the patient's massive recurrence of intrusive and disruptive memories. The patient's avoidance, which may be protective, needs to be separated from the clinician's avoidance based upon the inability to handle, in a therapeutic way, the profound affects raised by the terrible stories and ordeals encountered. It clearly helps if such history-taking comes in a therapeutic setting, that is, as part of an ongoing treatment for a chronic disorder. Not closing the diagnostic process is particularly important. Almost one half (46%) of our patients with PTSD have been diagnosed after they were in treatment for some time, often several years. The patient–therapist relationship over time allows for safe and open revelation of the trauma and its effects. Clearly, to determine accurately the presence of PTSD among Asians requires a sensitive interview, preferably in a therapeutic situation over time. The symptoms, the culture, and the clinician's bias all need to be recognized as important issues in the cross-cultural diagnosis of PTSD.

The Traumas of Indochinese Refugees

Severe, unusual traumatic events are required for the diagnosis of PTSD. The refugees from Southeast Asia suffered from several major types of events, and many refugees suffer from more than one of these. The major categories of traumas that are encountered clinically are described below.

The Pol-Pot Experience

From 1975 to 1979, the radical Marxist government led by Pol-Pot systematically destroyed all traces of traditional and Western influence: Buddhist monks, intellectuals, businessmen, and government officials were killed. Cities became nonexistent as the population was forced into agricultural "work camps." Families were separated. Children over the age of 6 were put into age-related camps. Through murder, torture, starvation, and disease about one fourth to one third of Cambodia's seven million people died (Becker, 1986; Hawk, 1982). Fifteen-hour work days, little food, constant fear of death, separation from family, constant death among friends and fellow workers, and the never-ending aspects of the threats lasted for 4 years. Even after the Vietnamese invaded in 1979, war and destruction continued and the escape process was dangerous.

The experiences for those who went to Thailand to refugee camps were often dangerous with both the Pol-Pot soldiers and the Thai guards sometimes exhibiting brutality and cruelty. The future typically remained very uncertain for many years. The refugees arrived in the United States with memories of past traumata, the loss of country, language, and religion, and having few friends. The experience of Nazi Holocaust victims most accurately parallels the Cambodians under Pol-Pot. However, there was not even a supportive network, such as the Jewish community had, to help integrate. Table 26.1 lists the traumata endured by a group of Cambodian adult patients and an adolescent population.

Effect of War on Civilians

As the war in Vietnam raged, the publicity was mostly on the effects of the combatants, particularly the American soldiers. Little publicity was given to the effects on the civilian Vietnamese population. Although there were a few clinical reports (Kleinman, 1987; Mollica, 1988), one must remember that Vietnam had been in a state of warfare almost continuously since the Japanese invasion in 1940. With the effects of World War II, overthrowing the French colonials, the civil war, and the American involvement, much of the countryside and the cities were involved in marked destruction of civilian housing, injuries, and death. Many patients described the houses being blown up, soldiers shooting in the streets, death of many friends and family members, and the ever-present corpses in the towns and fields. In addition, many had to go to the battlefields to help identify bodies, sometimes husbands and brothers. When the Communists took over in Vietnam, many people described being beaten by the Communists, several had

Table 26.1. Pol-Pot Concentration Camp Experiences

Population	Percentage	Traumatic stressor experiences
Adults (N = 75)		
74	99	Forced labor often 15 hours a day, 7 days a week, for 4 years
59	79	Separated from family
61	81	Went a long time without food
72	96	Death of family member (execution or starvation) or whereabouts unknown
Children (N = 40)		
25	63	Death or disappearance of fathers
15	38	Death or disappearance of mothers

relatives killed, and there were many brutalities in the "reeducation camp." These effects, although not as dramatic as those under Pol-Pot, are extremely severe and are long lasting.

Escape Process

The Vietnamese boat people, when escaping to Vietnam, often described brutal trauma. Leaving Vietnam, they were often chased or blown up by the Vietnamese Navy, or were exposed to the terrible atrocities of Thai and other pirates who beat, robbed, raped, and killed on the high seas. The traumata of these episodes are often extremely tragic and shameful to the survivors. Moreover, there also was the refusal to be accepted into foreign countries and many boats were pulled out to sea, which resulted in drowning and life-threatening sur-

vival situations. The risks at sea were many. Refugee boat people described starvation, and cannibalism was reported by several patients. The tribe people from Laos, especially the Mein, also reported much cruelty and brutality from many different militia in their flight to Thailand.

Trauma Unrelated to War

As in any population, traumata have occurred which were unrelated to war but occurred in context of daily life experiences. Some of these have been very brutal and have had lasting effects. Several patients were robbed at gunpoint, tied, gagged, and left in their own stores by thieves of their own country. Several patients described domestic violence usually by husbands or fathers. One girl described working as a servant and being beaten several times and raped at least once by her employer.

The various types of trauma reported by our patients from different ethnic groups are shown in Table 26.2.

Symptoms

In an early study (Kinzie, Frederickson, et al., 1984), our group reported on 12 cases of Cambodians with PTSD as a result of massive trauma. They all met the DSM-III criteria for PTSD, and most had a codiagnosis, usually of depression. The symptoms were consistent with DSM-III diagnosis with the exception of guilt (or its translated equivalent) which was not common; however, a sense of shame was very prevalent.

Later, our group undertook a systematic interview of 40 adolescents traumatized as children (Kinzie, Sack, Angell, Clarke, & Ben, 1986; Sack, Angell, Kinzie, Mason, & Rath, 1986). They were in concentration camps from an average age of 8 to 12. As shown previously in Table 26.1, they endured massive trauma. Intermittent depressive symptoms or dysthymia was very common. Half of the students qualified for the DSM-III diagnosis of PTSD. The major symptoms of a group of our patients

Table 26.2. Traumata Endured by Indochinese Clinic Patients with PTSD

Traumata	Cambodian	Vietnamese	Laotians	Mein
Pol-Pot concentration camp experiences	101 (100%)	—	—	—
War-related traumata most experienced as civilians	—	48 (55%)	12 (44%)	28 (44%)
Escape-related traumata	—	22 (25%)	4 (15%)	29 (45%)
Nonwar-related traumata	—	17 (20%)	11 (41%)	7 (11%)
Total (N = 279)	101	87	27	64

Table 26.3. Major PTSD Symptoms in Cambodian Patients with PTSD

Symptoms present in at least 75% of patients (N = 19)
Depressive symptoms with appetite and sleep disturbances
Avoidance of memories
Recurrent nightmares
Recurrent intrusive thoughts
Symptoms present in 50% to 75% of patients
Emotional numbing
Exaggerated startle response
Intensification of symptoms by exposure to events that symbolize traumata, or by stress

Symptoms in adolescent nonpatients (N = 40)
Symptoms in 50% to 75%
Recurrent nightmares
Exaggerated startle response
Shame about surviving
Avoided memories
Symptoms in 25% to 50%
Depressed feelings with sleep, interest, and appetite disturbances

and these students are shown in Table 26.3. Although half of the students did not meet criteria for PTSD, most were affected. Avoidance symptoms were very common. Indeed, both students and patients displayed a marked reluctance to talk about events of the past and clearly described a conscious attempt not to think about the past traumatic occurrences. In many ways, the difference between those students who met the criteria of PTSD and those students who did not was the success of the avoidance mechanism in preventing thoughts or reexperiencing thoughts and actions to reoccur.

In addition to the morbidity of depression, both populations (students and patients) were remarkable for the lack of other diagnoses, specifically alcohol use and antisocial behaviors, which were almost totally absent. Their symptoms and the terror that they experienced were personal, private, and subjective and were not express in acting out behavior or in any interpersonal conduct disorder in general.

Out of our first 100 Cambodian patients with PTSD, we diagnosed seven with psychosis indistinguishable from schizophrenia. Their behavior, however, was usually threatening and severely disruptive. All seven were hospitalized and needed antipsychotic medicine. None of the other 93 did. This group usually had a difficult treatment course. Sometimes when the psychosis was controlled, the PTSD symptoms remained. It is likely that a small group of people under severe trauma experience severe and chronic psychotic symptoms (Kinzie & Boehnlein, 1989).

The Vietnamese, Laotian, and Mein groups represented a continuing problem in the diagnosis of PTSD. When the trauma was severe, it was noted in the initial interview, and the diagnosis was usually correctly made. (In retrospect, all the psychiatrists on our team missed some obvious diagnoses.) Originally, we found only 13 of 92 Vietnamese patients with a diagnosis of PTSD, and 6 of 60 were Laotian and Mein patients. In March, 1988,

we systematically reviewed all clinic patients with respect to their traumas and PTSD symptoms. The results were shocking and troubling. We found 85% of 152 Vietnamese, Laotian, and Mein patients with a newly diagnosed but prior existing PTSD. Eighty-two percent of the PTSD diagnoses were missed in these groups prior to systematic interviewing. More importantly, it must be underscored that this was a group in treatment, usually for several years, whom we thought we knew well in terms of their relationships with the psychiatrists and the mental health workers. As the result of this new diagnosis, we have now found an extremely high rate of PTSD among Southeast Asian refugees. Among the 243 patients in established treatment over several years, we have found a rate of 92% of PTSD among Cambodians, an unexpectedly high 95% among the Mein, 65% among Laotians, and 58% among the Vietnamese. These results were shocking because of the high prevalence rates, and troubling because of the difficulty in making the diagnosis by a culture-sensitive and trauma-sensitive staff. Although these are chronic patients, and PTSD may contribute to the chronicity, we now feel that the prevalence is not overinflated but consistent with the needs of refugees seeking help at a psychiatric clinic. Since March of 1988, after we began to reinterview old patients, we found PTSD to be present in 67% of 79 new patients who were evaluated. This is very similar to the 74% found in the entire refugee population. Of the entire patient group of 333, only 15 (5%) had a previous diagnosis of PTSD (i.e., had symptoms of PTSD but recovered). For most refugees, PTSD is chronic and present for many many years.

The fact that such a high percentage of refugee patients have PTSD helps to explain the chronicity of their symptoms. The largest single codiagnosis is depression, and although the patients seem to benefit from the traditional therapies (i.e., antidepressant medications and group therapies), most have not totally recovered. The continued problems of being a refugee in a different country explains part of the chronicity. However, it is quite probable, that the presence of chronic PTSD symptoms, such as nightmares, startle reaction, intrusive reexperiencing of the trauma, poor concentration, vigilance, and other symptoms prevent full symptom reduction or decrease in the impairment. In other words, the patients remained impaired not because of depression or the problem of being a refugee but because of the symptoms of PTSD from severe trauma.

Course and Prognosis of PTSD among Refugees

Based on 11 years of experience with the treatment of refugees, we now have an increasingly clear picture of the possible courses of PTSD among Southeast Asians. More specifically, we conducted two major studies and worked extensively for 6 years with Cambodian refugees.

In our 1-year follow-up report (Boehnlein, Kinzie, Rath, & Fleck, 1985) of the original group of patients, we found that many had adapted well. Some no longer met the criteria for the diagnosis of PTSD (but in retrospect this was often because of not meeting the *numbing* requirement in DSM-III). At that time, we were fairly optimistic that the prognosis would be guarded but favorable. Subsequently, every one of our patients who improved had at least one complete relapse of the entire PTSD syndrome and depression. Indeed, symptoms universally responded in a *differential* fashion regardless of the type of treatment. Depressive symptoms responded to treatment most favorably with an increase in mood, sleep, and appetite. The intrusive symptoms, particularly nightmares and intrusive thoughts in the daytime, were next to abate. Irritability and signs of autonomic arousal improved as well. The avoidance symptoms, consciously not thinking about the events, avoiding experiences and events and news reports which may stimulate reexperiencing the past, amnesia for the events, social withdrawal, and not talking about the events in general did not improve by any treatment (Kinzie, 1989; Kinzie & Leung, 1991). Many Cambodians had a pervasive sense of shame about the events in Cambodia which was related to a concept of previous lives or *karma*. Consequently, it was stated that Cambodia must have done something very bad in its past to have this happen to it now. This sense of shame tended to stay despite treatment.

The most clinically relevant facet of the traumatized refugee is a sensitivity to ongoing life stress. A similar intolerance to stress has been found in both Vietnam and civilian PTSD patients (Burstein, Ciccone, Greenstein, *et al.*, 1988; Wilson, 1989). Despite how well the patients may appear (improved affect and lack of intrusive symptoms) under stress the entire syndrome returns. The range of stressors can vary from actual trauma, such as being robbed or having their house broken into, to *symbolic trauma*, such as a delayed welfare payment or a letter from a Cambodian friend describing the situation there. To a delayed income check often we would hear the statement "I will starve to death just as I about did in Cambodia." Children leaving for school or marriage brought back fears of abandonment and the PTSD symptoms would return. Other stressors, such as being involved in a traffic accident or surgery, provided recurrence of the symptoms. The symptoms which returned were most often intrusive nightmares or daytime thoughts, startle reaction, and irritability. Usually, the nightmares involved were the returning of the images of the Pol-Pot experience, being chased or tortured, or seeing people killed by the cadres. Even though the current stress caused return of nightmares, the nightmares themselves were those of the original trauma.

The most dramatic and disturbing example occurred when it appeared that our clinic would close. We told many patients that we might not be able to continue to serve them. All patients reported marked increase in PTSD symptoms, and when we talked, most looked visibly and profoundly disturbed with a combination of withdrawal and tremulousness. Later, two patients developed documented hypertension requiring emergency treatment. We began to realize the importance of our clinic in their lives and their extreme vulnerability to the lack of support. A sensitivity to stress, rejection, or loss remains one of the most profoundly disturbing symptoms of PTSD.

Nonpatient Studies on PTSD in Refugees

Generally, my work with refugees is from a clinical population and thus represents the prevalence of PTSD among patients seeking help. It may not be reflective of the community at large (i.e., the rates may be lower in those not seeking treatment). The number of community studies on Indochinese refugees is quite limited. Those that have been done often have involved symptom checklists (Lin *et al.*, 1979) and needs assessment (Rumbant, 1985; Gong-Guy, 1985). Although specific diagnoses were not usually made, a high level of distress is found among refugees. The Needs Assessment Study which did include PTSD items (done in California) showed that Cambodians had the most severe psychiatric needs. The results showed that psychiatric needs in each ethnic group was proportional to the prevalence of PTSD found in the clinic population. It is possible that the needs reflected in the community represent the prevalence of PTSD, in combination with other disorders, as a major source of their problems.

As mentioned before, a prevalence study of psychiatric disorders among Cambodian high school students showed the rates of depression and PTSD to be 50%. I received information on the students' family life through home visits by our Cambodian mental health worker. The Cambodian parents, both natural and foster, had high levels of stress, with more than one half of them reporting trouble sleeping, trouble concentrating, anxiety, fatigue, irritability, and sadness or feeling blue (Sack, 1986). Clearly, these Cambodian parents are highly symptomatic, and many of their symptoms are associated with PTSD.

We completed a 3-year follow-up study on Cambodian adolescents and they appeared less depressed and reported fewer depressive symptoms (Kinzie, Sack, Angell, Clarke, & Ben, 1989). However, 50% still had PTSD as they did in the previous study. More importantly, these 50% were not always the same individuals. Some had improved and no longer had the full PTSD syndrome. Others developed PTSD since the previous study. Another group remained at the same clinical diagnostic status. The avoidance symptoms of PTSD remained very high for all individuals, indicating that this was a more constant aspect of the syndrome. In this study, I concluded that, at least for some, the course of PTSD shows a variable remitting or cyclical quality similar to the patient group.

In summary, the prevalence of PTSD among the populations of Indochinese refugees is not known at this time. Clearly, it is high among those who were severely traumatized, specifically the Cambodians and the Mein tribes people. Based on our studies, it is possible that PTSD runs as high as 50% in the general Indochinese community and as high as 90% among treatment-seeking patients in a psychiatric clinic.

As I mentioned above, the adolescents who were studied showed very little antisocial or conduct disturbance behaviorally. These students had had about 8 years of "normal" family life before being traumatized and also had only been in the United States for about 2 years. Since that time, the Cambodian high school students are revealing more conduct disturbance, some antisocial behavior, such as drinking and dropping out of school, and less respect in the classroom. The students who were in high school from the years 1988 to 1989 often had no more than 2 years of normal family life before they were traumatized. Some even were born during the Pol-Pot regime. There were no appropriate role models, even for a time, nor was there adequate time to develop a basic sense of trust and autonomy. It is possible that not having the normal family life early on in psychosocial development did not prepare them for the more stressful periods of adolescence; thus, the symptom expression appeared as a conduct disturbance or as antisocial behaviors. If this is true, more evidence might be forthcoming about the impact of trauma on children and the subsequent types of symptoms that develop. Such a study is now being planned by our group.

Treatment Considerations

The treatment of a severely traumatized individual is a profound clinical challenge. Among refugees in a foreign country with a different language and culture, isolated from their main supports of society and religion, the therapeutic challenge is even greater. However, from our experience, general principles of therapy have developed. These approaches, which are tentatively stated and are continually evolving and evaluated, may give some useful guidelines for those clinicians working with traumatized refugees or other individuals. The general therapeutic approach to the refugee patient requires the understanding of the patient and therapist's cultural expectations.

The most frequent problems of therapy are the different expectations from treatment by the Indochinese refugees and the American physician or therapist. The Asians familiar with other doctors want the physician to be actively involved in diagnosis and expect a rapid reduction of symptoms, as occurs in treatment of infectious diseases. The therapist, on the other hand, may be passive and may expect the psychological treatment to be a long process without immediate results, which may lead to conflicts in the treatment process. A second problem is the use of interpreters in the psychotherapy, many of whom are untrained in mental health counseling and are uncomfortable when intense feelings are aroused by the patient's painful disclosures. The patients may feel embarrassed or "put down" or unaccepted by the interpreter.

The setting itself needs to be considered. In a small room with only males present, such as the psychiatrist and an interpreter, benign questions may stimulate painful memories of past interrogation. Several traumatized patients became silent after having been asked their names. Some family names marked people for execution in Cambodia. Even asking about trauma and symptoms may provide problems for the therapist that can range from insensitivity to the patient's culture or not recognizing specific stressors which have occurred in the lives of Cambodians, Vietnamese, and Laotians. A rigid therapeutic bias, such as traumatic symptoms or a reactivation of childhood trauma, can lead to a nonempathic impasse. Although the opposite view that Western psychiatry has nothing to offer to such patients and that they should be treated by their own native healers denies patients necessary treatment that modern techniques have to offer.

Countertransference feelings, resulting from hearing stories of human destructiveness, can lead to guilt or anger and cause the therapist to lose objectivity. Others may react with pity and push themselves as liberator to save the victim. Such therapeutic pressure can lead to frustration or anger on the part of both therapists and patients. (See Wilson, 1989, for a discussion of countertransference problems in posttraumatic therapy.)

With this background in mind, the most useful approach is for the clinician to take a thorough history of the patient's life before and after the trauma. As the traumatic story begins to unfold, listen quietly, waiting with warmth and empathy. Establish and maintain empathy with nonverbal communication, such as eye contact, closeness, and sensitivity to the patient's needs. The best reaction to a painful and difficult story is that it should be taken seriously, respectfully, and slowly. Patients are often only vaguely aware of their depressed feelings. Somatic complaints and an inability to function are often not connected to the trauma and losses. An explanation which summarizes the traumatic events and relates these to the symptoms gives meaning to the patient. It helps patients recognize that their reaction is not unique but rather a human reaction to an extreme loss.

It is necessary to have a long-term relationship for treatment of massive trauma. PTSD with refugees is a chronic illness, and long-term supportive therapy should be geared to this. There must be regular appointments which may be respected, and there must be continuity in the patient's therapeutic relationship. There is an expectation that the patient will get better, but there is no clear termination date. There is a need for humor, warmth, and a pleasant therapeutic encounter to reduce the stress and isolation.

It is important to reduce outside pressure on the patient. These include making sure financial stressors are minimized, obtaining housing, and getting in contact with relatives through Red Cross or the writing of letters. Ongoing case managers by our mental health workers have been very helpful; reinforcing traditional values has been very useful. Working with the Buddhist concept of acceptance, living for one's children, respect for the family, and hard work are useful coping strategies which fit in with most of the older refugees' culture. There must be flexibility on the therapist's part to ride up and down with these symptoms of this chronic disorder. A long-term perspective should be maintained. The therapist should not become too enthusiastic about immediate results or too pessimistic about exacerbations or regressions which occur (Kinzie, 1989). In my experience, avoidance is not only a major part of the syndrome to suppress intrusive thoughts but it works together with the quiet acceptance of one's fate, a traditional Asian concept. My co-workers and I have not found it a problem to treat this in individual therapy. Early in therapy it is probably valuable to support the patient's suppression (Kinzie & Fleck, 1987).

Psychopharmacology has a major role to play in the treatment of posttraumatic stress symptoms. Many medicines have been recommended (Bleich, Siegel, *et* al., 1986; Burstein, 1984; Falcon, Ryan, *et al.*, 1985; Friedman, 1988; Van der Kolk, 1983). The most successful treatment has been imipramine by most studies and indeed, in our experience, it or a similar tricyclic antidepressant has been very useful. It reduces predominantly the PTSD symptoms associated with depression: poor sleep, lack of energy, lowered mood, and nightmares. As has been pointed out by several authors, some of the DSM-III-R PTSD symptoms, particularly those of hyperarousal, vigilance, startle reaction, irritability, and perhaps nightmares, are consistent with central nervous system adrenergic hyperactivity (Kolb, 1987). Because of this, clonidine, which acts centrally to reduce norepinephrine, has been suggested. Our experience is that the drug is extremely valuable for patients in conjunction with imipramine. Our usual treatment modality is to start depressed PTSD patients with imipramine. When a satisfactory blood level is obtained, usually after a month, and if there are continued symptoms, clonidine is added to the treatment, initially in 0.1 mg BID dosages. This combination has been very well tolerated.

In a study of 68 PTSD patients, 43 of them, after 6 months, were on both medicines, antidepressants and clonidine. Eighteen were only treated with tricyclic antidepressants whereas 6 were given clonidine (one was on no medicine at the time). Clonidine is particularly useful in reducing a sense of anxiety, startle reactions, and nightmares. In a prospective study, we found that the depressive symptoms, sleep disorder, and nightmares were improved as a result of the antidepressant tricyclic clonidine combination (Kinzie & Leung, 1991). However, avoidance behaviors were not changed by the im0 ipramine–clonidine treatment. Imipramine and clonidine are very useful for some but not all symptoms of PTSD.

Group therapy is an unusual undertaking for Asians because they tend to be very private and keep thoughts to themselves or within the family network. However, for several years now, we have had group therapy of a particular type with Southeast Asians; one that has emphasized the socialization experience, traditional ethnic activities, and practical information (Kinzie *et al.*, 1988). At the time of these activities, psychological issues, such as losses, conflicts, relationship to children, and adjusting to the culture, as well as the meaning of somatic symptoms, were voiced and discussed easily throughout the activities. This was found to be very useful to decrease the sense of isolation and loneliness and to share experiences with each other.

For the Cambodian groups, we began a once-a-month meeting in a formal American-style group therapy with no activities in order to simply discuss issues. For the first year, the meetings were dominated by the losses and traumas of the Pol-Pot regime. This was accompanied by a great deal of affect, anguish, and subsequent exacerbation of symptoms. Patients became more reluctant to come to these meetings, although they found something meaningful was being done. Over time, the affect and the pressured quality of these meetings has diminished greatly and now, after two years, there is an ability to look at some of the issues and experiences in a less intense manner. It seems that the patients have become somewhat desensitized to their severe experiences and are not having the autonomic, personal, psychological, and physical reactions that were present previously.

Our experience would indicate that an individual relationship with the patient is essential in working with traumatized refugees. It establishes a relationship, a safe place to review the therapeutic history, and a place for an individual to talk about personal feelings, losses, traumas, and to gain support. Medication has a role in reducing some of the major symptoms, especially those of depression and intrusive aspects of posttraumatic stress disorder. Imipramine and clonidine combinations offer good relief of some symptoms. Group therapy is a process which is difficult to evaluate but seems to help with social isolation and the reduction of avoidance behaviors over time.

Further Research Questions

The horrors of Southeast Asian warfare are just beginning to be understood in their complexity. We know some things about the effects of trauma from this experience but we really are just beginning to address the right questions. We now recognize the effects of wars and systematic traumata on civilians which can cause long-term chronic effects, the most apparent, for example, being PTSD. What we do not know is enormous and includes: (1) How many people are affected? (2) Why are some people scarred for life and others apparently unaffected? (3) Why do some people improve after many years while others develop full symptoms for the first time long after the trauma has ended? (4) What is the course of the trauma? (5) Do all people remain vulnerable forever? (6) With time, will we continue to see more cases of PTSD among refugees? (7) What are the effects of age on the trauma? (8) Do young people do better or are the symptoms different? (9) Are there gender differences? (10) What are the physiological responses to trauma? (11) Are there changes in the central nervous system of norepinephrine that can be measured? (12) What is the response to treatment? (13) Does individual psychotherapy which emphasizes the past make PTSD worse? (14) Does group therapy increase or decrease the symptoms? (15) Do the pharmacological treatments provide permanent effects or only symptomatic relief? (16) What are the second generation effects, that is, the effects on children of those who suffered?

Clearly, much more needs to be known and these are possible research questions which can provide answers. The tragedy of Indochina may help bring knowledge on these issues for the betterment of mankind.

Concluding Remarks

From what we know about Southeast Asians and trauma we can generalize these results:

1. People of cultures vastly different from the West have similar reactions and syndromes as described for Western cultures in experiencing massive trau-

ma (i.e., PTSD and associated syndromes and features).

2. Not everyone with massive trauma is affected. After a severe trauma, more individuals are pathologically affected and the effects possibly last longer.

3. With severe trauma, more individuals have the numbing and avoidance symptoms of PTSD even if the full syndrome is not evident.

4. The major PTSD symptom clusters of intrusive re-experience and hyperarousal can be exacerbated but seem to function in relation to the severity of the avoidance behaviors.

5. The more biological aspects of PTSD include poor sleep, nightmares, startle reaction, hyperarousal, intrusive thoughts, and cause much impairment. However, they can be treated with medication.

6. Depression is strongly associated with PTSD and probably relates to many people becoming patients in mental health facilities.

7. When trauma occurs in early life, the trauma-associated symptoms which develop later may have a behavioral or conduct disturbance quality than those which develop in a more mature personality in adulthood.

8. A small group of persons may develop a severely disturbing psychosis with PTSD that is difficult to treat.

9. Refugees who had to leave their homeland under conditions of warfare, concentration camp, evacuation, and escape processes are at high risk for developing trauma and subsequent PTSD.

References

Becker, E. (1986). *When the war was over: The voices of Cambodian revolution and its people.* New York: Simon & Schuster.

Bleich, A., Siegel, B., Garb, R., & Lerer, B. (1986). Post-traumatic stress disorder following combat exposure: Clinical features and psychopharmacological treatment. *British Journal of Psychiatry, 1949,* 365–369.

Boehnlein, J. K., Kinzie, J. D., Rath, B., & Fleck, J. (1985). One year follow-up study of post-traumatic stress disorder among survivors of Cambodian concentration camps. *American Journal of Psychiatry, 142,* 956–960.

Burstein, A. (1984). Treatment of post-traumatic stress disorder with imipramine. *Psychosomatics, 25,* 681–687.

Burstein, A., Ciccone, P. E., Greenstein, R. A., Daniels, N., Olsen, K., Mazarek, A., Decatur, R., & Johnson, N. (1988). Chronic Vietnam PTSD and acute civilian PTSD: A comparison of treatment experiences. *General Hospital Psychiatry, 10,* 245–249.

Falcon, S., Ryan, C., Chamberlain, K., & Curtis, G. (1985). Tricyclics: Possible treatment for post-traumatic stress disorder. *Journal of Clinical Psychiatry, 46,* 385–388.

Friedman, M. (1988). Toward rational pharmacotherapy for post-traumatic stress disorder: An interim report. *American Journal of Psychiatry, 145,* 281–285.

Gong-Guy, E. (1985). California Southeast Asian Mental Health Needs Assessment. Oakland Asian Community Mental Health Services, California State Department of Mental Health Contract 85-76282A-2.

Hawk, D. (1982). The killing of Cambodia. *New Republic, 187,* 17–21.

Kinzie, J. D. (1989). Therapeutic approaches to traumatized Cambodian refugees. *Journal of Traumatic Stress, 2,* 75–91.

Kinzie, J. D., & Boehnlein, J. K. (1989). Post-traumatic psychosis among Cambodian refugees. *Journal of Traumatic Stress, 2,* 185–198.

Kinzie, J. D., Boehnlein, J. K., Leung, P. K., Moore, L. J., Riley, C., & Smith, D. (1990). The prevalence of posttraumatic stress disorder and its clinical significance among Southeast Asian refugees. *American Journal of Psychiatry, 147,* 913–917.

Kinzie, J. D., & Fleck, J. (1987). Psychotherapy with severely traumatized refugees. *American Journal of Psychotherapy, 41,* 82–94.

Kinzie, J. D., Fredrickson, R. H., Ben, R., Fleck, J., & Karls, W. (1984). Post-traumatic stress syndrome among survivors of Cambodian concentration camps. *American Journal of Psychiatry, 141,* 645–650.

Kinzie, J. D., & Leung, P. (1989). Clonidine in Cambodian patients with post-traumatic stress disorder. *Journal of Nervous & Mental Diseases, 177,* 546–550.

Kinzie, J. D., Leung, P., Bui, A., Ben, R., Keopraseuth, K. O., Riley, C., Fleck, J., & Ades, M. (1988). Group therapy with Southeast Asian Refugees. *Community Mental Health Journal, 24,* 157–166.

Kinzie, J. D., & Manson, S. M. (1983). Five years experience with Indochinese refugee patients. *Journal of Operational Psychiatry, 14,* 105–11.

Kinzie, J. D., Sack, W., Angell, R., Clarke, G., & Ben, R. (1989). Three-year follow-up of Cambodian young people traumatized as children. *Journal of the American Academy of Child and Adolescent Psychiatry, 28,* 501–505.

Kleinman, S. (1987). Trauma and its ramifications in Vietnamese victims of piracy. *Jefferson Journal of Psychiatry, 5,* 3–15.

Kolb, L. C. (1987). A neuropsychological hypothesis explaining post-traumatic stress disorders. *American Journal of Psychiatry, 144,* 989–995.

Lin, K. M., Tozuma, L., & Masuda, M. (1979). Adaptional problems of Vietnamese refugees. *Archives of General Psychology, 36,* 955–961.

Mollica, R. F. (1988). The trauma story: The psychiatric case of refugee survivors of violence and torture. In F. Ochberg (Ed.), *Post-traumatic therapy and victims of violence* (pp. 295–314). New York: Brunner/Mazel.

Nguyen, S. D. (1982). The psychosocial adjustment and mental health needs of Southeast Asian refugees. *Psychiatric Journal of University of Ottawa, 7,* 26–35.

Owen, T. C. (Ed.). (1985). *Southeast Asian mental health: Treatment, prevention, service, training, and research.* Washington, DC: National Institute of Mental Health.

Rumbant, R. G. (1985). Mental health and the refugee experience: A comparative study of Southeast Asian refugees. In T.C. Owens (Ed.), *Southeast Asian mental health: Treatment, prevention, service, training, and research.* Washington, DC: National Institute of Mental Health.

Sack, W., Angell, R., Kinzie, J. D., Mason, S., & Rath, B. (1986). The psychiatric effects of massive trauma on Cambodian children. II: The family and school. *Journal of American Academy of Child Psychiatry, 25(3),* 377–383.

Van der Kolk, B. A. (1983). Psychopharmacological issues in post-traumatic stress disorder. *Hospital Community Psychiatry, 34,* 683–691.

Westermeyer, J. (1988). DSM-III psychiatric disorders among Hmong refugees in the United States: A prevalence study. *American Journal of Psychiatry, 145,* 197–202.

Williams, C. L., & Westermeyer, J. (Eds.). (1986). *Refugee mental health in resettlement countries.* New York: Hemisphere Publishing.

Wilson, J. P. (1989). *Trauma, transformation and healing.* New York: Brunner/Mazel.

CHAPTER 27

Immediate and Long-Term Effects of Traumatic Combat Stress among Israeli Veterans of the Lebanon War

Zahava Solomon

Introduction

The Lebanon War, Israel's longest and most controversial war, broke out on June 6, 1982. Following heavy bombardment of Israeli towns in the North, Israeli soldiers crossed the Lebanese border and fought against Palestine Liberation Organization (PLO) and Syrian troops. Although the heavy fighting lasted only through several weeks of the summer of 1982, the cease-fire signed in August of that year did not put an end to all hostilities. Israeli soldiers remained in Lebanon, where periodic flareups continued to occur. These soldiers remained at high risk; many lost their lives and others were wounded.

Just as soldiers in other wars, the fighters in Lebanon were exposed to an extremely traumatic experience. The palpable threat to life and limb was doubtless the single most stressful component, but other stresses included the injury or death of fellow fighters, exposure to horrible sights, and the lack of food, sleep, drink, and other basic physical amenities. These stresses were aggravated by loneliness, lack of social support, social and sexual deprivation, and lack of privacy (Stauffer, Lumsdaine, & Lumsdaine, 1949; Titchener & Ross, 1974).

In the Lebanon War, there were also additional stresses. A major concern was the confusion engendered by the inability, in many cases, to clearly distinguish between friend and foe. Guerrilla tactics in which

fire could come at any time, from any direction, and by nonuniformed men, made it difficult for Israeli troops to identify the enemy, who sometimes included women and children.

These uncertainties were compounded by the fact that the identity of the enemy changed in midcourse. When Israeli troops first crossed into Lebanon, the farmers in the south welcomed them as liberators from the oppressive domination of the Palestinians, whom they saw as alien intruders. As the war dragged on, however, the same farmers became hostile, and before very long they, too, were shooting at Israeli forces.

Criticism of the war on the homefront also created stress, not unlike that of the anti-Vietnam War movement (Wilson, 1978). The Lebanon War was the first war Israel fought that many people considered a war of choice. Although certain segments of the population believed that the war was necessary and justified to rid Israel of the constant threat of Palestinian aggression, others regarded it as uncalled for and wasteful of human life and effort. The stresses particular to the Lebanon War created an extremely anxiety-provoking ambience, which compounded the stress of combat and increased the risk for psychological breakdown.

The Seven National Wars of Israel

The Lebanon War was not the first, but the seventh Israeli war in the 40 years of this country's existence. Yet there were many questions regarding human response to the stress of combat for which we did not have satisfactory answers on the basis of the current literature. Although the acute pathology of combat stress reaction (CSR) is well documented, information on this subject is

Zahava Solomon • Research Branch, Department of Mental Health, Medical Corps, Israel Defence Forces, Military P.O. Box 02149, Israel.

International Handbook of Traumatic Stress Syndromes, edited by John P. Wilson and Beverley Raphael. Plenum Press, New York, 1993.

based primarily on clinical impressions, and there are very few systematic empirical studies. Moreover, only a small number of studies have singled out the long-term sequelae of a psychiatric breakdown on the battlefield, and those which have yielded inconsistent findings (Solomon, 1989). Disorders of this type generally gain attention at the outbreak of war and immediately afterward with very little in the way of sustained long term follow-up. Thus, the knowledge in this field is quite fragmented; and lessons learned in one war are easily forgotten in the next (Mangelsdorff, 1985).

The issue of the psychological toll of war is particularly pressing in Israel, however, owing to the almost unremitting state of warfare between this country and its neighbors ever since the country's inception. The army is thus viewed as crucial for Israel's continued existence. There is a compulsory draft of all young men and women for 2 or 3 years after high school, even after that, men continue to serve at least 1 month per year in the reserves. Most able-bodied Israeli men have fought in at least one war; many have fought in two, and not a few in three or more. The society as a whole, and the military in particular, are necessarily concerned with all the implications of the protracted state of belligerency. A full understanding of the effects of exposure to combat stress is thus of vital importance for the functioning of Israeli society as a whole.

During and immediately after the Lebanon War, the Israeli Defense Forces (IDF) had several hundred psychiatric casualties, who suffered a psychological breakdown on the battlefield, termed *combat stress reaction* (CSR), also known as *battle fatigue* or *battle shock*. In the years since the 1982 Lebanon War, the number of psychiatric casualties has doubled because of the emergence of delayed reactions. Concerned with the well-being of its soldiers, the Israeli army initiated an extensive multi-cohort longitudinal research project to examine many aspects of the disorder, ranging from its causes through its diagnosis, course, correlates, and treatment.

In this chapter, I will present some of the major findings of this 7-year project and will examine the characteristic clinical picture of CSR during the Lebanon War, and will also present the results of a 3 year follow-up of CSR and non-CSR veterans. Finally, I will look at the phenomena of reactivated and delayed stress reactions.

Combat Stress Reaction

The most common and conspicuous immediate psychological disturbance of war is combat stress reaction, as described in the above case example. Also known as *shell shock*, *combat exhaustion*, or *war neurosis*, CSR is a breakdown on the battlefield. It is a labile, polymorphic phenomenon, and the afflicted soldier may run amok or withdraw into a quasiparalytic state; he may tremble or faint, vomit or defecate, or simply sit or wander around in a daze. Unlike most other psychiatric disturbances, however, it is not diagnosed via a fixed and clearly defined symptom pattern. Kormos (1978) suggested the following definition:

Combat reaction consists of behavior by a soldier under conditions of combat, invariably interpreted by those around him as signalling that the soldier, although expected to be a combatant, has ceased to function as such.

This definition is rather general, and functional in nature, and is based primarily on clinical observations. To the best of our knowledge, no systematic studies of the characteristics of CSR have been conducted to date. It was thus considered important to study the typical clinical picture among casualties diagnosed during the 1982 Lebanon War as suffering from CSR.

For the purposes of this study, a random sample of 104 male subjects was drawn from a subsample of soldiers who fought on the front line during the 1982 Lebanon War and were identified by Israel Defence Forces mental health personnel as CSR casualties.

Approximately 1 year after their participation in the war, subjects were interviewed. The interview transcripts were then subjected to content analysis which revealed 25 different types of affective, behavioral, cognitive, and somatic manifestations of the CSR episode (Solomon, Mikulincer, & Benbenishty, 1989).

Factor analysis yielded 6 principal factors with eigenvalues higher then 1, which explain 62% of the total variance. The factors were labeled as follows:

1. *Psychic numbing* (20% of total variance): Numbing of responsiveness or reduced involvement with the surrounding, seeking relief by mentally escaping from the combat situation, and thinking about civilian life experiences
2. *Anxiety reactions* (11% of total variance): Anxiety, fear of death, ruminations about death, and sleep disturbances because of nightmares and fear
3. *Guilt about functioning* (9% of total variance): Guilt feelings, ruminations about one's functioning, and fatigue
4. *Depressive reactions* (8% of total variance): A sense of helplessness, and feelings of loneliness and isolation
5. *Psychosomatic reactions* (7% of total variance): Crying, diarrhea or vomiting, and screaming or running amok
6. *Psychotic-like states* (6.5% of total variance): Disorientation, fainting, and tremors.

Taken as a whole, this taxonomy of CSR is quite similar to earlier theoretical classifications (e.g., Cavenar & Nash, 1976; Grinker, 1945) despite the fact that it was made in a different culture, for a different population, and following a different war. This strong resemblance has a major implication for the analysis and conceptualization of CSR: It emphasizes the universality of CSR manifestations, whatever the phenomenon may be called.

Does the War End When the Shooting Stops?

But what happens when the fighting ends? Is CSR a superficial disturbance that passes when the war ends, or does it leave scars and stress residues? If the latter is the case, are these stress residues manifested in a specific psychiatric syndrome, such as PTSD, or in other psychiatric symptomatology? Do these stress residues of war have implications for the veteran's subsequent social functioning in civilian life? Are they limited to psychiatric problems, or are stress residues reflected also in somatic disturbances?

In order to answer these questions, we followed up two groups of veterans for 3 years after the Lebanon War. The veterans who participated in the study were sampled from two populations. The CSR group consisted of frontline soldiers in the Lebanon War who were diagnosed with CSR on the battlefield by IDF mental health professionals. These subjects showed neither indication of serious physical injury nor indication of other combat-related disorders. The control group consisted of frontline soldiers of the Lebanon War who had not been treated for CSR. They were chosen from the same units as the CSR group and were pairwise matched with them for age, education, military rank, and assignment. At all three times, 213 CSR soldiers and 116 control soldiers participated (for a full description of the sample, see Solomon, 1989). Although the study was conducted after the war, we had access to IDF computerized data banks and were able to compare baseline data used by the IDF in premilitary screening of candidates for combat units. No differences between the CSR and non-CSR groups in prewar psychological adjustment or physical health were found.

Approximately 1, 2, and 3 years following their participation in the Lebanon War, CSR and control subjects were asked to report to the headquarters of the Surgeon General of the IDF. The request was accompanied by a personal letter explaining that they had been selected to participate in a periodic health assessment conducted by the Medical Corps.

Data were gathered using a series of questionnaires. Trauma-related psychopathology was examined via the PTSD inventory (Solomon, 1989) aimed at diagnosing PTSD and examining the intensity of PTSD symptomatology. The veterans' psychosocial status was assessed using measures of general psychiatric symptomatology (SCL-90; Derogatis, 1977), problems in social functioning (Solomon & Mikulincer, 1987a), and somatic health (Solomon & Mikulincer, 1987b).

Posttraumatic Stress Disorder

Assessment of PTSD rates via the PTSD inventory demonstrated that for a large proportion of Israeli combatants, the trauma of war left enduring and disruptive sequelae. Among the identified CSR casualties, PTSD rates were quite high throughout all 3 years of the study: 62% 1 year after Lebanon, 56% 2 years after, and 43% 3 years after (see Table 27.1). In other words, nearly half of those soldiers who sustained a CSR on the battlefield were still suffering from pervasive diagnosable disturbances 3 years after their participation in battle. Clearly then, for a large proportion of combatants, the war does not end when the shooting stops.

Since the literature does not offer norms for comparison to CSR casualties of other wars, it is difficult to gauge how representative these rates are. Recent studies of Vietnam veterans have found PTSD rates ranging from 15% to 48% (e.g., Center for Disease Control, 1988), but these calculations were made without reference to whether or not the subjects had sustained a prior CSR. What can be stated, though, is that for the majority of CSR casualties of the Lebanon War, the wartime breakdown was not just a transient episode, but was rather crystalized into chronic posttrauma from which recovery, if it came at all, was slow (Solomon, 1989).

The control group also showed substantial, if not nearly as dramatic, PTSD rates: 14% the first year after Lebanon, 17% the second, and 10% the third (see Table 27.1). These figures point to the detrimental impact of war on men who weathered the immediate stress of combat without a visible breakdown and resumed their lives without ever applying to a mental health agency. Undoubtedly, many were not aware that they had a definable disorder, or believed that their symptoms were a natural and inevitable outcome of their harrowing experiences on the front. Others were reluctant to seek help. They were aware of their distressing symptoms, yet they perceived them not as a psychiatric disorder, but as a natural and inevitable reaction to the stress of war. In other cases, the reluctance to seek help may be related to the social and emotional price that psychiatric care entails. In Israel, masculine identity is very strongly linked with military service. Identifying oneself as a PTSD casualty may well cost some men a heavy price in both self-esteem and social acceptance. Similar reluctance to seek treatment has been found among psychiatric casualties of the Vietnam War (Kadushin & Boulanger, 1981). It is all too likely that these silent PTSD veterans signify a much larger number of psychiatric war casualties whose distress is similarly unidentified and untreated.

Of all the PTSD veterans, the ones who had also sustained a CSR were the most seriously disturbed. Not only were their PTSD rates overwhelmingly higher, but as can be seen from Table 27.1, they also had significantly more symptoms. The greater severity of PTSD among CSR casualties might be indicative of this group's greater initial vulnerability. However, the fact that the CSR and control groups were carefully matched and did not differ in premilitary personality and adjustment variables suggests that the differences were caused by the CSR itself rather than by any precombat difference in vulnerability. Veterans who sustain a CSR have to contend with the implications of their breakdown, with the shame and guilt of having let down their buddies and betraying the trust placed in them by nation and family. Considering the great importance attributed to the army in Israel, their sense of failure, and the injury to their manhood and self-esteem, must weigh very heavily and exacerbate their posttrauma.

By the third year of the project, both the PTSD rates and the number of symptoms decreased significantly in both study groups. Time and circumstances seem to have combined in fostering healing. Similar improvements over time have been found in the posttraumatic symptoms of survivors of the Nazi Holocaust and other

Table 27.1. Means of Trauma-Related Symptomatology and Psychosocial Status for CSR and Non-CSR Veterans

	CSR			Non-CSR		
	Time 1	Time 2	Time 3	Time 1	Time 2	Time 3
PTSD inventory						
PTSD rates	0.63	0.57	0.43	0.14	0.16	0.10
PTSD intensity	6.86	6.44	5.01	2.59	2.45	1.47
SCL-90						
Global severity	1.10	1.12	1.10	0.46	0.45	0.43
Somatization	0.96	1.01	0.98	0.46	0.47	0.46
Depression	1.13	1.13	1.09	0.44	0.42	0.39
Phobia	0.75	0.80	0.80	0.19	0.25	0.23
Obsession	1.40	1.36	1.35	0.67	0.63	0.51
Anxiety	1.35	1.44	1.34	0.51	0.50	0.47
Paranoia	0.96	1.01	0.99	0.50	0.53	0.45
Interpersonal	1.02	1.04	1.04	0.49	0.46	0.46
Hostility	1.23	1.26	1.22	0.47	0.40	0.42
Psychoticism	0.85	0.83	0.86	0.34	0.32	0.28
Social functioning						
Work	0.44	0.42	0.42	0.18	0.24	0.17
Family	0.44	0.40	0.37	0.12	0.19	0.13
Sexual	0.39	0.38	0.36	0.08	0.19	0.13
Social	0.45	0.42	0.42	0.17	0.19	0.15
Motivation	0.54	0.49	0.50	0.18	0.18	0.17
Satisfaction	0.32	0.37	0.37	0.13	0.22	0.14
Independence	0.26	0.25	0.24	0.08	0.14	0.11
Somatic problems						
Absenteeism	0.06	0.41	0.46	0.05	0.17	0.22
Alcohol	0.16	0.16	0.21	0.03	0.08	0.07
Smoking	0.44	0.42	0.41	0.21	0.17	0.21
Hypertension	0.09	0.13	0.07	0.06	0.08	0.04
Digestive problems	0.16	0.13	0.13	0.06	0.09	0.02
Chest pains	0.29	0.30	0.21	0.12	0.09	0.08
Back pains	0.33	0.36	0.23	0.24	0.24	0.18

Note. Higher scores in the PTSD inventory, SCL-90, and SPF reflect more severe psychopathology and more problems in social functioning.

catastrophic events (Davidson, 1979). Moreover, just before the third wave of questionnaires was administered, Israel finally pulled most of its troops out of Lebanon. Since the IDF is a largely civilian army, with all men up through age 55 serving in the reserves, it was only at this juncture that the very real threat of being sent back to the front was lifted, and many PTSD veterans could breathe a sigh of relief and embark on the road to recovery. But these are the luckier ones. Forty-three percent of the CSR group and 10% of the controls continued to suffer from PTSD.

With regard to the profile of PTSD symptomatology (see Solomon, 1989), it was found that guilt feelings and reduced expression of anger did not play the prominent role that they repeatedly have in other forms of trauma (Glover, 1984; Haley, 1974). There are several possible explanations. One is that guilt and reduced anger are perhaps not necessary components of combat-related PTSD. Another is that the particular circumstances of the Lebanon War mitigated against guilt feelings. Unlike the Vietnam War, Israeli soldiers committed virtually no atrocities in Lebanon, but, on the contrary, went to great

lengths to protect civilian life, often at risk to their own. More importantly, since large parts of the Israeli population objected to the Lebanon War, public opinion permitted the expression of anger and dictated against expressions of guilt. Lastly, whatever the civilian population's feelings about the war, they heavily supported their soldiers.

General Psychiatric Symptomatology

The fact that the DSM-III (American Psychiatric Association, 1980) provides standardized uniform criteria for the diagnosis of PTSD has done a great deal to make possible objective research with fairly generalizable results. But this very standardization is also something of a disadvantage. To obtain it, the diagnostic criteria include only the symptoms common to the posttraumatic responses for all the events that were considered, whereas the symptoms particular to only one or even several events, such as anxiety, depression, and hostility, were considered as not essential to PTSD diagnosis. In this way, the exclusion of particular features of PTSD makes any instrument based on DSM-III criteria unable to provide a refined or detailed picture of the posttraumatic reaction following specific traumatic events.

On this basis, we decided also to obtain a more detailed clinical picture of PTSD among Lebanon War CSR casualties by assessing their psychiatric symptomatology, using the Symptom Checklist-90 (SCL-90) (Derogatis, 1977). Results indicated that soldiers who had wartime CSR showed greater psychiatric distress than their control counterparts. CSR casualties positively endorsed a greater number of symptoms, and rated them with a higher level of severity 1, 2, and 3 years after the war (see Table 27.1). They also showed more severe symptomatology on most of the SCL-90 symptom subscales at all three times of measurement than soldiers without CSR (see Table 27.1). These differences were especially marked with regard to depression, anxiety, obsessive-compulsive problems, and paranoid ideation.

Results also indicated that of all the SCL-90 symptoms, anxiety and depression are the most salient features associated with CSR in our sample. From a psychodynamic perspective, CSR is defined as an acute reaction to threatening events in which the individual is flooded with uncontrollable anxiety (Kardiner, 1947). In CSR soldiers who have PTSD after the war, this anxiety reaction may be reinforced by the intense trauma-related imagery and thoughts, and may finally crystallize despite the passage of the original threatening events. In these casualties, anxiety may take the form of phobic reactions, usually related to situations reminiscent of the original traumatic experience (Solomon, Garb, Bleich, & Grupper, 1987).

The finding that depression is a major symptom associated with CSR among Israeli veterans is consistent with observations of survivors of other catastrophes, including concentration camp survivors (Eitinger, 1969), prisoners, and combat veterans (Solomon, Garb, Bleich, & Grupper, 1987). Depression may derive from uncompleted mourning for friends who have died (Haley, 1974); it may also reflect the veterans' mourning over what they consider lost parts of themselves.

Among soldiers who had a CSR episode, depressive mood and ideation can be understood as a reaction to the CSR itself. The depressive mood could stem from severe shame over having collapsed during battle. The afflicted soldier may interpret his CSR episode as a failure to maintain the combatant role. Moreover, with crystallization of CSR into PTSD, the veteran's inability to restore his self-esteem and to improve his present life situation may add yet further cause to feel depressed.

Hostility, often explosive, was also found to be highly prevalent among Israeli veterans with CSR. This is consistent with numerous reports of high hostility among Vietnam veterans (Figley, 1978). The elevated level of hostility among CSR veterans may be explained in several ways. One possible explanation has to do with the comparatively high level of fear with which CSR casualties, as opposed to control veterans, had to cope during the war. During wartime, aggression is channeled against the enemy not only as an obvious means of survival but also as a way of coping with fear. After the war, the aggression, which had served to dampen

fear, remains and is generalized to peacetime situations. It may be that CSR casualties, who are experiencing a high level of stress as a result of their psychiatric condition perceive civilian life as an extension of the war, and try to cope with it in the same way.

The finding that obsessive-compulsive features are highly prevalent in our sample is not surprising. Such features are consistent with the second DSM-III criteria for diagnosis of PTSD; that is, repetitive reexperiencing of the traumatic event. The finding is also consistent with Horowitz, Wilner, and Alvarez's (1979) contention that a variety of repetitive behaviors are common manifestations of PTSD.

Social Functioning

Combat stress has been found to have long-lasting effects on the social aspects of the veteran's life (De Fazio, 1980; De Fazio, Rustin, & Diamond, 1975; Figley, 1978; Wilson, 1978). The DSM-III points out that in addition to psychiatric symptoms "PTSD may result in occupational or recreational impairment and psychiatric numbing may interfere with interpersonal relationships." Moreover, research findings indicate that social dysfunctioning is an important outcome of the experience of a traumatic event. Problems in social functioning have been found among concentration camp survivors (Chodoff, 1962), survivors of natural disasters (Gleser, Green, & Winget, 1981; Titchener & Kapp, 1976), and rape victims (Burgess & Holmstrom, 1974).

Nevertheless, most of the research to date has concentrated on the formation of intrapsychic psychiatric symptomatology following war, giving only limited attention to the interpersonal component of the disorder. Moreover, the available literature is inconsistent and sometimes conflicting. Some studies of Vietnam veterans (e.g., Egendorf, Kadushin, & Laufer, 1981; Wilson, 1978) have found them to have problems in intimacy and strong feelings of detachment from others, whereas other investigations (e.g., Borus, 1973; Worthington, 1977) found only a small and nonsignificant deterioration in social functioning.

In addition, few studies have examined the relationship between PTSD and social functioning (Carroll, Rueger, Foy, & Donahoe, 1985; Roberts, Penk, Gearing, Rabinowitz, Dolan, & Patterson, 1982). Their results indicate that the non-PTSD combat veterans do not differ in any measure from noncombat veterans; that is, problems in interpersonal adjustment because of combat have been found only among those soldiers who exhibited concomitant PTSD.

In order to assess the relationship between CSR and PTSD on the one hand, and problems in social functioning on the other, we employed the Social Functioning Problems scale (SFP), which queries about problems in seven facets of social life: work performance, family functioning, sexual functioning, social functioning, social motivation, social satisfaction, and social independence (for a detailed item description and information regarding psychometric properties, see Solomon & Mikulincer, 1987a).

The current data show that CSR casualties reported more problems in social, family, sexual, and work functioning than controls 1, 2, and 3 years after the war (see Table 27.1). The poorer social functioning of CSR veterans may be related to social rejection in the wake of their breakdowns. Their comrades in arms may have rejected the CSR casualties as cowards or as disloyal in the battlefield. This social rejection during the war may have further contributed to their vulnerability when they came home. Then, at home, when they were unable to adequately meet the requirements of civilian life, they may again have encountered negative attitudes. These rejections may have helped to create a self-perpetuating cycle of psychopathology and social rejection.

The findings also indicate that social dysfunctioning is strongly associated with the presence of PTSD 1, 2, and 3 years after the war (see Table 27.1). It is likely that a number of PTSD symptoms, such as numbing of responsiveness, reduced involvement with the external world, diminished interest in previously enjoyed activities, feelings of detachment from others, alienation, and constricted affect, may directly hinder social functioning, getting in the way of both intimate and more casual relationships, and so damper social interest. When they are combined with other PTSD symptoms—difficulties in concentration, memory, and sleep—problems could be expected to arise in functioning at work, too.

In addition, the elevated levels of hostility in PTSD veterans may have severe repercussions in both their family relations and less intimate social situations. Aggressive impulses and aggression control may affect the veteran's functioning in his numerous roles at work and as husband and father (see Williams, 1980).

Furthermore, veterans suffering from PTSD may employ considerable psychic energy in dealing with their avoidance and intrusion, drawing energy away from their social lives—whether this means maintaining normal family life or creating new social relationships.

Somatic Complaints

The manifestations of CSR and PTSD are not restricted to psychiatric symptomatology, but may be manifested in somatic disturbances as well. The DSM-III points out that in addition to psychiatric symptoms, PTSD may be linked with somatization and physical complaints. Moreover, research findings indicate that somatic complaints may be an important outcome of combat-related trauma (Rahe, Gunderson, & Arthur, 1970; Rubin, Gunderson, & Arthur, 1972; Rubin, Gunderson, & Doll, 1969).

In order to evaluate the veterans' physical health, this study employed a specially designed health questionnaire which inquired about the onset of illness in the past year as well as changes in a number of health-related behaviors (see Solomon, 1989). It was found that soldiers who had CSR during the war reported more health problems 1, 2, and 3 years after the war than controls (see Table 27.1). This finding may indicate the cumulative impact of stress. It may be that soldiers who contracted wartime CSR experience more distress during war and have fewer coping resources than soldiers who did not contract CSR. Their comparatively worse

physical health may thus reflect the greater distress they experience. Alternatively, the difference in the health reports of the two groups may stem from a difference in attitudes to somatic problems. Perhaps just as CSR soldiers are more aware of their psychological problems, they are also more aware than others of their somatic difficulties, and may therefore tend to overrate them.

Our findings also show that the number of endorsed PTSD symptoms was positively related with more health problems (see Table 27.1). It is possible that PTSD in and of itself exerts a great deal of pressure (Horowitz, 1982), and that the soldiers' somatic problems derive from the effects of that pressure (Engel, 1968). Unlike the non-PTSD soldier, the PTSD soldier has to deal with a whole range of emotional and behavioral difficulties. Doing this requires the allocation of considerable energy and inner resources, which, in turn, weakens the soldier and renders him more vulnerable to somatic disorders (Engel, 1968).

Research has shown a rise in the number of health problems during battle (Rubin et al., 1972), so it may be possible that soldiers with PTSD may simply continue to suffer from the somatic disorders that began during battle, just as they continue to suffer from the psychological problems that started there.

On the other hand, Titchener (1986) claimed that following psychological trauma, a growing hypochondria takes over, and somatic symptoms become the focus of the person's life. PTSD symptoms, including withdrawal from previously enjoyed activities, lead to isolation and to preoccupation with the physical self.

From another perspective, somatic disturbances may be considered an integral part of both CSR and PTSD (Titchener & Ross, 1974). Both CSR and PTSD have somatic components. CSR is often characterized or accompanied by diarrhea, vomiting, nausea, enuresis, chest pains, hyperventilation, and other physical symptoms (Kardiner, 1947). PTSD, according to DSM-III, is marked by an increase in somatization.

The current findings also show increased cigarette and alcohol consumption in CSR casualties in comparison to controls (see Table 27.1). This pattern of findings is consistent with results of earlier American studies (e.g., Egendorf et al., 1981; Figley, 1978). This change in health-related habits in CSR and PTSD casualties may also help explain in part why they have more somatic problems. Heavy drinking has been implicated in blackouts, job and school problems, and automobile accidents (Figley, 1978).

A number of methodological issues arise. One of the major methodological factors in this research was that the health data were collected without concomitant physical examinations. This may have numerous implications for the interpretation of the results. It is possible that soldiers suffering from PTSD reported a large number of health problems even if they were actually in good health. If such soldiers regard themselves as sick, it stands to reason that they would interpret whatever health problems they do have as more serious than they really are. Moreover, an exaggerated report of health problems may stem from the desire of PTSD soldiers to gain social support.

Longitudinal Analysis

In general, the longitudinal analyses revealed that the passage of time had no effect on the psychiatric symptomatology, social functioning, and somatic complaints in either of the two study groups. In neither the CSR nor the control groups did the psychiatric, social, and somatic status of the veterans undergo any significant change over the 3 years. It follows that the differences in these measures in the CSR and control groups were stable throughout the 3 years of the study. These results demonstrate the long-term detrimental effects of combat-related psychopathology. They further show that these psychopathological effects are not limited to psychiatric damage but are evidenced in social and somatic problems as well.

The stable psychiatric, social, and somatic status of the CSR casualty over the 3 years of the study contrasts with the observed decline in PTSD in the third year. Apparently, as the interval from the war increased, there was a shift from trauma-related symptoms to more general symptomatology. In other words, the decline in PTSD symptomatology does not necessarily mean that the CSR veterans were getting well. The observed reduction in PTSD does not imply an evaporation of psychopathology, but a crystallization of a different psychopathological entity.

Effects of Repeated Exposure to Combat

Israel's many wars have made it important to know the impact of recurrent combat exposure. Since most countries are fortunate enough not to have to require the same soldiers to fight in repeated wars, the literature on combat stress has little to offer on this subject. The only basis for prediction at the time of the current study derived from studies of psychological and somatic responses to adversity in general. These offer three alternative perspectives: (1) The *vulnerability perspective* (Coleman, Burcher, & Carson, 1980; Wilson, 1978) considers repeated exposure to stressful events to be a risk factor, since it drains a person's coping resources and thereby makes him more vulnerable. (2) The *stress inoculation perspective* (Epstein, 1983) holds that repeated stress serves as an "immunizer" in that it fosters the development of effective coping strategies and promotes adaptation. (3) The *stress resolution hypothesis* postulates that what matters is not so much the fact that a person was exposed to a particular stress, but how he coped with it. According to Block and Zautra (1981), successful coping leads to a feeling of well-being and to an increase in coping ability, while unsuccessful coping leads to increased distress and decreased coping ability.

To assess the applicability of these theories, we presented the subjects described in the previous section a list of seven Israeli wars and, for each, asked them to indicate whether or not they had participated in the fighting and whether or not they had sustained a combat stress reaction (Solomon, Mikulincer, & Jakob, 1987).

The highest CSR rates in the Lebanon War were among soldiers who had had a prior stress reaction (66%), lowest among soldiers who had fought previously without a stress reaction (44%), and in between among soldiers with no prior war experience (57%). The figures suggest that the successful resolution of previous stress indeed helps soldiers to cope with subsequent battle. But they also indicate that novice soldiers are better off than those who broke down in a prior war. Although not every soldier who sustains a combat stress reaction is doomed to a second breakdown under similar circumstances, it is clear that a combat stress reaction leaves most of the casualties more vulnerable the second time around.

The detrimental impact of combat becomes all the more apparent when the number of previous wars is taken into account. Among soldiers with a prior stress reaction, CSR rates in Lebanon increased linearly with the number of prior war experiences: 57% after one war, 67% after two; and 83% after three. Among soldiers who had fought without a prior stress reaction, CSR rates in Lebanon were curvilinear. Soldiers who actively participated in one or three previous wars showed higher CSR rates (50% and 44%, respectively) than soldiers who participated in two (33%).

Altogether, these figures again show that traumatic experiences scar the traumatized individual and weaken his resilience to future stress. They also suggest that whatever the possible benefits of successful stress resolution, repeated battery will eventually fell even the hardiest souls.

Reactivation of Posttraumatic Stress Disorder

Titchner and Ross (1974) likened the traumatic experience to the flooding of a piece of land. In some cases, when the water recedes, it leaves visible and massive damage. In other cases, the preflood order soon reappears, leading to the feeling that whatever damage has occurred can be rectified. In some of these cases, though, this may be deceptive since there can be invisible structural flaws that made the area more vulnerable to subsequent stresses.

This may also be the case with CSR. Even when the casualty seems to recover, he remains more vulnerable than other veterans to late stresses. As my colleagues and I were going through the files of the second-time casualties in Lebanon, we found ourselves reading more and more about their experiences in the 1973 Yom Kippur War, when most of them had suffered their first combat stress reaction. Far from being fresh episodes, their second reactions echoed the content and context of their Yom Kippur War experiences 9 years earlier. There were even soldiers who said outright that their Lebanon CSRs were triggered by associations with Yom Kippur battles 9 years earlier.

Reactivation of stress reactions is a well-known phenomenon. Widows have been found to have reactivated grief reactions after being reminded of their loss (Lindemann, 1944; Weiner, Gerber, Baltin, & Arkin, 1975), and rape victims to experience a similar reactivation of their response to the original trauma when they are reminded of it (Burgess & Holmstrom, 1974). Holocaust survivors and American World War II veterans have reported reactivated wartime traumas in conjunction with the losses associated with aging (Archibald & Tuddenham, 1965; Christenson, Walker, Ross, & Malthie, 1981). Vietnam War veterans have been found to respond with reactivated symptomatology when they attended war memorials and other public ceremonies that reminded them of their combat experience (Faltus, Sirota, Parsons, Daamen, & Schare, 1986).

At the time we were studying our own files, we found several dozen cases of reactivated or exacerbated CSR, though more have come to our attention since, as veterans with delayed-onset PTSD sought treatment. Thirty-five of these cases were evaluated by a team of four mental health professionals, including myself (Solomon, Garb, et al., 1987). The cases were then placed along a spectrum ranging in severity from very mild to extreme behavioral and functional disability.

Uncomplicated Reactivations

At one end of the spectrum are what might be called *classic reactivations*. Twenty-three percent of the veterans in question seemed to have completely recovered from their Yom Kippur combat reactions. They were virtually symptom-free between the wars. The first indication that all was not well came with their combat stress reactions in the Lebanon War, which were generally precipitated by a threatening incident directly reminiscent of their Yom Kippur experience. For example, one tank driver sustained his first CSR in the Yom Kippur War when a grenade that was thrown into his armored personnel carrier (APC) killed all the crew members except himself, and his second reaction in Lebanon when one of the tanks in a convoy he was in sustained a similar direct hit.

The remainder of the cases, which constitute about three quarters of our sample, are more aptly termed *exacerbated* PTSD. Here the Yom Kippur stress reaction left more visible residuals, and the veterans continued to suffer from PTSD symptoms of a greater or lesser severity. Symptoms became intensified during reserve duty, and the call-up notice to Lebanon provoked considerable anticipatory anxiety. Moreover, these men were sufficiently vulnerable for their second reactions to have been triggered by an incident unrelated to their Yom Kippur trauma and, in many cases, one that did not pose a direct or immediate danger. The exacerbated PTSD cases can be subdivided into the following three groups.

Heightened Vulnerability

The first group (51%) consists of men who suffered from mild, diffuse PTSD symptoms which did not interfere with their day-to-day functioning, and from heightened sensitivity to military stimuli. During reserve duty, they tended to be tense and withdrawn and to have other stress symptoms, such as nausea, depression, and the like; but as long as their tours of duty were uneventful, they functioned adequately. Their residual or subclinical PTSD developed into a full-blown syndrome when they were exposed in the Lebanon War to a direct military threat, often similar to that which had provoked their Yom Kippur breakdowns.

Moderate Generalized Sensitivity

Further along the spectrum are veterans who showed moderate generalized sensitivity in their civilian as well as in their military lives (9%). They suffered from sleep disturbances, nightmares, irritability, and uncontrollable outbursts of anger, which somewhat impaired their functioning. To cope with their distress, some resorted to drugs and alcohol, others to phobic responses. There were casualties, for example, who refused to ride on public buses, where terrorists might attack, others who shied away from dark places, and yet others who did everything in their power to avoid contact with weapons, tanks, and other military accoutrements even while they were in reserve duty. During the Lebanon War, the men in this group went to the front but soon developed CSR in response to relatively minor military stimuli, and many were discharged before they saw actual combat.

Severe Generalized Sensitivity

The most seriously ill veterans (17%) suffered from severe generalized sensitivity throughout the entire interwar period. Their lives were dominated by their PTSD, and their behavior was so bizarre and phobic that even though they are still being listed on the IDF's active roster, it could only be regarded as an oversight. There were men in this group who kept guns under their beds or who walked down the street keeping their eyes open for places that would serve for hiding in case of a terrorist attack. For such veterans, the mere arrival of the call-up order to Lebanon brought on an immediate and severe stress reaction. Many of them never saw combat or even reached the front before having their second stress reaction.

What should be emphasized is that all the casualties identified with reactivated or exacerbated PTSD in Lebanon had put a great deal of effort into their functioning in the 9 years following the first reaction, and generally succeeded. By selectively utilizing such psychological coping mechanisms as repression, denial, and avoidance in relation to their experiences, most of them married, started families, and kept down jobs—some even did very well professionally. None were hospitalized. All continued to serve in the reserves, despite the fact that their symptoms were intensified in the presence of military stimuli. Many hid their symptoms from their friends, families, and army commanders.

Their second reactions revealed the psychological damage that the first breakdowns had created, and deepened it. In general, there were more symptoms following the second reaction than the first, and the symptoms were more intense and debilitating (Solomon et al., 1987). Veterans who had become withdrawn and antisocial after their first reaction tended to become even more immersed in themselves after the second. Men who had been short-tempered and impatient after one CSR became violent after two; those who had already been violent tended to strike out even more. Many second-time casualties who had previously functioned without medication now required it; those who had previously overcome their anxieties so as to serve in the reserves could no longer bear to be in a military environment; and those who had previously been able to hide their symptoms could no longer keep them under cover.

Delayed PTSD

Psychiatric consequences of trauma sometimes are, or seem to be, delayed. Delayed onset can be said to occur when an individual at first appears to respond adaptively to traumatic stress but then develops symptoms after an asymptomatic latency period (see Christenson *et al.*, 1981; Figley, 1978; Van Dyke, Zilberg, & McKinnon, 1985). Delayed PTSD has been described among World War II veterans (Archibald & Tuddenham, 1965), concentration camp survivors (Chodoff, 1962), and Vietnam veterans (Laufer, Gallops, & Frey-Wouters, 1984). At the same time, the validity of this diagnosis has been questioned as some clinicians claimed that malingering, factitious symptoms, drug abuse, and precombat psychopathology were mistakenly diagnosed as delayed PTSD (Atkinson, Henderson, & Sparr, 1982; Sparr & Pankrant, 1983). Others (Pary, Turns, & Tobias, 1986) argued that the time lapse was not a true latency period since there were usually unacknowledged and untreated residual symptoms. The identification, rather than the onset, was delayed.

The many difficulties of carrying out retrospective research with a large, mobile, and dispersed population are often compounded by veterans' reluctance to cooperate. Several unique characteristics such as Israel's small size, the fact that most men continue to serve in the army after the war, and the IDF psychiatric register allowed for this study.

For the present study we utilized our psychiatric register which contains clinical information on all CSR casualties treated in IDF mental health outpatient clinics. Out of several hundred veterans who applied for treatment with combat-related disorders at least 6 months after the Lebanon War, 150 were selected at random and carefully reviewed by our research team, which consisted of four experienced IDF clinicians. Each clinician in the research team reviewed each file to confirm the diagnosis of PTSD and to establish the time of onset. Both PTSD diagnosis and delayed onset were confirmed using DSM-III criteria (for more details, see Solomon, Kotler, Shalev, & Lin, 1989).

Assessment of the files revealed a spectrum of symptoms ranging in intensity, severity, time of onset, and duration. Surprisingly, delayed PTSD was not the most common category, but, on the contrary, the least common among the combat-related disorders. Specifically, five categories were delineated: (1) delayed-onset PTSD (10%), (2) delayed help-seeking for chronic PTSD (40%), (3) exacerbation of subclinical PTSD (33%), (4) reactivation (13%), and (5) other disorders (4%).

Exacerbation of Subclinical PTSD

Of the sample, 33% experienced exacerbation of subclinical PTSD. These individuals were traumatized on the front in 1982 and suffered uninterruptedly from *mild* residual PTSD symptoms until accumulated tensions or exposure to subsequent adversity, either military or civilian, resulted in a full-blown PTSD syndrome. Reserve duty was the major military trigger. Other triggers included such life events as marriage and the birth of a child. The veterans in this group sought professional help when their subclinical symptoms were exacerbated.

Delayed Help-Seeking for Chronic PTSD

Of the sample, 40% were already suffering from *chronic PTSD* which the DSM-III defines as PTSD having a 6-month or longer duration, when they sought psychiatric help. Unlike the soldiers in the previous group who had mild, subclinical symptoms throughout the so-called latency period, these subjects suffered from the full-blown syndrome right from around the time they fought in Lebanon. They sought help not when an external trigger exacerbated their symptoms, but when they could no longer bear their distress usually during reserve duty. These soldiers put a great deal of effort into containing a relatively severe and disruptive disturbance before they finally gave up trying to cope with it on their own. Not infrequently, treatment was initiated by a family member who could no longer endure the pressure that the casualty's symptoms created.

Delayed-Onset PTSD

Ten percent of our sample, consisting of soldiers who came through the Lebanon War with no apparent psychiatric disturbance, were asymptomatic and functioned well during and for some time after the war. The latency period lasted from several weeks to several years. Then following exposure to stressful stimuli, their latent disturbance surfaced and they applied for treatment.

Other Psychiatric Disorders

Four percent of the soldiers had mild, transient, prewar psychiatric disturbances. They sought help for underlying problems which were either triggered or colored by their war experiences, but which were not originally induced by military events.

Reactivation

Of the sample, 13% showed reactivation of an earlier CSR episode. These veterans were also asymptomatic for a certain period following their participation in the Lebanon War. Most of them experienced a reawakening of their earlier trauma in connection with threatening military stimuli, such as a call-up to the reserves or a change in military unit. In other cases there was no single trigger but rather the accumulated stress of repeated military exposure to both actual warfare and periodic reserve duty.

In general, our results showed that the genuinely delayed onset of CSR was quite rare in our sample. By far the most prevalent phenomenon was delayed help-seeking for ongoing combat-induced disorders of various degrees of severity. The relatively low rates of delayed PTSD can be attributed to the relatively short follow-up period. It is possible that a longer follow-up of our sample would reveal a higher rate of delayed PTSD following a longer latency period and with aging.

These findings should be considered in light of the social context in which the traumatic event took place. In Vietnam, where the highest rates of delayed PTSD were reported, the wide use of drugs and alcohol may have masked immediate CSR. In Lebanon, however, substance abuse was relatively rare among Israeli troops and did not play a significant role in masking or delaying distress.

Another major contextual difference has to do with the dead and the consolation of the bereaved, which bring comfort and relief that help survivors to complete the mourning process. In the Holocaust, the Nazis pointedly disallowed these rites as part of their overall attempt to dehumanize their victims. In Vietnam, the rites of mourning were not observed on account of the relatively long tours of duty (1 year) and the fact that the soldiers were far from home. It might be that the unresolved grief of both Holocaust survivors and Vietnam veterans contributed to their subsequent vulnerability wherein reminders of their loss or other stressors would more readily trigger a reaction at a later date.

In Lebanon, on the other hand, as in other Israeli wars, the IDF made a concerted and well-organized effort to encourage the full mourning process. Every possible effort was made to evacuate the dead and bring them to burial in Israel; soldiers knew that nobody would be abandoned on the battlefield; and a special Rabbinical unit was in charge of seeing to the proper rites. Soldiers were routinely given leave to attend funerals and pay consolation calls. The ability to mourn and resolve their grief may have made the soldiers in our sample less vulnerable to the triggering effect of subsequent stressors.

From a different point of view, Horowitz and Solomon (1978) suggested that delayed onset may occur only after circumstances allow the individual to sufficiently relax his defenses. Both the long, 1-year tours of duty in Vietnam and the constant, unalleviated danger of the Holocaust made it extremely unsafe for people to down their guard during the events themselves. In Israel, on the other hand, wars are fought very close to home, allowing soldiers frequent home leaves. It may be that the warmth, comfort, and security of the home environment enabled repressed traumatic contents to surface while the soldiers were still serving in the army.

Furthermore, for the veterans of Lebanon, homecoming at the end of the war was by and large a positive event. Although public opinion on the war was divided, the men who had fought it were welcomed back with respect and affection as brave sons who had risked their lives in defense of the country. For both Vietnam veterans and Holocaust survivors, however, the postwar periods continued to be traumatic. Not only were Vietnam veterans denied a hero's welcome, but they came back to a country that had disowned them, to mass antiwar demonstrations. As for Holocaust survivors, they had no place to come back to. Most of their families and communities had been exterminated, their homes and property had been appropriated, and the communities where they had once lived were hostile and rejecting.

Then, when many of them finally immigrated to new countries, they had to overcome substantial adversity in rebuilding their lives. In both these groups, the accumulation of stress may have eventually led to the delayed onset of their latent disorder.

Conclusions

Our studies show that while many combatants cope well with the terrors of war, some of them do not fare as well and they suffer a psychological breakdown. We found the clinical manifestations of this breakdown to be labile and polymorphic, as had been previously suggested on the basis of clinical observations. It is extremely difficult to study immediate reactions in real time—that is, when traumatic events are actually taking place. Our study therefore makes a unique contribution.

The main focus of our work has been to follow-up the long-term effects of combat stress reaction. Our findings show that the war leaves quite marked stress residues among combatants. Moreover, for those soldiers who sustain a CSR, it appears that the war does not end when they cease to be exposed to the traumatic event. Many of these veterans suffer from a variety of posttraumatic residues that include—but are not limited to—PTSD. On the whole, we observed a decline in specifically trauma-related symptomatology over time, whereas general psychiatric symptomatology remained stable and was accompanied by impaired functioning at home, at work, and with friends, and by an increase in somatic complaints. We may summarize by stating that the war that took place outside becomes internalized and continues to cast a shadow on the lives of many posttraumatic veterans.

The harsh Israeli reality that exposes many men to more than one war can extract a heavy price, especially from those who sustained a CSR and recovered sufficiently to participate in combat again. Our studies show not a "corrective emotional experience," but rather a deepening of trauma. In cases of reactivated PTSD, a second trauma is more severe and more limiting than a first.

Another clinical aspect that we examined was the delayed syndrome. Results showed that those soldiers who return home from the war and resume their lives apparently unimpaired, only to develop a disorder at a later date, are actually a small minority of those who apply for treatment. In most cases, it was not the disorder that was delayed but the help-seeking. This pattern of avoiding treatment and postponing help-seeking, until the point of severe crisis, is in our estimation related to sociocultural factors. Israeli society gives less legitimacy to seeking treatment for emotional problems than does American society, for example, and this is especially true in regard to combat-related emotional disorders. In Israel, where masculinity is strongly tied to military service, psychiatric injury in the army is perceived as a painful and shameful failure. The issue of untreated PTSD has received only limited attention in the scientific literature. Future research, therefore, should follow-up untreated populations and document their coping in the community and its clinical outcome.

In summary, our studies contribute to a growing body of knowledge regarding the consequences of trauma. It would be wise to remember the words of Mangelsdorff (1985) and to do our utmost so that this knowledge will not be forgotten by the time of the next catastrophe. Regrettably, we are unable to put an end to war, but what we can do is to try and learn as much as we can about the many detrimental effects of trauma, in order to inform policy planning and clinical practice for the purpose of reducing the suffering caused by human violence.

References

American Psychiatric Association. (1980). *Diagnostic and statistical manual of mental disorders* (3rd ed.). Washington, DC: Author.

Archibald, H. C., & Tuddenham, R. D. (1965). Persistent stress reaction after combat. *Archives of General Psychology, 12*, 475–481.

Atkinson, R. M., Henderson, R. G., & Sparr, L. F. (1982). Assessment of Vietnam veterans for post-traumatic stress disorder in Veterans Administration disability claims. *American Journal of Psychiatry, 139*, 118–1121.

Block, M., & Zautra, A. (1981). Satisfaction and distress in a community: A test of the effects of life events. *American Journal of Community Psychology 9*, 165.

Borus, J. F. (1973). Re-entry II: "Making it" back in the States. *American Journal of Psychiatry, 130*, 850–854.

Burgess, A. W., & Holmstrom, C. C. (1974). Rape trauma syndrome. *American Journal of Psychiatry, 131*, 981–986

Carroll, E. M., Rueger, D. B., Foy D. W., & Donahoe, C. P. (1985). Vietnam combat veterans with post-traumatic stress disorders: Analysis of marital and cohabitation adjustment. *Journal of Consulting and Clinical Psychology, 94*, 329–337.

Cavenar, J. O., & Nash, J. L. (1976). The effects of combat on the normal personality: War neurosis in Vietnam returnees. *Comprehensive Psychiatry, 17*, 647–653.

Center for Disease Control: Vietnam Experience Study. (1988). Health status of Vietnam veterans. 1: Psychosocial characteristics. *Journal of the American Medical Association, 259*, 2701–2702.

Chodoff, P. C. (1962). Late effects of the concentration camp syndrome. *Archives of General Psychiatry, 8*, 323–342.

Christenson, R. M., Walker, J. L., Ross, D. R., & Malthie, A. A. (1981). Reactivation of traumatic conflicts. *American Journal of Psychiatry, 138*, 984–985.

Coleman, J. C., Burcher, J. N., & Carson, R. C. (1980). *Abnormal psychology and modern life* (6th ed.). Glenview, IL: Scott, Foresman.

Davidson, S. (1979). Massive psychic traumatization and social support. *Journal of Psychosomatic Research 23*, 395–401.

Derogatis, L. (1977). *The SCL—90 manual: Scoring, administration, and procedure for the SCL-90.* Baltimore: Johns Hopkins University, School of Medicine.

De Fazio, V. J., Rustin, S. X., & Diamond, A. (1975). Symptom development in Vietnam era veterans. *American Journal of Orthopsychiatry, 45*, 158–163.

Egendorf, A., Kadushin, C., & Laufer, R. (1981). *Legacies of Vietnam—comparative adjustment of veterans and their peers.* New York: Center for Policy Research.

Eitinger, L. (1969). Psychosomatic problems in concentration camp survivors. *Journal of Psychosomatic Research, 13*, 183–189.

Engel, G. H. (1968). A life setting conductive to illness: The giving in-giving up complex. *Annual International Review of Medicine, 69*, 293–300.

Epstein, S. (1983). Natural healing processes of the mind: Graded stress inoculation as an inherent coping mechanism. In D. Meichenbaum & M. E. Yarenko (Eds.), *Stress reduction and prevention* (pp. 39–66). New York: Plenum Press.

Faltus, F. J., Sirota, A. D., Parsons, J., Daamen, M., & Schare, M. L. (1986). Exacerbation of post-traumatic stress disorder symptomatology in Vietnam veterans. *Military Medicine, 151*, 648–649.

Figley, C. R. (1978). Psychosocial adjustment among Vietnam veterans: An overview of the research. In C. R. Figley (Ed.), *Stress disorders among Vietnam veterans: Theory, research, and treatment* (pp. 57–70). New York: Brunner/Mazel.

Gleser, G. C., Green, B., & Winget, C. (1981). *Prolonged psychosocial effects of a disaster: A study of the Buffalo Creek.* New York: Academic Press.

Glover, H. (1984). Survivor guilt and the Vietnam veteran. *Journal of Nervous and Mental Diseases, 172*, 393–397.

Grinker, R. P. (1945). *Men under stress.* Philadelphia: Blakiston.

Haley, S. A. (1974). When the patient reports atrocities. *Archives of General Psychiatry, 30*, 191–196.

Horowitz, M. J. (1982). Psychological processes induced by illness, injury, and loss. In T. Millon, C. Green, & R. Meagher (Eds.), *Handbook of clinical health psychology* (pp. 53–68). New York: Plenum Press.

Horowitz, M. J. & Solomon, G. F. (1978). Delayed stress response syndromes in Vietnam veterans. In C. R. Figley (Ed.), *Stress disorders among Vietnam veterans: Theory, research, and treatment* (pp. 269–280). New York: Brunner/Mazel.

Horowitz, M. J. Wilner, N., & Alvarez, W. (1979). Impact of event scale: A measure of subjective stress. *Psychosomatic Medicine, 41*, 209–218.

Kadushin, C., & Boulanger, G. (1981). *Legacies of Vietnam: Comparative adjustment of veterans and their peers* (Vol. 4). New York: Center for Policy Research.

Kardiner, A. (1947). *War stress and neurotic illness.* New York: Paul B. Hoeber.

Kormos, H. R. (1978). The nature of combat stress. In C. R. Figley (Ed.), *Stress disorders among Vietnam veterans: Theory, research, and treatment* (pp. 3–22). New York: Brunner/Mazel.

Lindemann, E. (1944). Symptomatology and management of acute grief. *American Journal of Psychiatry, 101*, 141–148.

Laufer, R. S., Gallops, M. S., & Frey-Wouters, E. (1984). War stress and post-war trauma. *Journal of Health and Social Behavior, 25*, 65–85.

Mangelsdorff, A. D. (1985). Lessons learned and forgotten: The need for prevention and mental health interventions in disaster preparedness. *Journal of Community Psychology, 13*, 239–257.

Pary, R., Turns, D., & Tobias, C. R. (1986). A case of delayed recognition of post-traumatic stress disorder. *American Journal of Psychiatry, 143*, 941.

Rahe, R. H., Gunderson, E., & Arthur, C. R. (1970). Demographic and psycho-social factors in acute illness reporting. *Journal of Chronic Disease, 23*, 245–255.

Roberts, W. R., Penk, W. E., & Gearing, M. L. (1982). Interpersonal problems of Vietnam combat veterans with post-traumatic stress disorders: Analysis of marital and cohabitating adjustment.

Rubin, R. T., Gunderson, E., & Arthur, C. R. (1972). Life stress and illness patterns in the U.S. Navy: Environmental, demographic, and prior life change variables in reaction to illness onset in naval aviators during combat cruise. *Psychosomatic Medicine, 34,* 445–452.

Solomon, Z. (1989). A three-year prospective study of PTSD in Israeli combat veterans. *Journal of Traumatic Stress, 2,* 59–73.

Solomon, Z., & Mikulincer, M. (1987a). Combat stress reaction, PTSD, and social adjustment—A study of Israeli veterans. *Journal of Nervous and Mental Disease, 175*(5), 277–285.

Solomon, Z., & Mikulincer, M. (1987b). Combat stress reactions, post-traumatic stress disorder and somatic complaints among Israeli soldiers. *Journal of Psychosomatic Research, 31*(1), 131–137.

Solomon, Z., Garb, R., Bleich, A., & Grupper, D. (1987). Reactivation of post-traumatic stress disorder. *American Journal of Psychiatry, 144,* 51–55.

Solomon, Z., Mikulincer, M., & Jakob, B.R. (1987). Exposure to recurrent comat stress: Combat stress reactions among Israeli soldiers in the 1982 Lebanon war. *Psychological Medicine, 17,* 433–440.

Solomon, Z., Kotler, M., Shalev, A., & Lin, R. (1989). Delayed onset PTSD among Israeli veterans of the 1982 Lebanon war. *Psychiatry, 52,* 428–436.

Solomon, Z., Mikulincer, M., & Benbenishty, R. (1989). Combat stress reaction—Clinical manifestations and correlates. *Military Psychology, 1,* 35–47.

Sparr, L., & Pankratz, L. D. (1983). Factitious post-traumatic stress disorder. *American Journal of Psychiatry, 140,* 1016–1019.

Stauffer, S. A., Lumsdaine, A. A., & Lumsdaine, M. H. (1949). *The American soldier, Vol. III: Combat and its aftermath.* Princeton: Princeton University Press.

Titchner, J. L. (1986). Post-traumatic decline: A consequence of unresolved destructive drives. In C. R. Figley (Ed.), *Trauma and its wake. Vol II: Traumatic stress—theory, research, and intervention.* New York: Brunner/Mazel.

Titchener, J. L., & Kapp, F. (1976) Family and character change at Buffalo Creek. *American Journal of Psychiatry, 133,* 295–299.

Titchener, J. L., & Ross, W. D. (1974). Acute or chronic stress as determinents of behavior, character, and neurosis. In S. Arieti & E. B. Brody (Eds.), *Adult clinical psychiatry: American handbook of psychiatry.* New York: Basic Books.

Van Dyke, C., Zilberg, N. J., & McKinnon, J. A. (1985). Post-traumatic stress disorder: A thirty-year delay in World War II veterans. *American Journal of Psychiatry, 142,* 1070–1073.

Weiner, A., Gerber, I., Baltin, D., & Arkin, A. M. (1975). The process and phenomenology of bereavement. In I. Gerber, A. Weiner, A. H. Kutscher, D. Peretz, & A. C. Carr (Eds.), *Bereavement: Its psychological aspects.* New York: Columbia University Press.

Williams, C. M. (1980). The veteran system—With a focus on women partners: Theoretical considerations, problems, and treatment strategies. In T. Williams (Ed.), *Post-traumatic stress disorders of Vietnam veterans* (pp. 93–124). OH: Disabled American Veterans.

Wilson, J. P. (1978). *Identity, ideology, and crisis: The Vietnam veteran in transition.* OH: Disabled American Veterans.

Worthington, E. R. (1977). The Vietnam-era veteran, anomia, and adjustment. *Military Medicine, 142,* 123–134.

CHAPTER 28

Psychiatric Morbidity Due to War in Northern Sri Lanka

Daya J. Somasundaram

Introduction

The psychological sequelae to war and other types of civilian violence have not been adequately assessed despite rapid advances is recent years. Admission rates to mental hospitals and suicide rates were reported to have dropped during times of war, as in the Franco-Prussian War of 1870 (Legrand du Saulle, 1871, cited in Lyons, 1971); World War I (Emzlie, 1915; Lyons, 1971; Smith, 1916–1917, cited in Lyons, 1971); the Spanish Civil War (Miru, 1939); and World War II (Dohan, 1966; Lewis, 1942; Odegaard, 1954). However, during World War II, there was a slight increase in the relative incidence of neurotic reactions in England (Lewis, 1942), and a marked increase among males of acute psychotic reactions in Norway (Odegaard, 1954), and of schizophrenia in the United States (Dohan, 1966). With respect to civilian violence, there was no increase in admissions to mental hospitals following the racial riots in Kuala Lumpur during 1979 (Tan & Simmons, 1973) and in the civil war in Lebanon during 1975–1976 (Nasr, Racy, & Flaherty, 1983), but there was a "rebound" increase in outpatient attendance. In reviewing the studies on the effects of civil violence in Northern Ireland, Curran (1988) concluded that "judging from hospital referrals and admission data, suicide and attempted-suicide rates, the practices of psychoactive drug prescriptions, and community based studies, the campaign of terrorist violence does not seem to have resulted in any obvious increase in psychiatric morbidity." The usual explanation given for this apparent benign effect of war on society as opposed to soldiers is that, in times of war,

culture comes together against a common foe and this united purpose and cohesiveness protects against "mental breakdown" (Curran, 1988; Lyons, 1979). Building on Durkheim's (1951) original observation on the reduction in suicide rates during war, some have postulated that the opportunity to "externalize aggressive behavior" during civilian violence reduces the incidence of suicide and depression, which are believed to be a result of aggression turned inward (Lyons, 1972), and that despite adverse effects on a small minority of unlucky victims, there is a "state of rebound psychological well-being in the rest of the community" (Curran, 1988).

Limitations of Previous Research on War Stress Effects

There were, of course, several methodological shortcomings in these early studies that should be considered before drawing any definitive conclusions about the psychological consequences of war. First of all, it must be realized that it is extremely difficult to carry out dispassionate, empirical, scientific analysis during conditions of war. Priorities would dictate that more urgent survival issues take precedence. As Lifton (1967) noted after the atomic bombing of Hiroshima, research workers were so struck by the depth of human suffering experienced that they ceased their studies and dedicated themselves to much needed welfare programs. In addition, the general chaos and disruption would mean that the mental health staff and other services were disorganized, understaffed, and functioning irregularly, if at all. Moreover, the population itself would be in a state of tension and fear, perhaps on the move as refugees or seeking temporary shelter and generally not available or willing to be studied, not to mention the risk involved in carrying out such "nonessential" tasks. Second, gross admission rates to mental hospitals may not be the best

Daya J. Somasundaram • Department of Psychiatry, University of Jaffna, Jaffna, Sri Lanka.

International Handbook of Traumatic Stress Syndromes, edited by John P. Wilson and Beverley Raphael. Plenum Press, New York, 1993.

indicator of psychiatric morbidity caused by war. As Lewis (1942) pointed out, "It is not easy to decide whether a mental disturbance—neurotic or otherwise—is directly attributable to war conditions." Apart from difficulties in etiological attribution, there are bound to be many confounding variables, not least because of the secondary stressor effects of war itself—displacement, separation from family, unemployment, malnourishment, epidemics, infection, injuries, and bereavement. It must be remembered that the majority of admissions to mental hospitals, at least in third world countries, are for psychoses (Ihezue, 1983). Such major psychoses as schizophrenia have a relatively constant incidence of onset and prevalence rates all over the world (Cooper, 1978) and could not be expected to be affected by such short-term stresses as war. Psychological trauma can be expected to increase the incidence of neurotic illnesses, which may present at outpatient clinics, general practice, indigenous and other alternate treatment centers, or as unrecognized psychosomatic conditions. Another common problem with war conditions is disruption of transport and problems of security for patients traveling to reach psychiatric services. In times of war and other disasters, physical problems of injury, safety, shelter, and basic survival will take precedence over emotional problems which may be ignored or supressed by the patient. Furthermore, the emotionally unstable and vulnerable may be the first to evacuate from areas of threatened trouble, leaving the more resilient population behind. Conversely, medical priorities may dictate that mental complaints not be encouraged or entertained while acute physical problems are the focus of triage. Thus, in many ways, the war situation will act to reduce the apparent number of patients seen by mental health workers. There may then be the well-documented phenomena of "rebound" increase in psychological problems once the acute emergency of a war is over.

The only way to establish the psychological sequelae to war is by population surveys with sensitive, valid, and reliable instruments. But studies in the aftermath of disasters, carried out in a variety of settings, have brought to light the immense problem of posttraumatic stress disorders (PTSD) (Raphael, 1986). In addition, the development of refined techniques for assessing posttraumatic reactions has meant that more sensitive research was possible. Thus, after World War I, only 2% of the combatants were thought to have had posttraumatic neuroses, whereas the figure had risen to 10% by World War II (Coleman, 1975), and 50% for the Vietnam War veterans (Walker, 1981; Wilson, 1988). A limited study of Falklands War veterans (see Chapter 25, in this volume, for a discussion) reported 65% with posttraumatic stress disorders (Orner, 1988). The development of such instruments as the General Health Questionnaire (GHQ) (Goldberg, 1972), rating scales such as the Impact of Event Scale (IES) (Horowitz, 1986), and operational diagnoses, such as the DSM-III-R PTSD (American Psychiatric Association, 1987) has meant more reliable and valid assessment of subjects (see Chapters 14 and 15, in this volume).

It should be noted that many of the studies were not carried out in situations approaching "complete" war conditions which include invasion and occupation. Death and destruction, life-threat and injury, displace-

ment, social chaos, separation, loss, and the like, are the realities of war that makes for devastation and human misery on unprecedented scales (Wilson, 1988). The existing life-events schedules used to assess the degree of stress are inadequate when applied to war stresses (Curran, 1988). Studies of the psychological consequences to Hiroshima victims and to the Holocaust survivors make abundantly clear the reality of the extreme stress of war. Thus, the "Survivor Syndrome" consisting of "recognizable pattern of chronic anxiety, depression, social withdrawal, nightmares, sleep disturbances, somatic complaints, and, often, fatigue, emotional lability, loss of initiative, and general personal, sexual, and social maladaption" have been found in a large percentage of those who survived the Nazi concentration camps and Hiroshima (Raphael, 1986; Wilson, Harel, & Kahana, 1988). Studies focusing on particular groups, such as children in Mozambique (Richman, Kanji, & Zinkin, 1988), Latin America (Allodi, 1980), and the Philippines (Children's Rehabilitation Center, 1986), or in torture victims (Somnier & Genefke, 1986) show the long-term consequences of war. Forty years after World War II, 71% of a sample of Australian veterans who had been Japanese prisoners of war and 46% of combatants who had served in the Asian and Pacific theaters were found to have significant psychiatric morbidity, namely anxiety disorders, depression, and alcohol abuse and dependence (Tennant, Goulston, & Dent, 1986). Long-term, transgenerational effects on the children of Holocaust survivors and World War II combat veterans have been described (Coleman, 1975; Rosenheck, 1986). Thus, the psychological consequences of war cannot be considered inconsequential by any means.

Cultural Limitations in Understanding Psychiatric Effects of War and Violence

One has to consider the perceptions and the motives of the researchers themselves and their attitudes toward violence and war. Invariably the professionals allowed to conduct the studies are part of the administrative system or establishment that is waging war. In such acute emergencies, when the very existence of a society or a cherished system is threatened, the need of the hour is to maintain public morale, to continue the public's belief and faith in the system that is operating and in the political ideology for the violence or the warfare. As Lewis so clearly put it:

Attention to signs of impaired morale in the population concerns itself chiefly with the premonitory and early signs of neurosis, such as are shown by people who cannot talk of anything else but the bombs for weeks after a raid; paranoid people who suspect strangers of being spies; depressive pessimists who see no chance of their town reviving after all the destruction; anxious worriers about the imminence of the next raid. . . . Investigations of all these matters is desirable since they affect public safety and public health. [He concludes after a survey conducted in Britain during World War II] Air-raids have not been responsible for any striking increase in neurotic illness. (Lewis, 1942)

Anxiety and other emotional problems that would be considered abnormal in other times, are classified as "normal anxiety," "appropriate to the situation," the "fear we all have," and the like. Obviously, what is pathological is the war and not the reactions to it. But awareness of the psychological effects of war may change attitudes and make people question the war effort. These "normal" reactions may in fact reflect the true psychiatric morbidity to war. Furthermore, many of the psychological studies on war have been by a generation of western or western-trained workers, who come from a culture where aggression has a positive value, and violence and war is considered inevitable (Sharp, 1978). Thus, the negative consequences of aggression tend to be played down, while the impulses towards such behavior is not strongly condemned, if not encouraged, influencing the "mental set" of the researchers. What is often described as resiliency and adaptiveness is apparent normalcy in a very abnormal situation. The coping process may mask an inestimable strain as well as create a stress of its own which may not become apparent until the burden of coping is lifted (Heskin, 1980).

War as a Disaster

An understanding of the psychological responses to war can be gained through looking at disaster studies. War can be seen as a more severe and prolonged form, or a sequence of repeated disasters overlapping one another and going on indefinitely. For any one village or individual, a particular event, such as a bombing raid or a search-and-destroy operation, could take on the dimensions of a disaster. Raphael wrote in her comprehensive treatise on disasters that

> the greatest death and destruction, loss and grief, dislocation and relocation are associated with the man-made disasters that have occurred through warfare. The slaying of man by man in either direct combat or through sophisticated weaponry bring cruel mutilating injuries and sudden, untimely, and violent deaths. Such deaths bring little opportunity for the healing process of physicians or the healing rituals of grief. And, of course, warfare destroys the houses and habitants, the livelihoods, and even lives of many non-combatants. . . . Mankind's capacity to create psychic trauma through war, to create horrifying forms of warfare, has increased exponentially. (Raphael, 1986, p. 18)

Psychodynamically, war is a form of severe stress that can cause temporary personality decompensation, even in previously stable personalities, leading to transient stress reactions. The decompensation may be acute or sudden as in the case of an individual exposed to an overwhelming experience of death and destruction, such as a bombing; or chronic and gradual, as in the case of a person who has been subjected to being a refugee or living under conditions of constant but unpredictable shelling. Usually, the individual shows good recovery once the stress situation is over, although in some cases there is residual damage to the personality and increased vulnerability to stress. In the case of individuals who are marginally adjusted to begin with or who are

predisposed to mental illness, the war stress may precipitate more serious psychopathology, neurotic or psychotic illness. In others, stress may lead to adaptation and provide the impetus for personality development and increased stress tolerance.

The War in Sri Lanka

My present study is an attempt to show the wide variety of psychological reactions to the stress of war by selecting illustrative case histories to demonstrate the mental processes involved. Unfortunately, some of the shortcomings mentioned previously were unavoidable in this study, owing to the prevailing situation of an ongoing war. From July, 1983 to July, 1987, the civilian population in the North and East of Sri Lanka, which is predominantly Tamil, have been exposed to the stress of a chronic civil war between Tamil militants and the Sri Lanka State. Ethnic conflict between the majority Sinhalese and minority Tamils had been growing for some time before that, resulting in considerable civil strife. The war itself has been characterized by a mixture of civil violence, guerrilla attacks and reprisals, and direct, conventional military fighting. There has also been increasing internal conflict within the Tamil community, resulting in internecine killings between the several Tamil militant groups. Following the signing of an accord between Sri Lanka and India in July, 1987, this area, mainly the Jaffna peninsula, experienced an acute war between the Indian army and the dominant Tamil militant group from October to December, 1987.

The purpose of this chapter, then, is to analyze and record a summary of the psychological sequelae to the various military conflicts during this period in the form of clinical cases who presented to me while I was working in the area. A more detailed description of the psychological causes and effects of the war are reported elsewhere (Somasundaram, 1992).

The psychiatric facilities for the Northern Sri Lanka, serving a catchment population from the Districts of Jaffna (population of 831,112), Mannar (106, 904), Vavuniya (95,904), and Mullaithivu (77,512) (Department of Census and Statistics, 1986) included daily outpatient clinics at the General (Teaching) Hospital in Jaffna and the Base Hospitals in Tellipallai and Point Pedro, and inpatient units of 60 beds at Base Hospital, Tellipallai, and 40 beds at Base Hospital, Point Pedro. As there were no psychiatrists in the Eastern province during this period, a proportion of patients from the Trincomalee District (population 256,790) and some patients from the Batticoloa District (303,899) sought treatment in the North. The clinical material presented here is based on the mental illnesses induced by the prevailing war situation, treated at the psychiatric units functioning in the area, and thus reflect the psychiatric morbidity due to war.

Methodology

Patients seen at the outpatient clinics and those admitted to the inpatient facilities in the North during the period of war, 1983–1988, formed the subject matter of the study. In addition to the overall statistics, representative case histories were selected to illustrate the range of psychiatric disorders that were caused or precipitated by the prevailing war stresses. Although the current situation has, in time, affected the whole local population, including the mentally ill, in one way or another, the sample is chosen from those for whom the war stress played a central, etiological role in their illness. Experience gained from general medical clinics held at refugee camps and some general observations from the period as a whole are also included. In general, the diagnostic categories from the *International Classification of Diseases*—Ninth Revision (ICD-9) (World Health Organization [WHO], 1978) have been used, though patients did not always fit into distinct categories, there being considerable overlap. Thus, a more phenomenological and descriptive approach in the form of case histories has been adopted.

Results and Discussion

Overall Statistics

The admission rates, new cases, and follow-up cases seen at the outpatient clinics at the psychiatric units in Jaffna, Tellipallai, and Point Pedro for the years 1976 to 1986 are given in Table 28.1, whereas the totals for the region as a whole are plotted in Figure 28.1. It is difficult to interpret these data as there are several confounding variables. There would appear to be a general tendency for an increase in admissions and new outpatients, reaching a peak in 1982–1983, and maintained at that level during the actual war years. The improving psychiatric services, changing public attitudes to western psychiatric treatment, together with the increasing stress of ethnic conflict and civil strife, may have influenced this trend. However, the war itself does not seem to have caused a significant increase in admission rates and new or follow-up cases in the outpatient clinics.

The psychiatric facilities in Northern Sri Lanka (see Figure 28.2) markedly improved in 1982 with the setting up of the University Psychiatric Unit. Three consultant psychiatrists with daily outpatient clinics were available. In addition, public attitudes to mental illness has been gradually changing with increasing numbers of patients seeking western psychiatric treatment. These factors would have caused the increase in the use of psychiatric services noted above.

War as a form of severe environmental stress can cause posttraumatic stress disorder, transient stress reactions, neurotic illness but not the major psychotic illnesses, though transient reactive psychoses can be precipitated in those patients with vulnerability to such reactions as will be reported later. The psychoses form the major proportion of admissions (85%) to the inpatient unit (Somasundaram, Yoganathan, Ganesvaran, & Mahadevan, 1985), and the majority of those seen at the outpatient clinics (65%) (Ganesvaran & Rajarajeswaran, 1988), as in other developing countries (Ihezue, 1983). Patients with neurotic illness or stress reactions rarely seek western psychiatric help in our cultural setting. The stigma attached to mental illness would mean that only the more severe, psychotic illnesses would seek western treatment, and that only as a last resort. Leff (1981) pointed out that patients from developing countries lack psychological awareness and tend to "somatize" their psychological problems through bodily complaints. All these patients would seek treatment from hospital outpatient units, general practice, physicians, or the native healers (Shamans). Thus, the current period of stress could not be expected to cause a marked increase in admissions and new cases seen at psychiatric clinics.

It is noteworthy that the peak in admissions and new outpatients was reached in 1982–83, just before the actual war broke out. It is probable that the increasing tension and threat of violence (and occurrence of racial riots elsewhere in the country) because of escalating ethnic conflict may have created more stress. In analyzing the pattern of admission and referral rates following civil violence in Belfast, Fraser (1971) concluded that "stress productive of psychiatric morbidity appears to be maxi-

Table 28.1. Psychiatric Outdoor (Clinic) and Indoor (Ward) Statistics (1976–1986)

| | Tellipallai Hospital | | | Jaffna Hospital | | Point Pedro Hospital | | |
| | Outdoor (clinic) | | Indoor (ward) | Outdoor (clinic) | | Outdoor (clinic) | | Indoor (ward) |
Year	New cases	Follow-up	Admissions	New cases	Follow-up	New cases	Follow-up	Admissions
1976	390	4,154	412	357	10,522	381	n.a.	n.a.
1977	338	6,856	736	326	9,683	210	n.a.	n.a.
1978	446	7,886	754	615	10,496	420	n.a.	628
1979	360	7,463	993	524	7,340	339	n.a.	502
1980	358	5,578	1,072	492	8,728	339	n.a.	462
1981	305	4,879	872	734	6,366	219	n.a.	371
1982	552	4,795	1,352	725	9,079	196	n.a.	326
1983	625	5,786	1,036	983	8,894	178	2,897	316
1984	319	4,022	1,113	884	9,012	168	2,625	371
1985	594	5,980	1,188	865	14,000	178	2,257	264
1986	342	2,919	1,183	748	10,411	180	2,581	372

Note. n.a. = not available.

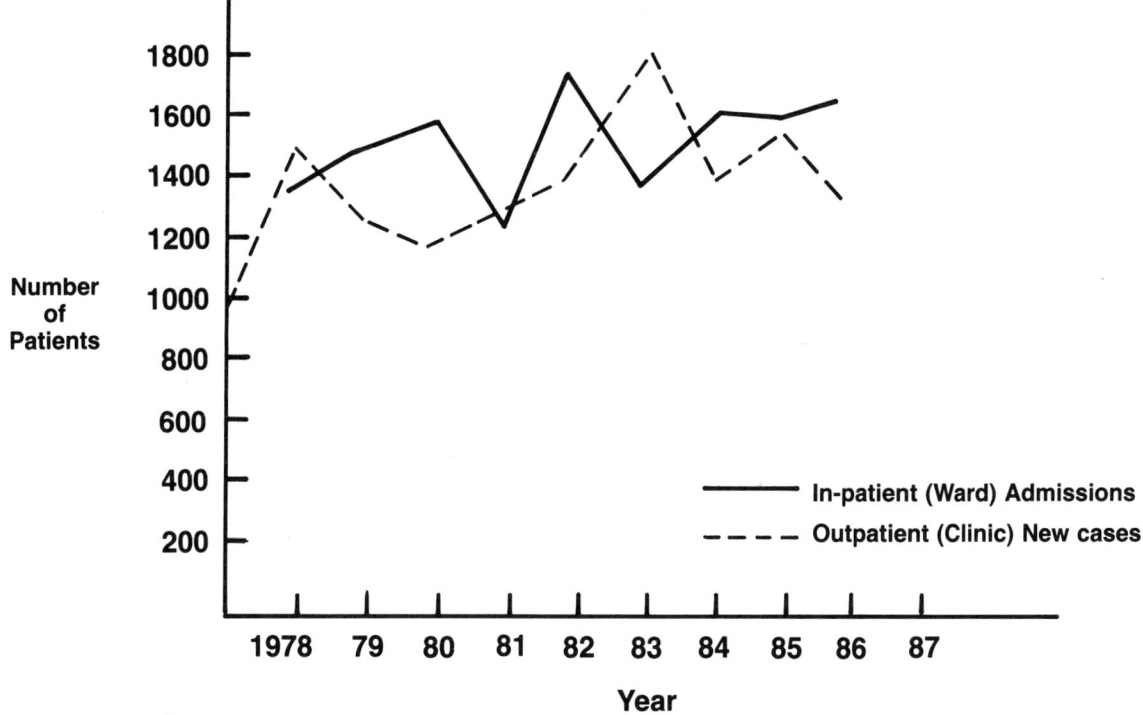

Figure 28.1. Total psychiatric admissions and new cases (clinic), North Sri Lanka (1978–1986).

mal in areas under threat of upheaval or attack, rather than in those areas where there is active combat or direct risk to life and property." Furthermore, stress tends to be much more disruptive initially, whereas prolongation of stress leads to habituation or to adaptation by the organism through defense mechanisms, such as denial or emotional numbing as a form of insulation against outer stress. Thus, there was a high incidence of psychiatric reactions to the first bombing attacks, as described later. In time, people adapted by building air-raid shelters or adopting a philosophical attitude as a form of rationalization. In 1982, it could be observed that a single shooting incident resulted in a tense atmosphere that prevailed for over a month and kept people indoors. By 1986–1987, one could observe people going about their daily routine and passenger buses plying on the very next street while helicopter strafing was in progress nearby. A degree of apathy and ennui was perceptible in the population as a whole toward the end of this period (Somasundaram, 1992).

Acute Stress Reaction

Acute stress reactions are transient reactions to a severely traumatizing experience that usually subside spontaneously once the stress is over or within a few days or weeks. Some common stress factors that were generated by the various military operations are listed in Tables 28.2, 28.3, and 28.4. Tables 28.3 and 28.4 are for relatively short-term acute operations; Table 28.1 reflects more long-term, chronic war stresses. From inspection of the tables it becomes obvious that the brunt of the war

has fallen on the civilian population. A significant phenomenon during the war was the large number of civilians who were displaced—*refugees* as they were referred to locally. During the chronic civil war (see Table 28.1), the number of refugees was estimated at 562,145 or 25% of the *total* local population of 2,084,660 in the North and East of Sri Lanka (Department of Census and Statistics, 1986). Although some refugees would have been from outside the North and the East, others would have emigrated without claiming refugee status.

In relief medical clinics held at refugee camps, the majority of cases, apart from skin conditions (like scabies), gastrointestinal disturbances (like diarrhea and peptic ulcer), and upper respiratory tract infections, were found to suffer from transient stress reactions, reactive depression, and anxiety. They manifested with somatic symptoms, of which the following were common: headache, dizziness, dyspnea, palpitation, chest pain, paresthesias, dyspepsia, and other multiple somatic complaints for which no obvious organic cause could be found. On questioning, sleep disturbances with nightmares, irritability, loss of appetite, fear, and uncertainty were elicited. In some cases, psychological stress was increased by physical complications, such as injury, mutilation, or physical handicap arising from, for example, the loss of a limb.

Flight or fight is the normal neurophysiological reaction of an organism to threatening stimuli. Of these, flight is the common response, particularly when the threat is severe and an escape route is available. Chronic, continuous danger leads people to flee home to seek safe refuge. Refugee status creates a feeling of homelessness and helplessness with loss of traditional

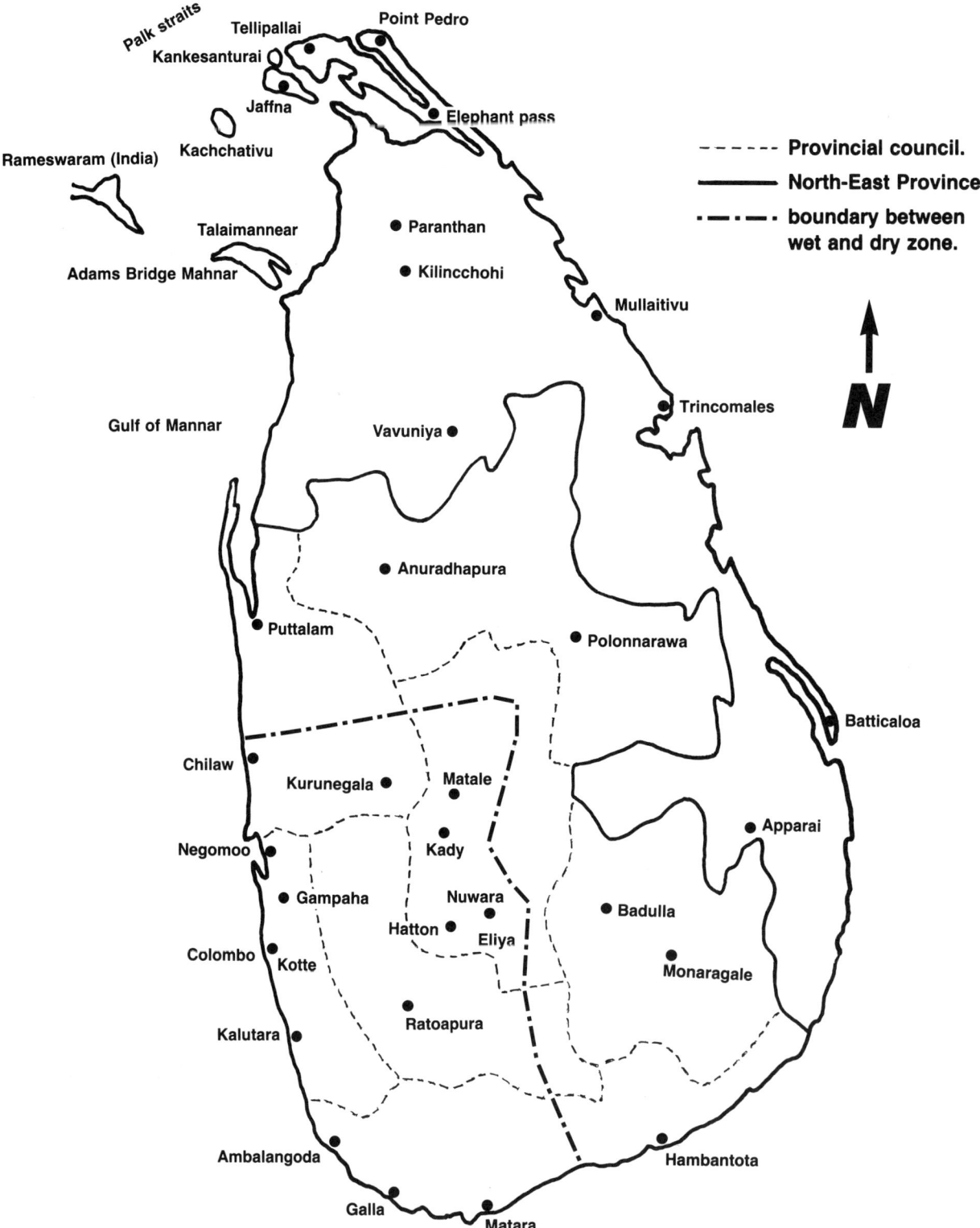

Figure 28.2. Sri Lanka.

Table 28.2. Stress Factors in North and East Sri Lanka (1981–1987) (Sri Lankan Forces)[a]

Description	Year	Months	N	Source[b]
Deaths (caused by ethnic violence)				
Civilians				
Tamils (total)	1981–1987	Up to July 1987	16,994	T.R.R.O.
	1981	Jan.–Dec.	840	H.H.R.
	1982	Jan.–Dec.	1,380	H.H.R.
	1983	Jan.–Dec.	3,670	H.H.R.
	1984	Jan.–Dec.	3,301	H.H.R.
	1985	Jan.–Dec.	2,935	H.H.R.
	1986	Jan.–Dec.	2,803	H.H.R.
Sinhalese	1987	Jan.–June	337	H.H.R.
Combatants				
Security forces	1980–1987	Up to July 1987	689	Sri Lankan government (quoted from Elanadu, Sept. 13, 1987)
Militants (LTTE)	1987	Up to Aug. 1987	631	LTTE (quoted from Uthayan, Aug. 28, 1987)
Missing and disappeared	1985	Jan.–Dec.	529	H.H.R.
	1986	Jan.–Dec.	199	H.H.R.
	1987	Jan.–July	550	T.R.R.O.
Injuries (admission to hospital)	1986	Jan.–Dec.	2,103	H.H.R.
	1987	Jan.–July	3,168	H.H.R.
Refugees				
Internal				
In camps	1987	July 15	110,680	T.R.R.O.
Outside camps	1987	July 15	226,465	T.R.R.O.
External (abroad)				
India	1987	Up to July	150,000	Indian government, Observer (May 16, 1987) estimated
Outside India—Europe	1987		50,000	
Other (Canada, Australia)	1987		25,000	
Total			562,145	
Nonrefugee emigration	No data available			
Arrests	1985	Jan.–Dec.	10,068	H.H.R.
	1986	Jan.–Dec.	36,667	H.H.R.
	1987	Jan.–July	16,905	H.H.R.
Released from detention	1986	Jan.–Dec.	20,336	H.H.R.
camps	1987	Jan.–June	4,936	H.H.R.
Damage to property	1987	Up to July	RS 60,000 Tril	Ronnie De Mel, Minister of Finance (quoted from Elanadu, Aug. 7, 1987)
Houses destroyed in Jaffna	1983–1987	July to July	2,362	
Loss of livelihood	No data available			

[a]Compiled by V. Kamalanathan, Alaveddy Citizen Committee.
[b]Reliable statistics were difficult to come by during this period. Sources quoted include the Tamil Refugee and Rehabilitation Organization (T.R.R.O.) and the Home for Human Rights (H.H.R.), which are nongovernmental organizations (NGOs) functioning in the North and East. Information was mainly obtained through citizen committees of the area, usually in the form of affidavits from those affected. The T.R.R.O. is headed by a respected academician, K. Sinathamby of the University of Jaffna and the H.H.R. by J. Xavier, attorney-at-law. Newspaper reports are much less reliable. Liberation Tigers of Tamil Elam (LTTE) is the main militant group.

support, collapse of the world they knew, and the regular routine that was the framework of their daily lives. The psychological consequences of displacement begin with the handicaps of the initial trauma with its attendant loss and grief, death and destruction, and other stressors. The immediate needs are safety and shelter which are often sought with relations and friends or in refugee camps. These temporary arrangements, especially if prolonged, can become extremely stressful in themselves (Raphael, 1986). The crowded conditions, sharing of inadequate facilities, inconvenience and poor sanitation, lack of privacy and other activities, concerns and worries of the inmates, ongoing war and the consequent fear and uncertainty, all can produce tensions and conflicts within the refugee population. Thus these multifactorial stressors could be expected to produce considerable psychosocial problems among refugee populations. The finding that patients from developing countries tend to "somatize" their psychological problems (Leff, 1981) could explain the high incidence of

Table 28.3. Operation Liberation in the Vadamarachi Area by Sri Lankan Forces[a]

Description	Year	Month or period	N	Source[b]
Deaths				
Civilians				
Tamils	1987	May to June	600	T.R.R.O.
Sinhalese				
Combatants				
Security forces	1987	May to June	92	H.R.R.
Sri Lankan Army				
Militants	No data available			
Missing and disappeared	1987	May to June	23	H.R.R.
Injuries	1987	May to June	229	T.R.R.O.
Arrests	1987	May to June	9,183	H.R.R.
	1987	May to June	2,673	Government communique, Minister of Defence, Lalith Athulath Mudali
Released	1987	May to June	3,005	H.R.R.
Damage to public property	1987	May to June	4	T.R.R.O.
Damage to private property	1987	May to June	196	T.R.R.O.

[a]Operation Liberation is a short-term, acute military operation that was undertaken by the Sri Lankan Forces to recapture Vadamarchi (Point Pedro).
[b]T.R.R.O. = Tamil Refugee and Rehabilitation Organization; H.R.R. = Home for Human Rights.

psychosomatic complaints reported above. Owing to a lack of awareness of the psychological antecedents of the condition, many patients would have been treated by traditional pharmacological approaches. Most of the patients seen at the refugee clinics made a spontaneous recovery on returning to their homes and ceased to be fearful and tense.

Some patients who presented to the psychiatric unit following acute stress reactions were found to be suffering from recognizable psychiatric disorders that met the traditional diagnostic categories to be discussed later. For example, sudden overwhelming stress was found to produce a more dramatic reaction and bring out underlying psychopathology.

CASE 1—LIFE-THREATENING ATTACK

Mrs. T., aged 65 years, was admitted to the psychiatric unit in Tellipallai in a state of excitement. The history was that she had been normal up to 10 days prior when she had been traveling by boat, the *Kumuthini*, from the Island of Delft. It had been stopped by navy personnel and all aboard were cut by swords and knives. She had seen her son and close kinsmen cut to death in front of her and she received serious cuts. She was treated at the general hospital neurosurgical unit for 10 days. Concussion or head injury had been ruled out, though she had superficial scalp injuries and diminution of vision. During her stay at the neurosurgical unit she had been confused and restless, and was constantly sedated and confined to her room. On discharge her wounds had healed but her mental condition remained disturbed. On admission to the psychiatric unit she was in an extreme state of agitation and highly suicidal—attempting to run and jump into a well. She was dishevelled, shouting, and crying while repeating the names of those who died. She was disoriented as to place and time, though she appeared to know her relations who had brought her. Due to the agitation and restlessness, she was immediately sedated and then put on amitriptyline with chlorpromazine because agi-

tated depression was the preliminary diagnosis. She calmed down while in the ward but continued to get attacks of restless, agitated, and suicidal behavior, though with decreasing frequency. She continued to be disoriented and confused in her general behavior. As she showed improvement and was stable, the relations discharged her early, believing that she would settle down in her familiar surroundings at home in Delft. She is reported to have improved gradually over the months and is able to do work and look after herself, though mild confusional symptoms and diminution of vision persisted.

Anxiety States

Anxiety disorder is basically a fear reaction that has become incapacitating. As fear was the prevalent emotion during this time, anxiety states were very common and could be considered almost "normal" (Miru, 1939) and appropriate under the circumstances. Patients reported intense apprehension, fear, a feeling of impending doom or death, and were found to be tense, edgy, irritable, vigilant, and easily startled. Dyspnea, palpitation, chest pain, choking sensation, sweating, abdominal pain, loose bowels, and increased frequency of micturition were common complaints. Some reported frequent panic attacks particularly during shelling, gunfire or on seeing the army. Children were reported to run and cling to their parents or hide under beds. Many had sleep disturbances, such as difficulty in falling asleep, interrupted sleep, anxiety dreams where they see themselves being injured or chased by the army but are unable to escape, night terrors, and fitful sleep with fatigue on awakening. Patients with previous history of angina pectoris developed anginal pain during these anxiety attacks. It was observed that some instinctively resorted to repeating mantras or short prayers which have been shown to work as relaxation techniques that alleviate anxiety.

Table 28.4. Stress Factors in Operation of the Indian Peace-Keeping Force (IPKF)

Description	Year	Month or period	N	Source[a]
Deaths				
Civilians				
Tamils (Jaffna area)	1987	Oct. to Dec.	1,320	T.R.R.O.
Total	1987–1988	Oct. 1987 to July 1988	1,990	H.R.R.
Other areas	1987	No data available		
Sinhalese	1988	Jan. to July	473	H.R.R.
	1987	Oct. to Dec.	215	H.R.R.
	1988	Jan. to July	126	H.R.R.
Combatants				
Sri Lankan forces	1987	Oct. to Dec.	39	H.H.R.
	1988	Jan. to July	38	H.H.R.
I.P.K.F. forces	1987	Oct. to Dec.	350	*Sunday Times* (Jul. 10, 1988)
Total	1987–1988	Oct. 1987 to July 1988	511	K. C. Pant, Indian Defense Minister (Jul. 28, 1988)
Militants (L.T.T.E.)	1987–1988	Oct. 1987 to July 1988	500	*Sunday Times* (Jul. 10, 1988)
Injuries				
I.P.K.F.	1987–1988	Oct. to July	1,526	K.C. Pant, in Rajya Sabha (Jul. 25, 1988) *Takmil Times* (Aug. 1988)
Captured				
L.T.T.E.	1987–1988	Oct. 1987 to July 1988	2,000	*Sunday Times* (Jul. 10, 1988)
Missing and disappeared				
Jaffna area	1987	Oct. to Dec.	1	H.R.R.
	1988	Jan. to July	11	H.R.R.
Other areas	1988	Jan. to July	49	H.R.R.
Torture	1987	No data available		
	1988	Jan. to July	26	H.R.R.
Injuries	1987	Oct. to Dec.	555	H.R.R.
	1988	Jan. to July	458	H.R.R.
Arrests	1987	Oct. to Dec.	1,667	H.R.R.
Jaffna area	1988	Jan. to July	1,625	H.R.R.
Other areas	1988	Jan. to July	4,343	H.R.R.
Released	1987	Oct. to Dec.	32	H.R.R.
	1988	Jan. to July	1,942	H.R.R.
Damage to property (Jaffna area)	1987	—	3,149	—

[a]Sources quoted include the Tamil Refugees Rehabilitation Organization (T.R.R.O.) and Home for Human Rights (H.H.R.). Information was mainly obtained through Citizen Committees of the area, usually in the form of affidavits from those affected.

Many who presented to the outpatient clinic requesting medical certificates for absence from work were found to be having signs and symptoms of phobic anxiety. Usually these patient had come from outstations and because of some incidents which occured there, were unable or afraid to go back to work. Typically, they reported fear and apprehension on thinking of going back, together with sweating, tremor, insomnia, anorexia, and constant worry. But they were not willing to accept that they had a mental condition and only wanted a note to cover their absence from work. Others developed phobic anxiety when their place of work was directly affected by military activity.

CASE 2—EXPOSURE TO WAR STRESSORS

Dr. S., aged 28 years, was working in a district hospital. The area around the hospital had come under heavy shelling and helicopter strafing and people around the hospital had evacuated to safer places. The hospital had been hit while she was on night duty. She had become very anxious about coming to work and described mounting fear when walking to the hospital. While at work, she was in a constant state of tension and was anxious to finish her work and leave the hospital. Night duty had become very difficult as there was only a skeleton staff and constant sound of explosions around the hospital. Even thinking of coming for night duty caused palpitation, tremor, sweating, loose bowels, and an unbearable dread. Since she was having her first pregnancy, she was worried about her unborn child and feared an abortion. As the situation deteriorated she became depressed and was unable to continue working.

Several patients who had undergone torture presented as severe anxiety states.

CASE 3—TORTURE AND INTERROGATION

Mr. S., aged 24 years, was a computer salesman working in the Middle East who had come home to get registered for marriage. According to his history, on his way back at the Katunayake Airport, after having cleared customs and immigration and while waiting in the departure lounge, he was "taken in" by plain clothes policemen (CID), unknown to his relations who assumed he had boarded the plane and departed. He was taken to the 4th floor in the police headquarters and questioned for three days without sleep or proper food and with frequent assaults. He was later removed to Welikade where he was put in with 70 other detainees in a room. While there, batches of five prisoners were taken to a room and each in turn was made to sit in a chair and a head band with a wire attached to a machine was applied around the temples. A little later the prisoner was seen to have a "fit," the description of which fitted a grand-mal seizure. This "treatment" was repeated for each while the others watched. Altogether he said that he received four such "treatments." At the end of three weeks, he was again taken to the airport to the waiting lounge and allowed to board the plane and proceed as before. On reaching Bombay, he felt too ill to proceed and was warded there and treated mainly for the contusions and bruising due to assault. Later, feeling apprehensive and anxious, he had decided to return to his home and presented at the consultant practice with florid anxiety neurosis. He was treated with anxiolytics and antidepressants and had improved gradually. On follow-up he had migrated to Canada. It is well known that electroconvulsive shock can make an anxiety state worse, or even precipitate it in a predisposed neurotic personality. Interestingly, ECT itself may not be a torture to the individual receiving it, as there is immediate loss of consciousness and amnesia for the event, but may appear frightening to those watching and as torture to those applying it. Thus, future applications could then take on a threatening torture-like quality, despite its effects.

Grief Reaction

Grief reactions were very common; this could be considered the phenomenon of the times in view of the large number of sudden and unexpected deaths (see Tables 28.2, 28.3, and 28.4). Owing to the psychologically traumatizing circumstances surrounding these unnatural deaths of loved ones (the noise, blood, mutilating injuries, pain, lack of medical attention, standing helpless as loved ones suffered and died, not being able to see the body or seeing the bloated and disfigured body, lack of funerals, etc.), there was an increased incidence of the more severe reactions and several with atypical features presented to the psychiatric unit.

CASE 4—THE SHOOTING OF A SPOUSE

Mrs. J., aged 30 years, was an assistant medical practitioner who had recently been married to Mr. J., an engineer. While traveling by passenger coach, Mr. J. had been shot at an army check point and succumbed to his injuries two days later. His wife developed a severe form of typical grief reaction with waves of crying spells and acute sorrow. She had strong guilt feelings over not immediately rushing to the husband's side and helping in his treatment. Further, she felt guilty that she had not stayed with her husband much longer after marriage so that she could have conceived before his death. She developed extreme social withdrawal and was unable to leave her room and meet people. Her symptoms have been very incapacitating, preventing her return to work. Her acceptance of her husband's death and working-through of her grief has been retarded and her recovery slow.

CASE 5—WITNESSING AN ATROCITY

Miss P., aged 18 years, had seen her brother, to whom she was very attached, shot and killed by army personnel in their home compound. The vision of him lying in a pool of blood used to repeatedly intrude into her mind, causing a restless, agitated behavior with crying spells. At times, she used to become extremely paranoid that the army was coming to kill them or that her father was going to hand her over to the army. She was put on antidepressant medication but showed no improvement. Later, characteristic delusions of persecution and auditory hallucination in third person were elicited and a diagnosis of schizophreniform reaction was made. She improved dramatically on phenothiazines and electroconvulsive therapy and continues to do well on follow-up.

CASE 6—THE SHOOTING OF HIS CHILDREN

A middle-aged engineer whose three children and mother-in-law had been pulled out of their homes and *shot dead* on the street by Indian jawans, developed a severe grief reaction with secondary alcoholism. He spent his days in deep sorrow with attacks of crying spells, the pangs of grief buffeting him like waves. His mind was preoccupied with thoughts of his children. He complained of loss of purpose in life with suicidal ruminations. His nights were particularly bad with recurrent nightmares about his children and their suffering, especially his pretty daughter. The soldier had lifted up her frock and shot her through the groin, so that she could not walk and had to drag herself along the road, to finally bleed to death for lack of medical attention. The image of this incident kept recurring in his mind. He said, "She was deeply loved, and I brought her up without a care. And now she had to suffer like this. . . . It is unbearable," and he would break into sobs. Hostility, a feature of typical grief reaction, was apparent in his want for revenge: "I will personally kill those soldiers." His wife, too, was unconsolable and he expressed a fear that she would cry herself to death. Both of them felt that without their children life had lost its meaning. Previously an occasional drinker, he had now started drinking heavily and was in a state of intoxication most of the day and night.

In some cases, multiple deaths of close relations precipitated decompensation. A nurse, previously of jovial personality, developed a severe depressive illness when several of her close relations were killed. She needed intensive treatment before she gradually recovered. A young mother lost her child and then her husband in quick succession to shelling. She developed a reactive psychosis that responded to treatment.

Reactive Depression: Reaction to Loss and Trauma

A large number of patients with depression secondary to losses sustained because of the prevailing war situation presented to the outpatient clinic and for inpatient treatment. In addition to the grief reactions that were due to loss of loved ones, some patients' responses merged into true depressive illness. Loss of a bodily part such as a limb; loss of one's house and property on account of shelling or bombardment; loss of employment or other source of livelihood (commonly affected groups included fishermen and farmers); loss of self-esteem and humiliation as a result of detention, assault, or torture; and also, loss of virginity or chastity by rape was found to cause the development of depressive illness. In some cases, wives presented with reactive depression when their husbands were taken in for questioning and assaulted or, conversely, husbands developed loss of libido and other depressive symptoms when their wives were raped.

CASE 7—REPEATED TORTURE

Mr. R. was a 22-year-old healthy helper in a local militant group. After his group had been "prescribed" by a rival group, he had been arrested by the other group. According to his history, he had been tortured for 2 weeks and held altogether for 3 months. He had been beaten all over the body with hands, legs, knees, poles, and iron rods and trampled on till he lost consciousness. He had been hung up by his two thumbs (so called "helicopter" treatment) and also upside down by his ankles and beaten on his soles. At various times his face and other parts were swollen from the beating, with bleeding from the ear and hematemesis. Two needles had been driven through his fourth finger. They were given one meal and three tumblers of water for all their needs for a day, which left them in a continuous state of hunger and thirst. He had been asked to sign a confession but had resisted. Others who had signed had been executed. After his release, he complained of pain all over the body, dyspnea, backache, difficulty in using his hands, dyspepsia, vertigo, and paresthesia. His mother had found him getting up screaming in the night, drenched in sweat. He felt weak and sleepy and could not do much activity. He was socially withdrawn and tended to brood and cry at times. He said that sometimes an irresistible desire to "eat" his captors overwhelms him. On examination, physically there was limitation of movement of several joints, particularly the first metacarpophalangeal, lumbosacral, and knee joints. Mentally, there was psychomotor retardation with marked disillusionment. Routine investigations and X rays were ordered and he was started on analgesics, antidepressants, and psychotherapy but left the ward in a short time saying that he was better.

In the brief period the Indian army has been in Sri Lanka, it appears that they have not yet adopted the more psychologically damaging torture methods. Thus, we have not seen the degree of psychological sophistication and the systematized prolonged torture of victims resorted to by the Sri Lanka forces, which resulted in short- and long-term neuropsychological symptoms. Torture by the Indian army tended to be short-term with the specific purpose of obtaining information. Although physical damage was sometimes severe owing to the brutal beatings resulting in fractures and even death, psychological sequelae presented a varied pattern.

CASE 8—INTERROGATION AND TORTURE

A foreman at a local factory was taken in for mistaken identity and tortured by being hung by the legs and beaten on the soles and back. Electrical current was passed into the sensitive mucous membranes of the tongue and penis, causing severe burns; and the burning end of a cigarette was applied to the arms. On his identity being established the next day, he was released. Despite painful physical injuries, he did not have any psychological sequelae on mental state examination. Denial of the trauma needs to be ruled out. In contrast, an engineer who was taken in by the Sri Lanka army about the same time was tortured systematically for a prolonged period, including, according to the patient, repeated passage of current through his head. Though physical damage was minimal, he suffered a complete psychological breakdown and was admitted to the psychiatric unit muttering irrationally and irrelevantly, extremely decompensated. It was only after vigorous treatment that he slowly recovered and was able to tell his story.

The Escalation of Torture Practices

As time goes on, the Indian army has started to use more sophisticated forms of torture, decreasing the physical scars, but increasing the efficiency with which they inflict psychological damage. Perhaps more pathogenic, the local militant groups have also resorted to these self-same "sophisticated" techniques of torture, used by the Sri Lankan and Indian armies, on each other.

Psychic Effects of Torture

A survey of 160 released detainees in the North found that *all* had been severely tortured. The common psychological symptoms reported by the torture victims and signs observed during the interview are given in Table 28.5. The study found predominance of affective disorders in the sample, namely, 69% were suffering from moderate to severe depression, 66% had anxiety disorder, and 85% had PTSD. The social problems that the torture victims faced included unemployment owing to easy fatigability, weakness, debilitating bodily pain, and low self-esteem. Difficulties with interpersonal relationships, particularly within the family because of anger (74%), irritability (62%), social withdrawal (38%), suspicion (53%), and rudeness (46%) as well as indebtness and threatening environment on account of risk or fear of rearrest and torture were all found to be causing marked handicap and impeding rehabilitation and recovery (Puvinathan, Schanmugavajah, Lakshman, & Doney, 1989).

Table 28.5. Psychological Signs and Symptoms Following Torture

Signs and symptoms	Number	Percentage
General tiredness	139	86
General nervousness	135	84
Recurrent intrusive memories	128	83
Memory impairment or poor concentration	125	79
Loss of appetite	110	69
Intensification of symptoms by symbolic association with trauma	108	88
Extreme fear	106	66
Headache, giddiness, fainting	103	65
Low self-esteem	92	59
Nightmares and sudden awaking	91	56
Extreme mistrust and suspiciousness	80	50
Irritability and aggressiveness	74	40
Sweating during interview	74	40
Suicidal thoughts	61	38
Social withdrawal	61	38
Crying or watering of eyes during interview	48	30
Sexual dysfunction	40	25
Suicide attempts	1	0.5

Trautman (1964) stated that human beings placed under extreme and prolonged existential stress, fear, and anxiety undergo an extensive adaptive change of mental and biological functioning. In his view, psychological sequelae should be seen as meaningful reactions of a sound and forceful constitution that makes survival possible in a very pathological situation, such as torture. Psychiatrists working in the International Rehabilitation and Research Centre for Torture Victims at Copenhagen (see Chapter 64, in this volume) have found that short-term and long-term neuropsychological symptoms following torture are common with no tendency to spontaneous recovery but respond to psychotherapy and rehabilitation (Somnier & Genefke, 1986).

Rape Trauma: Dual Layers of Victimization

Another important traumatizing experience associated with war that commonly leads to depression is rape. From time immemorial, plunder and rape have been considered the spoils of war. A kind of psychopathic liberation resulting in looting, rape, and heavy drinking has been reported to follow major stressful events (Kinston & Rosser, 1974). What is said about violence in general is applicable to sexual violence. However, aggressive sexual assault has its own unique characteristics and consequences. Thus, *rape* is a violent crime in which sexuality is used to express power, anger, and aggression, with a core meaning of devaluation, humiliation, sheer terror, and most intimate violation of the self for the victim (Mezey, 1985).

In the local traditional culture, sexual violence takes on a more serious significance and has a severe psychologically traumatizing effect on the victim and her close relations, including her husband. Chastity is traditionally considered to be one of the supreme virtues of women, to be safeguarded with the same diligence as their lives. Thus, some of the victims attempted to commit suicide after they had been raped. Loss of virginity in a young girl, even if it was against her will, meant that she could not aspire to marriage in the Tamil society and, if already married, there was a good chance that she would be abandoned. All rape victims were socially ostracized and this usually extended to the family as well. It was not surprising that rape victims were not forthcoming to report such incidents and usually swallowed the suffering and injury silently. Indeed, it was the fear of pregnancy that drove many victims or their mothers to seek medical help in the form of reassurance that there was no pregnancy through pregnancy tests and medical examination. In some cases, abortion was requested.

The psychological impact on the rape victim and her immediate family was quite severe. Initially, there was a period of shock, lasting from a few hours to a day or two, when she was unable to speak, choking and gasping. Later, a deep depression set in with withdrawal, quietness, and crying. Usually the incident left a permanent scar and many were unable to rejoin the mainstream of social life. The effects of rape often extended beyond the victim and her immediate family to include the whole of society. During the Indian offensive when raping reached epidemic proportions in Jaffna, a generalized, pervasive sexual anxiety among women was observable in the months of October and November, 1987. They reported feeling exposed and vulnerable; many fled to safer areas, while others took precautionary measures (Somasundaram, 1992).

Rape can be seen as a "loss event" for the victim where she loses her trust in others, self-respect, sense of security, chastity or virginity, social identity and acceptance, and becomes liable to secondary victimization because of social norms and values. It has been found that the long-term consequences of rape include depression in 40% of victims, psychosomatic problems, sexual dysfunction, specific rape-related phobias, impaired task performance and social adjustment, and risk of suicide attempts (Mezey, 1985).

Suicide

Suicide rates show a marked fall during major wars (Durkheim, 1951; Kreitman, 1978). Theoretically, this may be due to war providing an alternate channel for suicidal behavior (Burvill, 1980) or an opportunity to externalize aggression (Lyons, 1979). However, suicide rates were found to be high in certain groups after a war, as in Vietnam War veterans (Wilson, Harel, & Kahana, 1988). A study of suicide in Jaffna in the year 1982 has shown a high suicide rate (Ganesvaran, Subramaniam, & Mahadevan, 1984). Whereas suicide is common in the elderly elsewhere in the world (Krietman, 1978), this study showed the highest risk in the 15–34-year group. The authors concluded that this phenomenon may be related to ethnic violence and revolt among youth. Dissanayke and De Silva (1974) found a similar high risk for suicide and attempted suicide in the youth of Sri Lanka as a whole and attributed it to unemployment among educated youth and youth unrest as manifested in the 1971 insurgency. Attempted suicide in Jaffna was also found to be high among youth in 1984 and commonly followed stress (Ganesvaran & Rajarajeswaran, 1988).

A unique form of suicide that was not recorded in the above quoted statistics was the use of cyanide capsules by the militants in the event of imminent capture. An estimated one third to one half of their combat deaths (Table 28.1) were by this method. This pattern of suicide is similar to what the sociologist Émile Durkheim (1951) called *altruistic suicide*, in which the individual feels so closely identified with a group or committed to the cause that he is willing to sacrifice himself for the greater good. Suicide squads similar to the Japanese *Kamikaze* were seen and death fasts, some without even water. This may well have been the zenith of self-sacrifice for a political cause.

Psychosomatic Disorder

The relationship between psychological stress and organic illnesses like eczema, bronchial asthma, hypertension, peptic ulcer, and mucous colitis is well documented and has been shown to be quantifiable (Kinston & Rosser, 1974). War stress can be expected to cause an increase in morbidity and mortality. Psychosomatic disorders are usually treated in outpatient clinics by general practitioners, physicians, or shamans and rarely present to a psychiatrist. Psychosomatic symptoms like dyspepsia, tension headaches, backaches, hyperventilation, and palpitation were reported to have an increased incidence during this period (Nageswaran, personal communication, 1987).

Sadistic Aggression during Atrocities

Reports of disatisfaction, indiscipline, and suicide in army personnel may be related to motivation which was primarily economical, and may not have quite counterbalanced the risk to life, thus setting up a classical approach–avoidance conflict (Lyons, 1979). There were several authenticated instances of combatants, on both sides, going berserk and indulging in a frenzy of killing civilians as on the boat *Kumuthini*, at Anuradhapura and whole villages in the East. Victims of torture reported that their captors appeared to enjoy themselves while torturing, drinking, and laughing in the process. It has been postulated that war provides ample scope for sadistic personalities to derive pleasure from acts of violence, cruelty, and torture of hapless victims.

The Remission of Psychotic Symptoms during War Stress

The negative type of schizophrenic illness with apathy and indifference to external stimuli can protect against stress in some cases. When the Tellipallai Hospital was evacuated to a nearby hospital because of army action in the area, some of the schizophrenic patients in the psychiatric ward refused to budge and the unit had functioned throughout that critical period. They appeared well-insulated against all that was going on around them and were observed to be quite indifferent to the loud explosions. Their withdrawal into themselves may have been a defensive mechanism against external stress (Wing, 1978). Interestingly, for some psychotic patients who had been handicapped by a chronic illness, the period of stress proved to be therapeutic, similar in effect to shock treatment leading to normal behavior.

Forms of Dissociation and Personality Alteration

A brief description is given of a type of behavior seen during war which is called here, for want of a better term, *combat psychosis*, though *hysterical psychosis* may be more appropriate. It refers to a condition observed in combatants, usually after prolonged combat or a tense and stressful situation involving deaths of comrades, where they suddenly go out of control, killing bystanders in a "frenzy." Many examples, such as on the boat *Kumuthini*, whole villages in the East, the Killinochi railway station, the Murukundy post office, the Kent and Dollar farm, Chetiikulam, Kokadicholai, and Anuradhapura were reported during the war in Sri Lanka, occuring in combatants of all sides. There were reports of men under tension in camps suddenly going out of control, killing their comrades, officers, and then themselves. Eyewitnesses often attributed the behavior to the effects of drugs. An educated mother who had seen her children mowed down in front of her and an experienced physician described the behavior of the men as that of those under the influence of drugs. Two similar conditions are described in transcultural psychiatry, namely, "running amok" in Malays and going "berserk" in Germans. The author had an "opportunity" to observe the behavior on two occasions, once during the internecine war between the local militants and the other during the Indian offensive. On both occasions, the behavior was similar and suggested a hysterical dissociation under stress: Eyes appeared dazed, speech terse and vague, movements automated, consciousness narrowed with mild disorientation, all characteristic of twilight states found in hysteria or epilepsy. The term *psychosis* was chosen on account of the serious consequences to society in terms of massacres of the innocent and the alteration in consciousness of the twilight state indicative of a transient break with reality. The popular explanation is that it is a form of rage reaction, as revenge for the killing of comrades or as deliberate policy of the higher authorities. A jawan confessed simply, "When one of our comrades is killed, our blood starts boiling, and we don't know what we are doing," which is suggestive of hysterical dissociation under stress.

Childhood Disorders

Children's reactions must be understood within the context of the family. Their reactions are a function of the way in which reality is interpreted to them by those around them and thus commonly mirror their parents' reaction rather than relating directly to the event. Among the major fears of childhood is separation from parents. If this does not happen, and if the parents cope with the situation, children show little awareness of danger and minimal anxiety. However, if the parents react with fear and anxiety, lose control and discipline, or the child's regular and ordered world is changed frequently, or if the parents themselves are missing, the child will commonly present with disturbances in physical function (such as enuresis, functional diarrhea), emotion (such as crying spells, withdrawal), or behavior (such as clinging, temper tantrums).

Variations in Stress Response among Children

All children were not uniformly affected by the stress. It was noticed that after showing some initial fear and clinging behavior that was due to exploding shells and rattle of machine guns, some were quite undisturbed and took things in their stride. At refugee camps, children could be observed playing, making a huge racket, enjoying themselves, oblivious to the tension of the adults and the war. Others reacted badly, showing signs of anxiety and other emotional disturbances even after things had settled down or the family had moved to a safer place. To some extent, the child's reaction was dependent on the severity of the stress gone through and the reactions of the parents. Children of parents who were tense and anxious showed anxiety and fear. Parents reported that children were having disturbed sleep patterns and awakening frequently after nightmares and night terrors. Children were found to wake up screaming in the night, drenched in sweat. In some cases, parents had to stay with the children when they fell asleep and be by their sides whenever they awakened.

CASE 9—SLEEP TERROR AND SLEEPWALKING

Mr. R. was a well-to-do engineer with two sons, aged 6 and 8 years. One night, a local group came to their house and killed the father after assaulting him with chains in front of the children. Subsequently, both children used to get up in their sleep, screaming in terror and drenched with sweat. A benzodiazepine was prescribed for the night and the children got over their night terrors but any permanent scar on their development was difficult to assess.

The reliving of the traumatic experience in dreams may serve as a kind of natural abreactive process whereby the individual is able to work-through and come to terms with the distressing experience which he is unable to face while awake (Bleich, Garb, & Kottler, 1986).

Long-Term Developmental Effects on Children

Although children may show transient behavioral and emotional disturbances under stress, more permanent effects on the development of personality are difficult to assess. Studies of children born under war conditions or children of parents who survived concentration camps show permanent scarring. Transgenerational transmission of the effects of war was demonstrated in the grown up children of World War II combat veterans. This

continuing legacy of war time trauma was apparent in the adult lives of many of these offsprings. . . . in symptoms of their own, and in their choice of marital partners, careers, and life styles, these children seem to show the destructive stamp of their relationship with their fathers, and their fathers' PTSD. (Rosenheck, 1986)

Studies of children exposed to stress have revealed a marked change in orientation to the future, particularly a sense of foreshortened future and a tendency to magical and "omen" thinking (see Chapter 53, in this volume, for a review).

It is likely that exposure of children, during their formative years, to insecurity, homelessness, violent deaths of loved ones, other cruel and aggressive actions, and to the full paraphernalia of war with its instruments of destruction will permanently influence their development. Indications of this influence are quite evident in the Tamil society today. Children have become familiar with the military lingo and show preference for the plethora of war toys and games; this is encouraged and reinforced by parents and society. When a child was presented with an "educational" toy for his birthday, his mother, a doctor, protested saying "What good is that, you should have brought a toy machine gun." In another instance, a child was given some building blocks to play with. She immediately proceeded to build a "chain block" (tank) and a helicopter.

The children themselves have become completely saturated with the atmosphere of war and are growing up without knowing any other world. This trend is not helped by the increasing practice of involving and recruiting younger and younger children into military activities, at an age, when they cannot realize the meaning of their actions or their long-term consequences.

Bandura and Walters (1963) have shown that aggressive behavior is readily learned through observation and imitation of aggressive models and that it can be reinforced and maintained by a variety of conditions. Thus, aggression becomes a learned way of solving problems when the aggressor is rewarded by social recognition or the victim is seen to suffer. In turn, this shapes social behavior of children where conflicts are solved by aggression and the usual restraints (guilt, conscience) on aggression are reduced, while aggression is morally justified and encouraged (Hilgard, Atkinson, & Atkinson, 1979). Lyons (1979) concluded his comprehensive study of civil violence in Northern Ireland with the gloomy prognosis:

> The normal child in the short term enjoys the group activity and excitement, but in the longer term he has learned that violence is an acceptable and successful way of life and this will have a disturbing effect on his personality development in the future.

Conclusions

As wars go, the war in Sri Lanka never reached the degree or intensity of a conventional war. Nevertheless, for the small local population in the North and East Provinces of Sri Lanka, it was and continues to be a severely traumatizing experience. As the only functioning psychiatric units in the war zone, a representative sample of patients exhibiting a variety of the more severe psychological reactions were seen. A selection from these clinical cases has been presented to illustrate the pattern of psychiatric morbidity that followed a war and some general observations have been included to give a picture of psychological reactions. Although all the categories of psychiatric disorders reported here can be caused or precipitated by other forms of stress and the overall statistics do not establish a significant increase in psychiatric morbidity, the unique pattern that emerges from the study as a whole, specifically a higher incidence of stress reactions, phobic anxiety states, grief reactions, and reactive depressions, can only be a sequelae to a war. The study does establish the variety of psychological reaction that can be caused by war. Perhaps, the most disconcerting consequence of the climate of fear and the cult of violence that has been unleashed on this once peace-loving society is the long-term implications for the development of children. By all appearances, violence, aggression, and nonrespect for individual rights and human life itself is fast becoming part and parcel of the Tamil society and a way of life for the next few generations.

Throughout history, the cost of war in terms of death, mutilation, torture, grief, destruction of material resources and property, privation, and social disorganization has been enormous. The continued occurrence of war, the presence of standing armies, and the manufacture and stockpiling of costly weapons of limitless destructive power show humankind's incompetence at solving its problems in peaceful ways and its drive to power by aggression and force. Apart from the death and mutilating injuries, it is the psychological trauma to those who survive that is most poignant but least realized.

The purpose of this chapter has been to bring out the psychiatric morbidity that is due to war, using Sri Lanka as a case study. As Leff (1981) pointed out, the forms of the psychiatric symptoms remain the same all over the world; only the contents change from culture to culture on account of the pathoplastic effect.

ACKNOWLEDGMENT

I gratefully acknowledge the valuable comments and suggestions from their clinical experience during the war contributed by T. Ganesvaran and A. Selvaratnam, consultant psychiatrists, and for allowing access to clinical cases under their care. S. Yoganathan and K. Sivayoganathan, together with the Kanagaratnams and the staff of the psychiatric unit, assisted in obtaining information and statistics and in the treatment of those affected by war. Last but not least, I extend my gratitude to my patients, who are the real source of this study.

References

Allodi, F. (1980). The psychiatric effects of political persecution and torture in children and families of victims. *Canada's Mental Health, 28,* 8–10.

American Psychiatric Association. (1987). *Diagnostic and Statistical Manual of Mental Disorders* (3rd ed., rev.). Washington, DC: Author.

Bandura, A., & Walters, R. (1963). *Social learning and personality development.* New York: Holt, Rinehart, & Winston.

Bleich, A., Garb, R., & Kottler, M. (1986). Treatment of prolonged combat reaction. *British Journal of Psychiatry, 148,* 493–496.

Burvill, P. W. (1980). Changing patterns of suicide in Australia 1910–1977. *Acta Psychiatrica Scandinavica, 62,* 258–268.

Children's Rehabilitation Center. (1986). *Psychological help to children-victims of political-armed conflict.* Manila, Phillipines: Author.

Coleman, J. C. (1975). *Abnormal psychology and modern life.* Bombay, India: D. B. Toraporevala Sons.

Cooper, J. E. (1978). Epidemiology. In J. K. Wing (Ed.), *Schizophrenia: Towards a new synthesis* (pp. 32–36). London: Academic Press.

Curran, P. S. (1988). Psychiatric aspects of terrorist violence: Northern Ireland 1969–1987. *British Journal of Psychiatry, 153,* 470–475.

Department of Census and Statistics. (1986). *Statistical pocket book of the Democratic Socialist Republic.* Colombo, Sri Lanka: Author.

Dissanayke, S. A. W., & De Silva, W. P. (1974). Suicide and attempted suicide in Sri Lanka. *Ceylon Journal of Medical Science, 23,* 10–17.

Dohan, F. C. (1966). War time changes in hospital admissions for schizophrenia. *Acta Psychiatrica Scandinavica, 42,* 1–23.

Durkheim, É. (1951). *Suicide.* (J. A. Spaulding & G. Simpson, Trans.). Glencoe, Illinois: Free Press.

Emzlie, I. (1915). The war and psychiatry. *Edinburgh Medical Journal, 14,* 359–367.

Fraser, R. M. (1971). The cost of commotion: An analysis of the psychiatric sequelae of the 1969 Belfast riots. *British Journal of Psychiatry, 118,* 257–264.

Ganesvaran, T., & Rajarajeswaran, R. (1983). *Consultation in outpatient psychiatric clinic in General Hospital, Jaffna.* Paper presented at the Jaffna Medical Association 2nd Annual Session, Jaffna.

Ganesvaran, T., & Rajarajeswaran, R. (1988). Deliberate self-harm in Jaffna. *Jaffnamedical Journal, 23.*

Ganesvaran, T., Subramaniam, S., & Mahadevan, K. (1984).

Suicide in a northern town of Sri Lanka. *Acta Psychiatrica Scandinavica, 69,* 420–425.

Goldberg, D. P. (1972). The detection of psychiatric illness by questionnaire. *Maudsley Monograph 21.* London: Oxford University Press.

Heskin, K. (1980). *Northern Ireland: A psychological analysis.* Dublin: Gill & MacMillan.

Hilgard, E. R., Atkinson, R. L., & Atkinson, R. C. (1979). *Introduction to psychology.* New York: Harcourt Brace Jovanovich.

Horowitz, M. J. (1986). *Stress response syndromes.* New York: Jason Aronson.

Ihezue, U. H. (1983). Psychiatric in-patients in Anambra State, Nigeria. *Acta Psychiatrica Scandinavica, 68,* 277–286.

Kinston, W., & Rosser, R. (1974). Disaster: Effects on mental and physical state. *Journal of Psychosomatic Research, 18,* 437–456.

Krietman, N. (1978). Suicide and parasuicide. In A. D. Forrest, J. W. Affleck, & A. K. Zealley (Eds.), *Companion to psychiatric studies* (pp. 30–42). Edinburgh: Churchill Livingstone.

Leff, J. (1981). *Psychiatry around the globe: A transcultural view.* New York: Marcel Dekker.

Legrand Du Saulle, H. (1871). De l'état mental des habitants de Paris pendent les évènements de 1870–71. *Annales Médico-Psychologiques, 2,* 222–241.

Lewis, A. (1942). Incidence of neurosis in England under war conditions. *Lancet, 2,* 175–183.

Lifton, R. J. (1967). *Death in life: Survivors of Hiroshima.* New York: Random House.

Lyons, H. A. (1971). Psychiatric sequelae of the Belfast riots. *British Journal of Psychiatry, 118,* 265–276.

Lyons, H. A. (1972). Depressive illness and aggression in Belfast. *British Medical Journal, i,* 342–345.

Lyons H. A. (1979). Civil violence—The psychological aspects. *Journal of Psychosomatic Research, 23,* 373–393.

Mezey, G. C. (1985). Rape—Victimological and psychiatric aspects. *British Journal of Hospital Medicine, March,* 152–158.

Miru, E. (1939). Psychiatric experience in the Spanish war. *British Medical Journal, 1,* 342–345.

Nasr, S., Racy, J., & Flaherty, J. A. (1983). Psychiatric effects of the civil war in Lebanon. *Psychiatric Journal of the University of Ottawa, 8,* 208–212.

Odegaard, O. (1932). Emigration and insanity. *Acta Psychiatrica Scandinavica* (Suppl. 4).

Odegaard, O. (1954). The incidence of mental disease in Norway during World War II. *Acta Psychiatrica et Neurologica Scandinavica, 42,* 1–23.

Orner, R. (1988, August-September). *Traumatic stress response in Falkland war veterans.* Paper presented at the First European Conference on Traumatic Stress Studies, Lincoln, England.

Puvinathan, S. A., Shanmugavajah, H., Lakshman, M., & Doney, A. (1989). *Jaffna Medical Journal, 24,* 94.

Raphael, B. (1986). *When disaster strikes.* New York: Basic Books.

Richman, N., Kanji, N., & Zinkin, P. (1988). *Report on psychological effects of war on children in Mozambique.* London: Save the Children Fund.

Rosenheck, R. (1985). The malignant post-Vietnam stress syndrome. *American Journal of Orthopsychiatry, 55,* 319–332.

Rosenheck, R. (1986). Impact of postraumatic stress disorder of World War II on the next generation. *Journal of Nervous and Mental Diseases, 174*(6), 319–326.

Sharp, G. (1978). *The politics of non-violent action.* Boston: Extending Horizon Books.

Smith, R. P. (1916–1917). Mental disorders in civilians arising in connection with the war. *Proceedings of the Royal Society of Medicine, Section of Psychiatry, 10,* 1–20.

Somasundaram, D. J. (1992). *Scarred mind.* New Delhi: SAGE Publications.

Somasundaram, D. J., Yoganathan, S., Ganesvaran, T., & Mahadeven, K. (1985). Psychosocial profile of psychiatric admissions in northern Sri Lanka. *Jaffna Medical Journal, 20*(2), 84–85.

Somasundaram, D. J., Yoganathan, S., & Ganesvaran, T. (1992). Schizophrenia in Sri Lankan Tamils—A descriptive study. *Ceylon Medical Journal,* December.

Somnier, E. E., & Genefke, I. K. (1986). Psychotherapy for victims of torture. *British Journal of Psychiatry, 149,* 323–329.

Tan, E.-S., & Simons, R. C. (1973). Psychiatric sequelae to a civil disturbance. *British Journal of Psychiatry, 122,* 57–63.

Tennant, C., Goulston, C., & Dent, O. (1986). Clinical psychiatric illness in prisoners of war of the Japanese: Forty years after release. *Psychological Medicine, 16,* 833–839.

Trautman, E. C. (1964). Fear and panic in Nazi concentration camps: A biosocial evaluation of the chronic anxiety syndrome. *International Journal of Social Psychiatry, 10,* 134–141.

Walker, J. (1981). The psychological problems of Vietnam veterans. *Journal of American Medical Association, 246,* 781–782.

Wilson, J. P. (1988, August-September). *Combat trauma in war veterans.* Remarks by the Chairperson in the First European Conference on Traumatic Stress Studies, Lincoln, England.

Wilson, J. P., Harel, Z., & Kahana, B. (Eds.) (1988). *Human adaptation to extreme stress: From the Holocaust to Vietnam.* New York: Plenum Press.

Wing, J. K. (Ed.). (1978). *Schizophrenia: Towards a new synthesis* (pp. 254–261). London: Academic Press.

World Health Organization. (1978). *Mental disorders: Glossary and guide to their classification in accordance with the ninth revision of the Classification of Diseases.* Geneva, Switzerland: Author.

CHAPTER 29

The Psychiatric Effects of War Stress on Afghanistan Society

Abdul Wali H. Wardak

Introduction

Wars have been the scourge of humanity throughout history. The impulse to war seems deeply rooted in human nature. Nations war for a variety of reasons, including power, honor, aggression, supremacy, envy, defense, protection, and survival (Zargar, 1989).

Wars are often caused by nations rather than individuals, but individuals normally pay the price of the war. Since World War II, there have been more than 145 localized conflicts. In the last 25 years, since the Algerian War of Independence, there have been or are currently conflicts affecting 33 countries. At the present time, 10 countries in the world are involved in war or regional conflicts, and Afghanistan is one of those countries which has sustained material damage and endured an enormous number of human casualties. Furthermore, these wars have produced a massive exodus of people who have unwillingly left their homeland to take shelter in other countries (because of fear of persecution, torture, and execution). As a result of this inhumanity, there are over fifteen million displaced people in the world today, living in confusion and misery, not knowing what the future holds for them.

War situations produce unique traumatic experiences and multiple stresses such as injuries, loss of property, and loss of loved ones and leave a legacy in the psyche of those who are involved in them. It is generally believed that those who experience such atrocities as killing and large-scale destruction may retain a lasting imprint in their memory which may have adverse effects on their sense of humanity and dignity (Wilson, 1988).

The psychic impairment induced by war may range from fairly mild transient disequilibrium to profound psychological disorders, culminating in self-destructive outcomes such as suicide or spiritual annihilation (Milgram, 1986). The extent of psychic damage reflects the enormity of the devastation and material losses induced by war and is variously characterized by numbing, confusion, disorientation, shock, intense debilitating fears, anxiety, nightmares, and a sense of abandonment.

The relationship between war trauma and psychiatric disorder is discussed below. Investigations which delineate the distinguishing dimensions and characteristics of extremely traumatic experience and its aftermath are required. By definition, war is a very complex socioeconomic and sociopolitical phenomenon. It affects the entire culture of a country and has transgenerational consequences (Mansfield, 1982). The effects of war depend on the specific nature of the war (e.g., civil war, guerrilla war, nuclear war, or conventional war), the type of weapons, the duration, and the situation in which it occurred. These effects have been measured in various ways: loss of life, loss of property, devastation of the environment, economic decline, damage to the infrastructure, and the like. However, relatively little attention has been paid to the human consequences sustained by victims. My analysis will treat the dimensions and characteristics of the trauma experienced by Afghan refugees. In many armed conflicts, limited geographical and demographic zones are proclaimed as combat zones and hence are more susceptible to destruction, both material and human. In contrast, the situation in Afghanistan is an ongoing conflict in which almost everyone is involved, either as a combatant or, more likely, as a victim. War in Afghanistan, as everywhere else, has threatened the permanence of cherished entities, people, property, pursuits, institutions, norms, and values. More than one and a half million people have been killed; hundreds of thousands are amputees; villages and towns have been demolished; thousands of schools,

Abdul Wali H. Wardak • Department of Psychology, University of Hull, Cottingham Road, Hull HU6 7RX, England.

International Handbook of Traumatic Stress Syndromes, edited by John P. Wilson and Beverley Raphael. Plenum Press, New York, 1993.

hospitals, terraces, bridges, roads, and factories have been damaged. Education has been handicapped in most provinces, trade with foreign countries has been affected; both agricultural and industrial production have dropped to minimum levels and furthermore, over five million people have been forced to leave the country and take refuge in the neighboring countries of Pakistan and Iran.

War in Afghanistan is extremely damaging by all the criteria already referred to and represents a unique large-scale military experience with distinguishing characteristics comparable to the Vietnam war. The country has been the battleground between two warring forces (U.S.S.R. and Afghanistan forces versus the Resistance movement of the Mujahedin) with different sociocultural and ideological backgrounds. Moreover, the operation of war as a combination of ambushes, hand-to-hand fighting, guerrilla warfare, and confrontation with the enemy in a more conventional way at the front was itself a unique experience.

My aim in this study is to assess the degree and nature of psychiatric disorders that are induced by war trauma among Afghan refugees currently living in the refugee camps in the North-West Frontier Province (NWFP) region of Pakistan.

In this chapter attempts have been made to explore various aspects and characteristics of trauma resulting from the ten year war which ravaged the country by all measures commonly employed.

Such disasters as wars, terrorism, technological accidents, and also natural disasters offer unusual opportunities to examine the effects of traumatic stress on both the physical and mental state of human beings in these life-threatening situations.

I hope that in addition to aiding the development of a global theory of traumatic stress, this study may provide a basis for the development of mental health services for these afflicted people.

Dimensions of Trauma among Afghan Refugees

Attempts have been made to outline the specific feature of the Afghan refugee situation in Pakistan. The analysis is based on my observations and intimate knowledge of the culture and also my frequent visits to the refugee camps.

Exposure to Traumatic Experience

Since the eruption of conflict in Afghanistan in 1978, many people have been exposed to horrific events and a terrifying environment. They have witnessed the death of people in combat or bombardment, mutilations, the retrieval of bodies, and the complete devastation of houses, villages, and agricultural land. Some of them have actively participated in the killing of their enemies, in mortar bombing, ambush, hand-to-hand fights, assassinations, and interrogations. Many of them have been through the experience of a prolonged journey through mountains and very rough terrain. On this jour-

ney, they experienced fatigue, changes in diet and climate, and travel across time zones coupled with the constant fear of being caught, killed, or imprisoned.

A prolonged journey of this kind, characterized by exposure to extremely stressful conditions, is known to induce dissociative reactions and maladaptive behavior such as panic, suicide, or assault. Physiological disorders, for example, autonomic nervous system disorders, endocrine system disorders, and possible disorders of neurotransmitter functioning may also arise. These reactions have been observed in Vietnamese boat people (Barnes, 1980).

Reports and data provided by various organizations suggest that the Afghan refugees since the eruption of war suffer from a variety of emotional disorders ranging from minor anxiety or depression to full-blown psychoses compared to the prewar conditions of the society. Many of them report a complex picture of psychosomatic disorders, psychological distress, sociobehavioral disturbances, and outbursts of violence (Mufti, 1982).

Women and children constitute a group at greater risk and are often victims of bombing (United Nations High Commissioner for Refugees [UNHCR], 1988b), because when the shelling or bombing starts, they run into their houses for protection and are often caught by falling beams and roofs, or crushed by stone walls. Similarly, children are more likely than are adults to sustain injuries (in a frightening journey from the homeland, as a result of falling from a horse or camel used as a means of transport during their flight) during the journey through the jagged mountain passes (Daadfar, 1988).

Threat to Culture

Threat to Traditional Values and Functions

Entertainment of guests, provision of food and shelter for strangers, helping the needy, and showing generosity are matters of prestige and constitute very important social values that function within the Afghan sociocultural network. Enacting these traditions has been severely damaged, sometimes entirely thwarted, owing to the circumstances of refugee life.

Separation from Homeland

Traditionally, Afghans hold a special love and affection for their country, the "Fatherland," which has a central meaning in their lives. Afghan literature is full of proverbs and poems reflecting this sentiment. The separation from fatherland is therefore another catastrophic event in the lives of these people. Furthermore, their strong loyalty for their homeland puts them in a situation of severe moral conflict, created by the opposing needs to defend their country and protect themselves and their families.

Minority Status

By definition, refugees are stateless and homeless people. Whatever culture or race they came from, or whatever sympathy and support they receive from the host community, they are regarded by the natives as different and foreign (Tyhurst, 1981). Resentment is often shown by some members of the host community to the presence of refugees, and this may be particularly obvious in adverse economic conditions. Holding minority status and being regarded by some elements of the host society as intruders or being used by them as convenient scapegoats for their internal sociopolitical disputes are other stressful factors in the lives of Afghan refugees.

Threat to Social Network

Disruption of the Community Network

During the eruption of major disasters and the subsequent relocation of the victims in a new environment, it is difficult to preserve the natural support network of the people involved (Cohen & Ahearn, 1980). The case of the Afghan refugees is no exception.

Loss of proximity to friends and relatives is the most unhappy experience in the life of a displaced person (Korsching, Donnermeyers, & Burdge, 1980). The loss of the support network coupled with a new and unfamiliar environment can lead to social and emotional disorders (Hall & Landreth, 1975). In addition, the sense of uncertainty about the prospects of returning to the homeland and former neighborhood increases the level of stress among the evacuees (Western & Milne, 1979).

In the case of the Afghan refugees, social ties both within the total community and the local neighborhood have been damaged by the relocation of the family and the destruction of the environment where a variety of social events have traditionally been held. This destruction of the social network takes place at the very time when the need for it is especially great. A similar observation was made by Garrison (1983) regarding the Vietnamese.

The social structures of the rural population, based on strong ties with the extended family, lineage tribe, and ethnic community, may not have entirely disappeared, but have been severely damaged. Moreover, many people have lost their social status as defined initially within the sociocultural context of the Afghan society by their positions within the tribal genealogy and possession of wealth. In addition, wealth constitutes a basis for the fulfillment of various religious duties (e.g., paying alms, "zakat," and donating to other charities). These religious activities are handicapped because of the poverty, and this constitutes a major source of concern and guilt.

Disruption of the Family System

Another threat to the social system is via the destruction of the cohesive family structure, which is a distinguishing feature of the Afghan society. In many cases, the family is disintegrated; some of its members are either killed or have disappeared or been hospitalized because of injuries or separated from their families to live in another country. Experts on Afghanistan affairs believe that this form of disruption of the family network has disastrous consequences for both the men-

tal and physical health of the victims within the sociocentric cultural structure of the Afghan society and increases the chances of psychiatric morbidity. Some families are entirely without visits from friends, relatives, and neighbors. Most of the people have lost their customary work, hobbies, and recreation and hence the social contacts associated with these activities. Moreover, they have lost their neighbors and their neighborhood acquaintances—the comforting sense of familiar faces and familiar places.

Traditionally, youngsters are expected to show a great deal of respectful obedience to parents and other families and community elders, and to practice those traditional values which distinguish Afghan identity. This trend is somewhat damaged because of the disruption of the social structure and order, lack of education, and socioeconomic hardships. There is increased parental fear and apprehension about the potential social mobility of the new generation and a further disintegration of the traditional family. These fears are justified by some evidence that the traditional moral code of behavior is threatened as a result of which some youngsters have become undisciplined and delinquent (United States Committee for Refugees [USCR], 1985).

Social Isolation

The disruption of the previous social support system and the inability to form new relationships within the new neighborhood lead to the isolation of the refugees, with the resulting problems of alienation (Liu, Lamanna, & Murata, 1979). In other words, individuals feel neither protection from the community nor a sense of belonging to it.

Loss of Consistent Social Status

Many refugees lost their established social status after flight into exile, and as a consequence they have been compelled to accept lower status and perform jobs inappropriate to their qualifications and professional or social status in their home country. This discrepancy between self-concept or self-expectation and the existing reality, called a *status inconsistency*, leads to a sense of deprivation, humiliation, and insecurity and constitutes an important stressor in the life of the displaced person (Abramson, 1966).

Loss and Grief

Afghan refugees have sustained multiple losses, including tangible ones, for example, properties, businesses, social and professional status, life style, and family members. But there are also internal and less obvious losses, for example, loss of confidence in self and others, loss of self-esteem, and loss of identity. It would be expected that multiple losses combined with a range of other grievances would eventually constitute an enormous challenge to the mental state of the refugees and substantially affect their psychological equilibrium.

Many families have among their members those who have sustained severe physical injuries and consequently became permanently handicapped. This group of victims was recently estimated at around a half million (UNHCR, 1989b). Because there are not enough medical institutions to look after them and provide them with rehabilitation services, their families are compelled to provide the handicapped member with day-to-day care, thus increasing their emotional burdens.

For Afghan people, grief is often in private and, for cultural reasons, may not be revealed to outsiders. It is argued that this pattern of private grief and internalization of conflict, rage, and aggression may later on be reflected in the form of psychosomatic disorders as is the case in many Oriental cultures (Munger, 1986).

Environmental Stress

Weather in Afghanistan, with the exception of some areas, is agreeable with the temperature around 30°C and a very low degree of humidity in the summer season. In contrast, the geophysical conditions in the country of resettlement are quite different in most areas where the refugees are located. The hot season of summer lasts for a long period with the temperature well over 40°C and humidity around 80%. In the winter the temperature sometimes drops to zero. Most of the refugees, being inhabitants of cold dry areas, are not used to such a high temperature and humidity which affects their health (UNHCR, 1988a, 1989a).

Moreover, unfavorable living conditions, including shortage of drinking water, poor primary sanitation, malnutrition, and poor preventive medicine, combined with geophysical and environmental factors, represent important stressors which almost certainly have adverse effects on the health of the refugees. Children represent the group most susceptible to the effects of climatic variation and diverse environmental factors which have a negative influence on their physical and mental growth (Daadfar, 1988; UNHCR, 1989a).

Furthermore, because of lack of facilities, a great majority of children cannot receive proper education. Shortage of schools and educational facilities, lack of encouragement and stability in the camp life, illiteracy of most of the parents, and frustration and helplessness have left most of the children deprived of education. This constitutes one of the major concerns of parents regarding their children's future.

Adaptation

Refugees' Appraisal of Trauma

Despite the fact that the relief operation and general administration of the Afghan refugees is one of the best in the world (UNHCR, 1988a; USCR, 1982), the series of traumatic events subsequently followed by their displacement is negatively perceived by the great majority of the refugees. They feel humiliated, degraded, and dehumanized. This sense of degradation could be attributed to their historical pride, the glorious past, high self-esteem, and an awareness of themselves as former rulers of the region in which they are now refugees dependent on the aid and assistance of others. This nega-

tive perception of threat to themselves made them vulnerable to a variety of emotional disorders with different degrees of severity (Mufti, 1982; Daadfar, 1988).

It is broadly understood that the perception of threat determines the individual's response to traumatic stress and plays an important role in determining the short and long-term consequences of exposure to traumatic conditions (Kates, 1977). Moreover, cognitive appraisal of stressful situations is regarded as a very important factor in determining stress and anxiety responses (Lazarus, 1966).

Adjustment to a New Life-Style and Acculturation

The dramatic change in the life-style consequent upon the sociopolitical events in their homeland is likely to render Afghan refugees vulnerable to emotional disequilibrium. Cultural conflicts arising from the differences in two different life-styles (rural refugees and urban Pakistanis) tend to perpetuate and cause confusion and "intrapsychic turmoil" (Derbyshire, 1969). This psychic turmoil created by adaptation to the new environment and acculturation of the new way of life plus grief over tremendous loses is manifested in some refugees in various pathological terms (e.g., anxiety, depression, reactive depression, psychosomatic disorders, etc.) (Wardak, 1988a).

Posttrauma Adaption Efforts

After the reality of migration filters through, despite their strong commitment and belief in their cause, it is inevitable that the refugees will sometimes think about their lost identity, changed role, and shift from a perception of independence to a perception of dependence. Afghan refugees, like refugees everywhere else, face a new reality of harsh experience. They must come to terms with the strange and difficult environment of resettlement and strive to mobilize their own resources in order to suit the requirements of a new life.

The negative feelings of refugees, created by traumatic conditions preceding migration, such as loss of confidence, hostility, aggression, and humiliation, are reinforced and worsened by other unpleasant experiences in the new environment (e.g., discrimination, unemployment, and guilt). The traumatic experience of confrontation with destruction, death, and violence followed by utter helplessness is deeply imprinted in the memory of victims and may accompany them throughout their lives (Wardak, 1988b).

Many Afghan refugees experience compulsive flashbacks at anniversaries of traumatic events or when anything arouses memories of the horrors they have experienced. Others experience intrusive distressing recollections of the events without any external triggering stimulus (Daadfar, 1988; Mufti, 1982). These painful images and recollections are difficult to deal with in the conditions of resettlement. The process of adaptation is facilitated by a stable and supportive environment. The resettlement situation is therefore likely to prolong grief and impair adaptation.

War Trauma and Psychiatric Disorders

It is widely believed that those who have suffered such catastrophic events as the loss of a loved one, bereavement, torture, threat to life, serious illnesses, or injuries experience emotional disturbances. The pioneering contribution of Holmes and Rahe (1967) in the development of methodology and instruments for the assessment of life events has been a major breakthrough for scientists in this field, enabling researchers to explore more systematically the role of life events in the etiology of both mental and physical disorders. Since then, an enormous number of studies have been published, yielding considerable confirmatory evidence of the vital role of life events in the etiology of various mental and somatic disorders (Dohrenwend & Dohrenwend, 1974; Paykel, 1976).

Studies carried out in the field of life events and their relations to serious illnesses suggest that there is a positive correlation between the occurrence of traumatic life events and the onset of diseases (Lepowski, 1975). The unfortunate experience of war is always characterized by the commission of acts of violence or witnessing the consequences of others' tragedies. Despite the frequent occurrence of wars, the psychic wounds induced by war were not recognized until World War II. Previously, symptoms reported by victims were always identified as having physical origins, probably for cultural reasons (e.g., the association with weakness, cowardice, and lack of patriotism).

Recent investigations suggest that nearly everyone, when exposed to extreme stress, will manifest some acute stress-response syndromes. In their studies, Hendin and Hass (1984) and Hendin, Hass, Singer, Gold, and Trigos (1983) discovered that people with a higher capacity for stress tolerance will break down only if the level of stress is higher: A lower degree of stress may not be enough to induce stress syndromes.

Studies indicate that individuals with previous neurotic conflicts or a predisposition to certain type of stress may respond to a lower level of external stress. This finding was supported by Brill (1967), who observed that soldiers with previous neurotic symptoms had a seven to eight times higher chance of developing psychiatric problems compared with those with normal personality characteristics.

Krupinski (1984), in a study carried out among various migrant and refugee groups (e.g., Indians, Jewish, Russian, Polish, Ukrainian, Mediterranean, Lebanese, and Indochinese), found that physical morbidity of the migrants was related to imported diseases, change in physical and social environment, and change in overall habits. Psychiatric disorders were found to be associated with exposure to traumatic experiences preceding migration and postmigration adaptation.

Bonan and Eduards (1984), in a survey carried out on a clinical population in Australia among Indochinese refugees victimized by decades of war, reported severe psychiatric dysfunctioning, especially among those who lacked social support or suffered social dislocation. The survey also focussed on subsequent problems reported by refugees in the country of resettlement (e.g., persistent feeling of guilt, bewilderment, pining, difficulties in marriage, employment, and education).

Fakhr-el-Islam and Hussain (1969), in a little-known study conducted in Egypt among civilians evacuated from the military operation zone in the 1967 Arab–Israeli War and subsequently seeking psychiatric care in the Kasr-el-Aini psychiatric clinic in Cairo, indicated that exposure to the extremely stressful events of war, separation from families, and adaptation to the resettlement conditions were the main factors precipitating or exacerbating psychiatric disorders.

A brief account is now offered of specific symptomatology associated with the stress of war.

Association between traumatic or threatening conditions and anxiety is documented in various studies, such as combat situations (Grinker & Spiegel, 1945), tornados (Moore, 1958), and rape (Kilpatrick, Veronen, & Best, 1985). Various studies of different orientations, for example, psychoanalytic (Solnit & Kris, 1967), cognitive (Horowitz, 1979), and behavioral (Kilpatrick et al., 1985) have attached a significant role to the initial anxiety associated with the evolution of trauma in the development of subsequent short- and long-term pathological reactions.

Studies carried out with subjects who have endured major life events postulated that life events play a precipitating role in the onset of depressive disorders (Paykel et al., 1969; Uhlenhuth & Paykel, 1973). Similarly, the prevalence of depression is reported in a number of studies carried out with refugee populations traumatized by war conditions, for example, Cambodia (Kinzie, Tran, Breckenridge, & Bloom, 1980), Afghanistan (Mufti, 1982; Wardak, 1988a), Ethiopia (Wardak, 1988b), and Vietnam (Aylesworth, Ossorio, & Osaki, 1979; Kinzie et al., 1982).

There have been relatively few studies looking at the incidence of schizophrenia among populations who have suffered stressful conditions. However, it has been suggested by a number of researchers and clinicians that stressful life events may provoke schizophrenic disorders in nonpredisposed individuals (B. P. Dohrenwend, 1975; Kohn, 1973; Steinberg & Durell, 1968). The well-prepared study of Brown and Birley (1968) in this respect revealed that life events had causal effects in approximately 505 schizophrenic patients. Similarly, a significant correlation between stressful life events and onset of schizophrenia was reported by Schwartz and Myers (1977). Schizophrenia associated with war conditions is pointed out in a number of studies (Odegaard, 1932; Pedersen, 1949; Verdonk, 1979; Yesavage, 1983). A recent study carried out in Lebanon reported a dramatic increase in schizophrenic illness among the population affected by war trauma compared to the prewar era (Yakteen, 1988).

The prevalence of paranoid symptoms among uprooted people is well documented in the work of many researchers (Copeland, 1968; Kendler, 1982; Kino, 1960; Mezey, 1960a,b).

Observations made with victims of World War II suggest that isolation from the native culture, persecution of close relatives, and other war-related traumatic conditions were the main precipitating factors in the development of paranoid psychosis (Kumasaka & Saito,

1970; Retterstol, 1968; Tseng, 1969; Westermeyer, 1986).

The relationship between extreme stress and somatic illnesses has also been shown in a number of studies (Allodi, 1982; Eitinger, 1960; Kinzie *et al.*, 1982; Lin, Tazuma, & Mazuda, 1979; Naguyen, 1982; I. Tyhurst, 1951). These studies, carried out with victims of organized violence and refugees in various cultures, indicated that emotional distress arising from exposure to prolonged traumatic conditions plays a crucial role in the development of somatic illness.

The Study

This study with relatively small scope has limited aims from which limited conclusions can be drawn. The principal aim was to investigate the nature and degree of psychological impairment in Afghan refugees. Secondary aims were to comment on the role of culture (social support network) and explore the effects of age (maturity) and length of stay in refugee camps as these specific factors were believed to influence the relative success of individuals' adaptation. The independent variables in this study are traumatic stress of the war, the age of the subjects, and length of exile. The dependent variables are the psychiatric questionnaire responses. Afghans were chosen as the experimental (stressed) group for the reasons already outlined in the introduction. However, it was not possible to choose a control group from the Afghan population because of the overwhelming nature of the trauma prevailing in the country. Therefore, Pakistanis of the SWAT district of the NWFP region were chosen as a control group because of the proximity to Afghan people in ethnicity, language, religion, and traditions. The aim was to find a comparison group as similar to the Afghan people as possible but before the occurrence of the recurrent conflict.

After reviewing the traumatic stress literature and looking at the global experience of war in various countries the following general hypotheses have been formulated: (1) members of the experimental sample will have higher scores on questionnaires assessing emotional and psychiatric dysfunction; (2) members of the short stay subgroups in the experimental sample will indicate greater severity of stress-related psychiatric symptoms, compared to long-stay subgroups; (3) adolescents of the experimental group will manifest less stress-related symptoms compared to older age groups; and (4) young adults of the experimental sample whose ages are between twenty and thirty years will have a higher range of psychological disturbances than the mature adult group.

Methodology

The population sample of this study consisted of 240 subjects divided into two main groups—experimental (*n* = 120) consisted of Afghan refugees and control (*n* = 120) derived from the native Pakistani people of the NWFP in Pakistan. Each of these two groups was further divided into three subgroups on the basis of age as follows:

A. Adolescents, aged 13–16 years (*n* = 40), drawn from primary schools in the region
B. Young adults, aged 20–30 years (*n* = 40), drawn from colleges, training centers, and the University
C. Mature adults, aged 40 and above (*n* = 40), illiterate peasants drawn from refugee camps, basic health units (experimental group), and factory workers in the NWFP (control group)

In both groups, experimental and control, the sample was confined to males selected from a variety of settings (e.g., schools, factories, universities). All subjects except young adults of the lower middle class belonged to the lower socioeconomic class and to the same race, religion, culture, and language. The young adults, Group B, in both experimental and control groups were not married. In contrast, all subjects in Group C, experimental and control, were mature adults who were married and living with their families. Experimental groups in all three categories were divided into two subgroups: (1) SS (short stay), subjects who had spent less than 2 years in refuge; and (2) LS (long stay), subjects who had spent more than 2 years in refuge.

Instruments

Adults Category

All subjects with the exception of some university students were personally interviewed.

State-Trait Anxiety Inventory (STAI)

This test was designed by C. D. Spielberger in 1968–1970. It consists of 40 items and measures and distinguishes between state anxiety, a transitory condition of perceived tension, and trait anxiety, a relatively stable condition of anxiety proneness. The form (X-1) consists of 20 items and measures state anxiety, whereas the form (X-2) contains 20 items and is designed to assess trait anxiety (Spielberger, 1980).

Beck Depression Inventory (BDI)

This self-rating inventory was devised by Beck (1961) to measure depression. It also provides a useful tool for eliciting problems from patients who have difficulty in focussing on distressing symptoms or life situations. The inventory consists of 21 items and is widely used in academic and therapeutic settings.

Crown-Crisp Experiential Inventory (CCEI)

The Crown-Crisp Experiential Index (Crown & Crisp, 1979) was previously named the Middlesex Hospital Questionnaire. The scale is a self-report inventory which measures clinically recognized psychoneurotic disorders. It is composed of 48 items divided equally into 6 subscales, measuring Free-Floating Anxiety (FFA), Phobic Anxiety (PHO), Obsessionality (OBS), Somatic Anxiety (SOM), Depression (DEP), and Hysteria (HYS).

355

General Health Questionnaire (GHQ)

This 30-item test was devised by David Goldberg in 1969/1972 for adults. It is a self-administered screening test, which aims to detect psychiatric disorders among respondents in community settings, such as primary care or among general medical outpatients. The test is concerned with two major classes of phenomena: inability to continue to carry out one's normal "healthy" functions, and the appearance of new phenomena of a distressing nature. This test is especially concerned with the transitional phase between psychological sickness and psychological health. This test was found suitable for youngsters and consequently was administered to the adolescent group in this study (Goldberg, 1978).

Adolescents Category

State-Trait Anxiety Inventory for Children (STAIC)

This test, which was devised by C.D. Spielberger (1973), consists of 40 items and aims to investigate anxiety among youngsters. It includes two separate self-report scales for measuring state anxiety (C-1, 20 items) and trait anxiety (C-2, 20 items).

The Face Valid Depression Scale for Adolescents (FVDSA)

This scale was devised by Ada and Juan Mezzich (1979; also Mezzich, 1979) to measure depression among adolescents. It consists of 35 items, 14 of which were derived from the Minnesota Multiphasic Personality Inventory (MMPI) D scale and the remainder extracted from other scales.

Results

In support of Hypothesis 1, all experimental subjects in the two older age groups scored higher than control subjects on all measures. With respect to Hypothesis 2, no consistent significant differences were revealed between short-stay and long-stay subjects in all three groups. With respect to age differences, the results were not entirely as expected (Hypotheses 3 and 4). As predicted, the results supported Hypothesis 3, whereas no significant differences except for GHQ measure were found between experimental and control group adolescent subjects (see Table 29.1). The statistical analyses utilized in this study follow.

Adolescents (Group A)

All means for Group A can be found in Table 29.1. Using t test, no significant differences were found between the experimental and control groups or between the two subgroups, short stay and long stay except for GHQ where the experimental group scored significantly higher ($t = -2.33$, df 76, $p < .05$).

Young and Mature Adults (Groups B and C)

The results for each measure are presented in turn. Two analyses of variance were conducted on the data for each measure. First, a two-way ANOVA was carried out on the entire adult sample ($N = 160$), factors being group (experimental vs. control) and age (young adults vs. old adults). Second, the data from only the experimental group was considered ($n = 80$). Two-way ANOVAS were applied to assess the effects of age (young vs. older adults) and length of stay (short stay vs. long stay).

State-Trait Anxiety Inventory (STAI)

State Anxiety

Experimental subjects were found to be more anxious than control subjects ($F[1, 156] = 53.46$, $p < .001$). Comparing short-stay subjects with long-stay subjects, no significant differences were found for the variables age and length of stay in refuge.

Table 29.1. Test Results of Exposure to Trauma of Group A (Adolescents)

| | STAI | | | | GHQ | | FVDSA | |
| | State | | Trait | | | | | |
Length of stay in refuge	M	SD	M	SD	M	SD	M	SD
				Experimental group				
SS n = 20	27.65	8.33	36.95	8.41	17.45	14.34	11.90	6.47
LS n = 20	25.30	7.83	39.20	7.90	21.80	12.91	14.70	6.07
Total N = 40	26.47	8.10	38.10	8.13	19.62	13.65	13.30	6.35
				Control group				
Total N = 40	28.73	7.48	37.78	6.42	13.35	10.17	11.80	5.59

Table 29.2. Test Results of Exposure to Trauma of Group B (Young Adults)

	STAI							
	State		Trait		GHQ		BDI	
Length of stay in refuge	M	SD	M	SD	M	SD	M	SD
	Experimental group							
SS n = 20	33.60	8.76	53.30	8.38	38.55	14.35	18.40	8.36
LS n = 20	37.05	10.01	45.7	8.09	35.05	17.70	15.20	6.89
Total N = 40	35.33	9.45	49.50	8.99	36.80	16.10	16.80	7.73
	Control group							
Total N = 40	25.40	5.55	37.72	7.21	13.30	7.97	4.62	4.39

Trait Anxiety

On the Trait anxiety scale of the STAI, the experimental group reported a higher degree of anxiety ($F[1, 156] = 113.59$, $p < .001$). Comparison within experimental group revealed that short-stay subjects tend to be more anxious than the long-stay subjects ($F[1, 76] = 4.75$, $p < .05$).

Beck Depression Inventory

Experimental groups were found to be significantly more depressed than the control subjects ($F[1, 156] = 195.5$, $p < .001$) and this trend was higher in mature subjects ($F[1, 156] = 120.73$, $p < .001$). A significant interaction was found for length of stay and age within the subgroups (short-stay and long-stay) of the experimental subjects. Long-stay mature subjects were signifi-

cantly more depressed than the long-stay young subjects ($F[1, 76] = 6.12$, $p < .05$).

General Health Questionnaire

The experimental groups scored significantly higher than the control group ($F[1, 234] = 147$, $p < .001$). A highly statistically significant interaction between age and group ($F[1, 234] = 16.81$, $p < .001$) indicates that effects of conditions varied over the ages (see Tables 29.1 and 29.2). Within the control group there was no difference in the GHQ scores with age ($F[2, 234] = 2.41$, ns) while within the experimental group there was a highly significant effect of age ($F[2, 234] = 24.71$, $p < .001$) with adolescents scoring lower than the other two age groups. Comparing short-stay subjects with long-stay subjects, adolescents scored lower than the two older

Table 29.3. Test Results of Exposure to Trauma of Group C (Mature Adults)

	STAI							
	State		Trait		GHQ		FVDSA	
Length of stay in refuge	M	SD	M	SD	M	SD	M	SD
	Experimental group							
SS n = 20	32.85	7.17	49.65	9.49	34.05	10.52	17.40	4.80
LS n = 20	35.55	12.39	48.10	10.86	35.90	17.35	20.65	9.60
Total N = 40	34.20	10.08	48.87	10.30	34.98	14.20	19.02	7.67
	Control group							
Total N = 40	24.77	6.99	32.06	7.09	8.23	7.30	4.03	4.15

Table 29.4. CCEI Results of Exposure to Trauma of Group B (Young Adults)

Length of stay in refuge	Anxiety		Obsession		Depression		Phobia		Somatic		Hysteria	
	M	SD	M	SD	M	SD	M	SD	M	SD	M	SD
Experimental group												
SS *n* = 20	8.70	2.98	13.65	1.84	11.30	2.87	6.85	3.56	8.00	3.11	7.60	2.72
LS *n* = 20	7.35	3.13	12.30	2.20	8.90	3.80	7.65	2.76	6.35	2.89	7.30	3.18
Total *N* = 40	8.03	3.09	12.98	2.11	10.10	3.54	7.25	3.17	7.18	3.07	7.45	2.93
Control group												
Total *N* = 40	3.48	2.72	11.35	1.93	3.48	2.17	5.65	1.93	3.53	3.05	6.28	2.08

groups ($F[2, 114] = 16.38$, $p < .001$). No significant interaction was found.

Crown-Crisp Experiential Inventory

Anxiety (A)

The difference between the experimental and the control groups was found to be very highly statistically significant with the experimental group scores being twice as high as those of the control ($F[1, 156] = 114.3$, $p < .001$). No significant differences were found between short- and long-stay subjects of the experimental group. However, anxiety was higher in younger subjects ($F[1, 76] = 4.26$, $p < .05$). No statistically significant interaction was revealed ($F = .88$).

Obsession (O)

The comparison between groups indicated that the experimental group scored higher than the control group ($F[1, 156] = 15.22$, $p < .001$). No significant differences were found between short-stay and long-stay subjects of the experimental group or between age groups.

Depression (D)

The experimental group was found to be significantly more depressed than the control group ($F[1, 156] = 266$, $p < .0001$). A statistically significant interaction with age ($F[1, 156] = 4.3$, $p < .05$) is caused by a tendency for depression to be greater in the older experimental group than in the younger, and for depression to be lower in the older control group than in the younger. Neither of these differences were in themselves statistically significant ($F[1, 156] = 2.39$, 1.92, ns, respectively). Comparing short-stay subjects with long-stay subjects, neither main effects nor the interaction reached statistical significance.

Phobia (P)

The experimental group score was significantly higher than that of the control group ($F[1, 156] = 30.41$, $p < .001$). No significant interaction was reported. Similarly, no difference was found between short-stay and long-stay subjects or between age groups (B and C).

Table 29.5. CCEI Results of Exposure to Trauma of Group C (Mature Adults)

Length of stay in refuge	Anxiety		Obsession		Depression		Phobia		Somatic		Hysteria	
	M	SD	M	SD	M	SD	M	SD	M	SD	M	SD
Experimental group												
SS *n* = 20	7.05	3.28	12.30	2.45	11.05	2.46	8.20	3.25	8.35	2.85	5.10	1.52
LS *n* = 20	7.95	3.65	11.90	2.47	11.10	2.97	7.80	2.44	9.60	2.72	6.40	2.48
Total *N* = 40	7.50	3.45	12.10	2.44	11.08	2.69	8.00	2.85	8.98	2.82	5.75	2.13
Control group												
Total *N* = 40	2.08	2.43	11.22	1.51	2.60	2.70	5.15	2.05	3.18	2.93	4.80	2.20

Somatic (S)

The experimental group scored significantly higher than the control group ($F[1, 156] = 101.06$, $p < .001$). Also, a statistically significant interaction was found ($F[1, 156] = 5.23$, $p < .05$), which reflects a tendency for somatic complaints to be greater in older experimental group than the younger ($F[1, 156] = 7.33$, $p < .01$) and to be lower in older control group, whereas the age groups in the control subjects are undifferentiated on this measure ($F[1, 156] = 0.28$, ns).

Comparing short-stay subjects with long-stay subjects on the same scale, somatic complaints were found to be higher in older group than in the younger ($F[1, 76] = 7.72$, $p < .001$). The younger short-stay subjects were found with more somatic complaints by contrast with younger long-stay subjects.

Hysteria (H)

Comparing the experimental group with the control group a significant difference was found between two groups ($F[1, 156] = 8.10$, $p < .001$) and younger subjects scored higher than older ($F[1, 156] = 18.8$, $p < .001$). No significant interaction was found. Comparing short-stay subjects with long-stay subjects on the same scale, younger subjects scored higher than older ($F[1, 76] = 8.9$, $p < .001$). However, there was no difference between short-stay and long-stay younger subjects. No significant interaction was found.

Physical Illness Factors among Afghan Refugees

This study utilized data obtained from the UNHCR resources (see Figures 29.1 and 29.2) to indicate the extent of both physical and mental disorders, as well as data from specialized psychiatric clinics based in Peshawar, Pakistan, such as the Islamic Relief Agency (ISRA) and Psychiatry Center for Afghans (PCA) (Daadfar, 1988). Although these data represent the annual workload of the aforementioned organizations, it indicates tendencies and patterns of diseases which could be used to compliment the empirical data.

Discussion

The results of this study shed light on the nature and degree of various kinds of emotional dysfunctions experienced by Afghan people, as a result of their exposure to traumatic conditions. The overall findings indicate that experimental groups scored significantly higher on all measures applied in the study compared to the control groups.

As was expected, adult experimental groups, both young and mature, showed a significantly higher degree of state and trait anxiety compared to the control groups. However, surprisingly, trait anxiety scores in the experimental groups were relatively higher than were state anxiety scores. This trend in reporting anxiety symp-

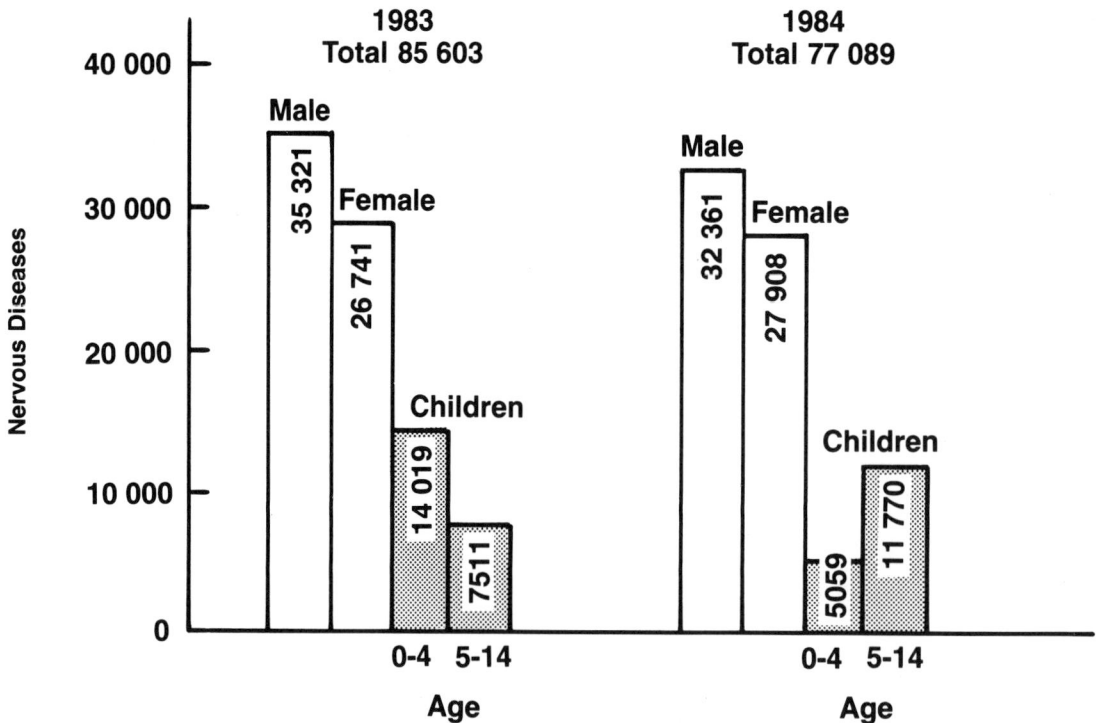

Figure 29.1. Distribution of nervous diseases among different age groups of Afghan refugees as reported by UNHCR medical office, 1985.

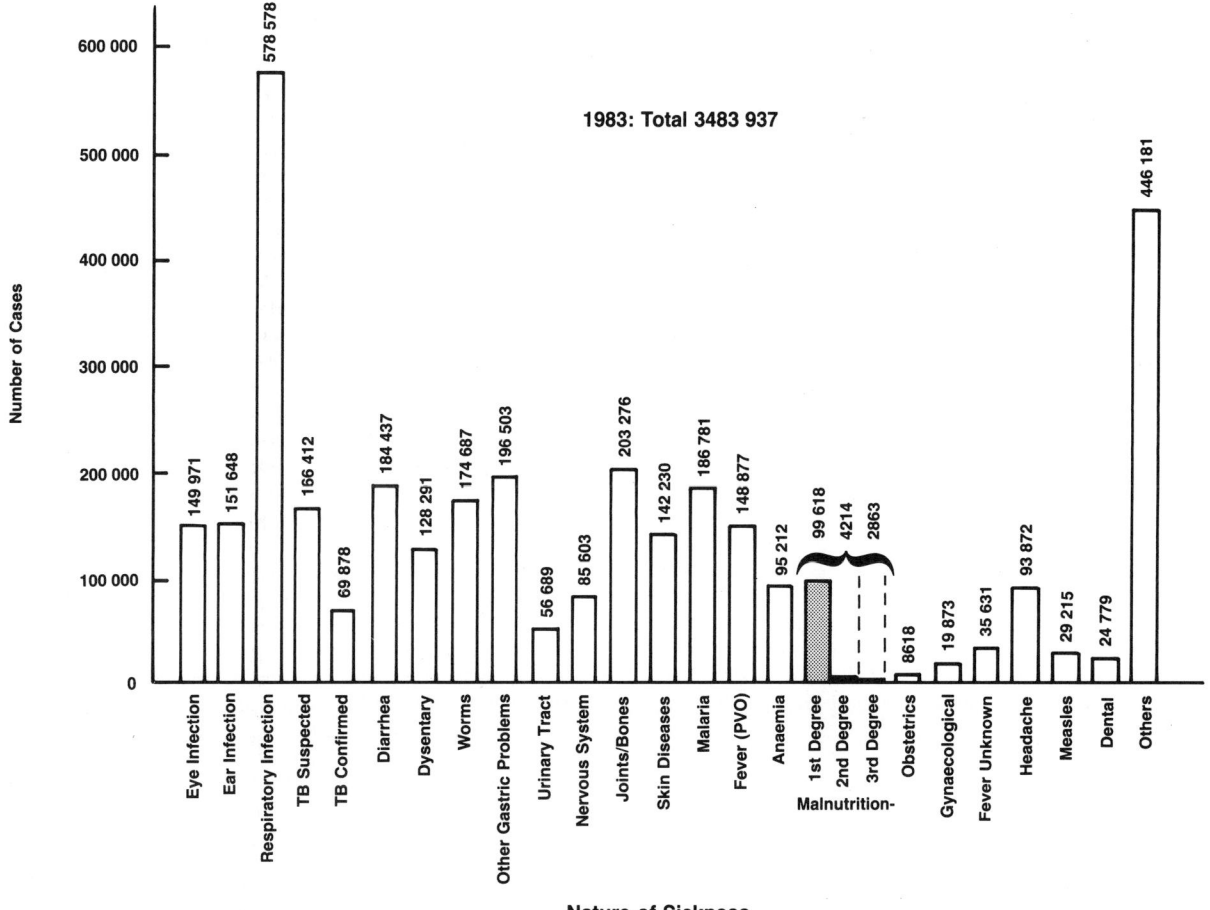

Figure 29.2. Distribution of diseases among different age groups of Afghan refugees as reported by UNHCR medical office, 1983.

toms could be attributed to the refugees' persistent exposure to stress both in the homeland and then in exile. Anxiety only decreases after the trauma has ended when cognitive assimilation takes place (Horowitz, 1979) and events are endowed with meaning (Lifton, 1983). This assimilation has not been possible; therefore, trait anxiety is higher for the refugees. With respect to state anxiety, more subjects reported feeling relaxed and secure during the interview with the researcher. This might have affected their responses to state anxiety inventory, resulting in lower scores than expected. The same argument could be applicable to short-stay and long-stay subjects; specifically, short-stay subjects have been exposed to stressful conditions over a long period of time in their homeland. In this respect the classification of short-stay and long-stay subjects was not very meaningful.

The results of this study indicated that all adult subjects in the experimental groups (young and mature adults) scored significantly higher on the Beck Depression scale (BDI) compared to control subjects. Studies carried out among Afghan refugees and available data from psychiatric clinics indicate that the ratio of depression is much higher than that among the native Pakistanis of the NWFP (Mufti, 1982; Daadfar, 1988; Wardak, 1988a). This could be due to the fact that Afghans are very proud and independent people with high self-esteem and a glorious past. This perception of self is damaged in the current tragic conditions and, as a consequence, they feel guilty, humiliated, and dehumanized, which lowers their self-esteem and contributes to the occurrence of depressive disorders. The significant role of self-esteem in the etiology of depressive disorders is well documented in the work of Bibring (1953). Another factor is the enormous losses the Afghans have endured during the last 10 years. The role of loss in the induction of depression is reported in several studies (e.g., Brown & Harris, 1978).

Although the present data cannot directly comment on changes over time, it is probable that initially when individuals were exposed to life-threatening situations in the war, greater psychic priority was attached to the fear of annihilation compared to the mourning over losses. Thus, anxiety dominated over other emotional problems. Following exile, however, annihilation anxiety diminished and grief and mourning over the experience of loss became more predominant, resulting in depression symptomatology. This assumption is quite consistent with research of Finlay-Jones and Brown (1981), who found a correlation between threatening experience and anxiety and loss and depression, respectively.

Certain symptoms reported by Afghans, such as severe dysphoria, sleep disturbances, and loss of appetite, are similar to those reported in Western cultures. Other symptoms (e.g., crying spells, feeling of guilt, suicidal thoughts and acts) are largely inhibited by sociocultural factors. Men and young boys are not supposed to cry; this is believed to be appropriate only for girls and women (Wardak, 1988a). Similarly, feelings of guilt and suicidal tendencies and acts are determined by religious values and social norms. Since Islam, like Judaism and Christianity, frequently emphasizes the idea of sin, a high frequency of guilt feelings as these data show is not strange to the Afghan sociocultural framework of the society. However, Islam strictly prohibits the act of suicide and regards it as a criminal act, neither does it condone death wishes. Suicidal thoughts are very rare among Afghans and I have never come across or heard of the act of suicide committed by a member of the community during several years of close contact with them. This impression is supported by epidemiological data (Gobar, 1970) which show a very low ratio of suicide in Afghanistan 0.25/100,000. Another possible reason is that Afghans externalize their aggression rather than internalize it. This is very consistent with the rather higher incidence of homicide compared with suicide in the country (Gobar, 1970). However, the incidence of domestic homicide is relatively low compared to other cultures.

In addition, the social familial cohesive character of the society, the care and respect for others, including strangers and people in crisis, are other factors which influence the lower occurrence of suicide. Patients, elderly, and those in crisis receive love and affection from friends, neighbors, distant and close relatives, even from strangers, and they never experience abandonment, isolation, or neglect. This helps them to maintain their sense of self-esteem, tolerance, peace, and security and enables them to cope successfully with life events.

Higher scores for obsessive compulsive neurosis were reported in both Afghan and Pakistani samples compared with other scales of the CCEI. This may arise because of the conservative style of culture with the numerous taboos, harsh rules, and norms imposed from childhood, plus the relatively poor standard of living rather than the current tragic conditions of war. This is amply evidenced by the higher frequency of these symptoms among Pakistanis who were not victimized by the war and conditions.

Although this study did not utilize specific scales for measuring PTSD, it has been observed that subjects indicated symptoms matching the criteria of PTSD symptoms as defined in the third edition of the *Diagnostic and Statistical Manual of Mental Disorders* (DSM-III) (American Psychiatric Association [APA], 1980) (e.g., nightmares, intrusive thoughts and memories, numbing of responsiveness to the external world, sudden acting or feeling as if the traumatic events were recurring, etc.) (Daadfar, 1988a; Mufti, 1982; Wardak, 1988a).

Although the present data clearly show that refugees experience psychoneurotic disturbance, these figures are probably underestimates of the magnitude of the impairment. Emotional problems are likely to be converted to physical disorders manifested in the form of headache, diarrhea, hypochondriasis, back pain, and

the like. Conversion to somatic problems is in keeping with the traditional conservative framework of the culture and constitutes a common ground for other neurotic disorders in almost all Oriental cultures. For example, the higher incidence of respiratory diseases among Afghan refugees in addition to such physical causes as anemia, tuberculosis, and malnutrition could be related to psychological factors (e.g., anxiety, panic attacks, hysteria, etc.). Because the diagnosis is done by general physicians with limited knowledge of psychiatry, it is possible that, hyperventilation which is associated with anxiety, hysteria, and PTSD (Gelder, Gath, & Mayou, 1985; Nixon, 1988) and chronic bronchitis which is associated with depression are being regarded as respiratory disorders. Moreover, emotional problems may provoke asthmatic attacks among those with established asthma (King, 1980).

Unless signs and symptoms of full-blown psychosis are observed, there is a tendency to attribute emotional problems to physical disorders. Consequently, the ratio of psychiatric disorders may appear less than is actually the case.

Afghans, like other Orientals, tend to somatize emotional problems. The conservative nature of their culture tends to discourage direct expression of their emotional problems and, as a consequence, they grieve privately, which may lead to the manifestation of grief in the form of physical complaints (e.g., headache, back pain, sleep disturbances, tensed shoulders, etc.). In my conversations with a number of physicians in various medical settings, they estimated that over 50% of their patients may be suffering from emotional disturbances manifested in the form of physical disorders, but the diagnosis and treatment are beyond their expertise, time, and the available facilities. It is reasonable to conclude that the higher incidence of various physical disorders compared to the prewar conditions in the homeland could also be partly attributed to emotional disorders prevailing among the nation (Wardak, 1988a).

A remarkable increase in epileptic cases, highlighted in the annual report of the PCA (Daadfar, 1988), seems to be due to genetic causes, although the triggering role of the appalling conditions could be important.

Afghan adolescents did not indicate symptoms of psychopathology different from those in the Pakistani adolescent group on the measures used in the study. Two factors may explain this result. First, the Afghan adolescents experience a higher degree of protection and security in the extended family system. Although they are aware of what is going on around them, their appraisal of the trauma may be lower than that expected in other cultures. Second, individuals in the control group are witnessing a period of rapid sociocultural change in their community in which liberal Western values are conflicting with the traditional values of their own society. This results in discord within the family and feelings of frustration. This view was expressed by a number of headmasters in the schools from which the control group subjects were drawn.

This study did not consider investigation of drug addiction; nevertheless, it is worth mentioning the extent of drug-related problems. Observations made by health professionals have raised apprehension about the increasing amount of drug abuse among youngsters in the homeland, which could be attributed to the weakening of spiritual traditions and religious values and the decreasing role of the family. Similar findings were reported by Nasr (1983) in the Lebanese Civil War. He revealed a distinct increase in abuse by youngsters of alcohol and drugs, such as heroin, morphine, cocaine, amphetamines, and other psychoactive substances.

Young people are more at risk of developing drug-abuse problems as reported by Du Pont (1989), the former head of the National Institute on Drug Abuse in the United States. He pointed out in his book that virtually all drugs are first used between the ages 12 and 20, and the age group most likely to abuse drugs is the 18 to 25 year olds.

Nevertheless, the overall social change and shift in values produced by the war culture, the lack of social support, the lack of sociofamilial cohesiveness as a major organizing force in the society, in addition to the painful episodes of conflict play a significant role in drug abuse and other forms of deviancy among the younger generation. Furthermore, the relationship between stressful conditions and substance abuse is well documented in the work of other researchers (Cooke & Allen, 1984; Smail, Stockwell, Hodeson, & Canter, 1984; Wanberg, 1969).

The conditions of youngsters within the family network in the refugee camps are better than those of young people living in the big cities in the homeland. The sociofamilial system, despite the damage it has sustained, is believed to be better in the refugee community, supported by religious values and traditions. In addition, it is believed that the degree of stress and exposure to life-threatening conditions is lower compared with the situation in the homeland. Thus, the constant exposure to traumatic conditions, the weakening of sociofamilial roles, isolation, fear, and other socioeconomic grievances could be reasons for the excessive substance abuse among youngsters in the homeland.

Trauma in Afghanistan as in all major catastrophes is individual and communal. The overwhelming nature of trauma represented in vast destruction and enormous loss of life has affected the life of each citizen in the country and in many cases shaken their psychological equilibrium, resulting in deep dysphoria, apathy, withdrawal anxiety and other emotional problems. It was collective because it has fractured the traditional cohesive framework of the social fabric and support system. This impairment, as documented in Erikson's (1976) work, did not occur suddenly as in the case of individual trauma, but developed as a result of continued chaotic upheaval of the country during the last 10 years of war, leading to an internal and external separation and displacement on a vast scale. In many cases, members of one family are separated in three or four different countries and have minimal contact with each other. Separation within the country is common in cases of some members of the family supporting the government and others joining the guerrillas (Mujahedin). Tens of thousands of people never returned from their prison and left behind them grieving families.

Psychic impairment sustained by Afghans could be partly attributed to the fragmentation of communality. But, more importantly, it is due to the deep sense of loss, both human and material, forced displacement, and the resulting demoralization. However, destruction of the community, the social support network, and separation from meaningful familiar places and faces has made it difficult for individuals to recover from their losses and from demoralization. The negative appraisal of the trauma is a very interesting and distinct feature within the sociocultural framework of the Afghan society. Despite the strong faith of the victims in the justness of their cause and their commitment to achieve their goals, their unwilling uprootedness both within and without the country was negatively perceived because the love of and attachment to the fatherland means much more than it does in some other cultures. The homeland is not merely the place of birth and living, it is the place of ancestors, honor, and historical pride from which they ruled the area for centuries. Thus, forced flight from home and fatherland is a humiliating experience which challenges the psychological equilibrium of the people and has major consequences for their well-being.

Perceived threat is believed to play a significant role in associating traumatic conditions with their long- and short-term psychological consequences and determines individual's reactions (Kates, 1977). Furthermore, cognitive appraisal of stressful situations determines stress and anxiety reactions (Lazarus, 1966; Spielberger, 1972). Paykel, Myers, Dienalt, Klerman, Lindenthal, and Pepper (1969), in their study of the situational precipitating factors in clinical depressive states, found that the critical factor was not the frequency of undesirable events, but the meaning of events to patients.

The psychological adjustment of Afghan refugees in Pakistan is believed on the whole to be better compared to that of those who migrated to the United States and European countries, for two reasons. First, the native inhabitants of the NWFP and Baluchistan regions, where the refugee are resettled, speak the same language, belong to the same religion, and are descendants of the same ethnic groups. Furthermore, they share the same traditional code of norms, values, and customs. The combination of these factors decreases the degree of cultural shock experienced by the refugees. Second, Afghan refugees in Pakistan have managed to restructure their traditional social support system and sociocultural institutions. This, in addition to the encouragement and hope provided by their brethren of the host communities, has enabled a more positive social environment compared to that of the more isolated refugees living in "alien" Western cultures.

The Afghans' sentimentality, love of family, the cohesive structure of their family and social groups, and their interpersonal orientation render them out of tune with the Western style of life. Their loyalty and deep attachment to their fatherland and thoughts of relatives left behind, together with problems associated with transplantation into an alien culture and environment (e.g., unemployment, incompetency in English, welfare dependence, low income, and sociocultural gap between the society of origin and the host country) increase their anxiety and doubts. Observations made by Afghan academics, professionals, and other experts have revealed a variety of psychosocial problems among Afghan refugees in the United States (USCR, 1985) arising from premigration traumatic conditions followed by problems faced in the country of resettlement. However, the full account of psychiatric impairment is not yet known.

Conclusion

The pattern of emotional disorder among Afghan people as documented in this and other studies (e.g., Daadfar, 1988; Mufti, 1982) is remarkably similar to clinical descriptions of war neuroses as initially described by Kardiner and Spiegel (1941).

Somatization among Afghans as in other Oriental nations is a way of expression for emotional problems and is likely to be a major component of PTSD as reported in the Horowitz (1979) model among Afghan subjects. Finally, war in Afghanistan has fractured the structure of the society to an extent which may need the efforts of future generations to cure its legacy. However, the postwar era, if properly utilized, provides a unique opportunity for modernization and rapid development of the Afghan society.

References

Abramson, J. H. (1966). Emotional disorders, status inconsistency and migration. *Millbank Memorial Fund Quarterly, 44,* 23–48.

Allodi, F. (1982). Psychiatric sequelae of torture and implication for treatment. *World Medical Journal,* 71–75.

American Psychiatric Association. (1980). *Diagnostic and statistical manual of mental disorders* (3rd ed.). Washington, DC: Author.

Aylesworth, L. S., Ossorio, P. S., & Osaki, L. T. (1979). Stress and mental health among Vietnamese in the U.S.A. In R. Endo, S. Sue, & N. Wanger (Eds.), *Asian-Americans: Social and psychological perspectives.* Palo Alto, CA: Science & Behavior Books.

Barnes, F. (1980). A psychiatric unit serving an international community. *Hospital and Community Psychiatry, 31,* 756–758.

Beck, A. T., Ward, C. H., Mendelsohn, M., Mock, J., & Erbaugh, J. (1961). An inventory measuring depression. *Archives of General Psychiatry, 4,* 561–571.

Bibring, E. (1953). The mechanism of depression. In P. Greenacre (Ed.), *Affective disorders* (pp. 17–47). New York: International Universities Press.

Bonan, B., & Eduards, M. (1984). The Indochinese refugees: An overview. *Australian and New Zealand Journal of Psychiatry, 18,* 40–52.

Brill, N. Q. (1967). Gross stress reaction II: Traumatic war neuroses. In A. M. Freedman & H. J. Kaplan (Eds.), *Comprehensive textbook of psychiatry* (pp. 1031–1035). Baltimore: Williams & Wilkens.

Brown, G. W., & Birley, J. L. T. (1968). Crisis and life changes and the onset of schizophrenia. *Journal of Health and Social Behavior, 9,* 203–214.

Brown, G. W., & Harris, T. O. (1978). *Social origin of depression.* London: Tavistock.

Cohen, R. E., & Ahearn, F. H. (1980). *Handbook for mental health care of disaster victims.* Baltimore: Johns Hopkins University Press.

Cooke, D. J., & Allen, C. A. (1984). Stressful life events and

alcohol abuse in women: A general population study. *British Journal of Addiction, 79*(4), 425–430.

Copeland, J. R. M. (1968). Aspects of mental illness in West African students. *Social Psychiatry, 3,* 7–13.

Crown, S, & Crisp, A. H., (1979). *Crown-Crisp Experiential Index (Manual).* North Pomfret, VT: Hodder & Stoughton.

Daadfar, M. A. (1988). *Psychiatry Centre for Afghan refugees (PCA), Annual Report,* Peshawar, Pakistan.

Derbyshire, R. (1969). Adaption of adolescent Mexican-Americans to the United States society. In E. Brody (Ed.), *Behavior in new environments.* Beverly Hills: Sage Publications.

Dohrenwend, B. P. (1975). Sociocultural and sociopsychological factors in the genesis of mental disorders. *Journal of Health & Social Behavior, 16,* 365–392.

Dohrenwend, B. S., & Dohrenwend, B. P. (1974). *Stressful life events: Their nature and effects.* New York: Wiley.

Du Pont, R. A. (1989, September). Illegal drugs, who's responsible? *The Plain Truth Magazine,* p. 4.

Eitinger, L. (1960). Psychiatric investigations among refugees: Patients in Norway. *Mental Hygiene, 44,* 91–106.

Erikson, K. T. (1976). *Everything in its path.* New York: Simon & Schuster.

Fakhr-el-Islam, M., & Hussain, A. Z. (1969). Evacuees presenting to the psychiatric clinic. *Journal of the Egyptian Medical Association, 52,* 333–340.

Finlay-Jones, R., & Brown, G. W. (1981). Types of stressful life events and the onset of anxiety and depression disorders. *Psychological Medicine, 11*(5), 803–815.

Garrison, J. (1983). *Mental health issues in relocation.* National Institutes of Health. Unpublished manuscript.

Gelder, M., Gath, D., & Mayou, R. (1985). *Oxford textbook of psychiatry.* Oxford Medical Publication.

Gobar, A. H. (1970). Suicide in Afghanistan. *British Journal of Psychiatry, 116,* 493–496.

Goldberg, D. (1978). *Manual of the General Health Questionnaire.* Windsor, U.K.: NFER-NELSON.

Grinker, R. R., & Spiegel, J. P. (1945). *Men under stress.* Philadelphia: Blakiston.

Hall, P. S., & Landreth, P. W. (1975). Assessing some long term consequences of a natural disaster. *Mass Emergencies, 1,* 55–61.

Hendin, H., & Hass, A. P. (1984). Post-traumatic stress disorders in veterans of early American wars. *Psychohistory Review, 12,* 25–30.

Hendin, H., Hass, A. P., Singer P., Gold, F., & Trigos, G. O. (1983). The influence of pre-combat personality on post-traumatic stress disorder. *Comprehensive Psychiatry, 24,* 530–534.

Holmes, T., & Rahe, R. (1967). The Social Readjustment Rating Scale. *Journal of Psychosomatic Research, 11,* 219–225.

Horowitz, M. J. (1979). Psychological response to serious life events. In V. Hamilton & D. M. Warburton (Eds.), *Human stress and cognition* (pp. 335–363). New York: Wiley.

Kardiner, A., & Spiegel, H. (1941). The traumatic neurosis of war. *Psychosomatic Medicine Monograph.* New York: Paul Hoeber.

Kates, R. W. (1977). Natural hazard in human ecological perspective: Hypothesis and models. *Economic Geography, 47,* 438–451.

Kendler, K. S. (1982). Demography of paranoid psychosis (delusional disorder): A review and comparison with schizophrenia and affective illness. *Archives of General Psychiatry, 38,* 890–902.

Kilpatrick, D. G., Veronen, L. J., & Best, C. H. (1985). Factors predicting psychological distress among rape victims. In C. R. Figley (Ed.), *Trauma and its wake: The study and treatment of post-traumatic stress disorders* (pp. 113–141). New York: Brunner/Mazel.

King, N. J. (1980). The behavioral management of asthma and asthma-related problems in children: A critical review of the literature. *Journal of Behavioral Medicine, 3*, 169–189.

Kino, F. F. (1960). Alien's paranoid reaction. *Journal of Mental Science, 79*, 589–594.

Kinzie, J. D., Tran, K. A., Breckenridge, A., & Bloom, J. D. (1980). An Indochinese refugee psychiatric clinic: Culturally accepted treatment approaches. *American Journal of Psychiatry, 137*, 1429–1432.

Kinzie, J. D., Manson, S. M., Do, T. V., Nguyen, T. T., Bui, A., & Than, N. P. (1982). Development and validation of Vietnamese language Depression Rating Scale. *American Journal of Psychiatry, 139*, 1276–1281.

Kohn, M. (1973). Social class and schizophrenia: A critical review and reformation. *Schizophrenia Bulletin, 7*, 60–79.

Korsching, P. F., Donnermeyers, J. F., & Burdge, R. J. (1980). Perception of property, settlement, payments and replacement housing among displaced persons. *Human Organization, 39*(4), 332–338.

Krupinski, J. (1984). Changing patterns of migration to Australia and their influence on the health of migrants. *Social Science and Medicine, 18*, 927–937.

Kumasaka, Y., & Saito, H. (1970). Kachizumi: A collective delusion among the Japanese and their descendants in Brazil. *Canadian Psychiatric Association Journal, 15*, 167–175.

Lazarus, R. S. (1966). *Psychological stress and the coping process.* New York: McGraw-Hill.

Lepowski, Z. J. (1975). Psychiatry of somatic diseases: Epidemiology, pathogenesis, classification. *Comprehensive Psychiatry, 16*, 105–124.

Lifton, R. J. (1983). *The broken connection.* New York: Basic Books.

Lin, K. M., Tozuma, L., & Masuda, M. (1979). Adaptional problems of Vietnamese refugees. *Archives of General Psychology, 36*, 955–961.

Liu, W. T., Lamanna, M., & Murata, A. (1979). *Transition to nowhere: Vietnamese refugees in America.* Nashville: Charter House.

Mansfield, S. (1982). *The Gestalts of war.* New York: Dial Press.

Mezey, A. G. (1960a). Personal background, emigration and mental disorder in Hungarian refugees. *Journal of Mental Science, 106.*

Mezey, A. G. (1960b). Psychiatric illness in Hungarian refugees. *Journal of Mental Science, 106*, 628–637.

Mezzich, J. E. (1979). A data based typology of depressed adolescents. *Journal of Personality Assessment, 43*, 1971.

Mezzich, A. C., & Mezzich, J. E. (1979). Symptomatology of depression in adolescence. *Journal of Personality Assessment, 43*, 267–275.

Milgram, N. A. (1986). *Stress and coping in the time of war.* New York: Brunner/Mazel.

Moore, H. E. (1958). *Tornados over Texas.* Austin: University of Texas Press.

Mufti, K. (1982). *Psychiatric problems among Afghan refugees.* Peshawar, Pakistan: Lady Reading Hospital. Unpublished manuscript.

Munger, R. G. (1986). Sleep disturbances and sudden death of Hmong refugees. In G. L. Hendricks *et al.* (Eds.), *The Hmongs in transition centre for migration study* (pp. 379–398). New York.

Naguyen, S. D. (1982). Psychiatric and psychosomatic problems among South East Asian refugees. *Psychiatric Journal of the University of Ottawa, 7*, 163–172.

Nasr, S. (1983). Psychiatric effects of civil war in Lebanon. *The Psychiatric Journal of the University of Ottawa, 8*(4), 208–212.

Nixon, C. (1988, August). *Psychophysiology of efforts.* Paper presented at the First European Conference on PTSD, Lincoln, England.

Odegaard, O. (1932). Immigration and insanity: A study of mental disease among the Norwegian born population of Minnesota. *Acta Psychiatrica et Neurologica Supplementum, 4*, 1–206.

Paykel, E. S. (1976). Life stress, depression and suicide. *Journal of Human Stress.*

Paykel, E. S., Myers, J. K., Dienalt, M. N., Klerman G. L., Lindenthal, J. J., & Pepper, M. P. (1969). Life events and depression. *Archives of General Psychiatry, 21*, 753–760.

Pedersen, S. (1949). Psychopathological reactions to extreme social displacements (refugee neurosis). *Psychoanalytic Review, 36*, 344–354.

Retterstol, N. (1968). Paranoid psychosis associated with unpatriotic conduct during WW II. *Acta Psychiatrica Scandinavica, 44*(3), 261–279.

Schwartz, C., & Myers, J. (1977). Life events and schizophrenia: Parts I & II. *Archives of General Psychiatry, 34*, 1238–1248.

Smail, P., Stockwell, T., Hodeson, R., & Canter, S. (1984). Alcohol dependence and phobic anxiety states. *British Journal of Psychiatry, 144*, 53–75.

Solnit, A. J., & Kris, M. (1967). Trauma and infantile experiences: A longitudinal perspective. In S. S. Furst (Ed.), *Psychic trauma* (pp. 175–220). New York: Basic Books.

Spielberger, C. D. (1972). Anxiety as an emotional state. In C. D. Spielberger (Ed.), *Anxiety: Current trends in theory and research* (Vol. 1). New York: Academic Press.

Spielberger, C. D. (1973). *Manual for the State-Trait Anxiety Inventory for Children.* Paper presented at the Seventh SIETAR Annual Conference, Vancouver, B.C., Canada.

Spielberger, C. D. (1980). *Manual for the State-Trait Anxiety Inventory.* Palo Alto, CA: Consulting Psychologists Press.

Steinberg, H. R., & Durell, J. (1968). A stressful social situation as a precipitant of schizophrenic symptoms: An epidemiological study. *British Journal of Psychiatry, 114*, 1097–1105.

Steiner, M., & Neumann, M. (1982). War neuroses and social support. In C. D. Spielberger & I. G. Sarason (Eds.), & N. A. Milgram (Guest Ed.), *Series in clinical and community psychology: Vol. 8. Stress and anxiety* (pp. 139–142). Washington, DC: Hemisphere.

Tseng, W. S. (1969). A paranoid family in Taiwan: A dynamic study of folie en famille. *Archives of General Psychiatry, 21*, 55–65.

Tyhurst, I. (1951). Displacement and migration: A study in social psychiatry. *American Journal of Social Psychiatry, 107*, 561–586.

Tyhurst, L. (1981). *Coping with refugees, a Canadian experience: 1948–1981.*

Uhlenhuth, E. H., & Paykel, E. S. (1973). Symptoms configuration and life events. *Archives of General Psychiatry, 28*, 743–748.

United Nations High Commissioner for Refugees. (1983). *Annual report on Afghan refugees.* Islamabad, Pakistan: Author.

United Nations High Commissioner for Refugees. (1985). *Annual report on Afghan refugees.* Islamabad, Pakistan: Author.

United Nations High Commissioner for Refugees. (1988a). *Annual report on Afghan refugees.* Islamabad, Pakistan: Author.

United Nations High Commissioner for Refugees. (1988b). *Refugee children around the world.* Geneva, Switzerland: Author.

United Nations High Commissioner for Refugees. (1989a). *Annual report on Afghan refugees*. Islamabad, Pakistan: Author.

United Nations High Commissioner for Refugees. (1989b). *Journal of refugees*. Islamabad, Pakistan: Author.

United States Committee for Refugees Publication. (1982/1985). *About Afghan refugees*. Washington, DC: U.S. Government Printing Office.

Verdonk, A. (1979). Migration and mental illness. *International Journal of Social Psychiatry, 25,* 295–305.

Wanberg, K. (1969). Prevalence of symptoms found among excessive drinkers. *International Journal of Addiction, 4,* 169–185.

Wardak, A. W. H. (1988a). *The investigation of some psychiatric and physiological effects of traumatic stress*. Unpublished doctoral thesis, University of Hull, U.K.

Wardak, A. W. H. (1988b). *Neurotic disorders, social support and trauma perception among Ethiopean refugees*. Unpublished manuscript, Department of Psychology, University of Hull, U.K.

Westermeyer, J. (1986). Migration and psychopathology. In C. L. Williams & J. Westermeyer (Eds.), *Refugee mental health in resettlement countries*. New York: Hemisphere Publishing.

Western, J. S., & Milne, G. (1979). Some social effects of a natural hazard: Darwin residents and Cyclone Tracy. In R. L. Heathcote & B. G. Thom (Eds.), *Natural hazards in Australia*. Canberra: Australia Academy of Science.

Wilson, J. P. (1988). Understanding the Vietnam veteran. In F. Ochberg (Ed.), *Post-traumatic therapy and victims of violence* (pp. 225–254). New York: Brunner/Mazel.

Yakteen, U. S. (1988). *Traumatic war stress and schizophrenia in Lebanon*. Paper presented in the First European Conference on PTSD, Lincoln, U.K.

Yesavage, J. A. (1983, June). Differential effects of Vietnam combat experiences vs. criminality on dangerous behavior by Vietnam veterans with schizophrenia. *Journal of Nervous and Mental Disease, 171*(6), 382–384.

Zargar, A. (1989, May 16–18). *War as a disaster*. Paper presented in the Second Workshop on War and Reconstruction, University of York, England.

CHAPTER 30

Stress, Coping, and Political Violence in Northern Ireland

Ed Cairns and Ronnie Wilson

Introduction

Since the late 1960s, Northern Ireland has been a relatively well-researched part of the world. Darby (1986) has noted that at least one bibliography on the Northern Irish conflict contains more than three thousand references. However, the question of the relationship between stress and political violence has not attracted the same level of interest. Indeed, apart from a flurry of activity in the 1970s, largely owing to the efforts of one researcher (Lyons, 1979), relatively little investigation has been carried out in this area. Furthermore, what research has been conducted has employed widely differing approaches. For this reason, the work to be reviewed here will be classified mainly in terms of the data-gathering methods used—primarily official statistics, such as admission and referral rates, clinical studies, and community-based studies. Under each of these headings, the existing research will be divided into two main areas focussing either on adults or on children.

The Violence in Perspective

Before examining the evidence relating stress and political conflict in Northern Ireland, it is important to place the violence in some sort of perspective. In order to do this, it is important to realize that before the political violence began, Northern Ireland was a relatively law-abiding society. For example, in the major conurbation, the Greater Belfast area, the number of murders in

the 1960s did not reach double figures, and in the period from 1960 to 1964 only one murder was reported in the city. Furthermore, since the onset of political violence, "ordinary" violence has increased steadily; however, it has consistently remained substantially lower than that in other parts of the United Kingdom (England, Wales, and Scotland).

Second, it is also important to remember that political violence is not the only problem that Northern Irish society has to contend with. The major problem, many would claim, is that it is one of the least affluent regions of Western Europe, with substantially lower average incomes, higher levels of unemployment, and larger families than the rest of the United Kingdom. These economic problems also predate the current economic unrest.

Finally, it is worth noting that the single biggest cause of death in Northern Ireland, aside from natural causes, is not political violence but road traffic accidents. In any year, residents of Northern Ireland are about twice as likely to be killed in a road traffic accident as they are to be killed by being the victim of political violence.

Background to the Violence

In order to understand any possible relationship between political violence and stress in Northern Ireland, it is necessary to understand something of the violence itself. If one uses 1969 as a starting date for the current political unrest in Northern Ireland, then since that date until the end of 1988 some 2,710 people have died directly as a result of political violence and almost 30,000 have been numbered among the official statistics as "injured." What these statistics do not reveal, however, is the complexity of the violence and, in particular, they do not allow the casual reader to understand that since 1969 violence in Northern Ireland has varied in three impor-

Ed Cairns and Ronnie Wilson • Department of Psychology and Centre for the Study of Conflict, University of Ulster, Coleraine, Londonderry BT52 1SA, Northern Ireland.
International Handbook of Traumatic Stress Syndromes, edited by John P. Wilson and Beverley Raphael. Plenum Press, New York, 1993.

tant ways: (1) temporally, (2) spatially, and (3) qualitatively.

Variations in Patterns of Violence

Temporal Variations

In the first year of the "troubles," only 13 people died, but this figure rose quickly to an all time high of 467 in 1972. After this, a slight drop occurred but deaths *per year* still averaged around 250 for the period 1973 to 1976. They then dropped again to an average of about 90 per year for the next 5 years and then declined over the subsequent 5 years to just below 70 per year, reaching the lowest level (54 deaths) since 1970 in 1985. However, over the last 3 years, the signs are that the graph is again moving in an upward direction.

Spatial Variations

Not only has the violence varied in intensity from year to year but it has also varied in terms of its geographical location. Perhaps this is best illustrated in data reported by Poole (1983). He examined deaths per thousand attributed to political violence over the period 1969 to 1981 for 27 towns in Northern Ireland with a population greater than 5,000 and reported a range from a maximum of 1.91 per 1,000 to a minimum of zero. He was able to record that 7 towns had recorded one or more deaths per thousand in this period while 4 had experienced no fatalities at all. The detailed explanation for these variations is beyond the scope of this chapter. However, in the light of data to be presented later, it is worth noting that Poole (1983) concluded that the ethnic composition of an area is an important factor, particularly the size of the local Catholic population vis a vis to the local Protestant population, such that those areas with a relatively larger Catholic population are more likely to have experienced greater levels of violence.

Qualitative Variations

The changes noted above in terms of time and space have also been accompanied by changes in the type of violence that has occurred over the last 20 years in Northern Ireland. In the beginning, *street rioting* was by far the most common form of violence, though this period only lasted for about 2 to 3 years. Since then, some form of confrontation between the security forces and the paramilitary organizations has become the norm. Also, the form that these confrontations have taken have changed over time. For example, *bombs* were rather more common in the late seventies, often directed at "economic" targets, such as shops, hotels, or pubs. More recently, *assassination attempts*, especially with members of the security forces as prime targets, have become more common. This is illustrated by the fact that, according to Pockgrass (1987), from 1972 to 1974 some 74% of the fatalities were civilians but that this figure dropped to 56% in the period from 1978 to 1983. As a result, today fewer people are probably directly involved in the violence compared to earlier periods. On the other hand, the violence has now spread beyond the one or two highly urbanized centers of the early period to include more rural locations.

Adults

Psychiatric Admission and Referral Rates

General Trends

The first study to examine the psychiatric impact of the political violence in Northern Ireland was that by Fraser (1971), which examined psychiatric admission rates and outpatient referrals in the city of Belfast—the area where the violence, largely in the form of street rioting, predominated at that time. For the purposes of this study, Fraser divided the city into three areas: one where the worst violence had occurred, one where "signs of tension" were present but where violence was not widespread, and the remainder of the city. The results led Fraser to conclude that stress productive of psychiatric morbidity appeared to be maximal in areas that were under threat of attack as opposed to those where there was a more obvious risk.

Orbell (1988) conducted an analysis of psychiatric inpatient statistics in Northern Ireland for 1981 in order to make comparisons with similar statistics from England and Scotland. These data were based on ICD-9 criteria—excluding admissions for mental retardation and admission for children under 15 years of age.

The data were collected into 10 diagnostic categories and for each area, age- and sex-specific rates of first and all subsequent admissions were calculated, and a direct age/sex standardization was carried out. Her results suggested that first admission rates in Northern Ireland were slightly higher, for both sexes, than those in Scotland and substantially higher than in England.

Perhaps the most ambitious use of official statistics to date has been that made by Murphy (1984), who divided Northern Ireland into four areas—Belfast, rural south, rural west, and rural east—and attempted to compare admission rates for a total of four diagnostic categories (affective disorders, alcoholism, neurotic disorders, and schizophrenia) with the level of political violence to which each of these areas had been exposed during the years 1971 to 1973. Based on an examination of Catholic/other ratios, he concluded that there appeared to be no particular relationship between hospitalization patterns and violence. However, he did speculate that there could be an interaction between segregation levels and violence which meant that where the minority "appears to be winning . . . and is largely segregated its admission rates drop."

Neurotic Disorders

What struck Orbell about her admission rate data for neurotic disorders was the remarkable difference between the rates for Northern Ireland and those for Scotland. In fact, she noted that this was the only category for which the rate in Scotland was more akin to that in England than in Northern Ireland. In particular, the rate of first admissions for males in Northern Ireland, was around *four times* that in Scotland or in England. Furthermore, Orbell was able to show that only in Northern Ireland were male and female admission rates for neurotic disorders relatively similar.

To a certain extent, this information appears at odds with that provided by Murphy (1984) who also commented on admission rates for neurotic disorders, this time for two different time periods, 1965 to 1966 (before the violence had begun) and 1970 to 1972 (the first years of the present "troubles"). The interesting observation that he made was that he detected a *shift* away from neurotic disorders toward affective diagnoses, especially for Catholic males, which he surmised might represent a genuine increase in the intensity of depressive reactions. However, these differences may represent a real change over the ten year interval separating Murphy and Orbell's data.

Depressive Illness

Lyons (1972) examined the incidence of depressive illness in Belfast, comparing mean rates from the period 1964 to 1968 with those for September 1969 to August 1970. This analysis indicated a significant decrease in depressive illness during this latter period, and Lyons noted that this reduction was most marked in males, those with endogenous depression, those over 40 years of age, and those in Social Classes IV and V.

This study also divided the city into different areas—this time into four quadrants plus an inner and outer zone—and reported the number of cases of male depression for four of these areas: the inner west, the outer west, the inner south, and the outer south because these segments contrasted most in terms of the amount of violence they had experienced (West Belfast had experienced the most as had the inner city). All these areas showed a reduction in the number of cases of male depression over the 1969 to 1970 period, and these reductions were statistically significant in all but the outer south area. In contrast, the rural region bordering on the outer south area of Belfast showed a significant increase in the number of cases of male depression.

Lyons thus concluded that reductions in levels of depression in Belfast but not in the neighboring rural area had been due to the greater opportunities to externalize aggression in Belfast at this time. However, as Heskin (1980) pointed out, this conclusion is not tenable because Lyons's own data show that the reduction in depression had been as great in South Belfast, where virtually no rioting had occurred, as it had been in West Belfast, where most of the rioting had occurred. Cairns and Wilson (1985) have also pointed out that if the externalization of aggression explanation offered by Lyons had been correct, one would have expected the reductions in depression to occur in younger males, not those over 40. Instead, they suggested that if Lyons documented a real phenomenon—the reduction of depression in Belfast in 1969 to 1970—then this was more likely to be due to migration out of the city of Belfast and into the neighboring, rural areas which was common at this time (Darby, 1986).

Finally, King, Griffiths, Reilly, and Merret (1983) provided data which they claim reveals that over the period 1966 to 1980 first admissions for all depressive illnesses in Northern Ireland declined steadily. In fact, the data suggest that total admissions actually peaked in 1970 and then dropped dramatically until 1975, rose slightly again, and declined once more. The authors suggested that this decline was due to the greater use of antidepressants by family doctors.

Suicide and Attempted Suicide

Lyons (1972, 1979), in a series of studies which examined suicide rates for Northern Ireland over the period 1964 to 1977 reported a decrease during the period 1970 to 1972 (the time when civil disturbances, particularly rioting, were at their height). The rate then rose again as rioting tailed off. Furthermore, this fall occurred at all ages but was most marked in the 15 to 24 age group. However, Cairns and Wilson (1985) have pointed out that a study (Dean, Adelstein, & Spooner, 1976) which compared suicide rates in Scotland, England, Wales, the Republic of Ireland, and Northern Ireland suggests that suicide rates in England and Wales also dropped during the early 1970s as they did in Northern Ireland.

The claim that increased political violence led to a decrease in suicides must also be balanced against the argument by O'Malley (1972) that there had been a striking increase in admissions owing to attempted suicide over approximately the same period. Lyons and Bindall (1977), however, found in a further study that rising admissions because of attempted suicide were common in almost every year and that this could be better explained as part of the general increase being observed throughout the rest of the British Isles. When Lyons and Bindall went on to examine the precipitating factors in each case, they found that in "no case was intimidation or being the victim of terrorist activity given as a cause."

A further problem in trying to make sense of suicide rates in Northern Ireland is that because of the strong religious views in the society concerning suicide, particularly among members of the Catholic community, it is always possible that suicides are actually under-recorded. Curran, Finlay, and McGarry (1988) noted therefore that when they combined suicide rates with "accidental" and "undetermined" deaths, the fall in the rate for the early 1970s was much less dramatic. They also reported that since then (the early 1970s) there has been a steady rise in suicides in Northern Ireland so that by 1986 the rate per million was at its highest since 1960 and exceeded that for England and Wales for the first time since that date.

Closer analysis of these data by Curran *et al.* (1988) revealed that this increase has been mainly a male phenomenon and confined to the under 45 age groups. Also hanging and firearms have become the most common two methods of suicide during this time. This latter point is of interest because there has been considerable media speculation that the rise in the suicide rate is largely the result of an increase in the number of young policemen who are taking their own lives. Curran *et al.* (1988) therefore compared rates per million for the general male population and for the male police population. The data revealed that although in absolute terms, the number of police suicides per year is small for the period

1980 to 1986, the rate had reached 32.9 per million among male policemen compared to 13.3 for the general population.

Psychosomatic Illnesses

Given that the amount of obvious psychiatric illness in the Northern Irish community appears to have been limited, it is perhaps surprising that researchers have not attempted to explore the relationship between other disorders, where the relationship with stress is rather less obvious, such as the whole range of psychosomatic illnesses.

To date only three papers have been published in this area. These (Clyde *et al.*, 1975; Hadden & McDevitt, 1974; Parkes, 1977) have reported attempts to link the political violence to thyrotoxicosis, peptic ulcers, and coronary heart disease. None of these studies is particularly wideranging or indeed methodologically sophisticated. All are in agreement, however, in that they found no relationship between the political violence and the particular illness they were investigating. And this failure to find any link between psychosomatic illness and the violence in Northern Ireland is reinforced by comments made by other authors. For example Lyons (1974), in his examination of bomb victims, noted that "somatic symptoms were not as frequent as might have been expected," while Bell, Kee, Loughrey, Roddy, and Curran (1988) noted that among their posttraumatic stress disorder (PTSD) patients there was "a low frequence of . . . psychosomatic manifestations."

Alcohol-Related Disorders

There has been at least one major epidemiological study of problem drinking in Northern Ireland (Blaney & Mackenzie, 1980). Unfortunately, this study made no attempt to examine the possibility that problem drinking in Northern Ireland might be related to the ongoing political violence. However, the authors noted that problem drinking was most prevalent in the eastern part of the province and especially among Catholic males in the age group of 18 to 29 years. This, they suggested, may reflect a lack of enforcement of liquor-licensing legislation in Catholic areas, especially at this time in Belfast. This finding replicated research by Harbison (1983) and by Murphy (1984) who, in his comparison of admission rates in 1965 to 1966 and 1970 to 1972, noted a "marked rise" in Catholic admissions for alcoholism among females. He suggested this could be explained in two ways: either a greater readiness on the part of Catholics to accept shelter, or, of course, to a genuine increase in alcohol-related problems.

As a result of an examination of admission rates for alcohol-related disorders in one year (1981), Orbell (1988) reported that rates in Northern Ireland are similar to those in Scotland, both of which are higher than those in England. Harbison (1983) also compared data from Northern Ireland, the Republic of Ireland, Scotland, England, and Wales for first-admissions rates for alcoholism or alcoholic psychosis per 100,000 over the period from 1967 to 1978. Results show that rates in the Republic of Ireland were the highest whereas those in Northern Ireland were broadly comparable to those in Scotland. However, although the Scottish rate showed an increase of 44% over this time period, the Northern Irish rate showed an increase of 67%.

Harbison (1983) also reported data on deaths from liver cirrhosis for the period 1968 to 1978 which revealed a 28% increase over this time compared to a 6% increase for the Republic of Ireland and a 30% increase in Scotland.

What is important however, is that all these figures assume a special significance when one remembers that various surveys have revealed (see Harbison, 1983, for a review) that a significant proportion of the adult population in Northern Ireland remains totally abstinent. This finding must mean as Harbison (1983) pointed out "that within the drinking group of Northern Irish adults a considerable proportion appear vulnerable to the development of alcohol related problems."

Psychotropic Drug Prescriptions

In the first study in this area, Fraser (1971) examined the prescribing rates for hypnotics, tranquilizers, and antidepressants in the city of Belfast for the months of August and September in 1968 and 1969 and reported no change for hypnotic and antidepressant prescribing but a significant increase in tranquilizer prescribing from 1968 to 1969.

This study also reported prescribing rates from two general practices located in each of these three areas, this time finding a significant increase for tranquilizer prescribing but only for the practices located in the area where violence was occurring.

It is difficult, however, to interpret this information because the study also reported increases in tranquilizer prescribing over the same period of time for three provincial towns situated some distance from Belfast, and indeed for the whole of Northern Ireland.

A more accurate picture of the complexity of research in this area has been well provided by a series of studies by King, McMeeking, and Elmes (1977) and King, Griffith, Reilly, and Merret (1982). The first of these studies reported an analysis of antidepressant prescribing in Northern Ireland for the period 1966 to 1975, showing a massive increase over this time. However, the authors argued that this was almost certainly not related to the development of political violence over this period because it was mirrored by a similar increase in England over the same time period.

The second study consisted of a much more sophisticated report of all psychotropic drug prescribing in Northern Ireland for the years 1966 to 1980. Again the authors concluded that tranquilizer prescribing bore no relationship to the political violence.

A detailed comparison between prescribing in Great Britain and Northern Ireland for the year 1978 revealed that there was significantly less hypnotic and antidepressant prescribing in Northern Ireland that year although there was significantly more prescribing of minor analgesics, antimimetics, and tranquilizers.

This study also reported a more detailed examination of psychotropic drug prescribing for the year 1978 within Northern Ireland. This finding demonstrated a link between certain categories of drugs and various sociodemographic variables, such as age, the proportion of women in the sample, and the degree of overcrowding in the home. Finally, this report also made comparisons between Northern Ireland and other European countries which showed that Northern Ireland ranked third (behind Iceland and Denmark) in 1980 for benzodiazepine tranquilizing drugs prescribed in terms of a defined daily dose per thousand population per day.

Clinical Studies

An insight into the type of patient seen in general practice for "psychiatric reasons" in the early days of the violence is provided by a follow-up study of 217 patients from three general practices in the central riot area of Belfast in August/September, 1969 (Lyons, 1971). The majority were women (79%) for whom the common diagnoses were related to what the author described as "normal anxiety" with only 19% referred to a psychiatrist at the time of the study. Also, even though only 13% had a history of psychiatric in- or outpatient treatment, 50% had been seen before by the physician for psychiatric reasons, suggesting that those with a previous history were more likely to show signs of stress at this time.

Information about a more specialized type of patient comes from the study by Lyons (1974) (noted above) which reported on 100 people who had been directly involved in a bomb explosion. These patients, Lyons noted, were likely to develop several symptoms. In the vast majority of the cases (92%), some type of affective disturbance was present, the commonest of these being anxiety *per se* or anxiety with various phobic symptoms. Of the phobic symptoms, the commonest was agoraphobia. Depression was also a symptom in 22% with irritability present. These adults also showed exaggerated startle reactions to loud noises and, in particular, their symptoms were apparently often intensified if they heard explosions or gunfire coming from other parts of the city.

The vast majority of these patients were treated as outpatients with only 6 requiring inpatient treatment. Also, there was a tendency for females to show more disturbance and a statistically significant trend for more disturbance to be present with increasing age. Overall, there was a fairly rapid rate of recovery among these Belfast patients, which, Lyons noted, is surprising given that the majority were still living in the same sort of environment that had originally precipitated their illness and that the original incidents had all been relatively serious with over half involving loss of life, sometimes of a relative. Overall, Lyons concluded that this was evidence of the development of "a remarkable resilience and tolerance" for this particular type of stress.

Hadden, Rutherford, and Merrett (1978) reported that there were no records of severely physically injured patients showing signs of emotional shock and, furthermore, that it was their impression that "badly injured patients were usually calm and cooperative." Their report was concerned with 1,532 consecutive patients who had been admitted to the accident and emergency unit of one of the major Belfast hospitals because of their exposure to a bomb explosion. The main focus of their report was with physical symptoms and treatment. However, the authors provideed some information

which is of interest here under the heading of "emotional shock." And what they noted is that some 50% ofthese patients were recorded as having sustained psychological shock, the vast majority of these being women (82%). Furthermore, only 23% of the female emotionally shocked sustained any physical injuries compared to 54% of the males who were so classified.

The information from these earlier studies has now been brought up to date by a series of reports describing individuals who were referred for medicolegal psychiatric assessment in the years from 1979 to 1984 (Bell *et al.*, 1988; Kee, Bell, Loughrey, Roddy, & Curran, 1987; Loughrey, Bell, Kee, Roddy, & Curran, 1988). This series is of particular interest because it includes not only victims of political violence but victims, for example, of sexual and common assault. These two categories combined accounted for some 21% of those referred while the remainder were classified as follows: (1) casual witness (at risk) 31%, (2) assassination attempt 13%, (3) hostage/captive 12%, (4) casual witness (no risk) 9%, (5) violent threat 9%, and (6) violent personal assault 5%. Examining the records of those patients over 16 years of age only, Kee *et al.* (1987) reported that 23% could be identified as suffering from posttraumatic stress disorder (PTSD) as defined by the DSM-III (American Psychiatric Association, 1980).

Remarkably, when the type of incident the patient was involved in was classified as noted above, there was no significant difference in the rate of PTSD resulting from *different* types of incidents. Nor indeed did the authors find any link between PTSD and the fact that the particular incident resulted in death to another individual. In fact, the only differences found between the PTSD group and the other patients was that the former were more likely to be women who were older and widowed and to have had marital disharmony and depressive features following the particular incident.

Community Studies

The few community-based studies that have been carried out in Northern Ireland have all used the same measure of psychiatric morbidity—the General Health Questionnaire (GHQ) (1978)—and have all been carried out within the last 5 years.

Cairns and Wilson (1985) provided some details of the first of these studies which were quota sample-based surveys of around 600 people chosen to represent the population of Northern Ireland in both 1983 and 1984. The mean score obtained in both years was somewhat higher than that obtained in similar studies in Australia and England. However, they do note that both their surveys were carried out in midwinter. Better evidence has come from a recent survey on health and life-style (Barker *et al.*, 1988) which involved administering the GHQ to a sample ($N = 547$) drawn at random to represent the Northern Irish population. These researchers noted that about 22% of their sample scored at or above the 80th percentile on the 30-item GHQ. This is about the same level as that reported by Cairns and Wilson (1984) from a random sample of two towns in Northern Ireland and is actually a little lower than the same statistic reported from a large random sample of the population of Great Britain (Huppert, Roth, & Gore, 1987).

In an attempt to provide more accurate data on levels of mental illness in Northern Ireland, Cairns, Wilson, McClelland, and Gillespie (1986) validated the GHQ against the PSE (Present State Examinations) using a Northern Irish community sample. The resulting information allowed Cairns and Wilson (1987) to estimate "true" prevalence rates for eight different random samples gathered over the period from 1983 to 1987. And what this study suggested is that the mean prevalence level is around 12% with a range from 9% to 13%.

Barker and her associates (1988) reported that in their study the group who scored highest on the GHQ were the unemployed. This is confirmation of the finding reported by Cairns and Wilson (1985) who, using multiple regression, were able to say that the best predictors of mild psychiatric morbidity were employment status, family size, and marital status in 1983. However, of particular interest here is the fact that, in 1984, when additional information about individual's perception of the level of violence in his or her own neighborhood was added, this was also identified as a statistically significant predictor of GHQ score, but only added a further 2% to the socioeconomic variables identified in 1983.

Evidence confirming the relationship between psychological well-being and the way in which the political violence is perceived came from a second study carried out by Cairns and Wilson (1984). This research involved comparing random samples of residents of two towns in Northern Ireland, which were similar in most respects, except that one town had suffered considerably more violence than the other. As expected, those who lived in the more violence-prone town scored at a significantly higher level on the GHQ. Also, regardless of which town they lived in, those who *perceived* that their town had experienced a good deal of violence scored higher compared to those who perceived that their town had experienced comparatively little or no violence. Finally, there was a significant interaction such that those who perceived more violence in their area, and also actually lived in the more violent town, scored more highly on the GHQ.

Coping with Violence

This last result, noted above, led Cairns and Wilson (1984) to speculate that denial might be playing an important role in coping with violence in Northern Ireland. They reached this conclusion because they noted that the majority of people who lived in the high violence town did not rate their town as having a particularly high level of violence. Further, this group of people, in turn, scored at a lower level on the GHQ than the minority of people in the high violence town who accurately reported that indeed they lived in a town where there had been "a lot" of violence. In other words, Cairns and Wilson suggested that perhaps people in Northern Ireland dealt with the stress generated by the violence by denying the existence of the violence going on around them.

In an attempt to provide further evidence to support this denial hypothesis, Giles and Cairns (1979) carried out a quasi-experimental study involving three groups of students: (1) English students temporarily resident in

Northern Ireland, (2) Northern Irish students who were permanent residents of Northern Ireland, and (3) a control group of English students permanently resident in England. All these young people undertook the same Stroop-like task which required them to name the colors of ink used to print a series of words related to the political violence in Northern Ireland. Previous studies by other researchers using such groups as spider phobics had indicated that interference with such emotional words can result even when the individual concerned denies the particular problem. However, contrary to the hypothesis, the group which took longest to name the violence-related words were the English in Northern Ireland. From this finding, the authors concluded that compared to these English students who were newly resident in Northern Ireland, the Northern Irish natives had become *habituated* to the violence and therefore reacted in the same way as the control group.

This result is interesting because the other major mechanism invoked to explain the relatively low levels of stress induced by the political violence in Northern Ireland has been *habituation*. As McWhirter (1987) put it, the "abnormal" features of the violence have become "normal" in that the political violence has "become an accepted part of the backcloth of events in Northern Ireland."

In the only other study carried out in this area, Cairns and Wilson (1989) asked a quota sample of people from two towns with contrasting levels of violence to complete two scales, Distancing and Seeking Social Support, from the Folkman and Lazarus Ways of Coping Questionnaire. This was done in order to find out how these people reacted when "the last serious incident" occurred. People were also asked how they rated the level of violence in their own town. The results indicated that those who perceived the violence *locally* to be more serious used *less* distancing while they also reported seeking the most social support. Most importantly, those who lived in a *high-violence* area were more likely to report using distancing than were those from a less violence prone area. Cairns and Wilson (1989) therefore concluded that some form of denial may indeed be the main form of coping and that this was, in turn, related to the appraisal of violence as well as to actual levels of violence.

Children

Hard evidence of the degree to which children in Northern Ireland have become embroiled with the political violence is difficult to come by. This is because there is no breakdown available of the casualties' figures by age. Cairns (1987) estimated that between 1969 and 1983 some 150 children under the age of 14 years had been killed or injured directly as a result of political violence.

Furthermore, there are clear indications that children in Northern Ireland have had widespread experience of the political violence in its variety of manifestations. The earliest survey of experience of the troubles among children was a study by McKeown (1973) of harassment on the way to school. In this survey, all of the postprimary schools in the province were contacted and a substantial majority agreed to take part; of these, 51% reported that a degree of harassment had occurred, and the data also showed that 50 children had been seriously injured and 1 child was killed.

In more recent years, as Cairns (1987) has pointed out, "hundreds of children in Northern Ireland have had to witness their father's murder and, on occasion, school teachers or school bus drivers have been murdered in front of the children in their care." More indirect experiences of the violence have included having a friend or relative killed or injured. The occurrence of an incident in one's home town may be stressful to vulnerable children even if no one they know has been involved.

Quantitative data on these types of experiences among children have been reported by McGrath and Wilson (1985). In a province-wide survey, 522 10- and 11-year-old children were sampled randomly from elementary school registers and interviewed about several areas of their lives and their mental health. Almost 20% of the children reported that they had been in or near a bomb explosion, 20.1% reported that they had a relative or friend injured or killed because of the troubles, and 12% said that they felt that their area was not safe to live in.

It would appear, therefore, that there has been a substantial level of both direct and indirect experience among children of the violence and its consequences. The remainder of this section will review the evidence in an attempt to decide if this experience has been associated with any adverse psychological effects.

Psychiatric Admission and Referral Rates

Only one study has actually made use of such information related to children (McCauley & Troy, 1983). This involved the examination of the records of children referred to a Child Psychiatric Clinic in Belfast in the years 1968 (i.e., before the "recent" outbreak of violence), 1972, 1976, and 1980. What this exercise revealed was that in 3 of the 4 years, around 400 children were referred annually. However, in 1972, the most violent year so far, only 229 children were referred.

McCauley and Troy also carried out a detailed examination of the case notes of a random sample of the children referred during these 4 years for reasons other than psychometric examination or for litigation purposes—approximately a 1:3 sample in each year. They noted that the children referred in each year were fairly well matched in terms of age (mean 10 years) and gender (around 60% were boys). Also, in 2 out of every 10 cases, at least one of the parents had had a previous psychiatric consultation and in 1 out of every 4 the family had moved the household in the preceding 2 years.

In general, over the 4 years, about one third of the cases examined were considered to have no abnormality in the sense of exhibiting a disorder which was sufficiently marked and prolonged to cause handicap to the child or his or her parents. With these mild or transient disorders excluded, the most common diagnosis was neurotic disorders followed by antisocial disorders. One change that is of particular interest is that there was a rise in the number of emergency referrals over time and that usually this was due to children making parasuicide attempts.

What the authors consider to be most surprising is that in the 4 separate years they examined, which covered a 12-year span, few changes had occurred in the pattern of referrals. As they noted, when one considers the changes in Northern Irish society over this period, both social and economic, including referral habits and diagnostic practices, this result was most unexpected.

The one major change that they recorded is that close examination of the case notes for any mention of the political violence revealed that in 1972 and 1976 about 30% of the records contained such a mention but that this dropped to around 10% in 1980. They also noted that in 1972 such a reference to the violence was most likely to be a general reference, whereas in 1976 and in 1980 it was more likely that mention of the violence would be of a specific event, such as a bombing or a shooting.

Overall, therefore, these authors cautiously concluded that their research provided no evidence for a direct link between child psychiatric disorders (strictly defined) and the political violence.

Clinical Studies

The only detailed clinical picture of those children whose mental health was adversely influenced by the political violence has been given by Fraser (1974). According to Fraser, the typical child victim of this time fell into a narrow age band of 8 and 13 years, who had been exposed to a particular violent incident which, at the time, had led to such things as a fainting fit, an asthma attack, or a sleep disturbance. Furthermore, these problems tended to continue after the precipitating event and often became worse with the passage of time. Indeed, the original phobic anxiety attack often generalized to other stimuli.

Some additional details can be gleaned from a report by Lyons (1974). This information comes in the course of a study which reported on 100 patients referred for psychiatric opinion who had been directly involved in bomb explosions. In the course of this report, Lyons noted that the age range of these victims was from 1.5 years to 73 years. Although unfortunately he does not say exactly how many children are affected, we are told that 27% were in the age range 0–19 years.

According to Lyons the children in his study showed various manifestations of anxiety, which could be grouped under the term *behavior disorder*. This included such things as enuresis, regression of speech, development of a stammer, and, in two children under 3 years of age, a refusal to eat for a period of 48 hours.

Community Studies

To date, just four community-based surveys have been carried out in order to explore the relationship between stress and political violence among children in Northern Ireland. The first two of these (Fee, 1980, 1983) involved the administration of a teacher-rating instrument which has been used extensively in epidemiological research on childhood disorders in Britain—the Rutter Teacher Questionnaire. Rutter (1967) argued that about 60% of children who score above the cutoff point for "disturbance" on the scale would normally be confirmed as disturbed when interviewed by a psychiatrist.

The surveys reported by Fee were carried out in 1975 and 1981, and in both the respondents were 11-year-old children living in Belfast (5,000 in the first survey and 7,000 in the second). In the first survey, some 15% of the children scored above the cutoff point on the questionnaire and in the second this had fallen to almost 9%. These results are of particular interest because they can be compared with those reported by (Rutter, Cox, Tupling, Berger, & Yule, 1975) for surveys carried out in the Isle of Wight and in 10 inner London boroughs, respectively, and also with two other similar surveys, one reported by Vikan (1985), carried out in Norway and the other reported by McGee et al. (1985), and carried out in New Zealand.

Although the prevalence in Belfast fell between 1975 and 1981, it was substantially higher in both years than that found in the Isle of Wight (6.8%), in Norway (5%), and in New Zealand (6%). The Belfast figure is, however, much lower than that found in the inner London boroughs (25%), but it should be pointed out that the London sample was drawn from areas which had a much higher level of multiple deprivation than would be the case in a general sample of Belfast.

The third survey carried out in this area so far is that reported by McWhirter (1983) involving a stratified, non-random sample of 1,000 children from "troubled" and relatively "peaceful" parts of Northern Ireland, who were compared to 210 children from the North of England. All the children completed two standard personality tests: the Junior Eysenck Personality Questionnaire (JEPQ), which assesses the higher-order personality constructs of extraversion, neuroticism, and psychoticism; and the Spielberger State-Trait Anxiety Inventory for Children (STAIC), which measures a similar construct to that tapped by the neuroticism scale of the JEPQ.

A complication in McWhirter's design is that the Northern Irish sample consisted of two age groups, 10-year-olds and 14-year-olds, whereas the English sample had only 14-year-olds. For this reason, her conclusions regarding the younger sample were based on comparisons with JEPQ norms, whereas those regarding the older sample were based on comparisons with norms and her own English sample. Using this approach, McWhirter reported that Northern Irish children did not score any higher on the trait anxiety scales compared to the British or American norms or indeed compared to her English sample. Nor were there any differences between Northern Irish children from peaceful and troubled areas in terms of trait anxiety.

Thus, McWhirter's data appear to confirm that children from Northern Ireland are not experiencing high levels of stress compared to English children, nor are children from areas which have been exposed to more political violence under more stress than children from more peaceful areas. However, a major problem in accepting this conclusion arises from the instruments used to measure anxiety. The JEPQ and the STAIC measure trait neuroticism, a stable personality construct, rather than anxiety that arises from environment stress, usually referred to as *manifest* or *state anxiety*. Second, McWhirter's study simply compared mean levels of trait anxiety in different subgroups, and did not try to answer the crucial question: How is the actual experience of the political violence related to stress in children?

The most recent survey to be carried out in this area is that reported by McGrath and Wilson (1985). This is a particularly important work because it is the first to attempt to survey the general population of children in Northern Ireland and to do so using random sampling. Also, it is the only survey in which an attempt has been made to relate children's stress levels to their experiences with political violence.

Three instruments were used to assess various manifestations of stress; namely, standardized scales to assess depression (Birleson, 1981) and manifest anxiety (Castaneda, McCandless, & Palermo, 1956) and the Rutter scale as used by Fee (see above). Multiple correlation analyses were used to explore the relationships between violence-related experiences and stress.

The overall percentage of children who scored above the cutoff point on the Rutter scale was 11%. These data are thus in agreement with Fee's results in showing that Northern Ireland has a somewhat higher Rutter scale score than similar populations. Further analysis can break down the Rutter scale into different subscales, and McGrath and Wilson's findings are also in agreement with those of Fee in that the subscale which taps antisocial behavior and conduct disorder is that which seems to account for the higher overall scores. This result parallels one of McWhirter's (1983) findings that Northern Irish children scored higher on the *psychoticism* subscale of the JEPQ compared to her English sample and is of interest because it is now generally recognized that this particular subscale taps mainly antisocial behavior and psychopathy.

McGrath and Wilson (1985) also reported that they detected a moderate, but statistically significant, amount of variation in the Rutter scale score associated with self-reports of actual violence-related experiences. At the level of individual experiences, children who had had a relative or friend injured in the troubles, and children who thought that their area was "not safe to live in," tended to have higher Rutter scores. Once again, McWhirter (1983) reported a parallel finding, in that children from the more violence prone areas in her study had a higher psychoticism score on the JEPQ compared to children from the more peaceful areas.

Surprisingly none of the reports of violence-related experiences were linked to depression, but a significant multiple correlation between these reports and manifest anxiety was found. In particular, children who had had a friend or relative injured, or who thought their area was unsafe to live in, were more likely to report symptoms of anxiety than were children who did not report having these experiences.

The broad pattern of results from these community surveys are therefore in agreement and support the conclusion reached by Cairns (1987) after a comprehensive review of the literature: that although a proportion of children in Northern Ireland have had personal experience with political violence, and some feel anxiety symptoms as a result, nevertheless, most of these children seem to be able to cope and do not suffer serious psychological impairment, at least in terms of depression. However, there are worrying indications that the political violence may be linked to variations in the level of certain aspects of antisocial and sociopathic behavior (see Chapter 52, in this volume, for a discussion of war trauma on children).

Coping with Violence

This is an area in which there has been virtually no empirical research. However, Fraser (1974) suggested that the way in which the children he studied managed to cope with stress was related to their own coping styles and to the emotional climates in the home. Fraser suggested that this emotional support was important both before and after the incident that precipitated the stress reaction. In particular, he found that children who experienced a severe stress reaction were more likely to show "an earlier tendency to nervous symptoms." He also found that one or more of the parents of these children was likely to have also been suffering from stress reactions.

Admittedly writing at a much later time in the history of the political conflict in Northern Ireland than Fraser, McWhirter (1984), proposed that children in Northern Ireland have coped with political violence because they have become habituated to it. So far she has reported only one attempt to substantiate this hypothesis based on comparisons of ratings of stressful life events made by children in Northern Ireland and the north of England. What she found was that there were no differences between the two groups of children in the types of events which they reported that they would find the most stressful. More importantly, events associated directly with the political violence were assessed as least stressful by the Northern Irish children. Certainly, these results are intriguing, but it is important to note that they only assess children's perceptions of the potential stressfulness of the events. They do not provide information on the actual experience of the events, or, indeed, if this experience is related to stress levels. Unfortunately, they do not provide a clear test of her hypothesis.

Issues and Implications

In order to decide if the political violence has led to increased levels of stress among the population in Northern Ireland, it is necessary to have data which cover the period before and after the onset of the current unrest. The data on admission and referral rates can meet this requirement and should therefore have been able to provide the necessary information. However, the research that has made use of this particular source has not, in the main, been of a particularly high standard. As Heskin (1980) noted, most of the early work by Lyons and Fraser was "frankly repetitive and methodologically limited." Indeed, only Murphy's work has begun to approach the task of analyzing these data with anything like the sophistication that is necessary, taking into account factors such as age, social class, and marital status. However, even he failed to take into account local factors, such as the fact that the provision of psychiatric beds differs markedly across different parts of Northern Ireland. Unfortunately, changes in policy regarding the hospitalization of the mentally ill means that future studies in this area will contain too much "noise" to produce any worthwhile information.

In a similar vein, the clinical case studies and the data on psychiatric referral rates for children, though by no means conclusive, indicate that there is little evidence of a direct influence of the violence on stress in children. One problem with these data is that many transient instances of impaired psychological well-being in children are seen by parents as simply "problems of growing up." In most cases, they are managed within the child's own family and are not brought to the attention of professionals. Thus, there may still be widespread effects of the troubles on children which are not reflected in clinical caseloads. However, such effects are difficult to assess because of the sensitivity of asking children direct questions about their troubles, and also because of difficulties surrounding the whole issue of assessing behavior problems in children.

The evidence from two other sources, *prescribing rates* and *alcohol-related disorders*, are available over time and appear to be on a sounder footing. Taken at their face value, both of these appear to provide evidence which, it could be argued, indicate an increase in levels of stress with the onset of the violence. However, it is interesting that researchers in both areas have offered alternative explanations for the increases they have described, although in neither case did they test directly the proposition that violence had a role to play.

The data on increasing suicide episodes also appear, when taken at face value, to fit in with the hypothesis that stress levels have been increasing in Northern Ireland. Once again, however, a more sophisticated analysis is required. For example, it is known that the population of Northern Ireland contains proportionately more younger people compared to the rest of the United Kingdom. Therefore, it may well be that a comparison involving age standardized rates would reveal that the increase in the suicide rate in Northern Ireland is not as dramatic as the raw data suggest.

The suicide statistics are also interesting because superficially they appear to support the ideas of Lyons (1972) about the relationship between depression, suicide, and aggression. He had suggested that with the opportunity to externalize aggression (in the street rioting of the early 1970s) depression levels fell and so did suicides. It could therefore be argued that the increase in suicide rate fits in with this hypothesis as, at the same time, communal violence has become relatively rare. It is important to note that the reduction in suicide rates in the early 1970s was simply not restricted to Northern Ireland as Cairns and Wilson (1985) pointed out. Furthermore, it is important to understand (Cairns, Peterson, & Neckerman, 1988) that recent research is now showing that "violent acts and suicidal behavior are not mutually exclusive; to the contrary they covary in a significant number of adolescents."

This finding raises an interesting new possibility that suicide is increasing among young men in Northern Ireland, not because they now have fewer opportunities to engage in overt aggression but, rather, because they are becoming more aggressive. This latter hypothesis finds some support in the community studies involving children, which were reviewed above. Here the evidence is quite consistent that antisocial and/or aggressive behavior by children, as reported by teachers, is on the increase in Northern Ireland since the early 1970s, despite the apparent fall in the actual level of violence since then.

The community surveys appear to have provided the best attempt to test empirically the relationship between violence and stress, and here the evidence is apparently quite consistent. For example, where children are concerned, as Cairns (1987) has pointed out, the drop in the proportion of children above the cutoff score from 1975 to 1981, as reported by Fee, could well have been related to a drop in the level of violence over this same period. Furthermore, the fact that McGrath and Wilson then reported a rise again in 1984 could again be linked to the fact that there has been an increase in violence over the period from 1981 to 1984. These findings, combined with the fact that Rutter scores also appear to be correlated with variations of experience of the violence among individual children, suggest that Rutter scores have in fact proved to be sensitive to changing trends in violence levels as well as in individual experiences.

The community studies which have focussed on adults, it can be claimed, have provided the best insights into the relationship between political violence and stress in the general population of Northern Ireland. Here the evidence suggests that increases in "normal" level of stress in areas where the violence is greatest or at times during which the violence is particularly marked. These studies have added the important proviso that how an individual *perceives* the violence in his or her neighborhood may be an important factor, interacting with actual levels of violence.

This work on the appraisal of violence is important from a theoretical viewpoint because it has links to the ideas of Lazarus and Folkman (1984) on coping and indeed has raised the whole issue of coping with stress because of the political violence in Northern Ireland. In particular, the whole issue of cause and effect will require some disentangling. One suggestion has been that the failure to deny or at least to distance oneself from high levels of violence in one's neighborhood leads to lower levels of psychological well-being. It is equally possible to turn this statement on its head and to suggest that it is those who are experiencing more psychological stress who are likely to report greater levels of violence. Here the research to date has undoubtedly been hampered by the use of cross-sectional designs. These, of course, do not make it possible to do justice to the dynamic nature of coping as envisaged by Lazarus and his colleagues. It would appear, therefore, that if theoretical considerations concerned with coping are to be advanced, this progress will depend on the use of longitudinal research designs allied to more sophisticated statistical techniques.

Recently, Loughrey and Curran (1987) extended this line of thinking by suggesting that the level of stress experienced by someone in Northern Ireland may well depend not upon their perception of the level of violence, as suggested by Cairns and Wilson (1984, 1989), but rather upon their perception of the outcome of the violence in political terms. In other words, to one individual in Northern Ireland an explosion in which, for example, members of the security forces are killed, may be an atrocity, whereas to another individual it may be a military victory. Therefore, Loughrey and Curran have suggested that, depending on the actual circumstances, the politically motivated on one side may actually feel better after a particular violent incident whereas those on the other may side feel worse. Thus, these opposite reactions will cancel each other out and this, they contend, may account for the failure of research to find a marked effect of violence on the mental health of the population of Northern Ireland. To date, however, Murphy (1984) has been the only researcher who has even attempted to incorporate this particular variable in his work, and it is of interest that his results can be construed as supporting Loughrey and Curran's hypothesis.

Conclusion

The research reviewed above points to the conclusion that only a very small proportion of the population not directly involved in the civil violence of Northern Ireland have become psychiatric casualties as a result of the political violence. Instead, the evidence suggests that a greater proportion of the population have probably suffered from mild forms of stress but that this has probably been relatively short-lived. These conclusions appear to apply equally to children and to adults. There is also some evidence from studies of psychotropic drug prescribing and from community studies, that other social stressors, particularly those associated with unemployment and general financial hardships, may have had a somewhat greater impact on the population of Northern Ireland than has the political violence.

It appears, therefore, that people in Northern Ireland have coped well with the stress of living in the midst of political violence. However, research has not made clear how this has been accomplished. Thus, it seems likely that this is an area which will come under increasing attention from researchers as the focus shifts from asking how many people have been harmed psychologically by the violence in Northern Ireland to asking them how this has been accomplished. In the future, what researchers will also have to determine is if "the coping process may be masking an inestimable strain as well as providing a stress of its own" in that "the very process of coping with and adapting to the stress of communal violence and turmoil may have a latent effect which will not become apparent until the burden of coping is lifted" (Heskin, 1980).

References

American Psychiatric Association. (1980). *Diagnostic and statistical manual of mental disorders* (3rd ed.). Washington, DC: Author.

Barker, M., McClean, S. I., McKenna, P. G., Reid, N. G., Strain, J. J., Thompson, K. A., Williamson, A. P., & Wright, M. E. (1988). *Diet, lifestyle and health in Northern Ireland: A report to the health promotion research trust*. Coleraine, Northern Ireland: Centre for Applied Health Studies, University of Ulster.

Bell, P., Kee, M., Loughrey, G. C., Roddy, R. J., & Curran, P. S. (1988). Post-traumatic stress disorder in Northern Ireland. *Acta Psychiatrica Scandinavica, 77*, 166.

Birleson, P. (1981). The validity of depressive disorder in childhood and the development of a self-rating scale: A research report. *Journal of Child Psychology and Psychiatry, 22*, 73–88.

Blaney, R., & Mackenzie, G. (1980). The prevalence of problem drinking in Northern Ireland: A population study. *International Journal of Epidemiology, 9*, 159.

Cairns, E. (1987). *Caught in crossfire: Children and the Northern Ireland conflict.* New York: Syracuse University Press.

Cairns, E., & Wilson, R. (1984). The impact of political violence on mild psychiatric morbidity in Northern Ireland. *British Journal of Psychiatry, 145*, 631.

Cairns, E., & Wilson, R. (1985). Psychiatric aspects of violence in Northern Ireland. *Stress Medicine, 1*, 193.

Cairns, E., & Wilson, R. (1987). *Psychiatric morbidity in Northern Ireland: A community based approach.* Paper presented at the Annual Conference of the Royal College of Psychiatrists, Belfast.

Cairns, E., & Wilson, R. (1989). Coping with political violence in Northern Ireland. *Social Science and Medicine, 28*(6), 621–624.

Cairns, E., Wilson, R., McClelland, R., & Gillespie, K. (1986). *The validity of the GHQ in a community setting in Northern Ireland.* Unpublished manuscript.

Cairns, R. B., Peterson, G., & Neckerman, H. J. (1988). Suicidal behavior in aggressive adolescents. *Journal of Clinical Child Psychology, 17*(4), 298–309.

Castaneda, A., McCandless, B. R., & Palermo, P. S. (1956). The children's form of the manifest anxiety scale. *Child Development, 27*, 317–325.

Curran, P. S., Finlay, R. J., & McGarry, P. J. (1988). Trends in suicide: N. Ireland 1960–86. *Irish Journal of Psychological Medicine, 5*, 98–102.

Darby, J. (1986). *Intimidation and the control of conflict in Northern Ireland.* Dublin: Gill & Macmillan.

Dean, G., Adelstein, A., & Spooner, J. (1976). Suicide and self-poisoning in Great Britain and Ireland. *International Journal of Epidemiology, 5*, 145.

Fee, F. (1980). Responses to a behavioral questionnaire of a group of Belfast children. In J. Harbison & J. Harbison (Eds.), *A society under stress: Children and young people in Northern Ireland.* Somerset, England: Open Books.

Fee, F. (1983). Educational change in Belfast school children 1975–81. In J. Harbison (Ed.), *Children of the troubles: Children in Northern Ireland.* Belfast: Stranmillis College Learning Resources Unit.

Fraser, M. (1974). *Children in conflict.* Harmondsworth, Middlesex, England: Penguin Books.

Fraser, R. M. (1971). The cost of commotion—Analysis of psychiatric sequelae of 1969 Belfast riots. *British Journal of Psychiatry, 118*, 257.

Giles, M., & Cairns, E. (1979). Colour naming of violence-related words in Northern Ireland. *British Journal of Clinical Psychology, 28*(1), 87–88.

Hadden, D. R., & McDevitt, D. G. (1974). Environmental stress and thyrotoxicosis. *Lancet, ii*, 577.

Hadden, W. A., Rutherford, W. H., & Merrett, J. D. (1978). The injuries of terrorist bombing: A study of 1,532 consecutive patients. *British Journal of Surgery, 65*, 525.

Harbison, J. J. M. (1983). *Factors associated with alcohol consump-*

tion in Northern Ireland. Unpublished doctor of philosophy thesis, New University of Ulster, Coleraine, Northern Ireland.

Heskin, K. (1980). *Northern Ireland: A psychological analysis.* Dublin: Gill & Macmillan.

Huppert, F. A., Roth, M., & Gore, M. (1987). Psychosocial factors. In B. D. Cox, M. Blaxter, L. J. Buckle, *et al.* (Eds.), *The health and lifestyle survey.* London: Health Promotion Trust.

Kee, M., Bell, P., Loughrey, G. C., Roddy, R. J., & Curran, P. S. (1987). Victims of violence: A demographic and clinical study. *Medicine, Science and the Law, 27*, 241.

King, D. J., McMeeking, C., & Elmes, P. C. (1977). Are we as depressed as we think we are? *Ulster Medical Journal, 46*, 105.

King, D. J., Griffith, K., Reilly, P. M., & Merret, D. J. (1982). Psychotropic drug use in Northern Ireland 1966–80: Prescribing trends, inter- and intra-regional comparisons and relationships to demographic and socioeconomic variables. *Psychological Medicine, 12*, 819.

King, D. J., Griffith, K., Reilly, P., & Merret, D. J. (1983). *Patterns of psychotropic drug prescribing in Northern Ireland.* Paper presented at the Conference on Health and Vulnerability in Northern Ireland, Belfast.

Loughrey, G. C., & Curran, P. S. (1987). The psychopathology of civil disorder. In A. M. Dawson & G. M. Besser (Eds.), *Recent advances in medicine.* Edinburgh: Churchill Livingstone.

Loughrey, G. C., Bell, P., Kee, M., Roddy, R. J., & Curran, P. S. (1988). Post-traumatic stress disorder and civil violence in Northern Ireland. *British Journal of Psychiatry, 153*, 554–560.

Lazarus, R. S., & Folkman, S. (1984). *Stress, appraisal and coping.* New York: Springer Publishing.

Lyons, H. A. (1971). Psychiatric sequelae of the Belfast riots. *British Journal of Psychiatry, 118*, 265.

Lyons, H. A. (1972). Depressive illness and aggression in Belfast. *British Medical Journal, 1*, 342.

Lyons, H. A. (1974). Terrorist bombing and the psychological sequelae. *Journal of the Irish Medical Association, 67*, 15.

Lyons, H. A. (1979). Civil violence—The psychological aspects. *Journal of Psychosomatic Research, 23*, 373.

Lyons, H. A., & Bindall, K. K. (1977). Attempted suicide in Belfast: A continuation of a study in a district general hospital. *Irish Medical Journal, 70*, 322.

McCauley, R., & Troy, M. (1983). The impact of urban conflict and violence on children referred to a child guidance clinic. In J. Harbison (Ed.), *Children of the troubles: Children in Northern Ireland.* Belfast: Stranmillis College Learning Resources Unit.

McGee, R., Williams, S., Bradshaw, J., Chapel, J. L., Robins, A., & Silva, P. A. (1985). The Rutter Scale for completion by teachers: Factor structure and relationships with cognitive abilities and family adversity for a sample of New Zealand children. *Journal of Child Psychology and Psychiatry, 26*, 727–739.

McGrath, A., & Wilson, R. (1985). *Factors which influence the prevalence and variation of psychological problems in children in Northern Ireland.* Paper presented at the Annual Conference of the Developmental Section of the British Psychological Society, Belfast.

McKeown, M. (1973). Civil unrest: Secondary school survey. *Northern Teacher, 1*(1), 39–42.

McWhirter, L. (1983). *How "troubled" are children in Northern Ireland compared to children who live outside Northern Ireland?* Paper presented at the Annual Conference of the Psychological Society of Ireland, Athlone.

McWhirter, L. (1984). *Is getting caught in a riot more stressful for children than seeing a scary film or moving to a new school?* Paper presented at the Annual Conference of the Northern Ireland Branch of the Psychological Society, Portballintrae.

McWhirter, L. (1987). Psychological impact of violence in Northern Ireland: Recent research findings and issues. In N. Eisenberg & D. Glasgow (Eds.), *Recent advances in clinical psychology* London: Gower.

Murphy, H. B. M. (1984). *Minority status, civil strife and the major disorders: Hospitalization patterns in Northern Ireland.* Unpublished manuscript.

O'Malley, P. P. (1972). Attempted suicide before and after the communal violence in Belfast, August 1969: A preliminary study. *Journal of the Irish Medical Association, 65,* 109.

Orbell, S. D. M. (1988). *Living with conflict in Northern Ireland.* Unpublished doctoral thesis, Queen's University of Belfast, Northern Ireland.

Parkes, W. E. (1977). Stress factors in Northern Ireland as seen from a coronary care unit. *Practitioner, 138,* 409.

Pockgrass, R. M. (1987). Terroristic murder in Northern Ireland: Who is killed and why? *Terrorism, 9*(4), 342–359.

Poole, M. (1983). The demography of violence. In J. Darby (Ed.), *Northern Ireland: The background to the conflict.* Belfast: Appletree Press.

Rutter, M. (1967). A child's behavioral questionnaire for completion by teachers: Preliminary findings. *Journal of Child Psychology and Psychiatry, 8,* 1–11.

Rutter, M., Cox, A., Tupling, C., Berger, M., & Yule, W. (1975). Attainment and adjustment in two geographical areas: I. The prevalence of psychiatric disorder. *British Journal of Psychiatry, 126,* 520–533.

Vikan, A. (1985). Psychiatric epidemiology in a sample of 1,510 ten-year-old children. *Journal of Child Psychology and Psychiatry, 26,* 55–75.

CHAPTER 31

Posttraumatic Stress Disorder and Civil Violence in Northern Ireland

G. C. Loughrey, Peter S. Curran, and P. Bell

Introduction

Historical Antecedents of Civil Violence and Political Conflict

Some 70 years ago, after the War of Independence and a bloody civil war, Ireland was partitioned with the 6 Northern counties, from a total of 32, remaining British counties within the United Kingdom. Eventually, the other 26 counties became the independent Republic of Ireland. In Northern Ireland, a local Parliament *Stormont* governed the Northern State with a guaranteed majority of Loyalists committed to the union with Great Britain. Approximately two thirds of Northern Ireland's population were of the Protestant faith (Loyalist/Unionist) and one third were Catholics (Republican/Nationalist). Over the decades, there were periodically modest Republican campaigns of violence waged against the Northern State, usually waning through lack of support from the existing Nationalist minority in Northern Ireland.

In the late 1960s and borrowing from the successful civil rights movement in the United States, there emerged in Northern Ireland an active Civil Rights Group, campaigning against the gerrymandering of local government boundaries, unfair housing allocations, and social injustices. However, this popular nonsectarian movement soon provoked old sectarian tensions, the existing Unionist majority seeing this campaign as again inspired by Republicans. Events came to a head in 1969 with widespread street rioting, pogroms, and shootings as traditional sectarian hatreds emerged. Republican paramilitary movements were reactivated but only to be met by Loyalist paramilitary groupings and the security forces of the state.

For 20 years now, Northern Ireland has had its own internal war which has not been stemmed by various political initiatives. Almost 3,000 people have been killed and countless thousands injured—this in a country of merely 1.5 million people, one large city (Belfast) with a population of 300,000, 20 smaller country market towns, and a largely rural community, much of it centered along a meandering border with the Republic of Ireland.

The litany of terrorist and sectarian incidents is endless: successful and failed internecine assassinations, bombings of large public buildings and selected targets, many shooting incidents, pogroms, and massive public gatherings. However, the nature of the violence has changed with time. The current Republican policy is selectively aimed at members of the security forces and opposing terrorist groupings, but the effect has been to provoke Loyalist terrorist gangs, alienation of the two communities, and the promotion of widespread sectarianism. The violence is largely curtailed to working-class areas and inner-urban zones. High unemployment and poor social conditions foster embitterment and guarantee new recruits to what is a historically old problem.

The population appears resigned to the inevitable possibility that "there is no solution" and perhaps coming to terms with that situation has allowed life to continue as "normal." We (Bell, Kee, Loughrey, Roddy, & Curran, 1988; Curran, 1988; Kee, Bell, Loughrey, Roddy, & Curran, 1987; Loughrey, Bell, Kee, Roddy, & Curran, 1988; Loughrey & Curran, 1987) have previously written of our experiences as psychiatrists in this situation, but our main interest in this chapter is to detail our experi-

G. C. Loughrey, Peter S. Curran, and P. Bell • Mater Infirmorum Hospital, Crumlin Road, Belfast BT 14 6 AB, Northern Ireland.

International Handbook of Traumatic Stress Syndromes, edited by John P. Wilson and Beverley Raphael. Plenum Press, New York, 1993.

ences of working with posttraumatic stress disorder (PTSD).

Victims of violence in Northern Ireland are entitled to seek compensation for their injuries, whether physical, psychological, or both. Irish law is basically adversarial, each side, plaintiff and respondent (defendant), gathering its own independent medical evidence for adjudication by the courts. Most of our research experience has been through such professional employment— assessing the type, degree and duration of "nervous shock" or psychological injury. However, in this chapter, we seek to describe selectively our experience of the clinical syndrome of PTSD in survivors of assassination attempts, paramilitary punishment shootings and beatings, violent assaults, intimidation, and exposure to bombings and shootings. Clearly these stressor experiences more than meet the minimal criteria set forth in *Diagnostic and statistical manual of mental disorders* (DSM-III-R) of the American Psychiatric Association (APA) (1987) as events that would lead to the development of PTSD.

Issues in PTSD Diagnosis

Horowitz (1976) described posttraumatic reactions in terms of two mental states: one of *intrusion*, characterized by intrusive repetitive thoughts, sleep disturbance including nightmares, hypervigilance, and pangs of strong emotion, and one of *denial*, characterized by inattention, amnesia, constriction of thought processes, and emotional numbing. Laufer, Brett, and Gallops (1984) have used this model in their work. They linked exposure to combat and the witnessing of abusive violence to denial symptoms. They stated on the basis of this work that "PTSD may not be the comprehensive phenomenon specified in the DSM-III" and that "PTSD may be a disorder in which one of two descriptions dominate the clinical picture." Other workers drew a distinction between PTSD after war trauma and PTSD after other forms of trauma. Silver and Iacono (1984) reported that Vietnam veterans differ from non-Vietnam veterans in that the former have a greater intensity of aggression and detachment and more intense reexperiencing. Burstein (1988) described different reexperiencing phenomena in Vietnam veterans compared with civilians with PTSD as being one of the clinical variables that distinguish these groups; others include the nature of the stressor, the chronicity, and substance abuse. More recently, Wilson (1989) reviewed the field and developed a conceptual model which integrates these disparate findings.

Concurrent Diagnosis of Depression

Among the concurrent diagnoses which can be made in the presence of PTSD are personality disorder, substance abuse, and depression. The links between depression and PTSD are very strong. Many of the characteristic symptoms of PTSD may also be those of depressive illness. There is a variety of figures for the frequency for which depression can be diagnosed in the presence of PTSD, for example; 41% (Davison, Swartz, Storck, Krishnan, & Hammette, 1985), 72% (Sierles, Chen,

McFarland, & Taylor, 1983), and 100% (Birkheimer & Devane, 1985).

In a recent detailed study of PTSD and other findings in male alcoholic Vietnam veterans, Van Kampen, Watson, Tilleskjor, Kucala, and Vassar (1986), besides confirming the strong link between PTSD and depression, questioned the validity of feelings of detachment from others and constricted affect as being characteristic symptoms of PTSD, since the DSM-III-R manual refers to "emotional anesthesia" or "psychic numbing," and there is increasing evidence in the literature of the importance of depressed mood.

In a review article which raised several questions about PTSD, Breslau and Davis (1987) remarked on the overlap of emotional states in the DSM-III Criterion C symptoms because loss of interest can be due to depression as well as to emotional numbing. Commenting on this, Lindy, Green, and Grace (1987) stated that although depression can occur as part of an individual's reaction to PTSD, it does not form part of the core symptoms. In a further comment, Ursano (1987) stated that this correlation required further clarification.

Following early reports of the efficacy of tricyclic antidepressants and monoamine-oxidase inhibitors in PTSD (Blake, 1986; Hogben & Cornfeld, 1981), recent work has indicated a variable response suggesting that depression is only one of the mood states which may be found in PTSD. The finding of an abnormal dexamethasone suppression test in 50% of the veterans with PTSD and Research diagnostic Criteria (RDC) major depression and in only 6% of veterans with PTSD but without depression bears this out (Kudler, Davidson, Meador, Lipper, & Ely, 1987). There is doubt as to whether antidepressants have an effect on depressed mood, on panic attacks, on REM sleep, or on overarousal (Friedman, 1988; van der Kolk, Greenberg, Boyd, & Krystal, 1985).

Associated Features and Complications

There have been four studies of these using DSM-III criteria. Two of these (Atkinson, Henderson, Sparr, & Deale, 1982; Boman, 1985) have used a control group to separate the effects of exposure to combat *per se* from the specific effects of the syndrome. In two uncontrolled studies (Escobar *et al.*, 1983; Sierles *et al.*, 1983), both of Vietnam veterans, high rates of impulsive violence, suicide attempts, antisocial behavior, and alcohol and drug abuse have been noted. In the controlled study by Atkinson and co-workers, American Vietnam veterans with PTSD had no significantly greater rate of violent outbursts or nonviolent impulsive behavior than veterans without PTSD. Similarly, Boman (1985) examined Australian Vietnam veterans and compared a group with severe combat experience who developed PTSD. He found no significant difference in the postcombat incidence of alcohol abuse, drug abuse, impulsive violence, suicide attempts, or marital disruption, separation, or divorce.

Recently, Van Putten and Yager (1984) questioned the specificity of the relationship between postcombat difficulties and PTSD and its reported complications and associated features.

Civil Violence and Psychiatric Sequelae

The purpose of these studies was (1) to ascertain the frequency of the characteristic symptoms of PTSD and its certain associated features and complications, (2) to evaluate the ICD-9 diagnosis of depression, and (3) to provide evidence for the validity of PTSD by face validity as evidenced by the presence of PTSD after acts of civil violence and predictive validity as evidenced by duration of syndrome and entry into psychiatric treatment of those with PTSD.

Methodology

All the population had been referred to and examined by a member of the research team (PSC) for medicolegal assessment between January, 1979 and December, 1984. In total, there were 499 consecutive referrals. The inclusion criteria were that each individual had to be aged 16 or over at the time of the incident, the individual had to be seeking compensation under the Criminal Injuries order (Northern Ireland) 1977, and the individual's psychiatric complaints had to result from an act of civil violence.

In terms of the clinical evaluation process, there was at least one report that provided a full psychiatric history and examination of mental state together with a detailed list of all reported symptoms following the incident irrespective of whether or not they had cleared up by the interview date. Other reports, psychiatric, medical, and surgical were also analyzed. The interval between the incident and the final psychiatric examination varied. In 319 cases (64%), this interval was 1 year or longer; in 105 cases (21%), 6 months to 1 year; in 46 cases (9%), 3 to 6 months; and in 29 cases (6%), less than 3 months. The clinical data available to us also disclosed an ICD-9 diagnosis and gave an account of the duration of the syndrome and included details of any psychiatric treatment in the interval between the incident and the final examination.

A comprehensive symptom checklist that included the characteristic and associated symptoms of PTSD (APA, 1980) was used and subjected to computer analysis which identified those with or without PTSD. The research team studied all case notes and reached a consensus conclusion as to whether a symptom was present or had been recorded at any stage by any clinician, irrespective of duration or severity of the symptom. The DSM-III gives no guidelines or minimum threshold for the recognition of such symptoms.

Sample Characteristics

Of the population, 264 (53%) were women and 235(47%) were men with the mean age for the entire sample at the time of the incident of 37.3 years (SD = 13.43). Eighty-seven (17.4%) were considered to be at special risk because of their occupations, 20 being soldiers and 41 being policemen. Thirty-three (6.6%) had a past psychiatric history and there was a family history of psychiatric illness of any type in a first-degree relative in

82 (16.4%). More complete details of the population are available (Loughrey et al., 1988).

Nature of Traumatic Stressors

All incidents were clearly related to the civil violence in Northern Ireland and all were significantly threatening. In 90 (18%) cases, the victims survived assassination attempts. In 34 (6.8%) cases, the incident had been a violent personal assault such as a punishment shooting where the victim was a selected target. In 75 (15%) cases, the subject was held captive by terrorists, usually within his own house. There were 57 (11.4%) incidents where the subject had been the victim of personally directed threats, usually involving a firearm but without physical injury. In 191 (38.3%) cases, they *witnessed* a violent incident in which they or a significant other was at personal risk of injury; and 52 (10.4%) subjects *witnessed* a violent incident in which there was no such risk. Injuries were sustained by 141 (28.3%), with 11 (2.2%) suffering a concussional injury and 5 (1%) with permanent brain or spinal damage. In 31 victims (6.2%), there was loss of limb or impaired limb function, and in 27 (5.6%) patients, there was conspicuous and disfiguring scarring. Eighty-five subjects (17%) had *witnessed* someone being *killed* in the incident. In 58 (11.6%) cases, the fatality was of a colleague or a close friend.

Results

The results are summarized in Tables 31.1, 31.2, and 31.3. In all these tables results for men and women are combined. The statistical significance of the results was not altered by considering men and women separately. Significantly, more men than women, whether or not they had PTSD, had an increase of alcohol or drug abuse. Otherwise, there were no differences between the sexes in any of the indices measured.

Table 31.1. Percentage of Frequency of Characteristic Symptoms of Posttraumatic Stress Disorder

Item	PTSD present (n = 116)	PTSD absent (n = 383)
Recognizable stressor	100.0	100.0
Recurrent intrusive recollections	84.5	46.5
Recurrent dreams	52.6	33.9
Acting or feeling "as if"	0.0	1.0
Markedly diminished interest	98.3	13.3
Detachment or estrangement	10.3	1.6
Constricted affect	12.9	2.3
Hyperalertness or exaggerated startle response	66.4	53.3
Sleep disturbance	96.3	84.6
Survivor guilt	6.9	1.3
Concentration or memory impairment	37.9	18.3
Avoidance of trigger stimuli	53.4	36.6
Intensification by exposure	77.6	55.9

Table 31.2. Percentage Frequency of Features Associated with Posttraumatic Stress Disorder

Item	PTSD present ($n = 110$)	PTSD absent ($n = 383$)	
Explosive outbursts	6.0	4.2	$\chi^2 = 0.34$; NS
Impulsive behavior	0.0	1.6	$\chi^2 = 0.76$; NS
Substance abuse	7.8	8.6	$\chi^2 = 0.01$; NS
Attempted suicide	4.3	1.0	$\chi^2 = 3.67$; $0.05 < p < 0.1$
	($n = 80$)	($n = 270$)	
Disharmony	46.3	23.3	$\chi^2 = 18.92$; $p < 0.001$

Table 31.1 shows that 116 (23.2%) of 499 subjects met the diagnostic criteria for PTSD. Tables 31.1 and 31.2 show the percentage frequency of characteristic symptoms and of associated features and complications. No significant correlation was found between the presence of PTSD and explosive outbursts, nonviolent impulsive behavior, or substance abuse. There was a strong link between the presence of marital disharmony and PTSD and a somewhat weaker link between the presence of attempted suicide and PTSD. There were statistically significant correlations between the longer duration of PTSD, entry into psychiatric treatment and the diagnosis of an ICD-9 depressive syndrome. Regarding the duration of the syndrome, the 3-month duration was chosen because of the time interval between the incident and the final examination; if a 6-month interval had been chosen, some cases would have been unclassifiable because for these, although examinations were carried out at 3 months, there would have been no reexamination at 6 months.

In conclusion, this study shows that in a population subject to acts of civil violence, 23.2% had PTSD. The obtained results are similar to the incidence of PTSD following such stresses as the Vietnam War and natural disasters. This study is one of the first to evaluate PTSD after incidents of civil and terrorist violence. Additionally, the sample is larger than is typically the case in many other studies that record individual symptom frequencies. It differs from much other work (e.g., the Vietnam War, Australian bushfires, and Israeli combat veterans) in that both genders were studied and evaluated for PTSD symptoms.

Discussion

Issues of Methodology

To minimize individual rater error, the research team reviewed the ethical notes jointly. For this session, tests of interrater reliability were not possible. It was felt that test-retest reliability could not be measured because many of the case notes had such a dramatic content that they could be readily identified. We would argue that, even though case control studies are often unreliable, information variance was low in this type of study since there was at least one full documented history of examination by one single psychiatrist, and that criterion variance was reduced by the use of the DSM-III manual and its explicit criteria. Scales that are now available for the measurement of PTSD were not available to us at the time the patients were seen (Blanchard, Kalb, Pallmeyer, & Gerardi, 1982; Friedman, Schneiderman, Nest, & Corson, 1986).

Since this study is of a litigant population, it leads to a potential risk of suggestion and overreporting. Nevertheless, findings reflect the low frequency of certain types of symptoms. Moreover, other than the recorded frequency of PTSD, comparisons were being made of subpopulations assessed in the same way so any overreporting may have acted equally between the two groups. Litigants or people who otherwise gain financially with declaration of symptoms are commonly studied in research on posttraumatic reactions and the difficulties in doing this have been reviewed by Wilson (1989). In retrospective studies of trauma, the time-since-

Table 31.3. Association between Posttraumatic Stress Disorder and Duration of Syndrome, Need for Psychiatric Treatment, and Diagnosis of an ICD-9 Depressive Syndrome

	PTSD present ($n = 116$)	PTSD absent ($n = 383$)	
Syndrome lasting longer than 3 months	92.2	74.7	$\chi^2 = 22.46$; $p < .001$
Consultation with psychiatrist (other than medicolegal)	44.8	21.7	$\chi^2 = 23.00$; $p < .001$
Diagnosis of an ICD-9 depressive syndrome	34.5	11.7	$\chi^2 = 30.90$; $p < .001$

event effect is important to note. This phenomenon could lead to difficulty with the reliability of assessment of characteristic symptoms if there is a latency period or of associated features and complications if a long time interval is necessary for their development. However, in the present study, there was no significant difference in duration of follow-up time between the group with PTSD and the group without PTSD.

Characteristic Symptom Patterns

With respect to individual symptom frequencies, it was clear that symptoms linked to overarousal, for example, startle reaction and sleep disturbance, were very common in both groups with and without a PTSD diagnosis. This is to be expected because they are a universal finding in the aftermath of severe stress. These symptoms, together with the phenomenon of "intensification by exposure," reflect a strong link between the symptoms and the stressful incident—which is acknowledged in the DSM-III but has gained less emphasis in ICD-9 manual definitions. Thus, intensification by exposure was frequently the most *persistent* PTSD symptom, despite the latency to assessment and evaluations.

The PTSD symptom of suddenly acting or feeling as if the event were reoccurring was not found in *any* of our cases of PTSD. Since this is a dramatic and distressing symptom, underreporting is unlikely. It has been suggested that there may have been underreporting of this symptom in combat veterans (Brett & Mangine, 1985), although elsewhere the DSM-III reports that this symptom is rare and that "such states have been reported in combat veterans" as dissociative reactions. Burstein (1988), who has reported extensively on this subject, drew the distinction between Vietnam combat veterans and survivors of other extreme stress with PTSD in that, referring to flashbacks, "these patients report a much more global experience, not reported by patients with acute PTSD," in which they dissociatively relive the trauma.

The infrequency of survivor guilt would be expected from the nature of the incidents endured by the litigants in that there were comparatively few fatalities compared with combat stress or severe disaster. In an epidemiological study of PTSD following a variety of severe stresses including war combat, Helzer, Robins, and McEvoy (1987) found survivor guilt to be rare. Similarly, MacFarlane (1988) noted survivor guilt was not prevalent in male fire fighters after a bushfire in Australia. Glover (1984) identified how survivor guilt can arise from specific aspects of a severe stress, such as war combat or the Holocaust (see also Wilson, Harel, & Kahana, 1988). Moreover, in the cases of both suddenly acting and feeling as if the event is reoccurring and of "survivor guilt," the frequency seems to be low because of the type of stress, even though the stress was severe enough to satisfy the first criterion of PTSD. Once the stressor criterion has been fulfilled, the symptoms should be as far as possible independent of the special characteristics of the stress. Otherwise, the usefulness of PTSD as a universally applicable syndrome is weakened.

The relative infrequency of feelings of detachment or estrangement from others or constricted affect was, we believe, in part consistent with the work of Laufer, Brett, and Gallops (1985), whose model subdivides PTSD symptoms into clusters of experiencing and symptoms of denial. They link symptoms of reexperiencing with either simple combat exposure or witnessing acts of abusive violence, whereas denial symptoms are associated primarily with participation in acts of atrocity. The trauma to which our population was subject is clearly more like the former, so this model should predict a high frequency of reexperiencing symptoms and a low frequency of denial symptoms. In their work, Laufer *et al.* (1985) studied 251 Vietnam War veterans who differed clearly from our group in that they were all Americans (182 whites and 68 blacks) and all male. They were chiefly from middle-income families and were in their late 20s or early 30s at the time of the interview, although the war had been over for at least 5 years at the time of the study (Laufer *et al.*, 1981). This group was different demographically from our sample therefore, in terms of country of origin, sex ratio, and age at the time of stress. The reexperiencing symptoms described by Laufer *et al.* (1985) included intrusive thoughts, dreams or nightmares, insomnia, and startle reaction; these symptoms were all frequent in our study. The denial symptoms included loss of interest, emotional detachment, constriction of affect, concentration difficulties, and phobic avoidance, which Laufer *et al.* found low in frequency; we found similarly for emotional detachment and constriction of affect. The very high frequency of loss of interest in activities, was not predicted by this model. These three symptoms together make up Criterion C of PTSD, which is diminished responsiveness to the external world usually referred to as *psychic numbing* or *emotional anesthesia* (DSM-III-R). Although loss of interest may be caused by this mood state, it may also be caused by depressed mood which, as shown by the high frequency of an ICD-9 depressive diagnosis, was common in our sample with PTSD. As the results indicate, there was a significant association between the diagnosis of PTSD and the diagnosis of an ICD-9 depressive syndrome.

Two other reasons may explain the low frequency of emotional detachment and constriction of affect. First, people with these symptoms may not be seeking compensation. In terms of our analysis, this would only present a problem if the symptoms of emotional withdrawal were present in the *absence* of symptoms of overarousal or reexperiencing. Second, these symptoms might not have been sufficiently probed or reported on in the interview. However, we would argue that they would be evident clinically even if not directly expressed by the patient. Birkheimer and Devane (1985) suggested that there may be underreporting of these symptoms since these features can become chronic and therefore on longer ego-alien. This sample, in comparison with Vietnam War veterans, is composed of more acutely ill individuals, so this is unlikely to be problematic. MacFarlane (1988), reported on a small group of male fire fighters who had been exposed to a bushfire, declaring that, even among those with PTSD, there was increased communal identity and involvement following the disaster. He observed that different stressors caused different effects on personal relationships. It was our impression that this is a pattern among most victims of violence in Northern Ireland.

Based on the finding of high frequency of loss of interest in significant activities, we believe that it is due to *depression* rather than to the defense mechanism of denial. Criterion C in PTSD seems to identify two emotional states; one of psychic numbing or emotional anesthesia and the other of depression which is the more common emotional state in our study. The high frequency of concentration difficulties and phobic avoidance is also consistent with our conclusion that depressive mood accounts for the apparently high frequency of some denial symptoms. These findings would also explain the variability of diagnosis of depression concomitant with PTSD.

Associated Features and Complications

We failed to find an association between PTSD and explosive outbursts or nonviolent impulsive behavior. Their absence may be due to observer error, although this is unlikely since such symptoms are readily documented. Second, in our sample, both genders had a low frequency of previous criminal record. Thus, these may be alternative explanations for the low incident of explosive behaviors of impulsiveness, including cultural sanctions against such acts if acted out in antisocial ways. Finally, many of those with PTSD (34.5%) had received prior psychiatric treatment. We tentatively suggest that prompt psychiatric treatment may have led to a reduction in frequency of impulsive nonviolent behavior and explosive outbursts, although other complications were not similarly prevented (Lindy *et al.*, 1987).

The low frequency of alcohol or drug abuse is unlikely simply to be due to underreporting. Psychiatrists in Northern Ireland are sensitive to the risks of alcohol abuse while abuse of other drugs is rare in this population. Reasons for the low rates and absence of association may be due to gender differences and the relatively high mean age of the sample. Combat exposure may have a direct link with substance abuse, irrespective of the presence of posttraumatic symptoms, or the prescription of psychotropic medication may reduce the incidence of self-medication with alcohol or illicit drugs (see Wilson *et al.*, 1988).

The low frequency but significant association between PTSD and suicidal behavior seems surprising because of the high frequency compared with those of war-veteran studies. However, previous studies show that an increase in the frequency of attempted or completed suicide during civil violence and the effects of an individual's depressed mental state may be balanced by those social factors particular to civil violence that militate against suicidal acts (Loughrey & Curran, 1987). Nevertheless, the rate of suicide attempts was four times greater in the PTSD positive group in comparison to those without such a diagnosis (see Table 31.2). Finally, it is noteworthy that there was a significant relationship between PTSD and marital conflict (i.e., "disharmony").

Validity of Diagnosis

The validity of diagnosis was considered with particular relevance to DSM-III by Spitzer and Williams (1985). They described in turn the face, descriptive, predictive and constructive validities. The face validity of the diagnosis may be questioned if PTSD consists of two distinct syndromes even though, as pointed out by Spitzer and Williams, complete homogeneity is not necessary. Face validity would be enhanced if PTSD were found after a wide range of severe stressors.

Of our sample, 23.2% had PTSD; thus, this syndrome can be identified in a mixed sex population that is subject to acts of civil violence. This extends the range of stressors which can elicit the syndrome and offer support to its face validity. The high frequency of the diagnosis of concurrent depressive illness and the low frequency of some characteristic symptoms reported in the introduction question the validity of the syndrome.

So far, there is little evidence on the predictive validity or construct validity of PTSD. The association between the presence of PTSD and the duration of the syndrome would support the predictive validity of this diagnosis. The data on entry into treatment also support the predictive validity of PTSD, especially since PTSD is not a diagnosis in common use in Northern Ireland and therefore would not of itself be used as a criterion for entry into psychiatric treatment in such a way that would make the reasoning behind this test of predictive validity tautological.

Conclusions

Our results show that PTSD can be identified in a population stressed by civil violence. We question whether some characteristic features and associated features and complications are too dependent on the special kind of population studied or on the special kind of stressors. The validity of most of the characteristic symptoms is accepted, although the emotional state identified using the diagnostic criteria may not be homogeneous.

Our findings give face validity to the concept of PTSD. The association between the diagnosis of PTSD and entry into treatment and the longer duration of the syndrome offer evidence in support of the predictive validity of PTSD.

References

American Psychiatric Association. (1980). *Diagnostic and statistical manual of mental disorders* (3rd ed.). Washington, DC: Author.

American Psychiatric Association. (1987). *Diagnostic and statistical manual of mental disorders* (3rd ed. rev.). Washington, DC: Author.

Atkinson, R. M., Henderson, R. G., Sparr, L. F., & Deale, S. (1982). Assessment of Vietnam veterans for post-traumatic stress disorder in Veterans administration disability claims. *American Journal of Psychiatry, 139,* 1118–1121.

Bell, P., Kee, M., Loughrey, G. C., Roddy, R. J., & Curran, P. S. (1988). Post-traumatic stress in Northern Ireland. *Acta Psychiatrica Scandinavica, 77,* 166–169.

Birkheimer, L. J., & Devane, C. L. (1985). Post-traumatic stress disorder characteristics and pharmacological response in the veteran population. *Comprehensive Psychiatry, 26,* 304–310.

Blake, D. J. (1986). Treatment of acute post-traumatic stress disorder with tricyclic anti-depressants. *Southern Medical Journal, 79*, 201–204.

Blanchard, E. B., Kolb, L. C., Pallmeyer, T. P., & Gerardi, R. J. (1982). A psychophysiological study of post-traumatic stress disorder in Vietnam veterans. *Psychiatric Quarterly, 54*, 220–229.

Boman, B. (1985). Post-traumatic stress disorder and concurrent psychiatric illness among Australian Vietnam veterans: A controlled study. *Journal of the Royal Army Medical Corps, 131*, 128–131.

Breslau, N., & Davis, G. C. (1987). Post-traumatic stress disorder. The stressor criterion. *Journal of Nervous and Mental Disease, 175*, 255–276.

Brett, E. A., & Mangine, W. (1985). Imagery and combat stress in Vietnam veterans. *Journal of Nervous and Mental Disease, 173*, 309–311.

Burstein, A. (1988). Differences among patients with post-traumatic stress disorder [Letter to the editor]. *American Journal of Psychiatry, 145*(6), 770–771.

Curran, P. S. (1988). Psychiatric aspects of terrorist violence. Northern Ireland 1969–1987. *British Journal of Psychiatry, 153*, 470–475.

Davidson, J., Swartz, M., Storck, M., Krishnan, R. R., & Hammette, E. (1985). A diagnostic and family study of post-traumatic stress disorder. *American Journal of Psychiatry, 142*, 90–93.

Escobar, J. I., Randolph, E. T., Puente, G., Spinak, F., Asamen, J. K., Hill, M., & Hough, R. C. (1983). Post-traumatic stress disorder in Hispanic Vietnam veterans. *Journal of Nervous and Mental Disease, 171*, 585–596.

Friedman, M. J. (1988). Towards rational pharmacotherapy for post-traumatic stress disorder: An interim report. *American Journal of Psychiatry, 145*, 281–285.

Friedman, M. J., Schneiderman, C. K., Nest, A. N., & Corson, J. A. (1986). Measurement of combat exposure. Post-traumatic stress disorder and life stress in Vietnam combat veterans. *American Journal of Psychiatry, 143*, 537–539.

Glover, H. (1984). Survival guilt and the Vietnam veteran. *Journal of Nervous and Mental Disease, 172*, 393–397.

Helzer, J. E., Robins, L. N., & McEvoy, L. (1987). Post-traumatic stress disorder in the general population. *New England Journal of Medicine, 317*, 1630–1634.

Hogben, G. L., & Cornfield, R. B. (1981). Treatment of traumatic war neurosis with phenelzine. *Archives of General Psychiatry, 38*, 440–445.

Horowitz, M. J. (1976). *Stress response syndromes.* New York: Jason Aronson.

Kee, M., Bell, P., Loughrey, G. C., Roddy, J. R., & Curran, P. S. (1987). Victims of violence: A demographic and clinical study. *Medical Science Law, 27*(4), 241–247.

Kudler, H., Davidson, J., Meador, K., Lipper, S., & Ely, T.

(1987). The DST and post-traumatic stress disorder. *American Journal of Psychiatry, 144*, 1068–1071.

Laufer, R. S., Brett, E., & Gallops, M. S. (1984). Post-traumatic stress disorder reconsidered: Post-traumatic stress disorder among Vietnam veterans. In B. van der Kolk (Ed.), *Post-traumatic stress disorder: Psychological and biological sequelae.* Washington, DC: American Psychiatric Press.

Laufer, R. S., Brett, E., & Gallops, M. S. (1985). Symptom pattern associated with post-traumatic stress disorder among Vietnam veterans exposed to war trauma. *American Journal of Psychiatry, 142*, 1304–1311.

Lindy, J. D., Green, B. C., & Grace, M. C. (1987). Commentary. *Journal of Nervous and Mental Disease, 175*, 269–272.

Loughrey, G. C., Bell, P., Kee, M., Roddy, R. J., & Curran, P. S. (1988). Post-traumatic stress disorder and civil violence in Northern Ireland. *British Journal of Psychiatry, 153*, 554–560.

Loughrey, G. C., & Curran, P. S. (1987). Psychopathology of civil disorder. In A. M. Dawson & G. M. Besser (Eds.), *Recent advances of medicine.* New York: Churchill Livingstone.

MacFarlane, A. C. (1988). The phenomenology of post-traumatic stress disorders following a natural disaster. *Journal of Nervous and Mental Disease, 176*, 22–29.

Sierles, F. S., Chen, J. J., McFarland, R. E., & Taylor, M. A. (1983). Post-traumatic stress disorder and concurrent psychiatric illness. *American Journal of Psychiatry, 140*, 1177–1179.

Silver, S. H., & Iacono, C. U. (1984). Factor analytic support for DSM-III post-traumatic stress disorder for Vietnam veterans. *Journal of Clinical Psychology, 40*, 5–14.

Spitzer, R. S., & Williams, J. B. W. (1985). Classification of mental disorders. In H. I. Kaplan & B. J. Sadlock (Eds.), *Comprehensive textbook of psychiatry* (4th ed., Vol. 1). Baltimore: Williams and Williams.

Ursano, R. J. (1987). Commentary. *Journal of Nervous and Mental Disease, 175*, 273–275.

van Der Kolk, B. A., Greenberg, M., Boyd, H., & Krystal, J. (1985). Inescapable shock, neurotransmitters and addiction to trauma: Toward a psychobiology of post-traumatic stress. *Biological Psychiatry, 20*, 314–325.

Van Kampen, M., Watson, C. G., Tilleskjor, C., Kucala, T., & Vassar, P. (1986). The definition of post-traumatic stress disorder in alcoholic Vietnam veterans. *Journal of Nervous and Mental Disease, 174*, 137–144.

Van Putten, T., & Yager, J. (1984). Post-traumatic stress disorder. *Archives of General Psychiatry, 41*, 411–413.

Wilson, J. P. (1989). *Trauma, transformation, and healing.* New York: Brunner/Mazel.

Wilson, J. P., Harel, Z., & Kahana, B. (1988). *Human adaptation to extreme stress: From the Holocaust to Vietnam.* New York: Plenum Press.

World Health Organization. (1978). *Mental disorders: Glossary and guide to their classification in accordance with the ninth revision of the International Classification of Diseases* (ICD-9). Geneva: Author.

CHAPTER 32

Effects of Postshooting Experiences on Police-Authorized Firearms Officers in the United Kingdom

Mary Bernadette Manolias and Arthur Hyatt-Williams

Introduction

Over the past few years, there has been a substantial increase in the number of incidents involving armed police officers in the United Kingdom (U.K.). This trend has been a cause of concern to police and to public alike. Whenever such incidents occur, they have invariably attracted a great deal of media attention, which sometimes portrays the police action in an unfavorable light.

Unlike the United States, the firearms officer in England is not only expected to perform a distasteful, dangerous, and highly stressful duty for the protection of society, but also in carrying out that duty is subjected to unreasonable pressures and criticisms by many sections of that same society. The effect of a shooting incident on the officer involved can be traumatic and occasionally results in permanent psychic damage.

The police staff associations, prompted by concern for these officers, approached the Home Office to request assistance in investigating the problem. The Home Office directed the Scientific Research and Development Branch (SRDB) to undertake a detailed investigation of the reactions of armed police officials in using their weapons to wound or take the life of a civilian. The primary aim of the exercise was to produce a set of guidelines to be used in the treatment and support of officers who become involved in shooting experiences.

Background Information

A review of the literature on PTSD (posttraumatic stress disorder) was carried out as a separate study (Cox & Hillas, 1986). A synopsis of its main findings is given below. Further background information was obtained through visits to a number of establishments with related interests including (1) the Home Office Antiterrorist Division, (2) the Metropolitan Police (Force Firearms Unit), (3) the Royal Ulster Constabulary, (4) the FBI Academy in Quantico, Virginia, (5) the Army Personnel Research Establishment, (6) the Royal Army Medical College, (7) the Queen Elizabeth Military Hospital in Woolwich, (8) the Sandhurst Royal Military Academy, and (9) the Northern Ireland Tactical Arms Training Establishment.

Visits to Antiterrorist Organizations

The visits to the Antiterrorist Division helped to clarify current Home Office policy on the issue of firearms and the police. They were also able to supply records of the total number of operations in which firearms were issued in each force for the period between 1980 and 1983, and similar figures for the Metropolitan Police for the period between 1970 and 1983. The latter also include figures for the number of occasions on which the weapons were fired, and the number of resultant deaths and injuries.

Mary Bernadette Manolias and Arthur Hyatt-Williams • Scientific Research and Development Branch, Home Office, Research and Planning Unit, Queen Anne's Gate, London SW1H 9AT, England.

International Handbook of Traumatic Stress Syndromes, edited by John P. Wilson and Beverley Raphael. Plenum Press, New York, 1993.

Researchers in the Metropolitan Police were making a study of the selection and assessment of firearms officers, and discussions with them were useful in establishing a common outlook. The contacts with the armed forces provided a wider context for the study by giving a more general impression of attitudes and policies toward the use of firearms. They also served to underline the very real differences between the armed fighting man and the armed police officer. Even with those soldiers trained for service in Northern Ireland, there were more contrasts than similarities (e.g., attitudes toward public safety and operational strategy).

Visits to the FBI Academy and the Royal Ulster Constabulary were helpful in understanding how carrying a weapon is reconciled with normal police work and traditional policing standards, as well as the special problems and the conflicts that are created by this aspect of the work. These visits not only provided a broad overview of the practicalities of weapons usage and training, but they also threw some light on the philosophies and intentions behind this. More importantly, they served to underline the unique position of the British Police with respect to firearms.

Differences between Police Officers and Armed Forces Personnel

There are essential differences between the army and the police and between the permanently armed police officer and the British firearms officer. Police officers, in general, differ from the armed services in the following ways:

1. Police weapons are carried mainly as a defense for themselves and innocent members of the public. The police officer's gun is intended primarily as a deterrent and will be used only as a last resort. The officer is nearly always armed with a handgun, which is kept in its holster unless there is a strong likelihood that it will be required to be used. In comparison with larger guns, the handgun is inaccurate and not very powerful.
2. For the armed forces, the purposes of a gun is destruction rather than the deterrence of an identifiable but impersonal enemy. Weapons are usually carried openly and in the fire-ready position whenever there is any chance of action. In a battle situation, the soldier is generally expected to kill repeatedly and indiscriminately, and his weapons are selected for accuracy and power. The probability of any western police officer being required to shoot at any time during his career is normally extremely low. When he does shoot, his stated aim in most cases is to stop his adversary. (It is understood that West Germany has attempted to train police officers to aim for an adversary's arms or legs.) Any deaths caused by police shooting must therefore be considered incidental rather than intentional.
3. The professional soldier shoots with the full backing of the army. He is normally one of a group, so it is rare for him to know whether he has been responsible for a particular death. His adversary is

most likely to be another professional soldier (Northern Ireland being a notable exception).
4. When a police officer shoots, there is a possibility that he may be on his own or with one partner. His adversary will typically be a civilian with possibly little previous experience with weapons.
5. The conditions under which the British firearms officer operates are different again. These individuals spend most of their working life unarmed (there are exceptions for special duties such as diplomatic protection where guns are always carried). Because he does not habitually carry a gun, he cannot have the same familiarity with his weapons as police officers from other countries. Neither will he have the ongoing practice in decision-making over using that weapon. Weapons are not issued except when there is a proven requirement. In consequence, officers will go to an incident anticipating that they may have to shoot.[1] It is against this background that the findings of the current study must be viewed.

Brief Literature Review

Nearly all the information on the police experience of shooting comes from American sources. Most of the literature takes the form of straightforward, often autobiographical accounts, of the experiences which have appeared in popular American police publications such as *Police Chief*, *The Trooper*, or *Police Stress*. They are of interest because collectively they confirm the existence of common behavioral patterns. However, there have also been a number of systematic studies based on case history data. The most notable examples are found in the work of Neilson (1981) and in Stratton, Parker, and Snibbe (1984). Another researcher, Wittrup (1985), has analyzed records of over 1,000 police officers who were interviewed after a shooting experience but has so far failed to publish his results.

There is broad agreement between these researchers and others who have carried out studies in this area on most aspects of the shooting experience, including the proportion of officers adversely affected, the severity and pattern of reactions, and the recommended treatment. There is also agreement from general stress studies that most American police officers view shooting as the most stressful event they could experience during their careers as police officers.

Not all officers involved in a shooting incident will suffer seriously adverse effects. Their reactions to the experience are governed by a combination of individual and situational factors. They include the degree of surprise, the individual's perception of the event, his current state of vulnerability both in the mental and physical spheres, and his use of coping mechanisms. The degree of the reaction can range from mild shock to severe posttraumatic stress disorder (PTSD).

---

[1] Most police officers consider firearms to be alien to the British police tradition. The officer who is prepared to carry a gun may be viewed by others as not being a proper policeman.

Posttraumatic stress disorder was first listed as a separate category of mental disorders in the *Diagnostic and Statistical Manual of Mental Disorders* (DSM-III) (American Psychiatric Association, 1980). It is most commonly observed in soldiers after prolonged exposure to battle situations and in the victims of major disasters where there is a large-scale loss of life and/or destruction that completely alters the victims' pattern of living (e.g., earthquakes, severe floods, etc.). The stressor may vary but must be of a type that exposes the individual's vulnerability and undermines his confidence in the continuity of life. Although each case is unique, certain characteristic symptoms are associated with the disorder (see also Chapter 78, in this volume, on the treatment of PTSD that is duty-related).

The shooting experience clearly lies on the borders of such extreme ordeals. Although it nearly always contains a very real threat to life, the situation is one which is rapidly resolved in one way or the other (usually by the death of one party). Nevertheless, the researchers found that nearly one third of the officers (33%) in the samples they studied had experienced the symptoms of severe PTSD. Of the remainder, approximately one half showed a moderate degree of reaction whereas the remainder suffered only mild shock. According to one study (Stratton *et al.*, 1984), all the officers interviewed had experienced recurring thoughts or flashbacks after the incident.

The consensus of advice from American researchers is that police shootings should always be regarded seriously by the police management because of the possible consequences to the officer concerned. Extreme reactions can often be avoided by timely treatment (see Chapter 76, in this volume, on critical stress incident debriefing).

The police experience of PTSD is complicated by the common use of denial or psychic distancing as a coping mechanism for dealing with the more unpleasant aspects of police work. This mechanism is only effective within certain limits and gives no protection against the impact of truly traumatic events, such as a shooting. Once the officer recovers from the immediate impact of the situation, the barriers are often rapidly reerected, and he may be ready to assert that the incident has had no effect. It is particularly important that psychological intervention occur during the time the officer is consciously aware of his full vulnerability. If intervention is delayed, the condition may no longer be readily accessible to treatment (Wittrup, 1985). Denial of the condition is often maladaptive. The adverse effects may be suppressed and ultimately lead to long-term damage. Finally, it has been observed that the prognosis is good if the onset of the reaction occurs within 6 months of the event and does not take more than 6 months to resolve. Beyond these time limits, the psychic damage may become permanent.

Perceptual Distortions

In the majority of cases, exposure to a life-threatening situation was found to have triggered a variety of perceptional distortions, a consequence of the primitive alarm reaction. By far the most common of these was the experience of time slowing down as if in a slow-motion film, although a few described time seeming to speed up. Other commonly reported distortions were tunnel vision and auditory blocking.

Among those officers experiencing some degree of PTSD, the most widely reported symptoms included thought intrusions (i.e., not being able to get thoughts about the event out of one's mind), depression, anxiety, sleep disturbances, fatigue, and an inability to focus thoughts. In most cases, the onset of PTSD was within 3 days of the incident (Loo, 1984). Emotional disturbances following a nonfatal shooting were usually found to be resolved fairly quickly, the average time being around 2 weeks. However, the aftereffects of a fatality could often last well over a year.

According to one study, the pattern of recovery follows through five main stages (Carson, 1982). These are denial, followed by anger and resentment, bargaining (fantasies about a different outcome), depression, and finally acceptance. Moreover, the responsibility for having taken a life frequently leads to feelings of guilt. In fact, there are many accounts of officers apologizing to the family of the deceased or trying to make some form of retribution for what has happened. There are several cases on record where the officer has provided financial support to the bereaved family and even attempted to take on the dead man's parental responsibilities.

Secondary Stressors

Some researchers have also made observations about the effect of the work environment on the officer involved in a shooting incident. Stratton and colleagues (1984) observed that fellow officers could be an additional source of stress through misplaced attempts to offer support (e.g., making jokes about the incident or treating it as a heroic exploit). Similarly, the effects of the incident could be instigated or exacerbated by significant others; a category that generally includes colleagues, senior officers, and members of the officer's own family. Additionally, the removal of the officer's gun, the legal consequences of the incident, the reactions of the media, and threats of reprisal to the officer's family were all mentioned as additional sources of stress.

Subjects

All the subjects who took part in this study did so on a voluntary basis. A personal approach was made to each individual by the chief constable of his force asking whether he would be willing to take part in a study of postshooting experiences. The names of those who agreed together with details of the incidents in which they had been involved were then forwarded to the SRDB researcher. After this, the researcher contacted each officer by telephone to explain the details of the experiment. The verbal arrangements were later confirmed by letter.

Of the original 25 officers ($N = 25$), 2 later chose to

withdraw from the experiment for personal reasons. However, they were replaced by 2 late volunteers. The first was told about this study by one of the subjects who was a close colleague. He approached the author directly to ask if he could take part. The second man had been responsible for a shooting accident during training, and the deputy chief constable asked the author to approach him. In this case, the injured officer was also interviewed along with the wives of both men.

Methodology

The study was conducted almost entirely through interview procedures with the volunteer subjects. Each officer was interviewed twice. The first interview, which was completely unstructured, was carried out by the consultant psychiatrist and lasted between 1 and 1.5 hours. The second interview, conducted by the government researcher, generally took longer (i.e., 1.5 to 2.5 hours) and was based on the topics listed in Table 32.1. The two researchers compared casenotes at frequent intervals throughout the study. All respondents also completed the Reaction Index, which yielded a measure of the PTSD resulting from the shooting experience. Twenty-four of the 25 subjects also agreed to complete the Sixteen Personality Factors Questionnaire.

Reaction Index (PTSD)

This questionnaire was designed by Calvin Frederick, Professor of Psychiatry and Behavioral Sciences at the University of California (Los Angeles) and Chief Psychologist at the Veterans Administration Medical Center. The test was initially developed to provide a straightforward measure of PTSD for members of the American Armed Forces who had suffered from psychiatric disorders after involvement in the Vietnam War. Subsequently, the test was proved to have a wider application and may be used as a diagnostic aid in conjunction with any traumatic experience.

Sixteen Personality Factors Questionnaire

The Personality Factors Questionnaire (designed by Cattell and Webster) is one of the most established psychological selection tests for police officers in the United States. It is also one of the tests suggested for the selection of firearms officers in a 1983 report on the Police Use of Firearms in the U.K.

Results

The results of the interviews are presented in the form of summarized extracts from the individual case histories which have been arranged under the following headings: (1) Attitudes toward Firearms, (2) Training, (3) Reactions in Shooting Officers, (4) Perceptual Distortion during the Shooting, (5) Official Actions and Senior Officers' Attitudes, (6) Attitudes of Colleagues, (7) Press

Table 32.1. Checklist for Interviews with Firearms Officers

General background

1. Marital status
2. Education
3. Religious convictions
4. Attitude to violence
5. Attitude to killing—just and unjust
6. Views of the police service on justifiable homicide (as they understood them before the event)

Preparation

1. Why did they undertake firearms training?
2. Were they asked if they felt able to shoot to kill?
3. Did they really think about having to carry out a killing?
4. Did they think they would be able to?
5. Did they discuss this with anyone: spouse, colleague(s), other?
6. Did the training prepare them for the real event? If so, how?
7. How did they feel when they were first told of the assignment?
8. Had they been on any similar assignments previously?
9. What were their feelings during the build-up to the incident?

Shooting

1. What were their feelings about the danger to self?
2. Training—did it help?
3. Perceptions—was there any alteration in perception, for example, time slowing down?
4. What were their immediate reactions after the event?
5. Did they see the person they had shot? What were their feelings toward him or her? Then? Now?

Aftermath

1. What were the immediate reactions from colleagues and commanding officers? Were the firearms officers congratulated, reprimanded, debriefed, questioned at length, isolated, sent home?
2. Did anyone in the force understand how they felt, or try to help them? How did they feel about the way they were treated? Then? Now?
3. Have they subsequently discussed the experience in detail with anyone? Who? How soon after?
4. What were their colleagues' reactions?
5. Those of their families?
6. Their friends?
7. Were the media involved? How did this affect the situation?
8. What has been the effect on their marital relationship? On their relationships with children? On their relationship with friends at work?

Personal effects

1. Were there any physical disturbances, for example, sleep patterns, sweating or trembling, eating and digestion, sexual performance?
2. Were there any psychological effects, such as flashbacks? How realistic? Visual? Olfactory? Nightmares, phobias, anxiety, depression, and the like?
3. Were there any noticeable behavioral changes, for example, withdrawal, unprovoked outbursts of anger, heavy drinking, gambling, extramarital affairs?
4. Have they come to terms with the experiences? If so, how?
5. Are they still firearms officers? If not, why?

and Public, (8) Reactions of Families of Officers, and (9) Legal Litigation and Appearance in Court.

Some caution must be urged in accepting these results at face value since they are based on subjective accounts of a highly emotional experience that, in most cases, had occurred some considerable time previously; furthermore, the memory of most events becomes modified over time. This is particularly true when it concerns a potentially painful incident of the type being investigated here. In such cases, there is an unconscious tendency to revise or reappraise the event to a more acceptable form. Given the circumstances of the investigation it would have been inappropriate to attempt to probe hidden memories and risk upsetting an individual's equilibrium after he had managed to come to terms with the experience.

The results from the PTSD Reaction Index and the 16-PF test are not included in the report for reasons of confidentiality and ethicality under the auspices of the Home Office in London.

Attitudes toward Firearms

The main reason given for carrying a firearm was self-protection and the protection of others. Quite a few of the officers who gave this reason had been attracted to working in a specialist area where a firearms license was either a requirement or a desirable attribute. The majority of these men said that they disliked guns. The second most common reason was a special interest in firearms and competitive marksmanship.

It seems that only a few officers had seriously considered the possibility of having to kill another human being prior to taking up firearms duties. The majority seem to have regarded it as too remote a possibility to require any deep thought at that stage, whereas one or two said that it was not advisable to think too closely about such things. Again, very few had actually discussed their decision to become firearms officers with their wives or anyone else.

Training

Officers were asked how well they thought their training had prepared them for the reality of the situation. Only one man said he felt insufficiently trained for his actions to be instinctive. The remainder felt that their weapons handling was adequate or better. At least one third of the men in this sample were very well trained and above average marksmen. Either they had trained for special duties, or had been in the army, or were interested in target shooting as a leisure activity. However, there were criticisms of the training. A few men said they were totally unprepared for such aspects of shooting as the actual effect of their weapon on a human body and the sound of the gunshots. All said that they had been asked at the start of their firearms training course to consider whether they would be able to shoot another person if required. In some cases, this had seemed almost a formality. In no case did the psychological aspects of killing or being involved in a life-threatening situation form a part of the course.

Reactions in Shooting Officers

Despite individual differences in temperament, the degree of anxiety that the men experienced prior to the actual shooting seems to have been mainly dependent on the circumstances surrounding it. Not all officers came under direct life threat or, if they did, did not have time to realize the gravity of the situation. There was little sense of fear under these conditions. When there was time to anticipate the event and they were in a passive or vulnerable situation, there was generally a great build up of tension and anxiety. At the point of greatest danger, most men became extremely calm and clear-headed, although four of them reported feelings of intense fear, which were rapidly replaced by overwhelming anger. Only one man reported feeling terrified throughout the incident. This affected his performance to the extent of putting him in grave danger, that is, he fired several bullets into the swing door in front of him and his hands were trembling so much that he had difficulty in reloading his weapon. Despite his fears he acted with great bravery.

After the shooting, immediate reactions varied from feelings of relief or even elation that it was over, to quite serious shock. It is believed that most men, certainly all those who had been under direct life threat, experienced some form of shock although they were not necessarily able to recognize it in themselves. Among the milder symptoms that were described were excessive talking and the sensation of having a dry mouth. One man said that he felt quite calm but when he attempted to write a statement shortly afterward, he found he was unable to control his hand. Other men reported feeling shocked and shaken or completely drained.

About half the officers interviewed said that they had no regrets about the shooting. They felt the action had been necessary and that they were justified in taking it. One or two of these officers, however, said that they felt sorrow for the dead man's family. The remainder felt sad or guilty about the wounding or death they had caused but had eventually been able to come to terms with this. In one instance, an officer had attempted to resuscitate the man he had killed. He remained very distressed about the killing for a long time.

The interviews indicate that around two thirds (67%) of the officers in the sample had a marked emotional reaction after the incident. The onset of the condition started several hours after the incident, with the most commonly reported symptoms being that of thinking over the incident repeatedly and continuously for days at a time. Other common experiences were sleep disturbances, which included sleeplessness, sudden waking, cold sweats, and nightmares. Bouts of crying were also quite usual. Some officers also reported digestive upsets and loss of appetite, and one man claimed that some of his hair had turned gray as a direct result of the experience. Feelings of anxiety and depression accompanied by some degree of social withdrawal were also common. In most cases, the difficulties resolved themselves between several weeks and several months of the incident, but in a few exceptional cases they lasted much longer. There were at least three cases of severe PTSD according to the DSM-III diagnosis criteria. In addition to the classic symptoms of PTSD, these men suffered other effects as well:

1. Officer A reported that the shooting had had a permanent effect on him. He still has occasional bouts of weeping. The incident took place 12 years ago.

2. Officer B reported that he had no feelings or regret about the man he had wounded. However, he found the act of shooting was so repellent to him, because it was the complete antithesis of all he felt policing stood for, that he experienced a dramatic psychosomatic reaction. This took the form of a migraine headache that persisted continuously for several months together with a partial loss of sensation in the right side of his body.

3. Officer C suffered from severe depression for a period of around 2 years and became completely withdrawn from his family and colleagues. He also suffered from continuous digestive upsets. In order to distract himself in his isolated state he spent a great deal of his time playing the one-armed bandits at the police club and lost a lot of money. The large debt he incurred finally prompted him to seek help for his problems.

Perceptual Distortion during the Shooting

Around 60% of the officers interviewed reported experiencing some form of perceptual distortion during the incident, a finding supported by most American studies of this area. The most usual manifestation was that of time seeming to slow down. Other forms of perceptual distortion described were tunnel vision, apparent exaggeration of size or distance, and distortions in hearing such that some sounds seemed very loud while others were not registered at all.

Perceptual distortions were experienced mainly by those officers who felt their lives to be under direct threat. One officer explained that there had been no perceptual distortion in his case during the shooting incident because he was not in any real personal danger, but that he had encountered the sensation of time slowing down some time previously when he fell in a mountaineering accident. Officers not reporting perceptual distortions generally said that the incident was over too quickly for them to feel any real fear.

The sensation of time slowing was generally accompanied by a feeling of detachment and the conviction that there was ample time to consider all the implications of the situation and arrive at the correct decision. Most officers who had experienced this sensation described being able to think very clearly and faster than usual, and some were able to recall all the thoughts that went through their minds at the time. However, after they had discharged their weapons, this same phenomenon became a cause of alarm because the effects of the shot also seemed to be delayed, and they became convinced that their guns had failed to work. For one officer, time slowing *altered* to time speeding-up *after* the gunman had fallen to the ground and then returned again to normal. Several officers also described distortions in size or distance. In some cases, size became exaggerated. To one officer the end of his adversary's shotgun looked like a "pair of binoculars." Size could also appear to be reduced, and, in the excitement of giving chase, another man scaled a 15-foot fence which had seemed to be only

waist high at the time. Distances could also be affected, and there were two reports of officers' thinking themselves to be much further away from the gunman than was the case. Later checks proved the distance to be about one third of what they had estimated.

There were two instances when gunshots had not been heard, and another when an officer had not heard his colleague shout the required warning. There was also one case reported where the officer had hardly registered the sound of his own gun firing, but that of his partner seemed so loud that it was ringing in his ears for hours after. Several officers described the experience of tunnel vision. One man said that everything except the gunman seemed to disappear, whereas another did not realize until after the incident, that there was a bus standing alongside the patrol car.

The emotional reactions that were found to be closely associated with the experiences described here are particularly noteworthy. Four of the officers described feelings of intense fear being replaced by extreme anger. None of the men affected had ever before felt such an overwhelming fury (i.e., from fear to rage). No published reports of this type of behavior have been found in the American literature, although it appears to be known to the researchers working in this area.

Official Actions and Senior Officers' Attitudes

In the majority of cases, it appeared that senior officers were supportive and reassuring. However, there were some notable exceptions. In at least two instances, the firearms officer reported that senior officers had distanced themselves until they were certain that the shooting had been carried out in an acceptable manner and would not reflect badly on themselves or the force. This was a source of deep resentment. Quite a number of officers of ACPO seem to have gone out of their way to congratulate firearms officers or assure them of support. In one instance, an ACPO rank officer accompanied a wounded man to the hospital and refused to leave until his relatives arrived. In every case, these demonstrations of concern left a lasting impression on the recipient. ACPO ranking officers are also in a position to cause great resentment through unthinking actions. This happened in only one instance. The officer in question together with others involved in the same firearms incident were arbitrarily removed from firearms duty. They were informed of this decision via a typed memorandum sent to their senior officers. No explanation for this action was ever given, and the affected officer reported that his feelings of anger and frustration lasted for around 18 months. Another man who was also removed from firearms duty reported that his clothing had been taken away and not returned although it was of no use for forensic purposes.

Quite frequently, little consideration seems to have been shown about the welfare of the firearms officers. One man, following an incident that was very successfully concluded (i.e., no one was really hurt), was locked in a room alone for 2 hours to write his statement without even being offered a cup of tea. Other men reported that they had driven themselves back to the police station and/or home later. One man said he had not been allowed to telephone his wife to let her know everything was all right.

Attitudes of Colleagues

Almost invariably, colleagues acted in an overtly supportive manner immediately following a shooting incident. Despite this, most firearms officers thought that very few people were interested in their feelings or were able to understand them (see also Chapter 76, in this volume, on critical incident debriefing). General reactions at the police station were frequently inappropriate with jokes or unthinking remarks in poor taste. This was particularly marked when a dangerous criminal had been brought down after a prolonged police search and there was a very natural feeling of elation at the police station. Where an incident had gone wrong, there was generally very genuine sympathy and concern for the firearms officer and real efforts were made to reassure him. The colleagues of one man who was suspended for some considerable time made a point of meeting him regularly in a local pub to ensure that he did not feel "cut-off."

In a number of instances, colleagues gave valuable psychological first aid. One example cited was that of a close colleague sitting with the firearms officer while they waited for an ambulance to arrive at the scene and then accompanying him back to the police station. Mutual support at this stage was found to be equally valuable. In one instance, two other firearms officers who had also been involved in the incident went home with the shooting officer and stayed drinking and talking together until 3 A.M. In another, the firearms team met up in a pub the following evening, but they did not discuss the incident. It was enough to know that they had all shared in the same experience.

Although they are generally ready to respond to the obvious needs of colleagues, police officers often seem to be unaware of long-term problems or perhaps are unwilling to appear as interfering in another's personal affairs. One officer who suffered from long-term depressive illness as a result of his shooting experiences said that although he had changed from being very outgoing and friendly, and had become withdrawn, his behavior was completely ignored by the people he worked with. In the long-term work situation, fellow officers can sometimes be a source of annoyance to the firearms officer who has been involved in a shooting incident. Colleagues may be curious about an event he would prefer to forget, or make jokes or remarks about it that show ignorance and tactlessness.

Press and Public

Nearly all the incidents discussed in this study attracted considerable news coverage. For the most part, the names of the officers involved were not divulged to the press until after the court case by which time media interest had died down. In three cases where officers' names were released prematurely, the men and their families were subject to considerable harassment. One man said that he and his family were unable to leave the house for a week and that all telephone calls had to be intercepted.

Some officers felt that the press accounts of their own incident were fair but many found them inaccurate and hurtful (see Chapter 38, in this volume, for a similar description in disasters). It was generally thought that letters from the public published in the newspapers displayed little understanding of the true situation. The officers felt angry and frustrated at being unable to reply. One officer is still hoping for the opportunity to tell his side of the story 6 years later. Two officers said that they were particularly angered by the appearance of politicians on television using the incident as an opportunity to further their own political ends.

Reactions of Families of Officers

The effects of the shooting incident were found to have spread to all immediate family members, that is, wives, children, and parents. It seemed that only about half of the officers interviewed had chosen to consult their wives before assuming firearms duties. In one instance, the wife was completely unaware that her husband carried a gun until he was involved in a very dangerous shooting incident. The officer concerned believes that the resulting shock was so great that it caused her to have a serious stroke shortly afterward. He had not previously realized how much she had always worried over his safety, particularly when he was on night duty. He has had mixed feelings of resentment over the incident and personal guilt ever since.

In many cases, the officers' wives were understandably very distressed by their husbands' involvement in a shooting, but were still able to offer them valuable support. Those men who were willing to discuss the experience and share their feelings about it with their wives said that this had helped considerably. At least two of them believed that the experience had helped to strengthen their marriages. A few men who said that they did not normally discuss work matters with their spouses had made an exception on this occasion. However, this still left quite a number of men who chose to keep their experience to themselves (without interviewing the wives it is difficult to comment on what effect this might have had on them). One officer rejected the comfort offered by his wife because he felt he could not cope with her emotions as well as his own. He wanted mental privacy in order to work through his feelings for himself. Another officer who suffered a very severe depression after the shooting alienated himself from his wife and children for around 2 years. He has since explained his behavior to his wife, but they have never been able to discuss his experience in depth.

In most families, it had been impossible to keep the knowledge of their father's involvement in a shooting from the children. The children's reactions ranged from curiosity to attempting to comfort their father. In most cases, the parents dealt with the matter in a straightforward and practical way giving the children as much information as necessary. There were no reports of any serious effects on an officer's children.

Parents and in-laws of the officers frequently had reacted with shock or distress (sometimes there was also justifiable pride in their son's bravery), but in all instances they were very supportive. For one officer, the shooting incident followed very closely the death of his father. The cumulative effect of the two shocks was overwhelming for his mother and completely demolished her efforts to retain any semblance of composure.

Legal Litigation and Appearance in Court

Court cases and litigation invariably caused a great deal of additional anxiety and, in certain respects, were a greater ordeal than the shooting itself. The worst aspects seem to have been the length of time spent waiting for the case to come to court and the uncertainty about the outcome. In two separate instances, officers were not kept informed about the inquest file. One man said that this worried him so much that he had recurring nightmares and kept waking throughout the night.

Discussion

It was found that both the immediate and long-term reaction patterns described in the previous sections closely coincided with those reported in the American studies. The majority of those interviewed had had little difficulty in coming to terms with having had to take a life. This was easiest in straightforward situations where the officer was presented with a clear choice between his own life (or that of a threatened civilian) and that of the gunman. In such cases, it was quite possible to justify the killing to himself however distasteful he found the act. Not all the incidents were resolved in this clearcut way (e.g., the gunman turned out to be using a replica weapon, the shooting had resulted in the permanent paralysis of the man shot, and, in a further instance, an unarmed civilian was fatally wounded by the armed officer). The distress and guilt feelings associated with such outcomes were difficult and sometimes impossible for the officer to resolve without suitable assistance and often resulted in long-term psychological disturbances.

Treatment of Postshooting Reactions

American studies show that nearly all officers directly involved in shooting incidents suffer some degree of shock. It was difficult to confirm whether or not this was also true for the British officers since the researchers were dependent on the evidence from retrospective interviews, but it would seem a sensible precaution if a routine medical check was introduced for all such cases.

In some forces in the United States, it is also common practice for an officer who has been actively involved in a shooting incident to be seen by the police psychologist as soon as possible and before he is asked to complete a statement or is interviewed by the investigating team. The psychologist's intervention can assist him in diffusing the initial feeling triggered by the incident and in recovering his composure and ordering his thoughts before the interview. Clearly, such procedures

may raise questions about collusion but such objections are somewhat unrealistic. It has to be emphasized that almost every officer who goes through this particular experience will be in a state of shock for several hours afterward. A statement taken during this time will be confused and unclear, and the procedure will have to be repeated after he has had time to recover from the initial effects of the incident (see critical incident debriefing, in Chapter 76, in this volume).

Counseling help can be called up for immediate care after a shooting, but this might not provide the most appropriate source of first-line assistance. Probably, the officer will feel most comfortable with a close colleague or another member of the firearms team. Support from these sources is likely to be readily available, and their value and acceptability were confirmed by officers interviewed in this study.

Training in practical first-line supporting skills could easily be incorporated into the firearms training course. Alternatively, the services of the welfare officer or local federation representative might be utilized as well. Furthermore, it is also desirable that each officer be referred to a mental health professional (i.e., a clinical psychologist or psychiatrist for a check-up interview within 2 to 3 weeks of the incident). The results of this interview would remain confidential and any arrangements for subsequent treatment would ideally remain a matter between the officer and the consultant.

Management Support

It must be emphasized that the firearms officer is often in an emotionally vulnerable condition during the period immediately following an incident and that the reactions of those in close contact with him at this time can have a profound and lasting effect. If possible, coworkers should be advised to respect his feelings. Simple congratulations or expressions of support are in order depending on the outcome, but no event which has resulted in a death or serious wounding should be turned into a celebration. The officer responsible will not be happy at being treated as a "conquering hero." Platitudes such as "I know how you feel" or "He deserved everything he got" are likely to irritate and should be avoided since they minimize the complexities of what occurred during the shooting incident.

The attitudes of senior officers are equally important. Thoughtless or inconsiderate actions on their part can provoke lasting anger and resentment. The main contribution of senior officers at this time might be to provide reassurance. Regardless of the outcome of the incident and its future consequences, the firearms officer still deserves the full support of the service.

The case histories contained several examples of supportive behavior on the part of senior officers that was obviously helpful and greatly appreciated by the recipients. The evidence from the interviews indicated that this had almost invariably been the case when an incident had gone awry and where the officer was likely to face serious consequences. Unfortunately, there were also a number of instances of what appeared to be callous or even cruel treatment. For example, an apparent interpersonal distancing from the firearms officer was not unusual, but it is in fact unlikely that this behavior was in any way deliberate. A police shooting is a very rare event in the U.K., and such reactions probably stemmed directly from uncertainty and a lack of knowledge on the correct procedures to be followed under those unfamiliar conditions. They would be further complicated by an understandable anxiety over adverse publicity and the possible legal implications of the incident. It should be obvious that the firearms officer will be subject to similar and even greater anxieties; yet despite this, there had been several instances where no effort had been made to explain the legal position to him or how he would be affected by the discipline code. Such defects are simple to remedy and it could be made a part of routine procedure for the local federation representative or other suitable persons to advise the officers on these topics and related matters. Most of the common mistakes made in the treatment of firearms officers following a shooting incident could be avoided if each force were to issue clear guidelines on the treatment of firearms officers following a shooting incident. Ideally, such guidance material would include an explanation of the effects of PTSD as well as advice on practical procedures (see Chapter 76, in this volume, for an extensive discussion of these issues).

Managements' responsibilities for the welfare of the firearms officers have never been clearly defined and, consequently, there have been some rather obvious oversights. Those included allowing the officer to drive while he was probably in a state of shock, and not allowing him to telephone home to explain the situation to his wife before she heard the news from other sources. The interviews showed that the company of a close or sympathetic colleague could be a source of great reassurance but the majority of officers were left without any form of support. Supervising officers could ensure that such support is always provided. They should also check that the officer has an adequate social support system at home (e.g., wife, girlfriend, or parents). If the officer is living on his own, it is suggested that a close colleague should be assigned to accompany him home and be prepared to spend time with him if necessary.

Supervisors should also consider giving the officer some time at home with his family following a shooting incident. Some officers may welcome the opportunity to take time off to readjust and work through the likely reactions with those who are emotionally closest to them. Others will prefer to keep themselves occupied with routine duties. Time off should not be made compulsory since this might possibly be construed as a punitive measure.

Occasionally, an officer will have to be suspended from duty as the result of his actions during the incident. In the cases described in this study, the reasons were generally well understood and accepted by the officers concerned and all said they felt the matter had been handled in a sympathetic manner. However, the reality of suspension and the length of time waiting for the case to be heard were an additional source of strain. Psychiatric support should be made available in such cases, but management can also assist more directly by ensuring that the officer is kept fully informed about all aspects of the case.

Training

Almost all the officers interviewed thought that their training had been adequate for their shooting experience, but it is clear that British firearms officers have less opportunity to become familiar with their weapons than their counterparts in other countries. Several men mentioned this as a serious cause for concern. One suggestion put forward for overcoming the difficulty was that officers could be given the opportunity to become familiar with their weapons by being given the access to them within the confines of the police station. It was felt that constant practice in loading and unloading could go a long way toward increasing confidence in this area.

Training for a hazardous task of this kind should not only aim to ensure that the officer's competence is far superior to that of his adversary but that he himself feels confident that it is. It is suggested that basic weapons training should concentrate on weapons handling, target practice, and safety procedures up to the point where those become reflex before any element of tactical training or higher level decision skills are introduced.

Recommendations

1. Immediate psychological support should be provided. Where possible, access to a mental health professional should be offered at this time. The officer's physical condition should also be checked.

2. The officer is likely to be in a state of physical and mental shock and suffering some degree of confusion. Statements taken under these conditions may be of limited forensic value. Some way of delaying the formal investigating procedure should be considered in order to give the officer the time and opportunity to recover from the initial effects of his experience.

3. It should be standard practice for a shooting officer to be interviewed by a clinical psychologist or a psychiatrist as soon as possible following an incident.

4. Whatever the outcome of the shooting incident, the officer responsible should not be made to feel he is ostracized by the force.

5. It is important to ensure that the officer has an adequate social support system outside the service. If the individual lives on his own, his supervising officer should assign a close colleague to spend some time with him during off-duty hours and to remain in close contact during the week following the incident.

6. The force should extend its support to the officer's family. The officer's wife should be alerted to the possible psychological consequences of the incident and should be offered an opportunity to discuss the situation with the force's selected mental health consultant.

7. Precautions should be taken to protect the officer and his family from unwanted publicity.

8. The officer should be kept fully informed of all developments connected with inquests or court cases.

9. If suspended, the officer should have access to close personal friends in the service.

10. Firearms training should prepare officers for the realities of a shooting and its consequences. Issues connected with the taking of life should be discussed. Train-

ing in human awareness skills and appropriate colleague support skills should form part of the firearms training course.

Conclusions

In the main, the results of this study were found to be in close agreement with American research in this area. The mental and physical reactions experienced by British officers as a result of firearms incidents were broadly similar both in the short- and long-term sequence to those described by their American colleagues. However, there was a very marked contrast between the circumstances surrounding the incidents in the two countries which serves only to emphasize the unique position of the British firearms officer.

References

American Psychiatric Association. (1980). *Diagnostic and statistical manual of mental disorders* (3rd ed.). Washington, DC: Author.

Carson, S. (1982, October). Post shooting stress reaction. *Police Chief*, October, pp. 66–68.

Loo, R. (1984). The role of human factors in police shooting incidents. *Proceedings of the 1984 International Conference on Occupational Ergonomics* (pp. 108–112).

Neilson, E. (1981). *The law enforcement officer's use of deadly force and post-shooting trauma*. Unpublished doctoral dissertation, University of Utah.

Stratton, J. G., Parker, D. A., & Snibbe, J. R. (1984). Post-traumatic stress: Study of police officers involved in shootings. *Psychological Reports, 55*, 127–131.

Wittrup, R. (1985). *Problems in post-critical incident psychological reaction*. Paper presented at NATO Advanced Study Institute of Police and Psychology, Skiathos, Greece.

Trauma Related to Disasters of Natural and Human Origin

Part IV contains thirteen chapters concerned with the traumatic aftermath of involvement in disasters of natural and human origin. These disasters span the spectrum from bushfires in Australia to the nuclear reactor meltdown at Chernobyl in the Soviet Union. Included in Part IV, then, are investigations of the traumatic consequences of disaster impacts on the individual psyche and to entire communities. More specifically, the disasters studied include: (1) technological accidents through biospheric contamination, (2) bushfires in Australia of enormously high temperatures, (3) the nuclear disaster at Chernobyl, (4) the Buffalo Creek Dam disaster, (5) the Kings Cross Underground Railway station fire in London, England, (6) two major oil rig disasters in the North Sea, (7) the sinking of the *Herald of Free Enterprise*, also known as the "Zeebrugge disaster," (8) earthquakes in China and Japan, (9) motor vehicle accidents, (10) rape victims, and (11) HIV autoimmune disease (AIDS). These studies are summarized in Table IV.1.

In Chapter 33, Elizabeth M. Smith and Carol S. North discuss PTSD in natural disasters and technological accidents. This chapter presents a comprehensive survey of the current literature on the relationship between the types of disaster and the prevalence of PTSD as a diagnosis, or the presence of symptoms of the stress syndrome that are associated with the various stressors experienced during the event. To accomplish this, Smith and North first present a conceptual organization of disaster research as well as noting the methodological problems in obtaining reliable data. Their discussion of research methodology echoes the recommendations made by Baum, Solomon, Ursano, and their colleagues in Chapter 10 and point out how difficult it is to establish accurate estimates of the prevalence of PTSD if the research design limits the ability to draw inferences about psychiatric sequelae or to determine complex interaction effects between the person, the type of trauma, and the nature of the stress reactions exhibited. For example, in commenting on one study of a tornado and on another of a plane crash into a hotel, the authors state:

> Because the methodology was exactly the same for these two studies, the large difference in rates of PTSD between the two sites must be due either to the type of the disaster agent or to different predisposing characteristics of the two populations studied, or to some combination of these factors.

Table IV.1. An Overview of Research on Trauma Related to Disasters of Natural and Human Origin

Chapter/study and authors	Population studied	Median age and related features	Measures used and time period assessed	Symptoms evident	Major findings
33 Technological accidents Smith and North	Comprehensive literature review	Victims of disaster	MMPI Clinical interviews Survey GHQ SCID	Anxiety Depression PTSD symptoms Somatization Intrusive recollections	PTSD rates vary by disaster PTSD diagnosis rates are low but symptom levels are high
34 Bushfire McFarlane	N = 469 survivors of bushfire (Australia)	Firefighters and others	Diagnostic Interview Schedule (DIS)	PTSD symptoms Depression Anxiety Intrusive recollections Sleep disturbance	Single diagnosis rare; high rates of comorbidity Premorbid factors prevalent
35 Chernobyl Lundin, Mårdberg, and Otto	Swedish citizens affected by nuclear fallout	N = 840 adults living in Sweden N = 216 in high-risk area	Telephone interviews Threat index Coping index General questionnaire	Concern about radiation Depressive symptoms	Premorbidity associated with less fear of fallout Coping moderated perception of threat
36 Buffalo Creek disaster Grace, Green, Lindy, and Leonard	Buffalo Creek survivors	14-year follow-up study N = 195	SCID-PTSD Clinical interviews SCL-90-R IES Psychiatric Evaluation Form Flood Stressors Measure 1974–1988	Anxiety Depression PTSD symptoms	63% PTSD rate (lifetime) 23% PTSD rate (current) PTSD comorbid with depression and generalized anxiety disorder 11% delayed onset of PTSD Stressor meausres predict PTSD
37 Underground Railway station fire Turner, Thompson, and Rosser	Kings Cross Underground Railway station fire survivors	N = 50 (total) N = 22 (passengers) N = 18 (EMS) N = 8 (workers) N = 2 (others)	GHQ IES Eysenck Personality Inventory (EPI)	Anxiety Depression PTSD symptoms	65% psychiatric caseness IES scores high and suggest PTSD
38 Piper Alpha oil rig disaster Alexander	Workers on rig who survived (N = 62 of 226)	Adult males who worked on oil rig	1988–1989 Clinical interviews Hospital treatment Case follow-up	PTSD symptoms Anxiety Depression Anger Grief Mistrust	Developed treatment plan to aid victims Strategies for management discussed

Disaster / Author	Population	Design	Symptoms	Findings
39 North Sea oil rig disaster Holen	Workers on rig who survived (N = 123 of 212)	Studied in 1980, 1981, 1984, and 1988 DSM-III PTSD criteria Dissociative symptoms Cognitive and social functioning	PTSD Anxiety Depression Grief	33% poor psychiatric outcomes 40% reduced cognitive functioning 67% had dissociative reaction during trauma Proneness to dissociate predictive of PTSD
40 Zeebrugge disaster Johnston	Survivors of the *Herald of Free Enterprise* Treatment-seeking population (N = 352)	No formal measurements (1987–1989)	PTSD Anxiety Depression Grief Mistrust	Developed treatment plan to aid victims Strategies for management discussed
41 Earthquake in Japan Odaira, Iwadate, and Raphael	N = 7,129 (Study 1) N = 525 (Study 2) General population (S1) Patients and staff of hospital (S2)	1968 and 1978 psychiatric symptoms Physical reactions	Body swaying Trembling Anxiety Fear Irritability Depression	Symptoms dissipated in 2 weeks Mental patients reacted differently than normals
42 Earthquake in China McFarlane and Hua	Random sample of ethnic Chinese Cross-section of population N = 1,258	GHQ DIS-PTSD EPI	Anxiety Depression PTSD symptoms	50% caseness rate PTSD prevalent High comorbidity rates Cultural factors affected attributions of causality
43 Motor vehicle accidents Horne	Automobile accident victims N = 7 adults	Clinical interviews and behavioral treatment for 6–14 sessions	Anxiety Phobias Depression PTSD symptoms	43% PTSD rate 57% phobic
44 Rape victims Hartman and Burgess	Rape victims Adult females	Clinical interviews	Anxiety Anger/rage Depression PTSD symptoms	Outline treatment approaches PTSD rates high Depression comorbid with PTSD
45 AIDS Kelly and Raphael	N = 35 AIDS victims Ages 16–65 HIV-infected	Studied for 3 years IES Beck Depression Inventory GHQ EPI	Anxiety Fear Alienation Stigmatization PTSD symptoms Depression	50% caseness on GHQ PTSD prevalent

In the balance of the chapter, the authors review the strengths and limitations of the most current studies and draw a general set of conclusions about PTSD and symptom prevalence as related to both natural and technological disasters. Directions for future research are indicated and will aid investigators in designing and carrying research projects into disaster impacts.

In Chapter 34, Alexander Cowell McFarlane discusses the Ash Wednesday bushfire disaster in Southeastern Australia, which occurred on February 16, 1983. Dry weather had created the ideal conditions for a bushfire explosion in the area. Once the fires began, because of a confluence of precipitating factors, they were nearly impossible to contain; the flames soared over 800 feet high in zero-visibility conditions, with the temperatures rising to several thousand degrees Fahrenheit. When it was all over, the earth was scorched black. Seventy-two people died in the fire, 2,000 homes were destroyed, and over 300,000 sheep and cattle were lost.

McFarlane studied 469 individuals involved in the fire to determine the prevalence and duration of psychiatric symptoms among subgroups of individuals. He states that

> forty-two months after the disaster all those who had developed significant symptoms were interviewed. Of the 58 who were found to have a posttraumatic stress disorder, only 16 had it as a single diagnosis. Of 22 firefighters who had an anxiety disorder diagnosis, 13 also had a PTSD. Of the 34 who satisfied the diagnostic criteria for major depression, 29 also had a PTSD and 30 also had another anxiety disorder diagnosis.

These findings suggest that the spectrum of traumatic reactions is not limited to PTSD, but comorbid conditions exist as well which predictably involve anxiety and depressive reactions.

Since the issue of pretrauma personality and background factors is almost always relevant to a complete scientific understanding of the interaction effects of the nature of the person, trauma, and recovery environment, McFarlane attempted to ascertain the degree to which these factors contribute to the psychiatric sequelae among a subsample of the disaster victims. Using the Diagnostic Interview Schedule (discussed by Smith and North in Chapter 33), McFarlane found that

> the acute PTSD group had no major vulnerability factors and seldom had a coexistent psychiatric disorder. In contrast, the chronic PTSD group scored significantly higher on a number of vulnerability factors, such as concurrent psychiatric disorder, a positive family history for psychiatric disorder, avoidance as a personality trait, as well as being older and having panicked more during the disaster.

These findings parallel those discussed by Weisaeth and Eitinger in Chapter 6 who classified *risk-proneness* into three categories: (1) high-risk *situations*, (2) high-risk *persons*, and (3) high-risk initial *reactions* to trauma. Thus, McFarlane's study appears to be identifying all three types of risk-proneness in his population of survivors. He concludes his discussion of the many interesting findings in the chapter by noting that

> The study of disasters examines the impact of a state of terror that may last for only seconds in contrast to the prolonged exposure of a soldier in battle to the threat of death. The similarities and different effects of such stressors in the etiology of posttraumatic stress disorder has been given little attention but is important to an understanding of the etiology of PTSD.

The advent of the nuclear age created the opportunity for new technologies to be applied to the production of energy by the use of nuclear reactors. Although the prospect of using nuclear reactors to produce electric power was appealing, many people feared the potential danger if a "meltdown" condition was to occur which would release radioactive material into the environment. Just such a scenario occurred on April 26, 1986, when a nuclear power unit was destroyed by an explosion and a fire at Chernobyl in the Soviet Union. Approximately 135,000 persons were displaced from the immediate community; 18,000 were treated medically; nearly 300 became inpatients in hospitals in Moscow; and at least 26 died as a result of the disaster by June, just two months later. Furthermore, nuclear radioactive material was swept up into the atmosphere and carried by winds over parts of Sweden, Poland, and Finland.

Chapter 35, by Tom Lundin, Bertil Mårdberg, and Ulf Otto, reports on the psychological effects of the nuclear fallout in Sweden, where nuclear activity was registered 100 kilometers north of Stockholm. They state:

> Reactions of confusion and anxiety developed slowly in the Swedish population. The event was unique and unlike any previous disaster in Sweden. Fallout cannot be seen or detected by most sensory mechanisms. It is known to produce long term medical reactions. It cannot be removed from huge areas, such as a country, by any technical means or human effort. Furthermore, from the Swedish point of view, the Chernobyl disaster became a threat to the overall welfare of the nation because of the expected effects of the radiation in persons, food, water, and on the environment in general.

To study the psychological effects of nuclear radiation fallout in Sweden, Lundin and his associates sampled 840 persons from the entire country who were older than 17 years. A structured interview was conducted by telephone and included measures of threat and coping.

The results revealed that most people in Sweden had good information about the situation, that concerns about well-being were widespread, and that unpleasant thoughts about the disaster were common. Among the many intriguing findings in this study is that the perception of threat was associated with negative feelings toward the accident and nuclear power in Sweden, and greater concern about the safety and well-being of loved ones. Moreover, individuals with a prior psychiatric history were less concerned about radiation effects but were simultaneously more depressed. Using a latent profile analysis, Lundin et al. were able to discern nine profiles of reactions and classify subjects in the sample accordingly. Each of these profiles is discussed. In their conclusion, the authors state that "negative emotional reactions and the perception of the Chernobyl threat to individuals were also predicted by living in a high-risk zone, gender, education level, structuring ability, general threshold for threat perception, and coping potential."

In 1972, along a 16-mile hollow known as Buffalo Creek in Logan County, West Virginia, a man-made slag dam that was poorly constructed gave way and unleashed a devastating flood that careened through the Appalachian valley. One hundred and twenty-five persons were killed and nearly 5,000 were displaced from their homes. Eventually, a lawsuit followed by the survivors against the Pittston Corporation; questions of psychological damage were carefully studied by both sides of the litigation.

In 1981, the first comprehensive examination of the flood was published by Gleser, Green, and Winget under the title *Prolonged Psychosocial Effects of Disaster: A Study of Buffalo Creek*, a landmark work because of the methodological rigor with which the research was conducted. In Chapter 36, Mary C. Grace, Bonnie L. Green, Jacob D. Lindy, and Anthony C. Leonard present a 14-year follow-up on the survivors of the Buffalo Creek disaster.

These researchers from the University of Cincinnati returned to Buffalo Creek in 1986 to conduct interviews with as many of the original subjects as they could find. Additionally, several psychiatric measures were employed, including the Structured Clinical Interview for DSM-III-R (SCID) (discussed in Chapter 15), the Psychiatric Evaluation Form (PEF), the Symptom Checklist (SCL-90R), the Impact of Event Scale (IES), and measures of flood stress.

The authors located and interviewed 39% of the original 381 survivors previously studied. About one third of the original subjects had moved out of state and about one third refused to be interviewed (36%) or could not be located (32%).

There was a host of important findings in this study which shed light on the long-term effects of traumatization. First, whether the subjects participated in the lawsuit or not made no difference in the global measures of psychopathology. In comparison to a control group, the Buffalo Creek survivors had more depression and anxiety. Perhaps more important is the finding that 63% of the Buffalo Creek survivors had a *lifetime* disaster-related diagnosis of PTSD as well as a generalized anxiety disorder and major depression. Moreover, in looking at predictors of psychopathology, the stressors of life threat and bereavement were most strongly associated with the mental health outcome measure. In their conclusion, the authors state:

> It is seen as a historical marker for the entire community with events, including births, deaths, marriages, and so forth being classified as "before the flood" or "after the flood." Such daily reminders serve as renewed stressors, with some residents being moved to tears when thinking about the flood again.

As many observers of disaster have noted, there are many dimensions to such horrific events. The speed of onset is one such dimension and is among the central features of the fire disaster at the Kings Cross Underground Railway station in London, England, on November 18, 1987. Thirty-one people were killed in this tragedy, which occurred during the evening rush hour, and hundreds were injured and adversely affected by the fire which began five stories below the ground in the ascending escalators. People became trapped as the escalator was switched off; smoke and fire spread rapidly throughout the complex. It took $2^{1}/_{2}$ hours to contain the fire and restore control over the situation. The Phase-One disaster intervention was well prepared and the victims were treated at the University College Hospital. However, the Phase-Two, long-term care for the victims had to be developed and implemented. In Chapter 37, Stuart W. Turner, James Thompson, and Rachel M. Rosser report on the early psychological reactions and their implications for organizing the long-term treatment of the survivors.

In their chapter, they also present research data on 50 survivors of the fire (22 passengers, 18 emergency medical service personnel, 8 Underground staff members, and 2 others). These subjects were interviewed and administered the General Health Questionnaire (GHQ), the Impact of Events Scale (IES), the Eysenck Personality Questionnaire (EPQ), and a special measure of involvement in the disaster.

The results indicated that 33 of the 50 (65%) had scores on the GHQ indicating psychiatric caseness. The scores on the IES were high and consistent with those known for persons suffering from PTSD. In terms of their role in the fire, those with high subjective ratings of exposure had more psychiatric symptoms.

Based on all their significant findings pointing to powerful posttraumatic stress reactions, the authors go on to discuss the development of Phase-Two response which specifies intervention strategies for each segment: (1) the immediate aftermath, (2) the reactive period, and (3) the formal outreach.

On July 6, 1988, at 10:00 P.M., the world's worst oil rig disaster began at the *Piper Alpha* structure in the North Sea, about 200 kilometers northeast of Aberdeen, Scotland. In Chapter 38, David Alan Alexander chronicles this disaster and the mental health response he supervised throughout the ordeal which killed 164 (72%) of the 226 men on board. All survivors were treated at the Aberdeen Royal Infirmary in Scotland.

Throughout his chapter, Alexander describes the different phases of response to the disaster, both by the survivors themselves and by the victims' families. This review of the Phase-One and Phase-Two responses to the disaster is very important because it illustrates the multifaceted issues that emerge in the course of dealing with the crisis. Included are such topics as (1) the initial plan for intervention and counseling, (2) the "rule" of the psychiatric team (e.g., be low-key, flexible, proactive, and authentic), (3) the accident and emergency department, (4) the burn unit staff problems, (5) the nursing staff difficulties, (6) the temporary morgue, and (7) the survivors' reunion gathering. In his conclusion, Alexander states:

> A major trap seems to be that helpers become pedlars [*sic*] of gloom and miserable statistics about the prevalence of posttraumatic stress symptoms. However awful the circumstances of a disaster, it is imperative that a positive approach be maintained. People do cope with adversity, and even in the worst tragedies one can (and should) find the positive gains. In the case of the *Piper Alpha* oil rig disaster, these included individuals who found themselves to have resources and strengths of which they were unaware, new ways of dealing with difficult technical problems were established, and there were many cases of reaffirmation of important relationships or the development of new ones.

In Chapter 39, Are Holen presents a study of another oil rig disaster in the North Sea. This time, a leg broke off the huge floating residential structure, known as the *Alexander L. Kielland*, at 7:50 P.M. on March 27, 1980, causing the unit to tilt, then gradually capsize into the frigid, turbulent waters below. Of the 212 men on board, 123 (57%) were killed.

In this chapter, Holen reports on the psychiatric effects of the disaster on the 89 survivors. Four studies were conducted: the first in 1980 and the others in 1981, 1984, and 1988. The survivors were compared to a matched control group on a variety of measures which included the DSM-III PTSD criteria, the IES, and measures of cognitive and social functioning.

As expected, the results produced a number of significant findings. About 40% of the sample had reduced cognitive functioning in terms of decision-making ability and the capacity to understand what happened to them. Similarly, about two thirds of the sample experienced dissociative reactions at the time of the event and less so over the next 8 years. Likewise, other stress-response symptoms decreased with time, achieving a stable level within about 1 year. In summarizing the study, Holen states:

> The subjective components tended to be associated with the long-lasting posttraumatic problems, whereas the objective components were more related to problems of a shorter duration, which indicates the relevance of the stressor criterion. However, regarding the prolonged posttraumatic problems, one may speculate that there are correlations with certain personality traits, and that the stressor represents the necessary precipitating event . . . the tendency to dissociate may define a vulnerability factor in the personality with regard to traumatic stress.

In Chapter 40, Janet Johnston reports on a maritime disaster in which the British ferry, the *Herald of Free Enterprise*, capsized in the English Channel after departure from the port of Zeebrugge in Belgium on March 6, 1987. In all, 193 people were killed; 352 others, including the crew, were subjected to a terrifying ordeal as the ferry listed to port and lost electricity. By luck, the ferry sank onto a sandbar or else the scale of the tragedy would have been much greater.

In this chapter, Johnston chronicles the efforts of the social services department of Kent County in England to provide psychological assistance and counseling to the survivors. In a manner similar to that of Alexander in Chapter 38, Johnston describes the different phases of response to the Zeebrugge disaster. She begins with a clear and informative description of the ship's collapse and the various stressors experienced by the passengers and crew on board. Since the ferry's home port was Dover, England, the emergency intervention efforts were located there, and the Kent social service workers had to devise a plan of intervention. Within 1 week, they created a specialist team, set up a telephone hotline, identified who was severely affected, and began formal counseling. Similar to Alexander's team in the *Piper Alpha* disaster, the Kent social workers took a proactive and flexible approach to helping the survivors. However, even with the resourcefulness and dedication of the team of specialists, the work with trauma victims exceeded anything they had ever encountered before. As Johnston states, "though we were prepared . . . for the symptoms of posttraumatic stress disorder, nothing could have prepared us for the sheer intensity of the horror of the survivors' experience." As is expectable in work with PTSD, countertransference reactions were strong among the counselors; steps had to be taken to address the powerful affective reactions in order to maintain effective functioning.

In the long-term, Phase-Two planning, a three-stage process was evident: (1) identification of the client's feelings and PTSD symptoms, (2) validation of the postdisaster reactions, and (3) aiding the recovery process. Through these stages, the counselors were able to develop trust with survivors—a trust and sense of security that were essential to the therapeutic alliance and the working-through of the unresolved traumatic material.

In Chapter 41, by Odaira, Iwadate, and Raphael, and in Chapter 42, by McFarlane and Hua, are presented results of studies of two earthquakes that occurred in Japan and China, respectively. These two chapters present interesting data on how individual and cultural variables moderate posttraumatic reactions.

In Chapter 41, the authors examine reactions to two major tremors that occurred 10 years apart, known respectively as the Miyagi-oki and the Tokachi-oki earthquakes. In the first study, 7,129 individuals in the Miyaki Prefecture were surveyed; 5,474 completed the questionnaire. The sample included primary and secondary school children as well as adults. The major findings indicated acute anxiety reactions and indications of increased autonomic nervous system activity which were not prolonged.

In the second study of the Tokachi-oki earthquake, which measured 7.8 on the Richter scale, 525 individuals responded to a survey questionnaire. These included 217 psychiatric patients, 99 tuberculosis patients, 42 medical patients, and 167 normal adult male and female subjects. The results indicated that bodily sensations (e.g., body swaying, trembling) were nearly uniform among the comparison groups.

Among the nonpsychiatric population, the psychological reactions that were present included feelings of uneasiness, fear, decreased efficiency, sorrow, and worry about the future. An unexpected result was also obtained from the psychiatric population, which exhibited far less agitation during the earthquake and afterward than was anticipated.

In their conclusion, the authors state that "it is clear . . . that there is a substantial reaction to the stress and trauma of earthquakes. The reaction encompasses bodily complaints as well as psychological indications of anxiety and is maximal immediately after the tremors, rapidly declining 1 to 2 weeks later."

In Chapter 42, Alexander Cowell McFarlane and Cao Hua report on the psychological effects of a massive earthquake in the Yunnan Province of Southwestern China which occurred on November 6, 1988. The quake measured 7.6 on the Richter scale and directly affected 81,000 families and 430,144 people within 2,141 square miles. In all, 643 people were killed in the disaster and 3,558 were injured.

To assess the psychiatric sequelae of the quake, three representative villages were chosen for investigation. The subjects were randomly sampled and interviewed by ethnic Chinese. Additionally, they were administered the General Health Questionnaire (GHQ), the Impact of Events Scale (IES), the Eysenck Personality Inventory (EPI), and the PTSD module of the Diagnostic Interview Schedule (DIS). A control group not affected by the earthquake was used for comparison purposes.

The results indicated that nearly 50% of the subjects met the criteria for "caseness" on the GHQ, indicating high levels of distress. However, when asked about the cause of their symptoms, a common attribution made by these poor and uneducated people was that

> the great dragon wanted the earth to turn over because the dragon was unhappy and angry. They also believed that the dragon had people trapped under the earth who he was wanting to let out to replace the people on the earth's surface.

Clearly, this interpretation illustrated well how cultural differences can affect the perception and processing of a disaster and therefore has important implications for intervention and treatment. Finally, the incidence of psychiatric "caseness" found in this study is consistent with that found in other disasters, such as the Australian bushfires and the Kings Cross Underground Railway station fire in London, England. Thus, there is a remarkable constancy to posttraumatic psychological reactivity across different disasters.

Although we tend to think of disasters in terms of such events as tornadoes or earthquakes, it is also true that in the United States and elsewhere tens of thousands of people are killed each year in automobile accidents. In Chapter 43, David J de L Horne examines the posttraumatic consequences of automobile accidents for seven patients who were seriously injured in crashes. Detailed clinical assessments were made for each patient; three fully met the DSM-III-R diagnostic criteria for PTSD, and the other four individuals all developed phobic disorders. Moreover, the persons suffering from PTSD were all likely to have phobic symptoms as well. For each case history presented, Horne discusses six issues that confront the therapist: (1) the nature and source of referral, (2) the initial problems encountered, (3) the assessment and definition of the patient's clinical problem, (4) the formulation of a plan for intervention, (5) the implementation of therapy, and (6) the evaluation of the effectiveness of therapy, termination of treatment, and continuing long-term management. Thus, the structure of the case presentations is quite useful and heuristic because it indicates that different therapeutic interventions may be required to properly treat the patient. For example, whereas systematic desensitization (graded approach) may be quite successful with a phobic reaction to trauma, it is potentially harmful to a person in the intrusion phase of PTSD since the technique of desensitization may actually cause increased affective flooding and psychic overload. In summary, Horne's chapter is important because it is one of the first attempts to understand posttraumatic functioning resulting from such ordinary, yet threatening events as automobile accidents.

In Chapter 44, Carol R. Hartman and Ann W. Burgess present a comprehensive analysis of rape and its psychological consequence to the victim of this violent crime. They begin by noting that in 1988 in the United States there were over 90,000 cases of rape reported although prevalence estimates suggest that the actual number may well approach 200,000. By any standard of determination, rape is a serious societal problem.

In their chapter, Hartman and Burgess begin by reviewing the research literature of the phases of rape trauma which include (1) the pretrauma history, (2) the traumatic event stage, and (3) the posttraumatic stress reactions. Once they have established these phases and the problems faced by the rape victim within each phase, the principles of intervention and treatment are examined. Three major approaches to working with women psychically scarred by rape are explicated: crisis intervention, cognitive-behavioral techniques, and traditional modes of psychotherapy. The authors note that "the three models of treatment support the clinical belief that fearful responses can be modified effectively when the structure of the cognitive defense and emotional arousal is addressed and when resource and skill training is provided." Also included in this densely packed chapter are discussions of differential diagnosis, issues involved in litigation, and the long-term effects of rape trauma.

Part IV concludes with Chapter 45, which examines the psychological impact of acquired immune deficiency syndrome (AIDS), one of the most serious health problems of our time. Brian Kelly and Beverley Raphael first discuss the epidemiology of AIDS and note, for example, that it is a major cause of death among young men and women in New York City.

What are less known at this time are the psychiatric complications for the AIDS victim, since a positive diagnosis of HIV infection is presently tantamount to a death sentence. Clearly, many questions come to mind about those so infected. Do they develop a psychiatric disorder? Do they suffer from a traumatic stress reaction? Do they feel stigmatized and tainted by the presence of the disease? Do their interpersonal relations and sources of social support suffer and deteriorate? How do they cope with the specter of death and possibly those others they might have infected?

To begin an initial empirical inquiry into these questions, Kelly and Raphael gathered together 35 homosexual and bisexual men with HIV infection who were attending outpatient hospitals in Brisbane, Australia, and administered to these patients various testing instruments.

The results indicated that about 50% of the sample met psychiatric caseness on the General Health Questionnaire (GHQ), indicating severe psychiatric morbidity. The Impact of Events Scale (IES) revealed high levels of both intrusive and avoidant symptoms of PTSD. Associated with psychiatric morbidity were feelings of depression, helplessness, fatalism, and anxious preoccupation with the state of their health. In their conclusion, the authors observe that

> fears of death may form an early and persistent component of distress and psychological morbidity. Additionally, such fears and responses to them may have an important role in the motivational factors influencing an individual's health-related behavior. . . . In the setting of such a serious illness, simply defining the levels of depression or anxiety may not sufficiently highlight the specific features of the psychological response to this adversity.

CHAPTER 33

Posttraumatic Stress Disorder in Natural Disasters and Technological Accidents

Elizabeth M. Smith and Carol S. North

Introduction

It is almost impossible to listen to a news broadcast or to pick up a newspaper without learning of yet another catastrophic event. As modern society becomes increasingly technologically based, it can be anticipated that the frequency of disasters will grow, and the types of disasters that occur will change. Disaster events of ages past were primarily natural occurrences, such as floods, volcanic eruptions, and tornadoes. Recent science has provided us with new potential disaster agents, such as nuclear power plants, jumbo jets, and toxic substances. For an excellent historic overview, the reader is directed to a comprehensive discussion in Raphael (1986).

A disaster area is a logical place to study posttraumatic stress disorder (PTSD). There is no shortage of disaster events upon which such studies can be based. Established figures describing the frequency of traumatic events around the world include recent estimates that almost two million households annually experience damages and/or injuries from fire, floods, hurricanes, tornadoes, and earthquakes (Rossi, Wright, Weber-Burdin, *et al.*, 1983). The number of potentially hazardous chemical dumps was recently estimated at 30,000 (Cohn, 1980).

Only carefully designed and implemented systematic data-oriented studies can clarify the nature of PTSD and illuminate the mechanisms by which severe traumatic events evoke such a response. In recent years, several methodologically sound studies have begun to untangle the factors involved and their interactions.

Background to Posttraumatic Stress Disorder

Most of what is known about PTSD derives from research studies on Vietnam veterans. Only recently has PTSD been systematically studied in the context of a disaster setting. The literature of the last decade contains a small collection of data on the frequency of disaster-related PTSD and a larger body of material relating to individual symptoms of PTSD, such as insomnia, nightmares, and recurrence of symptoms with reminders of the disaster event.

The diagnosis of PTSD is a relatively new one on the psychiatric horizon, having made its first official appearance in the third edition of the *Diagnostic and Statistical Manual of Mental Disorders* (DSM-III) (American Psychiatric Association [APA], 1980). Previously, the syndrome of pathological response to catastrophic trauma was delineated as "transient emotional disturbance" in the DSM-II (APA, 1968) and as "gross stress reaction" in the first edition of the DSM (APA, 1952). Given this history, it is clear that not until 1980 could systematic research on PTSD proceed, because prior to that time, the syndrome to be studied had not even been defined.

The DSM-III-R (APA, 1987) refined the DSM-III criteria for PTSD to reorganize the criterion symptoms around three dimensions of the stress experience: (1) reexperiencing the trauma, (2) avoidance and numbing, and (3) physiological arousal.

Symptoms added to PTSD in DSM-III-R that were not present in DSM-III include criteria with additional detail about avoidance responses, amnesia, and a sense

Elizabeth M. Smith and Carol S. North • Department of Psychiatry, Washington University School of Medicine, St. Louis, Missouri 63110.

International Handbook of Traumatic Stress Syndromes, edited by John P. Wilson and Beverley Raphael. Plenum Press, New York, 1993.

of foreshortened future. Survivor guilt was eliminated from PTSD criteria in DSM-III-R. DSM-III-R contains an additional stipulation that the symptoms be present for at least 1 month in order to make the diagnosis. Although PTSD is classified with the anxiety disorders, some argue that it should be reclassified as a dissociative disorder owing to prominent dissociative symptoms contained in the criteria. The ongoing evolution of the definition of PTSD makes comparison of data between systematic studies using nonidentical diagnostic criteria somewhat difficult.

Current criteria for PTSD require that qualifying symptoms must be specifically related to the traumatic event in the mind of the subject reporting it. Solomon and Canino (1989) showed that this requirement might underestimate rates of reported symptoms, because subjects may either fail to associate symptoms, such as depression and anxiety, with the disaster, or they may report these symptoms but deny that the event was upsetting to them.

By definition, there are a wide variety of traumatic events that may evoke symptoms of PTSD. Although such personal traumas as rape, robbery, or assault are also recognized as associated with the occurrence of PTSD, in this chapter we will confine our discussion to PTSD that occurs in the collective stress setting of community disasters.

Literature Review

Typology of Disasters

Community disasters may be classified as accidental or intentional. Discussion in this chapter will be confined to traumatic events that are accidental. Intentional disasters, such as acts of kidnapping, other terrorism, and war are beyond the scope of this chapter and are reviewed in other sections of this book. Accidentally caused disasters may be subdivided into those that are natural, such as tornadoes, earthquakes, and "acts of God," and those that are technological, such as toxic spills and plane crashes.

Unfortunately, the boundaries between the different kinds of disasters within this typology are not always clear, a shortcoming recognized by others in the field (Beigel & Berren, 1985; Lindy, 1985; Quarantelli, 1985). It is not always easy to determine whether a catastrophic event represents a natural disaster or a technological accident. Some disaster events may have both natural and technological attributes simultaneously. For example, when a commercial building collapsed last year in Brownsville, Texas, due to unusually severe torrential rains, it appeared at first glance to represent a natural disaster. It was only later determined that part of the reason for the structural collapse lay with problems in the design of the roof. This discovery imposed elements of a technological nature on this event, making it a disaster of mixed typology.

The initial response to the crash of a commercial aircraft over Lockerbie, Scotland, was to assume a mechanical failure, which would place the event in the technological category. When more evidence was gath-

ered, however, it was determined that this event represented an act of terrorist bombing. Initial responses of the victims to these events might have been colored by their perceptions of the type of disaster agent involved. Other researchers have suggested that different types of disasters evoke different responses (Baum, Fleming, & Davidson, 1983; Beigel & Berren, 1985; Gleser, Green, & Winget, 1981). That disasters frequently contain mixed typological elements makes study of their differential effects even more difficult.

Methodological Considerations

The wide variety of psychological symptoms and emotional responses that have been reported make the comparison of studies of PTSD in disaster victims difficult. These responses have ranged from reports of hostility (Green, Grace, J. D. Lindy, Titchener, & J. G. Lindy, 1983), distrust for authorities (B. P. Dohrenwend, B. S. Dohrenwend, Warheit, et al., 1981), demoralization (Baum, Gatchel, & Schaeffer, 1983; Erikson, 1976), guilt (Boman, 1979; Lifton & Olson, 1976; Titchener & Kapp, 1976), and nightmares (Henderson & Bostock, 1977; Maida, Gordon, Steinberg, & Gordon, 1989; McCammon, Durham, Allison, & Williamson, 1988; Miller, Turner, & Kimball, 1981; Ploeger, 1977; Sloan, 1988) to nonspecific syndromes such as "neurosis" (Boman, 1979; Hoiberg & McCaughy, 1984). It is impossible to relate the finding of "distrust for authorities" in one study to rates of PTSD symptoms in another.

Even when studies examine the same kinds of psychopathology, the diagnostic instrument used in gathering the data will have a crucial bearing on the findings. For example, a diagnosis of depression inferred by Minnesota Multiphasic Personality Inventory (MMPI) results would provide a very different set of data than the same diagnosis achieved by using the Diagnostic Interview Schedule (DIS) (Robins, 1983) with DSM-III criteria. Studies reporting mean scores on a scale do not allow effective comparison with studies presenting rates of specific disorders.

Only with the benefit of the relatively recent formal definition for the syndrome of PTSD has it been possible to develop a structured interview, such as the DIS, and to use this interview to collect diagnostic data systematically. Hartsough (1985) condemned the use of homemade questionnaires and inventories in conducting disaster research and championed those who have exercised the foresight to choose a standardized instrument of measure in designing disaster studies. One problem with using standardized instruments is that their intrinsic specificity and sensitivity may be undesirably low (Bromet & Schulberg, 1988). The use of several instruments or data collection methods, however, may address the disadvantages of structured interviews (Hartsough, 1985).

Psychiatric symptomatology may vary greatly over time, and, thus, the timing of psychiatric assessment may be crucial to the results. This may be particularly true for PTSD, where symptoms may recede rapidly with time, and may or may not reoccur, or may possibly occur in a delayed syndrome months or even years later. For example, Green's group reported a 44% prevalence rate of PTSD as late as 18 to 26 months after the Buffalo Creek dam collapse (Green, Grace, Lindy, et al., 1989). Fourteen years later, Green found the PTSD rate had dropped to 28% (Green, Lindy, Grace, et al., 1989). During that period, however, 11% of victims without PTSD had later gone on to develop a delayed-onset case. Unfortunately, because different methods of assessment were used for the two interviews, we cannot know how much of this drop in rates over time purely represents the effects of the passage of time. The use of a structured interview only at the second assessment would be expected to have yielded lower rates because of the low sensitivity ascribed to structured instruments.

No particular standard for the best time of assessment has been established, and studies vary widely on their timing. This variability further limits our ability to accomplish an adequate cross-study comparison. It is particularly difficult to mount a well-designed, large-scale research strategy to obtain data in the immediate postdisaster period; hence there are few large systematic studies of acute postdisaster mental health. Depending on the focus of the research, the interval between the event and the interview might vary considerably, the acute phase might not be included, or, conversely, several points in time could be used for the interview.

There have been few systematic studies providing assessments of PTSD symptoms at multiple points in time. Two notable exceptions are the previously mentioned study by Green et al. (1989) and the Steinglass and Gerrity (1989) study in which the DIS was administered at two points in time. A study by Bromet's group (Bromet, Parkinson, Schulberg, Dunn, & Gondek, 1982) was noteworthy for using a multiple-point evaluation, though the study preceded the definition of PTSD.

Only rarely has there been an opportunity to obtain pre- and postdisaster data prospectively, and two studies that have managed to attempt this have suffered from relatively low numbers (Canino, 1989; Robins, Fischbach, Smith, Cottler, & Solomon, 1986). Most studies that have examined predisaster information have had to rely upon retrospective reporting, which could present problems with reliability, or upon medical records, which may be marred by incompleteness or may have been destroyed in the disaster.

Undoubtedly, there are many factors that affect a researcher's selection of a specific disaster for study. Among these are availability of cooperative survivors, geographic location, and severity and nature of the event. The act of selecting a particular event to study may in itself have an impact on the findings. For example, it has been said that technological disasters are associated with higher rates of psychopathology than natural disasters (Baum, Fleming, & Davidson, 1983). Subject selection presents additional difficulties. Much of the earlier disaster literature is composed of anecdotal reports based on very small samples, prohibiting data analysis. Fortunately, few disasters seriously affect large enough populations to provide sufficient statistical power for significant findings. This is particularly relevant for examination of specific outcome variables, such as rates of diagnosis of PTSD, because PTSD may affect only a fraction of those exposed to a disaster. Even in disasters affecting large numbers, obtaining a truly random or representative sample is fraught with difficulty.

Survivors may have already scattered (as in a commercial plane crash or in victims relocated after their homes are destroyed); information as to location or identification of persons may have been destroyed in the disaster; and key informants with knowledge of survivors' whereabouts may be very disorganized themselves in the acute postdisaster period. Because of these problems, investigators have had to rely on samples of convenience or on special populations, such as emergency rescue workers, who are more readily accessible.

Efforts to widen the subject base may lead researchers to include subjects who were not as severely affected by the disaster (e.g., subjects who were merely peripheral to the disaster impact, or who were only indirectly or vicariously affected via friends or family members). Bolin (1985) defined victims as either *primary* (directly exposed) or *secondary* (indirectly affected). This variation in exposure level results in further difficulties in comparing responses to different disasters. Other studies have examined emergency workers who may represent another class of victim sample with propensity to react differently to disaster situations. Some studies have combined the different victim groups into one analysis, making it even more difficult to interpret the data (e.g., Wilkinson, 1983).

If identifying a proper group of study subjects is difficult, identifying an appropriate control group is even more difficult. Earlier work in disaster research was anecdotal and descriptive, and controls were typically omitted altogether. The crux of the problem is to identify an appropriate control group which is as similar as possible to the study group in every way except, of course, that they were not exposed. Theoretically, this would be nearly impossible because such a group would best be sampled from another part of the affected community or a nearby location; but in studying a disaster of the magnitude required to achieve high enough numbers for statistical significance, the entire community will generally be affected in one way or another—via friends, neighbors, and the like. Thus, a similar comparison group will generally constitute an indirectly affected population, or, if not, it may be different from the victim group in important ways.

There is often disagreement over what constitutes the best choice of control group. For example, in the Indianapolis hotel jet crash, contenders for a potential comparison group included employees of the hotel who were not at the scene of the crash ("off-site"), employees of a nearby hotel, and employees of another hotel of the same chain in a different area of the city. Use of each group would have its own advantages and disadvantages. The off-site employees of the damaged hotel would be most similar to the victims, but they themselves were indirectly affected to various degrees through loss of colleagues, personal possessions, and their jobs. Melick (1985) reported that even nonvictim control groups may experience stress as a result of the disaster. Employees of other hotels would have limited or no exposure, the degree depending on geographical proximity or belonging to the same hotel chain; on the other hand, they might be less similar to employees of the affected hotel. There is some question as to whether or not a control group would even be necessary for certain purposes. For example, when investigating disorders which have low prevalence rates in the general population, such as PTSD, general population data such as that available from the ECA study can provide general rates for comparison.

Individuals at risk to experience a disaster may have unique characteristics that accompany this risk, such as lower socioeconomic status. It has been demonstrated that the likelihood of an individual's being exposed to a significant life event is related to such individual characteristics as demographic factors, personality, and psychiatric history (Fergusson & Horwood, 1987; Seivewright, 1987; Tennant & Andrews, 1977). Extending this work to the area of disaster research, others have observed that personal characteristics, such as educational achievement, use of alcohol, and history of childhood behavioral problems, predict risk for experiencing a disaster and for the degree of the individual's exposure to it (Helzer, 1981; Helzer, Robins, & McEvoy, 1987; Smith, 1989; Smith, Robins, Przybeck, et al., 1986). The nonaffected comparison group should be selected as carefully as possible to control for socioeconomic level. Because lower socioeconomic groups tend to have higher rates of psychopathology, differences found between two socioeconomically discrepant groups could represent merely a reflection of their socioeconomic level and not the result of the disaster experience in the exposed group. Two researchers (Baum, Gatchel, & Schaeffer, 1983; Bromet, Parkinson, Schulberg, Dun, & Gondek, 1980) have exercised ingenuity in dealing with this problem by choosing control groups living near undamaged nuclear plants to compare with their Three Mile Island study victims. By doing this they were able to document greater psychopathology in the victim group and attribute it more probably to effects of the nuclear accident itself. Similarly, Hoiberg and McCaughey (1984) documented higher rates of neuroses after a maritime collision in the disaster survivors compared to controls from an unrelated ship on a similar mission but without an accident.

Studies of PTSD in Disaster Victims

Table 33.1 summarizes the methodology of all the studies described in the current review. We are aware of 13 studies which have reported rates of PTSD in the context of disaster by using well-established criteria, and these are listed in Table 33.2. Four of these studies used the DIS or the Diagnostic Interview Schedule/Disaster Supplement (DIS/DS) (Robins & Smith, 1983) which makes diagnoses by DSM-III criteria. Most of the other studies used DSM-III criteria.

Table 33.2 demonstrates that studies using the DIS have generally reported lower rates of PTSD than studies using less structured data collection. Compared to natural disasters, disasters of a technological nature were generally associated with higher rates of PTSD. Review of Table 33.2 reveals that those studies of *technological* disasters *not* using structured interviews tend to report the highest rates of PTSD, and the highest rate on this table occurred in the study by Newman and Foreman (1987) which is a study with both of these characteristics. Reports on *natural* disasters using *structured* interviews such as the DIS generally show the lowest

rates. Indeed, the lowest rates on the table are reported in the studies by Shore's group (Shore, tatum, & Vollmer, 1986) and by us (North, Smith, McCool, & Lightcap, 1989), both reporting the same low rate of 2.3%, and both having these characteristics.

A study conducted by one of us (Smith et al., 1986) examined individuals residing in a semirural area near St. Louis that was affected by both floods and toxic contamination from dioxin. The combination of both events occurring in the same area afforded a unique opportunity to examine the differential effects of a natural disaster and a technological accident. Data were collected approximately a year after the disasters by structured interview using the DIS/DS.

Of the exposed population within the area, 173 individuals were directly affected by the disasters, 75 by the flooding only, 29 by dioxin only, and 69 by both flooding and dioxin; 189 unexposed and 139 indirectly exposed subjects served as comparison groups. The flood killed five individuals and left thousands homeless. Most of the dioxin victims were permanently displaced from their homes.

Rates of psychiatric disorders were not high, and PTSD was the only diagnosis that was significant as a new psychiatric problem in the exposed group compared to the unexposed group after the disaster (i.e., in the absence of predisaster psychopathology). The type of disaster experienced (i.e., flood vs. dioxin) did not affect the rates of PTSD, and all exposed groups ranged between 4% and 7% (compared to 0.5% in the nonexposed group). Rates of individual symptoms of PTSD were much higher than rates of diagnoses, however, and these will be discussed below under the section on symptoms. The low rate of diagnosable PTSD in these disaster victims was ascribed in large part to the relative mildness of the disaster agents.

We have studied survivors of two additional disaster events, one a natural occurrence (a tornado) (North *et al.*, 1989) and the other technological (a plane crash into a hotel lobby) (Smith, North, McCool, & Shea, 1989). Both disasters entailed fatalities and serious injuries, and the experience of horror and terror. Identical methodology was used in both studies: Subjects were sampled randomly, they were interviewed with the DIS/DS, and the timing of the interviews was at approximately 1 month after the disasters. Of the 42 tornado victims interviewed (one representative subject of all households in the path of the tornado), only one case of PTSD was diagnosed. Of all interviewed employees of the hotel that suffered the plane crash ($N = 46$), 29% of the 17 directly exposed victims met criteria for PTSD, compared to 17% of the 29 employees who were not in the hotel at the time of the crash.

Because the methodology was exactly the same for these two studies, the large difference in rates of PTSD between the two sites must be due either to the type of the disaster agent or to different predisposing characteristics of the two populations studied, or to some combination of these factors. There was a significantly greater history of preexisting psychiatric disorder in the hotel–plane crash population, the group which also reported the higher postdisaster rate of PTSD. Other factors of potential influence include severity of the disaster agent, the technological element, and the degree of ter-

Table 33.1. Methodology of Studies of PTSD and Disaster

Authors	Year	Event	Location	Subjects	N^a	Controls	Instrument/methods[b]	Timing
Adler	1943	Nightclub fire	Cocoanut Grove, Boston	Hospitalized with injuries	131	No	Observation	First weeks through 11 months
Leopold & Dillon	1963	Marine collision and explosion	Delaware	All crew of one ship	36	No	Observation and anecdotal	11–13 days; follow-up 3½–4½ years
Popovic & Petrovic	1964	Earthquake	Macedonia	Unspecified		No	Observation and anecdotal	22 hours through 5 days
Fairley	1984	Cyclone	Fiji		75	No	GHQ and interview	
Lifton & Olson	1976	Dam break and flood	Buffalo Creek	Litigants	22	No	Interview, anecdotal	1–2 years
Titchener & Kapp	1976	Dam break and flood	Buffalo Creek	Litigants	654	No	Psychoanalytically oriented interviews	2 years
Henderson & Bostock	1977	Shipwreck	Australia	All	7	No	Group interview, individual	5 days; follow-up 12–24 months
Parker	1977	Cyclone Tracy	Darwin, Australia	All evacuees	68	No	GHQ	5–8 days; follow-up 10 weeks and 14 months
Ploeger	1977	Mine explosion	Granville	Miners	10	No	"Clinical observations," anecdotal	10 years
Boman	1979	Train wreck		Not specified		No		Up to 18 months
Perlberg	1979	Jet collision	Canary Islands	All survivors agreeable to participate	8	No	MMPI, TAT, Rorschach, interview	5 months
Wert	1979	Nuclear accident	Three Mile Island	Employees of local business	1,435	No	Postal questionnaire	2 weeks
Ahearn	1981	Earthquake	Managua, Nicaragua	Psychiatric patients	17,160	Yes	Hospital records	
Gleser, Green, & Winget	1981	Dam collapse/flood	Buffalo Creek	Litigants	242	No	Sleep disruption questionnaire	
Miller, Turner, & Kimball	1981	Flood	Big Thompson Canyon, CO	Not specified	162	No	Interview	1 year

(*continued*)

Table 33.1. (*Continued*)

Authors	Year	Event	Location	Subjects	N^a	Controls	Instrument/methods[b]	Timing
V. Patrick & W. R. Patrick	1981	Cyclone '78	Sri Lanka	Household sample	100	Yes	Questionnaire	1 month
Bolin & Klenow	1982–1983	Tornadoes	Texas	Victims seeking disaster assistance (random)	302	No	Questionnaire	2 weeks
Wilkinson	1983	Hyatt-Regency skywalk collapse	Kansas City	Injured (mailing respondents)	102	No	Symptom questionnaire (DSM-III)	≥ 1 week
Weisaeth	1985 1989	Paint factory fire	Norway			Yes		1 week 7 months
P. R. Adams & G. R. Adams	1984	Volcano eruption	Mt. St. Helens	Area population		No	Medical and legal statistics	1–8 months
Lopez-Ibor, Canas, & Rodriguez-Gamazo	1985	Toxic oil poisoning	Spain	Psychiatric referrals	2,926	Not for symptom data	Unified clinical record (?)	Unspecified
McCaughey	1985	Marine collision	Chesapeake Bay	Crew of Navy ship	16	No	Questionnaire	≤ 3 days
McFarlane	1986	Bushfires	South Australia	Victims seeking psychiatric treatment	36	No	Anecdotal (DSM-III criteria)	1–2 years
Shore, Tatum, & Vollmer	1986	Volcano eruption	Mt. St. Helens	Had damaged households	548	Yes	DIS	3–4 years
Smith, Robins, Przybeck, Goldring, & Solomon	1986	Flood, dioxin flood, and dioxin tornadoes	St. Louis area	Random sample	75 29	Yes (ECA)	DIS/DS	1 year
Conyer, Amor, Medina-Mora, Caraveo, & De la Fuente	1987	Earthquake	Mexico City	In shelters	524	No	Interview based on SCID and DIS	1–2 months
Lima, Pai, Santacruz, Lozano, & Luna	1987	Volcano eruption	Armero, Colombia	Shelters and camps	200	No	SRQ	7 months
Newman & Foreman	1987	Plane crash into shopping mall	Sun Valley	Employees, shoppers, rescue workers	50	No	Questionnaire, HIES	6 months 12 months 18 months

Study	Year	Disaster	Location	Sample	N	Control group	Instrument	Time of assessment
McCammon, Durham, Allison, & Williamson	1988	Apartment explosion	North Carolina	Rescue workers, hospital staff	53 26	No	Questionnaire	3 months 3 months
		Tornado		Rescue workers, hospital staff	28 92			5 months 5 months
Sloan	1988	Airplane crash landing	Tennessee	Male basketball team passengers	30	No	Structured interview, checklist (DSM-III)	12 days; follow-up at 1 year
Canino	1989	Torrential rains, mudslides	Puerto Rico	Random sample	321	Nonexposed	DIS/DS	
Green, Grace, Lindy, Gleser, Leonard, & Kramer	1989	Dam break and flood	Buffalo Creek	Litigants	381	Nonlitigants and recruited unexposed	PEF, symptom checklist	18–26 months
Lima, Chavez, Samaniago, Pompei, Pai, Santacruz, & Lozano	1989	Earthquakes	Ecuador	Primary care clinics (random)	120 150	No No	SCID SQR	14 years 3 months
Maida, N. S. Gordon, Steinberg, & G. Gordon	1989	Fires	Baldwin Hills	Mailing respondents	25	No	DIS/DS	2–4 months
North, Smith, McCool, & Lightcap	1989	Tornado	Madison, FL	All affected	42	No	DIS/DS	1 month
Smith	1989	Dioxin, flood	St. Louis, MO area	Random sample	345	Nonaffected area nearby	DIS/DS	3.5–4 years
Smith, North, McCool, & Shea	1989	Plane crash at Ramada Inn	Indianapolis	All employees	17	Yes (employees not at hotel)	DIS/DS	1 month
Steinglass & Gerrity	1989	Tornado Flood	Albion, PA Parsons, WV	Displaced from homes	39 76	No	DIS, HIES	4 months 16 months

aN = number of victims.
bBNDC = Before and Now Disaster Checklist; DIS/DS = Diagnostic Interview Schedule/Disaster Supplement; GHQ = General Health Questionnaire; HIES = Horowitz Impact of Events Scale; HSCL = Hopkins Symptom Checklist; MMPI = Minnesota Multiple Phasic Inventory; PEF = Psychiatric Evaluation Form; SADS-L = Schedule for Affective Disorders and Schizophrenia-Lifetime version; SCID = Structured Clinical Interview for DSM-III; SCL-90 = Symptom Check List of Derogatis; SRQ = Self-Report Questionnaire; TAT = Thematic Apperception Test.

Table 33.2. Rates of PTSD Diagnosis

Authors	Year	Event	Rates of PTSD (%)	Diagnostic criteria (instrument)
Fairley	1984	Cyclone	8	DSM III
McFarlane	1986	Bushfires	53	DSM-III
Shore, Tatum, & Vollmer	1986	Volcano	2.3	DSM-III (DIS)
Smith, Robins, Przybeck, Goldring, & Solomon	1986	Floods and dioxin	4–7	DSM-III (DIS/DS)
Conyer, Amor, Medina-Mora, Caraveo, & De la Fuente	1987	Earthquake	32	DSM-III
Newman & Foreman	1987	Plane crash into shopping mall	50–100	DSM-III
Sloan	1988	Airplane crash landing	54	DSM-III
Canino	1989	Torrential rain and mudslides	3.7	DSM-III (DIS/DS)
Green, Lindy, Grace, Gleser, Leonard, Korol, & Winget	1989	Dam break flood	44 (at 18–26 months) 28 (at 14 years)	DSM-III approximation DSM-III (SCID)
North, Smith, McCool, & Lightcap	1989	Tornado	2.3	DSM-III (DIS/DS)
Smith	1989	Floods and dioxin	4–8	DSM-III (DIS/DS)
Smith, North, McCool, & Shea	1989	Plane crash into hotel	29	DSM-III (DIS/DS)
Steinglass & Gerrity	1989	Tornado	21 (prevalence in 16 months)	DSM-III (DIS)
		Flood	14.5 (at 4 months) 4.5 (incidence at 16 months)	

ror and horror, all of which were strongly present in the hotel–plane crash disaster. Important secondary sequelae, such as bereavement, loss of employment, and disruption of social networks, probably all contributed to overall morbidity in this group. Another confounding variable that appeared operative in the hotel–plane crash event was the lack of a strong cohesive community to lessen the impact of the disaster.

Steinglass and Gerrity (1989) also found very different rates of PTSD symptoms in two disaster sites using the same methodology in both studies. They suggested that interrelationships between victims and the affected communities might account for this difference.

We are aware of several completed studies of PTSD in disaster victims that are as yet unpublished (e.g., Holen, 1987; Stewart & Healy, 1987; Weisaeth, 1984; also J. P. Wilson, personal communication, 1989), and a number of additional studies are published in other chapters of this volume.

Studies of PTSD-Like Syndromes

Prior to the arrival of the current definition of PTSD as we know it today, extreme responses to traumatic events were studied without the benefit of a clear definition. Other investigators termed the syndrome "posttraumatic reaction," "disaster syndrome," "reactive disaster syndrome," "survivor syndrome," "traumatic neurosis," and event-specific names such as the "Buffalo Creek Syndrome." Leivesley (1984) commented on the wide variety of terms used to describe postdisaster reactions in the literature, and the frequent lack of adequate definition of such terms as "emotional parturition" or "psychic numbing" appearing in these reports. Without the benefit of specified criteria, it has not been possible to examine these postdisaster syndromes except anecdotally and without systematic data collection. Reported rates of these PTSD-like syndromes ranged between 11% and 100% (see Table 33.3).

PTSD Symptoms in Disaster Victims

Rates of individual *symptoms* of PTSD reported after disasters are listed on Table 33.4. Frequencies range widely. Percentages of subjects reporting one or more PTSD symptoms, for example, range from 16% to 100%. Rates of individual PTSD symptoms reflect this wide spread as well. For example, insomnia was reported in rates of 0 to 92%. This general disagreement in rates of PTSD symptoms across studies is striking, though not too surprising given the methodological difficulties in this research described earlier in this chapter. Table 33.4 generally shows the same pattern for PTSD symptoms as that seen in Table 33.2 for diagnoses of PTSD, in that rates of symptoms were generally highest in studies using unstructured data collection and in studies of technological events.

It might be expected that symptom profiles would

Table 33.3. PTSD-Equivalent Syndromes

Study	PTSD-equivalent syndrome
Adler, 1943 Cocoanut Grove fire	Posttraumatic neurosis, fear neurosis 54%
Lifton & Olson, 1976 Buffalo Creek dam collapse and flood	Survivor syndrome
Titchener & Kapp, 1976 Buffalo Creek dam collapse and flood	Traumatic neurosis
Parker, 1977 Cyclone Tracy	Disaster syndrome 100%
Boman, 1979 Granville train wreck	Postdisaster syndrome
Perlberg, 1979 Tenerife jet crash	Traumatic neurosis
Ahearn, 1981 Nicaragua earthquake	Neurotic symptoms, postdisaster stress
Gleser, Green, & Winget, 1981 Buffalo Creek dam collapse and flood	Buffalo Creek syndrome
V. Patrick & W. R. Patrick, 1981 Sri Lanka cyclone	Disaster syndrome 23%
Weisæth, 1985, 1989 Norway paint factory fire	Traumatic anxiety syndrome
P. R. Adams & G. R. Adams, 1984 Mt. St. Helens volcano eruption	Postdisaster stress reaction
Lopez-Ibor, Canas, & Rodriguez-Gamazo, 1985 Toxic oil poisoning	Reactive psychological disaster syndrome

differ following various types of disasters. From Table 33.4, however, there does not appear to be any particular pattern of symptoms occurring more frequently in specific kinds of disaster events. Toxic disasters with no tangible sensory experience might be expected to produce different symptomatology than plane crashes with strong and horrible sensory experiences. The visual experience of gruesome occurrences could be expected to recur in the form of intrusive visual memories or flashbacks. It is perhaps these gruesome sensory experiences that are the essence of the phenomena of terror and horror frequently described in the literature. Several investigators (Bolin, 1985; Erikson, 1976; Lifton & Olson, 1976; Taylor & Frazer, 1982) have suggested that the elements of terror and horror contribute to a disaster's severity (and therefore its impact). In this way, severe sensory experiences could play a part in evoking symptomatology.

Wilkinson's study of the Hyatt Regency skywalk collapse (Wilkinson, 1983) had the highest symptom rates of practically any study on Table 33.4. This was a disaster with extremely gruesome sensory experiences described as "bodies literally exploding," amputated

limbs strewn around, a man's stomach protruding through his mouth, a body cut neatly in half just below the thorax, people crushed beyond recognition, and victims pinned under piles of steel with water and blood flowing all around and creating "a penetrating odor that seemed to last forever." Such experiences are the basis for the "death imprint" described by Lifton and Olson (1976), and the material of flashbacks.

In comparison, the plane crash into a hotel which we studied (Smith *et al.*, 1989) was also marked by extreme terror and horror of all the senses: visual (seeing individuals wrapped in flames), auditory (hearing the screams of co-workers as they perished in the fire), tactile (intense heat), and olfactory (the smell of jet fuel mixed with smoke). This study also revealed very high rates of symptoms, and individuals specifically reported intrusive memories and nightmares of plane crashes as well as feelings of fear and panic whenever airplanes flew near. Despite the differences in methodology between these two studies, the fact that they both had high rates of symptoms might suggest that symptomatology could be linked to the elements of terror and horror.

In contrast, a tornado we studied (North *et al.*, 1989) was associated with considerably less terror and horror partly because it struck so quickly and without much warning, and it was over before most people knew what was happening. There were also fewer injuries and fatalities associated with the tornado than with the hotel plane crash. Although the tornado victims reported a recurrence of symptoms with threatening weather or strong winds, symptom rates were much lower after the tornado compared to the hotel plane crash. Again, a possible explanation for the dissimilar symptom rates in these two studies using identical methodology might be that the more extreme terror and horror in the plane crash may have evoked more symptoms.

Studies of toxic events, such as radiation and chemical spills, might be expected to evoke fewer PTSD symptoms. These "invisible" events lack the sensory components classically associated with PTSD symptoms, such as vivid memories and nightmares. It is likely that other kinds of symptoms such as somatoform symptoms might occur with toxic events. For example, in the study by Smith's group (1986), when dioxin-exposed individuals learned of the event years later, many of them attributed ordinary health problems to the exposure, and others developed many of the symptoms that were reported by the press as being associated with this chemical in its most concentrated form in studies of laboratory animals.

The complexity of disaster events and the differences in the involved populations, coupled with widely varying methodology, have been shown to contribute to the lack of precision which is reflected in broadly ranging symptom rates seemingly without an identifiable pattern as found in Table 33.4. For further discussion of methodologic issues, the reader is referred to Chapter 8 in this volume.

PTSD Risk Factors

In addition to the elements of terror and horror, a number of variables have been described in association

Table 33.4. Rates of PTSD Symptoms

Study and year	a	b	c	d	e	f	g	h	i	j	k	l	m	n	o	p	q
Adler, 1943		19															
Leopold & Dillon, 1963										77.7							
Popovic & Petrovic, 1964		23															
Henderson & Bostock, 1977		29								43	29	14			14		57
Ploeger, 1977		90									90						
Wert, 1979												55.8					
Gleser, Green, & Winget, 1981		70.7								92.1							
Miller, Turner, & Kimball, 1981																	
Parents		22								32		24			17	27	
Elderly										37		37			<10		
Bolin & Klenow, 1982–1983		30.5					13										
Wilkinson, 1983	88.2	52.0		37.2	40.2	88	34.3	29.4	36.3	50.0	35.3	44.1		45.1	44.1	27.4	
Lopez-Ibor, Canas, & Rodriguez-Gamazo, 1985						3			5	57		20				22	
McCaughey, 1985		18.8								12.5	37.5	37.5					
Smith, Robins, Przybeck, Goldring, & Solomon, 1986																	
Flood		1.5[a]	6.7	4.8	6.7		4.8[b]			12.5		10.6[c]	6.7		1.9		29.8
Dioxin		3.1[a]	1.0	4.1	2.0		5.1[b]			6.1		4.1[c]	1.0		0		28.9
Tornado		0[a]	0	4.8	0		0[b]			4.8		0[c]	0		0		4.8
Radioactive water		0[a]	0	0	0		0[b]			0		0[c]	0		0		0
Lima, Pai, Santacruz, Lozano, & Luna, 1989					36	35	27[b]			42							
Conyer, Amor, Medina-Mora, Caravao, & De la Fuente, 1987	53	33[a]	60					28	19	32		20[c]	51		31		

Study	a	b	c	d	e	f	g	h	i	j	k	q
Newman & Foreman, 1987												
Shoppers	74	6	6	0	4	0	2	2	2	8	0	59
Employees	67	32	11	4	7	4	4	4	4	15	11	18
Rescue workers	46	0	8	4	4	0	0	0	0	0	0	13–23
McCammon, Durham, Allison, & Williamson, 1988	85	23	30	4	6	4	9		10	15	0	71
Sloan, 1988	74	50	54	68	79	82						100 (12 days); 41 (1 year)
Lima, Chavez, Samaniago, Pompei, Pai, Santacruz, & Lozano, 1989	16.7											43.3
Maida, N. S. Gordon, Steinberg, & G. Gordon, 1989	33[a]	25	44	11	67	56	0					12
North, Smith, McCool, & Lightcap, 1989	17[a]	10	21	10	2[b]	31	29	29	7	38		12
Smith, 1989												
Flood — Parents	8.4[a]	2.6	8.9	10.5	6.8[b]	17.3	13.1[c]	6.3	0.5			23.0
Flood — Adult children	11.8[a]	0	7.8	13.7	7.8[b]	15.7	13.7[c]	3.9	2.0			16.3
Dioxin — Parents	3.6[a]	1.4	7.9	7.9	7.2[b]	10.1	8.6[c]	2.9	0.7			25.9
Dioxin — Adult children	2.6[a]	0	2.6	2.6	2.6[b]	5.3	5.3[c]	2.6	0			18.9
Smith, North, McCool, & Shea, 1989	94[a]	59	71	65	29	88	59	82	41			100
Steinglass & Gerrity, 1989												
Flood (4 months)	45[a]	24	20	22[b]	63	42[c]	24					3
(16 months)	15[a]	3	11	17[b]	12	11[c]	6					2

Key: a = intrusive recollection, b = dreams, c = recurring, d = reminder distress, e = avoid reminders/activities, f = amnesia, g = loss of interest, h = detachment/estrangement, i = constricted affect/numb, j = insomnia, k = irritable/anger, l = impaired concentration, m = jumpy, n = physiologic reactivity at reminder, o = survivor guilt, p = memory problem, q = *any* PTSD symptom.
[a] Combined nightmares/intrusive recollections as elicited by DIS.
[b] Combined nightmares/intrusive recollections per DIS.
[c] Combined impaired concentration/memory disturbance per DIS.

with PTSD. A study of an apartment explosion and a tornado by McCammon's group (1988) and of an earthquake by Lima et al. (1989) both reported a response effect related to the magnitude of the disaster agent. Several groups (Fairley, 1984; Maida et al., 1989; Miller et al., 1981; Shore et al., 1986; Wilkinson, 1983) have reported that psychiatric morbidity increases with increasing exposure or proximity of the individuals to the disaster agent. McFarlane and Frost (1984), however, did not find that intensity of exposure was predictive of PTSD in firefighters. A related factor, personal injury, was associated with psychiatric problems after a cyclone (Parker, 1977) and after a volcano and an earthquake (Lima, Pai, Santacruz, Lozano, & Luna, 1987; Lima et al., 1989) but not after a nightclub fire (Adler, 1943).

Parker (1977) found the element of terror (i.e., perceived threat of personal injury or death) to have a strong effect, and Lima's group (1987) noted the contribution of the experience of horror (i.e., experiencing grotesque or mutilating events). Bereavement was felt to be an important modifier of the disaster response by Gleser et al. (1981), McFarlane (1986), Newman and Foreman (1987), and Shore et al. (1986), whereas Adler (1943) did not observe any ill effect from bereavement. Social support was found to be an important ameliorating factor by Newman and Foreman (1987), Fleming, Baum, Gisriel, and Gatchel (1982), Bromet's group (1982), and Madakasira and O'Brien (1987).

Subjects sustaining the greatest property damage or who lost their homes were noted to have a poorer outcome than those without these problems in studies by McFarlane (1986), Parker (1977), and Lima et al. (1989), but the study by Madakasira and O'Brien (1987) did not support this. Maida's group (1989) found that loss of personal property and homes was associated with symptoms of depression but not with PTSD. Individuals who evacuated their homes reported more distress than those who remained in two studies (Gleser et al., 1981; Miller et al., 1981). Part of the psychopathology in technological disasters may be related to the presence of a party that is held responsible for the event and therefore potentially a subject of litigation. On the other hand, you can't sue God.

Certain individual characteristics have been associated with psychiatric symptoms, particularly the female gender (Fairley, 1984; Gleser et al., 1981; Kasl, Chisholm, & Eskenazi, 1981; Lopez-Ibor, Canas, & Rodriguez-Gamazo, 1985; Moore & Friedsam, 1959; Parker, 1977; Shore et al., 1986; Steinglass & Gerrity, 1989; Weisæth, 1984; but not Madakasira & O'Brien, 1987). Lower socioeconomic level or lesser educational attainment was associated with greater symptom rates in studies by Gleser's group (1981) and Lopez-Ibor's group (1985), but not in the studies by Miller and co-workers (1981) and Madakasira and O'Brien (1987). Being currently married was a predictor of distress in the Lopez-Ibor study, but Lima's group (1989) found that being single was a risk factor. Madakasira and O'Brien (1987) found no relationship of marital status and PTSD. Gleser's group (1981) reported that adult victims were more psychologically affected than children, and the preponderance of studies indicates that older and elderly subjects are at highest risk (Leopold & Dillon, 1963; Lima et al., 1987; Lopez-Ibor et al., 1985; Parker, 1977; Shore et al., 1986; Wilkin-

son, 1983). Madakasira and O'Brien (1987) found no relationship between age and PTSD. Caucasians were more at risk than nonwhites in one study (Gleser et al., 1981).

An important variable which has been identified as a predictor of postdisaster psychopathology is preexisting psychiatric morbidity (Bromet et al., 1982; Lopez-Ibor et al., 1985; McFarlane, 1986; Weisæth, 1985), although this point has been argued conversely (Madakasira & O'Brien, 1987; Parker, 1977; Wilkinson, 1983). Weisæth (1985) found higher rates of PTSD in disaster victims with a history of prior adaptational problems, high psychosomatic reactivity, and character pathology. Family history of psychiatric problems was also found to be more prevalent in those with PTSD than in those without this disorder (McFarlane, 1985). Weisæth (1985) found that the best predictor of long-term psychopathology (at 4-year follow-up) was the intensity of acute PTSD.

It is worthwhile to note that though we are confining our discussion to PTSD, this disorder does occur within a broader context of psychopathology. For example, Helzer's group (1987) found that in a general population sample, subjects meeting criteria for PTSD had twice as much risk for another lifetime psychiatric diagnosis as did individuals who had never experienced PTSD. The greatest increase in risk was for obsessive-compulsive disorder, dysthymia, and manic-depressive disorder. In victims of the hotel plane crash, PTSD occurred in conjunction with either depression or generalized anxiety disorder four times more frequently than it did alone (Smith et al., 1989). Smith and co-workers (1986) found that 89.4% of their sample with PTSD also met criteria for another lifetime psychiatric diagnosis. A study of Vietnam veterans with PTSD revealed that 84% had coexisting psychiatric conditions, especially alcoholism, antisocial personality, drug abuse, depression, and anxiety (Sierles, Chen, Messing, Besyner, & Taylor, 1986). Subjects for that study, however, were selected from stress disorder treatment groups, and could be expected to have high rates of comorbidity. In Mt. St. Helens survivors, Shore's group (1986) found that of eleven subjects with PTSD, only two met PTSD criteria in the absence of major depression or generalized anxiety disorder.

This comorbidity may have implications for future conceptualization of the PTSD syndrome. Indeed, there is considerable overlap between criterion symptoms of PTSD with major depression (e.g., sleep disturbance), anxiety disorder (e.g., hyperalertness), and dissociative disorder (e.g., numbing or detachment). Madakasira and O'Brien (1987) found significant associations between severity of PTSD and indicators of depression and somatization. Green, Lindy, and Grace (1985) and Solomon and Canino (1989) have questioned the usefulness of PTSD as a diagnostic entity as it now stands. Green suggests examining the relationship of PTSD to character pathology in trying to clarify this issue.

Discussion

This chapter has attempted to review all available studies of PTSD and related symptoms following disaster events. Some of the limitations in completing this review were that PTSD is only a recent diagnostic entity that is still evolving, that there was little uniformity in methodology across studies, and that each disaster event and each affected community have unique characteristics.

It is important to study PTSD in populations other than in Vietnam veterans, where most of the work on PTSD has been accomplished, and other than in settings of personal trauma, such as rape and assault. Just as natural and technological events are thought to induce differential responses, these events would also be expected to have different symptomatology associated with them than with war or rape.

It was found that rates of diagnosable disorders are generally low after disasters. Symptoms, however, are plentiful. That symptoms abound but do not cluster into diagnosable syndromes within the current system of psychiatric classification might suggest that symptoms may actually cluster into some as yet undefined grouping. Table 33.4 was an attempt to examine postdisaster symptoms for obvious patterns, but due to the limitations described above no such clusters emerged. The only suggestion of any tendency was that rates of PTSD symptoms reported seem higher in studies of technological disaster and those utilizing unstructured data collection.

In order to learn more about PTSD and disaster response, future studies must be done in a systematic manner with reliable instruments using valid criteria which will be expected to evolve as this work progresses. Ideally, bodies of systematic data collected from a variety of disasters with the same methodology should be merged to yield a large mass of data with a variety of characteristics. This will allow sophisticated analysis of data to untangle the numerous variables characterizing disaster agents, populations, and communities affected. It will also point to significant risk factors to help identify those in greatest need of services.

Although there is no way to prevent disasters from occurring, there is much that can be done to assist survivors by identification of their risk for postdisaster symptomatology and describing their process of recovery. This will allow the limited resources available in postdisaster periods to be focused on specific individuals at risk. Future funding for research is needed for studies that can translate the research findings into intervention measures. As the future sees increasing rates of technological disasters, this knowledge will become increasingly important. As new and different types of disasters continue to evolve, research must continue to keep up with understanding of the unique kinds of responses that these different events may be expected to evoke.

References

Adams, P. R., & Adams, G. R. (1984). Mount St. Helens's ashfall: Evidence for a disaster stress reaction. *American Psychologist, 39*(3), 252–260.

Adler, A. (1943). Neuropsychiatric complications in victims of Boston's Cocoanut Grove disaster. *Journal of the American Medical Association, 123*, 1098–1101.

Ahearn, F. L., Jr. (1981). Disaster mental health: A pre- and post-earthquake comparison of psychiatric admission rates. *Urban and Social Change Review, 14*(2), 22–28.

American Psychiatric Association. (1952). *Diagnostic and statistical manual of mental disorders.* Washington, DC: Author.

American Psychiatric Association. (1968). *Diagnostic and statistical manual of mental disorders* (2nd ed.). Washington, DC: Author.

American Psychiatric Association. (1980). *Diagnostic and statistical manual of mental disorders* (3rd ed.). Washington, DC: Author.

American Psychiatric Association. (1987). *Diagnostic and statistical manual of mental disorders* (3rd ed., rev.). Washington, DC: Author.

Baum, A., Fleming, R., & Davidson, L. M. (1983). Natural disaster and technological catastrophe. *Environment and Behavior, 15*, 333–354.

Baum, A., Gatchel, R. J., & Schaeffer, M. A. (1983). Emotional, behavioral, and physiological effects of chronic stress at Three Mile Island. *Journal of Consulting and Clinical Psychology, 51*, 565–572.

Beigel, A., & Berren, M. (1985). Human-induced disasters. *Psychiatric Annals, 15*(3), 143–150.

Bolin, R. (1985). Disaster characteristics and psychosocial impacts. In B. J. Sowder (Ed.), *Disasters and mental health: Selected contemporary perspectives* (pp. 3–28). Rockville, MD: National Institute of Mental Health.

Bolin, R., & Klenow, D. (1982–1983). Response of the elderly to disaster: An age-stratified analysis. *International Journal of Aging and Human Development, 16*(4), 283–296.

Boman, B. (1979). Behavioural observations on the Granville train disaster and the significance of stress for psychiatry. *Social Science and Medicine, 13*, 463–471.

Bromet, E. J., Parkinson, D. K., Schulberg, H. C., Dunn, L., & Gondek, P. C. (1980). *Three Mile Island: Mental health findings.* NIMH Contract No. 278–79–0048 (SM). Final report. Rockville, MD: National Institute of Health.

Bromet, E. J., Parkinson, D. K., Schulberg, H. C., Dunn, L. O., & Gondek, P. C. (1982). Mental health of residents near the Three Mile Island reactor: A comparative study of selected groups. *Journal of Preventive Psychiatry, 1*, 225–276.

Bromet, E. J., & Schulberg, H.C. (1988). Epidemiologic findings from disaster research. In R. E. Hales & A. J. Frances (Eds.), *Psychiatric Update: American Psychiatric Association Annual Review* (Vol. 7). Washington, DC: American Psychiatric Press.

Canino, G. (1989). *Psychiatric reactions to disaster stress: A retrospective and prospective description.* Paper presented at the World Psychiatric Association, Section of Epidemiology and Community Psychiatry, Toronto, Canada.

Cohn, V. (1980, June 7). Waste sites may invade water supply, subcommittee told. *The Washington Post,* p. A2.

Conyer, R. C. T., Amor, J. S., Medina-Mora, E. M., Caraveo, J., & De la Fuente, J. R. (1987). Prevalence of post-traumatic stress syndrome in survivors of a natural disaster. *Salud Público de Mexico, 29*(5), 406–411.

Dohrenwend, B. P., Dohrenwend, B. S., Warheit, G. J., Bartlett, G. S., Goldsteen, R. L., Goldsteen, K., & Martin, J. L. (1981). Stress in the community: A report to the President's Commission on the Accident at Three Mile Island. *Annals of the New York Academy of Sciences, 365*, 159–174.

Erikson, K. T. (1976). Loss of community at Buffalo Creek. *American Journal of Psychiatry, 133*, 302–305.

Fairley, M. (1984). *Tropical cyclone Oscar: Psychological reactions of a*

Fijian population. Paper presented at the Disaster Research workshop, Mt. Macedon, Victoria, Australia.

Fergusson, D. M., & Horwood, L. J. (1987). Vulnerability to life events exposure. *Psychological Medicine, 17,* 739–749.

Fleming, R., Baum, A., Gisriel, M. M., & Gatchel, R. J. (1982, September). Mediating influences of social support on stress at Three Mile Island. *Journal of Human Stress,* 14–22.

Gleser, G. C., Green, B. L., & Winget, C. N. (1981). *Prolonged psychosocial effects of disaster: A study of Buffalo Creek.* New York: Academic Press.

Green, B. L., Grace, M. C., Lindy, J. D., Gleser, G. C., Leonard, A. C., & Kramer, T. L. (1989). *Buffalo Creek survivors in the second decade: Comparison with unexposed and non-litigant groups.* Unpublished manuscript.

Green, B. L., Grace, M. C., Lindy, J. D., Titchener, J. L., & Lindy, J. G. (1983). Levels of functional impairment following a civilian disaster: The Beverly Hills Supper Club fire. *Journal of Consulting and Clinical Psychology, 50,* 573–580.

Green B. L., Lindy, J. D., & Grace, M. C. (1985). Posttraumatic stress disorder: Toward DSM-IV. *Journal of Mental Diseases, 173,* 406–411.

Green, B. L., Lindy, J. D., Grace, M. C., Gleser, G. C., Leonard, A. C., Korol, M., & Winget, C. (1989). *Buffalo Creek survivors in the second decade: Stability and change of stress symptoms over 14 years.* Unpublished manuscript.

Hartsough, D. M. (1985). Measurement of the psychological effects of disaster. In J. Laube & S. Murphy (Eds.), *Perspectives on disaster recovery* (pp. 22–60). Norwalk, CT: Appleton-Century-Crofts.

Helzer, J. E. (1981). Methodological issues in the interpretation of the consequences of extreme situations. In B. S. Dohrenwend & B. P. Dohrenwend (Eds.), *Stressful life events and their contexts: Monographs in Psychosocial Epidemiology 2* (pp. 108–129). New York: Neale Watson Academic Publications.

Helzer, J. E., Robins, L. N., & McEvoy, L. (1987). Posttraumatic stress disorder in the general population: Findings of the Epidemiologic Catchment Area Survey. *New England Journal of Medicine, 317*(26), 1630–1634.

Henderson, S., & Bostock, T. (1977). Coping behavior after shipwreck. *British Journal of Psychiatry, 131,* 15–20.

Hoiberg, A., & McCaughey, B. G. (1984). The traumatic aftereffects of collision at sea. *American Journal of Psychiatry, 141,* 70–73.

Holen, A. (1987). "Health and pain in survivors of an oil rig disaster." Presentation to the Society for Traumatic Stress Studies, Baltimore, MD, October.

Kasl, S. V., Chisholm, R. E., & Eskenazi, B. (1981). The impact of the accident at Three Mile Island on the behavior and well-being of nuclear workers. *American Journal of Public Health, 71,* 472–495.

Leivesley, S. (1984). Psychological response to disaster. In J. Seaman, S. Leivesley, & C. Hogg (Eds.), *Epidemiology of natural disasters: Contributions to epidemiology and biostatistics* (Vol. 5). Farmington, CT: S. Karger.

Leopold, R. L., & Dillon, H. (1963). Psychoanatomy of a disaster: A long-term study of posttraumatic neuroses in survivors of a marine explosion. *American Journal of Psychiatry, 119,* 913–921.

Lifton, R. J., & Olson, E. (1976). The human meaning of total disaster: The Buffalo Creek experience. *Psychiatry, 39,* 1–18.

Lima, B. R., Pai, S., Santacruz, H., Lozano, J., & Luna, J. (1987). Screening for the psychological consequences of a major disaster in a developing country: Armero, Colombia. *Acta Psychiatrica Scandinavica, 76,* 561–567.

Lima, B. R., Chavez, H., Samaniego, N., Pompei, M. S., Pai, S., Santacruz, H., & Lozano, J. (1989). Disaster severity and emotional disturbance: Implications for primary mental health care in developing countries. *Acta Psychiatrica Scandinavica, 79,* 74–82.

Lindy, J. D. (1985). The trauma membrane and other clinical concepts derived from psychotherapeutic work with survivors of natural disasters. *Psychiatric Annals, 15*(3), 153–160.

Lopez-Ibor, J. J., Jr., Canas, S. F., & Rodriguez-Gamazo, M. (1985). Psychological aspects of the toxic oil syndrome catastrophe. *British Journal of Psychiatry, 147,* 352–365.

Madakasira, S., & O'Brien, K. F. (1987). Acute posttraumatic stress disorder in victims of a natural disaster. *Journal of Nervous and Mental Disease, 175*(5), 286–290.

Maida, C. A., Gordon, N. S., Steinberg, A., & Gordon, G. (1989). Psychosocial impact of disasters: Victims of the Baldwin Hills Fire. *Journal of Traumatic Stress, 2*(1), 37–48.

McCammon, S., Durham, T. W., Allison, E. J., & Williamson, J. E. (1988). Emergency workers' cognitive appraisal and coping with traumatic events. *Journal of Traumatic Stress, 1*(3), 353–372.

McCaughey, B. G. (1985, Spring). U.S. Coast Guard collision at sea. *Journal of Human Stress,* 42–46.

McFarlane, A. C. (1985). *The etiology of posttraumatic stress disorders following a natural disaster.* Unpublished manuscript, Department of Psychiatry, Flinders University of South Australia.

McFarlane, A. C. (1986). Posttraumatic morbidity of a disaster: A study of cases presenting for psychiatric treatment. *Journal of Nervous and Mental Disease, 174*(1), 4–13.

McFarlane, A. C., & Frost, M. E. (1984). *Posttraumatic stress disorder in firefighters: Ash Wednesday.* Unpublished manuscript, Department of Psychiatry, Flinders University of South Australia.

Melick, M. E. (1985). The health of postdisaster populations: A review of literature and case study. In J. Laube & S. Murphy (Eds.), *Perspectives on disaster recovery* (pp. 179–209). Norwalk, CT: Appleton-Century-Crofts.

Miller, J. A., Turner, J. G., & Kimball, E. (1981). Big Thompson Flood victims: One year later. *Family Relations, 30,* 111–116.

Moore, H. E., & Friedsam, H. J. (1959). Reported emotional stress following a disaster. *Social Forces, 38,* 135–138.

Newman, J. P., & Foreman, C. (1987). "The Sun Valley Mall Disaster study." Presentation to Society for Traumatic Stress Studies, Baltimore, MD, October.

North, C. S., Smith, E. M., McCool, R. E., & Lightcap, P. E. (1989). Acute post-disaster coping and adjustment. *Journal of Traumatic Stress, 2*(3), 353–360.

Parker, G. (1977). Cyclone Tracy and Darwin evacuees: On the restoration of the species. *British Journal of Psychiatry, 130,* 548–555.

Patrick, V., & Patrick, W. R. (1981). Cyclone '78 in Sri Lanka—The mental health trail. *British Journal of Psychiatry, 138,* 210–216.

Perlberg, M. (1979, April). Trauma at Tenerife: The psychic aftershocks of a jet disaster. *Human Behavior,* 49–50.

Ploeger, A. (1977). A ten-year follow-up of miners trapped for two weeks under threatening circumstances. In C. D. Spielberger & I. G. Sarason (Eds.), *Stress and anxiety* (pp. 23–28). New York: Wiley.

Popovic, M., & Petrovic, D. (1964, November 28). After the earthquake. *Lancet, 2,* 1169–1171.

Quarantelli, E. L. (1985). What is disaster? The need for clarification in definition and conceptualization in research.

In B. J. Sowder (Ed.), *Disasters and mental health: Selected contemporary perspectives* (pp. 41–73) (DHHS Publication No. ADM 85–1421). Rockville, MD: National Institute of Mental Health.

Raphael, B. (1986). *When disaster strikes*. New York: Basic Books.

Robins, L. N. (1983). The development and characteristics of the NIMH Diagnostic Interview Schedule. In M. M. Weissman, T. M. Myers, & C. C. Ross (Eds.), *Epidemiologic community surveys*. New Brunswick, NJ: Rutgers University Press.

Robins, L. N., Fischbach, R. L., Smith, E. M., Cottler, L. B., & Solomon, S. D. (1986). The impact of disaster on previously assessed mental health. In J. H. Shore (Ed.), *Disaster stress studies: New methods and findings* (pp. 22–48). Washington, DC: American Psychiatric Press.

Robins, L. N., & Smith, E. (1983). *The Diagnostic Interview Schedule/Disaster Supplement*. St. Louis: Department of Psychiatry, Washington University School of Medicine.

Rossi, P. H., Wright, J. D., Weber-Burdin, E., & Pereira, J. (1983). Victimization by natural hazards in the United States, 1970–1980: Survey estimates. *International Journal of Mass Emergencies and Disasters*, 1(3), 467–482.

Seivewright, N. (1987). Relationship between life events and personality in psychiatric disorder. *Stress Medicine*, 3, 163–168.

Shore, J. H., Tatum, E. L., & Vollmer, W. M. (1986). The Mount St. Helens stress response syndrome. In J. H. Shore (Ed.), *Disaster stress studies: New methods and findings* (pp. 7–97). Washington, DC: American Psychiatric Press.

Sierles, F. S., Chen, J. J., Messing, M. L., Besyner, J. K., & Taylor, M. A. (1986). Concurrent psychiatric illness in non-Hispanic outpatients diagnosed as having posttraumatic stress disorder. *Journal of Nervous Mental Disease*, 174(3), 171–173.

Sloan, P. (1988). Posttraumatic stress in survivors of an airplane crash-landing: A clinical and exploratory research intervention. *Journal of Traumatic Stress*, 1(2), 211–229.

Smith, E. M. (1989). *Impact of disaster on children: Dioxin and flood* (Final Report, MH40025). Washington, DC: Department of Health and Human Services. Unpublished manuscript.

Smith, E. M., North, C. S., McCool, R. E., & Shea, J. M. (1989). Acute post-disaster psychiatric disorders: Identification of those at risk. *American Journal of Psychiatry*, 147(2), 202–206.

Smith, E. M., North, C. S., & Price, P. C. (1988). Response to technological accidents. In M. Lystad (Ed.), *Mental health response to mass emergencies: Theory and practice* (pp. 52–95). New York: Brunner/Mazel.

Smith, E. M., Robins, L. N., Przybeck, T. R., Goldring, E., & Solomon, S. D. (1986). Psychosocial consequences of a disaster. In J. H. Shore (Ed.), *Disaster stress studies: New methods and findings* (pp. 50–76). Washington, DC: American Psychiatric Press.

Solomon, S., & Canino, G. (1989). *Appropriateness of DSM-III-R criteria for posttraumatic stress disorder*. Unpublished manuscript.

Steinglass, P., & Gerrity, E. (1989). Natural disasters and posttraumatic stress disorder: Short-term vs. long-term recovery in two disaster-affected communities. *Journal of Applied Social Psychology*, 20, 1746–1765.

Stewart, A., & Healy, J. (1987). Presentation at the Annual Meeting of the Society for Traumatic Stress Studies, Baltimore, MD.

Taylor, A. J. W., & Frazer, A. G. (1982). The stress of post-disaster body handling and identification work. *Journal of Human Stress*, 8, 4–12.

Tennant, C., & Andrews, G. (1977). A scale to measure the cause of life events. *Australia and New Zealand Journal of Psychiatry*, 11, 163–167.

Titchener, J. L., & Kapp, F. T. (1976). Family and character change at Buffalo Creek. *American Journal of Psychiatry*, 138, 14–19.

Weisæth, L. (1985). Posttraumatic stress disorder after an industrial disaster. In P. Pichot, P. Berner, R. Wolf, & K. Thau (Eds.), *Psychiatry—The state of the art* (Vol. 6, pp. 299–307). New York: Plenum Press.

Weisæth, L. (1989). The stressors and the posttraumatic stress syndrome after an industrial disaster. *Acta Psychiatrica Scandinavica*, 80(Suppl. 355), 25–37.

Wert, B. J. (1979). Stress due to nuclear accident: A survey of an employee population. *Occupational Health Nursing*, 27(9), 16–24.

Wilkinson, C. B. (1983). Aftermath of a disaster: The collapse of the Hyatt Regency hotel skywalks. *American Journal of Psychiatry*, 140, 1134–1139.

CHAPTER 34

PTSD: Synthesis of Research and Clinical Studies

The Australia Bushfire Disaster

Alexander Cowell McFarlane

Introduction

The incorporation of posttraumatic stress disorder (PTSD) in the DSM-III (American Psychiatric Association, 1980) has acted as a major catalyst for clinical observation and research into the effects of traumatic stress. Prior to its definition, it was as if the psychiatric community had to rediscover the importance of traumatic neurosis after every major war and calamity (Lindy, Green, & Grace, 1987). Now there appears to be a stable foundation on which future knowledge can be built. However, a number of controversies remain about the etiology, phenomenology, and treatment of PTSD. For example, Breslau and Davis (1987) suggested that the literature on disasters, civilian and wartime, and on more ordinary life events does not support the view that extreme stressors form a discrete class of events in terms of the probability of psychiatric sequelae or the distinctive nature of subsequent psychopathology. On this basis, they questioned the validity of the diagnosis of PTSD as it was defined in the DSM-III.

The extent and nature of psychological reactions to natural disasters have also been specifically questioned. Quarantelli (1985) has gone so far as to suggest that "in our judgement, the individual trauma approach is still at the mythological stage that most social and behavioral disaster researchers were at about two decades ago" (p. 204). Although there are many who would disagree with this opinion, it is difficult to generalize from much of the disaster literature because of the methodological deficiencies of much of the research which has examined the psychological effects of disaster (Green, 1982).

In this chapter, I will explore some of these controversies in the light of a series of studies that were conducted into the effects of a massive bushfire disaster that affected large areas of Southeastern Australia on February 16, 1983 (McFarlane & Raphael, 1984). These fires provided an unusual opportunity to study the acute and long-term psychological effects of a disaster because the populations affected were easily identified and tended to remain and rebuild within the disaster area rather than move to unaffected locations. As well, the victims who did not develop psychiatric symptoms, could be studied to elucidate the patterns of reaction that differentiated the people who remained relatively immune to long-term effects of the experience. This comparison group also meant that it was possible to examine carefully the phenomenology of the trauma response and what characterized the pathological outcomes. Against this background, the current diagnostic criteria for posttraumatic stress disorder (American Psychiatric Association, 1987) will be examined with an analysis of their validity and discriminatory ability. As well, the etiology and longitudinal course will be examined against the background of these uncertainties.

Stressor Criterion

Posttraumatic stress disorder (PTSD) was included in the DSM-III because of the belief that a unique pattern of symptoms followed the experience of extremely stressful events. This evidence was accumulated from a variety of settings including World Wars I and II (Brill &

Alexander Cowell McFarlane • Department of Psychiatry, University of Adelaide, Gilles Plains, South Australia 5086, Australia.

International Handbook of Traumatic Stress Syndromes, edited by John P. Wilson and Beverley Raphael. Plenum Press, New York, 1993.

Beebe, 1955; Slater, 1943), the Vietnam War (Figley, 1978), Hiroshima (Lifton, 1967), the Holocaust (Eitinger, 1961), and various natural and manmade disasters (Gleser et al., 1981). However, Breslau and Davis (1987) stated that there is "insufficient data to show that the set of symptoms characteristic of PTSD is strongly and uniquely with extraordinary stressors." They emphasized that previous studies examining survivors of various disasters and wars have focused on a wide range of psychological problems and psychiatric symptoms.

The divergence of opinion about the definition of the stressor criterion has made attempts to characterize the central features of these catastrophic events a highly controversial and difficult task. The DSM-III-R (American Psychiatric Association, 1987) states that the type of events that lead to PTSD are those experiences outside the range of usual human experience that would be markedly distressing to almost anyone. There are some who believe that the current criteria are too restrictive, whereas other clinicians are concerned that the diagnosis will lose its utility if the category is widened. The use of PTSD in personal injury claims means that a precise definition is an important issue. The application of these criteria with the bushfire victims allowed a series of observations about the problems with and utility of this definition.

Criteria for Disease, Disorder, and Distress

First, the definition of an event that is markedly distressing to almost everyone has a number of associated problems. To begin with, the DSM-III-R does not provide a definition for the term distress and no major psychiatric textbook discusses this concept at all despite its importance to psychiatric diagnosis. It seems to be a phenomenon which everyone knows about but one that presents many definitional problems. The word *distress* was not differentiated from *disease* until the fifteenth century, emphasizing the blurred boundaries of the concept (Ingham, 1981). In fact, the problem of separating minor symptoms of sadness and worry from clinically significant depression and anxiety has been given remarkably little attention in the literature (McFarlane, 1985). This is partly because behavioral and psychodynamic theories of etiology do not distinguish between clinical disorder and the minor psychopathology of everyday life, which is more akin to distress. This problem of definition is an important issue for epidemiological psychiatry because of the problem of interpreting the clinical significance of short-lived symptoms triggered by the experience of minor adversity. Examination of such questions is important to an understanding of PTSD. Quarantelli (1985) argued that disasters are a potent cause of distress but not disorder. This leads him to the view that mental health professionals have little role in these settings, further challenging the use of the term *distress* in the definition of PTSD.

Although Horowitz (1986) extensively explored cognitive and affective processing of traumatic events using an information-processing model, he essentially avoided an explicit discussion of normal distress. Many of his observations about the impact of traumatic events are perhaps more relevant to the understanding of the normal distress response than to the psychopathology of PTSD. Essentially, he proposed that there are two dimensions to this pattern of response where the individual is, on one hand, haunted and preoccupied by intrusive memories of the trauma while simultaneously attempting to avoid them and the distress they evoke. These images occur because the event is new information which the individual must integrate into his or her preexisting view of the self, others, and the world. The cognitive and affective reworking fluctuates between the intrusion and denial in an attempt to process the information without the individual's becoming overwhelmed by the enormity of the trauma. As the trauma recedes into the past, these involuntary recollections decrease until an equilibrium is reached where the person incorporates the experience into a world view. Brett and Ostroff (1985) suggested that this two-dimensional framework be used to characterize the symptoms of PTSD. None of the clinical accounts which they reviewed of these phenomena in victims of traumatic stress have attempted to differentiate this pattern of response in those who manage to adapt successfully after these events from those who develop stress disorders.

Stress Reactions after a Bushfire in Australia

The available evidence fails to demonstrate that this pattern of response is unique to people who develop PTSD after catastrophic stress but would rather suggest it is a universal reaction. This is supported by a series of observations of the three different groups after the bushfire (McFarlane, 1986, 1988a). There were many adults and children who experienced intense and intrusive images soon after the disaster and also used a same range of strategies to avoid their thoughts and affects but who did not go on to develop symptoms of pathological anxiety (McFarlane, 1988b,c). In general, the more intense and prolonged the exposure to the disaster, the greater the intensity of these phenomena. Although these images tended to decrease in frequency fairly quickly after the disaster, people who did not have a PTSD continued to have intrusive thoughts for many years after the disaster, particularly if the weather conditions were similar.

This suggests that the phenomena described by Horowitz (1986) and Brett and Ostroff (1985) are not a pathological pattern of response to a stressor but rather the normal distress response. If the distress were defined using this information-processing model in the diagnostic criteria for PTSD, it would allow an observable and quantifiable criterion for characterizing the type of events that were likely to lead it.

The stressor criterion also implies that PTSD is particularly likely to follow an event that would be markedly distressing to almost anyone. One study conducted after the fires examined the onset and course of psychiatric morbidity in a group of 469 firefighters who had a particularly intense exposure to the disaster (McFarlane, 1988b). Forty-two months after the disaster, all those who had developed significant symptoms were interviewed. Of the 58 who were found to have a post-traumatic stress disorder, only 16 had it as a single diagnosis. Of 22 firefighters who had an anxiety disorder diagnosis, 13 also had a PTSD. Of the 34 who satisfied the diagnostic criteria for major depression, 29 also had a PTSD and 30 also had another anxiety disorder diagnosis. The group who only developed PTSD did not have a more intense exposure to the disaster in terms of physical injury, bereavement, or exposure but did sustain greater property losses. In other words, PTSD was not predicted by the threat experienced during the height of the disaster but rather by the more chronic distress caused by secondary stressors, such as the destruction of farms and the death of stock (McFarlane, 1988c). These data suggest that the nature of the experience alone may be an inadequate predictor of the pattern of symptoms after such an event and that PTSD is not a unique syndrome in the setting of a disaster.

The nature of the relationship between the fires and the onset of symptoms was also examined in a series of correlational analyses. Even 4 months after the fires, the disaster only predicted 5% of the variance of the symptoms in the firefighter population, and this was very similar to the 4% of the variance predicted by other life events that had occurred prior to and independent of the disaster. By 29 months after the disaster, it no longer acted as a predictor of symptoms in this population (McFarlane, 1989a). This implied that the disaster experience and the magnitude of the losses were a relatively poor predictor of symptoms in this population. This issue was also examined in a study of all the registered disaster victims. Again, the disaster only accounted for 4% of the variance of symptoms, suggesting that the small size of this relationship was not due to a Type 2 error in the analysis. A study of 808 primary school children also affected by this disaster failed to find a strong correlational relationship between the disaster and the onset of symptoms.

The onset of symptoms after this disaster were not predicted to any greater degree by the nature of the experience than after other types of adversity. Evidence from well-conducted studies examining the impact of the adversity of everyday life have similarly found that life events account for less than 10% of the variance of disorder (Tennant, 1983). This does not support the hypothesis that there is a strong and direct relationship between the experience of inescapable horror of a natural disaster and the onset of PTSD; but there appeared to be a more complex interaction between the meaning of the event, the individual's previous life experience, and personality style. The importance of the personal meaning of the event as the central determinant of the onset of symptoms was particularly apparent in the patients seen after the disaster (McFarlane, 1986). The constant reinterpretation of the images of the disaster in terms of personal conflicts and responsibilities seemed to be critical in determining the ongoing distress and extent of chronically disturbed arousal. Many of these people seemed to lose the ability to form symbolic representations of events that followed the disaster (Lifton, 1967, 1973). These events repeatedly recaptured the victims' preoccupation with their losses, their sense of vulnerability, and the fragility of their control. However, if this issue of personal meaning was included into the stressor criterion, it would create many problems by introducing the concept of *personal vulnerability*.

Thus, the systematic studies of this disaster did little to clarify the borderline of the stressors that are likely to cause PTSD. Equally, even though PTSD emerged as the most frequent diagnosis, major depressive disorder and anxiety disorders were almost as frequently triggered by the disaster, suggesting that the specificity of the trauma is not as great as the diagnostic criteria would imply—results similar to the findings of other groups (Davidson, Schwartz, Storck, Krishnan, & Hammett, 1985; Escobar et al., 1983; Sierles, Chen, McFarland, & Taylor, 1983).

Reexperiencing Phenomenon

Mental health professionals are required to differentiate the various states of cognitive and affective disturbance which occur after extremely traumatic events for several practical reasons. First, after a major calamity when the available services would be unable to meet the demand for treatment, some form of triage would be necessary. This means that services would need to be directed to the high-risk group of victims whose distress was not likely to subside and those whose symptoms were likely to be a major source of disability and handicap in the long term. Second, following events where negligence results in personal injury claims, mental health professionals are legally obligated to make precise definitions of patients' mental states. In Australia, financial compensation will only be paid if the individual experiences a diagnosable disorder in contrast to a state of nonspecific distress or interruption to an individual's projected developmental path. Third, administrators and health care planners can be assisted in developing services if it is possible to define morbidity that can be directly attributed to the stressor, in contrast to psychiatric illness that would already exist within the affected community.

When the specificity and sensitivity of the various diagnostic criteria for PTSD were examined, the reexperiencing phenomena were found to have the lowest specificity of all phenomena (McFarlane, 1986). For example, the intrusive imagery had a specificity of only 39% 8 months after the disaster and the triggering of intrusive images was an almost universal phenomenon. The frequency, intensity, and extent of the triggering of memories was significantly greater in the people with PTSD. Nightmares and feelings as if the event were recurring were highly specific but only occurred in a minority of the subjects. Dreams of a less frightening quality were more common and also specific.

Thus, these phenomena are as much a marker of the fact that an individual has had an extremely traumatic experience as they are of psychopathology. On the other hand, in a typical outpatient setting, such imagery would be a highly specific marker for PTSD because very few patients would have been exposed to extremely stressful life events. These findings might suggest that the discriminant value of these phenomena could be improved if the diagnostic criteria stated that these symptoms had to occur on a certain number of occasions within a given time period. However, the longitudinal investigation of the victims of this disaster found that the frequency of the intrusive memories and dreams tended to decrease significantly in the first four years after the event and that the rate of decay of these symptoms was similar in victims who developed PTSD and those who remained well. The only differentiation was that the disordered group had significantly more symptoms immediately after the event. As well, a number of people who had a severe disorder of arousal but had adapted by the extensive use of avoidance only infrequently had intrusive memories. However, when the disaster was brought to awareness, these people were particularly distressed by their memories. Thus, the inclusion of a frequency threshold for these phenomena in the diagnostic criteria would lead to the exclusion of a number of people who had severe posttraumatic reactions.

Although intrusive memories and images of the traumatic event are obviously a central experience of people with PTSD, the fact that they are also a part of the normal distress response creates some difficulty when using them as "symptomatic" criteria. A more detailed examination of the role of these phenomena demonstrated that the intensity of the distress response was the intervening process between the individual's experience of the disaster and the onset of a disordered pattern of arousal. This was demonstrated both cross-sectionally (McFarlane, 1988a) and longitudinally (McFarlane, 1987a). The avoidance phenomena did not play a role in the onset of symptoms but rather were a reactive strategy to the intensity of the distress experienced.

Thus, the experience of these phenomena, in close temporal proximity to the disaster, was a much better predictor of who was at risk of developing a psychiatric disorder than the extent of the losses sustained or the intensity of the individual's confrontation with death or injury. This finding suggests that preventive programs provided in the setting of a disaster may be better aimed at those who are very distressed by their experience and whose distress does not rapidly resolve rather than targeting the victims who had a particularly intense exposure.

Once anxiety symptoms and/or depression have become established, a feedback effect begins to occur where the intensity and frequency of the memories of the disaster are increased. In both the adults and children studied after this disaster, once a pattern of symptoms has become established, depression and anxiety symptoms are as important determinants of the intrusive memories as is the reverse where the memories lead to anxiety and depression. This is a clinically important observation because of the onset of a coexistent anxiety disorder or major depression that plays a major role in determining the intensity of the patient's nightmares and intrusive memories (Davidson et al., 1985). The identification and treatment of a concurrent depressive episode are often critical to the successful management of the individual's posttraumatic stress disorder as is the specific treatment of traumatic memories. In the longitudinal investigation of 469 firefighters, one important factor which differentiated subjects with chronic PTSD from those with more short-lived symptoms was the experience of concurrent disorders.

Trauma Impact on Family Systems

Following a natural disaster, more than one family member may develop a PTSD. A series of important interactions can occur between individuals which can have a significant bearing on the adjustment of other family members and relatives. To begin with, if one person has been particularly adversely affected, this will be a constant reminder of the effects of the disaster and prevent the family from working through the experience. Frequently, the intensity of preoccupation resonates between family members and affects many interactions, such as the pattern of parenting (McFarlane, 1987b). Children quickly pick up their parents' anxiety and react to any overprotection with an increase in their fear about various dangers, including the possibility of a recurrence of the disaster. In this way, the reexperiencing symptoms of PTSD can be an important indicator of the family's pattern of response as well as the extent of individual traumatization.

Avoidance and Numbing

The ability of people to tolerate their traumatic memories varied widely in the victims of this disaster. This issue confronts both the clinician and researcher in these settings. To begin with, the return rates from epidemiological surveys tends to be much lower than in many other settings and tend to skew the response of those less affected. Subsequent conversation with many of the victims who did not respond to the survey which examined all the registered victims indicated their irrational anger about this inquiry because it was experienced as a major challenge to their attempts to put the experience out of their mind. Similar attempts to collect data from patients was not infrequently met with a refusal because they could not face the effort of reporting aspects of their experience without the support of the clinician.

The extent of the avoidance was also demonstrated by the low rates of diagnosis of psychiatric disorder in the victims by their general practitioners (McFarlane, 1986). This was despite the fact that a series of physical symptoms were often presented. The length of time that elapsed between the presentation of these complaints and the disaster meant that a possible link with the fires and these symptoms was frequently overlooked. Rather it was the lawyers who were managing the victims' property-damage claims who often identified the extent of the victims' ongoing but partially hidden distress. They observed that there were unusual difficulties in getting the victims to complete the necessary paper work for the lodgement of claims. In fact, a significant number of victims had chosen not to lodge damages claims because they could not face the distress this would cause, and others accepted unreasonably low offers for damages to avoid the need to continue thinking about the disaster because of the continuing legal proceedings.

The intensification of symptoms following an assessment interview was another important manifestation of the degree to which avoidance was used by these patients to contain their ongoing distress. It was important to acknowledge this issue and not to evoke a degree of catharsis that would leave the person feeling threatened and out of control. Only a small proportion of the people with clinically significant and disabling symptoms sought professional help despite the fact that many continued to have problems 6 years after the fire.

Many problems would appear to exist in the reliable definition of the avoidance and interpersonal estrangement. Particularly in an instrument such as the Diagnostic Interview Schedule (Helzer, Spitznagel, & McEnvoy, 1987), these phenomena are elicited using direct questions that require yes/no answers. Symptoms, such as constricted affect and emotional numbing, require considerable exploration and description before they can be definitely said to be present. Therefore research interviews that depend on a structured format are likely to underdiagnose PTSD. The extent to which the symptoms interfere with people's lives are also often disguised by the use of business in work and trivial activities. Rather, people lose the ability to relax and use their time in a relatively unstructured manner. As a consequence, they find it difficult to pursue recreational interests or spend time with spouses and children.

In essence, many of the phenomena included in this set of diagnostic criteria represent the disabilities and handicaps that arise from the impact of traumatic stress (McFarlane, 1988c). They describe the various behavioral and interpersonal strategies which can be put in place to contain the intrusive memories and the emotional lability, anxiety, and disturbed concentration. In part, they serve an adaptive purpose but they also become a source of distress and regret. They tend to be less prominent in the early stages after the trauma and slowly emerge as the individual copes with the continuing disruption caused by his symptoms. In the longitudinal study of the firefighters conducted after this disaster, a subgroup of 50 subjects were interviewed at 8 months and then again at 42 months (McFarlane, 1988b). Of the 5 subjects who were found to have a borderline disorder at 8 months, 3 were found to have a definite diagnosis at 42 months. At 8 months the lack of constricted affect, numbing, and estrangement were not present but emerged during the next 34 months. Thus, these diagnostic criteria have questionable validity particularly in close proximity to the triggering event.

The likelihood of a traumatized individual demonstrating these phenomena is also influenced by his premorbid character. A person who is an extrovert is less likely to respond by withdrawing socially and may do the reverse of being drawn into a variety of social supports in an attempt to resolve his or her distress. In contrast, the introvert who is naturally shy and inhibited in social settings is much more likely to withdraw after a traumatic event. The introvert's characteristic behavior pattern is also partly portrayed by these phenomena, meaning that there is a greater probability of satisfying these diagnostic criteria. Similarly, people who tend to avoid conflict as a characteristic coping strategy are also more likely to fulfill these criteria. Therefore, the probability of satisfying this group of diagnostic criteria is partly dependent on the individual premorbid personality.

Finally, the nature of the traumatic experience also

influences the extent to which the individual resorts to the use of avoidance. In this disaster, the range of experiences was considerable. Some people came close to losing their lives after being trapped in the enormous firestorm that produced flames over 800 feet tall and with winds strong enough to flatten radiata pine trees with trunks 3 feet in diameter. In contrast, others were involved in situations where people died. On occasions, this latter group often had thoughts that their behavior had contributed to the death in some way. For example, one man found human remains on the front of his car after driving along a road through smoke and flames that completely obscured his vision. He subsequently found out that a person had been found burned to ashes on the road he had driven along. He could not bring himself to discuss this situation with anyone and had changed general practitioners when one doctor began to inquire about his posttraumatic symptoms. Thus, the degree to which a person feels his behavior is culpable in a traumatic situation will also influence the extent of the use of avoidance and interpersonal estrangement. This means that this set of phenomena are not just a measure of the individual's experience but also an indicator of the nature of the traumatic experience and may decrease the likelihood of the diagnosis following events that do not involve personal violence or feelings of responsibility for the death or injury of others.

Disordered Arousal and Attention

In contrast to the low specificity of traumatic imagery, the disturbance of attention and arousal appeared to discriminate more precisely between those victims with and those without PTSD. At 8 months, the disturbance of concentration was found to have a specificity of 81%. Disturbed concentration at 8 months after the fire was the one symptom that predicted the continued presence of PTSD 3 years later. At 42 months, all the firefighters in this study who had experienced significant symptoms on any of the previous four sampling stages were interviewed using the Diagnostic Interview Schedule (Helzer et al., 1987). The role of these attention related phenomena was specifically investigated by a series of questions focusing on distractibility. Factor analysis was used to characterize the pattern or grouping of phenomena incorporated in the existing diagnostic criteria. The first factor was characterized by a disturbance of attention, suggesting that these impairments best distinguished people with PTSD from those who did not have the disorder. Two other factors were identified: one characterized by irritability and intrusive memories and the third by dreams and flashbacks.

These data did not find that posttraumatic phenomena fell on two polarities of intrusion and avoidance as suggested by Horowitz (1986) or Brett and Ostroff (1985). The findings from this study are supported by the factor analytical study of Silver and Iacono (1984), in which trouble concentrating was the first item loading on their first factor, although they regarded it as an indicator of depression. The subtlety of the occurrence of disturbed attention in PTSD may explain why sufferers do not complain of this phenomenon more readily, in contrast to cognitive and affective intrusion of traumatic imagery (Nisbett & Wilson, 1977).

The importance of disturbed arousal as a central element of PTSD was also suggested by the landmark longitudinal investigation of Weisaeth (1984) of a factory fire where he found that anxiety symptoms and sleep disturbance in close proximity to the disaster were the best predictors of long-term disorder. A similar observation was made in the longitudinal study which examined the posttraumatic reactions of 808 primary school children. Here the data indicated that distractibility and restlessness, akin to poor concentration and memory in PTSD, were consistent predictors of children with clinically significant levels of symptoms 26 months after the disaster.

This attentional abnormality is currently being investigated using cortical evoked potentials. Preliminary findings have demonstrated that PTSD subjects have significantly excessive responses to a range of background stimuli, but particularly to distractors. This attentional deficit appears to be improved by the prescription of tricyclic antidepressants which decrease the attention devoted to irrelevant stimuli but increase attention involved in the processing of target stimuli. Thus, tricyclic antidepressants may exert their beneficial effects in this disorder by altering the information-processing abnormality which appears to exist in this disorder.

The memory disturbance which was included in the original DSM-III diagnostic criteria (American Psychiatric Association, 1980) would appear to be related to this attentional abnormality. It appears to be a consequence of the sufferer's not being able to discriminate and register relatively minor events and is probably due to a failure to define the salience of a relevant stimulus in comparison to other background environmental information. Similarly, the exaggerated startle response in PTSD is probably a direct consequence of the sufferers' inability to shut out background environmental noise and happenings that have little or no relevance to these individuals. It is as though their sensory gate is open and unable to filter much of the irrelevant stimulation from the environment. This phenomenological observation may provide some insight into some of the proposed neurobiological abnormalities in PTSD.

The work of Kolb (1987), van der Kolk (1987), and others (Wilson, 1989) have focused extensively on the possibility that PTSD involves a depletion of noradrenaline in the projections from the *locus coeruleus*. They have suggested that the animal model of learned helplessness following inescapable electric shocks may provide important insights into the neurobiology of PTSD (Wilson, 1989). In particular, learned helplessness has long been associated with noradrenaline depletion, particularly in the coeruleal noradrenaline system, and this has been postulated to result from the failure to replenish noradrenaline after a large increase in turnover produced by stressors, such as unpredictable, unavoidable electric shocks.

The accumulated evidence in both humans and animals suggests that noradrenaline plays a central role in the process of attention by modulating forebrain activity (Robbins, 1984). In particular, the dorsal noradrenergic ascending bundle is necessary for the discrimination of relevant environmental information and turnover is increased by both noxious and not obviously aversive or stressful stimuli. Locus coeruleus activity correlates positively with attention, but perceptual, motor, or emotional states and any abnormality of its activity will be reflected in an individual's capacity to attend. This role of noradrenaline in the attention process has not been discussed in relation to PTSD. Thus, the disturbance of concentration and hypervigilance may be a manifestation of this abnormality of noradrenaline production.

Therefore, the disturbance of this neurophysiological process may be the phenomenon which best accounts for the nature of the symptoms of posttraumatic stress disorder and its differentiation from other disorders and states of distress following a severe stressor. That is not to say that the other phenomena do not play an important role in the formation of this pattern of response. However, the vulnerability to develop a disturbance of noradrenaline production following an extreme trauma may be a biological predisposing factor that plays an important role in the onset of chronic posttraumatic symptoms. The fact that more than 50% of posttraumatic stress disorder patients have a family history of psychiatric disorder (Davidson et al., 1985) suggests that this may partly relate to an inherited predisposition related to cerebral catecholamine production. The study by Davidson et al. (1985) found an incidence of depression and anxiety very similar to the relatives of patients with generalized anxiety disorders; also, unpublished data from the firefighters' study found that a family history of psychiatric disorder was particularly associated with a chronic course. These observations further suggest that PTSD in its more chronic forms may be related to some underlying disturbance of neurotransmitter modulation of cortical function (Wilson, 1989).

The possible role of such a biological disturbance is further suggested by the frequent coexistence of posttraumatic stress disorder with other disorders. The concurrence of PTSD has now been studied in several patient populations and more than 50% are found to be suffering from another psychiatric disorder (Davidson et al., 1985; Escobar et al., 1983; Sierles et al., 1983). As previously described, this degree of concurrence has also been found in the sample of firefighters described (McFarlane, 1989a), suggesting that this finding in patient populations is not simply the product of concurrent disorders' increasing the severity of symptoms and increasing the likelihood of the individual becoming a patient. These data suggest that PTSD probably shares common etiological processes with both the anxiety disorders and depression and hence may share some of the same vulnerabilities. This raised the important and unanswered question about whether similar etiological pathways exist in PTSD.

From a clinical perspective, there is considerable evidence that the sleep disturbance, hypervigilance, and disturbed concentration are significantly worsened if the person develops a coexistent disorder. In fact, a number of patients initially present with PTSD at times when they develop major anxiety or depressive symptoms. Similarly, the patients' intrusive thoughts often become much more distressing and frequent if there is an intensification of their depression. Equally subsequent adversity also can play an important role in intensifying the disturbed arousal and the attentional abnormalities in PTSD. Thus, a complex web of psychodynamic, biological, and environmental factors influence the intensity of this aspect of the phenomenology of PTSD.

Etiology and Longitudinal Course

The role of personality and vulnerability factors is another major controversy that has surrounded the psychological effects of extremely traumatic events.

The classification of psychiatric disorders which follow in the wake of such events has been greatly influenced by the uncertainty about the role of personality and other predisposing factors in the etiology of these disorders. The inclusion of posttraumatic stress disorder (PTSD) in DSM-III (American Psychiatric Association, 1980) arose from a consensus view that the nature and intensity of the stressor was the primary etiological factor determining the symptoms which people develop in the setting of extreme adversity (Breslau & Davis, 1987).

In contrast, earlier systems of classification separated the issues involved in the development of acute symptoms from more enduring patterns of psychopathology. For example, the previous systems of classification tended to assume that symptoms would be time limited unless some preexisting character pathology was present which would contribute to their maintenance (Green, Lindy, & Grace, 1985). This implied that the stress response was transient in nature unless the individual had some particular preexisting vulnerability. Thus, the notion that very traumatic events in adult life could have prolonged adverse psychological consequences represents a recent change in the formulation of the effects of traumatic stress.

This issue was investigated in two ways in a longitudinal study of the 469 firefighters. When the relative contribution of the disaster experience and vulnerability factors to the symptoms in this group were compared over time, the role of the threat experienced and the losses incurred progressively decreased over a 29-month period (McFarlane, 1989a). In contrast, the longer the symptoms of posttraumatic morbidity remained, the greater the role played by several vulnerability factors, such as neuroticism, a family or personal history of psychiatric illness, and a tendency not to confront conflicts. Because the measures used in this study had also been used in several other epidemiological studies in Australian populations, it was possible to compare the contribution of these vulnerability factors to the development of symptoms in populations unaffected by disaster. The contribution of neuroticism to symptoms was less than half the size of that found in an average urban population, suggesting that the role of vulnerability factors plays a significantly smaller role in the onset and maintenance of posttraumatic morbidity than in the other types of psychiatric impairment more commonly present in nontraumatized populations.

A selected subsample of this population was interviewed using the Diagnostic Interview Schedule (Helzer et al., 1987) and the determinants of acute, delayed onset, and chronic PTSD were examined. The acute PTSD group had no major vulnerability factors and seldom had a coexistent psychiatric disorder. In contrast, the chronic PTSD group scored significantly higher on a number of vulnerability factors, such as concurrent psychiatric disorder, a positive family history for psychiatric disorder, avoidance as a personality trait, as well as being older and having panicked more during the disaster (McFarlane, 1988c). The combined data from this study suggest that even though the disaster event plays a critical role in the onset of PTSD, its chronicity is predicted to a significant degree by a variety of premorbid factors but that these probably exert a lesser impact than in other psychiatric disorders.

These findings were similar to the Weisaeth (1984) study where he successfully followed up all the victims of a huge Norwegian paint factory fire in an investigation which commenced several days after the accident. He found that the prevalence of acute PTSD was determined by the initial intensity of the exposure. However, the prognosis at 4 years was more influenced by the preaccident psychological functioning than the intensity of exposure to the explosion. On the other hand, Green, Grace, and Gleser (1986) found that PTSD in the victims of a supper club fire was largely accounted for by the traumatic experience of the disaster (60% of the variance), with vulnerability factors playing a minor role. However this investigation had examined only 117 out of the 2,500 affected people and the representativeness of the sample could not be defined.

Continuing Controversy

On balance, the data collected after disasters raise a number of questions about the relationship between PTSD and other psychiatric disorders produced by such events. The division between PTSD, major depression, generalized anxiety disorder, and panic disorder is not as clear-cut as much of the recent literature would suggest, particularly as the triggering event recedes into the past. On balance, it would seem that many of the controversies that existed about the effects of traumatic stress at the end of World War II still require further clarification (Palinkas & Cohen, 1987; Rahe, 1988). The doubts raised by Breslau and Davis (1987) are certainly not dispelled by the data examining the impact of this disaster, particularly whether the extremely traumatic events do have a qualitatively different relationship with subsequent morbidity. Similarly, they do little to solve the question of whether PTSD is best classed as an anxiety disorder, which is the case in the DSM-III-R. On the other hand, there would appear to be little evidence to support the Horowitz, Weiss, and Marmar (1987) proposal that PTSD should be classed in a category of stress-response syndromes, particularly in the light of the role of various vulnerability factors. As well, only one case of a brief reactive psychosis was identified in over 300 of the victims who had the most intense exposure to the disaster, and this person went on to develop a major depressive disorder, suggesting that many questions remain about the etiology of psychotic symptoms which begin in close proximity to a catastrophic event.

The systematic examination of the impact of this disaster does demonstrate that there is a significant increase in psychiatric morbidity in the victims. When all the registered victims were surveyed 12 months after the fires, 42% had levels of symptoms similar to psychiatric patients. This study used the General Health Questionnaire which has been extensively utilized in a series of epidemiological studies of Australian populations (Henderson, Byrne, & Duncan-Jones, 1981). Using these studies as comparison groups suggested that the disaster-affected population had twice the level of morbidity expected. These data were significant because this level of morbidity was found when the acute perturbation caused by the property losses and grief had resolved. When the GHQ was validated against a structured interview, the majority of people were suffering from PTSD and their symptoms were proving to be an important source of disability. Similarly, in the study examining all the primary school children in one area that experienced a particularly destructive conflagration, twice the level of clinically significant symptoms were demonstrated 26 months after the disaster. Furthermore, these symptoms were shown to have a detrimental impact on the academic performance of the children affected.

Thus, the claims made by Quarantelli (1985) that disasters are important causes of distress but not of psychiatric illness were disproved after this disaster by using widely accepted questionnaires and an epidemiological method. At the same time, these studies found that more than half the population demonstrated remarkable resilience in the face of considerable threat and deprivation. Even those who were adversely affected from a psychological perspective were very reluctant to admit to their predicament and only a minority sought psychiatric treatment and only then with considerable ambivalence. Psychiatric services provided in the postdisaster period need to take account of people's desire for independence while ensuring that their denial and avoidance are confronted appropriately. There is a significant danger that services provided in an excessively intrusive manner which overdramatizes the victim's distress and helplessness in the early days after a disaster can ultimately alienate the latter need for mental health interventions (McFarlane, 1989b). Although clinical issues of treatment are important, they are discussed more fully in Part V of this volume.

Conclusion

Although the definition of PTSD in the DSM-III (American Psychiatric Association, 1980) has led to an explosion of research into the effects of traumatic stress, many uncertainties remain about this disorder. The studies of the bushfire disaster pointed to a number of issues which require continued investigation including the relationship between PTSD, panic disorder, and major depressive disorder, and the borderline between PTSD and normal distress, and the role of primary prevention. Similarly, the role of personality and other vulnerability factors was found to be more important in the etiology of PTSD in this group of victims than in many other recent studies. These data cannot simply be dismissed as an exception because these studies examined

representative samples who were studied in considerably closer temporal proximity to the trauma than most other research. The failure to demonstrate a strong relationship between the intensity of the trauma and the severity of posttraumatic symptoms in three studies raises important doubts about the stressor criterion which again must be answered because of the intensity of this disaster. On the other hand, the current formulation of PTSD, which deemphasizes the responsibility of the individual and focuses on the critical organizing role of the trauma, has a number of clinical advantages. The extent to which these data can be generalized requires clarification.

Most disaster and traumatic stress research has examined events that affect relatively small groups, in contrast to the disasters that often are experienced in the third world which may involve hundreds of thousands of victims. The extent to which the results of the research in these more minor events can be applied to these more devastating situations is an important issue for theoretical and for humanitarian reasons. Furthermore, the study of disasters examines the impact of a state of terror that may last for only seconds in contrast to the prolonged exposure of a soldier in battle to the threat of death. The similarities and the different effects of such stressors in the etiology of posttraumatic stress disorder has been given little attention but is important to an understanding of the etiology of PTSD.

Finally, the growth of knowledge into the effects of traumatic stress has meant future studies will need to be considerably more sophisticated if they are to provide new information. Disaster research has often been poorly planned and has repeatedly asked the same questions, partly because disasters infrequently occur in the same region, meaning that each event brings a new group of researchers. This raises important ethical issues about informed consent and the ethical clearance of disaster research protocols. The victims of disasters are therefore in some need to having their privacy protected and to ensuring that only research that will contribute to the growth of knowledge is permitted. Thus, collaborative disaster research has much to recommend it, particularly where groups can decide on uniform measures to investigate well-formulated questions.

References

American Psychiatric Association. (1980). *Diagnostic and statistical manual of mental disorders* (3rd ed.). Washington, DC: Author.

American Psychiatric Association. (1987). *Diagnostic and statistical manual of mental disorders* (3rd ed., rev.). Washington, DC: Author.

Breslau, N., & Davis, G. C. (1987a). Post-traumatic stress disorder: The etiologic specificity of wartime stressors. *American Journal of Psychiatry, 144*, 578–583.

Brett, E. A., & Ostroff, R. (1985). Imagery and post-traumatic stress disorder: An overview. *American Journal of Psychiatry, 142*, 417–424.

Brill, N. Q., & Beebe, G. W. (1955). *A follow-up study of war neuroses.* Washington, DC: Veterans Administration Medical Monograph.

Davidson, J., Swartz, M., Storck, M., Krishnan, R. A., & Hammett, E. (1985). A diagnostic and family study of post-traumatic stress disorder. *American Journal of Psychiatry, 142,* 90–93.

Eitinger, L. (1961). Pathology of the concentration camp syndrome. *Archives of General Psychiatry, 5,* 371–379.

Escobar, J. I., Randolph, E. T., Pruente, G., Spiwak, F., Asanen, J. K., Hill, M., & Hough, R. L. (1983). Post-traumatic stress disorder in Hispanic Vietnam veterans. *Journal of Nervous and Mental Disease, 171,* 585–596.

Figley, C. R. (Ed.). (1978). *Stress disorder among Vietnam veterans.* New York: Brunner/Mazel.

Gleser, G., Green, B. L., & Winget, C. (1981). *Prolonged psychosocial effects of disaster: A study of Buffalo Creek.* New York: Academic Press.

Green, B. L. (1982). Assessing the levels of psychiatric impairment following disaster. *Journal of Nervous and Mental Disease, 170,* 544–552.

Green, B. L., Grace, M. C., & Gleser, G. C. (1986). Identifying survivors at risk: Long-term impairment following the Beverly Hills Supper Club Fire. *Journal of Consulting Clinical Psychology, 53,* 672–678.

Green, B. L., Lindy, J. D., & Grace, M. C. (1985). Post-traumatic stress disorder: Toward DSM IV. *Journal of Nervous and Mental Disease, 173,* 406–411.

Helzer, J. E., Spitznagel, E. L., & McEvoy, L. (1987). The predictive validity of lay diagnostic interview schedule diagnoses in the general population. *Archives of General Psychiatry, 44,* 1069–1077.

Henderson, S., Byrne, D. G., & Duncan-Jones, P. (1981). *Neurosis and the social environment.* Sydney: Academic Press.

Horowitz, M. J. (1986). *Stress response syndromes.* New York: Jason Aronson.

Horowitz, M. J., Weiss, D. S., & Marmar, C. (1987). Commentary: Diagnosis of post-traumatic stress disorder. *Journal of Nervous and Mental Disease, 175,* 267–268.

Ingham, J. (1981). Neurosis: Disease or distress? In J. K. Wing (Ed.), *What is a case? The problem of definition in psychiatric community surveys.* London: L. M. Grant McIntyre.

Kolb, L. C. (1987). A neuropsychological hypothesis explaining post-traumatic stress disorders. *American Journal of Psychiatry, 144,* 989–995.

Lifton, R. J. (1967). *Death in life: Survivors of Hiroshima.* New York: Random House.

Lifton, R. J. (1973). *Home from war.* New York: Simon & Schuster.

Lindy, J. D., Green, B. L., & Grace, M. C. (1987). Commentary: The stressor criterion and post-traumatic stress disorder. *Journal of Nervous and Mental Disease, 175,* 269–272.

McFarlane, A. C. (1985). The effects of stressful life events and disasters: Research and theoretical issues. *Australian and New Zealand Journal of Psychiatry, 19,* 409–421.

McFarlane, A. C. (1986). Post-traumatic morbidity of a disaster: A study of cases presenting for psychiatric treatment. *Journal of Nervous and Mental Disease, 174,* 4–14.

McFarlane, A. C. (1987a). Post-traumatic phenomena in a longitudinal study of children following a natural disaster. *Journal of American Academy of Child and Adolescent Psychiatry, 26,* 764–679.

McFarlane, A. C. (1987b). The relationship between patterns of family interaction and psychiatric disorder in children. *Australian and New Zealand Journal of Psychiatry, 21,* 383–390.

McFarlane, A. C. (1988a). Relationship between psychiatric impairment and a natural disaster: The role of distress. *Psychological Medicine, 18,* 129–139.

McFarlane, A. C. (1988b). The phenomenology of post-traumatic stress disorder following a natural disaster. *Journal of Nervous and Mental Disease, 176,* 22–29.

McFarlane, A. C. (1988c). The aetiology of post-traumatic stress disorder following a natural disaster. *British Journal of Psychiatry, 152,* 116–121.

McFarlane, A. C. (1989a). The aetiology of posttraumatic morbidity: Predisposing, precipitating and perpetuating factors. *British Journal of Psychiatry, 154,* 221–228.

McFarlane, A. C. (1989b). The prevention and management of the psychiatric morbidity of natural disasters: An Australian experience. *Stress Medicine, 5,* 29–36.

McFarlane, A. C., & Raphael, B. (1984). Ash Wednesday: The effects of a fire. *Australian and New Zealand Journal of Psychiatry, 19,* 913–921.

Nisbett, R. E., & Wilson, T. D. (1977). Telling more than we can know: Verbal reports on mental processes. *Psychological Review, 84,* 231–259.

Palinkas, L. A., & Coben, P. (1987). Psychiatric disorders among United States Marines wounded in action in Vietnam. *Journal of Nervous and Mental Disease, 175,* 291–300.

Quarantelli, E. L. (1985). An assessment of conflicting views on mental health: The consequences of traumatic events. In E. Figley (Ed.), *Trauma and its wake* (pp. 173–215). New York: Brunner/Mazel.

Rahe, R. H. (1988). Acute versus chronic psychological reactions to combat. *Military Medicine, 153,* 365–372.

Robbins, T. W. (1984). Cortical noradrenaline, attention and arousal: Functions of the dorsal noradrenergic ascending bundle. *Psychological Medicine, 14,* 13–21.

Sierles, F. S., Chen, J., McFarland, R. E., & Taylor, M. A. (1983). Post-traumatic stress disorder and concurrent psychiatric illness: Preliminary report. *American Journal of Psychiatry, 140,* 1177–1179.

Silver, S. M., & Iacono, C. V. (1984). Factor-analytic support for DSM-III'S posttraumatic stress disorder for Vietnam veterans. *Journal of Clinical Psychology, 40,* 5–14.

Slater, E. (1943). The neurotic constitution. *Journal of Neurological Psychiatry, 6,* 1–6.

Tennant, C. (1983). Life events and psychiatric morbidity: The evidence from prospective studies. *Psychological Medicine, 13,* 483–486.

van der Kolk, B. A. (1987). *Psychological trauma.* Washington, DC: American Psychiatric Press.

Weisaeth, L. (1984). *Stress reactions in an industrial accident.* Unpublished doctoral thesis, Oslo University, Oslo, Norway.

Wilson, J. P. (1989). *Trauma, transformation, and healing: An integrative approach to theory, research, and post-traumatic therapy.* New York: Brunner/Mazel.

CHAPTER 35

Chernobyl: Nuclear Threat as Disaster

Tom Lundin, Bertil Mårdberg, and Ulf Otto

Introduction

Within the field of disaster studies, several aspects of normal psychological reactions and psychiatric disorders have been investigated. Most studies have been initiated after a specific disaster. There are prospective and retrospective investigations concerning directly and indirectly affected persons. It is well known that bereavement (Brown, 1986; Glick, Weiss, & Parkes, 1964b, 1972; Lundin, 1984a, 1987; Maddison & Walker, 1967; Parkes, 1964b, 1972; Raphael, 1983) and especially sudden and unexpected bereavement (Cowan & Murphy, 1985; Lundin, 1984b, 1987; Parkes & Weiss, 1983; Singh & Raphael, 1981) can cause increased somatic and psychic morbidity. There are also many studies of postdisaster effects among survivors (Bennet, 1970; Boman, 1977; Green, Grace, & Gleser, 1985; Green, Grace, Lindy, Titchener, & Lindy, 1983; Lifton & Olson, 1976; McFarlane & Raphael, 1984; Titchener & Kapp, 1976; Weisæth, 1984), which show an increased rate of mental illness or posttraumatic stress disorders (PTSD). Rescue and health care personnel (Holen, Sund, Weisæth, & Alexander, 1983; Lindstrom & Lundin, 1982; Raphael, 1986; Raphael, Singh, Branbury, & Lambert, 1983–1984) are also indirectly affected groups at risk. Threat and coping (Bennet, 1970; Grinker & Spiegel, 1945; Lazarus, 1966; Menninger, 1952; Weisæth, 1984) as well as anticipation of a disaster, including warnings, response, and preparedness (Raphael, 1986) are important factors for the psychological outcome in mental health (Green *et al.*, 1983; Gleser, Green, & Winget, 1981; Lopez-Ibor, Soria, Canas, & Rodriguez-Gamazo, 1985).

With regard to nuclear threat, several aspects of the impact of the Three Mile Island accident have been studied. Sills, Wolf, and Shelanski (1982) stated that public fear of nuclear power should not be viewed as irrational and they pointed out that management of nuclear power must be based upon an understanding of how people think about such risks. Reactions following an accident can be seen as an effect of the assessment of nuclear risks and the fundamental thought processes that determine perceptions of risk. The amount of stress experienced by people living near Three Mile Island was supposed to be a function of the perceived amount of threat to physical safety and the reliability of the information being used to ascertain the degree of danger.

The effects of social support on stress after the disaster were studied one year after the accident (Fleming, Baum, Gisriel, & Gatchel, 1982). Higher levels of psychosocial support were associated with fewer psychological and behavioral symptoms of stress. Moreover, three affected groups were studied 9 to 12 months after the Three Mile Island accident (Goldsteen & Schorr, 1982): mothers of preschool children, nuclear power-plant workers, and community mental health system clients were compared with three control groups. The investigators had personal contact with all participants in a structured interview. The mothers of Three Mile Island had a significant higher risk of experiencing episodes of anxiety and depression during the year after the accident. These episodes were not associated with other stress factors. Those with prior mental health problems had significantly more symptoms. Among the plant workers, there were differences in frequency of clinical disorders after the accident. The mental health clients in Three Mile Island who perceived the accident as dangerous and the community as unsafe had higher anxiety scores. Furthermore, a study on children's reactions following the Three Mile Island accident was initiated during the first month (M. Schwebel & M. A. Schwebel, 1981). Questionnaires with four open-ended items were answered by 368 children from 10 school

Tom Lundin, Bertil Mårdberg, and Ulf Otto • Department of Psychiatry, University Hospital, S-58185 Linköping, Sweden.
International Handbook of Traumatic Stress Syndromes, edited by John P. Wilson and Beverley Raphael. Plenum Press, New York, 1993.

districts. The questions were: Do I think there will be a serious nuclear accident? Do I care? What do I think will happen if there is a serious nuclear accident near my home? What should be done about nuclear plants? The respondents were grouped according to three age levels: 10–12, 13–14, and 15–18 years. There were significant differences between age groups concerning the first question: The two older groups were more pessimistic. The younger group had a higher percentage of yes responses to the second question. Similar differences could be seen concerning the third and fourth questions.

During the last decades, there have been relatively few large-scale accidents and disasters in Scandinavia. Some of these (Bjorklund, 1991; L. Carlstedt & B. Carlstedt, 1985; Holen *et al.*, 1983; Larsson, 1986; Lindstrom & Lundin, 1982; Lundin, 1987; Lundin & Otto, 1991; Shalit, 1986; Syren, 1981; Weisæth, 1984) have been investigated and referred to earlier (Holen *et al.*, 1983; Lindstrom & Lundin, 1982; Lundin, 1987; Shalit, 1986; Weisæth, 1984). Therefore, it was thought to be especially important to exclude disaster research and to develop instead a greater understanding of risk and threat aspects, and, in particular, any aspects relevant to nuclear disaster because of the high reliance in Sweden and in Europe on nuclear power.

The aim in this chapter is to investigate the psychological reactions in the Swedish population to the threat of the Chernobyl accident. What was the magnitude of the reactions? Which background variables accounted for the variance or differences? Which reaction patterns are shown in the population?

Background

On April 26, 1986, one of the four nuclear reactor aggregates at the plant at Chernobyl in the USSR was destroyed as a consequence of an explosion and a disastrous fire. A great amount of nuclear active material was carried up to an altitude of 1000 m and blown by the winds over Poland, Finland, and the eastern and northern parts of Sweden. Two days after the disaster, an increased level of nuclear activity was registered at a routine control station around the nuclear plant at Forsmark, 100 km north of Stockholm. It was soon evident that the nuclear material did not come from any plant in Sweden or from a nuclear weapon. Some days later, the disaster was confirmed by Soviet authorities.

It was estimated that around 135,000 persons living in the Chernobyl area were evacuated during the first two days. Eighteen thousand were given medical examinations and 299 were treated as inpatients in Moscow. Of these patients, 26 had died by the beginning of June, 1986.

The Swedish Situation

Rather soon, it was evident that at least the eastern parts of Sweden were at high risk for nuclear fallout. Because of changes in the wind directions, there was different information about the risks from one day to the next. During the first weeks, no special attention was paid to the importance of nuclear rain. The authorities in Sweden had different opinions about the risks for several months after the disaster.

The Chernobyl disaster was a special threat for people living in Sweden. During the last decade, there has been an intense debate with regard to the Swedish nuclear power program, including a referendum resulting in a great amount of information on nuclear power issues and a polarization for and against the program among the populace.

Reactions of confusion and anxiety developed slowly among the Swedish population. The Chernobyl event was unique and unlike any previous disaster in Sweden. Fallout cannot be seen or detected by most sensory mechanisms. It is known to produce long-term medical reactions. It cannot be removed from huge areas, such as a country, by any technical means or human effort. Furthermore, from the Swedish point of view, the Chernobyl disaster became a threat to the overall welfare of the nation because of the expected effects of the radiation on persons, food, water, and on the environment in general. However, nobody was immediately and visibly hurt. Actually, the threat was very diffuse with no direct manifestations of damage and, in the first place, it generated mostly worry and anxiety. Official information about what was actually happening and the risks involved was very ambiguous. The theoretical complexity of the subject did not make the issue clearer. The situation remained potentially threatening because of (1) the uncertainty as to the immediate effects on those affected by radiation fallout from Chernobyl, and (2) long-term, damaging effects on the food chain and environment and their eventual secondary effects on the population.

Methodology

A representative sample of 840 persons (aged > 17) was selected from the whole of Sweden. Another representative sample of 216 persons (aged > 17) was obtained from a high-risk area (the county of Gavle). The persons selected were interviewed by telephone 2 weeks after the disaster. The interview was structured and followed partly the international guidelines (Raphael, Lundin, & Weisæth, 1988) and was supplemented by a special set of questions on threat and coping compiled by the National Defence Research Institute. This *threat index* comprises eight separate items. The respondents were asked to indicate their perception of threat in each of the following: (1) inability to manage well in life; (2) inability to solve a serious problem in the family; (3) inability to trust family members; (4) exposure to physical suffering; (5) loss of a family member; (6) the repeated violation of Sweden's frontiers; (7) that Sweden as a democracy should be called into question; and (8) limitation by the United States or Soviet Union of the freedom of action of the Swedish government.

In the analysis of the data the threat questions constituted a threat index (1 = low, 2 = medium, 3 = high). The questionnaire also contained sociodemographic background variables. There were 50 items including questions on comprehension of information provided by radio, TV, and newspapers and knowledge about the risks for radiation injuries. Additional variables for the statistical analysis were: coping index, knowledge about the situation, emotional reaction, anxiety, the Chernobyl threat, abolition of nuclear power, guidance, confidence, changing of habits, and being outdoors.

The statistical analyses were performed with the help of Student's t-test, analysis of variance (ANOVA), and cluster analysis. Latent profile analysis was used for classifying different patterns of reactions in the representative sample from the whole of Sweden ($n = 840$).

Results

The population in Sweden had a good comprehension (73.5%) of the information from the mass media, but only 55.3% had high confidence in this information. A high percentage of the persons interviewed were concerned about radiation injuries to themselves (41.3%) and to their close relatives (60.5%). More than one third (38.9%) of the population had unpleasant thoughts about the disaster. Less than 10% had changed their habits or developed feelings of depression.

There were no significant differences in sociodemographic background variables between Sweden ($n = 840$) and Gavle ($n = 216$) except concerning the level of education. In this respect, the level in Gavle was significantly ($p < .05$) lower. Furthermore, the interviewees from the Gavle area understood significantly ($p < .01$) less of the information from the mass media and had less ($p < .05$) knowledge about self-protection against nuclear radiation. They had less ($p < .001$) confidence in information from authorities. These persons and their children were outdoors ($p < .001$) less than the respondents from the whole of Sweden during the weeks after the disaster. Concerning unpleasant thoughts, preoccupation by thoughts and feelings about the disaster, subjective estimation of ability to overcome unpleasant thoughts about the disaster, and depressive feelings, there were no differences between Gavle and Sweden as a whole (see Table 35.1).

In the analysis of relations between combinations of background variables, and a group of effect-variables, some differences were found. Change of personal habits, unpleasant thoughts, and feelings of depression were significantly ($p < .05$) more pronounced among highly educated persons in the Gavle area. Moreover, elderly people in this area had significantly more unpleasant thoughts ($p < .05$). Married women with small children in Gavle were ($p < .01$) outdoors significantly less.

It was found that people with a moderate level of education and especially women, both in Gavle and in Sweden, were significantly more ($p < .05$) preoccupied by unpleasant thoughts and feelings. Furthermore, people in the Gavle area with high educational level were significantly ($p < .05$) more depressed. Moreover, there were important differences between age groups in Sweden concerning variables of information, reaction, and acting (see Table 35.2).

All variables of information, reaction, and feelings of being discriminated against were significantly

Table 35.1. Percentage of Differences between Sweden and Gavle for Some Important Variables

Item	Sweden ($n = 840$)	Gavle ($n = 216$)	Difference
Negative about nuclear power in referendum 10 years earlier	33.7	28.8	
Earlier psychological problems	10.0	11.5	
Somatic health problems	15.4	16.6	
Good comprehension of information from mass media	73.5	61.6	$p < .01$
Good knowledge on self-protection against nuclear radiation	39.2	28.4	$p < .05$
High confidence in information	55.3	41.3	$p < .001$
Concerned about radiation injuries to oneself	41.1	39.8	
Concerned about radiation injuries to close relatives	60.5	64.5	
Unpleasant thoughts about the disaster	38.9	35.9	
Preoccupation by thoughts and feelings	36.4	42.6	
Feeling of being able to overcome unpleasant thoughts	41.7	42.5	
Depressive feelings	6.2	8.2	
Being less outdooors after the disaster	5.5	14.0	$p < .001$
Allowing children to be less outdoors	10.0	27.4	$p < .001$
Abolition of nuclear power as soon as possible	61.5	70.1	$p < .05$

different between men and women. Women were more negative than men to the official information, changed their personal habits more, and had more negative thoughts and feelings (see Table 35.3).

There were significant differences between the threat index (measured as low, medium, and high) versus how the threat was perceived, the level of comprehension, and the degree of depression. A *high perception of threat* was associated with negative feelings about the accident and the Swedish nuclear power program; there was more concern about close relatives and with bad comprehension and knowledge about the disaster (see Table 35.4).

People with previous mental health problems were significantly ($p < .01$) less concerned with radiation injuries to themselves, but had more ($p < .01$) depressive

Table 35.2. ANOVA for Age Groups in Sweden Concerning Variables of Information, Reaction, and Acting[a]

Item	Age				Difference
	To 29	30–49	50 64	65+	
Comprehension of information from mass media	2.84 (n = 166)	2.98 (n = 333)	2.81 (n = 159)	2.82 (n = 166)	$p < .01$
Knowledge on self-protection against nuclear radiation	2.23 (n = 165)	2.33 (n = 339)	2.17 (n = 160)	1.89 (n = 159)	$p < .001$
Estimate of the quality of the information	2.12 (n = 155)	2.38 (n = 327)	2.42 (n = 155)	2.46 (n = 142)	$p < .01$
Preoccupation by thoughts and feelings	1.28 (n = 167)	1.37 (n = 340)	1.43 (n = 162)	1.38 (n = 169)	$p < .05$
Abolition of nuclear power as soon as possible	1.57 (n = 167)	1.57 (n = 340)	1.67 (n = 162)	1.70 (n = 169)	$p < .01$

[a]Only significant differences are reported.

thoughts and a higher ($p < .05$) degree of depression. People with mental health problems in the Gavle area had significantly ($p < .05$) more unpleasant thoughts about the disaster, were more depressed, and they spent less time outdoors after the disaster (see Table 35.5).

Patterns of Reactions

With the use of the latent profile analysis (Gibson, 1959), nine patterns of reactions (profiles) for Sweden were found (see Table 35.6). These profiles had the following specific characteristics.

Table 35.3. Differences between Sexes in Sweden Concerning Variables of Information, Reaction, and Acting[a]

Item	Range	Men	Women	Difference
Comprehension	1–4	3.02 n = 369	2.78 n = 546	$p < .001$
Knowledge on self protection against nuclear radiation	1–4	2.39 n = 368	2.04 n = 456	$p < .001$
Estimation of the quality of the information	1–4	2.47 n = 356	2.26 n = 425	$p < .01$
Confidence in information	1–4	2.65 n = 358	2.49 n = 432	$p < .01$
Abolition of nuclear power as soon as possible	1–2	1.47 n = 375	1.73 n = 465	$p < .001$
Concerned about radiation injuries to oneself	1–2	1.35 n = 375	1.46 n = 465	$p < .001$
Concerned about radiation injuries to close relatives	1–2	1.52 n = 375	1.67 n = 465	$p < .001$
Affected by thoughts and feelings	1–2	1.87 n = 375	1.96 n = 465	$p < .001$
Preoccupation with thoughts and feelings	1–2	1.28 n = 375	1.43 n = 465	$p < .001$
Depressive thoughts	1–2	1.25 n = 375	1.37 n = 465	$p < .001$
Unpleasant thoughts about the disaster	1–3	1.93 n = 371	1.57 n = 461	$p < .001$
Feeling of being able to overcome unpleasant thoughts	1–4	2.27 n = 89	2.75 n = 160	$p < .001$
Degree of depression	1–4	1.36 n = 366	1.64 n = 447	$p < .001$
Changing of personal habits	1–2	1.16 n = 375	1.33 n = 465	$p < .001$
Being outdoors less after the disaster	1–2	1.97 n = 369	1.92 n = 457	$p < .01$

[a]All variable show significant differences.

Table 35.4. Differences in Sweden between Threat Index
and Variables of Perception and Experience[a]

Item	Range (n = 246)	Low (n = 281)	Medium (n = 313)	High	Difference
Comprehension	1–4	2.98	2.88	2.82	$p < .05$
Knowledge of self-protection	1–2	2.40	2.17	2.06	$p < .001$
Abolition of nuclear power as soon as possible	1–2	1.50	1.65	1.67	$p < .001$
Concerned about radiation injuries to close relatives	1–2	1.51	1.63	1.66	$p < .001$
Affected by thoughts and feelings	1–2	1.86	1.93	1.96	$p < .001$
Preoccupation with thoughts and feelings	1–2	1.29	1.36	1.43	$p < .01$
Depressive thoughts	1–2	1.23	1.31	1.38	$p < .001$
Unpleasant thoughts about the disaster	1–3	1.93	1.71	1.59	$p < .001$
Feeling of being able to overcome unpleasant thoughts[a]	1–4	2.22	2.60	2.73	$p < .05$
Degree of depression	1–4	1.32	1.50	1.67	$p < .001$
Estimation of threat from the Chernobyl accident	1–3	2.30	2.59	2.73	$p < .001$

[a]The result for this item is based on fewer respondents: low: $n = 54$, medium: $n = 82$, high: $n = 113$.

Profile 1 (n = 43)

In this group people wanted to abolish nuclear power as soon as possible. They had unpleasant thoughts and feelings and spent less time outdoors. They had changed their personal habits.

Profile 2 (n = 164)

The persons in this group did not want to abolish nuclear power. Only a few persons had depressive thoughts. They were not concerned about radiation injuries to themselves or to close relatives. Although they had few unpleasant thoughts and feelings, they did not find the Chernobyl accident to be a threat. They did not change their personal habits.

Profile 3 (n = 134)

This group was average in all variables except three, which were higher than mean values: unpleasant

Table 35.5. Differences in Some Variables between People
with and *without* Previous Mental Health Problems[a]

Item	Space	Previous mental health problems		Difference
		Yes	No	
		Sweden		
Concerned about radiation injuries to oneself	1–2	1.28 n = 83	1.43 n = 738	$p < .01$
Depressive thoughts	1–2	1.44 n = 82	1.31 n = 738	$p < .01$
Degree of depression	1–4	1.69 n = 81	1.49 n = 722	$p < .05$
		Gavle		
Unpleasant thoughts about the disaster	1–3	1.50 n = 24	1.75 n = 182	$p < .05$
Degree of depression	1–4	2.08 n = 24	1.53 n = 181	$p < .001$
Being outdoors less after the disaster	1–2	1.71 n = 24	1.88 n = 180	$p < .05$

[a]Only significant differences are reported.

Table 35.6. Patterns of Reactions Found by Help of Latent Profile Analysis[a]

Profile	Unpleasant thoughts and feelings	Depressive thoughts	Threat experience	Concerned about radiation injuries to oneself	Close relatives	Knowledge on self-protection	Estimation of the quality of information	Being less outdoors	Changing of habits	Abolition of nuclear power program
1 (n = 43)	+							+	+	+
2 (n = 164)	−	−	−	−	−				−	−
3 (n = 134)	+	+							+	
4 (n = 114)	−		+	−	−					−
5 (n = 177)				+	+				−	
6 (n = 72)		+		−					−	+
7 (n = 19)		−	+	−	+	+	+			
8 (n = 84)		−	+	−		−	−		−	+
9 (n = 33)	+	−	+	+	+	−	−			

[a]Differences between profiles and total means more than 40 in standardized scores are marked by + or −, respectively.

thoughts and feelings, depressive thoughts, and change of personal habits.

Profile 4 *(n = 114)*

The people in this group were characterized by no anxiety or unpleasant thoughts; they did not want to abolish nuclear power. Even though they experienced an overwhelming threat from the Chernobyl accident, they were not concerned about radiation injuries to themselves or to their close relatives.

Profile 5 *(n = 177)*

People in this group were strongly concerned about radiation injuries to themselves or to their close relatives. None had changed their personal habits after the accident.

Profile 6 *(n = 72)*

These persons wanted to abolish nuclear power as soon as possible. They were less concerned about being injured than the average person, but they had a high degree of depressive thoughts. Not one had changed his or her personal habits.

Profile 7 *(n = 19)*

People in this group had a good knowledge of self-protection and found the information sufficient. They were not especially concerned about radiation injuries to themselves, but were more concerned about their close relatives. The variable "depressive thoughts" was scored low, but the threat from Chernobyl was perceived as rather high.

Profile 8 *(n = 84)*

This particular group was characterized by a wish to abolish nuclear power as soon as possible. These people had poor knowledge of self-protection and found the information negative. They were not concerned about injuries and had a low degree of depressive thoughts. Although the threat from Chernobyl was perceived as high, only a few had changed their personal habits.

Profile 9 *(n = 33)*

People in this group had poor knowledge of self-protection. They found the information negative and were very concerned about radiation injuries to themselves and to their close relatives. They had unpleasant thoughts and feelings but no depressive thoughts. The Chernobyl accident was perceived as threatening.

Discussion

The attitude in Sweden toward nuclear power is influenced by the current political situation and the rela-

tively great possibility of using hydroelectric power. Many peace organizations have pointed out the connections between nuclear power and nuclear weapons. Also, many people in Sweden experience an impending threat from air and water pollution. The discussions in the mass media and among individuals have fluctuated in intensity since the referendum on the Swedish nuclear power program.

It is of interest to note that the first indications of the Chernobyl accident outside the USSR came from the measurement of an increase in nuclear activity around one of the Swedish nuclear power plants. This news reactivated the feeling of threat for a great many people. Another rationale for investigating the psychological and psychiatric effects in Sweden were the special circumstances: The threatening agent was introduced from abroad and there was no possibility to avoid the disastrous situation. The fallout of nuclear material has also special psychological implications because it cannot be registered by a person's sense organs. The experience of threat will therefore be an effect of the information provided by the government and by other authorities, mostly that presented by the mass media.

One aim of this study was to try to compare a high risk area with the whole of Sweden. It was difficult, however, to find any outstanding differences, except for those in educational level and those attributable to the very unclear official information that was released during the first weeks after the Chernobyl accident. The importance of the reliability of the information was significantly lower in the high-risk area of Gavle, which might be an effect of the lower level of education of the county's people and can be compared with the findings (Baum, Gatchel, & Schaeffer, 1983) that living near a nuclear power plant resulted in a higher frequency of reported symptoms of distress and anxiety. More adequate information is needed when the stress level is high; the information provided could not meet this need.

In the Gavle area, parents with small children allowed their children to be outdoors less. A similar result was reported (Bromet, Parkinson, Schulberg, Dunn, & Gondek, 1982) after the Three Mile Island accident, where mothers of preschool children had more episodes of anxiety and depression. Furthermore, middle-aged individuals seemed to have the best comprehension of information from the mass media and the best knowledge about self-protection against nuclear radiation. It is also interesting to note that elderly people were more emotionally affected. It is well known that elderly people constitute a high-risk group in disaster situations (Green *et al.*, 1985; Maddison & Walker, 1967; Parkes, 1972; Raphael, 1983, 1986). The most outstanding differences concerning variables of information reaction and acting were found between gender, which is consistent with other studies on bereavement (Lundin, 1984a, 1987; Parkes, 1964a; Raphael, 1973, 1986) and threat (Lindstrom & Lundin, 1982; Lundin & Otto, 1991; Weisæth, 1984). Thus, a high threat index might be the result of low education and poor knowledge as well as a result of high vulnerability to threat and psychological trauma. Psychological reactions among these individuals might have been overdetermined by previous personal crises. This hypothesis might explain the higher preoc-

cupation with thoughts and feelings, with more unpleasant thoughts, and with the higher degree of depression. For example, those interviewees who had
previous mental health problems were generally more
affected by the Chernobyl disaster. Such circumstances
have earlier been reported by other authors (Green *et al.*,
1985; Lundin & Otto, 1991; Pilowsky, 1985; Raphael,
1983; Shalit, 1986; Shore, Tatum, & Vollmer, 1986).

These patterns of reactions emerged with latent profile analysis and might provide a way to identify groups
at risk and under threat after a disaster. They should be
helpful as well for planning the prevention of inappropriate behavior during a disaster and ineffective coping methods afterward.

Conclusions

The aim of this investigation was to show the relationships between (1) emotional reactions of people to
the Chernobyl accident and living in a high-risk area,
and (2) the emotional reactions of these people to the
accident and the variables of gender, educational level,
structuring ability, general threshold for threat perception, and coping potential.

Negative emotional reactions and the perception of
Chernobyl's threat to individuals were predicted by living in a high-risk zone, gender, educational level, structuring ability, general threshold for threat perception,
and coping potential.

People in the high-risk zone of Gavle showed
stronger negative reactions to the accident and higher
frequencies of changed personal habits than did people
in the whole country of Sweden, indicating the effect of
the objectively registered high-risk situation. Furthermore, women showed stronger negative reactions
against the accident than did men. A possible speculation is that stronger association with children, pregnancy, and other biological life processes generate a greater
emotional sensitivity to life-threatening events in wom-
en, particularly events of this kind. It was, however,
mostly women who, although feeling more anxious than
men, tended to cope actively with the Chernobyl threat.

There are also other possible reasons for the differences between men and women: (1) different attitudes
with regard to what kind of information is relevant;
(2) different traditions in viewpoints about the importance of new techniques in society; and (3) different
technical knowledge about nuclear processes because of
differences in education.

It seemed possible to predict the level of the reaction
to specific threat on the basis of a general disposition
toward the perception of the threat. For people in the
high-risk zone, educational background affected the adequacy of available information. All groups at the university level of education tended to perceive the threat
as less threatening than people with lower educational
levels. In a related finding, structuring ability turned out
to be an effective variable in predicting the reactions to
the accident: the poorer inferred structuring ability, the
stronger the negative reactions.

Although the study was performed only two weeks
after the accident, it has to be assumed that people had

time to analyze different cognitive aspects of the accident, and that they tried to reduce emotional reactions
by looking for more information and relating to alternative coping strategies.

References

Baum, A., Gatchel, R. J., & Schaeffer, M. A. (1983). Emotional,
behavioral and psychological effects of chronic stress at Three
Mile Island. *Journal of Consulting and Clinical Psychology, 51*(4),
565–572.
Bennet, G. (1970). Bristol floods 1968. Controlled survey of
effects on health of local community disaster. *British Medical
Journal, 3*, 454–458.
Bjorklund, B. (1991). The landslide in Tuve: The families and
their dwellings [Swedish text with a summary in English].
Disaster Studies, Uppsala University, Sweden.
Boman, B. (1977). Behavior observations on the Granville train
disaster and the significance of stress for psychiatry. *Social
Science Medicine, 13*, 463–471.
Bromet, E., Parkinson, D. K., Schulberg, H. C., Dunn, L. O., &
Gondek, P. C. (1982). Mental health of residents near the
Three Mile Island reactor: A comparative study of selected
groups. *Journal of Preventative Psychiatry, 1*(3), 225–876.
Brown, J. T. (1986). Grief response in trauma patients and their
families. *Advances in Psychosomatic Medicine, 16*, 93–114.
Carlstedt, L., & Carlstedt, B. (1985). Perception and coping dur-
ing the Karlskoga gas accident [Swedish text with a summary
in English]. FAO Report C 50031-H3, Stockholm, Sweden.
Cowan, M. E., & Murphy, S. A. (1985). Identification of
postdisaster bereavement risk predictors. *Nursing Research,
34*(2), 71–75.
Fleming, R., Baum, A., Gisriel, M., & Gatchel, R. J. (1982, September). Mediating influences of social support on stress at
Three Mile Island. *Journal of Human Stress*, 14–19.
Gibson, W. A. (1959). Three multivariate models: Factor analysis, latent structure analysis and latent profile analysis. *Psy-
chometrica, 24*, 229–252.
Gleser, G. C., Green, B. L., & Winget, C. (1981). *Prolonged
psychosocial effects of disaster: A study of Buffalo Creek*. New York:
Academic Press.
Glick, I. O., Weiss, R. S., & Parkes, C. M. (1974). *The first year of
bereavement*. New York: Wiley.
Goldsteen, R., & Schorr, J. K. (1982). The long-term impact of a
man-made disaster: An examination of a small town in the
aftermath of the Three Mile Island nuclear reactor accident.
Disasters, 6(1), 50–59.
Green, B. L., Grace, M. C., Lindy, J. D., Titchener, J. L., &
Lindy, J.G. (1983). Levels of functional impairment following
a civilian disaster: The Beverly Hills Supper Club fire. *Journal
of Consulting and Clinical Psychology, 51*(4), 573–580.
Green, B. L., Grace, M. C., & Gleser, G. C. (1985). Identifying
survivors at risk: Long-term impairment following the Bev-
erly Hills Supper Club fire. *Journal of Consulting and Clinical
Psychology, 53*(5), 672–678.
Grinker, R. R., & Spiegel, J. (1945). *Men under stress*. Phila-
delphia, PA: Blakiston.
Holen, A., Sund, A., Weisæth, L., & Alexander, L. (1983).
*Kiellandkatastrofen 27 mars 1980. De over levende og redningsper-
sonellet*. Division of Disaster Psychiatry, Oslo University,
Oslo, Norway.
Larsson, G. (1986). *Stress reaction among civilians and rescue per-*

sonnel at the gas accident in Karlskoga in 1985 [Swedish text with a summary in English]. FAO Report C 50035-H3, Stockholm, Sweden.

Lazarus, R. (1966). *Psychological stress and the coping process.* New York: McGraw-Hill.

Lifton, R. J., & Olson, E. (1976). The human meaning of total disaster: The Buffalo Creek experience. *Psychiatry, 39*, 1–18.

Lindstrom, B., & Lundin, T. (1982). Occupational exposure to disaster [Swedish text with summary in English]. *Nordisk Psykiatrika tidskrift, 36*: Supplement 6.

Lopez-Ibor, J. J., Jr., Soria, J., Canas, F., & Rodriguez-Gamazo, M. (1985). Psychopathological aspects of the toxic oil syndrome catastrophe. *British Journal of Psychiatry, 147*, 352–365.

Lundin, T. (1984a). Long-term outcome of bereavement. *British Journal of Psychiatry, 145*, 424–428.

Lundin, T. (1984b). Morbidity following sudden and unexpected bereavement. *British Journal of Psychiatry, 144*, 84–88.

Lundin, T. (1987). The stress of unexpected bereavement. *Stress Medicine, 3*, 109–114.

Lundin, T., & Otto, U. (1991). Acute post-traumatic stress reactions to an industrial gas-leakage disaster. Unpublished manuscript.

Maddison, D., & Walker, W. (1967). Factors affecting the outcome of conjugal bereavement. *American Journal of Psychiatry, 113*, 1057–1067.

McFarlane, A. C., & Raphael, B. (1984). Ash Wednesday: The effects of a fire. *Australian and New Zealand Journal of Psychiatry, 18*, 341–351.

Menninger, W. C. (1952). Psychological reactions in emergency. *American Journal of Psychiatry, 109*, 128.

Parkes, C. M. (1964a). Recent bereavement as a cause of mental illness. *British Journal of Psychiatry, 110*, 198–204.

Parkes, C. M. (1964b). The effects of bereavement on physical and mental health: A study of the medical records of widows. *British Medical Journal, 2*, 274–279.

Parkes, C. M. (1972). *Bereavement: Studies of grief in adult life.* London: Tavistock.

Parkes, C. M., & Weiss, R. S. (1983). *Recovery from bereavement.* New York: Basic Books.

Pilowsky, I. (1985). Cryptotrauma and "accident neurosis." *British Journal of Psychiatry, 147*, 310–311.

Raphael, B. (1983). *The anatomy of bereavement.* New York: Basic Books.

Raphael, B. (1986). *When disaster strikes: How individuals and communities cope with catastrophe.* New York: Basic Books.

Raphael, B., Lundin, T., & Weisæth, L. (1989). A research method for the study of psychological and psychiatric aspects of disaster. *Acta Psychiatrica Scandinavica, 80*,000–000.Raphael, B., Singh, B., Branbury, L., & Lambert, F. (1983–1984). Who helps the helpers: The effects of a disaster on the rescue workers. *Omega, 14*, 9–20.

Schwebel, M., & Schwebel, M. A. (1981). Children's reactions to the threat of nuclear plant accidents. *American Journal of Orthopsychiatry, 51*(2), 260–270.

Shalit, B. (1986). *The perception of threat by a noxious gas accident and the reported coping style.* FAO Report C 50036-H3, Stockholm, Sweden.

Shore, J. H., Tatum, E. L., & Vollmer, W. M. (1986). Psychiatric reactions to disaster: The Mount St. Helens experience. *American Journal of Psychiatry, 143*(5), 590–595.

Sills, D. L., Wolf, C. P., & Shelanski, U. B. (Eds.). (1982). *Accident at Three Mile Island: The human dimensions.* Boulder, CO: Westview Press.

Singh, B., & Raphael, B. (1981). Postdisaster morbidity of the bereaved. *Journal of Nervous Mental Disorder, 169*(4), 203–212.

Syren, S. (1981). *The Tuve landslide: Organized activities* [Swedish text with a summary in English]. *Disaster Studies*, Uppsala University, Sweden.

Titchener, J., & Kapp, F. (1976). Family and character change at Buffalo Creek. *American Journal of Psychiatry, 133*(3), 2195–2199.

Weisæth, L. (1984). *Stress reactions to an industrial disaster.* Unpublished doctoral thesis, Oslo University, Oslo, Norway.

CHAPTER 36

The Buffalo Creek Disaster

A 14-Year Follow-Up

Mary C. Grace, Bonnie L. Green, Jacob D. Lindy, and Anthony C. Leonard

Introduction

The collapse of the Buffalo Creek dam and subsequent flood disaster has received a great deal of attention in the literature since its occurrence in 1972. Previous reports of that disaster covered its legal (Stern, 1976), sociological (Erikson, 1976), and psychological (Gleser, Green, & Winget, 1981; Titchener & Kapp, 1976) aspects.

Initial accounts of the event showed high levels of psychological symptomatology and impairment present among the 381 adult survivors who sued the Pittston Coal Company, which built the dam, at a point 2 years after the flood. A subset of these survivors who were followed up to 5 years after the disaster demonstrated reduced but clinically significant impairment (Gleser et al., 1981). Based on these findings, we were extremely interested in determining how the group was faring many years later.

Our purpose then in this chapter is to describe our efforts to locate and conduct follow-up interviews with these survivors some 14 years after the disaster to determine whether or not there were long-lasting psychological effects of the dam collapse over a decade later.

Mary C. Grace, Jacob D. Lindy, and Anthony C. Leonard • Traumatic Stress Study Center, Department of Psychiatry, University of Cincinnati College of Medicine, Cincinnati, Ohio 45267–0539. Bonnie L. Green • Department of Psychiatry, Georgetown University School of Medicine, Washington, DC 20007–2197.

International Handbook of Traumatic Stress Syndromes, edited by John P. Wilson and Beverley Raphael. Plenum Press, New York, 1993.

Long-Term Psychological Consequences of Disaster

Literature on long-term effects of catastrophic events has its roots in studies of World War II survivors. Krystal (1968) and Niederland (1968) both wrote extensive clinical accounts detailing the chronic problems of holocaust survivors. Following these came more systematic studies which demonstrated that holocaust survivors, although not necessarily suffering severe impairment, did show continued psychological effects of their earlier experiences (Eaton, Sigal, & Weinfield, 1982; Matussek, 1975). Similarly, POWs from World War II were shown to have high rates of posttraumatic stress disorder (PTSD) (32% of moderate or marked) over 40 years after their war experience (Elder & Clipp, 1988).

Reports on long-term survivors of nonwar traumatic events also have shown chronic psychological effects of these events, such as a marine collision (Leopold & Dillon, 1963) and a mine collapse (Ploeger, 1972). Beginning in the early 1980s, a number of studies reported on the long-term psychological consequences of the Vietnam War, which had concluded in 1975. Combat veterans were repeatedly shown to have a greater number of psychological problems than did their peers who had not seen combat (cf. Card, 1983; Kulka, Schlenger, Fairbank, Hough, Jordan, Marmar, & Weiss, 1988; Laufer, 1985). Several of these studies were also able to link aspects of the soldiers' combat experience to specific types of psychological impairment, including posttraumatic stress disorder (Foy, Sipperelle, Rueger, & Carroll, 1984; Green, Lindy, Grace, & Gleser, 1989; Green, Grace, Lindy, Gleser, & Leonard, 1991; Laufer, Gallops, & Frey-Wouters, 1984).

Longitudinal studies of survivors of catastrophic events are less prevalent in the trauma literature than cross-sectional, descriptive studies. Those that have been done have not, for the most part, focused on long-term follow-up to assess the chronic effects of the traumatic event and explore differential symptom patterns at different phases of the recovery process. Nonetheless, the studies that do exist provide some evidence for decrease in psychological problems over time. For example, survivors of Cyclone Tracy were found to evidence a significantly decreased percentage of probable psychiatric cases in the period from 1 week to 14 months (Parker, 1977) even though, compared to the non-traumatized population, they sustained a higher psychiatric morbidity over time. A longitudinal study of Israeli combat veterans found a significant decrease in overall stress response symptoms from 1 to 2 years in addition to a decline in intrusive symptoms for the same period (see Chapter 27, in this volume, for a description of these reactions).

Previous studies by the University of Cincinnati Traumatic Stress Study Center on first-decade effects of the Buffalo Creek dam collapse (Gleser *et al.*, 1981) as well as the Beverly Hills Supper Club fire (Green, Grace, & Gleser, 1985) showed a general decrease in psychopathology over time. However, it was also the case that several specific types of pathology (e.g., hostility, alcohol abuse) actually increased from the first to the second assessment.

A number of other studies have also observed these phenomena of a decrease in some symptoms and an increase in others over time (Sales, Baum, & Shore, 1984; Tierney & Baisden, 1979). Most of these studies show that groups of survivors do not return to nonclinical levels of impairment in all aspects of psychological functioning, even after a number of years (McFarlane, 1988; Phifer, Kaniasty, & Norris, 1988). These findings suggest a potential latency period for some specific types of distress (i.e., hostility, alcoholism) as well as a potential waxing and waning of distress throughout the recovery process.

Taken together, there is some evidence from these studies that there is a natural history of stress response in the first several years following a disaster and that in general this includes a tendency for most symptoms to decrease over time. It remains unclear if and for whom this decline in psychopathology persists through the second decade. Thus, our intent is to take up that question as it applies to the 14-year follow-up of the adult survivors of the Buffalo Creek dam collapse and flood.

Methodology

Background to the Present Study

The Disaster and the Lawsuit

Buffalo Creek is a small mining community located on an 18-mile valley in Logan County, West Virginia. In February of 1972, it had been raining for several days, and there was concern about the safety of the slag dam at the top of the valley, which had been built by a mining company. The coal company had assured residents that there was nothing awry. Early Saturday morning, the

26th, the dam gave way, pouring millions of gallons of water and black sludge into the narrow valley below. It was several hours before the last of the flood waters had emptied into the Guyandotte River, leaving 125 people dead and several thousand homeless. Many weeks later, the worst of the debris was still being cleared away. Ill-conceived relocation efforts also compounded the trauma and probably increased the risk for subsequent problems (Drabek, 1986). These included the separation of kin and nuclear families, multiple relocations, and the decision of the West Virginia government to build a new highway up the middle of the valley, preventing many people from returning to their land. The situation in the valley did not fully stabilize until several years later.

A number of residents blamed the Pittston Corporation for building a poorly constructed slag dam in a negligent manner. They joined in a lawsuit against the company which included claims of "psychic impairment" as well as property damage and wrongful death. The Department of Psychiatry of the University of Cincinnati participated in this suit on the side of the plaintiffs and conducted extensive diagnostic psychiatric interviews with 381 adults and 207 children. A psychiatrist for the defense examined all parties as well. The interviews were conducted between 18 and 26 months postflood. The two sets of reports based on these interviews were rated by our research team for psychopathology. A self-report checklist was also collected. An extensive account of the levels of psychopathology, as well as the prediction of that pathology from certain aspects of the experience (e.g., extent of bereavement, life threat) for both adults and children can be found elsewhere (Gleser *et al.*, 1981; Green & Gleser, 1983).

In the summer of 1974, the suit was settled out of court (Stern, 1976) and awards for psychological damages were made to the plaintiffs. Research teams from the Traumatic Stress Center made four trips back to Buffalo Creek after the settlement (1975–1977) to assess the status of a subset of the plaintiffs.

In 1986, with support from a grant from the National Institute of Mental Health (NIMH), we returned to reinterview many of the original 381 adults. This report describes the residents we were able to locate and who agreed to participate in the study and specifically addresses the changes that occurred in these residents during the past 14 years.

Procedure

Four trips were made to the Buffalo Creek valley and one trip to the Cabin Creek–Big Coal River area to collect research data. This latter area was used as a comparison sample of an Appalachian coal-mining community which had not had a flood. The trips were made between February and July of 1986 and lasted from 6 to 9 days each. The follow-up included individuals living in the valley as well as some who had moved within a 60-mile radius. Interviews were conducted in the subjects' homes or in the local health center. Because of the potential for arousing distress, subjects were provided referral information about the local mental health clinic when appropriate.

Interviewers

Interviewers were seven women and four men. Six were students in clinical psychology. Extensive interviewer training was conducted, including sensitization to the culture and general trauma experience of the survivors, training in administration and scoring of the SCID (see Chapter 15, in this volume, for a review), the Psychiatric Evaluation Form (PEF), and the Impact of Events Scale (IES), and practice interviews among the interviewers and with patients from our outpatient clinic. Each interviewer made at least two of the five data-collection trips, and six interviewers made all five trips.

Instruments

Structured Clinical Interview for DSM-III (SCID) (Spitzer & Williams, 1986). This diagnostic interview is designed to be used by individuals with clinical training. It covers all major Axis I diagnoses and has been modified to address most of the DSM-III-R criteria. The version we used contained all of the III-R symptoms for PTSD except sense of foreshortened future (denial criterion, C) and physiological reactivity (increased arousal, D). Consequently, only two "C" symptoms and one "D" symptom were required for a diagnosis of PTSD. The PTSD module was modified somewhat by our research team after several trials, since the original did not effectively distinguish between intrusive images and voluntary recollections. Our modified version, with the additional symptoms (DSM-III-R), was subsequently adopted in the general interview schedule and was used in the validation portion of a national study of Vietnam veterans (Kulka *et al.*, 1988).

The diagnosis of posttraumatic stress disorder in 1974 was made retrospectively based on a review of the diagnostic reports described earlier. Although there was no PTSD diagnosis in 1974, diagnosticians from both sides of the lawsuit were investigating the presence of transient stress reactions and traumatic neurosis. In order to receive a diagnosis in the present study of PTSD, we required evidence of one intrusion symptom, two avoidant or numbing symptoms, and one physiological arousal symptom from the earlier reports obtained in 1974.

Psychiatric Evaluation Form (PEF) (Endicott & Spitzer, 1972). The PEF consists of 19 clinical rating scales of different symptoms (e.g., anxiety, depression, suicidal thoughts, grandiosity, etc.) as well as a scale of overall severity. The scales range from one to six (none to extreme impairment). Ratings were made by the interviewer following the full SCID interview, and covered behavior and functioning in the past month. A few scales were dropped because of low interrater reliability or because they measured more severe pathology (e.g., grandiosity, inappropriate affect or behavior) and were rated "none" for virtually all subjects. Interrater reliability on the remaining scales ranged from .58 on anxiety to .90 for suspicion-persecution, with a figure of .66 for overall severity.

Symptom Checklist-90R (SCL-90R) (Derogatis, 1983). The SCL-90R is a 90-item self-report symptom inventory on which subjects indicate the degree to which they have been bothered by the symptoms during the past week. Nine subscale scores are calculated along with the Global Severity Index, a measure of average symptom distress. A 48-item precursor of the instrument, the Hopkins Symptom Checklist (Derogatis, Covi, Lipman, Davis, & Rickels, 1971), was used in the 1974 investigation. Several items from this instrument were added to the SCL-90 for the 1986 investigation so that direct comparisons could be made.

Impact of Events Scale (IES) (Horowitz, Wilner, & Alverez, 1979). This instrument consists of 15 statements which the subject is asked to rate in terms of their response to a stressful life event. The statements are divided into intrusion and avoidance subscales along the lines of the theoretical model proposed by Horowitz of the stress-response syndrome. The instrument has been used in a number of studies and has good reliability and validity.

Measures of Flood Stress. Ratings of various aspects of the individual's stressor experience during the dam collapse were made from information in the 1974 reports (bereavement, life threat, displacement) as well as from new information collected in 1986 which focused on more specific aspects of exposure (being blocked in escape, seeing dead bodies, exposure to elements).

Results

Characteristics of the Follow-Up Sample

Our first task was to locate and interview as many of the original 381 survivors as possible and to investigate the integrity of the original sample at a point approximately 14 years since the dam collapse. We were particularly interested in the question of selective attrition, determining whether or not specific demographic characteristics or stressor experiences influenced subjects' willingness or availability to participate in our follow-up interview (Green & Grace, 1988). One hundred twenty-one of the original 381 adult plaintiffs were located and completed a valid interview. Since 52 of the original plaintiffs had died, this figure represented 39% of the living survivors. Of those living survivors not interviewed, 33% were known to have moved out of state, 36% refused, and 32% were either not able to be accounted for, were never contacted, or were unable to be scheduled for an interview (Green & Grace, 1988).

When comparing demographic characteristics of completers versus refusers, there were no significant differences between the two groups with regard to age or education; however, there was a higher proportion of blacks from the original sample who participated in the follow-up. On the other hand, both age and education differentiated those who had moved away from the valley (they were younger and better educated at the time of the flood than those who remained). With regard to stressor experiences, bereavement (loss) scores were significantly higher for those who refused participation in the follow-up compared with those who participated. No differences were found with regard to other aspects of the stressor experience. With regard to psychopathology as assessed in 1974, there were no differences on any of the original psychopathology measures between those who were interviewed in 1986 and those who refused participation.

These findings suggested to us that those who volunteered in 1986 were a fairly representative subsample of the original sample. Concerns that only the sickest people might be interested in follow-up participation seem unwarranted.

Comparison of Litigant Survivors with Nonlitigant and Unexposed Groups

In order to investigate the potential differential effects of participation in legal activities on long-term psychological functioning, we located a sample of 78 individuals in Buffalo Creek who were exposed to the disaster but did not participate in the original lawsuit. In addition, a nonexposed group of 50 subjects from a geographically and culturally similar neighborhood were interviewed to serve as a comparison sample. Demographic characteristics of these three samples are included in

Table 36.1. Detailed comparison of these three samples are reported elsewhere (Green, Grace, Lindy, Gleser, Leonard, & Kramer, 1991).

Results indicated that Buffalo Creek residents did not differ based on their status regarding participation in the lawsuit, either demographically or on the global measures of psychopathology. Likewise, information obtained on degree of loss, life threat, and geographic displacement (stressor variables) did not significantly differentiate the two groups.

Because these two Buffalo Creek samples were similar, they were combined and compared to the Coal River/Cabin Creek comparison sample. This was done for white subjects only as there were no black subjects in the comparison sample. The Coal River group differed from Buffalo Creek survivors on age (older), education (greater), and percentage employed (greater). Since these demographic variables were slightly related to outcome, they were controlled for statistically in examining differences in psychopathology between the groups.

Tables 36.2 and 36.3 summarize significant findings with regard to type and level of psychopathology for the Buffalo Creek–Coal River comparison. On the clinically rated PEF, the Buffalo Creek survivors indicated significantly more depression and anxiety, as well as overall severity. On the self-report symptom checklist, differences were also in the areas of anxiety and depression with the exposed sample scoring higher. The SCL-90

Table 36.1. Demographic Variables by Percentage of Flood-Status Group

Variable	Litigants (n = 121)	Nonlitigants (n = 78)	Litigants and nonlitigants (whites only) (n = 145)	Nonexposed (n = 50)
Sex				
Male	39	31	34	48
Female	61	69	66	52
Race				
White	76	84	100	100
Black	24	16	0	0
Age	X̄ = 53.2	X̄ = 52.6	X̄ = 50.7	X̄ = 55.6[a]
	SD = 15.4	SD = 15.4	SD = 14.6	SD = 13.7
Marital status				
Married	73	64	75	77
Divorced/separated	5	4	5	4
Single	6	4	2	0
Widowed	16	28	18	19
Education				
No high school diploma	70	62	68	36
High school diploma	18	29	23	36
College+	12	9	9	28
Employment				
Employed	29	30	31	44
Disabled	19	8	13	18
Retired	12	9	10	24
House spouse	37	46	44	14
Other	3	7	2	0
Income				
Family	X̄ = 20,659	X̄ = 17,891	X̄ = 22,192	X̄ = 26,467
	SD = 14,201	SD = 11,965	SD = 14,220	SD = 17,228

[a]Category differed between combined Buffalo Creek group (white subjects only) and nonexposed group at p .05.

Table 36.2. Mean Psychiatric Impairment
for Buffalo Creek and Big Coal River Samples[a]

Selected PEF scales[b]	Buffalo Creek (n = 136)	Big Coal River (n = 50)	E[c]
Suicide	1.16	1.06	.02
Somatic	1.36	1.14	1.75
Social isolation	1.37	1.12	.73
Belligerence-negativism	1.08	1.04	.04
Anxiety	1.97	1.26	6.36*
Suspicion-persecution	1.14	1.08	.22
Denial of illness	1.09	1.12	.66
Depression	2.01	1.20	7.50*
Overall severity	1.89	1.17	5.24*

[a]1 (none) to 6 (extreme); white subjects only.
[b]Unadjusted means presented in table.
[c]Analysis of covariance (controlling for age, education, and employment).
*p .05.

Table 36.3. Mean Symptom Distress
for Buffalo Creek and Big Coal River Samples[a]

SCL-90R scales[b]	Buffalo Creek (n = 133)	Big Coal River (n = 48)	F[c]
Somatic	.99	.73	.39
Obsessive-compulsive	.95	.64	.75
Depression	.97	.52	1.70
Anxiety	.85	.46	1.30
Hostility	.61	.30	1.04
Phobic anxiety	.55	.13	3.39*
Psychoticism	.42	.21	.72
Paranoid ideation	.70	.47	.27
Interpersonal sensitivity	.65	.40	.17
Global Severity Index	.81	.48	1.34

[a]0 (not at all bothered) to 4 (extremely bothered); white subjects only.
[b]Unadjusted means presented in table.
[c]Analysis of covariance (controlling for age, education, and employment).
*p .07.

Global Severity Index (GSI) for the Coal River group was quite similar to a normative sample (Derogatis, 1983), whereas the GSI for the Buffalo Creek survivors fell between means reported for normals and psychiatric outpatients. Table 36.4 provides diagnostic information for the two groups. With regard to current diagnoses, Buffalo Creek survivors had significantly more depression and anxiety diagnoses. Approximately 65% of the Buffalo Creek survivors had a lifetime prevalence of a disaster-related diagnosis (PTSD, general anxiety disorder, and major depression) whereas only 36% of the comparison valley subjects had a lifetime prevalence of one of these three.

Stability and Change of Stress Symptoms over Time

In keeping with the longstanding interest among scientists in whether traumatic events can have psychological effects that last years or even decades, we were interested in tracing the natural history of the survivor's response to the stress of the flood into the second decade, focusing on longitudinal stability and change. As noted earlier, there is evidence in the literature that the natural history of stress reactions in the first several years includes a tendency for most symptoms to decrease over time. However, not all symptoms may decrease during this time for all groups of survivors and there is some question as to whether symptoms which increase in the short term can be expected to decrease later on. Longitudinal information on groups of survivors can begin to answer some of these questions.

It is these questions that were examined using the data we had on 121 survivors both in 1974 and 1986. In addition, for a subset of these survivors, there was an additional assessment 2 to 5 years postflood. These findings are reported in detail elsewhere (Green et al., 1990).

Results indicated that there were highly significant changes over the 12-year period with symptoms decreasing in all cases. On the PEF, the overall severity

ratings and the anxiety, depression, and belligerence cluster scores all decreased significantly for men and women. Self-reported symptom checklist scores for the 47 items administered at both points in time also showed a significant decrease. The reported rate of PTSD was 44% of the sample in 1974 and declined to 28% of the sample in 1986.

Focusing on the PTSD diagnosis, 28% of the sample went from having the diagnosis in 1974 to not having it in 1986, which fits well with the overall finding of decreased pathology over time. A group with "delayed" PTSD (11%) was also identified (no PTSD in 1974; met criteria in 1986) (Green et al., 1990).

When the data were analyzed by sex, it was found that the proportion of current PTSD decreased significantly from 1974 to 1986 for the women (21% decline) but

Table 36.4. Current Diagnostic Categories
by Percentage for Buffalo Creek
and Big Coal River Samples[a]

Diagnosis	Buffalo Creek (n = 135)	Big Coal River (n = 50)	F[b]
Major depression	21	2	4.04*
Dysthymic disorder	6	2	.55
Panic disorder	2	0	1.07
Social phobia	4	4	.10
Simple phobia	15	10	.03
Generalized anxiety disorder	18	2	3.98*
Substance abuse	5	6	.46
PTSD—current	23	8	.42
PTSD—lifetime	63	24	11.54*

[a]Based on the Structured Clinical Interview for DSM-III-R; white subjects only.
[b]Analysis of covariance (controlling for age, education, and employment).
*p .05.

not for the men (9% decline). Women also scored higher than men initially (1974) on both the clinical ratings and self-report, with the exception of belligerence and alcohol abuse. By 1986, however, scores for the two genders were nearly identical for the clinical ratings and women were slightly lower on the symptom checklist. Thus, the changes for women were more pronounced than those for the men.

Longitudinal Trends

As noted earlier, there was a subsample of 39 survivors on whom we had more than two follow-up interviews. In that subsample, the 1974 and 1986 data points were identical to the total group of 121 litigants suggesting that longitudinal trends observed for the subsample were probably applicable to the larger sample. Clinically rated PEF cluster scores showed a gradual decline from the 1974 presettlement period to the postsettlement period (1975–1977) to the 1986 evaluations. The overall severity rating decreased more sharply from pre-· to postsettlement and then more gradually from 1976 to 1986.

Changes in the self-report symptom checklist were similar to the Overall Severity rating with the greatest decline occurring between the settlement and the first follow-up, although there was additional significant decline through 1986.

Prediction of Psychopathology from Stressor Experiences

A major goal of our investigation was to delineate specific aspects of an individual's stressor experience and examine the degree to which these experiences predicted psychological impairment (both type and intensity) at a point 14 years following the Buffalo Creek slag dam collapse.

Stress ratings were assigned to the 381 original survivors in 1974 on the basis of a family narrative of the flood experience recounted in the reports of the University of Cincinnati examining team (on behalf of the litigants suing the coal company) and in the individual narratives provided in the examinations by the psychiatrist for the defense (on behalf of the coal company). Scales were: Bereavement (loss of friends, family, and possessions), S1 (the immediate life threat to the individual), S2 (the extent and duration of physical and psychological traumata within 2 weeks postflood), and displacement (geographically from home and community). Each of these stressor experiences was shown to be positively related to measures of psychopathology in 1974. The combined stress ratings accounted for almost 20% of the variance in overall severity 2 years after the flood. With respect to specificity of symptoms, depression and anxiety were predicted by bereavement and Sl for women, whereas only depression was correlated with bereavement for the men. In general, correlations with stress scales tended to be lower for men than for women.

Attempts to scale the immediate impact of the flood stress (S1) and the physical hardships of the two weeks following the flood (S2) were somewhat global in 1974,

resulting in low but significant correlations with psychopathology. Consequently, in the 1986 investigation, additional flood-experience data were collected from survivors which would more comprehensively delineate the various aspects of their flood experience. Using the new data as well as the two 1974 reports, 16 new stressor variables were created which could be grouped into *life threat* variables (i.e., amount of warning, injury, being blocked, exposure to extreme danger), *loss* (i.e., household members, immediate family, relatives, nonfamily members), and *exposure to the grotesque* (i.e., seeing or having contact with dead bodies). Reliability studies using these new stressor variables were successfully completed, and all 121 original litigants who participated in the current investigation as well as the 78 nonlitigants were rated.

Although there were numerous measures of psychopathology included in the 1986 investigation, preliminary analysis of the prediction of psychological status from stressor experience has been limited to intrusion and avoidance symptoms, seen as the hallmark of a traumatic stress response, and the presence of a current (1986) diagnosis of PTSD.

Correlations of individual stressor experiences with these outcomes are presented in Table 36.5. Since the stressor experiences were at least modestly related to each other, multiple regression analyses were used to obtain the weights of each type of stressor experience with the others held constant. The multiple regression analyses for the various flood stressors and psychopathology outcomes are presented in Table 36.6. The analyses were done in sets of variables using a hierarchical procedure with the life-threat set of variables entering first.

A number of points can be made from these data. The most striking finding is that certain aspects of the flood experience continue to be predictive of stress-response symptoms even after a period of 15 years. The various activities which pose a threat to the survivor's

Table 36.5. Relationships of 1986 Stressors with PTSD and Related Symptoms[a] for Litigants and Nonlitigants

Stress scale	Current PTSD	IES Intrusion	IES Avoidance
Life threat			
Amount of warning	10	6	11
In water during escape	13	8	20**
Blocked in escape	10*	13	16*
Injured	21**	14	14
Exposed to elements	30**	20**	15*
Loss			
Nonfamily members	−15*	−10	−8
Loss of household member	16*	17*	13
Loss of large number of people	5	8	7
Grotesque			
Saw dead bodies	20*	23**	14

[a]n = 198; decimals omitted.
*p .05.
**p .01.

Table 36.6. Regression Analyses for Selected Psychopathology Outcomes ($n = 180$)

Independent variable	Current PTSD	IES Intrusion	IES Avoidance
1986 life threat			
Multiple R (including life threat)	.33	.23	.23
R^2 (% variance explained)	11%	5%	5%
1986 loss			
Multiple R (including loss and life threat)	.36	.27	.25
R^2 (% variance explained)	13%	7%	6%
Grotesque			
Multiple R	.37	.30	.29
R^2 (% variance explained)	13%	9%	8%

life (exposure, injury, being blocked during escape) show the strongest associations with the diagnosis of PTSD. Bereavement (particularly loss of a household member) remains a significant predictor of outcome, both for PTSD diagnosis and for intrusion symptoms. Current avoidant symptoms, on the other hand, are not related to loss at the time of the flood, but are predicted by the degree of life threat, especially being in the water during escape or suffering extreme exposure to the elements. Seeing dead bodies, one of the grotesque experiences coded from the stressor data, was the best predictor of intrusive symptoms. When the various sets of stressor variables are considered in the regression analysis, the threat to life variables accounted for the major proportion of the variance. The actual amount of variance accounted for by these variables, however, is quite modest (PTSD 11%, Intrusion 5%, Avoidance 5%). Adding the loss variables and the exposure grotesque variable enhances these figures only slightly. It seems likely that over the course of 14 years, a number of other intervening variables (subsequent life events, coping styles) come into play in explaining the maintenance of symptoms.

These results do indicate that the natural history of response to trauma is a decrease in symptoms over time, although it is clear from the earlier results that subjects still had notable problems. The best predictors of current stress-response symptoms are the experiences associated with the threat to one's life and body integrity. These individual effects are modest in this sample but can be detected in the second decade in spite of the common stressors and recovery characteristics that all survivors experienced.

Discussion

Results of the 14-year follow-up study provide evidence that there is a gradual decrease in symptom distress as well as improvement in functioning among survivors of a man-made disaster over a 12-year period. These findings are in keeping with other reports in the literature (Green et al., 1981; Phifer et al., 1988; Sales et al., 1984), which have found a decrease in psychologic distress over shorter periods of time, and expand our understanding of survivors' responses over longer inter-

vals. They also provide evidence for the persistence of some amount of trauma-related psychopathology into the second decade. Several unique aspects of the current study allow a number of related issues to be addressed as well. One of these concerns the role of participation in a lawsuit as a factor which may affect psychological reaction to disaster.

As mentioned previously, many but not all members of the Buffalo Creek Community in the dam collapse were involved in the lawsuit. An early investigation of litigants and nonlitigants in 1974 found no differences in these groups with regard to level of pathology. As noted in this report, when litigants were again compared to a nonlitigant sample in 1986, no significant differences were found. One possible explanation for this finding is that the activity of the lawsuit, including visits to the valley by teams of expert interviewers and the giving of depositions kept the experience of the flood alive for everyone in this small, tightly knit community. It was also the case that a number of nonlitigants chose to be financially compensated in out-of-court settlements by the Pittston Coal Company in lieu of participation in the lawsuit. This decision was probably not based on a lack of psychological distress caused by the flood but rather an impatience with or lack of hopefulness in the legal process. Another possible explanation is that the ongoing community disruption caused by the relocation of housing and rebuilding of roads were a continued stressor for all members of the community, regardless of their legal status. It will be important in future studies of disasters that involve litigation to see if these findings extend to events which affect various types of socioeconomic communities similarly affected by a major disaster.

It should be noted, however, that there does seem to have been some benefit to participation in the lawsuit early in the course of recovery. Among the litigants who were followed at a 4-year postflood and a 2-year postflood settlement there was clearly some relief in symptoms following the settlement of the lawsuit with many survivors attributing their improved psychological functioning to the successful resolution of the lawsuit.

The current report also sheds new light on the question of who is willing to participate in follow-up studies of disaster survivors over a long period of time. Although no differences were found when completers were compared to refusers in terms of their initial distress scores (1974), there were differences found with regard to specific aspects of the individual's stressor experience. Specifically, this had to do with those survivors who had greater bereavement being more likely to refuse a follow-up interview in 1986. This finding points to the potential long-lasting effect of the death of a loved one on later functioning. It also suggests that people with extreme stressor experiences may decline participation in order to avoid reexposure to memories of the traumatic event. In any case, it seems clear that those who volunteer for continued follow-up are not necessarily the most stressed or the most impaired of the initial sample.

Demographic characteristics also determined who would be available for follow-up in the Buffalo Creek community. Education and age were both significant predictors of those who were unable to be followed up because they had moved from the valley. Probably this is due to the decrease in job opportunities in the coal-mining industry so central to Buffalo Creek. In many cases, younger people left the Buffalo Creek valley to find careers and jobs less dependent on mining which they perceived as both dangerous and limited in terms of future career opportunity.

Most important, however, is the notable decrease in distress and the improvement in functioning found in survivors followed over such a long period of time. Rates of PTSD decreased significantly, as did measures of subjective distress and clinically rated impairment. Nonetheless, when compared to a group of nonexposed residents in a comparison valley, it is clear that the effects of the flood are still present in some survivors. There are a number of possible explanations for this. To a small degree, the slag dam collapse and flood remains alive in Buffalo Creek even today. Residents of the valley continue to include discussions of it in their conversation. It is seen as a historical marker for the entire community with events, including births, deaths, marriages, and so forth, being classified as "before the flood" or "after the flood." Such daily reminders serve as renewed stressors, with some residents being moved to tears when thinking about the flood again. Given the small and somewhat tightly knit nature of the Buffalo Creek community, it is hard for residents to put their experiences of the flood completely behind them. An additional feature that may help explain the lack of complete recovery among survivors is the restricted range of social supports and coping strategies available to the residents. Since nearly everyone in the valley had been touched by the flood experience, it was difficult to find friends and relatives to turn to who were not also burdened by their own losses and traumata. Given the almost total destruction of the community, there were limited actions residents could take to improve their situations; rather they had to stand by helplessly and wait for the outside agencies to intervene on their behalf. All these factors would conceivably limit the possibility of complete recovery for some. Given the idiosyncratic nature of the Buffalo Creek community, it seems important to conduct long-term follow-up studies of other groups of survivors to see if similar patterns of recovery are found. Only in that way can we achieve greater understanding of chronic effects of major traumatic events.

References

Card, J. J. (1983). *Lives after Vietnam: The personal impact of military service*. Lexington, MA: D. C. Heath.

Derogatis, L. R. (1983). *SCL-90 revised version: Manual I*. Baltimore, MD: Johns Hopkins University.

Derogatis, L. R., Covi, L., Lipman, R. S., Davis, D. M., & Rickels, K. (1971). Social class and race as mediator variables in neurotic symptomatology. *Archives of General Psychiatry, 25*, 31–40.

Drabek, T. E. (1986). *Human system responses to disaster: An inventory of sociological findings*. New York: Springer-Verlag.

Eaton, W. W., Sigal, J. J., & Weinfeld, M. (1982). Impairment in Holocaust survivors after 33 years: Data from an unbiased community sample. *American Journal of Psychiatry, 139*, 773–777.

Elder, G. H., & Clipp, E. C. (1988). Wartime losses and social bonding: Influence across 40 years in men's lives. *Psychiatry, 51*(2), 177–198.

Endicott, J., & Spitzer, R. (1972). A diagnostic interview: The Schedule for Affective Disorders and Schizophrenia. *Archives of General Psychiatry, 35*, 837–844.

Erikson, K. T. (1976). *Everything in its path: Destruction of community in the Buffalo Creek flood*. New York: Simon & Schuster.

Foy, D., Sipperelle, R., Rueger, D., & Carroll, E. (1984). Etiology of post-traumatic stress disorder in Vietnam veterans: Analysis of premilitary, military, and combat exposure influences. *Journal of Consulting and Clinical Psychology, 52*, 79–87.

Gleser, G., Green, B. L., & Winget, C. (1981). *Prolonged psychosocial effects of disaster: A study of Buffalo Creek*. New York: Academic Press.

Green, B. L., & Gleser, G. C. (1983). Stress and long-term psychopathology in survivors of the Buffalo Creek disaster. In D. Ricks & B. S. Dohrenwend (Eds.), *Origins of psychopathology*. New York: Cambridge University Press.

Green, B. L., & Grace, M. C. (1988). Conceptual issues in research with survivors and illustrations from a follow-up study. In J. P. Wilson, Z. Harel, & B. Kahana (Eds.), *Human adaptation to extreme stress: From the Holocaust to Vietnam*. New York: Plenum Press.

Green, B. L., Grace, M. C., & Gleser, G. C. (1985). Identifying survivors at risk: Long-term impairment following the Beverly Hills Supper Club fire. *Journal of Consulting and Clinical Psychology, 53*, 672–678.

Green, B. L., Grace, M. C., & Gleser, G. C. (1989). Multiple diagnosis in post-traumatic stress disorder: The role of war stressors. *Journal of Nervous and Mental Disease, 177*, 329–335.

Green, B. L., Lindy, J. D., Grace, M. C., Gleser, G. C., Leonard, A. C., Korol, M., & Winget, C. (1990). Buffalo Creek survivors in the second decade: Stability of stress symptoms. *American Journal of Orthopsychiatry, 60*, 43–54.

Green, B. L., Grace, M. C., Lindy, J. D., Gleser, G. C., & Leonard, A. C. (1991). Risk factors for PTSD and other diagnoses in a general sample of Vietnam veterans. *American Journal of Psychiatry*.

Green, B. L., Grace, M. C., Lindy, J. D., Gleser, G. C., Leonard, A. C., & Kramer, T. L. (1990). Buffalo Creek survivors in the second decade: Comparison with unexposed and non-litigant groups. *Journal of Applied Social Psychology, 20*, 1033–1050.

Horowitz, M. J., Wilner, N., & Alvarez, W. (1979). Impact of Event Scale: A measure of subjective distress. *Psychosomatic Medicine, 41*, 209–218.

Krystal, H. (Ed.) (1968). *Massive psychic trauma*. New York: International Universities Press.

Kulka, R. A., Schlenger, W. E., Fairbank, J. A., Hough, R. L., Jordan, B. K., Marmar, C. R., & Weiss, D. S. (1988). *National Vietnam veterans readjustment study (NVVRS): Description, current status, and initial PTSD prevalence rates*. Research Triangle Park, NC: Research Triangle Institute.

Laufer, R. S. (1985). War trauma and human development: The Vietnam experience. In S. M. Sonnenberg, A. S. Blank, & J. A. Talbott (Eds.), *The trauma of war: Stress and recovery in Vietnam veterans*. Washington, DC: American Psychiatric Press.

Laufer, R. S., Gallops, M., & Frey-Wouters, E. (1984). War stress and trauma: The Vietnam veteran experience. *Journal of Health and Social Behavior, 25*, 65–85.

Leopold, R. L., & Dillon, H. (1963). Psychoanatomy of a disaster: A longterm study of post-traumatic neuroses in survivors of marine explosion. *American Journal of Psychiatry, 119*, 913–921.

Matussek, P. (1975). *Internment in concentration camps and its consequence*. New York: Springer-Verlag.

McFarlane, A. C. (1988). The longitudinal course of post-traumatic morbidity: The range of outcomes and their predictors. *Journal of Nervous and Mental Disease, 173*, 406–411.

Niederland, W. G. (1968). The problem of the survivor. In H. Krystal (Ed.), *Massive psychic trauma*. New York: International University Press.

Parker, G. (1977). Cyclone Tracy and Darwin evacuees: On the restoration of the species. *British Journal of Psychiatry, 130*, 548–555.

Phifer, J. F., Kaniasty, K. Z., & Norris, F. H. (1988). The impact of natural disaster on the health of older adults: A multiwave prospective study. *Journal of Health and Social Behavior, 29*, 65–78.

Ploeger, A. (1972). A ten-year followup of miners trapped for 2 weeks under threatening circumstances. In C. Spielberger & I. Sarason (Eds.), *Stress and anxiety (Vol. 4)*. New York: Wiley.

Sales, E., Baum, M., & Shore, B. (1984). Victim readjustment following assault. *Journal of Social Issues, 40*, 117–136.

Tierney, K. J., & Baisden, B. (1979). *Crisis intervention programs for disaster victims: A source-book and manual for smaller communities* (U.S. Department of Health, Education and Welfare Publication No. ADM 79–675). Washington, DC: U.S. Government Printing Office.

Titchener, J., & Kapp, F. T. (1976). Family and character change at Buffalo Creek. *American Journal of Psychiatry, 143*, 1443–1446.

Spitzer, R. L., & Williams, J. W. (1986). *Structured clinical interview for DSM-III: Non-patient version (SCID-NP-11-1-86)*. New York: Biometrics Research Department.

Stern, G. M. (1976). *The Buffalo Creek disaster: The story of the survivor's unprecedented lawsuit*. New York: Random House.

CHAPTER 37

The Kings Cross Fire

Early Psychological Reactions and Implications for Organizing a "Phase-Two" Response

Stuart W. Turner, James Thompson, and Rachel M. Rosser

Introduction

On November 18, 1987, at the end of the evening commuter rush hour, there was a major fire at Kings Cross Underground Railway station in London, England. Thirty-one people died, several hundred were present, and many more were affected by the experience. In the aftermath of this disaster, and in collaboration with the London Borough of Camden and local volunteer groups, we initiated a program of psychosocial responses for the survivors and the bereaved.

In this chapter, we present the circumstances of the fire, the development of this "phase-two" response to the psychosocial needs of the victims, and a description of the early psychological problems.

The Fire

The Underground Railway station at Kings Cross in London occupies a network of tunnels that serves five independent underground rail lines (the Piccadilly, the Victoria, the Northern, the Metropolitan, and the Circle

lines). Above the Underground station complex, there are connections to the overground railway system via three separate stations (Kings Cross, St. Pancras, and Thameslink). The underground station is unique in that it was built at five different levels below ground. At the time of the fire, it was the busiest station on the London Underground network. On an average weekday, over 250,000 passengers used the station, about 100,000 passing through each evening rush hour, between 4:00 P.M. and 6:30 P.M.

There are two features of the structure which require explanation. First, although at track level, the Piccadilly and Victoria lines appear to be some distance from each other, the exit (up) escalators from both services enter the same booking hall. In other words, they converge at the next higher level.

Second, the escalators on the Piccadilly line were of an old wooden construction. Below the tracks, there was an accumulation of grease and detritus which later tests demonstrated to be flammable. At the official inquiry, it was revealed that small-scale fires on this type of escalator were not unusual. In an earlier report, following a serious fire as long ago as 1947, it was disclosed that there had been 77 fires on this type of escalator between 1939 and 1944. As a consequence, water-fog equipment was fitted to many of the wooden escalator systems and was used initially on a daily basis, not as a major fire extinguisher, but rather to dampen the wooden structures and so extinguish any smoldering. Unfortunately, it was subsequently discovered that this caused excessive corrosion of the equipment. The practice was changed to a fortnightly spray which had become rather more infrequent in recent years.

Stuart W. Turner, James Thompson, and Rachel M. Rosser • Department of Psychiatry, University College and Middlesex School of Medicine, Wolfson Building, Middlesex Hospital, London W1N 8AA, England.

International Handbook of Traumatic Stress Syndromes, edited by John P. Wilson and Beverley Raphael. Plenum Press, New York, 1993.

These, then, are the events which took place on the fateful night on November 18, 1987. The timing and the detail in this description are taken from the official report into the Kings Cross fire (Fennell, 1988).

At 7:29 P.M., a passenger travelling on the up escalator from the Piccadilly line noticed a small fire and reported it to London Underground staff, who proceeded to investigate. At about 7:30 P.M., another passenger pressed the emergency button to stop these escalators and shouted to people to vacate the area. A policeman on duty in the underground station decided to call the fire service but as his radio was ineffective below ground, he had to travel to the surface to make his call (7:33 P.M.). Within three minutes of his call, London Fire Brigade had despatched four pump appliances, a turntable ladder and two control units (7:36 P.M.).

Meanwhile, the escalator was taped off, and at 7:39 P.M., the police officers in the station decided to evacuate the area. Passengers were directed to leave the Piccadilly line platforms and to travel by a normal communicating tunnel to the escalators serving the Victoria line. It was not appreciated that this would take them directly to the booking hall above the fire. At 7:40 P.M., the London Underground staff instructed trains not to stop at Kings Cross, and from 7:41 P.M., tickets were no longer sold. In fact, trains continued to stop and let out passengers until 7:43 P.M. on the Piccadilly line and 7:48 P.M. on the Northern line.

The first London Fire Brigade pump appliance arrived at 7:42 P.M. and the Fire Brigade Officers found a fire about the size of a large cardboard box on the Piccadilly line up escalator but with flames licking up the escalator handrail. Firemen with breathing apparatus and a jet were told to respond to the fire. Very rapidly, however, the ticket hall at the top of the escalator became engulfed in intense heat and filled with thick black smoke. At 7:45 P.M. there was a sudden flashover in the ticket hall. Witnesses saw a jet of flames shoot up the escalator shaft, and the hall was hit by a fireball. This was probably caused by an aerodynamic process (now called the *trench effect*) in the escalator system.

Entrapment and Trauma in the Underground

Passengers who had been directed away from the Piccadilly line escalators and who were instead advised to use the Victoria line escalator system had entered the same booking hall. This was the area where most of the deaths occurred.

In fires, there is a tendency for people to use familiar routes and exits and to assume familiar roles. In evacuating buildings on fire, people choose the way out they know best, run away from smoke, tend to follow a leader, head toward brighter places, such as windows, and some will shut themselves in a room after successfully evacuating (Canter, 1990). At Kings Cross, there were the additional disorientating factors of being underground and of being inside a structure which was highly complex and only small parts of which were known to most people. Evacuation plans were sketchy and conflicting. There was a low level of emergency training.

Nonetheless, it was a matter of subsequent regret and guilt for some of the officials that passengers had been mistakenly directed into the heart of the disaster.

No water had been directed on to the fire during this period and the water-fog system had not been used. At the time of the fire, a temporary wooden hoarding had been erected which sealed off part of the booking hall including access to an emergency stair case, a fire hydrant and hose, and one of the London Fire Brigade plan boxes (containing a detailed plan of the station for use in emergencies). Attempts had been made to use a small fire extinguisher, but the fire was too fierce for this to be a practicable measure.

The fire was not controlled until 9:54 P.M. and it was not until 1:46 A.M. that the fire was finally extinguished. Following the flashover, some of the survivors were trapped below ground and several hundred were subsequently evacuated by stopping a train and leaving in that way.

Disaster Intervention: Phase One

The emergency services and local hospitals had prepared contingency plans to deal with the immediate life-threatening injuries of the survivors. This "phase-one" response was effective and at University College Hospital, the Accident and Emergency staff were able to offer immediate assistance to many of the injured, some of whom have required prolonged inpatient and outpatient treatment under the care of the plastic surgical team. However, it very soon became apparent that there were no plans to meet the longer term psychosocial needs of the victims of the Kings Cross fire. Usually, this phase-two response has been given a low priority in disaster planning in the United Kingdom. There are now strong arguments for believing that it should be an essential component of all coordinated major incident plans.

Immediate Aftermath

Hitherto, the scale of the psychological impact of a disaster had been neglected. Following the Kings Cross fire, twelve thousand people were sufficiently concerned to telephone the police inquiry service in the first three days. To some degree, all these people had been touched by the psychological fallout of the disaster.

Gathering of Volunteers

On the evening of the disaster, a member of the psychiatry team visited the Accident and Emergency (A&E) Department at University College Hospital to offer help; others contacted the department by telephone. The psychiatrist on site was asked to deal with the other psychiatric emergencies, people who had presented in the usual way, and thus take the pressure off the A&E staff. There were no emergency plans for the psychosocial needs of the fire victims.

The following morning, there was still a haphazard

response from many individuals within the hospital mental health and counseling services. We decided that we should visit all the key units to make contact, to determine early needs, and to try and coordinate the health service psychosocial response. We spoke to the A&E Department consultants who had been on duty the previous evening and to the senior nurses; we consulted the plastic surgeon, the surgical registrars, the nursing tutors, the Divisional and Unit General Managers, the Divisional nursing officer, the Staff Counseling Service and many others. A decision was taken to form a specific disaster unit and a temporary coordinator was appointed. The mental health service was formally alerted and a meeting was called for all trained volunteers, including many capable of working in more than one language.

Contact was also made with the local governmental authority, the London Borough of Camden, which was initiating an outreach service to the general public. A 24-hour telephone service, staffed by local authority social workers and lay counselors from the many local voluntary agencies, was opened within 48 hours of the fire. An early decision was made that there should be a single agency, the Kings Cross Support Team (KCST), which would meet regularly and act as a steering committee to coordinate the many agencies and ventures developed in response to the fire.

One of the first tasks was to produce, with little or no prior planning and without committed funding, an appropriate response to the psychosocial needs of the victims (Turner, Thompson, & Rosser, 1989). In starting to coordinate these responses, a knowledge of the academic literature was of considerable help.

Types of Victims

In the very early planning stages, it was recognized that there were many categories of people likely to be affected by a disaster. For example, Taylor (1987) described six classes of victims. These include (1) those directly exposed to a large-scale catastrophe, (2) those with close family and personal ties to the primary victims and the dead, (3) those whose occupations and duties require them to respond to the disaster and to assist in subsequent restoration and rehabilitation, plus three other miscellaneous groups. This emphasizes that not only do the needs of the survivors and the immediate families of the dead have to be considered, but also their social networks and the emergency service personnel. Ultimately, those who become involved in running the phase-two response may themselves become victims.

Types of Psychological Responses

Similarly, it was possible to take account of the literature on traumatic stress reactions. Work with survivors of the Holocaust and with the Far East prisoners of war since the 1940s (Kinston & Rosser, 1974), torture survivors (see Chapter 58, in this volume), and the veterans of the Vietnam War in the 1970s and 1980s (Wilson, 1989) has led to increasing attention being paid to the role of severe external trauma in adulthood as a cause of dis-

tress in otherwise normal people. In 1980, the American Psychiatric Association introduced the diagnosis of post-traumatic stress disorder (PTSD) into the *Diagnostic and Statistical Manual of Mental Disorders* (DSM-III) (American Psychiatric Association, 1980) and further refinement has taken place in the definition that is used in the revised form (DSM-III-R) (American Psychiatric Association, 1987). It is recognized that PTSD may coexist with other psychological reactions, for example, anxiety or depressive disorders, and may constitute only a part of the reaction to severe trauma. Its importance is chiefly as a specific consequence of major trauma; the content of many of the phenomena (e.g., flashbacks or avoidance behavior) seen in PTSD relates directly to the traumatic event. Thompson (1990) discussed how such reactions to trauma fit in to more general models of stress.

Types of Disasters

Classifications of disaster have also been formulated (Green, 1982; Taylor, 1989). These include such features as type, duration, scope, speed, and personal impact of the disaster as well as more general features, such as social preparedness, potential for recurrence, and control over future impact. Thompson (1990) argued that the main factors are always threat and loss, regardless of the disaster type. Although these factors often fulfill a purely descriptive function, it has also been suggested (Green, 1982) that degree of impairment is likely to be related to such factors as the degree of life threat, degree of bereavement, prolongation of suffering, amount of geographical displacement, proportion of the community affected, and the cause of the disaster (whether natural or man-made). These may help in predicting the scale of psychological distress and also bring out the difficulties in mounting a coordinated response following disasters which have high levels of geographical dispersal or displacement. Transportation disasters often share a number of these complicating factors and may be associated with high levels of postdisaster psychological morbidity (Hodgkinson, 1988).

Experience of Other "Phase-Two" Responses

The psychosocial intervention program following the fire in the Bradford City football stadium (Crook & Baugh, 1986; Eaton, 1985) was an important step in the development of an effective policy in the United Kingdom, and more experience has been gained subsequently in the aftermath of other disasters, for example, the sinking of the *Herald of Free Enterprise* ferry (Hodgkinson & Stewart, 1988). This was of considerable value in helping to inform the group of professionals and volunteers who met following the Kings Cross fire, but it is clear that yet more work is required to establish which are the essential elements which must be included in the planning process.

Developing "Phase-Two" Responses

Having accepted that there was a need to respond to the victims likely to be affected by this event, services were tailored for each of the main groups of potential victims.

The severely injured, who required admission to University College Hospital, were all offered support by a psychiatrist. Most patients took up this offer, either immediately or at some point in the ensuing year, and found it useful. Their immediate relatives were similarly allocated to named social workers and experienced senior psychiatric nurses were also involved.

The bereaved were approached by representatives of the Kings Cross Support Team (KCST) and offered support. In 28 of the 30 identified families, the team was asked to counsel one or more members of the extended family or friends of the dead person.

The London Underground staff, the emergency services personnel, and the hospital staff who had to receive the dead and injured were also among the potential victims. With the permission of their managers, 250 hospital staff were contacted (most were seen in person), seminars were organized, and leaflets were distributed, offering help and describing the typical responses to stress of this nature. In the case of the emergency services and Underground staff, initial contact was established with the welfare agencies and senior staff, letting them know about the facilities available for anyone affected by the fire.

The general public formed the largest group of people who were affected. An emergency telephone service and an outreach program were instituted. One of the features of the typical postdisaster condition was the fragmentation and incoordination of responses. Although the KCST was rapidly instituted (during the first 2 days after the fire) with contributions from health care professionals, and social work and volunteer groups, a preliminary analysis of the early responders indicates that some survivors had to face questions from many other groups and organizations. There is a need to resolve the difficult issue of how such groups, often with very different functions, should work together to the benefit of the affected population.

Difficulties in Planning

As contingency planning had not included the psychosocial needs of the victims, all arrangements had to be made in an *ad hoc* fashion in the period immediately after the fire. Inevitably, this led to the diversion of energy away from direct relief into the work of forming a cohesive team approach. In view of the diversity of styles and approaches, this was hardly surprising but it constituted a major distraction that hampered our work.

Although local authorities in the United Kingdom are charged with the responsibilities of planning for, and dealing with, such specific events as nuclear disasters, no one appeared to have any statutory duty to respond to the usual range of civil disasters like the Kings Cross fire. Such statutory responsibility may not, however, offer the best solution. What may be needed is a variety of patterns of local planning, each designating leadership to one or more named individuals with relevant expertise. The present system depends on natural or emergent leadership and carries the risks of conflict on the one hand and a leadership vacuum on the other

hand, both being formulas for the wastage of human resources.

One of the organizational priorities was the early identification of potential victims. The collection of names before people disperse, the immediate availability of a helpline number for release to the media, and the urgent need to produce posters and leaflets are all important in this regard. If this opportunity is missed, the rest of the work of tracing people is made so much more difficult. Following the Kings Cross fire, many of the difficulties arose directly from the lack of prior planning for this single process.

Another of the major problems was the need to make contact with so many other groups and organizations who were also interested in the survivors. Perhaps this was a larger problem for a group working in the inner city than it has been in rural areas. Not only has each of our patients been in touch with many other agencies, the KCST has also had to deal with many of these and other groups.

Finally, there is no natural source of funding for the phase-two response. The London Borough of Camden was able to identify a small sum of money to fund a coordinator and her secretary. The Academic Department of Psychiatry (University College and Middlesex School of Medicine, London) had raised a little charitable funding to take on a temporary secretary/coordinator. The disaster fund appeal later added a small contribution so that the service could continue. There is a vital need to consider funding as an integral part of the phase-two plan.

Psychological Reactions

A range of different therapeutic styles and approaches have been adopted in previous work varying from informal group meetings with adults or children to specialized psychotherapy. In view of the large numbers involved, the KCST made an early decision to use a screening questionnaire, both to identify those most severely affected and also to allow the evaluation of the work by follow-up examination. In any setting where resources are limited and large numbers of people may be in need of varying degrees of help, some sort of screening approach is likely to be inevitable.

Psychological Measures of the Disaster Impact

A booklet was prepared which included the 28-item form of the General Health Questionnaire (GHQ-28) (Goldberg & Hillies, 1979), the Impact of Event Scale (IES) (Horowitz, Wilner, & Alvarez, 1979), the Eysenck Personality Questionnaire (EPQ) (H. J. Eysenck & S. B. Eysenck, 1976), and a specific Kings Cross Event Schedule, which sought information about location and involvement in the disaster. Lay volunteers assisted each person who had contacted or been referred to the helpline service to complete the questionnaire and also made their own assessment of urgency and need for help. Later, a short form of this questionnaire was sent with the permission of Desmond Fennell, chairman of the Kings Cross Enquiry, to all those who had made witness statements. Only the preliminary helpline data are presented here.

This group of 50 people comprised 22 passengers, bereaved and injured, 18 emergency services personnel (police, ambulance, fire services), 8 Underground Transport staff, and 2 whose role was not known. There were 34 men and 16 women, and the mean age of the whole group was 36.2 (SD 13.3). The interviews took place between 1 and 12 months after the fire.

The group contained many people with evidence of psychological distress. Mean scores on the GHQ-28 (using the standard scoring method) were 10.0 (SD 7.7). Scores above 4 are often considered to be indicative of probable caseness (sensitivity 88%, specificity 84%) (Goldberg & Hillies, 1979). In this sample, 33 had scores above this value. Similarly, for the IES, mean scores of 16.9 (SD 9.3) for the intrusion scale and 14.1 (SD 10.2) for the avoidance scale were moderately high. The total IES score was 31.0 (SD 18.4).

The 20 subjects who had contacted their family doctors following the fire had significantly higher total GHQ and IES scores (e.g., for the GHQ, mean scores were 13.1 and 7.2, $t = 2.8$; $p < .001$; $n = 47$). This may be taken as relatively crude evidence supporting the validity of the scales. Those who had decided that they needed to obtain medical assistance also scored highly on subjective distress on the screening instrument. The IES total had a moderately high correlation with the GHQ ($r = .60$, $p < .001$, $n = 49$). The coefficient of determination (r^2) was therefore 0.36 suggesting that scores on one measure explained only a third of the variance in the other, a result compatible with the view that the two scales are measuring overlapping but different psychological constructs.

Perhaps the most important results came from the event schedule. The initial analyses suggested that those who had been able to talk about what had happened soon after the fire had lower GHQ and IES scores. Examining the data in more detail, however, revealed that very few did not have the opportunity to talk soon after the fire, and these differences were not robust. On the other hand, those who did talk thought it helped them. Of the 43 people who were able to talk about the disaster soon afterward, 81% reported that they found it helpful. Of the 24 subjects who were able to talk in considerable detail, 92% reported subjective benefit. Thus, early debriefing may be a valuable component of the disaster response, although at this stage objective evidence is lacking.

Work on the processing of emotional material suggests that the majority of individuals are able to overcome traumatic events in ordinary life. The failure to do so on the part of a minority has enormous consequences, and may be partly explicable by a maladaptive cognitive strategy which impedes the natural recovery process (Rachman, 1980). More recent work (Pennebaker & Beall, 1986) suggested that even a relatively small intervention which allows subjects to recall the emotions surrounding traumatic events can significantly reduce their illness behavior and subsequent consultation rates.

Following the Mount St. Helens volcanic eruption in 1980, three psychiatric disorders (single episode depression, generalized anxiety disorder, and PTSD) were identified with increased frequency in the affected population. Systematic research (Shore, Tatum, & Vollmer, 1986) demonstrated both exposure-related onsets for these disorders and also a significant "dose-response" pattern. Those in the high-exposure group had significantly higher levels of morbidity. Most symptoms of depression and anxiety had abated by the third year although symptoms of PTSD tended to persist longer.

In the Kings Cross sample, subjective ratings of exposure were associated with higher GHQ scores, initially suggesting a similar dose-response relationship. For example, the 23 subjects who reported that during the episode they had felt that their life was at risk had higher GHQ scores (mean scores were 12.3 versus 5.5; $t = 3.4$; $p < .01$; $n = 43$). However, reports of seeing smoke, or witnessing dead bodies were not associated with significantly higher GHQ scores, and even the 19 people who reported seeing flames only had a trend toward higher GHQ scores (mean scores were 11.84 versus 7.6; $t = 1.96$; $p = 0.06$; $n = 44$).

There are two likely, and not mutually exclusive, explanations for these effects. There may be a true dose-response relationship with greater levels of exposure to trauma producing greater subsequent distress. On the other hand, it may be that high levels of current psychological distress affect a subject's recall of the event. Those who have worked through more of the trauma may remember the fire without the high levels of intrusive distress experienced by those with a more persistent or more severe traumatic stress response; they may therefore report fewer memories of subjective fears when describing the incident.

In further analyses, present anger about the fire or persistent fear of another fire were both positively correlated with GHQ score (Spearman rho = 0.59, $p < .001$ and .39, $p < .01$, respectively). Similarly persistent avoidance of Kings Cross station since the fire ($n = 17$) was associated with higher GHQ scores (mean scores were 14.1 versus 7.0; $t = 3.39$; $p < .01$; $n = 46$). Hence it is likely that subjective recall of the events and degree of risk at the time of the fire are at least being colored by present emotional state.

MacFarlane (1987, 1988) has already called into question this overriding effect of exposure to trauma and has reported that, in a sample of Australian fire fighters, introversion, neuroticism, and a past history and family history of psychiatric disorder were of more importance. In this group of Kings Cross fire survivors, GHQ score had positive correlations with EPQ neuroticism ($r = .46$, $p < .01$, $n = 47$) and L-scale scores ($r = .25$, $p < .05$, $n = 47$), both standardized for age, but there were no significant correlations with introversion or psychoticism scores.

As a final note of caution in this as in many other disaster responses, the competing needs of research and clinical service provision make it impossible to control for all the key variables. For example, in this case, people presented to the helpline service at different times after the fire and for different reasons. A full analysis of the data set will require that these and other potentially confounding variables be taken into account.

In summary, these preliminary results, in 50 people presenting to a helpline service, provide evidence of emotional disturbance following the Kings Cross fire. There were high levels of intrusion, avoidance, and general distress. Both environmental (amount of traumatic exposure) and personality (EPQ neuroticism and L-scale scores) factors were investigated in relation to the total GHQ scores. Being able to talk about the fire shortly afterward was quantitatively associated with subjective benefit, although objective results were less easy to demonstrate. It is anticipated that more detailed analysis of the full data set will allow some of these questions to be explored in more detail.

Recommended Components of the Phase-Two Plan

The planning of the phase-two disaster response is an important area of concern. Ideally, it should be tackled in advance of a major incident, and include plans for rapid assembly of key people as soon as there is an alert. The phase-two disaster plan may be conceptualized within several time periods: (1) the immediate aftermath, (2) the reactive period, and (3) the formal (proactive) outreach program.

The Immediate Aftermath

In the first few hours, there are four main tasks: (1) the provision of comfort and support, (2) meeting the social needs of victims facing homelessness or displacement, (3) the identification of all involved, and (4) the institution of a telephone support and counseling service.

Comforting the distressed and the bereaved is likely to be important for several reasons. There is the obvious value of offering support to people in distress; it may free other staff to deal with the injured. Also, it will alert people to the presence, even at such an early stage, of a support team. By setting a model, it may make it easier for others to reveal their own distress to family and friends, thus undergoing a form of debriefing. The group best able to take a leadership role here will often be religious and community leaders. They are likely to require assistance if the numbers are large and professional backup for the occasional person who presents as a psychiatric casualty of the disaster.

Depending on the nature of the disaster, there may be problems of homelessness or loss (death or incapacity) of spouses and parents. Rapid access to a source of funds would be of great benefit and should be a matter for government policy. There will often be an important role for social casework or relief.

Next, there is the matter of attempting to identify all those involved. This relatively small action must take a very high priority. All emergency service and hospital personnel should be asked to log their names when leaving the disaster-affected area. Without being overintrusive, as many witnesses, survivors, and injured as possible should be asked for their names, addresses, and telephone numbers. The representatives of the media,

who should also be identified, may already be collecting this information for future reporting and may be willing to supply these details in confidence. Once the dead are identified, the names and addresses of relatives should also be obtained.

In practice, this aspect of the immediate phase-two response is likely to be ignored unless a simple system is adopted and rehearsed in advance of a disaster. All personnel must be educated about the reasons for and importance of this record. Material for record-keeping must be available as part of the disaster equipment.

Finally, a high priority must be given to the rapid institution of a 24-hour telephone helpline service for anyone to use who is experiencing distress. This single phone number, with several lines, should have been planned in advance of the disaster. There is a need for a rota of volunteers to staff the telephones; these will usually be lay counselors with some professional support.

The Reactive Period

In the next few days or weeks, the service will continue to be largely reactive. At crucial times, such as the publication of an inquiry report, the inquest and the first anniversary of the disaster, the service will become reactive once again. It may be helpful to reopen the helpline service at such times and to publicize the work of the support team once again.

Those already identified as particularly distressed, and those who come forward asking for help in this period, should continue to receive help. In addition, key named personnel should be identified for psychiatric liaison with medical and surgical patients kept in the hospital, social casework with their relatives and the relatives of the dead, and early contact, in conjunction with staff welfare agencies, with groups of health care and emergency services personnel.

Where people are congregated together, it has been suggested that the early use of Critical Incident Debriefing is helpful (Dyregrov, 1989). People are seen in groups, within the first few days after the disaster, and given the opportunity to discuss the events and their own feelings about what happened. In a major transportation disaster such as the Kings Cross fire, the geographical dispersal may make this approach impossible with the primary victims. Others may reject this approach, fearing for the confidentiality of their disclosures. However, in our work with the health care staff, we often used a group approach which was helpful for two reasons. It made manageable the task of seeing large numbers of people quickly. It also made it easier for staff members to see this as a routine response, hence avoiding some of the stigma associated with talking about feelings and distress.

There are significant areas of overlap in the interests of the support team and the media; for example, the need to publicize the helpline telephone number. These issues should be considered in advance of a disaster. Besides offering publicity for the support service and its telephone line, there may be opportunities to describe the ways people respond to disaster, emphasizing the normality of an emotional response and the value of acknowledging these feelings in early discussions with family and close friends. During this period, posters advertising the support team may be displayed in appropriate places. A comprehensive collection of press cuttings should be started.

A leaflet has been distributed in many of the recent disaster programs and this has been an additional way of communicating with large numbers of people rapidly in the early stages after the incident. This procedure was first used following the Ash Wednesday bushfires in Australia (Valent, 1984) and has been adapted for use in subsequent disasters in the United Kingdom. It has an educational content, outlining normal reactions to trauma as well as offering advice on the services available.

A previously developed computerized disaster database capable of bearing all the names of potential victims should be immediately available and the names already obtained should be entered. It should be possible to extract lists of people present in the different areas of the disaster scene for ease of contact tracing later.

The opportunities of this period should not be overlooked. For example, it may be helpful for later work to have photographs of all the dead. Wherever possible, relatives should be encouraged to see and touch remains or possessions. But inevitably, some relatives will have been unable to see the body and the photograph may be a useful substitute in selected cases. Similarly, a member of the team should attend any inquiry or inquest. This is important for identification of victims and also to raise the profile and the credibility of the support team.

However, the fundamental organizational elements concern management and funding. These vital aspects of the work will depend to some degree on local opportunities and current policies of local and central government and they will be considered in more detail later. The need to identify a management structure which includes adequate support for the managers and the counselors cannot be emphasized too strongly. Similarly, the recognition that an effective service has financial requirements is essential for the long-term survival of the project. It cannot be assumed that an effective professional large-scale response can be mounted relying only on voluntary funding.

The Formal Outreach Program

Gradually, the psychosocial work changes in its emphasis from being largely reactive to being fully proactive. This last period of the phase-two response will last from 1 month to several years after the disaster. The main work of the phase-two intervention team will be to organize and lead a formal outreach program. A coordinated response should be made to each involved individual. This will require the accurate identification of all those present or otherwise directly or indirectly involved in the disaster. An at-risk register should be compiled using the computer database system already prepared. Anyone contacted by the team should be asked for names of other people they knew to be present or involved so that, in this way, a comprehensive register will be obtained. This should be the basis of a proactive outreach program in which people are contacted sensitively and made aware of appropriate help.

As described earlier, the Kings Cross screening instrument which was based on standard and well-validated psychometric procedures, was used to identify people particularly likely to need formal professional assistance. Although it is important to acknowledge that most normal people have emotional reactions to extreme trauma, in the case of a service with limited resources, it is important to be able to target those people in most need of specialized help. A large majority of victims may be dealt with competently by lay counselors. Pressures of time and other work may make full training in basic counseling skills less appropriate after a disaster; it is often more helpful to identify and select those volunteers who already have these skills. On the other hand, education about the specific aspects of postdisaster counseling is often helpful and continued support is essential.

The optimal content of the therapeutic intervention remains uncertain. There is a need to evaluate in controlled trials, different therapeutic options. Some survivors may require pharmacological methods of treatment, including antidepressants; others will be helped by a psychological intervention. On the basis of present knowledge about emotional processing (Rachman, 1980), it seems preferable to offer a smaller number of long sessions in which unpleasant emotional material is recalled and undergoes habituation; the risk of many brief interventions (perhaps by multiple agencies) is that the individual will be sensitized to the events and may experience more emotional distress as a result.

Recommended Organization of the Phase-Two Plan

If there is to be an informed and effective approach to future civil disasters in the United Kingdom, a national policy is required. This should address the issues of local responsibility, funding obligations, and the need for a resource base, which should include information about international approaches and agencies.

The work of the first few hours must be carried out locally and will depend on prior arrangements made with the emergency services (including health and social services). The national policy should clarify the extent of the responsibility of the individual services for carrying out or organizing the separate elements of this stage of the response. It should also offer advice about the need for rehearsals to include the early components of a phase-two response.

At the moment there is a procedure in the United Kingdom for announcing a police telephone number for inquiries about those who may have been caught up in a disaster. A similar procedure should be used to announce a helpline service for all those who require support. The number should be (1) reserved in advance, (2) simple to remember, and (3) able to support several lines quickly.

This should be followed rapidly by the activation of a planned steering group. However, it is important to examine two conflicting interests before coming to a recommendation on the composition of this group. It has already been demonstrated that following the fire at Kings Cross, survivors were often in contact with multiple agencies, including hospital and community health workers, the support team, the trust fund assessors, the media, the police and the official inquiry, staff welfare groups, the coroner and his staff, and sometimes many others. Working on the principle that frequent short or uncoordinated interviews may serve to sensitize people even further to disaster-linked material, it seems best to offer a coordinated approach with pooling of information between agencies while safeguarding confidentiality. This would allow the victim to supply information for any essential purposes but, at the same time, make it possible for the interviewer to spend the time needed to try and work through some of the painful memories and associated feelings.

On the other hand, there is a need to demonstrate the independence of the service from employers. It is easier for a person in one of the emergency services to come to an independent and confidential counseling unit than to visit the staff welfare service. Similarly, problems may arise if the distinct functions of the disaster fund assessment, the statement needed for the official inquiry, and the initial therapeutic assessment are blurred.

We believe that there is scope for further experimentation in this area, looking to the responses obtained from the users of the service to guide future planning. One option would be to divorce the work of the steering group from the day-to-day work of counseling. Members of the group would then come from all interested agencies and would plan ways of coordinating contacts without necessarily pooling confidential information obtained from clients. The manager of the support team would be answerable to the steering group but would withhold specific information from the whole group; sharing of information between agencies would take place only with the full consent of the individual client. Those representatives of the health, social work, and lay counseling services on the steering group might meet as a subcommittee to supervise the more confidential and therapeutic aspects of the work and individuals would only be identified for essential and unavoidable reasons.

An at-risk register would be compiled with contributions from all the member agencies of the steering group. This would be based on lists of names of those present, injured, or bereaved at the disaster, and the emergency services' staff involved in the response. Only people contacting the support service directly would be excluded from the main list until their permission had been obtained. Files on those who had given information and who were prepared for this to be used by some or all of the other agencies would be made available as appropriate. Anyone wishing to contact an individual would first consult the register. This would include coordinators of self-help groups.

If it is possible to arrange such a clear separation between the availability of detailed confidential information and the planning and coordination roles of the steering group, we would recommend that all interested agencies should be represented. These should include central government (disaster coordination), local authority social services, local health authority, disaster fund, local voluntary agencies, emergency services, other local religious or community groups, and the victims' self-help group. The steering group should expect to function for at least 2 years. Ideally, a large proportion of the group members should be selected prior to the occurrence of a disaster. Either a national disaster unit is needed or assistance would be required from one of the centers experienced in responding to disasters. This task will be made easier in areas where local academic departments have already gathered a theoretical knowledge base.

The steering group will be charged with the duty of providing the remaining services required in the phase-two plan. It will normally discharge its responsibilities by appointing a chairperson with managerial authority and a core team of professional and lay counselors, some of whom will be seconded from local voluntary and statutory agencies. It will have to give a high priority to the support and supervision of its team of workers to prevent them from joining the list of victims (Hodgkinson & Stewart, 1988). The manager will be required to keep records on all those on the at-risk register. A formal screening program should be undertaken based on standard psychometric principles. Progress should be evaluated within 1 year of the disaster.

Finally, the question of funding should be addressed in a national policy. As large-scale disasters are sporadic events, there would be advantage in holding the responsibility for funding centrally with allocation by publically agreed formulas. This would also mean that one agency would be involved in several areas and would have an interest in evaluation and the development of an efficient service. If local agencies were required to carry the costs of the phase-two response, there should be a central policy about the appropriate budget to be charged. This should be reflected in local contingency planning.

Implications for Future Disasters

There is an urgent need to evaluate the work of a postdisaster counseling service. There is now a tendency for services to converge on the scene of a major incident and to believe that psychosocial assistance will do more good than harm. However, the evidence on this important matter is minimal.

The theoretical grounds for presuming that a cognitive-behavioral style of intervention may be valuable to previously healthy survivors of disaster have already been discussed, although for those with previous histories of trauma and early deprivation, a deeper exploration may be unavoidable. Following the Kings Cross fire, a treatment intervention study is underway to shed new light on some of these points. In the meantime, we would argue that policies, based upon best available current information, should be in place in advance of a major disaster and that these should routinely include a phase-two psychosocial program for at least 2 years after the event.

ACKNOWLEDGMENTS

We gratefully acknowledge Marks and Spencer plc for financing the appointment of a secretary to the project; the London Borough of Camden for financing the coordinator and secretary to the support team; S. Dewar for his assistance in analyzing the data; and our many colleagues in Bloomsbury and Islington and in Camden who offered their help to the victims of the Kings Cross Fire.

References

American Psychiatric Association. (1980). *Diagnostic and statistical manual of mental disorders* (3rd ed.). Washington, DC: Author.

American Psychiatric Association. (1987). *Diagnostic and statistical manual of mental disorders* (3rd ed., rev.). Washington, DC: Author.

Canter, D. (1990). *Fires and human behaviour* (2nd ed.). London: David Fulton.

Crook, J., & Baugh, S. (1986, November). *The Bradford fire disaster*. Annual Conference of the Society of Psychosomatic Research, London, England.

Dyregrov, A. (1989). Caring for helpers in disaster situations: Psychological debriefing. *Disaster Management, 2,* 25–30.

Eaton, L. (1985). Bringing balm to Bradford. *Social Work Today, 24,* 15–17.

Eysenck, H. J., & Eysenck, S. B. (1976). *Manual of the EPQ (Eysenck Personality Inventory)*. San Diego: Educational and Industrial Testing Service.

Fennell, D. (1988). *Investigation into the King's Cross Underground Fire*. London: Her Majesty's Stationery Office.

Goldberg, D. P., & Hillies, V. F. (1979). A scaled version of the General Health Questionnaire. *Psychological Medicine, 9,* 139–145.

Green, B. L. (1982). Assessing levels of psychological impairment following disaster: Consideration of actual and methodological dimensions. *Journal of Nervous and Mental Disease, 170*(9), 544–552.

Hodgkinson, P. E. (1988). Psychological aftereffects of transportation disasters. *Medical Science Law, 28,* 304–309.

Hodgkinson, P. E., & Stewart, M. (1988). Missing, presumed dead. *Disaster Management, 1,* 11–14.

Horowitz, M., Wilner, N., & Alvarez, W. (1979). Impact of Event Scale: A measure of subjective stress. *Psychosomatic Medicine, 41*(3), 209–218.

Kinston, W., & Rosser, R. M. (1974). Disaster: Effects on mental and physical state. *Journal of Psychosomatic Research, 18,* 437–456.

MacFarlane, A. (1987). Life events and psychiatric disorder: The role of a natural disaster. *British Journal of Psychiatry, 151,* 362–367.

MacFarlane, A. (1988). The aetiology of post-traumatic stress disorders following a natural disaster. *British Journal of Psychiatry, 152,* 116–121.

Pennebaker, J. W., & Beall, S. K. (1986). Confronting a traumatic event: Toward an understanding of inhibition and disease. *Journal of Abnormal Psychology, 95,* 274–281.

Rachman, S. (1980). Emotional processing. *Behaviour Research and Therapy, 18,* 51–60.

Shore, J. H., Tatum, E. L., & Vollmer, W. M. (1986). Psychiatric reactions to disaster: The Mount St. Helens experience. *American Journal of Psychiatry, 143,* 590–595.

Taylor, A. J. (1987). A taxonomy of disasters and their victims. *Journal of Psychosomatic Research, 31*(5), 535–544.

Taylor, A. J. W. (1989). *Disasters and disaster stress*. New York: AMS Press.

Thompson, J. (1991). Theoretical issues in responses to disaster. *Journal of the Royal Society of Medicine. 84,* 19–22.

Turner, S. W., Thompson, J. A., & Rosser, R. M. (1989). The Kings Cross fire: Planning a "phase two" psychosocial response. *Disaster Management, 2,* 31–37.

Valent, P. (1984). The Ash Wednesday bushfires in Victoria. *Medical Journal of Australia, 141,* 291–300.

Wilson, J. P. (1989). *Trauma, transformation and healing*. New York: Brunner/Mazel.

CHAPTER 38

The *Piper Alpha* Oil Rig Disaster

David Alan Alexander

Introduction

The *Piper Alpha* oil rig disaster occurred about 9 months prior to the initial preparation of this chapter. It is, however, still a live and emotional issue for several reasons. First, the public inquiry has just begun and it is likely to continue for about 6 to 9 months or longer. Second, there is much uncertainty and disagreement about how best to dispose of the wreckage of the installation which now lies in over 140 meters of water. Third, there is much debate about the possibility of retrieving any more human remains from the site. Fourth, final judgments about litigation and compensation have yet to be reached.

For these and certain other reasons it is not possible to provide an objective and rigorously analyzed account of this tragedy. What follows is, therefore, a highly personal account since I was privileged to be involved in a number of ways. These include: (1) working in the accident and emergency department in the immediate aftermath; (2) spending several days on a firefighting ship with rescuers; and (3) working at the oil terminal during the retrieval of bodies from some of the wreckage of the *Piper Alpha*. As part of my routine psychiatric commitments, I have also treated a number of survivors, bereaved, and other victims.

This chapter contains five sections. First, to give the reader some idea of the nature of the tragedy there are descriptions of the *Piper Alpha* installation and the men who worked on it. Second, the accident itself is described, providing an insight into what the victims had to endure and what happened to them. Third, an outline is given of the general responses from local services as the tragedy unfolded. Fourth, the involvement of a small specialist psychiatric team is described in terms of its

contribution in different settings and stages of the disaster. Finally, the chapter ends with a general comment on what has been learned from this experience.

Background

The Piper Alpha *Installation*

Owned by the oil firm, Occidental Petroleum, the rig was designed to tap dry gas, wet gas, and oil from a field in the North Sea, 193 kilometers northeast of Aberdeen, which is a city of about a quarter of a million inhabitants, situated on the northeast coast of Scotland. The North Sea is one of the world's most inhospitable working environments, in which winds can rise to 160 kph and icy waters can generate waves up to 27 meters. The oil-drilling rig itself was enormous, weighing approximately 35,000 tons and standing nearly 152 meters tall. At any time, it housed a community of about 200 personnel, who worked 12-hour shifts on a two weeks on/two weeks off basis.

The Crew of the Piper Alpha

It is important to recognize some of the features of this group of men because they are quite different from those of a heterogeneous collection of individuals who might happen by chance to be together when, for example, a train or aircraft crashes. Clearly, these personal characteristics are relevant to understanding posttrauma reactions.

The crew was all-male, most of whom were used to working in harsh and uncompromising conditions. Many of them had worked in the oil industry or in the fishing industry for years, and for a substantial number the oil installation was their second home. Inevitably, their being confined to the rig for extended periods led to the development of a community spirit among the men and to the forging of strong bonds and morale among them. In some cases, it would appear that these

David Alan Alexander • Department of Mental Health, University of Aberdeen Medical School, Foresterhill, Aberdeen AB 2ZD, Scotland.

International Handbook of Traumatic Stress Syndromes, edited by John P. Wilson and Beverley Raphael. Plenum Press, New York, 1993.

relationships were more durable than their marital ones. Although the effect of being away from home may have been to strengthen some marital relationships, the shift system certainly imposed strains on some marriages. Thus, living for 2 weeks at a time in a hard and deprived environment led some men on their return to shore to seek various pleasures including alcohol (the rig being "dry"). It would have to be said, in all due respect, that some of the men had problems with alcohol and intimate relationships long before the tragedy. Since this is an important issue, it will be addressed later when considering the postdisaster consequences on adaptive behavior.

Given the nature of the work and the environment, these men were not strangers to adversity and, although probably none anticipated a major disaster, many of them had experienced a number of incidents which reminded them of the hazards of this kind of work. However, it should also be noted that only a minority of the men were employed directly by Occidental; the rest were employed by various subcontractors. Clearly, this status is relevant in terms of litigation and compensation issues which arose in the wake of the disaster.

The Tharos

In view of the key role played by the MSV *Tharos*, a brief description of this rescue vessel is merited. This multifunctional support vessel was crewed by about 50 men, and was specially designed with extensive firefighting, emergency support, and maintenance and diving capabilities. In particular, it could provide intensive care for 23 patients; general hospital facilities for 88 men suffering from shock, exposure, hypothermia, and mild burns, and stored medical supplies for over 300 individuals.

Disaster

Explosion

The world's worst oil rig disaster began at about 22:00 hours on Wednesday, July 6, 1988. At that time, there was an initial explosion which was to serve as a trigger for a series of explosions which culminated in the almost complete destruction of the installation above sea level.

The first explosions probably rendered useless the main control room, the generator, and the power distribution system, which resulted in the disabling of the essential and emergency services (including the emergency lighting and gas/fire detection systems). Moreover, all telecommunications and the internal and external alarm systems were incapacitated immediately.

Despite the efforts of support vessels, including the MSV *Tharos*, the fires extended until almost the entire installation was engulfed in a fireball. Initial control of the burning wells was not achieved until July 9, 1988, and they were only finally brought under complete control on September 4, despite the best efforts of an internationally acclaimed firefighting team.

The evidence from the interim report of the technical investigation suggests that no instructions were given to abandon the platform. Many men appear to have remained in the accommodation modules which were subsequently engulfed in flame and dense toxic fumes. Others sought escape either by jumping into the sea (in some cases from over 30 meters) or by clambering down ropes or the external structure to sea level. At the best of times the North Sea is a formidable refuge, but because areas of sea up to about 140 meters from the installation were ablaze with oil and gas, it became a dangerous and life-threatening cauldron of sea in which to attempt an escape. Some inflatable life rafts were launched but did not inflate properly and other survival crafts were not launched. Because of the density of the smoke and the intensity of the heat, it was not possible to deploy a helicopter from the MSV *Tharos*. Thus, the situation could be described as one of chaos and extraordinary difficulty in terms of either survival or rescue efforts.

Fortunately, the sea was relatively calm and, therefore, those who had escaped from the fire and toxic fumes were eventually able to be picked up by rescue craft. However, in some cases, the nature of their injuries (in particular, severe burns to the hands) and the design of the rescue vessels made it difficult for the survivors to clamber on board; a fact which added substantially to their pain and suffering.

Specific Stressors on the Rig and Environs

As the previous section has described, the men were faced in the early stages with fire, smoke, and toxic fumes, as well as with the risk of further explosions. Confusion and uncertainty reigned not only with regard to what had happened and was happening, but also about what should be done. Many men were uncertain as to whether they should follow their instincts or the training procedures they had been taught. Much frustration and anguish was also caused by the fact that rescue facilities were in sight but generally the craft could not approach close enough to effect a straightforward rescue. For example, at the time of the first explosion, the MSV *Tharos* was about 550 meters away but was unable to bring to bear its full firefighting and rescue capabilities for some time.

Although the sea was relatively calm, some of the survivors could not swim, and others had no life jackets or adequate clothing to shield them against the freezing water. There was, in addition, the constant fear of further explosions and sea-borne fires (two of the rescue workers were subsequently killed by one of the fires, having turned back to save more of the survivors).

Many of the men reported a profound sense of helplessness and despair because of the lack of firefighting and other facilities on the *Piper Alpha* in the face of the enormity of the disaster, the full scale of which became increasingly evident to them. The devastation, the ever-increasing conflagration, and the sights of injured and dead colleagues imprinted on their minds a thoroughly distressing scene, which was exacerbated by the sense of isolation that being on a rig in the middle of the North Sea inevitably created.

Additional stress was caused by the lack of medical facilities and expertise on some of the rescue craft. It was only after survivors had been transferred to the MSV *Tharos* that proper medical and surgical care could be provided. From there the survivors still had to face a helicopter flight of 60 to 90 minutes back to the Aberdeen Royal Infirmary.

Casualties and Survivors

Of the 226 men originally on board the *Piper Alpha*, 164 (72%) were killed and one subsequently died in the Aberdeen Royal Infirmary. Two men in a rescue vessel also lost their lives while trying to rescue others. All survivors were taken first to the Aberdeen Royal Infirmary where 21 were admitted for inpatient care. The majority of men suffered burns, particularly to the head, face, and hands, and were subsequently transferred to a ward specializing in the management of burns. When healthy enough, the men were discharged to their own regional hospitals. Only 22 of the survivors were local men. Most remained at the Aberdeen Royal Infirmary for a few days or weeks; only two faced an extensive period of stay of several months.

Responses to the Disaster

As a city in a region of fishing communities, Aberdeen was not completely unfamiliar with tragedy, such as occurs when a ship is lost, but Aberdeen awoke on the morning of July 7, 1988, faced with the daunting task of providing emotional and physical help to what seemed to be an endless succession of spouses, relatives, and friends, many of whom had traveled far to meet with or at least find out about their loved ones.

Early on Thursday morning, as survivors were still being brought in to the Accident and Emergency Department, a social work management team was set up to coordinate help for the survivors, the bereaved, and the families of the men who were still missing. Advice and information was obtained from agencies of other regions, such as Kent and Manchester, who had had recent experience of large-scale disasters. Following discussions with the Chief Constable of the Grampian Police Force, a 24-hour helpline was set up to provide information and support for anybody affected by the disaster. Links were also established with other local authorities to give them information about individuals from their areas. A leaflet offering information, advice, and comfort was widely circulated (see Chapter 82, in this volume, for a discussion of mental health intervention in disasters).

Professionals who had had experience of two earlier disasters in the United Kingdom were invited to address a large audience of representatives of professional and lay agencies forewarning them of some of the problems that might be encountered.

Coordination between the Social Work Department and the medical, psychiatric, and voluntary agencies was quickly established to decide on priorities and, in particular, which proactive steps should be taken. Coordination and cooperation were also facilitated by a series of meetings organized by Occidental Petroleum who readily made available financial and other resources.

Initial Plan for Intervention and Counseling

It was agreed that (1) all victims' families should be visited by a representative of the employer as soon as possible after they had been contacted by the police. (Empowered by the Scottish Home and Health Department, through the Local Government [Scotland] Act, 1973, it is the responsibility of the police to inform relatives of a sudden death.) (2) All families should have one "uninvited" visit by the social work team, with offers of more help if required. (3) Debriefing of all involved, including Occidental staff, should be carried out as soon as possible. (4) Those bereaved or survivors particularly at risk should be identified. In particular, individuals who might constitute "hidden" victims were identified. These included some of the Occidental staff and men of the backing crew of the *Piper Alpha* who would, but for chance, have been on the rig. Groups for these persons were run by the Clinical Psychology Department which made a valuable contribution to the welfare of various groups of victims. (5) There should be a memorial service in the following week. (6) Up-to-date records of "missing" and "dead" should be made available to specialist helping groups. Also, (7) back-up facilities should be provided for "helpers" should they themselves need some help.

The Social Work Department, through an outreach team, has continued to run a helpline and organize regular meetings, particularly for survivors and bereaved. Psychiatric back-up has been offered but so far has not been required. (See Chapters 76 and 82, in this volume, for an important review of these key issues of debriefing.)

Role of the Psychiatric Team

Early on Thursday, July 7, 1988, it was agreed that the initial response of the psychiatric services should be by means of a small team of senior and experienced clinicians, all of whom had had considerable experience of dealing with crises. The team comprised two consultant psychiatrists from the National Health Service, and two staff members from the University Department of Mental Health, the professor, and myself. The team decided that their contribution should be (1) low-key and undramatic, (2) readily available and flexible, (3) credible and realistic, and (4) proactive as well as reactive.

Since these were the features of their involvement throughout, some amplification is justified. There was quite enough drama and tension without the psychiatric teams appearing to overreact to the occasion. Instead of their having to be called out as an emergency, they decided they should have a continuous presence and involvement throughout the different stages of the aftermath of the disaster. Common sense suggested that a ponderous system of referrals and appointments would also be unhelpful. The team's first location, therefore, was a room in the Accident and Emergency Department at the Aberdeen Royal Infirmary. (It was not difficult to obtain a unanimous decision from the team that the room should not be called the "Bereavement Room" as had been proposed by certain authorities!) Although only four staff were initially involved, the arrangement was flexible in that, for example, as needs increased or changed, other colleagues were available to join the team. The credibility of the team, it was hoped, would be achieved by being seen to be publicly active and effective, and working in concert with other medical, nursing, and surgical colleagues. Although the prevailing needs to which the team had to react were extensive, it was also believed to be vital that a positive preventative approach be pursued. This was done, for example, by identifying individuals particularly at risk in different settings, and by being actively involved when various plans (e.g., those for the retrieval of bodies) were being discussed. Although psychiatric investment occurred at many stages of the response to the disaster, the team adopted a positive view, emphasizing the resilience of the individual and his or her ability to cope with the adversity.

As the following paragraphs indicate, the psychiatric team was most actively concerned with survivors and the police. It did, however, also provide a consultation service for Occidental who sought their opinion on a range of issues, including those pertaining to the retrieval of bodies and the timing of events, such as memorial services. A local psychiatrist also made an important contribution to planning for the bereaved by virtue of his status in the community.

Accident and Emergency Department

The team saw many of the survivors. Their problems ranged from basic ones (such as wanting to know how to contact their families or when they were going to be discharged) to having a florid, toxic, confusional state. Most, however, just wanted "a chat." Consequently, simple befriending was what was asked initially of the team. In some respects, this was a modest contribution but it proved to have important longer-term consequences. For instance, it defused much anxiety in the minds of survivors and their families about psychiatric contact and it now seems to be easier for them to seek and accept more formal psychiatric help. Even though their contact is quite often "social" and informal, the survivors have maintained their links with the team, forged during the early days in the Accident and Emergency Department. Thus, an informal support network was established.

After the initial crisis had abated, I also spent time meeting, quite informally, some of the nursing staff, sometimes at their own request and sometimes at the suggestion of one of the nursing officers. The concerns of the nurses were varied. A few had found aspects of the practical side of dealing with burns upsetting and distasteful. For others it was the nature and pressure of work which caused to surface latent doubts about their

motivation for nursing. For one nurse the intensity of the atmosphere had brought to light a long-standing but heavily disguised problem between herself and other colleagues. Only in the minority of cases, therefore, was the disaster *per se* the direct cause of the nurses' distress; more commonly, it merely exacerbated preexistent problems or raised latent ones.

Two further observations are worth noting. First, the nurse who had the most difficult time adapting to the consequences of the disaster was one who went off duty immediately before the initial surge of admissions had been completed. As she admitted and recognized, she missed out on the informal debriefing and winding down which took place over the next 2 to 3 days. The second is that it is easy to miss a "hidden victim." It was only thanks to an observant nursing officer that the needs of a receptionist did not go undetected. On reflection it is not difficult to see why this person would have had a torrid time having been faced quite unexpectedly, very early in the morning, by worried (and angry) relatives, injured survivors, the press corps, and more. Her example confirms the danger that those who have a "low profile" in the course of their normal duties may be individuals at risk when a crisis develops and their needs may go unnoticed.

Burns Unit

Survivors

Inevitably, the physical needs of the burned men commanded most attention from the medical and nursing staff, but psychological reactions emerged quickly. Indeed, most of the nursing staff expressed surprise at how quickly, and admitted some uncertainty about how best to deal with them. In general, however, for the first couple of days there were obvious signs of relief and euphoria among the survivors. They became the center of much public and media attention, to which a number of them responded quite enthusiastically. Interestingly, two survivors have since regretted their public "performance" on television, and wished steps had been taken to dissuade them from doing them. The mood in the ward changed as the death toll increased and when one of the survivors died in the Infirmary (the only one to do so). Bouts of tearfulness, irritability, generalized anxiety, and anxiety caused by anticipation of the problems likely to be encountered on discharge became more common. A depressive reaction was seen in two individuals.

Throughout, the psychiatric team maintained their contact with the men and with the families who visited (the "ripple" effect soon was evident among spouses and families once the initial sense of relief had passed). Sometimes the men merely chatted and "got things off their chests," but they suffered badly from uncertainties. For example, some became quite upset if the theater lists were changed or if their dates for discharge were not given with sufficient precision. Others did not tolerate well changes in staff or routine. Some would complain because a new nurse did not do their dressings exactly the way another nurse had done them. The psychiatric contribution often entailed providing a sympathetic ear or a link between the medical/surgical staff and the survivors. The team also tried to help by contacting the survivors' general practitioners or their regional psychiatric services prior to discharge.

Despite their difficulties, it was noticeable in the ward that the victims quickly emerged as a mutually supportive and cohesive group, presumably at least in part because there was already a fellowship or community spirit among them. There was also a good deal of "black" humor (used quite healthily) and some good-natured banter and rivalry (for instance, about whose burns were healing best). The helpful impact of these factors lessened as more men left the ward. It was most difficult for the two men who were most severely injured, when they were alone in the ward; we found that much more support was required for them.

Paradoxically, the cohesiveness of the group and the good atmosphere they created in the ward had two unfortunate consequences. First, it made discharge for some a very threatening experience. The prospect of leaving the support and security of the ward was a daunting one for several individuals. This raised various anxieties such as: "Will my children still love me when they see me?" "How can I face the wife of my friend who died?" and "How will I deal with all the questions people will ask me?" Second, a major oversight was committed. Nearly all the visiting professionals who came to the Infirmary to provide counsel and support forgot about another survivor who was alone in an orthopedic ward. Not only did he miss out on the advantages of the community spirit, which had developed in the Burns Unit, he did not receive as much support and other help as he might have had from certain professionals who were distracted from his needs by the attractive atmosphere in the Burns Unit. There are many reasons for becoming a "hidden victim."

Nursing Staff

Some months after the disaster, when all but two of the survivors had been discharged from the Infirmary, I interviewed a number of the nurses. None reported any long-standing adverse reactions to the work following the disaster. At the time, however, several had found it particularly "grueling" dealing with relatives, from whom came very awkward, if not impossible, questions, particularly in the case of wives whose husbands were still missing. The nurses also regretted they had had insufficient time to speak with the men; often their contact was confined to those occasions when they were changing dressings. It may be for this reason that the involvement of the psychiatric team was welcomed by the nurses. Another initial problem was that some of the nurses found it hard to unwind when they went home. Some felt guilty when they went off duty despite the fact most worked longer than their required shifts. Senior nurses confirmed these problems among their colleagues and emphasized the need for senior staff to take responsibility and say "enough is enough," without implying that their colleagues were in any way inadequate to their tasks. Interestingly, some of the part-time ancillary staff felt "hurt" and "resentful" of the fact that, during the peak of the crisis, their contribution had been applauded and welcomed, but when the pressure had

eased and they resumed their normal duties, the perceived value of their presence dropped. Some felt they had to "go back to the kennels" of lesser status.

In terms of their relations with the survivors, the nurses commented on some difficulties. They found it hard to deal with the men when they were angry. Several of them took the anger very personally and needed some persuasion that most of it was displaced anger. They also thought the men were oversensitive, for example, to changes in the mood or attitudes of the staff. Some of the nurses felt they always had to be friendly, supportive, and smiling however else they may have been feeling inside.

A strong division of opinion arose among the nurses about the merits of open visiting times, and about whether or not relatives should be allowed to help in the management of the survivors (e.g., by bathing their eyes or helping with patient feeding).

MSV *Tharos*

It was agreed by the team that I should fly out to this vessel (which at that time was moored alongside and fighting the fires on the remnants of *Piper Alpha*) to assess what were reported to be "stress problems" among some of the rescuers aboard.

My arrival on the vessel, on the Sunday after the disaster, provoked some suspicion and, indeed, some surprise and perhaps disappointment as a rumor had gone around that a young, female "stress counselor" was being flown out! On board at that time was a local general practitioner who had been one of the first medical staff to be flown out. His knowledge of the crew proved invaluable. Over a dozen of the crew were interviewed. These included individuals who had reported to the physician that they were feeling the effects of their recent efforts, as well as those whom the author and the physician thought might have been at risk (this included one man with a history of major depression). Although the setting itself was bizarre and thoroughly unpleasant, all efforts were made to make these interviews as casual and relaxed as possible. The word *counseling* was never used, and I was introduced merely as "a doctor who has an interest in stress and has come out to see how things are going." The situation was also helped by the fact that, at the same time, a number of police officers were also on board taking statements from the crew. Consequently being seen or being interviewed was not an extraordinary occurrence. In any case, to grace these encounters with the term *interview* is to disguise the fact that, although some took place in the comfort of a warm cabin or surgery, a number took place in a noisy cafeteria, or on a wet and windy gangway of a vessel in the middle of the North Sea, about 80 meters from blazing wellheads. There seemed to be some merit in seeing these individuals wherever they felt most comfortable.

Several factors had a bearing on how these sessions were conducted. In the first place, these men still had to work 12-hour shifts and their ability to be able to continue was an important consideration. Second, these were in the main a fairly hardy and down-to-earth group of men who would not easily have been able to say they were not coping. Third, even those at risk did, however, seem to be coping quite well. This does not mean that they had not suffered. A few reported flashbacks (intrusive imagery) of sights of burned faces; insomnia was quite common (although some of the men had worked for 32 hours nonstop); and one or two reported a generalized anxiety and "tension." Most admitted they could hardly absorb the full scale of the disaster and preferred to get on with work, which they rightly considered important, recognizing that "it would hit them" when they went on shore. None reported feeling depressed. It was noticeable but not surprising how disoriented many were with regard to time and it seemed to mean nothing to them.

Panic had not been reported when the disaster first broke, although some of the men "just walked away" from the immediate scene and could not face trying to retrieve the injured or the dead. Some were surprised at their own reactions and were concerned that they had been "callous" and "logical" in the way they dealt with the dead, dying, and injured. Nearly all were concerned about whether or not they had "done a good job," and wanted feedback about the welfare of their rescued colleagues. At that time, of course, communications with what was happening on shore and in the Infirmary were limited. The lack of good information may also have been responsible for some of the rumors which began to spread through the crew; rumors about how many had died, how they had died, and why they had died.

In terms of psychiatric help, reassurance and facts were the mainstay. These were required to convince the men that their reactions were within the bounds of "normality" and that they were doing and had done a "good job." In addition, Occidental Petroleum arranged thereafter that regular and frequent bulletins about the survivors should be issued to the *Tharos*. In part, their need to be convinced that they did a good job may have stemmed from the fact that the *Tharos* had not been able to engage the fires immediately and, consequently, many of its crew had had to watch helplessly much of the suffering of their colleagues from *Piper Alpha* and its disintegration.

Another factor which contributed to their need for reassurance was that one of the visiting "experts" was reported in the local press to have stated that a third of the rescuers would have psychological problems because of their efforts. In the intense and self-conscious atmosphere of the *Tharos* such information fueled concerns. Small wonder that one of the first comments made to me on my arrival was: "they needn't think I'm going to be a psychiatric wreck."

There were, however, positive signs. Most of the men had quite spontaneously spoken much about the previous 3 days, and some had convinced themselves that they had coped better than they would have anticipated: this was particularly the case for those who feared that they would "lose control" as the consequences of the disaster worsened.

Temporary Mortuary

A temporary mortuary was set up in Aberdeen to house the remains of the dead while the difficult task of postmortem examination and identification was carried out. It was under the control of the Chief Constable and was manned by 51 officers (men and women). At that stage, the psychiatric team was not directly involved but had offered their services should this have been necessary. These officers, however, are now involved in a follow-up study which will be described later in the section "Research and Follow-Up" (Alexander & Wells, 1991).

One observation which was regularly made, however, was that the officers felt at their worst when they had little to do. While they were purposefully active, the nature of their work troubled them much less.

The police had recommended that relatives not view the bodies because many had suffered the ravages of fire, explosion, seawater, and sealife. No relative insisted on seeing a body although relatives could have insisted on legal grounds that they examine the bodies once they had ceased to be the property of the police, which they were until cause of death had been established. Only one (a police officer) did identify a body and even then it was by means of a tattooed arm. In the early stages, an oil company representative viewed the bodies for identification but, thereafter, this was achieved by odontology, fingerprinting, clothing, and the like.

Flotta Oil Terminal

Some months after the disaster, 105 bodies were still missing. It was assumed that some would have been atomized in the intensity of the explosions, but reports from divers and survivors suggested that many had been entombed in the accommodation modules. The retrieval of these bodies constituted another stage in the disaster and, in turn, generated much emotion and debate. It also posed a major organizational and technical problem because the modules (one of which was the height of a three-story hotel) lay in about 140 meters of water.

However, after several postponements, the modules were raised from the seabed and were ferried by barge to an isolated island called Flotta in the Orkney archipelago, where Occidental Petroleum had an oil terminal. The delays because of inclement weather and technical problems caused much distress to the families awaiting the remains of their loved ones, and some anticipatory anxiety among those responsible for their retrieval.

Overall responsibility for this exercise rested with the Grampian Police Force. In view of the unpleasant nature of the task, it was decided to select volunteers who generally had had experience of dealing personally with death or at least were in a department which was commonly dealing with death. Other selection criteria were age (older officers were preferred) and a good sense of humor. All 23 officers involved were male although two females were employed in the administration team.

Flotta is an isolated and barren island and its isolation was increased by the exclusion zone and high security which had to be drawn around the whole site.

There the officers worked with others (e.g., divers) in shifts of about 12 hours. The duties of those handling the bodies were rotated and, except in the case of one of the most senior officers, no officer remained on Flotta for more than 7 days.

All individuals on site, irrespective of their duties, were given an intensive induction, during which particular attention was paid to safety, hygiene, security, and personal reactions (physical and emotional). The references to the latter were realistic, helpful, and undramatic. It was indicated on that occasion that two members of the team (a consultant psychiatrist, with extensive service experience, and myself) would be "around to see how things were going" and would be available if anybody wanted to have a word with us. We had also been involved in the planning of the exercise, and the psychological needs and possible reactions of those most intimately involved with the retrieval of the human remains were given serious consideration at each stage of the planning. Similar attention was shown at the daily briefing and debriefing sessions.

Nobody enjoyed the work but none reported persistent adverse reactions. There had been a marked enthusiasm (which suggested a high level of anticipatory anxiety) to enter the larger accommodation module once it had arrived at Flotta. However, in view of the rumors and air of mystery which had been created, and in view of the frequent postponements, such an initial reaction was not surprising. In fact, once they had started the work, despite the unpleasant and at times dangerous environment in which they were working, many of the officers commented that it was not as bad as they had feared. Only one person, an engineer, showed marked signs of stress but this was not due to the retrieval of bodies *per se*. Rather, it was due to the enormous pressure he had been under throughout the whole exercise which he had masterminded.

The preliminary evidence suggested that police negotiated their duties successfully without residual difficulties. None had contacted the psychiatric team or their own medical officer; none had taken time off work or reported to be showing impaired work performance since returning to normal duties. However, a more systematic follow-up is now being conducted, as is described in the section entitled "Research and Follow-Up."

There seemed to be a number of factors which may have reduced the likelihood of adverse reactions. First, the whole operation was very professionally organized and the men's needs were taken seriously. Second, the idea that this exercise was valuable (both to the bereaved and to the inquiry) was heavily emphasized. Third, there was an excellent *esprit de corps* among the various workers (even the divers, who are not renowned for the ease with which they mix, got on well with the police and others). The cohesiveness of the group may also have been strengthened by the fact that none of the men went home at the end of his shift, and they all therefore shared the same social and recreational facilities after work. Finally, a number of them had devised their own highly effective coping strategies. As one senior detective said to the author: "Sir, when I go in there [the accommodation module] as far as I am concerned I'm going into a spaceship looking for Martians." Any cognitive psychotherapist would be impressed.

Additional Involvement

Survivors' Reunion

One of the special features of the men of *Piper Alpha* was that they already constituted a community; they were not thrown together by fickle adversity. It was felt that this group spirit should be built upon since it seemed to have therapeutic potential. I arranged, therefore, to organize a reunion for all survivors in mid-December in a local hotel. Funding for this was obtained from the Aberdeen Town Council (some of the survivors indicated that they would not come if the money were to be provided by the oil firm). This finance provided full board and accommodation as well as vouchers for the men's travel. It was decided that the evening session should be confined to survivors because this had been the prevailing view of a sample surveyed before the event was organized. The only "staff" who were there were the Hospital Chaplain (who was well known and liked by the survivors) and myself and one of my colleagues from the psychiatric team. Ostensibly, we were in attendance only to ensure that the occasion went smoothly. Any professionals and lay groups who had been involved with the disaster were invited to meet the survivors on the following morning. The press were allowed to take only one photograph in the morning: no other media involvement was permitted.

With the individuals' permission, the names and addresses of all survivors were circulated among those attending in the evening in order that they could trace some of their friends and colleagues. Only about five individuals did not wish this information to be made available in this way.

Since it was the case that two thirds of the survivors were not local and because some were away working or were not living at their last known address (at least four had broken up with their wives) it was difficult to contact all the survivors personally, but of the 59 known to have received a written invitation only 6 declined to accept. None of these, however, thought that the idea was undesirable in principle, but only that he did not think attending such an event would have been helpful for him personally.

An important lesson was learned, however, about communication. Initially, I had written a carefully worded letter to each survivor inviting him to attend. The response was disappointingly low. However, almost all the men who had failed to reply indicated that they would be delighted to attend when I telephoned them personally. They admitted that they often did not bother to reply to "official" letters.

It was noticeable that the evening went well; there was much talk and reminiscing—not all about *Piper Alpha*. Although much alcohol was consumed (perhaps no more than oilmen might be expected to consume), there was only one incident which required my attention in the early hours of the morning, when an excess of alcohol had caused a survivor to "abreact." The open session in the morning was rather more stilted and, although the various helpers who came were obviously pleased to see the survivors and vice versa, the atmosphere was not particularly relaxed. Subsequent feedback from the men suggested that the morning was something of an anticlimax compared to the evening, and that they were more preoccupied with "going back to reality" at home. Nonetheless, the majority claimed that it was an enjoyable and valuable occasion and would welcome others, including occasions to which wives might be invited.

Routine Psychiatric Work

By means of the Aberdeen Psychiatric Case Register, it has been possible to establish that out of 22 local survivors, 10 have been referred to either the local psychiatric or clinical psychology services by April, 1989. Data are not yet available on those living outside the local area.

The public inquiry is currently in progress. Prior to the inquiry, I contacted personally all survivors indicating that I would be willing to see them at any time before, during, or after their giving evidence at the inquiry. So far five have accepted this invitation.

Research and Follow-Up

The psychiatric team was unanimous in their view that they should fulfil their clinical duties first before launching any kind of research project. This view was sharpened by several factors. First, a number of the survivors indicated that they were very sensitive about becoming research subjects, and were suspicious of the motives of those who conducted such projects. Second, the disaster was still a live issue because of such matters as the inquiry. Third, the whole issue of culpability, litigation, and compensation was far from resolved, and this factor was likely to bedevil much research.

However, the plans for a follow-up are now well advanced. (The term follow-up has been preferred to that of research.) A small steering committee has been set up to consider a number of projects and to coordinate research endeavors because it was considered neither ethical nor methodologically sound to have survivors, bereaved, or helpers being exposed to opportunistic or *ad hoc* research projects. It is intended shortly to appoint a senior research nurse (one already known to a number of the survivors) who will interview survivors and their families in their own homes or in a setting of their choosing. This will provide an opportunity for assessing the impact of the disaster on their health and on their social and family functioning.

One project which has already begun is that involving the police officers who were on duty at the mortuary and at Flotta. Quite fortuitously, I along with two other colleagues from the Medical School had begun about 2 years ago an extensive survey into occupational health in the Grampian Police Force. This was conducted by means of questionnaires, interviews, and rating scales. In particular, the project derived much information on sources of stress, impairment because of stress, and the officers' methods of combating stress reactions. Consequently, nearly all the officers involved in the *Piper Alpha* disaster took part in that study, providing an invaluable and highly unusual opportunity to make before-and-

after comparisons. Moreover, it will also be possible to compare their well-being and performance with a matched control group of officers from the same force who were not involved in such work.

Discussion and Summary

Following a tragedy of this magnitude, it is easy to be "wise" after the event, but what follows is a summary of some observations derived from the work of the psychiatric team. They will be discussed under three headings: (1) Organization, (2) Reactions, and (3) Traps.

Organization

In the so-called honeymoon phase, the local and outside response to the disaster was as overwhelming as it was genuine. The need for organizing the response became immediately evident. In such circumstances, however, the organization has to be flexible because it has to harness the response to needs which change over time as the different phases of the disaster emerge. Key contributions of the individuals organizing the response are those of identifying new needs as they appear, locating and directing the sources of help which might meet these needs, obtaining good information about the overall circumstances, and disseminating this information to those who need it. In the wake of this disaster, the survivors, the bereaved, and the helpers became the victims of "misinformation" or at least a lack of good information. Clearly, an anxiety-ridden situation is a fertile breeding ground for unhelpful rumor.

The organization must also be able to make the best use of outside "experts"; although their contribution can be considerable, their intrusive presence is likely to be resented by local helpers. Perhaps their knowledge and expertise should be used to facilitate and enhance the community response but should not be allowed to inhibit it or supplant it (see Raphael, 1986, for a discussion). Of course, this issue relates to the need to acknowledge not only the similarities between disasters but also their differences. The men of *Piper Alpha* were not the same as, for instance, an almost random assortment of passengers on a ferry. Also, one must consider idiosyncratic features of the local population. Generally, the inhabitants of the northeast of Scotland are very reticent individuals to whom the public expression of emotion, including suffering, is quite foreign. This had a marked bearing on what facilities and resources they made use of.

In organizing the response, the provision of continuity of care is essential. Without sounding skeptical, it is relatively easy to offer help at the early stages (partly because it is so much of a reflexive reaction) but it is much harder to maintain a commitment as needs continue to grow or change. What one does not want is a relative vacuum of care to follow in the wake of the flood of concern which characterizes the situation in the immediate aftermath. Albeit with good intentions, some individuals may become involved in the early stages of intervention but may find themselves unable to sustain their commitment. Unfortunately, help may be even more necessary in the later stages of the disaster when problems can be intensified or new ones can emerge. One of the sad features of this disaster is its prolongation by such factors as the retrieval of bodies, the demolition of the remnants of the installation, and accusation and counteraccusation about matters pertaining to culpability, the payment of wages, the disbursal of the Disaster Fund, and the efficiency of the rescue operation. For anybody trying to come to terms with the initial disaster back in July, such matters (highlighted, of course, by the media) constitute a painful and wearisome epilogue.

As a feature of the organization it is important to have managers at strategic phases or points of the intervention, who have the authority to withdraw people when they have given enough or are in "overdrive" and running the risk of mental and physical exhaustion. For committed helpers, it may be too much to expect them to be able to say for themselves "enough is enough" because they are likely to misperceive this as being "weak" or "selfish."

From a psychiatric point of view, it was felt that the early intervention had four main advantages. First, intimate, first-hand experience and knowledge of the disaster was gained which increased the credibility of the team in their later involvement. Second, their early presence allowed them to be seen as part of the medical/surgical team and not as a distant and rather threatening group to whom the "weak" were subsequently referred. Third, strong bonds emerged between the team and some of the victims and other helpers: bonds which proved to be invaluable later. Moreover, it was almost as though in the emotionally charged atmosphere in the early phase of the disaster a special bonding or "imprinting" took place. Fourth, it allowed the team to conduct psychological triage and to identify those particularly at risk.

One final comment about the organization of the response is that, particularly when offering help to those who are themselves members of well-organized and professional groups (as was the case here, for example, with the divers and the police officers), the response itself must be well-organized and professional.

Reactions

There were certain reactions which merit comment. On certain occasions (e.g., prior to the removal of the bodies from the modules at Flotta), there seemed to be a widespread and disproportionate anxiety. This seems to have had a number of causes. First of all, the media with their indefatigable propensity for finding or generating drama made much of the unpleasantness of the forthcoming task and the likely consequences for those involved. Also, there were many offers of "counseling" (including from private organizations) for all those involved; offers which were made quite without discussion with their potential consumers. However, a less obvious source of anxiety was later recognized to be "projected" anxiety from some of those in managerial positions who clearly became anxious about the exercise but imputed this anxiety to those at "the sharp end." After a while, some of the latter began to react to this.

Indeed, one police officer even said to me: "Is there something wrong with me because I don't feel that anxious?"

The whole issue of counseling on a broad scale is a contentious issue. There have to be concerns as to the competence of some who are keen to offer such a service after a disaster. Unfortunately, although well-intended, some such offers may merely harden the resistance of some individuals to the idea of accepting any kind of help. Understandably, some groups (particularly the divers and the police officers) felt that there was implied in these offers a belief that they would not be able to cope. The so-called macho image became too easy and cheap a target. The fact is that many of the divers and the police officers had had considerable experience in dealing with some of the less savory aspects of life and were fairly hardened individuals. This does not mean that they were "supermen" or that they would not have been distressed by some of their experiences, but it is important that acknowledgment should be given to the ability of such individuals to deal with difficult circumstances. They would be quite happy to tell you how they had coped, and they were quite happy with the notion of debriefing, but the suggestion that they would all *need* counseling was not well received, and for quite understandable reasons.

Another important reaction was noted among some of the survivors and other victims, with whom some helpers colluded. For certain individuals, the disaster became an explanation for a variety of almost completely unrelated problems, including alcohol and drug abuse, marital disharmony, violent behavior, and drunk-driving offenses. It was known that some of these men already had problems in their lives and that the *Piper Alpha* disaster merely exacerbated them or simply cast them in higher relief. It seemed to be an important aspect of helping these men to come to terms with the reality of the disaster that they were helped to acknowledge that the disaster could not be used to rationalize all subsequent misfortune or misdemeanor. Often this entailed helping their families to achieve the same degree of understanding.

Traps

Helping victims of disasters is not an easy task, as is already well known, but the experiences with the victims of *Piper Alpha* highlighted a number of traps or pitfalls for the unwary helper.

Victims are ordinary people; they are not saints, thus they have their good and bad points like everybody else. For some helpers, there seemed to be much frustration and disappointment which seemed to emanate from the fact they had an altogether unrealistic view of the individuals they were helping in terms of the kind of people they were and what could be expected of them. It was also observed how easy it was to create dependency among the victims and to be protective. The aim of intervention should be to help such victims to become self-determining individuals and to retrieve a sense of control over their own lives. On certain occasions, some of the medical staff might have been too protective because they were very reluctant to let some of the survivors meet with relatives who wanted news of their missing loved ones. It was my experience, however, that survivors generally were quite keen to impart such information, in part, because this was one way to deal with their "survivor guilt." Such meetings were often very emotional and professional support was usually found to be valuable. Overprotectiveness may also have underlined the tendency of some helpers to become embroiled in public causes involving, for instance, litigation and compensation. It may be that such tendencies are more likely to occur if helpers are dedicated full-time to their disaster. Perhaps those who are required to continue, at least to some extent, with their normal duties are able to regain a more balanced and realistic perspective. This may also make for easier disengagement when the disaster work is completed.

Finally, a major trap seems to be that helpers become peddlers of gloom and miserable statistics about the prevalence of posttraumatic stress symptoms. However awful the circumstances of a disaster, it is imperative that a positive approach be maintained. People do cope with adversity, and even in the worst tragedies one can (and should) find the positive gains. In the case of the *Piper Alpha* oil rig disaster, these included individuals who found themselves to have resources and strengths of which they were unaware, new ways of dealing with difficult technical problems were established, and there were many cases of reaffirmation of important relationships or the development of new ones. As the Roman poet Horace (65 B.C.) stated:

> Adversity has the effect of eliciting talents which in prosperous circumstances would have lain dormant.

References

Alexander, D. A., and Wells, A. (1991). Reactions of police officers to body-handling after a major disaster. A before and after comparison. *British Journal of Psychiatry, 159,* 547–555.

Raphael, B. (1986). *When disaster strikes.* New York: Basic Books.

CHAPTER 39

The North Sea Oil Rig Disaster

Are Holen

Introduction

Located halfway between the United Kingdom and Norway, the Ekofisk is the most highly developed of the oil fields of the North Sea. Approximately two dozen permanent and a few floating rigs are in operation there; some of them are interconnected by bridges. From the Ekofisk pipelines, crude oil is channeled to Teesside in England and gas to Emden in western Germany. The basic function of the Ekofisk fields is the supply of energy, made possible by the gigantic achievements of modern technology. Considerable attention has been given to safety issues, yet accidents and disasters have occurred.

On March 27, 1980, the weather conditions were extremely bad and were gradually getting worse throughout the day. By late afternoon, the wind was developing into near gale force, blowing with 16 to 20 meters per second. The water temperature was 4° centigrade, close to the freezing point, and waves were 6 to 8 meters high. Because of the dense fog, clear sight was only 30 meters. Under normal conditions, 800 meters clear sight was required for helicopters to fly. Shuttle helicopters to and from the pump and production rigs were not operating. For this reason, the rigs where people lived, were far more crowded than usual.

The *Alexander L. Kielland*—named after a nineteenth-century Norwegian author—was a floating rig where the oil workers dwelled when offshore. This rig would normally be connected with the adjacent *Edda* rig by a movable bridge. During bad weather the bridge would be pulled onto the *Kielland* and the distance between the two rigs would be widened by adjusting the anchoring wires.

Around 6:00 P.M. on March 27, 1980, the rig was rather busy; it was time for shifts to change, and one of the daily helicopter flights from the mainland was expected to arrive with new oil workers and take others back to shore. The widening of the distance between the two rigs was completed. Approximately half an hour later, the tragedy began: One of the five legs of the *Alexander L. Kielland* rig broke off. The structure immediately tilted to a 30° angle and temporarily stabilized, while starting to sink. After a couple of minutes, the electricity failed, and the situation on board became rather chaotic. During the next half hour the angle gradually increased to 45° and then the rig suddenly capsized.

No pictures or films could possibly be taken of the tragic event that took place on this stormy, cold, dark, and foggy evening way out in the North Sea, where 212 men were on board the fatal rig. The majority, 123, died; only 89 survived. There were no women on board.

The rescue operation was extremely difficult: The first lifeboat launched from the rig was devastated on its way down when it was hit by the waves and crushed against the legs of the tilted rig. Two other lifeboats were lost under similar conditions, and eyewitnesses saw people fall out of the boats. Only one boat was launched successfully; however, its top cover became partly broken. Another lifeboat was released after the rig had capsized; this boat emerged upside down, but individuals who were in the water managed to turn it right side up and enter. Because the unsuccessful launching of the lifeboats had made some rather hesitant about entering them, many men decided to stay on the rig and gathered in groups on the deck. However, the rig was not a safe place. Occasionally, containers and various debris would rush down the deck, and some men were hit fatally. Others managed to jump aside.

Nobody expected the rig to capsize at this early stage. It was thought that if the rig would sink, there would be sufficient time for those on board to be picked up by the organized rescue operation underway. It was soon realized, however, that the rig would capsize at any moment. Men started to jump into the water; most of them had life jackets on, but few wore survival suits.

Are Holen • Department of Psychiatry, University of Oslo, P.O. Box 85, Vinderen N-0319, Oslo 3, Norway.

International Handbook of Traumatic Stress Syndromes, edited by John P. Wilson and Beverley Raphael. Plenum Press, New York, 1993.

Of the survivors, seven men managed to swim across to the neighboring *Edda* rig and were pulled aboard by means of a basket. Most survivors managed to get into the lifeboats at some point before or after the rig capsized. Sixteen survivors had rafts as their refuge and seven others were rescued out of the sea by supply vessels. The helicopters picked up a few survivors directly out of the sea, but their most important role in the rescue operation was to locate the lifeboats and rafts and transport survivors back to safety.

People on the neighboring rig were witnessing this silent offshore drama while almost completely unable to help their fellow workers; the wind and waves were too strong. The many tragic scenes that they observed and the fact that they had limited opportunities to assist were felt as a tremendous burden. Later on, they, too, were in potential danger. It was feared that the capsized rig might collide with the *Edda*, and so this rig was ordered to be evacuated.

The Event in Perspective

The capsizing of the *Alexander L. Kielland* rig was for a long time the worst oil-rig disaster ever, until the explosion, in July 1988, on the *Piper Alpha* rig which left 167 dead. This rig was located off the northeast coast of Aberdeen, Scotland.

Maritime disasters differ from other cataclysmic events by the fact that the site of danger is constantly surrounded by yet another danger: the capricious sea. Even after having obtained a safe distance from the sinking or burning ship, or the capsized rig, the survivors' lives may still be in jeopardy.

Disasters not only bring about tremendous problems for the survivors themselves, but also for the involved families of both the deceased and the survivors. In addition, one may have to deal with problems among the rescuers and fellow workers. Employers, contractors, and those in charge of the rescue operation and its related health services are met with many challenges. The same applies to the medical and social scientists, and to the society at large.

Aid and Research Program

After the *Alexander L. Kielland* disaster, an aid and research program was initially supported by the Norwegian government. Later on, grants were provided by the Norwegian Research Council for Science and the Humanities, and the Phillips Petroleum Oil Company, Norway. It was decided that the research program should focus on the survivors. This decision was based on the view that there already existed several valid studies of loss and mourning, whereas an understanding of the psychological processes related to catastrophic stress left much to be desired.

The main focus of the research was on the survivors, and the chief purpose was to explore the long-term consequences of a major stressful event. The survivors were approached by different methods: semi-

structured interviews, standardized questionnaires, and behavioral tests. The health insurance records of the survivors were also examined. So far, the data have been collected at four different stages:

1. The first study (1980) was done in the months right after the disaster. It was carried out by means of a 90-minute semistructured interview and a few standardized questionnaires.
2. The second follow-up study (1981) was a questionnaire mailed to the survivors 1 year after the event.
3. Five years posttrauma (1985) the next follow-up study was made. It consisted of a 3-hour, in-depth, semistructured interview and several standardized questionnaires measuring personality traits and different aspects of symptom levels. At this time, a comparison group was chosen.
4. The last follow-up so far (1988) was made 8 years posttrauma by looking into the complete health insurance records of the survivors and the comparison group—covering the time both before and after the disaster.

Efforts to reach every survivor were given a high priority and gradually resulted in satisfactory cooperation. The participation of the survivors was 100% in 1980 and 1981, and well above 90% in 1985 and 1988.[1] There emerged an altruistic attitude related to participation in the program: By sharing their experiences, the survivors wanted to provide information that might be of help to others in similar situations.

Populations Involved

There are three populations involved in the research presented, all oil workers of Ekofisk: the survivors, a matched comparison group, and the deceased.

Comparisons between the deceased and the survivors were based on the general information given by the police about those on board the *Alexander L. Kielland* rig. Additionally, comparisons were made between the populations of survivors and unexposed oil workers, and within the population of survivors—contrasting those with a poor and a favorable outcome.

In general, offshore workers may be regarded as fairly healthy people both physically and psychologically, owing to the selection procedures used by the oil companies. Thus, a proper comparison group had to consist of oil workers and was recruited from the Ekofisk fields in 1984. They were matched for domicile, age, and sex and totaled 92 persons, all men.

Of the 89 survivors, 75 had their domicile in Norway. The remaining 14 consisted of 10 men from the United Kingdom, 2 from Spain, 1 from Portugal, and 1 from Finland. To avoid problems related to language, cultural differences, and the like, it was decided that the research program should focus on the 75 Norwegian survivors. The mean year of birth for the survivors was

---

[1]SPSS^X statistical software was used for data analyses reported in this chapter (SPSS, 1983).

1945 (SD = 8.9), the same as that of the comparison group (SD = 8.3).

None of the 75 survivors had ever been hospitalized for any kind of psychiatric morbidity prior to the disaster. Only four men reported ever to have had any consultation for minor problems related to psychiatry. In short, manifestation of psychiatric morbidity among the Norwegian survivors preceding the event was fairly moderate. Compensation issues did not play a central role in the life of many survivors. Generally, the situation in Norway is different from what seems commonplace in Anglo-American parts of the world, and the research program was not involved in these matters during the time of the data collection.

Consequently, the survivors from this disaster constituted a population of healthy men suddenly and unexpectedly involved in a major stressful event likely to evoke considerable distress in almost every one of them. They were all exposed to the same situation, an overwhelming death threat in a maritime disaster, a catastrophic stressor. In other words, the survivor population fulfilled the stressor criterion of the posttraumatic stress disorder (PTSD) in the *Diagnostic and Statistical Manual of Mental Diorders* (DSM-III) (American Psychiatric Association [APA], 1980) and in the revised manual (DSM-III-R) published 7 years later (APA, 1987).

Thus, it was not a sample but an unselected survivor population of men that was studied. The participation rate was close to 100%. The findings that described the survivors from the *Kielland* are therefore factual and not inferential. This allows more freedom for generalizations for the outcome of similar catastrophic events, and even to other areas of event-related pathology: the stress-response syndromes.

Survivors and Victims

From the sparse formal data about the deceased, it was possible to make certain relevant comparisons between those who survived and those who did not. The first computation was related to ethnic background. One may speculate whether belonging to a minority group might impede one's survival because of language barriers and by limiting the cooperation, the seeking of help, the understanding of orders, and so forth. Of the total on board, the majority, 173 persons (82%), were classified as belonging to the ethnic majority (Norwegian), whereas 39 persons (18%) were classified as ethnic minority (non-Norwegian) (see Table 39.1). However, no significant difference was found in the frequencies of deceased among those who were classified as native and those who belonged to the ethnic minority.

Poor and Good Outcome

A variety of outcome measures have been employed in the *Kielland* program: symptom checklists, diagnostic measures, behavioral tests, and the diagnoses and durations of sick leaves or occupational dysfunction. The

Table 39.1. Frequencies and Intraclass Percentages between Survivors and Deceased[a]

Ethnic background	Deceased		Survivors		Total on board	
Ethnic majority	98	(57%)	75	(43%)	173	(100%)
Ethnic minority	25	(64%)	14	(36%)	39	(100%)
Total	123	(58%)	89	(42%)	212	(100%)

[a]Differences not significant at .05 level.

measurements cover miscellaneous features of the posttraumatic manifestations, and the outcome depends somewhat on the means of assessment. Nevertheless, there is a reasonably good intercorrelation between the measures, and, with some variation, about one third of the survivor population seemed to be facing severe posttraumatic problems during the observed period.

For the sake of simplicity, the designations *good outcome* and *poor outcome* will be used. *Poor outcome* will refer roughly to one third of the population with psychological problems, and *good outcome* (or *favorable outcome*) will refer to the other two thirds of the population with minor or no such troubles at the time.

Components of the Stressor

There is a growing body of research establishing a dose-response relationship between the stressor and the stress responses. To define a stressor gradient seems relevant; the greater the impact of the stressor, the more psychological disturbances are expected. Thus, the extreme or catastrophic stressors may be regarded as an etiological factor for a certain group of psychiatric disorders that are occasionally labeled stress-response syndromes (Holen, 1991). Epidemiological research on traumatic stress seems fairly unavailing unless the stressor gradient is accounted for. Progress in contemporary stress research may be related to better scientific descriptions of the stressor. There is a need to make inquiries into both the *quantitative* and *qualitative* nature of the stressor in order to arrive at valid between-disaster or interstressor dimensions operable across different catastrophic events. However, at this stage a within-disaster exploration of relevant dimensions seems to be a major challenge; from here, future generalizations to between-stressor components may prove to be rewarding.

Lately, an increasing interest has developed for the psychological manifestations at the time of the event (i.e., during the impact phase). Likewise, there is an intensified search for structural or situational aspects of the stressor (i.e., components that may initiate particular posttraumatic developments).

Three areas that seem relevant for advances in psychological stress studies are mentioned here, of which the latter two will be addressed in this chapter: (1) establishment of a *stressor gradient*, (2) *subjective components* of the response to the stressor, and (3) situational or *objective components* of the stressor.

The establishment of a grosser stressor gradient for the oil rig survivors represented a minor problem; without exception, everyone had been exposed to the same catastrophic event. This fact brought about a favorable and rare opportunity to explore subjective and objective within-stressor components.

Subjective Components Related to Stressor

In disasters "markedly distressing to almost everyone," rescue personnel and clinicians have struggled with the cumbersome question: What early psychological signs and symptoms may be indicative of later poor or favorable psychosocial outcome? In other words: What defines an at-risk person? It is a major task for researchers to offer good answers.

In determining subjective components, Horowitz, Wilner, and Alvarez (1979) have offered a pioneering work in the Impact of Event Scale (IES). The IES has been successfully used in the *Kielland* program, but the results are not included here. Instead, some additional dimensions are presented; with varying precision, all of them have significantly indicated the psychosocial outcome of the survivors. It might be argued that these components represent various aspects of dissociative states—which might be correct—but dissociation will be dealt with under a separate headings below.

Initial Cognitive Functioning

How will people behave and react in a situation of overwhelming and life-threatening stress? The survivors were interviewed about their cognitive assessments, decisions, and actions during the very first minute of the disaster (i.e., about their functioning *immediately* after the rig had tilted to a 30° angle). The selected answers have to some extent been cross-checked and verified by fellow oil workers. For the results, see Table 39.2.

Apathy, Denial, or Warding Off

Beyond the first minute of the disaster, a certain lack of feeling or partial indifference seemed to be central in the mental state of many of the men on board the rig. This state will be labeled *apathy* and may be understood as an expression of denial or self-protection against what was really happening. The most extreme expressions of this apathy were observed in several of the men who died: Quietly, and with a blank expression, they walked singing into the waves, as if there were no danger. They immediately drowned. By a rough division of the survivors, three levels of apathy were defined.

A minor degree of apathy or none at all was reported by approximately 20%. This group also encompassed the highest representation of spontaneous leaders. The situation was so chaotic that no formal leadership functioned, but these men managed to organize the others constructively. Generally, those who were in this subgroup tended to have a favorable outcome.

Table 39.2. Initial Cognitive Functioning of Survivors (N = 75)

Reaction to trauma	Percentage of survivors
Assessment	
Reduced capacity to understand or perceive what really happened	37
Decision making	
Reduced capacity to plan one's moves in order to avoid dangers	40
Behavior	
Reduced capacity to act or implement plans when situations was understood	24
Markedly inadequate behavior	13

The 60% majority reported a moderate degree of apathy, and were able to comply with orders and tended to do what they had been trained to do or to follow what others did. In this subgroup, there was no clear direction toward a poor outcome.

The last group of individuals in this section, approximately 20%, displayed diverse but extreme reactions: They were agitated or extremely apathetic or were the *Rambos*. As a subgroup, they tended to have the poorest outcome. They all seemed to have in common a mental state of utmost distance to the overwhelming dangers of the here-and-now. Most of them reported being highly agitated either verbally, motorically, or both. A smaller number said they were extremely indifferent, "completely shut off from within." The *Rambos* tended to be loners in the disaster and, at some point, took the most uncalculated risks; some of them overlapped with those who were agitated. The distribution of these three groups is illustrated in Figure 39.1.

Subjective Death Threat

In the first interview a few months after the disaster, the survivors were asked how they perceived their risk of dying at the time of the disaster—the *subjective death threat*. Some felt quite convinced they would die; others reported a firm conviction that they would survive. After 5 years, the survivors were again asked the same questions; their answers at the later follow-up correlated well with their earlier responses. However, they correlated marginally with a gradient of exposure to the factual dangers in the situation. Thus, we were dealing with a measure of the subjective death threat. Interestingly, the more a person thought he would die in the disaster, the more he tended to be associated with a poor outcome.

Dissociative Phenomena

Dissociation may be defined as distortions in the perceptions of time, self, and situation. At the time of the disaster dissociation was found to be significantly associated with the general short-term outcome, less so

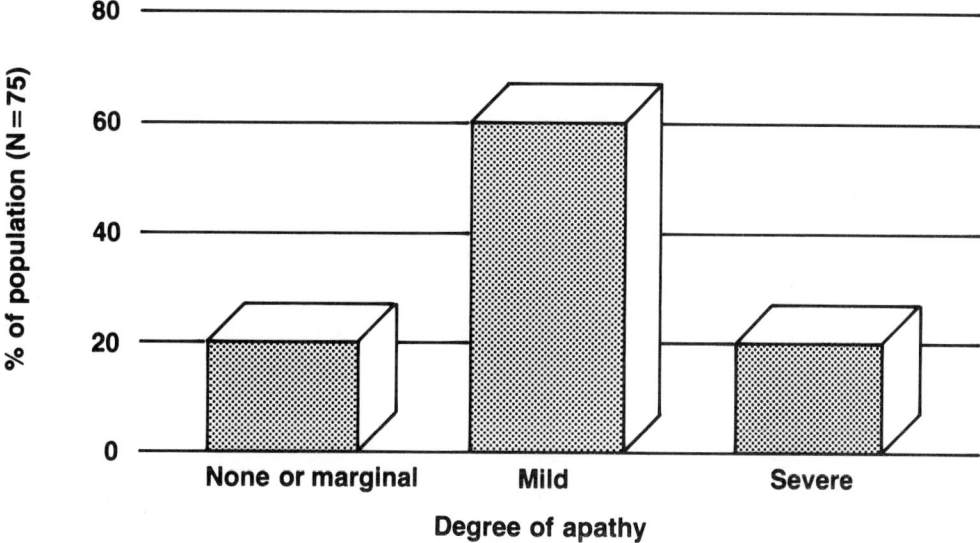

Figure 39.1. Degree of apathy.

in the long term, where it was found to be associated with the avoidance score on the Horowitz' scale (IES) (Horowitz, 1976, 1986). This led to speculations about the role of dissociation as a predictor. Is it true that the more a person dissociates, the more uncompleted will his processing of the traumatic experience be? Janet (1889/1973), the French psychiatrist, had some fascinating thoughts on the subject by the end of the last century. His views have been of considerable inspiration for parts of modern stress research.

Situational or Objective Components of the Stressor

Within the disaster situation itself, it was possible to distinguish between several components of the disaster situation representing different part-traumata that were associated with a poor outcome.

A person was rated under the *spectator trauma* if he reported to have witnessed particularly grotesque scenes during the disaster: Some saw fellow workers being swept overboard by a container rushing down the deck; others saw two persons get killed by a huge wire that came at full speed through the air. Almost everyone (71 persons) reported to have witnessed scenes of this kind. Such experiences influenced the symptom levels during the first weeks, but no impact was traced after 5 years.

Trauma of loss was related to the feeling of loss of a person in the disaster. A few of those on board did not know any of their fellow workers. The majority of the 68 survivors, however, reported a sense of loss in relation to their fellow workers in the immediate aftermath of the disaster. This disaster was not quite suitable for studying the outcome of traumatic losses, since very few lost a significant person. The degree of loss was found to effect the short-term outcome, but not the situation after 5 years.

A number (34 men) of the survivors were rescued in

lifeboats without having had to jump into the water. The rest spent some time in the water. Needless to emphasize, being immersed in the icy cold sea water represented an additional threat to life; their escape was met with a certain hindrance. Some survivors had to cope with completely different impediments: In the disaster situation, they got stuck in a room with no available exits, or with a heap of furniture on top of them. One person found himself squeezed against the wall with a big kettle of hot soup on his chest. All such situations where the survivors were stuck or in sea water, represent a kind of stressor which in this study was called *evacuation trauma*. It may resemble what has been described as "inescapable shock," where the individual has rather limited options to influence his situation. Evacuation trauma had a clear impact on the short-term outcome.

A few survivors suffered from heavy guilt feelings and severe self-blame. Survival guilt also occurred, but the core was a kind of moral conflict that haunted everyone who had been alone and had failed in their efforts to rescue a person, or who had to leave someone dying in the disaster. This has been called a *responsibility trauma*: The survivor saw himself as the major cause of the death of another human being.

After the rig had capsized, one person (here called *John*), was swimming in the direction of a lifeboat. John caught up with another person who said he could not make it anymore, who was freezing, and who had no more energy. Said John: "But I have sufficient energy for both of us. You hold on to me and we shall make it up to the lifeboat!" The person took a firm grip around John's hips. Slowly they were getting nearer. Then, all of a sudden, John felt the grip loosen. Quickly he turned round. The other fellow had disappeared. Hurriedly, John stuck his arm deep into the water and searched desperately. He got hold of the other person's hair and pulled with great force, but—in vain. He only felt the hair slip through his fingers.

In the aftermath, John was struggling with a severe depression and ruminating thoughts of this particular event: a responsibility trauma. His heavy self-accusations were related to the feeling of having caused this person's death. Only a few survivors had been exposed to this kind of constellation; that is, of being completely alone in their unsuccessful efforts to rescue another person. Without exception, each of them was depressed, burdened by merciless self-blame.

Concurrent Stress

At the time of the disaster, some of those on board were already involved in difficulties in their lives. A few had trouble with their spouses. Others reported financial difficulties, and some were in conflict with their superiors or fellow workers. Such events were considered indicative of concurrent stress at the time of the disaster and it tended to go along with a poor outcome. Those who were not burdened by such hazards were more likely to come up with a good outcome.

Childhood and Personality Traits

The quality of the childhood was measured by the Childhood Environment Scale (Vaillant, 1977). A poor childhood pointed in the direction of a poor outcome, particularly in the long-term perspective. The personality traits were detected by means of the Torgersen (1980) questionnaire, the Basic Character Inventory (BCI), which is standardized on a twin population. Its cluster of general neurotic traits seemed to point in the direction of a poor long-term outcome, whereas a high score on "sociability" and "aggressive verbal assertion" (oral aggression) pointed in the direction of a favorable outcome.

Health Insurance Records

Survivors and members of the comparison group who lived in Norway during the observation period,

from 1980 postdisaster until the end of June, 1988, were analyzed for occurrence and persistence of sick leaves. *Occurrence* expresses the number of individuals who within a certain year have been given certain diagnoses. *Persistence* is an expression of duration, that is, how many weeks sick leave a person has had within a year.

The source of the information was the official Norwegian health records, which contained exact data on sick leaves, hospitalizations, the main diagnosis, and the dates for the beginning and end of each sick leave. Baseline data from 2 years prior to the disaster showed no significant differences between the populations. The differences appeared after the disaster. Among the survivors, significant increases were found in both occurrence and persistence for the psychiatric and psychosomatic diagnoses, whereas the general somatic diagnoses, covering internal medicine and surgery, did not show significant differences. Survivors had a significantly higher frequency of casualties, which may be indicative of an increased accident proneness in victims of traumatic stress. Table 39.3 summarizes some of the findings that were published elsewhere (Holen, 1991).

PTSS-12: A Scale Measuring Stress Symptoms

The criteria of PTSD in the DSM-III (APA, 1980), and other items suggested in the literature as indicative of a person's exposure to traumatic stress, were separately tested in relation to occupational dysfunction 1 year after the disaster. The aim of these computations was to find which of the items could demonstrate separately a significant distribution with regard to occupational dysfunction. This was part of an effort to design a new questionnaire that would be brief enough for the disaster victims to complete within a few minutes, in order to give the clinician an indication of their current state. The common method of using factor analysis for the design of a questionnaire was avoided in order to obtain a clearer assessment of each item. The 12 items that passed the test were put together in the Post-traumatic

Table 39.3. Diagnoses during Sick Leaves

Group[a]	Psychiatric	Casualties	Psychosomatic	General somatic	Other
			Occurrence means[b]		
Survivors	12.3	5	13	5	2
Unexposed	1.5	3	8	4	2
p	.000	.03	(.07)	NS	NS
			Means of persistence[c]		
Survivors	4.10	0.69	2.00	0.54	0.07
Unexposed	0.20	0.18	0.52	0.20	0.06
p	.003	.05	.04	.12	NS

[a]Survivors ($n = 73$) and the unexposed comparison group ($n = 89$) compared during observation period from 1980 to 1988.
[b]Occurrence means indicating the average number of persons out of 100 per year with the different groups of diagnoses.
[c]Means of persistence indicating the average duration of sick leaves in weeks per year for different groups of diagnoses.

		Nowadays	
01.	Difficulties with sleep	Yes	No
02.	Nightmares about the event	Yes	No
03.	Depressed mood	Yes	No
04.	Tendencies to jump or startle at sudden noises or moves	Yes	No
05.	Tendencies to withdraw from contact with others	Yes	No
06.	Irritable feelings (easily getting irritable or angry)	Yes	No
07.	Unstable mood; frequent ups and downs	Yes	No
08.	Bad conscience, self-accusations, or guilt	Yes	No
09.	Fear of situations that may initiate memories of the event	Yes	No
10.	Tensions in the body	Yes	No
11.	Impaired memory	Yes	No
12.	Difficulties in concentrating	Yes	No
SUMMING UP: How many Yes		☐	

Figure 39.2. Post-traumatic Symptom Scale: Reactions to a Major Event (PTSS-12).

Symptom Scale (PTSS-12), shown in Figure 39.2. Initially, there was a 10-item version. Two items were marginally significant: difficulties in *concentrating* and in *remembering*. They have been included in the 12-item version of the PTSS.

Interpretation of the PTSS-12

Beyond the first 4 weeks of the event, a score of 6 yes or more served as an indication of a case with occu-pational dysfunction; a score of 3 to 5 yes accounted for a zone of uncertainty; and a score of 2 yes or less was not likely to go along with occupational dysfunction.

On the basis of information given during the first interview posttrauma, it was possible to make a retro-spective reconstruction of the PTSS-10 score (number of yes responses) at different intervals from the first week through eighth week, at the first interview, and after 1 year, as demonstrated in Figure 39.3. The reconstructed PTSS-10 scores showed a fairly rapid fall in symptom levels during the first four weeks. Then, it seemed to stabilize. As one may see, the average score was prac-tically the same at 4 weeks, at 8 weeks, at the time of the first interview, and 1 year posttrauma.

Discussion

None of the parameters applied showed significant differences in the proportionate rates of the deceased and the survivors, which may indicate that survival re-lated to ethnicity or age was fairly incidental in this di-saster. Such questions are sensitive, but highly relevant for e.g., in safety training, selection procedures, etc..

The survivors who were studied constituted an un-selected population. Generally, they were neither liti-gants seeking compensation nor referred psychiatric pa-tients as in many Vietnam War veteran studies. The question of compensation was not an issue during the first 5 years posttrauma, and the research program oper-ated independently of legal matters.

There were no problems related to the spatial dimensions of the disaster (i.e., whether the survivors were in the center or in the periphery of the event) (Malt, 1986). There was no such stressor gradient. With a response rate of almost 100% within the target group, no effort had to be made to infer from sample to popula-tion. The relevant question was rather to what extent

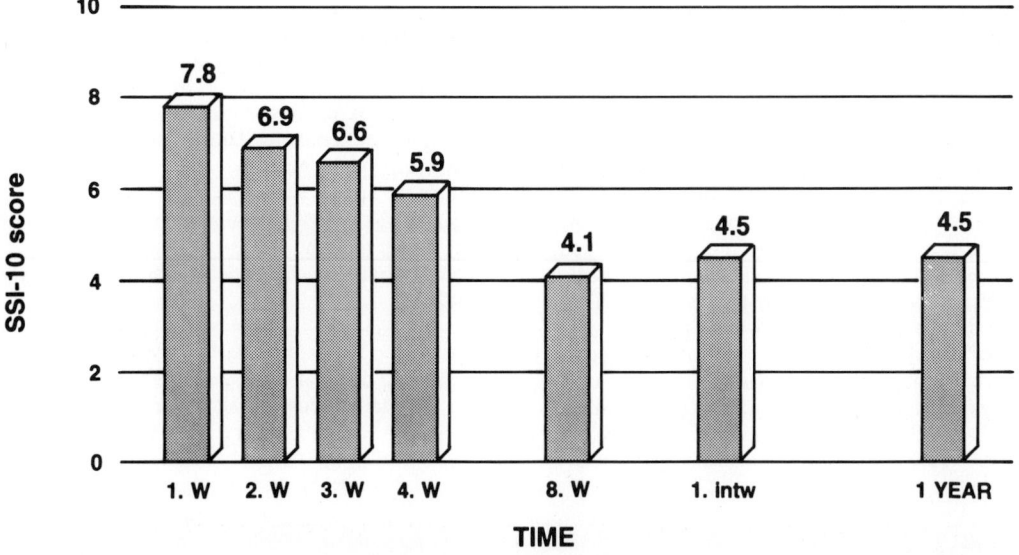

Figure 39.3. PTSS-10 reconstructed.

generalizations may be valid for similar catastrophic stressors. To some degree this depends on the comparison group. The current group were oil workers from the same oil fields, and matched for domicile, age and sex.

One third of the survivors had a poor outcome and two thirds were without such manifestations. This finding is much in line with those on similar populations (Raphael, 1986; Weisaeth, 1984). The fraction of persons with problems remains fairly constant after the initial weeks.

The subjective components tended to be associated with the long-lasting posttraumatic problems, whereas the objective components were more related to problems of a shorter duration, which indicates the relevance of the stressor criterion. However, regarding the prolonged posttraumatic problems, one may speculate that there are correlations with certain personality traits, and that the stressor represents the necessary precipitating event. If the subjective components are more or less parts of the dissociative phenomena in a broad sense, and they prove to predict outcome, we may have an important key for the search of relevant personality traits. The tendency to dissociate may define a vulnerability factor in the personality with regard to traumatic stress. The objective components may constitute another important variable in explaining the outcome.

Concurrent stress at the time of the disaster also points in the direction of a poor outcome. Those individuals who are already burdened by stress may have had less resources to cope with additional stress. However, one may also speculate whether it is not so much a question of the amount of stress as of the personality of the person involved.

The findings from the health insurance records of extensive psychiatric, psychosomatic, and even casualty-related problems in disaster survivors have implications for safety procedures and disaster help programs. The aim of such services will be to reduce the occurrence and persistence of posttraumatic manifestations of catastrophic stress. It is important to assess which therapeutic measures will prove conducive for the process to recovery.

The PTSS was first published only in Norwegian (Holen *et al.*, 1983). It is a simple and useful tool for monitoring stress symptoms: Higher scores have been associated with the loss of the ability to hold a job. Psychometric properties of the SSI scale will be published in a later paper. Figure 39.3, showing the average scores of the "former version, the PTSS-10 Reconstructed," may indicate a period which lasted the first 4 weeks posttrauma. This period is characterized by high symptom levels, but also by a rapid drop in those levels. These first 4 weeks may be called the *phase of spontaneous recovery*. When stabilized after 4 weeks, the average scores remained fairly stable; very few changes seem to occur thereafter during the first year. This finding supports the inclusion of the new criteria in the diagnosis of PTSD in the DSM-III-R, which requires the disturbance to have endured for at least 1 month.

ACKNOWLEDGMENTS

This study has been supported by grants from the Norwegian Research Council for Science and the Humanities and the Phillips Petroleum Company Norway. I am especially indebted to Tor Nome, Medical Director of Phillips Petroleum, for generous and benevolent support in every phase of the program. The Stavanger Police Department was very cooperative in supplying information on the deceased. My thanks are also extended to Marit Gilje Jaatun, who persistently collected a major part of the data in the early days of the program, as well as to the faculty members of the Division of Disaster Psychiatry at Gaustad and the Department of Psychiatry at Vinderen, University of Oslo, in Norway.

References

American Psychiatric Association. (1980). *Diagnostic and statistical manual of mental disorders* (3rd ed.). Washington, DC: Author.

American Psychiatric Association. (1987). *Diagnostic and statistical manual of mental disorders* (3rd ed., rev.). Washington, DC: Author.

Holen, A. (1991). A longitudinal study of the occurrence and persistence of post-traumatic health problems in disaster survivors. *Stress Medicine,7,* 11–17.

Holen, A., Sund, A., & Weisaeth, L. (1983). The Alexander L. Kielland disaster. Oslo, Norway: University of Oslo, Division for Disaster Psychiatry. (In Norwegian)

Horowitz, M. J. (1976, 1986). *Stress response syndromes*. New York: Jason Aronson.

Horowitz, M. J., Wilner, N., & Alvarez, W. (1979). Impact of Event Scale: A study of subjective stress. *Psychosomatic Medicine, 41,* 209–18.

Janet, P. (1973). *L'automatisme psychologique: Essai de psychologie expérimentale sur les formes inférieures de l'activité humaine.* Paris: Société Pierre Janet/Payot. (Original work published 1889)

Malt, U. (1986). Biopsychosocial aspects of accidental injuries. (Doctoral dissertation), University of Oslo, Department of Psychiatry, Oslo, Norway.

Raphael, B. (1986). *When disaster strikes.* London: Hutchinson.

Torgersen, S. (1980). Hereditary-environmental differentiation of general neurotic, obsessive, and impulsive hysterical personality trait. *Acta Geneticae Medicae et Gemellologiae, 29,* 193–207.

Vaillant, G. E. (1977). *Adaptation to life.* Boston: Little, Brown.

Weisaeth L. (1984). *Stress reactions to an industrial disaster.* Unpublished doctoral dissertation, University of Oslo, Division for Disaster Psychiatry, Oslo, Norway.

CHAPTER 40

Traumatic Stress Reactions in the Crew of the *Herald of Free Enterprise*

S. Janet Johnston

Introduction

On March 6, 1987, the British ferry, the *Herald of Free Enterprise*, with 545 passengers and crew on board, capsized in the English Channel shortly after leaving the Belgian port of Zeebrugge. One hundred and ninety-three people lost their lives in Britain's worst maritime disaster in peacetime since the sinking of the *Titanic* in 1912. Three bodies are still missing. In the immediate aftermath of the disaster, the Social Services Department of Kent County Council set up a special unit named (after the ferry) the *Herald Assistance Unit*. Its mission was to coordinate the caring response to all those affected by the disaster and to provide special coverage for Southeast Kent, where the crew and company were based.

It is as a member of that unit that I would like to describe the particular effect the disaster had on the 42 members of the ferry's crew of the 80 who survived, and the help that was given to them at the unit. What follows is not a scientific analysis but, I hope, an informative and enlightening account nevertheless.

Because it is an island nation, the sea and seafaring hold a particular place in the British imagination. For all 349 survivors of the disaster, March 6, 1987 was a dramatic reminder of the power of the sea and how vulnerable we are when things go wrong. But, for the members of the ferry's crew, whose lives revolved around the sea, the disaster brought a shattering blow and massive repercussions to their known world. They belonged to an

industry which is, to a large extent, a self-contained culture, bound together by a powerful camaraderie: the crew survivors referred to it as their "other family." In the wake of the disaster, they found that this family, in which they worked and socialized, did not in any way acknowledge or permit the expression of their feelings. There was no outlet for the overwhelming feelings of guilt, fear, and loss which they experienced, and this compounded a deep sense of shame. This was the context in which the Herald Assistance Unit sought to help the crew to find ways of coping with their posttraumatic experience.

The Disaster

Disaster struck the *Herald of Free Enterprise* suddenly and unexpectedly. The ferry had safely left Zeebrugge shortly after sunset on a routine sailing for Dover, England, only 76 miles away. The crew had left their manning stations, and passengers were sitting down to meals. The weather was fine and the atmosphere was relaxed. When just outside the harbor, the ferry suddenly listed to port (the left side of the ship). Crew members were not concerned; their initial reaction was that the ferry was swerving to avoid something and would right itself shortly. To their utter disbelief, the ferry continued to list and within 60 seconds had turned completely onto its port side. The lights went out and water poured in. Anything that was not bolted to the floor was thrown across the ship. For a moment, the lights came on again, illuminating for the passengers and crew the horrific scene before plunging them again into darkness. By a miracle, the ferry settled, half submerged, onto a sandbank, a factor that undoubtedly saved the lives of most of those who were on board.

S. Janet Johnston • Dover Counselling Centre, 9 Cambridge Terrace, Dover CT16 1YZ, England.

International Handbook of Traumatic Stress Syndromes, edited by John P. Wilson and Beverley Raphael. Plenum Press, New York, 1993.

Many of those who had been on the right side (starboard) of the ship managed to clamber through corridors and escape onto that side of the ferry. Most of the others were engulfed in freezing water without life jackets and in pitch darkness. Some managed to climb to safety, while others were left struggling to hold on amid floating debris and bodies. Members of the crew who made it out onto the side of the ferry immediately took responsibility for trying to rescue those who were still in the body of the ship. Nothing had prepared the crew for this eventuality: Their training had led them to believe that the ship would not sink by turning over and that in the event of an emergency they would have at least 15 minutes to disembark. Nevertheless, crew members began doing whatever they could. They smashed the windows on the side of the ship, lowered ropes into the darkness below, and hauled passengers out of the water. The temperature of the sea in March was so cold that they were racing against the onset of hypothermia. They had to make rapid decisions about who was alive and who was dead; they sorted bodies according to signs of life: dead to the right, alive to the left. One crew member related later: "Those that shouted got the help." They heard the voices of their colleagues crying for help—and worse—heard their crying stop. Crew members worked until they collapsed from exhaustion or were removed by the rescue services.

It did not take long for the rescue services to arrive, but the crew remained on the wreck as passengers were carried to safety. They were reluctant to leave while there was hope of rescuing more survivors. When they finally arrived on dry land, they were to have blazing lights, cameras, and microphones thrust into their faces. But they were not ready or able to respond to the intense media interest and strongly resented this intrusion into their personal experience. It was not until later when the surviving crew members were back in Zeebrugge that the enormity of what had happened gradually became evident to them. They began to realize how many people had died and how many of their friends and colleagues were still missing. Only half of the crew of 80 survived the disaster.

The next day, crew survivors reported to the Belgian authorities, before returning to Dover to face further interviews from the ferry company, government officials, the police, and the media. These inquiries indicated what was later confirmed at the official Department of Transport inquiry, that it was the failure to close the bow doors of the ferry, which are used for loading vehicles, that had been the cause of the disaster. Once the ship had left the harbor and hit the open sea, water had poured on to the car deck and capsized the vessel. The Department of Transport inquiry pointed to failures at all levels of management to institute proper and safe procedures that might have prevented the disaster. The lengthy coroner's inquest into the deaths, which followed the inquiry, returned a verdict of unlawful killing. This verdict weighed heavily on the surviving crew members. At the time of my writing, 2 years later, the Director of Public Prosecutions had just instituted criminal proceedings for manslaughter against the directors of the ferry company and three members of the crew. Guilt is a normal posttraumatic response, whether or not individuals actually see themselves as responsible for the incident concerned. In this case, the crew had to face the fact that they were implicated by association in the responsibility for the death of nearly 200 people.

Immediate Response and Intervention

The British response to the disaster naturally centered on Dover, the home of the ferry, the company, and many of the crew. Dover, like all major towns in Britain, has a disaster plan which it can bring into effect in an emergency. This plan was effective in coordinating responses to the physical and material requirements of the survivors. The local disaster plan, however, made no provision for the psychological effects of the disaster. In recent years, we have seen a growing awareness of and a need to respond to the emotional trauma experienced by survivors. The local Department of Social Services suddenly became aware that responsibility for this would fall to them. However, Kent social workers had no experience of providing for a disaster on this scale, nor were they prepared or resourced to meet the demands suddenly put upon them. There was a need to act quickly. In the event, specific advice came immediately from a British Department of Social Services which had experience of responding to a similar situation, and this was instrumental in helping the Director of Social Services in Kent to shape and coordinate his response. In the previous year, the Bradford Department of Social Services had to cope with the aftermath of a fire which swept through a spectator stand at Bradford City Football Ground, resulting in more than 50 deaths and many more injuries. Their advice was (1) to set up a specialist team, (2) to compile data on those who may have been affected, (3) to give these people a contact point for help, and (4) to reach out to those affected and not to wait for people to ask. Additional support and advice was freely given by CRUSE Bereavement Care, a voluntary organization with individuals who had counseling experience going back to the Aberfan disaster in October, 1966.

During the first week following the disaster, the Kent Department of Social Services was involved in setting up telephone help lines at the ferry company's headquarters and at the local Social Services Office for all the survivors with emotional as well as material needs. This was manned by local social workers who responded, on one level, to desperate requests by parents seeking their children, and on the other, to people anxious to have their lost duty-free purchases replaced. During this week, the crew members were seen in groups by a psychotherapist who was not linked to the local response, and, unfortunately, about whose work we know little, as she died shortly afterward. By day seven, March 13, 1987, formal counseling was being offered by the Social Services to the survivors, the bereaved, and to those directly involved in the aftermath. Among the first clients that a Social Services' colleague and I saw were senior masters who were anxious to show their crews that it was acceptable to ask for help, secretaries who typed lists of the dead and survivors (many of whom were known to them), as well as some of the surviving crew of the ferry. Our approach was to try to give them space to express their confusion and anguish.

On day 12, a meeting was arranged which was attended by representatives of all agencies involved in responding to the needs of those affected by the disaster. These included Dover District Council, Southeast Kent Health authority, the voluntary counseling organization CRUSE Bereavement Care, the shipping company, the Director of Kent Social Services, the Area Director of Southeast Kent Social Services, the Area Manager of Dover Social Services, and representatives from Bradford Social Services. At this meeting, it was agreed that since there were no local counseling services to meet the needs of those affected, the Herald Assistance Unit should be set up to coordinate the caring response. Subsequently, the unit was divided into two teams: a *Home Team* and an *Away Team*. The Home Team would help all those affected (including the crew survivors) who lived in Southeast Kent, and the Away Team would visit once those affected who lived in all other parts of the country in order to link them in to local help. The Home Team, which worked with the crew survivors, was led by Colin Weaver, previously Training and Staff Development Officer of Southeast Kent Social Services, with me, a generic social worker based in Maidstone, Kent, as his deputy. Colin and I had worked together for some years in bereavement counseling with CRUSE Bereavement Care in Maidstone. The other twelve team members, whom we recruited quickly, were all experienced counselors who had some knowledge of grief, and only two of these were social workers.[1] No professional psychiatric or psychological help was directly accessible to us until June, 1987, when our own psychologist was recruited.

First Work of the Unit

Our first task at the unit was making contact with our client group. We took on board the Bradford's Social Service advice to take a proactive stance and not to sit back and wait for requests for help. This was a period of intense anxiety for the crew survivors. In the aftermath of the disaster, they found themselves without work (it was weeks before any were reassigned to other vessels) and were under pressure from the media, the police, and the company. We were fortunate that the shipping company recognized that the crew needed the kind of support we were able to offer and they cooperated with the first phase of the unit's work by providing rooms at their headquarters for us to interview any of the staff about whom they were concerned or who wanted to see us. We had written to each surviving crew member within the first two weeks following the disaster, offering them the opportunity to discuss their feelings and reactions with a counselor. At the same time, we produced a leaflet (Kent County Council Social Services, 1987) which was given to all those who may have been affected by the disaster. It was issued by the Kent Social Services but

was based on a leaflet produced for the Bradford City Council. This leaflet set out the typical symptoms of posttraumatic stress disorder, and showed how others had reacted in similar situations. It encouraged them to help the normal healing process by working through their feelings and not suppressing them.

Within a month, the unit had its own premises, which became the organizational center for the total response. Administrative support was provided and computer software created to catalog information on the familial networks of all 349 survivors and those who had died. This software is now called the *Herald System* and has been used after many subsequent disasters. This was crucial in ensuring that all those needing help after the disaster were able to make contact with the unit. An additional and most important function of the unit, as far as the crew was concerned, was that its premises offered a readily accessible and safe environment.

Shortly after the disaster and before we had engaged the crew survivors in any meaningful work at the unit, a Royal Naval psychiatrist, Morgan O'Connell, and his team arrived in Dover, without consultation with the Department of Social Services in Kent. They saw crew survivors and their partners individually and in groups once, and carried out a questionnaire survey of the crew's experiences. There was little liaison between the Navy Team and the Herald Unit, and we received no direct feedback on the work done with the crew. However, they did recommend to crew survivors that they make use of the facilities at the unit.

Against this backdrop, we began to offer counseling on an individual basis. Our approach to this was to work from the basis that these people's experience was a normal reaction to an abnormal event. We did no "pathology hunting" but sought simply to provide a supportive environment within which thoughts and emotions could be shared and worked through. Although we were prepared, as a team, from what we had learned previously, for the symptoms of posttraumatic stress disorder, nothing could have prepared us for the sheer intensity of the horror of the survivors' experience. The *Herald* crew survivors were overwhelmed by the strength and the quality of feelings of which they had no previous conscious experience or knowledge of how to cope. A powerful example of this was the guilt they felt because some of their shipmates remained entombed in the capsized vessel, a feeling which was compounded by the fact that they were not permitted or even able to join the search.

As the scale of the task before us became apparent, it was a gruelling experience for us as counselors to provide a foil for so much raw emotion. We were very dependent on our own support and supervision and needed to adhere to a consistent pattern and approach to the work we were doing. The definition of counseling which follows, previously developed for our work in CRUSE, summed up the team's ethos:

> Counseling is a way of relating and responding to another person, so that that person is helped to explore his thoughts, feelings and behavior and to reach clearer self-understanding, and then is helped to find and use his strengths so that he copes more effectively with his life by making appropriate decisions or by taking relevant action.

---

[1] The Home Team comprised Frances Clegg, Liz Hubbard, Janice Benton, Janet Johnston, Sue Morrish, Mandy Gottschalk, Melanie Steers, Ann Palmer, Christine Smith, Penny Lewis, Colin Weaver, Kate Weaver, Valerie Cunningham, and Norma Prior.

Even so, it was difficult to convince crew survivors that this approach could be of value to them. Many of the crew could not, despite their evident distress, acknowledge the fact that they were eligible for help, nor were they prepared, as they saw it, to put themselves at risk by doing so. We had to compete with regular statements of "the bereaved need you more," or "talking about it makes it worse," and family advice to "forget about it." Some family doctors offered similar advice, encouraging them to get on with their lives before they forgot how. When crew survivors were reassigned to another vessel, the *Vortigan*, some weeks after the disaster, they found they were unable simply to get on with their lives; they found it impossible to put themselves in such responsible positions again. The effect of this was to drive the surviving crew closer together. They spent a great deal of their time in the company of one another in small groups. It was only among themselves that they felt they were understood, that they did not have to explain.

The majority of the surviving crew attended each of the 38 funerals of their dead colleagues, some of which took place 6 weeks later, after the last bodies were recovered from the wreck. As well as the funerals, there was the public inquiry, and the inquest, at which some of the crew were required to give evidence. It was alongside events such as these, and the continuous press coverage, events over which we had no control, that the unit struggled to provide a supportive presence.

Psychosocial Consequences among Crew Members

PTSD and Grief Reactions

As we interviewed the crew survivors, two inextricably intertwined strands to their experience emerged. First, they showed the acute symptoms of posttraumatic stress disorder (PTSD). Second, they were reacting to the severe losses they had suffered. These two strands were ultimately inseparable, since the experience of loss was itself part of the trauma. But the nature and circumstances of the disaster and its particular significance to the crew meant that the scale of each of these strands exceeded all expectations. On the one hand, the fact that the disaster happened so suddenly and was so far outside the crew's expectations, and the fact that they were implicated by association in the responsibility for the tragedy, combined to exacerbate the classical posttraumatic symptoms of intrusive recollection and survivor guilt. On the other hand, crew survivors experienced a catalog of loss: their friends, their ship, their employment and income, their normal community or other family, their assumptions and ways of coping, and their self-respect and self-confidence.

The crew survivors found that they were unable or unwilling to share these feelings with other colleagues or their families. Relationships in their community were dominated by a seafaring machismo, and signs of vulnerability were not tolerated. Consequently, these factors manifested themselves in their behavior. They underwent personality changes: gentle men became aggressive, aggressive men became withdrawn. Many were overcome by feelings that they could not cope and even that they were going mad, and that life had no meaning or purpose for them. Some left home, some started having affairs, three moved away from the area, and one emigrated to Australia. Family lives were disrupted. Frustration and anger were directed at wives, parents, and in some cases, children, as they found they were unable to live up to their perception of their role as provider or carer within the family. Many found that they could not handle being close to anyone, especially a new baby. And yet, they were afraid of being alone and of losing anyone else, particularly their partners, who suffered most as a result of their change of behavior. Some found they were unable to perform sexually. They suffered nightmares, an inability to sleep, intrusive recollections, and extreme sensitivity to anything that reminded them of the traumatic events. Some slept with the light on; many became hyperalert, being easily startled, restless, and agitated; they were liable to feel at any moment that the trauma was recurring. Physical sensations experienced at the time, such as the feeling of having wet feet, also recurred. Crew survivors went to extreme lengths to block out the memories of the disaster and their failure to cope with the emotional consequences, with alcohol abuse being a key method. They lost their appetites and their ability to relax; they lost weight and became physically drained.

The feelings of guilt were devastating to them: They felt that they could have done more at the time of the disaster to save the lives of colleagues and passengers, that they should have stayed on the wreck longer. They felt guilty because they had saved themselves first, and that their lives were spared at the expense of someone else's. They extended this assumed guilt to their behavior before the disaster, because they had felt, on occasion, that things were unsafe and they had done nothing about it. Some felt that they should have taken their safety training more seriously. There was, in addition, the feeling that the crew had let themselves and their company down.

Having accepted that they would never be able to return to the sea, many of the crew felt worthless, and, consequently, considered themselves unworthy of the attention of others. They felt they were a liability to their subsequent employers and to their families. Some felt that their families would be better off without them and that those who died were the lucky ones. Initiatives with regard to new careers faltered because of their lack of ability to concentrate, to apply themselves, to trust anyone enough to manage them, and to accept lower salaries. These negative components stirred deep anger at the ferry company for not offering them land-based jobs of equal status after the disaster, at new employers for not paying enough attention to safety of employees, and at themselves for not being able to go back to sea.

Long-Term Work of the Unit

For the first year, most of the work of the unit was carried out on an individual basis by a small team of counselors with experience of working with bereavement. Much of this work took place in the homes of the crew and involved helping partners and children to share and understand their experience. Our approach, which I will describe in detail when we look at group work, can be broken down into three stages: (1) Helping the survivors to sift through their feelings to *identify and contextualize* which of these were related to their experience as survivors and were preventing them from leading normal lives. (2) *Validating* those feelings, and helping survivors to find ways of managing them, with the emphasis throughout on helping the survivors to help themselves. (3) Since we had no influence or control over the crew survivors' environment, the only meaningful progress which could be made was dependent on the survivors themselves feeling that they were in control of their lives: They needed to take the *responsibility* for their own recovery.

Identification and Validation of Postdisaster Reactions

Although there was obvious merit in working on an individual basis with a survivor and his family, from an early stage we were aware that the identification and validation of feelings could be greatly assisted by bringing the crew together to share their experience in groups. What they were going through as individuals so undermined their usual methods of coping with problems that they found it very difficult to accept that their responses were normal reactions. We surmised that they needed to find this out from each other. However, our attempts to get some group work off the ground encountered resistance from the survivors, who were unable to believe that their colleagues were going through a similar experience and that they would find it acceptable if they opened up and shared these feelings together. There was an intense unwillingness to look at painful issues except individually. On top of this was the fact that the crew had at best a misleading impression of our function as carers and of the kind of work we wanted to do with them; privately, they termed us "the mind-benders."

Mistrust, Resistance of Counseling, and Denial

Initially, the only way we could get crew survivors to talk together about these issues was to offer them the use of a room at the unit to hold a regular meeting, on the understanding that none of the team would be present. This invitation, made in September, 1987, was done very informally so as to encourage them to view the meetings as more of a social event than a counseling session. These meetings were well attended, and those who came found the format and environment conducive to helping them work through their feelings. The wives of the crew survivors, however, did signal a desire to share their feelings in a structured group with counselors. By August, 1987, six of the wives were ready, with their counselors' help, to participate in some group work. Here, the grapevine, and the fact that the community was fairly close-knit, had worked for us rather

than against us. A further four wives came forward to participate in a second group.

The feedback that we received on the crew survivors' informal meetings, through individual counseling sessions, indicated to us that they needed help to look at the issues that most frightened them. There was a certain amount of denial and avoidance which needed to be confronted and teased out to help them make progress. Our breakthrough in this respect came just before the anniversary of the disaster. The unit was approached by a television company which wanted to interview the survivors for a program to commemorate the disaster. We put this to the crew survivors, and many were keen to take advantage of what they saw as an opportunity to "tell the world" what they were going through. They saw it as a way of counterbalancing the implicit criticism they had received from the media in the wake of the disaster. We were reluctant to allow the television company unrestricted access to the crew. We were well aware of the media's tendency, however honorable its intentions, to trample the individual's feelings in the process. The compromise we reached with the crew and the television company was that the crew survivors should be filmed being led through a discussion of their experience by two of the workers from the unit. Thus, excerpts from the first group work we did with crew survivors were broadcast on national television.

Those of the survivors who participated in the program and those who watched from the wings or at home felt the value of the group experience and wanted to do more. We began running a weekly group which was attended by 20 of the crew (17 men and 3 women) on and off during the course of the following year. Between October, 1987, and April, 1988, there were 146 individual attendances at the group, there being on average a group membership of at least six.

Our approach to the group work was essentially the same as the one we had taken toward the work with individuals, that is, helping the survivors to identify, validate, and manage their feelings. The most pressing need the survivors had was to make sense of their experience. During the disaster, they had very little control over what was happening to them and part of the hangover from the experience was a feeling of total helplessness. Their memories of what had happened were consequently random and incoherent; there was no clear connection between cause and effect. The stage of identification is one of making that connection, of identifying the causes of their reactions. By helping them and, most importantly, by their helping each other to put events together in some kind of sequence and order and to fill in gaps in their understanding of what took place, they began to develop a clearer, more logical memory of what had happened to replace the jumbled and frightening confusion. This explains the importance of building a clear picture of what had happened to them to enable them to manage their memories more effectively and provide a clearer context for their feelings. Some of them still have a craving for a precise "video record" of their experiences on that night.

A tool we found useful in the identification process was to ask crew survivors a series of questions as they talked through events: What were their reactions, their thoughts, their feelings, and their behavior. By applying this thoroughly, it helped to fill in gaps in their experience and to build up a detailed context for their reaction to events. It was especially important that every part of the experience that the crew regretted or felt guilty about was acknowledged. Initially, a few individuals were simply unable to bring to their conscious awareness some of the events of the disaster. One man, who found himself in the hold of the ship after the ferry capsized, had come across the body of a woman in the darkness and attempted to rescue her, although he did not know whether she was dead or alive. Eventually, he abandoned the body because he would have been unable to escape himself if he had continued with his attempt to rescue this person. For 2 years, he did not mention this to anyone, and rationalized the event by trying to convince himself that she must have been dead. Until he was able to talk this through and acknowledge his uncertainty and guilt, he was unable to find any relief.

Having built up a clearer understanding of what they had been through, the crew survivors were more able to distinguish between those feelings which were directly connected with events, and those which were not. They helped each other to sift through their feelings, to identify them, and to assign them appropriately. They were able to untangle their confused and overwhelming feelings and to build up a pattern of what they had been through at the time of the disaster and in the aftermath, and the feelings associated with it.

Emergence of Trust and Validation

By now, the second stage, the process of validation was under way. Crew survivors were able to see for themselves and confirm by observation of their colleagues that these were reasonable and normal responses. Once they began to open up and talk more freely about their experiences, they began to see that they were reacting in similar ways to their colleagues, that they were not alone in their distress and in finding it difficult to cope. As group leaders, we supported this process by acknowledging the strength of their feelings and the horror they had been through, as well as reinforcing their growing acceptance of the validity of their feelings. This was a process that brought back the intensity of their most extreme emotions and brought tremendous relief that their response was shared and understood by others.

Having identified and validated their feelings, the survivors had gone some way toward managing them. By contextualizing and understanding what they were going through, their feelings were less frightening and seemed less overwhelming. Fear of encroaching insanity receded. They were still vulnerable, however, to sudden and incapacitating periods of distress. Many suffered, and continue to suffer, nightmares, intrusive recollections, panic attacks, and outbursts of anger. The group shared their experience of these and helped each other to find ways of managing them. Again, part of this process was achieved by acknowledgment and sharing. Once a panic attack is understood by the sufferer, it is less likely to be experienced again. As group leaders, we offered information and contributed factual advice. For example, we encouraged crew survivors to keep diaries

of their nightmares; we taught basic principles of stress management; we suggested they put a certain amount of time aside each day to work through their feelings. We discouraged them strongly from using alcohol as a method of escape and helped them to see that it would be more likely to make their problems greater, rather than the reverse. All the time the emphasis was on the choice they had of aiding their own recovery by taking advantage of the opportunities provided. We suggested ways in which they might help themselves and supported them through their own discoveries. We felt very strongly that it would be inappropriate and counterproductive to try to pressure them to take certain paths because of our own convictions. It was crucial that the crew should discover their own way of dealing with their experience and should take responsibility for their own recovery, because we would not always be around to support them.

Countertransference Reactions among the Counselors

One of the most difficult areas we as carers had to deal with was the tremendous anger the crew expressed during these sessions. Looking back, I can see that, as clinicians, we were afraid of this, and that the management and control of their anger was the least satisfactory aspect of the work we dealt with. The work we did with intrusive recollections was more successful. We helped the crew to identify trigger factors, such as the noise of water faucets being turned on fast, or children screaming in a playground, or, the most powerful of all, seeing a widow of a colleague, and we looked at ways of preparing for these and managing them when they came. One man found it impossible to drive to work along a certain road because that was the road he had traveled to work with two of his friends who had both been killed on the ferry. Eventually, he learned to cope with this by spending a few minutes thinking of his colleagues and experiencing their loss before setting off along this road.

During the course of the year following the start of this group work, we began to see signs of recovery in the crew survivors. They began to look healthier, less hunched and drawn, and they began to put on weight. They became more open about expressing negative emotions, including grief, and were better able to control negative aspects of their behavior. Two years later (1989), life is still difficult for these people and some have fared better than others with jobs and relationships. There are several of the crew survivors who did not come to the groups or who moved away, and we know very little of how they coped with the experience or not as the case may be. It is a testament to the scale and trauma of the experience these people went through, that only two of the 42 crew survivors are still at sea.

Conclusion

Recently, the Herald Assistance Unit has become independent of the Kent Department of Social Services.

Renamed the Dover Counselling Centre, it now offers a wider service to the local community and is responsible for raising its own funding. A group of 10 members of the crew still meet monthly at the center. Having carried out or commissioned no empirical research into the effects of the disaster on the surviving crew or of their recovery, it is difficult to draw hard conclusions about the success of our methods. All we have is our belief in the value of counseling and the evidence of our eyes and ears as the distress and the horror of that night and its consequences in the lives of these people diminish.

We learned much during this work, and, looking back, we realize that there are things we could have done better. However, we have summarized what we feel were the main lessons in the hope that they will be of use to others who work with posttraumatic therapy:

- The importance of allowing people to take *responsibility* for their own recovery;
- the process of *identification, validation,* and *management* as a route to recovery;
- the training of carers to respond effectively to post-traumatic stress disorder;
- the importance of caring for carers—recognizing their physical and emotional needs—and also the effect of this work on carers' families;

- and, more specifically, the value of Critical Incident Stress Debriefing—a process we learned about some time after the disaster (Dyregrov, 1988) which we were able to put to good effect when a ferry carrying British school children sank in the Mediterranean the year after the *Herald of Free Enterprise* sank.

ACKNOWLEDGMENTS

I wish to acknowledge with thanks the help given to me by my eldest son, Jeremy James, in the writing of this chapter. I also wish to thank my other children, Stephen and Freya, for keeping my world in perspective during 1987 and 1988. Thanks also must go to Susan Hardaker for the personal supervision given to me during 1987 and 1988.

References

Kent Council Social Services. (1987). *Coping with a major personal crisis.* Kent, England: Author.

Dyregrov, A. (1988, August). *Critical incident stress debriefing.* Paper presented at the First European Conference on Post-Traumatic Stress, Lincoln, England.

CHAPTER 41

Earthquakes and Traumatic Stress

Early Human Reactions in Japanese Society

Tsunemoto Ōdaira, Toshiharu Iwadate,
and Beverley Raphael

Introduction

There have been few studies of immediate reactions to earthquakes and devastating disasters in many parts of the world. Historically, Japan suffers earthquakes and these have had severe effects on communities, as in the earthquake of 1923 when at least 200,000 died. In this chapter, we will report preliminary findings on two separate earthquakes that occurred 10 years apart.

The early reactions of different groups in the general population are important since they may define the capacity for life-saving and appropriate actions for mental health outcomes. They may also indicate impaired functioning immediately after, and this, of course, has significance in the tasks people may be called upon to perform for the safety and recovery of themselves and their communities. Symptom levels and mental and physical reactions may be transient effects of stress which need to be understood so that people can be properly treated. It is also critical to know whether vulnerable groups, such as the acutely or chronically ill, react in different ways and thus require special attention.

Miyagi-oki Earthquake

At 5:14 P.M. on June 12, 1978, the Miyagi-oki earthquake of magnitude 7.4 and seismic intensity 5 occurred in the Miyagi Prefecture, Japan. It affected the Pacific coastal area of the southern Tohoku district and caused deaths, injuries, and widespread damage and was concentrated in the city of Sendai and the surrounding areas. Since this could become a model case of urban disaster that includes both secondary and tertiary effects arising in relationship to complex urban functions, the effects of this earthquake are being investigated from many perspectives. In the Miyagi Prefecture, 7,129 citizens were subjects for a survey conducted concerning this disaster. The survey was conducted 1 week after the earthquake, from June 19 to the 26, 1978, and 5,474 individuals completed the questionnaire. The contents of items in the questionnaire were explained to the primary school students in the sample. Additionally, the survey sampled different age groups: from fifth graders to adults in their sixties. The sample was divided into four groups: primary school students (years 5 and 6), junior high school students (years 7 to 9), senior high school students (years 10 to 12), and adults (mostly parents of these pupils and students). In regard to geographical location during the quake, 24.7% of the sample were outdoors when the quake started, whereas almost half were (48.2%) when it ended (see Table 41.1).

In terms of initial emotional responses, 28% felt anxious during the quake. More detailed statistics show that the primary school girls suffered the most serious disturbance, followed by primary school boys, senior high school girls, junior high school girls, adult females, junior high school boys, adult males, and high school boys. A similar finding is reflected in the number of mental and physical complaints each group member made after they had experienced the earthquake.

In terms of distress reported, the average number of complaints per person was 3.7. The adults had the largest average number of complaints, followed by primary school pupils, junior high school students, and senior high school students. Further analysis revealed that the

Tsunemoto Ōdaira and Toshiharu Iwadate • Department of Psychiatry, School of Medicine, Tohoku University, Aoba-ku, Sendai 980, Japan.   **Beverley Raphael** • Department of Psychiatry, Royal Brisbane Hospital, University of Queensland, Herston 4029, Australia.
International Handbook of Traumatic Stress Syndromes, edited by John P. Wilson and Beverley Raphael. Plenum Press, New York, 1993.

Table 41.1. Number of Deaths and Injuries in Miyagi Prefecture

Area	Deaths (N)[a]	Injuries[b] Severe	Light	Total
Myagi Prefecture	27	262	10,700	10,962

[a]Main causes of death: crushed by concrete wall/fence (10 deaths), crushed by stone fence or gate posts (6 deaths), collapse of house (5 deaths), crushed by monument, roof, or earth/sand (3 deaths), caused by shock of earthquake (3 deaths). Of the those who died, 77.8% were either 60 or over or 12 and under.
[b]Of those injured, 65% were female and most were housewives; 72% of the injuries occurred indoors.

number of complaints per person was largest (5.6) in the group of adult females under 29, followed by fifth-year primary school boys, fifth-year primary school girls, and adult females over 60. Generally speaking, primary school pupils and females in other groups suffered the largest number of complaints. The groups with the fewest number of complaints were high school boys, followed by adult males in their fifties, and adult males in their forties (see Table 41.2).

Types of Complaints

When we examine the particular types of complaints, swaying of the body associated with the vibration of the earthquake was mentioned by the largest number of subjects, followed by vague feelings of anxiety. Other complaints widely reported included hypersensitivity, fear, lessening of efficiency, tiredness, anorexia, loose thinking, irritation, palpitation, loss of purpose, shaking of the body, worry, and melancholic feelings. The complaints observed in large numbers in all groups included swaying, vague feelings of anxiety, hypersensitivity, and fear. Clearly, these emotional reactions reflect heightened levels of autonomic nervous system arousal in response to the tremors produced by the quake (see Tables 41.3 to 41.6).

Tokachi-oki Earthquake

In the morning of May 16, 1968, the Tokachi-oki earthquake occurred while we were working in a psychiatric hospital in Hakodate City. We were able to witness the actions of psychiatric patients and were impressed

Table 41.2. Number of Respondents and Response Rate

Group	Level	Subjects (N)	Actual respondents (N) Male	Female	Total	Response rate
Primary school						
Kano Primary School	Year 5	208	98	105	203	97.6
	Year 6	182	93	88	181	99.5
Total		390	191	193	384	98.5
Junior high school						
Nagamachi Junior High School	Year 7	428	174	188	362	84.6
	Year 8	393	178	180	358	91.1
	Year 9	421	230	181	411	97.6
Total		1255	582	549	1131	90.1
Senior high school						
Sendai 2nd Senior High School	Year 11	366	300	—	300	82.0
Kogota Agricultural Senior High School	Year 10 and 12	471	363	—	363	77.1
Sendai 2nd Girls Senior High School	Year 11	372	—	323	323	86.8
Yamoto Senior High School	Years 10, 11, and 12	550	—	426	426	77.5
Total		1759	663	749	1412	80.3
Adults						
Families of Kano Primary School		865	134	558	692	80.0
Families of Nagamachi Junior High School		1126	203	590	793	70.4
Families of Sendai 2nd Senior High School		366	76	153	229	62.6
Families of Kogota Agricultural Senior High School		471	113	113	226	48.0
Families of Sendai 2nd Girls Senior High School		372	75	200	275	73.9
Families of Yamoto Senior High School		525	103	229	332	63.2
Total		3625	704	1843	2547	68.4
Totals		7129	2140	3334	5474	76.8

Table 41.3. "Did You Behave Calmly?" (Number/Percentage)

Groups/respondents	Calmly	Not calmly	As usual	Don't know	Unsure	No answer	Total
Male							
Primary school	111(58.1)	72(37.7)	2(1.0)	2(1.0)		4(2.1)	191(100.0)
Junior high school	405(69.6)	132(22.6)	11(1.9)	12(2.1)	6(1.0)	16(2.7)	582(100.0)
Senior high school	535(80.7)	73(110.0)	10(1.5)	15(2.3)	3(0.5)	27(4.1)	663(100.0)
Adults	495(70.3)	118(16.7)	18(2.6)	16(2.3)	7(1.0)	50(7.1)	704(100.0)
Subtotal	1546(72.2)	395(18.4)	41(1.9)	45(2.1)	16(0.7)	97(4.5)	2140(100.0)
Female							
Primary school	77(39.9)	112(58.0)	3(1.6)	1(0.5)			193(100.0)
Junior high school	283(51.5)	198(36.1)	21(3.8)	12(2.2)	2(0.4)	33(6.0)	549(100.0)
Senior high school	414(55.3)	275(36.7)	20(2.7)	13(1.7)	1(0.1)	26(3.5)	749(100.0)
Adults	1062(57.6)	536(29.1)	34(1.8)	33(1.8)	15(0.8)	163(8.8)	1843(100.0)
Subtotal	1836(55.1)	1121(33.6)	78(2.3)	59(1.8)	18(0.5)	222(6.7)	3334(100.0)
Male and female							
Primary school	188(49.0)	184(47.9)	5(1.3)	3(0.8)		4(1.0)	384(100.0)
Junior high school	688(60.8)	330(29.2)	32(2.8)	24(2.1)	8(0.7)	49(4.3)	1131(100.0)
Senior high school	949(67.2)	348(24.6)	30(2.1)	28(2.0)	4(0.3)	53(3.8)	1412(100.0)
Adults	1557(6.11)	654(25.7)	52(2.0)	49(1.9)	22(0.9)	213(8.4)	2547(100.0)
Total	3382(61.8)	1516(27.7)	119(2.2)	104(1.9)	34(0.6)	319(5.8)	5474(100.0)

Table 41.4. "Did You Sleep That Night?" (Number/Percentage)

Groups/respondents	Yes	No	No answer	Total
Male				
Primary school	97(50.8)	93(48.7)	1(0.5)	191(100.0)
Junior high school	422(72.5)	156(26.8)	4(0.7)	582(100.0)
Senior high school	574(86.6)	86(13.0)	3(0.5)	663(100.0)
Adults	428(60.8)	263(37.4)	13(1.8)	704(100.0)
Subtotal	1521(71.1)	598(27.9)	21(1.0)	2140(100.0)
Female				
Primary school	80(41.5)	112(58.0)	1(0.5)	193(100.0)
Junior high school	350(63.8)	195(35.5)	4(0.7)	549(100.0)
Senior high school	486(64.9)	256(34.2)	7(0.9)	749(100.0)
Adults	673(36.5)	1150(62.4)	20(1.1)	1843(100.0)
Subtotal	1589(47.7)	1713(51.4)	32(1.0)	3334(100.0)
Male and female				
Primary school	177(46.1)	205(53.4)	2(0.5)	384(100.0)
Junior high school	772(68.3)	351(31.0)	8(0.7)	1131(100.0)
Senior high school	1060(75.1)	342(24.2)	10(0.7)	1412(100.0)
Adults	1101(43.2)	1413(55.5)	33(1.3)	2547(100.0)
Total	3110(56.8)	2311(42.2)	53(1.0)	5474(100.0)

Table 41.5. Recollections of Day of Earthquake

Respondents	June 12 5:10–5:15 P.M. N(%)	June 12 4:00–6:00 P.M. (excluding I)[a] N(%)	Answers other than I and II N(%)	I and II[b] N(%)	No answer N(%)	Respondent numbers
Primary school	310(80.7)	55(14.3)	19(4.9)	365(95.1)		384
Junior high school	957(84.6)	124(11.0)	50(4.4)	1081(95.6)		1131
Senior high school	1138(80.6)	171(12.1)	103(7.3)	1309(92.7)		1412
Adults	2227(87.4)	248(9.7)	70(2.7)	2475(97.2)	2(0.1)	2547
Total	4632(84.6)	598(10.9)	242(4.4)	5230(95.5)	2(0.1)	5474

[a]I = correct; II = incorrect.
[b]The ratio of correct replies probably increases if the questions are answered at home because of the availability of information from the media. Accuracy probably depends on amount of media coverage and the interest held by respondent toward this.

Table 41.6. Comparison of Average Number of Reactions (Complaints) per Person

| | Immediately after | | | | | |
| | Male | | | Female | | |
Group	Total reactions	Respondents	Average reactions per person	Total reactions	Respondents	Average reactions per person
Primary school						
Year 5	517	98	5.3	514	105	4.9
Year 6	283	93	3.0	313	88	3.6
Junior high school						
Year 7	563	174	3.2	672	188	3.6
Year 8	464	178	2.6	603	180	3.4
Year 9	520	230	2.3	652	181	3.6
Senior high school						
Year 7	640	300	2.1	1221	323	3.8
Years 9, 10, 11, and 12	467	363	1.3	1413	426	3.3
Adults						
Under 30	45	14	3.2	303	48	6.3
In 30s	310	82	3.8	3947	648	6.1
In 40s	1250	494	2.5	4899	1069	4.6
In 50s	213	93	2.3	294	62	4.7
60 and over	88	21	4.2	77	16	4.8
Primary school	800	191	4.2	827	193	4.3
Junior high school	1548	582	2.7	1927	549	3.5
Senior high school	1107	663	1.7	2634	749	3.5
Adults	1926	704	2.7	9520	1843	3.5
Total	5381	2104	2.5	14908	3334	4.5

by the lack of confusion they exhibited. To see whether or not the reactions of these psychiatric patients to a sudden disaster was really unique and whether or not they were psychologically agitated by it, a survey was conducted in the form of a written questionnaire, which was administered to patients and a control group of persons without psychopathology.

The large-scale earthquake resulted in many deaths, disappearances, and destruction of houses. It occurred on the Pacific coast of the northeastern region of Hokkaido with a magnitude of 7.8 and a seismic intensity of 5.0. The aftershocks continued for about 5 weeks.

The quake began at 9:49 A.M. on May 16 with light tremors for 30 seconds to which large sidewaves and floor wave shocks were added for another 7 minutes. At the time, the authors were in the hospital on duty. We went outside during the most severe tremors. During the quake, the corridors were moving as though hit by waves and we were lucky to be able to walk without falling.

Methodology

There were 525 respondents to the survey covering five groups: psychiatric ($n = 217$), tuberculosis ($n = 99$), and medical patients ($n = 42$), and male ($n = 77$) and female ($n = 90$) nonpatients. One week after the earth-

quake, the survey was conducted in the form of a written questionnaire, during 3 days. The major purpose of the survey was to investigate psychological disturbances and helping actions. Questions were asked in interview form for those patients who could not write.

Outline of the Kashiwagi Hospital and Hakodate Nursing Home

Simple physical comparisons of the five groups was difficult because of differences in the configuration of the buildings in which they resided. However, the external conditions of the Kashiwagi Hospital, which housed the psychiatric patients, and the Hakodate Nursing Home, which housed the tuberculosis patients, are very similar. They are one-story timber buildings built in 1926. Despite reconstructions, both structures are fairly decrepit. In the Kashiwagi Hospital, there are three wards: male, female, and open wards. At the time of the earthquake there were 217 patients.

Characteristics of General Medical Patients and Normal Respondents

The normal male subjects came from the Hakodate Private University and were aged between 18 and 20.

Table 41.6 (*Continued*)

	At present				
	Male			Female	
Total reactions	Respondents	Average reactions per person	Total reactions	Respondents	Average reactions per person
259	98	2.6	261	105	2.5
184	93	2.0	177	88	2.0
295	174	1.7	286	188	1.5
219	178	1.2	298	180	1.7
211	230	1.9	270	181	1.5
280	300	0.9	543	323	1.7
216	363	0.6	947	426	2.2
19	14	1.4	140	48	2.9
206	82	2.5	2350	648	3.6
694	494	1.4	2825	1069	2.6
124	93	1.3	163	62	2.6
63	21	3.0	38	16	2.4
443	191	2.3	410	193	2.1
725	582	1.3	854	549	1.6
496	663	0.8	1490	749	2.0
1086	704	1.5	5516	1843	3.0
2750	2140	1.3	8270	3334	2.5

Most were located in a four-story reinforced concrete university building during the quake. The normal female subjects came from a kindergarten teacher training night school called Hakodate Kindergarten College and were aged between 19 and 21. At the time of the quake, they were in their various places of nighttime work. The general patients were acute medical patients suffering from a variety of diseases and illnesses.

Among the males, normal individuals suffered the most physical and mental reactions, followed by general medical, tuberculosis, and psychiatric patients in that order. Among the females, general medical patients suffered the most physical and mental reactions, followed by normal persons, tuberculosis, then psychiatric patients. The most common physical reactions among the normal subjects were body swaying (75%), hypersensitivity (56%), body trembling (20%), heavy head (17%), tiring easily (17%), palpitations (15%), body feeling strange (13%), dizziness (11%), eye tiredness (10%), and no desire to eat (9%). With the exception of body swaying (38%) and hypersensitivity (17%), the percentages were quite similar for the psychiatric group.

The most common mental reactions among the normal subject group were feelings of unease (47%), fear (34%), drop in efficiency (16%), sorrow (grief) (16%), worry about the future (16%), heavy feelings (15%), inability to gather thoughts together (14%), irritability (14%), depression (14%), unable to know what to do (11%), not feeling like oneself (8%), wanting to shout out

(7%), and feelings change easily (5%). With the exception of the feelings of unease (27%) and fears (24%), the percentages were quite similar for the psychiatric sample. Fear was less prevalent in tuberculosis patients than in psychiatric patients (11%), but heavy feelings (11%), inability to gather thoughts together (8%), and worry about the future (9%) were more prevalent in tuberculosis patients.

Although there was less agitation in the psychiatric group than expected, there was an 8.3% of "problem behavior" patients or those who acted in a way contrary to their usual adaptive behavior (51% were schizophrenic patients). The types of behavior included (1) hiding under the bed and making no attempt to move, (2) continually wiping up water flowing out of the tap at the washbasin and making no attempt to follow the nurses' instructions, (3) not moving and saying it would be better to die, (4) crying out very loudly, (5) going to hide in the toilet and coming out only after much persuasion, (6) finding a nurse and not letting the nurse out of sight, (7) going outside still holding a bucket of hot water obtained while in the bathroom, (8) returning back into the building to collect slippers that had been forgotten, (9) standing stock still after having picked up slippers, (10) going to get luggage but unable to escape outside, and (11) lying prostrate without moving at the refuge shelter.

There was almost no change in the number of psychiatric outpatients attending the Kashiwagi Hospital.

The only change was on the day of the earthquake when only one half of the normal number came in. There was only an increase in the number of regular neurosis outpatients who complained of body swaying and tiredness after the earthquake.

Summary

At first we described the early reactions of the genearl population (7,129 citizens) to the Miyagi-oki earthquake on June 12, 1978, and then we compared and discussed the reactions of 217 psychiatric patients, 77 normal males, 90 normal females, 99 tuberculosis patients, and 42 medical patients who experienced the Tokachi-oki earthquake in Hakodate City on May 16, 1968.

Compared with other groups, the percentage of psychiatric patients who escaped outdoors was the same, if not higher, than other groups and the percentage who acted calmly was high. However, their recollection of the date and time of the earthquake was extremely poor. They had few mental and physical reactions, and the type of reactions were slightly different to those in other groups.

We termed all the reactions at the time of the earthquake as "shock syndrome due to earthquake" and outlined the characteristics of reactions of the psychiatric patient group. As background to this we examined (1) effects of "sickness" characteristics of psychiatric patients, in particular, schizophrenic patients; (2) effects of long-term hospitalization; and (3) effects of locked psychiatric wards and the unease caused by the earthquake. However, the form of reactions in the psychiatric patient group had much to do with the effects of social factors as well as the effects of "sickness" characteristics.

Reactions of Psychiatric Patients

Throughout the earthquake the psychiatric patients appeared to show fewer reactions than others. Overall, they were "calmer." However, their memory of the date and time of the earthquake was poorer. Reaction numbers were similar to those of tuberculosis patients but, unlike these and other groups, their reactions tended to continue at a high level.

Conclusion

It is clear from our discussion that there is a substantial reaction to the stress and trauma of earthquakes. The reaction encompasses bodily complaints as well as psychological indications of anxiety and is maximal immediately after the tremors, rapidly declining 1 to 2 weeks later. The reactions are of such frequency as to affect more than half the population immediately, and to still be present to some degree for more than a quarter of the population 1 to 2 weeks later. These reactions show the earliest manifestations of traumatic stress effects which are normal for the population but still potentially serious. Whether or not they result in long-term problems is yet to be established, but it would seem that for the majority of those studied they are more likely to experience a reactive process which can be understood as normal and frequent after such a traumatic event.

References

Ōdaira, T., Katō M., Fukuda, M. (1974). Reactive attitudes of psychiatric patients to the Tokachi-oki earthquake (Japan). *Seishin Igaku, 16*, 31–39.

Ōdaira, T., Itō, F., Shingū, S., *et al.* (1979). Psychiatric study about reactions of the general population in the Miyagi-oki earthquake (Japan). *Bulletin of Miyagi Mental Health Center, 7,* 1–25.

Raphael, B. (1986). *When disaster strikes.* New York: Basic Books.

CHAPTER 42

Study of a Major Disaster in the People's Republic of China

The Yunnan Earthquake

Alexander Cowell McFarlane and Cao Hua

Introduction

Long-Term Effects of Disaster

There is continuing controversy about the nature and extent of psychological effects of major disasters (McFarlane, 1985; Quarantelli, 1985). The opinions range from those who state that disasters have little or no immediate effect (Melick, 1978; Quarantelli & Dynes, 1977) to those who state that disasters have significant long-term consequences (Gleser, Green, & Winget, 1981; McFarlane, 1988; Shore, Tatum, & Vollmer, 1986). This controversy may arise from a number of reasons. First, the research methodologies used to study disasters have many associated problems (Green, 1982). Often, highly selective subsamples of victims have been studied, for example, all the victims evacuated to one area (Parker, 1975). Not infrequently, poorly validated instruments have been used which make the interpretation and clinical significance of the results difficult to establish. Furthermore, many of the early studies failed to describe adequately the experience of the individual victims in the disaster or relate the levels of exposure to the intensity of symptoms. This is an important issue because certain characteristics of the disaster, such as the seriousness and level of the impact, the speed of the onset, the duration of the disaster, and social preparedness of the community to handle the disaster, may all be important determinants of the outcome (see Chapter 27, in this volume, for a discussion of these issues).

However, a number of these earlier deficiencies have been overcome in more recently conducted studies (McFarlane, 1988; Shore et al., 1986). The recent upsurge in interest into the effects of traumatic stress, which followed the definition of posttraumatic stress disorder in the DSM-III (American Psychiatric Association, 1980), has provided a major impetus for research into the effects of traumatic stress generally. This has served to provide a much more focused inquiry into the type of symptoms that are likely to arise from stressful events, as well as the general process of adaptation to traumatic events. As well, specific attempts have been made to develop instruments which have a demonstrated validity in the populations being examined (Lima, Santacruz, Lozano, & Luna, 1988). Despite these important improvements, there is still a paucity of data from proper epidemiologically conducted studies sampling the differential effects of exposure to natural disasters. Although the sophistication of the studies has been improving, practicalities have meant that systematic population samples are often not studied. For example, Maj et al. (1989) studied the prevalence of psychiatric disorders among general practice attenders from three regions differentially exposed to an Italian earthquake. Even though these data give some preliminary estimates, it clearly does not represent a population estimate as a number of other variables may influence attendance to a general practitioner. In contrast, McFarlane (see Chapter 34, in this volume) investigated the impact of a bushfire on an affected population. Shore et al. (1986), although not giving population estimates, studied the effects in specific communities with a differential exposure to the Mount St. Helen's volcanic eruption. Lima et al. (1987), in their study of the Amero Mud Slide, pointed out that

Alexander Cowell McFarlane • Department of Psychiatry, University of Adelaide, Gilles Plains, South Australia 5086, Australia.   Cao Hua • Department of Psychiatry, Flinders University of South Australia, Bedford Park, South Australia 5042, Australia.

International Handbook of Traumatic Stress Syndromes, edited by John P. Wilson and Beverley Raphael. Plenum Press, New York, 1993.

much of the disaster data generated has been from industrialized countries. They emphasized that the plight of developing countries has been largely ignored and that the experiences from developed countries may not necessarily be applicable.

The degree of technological development of a country may have implications for the study of disasters. Until 1986, excluding the United States, there were 2,392 disasters in the world, of which 86.4% had occurred in highly industrialized nations. Of the 42 million deaths that had occurred, 78% were in industrialized nations. The observed ratio between affected (exposed) to killed was 2.9 for developed nations. The comparative ratio of exposed/killed in underdeveloped countries is ten times greater (United States Agency for International Development, 1986). This higher prevalence of death to exposure may reflect the ability for more technologically sophisticated countries to create physically effective rescue and recovery mechanisms. Disasters, therefore, are not only disproportionately more frequent events in the Third World but are also responsible for a much higher proportion of victims who will need long-term assistance.

The growth of populations in developing countries has also meant that populations are frequently being forced to occupy areas that are vulnerable to a variety of natural hazards. For example, of the 1 billion 100 million people living in the People's Republic of China, it is estimated that 400 million live in flood-prone regions (*New China Daily*, 1989). Against this background, there is a major imperative to gain a better understanding of the impact of natural disasters in developing countries. The massive impact of many disasters in these countries is likely to place extreme demands on their health and welfare systems. As well, it is important to examine the predictors of disorder within these communities.

This chapter will focus on the impact of a major earthquake which affected Yunnan Province in Southwest China in 1988. China, being the most populated country, is also particularly prone to disasters. In recent history, this nation has been subject to a number of extremely catastrophic events. Floods and tidal waves in the Hwang-Ho River in 1931 claimed approximately 3.7 million lives. A more recent disaster was the earthquake in Tangshan in 1976, which took over 655,000 lives (Lystad, 1988).

Phenomenology of Traumatic Stress Reactions in Developing Countries

The study of traumatic events in developing countries has a further contribution to make to psychiatric research. For example, in the 1980s, posttraumatic stress disorder (PTSD) has occupied a central focus in psychiatric research. Much of the data have been generated from the investigation of United States Vietnam veterans (Wilson, 1988, 1989). This raises many questions about the extent to which the findings can be extrapolated to other populations, just as it is difficult to know how much it is possible to generalize from the studies of disaster (Green and Grace, 1988). Understandably, chronic attenders at veteran's affairs outpatient and inpatient services have been the particular focus of a generation of

researchers. Often, they have been symptomatic for 15 or more years, and the role of such factors as compensation, drug and alcohol abuse, and chronic patient status have come to affect their reasons for presentation and the pattern of symptoms. As well, a number of other groups of victims have been studied and results have found a number of differences when compared to the Vietnam veterans. Such issues as the relevant importance of premorbid personality to the etiology of posttraumatic stress disorder still require considerable clarification of different populations. Furthermore, the sensitivity and specificity of the diagnostic criteria for PTSD are liable to change according to the population examined and the duration of the disorder. There is considerable need for clarification of these issues (McFarlane, 1988a,b).

Investigations of these issues in an underdeveloped country would contribute significantly to the future refinement of the criteria of posttraumatic stress disorder in a revision of the DSM. For example, the definition of the *stressor criterion* in the DSM-III-R (American Psychiatric Association, 1987) is significantly influenced by factors that affect the perception of what is a traumatic event. The loss of property to an affluent community may have a different meaning than to an impoverished peasant farmer. The diagnosis of PTSD implies the existence of high levels of the distress generated by traumatic events. It is therefore particularly important that these hypotheses are examined critically and the developing countries offer an unusual opportunity in this regard. Equally, the distress response and its phenomenology are likely to be influenced by important cultural and ethnic influences. The relative importance of these issues is also likely to clarify whether or not a posttraumatic stress disorder can be legitimately seen as a universal pattern of trauma response.

Yunnan Earthquake

This chapter will describe a major disaster in Southern China and the methodology of a research project which aims to examine some of the issues outlined. A massive earthquake struck in Yunnan Province in Southwestern China on November 6, 1988. The affected county (province) is one of the poorest in the People's Republic of China, with 47.8% of the population living on the borderline of inadequate food supplies. In the area affected, 25% were of Chinese descent and origin. The majority of the population were made up of ethnic minorities, including the Lafu, a group related to the Burmese whose written language is Arabic symbols and the Dai people who are closely related to Thai people. In the Lanchang county, which was affected by the earthquake, the majority of the population are peasant farmers, 60% owning their own houses. The ethnic Chinese were responsible largely for the provision of government services and professional occupations, and they also ran the trading posts.

Nature of the Earthquake

The earthquake struck at 21:03 hours and measured 7.6 on the Richter Scale. In all, 81,000 families and

430,144 people were affected by the earthquake. Damage occurred over an area of 2,141 square miles, with 24.3% being seriously affected. The area of this seriously affected region was inhabited by 119,465 people.

Stressors and Impact of the Disaster

The numbers killed and injured were much smaller than may have been the case: 643 died and 3,558 people were injured, of whom one third sustained serious injuries. At the time of the Sunday night when the earthquake occurred, many farmers were still working, whereas the rest of the population were in open-air theaters. Furthermore, a small tremor heralded the major quake by 10 minutes, which meant that most people had gone outside for safety. Between November 6 and January, 1989, 5,020 aftershocks were experienced in the district.

Initial Rescue and Relief Efforts

The immediate relief was provided by the army, who occupied the district for 1 month and were involved in reconstruction work. They distributed clothes, blankets, and food, and the distribution was made according to need. However, there was considerable dissatisfaction among the community about the mechanism of distribution. The government gave no money directly to the peasants. However, the 1,000-yuan allotment distributed per person went to such public institutions within the district as schools and hospitals. Many complained that the clothes they were provided were old and dirty and often without buttons. Some of the area residents felt that they were slighted in the distribution of aid money following the earthquake.

Sample Characteristics

Villages Studied

Three villages were chosen for investigation. The first lay 20 kilometers from the epicenter of the earthquake and included 2,490 people, of whom 1,595 were ethnic Chinese. In this village, 18 people were killed and 162 seriously injured.

The second village to be studied lay 37 kilometers from the epicenter and consisted of 5,762 people, of whom 2,623 were ethnic Chinese. Nobody was killed in this village, although 45 were seriously injured and 30 sustained minor injuries. In this village, the earthquake was of an intensity that destroyed mud brick homes but only left structural damage of more substantial dwellings of fired bricks and reinforced concrete.

The third village lay 60 kilometers from the epicenter. In this district, the strength of the earthquake was only sufficient to crack walls and remove plaster. The exact population estimates of this village could not be ascertained, and approximately one third were ethnic Chinese.

Methodological Difficulties

In the disaster population, it was not possible to study the ethnic minorities because they did not speak the Mandarin dialect. Furthermore, it was extremely difficult to carry out a systematic investigation of the ethnic Chinese because no public records were available for the random selection of subjects. Rather, the main street of each village was surveyed. In each village, the primary schools, high schools, government offices, shops, post offices, banks, and hospitals were surveyed. Within each institution, the subjects were randomly sampled. The number working within each institution was also chosen so that the proportions in the total sample were similar between the two villages. In this way, there was an attempt to match the subjects in each village by sex and occupation. The investigation was hampered by the primitive communications in the district, and the data had to be collected prior to the monsoon season. Frequently, by May or June, the roads in the district became impassable because of the weather conditions.

Control Group Population

A population from a very similar community on the basis of the commerce in the district and the ethnic mix was also surveyed as a control population. This population was unaffected in the disaster. Subsequently, a group of ethnic minorities in the region was examined using a similar methodology. This subpopulation was examined to see what effects the ethnic differences had on the outcome from the disaster. As well, a subgroup of 50 disaster victims were interviewed using the complete Diagnostic Interview Schedule (DIS) to examine the comorbidity of posttraumatic stress disorder in this population.

Methodology

The subjects were initially given a questionnaire which consisted of a detailed inventory of their exposure and losses in the disaster based on that developed by McFarlane (1987) for the investigation of another disaster. The 28-item General Health Questionnaire (GHQ) (Goldberg, 1972), the Impact of Events Scale (IES) (Horowitz, Wilner, & Alvarez, 1979), and the Eysenck Personality Inventory (EPI) had previously been used for social psychiatric research in the People's Republic of China, and found to be appropriate measures. The questionnaires were given to the individual subjects by one of a team of five people. Three were psychiatrists from a local mental hospital, one was a doctor from the People's Liberation Army, and the fifth was Dr. Cao, who also coordinated the collection of data. The questionnaires were scored the following night, and those with a GHQ score of five or greater were interviewed using the Posttraumatic Stress Disorder section of the DIS (Robins, Helzer, Croughan, & Ratcliff, 1981) (see Chapter 15, in this volume, for a discussion of the DIS).

Preliminary Observations

The earthquake in Yunnan occurred after nightfall. Many people stated they saw a very bright blue light, which was likened to the color of fireworks burning. This phenomenon only accompanied the first earthquake. Subsequently, the sight of a similar colored light (e.g., from a welder) acted as a powerful trigger for post-traumatic memories. In the two villages closest to the epicenter, people were unable to stand, and the shock of the tremor made the ground visibly move and buildings sway.

Phobic anxiety was a commonly described symptom. For example, half the population interviewed stated they had not gone back to the open-air theaters following the earthquake because of their fear which was engendered at the height of the quake.

Cognitive Attributions of the Quake Tremors

The ethnic minorities appear to have been particularly perplexed by the experience. Some of them had no knowledge of the existence of earthquakes. Rather they had a mythical explanation that the tremor was due to a great dragon who was moving underneath the ground. They believed that the dragon wanted the earth to turn over because the beast was unhappy and angry. They also believed that the dragon had trapped people under the earth whom it wished to let out to replace the people on the earth's surface. For this reason, during the height of the quake, many of these people ran out of their homes shouting "I am here" to tell the dragon there were already enough people on the surface of the earth. Others believed that there were several dragons: the father, who was seen as being evil, and the son, who was good.

One group of ethnic minorities found it particularly difficult to manage in the period after the disaster. A group of approximately 20 individuals attempted mass suicide by eating an herbal preparation, although none of them died.

In the community, there was little overt complaint about psychiatric morbidity. Physical symptoms, such as palpitations, were a common focus of people's distress. Similarly, headaches were a frequent focus of complaint. The available medical services in the district were inadequate, and the nearest hospital was 78 kilometers away. Most of the local doctors were incompletely trained, having had but three years of graduate training.

The researchers were alerted to several cases of psychotic illness, triggered by the earthquake, among the subjects they examined. At the local psychiatric hospital, there was an increased number of admissions from the disaster area. This was of particular note because the scarce resources in this district meant that only the severely psychotic and behaviorly disturbed were admitted to the hospital. The increase in admissions was mostly accounted for by victims with schizophrenia, although there was also a concurrent increase in admissions with depressive illness. It was not possible to ascertain whether this reflected the true increase in the

incidence of these disorders, or whether it was simply that the disaster-affected community was less able to manage the mentally ill living in the region.

Results

At this stage, not all the data from the study have been analyzed. A total of 1,288 subjects were examined in the disaster region.

In the most severely affected village, 410 people were studied and 59.5% scored five or greater on the General Health Questionnaire. In the second village, where mud brick homes were destroyed but more stable structures were damaged but remained standing, 458 of the population were studied. Of these, 214 (46.2%) scored in the caseness range on the GHQ. In the third village, which only sustained minor damage, 180 of the 420 people scored in the caseness range. This represented 42.8% of the population. Overall, 49.5% of the population were scoring in the caseness range. The prevalence range from the control population are not yet available in any detail. However, 30.8% of this population scored five or greater on the GHQ. A preliminary analysis of this investigation demonstrated that, in the most severely affected regions of this disaster, there is approximately a doubling of the psychiatric morbidity rates, with 60% of the population scoring five or greater on the 28-item GHQ. These rates of morbidity were observed 6 months after the disaster, suggesting that they were detecting a more enduring pattern of psychiatric morbidity rather than the acute distress associated with a major disaster. By this time, most people were rehoused and the public services had been reinstituted. Thus, this psychiatric disorder could not be seen simply as a result of the immediate social hardships endured by the population.

Similar to the study of Shore *et al.* (1986), a *gradient effect* was found across these communities. In the least affected community, there were no injuries or deaths, and only minor damage was sustained. In contrast, in the most severely affected community, the majority of houses were either destroyed or severely damaged and a number of deaths had occurred. Despite the marked difference in the intensity of the quake and this destructiveness, there was only a 17% greater morbidity in the most severely affected community. This points to the role of a variety of other intrapsychic, biological, and social factors influencing the prevalence of morbidity within this disaster-affected community.

Discussion

The other major study which has examined the prevalence of psychiatric disorder, using an epidemiological method, found that 12 months after a major bushfire disaster in Australia, the affected community had approximately twice the prevalence of psychiatric morbidity anticipated (see Chapter 34, in this volume). Thus, the order of effect demonstrated in these disasters was very similar.

The findings of this current study are of particular note because they demonstrate a substantial rate of morbidity, considering the very large populations affected. This is likely to have particular importance on influencing the behavior and long-term rehabilitation of the affected population. The anecdotal observation that much of the posttraumatic morbidity was manifest as somatic symptoms, emphasizes the importance of alerting primary health care workers in developing countries of psychiatric morbidity.

Following the Bhopal disaster in India, one of the major steps taken to assist the victims was the development of a mental health education program for general practitioners. It was recognized that there were many deficiencies in undergraduate psychiatric education, and, as a result, a special manual and teaching program was developed (Murthy, Isaac, Chandrasekhar, & Bhide, 1987). Lima, Pai, Santacruz, Lozano, and Luna (1987) also investigated these issues extensively after the Amero Mud Slide in Colombia. They developed a screening instrument for detecting psychiatric morbidity in this population, as well as developing a model for assisting interventions by primary health care workers. Thus, the increased prevalence of psychiatric morbidity found in the current study is further justification for the development of such an approach. The focus of early inputs on the training of mental health workers is also of importance in developed countries (McFarlane, 1986). Disaster victims often wish to use their own resources and community health workers rather than turn to the relief agencies who come into their regions because they may be perceived as not being particularly understanding of their unique predicament.

The systematic collection of the data in this study and the careful sampling of the affected populations provide considerable weight to the findings. It is further evident that the view of Quarantelli (1985) that disasters cause no psychiatric morbidity requires significant modification. Many of the criticisms that he has correctly made of earlier studies have now been met by this and other more recent investigations. Particularly because compensation was not a possibility for the victims of this disaster, this variable cannot be seen as complicating these findings. If anything, the interviewers in this study were likely to have underscored the severity of people's reactions because of the relative lack of knowledge about posttraumatic stress disorder in the People's Republic of China.

Many questions arise from these preliminary analyses. The extent to which people's individual exposure to the disaster might predict the prevalence of morbidity will need to be examined in considerably more detail by comparing the impact of individual losses on the levels of symptomatology. This will provide some interesting insights into the definition of the stressor criterion in the DSM-III-R. In particular, it will be relevant to examine the relative prevalence of posttraumatic stress disorder in the most severely and least severely affected communities.

The pattern of symptomatic complaint in this underprivileged area of the People's Republic of China will also provide some important clues into the nature of posttraumatic phenomenology. For this reason, a special attempt is being made to interview members of the eth-nic minorities. Their belief about the role of the "dragon" during the earthquake will also be investigated to see how this influences the nature of their traumatic imagery and recollections.

Finally, this study highlights some of the ongoing difficulties of disaster research. Although these communities were relatively open to the investigations, the inadequacy and lack of availability of public records significantly hampered a more systematic attempt at sampling. The procedure of examining a carefully balanced selection of the institutions in the main streets of each town would appear to provide a viable comparison, although it is less adequate than the random selection of subjects from a census list. In a more detailed analysis, the matching of the samples will be checked to ensure that this did not inadvertently lead to any particular bias. In contrast to some other studies of disasters, the return rate in this investigation was 100%. This provides further support for the validity of the conclusions.

Finally, the report of the increased admissions to the mental hospital training may indicate an increase in the incidence of schizophrenia or major depression following this event. Conversely, it is quite probable that the ability of these communities to contain their mentally ill would have been severely taxed during the period of considerable hardships through the winter which followed this disaster, necessitating the admission of such patients to a hospital. Whatever the case, it does indicate that developing countries may have to prepare themselves for this increased rate of hospital admission, particularly when very large populations, in the order of hundreds of thousands, are affected. Furthermore, the attempted suicide by a large group of people from one of the ethnic minorities in this region demonstrates the intensity of despair that can occur following the communal disruption and disorganization after such a major event. It points to the importance of disaster organizations' understanding the potential for such despair and distress and providing immediate support and assistance for any particularly fractured or distressed community.

References

American Psychiatric Association. (1980). *Diagnostic and statistical manual of mental disorders* (3rd ed.). Washington, DC: Author.

American Psychiatric Association. (1987). *Diagnostic and statistical manual of mental disorders* (3rd ed., rev.). Washington, DC: Author.

Gleser, G. C., Green, B. L., & Winget, C. (1981). *The long psychosocial effects of disaster*. New York: Academic Press.

Goldberg, D. P. (1972). *The detection of psychiatric illness by questionnaire*. London: Oxford University Press.

Green, B. L. (1982). Assessing the levels of psychiatric impairment following disaster. *Journal of Nervous and Mental Disease, 170*, 544–552.

Green, B. L., & Grace, M. (1988). Conceptual issues in research with survivors and illustrations from a follow-up study. In J. P. Wilson, Z. Harel, & B. Kahana (Eds.), *Human adaptation to extreme stress: From the Holocaust to Vietnam* (pp. 105–123). New York: Plenum Press.

Horowitz, M. J., Wilner, N., & Alvarez, W. (1979). Impact of events scale, their measure of subjective distress. *Psychosomatic Medicine, 41,* 209–218.

Kinzie, J. D., Frederickson, R. H., Benn, R., Fleck, J., & Kail, W. (1984). Post-traumatic stress disorders amongst survivors of Cambodian concentration camps. *American Journal of Psychiatry, 141,* 645–652.

Lima, B. R., Pai, S., Santacruz, H., Lozano, J., & Luna, J. (1987). Screening for the psychological consequences of a major disaster in a developing country: Colombia. *Acta Psychiatrica Scandinavica, 76,* 561–567.

Lima, B. R., Santacruz, H., Lozano, J., & Luna, J. (1988). Planning for health-mental health integration in emergencies. In M. Lystad (Ed.), *Mental health response to mass emergencies* (pp. 371–393). New York: Brunner/Mazel.

Lystad, M. (1988). Perspectives on human response to mass emergencies. In M. Lystad (Ed.), *Mental health responses to mass emergencies: Theory and practice* (pp. xvii-xliii). New York: Brunner/Mazel.

Maj, M., Starace, F., Crepet, S., Lobrace, F., Veltro, F., DeMarco, F., & Kenali, D. (1989). Prevalence of psychiatric disorder amongst subjects exposed to natural disaster. *Acta Psychiatrica Scandinavica, 79,* 544–549.

McFarlane, A. C. (1985). The effects of stressful life events and disasters: Research and theoretical issues. *Australian and New Zealand Journal of Psychiatry, 19,* 409–421.

McFarlane, A. C. (1986). Post-traumatic morbidity of a disaster: A study of cases presenting for psychiatric treatment. *Journal of Nervous and Mental Disease, 174*(1), 4–14.

McFarlane, A. C. (1987). *Life events and psychiatric disorder: The role of the natural disaster, 151,* 362–367.

McFarlane, B. (1988a). The phenomenology of post-traumatic stress disorder following a natural disaster. *Journal of Nervous and Mental Disease, 176,* 22–29.

McFarlane, A. C. (1988b). The longitudinal course of post-traumatic stress morbidity: The range of outcomes and their predictors. *Journal of Nervous and Mental Disease, 176,* 30–39.

Melick, M. E. (1978). Life change and illness: Illness behaviour of males and the recover period of a natural disaster. *Health and Social Behavior, 19,* 335–342.

Murthy, R. S., Isaac, M. K., Chandrasekhar, S., & Bhide, A. V. (1987). *Bhopal disaster manual of mental health care for medical officers.* Bangalaw, India: National Institute of Mental Health and Neurosciences.

Parker, G. (1975). Psychological disturbance in Darwin evacuees following cyclone Tracy. *Medical Journal of Australia, 24,* 650–652.

Quarantelli, E. L. (1985). An assessment of conflicting views on mental health. In C. R. Figley (Ed.), *Trauma and its wake* (pp. 173–215). New York: Brunner/Mazel.

Quarantelli, E. L., & Dynes, R. R. (1977). Response to social crisis and disaster. *Annual Review of Sociology, 3,* 23–49.

Robins, L. N., Helzer, J. E., Croughan, J., & Ratcliff, K. S. (1981). National Institute of Mental Health diagnostic interview schedule: Its history, characteristics and validity. *Archives of General Psychiatry, 38,* 381–389.

Shore, J. H., Tatum, E. L., & Vollmer, W. M. (1986). Psychiatric reactions to disaster: The Mount St. Helen's experience. *American Journal of Psychiatry, 143,* 590–595.

Staff. (1989, May 26–29). Beijing: *New China Daily.*

United States Agency for International Development (1986). *Disaster history: Significant data on major disasters worldwide, 1900–1989.* Washington, DC: Office of U.S. Foreign Disaster Systems.

Wilson, J. P. (1988). Understanding the Vietnam veteran. In F. Ochberg (Ed.), *Post-traumatic therapy and victims of violence* (pp. 225–254). New York: Brunner/Mazel.

Wilson, J. P. (1989). *Trauma, transformation and healing: An integrative approach to theory, research with post-traumatic therapy.* New York: Brunner/Mazel.

CHAPTER 43

Traumatic Stress Reactions to Motor Vehicle Accidents

David J de L Horne

Introduction

The traffic problem is one of the most serious confronting the living organism. Deaths on the highway and on the city streets are increasing rapidly. The use of the automobile, a result of the highly developed human nervous system, also taxes that nervous system to its utmost because many of the activities of the individual bring him unexpectedly or uncontrollably into relationship with that moving, potentially homicidal object, the automobile. It is necessary for the individual to have perfect coordination in avoiding an automobile which is rapidly approaching him and to have perfect coordination in handling one. His psychosensory equipment must be adequate, so that he can sense and perceive traffic complications. (Selling, 1940, p. 385)

This passage was written 50 years ago and raises questions about what progress has really been made since then by human beings in their dealings with that "potentially homicidal object," the automobile. What happens when things go wrong with the delicate human "psychosensory equipment" and an "accident" occurs, has, of course, been the focus of considerable inquiry. Treatment of physical trauma has improved substantially, but is the same true for the treatment of psychological sequelae to road trauma? A literature search reveals very little. We know that general understanding of trauma and its psychological effects has improved immensely in the past 10 years, but it is strange that one of the most frequent of all traumatic events, road accidents, receives such scant attention (Kluch, Swinson, & Kirby, 1985; Walker, 1981). A handful of papers have appeared

during the 1980s pointing out that even when physical injury is relatively slight and good recovery has been made, people involved in motor vehicle and other common accidents can be left with residual, undetected, and untreated long-term psychological disturbances (Pilowsky, 1985). Thus, it does seem that people with psychological problems after a traffic accident receive far less attention than they deserve, and this has both personal and societal costs.

The incidence of fully developed posttraumatic stress disorder (PTSD) in road accident cases, as defined by the American Psychiatric Association's (APA) *Diagnostic and Statistical Manual of Mental Disorders*—3rd edition, revised (1987, pp. 247–251) (DSM-III-R)—is probably rare (Helzer, Robins, & McEvoy, 1987) but other psychological stress reactions, particularly phobic anxiety and panic symptoms, would often appear to go undetected and untreated (Kluch *et al.*, 1985). Also, more attention may need to be paid, than has been done in the past, to helping people with motor vehicle accident-induced whiplash injury learn how to cope with chronic pain (Porter, 1989).

In this chapter, I will argue, through the presentation and analysis of seven case histories, that the imbalance of attention to the psychological consequences of being a road accident victim needs to be redressed. From the limited findings to date, a good argument can be made that appropriate early assessment and treatment of the psychological consequences of being such a victim can significantly reduce the stress experienced and often speed up a return to a more normal and happier life.

Trauma Patients

The seven patients all suffered from long-term (more than 6 months) psychological problems. They were all treated by me. They did not form part of a

David J de L Horne • Department of Psychiatry, Clinical Sciences Block, University of Melbourne, Victoria 3050, Australia.
International Handbook of Traumatic Stress Syndromes, edited by John P. Wilson and Beverley Raphael. Plenum Press, New York, 1993.

systematic research project but careful analysis of the way they eventually came to receive therapy and the issues encountered in carrying out therapy did provide information that could lead to more effective intervention with these people in the future. This study also highlights areas where both research and education of the community needs to be improved. Upon referral, all seven individuals were carefully assessed against the APA's (1987) criteria for PTSD. The results are presented in Table 43.1.

Table 43.1. Analysis of Motor Vehicle Accident Cases

Diagnostic criteria of PTSD	Full PTSD cases (sex and age)			Other cases (phobic) (sex and age)			
	(1) Female 33	(2) Female 33	(3) Female 25	(4) Male 37	(5) Female 32	(6) Male 33	(7) Female 26
A. Person experienced that event outside the range of usual human experience and that would be markedly distressing to almost anyone.	+	+	+	+	+	+	+
B. Traumatic event persistently reexperienced in at least two of the following ways:							
1. Recurrent, intrusive, distressing recollections of the event	+	+	−	−	−	−	−
2. Recurrent, distressing dreams of the event	−	+	+	−	−	−	−
3. Sudden acting or feeling as if the traumatic event were recurring (reliving it, illusions, hallucinations, flashbacks)	−	+	−	−	−	−	−
4. Intense psychological distress at exposure to events symbolizing the trauma, including anniversaries	+	−	+	−	−	−	−
C. Persistent avoidance of stimuli associated with the trauma or numbing of general responsiveness in at least three of the following ways:							
1. Efforts to avoid thoughts or feelings associated with the trauma	+	+	+	−	+	−	−
2. Efforts to avoid activities or situations that arouse recollections of the trauma	+	+	+	+	+	+	+
3. Inability to recall an important aspect of the trauma	−	−	−	−	−	−	−
4. Markedly diminished interest in significant activities	+	+	−	−	−	−	−
5. Feeling of detachment or estrangement from others	+	+	+	−	−	−	−
6. Restricted range of affect	+	+	+	−	−	−	−
7. Sense of foreshortened future	−	+	−	−	−	−	−
D. Persistent symptoms of increased arousal, as indicated by at least two of the following:							
1. Difficulty falling or staying asleep	−	+	+	+	−	+	−
2. Irritability or outbursts of anger	+	+	+	−	−	+	−
3. Difficulty concentrating	+	+	+	−	−	+	−
4. Hypervigilance	+	+	+	+	+	+	+
5. Exaggerated startle response	+	+	+	−	−	−	−
6. Physiologic reactivity upon exposure to events that symbolize or resemble aspects of the traumatic event	+	+	+	−	−	−	−
Number of sessions seen	14	30	18	6	6	9	9
Months since accident before seen	40	22	25	7	7	18	45

The treatment of these cases will be described in some detail as a basis for discussion of points relevant to improving the future medicolegal processing and therapeutic intervention of road trauma victims. Issues to be considered include (1) the nature and source of referral to the therapist, (2) the initial problems encountered, (3) the assessment and definition of the patient's clinical problems, (4) the formulation of a plan for intervention, (5) the implementation of therapy, and (6) the evaluation of the effectiveness of the therapy, termination of treatment, and continuing long-term management.

From Table 43.1 it is clear that these seven patients formed two groups: those who met the formal DSM-III-R diagnostic criteria for PTSD (Cases 1 to 3) and those who had a more limited range of symptoms (Cases 4 to 7). This latter group will be considered first. They will be referred to as the *phobic reaction group*.

Phobic Reaction Group

All these patients meet the requirements for diagnostic category A; that is, being involved in a serious motor car accident is considered as experiencing

> an event that is outside the range of usual human experience and that would be markedly distressing to almost anyone, e.g., serious threat to one's life or physical integrity; serious threat or harm to one's children, spouse, or other close relatives and friends; sudden destruction of one's home, or community [and, perhaps one's car]; or seeing another person who has recently been, or is being, seriously injured or killed as a result of an accident or physical violence. (APA, 1987, p. 250)

In Category B, there were no symptoms. In Category C, with one exception, the only symptom reported was C(2), concerned with avoidance behavior. In Category D, symptom (4), hypervigilance, was universally present and the only symptom in two of the cases. The other two had a range of other symptoms, particularly Case 6.

It is often argued that quick intervention after a traumatic experience is ideal for preventing the development of long-term psychological problems. From Table 43.1 it can be seen that for this group the delay in treatment ranged from 7 to 45 months and that, although the small numbers limit generalization, those who were treated early required less therapy. None of these patients had had any prior psychotherapy before referral.

Actual treatment consisted of a program of systematic desensitization (SD) to the phobic anxiety associated with automobile travel. More specifically, this involved a combination of training in relaxation using guided imagery, imaginal SD in therapy, self-monitoring for severity of anxiety in phobic situations, using a Subjective Units of Distress (SUD) analogue scale (McCormack, Horne, & Sheather, 1988) where 0 equals no anxiety and 100 equals panic. Patients were also given a program of self-executed *in vivo* exposure to phobic situations between therapy sessions. All four patients responded very well. For example, in Case 5, SUD ratings for "traveling by car to parents' place across the city" dropped from 90 to 0, and all avoidance of automobile travel had disappeared. Even when SUD scores did not decrease quite as dra-

matically, as in Case 6, where "passing a truck on the inside in the rain," fell from 100 to 55, the avoidance behaviors were eliminated.

Also present initially were symptoms of depression (Cases 5 and 6), negative and avoidance thought patterns (Case 5), and sleep difficulties, anger, irritability, and concentration problems (Case 6). In Case 6, these were severe enough to constitute a real strain upon the patient's family and to lead to talk of ending the marriage. In both of these cases, additional cognitive-behavioral intervention for the depressive aspects proved to be very effective.

Thus, where phobic anxiety was the major psychological disorder subsequent to an automobile accident, treatment by cognitive-behavioral methods was quick and effective, even when some depression was present.

The accidents were not minor ones and included being knocked off a bicycle by a high-speed truck and receiving a fractured shoulder, ribs, and punctured lung (Case 4); a head-on collision at night time with minor injuries to the neck and sternum (Case 5); neck and shoulder bruising and a major gash in the leg from being knocked off a motorbike by a truck (Case 6); and a fractured sternum, spinal compression, and whiplash from a side-on collision with a car that failed to stop at a "stop-sign"-controlled intersection (Case 7). None of these cases received any form of head injury. The only medication used by any of them were minor anxiolytics and analgesics, as required.

PTSD Group

As can be seen in Table 43.1, three cases (1, 2, and 3) clearly met the criteria for a formal diagnosis of PTSD. Unlike the phobic reaction group, they all had Category B symptoms and a far greater frequency of Category C symptoms. With the exception of phobic patient Case 7, the PTSD group experienced far greater delay before treatment commenced. All three cases required many more treatment sessions, and the whole process of defining these patients' problems, carrying out appropriate assessment, and implementing therapy was much more complicated. Because of the heuristic value of these three cases, they are presented in some detail.

CASE 1

This was a 53-year-old woman who had previously been living a normal, well-adjusted life with her husband and three daughters who were in their teens and early twenties.

She was first seen 40 months after a car accident in which she was a front-seat passenger with one of her daughters' being the driver. There was a front-end collision, and she received a fractured left collar bone and soft tissue injury to the left shoulder and neck resulting in a permanent restriction in the use of her left arm. After the crash, smoke started entering the car and she had to pull free her daughter, who was conscious but had her feet trapped under the foot pedals. She was initially referred by her lawyers for assessment, but they agreed that she should undergo treatment.

On presentation her complaints were as follows: (1) she sees herself as an old person; (2) she "freezes" when she gets in a car and then mimics driving even though she is a passenger and has never driven a car; (3) her energy, memory, and concentration are all greatly decreased; (4) she is irritable and has a labile mood; she has lost all interest in cuddling and sex; (5) she is socially withdrawn and avoids many situations; her family life has been disrupted; (6) she has developed panics and fears, including a fear of her family getting hurt; and lastly (7) from Table 43.1, she shares all criteria for Category D symptoms except difficulty falling or staying asleep.

This client had had no previous psychological treatment at any time in her life. She was taking no medication and was reluctant to do so. In order to reduce high levels of tension, she was trained in relaxation using guided imagery and was able to produce a relaxing image for herself, "lying in the sun on a beach, watching clouds drifting across the sky."

A SD program was devised which involved both imaginal exposure to a hierarchy of car-travel scenes and home-based *in vivo* practice. However, as the SD progressed, it became apparent there were many other problems requiring attention. She was frequently tearful in therapy but said she avoided expressing emotion at home even though she often felt extremely angry. She also avoided all cuddling and love-making with her husband and when traveling in their car (on the rare occasions she did) would criticize him, while sitting rigidly in the front passenger seat mimicking his driving behaviors. She experienced severe panic and had an exaggerated startle response to the sound of skidding cars. Her avoidance of thinking about, discussing, and actually traveling itself (except by local public transport) was severe. Her whole outlook to the future was very negative.

Cognitive-behavioral therapy (CBT) was used intensively to treat her avoidance and depressive thoughts, feelings, and behaviors. Much time was spent in disputation of her beliefs (irrational) about the consequences of using avoidance as a coping technique. She was encouraged to express anger and not to bottle up feelings all the time, to be more assertive and, very importantly, to listen repeatedly to an audiotape of the sounds of a car skidding and crashing. By the end of fourteen therapy sessions she reported the following improvements: (1) She could travel anywhere within the Melbourne metropolitan area by car and use public transport with ease. Her SUD ratings for car travel still varied between 10 and 80 but, prior to treatment, they had never fallen below 60 on the rare occasion she had allowed herself to get into a car. (2) Her social and family life had greatly improved and she no longer had major feelings of irritability and anger. (3) She could talk about the accident and its aftermath without getting upset. (4) Her hyperalertness and noise sensitivity had greatly decreased. (5) She felt she had made real progress and was sometimes experiencing "great" days where she would find herself spontaneously whistling, feeling happy, and not having a single thought about the accident. She also stated that the future "looks great."

Some marriage difficulties did remain. She and her husband had been seen together on a couple of occasions during therapy but she felt she was so much better that she could manage on her own and wanted no further treatment.

CASE 2

This 33-year-old divorced musician was living with and caring for her teenage daughter. She was first seen 22 months after the fourth of a series of motor car accidents in the preceding 18 months. Accidents three and four were 5 months apart and more severe than the earlier two. After accident three, normal life was resumed but nightmares of being trapped in a blazing car were experienced. Accident four involved a head-on collision with an oncoming car with resultant concussion due to a knock on the right frontotemporal area and extensive bruising but no major physical injury. She was referred for treatment by a psychiatrist who had seen her for a medicolegal assessment.

On presentation her complaints were as follows: (1) her energy, concentration, and memory were all appalling; (2) she had periods of binge eating but no induced vomiting; (3) she experienced severe obsessional ruminations and compulsive checking; (4) she felt her mind was racing all the time; (5) she had flashbacks and nightmares about death and being trapped; (6) she was hypersensitive to light and noise; (7) she had nausea and headaches; (8) she was phobic of car travel; she does it but is very restricted in where she goes; (9) she feels "detached" from the world, as if "going through the motions"; (10) she has lost interest in relationships and sex; (11) she has become socially withdrawn; (12) she avoids listening to, teaching, and playing music; and lastly (13) she shares, from Table 43.1, all criteria for Category D symptoms.

Treatment was by a complex program of CBT involving 30 sessions over a 12-month period provided by a clinical psychologist (the author), with additional psychological support and antidepressant medication being provided by a psychiatrist colleague.

This patient often found it hard to adhere to the treatment program because of problems with lack of both energy and concentration. This was a new experience for her because prior to the last two accidents, life had been very easy and her career was highly successful.

Her memory and concentration problems were clinically severe and, combined with the fact she had received a minor head injury, provided the impetus for a full neuropsychological investigation. The results confirmed the presence of significant deficits and referral was arranged to a neurologist who organized a computer tomography brain scan. These further investigations produced no significant evidence of organic pathology but did provide useful feedback both in reassuring the patient and in motivating her to pursue the not always comfortable psychological therapy. Some specific issues which were dealt with during therapy and which seemed to be important milestones in achieving the eventual recovery were as follows: (1) exposure to recall of the accidents both through imagery while relaxed, talking about them, and playing the same audio tape (Case 1) of a motor car going into a skid and crashing; (2) writing down the nightmares about death and discussing them in therapy; (3) recalling, discussing, and dealing with an event that occurred in the same year as, but prior to, her fourth accident: this was the death of her former sister-in-law and her son in a "silly" car accident while they were shopping at a local supermarket; (4) exposure to music; although music had been her life until the last accident, she had been avoiding all contact with it and had developed strong resistance to becoming reinvolved with it. However, this was worked-through by talking about and, more importantly, by using SD and modeling to help her deliberately select and play audiotapes of music with particularly strong emotional significance; (5) legal and compensation issues had become complex and added to the stress she was experiencing but, in the end, they were resolved satisfactorily.

Thus, by the end of therapy, she reported she was "going very well." She still had the occasional nightmare and some concentration problems but no longer felt she had no future. Her energy had greatly improved and she was, in fact, pursuing an active career in music. Before treatment, listening to music had left her with feelings of "nothingness," and a foreboding that "I do not have much time left" (psychic numbing). Concentrating on music in therapy did result in her regaining her interest in and resuming a career in this field, albeit in a somewhat different manner than prior to the accident. She was also enjoying being interested in her daughter's schooling and social life and was greatly relieved there were no further compensation and legal issues to be dealt with.

CASE 3

A 25-year-old single woman initiated referral for therapy herself by exerting pressure upon her attorneys in order to convince them she needed more than a medicolegal assessment and actually required help.

She was first seen 26 months after a car accident. She had been the driver of a car that, at the time of the accident, was stationary, waiting to turn right from the center lane of a road [in Australia traffic travels on the left-hand side of the road] when a car ran into her from the rear. She heard the brakes squeal before impact. She received bruising to the right frontotemporal area of her head, was concussed, and felt that she was going to die. The police charged and successfully prosecuted the driver of the other car and she was exonerated of any blame. Prior to the accident, she had a history of enjoying life with good relationships with family and friends and a consistent work record as a business secretary. Since the accident she had only worked in temporary positions.

She presented as a fashionably dressed, pleasant, but obviously worried young woman. She was able to give a clear account of both her past and present state but was confused as to why she had not fully recovered from what seemed to be relatively minor injuries.

On presentation her complaints were as follows: (1) frequent, at times severe, neck and back pain; (2) recurrent headaches; (3) frequent, severe nightmares (e.g., "Water—a big ocean and people drowning, including babies. I am trying to save them but I am struggling to survive myself"); (4) intense distress upon hearing the sound of automobile tires/brakes squealing (a frequent sound in her residential environment); (5) avoidance of thinking or talking about the accident; (6) feeling numb inside, lacking in trust of others, and an inability to express feelings even though she was aware she had them deep inside; (7) having a deep feeling of "profound unhappiness inside, like an ugliness, whereas before I was known as a lovely, bubbly, very happy person"; (8) very

poor concentration and memory; doing "stupid" things; being vague and incredibly forgetful; and (9) from Table 43.1, all criteria for Category D symptoms.

The only previous treatment for injuries received from the accident had been physiotherapy for her back and neck pain and analgesics prescribed by a local general medical practitioner. In view of the marked difficulties with memory and concentration and the blow to the right frontotemporal area of the head, a full neuropsychological investigation was carried out. The results confirmed the presence of these problems, particularly the learning and recall of complex material. Because of these results and the fact that she had never had a neurological examination, one was organized. As with Case 2, the results proved normal, including electroencephalograph and computer tomography brain investigations.

Treatment followed similar CBT lines for the previous two cases, with training in relaxation, exposure to the same audiotape of a car crash, and encouragement of expression of feelings and thoughts normally avoided, both in association with the accident, and of general depression and anger. An active program of both imaginal and *in vivo* SD to travel was implemented, as was a graded approach to dealing with tasks that placed increasing demands upon memory and concentration.

She was seen with her boyfriend on two occasions to help him understand what was happening to her and to enlist his help with some of the between-therapy planned activities.

By treatment session 14 when therapy was terminated, she still had a number of problems, particularly concerning her career and relationships. She continued to have neck and back pain and occasional nightmares, but there had been a significant improvement in general psychological well-being. She was beginning to have good feelings again, with a definite improvement in motivation and energy and more stable mood. She was also much less phobic about travel and, for economic reasons, was getting rid of her car and thus would have to rely on previously anxiety-producing public transport. She saw this as a positive step to achieving a greater degree of independence and self-assertion. Very importantly, she had noticed a significant improvement in her memory and concentration. In spite of some major issues still to be resolved, including resolution of the legal and compensation aspects of her case, she was coping well and taking stock of what she wanted out of life in the future.

Discussion

"When you have an accident, there's so many people trying to prove you are all right you get to hiding pain when it occurs and pretending it's not there. You feel people are not going to understand you" (Case 1).

"I am just another crash-and-bash case and nobody is interested in me; doctors and solicitors especially" (Case 3). These quotations, from two of the patients discussed here, serve to capture the sense of confusion, and even helplessness, that they experience. One purpose of the discussion which follows is to suggest ways this situation may be ameliorated in the future.

Referral Issues

Perhaps the first question to be raised from the review of these cases is that of appropriate referral. It could be asked what would have happened to the phobic reaction group if the delay in referral for treatment had been as prolonged as that for the PTSD group? It is possible their symptoms could have worsened, perhaps to become as severe as those of the PTSD group. On the other hand, the phobic symptoms could gradually have gone into remission as a result of day-to-day experience. What is clear is that if phobic symptoms are detected early and treated through the well-tried behavior therapy technique of SD, then intervention is minimal and recovery rapid. It would also seem important to treat the PTSD group as early as possible. This might prevent their symptoms from becoming so severe as to meet the formal diagnostic criteria for PTSD; but, further research is required before this can be asserted with any degree of certainty.

One difficulty regarding referral seems to be lack of knowledge about both psychological sequelae to trauma and the effective psychological interventions that are available. Some medical and legal practitioners seem to be becoming more concerned that this group of accident victims have not only their psychological/psychiatric problems assessed for compensation purposes but also receive appropriate treatment as soon as possible. However, it is very much a matter of chance whether a particular victim is actually referred for treatment of psychological problems.

In Australia, at least, there are legal complications if a client/patient is referred directly for therapy to a psychologist. The relevant insurance agencies will pay the fees for therapy by a psychologist only if the patient is referred by a medical practitioner whereas costs for medical treatment are automatically recoverable. Referral by a lawyer simply for psychological assessment for compensation and litigation purposes is a different matter; such fees are recoverable. A consequence of these complexities is that the patient may continue longer than necessary on the "referral-to-specialist-circuit" for assessment, when treatment could already have been implemented.

Physical injuries are tangible and therefore are more easily dealt with at conceptual, legal, and medical levels than are psychological disorders. Thus, by the time patients of the type described above receive appropriate psychological intervention (if they are so lucky), they may well have learned to feel powerless in the system, angry, frustrated, and resigned to their lot, as conveyed in the quotations above.

Initial Problems Encountered

From the type of comments made so far, among the first things to accept and deal with in therapy for automobile accident victims are their feelings of confusion, of being pawns in some process over which they have no control, and even of being perceived as cheats or liars trying to rip off the system. The issues of malingering, factitious disorders, and secondary gain are complex

and reasonably well-explored in the literature. It could be argued that a litigious system for determining compensation reinforces some of these ultimately maladaptive strategies. However, it is probable (Brown, Conrad, & Quinn, 1987) that the vast majority of road accident victims really do wish to get better and back to normal as quickly as possible, regardless of financial gain. In all seven cases, some aspects of the legal and compensation ramifications were important but they were particularly stressful for the PTSD cases. In Case 2, once resolved, a great sense of relief was experienced; however, the improvement in psychological well-being clearly preceded settlement. Thus, compensation and, particularly, the legal processes, such as court appearances, are significant stressors. However, their removal and resolution does not account for the observed recovery because many patients still have significant symptomatology after this (Tarsh & Royston, 1985). Part of the cognitive-behavioral therapy can be devoted to preparing the patients to have a better perspective about the medicolegal aspects of their cases and to specifically prepare them for coping with legal interactions, including the courtroom.

Thus, the first step to successful treatment is to convey acceptance of the patient's complaints as being valid and this really is dependent upon the therapist initially sitting back and letting the patient talk. Before intervention is undertaken, it does seem essential to hear what the patient has to say. What to do about the problems once they are outlined is another matter, but if that initial acceptance is not present, it is unlikely the patient will persist in therapy and the necessary preliminary, more formal, assessment procedures.

Having clarified these issues and essentially provided a framework, or structure, that is agreeable to both patient and therapist by, in effect, establishing a contract, the next step is to carry out a detailed clinical assessment.

Assessment and Definition of Clinical Problems

As well as carrying out normal clinical procedures, specific reference to the diagnostic criteria presented in the DSM-III-R for PTSD (APA, 1987, pp. 247–251) does provide a useful and practical means of assessing the patient. If this were done earlier on in the merry-go-round of medicolegal assessment of road trauma patients, those with significant psychological problems could be detected and treated appropriately. There are theoretical and conceptual problems with a DSM-III-R diagnosis of PTSD but, it does, at least, have a face validity and is certainly of practical help in differentiating the primarily phobic from the more complex PTSD cases.

Of course, as described in Cases 2 and 3 above, further detailed investigations may be required, especially when there is the possibility of brain damage. When there is previous obvious head injury and brain damage after a road accident, intensive investigation and treatment will usually have to be undertaken; the physical is tangible and resources to deal with physical injuries are good in many societies. Cases with minimal head injury are more complex (Alves, Coloban, O'Leary,

Rimel, & Jane, 1986). In both Cases 2 and 3, where neuropsychological and neurological investigations were carried out, the extent and severity of memory and concentration difficulties were confirmed, but the likelihood of actual brain damage being present was virtually excluded.

The pursuit of such thorough investigations as an integral part of treatment and management served at least two purposes. First, it helped to formulate an accurate clinical picture of the patients' complaints as a basis for planning appropriate treatment. Second, it provided excellent feedback to patients to help reduce some of their concerns and to lead into a discussion of the rationale for the therapies to be undertaken.

Treatment

Details of treatment have been described in the presentation of the case histories. Case presentations by no means provide conclusive evidence for the efficacy of the specific techniques that were used. However, the actual components of therapy described here do not differ in any substantive way from descriptions of cognitive-behavioral interventions in the relevant literature. It is interesting that even after over 30 years of research since Wolpe's original (1958) description of SD for phobic anxiety, ignorance of the effectiveness of this technique, and its ready availability from psychologists, remains fairly widespread among medical practitioners and the legal profession, with the exception of some psychiatrists. Clearly, further education of these professions is required. The cost-effectiveness of early behavioral intervention for the large numbers of automobile accident trauma victims with phobic anxiety, although not systematically investigated, can hardly be doubted. This certainly is an area worth further research.

Reference was made to the role of psychotropic medication in the description of the cases. It would appear to have a limited but useful role (Bleich, Siegel, Garb, & Lerer, 1986) particularly, the appropriate prescription of antidepressants. In this case, close collaboration in therapy between the clinical psychologist and the psychiatrist was probably an important factor in successful outcome. Treatment of PTSD in any patient requires many skills and interprofessional collaboration can increase the likelihood of success. What does seem to be particularly important is that patients receive consistent messages from those involved in their therapy. These patients are already confused enough, for reasons discussed earlier, and do not benefit from any additional iatrogenically produced symptoms.

The effectiveness of a cognitive-behavioral approach to both phobic anxiety and to full PTSD is well established (Keane, Fairbank, Caddell, Zimering, & Bender, 1985) and was the main approach used here. However, this does not deny the validity of other psychological methods, such as more interpretative psychodynamic or family systems approaches. Although not highlighted in the cases that were presented above, the role of interpretation (and the conceptual framework that it provided) was very important, as was discussion of the impact of patients' problems on close associates, such as family

members. In all three PTSD cases, significant others were seen on at least one occasion during therapy. This helped them to understand what was happening to the patient and, in some instances, to take an active role in helping the patient carry out between-therapy-session tasks (e.g., accompanying the patient when he or she was deliberately exposing him- or herself to situations previously avoided at any cost).

There are further advantages to a cognitive-behavioral approach to treatment. The first is that treatment is a highly active process, and it has been shown, both for posttrauma phobias and PTSD, that active intervention is essential regardless of theoretical orientation (Scurfield, 1985). Second, an integral part of the approach is self-monitoring. This is not the place to explore the complexities of its role in therapy but to point out that it does lend itself to readily operationalizing and quantifying important aspects of the psychological problems being tackled. In all cases reported here, a diary of actual approach and avoidance behaviors, and accompanying SUD ratings, was kept by each patient more or less consistently. These records provided valuable feedback in therapy sessions and helped to identify both internal events, such as thoughts and images, and external cues that triggered high SUD ratings and other feelings of discomfort and distress. Such systematic recording and reporting of information by the patients throughout therapy allowed continuous monitoring of progress, or the lack of it, and systematic planning of each phase of therapy as well as helping to determine the point at which no further treatment was required. In the case of the phobic reaction group, results from such an approach were excellent. For the three PTSD patients, outcomes were also very good but, at the end of formal therapy, there were still considerable residual problems. However, in all three cases the desire was to finish with therapy, at least for the time being, and to get on with living a life free of visits to doctors, psychologists, and lawyers.

References

Alves, W. M., Coloban, A. R. T., O'Leary, T. J., Rimel, R. W. and Jane, J. A. (1986). Understanding post-traumatic symptoms after minor head injury. *Journal of Head Trauma—Rehabilitation, 1*, 1–12.

American Psychiatric Association. (1987). *Diagnostic and statistical manual of mental disorders* (3rd. ed., rev.). Washington DC.

Bleich, A., Siegel, B., Garb, R., & Lerer, B. (1986). Posttraumatic stress disorder following combat exposure: Clinical features and psychopharmacological treatment. *British Journal of Psychiatry, 149*, 365–369.

Brown, B., Conrad, P., & Quinn, J. (1987). *Assessment and treatment of post-traumatic stress disorder.* Workshop presented at the Tenth National Conference of the Australian Behaviour Modification Association, Gold Coast, Queensland.

Helzer, J. E., Robins, L. N., & McEvoy, L. (1987). Post-traumatic stress disorder in the general population: Findings of the epidemiologic catchment area survey. *New England Journal of Medicine, 317*(26), 1630–1634.

Keane, T. M., Fairbank, J. A., Caddell, J. M., Zimering, R. T., & Bender, M. E. (1985). A behavioral approach to assessing and treating post-traumatic stress disorder in Vietnam veterans. In C. R. Figley (Ed.), *Trauma and its wake: The study and treatment of post-traumatic stress disorder* (pp. 257–294). New York: Brunner/Mazel.

Kluch, K., Swinson, R. P., & Kirby, M. (1985). Post-traumatic stress disorder after car accidents. *Canadian Journal of Psychiatry, 30*, 426–427.

McCormack, H. M., Horne, D. J. de L., & Sheather, S. (1988). Clinical applications of visual analogue scales: A critical review. *Psychological Medicine, 18*, 1007–1019.

Pilowsky, I. (1985). Cryptotrauma and "accident neurosis." *British Journal of Psychiatry, 147*, 310–311.

Porter, K. M. (1989). Neck sprains after car accidents: A common cause of long term disability. *British Medical Journal, 298*, 973–974.

Scurfield, R. M. (1985). Post-trauma stress assessment and treatment: Overview and formulations. In C. R. Figley (Ed.), *Trauma and its wake: The study and treatment of post-traumatic stress disorder* (pp. 219–256). New York: Brunner/Mazel.

Selling, L. S. (1940). A neuropsychiatric study of traffic offenders. *Psychosomatic Medicine, 2*(4), 385–397.

Tarsh, M. J., & Royston, C. (1985). A follow-up study of accident neurosis. *British Journal of Psychiatry, 146*, 18–25.

Walker, J. I. (1981). Post-traumatic stress disorder after a car accident. *Postgraduate Medicine, 69*, 82–86.

Wolpe, J. (1958). *Psychotherapy by reciprocal inhibition.* London: Oxford University Press.

CHAPTER 44

Treatment of Victims
of Rape Trauma

Carol R. Hartman and Ann W. Burgess

Introduction

It was a warm spring morning. Because of a very sore throat, Mrs. Claven had a doctor's appointment. All proceeded smoothly until her throat was swabbed for a culture. Suddenly, Mrs. Claven became shaky, nauseated, grabbed the physician's arm, pulled the swab out of her mouth, and ran sobbing out of the clinic. She drove to her home and, after calming herself, telephoned the detective who had arrested her rapist of 3 years previous. She was totally unaware as to why she was calling this detective, but her fear was so great that she instinctively knew only that he would make her feel safe. She told him about her throat examination.

This is an illustration of the complex phenomena of the mind's attempt to master and deal with the life-threatening event of rape. Mrs. Claven's major defense was to dissociate from the rape, and parts of the assault were lost to memory. Three years later, the sensory and perceptual experience of the throat swab led to physiological responses, panic, and escape at the reexperiencing of danger. The detective called a rape consultant for assistance, sensing that Mrs. Claven's reaction was in some way related to the sexual assault. The consultant verified the delayed trauma response and talked with Mrs. Claven. Her bewilderment over the strong reaction began to dissipate as she was able to bear the emotion and relate, for the first time, this humiliating and terrifying aspect of the sexual assault which had previously been blocked and fragmented in her memory.

Carol R. Hartman • Department of Psychiatric Mental Health Nursing, Boston College School of Nursing, Chestnut Hill, Massachusetts 02167. Ann W. Burgess • Department of Psychiatric Mental Health Nursing, University of Pennsylvania School of Nursing, Philadelphia, Pennsylvania 19104.

International Handbook of Traumatic Stress Syndromes, edited by John P. Wilson and Beverley Raphael. Plenum Press, New York, 1993.

Background

In the United States, rape affects the lives of thousands of people each year. The Federal Bureau of Investigation (FBI) Uniform Crime Report indicates a 21% increase in reported forcible rape cases between 1979 and 1988. In 1988, there were over 92,486 cases of reported rapes with a 52% clearance rate by law enforcement indicating the high number of unapprehended assailants. Nine percent of the forcible rape clearances involved juveniles under the age of 18. To truly grasp the enormity of the problem, those figures must be doubled since it is estimated that at least 50% of violent crimes go unreported (President's Task Force on Victims of Crime, 1982) and criminal victimization surveys estimate between 40% to 50% of forcible rapes are not reported (LEAA, 1975).

The incidence of rape is strongly influenced by the definition of rape. When these calculations are realized as being based primarily on the legal definition of rape (which varies from state to state) and usually addresses lack of consent, force or threat of force, and sexual penetration, the clinical understanding of rape greatly expands these estimates. Since the extent of rape and its sequelae affect such a large population, it is imperative to gain some understanding of the nature of the event, its impact, and the factors influencing recovery.

Historically, the realization of rape as a violent act committed in a sexual context was the beginning of national efforts to address the problems inherent in this traumatic life event (Largen, 1985). Prior to the women's movement, avoidance and silence dominated the professional reactions to victims of rape. Given this pattern, the first efforts of feminists, women's groups, and professionals were to raise the awareness of others that rape was a criminal act not desired by the victim. Furthermore, the victim was not responsible for the behavior and choices of the predator; rather, the rapist was acting out of his own intentions and patterns of beliefs.

Rape trauma seriously taxes a victim's personal coping resources. The need for identifying variables and factors which influence recovery from rape is imperative. A descriptive data base is being accumulated which indicates that individuals who have been raped do not necessarily return to a prerape level of psychological functioning, though there is a return to social role functioning (Burgess & Holmstrom, 1978; Finkelhor, Hotaling, Lewis, & Smith, 1989; Jehu, 1989; Sales, Baum, & Shore, 1984; Veronen & Kilpatrick, 1983).

The following case history demonstrates the complexity of the traumatic response to rape and is presented for discussion of pretrauma history and trauma factors and their relationship to posttrauma functioning.

CASE EXAMPLE

Jennifer, a 19-year-old mother, attended a rock concert with her boyfriend. While the concert was in progress, a group of young men began to organize and dominate the aisle area in front of the performers. Jennifer and her friends became nervous and decided to leave. As they moved out of their seats and attempted to exit, the group of men surrounded them and pulled the couple away. Jennifer was simultaneously beaten, her clothes were torn off, and she was thrown to the floor. A tire iron was pushed into her vagina, and she was then forced to perform oral sex on a number of the assailants. She was vaguely aware of her boyfriend's being beaten and his cries and efforts to help her.

The initial interventions in this crisis is to secure a state of safety for the victim. Jennifer was acutely aware that a length of time elapsed before anyone interrupted the assault and came to the aid of herself and her boyfriend. Compounding her terror was the humiliation of the public rape and her nudity. She and her boyfriend were eventually wrapped in sheets, moved through the crowd, and taken by ambulance to a nearby hospital. While in the ambulance she became aware of a large bloodstain emerging from the sheet that covered her. This resurrected the painful memory of the steel object that penetrated her. She was stunned, bewildered, terrified, and coped with these emotions by periodically feeling she was not in her body but rather looking down at herself.

In the emergency room, the nurse asked her what had happened but Jennifer could not answer. She was in too much pain to be examined; thus, she was medicated and hospitalized for further examination and treatment.

One year later there was a criminal trial in which several of the assailants were convicted. Jennifer testified at the trial.

The important aspect of this case is that despite some short efforts at treatment, Jennifer did not identify subsequent aspects of adjustment as being related to the rape. She did proceed with a civil suit. It was in the process of this legal action that a determination had to be made as to whether she had any residual effects because of the rape or were they manifestations of prerape personality and situational states.

In this chapter, we will review research related to three areas: pretrauma history, trauma-related factors, and posttrauma factors specifically for their use in answering the causal question asked in civil litigation.

Research by Phases of Rape Trauma

Pretrauma History

To evaluate the impact of rape trauma over time, it is important to assess the client prior to the assault. This assessment of the pretrauma phase is done in a careful and tactful manner to avoid dismissing or diminishing the response to the traumatic event itself. A critical feature is the timing of eliciting this information. For the most part, it is best to defer extensive evaluation of pretrauma factors until there has been indications of reestablishment of the victim's personal coping resources. Some of the stabilization can be achieved by having victims recount how they have managed other crisis events prior to the rape. This is a way of supporting resources that can assist in coping with the trauma of rape and to offset dysfunctional conclusions regarding the rape itself.

Research on pretrauma history is not yet clear in terms of what factors increase risk, act as protective factors, or predict symptoms posttrauma. Early efforts to associate pretrauma variables of rape victims in response to crisis intervention and recovery found no association between usual demographic variables, such as marital status, employment, education, and religion. Some early studies suggest that younger women have more symptoms initially but of a short duration whereas older women have a more prolonged reaction (Sales *et al.*, 1984). Some preexisting psychological or developmental problems have been found to heighten the impact of the assault and compound recovery (Atkeson *et al.*, 1982; Burgess & Holmstrom, 1974; Krupnick & Horowitz, 1980; Sales *et al.*, 1984; Symonds, 1980).

Pretrauma coping styles are important in understanding the rate of recovery from rape and the impact of models of treatment, such as crisis intervention and psychotherapy. The Intrusive Imagery Scale of Horowitz (1975) distinguishes between avoidant mechanisms and intrusive thoughts (see Chapter 14, in this volume, for a review). He defined coping modes as containing appraisal and expectation patterns which bear heavily on the meaning ascribed to events and the subsequent organization and selection of internal and external responses. Evaluation of recovery according to avoidant/intensive modes has not been well explored. There is indication, however, that attributional styles and coping mechanisms influence the response to and recovery from rape (McCormick, Taber, & Kruedelback, 1989).

Following from the above discussion, the influence of pretrauma life-events on recovery is a complex matter. Again, there may be an interactional aspect operating in the interpretation of life event stressors on recovery. Mastery of prior life events may operate to help an individual handle another major stress. However, negative reactions to a subsequent life stressor may influence recovery. Burgess and Holmstrom (1978) found that 37% of rape victims experiencing unemployment, limited income, and need for outside support continued to have rape trauma symptoms 4 to 6 years after assault. Ruch and Chandler (1980) found a variation in responses according to the number of life stressors; those with a moderate number doing fairly well, whereas those with either major or minimal life stressors having the strongest reactions. These findings suggest that personal appraisals regarding the amount and intensity of life stressors or their absences plays a role in patterning expectations and perceptions of the assault and the meaning of survival. Burgess and Holmstrom (1978) also reported the impact of a prior victimization within a 2-year time period of the current rape as delaying recovery.

Efforts to evaluate victims' prior social network and social support system have relied on statements defining the number of people and a personal appraisal of the quality of the relationships. Social support and the quality of that support are associated with the rate of recovery and long-term symptoms (Burgess & Holmstrom, 1978; Norris & Feldman-Summers, 1981; Sales, Baum, & Shore, 1984). The quality of social support before the rape does not appear to be associated with the severity of symptoms at the immediate postassault phase (Sales et al., 1984).

Traumatic Event Phase

The critical variables of the trauma are the type of rape which includes the modus operandi of the victimizer and whether the rape was a blitz and sudden attack or one in which the confidence of the victim was betrayed (Burgess & Holmstrom, 1974). The interaction between victim and offender and the coping/survival behaviors employed by the victim are also important trauma variables.

Research on coping and survival strategies during the rape have focused primarily on what the victim did vis-à-vis the offender. A wide variety of reported behaviors emerge: the use of verbal strategies, physical action as a way to escape attack, and verbal negotiations (Burgess & Holmstrom, 1976). Recent investigation of coping strategies and the response of the rapist to them indicate that some of the violence toward the victim may be a function of the struggle to protect themselves during the rape. Of particular importance is the study by Hazelwood, Reboussin, and Warren (1989) who studied 41 serial rapists. Ten of these rapists reported an increased pleasure and an increase in violence toward their victims when they fought back. Another study that examined the amount of injury to the victim by type of rapist indicates that there are rapists who will inflict more harm if a strategy used by the victim is to defend themselves (Prentky, Burgess, & Carter, 1986).

Some studies have reported a longer time period for recovery associated with higher degrees of violence (Bard & Sangrey, 1980; McCahill et al., 1979; Peters, 1977). Other studies have found a mixed outcome when isolating the variables into threat, amount of physical abuse, the use of a weapon, and the type of penetration and have suggested some differential degree of symptom manifestation. Sales et al. (1984) found threat of death was associated with more symptoms initially; type and presence of sexual penetration was associated with strong reactions throughout the phases of recovery, whereas physical injury was associated with recovery; and multiple assailants contributed most to high levels of symptoms. When all these variables were combined

into an overall violence variable, it was associated with symptom severity. Sales and colleagues (1984) did not find supportive evidence that the victim–offender relationship is related to the symptom formation and recovery.

Posttrauma Response

Clinical research indicates that there are victims who withstand the assault, the immediate aftermath, and within 3 to 6 months return to social integration. A small portion, 17% to 25% report to be symptom-free 1 year postrape without any intervention (Burgess & Holmstrom, 1978; Veronen & Kilpatrick, 1983). However, the majority report some fear and anxiety symptoms above prerape functioning (Kilpatrick, Resick, & Veronen, 1981). Sales et al. (1984) suggested that there is an uneven course of recovery with the acute phase subsiding within a 6-month period only to exacerbate at a later period of time, perhaps at less an intense degree than immediately after the assault, but nevertheless with intensity. Their data suggest that there is "never" a return to a preassault state. Several studies indicate that rape victims experience significant long-term problems in the areas of psychological functioning (e.g., fear/anxiety, depression), social adjustment, and sexual behavior (Ellis, 1983; Holmes & St. Lawrence, 1983; Steketee & Foa, 1987). Furthermore, being a victim of rape may be associated with an increased risk of suicide (Kilpatrick et al., 1985; Kilpatrick, Veronen, Saunders, Best, Amick-McMullen, & Paduhovich, 1987). The results of one study indicated that 19.2% of completed rape victims had attempted suicide, a rate 8.7 times higher than the rate for nonvictims (Kilpatrick et al., 1985). Resnick (1987) suggested it was impossible to know how many victims kill themselves as a function of crime-induced trauma. In a study by Katz and Burt (1988), self-blame was correlated with a longer recovery; that is, the more the victims blamed themselves for the rape, the greater the likelihood that they had been psychiatrically hospitalized, the more suicidal they had been, and the lower their self-esteem.

In a sample of 372 nonpsychotic females, aged 18 or older with a history of one sexual assault, compared to a control group of no sexual assault history, victims showed disruption in early sexual response cycle, fear of sex, arousal dysfunction, and desire dysfunction (Becker, Skinner, Abel, & Cichion, 1986). In a large national representative survey of 2,626 adult Americans, men and women, who reported a history of childhood sexual abuse involving penetration were likely to report a disrupted marriage, dissatisfaction in sexual relationships, and a tendency to not practice their religion (Finkelhor et al., 1989).

The impact of rape on self-esteem has been reported to extend over a 2-year period of time postrape (Murphy et al., 1988). Where there is multiple incidence of rape, symptoms extend well over 2 years (Marhoefer-Dvorak, Resick, Hutter, & Girelli, 1988).

Regarding social support, it is important not only to identify, characterize, and estimate the strength of the social network support system, but to understand how victim responses interact to influence the response of the system over time and what is this interactional effect on symptoms and recovery. The strength of this variable is realized in the treatment that includes family members. Family members influence the amount of talk that surrounds the event and their patterns of expectations reflect anxiety over the prolonged effects. Personal guilt of family members combined with avoidance patterns can greatly influence the victim's response. Coates, Wortman, and Abbey (1979) concluded that victims face a complex dilemma in gaining social support because people tend to be rejecting of victimized people. Their work suggests that members of the support system rated rape victims as more maladjusted when they expressed negative affect and self-blame.

A time-differential response to social support has been noted by Sales *et al.* (1984) in that victims with close family ties had a greater amount of distress during the acute phase, whereas there was a diminution of symptoms on a long-term basis. This finding may support a different interpretation of what is initially termed *symptoms*. As suggested in the work of Horowitz (1975), the manifestation of intrusive thoughts may in fact be a necessary process in organizing traumatic experiences into long-term memory. This point will be discussed more under the section on intervention. There is evidence that the quality of the social support of the victim has a differential influence on psychological disruption over time.

A new emerging area of concern both for the victim and for subsequent long-term effects deals with medical complaints (Cunningham, Pearce, & Pearce, 1988). Victims are increasingly raising questions and concerns regarding sexually transmitted diseases, in particular AIDS (Baker, Burgess, Davis, & Brickman, 1990; Murphy, Kitchen, Harris, & Forster, 1989).

The impact of the judicial system on symptoms over time is mixed. Early studies that focus on the criminal court proceedings indicated that victims who went to trial tended to have more symptoms (Holmstrom & Burgess, 1978). Other investigators reported an inconsistent link between engagement with the court experience and symptoms (Sales *et al.*, 1984). Originally, two hypotheses were advanced: (1) that going to court prolongs the victim role, and (2) that there are subsequent demands made on the victim that create a crisis of their own and activate the trauma. This second hypothesis points to the need to examine two discrete phenomena. First, the court process itself and the type of intimidation and victimization that can occur in this process. The second is the maintenance of active reminders of the traumatic event. This latter point suggests that the constant involvement with the details of the traumatic event has a negative impact as opposed to a lessening of tension through the phenomenon known as *catharsis*. The unfortunate problem with the criminal court proceeding is that it proceeds before adequate recovery of personal resources are available for the victim to handle the traumatic consequences.

The emerging interest in court actions with regard to symptomatology is coming by way of victims' attempting to deal with their assaults through civil suits. There are mixed positions regarding how helpful civil suits are in reducing symptoms. Barbieri (1989) and Dawson (1989) wrote pros and cons on this issue.

Diagnosis of Rape Trauma

Although the official reporting agencies indicate an increase in reported rape, it should be remembered that not all victims will report sexual assault. Therefore, clinicians should be alert to situations in which the victim does not report immediately and those in which there is a delayed reporting time period. Examples of rape trauma, both immediately reported and not immediately reported, are included in the case discussion.

Immediate Reports of Rape Trauma

The clinical term *rape trauma* describes a clustering of sensory, perceptual, cognitive, behavioral, and interpersonal symptoms exhibited in varying degrees by a victim following nonconsenting, sexual activity. The symptoms and their organization can last and change over a long period of time. Most victims of forcible rape develop a pattern of moderate to severe symptoms described as *rape trauma syndrome*; a minority of victims report no or mild symptoms. This syndrome is an acute reaction to an externally imposed situational crisis (Burgess & Holstrom, 1974).

Generally, there is an immediate impact reaction to rape. Victims evidence a wide range of emotion in the hours and days following the rape, the most common of which are shock and disbelief. Two styles of emotions are often noted in victims: *expressed* and *controlled*. In the expressed style, the victim demonstrates such feeling as anger, fear, and anxiety. The style is noted by the victim's being restless during an interview, becoming tense when certain questions are asked, crying or sobbing when describing certain acts by the assailant, and smiling in an anxious manner when stressful issues are stated. In the controlled style, the feelings of the victim are masked or hidden, and a calm, composed, or subdued affect can be noted.

An acute phase of the syndrome, called *disorganization*, includes physical symptoms, especially skeletal muscle tension, gastrointestinal irritability, and genitourinary disturbance. Marked disruption may be noted in eating and sleeping patterns. There is a hyperaroused state with fluctuating mood swings and the development of flashbacks to the assault.

The second phase of the syndrome, the reorganization phase, includes increased motor activity. During this phase, a search for security necessitates changes in telephone and place of residence. There may be an increased need for family and social support. The development of fears and phobic reactions to the circumstances of the assault are common, as well as repeated frightening day- and nightmares.

The trauma of the victim results from the confrontation with a life-threatening or highly stressful situation. Some of the symptoms of the crisis that result when a person is raped are in the service of self-preservation.

Posttraumatic Stress Disorder

For many rape victims, responses during the rape and after the rape correspond to the critical symptoms of posttraumatic stress disorder (PTSD). Adjustment over time reveals that symptoms and patterns of adjustment can take on traits that reduce the capacity of the victim to trust in herself and in others.

Rape and Posttraumatic Stress Reactions

It has been increasingly important in the area of psychiatric mental health clinics to carefully scrutinize symptom patterns of women for a history of sexual abuse and rape. Many symptoms that have been assumed under personality disorders and other psychiatric diagnosis are better explained by the diagnosis of PTSD.

The early conceptualization of the stress-response patterns of rape victims (Burgess & Holmstrom, 1974; Sutherland & Scherl, 1970; Symonds, 1975), although not controlled systematic studies, provided important descriptive information and has prompted subsequent research which has confirmed the clinical observations. According to Resnick (1983), several large-scale studies that have been conducted yielded surprisingly consistent data.

Rape victim responses are consistent with the diagnostic criteria of PTSD of the DSM-III-R. The four cardinal criteria are:

1. The stressor must be of significant magnitude to evoke distinguishable symptoms in almost everyone. PTSD is defined by symptoms that have a temporal and presumably causal relationship to a stressor beyond human experience (Ochberg & Fojtik, 1984).
2. The victim reexperiences the trauma, which is most frequently evidenced by recurrent and intrusive recollection of the event.
3. There is numbing or responsiveness to or reduced involvement with the environment.
4. Two of the following symptoms are present that were not present prior to the rape: exaggerated startle response or hyperalertness, disturbance in sleep pattern, guilt about surviving or behavior during the rape, impairment of memory and/or power of concentration, avoidance of activities that arouse recollection, and increased symptoms to events that symbolize or resemble the traumatic event.

Three Major Approaches to Treatment of Rape Victims

Crisis Intervention

Three major models of treatment have been used with rape victims with varying degrees of success. The first, *crisis intervention*, is successful in the acute phase.

This model was first used by paraprofessionals at the rape crisis centers in the early 1970s and a strong advocacy framework was utilized (Largen, 1985). This model, used in the Boston study by Burgess and Holmstrom (1974) and designed as a counseling and research project, applies the tenets of crisis theory to a method of assisting victims. Most crisis counseling efforts have followed, in modified form, this type of outreach, emergency care, and advocacy assistance programming. The objective of the model is to validate the crisis nature of the event, carefully review the details of the rape, and focus on issues raised by the crisis. This focus is on the assault and its aftermath with an emphasis on assisting the person to achieve mastery over the life-threatening anxiety created by the rape, in identifying a supportive social network, and in seeking self-enhancing ways of solving problems related to the rape and subsequent events which occur.

Cognitive-Behavioral Intervention

The second model is a *cognitive-behavioral intervention* that subscribes to a wide variety of therapeutic techniques, based upon somewhat different conceptualizations. The techniques cover rational-emotive therapy, cognitive therapy, coping skills therapies, problem-solving therapies, self-instructional training, self-control processes, interpersonal skills training, to name a few. Among these approaches are various theoretical differences. These theories range from conditioning to cognitive information processing and social learning conceptualizations. Interventions and prescriptions are primarily directed toward interruptions of the cognition-affect-behavior-consequences complex. Even though these theories and techniques are implemented in a variety of ways (directly, collaboratively, indirectly), there are basic assumptions about style and behavior change.

With regard to style, interventions are usually active, time-limited, and fairly structured. There is a basic assumption that behavior and feeling are largely determined by the way an individual perceives and constructs meaning of the world and the self. The techniques are so designed as to enhance the person's awareness and control over the cognitions and the behavior responses.

Behavioral change is believed to be an outcome of interrelationships of the person's cognitive structures (schemata, beliefs, programs), internal cognitive processes (automatic thoughts, internal dialogue, images, kinesthetic experiences), internal states (moods, feelings, and their labeling), and external behaviors, which have interpersonal and intrapersonal consequences, feeding back to the internal processes.

Although there appears to be a strong difference in style with regard to psychoanalytic approaches, there is indication that from a therapeutic process and client outcome, the working-through of distorted perceptions, emanating from unconscious conflicts, converges with many of the activities of cognitive-behavioral approaches. Thus, the cognitive-behavioral model offers an integrative approach which prioritizes victim content regarding the rape, thus permitting therapist flexibility in dealing with the multiple facets of behavior and circumstances confronting a rape victim. In addition, it allows for an interpretive scheme of victim behavior that is not grounded in pathology, but respects the yet unclarified, natural processes put into play during crises and crises resolution.

Traditional Psychotherapy

The third model of treatment, *traditional psychotherapy*, has been less successful. Werner (1972) described a case where the patient, a graduate student in her twenties, was in the second year of therapy when the attack occurred. Werner conceptualized the attack as an external stress and spoke of the subsequent therapy material as resulting from an "actual tragedy rather than a fantasy." He emphasized how the rape interrupted therapy in two important ways: (1) the pace and content changed in that it was no longer a leisurely exploration of relationships and fantasies; and (2) new symptoms of insomnia, appetite loss, frequent crying, and fears of being alone gave a clinical picture suggestive of a severe grief reaction.

A Multidimensional Model of Intervention

The three models of treatment support the clinical belief that fearful responses can be modified effectively when the structure of the cognitive defense and of the emotional arousal is addressed and when resource and skill training is provided. The increasing awareness of the impact of trauma on the limbic system (van der Kolk, 1989) suggests that many of the symptoms associated with forcible rape represent an overriding of the human alarm system which impacts on memory, sleep, sexual functioning, and attachment. In essence, there has been a type of "trauma learning" which alters sensory, perceptual, cognitive, behavioral, and interpersonal regulatory patterns (Hartman & Burgess, 1988). The vulnerability of the rape victim to subsequent victimization and/or self-limiting lives underscores the need for a multidimensional approach to treatment.

The resolution of traumatic aftereffects is complicated in the case of rape. Kilpatrick and Veronen (1983) suggested that the amount of disorganization immediately after the attack is too much for the full participation of the victim. Moos and Billings (1982) stressed that there is a differential use of coping responses given the nature of the life stressor; they also indicated that there is a tendency for women to use more avoidant patterns than active patterns and that these are more highly associated with symptoms and depression. Bohart (1980) in investigating the therapeutic value of catharsis suggested that catharsis alone is often experienced as a noxious experience. However, when it is accompanied by strategies aimed at shaping cognitions, it is found useful. The theoretical question remaining for the development of a model of intervention is how to structure interventions so that they are compatible with the more immediate crises period.

The seminal works of Horowitz (1975) address in part this question. In his research on whether intrusive and repetitive thoughts after experimental stress are characteristic of certain individuals or whether they represent a general stress response tendency, he concluded that the "symptoms" of repetitive imagery, thoughts, sounds, and feelings are part of a general stress-response tendency and further can be understood by a model of information-processing.

The continued manifestation of intrusive imagery indicates then, that the victim, overwhelmed with new information, is attempting to place important information in storage, the first being recent memory. It is only relegated to long-term memory when more important information takes its place. Based on the propositions of Horowitz (1982), symptoms can now be understood as parts of a process of cognitive reorganization. Therapeutic techniques which address this process hold promise for victims.

A model which allows for the convergence of techniques that address sensory, perceptual, cognitive, behavioral, and interpersonal patterns is neurolinguistic programming (Bandler & Grinder, 1975; Dilts, Grinder, Bandler, Bandler, & DeLosier, 1980; Grinder & Bandler, 1976). This model addresses the structure of subjective experience. As such, based on the responses of the person, interventions are devised to disrupt patterns which impede flexibility. A major contribution of this model has been the memory storage of experience. This is particularly important in the assessment of how the victim processes trauma and how members of the social support system to the victim process the trauma (Hartman & Burgess, 1986). Overridding images, internal dialogue, and kinesthetic responses are recognized for their stimulus value. Strategies which address the symptom maintenance aspect of these images and internal dialogue can be devised to reduce the dysfunctional consequences. Fragments (internal and external) of powerful experiences act as an anchor, having a signal effect to trigger unwanted states or desired states. Techniques are aimed at broad patterns of the victim's beliefs, presuppositions, and criteria and are referred to as metaprograms, external behavior, internal states, and internal processes.

The value of this model is that it does not exclude different theoretical positions regarding causality. Rather it focuses on behavior change which is accomplished through different strategies and is tested in the space of intervention and outside. If it is incomplete, work is done until the desired outcome is achieved. Since the outcome is set in the terms of the person who is seeking assistance, motivation to persist until goals have been achieved is enhanced. This fits with the model of cognitive information-processing of Horowitz (1975).

The model develops and demands flexibility on the part of the clinician. If the change to be effective is too hard, then the task is broken down into smaller units. Thus, if during an acute state, immediately postassault, the victim is overwhelmed with emotion, the first step is to assist the person in gaining control over reducing and intensifying feeling states in the here and now. This not only establishes a sense of control but begins to address the connection between internal processes, such as images, sounds, and thoughts, with emotional arousal and the arousal potential of the assault.

If the person is numb and cut off from feeling and thoughts, the first step is to build a strong sense of comfort in the present by establishing an external cue for the state. Then gradually the patient is moved back in time, using the positive cue to reduce emotional arousal when it is too intense. Little by little the person gains personal control in the here and now. As these steps are taken, the emergent beliefs and presuppositions regarding the assault will be elicited and their power for symptom maintenance can be scrutinized. As personal control is experienced and increased, the person can focus more on the defensive cognitions and their alterations.

The important point is that therapeutic interventions are not prescribed but tailored made for the individual. The intervenor is active with the person. It does not exclude the social support system but does direct attention to the quality of that system's support. In the case of rape, since the social support network can be equally upset, attention needs to be given to how they cope with the new information and the behavior of the survivor.

In summary, a model of intervention has been proposed which can address a general stress-response pattern to the rape that occurs regardless of the past makeup of a person. The stress-response pattern requires sensory, perceptual, cognitive, and interpersonal reintegration. The coping abilities of the individual, as well as the type of rape and circumstances, and the coping abilities employed to survive bear heavily on the victim's recovery. Critical variables influencing recovery have been identified interacting with and influencing the reactions of the victim.

Case Analysis

To return to the case of Jennifer 9 years later. We find a young woman of 28 involved in a civil suit. The point of argument is that any limitations in her present functioning are a result of prior traumatic event personality characteristics or a direct consequence of the assault itself. The argument is at the core of research questions and treatment issues. In the analysis of Jennifer's situation, we wish to focus first on the traumatic assault itself.

Jennifer is the victim of a blitz type of rape (Burgess & Holstrom, 1974). There is no question as to the violent life-threatening features of this rape. The multiple offenders and the sexual and sadistic acts increase the likelihood of severe long-lasting symptomatology. In addition, the social context carries a traumatizing dimension. In a state of terrorizing helplessness with other people present, no one responds to protect Jennifer.

In assessing Jennifer, attention was paid to how she experienced the ongoing events and how she attempted to cope. This introduces the way Jennifer constructed thoughts, meanings, and purposes to both her actions and her inability to act. She remembers the horror of realizing that no one was responding to help her with the exception of her boyfriend. His cries and efforts to reach through to touch her were significantly important in maintaining a sense of connectedness to others. This was at the early phase of the assault. As she was brutalized and since the pain was excruciating, her attention was drawn to surviving the pain. The phenomenon of dissociation was clearly described as she experienced herself outside of her body watching herself. The thoughts focused on her living so that she could care for her child; no matter what happened, she must live. In eliciting this information, Jennifer was relieved that the questions were asked in a way in which she could reveal her fear and experiences. Her fear had been that if she told anyone about these experiences, she would be deemed insane. Her sense of participating in her own defense and survival was enhanced when she was assisted in recognizing the power of the psychological strategies she employed to save her life.

Reviewing the crisis period, medical records indicate that she had "abrasions and contusions to the face, neck, breasts, and legs; active bleeding from the vaginal orifice with increased pain." She had vaginal lacerations which required surgical repair. She suffered from a bladder infection. All through her hospitalization she felt "disgraced, humiliated, and hurt." At home, her depression continued. She became irritable and hostile. Small incidents that reminded her of the rape would precipitate crying spells. She constantly thought of the incident, and this preoccupation impaired her concentration and ability to relate to people. She also began suffering from acute episodes of intense anxiety, with shaking and palpitations. This reaction would occur when she encountered groups of people reminiscent of the assailants' ethnicity.

Jennifer tried to avoid reminders of the rape. Subsequent mood swings, night terrors, and depression were minimally understood as a reaction to the rape itself by Jennifer, her family, and her employers. The pervasive irritability, the diminished trust, the lack of a sense of future for herself, only a future for her child, an avoidance of prior spontaneous and pleasurable activities tended to be interpreted as a sign of personal weakness rather than protective maneuvers to avoid any stimulation that would revive memories of the assault itself. Prior to the rape, she was extroverted, independent, and enjoyed an ability to trust people. Years following the rape she is frightened, suspicious, constantly vigilant and ill at ease. She was totally preoccupied with the safety of her child. Although she married her boyfriend, the relationship deteriorated. She developed sexual problems which caused her to seek a counselor. While she described her inability to relate sexually, she was embarrassed when asked to go into details of her problems.

Her problems did not abate with time. Her fear of public places increased as did her difficulty in sleeping and in relating to people. Her response was to feel ashamed of her emotional reactions and to be embarrassed by the change of her attitudes toward minorities. She threw herself into her work and into the care of her child.

Serious consideration of her state of mind and various symptoms did not come about until the civil suit required that she be evaluated for psychological injury.

Civil Litigation and Assessing Injury

Psychological evaluation by examining experts agreed that Jennifer had suffered posttraumatic stress and rape trauma syndrome both immediately after the rape (first 6 months) and postrape (now almost 8 years later). In contrast, the defense experts referred to the rape as a "physical assault," and did not agree there was PTSD or rape trauma; rather, they attributed all of Jennifer's symptoms and responses to prior psychiatric and personality problems and presented a diagnosis of chronic dysthymic disorder.

Given this polarized view, what was the rationale for each? The defense argued that all the symptoms presented by the victim could be explained directly and simply by prior stressful life events and Jennifer's response to them. This included (1) childhood molestation attempts at age 5 by her maternal grandfather and by two uncles at age 6 and 8, and (2) a suicide attempt at age 16. The molestations were confirmed to be single episodes of sexualized rubbing through clothing of her chest and genitals. When Jennifer revealed these incidents, her mother responded by having the grandfather leave the house and by monitoring the behavior of other adult males. The suicide attempt followed a fight with her boyfriend, an angry retreat to her room, and the ingestion of 20 aspirin, and calling her mother as she started vomiting. She was taken to the hospital emergency room to have her stomach pumped, and admitted to a psychiatric unit for 10 days. She was given a diagnosis, at that point in time, of depression. This history coupled with her present presentation of depressive symptomatology was linked together to establish a basis for her responses postrape.

The experts on the plaintiff's side evaluated the response of Jennifer to the rape itself and to postrape behaviors. In addition, there was an examination of her prerape behavior and her relationships. A comparative analysis revealed considerable differences in personal and physiological states of well-being, an arousal of fear to certain perceptual cues and interpersonal experiences, shifts in beliefs regarding herself, others, and the future, and considerable disruption in interpersonal relationships compared to prerape relationships. Furthermore, examination of psychological tests, preassault and postrape, indicated dramatic differences in a range of symptomatology. Besides depression, there were specific symptoms of hyperarousal, numbing, intrusive images of the assault, and fear of men and places. An assessment of the length of time of depressed mood was done prior to the assault and afterward. Jennifer was quite clear that she was not burdened by prolonged days of dysphoria. Her present state was aimed at avoiding and shaking off thoughts and experiences that she associated to current states of sadness and depression. She was far more preoccupied with the anxiety-provoking responses.

An important pretrauma variable was Jennifer's coping and adjustment to the molestations and to her suicidal gesture. This assessment revealed capacities to sort out what had happened. For example, she was quite aware that her mother protected her. With regard to the suicidal gesture, her appraisal to it was that she made the attempt out of anger and she interpreted it as an attention maneuver, albeit it was a dangerous act. She did not want to die nor has she thought of repeating such an act despite her distress associated with the rape. She did not view the long-lasting effects of these two events as troublesome to her.

Posttraumatic Stress Disorder versus Chronic Dysthymic Disorder

The PTSD diagnosis is new to the DSM-III-R (American Psychiatric Association, 1987). Historically, the diagnosis has been present in both of the first two editions, but it has been the clinical research on victims of rape, sexual assault, and family violence as well as the Vietnam veteran that has brought the diagnostic category into the mainstream of treatment and to its current controversial position.

It appears there is division in the psychiatric mental health field on PTSD that evidences itself in two groups:

1. There are clinicians who believe the existing system of traditional nomenclature should be used and who give minimal attention to the posttraumatic stress disorder (PTSD) category. In cases in which there is a known trauma, these clinicians try to fit disparate information into a non-PTSD diagnostic framework.
2. Clinicians who work with trauma victims and who have participated in some of the latest research in this area adhere to a PTSD model. The traditional group tends to accuse those who utilize a model of PTSD of trying to take symptomatology that could be classified under the more traditional diagnostic categories as all fitting under PTSD.

One of the strongest arguments for adhering to the PTSD classification is because it does explain the multidimensional symptom patterns that have led to diagnostic confusion and misdiagnosis in the past. The traditional use of diagnostic nomenclature has in fact missed critical phenomenological presentations by the patient and as a result the interventions and treatments have been inadequate to the symptomatology of people following a traumatic event.

Of particular importance is the diagnostic confusion that comes about as the traumatized individual tries to accommodate moving from disrupted states of arousal to states of numbness. This has been the conundrum in the missed diagnosis area because we find symptoms that are both anxiety, arousal disorder, impulsivity, disruption in thinking and in relationships combined with avoidant, detached, numbing amnesic symptomatology. Often this mixed presentation has been so confusing to treating clinicians that a whole host of practice labeling goes on such as the client is manipulative, the client is dramatic, the client is falsifying, lying, or ingenious. In clinical terminology, this switching from one phenomenological state to another has resulted in other kinds of defensive labeling procedures, such as splitting, which is often then attributed to borderline personality. What the traditional classification system overlooks when it fails to consider a response to traumatic events is that traumatic events in fact override the alarm regulatory system within the individual and break down the capacity of the human being on a physiological and on a psychological level to regulate emotional states and consequently ideational cognitive states.

Many of the current methods of psychological testing of patients do not specifically address the stress response. Rather, the items are interpreted within a nosological framework that has come out of traditional past constructs. Some of these tests have not been updated to the current DSM-III-R criteria. Tests that have been updated, such as the Minnesota Multiphasic Personality Inventory, have identified subscale test scores to discern PTSD as a subdiagnostic category. Therefore, when one begins to examine the interpretation of existing psychological test data, it is interesting to note that though one might not ascribe to the notion of a PTSD diagnosis, the ambiguity in the interpretation of the results is there and, in fact, documents the arousal disruption and the numbing phenomenon. That is what will be identified in the reports that refute a PTSD diagnosis.

The legal outcome of this case was a settlement in the seven figure range. This case demonstrates an assessment of various stages associated with a rape assault. In addition, an assessment is made of preassault factors and their lifetime relevance to the victim and any point of interdiction with the present response to the rape. To simply operate from the notion that current responses to life events are solely dependent upon early childhood experiences is to distort the reality of traumatic events and what they impart.

Conclusion

This review of the relationship of rape trauma syndrome and posttraumatic stress response to acute rape experiences identifies research findings related to pretrauma history, traumatic event history, and posttrauma factors. It is important for clinicians to understand the historically strong professional bias against rape victims, holding them responsible for the acts committed against them. With new understandings of the traumatic nature of rape, it is hoped that clinicians will be attentive to the trauma and injury suffered by victims and that treatment efforts will be aimed at reducing symptomatology through careful diagnostic and therapeutic skills.

References

American Psychiatric Association. (1987). *Diagnostic and statistical manual of mental disorders* (3rd ed., rev.). Washington, DC: Author.

Atkeson, B. M., Calhoun, K. S., Resick, P. A., & Ellis, E. M. (1982). Victims of rape: Repeated assessment of depressive symptoms. *Journal of Consulting and Clinical Psychology, 50*(1), 96–102.

Baker T., Burgess, A. W., Davis, R. C., & Brickman, E. (1990). Rape victims concern over possible exposure to HIV. *Journal of Interpersonal Violence, 5*(1), 49–60.

Bandler, R., & Grinder, J. (1975). *The structure of magic* (Vol. 1). Palo Alto: Science and Behavior Books.

Barbieri, M. K. (1989). Civil suits for sexual assault victims: The down side. *Journal of Interpersonal Violence, 4*(1), 110–113.

Bard, M., & Sangrey, D. (1980). *The crime victim's book*. New York: Basic Books.

Becker, J. V.; Skinner, L. J.; Abel, G. G., & Cichon, J. (1986).

Level of postassault sexual functioning in rape and incest victims. *Archives of Sexual Behavior, 15*(1), 37–49.

Bohart, A. C. (1980). Toward a cognitive theory of catharsis. *Psychotherapy Theory, Research, and Practice, 17*(2), 192–201.

Brownmiller, S. (1975). *Against our will: Men, women and rape*. New York: Simon & Schuster.

Burgess A. W., & Holmstrom, L. L. (1974). Rape trauma syndrome. *American Journal of Psychiatry, 131*, 981–986.

Burgess A. W., & Holmstrom, L. L. (1976). Coping behavior of the rape victim. *American Journal of Psychiatry, 133*, 413–418.

Burgess A. W., & Holmstrom, L. L. (1978). Recovery from rape and prior life stress. *Research in Nursing and Health, 1*(4), 165–174.

Burgess A. W., & Holmstrom, L. L. (1979). Adaptive strategies and recovery from rape. *American Journal of Psychiatry, 136*, 1278–1282.

Burgess A. W., & Holstrum, L. L. (1986). *Rape: Crisis and recovery*. West Newton, MA: Awab, Inc.

Carmen (Hilberman) E., Rieker P. P., & Mills T. (1984). Victims of violence and psychiatric illness. *American Journal of Psychiatry, 141*(3), 378–383.

Cunningham, J., Pearce, T., & Pearce, P. (1988). Child sexual abuse and medical complaints in adult women. *Journal of Interpersonal Violence, 3*(2), 131–144.

Dawson, R. (1989). Civil suits for sexual assault victims: The up side. *Journal of Interpersonal Violence, 4*(1), 116–122.

Dilts, R., Grinder, J., Bandler, R., Bandler, L., & DeLosier, J. (1980). *The study of the structure of subjective experience. Neurolinguistic programming* (Vol. 1). Cupertino, CA: Meta Publications.

Ellis, E. M. (1983). A review of empirical rape research: Victim reactions and response to treatment. *Clinical Psychology Review, 90*, 263–266.

Federal Bureau of Investigation. (1988). *Crime in the United States: Uniform crime reports*. Washington, DC: U.S. Department of Justice.

Finkelhor, D., Hotaling, G., Lewis, I., & Smith, C. (1989). Sexual abuse and its relationships to later sexual satisfaction, marital status, religion, and attitudes. *Journal of Interpersonal Violence, 4*(4), 379–399.

Frank, E., Turner, S. M., & Duffy, B. (1979). Depressive symptoms in rape victims. *Journal of Affective Disorders, 1*(1), 269–277.

Gibbs, M. (1989). Factors in the vicitm that mediate between disaster and psycho-pathology. *Journal of Traumatic Stress, 2*(4), 489–514.

Gleser, G. C., Green, L., & Winget, C. (1981). *Prolonged psychological effects of disaster: A study of Buffalo Creek*. New York: Academic Press.

Grinder, J., & Bandler, R. (1976). *The structure of magic* (Vol. 2). Palo Alto: Science and Behavior Books.

Hartman, C. R. & Burgess, A. W. (1986). Child sexual assault: Generic roots of the experience. *Psychotherapy and the Family, 22*, 77–87.

Hartman, C. R. & Burgess, A. W. (1988). Information processing of trauma: Case application of a model. *Journal of Interpersonal Violence, 3*(4), 443–457.

Hazelwood, R. R., Reboussin, R., & Warren, J. I. (1989). Serial rape: Correlates of increased aggression and the relationship of offender pleasure to victim resistance. *Journal of Interpersonal Violence, 4*(1), 65–78.

Hilberman, E. (1976). *The rape victim*. New York: Basic Books.

Holmes, M. R., & St. Lawrence, J. B. (1983). Treatment of rape-induced trauma: Proposed behavioral conceptualization and review of the literature. *Clinical Psychology Review, 3,* 417–433.

Holmstrom, L. L. & Burgess, A. W. (1978). *The victim of rape: Institutional reactions.* New York: Wiley.

Horowitz, M. J. (1975). Intrusive and repetitive thoughts after experimental stress. *Archives of General Psychiatry, 32,* 1457–1463.

Horowitz, M. J. (1982). Stress response syndromes and their treatment. In L. Goldberger & S. Breznitz (Eds.), *Handbook of stress: Theoretical and clinical aspects* (pp. 711–732). New York: Free Press.

Jehu, D. (1989). Mood disturbances among women clients sexually abused in childhood: Prevalence, etiology, treatment. *Journal of Interpersonal Violence, 4*(2), 164–184.

Katz, B. L., & Burt, M. R. (1988). Self-blame in recovery from rape. In A. W. Burgess (Ed.), *Rape and sexual assault* (Vol. 2). New York: Garland.

Kilpatrick, D. G., Best, C. L., & Veronen, L. J. (1985). Mental health correlates of criminal victimization: *Journal of Consulting and Clinical Psychology, 53*(12), 866–873.

Kilpatrick, D. G., Resick, P. A., & Veronen, L. J. (1981). Effects of a rape experience: A longitudinal study. *Journal of Social Issues, 37*(4), 105–122.

Kilpatrick D. G., & Veronen L. J. (1983). Treatment for rape-related problems: Crisis intervention is not enough. In L. H. Cohen, W. Claiborn, & G. Specter (Eds.), *Crisis intervention* (pp. 181–202). New York: Human Sciences Press.

Kilpatrick, D. G., Vernonen, L. J., Saunders, B. E., Best, C. L., Amick-McMullen, A., & Paduhovich, J. (1987). *The psychological impact of crime: A study of randomly surveyed crime victims.* Washington, DC: National Institute of Justice.

Koss, M. P. (1985). The hidden rape victim. Personality, attitudinal, and situational characteristics. *Psychology of Women Quarterly, 9,* 193–212.

Krupnick, J. L., & Horowitz, M. J. (1980). Stress response syndromes: Recurrent themes. *Archives of General Psychiatry, 38*(4), 428–435.

Largen, M. A. (1985). The anti-rape movement. In A. W. Burgess (Ed.), *Rape and sexual assault: A research handbook* (Vol. 1). New York: Garland Publishing.

Lazarus, R. (1966). *Psychological stress and the coping process.* New York: McGraw-Hill.

Marhoefer-Dvorak, S., Resick, P., Hutter, C., & Girelli, S. (1988). Single-versus multiple-incident rape victims: A comparison of psychological reactions to rape. *Journal of Interpersonal Violence, 3*(2), 145–160.

McCormick, R., Taber, J., & Kruedelbach, N. (1989). The relationship between attributional style and post-traumatic stress disorder in addicted patients. *Journal of Traumatic Stress, 2*(4), 477–488.

Moos, R., & Billings, A. (1982). Conceptualizing and measuring coping resources and process. In L. Goldberger & S. Breznitz (Eds.), *Handbook of stress: Theoretical and clinical aspects* (pp. 212–230). New York: Macmillan.

Murphy, S., Amick-McMullen, A., Kilpatrick, D., Haskett, M., Veronen, L., Best, C., & Saunders, B. (1988). Rape victims' self-esteem: A longitudinal analysis. *Journal of Interpersonal Violence, 3*(4), 355–370.

Norris, J., & Feldman-Summers, S. (1981). Factors related to the psychological impacts of rape on the victim. *Journal of Abnormal Psychology, 90*(6), 562–567.

Ochberg, F. M. (1988). *Post-traumatic therapy and victims of violence.* New York: Brunner/Mazel.

Ochberg, F. M. & Fojtik-Stroud, K. M. (1984). A comprehensive mental health clinical service program for victims. *American Journal of Social Psychiatry, 4*(8), 12–23.

Prentky, R. A., Burgess, A. W., & Carter, D. (1986). Victim responses by rapist type: An empirical and clinical analysis. *Journal of Interpersonal Violence, 1*(1), 73–98.

Resnick, P. A. (1983). Sex-role stereotypes and violence against women. In *The stereotyping of women: Its effects on mental health* (Focus on women: Vol. 5). New York: Springer Publications.

Resnick, P. A. (1987). Psychological effects of victimization: Implications for the criminal justice system. *Crime and Delinquency, 33*(4), 468–478.

Ruch, L. O.; Chandler, S. M.; & Harter, R. A. (1980). Life change and rape impact. *Journal of Health and Social Behavior, 21*(3), 248–260.

Ruch, L. O., & Leon, J. J. (1983). Sexual assault and trauma change. *Women and Health, 8*(4), 5–21.

Ryan, G. (1989). Victim to victimizer: Rethinking victim treatment. *Journal of Interpersonal Violence, 4*(3), 325–341.

Sales, E., Baum, M., & Shore, B. (1984). Victim readjustment following assault. *Journal of Social Issues, 40*(1), 117–136.

Sutherland, S., & Scherl, D. (1970). Patterns of response among victims of rape. *American Journal of Orthopsychiatry, 40,* 503–511.

Symonds, M. (1975). The rape victim: Psychological patterns of response. *American Journal of Psychoanalysis, 35,* 19–25.

United States, President's Task Force on Victims of Crime: Final report. Washington, DC: The Task Force, 1982.

van der Kolk, B. A. (1989). The compulsion to repeat the trauma. *Psychiatric Clinic of North America, 12*(2), 389–411.

Veronen, L., & Kilpatrick, D. (1983). Stress management for rape victims. In D. Meichenbaum & M. E. Jaremko (Eds.), *Stress reduction and prevention* (pp. 341–374). New York: Plenum Press.

Werner, A. (1972). Rape: Interruption of the therapeutic process by external stress. *Psychotherapy: Theory, Research and Practice, 9,* 349–351.

CHAPTER 45

AIDS

Coping with Ongoing Terminal Illness

Brian Kelly and Beverley Raphael

Introduction

Acquired immunodeficiency syndrome (AIDS) has become a subject of major medical, social, and political concern. It was first reported in Africa in the late 1970s and this "new acquired cellular immunodeficiency" was first described in homosexual men in the United States in 1981 (Gottlieb, Schroff, Schanker, Weisman, Fan, Wolf, & Saxon, 1981; Masur, Michelis, Greene, Onorato, Vande Stouwe, Holzman, Wormser, Brettman, Lange, Murray, & Cunningham-Rundles, 1981).

The virus has been isolated from body fluids, particularly blood and semen, but also in saliva, tears, breast milk, and cerebrospinal fluid (Ho, Pomerantz, & Kaplan, 1987). Individuals using intravenous drugs and sharing needles, as well as persons engaging in sexual practices that facilitate transmission of the infection (e.g., anal intercourse), and those who have received infected blood by transfusion are most at risk.

The clinical syndromes resulting from the human immunosuppressive virus (HIV) infection include the immunodeficiency syndrome and opportunistic infection, the lymphodenopathy syndrome, and a subacute encephalitis referred to as *AIDS dementia complex* (Navia, Jordan, & Price, 1986). An acute febrile illness at the time of seroconversion has recently been described (Tindall, Barker, & Donovan, 1988). Other HIV-related disorders include Kaposi's sarcoma and the lymphodenopathy syndrome (Ho *et al.*, 1987).

Persons infected with HIV develop clinical signs and symptoms at a variable rate. All those infected with HIV are likely to progress to a stage of immunodeficiency in which life-threatening complications can be expected (Moss & Bachetti, 1989). Preliminary natural history data in Europe and in North America estimate that approximately 2% to 5% of HIV infected persons annually progress to AIDS (Piot, Plummer, Mhalu, Lamboray, Chin, & Mann, 1988) with a median time to progression of 7 to 10 years from infection (Moss & Bachetti, 1989). Once AIDS is diagnosed, the median survival is estimated in Australia to be 10.4 months (Whyte, Swanson, & Cooper, 1989). Therefore, most persons who reach this stage of AIDS will die from the disease in the following 12 months, although the duration from time of infection to the development of AIDS is as yet unclear.

Epidemiology of HIV Infection

Currently, AIDS is the leading cause of death among men aged 25 to 44 years and women aged 25 to 34 years in New York City, (Imperato, Feldman, Nayeri, & DeHovitz, 1988), and 50,000 cases overall in the United States between 1981 and 1987 (Curran, Jafe, Hardy, Morgan, Selik, & Donero, 1988). In Australia, as in the United States, the age group of 20 to 39 years accounts for the majority of cases (Piot *et al.*, 1988). The number of cases of AIDS reported to the National Health and Medical Research Council Special Unit for Epidemiology in Australia was, 1707 up to February, 1989 (Communicable Disease Intelligence, 1990). Estimation of the true prevalence of HIV infection relies on the notification of persons newly diagnosed and does not reflect the likely prevalence of persons with asymptomatic disease in the community. In Australia, 79.5% of documented AIDS cases were reportedly infected through homosexual transmission, 2.7% through needle sharing with the possibility of additional risk through homosexual contact, 4.7% through intravenous drug use (heterosexual), 6.0% through blood or blood products, 2.7% by

Brian Kelly and Beverley Raphael • Department of Psychiatry, Royal Brisbane Hospital, University of Queensland, Herston 4029, Australia.

International Handbook of Traumatic Stress Syndromes, edited by John P. Wilson and Beverley Raphael. Plenum Press, New York, 1993.

heterosexual transmission, and the remainder (4.2%) with undetermined mode of transmission (Communicable Disease Intelligence, 1990).

A major obstacle to obtaining accurate epidemiological data is that the reporting of AIDS cases may not reflect the true number of cases owing to the lag time between HIV infection and the appearance of reported cases, along with the largely unknown natural history of this infection (Novick, Benedict, & Lehman, 1988). Differing epidemiological patterns in the prevalence of HIV infection around the world have been described by geographically subgrouping nations and has been summarized by Piot et al. (1988). Pattern One countries, which include Australia and New Zealand, North America, some areas of South America, and Western Europe, are characterized by prevalence in homosexual/bisexual men (over 50% of homosexual men in some urban areas being infected) and intravenous drug users. Heterosexual transmission in this group of countries is at present limited although some have speculated that by the end of the 1990s AIDS is likely to be predominantly a heterosexual disease, as is the case in Africa (Moss & Bachetti, 1989).

Pattern Two countries include Africa, the Caribbean, and some areas of South America. In these regions, heterosexuals are the main population affected with up to 25% of the 20 to 40 year age group in some urban areas infected and up to 90% of female prostitutes. Transfusion of HIV-infected blood in these areas is a major public health problem along with the risks of perinatal transmission, with 5% to 15% of women HIV-1 antibody positive in some areas (e.g., Kinshasa, Zaire, and some rural parts of Uganda).

Pattern Three countries include areas of low seroprevalence where more recent introduction of the disease has occurred with spread among persons with multiple sex partners. This region includes Asia, the Pacific Region (minus Australia and New Zealand), the Middle East, and some rural areas of South America. This pattern of analysis of epidemiological data in HIV infection is that adopted by the WHO Global Programme on AIDS (GPA) (Chin, 1988).

Psychological Distress and Psychiatric Disorder

Studies to date suggest high levels of distress and disorder in those clinical and research assessments that have been done at various stages of the disease. Many researchers have concentrated on reports of morbidity in those hospitalized with AIDS (Dilley, Ochitill, Perl, & Volberding, 1985; Perry & Tross, 1984). The most common diagnosis appears to be adjustment disorder with depressed mood and a range of organic syndromes, particularly delirium in the setting of what is usually a multisystem disease (Buhrich & Cooper, 1987). Schizophrenia-like psychoses have also been reported in the absence of delirium (Buhrich & Cooper, 1988).

Findings published more recently, based on larger samples of HIV positive and negative homosexual bisexual men across the spectrum of stages of HIV infection, have used structured diagnostic interviews and have indicated a high lifetime prevalence of psychiatric disorder in both HIV positive and negative groups (Atkinson et al. 1988; Williams et al. 1991). Substance abuse, major depression, and anxiety disorders were prominent (up to 30% lifetime prevalence) and the findings indicate the combination of preexisting adversity and vulnerablity in these groups.

Although significant distress is likely to be present in persons across all diagnostic subgroups of HIV infection (asymptomatic but HIV-antibody positive, AIDS-Related Complex or ARC, and AIDS), depression, anxiety, and other forms of serious psychiatric morbidity may be more frequent in the less advanced disease groups (Chuang, Devins, Hunsley, & Gill, 1989; King, 1989). The reasons for this higher morbidity with less advanced disease may reflect the degree of uncertainty and fear associated with the asymptomatic state which may lessen with the final appearance of AIDS (Miller, 1987).

Factors that have been associated with psychiatric morbidity in men with HIV infection in all stages of disease include: bisexual orientation, younger age, lower socioeconomic status, absence of a confidant, and uncertainty about any past sexual contact with a person who subsequently developed AIDS (Ostrow, Monjan, & Joseph, 1989) although none are necessarily predictive of psychiatric morbidity. The similarity of early HIV-related symptoms (e.g., lethargy, psychomotor slowing) with those of depression and anxiety syndromes needs to be considered in clinical assessment.

Suicide rates in those with HIV infection have been estimated to be 36 to 66 times that of the general population (Marzuk et al., 1988). The complex associated psychopathology in AIDS (e.g., dementia, psychoses, organic affective syndromes, and delirium) may have their own attendant risks of suicide and operate in synergism with demographic and psychosocial factors with some specific to AIDS and others common to other chronic illness.

Whether or not morbidity may be related to specific stressor effects, such as the diagnosis of the disease itself, the life threat inherent in its diagnosis, or aspects of disease progression does not appear as yet to have been fully and carefully investigated. Consequently, this chapter explores further what is currently known and the research in progress, which may help clarify these aspects. Such considerations are important: if psychiatric morbidity does result, even in part, from traumatically stressful experiences associated with the disease, it may be better understood, prevented, and managed if traumatic stress concepts are utilized. Similarly, adjustment processes to the disease and its progress need to be investigated for evidence from the field of oncology to highlight the way that adjustment processes may influence the course of the condition.

Stress and Adjustment and Potential Sources of Stressors

The HIV infection causes the death of a group of predominantly young men in Pattern One countries and young men and women in Pattern Two countries. There is great uncertainty about prognosis and there may be anticipation of a protracted and wasting death. Death and the response of individuals and those close to them to the threat of imminent death are fundamental psychological themes in this disease.

HIV infection and AIDS are diseases primarily affecting disenfranchised groups (Ostrow *et al.*, 1989) and as such there exists the coincidence of infection with preexisting psychosocial stressors (Ermann, 1989).

The diagnosis of HIV infection and AIDS may place an individual at the focus of harsh social stigma and discrimination. All affected groups may be stigmatized by the community stereotypes of the AIDS sufferer (Cassens, 1985). The theme of the innocent and guilty victim is likely to heighten distress, particularly with increasing attention to the plight of those infected by transfusion who are seeking compensation.

An individual may be unable to share the news of the diagnosis with others because guilt, fear, and shame arise as well as concern over social repercussions of such news (e.g., loss of accommodation, employment, social network) (Cassens, 1985). Individuals may face a medical staff who have ambivalent and at times rejecting attitudes so that their own sense of hopelessness may come to be mirrored in the response of carers to them (Dilley *et al.*, 1985). There is likely to be a constriction of social network, loss of job opportunities, demands to alter patterns of sexual relationships, along with the exposure for some of previously undisclosed sexual behavior particularly as the illness becomes more disabling.

HIV infection is likely to have a profound impact on close relationships. Grief and reactions to loss are prominent issues. A unique aspect of HIV infection is the exposure to multiple loss, such as the death of friends and partners, creating a gradual erosion of social networks, with illness and death at a level comparable to a community disaster (Altman, personal communication). This disaster continues over many years both for individuals and for their communities. The impact on community of HIV infection is likely to have a considerable effect on the individual's psychological vulnerablity in efforts to cope with the distress of the loss of attachments and sources of social integration, as well as to deal with one's own disease and anticipated death. In many instances, there is protracted illness with increasing care often needed from family members or partners. These factors must be faced in addition to specific aspects of the disease, such as the fear of contagion that may be present in those caring for the infected person, the impact of the news of the affected person's membership in a group that is still seen by many as deviant, and the wide range of emotional responses to such issues. There is an altered intimacy of relationships, strong demands for alteration in patterns of sexual behavior, and conflict over the exposure of news of the diagnosis given its adverse social consequences. For some, the mode of acquisition of infection may evoke issues of infidelity in stable partnerships.

Psychosocial issues and adaptive demands are likely to alter with progression of the disease (Chuang *et al.*, 1989). Those at earlier stages, although unimpaired physically by the infection, may nevertheless experience considerable psychosocial disability. Preoccupation with physical symptoms may be prominent (Kessler, Obrien,

& Joseph, 1988) and the physical symptoms of anxiety and depression may be interpreted as the evidence of accelerated deterioration. This may also apply to the impaired concentration and the subjective sense of memory failure that often accompany depression and anxiety. These may be interpreted by the person with HIV infection as evidence of impending dementia. Such symptoms as depression, apathy, and psychomotor slowing may be indicative of HIV encephalopathy (Perry & Jacobsen, 1986). Similarly, the impact of psychosocial stress on apparent intellectual functioning needs to be considered in evaluating the clinical aspects of HIV-related brain disease (Eisenberg, 1989). The frequent central nervous system (CNS) complications may impair the patient's ability to adapt to stress and illness (Holland & Tross, 1985).

Individuals may lose their ability to work and an important source of gratification and satisfaction as well as social integration is lost. Work may also lose its sense of purpose or goal as the person searches for a way to create meaning and satisfaction with the limited time left to live. Equally, the workplace may highlight fears of rejection and stigma, particularly as the disease progresses and the presence of AIDS becomes evident.

Adaptations

Clinical studies in the earlier stages of the epidemic described themes and patterns observed with some patients at that time. Although these reports are interesting, they may not reflect the broad spectrum of adaptations that would be found in community studies of representative groups of infected persons. For instance, Nichols (1985) described the process of psychosocial reaction of persons with AIDS which includes an initial crisis, a transitional state characterized by self-devaluation, suicidal ideation and actual suicide with a review of one's past, a deficiency state with the formation of a "new, stable identity" and acceptance of what others have labeled *supportive denial*, and finally a preparation for death. Dilley and co-workers (1985) described some of the "psychological themes" relevant to adjustment that are encountered in working with these patients; the uncertainty surrounding the illness and its treatment with resulting anger and anxiety, and conflicting relationships between staff and patients in which these emotions and fears of social abandonment emerged strongly. Patients' guilt and perception of their illness as punishment were highlighted. The numerous fears and multiple losses (health, relationships, employability, friends and partners) became potent themes in response to a life-threatening illness.

Research Studies

The impact of HIV infection on seronegative as well as seropositive men has been explored in recent reports from the Multicenter AIDS Cohort Study in the United States (Ostrow *et al.*, 1989). Using the Center for Epidemiological Studies Depression Scale (CES-D), a self-report depression inventory, along with questionnaires to assess a broad set of psychosocial variables (e.g., social support, coping mechanisms, life-style), Ostrow and his co-workers reported that a primary predictor of an increase in depressive symptoms in their large cohort was the number of self-reported HIV-related symptoms at baseline assessment of a high-risk group who were unaware of their serostatus. Increase in depression was independent of whether the men were infected; fear of developing the illness was considered responsible for many of the depressive symptoms. These researchers reported an overall elevation of depressed affect subscale of the CES-D in their large cohort (both seronegative and seropositive) compared with other data of a sample of married men. They also highlighted that high-risk groups may experience a chronic state of concern about physical and emotional symptoms that may be prodromal to AIDS.

A recent report displayed the application of traumatic stress theory to the assessment of distress in persons with HIV infection. Jacobsen and Perry (1988) used the Impact of Event Scale (IES) to assess the "intrusive and avoidant coping responses" of a small group of men who were undergoing a double-blind placebo-controlled drug in the treatment of HIV infection. The nondrug group displayed a greater level of distress on a self-report of psychological symptom measures. This distress was significantly related to the perception that there was insufficient opportunity to discuss with a physician the results of HIV testing that was performed earlier. More importantly, the distress also was significantly associated with the higher level of intrusive coping as measured by the IES of the process of response rather than as a more specific variant of the distress itself.

Avoidant and intrusive thoughts and emotion about AIDS have been reported as forming important symptoms of AIDS-related bereavement in a large cohort of homosexual men in New York (Martin, 1988). In the group, those men who had experienced the loss of a lover or close friend because of AIDS exhibited a significantly greater degree of sedative and recreational drug use and referrals to psychological services because of their own AIDS concerns in addition to the posttraumatic stress symptoms about AIDS. Other reports also highlight the multiple stressors that are likely to impinge on the bereavement outcome in groups such as this (e.g., loss of job, accommodation, family reactions) (Kessler *et al.*, 1988).

Research documenting the features of adjustment needs to adopt a sufficiently broad approach to the dominant symptomatology in order to encompass the range of behavioral and emotional disturbances that may evolve, whether these represent reactive processes or categories warranting diagnosis as a disorder. The definition of *adjustment disorder* presents some problems in patients with HIV infection (Williams *et al.*, 1991). Ehrhardt, Stein, and Spitzer (1987) made the point that

> it is difficult to judge the distinction between normality and a maladaptive reaction to having a terminal illness, as is the case for many of those infected with the virus. Clearly more operational guidelines have to be developed for any meaningful use of this category in this population.

This observation applies even more in the instance of posttraumatic stress in HIV infection. Posttraumatic symptoms that occur in reponse to the personal trauma of diagnosis of a life-threatening illness is an area of limited exploration to date. This has been applied to the impact of the disease, specifically, the impact of news of the risk for premature heart disease (Horowitz, Simon, Holden, Connett, Billings, Borhani, & Benfari, 1983). A small group of those persons who were informed of their risk of disease, in a study of risk factors for cardiovascular disease, exhibited posttraumatic symptomatology in response to such news.

The importance of psychological adjustment in cancer patients has been emphasized in studies of the prevalence of psychiatric morbidity and the relationship that has been detected between psychological adjustment and level of distress (Watson, Young, Inayat, Burgess, & Robertson, 1988). Psychological adjustment is also important in patient's likelihood of compliance with chemotherapy (Gilbar & DeNour, 1989). Speculation has risen over the importance of such adjustment in the overall prognosis of the disease (Pettingale, Morris, Greer, & Haybittle, 1985; Morris & Pettingale, 1979).

Watson and colleagues (1988) described the relationship between different types of coping and distress in subjects with cancer. In their survey, they used the self-report instrument, the Mental Adjustment to Cancer Scale (MACS), in addition to measures of mood state. Three discrete subscales of this measure (anxious preoccupation, helplessness, and fatalistic responses) were associated with greater psychological symptom score. They concluded that these responses may form a negative coping style, the so-called fighting-spirit response, and may represent a more positive reaction that protects against psychopathology in view of the strong negative correlation between responses of this kind and overall levels of anxiety and depression.

The diagnosis of an illness, such as HIV infection, presents a threat to life after an interval of uncertain duration and with death of an uncertain nature. Symptoms relating to death then are likely to intensify with the passage of time. Such a threat of impending death may be present for years prior to the development of overt signs of illness and may become a form of chronic adversity compounding the physical or other disabilities of the disorder itself. These factors are compounded by the additional adversity and disadvantage that some individuals may encounter in the disclosure to others of their disease when its presence becomes obvious. The constant threat of premature death occurs for most such patients at a time in the life cycle when death is less of a tangible potentiality. As such, life-threatening illness at this stage may cut across the usually future-directed and goal-oriented phases of early adult life.

Fears of death are likely to be prominent from the earliest time following diagnosis and may also become a source of distress for those who see themselves at risk of this disease but are as yet uninfected. This latter point is becoming increasingly evident as the broader community impact of HIV receives increasing attention. Volunteer agencies who assist persons with AIDS are often staffed by persons who may have been or continue to be at risk of the disease. Observing the progressive disability and death of peers with whom one has a strong identification may become a potent source of fears for one's own vulnerability to death from this disease. The work of Lifton (1973) may be applicable to such groups who are affected most by HIV infection, emphasizing the role of death anxiety in the development of post-traumatic symptoms. Psychic numbing is viewed as a defense against the traumatic experience and the concomitant death anxiety and "death guilt," with traumatic intrusive images forming the expression of the "death imprint" left by the traumatic experience.

These anxieties concerning death may be exacerbated by the difficulties faced by AIDS carers (both professional and volunteer) in discussing such concerns. For medical and nursing staff, a denial of these issues may occur in part due to the distressing experience of helplessness in thwarting the progression of disease and, at times, a sense of having failed in their therapeutic role (Dilley et al., 1985). Such anxieties, in addition to the frequent hopelessness that may develop in treatment settings, may be represented in the often negative or prejudicial attitudes toward persons with AIDS in health professionals (Wallack, 1989) and may encourage an avoidance of the most distressing concerns for the patient, their families, and their partners.

Traumatic Stress and HIV Infection

In the following section, we offer a description of preliminary data from a prospective study of the correlates of psychiatric disorder in a person with HIV infection. This study has been devised as a multifaceted project with examination of biological, psychological, behavioral, and social aspects of the disease in three centers in Australia.

The data presented in this section concern the cross-sectional evaluation of the presence of traumatic stress symptoms in persons who have HIV infection and the association between posttraumatic phenomena and other measures of psychiatric morbidity. Additional aims include the association between such dependent variables and conventional measures of vulnerability to psychological morbidity. These early data, which are based on assessment of a relatively small group of subjects, are unable to fully examine the predictive value of measures of vulnerability.

A key interest in this project was to assess the applicability of conventional notions of posttraumatic stress symptoms (e.g., intrusive and avoidant images, thoughts, and affects) in the processes of adaptation to the chronic adversity of a life-threatening illness.

The chief hypotheses being examined in this phase of the study were that in those individuals with HIV infection, patterns of posttraumatic symptoms in response to the diagnosis of HIV infection would be present and would form an important component of the distress that is experienced. It was proposed that a key element of the traumatic aspect of this disease is likely to be the cognitive and emotional reactions to the threat of one's own death. It was also hypothesized that a positive correlation would be detected between such posttraumatic phenomena and the overall levels of psychological symptoms of distress, and that the presence of

such morbidity would correlate with the measures of vulnerability to psychiatric disorder.

Methodology

Homosexual and bisexual men with HIV infection who were attending outpatient clinics of the two major general hospitals and a government health department AIDS clinic in Brisbane, Australia, were approached to participate in this project. Participants were asked to complete a brief questionnaire and participate in a structured clinical interview and neuropsychological testing.

Data are presented here on 24 HIV antibody-positive men.

A true random sample could not be drawn and, as in most reports on homosexual populations, the representativeness of any sample is difficult to evaluate because there is no clear means of defining the overall homosexual population from which subjects in this and other similar projects are drawn (Kessler et al., 1988; Martin, 1988).

Measures

A modified version of the Impact of Events Scale (IES) (Horowitz, Wilner, & Alvarez, 1979) was used. This was presented in two forms: the first transformed the items of the IES to inquire about intrusive and avoidant phenomena concerning being told one has an HIV infection; the second was similarly constructed but examined intrusive and avoidant phenomena the focus of which was the response to the threat of death from HIV infection. Subjects were asked to report the frequency of these phenomena over the preceding 7 days from "not at all" to "often." Items chosen from the IES were selected on the basis of their ability to be transformed to a format applicable to HIV infection. A total of 14 of the original 15 items have been included. The deleted item ("I know I still have feelings about it") was considered to be less applicable in the setting of ongoing adversity such as HIV infection.

The Mental Adjustment to Cancer Scale (MACS) (Watson et al., 1988) was modified for use with persons with HIV infection. The original version of this measure is a self-report instrument examining a range of cognitive and emotional responses to cancer and has established validity and reliability in persons with a range of malignant disease. Developed from an interview based on an approach to the evaluation of discrete patterns of psychological adjustment, the self-report version has proven concurrent validity with clinician ratings of predominant patterns of coping. Scores are obtained on five subscales: Avoidance, Anxious Preoccupation, Fatalism, Helplessness/Hopelessness, and Fighting Spirit.

The items in this questionnaire were simply transformed to inquire about such a response to HIV infection rather than cancer. Each item presents a statement concerning a response to the disease (e.g., "I feel that nothing I can do will make a difference"), and the respondent is asked to indicate "How far it applies to you at present"

PART IV • DISASTERS OF NATURAL AND HUMAN ORIGIN

on a 4-point scale from "Definitely does not apply to me" to "Definitely does apply to me."

These instruments were used in addition to the 28-item General Health Questionnaire and the Beck Depression Inventory (Beck, Ward, & Mendelson, 1961) as conventional measures of psychological symptoms and, in the case of the GHQ, the probability that such symptoms in an individual may represent a psychiatric disorder.

Other instruments used included measures of vulnerability to psychological morbidity: the Eysenck Personality Inventory (EPI) short form (Andrews, G., personal communication), an abbreviated self-report form of the Interview Schedule for Social Interaction (Henderson, Byrne, & Duncan-Jones, 1981) as a measure of social support, and a brief life-events inventory.

Results

Sociodemographic characteristics of the sample are similar to the reported data from other research in this field which indicates that this group is similar in these characteristics to other groups of HIV antibody-positive homosexual and bisexual men (Kaslow, Ostrow, & Detels, 1987). The mean age was 32.8 years (range = 21–50, SD = 9.6). Eighty-six percent were born in Australia, 72% had at least 10 years of education, and the majority (74%) had never married. Only 50% of this group were in full-time employment. Ninety-two percent (92%) were in the early stages of the disease (CDC Group II) as defined by the infectious diseases physician who was responsible for their care and the mean duration in time since diagnosis was 30.9 months (range = 1–74, SD = 21.63).

Psychiatric Morbidity

The mean score on the General Health Questionnaire-28 was 6.8 (SD = 6.9), using a dichotomous scoring method. Using the standard cutoff point of greater than or equal to 4 for a community sample would indicate that approximately 49% of this group were likely to classify as psychiatric cases. If a higher cutoff point of greater than or equal to 11 is used, as has been applied to hospital inpatients (Bridges & Goldberg, 1981), the rate of caseness remains high (28%).

Traumatic Stress

On examination of the Impact of Events Scale with this group, a number of interesting findings emerge. All intrusive items were endorsed as "occurring sometimes or 'frequently'" by 25% to 65% and avoidance items in the range of 10% to 50%, indicating the relevance of these symptoms.

Table 45.1 provides data that employs simple Pearson correlation scores of the association between these subscales. Particularly important is the high correlation between the intrusive phenomena concerning HIV infection and those concerning death, which indicates the

Table 45.1. Pearson Correlation of Impact of Event Scale Subscales

Symptom	Death–I	Death–A
HIV–I	.89**	47*
HIV–A	.27	.84**

Note. I = Intrusion subscale; A = Avoidance subscale.
*$p \leq .05$; **$p \leq .001$.

salience of death-related anxiety in this group of patients. Clearly, a correlation at this level suggests that the same construct is being measured by these subscales.

Avoidance items were endorsed less frequently than intrusive items. The low correlation between the two subscales contrasts with the reports of Zilberg, Weiss, and Horowitz (1982) who reported a correlation of .45, suggesting a level of covariance between the two sets of phenomena. One explanation for the salience of intrusive symptoms in this group may lie in the phasic nature of traumatic stress reactions. Zilberg and colleagues described the state of being overwhelmed by trauma, with the experience predominantly of "undercontrolled intrusion states." The combination of this pattern alongside those with an oscillation over a week between high avoidance and high intrusion, in addition to persons with high avoidance alone, is likely to explain the low correlation overall between the intrusion and avoidance subscales. Such a mixture may characterize the psychopathological syndrome of posttraumatic stress disorder. These are the hypotheses proposed by Zilberg and co-workers (1982) to explain the variation in the subscale correlation.

The importance of intrusive posttraumatic phenomena is borne out in the correlation of the intrusive subscales of the IES with the GHQ score and the scores on the Eysenck Personality Inventory, which are detailed in Table 45.2. It appears that intrusive phenomena of both forms of the IES displayed a most significant correlation with overall psychiatric morbidity. This finding may simply be describing the interrelation of distress concerning HIV infection and death which are part of the same construct of distress that is being measured by the GHQ.

The failure of avoidance items to correlate with distress or symptom score suggests that it is the conscious preoccupation with thoughts and images of the disease and of death that covary with the level of distress, but that avoidance exhibits no consistent relationship with that distress. Neither age nor duration since time of diagnosis exhibited a significant relationship with GHQ score or IES subscale and total scores.

When examining the correlates of IES scores with measures of vulnerability, a clear relationship emerged between the EPI neuroticism and IES intrusive subscales concerning both HIV infection and death. It is interesting to note that the level of symptom scores on both the GHQ and the BDI did not exhibit a statistically significant relationship with either life-event score or perceived level of social support; yet this is observed with posttraumatic symptoms. As would be predicted, a robust positive correlation of EPI neuroticism with both GHQ and BDI were found.

Table 45.2. Correlation of Impact of Event Scale Subscales

Instrument	HIV–I	HIV–A	Death–I	Death–A
General Health Questionnaire	.78**	.31	.71**	.20
Eysenck Personality Inventory	.61*	.29	.58*	.22
Fatalism	.73**	.31	.68**	.18
Anxious Preoccupation	.56*	.23	.61*	.31
Helplessness/Hopelessness	.56*	.23	.57*	.02
Fighting Spirit	−.30	.19	−.31	.27
Avoidance	.23	.37	.10	.30

Note. Number of respondents varies between analyses due to missing data (range of 18–24 subjects).
$*p \leq .005; **p \leq .001.$

Although it is not possible to state categorically that this high correlation between the IES intrusion scale and the GHQ may be indicative of diagnosis of PTSD the GHQ has certainly been found to be a valid indicator in screening for PTSD in disaster populations (McFarlane, 1990). It seems likely that this high preoccupation with having been told of the disease (not related to time frame of diagnosis) and with the possibility of death reflects not only posttraumatic symptomatology but also PTSD in this population. Furthermore, aspects of the prospective study that include a diagnostic interview using the DIS should be helpful in clarifying this relationship.

The Mental Adjustment to HIV Scale (Mental Adjustment to Cancer Scale [MACS] modified for mental adjustment to HIV infection) shows further important data on adaptation.

On all measures of distress (i.e., GHQ, IES intrusive symptoms, and BDI scores), the subscales of helplessness, fatalism, and anxious preoccupation displayed a significant positive correlation with psychological morbidity, whereas the converse applied for the fighting spirit constellation. Details of these findings in a larger asymptomatic cohort have been reported elsewhere (Kelly *et al.* 1991). Table 45.2 displays the correlation between each section of the MACS and the four IES subscales used. Again, it is clear that it is with intrusive phenomena that the most pertinent relationships emerge.

Although the influence of state factors, such as depression and anxiety, on self-reported adjustment on the MACS needs to be borne in mind in interpreting these results, the clustering of posttraumatic symptoms with aspects of adjustment further emphasizes their relevance in attempting to describe and understand the processes of adaptation that occur. The prospective component of this research will address changes in these factors over time and the predictive validity of such measures of adjustment in terms of later morbidity.

Discussion

These findings represent the first phase of a prospective project which will examine the psychological adjustment to HIV infection. Invariably, this disease is fatal and has many important and unique psychosocial aspects that are likely to impinge on the tasks that confront the individuals with this disease.

As a disease with a broad range of manifestations, the interrelation between stages of disease severity and adaptation are important considerations. Although it is not a conventional practice to apply models of posttraumatic phenomena to the understanding of adaptation to chronic and changing stress of a life-threatening illness, this model may have substantial application in defining more clearly the changing cognitive and emotional processes that occur.

Fears of death may form an early and persistent component of distress and psychological morbidity. Additionally, such fears and responses to them may have an important role in the motivational factors influencing an individual's health-related behavior (e.g., in the case of HIV infection, their sexual behavior). In the setting of such a serious illness, simply defining the levels of depression or anxiety may not sufficiently highlight the specific features of the psychological response to this adversity. It is the understanding of such aspects of adaptation that is important in providing a more empirically based approach to the psychological care of persons who are affected by chronic and life-threatening illness and provide more substantial systematic basis for counseling and other therapeutic techniques. Models of adaptation need to be tested in this way to avoid misleading clinical folklore. For example, denial may be an appropriate and healthy defense at some stages of the illness if it protects against overwhelming distress; but if it impinges on illness behavior (e.g., failure to follow through with treatment or failure to present for care when symptoms arise), then its adaptiveness is limited. A multidimensional approach to the global concept of adaptation and the different demands that are entailed in the psychosocial adjustment to the disease and its threat to life are more likely to bring together more accurately this complex field.

References

Atkinson, J. H., Grant, I., Kennedy, C. J., Richmann, D. D., Spector, S. A., & McCutchan, J. A. (1988). Prevalence of psychiatric disorders among men infected with Human Immunodeficiency Virus. *Archives of General Psychiatry, 45,* 859–864.

Beck, A. T., Ward, C. H., & Mendelson, M. (1961). An inventory for measuring depression. *Archives of General Psychology, 4,* 561–567.

Borland, R., & Lewis, V. (1989). Changing behaviour to prevent the spread of the human immunodeficiency virus. *Medical Journal of Australia, 151,* 305–306.

Bridges, K., Goldberg, D. (1981). The validation of the GHQ-28 and the use of the MMSE in neurological inpatients. *British Journal of Psychiatry, 148,* 548–553.

Buhrich, N., & Cooper, D. A. (1987). Requests for psychiatric consultation concerning 22 patients with AIDS and ARC. *Australian and New Zealand Journal of Psychiatry, 21,* 346–353.

Buhrich, N., & Cooper, D. A. (1988). HIV infection associated with symptoms indistinguishable from functional psychosis. *British Journal of Psychiatry, 152,* 649–653.

Cassens, B. J. (1985). Social consequences of the acquired immunodeficiency syndrome. *Annals of Internal Medicine, 103,* 68–771.

Chin, J. (1988). *The global epidemiology and projected impacts of AIDS. WHO consultation on neuro-psychiatric aspects of HIV infection.* Geneva, Switzerland: World Health Organization.

Chuang, H. T., Devins, G. M., Hunsley, J., & Gill, M. J. (1989). Psychosocial distress and well-being among gay and bisexual men with the human immunodeficiency virus infection. *American Journal of Psychiatry, 146,* 876–879.

Communicable disease intelligence, Bulletin 90/3, February 12, 1990. Australian Commonwealth Department of Community Services and Health.

Curran, J. W., Jaffe, H. W. Hardy, A. M., Morgan, V. M., Selik, R. M., & Donero, T. J. (1988). Epidemiology of HIV infection and AIDS in the United States. *Science, 239,* 610–616.

Dilley, J. W., Ochitill H. N., Perl, M., & Volberding, P. A., (1985). *Findings in psychiatric consultation with patients with acquired immune deficiency syndrome.* American Journal of Psychiatry, 42, 82–86.

Dilley, J. W., Shelp, E. E., & Batki, S. L., (1986). Psychiatric and ethical issues in the care of patients with AIDS. *Psychosomatics, 27,* 562–566.

Eisenberg, L. (1989). Health education and the AIDS epidemic. *British Journal of Psychiatry, 159,* 754–767.

Erhardt, A. A., Stein, Z., & Spitzer, R., (1987). *HIV center for clinical and behavioural studies.* Book I. Core I, Psychiatric/Psychosocial Assessment Core, 10–25.

Erman, M. (Ed.). (1989). *Psychosocial and psychosomatic aspects of AIDS research, in interaction between mental and physical illness.* Berlin: Springer-Verlag.

Gilbar, O., & De-Nour, A. K. (1989). Adjustment to illness and dropout of chemotherapy. *Journal of Psychosomatic Research, 33*(1), 1–5.

Gottlieb, M. S., Schroff, R., Schanker, H. M., Weisman, D. O., Fan, P. T., Wolf, R. A., and Saxon, A. (1981). Pneumocystis carinii pneumonia and mucosal candidiasis in previously healthy homosexual men. *New England Journal of Medicine, 305*(24), 1425–1430.

Greer, S., Morris, T., & Pettingale, K. W. (1979). Psychological response to breast cancer: Effect on outcome. *Lancet, 2,* 785–787.

Henderson, A. S., Byrne, D. G., & Duncan-Jones, P. (1981). *Neurosis and the social environment.* Orlando, FL: Academic Press.

Ho, D., Pomerantz, R. J., & Kaplan, J. C. (1987). Pathogenesis of infection with human immunodeficiency virus. *New England Journal of Medicine, 317*(5), 278–283.

Holland, J. C., & Tross, S. (1985). The psychosocial and neuropsychiatric sequelae of the acquired immunodeficiency syndrome and related disorders. *Annals of Internal Medicine, 103,* 760–764.

Horowitz, M. J., Wilner, N., & Alvarez, W. (1979). Impact of Event Scale: A measure of subjective stress. *Psychosomatic Medicine, 41*(3), 209–218.

Horowitz, M. J., Simon, N., Holden, M., Connett, J. E., Billings, J. H., Borhani, N., & Benfari, R. (1983). The impact of news of risk for heart disease. *Psychosomatic Medicine, 45*(1), 29–37.

Imperato, P. J., Feldman, J. G., Nayeri, K., & Dehovitz, J. A. (1988). Medical students' attitudes towards caring for patients with AIDS in a high incident area. *New York State Journal of Medicine, 88*(5), 223–227.

Jacobsen, P. B., & Perry, S. W. (1988). Psychological reactions to individuals at risk for AIDS during an experimental drug trial. *Psychosomatics, 29,* 182–189.

Kaslow, R., Ostrow, D. G., & Detels, R. (1987). The multicenter AIDS cohort study: Rationale, organization, and selected characteristics of the participants. *American Journal of Epidemiology, 126,* 310–318.

Kelly, B., Dunne, M., Raphael, B., Buckham, C., Zournazi, A., Smith, S., & Stthan, D. (1990). Relationships between mental adjustment to HIV diagnosis, psychological morbidity and sexual behaviour. *British Journal of Clinical Psychology. 30,* 370–372.

Kessler, R. G., O'Brien, K., & Joseph, J. G. (1988). Effects of HIV infection, perceived health, and clinical status on a cohort at risk of AIDS. *Social Science Medicine, 27,* 569–578.

King, M. B. (1989). Psychosocial status of 192 outpatients with HIV infection and AIDS. *British Journal of Psychiatry, 154,* 237–242.

Lifton, R. J. (1973). *Home from the war: Vietnam veterans: Neither victims nor executioners.* New York: Simon and Schuster.

Lifton, R. J., & Olson, E. (1976). The human meaning of total disaster: The Buffalo Creek experience. *Psychiatry, 39,* 1–18.

Martin, J. L. (1988). Psychological consequences of AIDS-related bereavement among gay men. *Journal of Consulting and Clinical Psychology, 56*(6), 856–862.

Marzuk, P. M., Tierney, H. Tardiff, K., Gross, E. M., Morgan, E. B., Hsu, M. A., and Mann, U. U. (1988). Increased risk of suicide in persons with AIDS. *Journal of the American Medical Association, 259*(9), 1333–1370.

Masur, M., Masur, H., Michelis, M. A., Greene, J. B., Onorato, I., Vande Stouve, R. A., Holzman, R. S., Wormser, G., Brettman, L., Lange, M., Murray, H. W., & Cunningham-Rundles, S. (1981). An outbreak of community acquired pneumocystis carinii pneumonia. *New England Journal of Medicine, 305,* 1431–1438.

Mayou, R., & Hawton, K. (1986). Psychiatric disorder in the general hospital. *British Journal of Psychiatry, 149,* 172–190.

Miller, D. (1987). HIV counseling: Some practical problems and issues. *Journal of the Royal Society of Medicine, 80,* 278–281.

Moss, A. R., & Bachetti, P. (1989). Natural history of HIV infection. *AIDS, 3,* 55–61.

Navia, B. A., Jordan, B. D., & Price, R. W. (1986). The AIDS dementia complex: I clinical features. *Annals of Neurology, 19*(6), 517–524.

Nichols, S. E. (1985). Psychosocial reactions of persons with AIDS. *Annals of Internal Medicine 103,* 765–767.

Novick, L. F., Benedict, T. I., & Lehman J. S. (1988). The epidemiology of HIV in New York State. *New York State Journal of Medicine, 242,* 246.

Ostrow, D. G., Monjan, A., & Joseph, J. (1989). HIV-related symptoms and psychological functioning in a cohort of homosexual men. *American Journal of Psychiatry, 146*(6), 737–742.

Perry, S. W., & Jacobsen, P. (1986). Neuropsychiatric manifestations of AID-spectrum disorders. *Hospital and Community Psychiatry, 37*, 135–141.

Perry, S. W., & Tross, S. (1984). Psychiatric problems of AIDS inpatients at the New York Hospital: Preliminary report. *Public Health Reports, 99*(2), 200–205.

Pettingale, K., Morris, T., Greer, S., & Haybittle, J. L. (1985). Mental attitudes towards cancer: An additional prognosis factor. *Lancet, 1*(8431), 750.

Piot, P., Plummer, F. A., Mhalu, F. S. Lamboray, J. L., Chin, J., & Mann, J. M. (1988). AIDS: An international perspective. *Science, 239*, 573–579.

Tindall, B., Barker, S., & Donovan, B. (1988). Characterization of the acute clinical illness associated with human immunodeficiency virus infection. *Archives of Internal Medicine, 148*, 945–949.

Wallack, J. J. (1989). AIDS anxiety among health care professionals. *Hospital, Community Psychiatry, 40*, 507–510.

Watson, M., Greer, S., & Bliss, J. M. (1989). Mental adjustment to cancer, user's manual.

Watson, M., Greer, S., Young, J., Inayat, Q., Burgess, C., & Robertson, B. (1988). Development of a questionnaire measure of adjustment to cancer: The MAC scale. *Psychological Medicine, 18*, 203–209.

Whyte, B. M., Swanson, C. E., & Cooper, D. A. (1989). Survival of patients with the acquired immunodeficiency syndrome in Australia. *Medical Journal of Australia, 150*, 358–362.

Williams, J. B., Rabkin, J. G., Remein, R. H., Gorman, J. M., & Ehrhardt, A. A. (1991). Multidisciplinary baseline assessment of homosexual men with and without Human Immunodeficiency Virus Infection: II. Standardized clinical assessment of current and lifetime psychopathology. *Archives of General Psychiatry, 48*(2), 124–30.

Zilberg, N. J., Weiss, D. S., & Horowitz, M. J. (1982). Impact of Event Scale: A cross-validation study and some empirical evidence supporting a conceptual model of stress response syndromes. *Journal of Consulting Clinical Psychology, 50*, 407–414.

PART V

The Impact of Trauma on Children and Adolescents

A traumatic event can impact on any stage of life-cycle development. It is also known that the effects of trauma have both age- and stage-related consequences to psychosocial and epigenetic processes of ego differentiation and maturation.

In Chapter 46, Robert S. Pynoos and Kathi Nader discuss issues in the treatment of posttraumatic stress reactions in children and adolescents. They begin by observing that the treatment of traumatized children traverses several disciplines, such as neurobiology, psychodynamics, pediatrics, psychiatry, child psychology, and education. Their comprehensive chapter summarizes the relevant literature on PTSD in children and is organized into four sections: (1) prevention and psychological first aid, (2) the initial consultation, (3) brief therapy, and (4) long-term therapy.

In the past, there was a paucity of data to determine adequately if children manifest PTSD symptoms in the same way as do adults. Based on current studies, it is quite clear that children exhibit the full range of PTSD and its associated features, including dissociation, flashbacks, forms of denial, unconscious behavioral reenactments, psychic numbing, and states of overdriven hyperarousability (e.g., startle reactions).

Pynoos and Nader propose a twofold developmental model of external and internal threat as the core mechanisms underlying PTSD in children. In discussing this model, they state:

> In their conscious fantasies, children demonstrate a developmental hierarchy in their approaches and responses to the external danger. This hierarchy simultaneously incorporates changes in how they address internal dangers as well. For example, preschool children may desperately envision the need for outside help while invoking fantasies of superhuman powers primarily to protect themselves and their physical integrity against attack.

Thus, children are especially prone to *intervention fantasies*, which are attempts to deal with the painful memories of the trauma. Pynoos and Nader write, "because these intervention fantasies become inextricably associated in children's memory with the event, treatment approaches must include specific developmental means to explore these mental activities." The remainder of this highly detailed chapter provides a set of practical clinical principles by which to understand the nuances of working with children whose egos have been scarred by a trauma. In conclusion, Pynoos notes that "reworking is a complicated task with children because of their fantasy, their evolving development, and their reappraisals that accompany experiential growth and cognitive maturity."

In Chapter 47, Dora Black, Tony Kaplan, and Jean Harris Hendriks look at what happens to children in a family when the father kills the mother, a brutal act which is witnessed directly by about half of the children who are victimized by this event.

To study the psychiatric sequelae of an intrafamilial homicide, Black and her colleagues evaluated 49 girls and 46 boys between the ages of 8 and 15 years at the time of the killing. These children were referred by court authorities in the United Kingdom for evaluation; this afforded the opportunity to gather data.

Based on clinical interviews, various types of information were coded and subjected to statistical analysis. The results revealed that 44% of the children had witnessed the killing or heard it taking place. As would be expected, bereavement (48%) and emotional problems (70%) were common and were associated with conduct problems (44%), learning difficulties (48%), and conflict with peers (38%). PTSD was present in 26% of the children but was regarded as an underestimate of prevalence because of the lack of familiarity with the diagnosis by the professionals who first evaluated the children. Furthermore, children who had previously witnessed violence in the home were more likely to have behavioral problems (87%) than those who did not have this experience. A similar finding is reported in Chapter 53 by Harkness for the children of Vietnam veterans whose fathers had PTSD and were violence-prone.

The balance of the chapter discusses clinical issues in working with these children, including the necessity of finding the right placement for them in order to avoid long-term negative effects on psychosocial development. For example, they state:

> It is likely that untreated PTSD results in long-term problems. We have clinical examples of placements in which compliant children with constricted affect have been greeted with relief by troubled caretakers, a situation likely to lead to psychiatric disorders at a later time.

Children whose fathers kill their mothers are likely to suffer from PTSD, particularly if they witness the killing. They need urgent crisis intervention with skilled help to uncover what they experienced in order to minimize the risk of disorder in the future.

In Chapter 48, Rob Gordon and Ruth Wraith discuss the responses of children and adolescents to disaster. Since traumatic events are not alike and differ on a number of stressor dimensions, the authors begin by reviewing the literature on traumatic reactions in children and the characteristic effects of psychic trauma. Included here are the following considerations: (1) trauma is beyond normal experience; (2) a massive quantity of emotion is generated; (3) trauma violates normal psychological assumptions; (4) trauma ruptures expectations about the future; (5) trauma ruptures preexisting adaptations and meaning; (6) the trauma experience is placed outside time, and is constantly repeated in the present; and (7) trauma has an existential dimension.

Based on their work with children who were in the bushfires of Southern Australia (see Chapter 34), the authors have codified the nature of the short-, medium-, and long-term effects of disaster upon psychosocial development. During the first weeks, there are many expectable reactions, such as fear and insecurity, emotional lability, intrusive recollections and behavioral reenactments, regressed and disorganized behavior, hyperarousal states, and obsessive preoccupation with trauma-related issues. In the medium-term phase, some of the initial reactions may carry over. Relationship, mood, and attitude changes may be expressed in different ways (e.g., withdrawal, acting-out, loss of communication). Also, there may be signs of developmental arrestation, school problems, and changes in peer-group relations. Long-term psychological consequences of traumatization may begin to solidify the previous phasic reactions into personality changes, school failure, poor interpersonal relationships, and a struggle with identity and ideological views.

Once the central themes that define postdisaster functioning have been identified, the authors describe a variety of techniques designed to ameliorate the disruption to the life continuum and ego development. Among the many useful clinical insights contained in their chapter is that "effective strategies promote normal recovery by identifying vulnerabilities and interference from relationships or other areas of life and assist the child and the family to take control of them."

In Chapter 49, Arthur Green discusses childhood sexual and physical abuse. To begin, he notes that the essence of child abuse is the repeated infliction of physical and psychological injury to a child within the context of a pathological family system. The consequence of the continuous assault to the child's ego leads to defensive efforts, such as avoidance, distancing, numbing, and denial to attempt to seal over the narcissistic injury to the vulnerable and developing ego.

If the trauma is prolonged, it may lead to one of several alternative pathways of adaptation and defense, which include (1) identification with the aggressor; (2) masochistic behavior and passive identification; and (3) borderline-like states characterized by fragmentation of the ego, emotional lability, and identity confusion, depending on the type of trauma experience (e.g., physical punishment, sexual molestation, verbal belittlement).

In his densely packed chapter, Green systematically reviews the impact of physical and sexual abuse on children by content area and dimension of psychodynamic functioning. Thus, among the topics covered are anxiety and depression states, eating disorders, adult survivors of maltreatment, aggressive and assaultive behavior, sexual disorders, borderline personality disorder, multiple personality disorder, and long-term effects on life-course development.

Green notes that a variety of therapeutic interventions can aid the recovery process for the abused child. These include psychodynamic play therapy and psycho-educational techniques. As noted by Lindy in Chapter 68, the core of the focal therapeutic process is an empathic stance toward the child which enables rebonding through the therapeutic alliance—a consolidation—in which the victim transfers identification to the super-ego strength of the analyst or counselor.

In Chapter 50, Judith Lewis Herman discusses father–daughter incest, a traumatic event that ruptures the bond of trust between a parent and a child and the family system as well. Incest within families is often difficult to detect because there is very little that is unconventional about incestuous families; they come from all walks of life and social classes. However, what is common is the *paternal abuse of authority* and power inherent in the role of a provider and caretaker. As Herman notes:

> Incestuous fathers often attempt to isolate their families, restricting the mobility and social contacts of both their wives and their daughters. It is not unusual for survivors to report that their fathers discouraged their mothers from working outside the home, socializing, or even driving a car, that the family never had visitors in the home, or that the children were not allowed to participate in normal peer activities because of their fathers' jealousy and suspiciousness.

The portrait that emerges for the perpetrator, the incestuous father, is that of a highly egocentric, dominating person who has a special attitude of entitlement to female attention and service to meet his needs for power and control. Contrary to popular misconceptions, the incestuous father does not typically suffer from a mental illness or alcoholism. Although sociopathic, paranoid, and narcissistic personality characteristics have been noted, it is the preoccupation with his own fantasies and needs that leads him to dominate and exploit others, especially those who are vulnerable.

Herman explains that for incest to occur, the *secrecy principle* must exist:

> Secrecy becomes the dominant principle of family life, imposed by the father's need to preserve sexual access to his daughter. The sexual contact is rarely a single event, rather it is repeated over a period of months or years, ending only when the child finds the resources to escape.

Children who are victims of father–daughter incest frequently become symptomatic: there is bedwetting, insomnia, nightmares, fearfulness, social withdrawal, acting-out behaviors, and a range of somatic complaints. Many incest victims meet the diagnostic criteria for PTSD; often psychological distress increases in adolescents as demands continue and the fear of pregnancy becomes a reality.

Once the daughter discloses the secret of the sexual abuse, the potential for interventions and treatment exists. Herman details the issues of clinical approaches to working with victims of incest. Among the many principles noted (cf. the important one to all successful treatment of PTSD) is the necessity for a complete history with specific questions about what happened in the trauma. Many victims of PTSD go undetected for years because of a failure to uncover a traumatic event that produced psychic damage.

Once the incest is discovered, it puts the family into a crisis of major proportions. At first, the perpetrator may deny allegations but eventually, when faced with the specter of legal prosecution, will become more compliant and seek treatment. Herman states that at this point it is usually necessary for the father to leave the home and consent to undergo treatment under stringent legal guidelines with punishing consequences for noncompliance. Furthermore,

> during the crisis period, all family members are in great distress and need intensive support. The child needs to be assured that protective and responsible adults believe her story and will not allow her to be further exploited.

The successful treatment program needs to have three interrelated foci: (1) to empower the mother, (2) to provide psychotherapy for the daughter, and (3) to force court-ordered compliance for the treatment of the father. In her conclusion, Herman states that

> because the trauma of incest is profoundly social, so is the recovery process. A full resolution of the trauma involves the restoration of social bonds and a renegotiation of the patient's relationship with her family of origin.

In Chapter 51, Michael A. Simpson explores the effects of political repression, chronic unrest, and civil violence on children and adolescents, as well as their families, who live in South Africa. He begins by calling for a more comprehensive and holistic view of posttraumatic reactions.

> I want to bring to attention a number of usually neglected aspects of trauma and its results: such as the matter of community trauma and communal responses to trauma; the nature and effects of continuing and recursive violence; the necessity to recognize the political context of trauma and its effects; the interplay between multiple traumata; and the fact that structural violence, such as that inherent in oppressive systems, has potentially severe and continuing posttraumatic effects.

Following an insightful discussion of the limits of current conceptualizations of PTSD, Simpson shifts his focus to the children of South Africa. He argues that by many yardsticks of medical and psychological health, South Africa is a sick country. He notes, for example that "between 1984 and 1986 alone, 300 children were killed by the police, 1,000 wounded, 11,000 detained without trial, 18,000 arrested on charges related to protest, and 173,000 were held in police cells." Thus, at many, if not all, levels of South African society there exist conditions that engender fear, threat, and the on-going potential to be the victim of systematic repression with the loss of individual freedoms.

The long-term effect of these coercive conditions of society for the oppressed moves beyond the hassles and stresses of "normal" living to resemble protocols experimentally designed to generate traumatic states in laboratory animals.

Through case example and analysis, Simpson makes the point that the current literature lacks knowledge and good research findings that could be employed to understand the subtle, destructive, and pervasive emotional reactions to apartheid in South Africa. For example, he states:

> So little research has been done, and so little of this is well done, or useful, or justifies the weight of the conclusions that may be based on it. Most of the literature on disasters, war, and posttraumatic disorders simply ignores children and adolescents. If they look at children at all, many of the studies examine the impact of a single horrible event (such as an earthquake), and few study the effects of the sort of chronic, suppurating violence and unrest that afflict many parts of the world. Most of the emphasis is on short-term effects . . . except for some studies of Holocaust survivors, there has been little attention to the effects in adult life of exposure to horrors as a child.

What this seems to imply, of course, is the need to broaden the systematic scope of posttraumatic research programs, to undertake cross-sectional programs of research into the effects of single, multiple, and recurring and/or chronic stressors on the developmental pathways of epigenetic development.

Throughout the remainder of his chapter, Simpson systematically presents the research evidence of the effects of civil unrest, violence, detention, prejudice, encounters with death, and more. The result is one of the most massive compilations on posttraumatic stress reactions and psychiatric sequelae in children ever attempted. Written with passion and analytical clarity, its intrinsic and heuristic value is enormous; it will promote researchers, clinicians, and educators in directions for future studies which will continue to evolve at an exponential level.

In Chapter 52, Mona S. Macksoud, Atle Dyregrov, and Magne Raundalen examine the effects of exposure to and involvement in traumatic war experience on children. After a brief conceptual orientation to PTSD, trauma, and the research literature on children affected by war, the authors delineate the types of stressors that are indigenous to war trauma and explore their effects on intrapsychic functioning and psychosocial development. As noted by Bonnie L. Green in Chapter 11, it is important for researchers to attempt to discern the link between specific types of stressors and their contribution to posttraumatic reactions. In this regard, the authors categorize about 10 stressor events that are common to children who are traumatized by the events of warfare which include: (1) the violent death of a parent, (2) witnessing the killing of close family members, (3) separation and displacement, (4) terror, attacks, kidnapping, and life-threat, (5) participation in violent acts, (6) bombardment and shelling, (7) witnessing parental fear reactions, (8) physical injuries and handicaps, (9) extreme poverty and starvation, and (10) other acts of threat and fear that are not easily classified.

After reviewing how the stressor events affect the child's psyche, Macksoud and her co-authors examine the relationship of PTSD to developmental stages in terms of both the short- and long-term effects. Consistent with the findings of Rob Gordon and Ruth Wraith in Chapter 48, issues emerge from this analysis, such as the effect of traumata on moral development, personal identity, trust and feelings of vulnerability, pessimism about the future, school performance, and psychosocial development.

With these issues identified and explicated, the authors next discuss intervention and treatment and denote special types of emotional disturbance, such as the violent child, the child politician, the child refugee, and other forms of identity formation, coping, and adaptation. In their conclusion the authors state:

> We do not really know what happens to a generation of vulnerable children who have lost their sense of safety, who have acquired a high tolerance for violence, who are haunted by terrifying memories, mistrusting and cautious of others, and who hold a pessimistic view of the future.

At the most basic level of humaneness, we must ask the questions: What kind of adults will these children of war become and what will be their vision of leadership and authority? How will the war trauma affect their view of the future?

The accumulating body of clinical and empirical research in the Holocaust has shown that the adverse effects of the concentration camp experience for the survivor extended into his or her family system as well. Thus, the *second generation* was affected by their parents' difficulty in making peace with the traumata that happened to them.

Transgenerational effects of PTSD are now recognized as a distinct phenomenon and yet there are only a few studies which have attempted to delineate the mechanisms by which this occurs. Clearly, family systems theory is most relevant here in order to begin a conceptual framework with which to explore hypotheses as to how the psychological symptoms of the affected parent get transmitted within the family.

Laurie Leydic Harkness, in Chapter 53, examines the *transgenerational transmission* of war-related trauma among the children of Vietnam combat veterans. She begins by noting:

> The first tenet is that the family is a highly complex system which consists of a number of interlocking parts engaged in patterned interaction. The family must be viewed as a whole unit and cannot be reduced to the properties or characteristics of its individual members. The second tenet is that individuals influence each other through their interaction. This influence can either increase or decrease the frequency or intensity of certain behavior. In other words, what affects one part of the system (family) is felt by others in that system.

When considering the potential impact of parental PTSD on the family system, it is thus possible to construct an analogy to the effects of alcoholism: Co-dependent roles may be established; episodes of violence, unpredictability, unreliability, and emotional stability can adversely affect the children and the spouse. Furthermore, it is possible to have vicarious victimization and the development of PTSD symptoms among particular family members, especially those with the strongest bonds of affection and identification with the PTSD-affected parent.

In her chapter, Harkness uses the Salvador Minuchin terms of *enmeshment* and *disengagement* to explore how it is that PTSD affects the family system. She also hypothesizes that tendencies toward impulsivity and violence will have a powerful effect on the transmission of transgenerational emotional difficulties in development. To explore these ideas, Harkness studied 86 children from 40 families in which the father was a PTSD-positive Vietnam veteran. In addition to in-depth clinical interviews, each family member completed a set of questionnaires to assess family functioning and the children's performance at school and in terms of their mental health.

The results produced many interesting findings which supported her hypotheses. Among these was the tendency for some children to behave in a manner similar to that of the father:

> Many of the child behaviors reported by the parents resembled behaviors exhibited by the father (e.g., depression, anxiety, low frustration tolerance, and outbursts of anger). These behaviors might be the children's attempt to identify with their fathers or to understand their father's behavior; or these children are secondarily traumatized by having a father with PTSD. In working with these children, clinicians need to be sensitive to the presence of these behaviors in the fathers as they diagnose and treat the children.

Harkness concludes her chapter with a set of recommendations for treatment of the family system and the children in individual therapy.

In Chapter 54, Derrick Silove and Robert Schweitzer explore the effect of apartheid on children and adolescents in South Africa. They begin by noting a fact, not obvious to many Western clinicians and researchers, that

> it is a commonly held maxim among antiapartheid workers that to explain South African society convincingly to the outside world, one has to dilute the truth to make it plausible—the reality is so improbable that incredulity quickly takes over.

In a manner consistent with the research discussed in Chapter 51 by Michael A. Simpson, another South African psychiatrist, these authors clearly argue that the current society is *permeated* with multiple levels of stressors which are enduring (continuous), insidious, and often hidden in nature. It is the chronicity and periodicity of the trauma that have a devastating and often crippling impact on the psychosocial development and well-being of black children and adolescents. To this end, Silove and Schweitzer review the effects of racial prejudice in terms of physical health (e.g., pellagra at a 66% prevalence level), social consequences, and damage to ego development as a result of political abuse and torture. In summarizing the effects of these experiences, the authors state:

> It is possible that in comparison to natural disasters, human-engineered disasters like apartheid may have singularly damaging effects on the individual's long-term sense of social integration and feelings of fundamental trust, and that these effects may be particularly marked in the child. Because the aim of torture is explicitly to disintegrate and alienate the personality of the victim—an aim which is directly antithetical to that of psychiatric treatment—psychiatrists have a responsibility to demand effective action to prevent such atrocities.

Part V concludes with a chapter by Guus van der Veer on psychotherapy with young adult political refugees. The chapter is based on the author's work with refugees from countries in which political oppression and torture were instruments of control and social influence of ideological belief systems.

Van der Veer has identified five major themes that are common to traumatization and adolescent development, which are discussed in the beginning of the chapter: (1) loyalty, (2) future orientation, (3) need for recognition, (4) changing motivation, and (5) mistrust. Each of these themes is discussed in terms of a twofold conceptual paradigm: emergent developmental and epigenetic life-stage crises and the impact of trauma to the young adult and his or her family. For example:

> The feelings which young refugees have toward their parents are also complicated by other factors, such as political opposition to the government of their native country. In some instances, their political activities were the result of a *first independent choice*, or a *first act of rebellion* against their parents. But if the first independent step has such a disastrous or traumatic consequence, it may not be easy to take a second one on account of fear, anxiety, and uncertainty. Furthermore, if their parents have political sympathies with those who use torture as a political instrument, then this may profoundly influence their attitude toward their parents.

After van der Veer has discussed the psychosocial implication of the core themes that the young refugee adults struggle with in their new country, he reviews strategies for psychotherapy with a special emphasis on two techniques: the testimony method and interpretation of nightmares. He concludes his chapter by noting:

> The therapist who works with adolescent victims who are political refugees needs to be aware that traumatic experiences can intensify epigenetic developmental processes that are normative during adolescence, and that they may have an impact especially on the processes relevant to (1) identity formation, (2) separation-individuation, (3) future goals and values, (4) intimate relations, (5) parental relations, and (6) current motivational states.

CHAPTER 46

Issues in the Treatment of Posttraumatic Stress in Children and Adolescents

Robert S. Pynoos and Kathi Nader

Introduction

The treatment of traumatic stress responses in children raises issues that transverse the disciplines of neurobiology, psychodynamics, psychosocial influences, and behavioral and cognitive development. Here, the University of California–Los Angeles (UCLA) Neuropsychiatric Institute and Hospital, we have established a research and clinical prevention intervention program in the area of violence, trauma, and sudden bereavement in childhood. We have responded to requests for assistance from numerous communities after extreme acts of violence or disaster.

In this chapter, we will focus primarily upon children's exposure to single-incident violence and disaster but will also mention certain salient features of chronic trauma, including sexual or physical abuse. We will discuss four phases of treatment: (1) prevention and psychological first aid, (2) the initial consultation, (3) brief therapy, and (4) long-term therapy. We will examine four different sites of intervention (school, family, individual, and group) as they relate to specific stress responses.

Like adults, children respond to trauma with symptoms of reexperiencing, emotional constriction or avoidance, and increased arousal (Pynoos, Frederick, Nader, Arroyo, Steinberg, Eth, Nunez, & Fairbanks, 1987; Terr, 1979). Reexperiencing phenomena indicate how elements of the traumatic experience remain active in the child's mental life. The reexperiencing of traumatic phenomena is evidenced by traumatic play, behavioral reenactments, intrusive thoughts, images, sounds or smells, traumatic dreams, and psychological reactivity to reminders. Avoidant behavior and psychological numbing indicate how a child continues to restrict or regulate emotions or behavior in an effort to control the recurrent impressions and the associated affect. Children report becoming avoidant of specific thoughts, locations, concrete items, themes in their play, and human behaviors that remind them of the incident. They may exhibit reduced interest in usually pleasurable activities, a sense of aloneness, even estrangement from others, a fear of renewed overwhelming affects, memory disturbances, and temporary regressions or loss of acquired skills. Traumatic avoidance may selectively restrict daily activity or generalize to more phobic behavior. Furthermore, a profound change in future orientation may result, which may include more pessimistic appraisals, expectations of further harm or a foreshortened future, and altered views of future career, marriage, and family.

Increased states of arousal may include sleep disturbances, irritability and anger, difficulty concentrating, hypervigilance, exaggerated startle response, and physiological reactivity to reminders. Traumatic exposure may result in a temporary increase in risk-taking behavior. Exposure to cries of distress and witnessing mutilation often leads to unalleviated states of empathic arousal (Hoffman, 1979). Also, there may be associated feelings of guilt because children felt unable to provide aid, they escaped to safety while others were harmed, or they believed their actions endangered someone else.

Posttraumatic stress disorder (PTSD) is among stress responses a distillation of common traumatic reactions. The discussion of traumatic responses goes beyond this constellation of symptoms because of trauma's impact on a child's emerging personality and intrapsy-

Robert S. Pynoos and Kathi Nader • Program in Trauma, Violence, and Sudden Bereavement, University of California, Los Angeles, and Neuropsychiatric Institute and Hospital, Center for Health Sciences, Los Angeles, California 90024.

International Handbook of Traumatic Stress Syndromes, edited by John P. Wilson and Beverley Raphael. Plenum Press, New York, 1993.

chic life. For example, accompanying neurophysiological changes may not only alter behavior but may affect the child's self-concept. Changes in self-concept may then produce secondary behavioral changes and may potentially alter character formation.

Post-traumatic stress is not the only set of reactions to occur in the aftermath of a traumatic experience. A single event can lead to the experience of loss and grief or worry about a significant other and continued apprehensions, or it may serve as a reminder of a past experience and generate renewed symptoms or distress. Furthermore, one event, for example a disaster, may be associated with multiple adversities such as life threat, loss of a family member, loss of residence and relocation, involuntary unemployment of a parent, or change in the family's financial status. The chronic traumas inflicted by war also involve many adversities in addition to traumatic experiences (e.g., deprivation, malnutrition, family disruption, immigration, and resettlement). In general, multiple adversities increase the risk of co-morbidity, especially of major depressive disorder or general anxiety disorder (in young children, separation anxiety disorder) (Rutter, 1985). Therefore, strategies of intervention for children and adolescents, must include a multifocal approach to address each of these different sets of circumstantial reactions, to minimize adversities or to treat the multiple psychiatric disorders that may result.

Developmental issues influence children's experience, symptomatic presentation, course of recovery, and behavior in treatment. These developmental influences affect children's appraisals of threat, the intrapsychic meaning they attribute to the event, their emotional and cognitive means of coping, their capacity to tolerate their reactions, and their ability to address the secondary changes in their lives.

Childhood Traumatic Response: A Twofold Developmental Model of External and Internal Threat

In the discussion of childhood traumatic responses, a debate has continued over whether to emphasize objective factors about the external event or subjective perceptions including the appraisal of threat. In this chapter, we rely on Freud's (1926/1968) original model of traumatic helplessness, defining a traumatic situation as one where "external and internal, real and instinctual dangers converge" (p. 168). One key to intervention is ongoing attention to the reprocessing of both external and internal dangers. Choices about the type of intervention and duration often hinge on the amount of therapeutic attention that is needed to address each of these experienced dangers and on the differences by exposure, circumstance, phase-specific development, maturity, and past experience that determine the content and reaction to these dangers.

Developmental maturity and experiential growth have an impact on children's assessments of both external and internal threats. In general, very young children may gain partial protection from the traumatic impact because they do not understand the potential danger.

Early studies of traumatized children focused primarily on potential life-threatening situations, for example, air raids during World War II (Burt, 1943). As reported in these studies, young children's reactions frequently reflected parental attitude, behavior, and degree of anxiety.

This protective influence often fails, however, when real harm occurs. Even in the World War II studies, clinical researchers reported severe traumatic reactions in children when, for example, a bomb hit their house and injured family members. Furthermore, even though adults may protect children from stress by trying to appear unalarmed, there are many horrifying and catastrophic situations in which they cannot be expected to do so. In fact, children may be confused, disturbed, and potentially put in greater jeopardy by adults who minimize the obvious threat (Pynoos & Nader, 1988a). As children mature in their appraisal of life threat, they rely less on cues from their caretakers and more fully understand situations of potential threat. Adolescents, for example, may rely on their own appraisals and fully envision the threatened harm even when it is not carried out, for example, when a gun has been held on them during a robbery.

Internally, the child contends with a variety of threats: from his physical and affective responses, from a sense of helplessness and ineffectualness, from disturbances to his emerging self-concept, from intrapsychic dangers of abandonment, loss of love, castration anxiety, and superego condemnation, and from disturbances in impulse control and processes of identification. The child may not feel that he can regulate his physical response (e.g., "My heart was beating so fast, I thought it was going to break") or affective response (e.g., internally generated murderous impulses), or may be overwhelmed by the intensity of the psychodynamic threat. For example, the internal danger of abandonment when a parent is placed in a different lifeboat (Friedman & Linn, 1957), parental exclusion when yelled at not to enter the bedroom just before the mother is murdered (Bergen, 1958), castration anxiety when witnessing the use of a dildo in the sexual assault of his mother (Pynoos & Nader, 1988b) or self-condemnation for not being able to do more to protect himself or someone else (Pynoos & Nader, 1989b).

In their conscious fantasies, children demonstrate a developmental hierarchy in their approaches and responses to the external danger. This hierarchy simultaneously incorporates changes in how they address internal dangers as well. For example, preschool children may desperately envision the need for outside help while invoking fantasies of superhuman powers primarily to protect themselves and their physical integrity against attack. School-aged children may entertain conscious fantasies of intervening, for example, taking the gun out the assailant's hand, may evoke fantasies of special powers (as superman or he-man) in order to intervene without fear of harm, or may employ phase appropriate post-Oedipal fantasies of rescue and exile to seek safety for themselves or others. Preteen boys may become more specific in the manner in which they would intervene, such as the 11-year-old boy who wished he had used his martial arts training to stop his mother's rapist and who proceeded to further perfect his martial arts skills. With maturity, adolescents more fully appraise the circumstances and opportunities for intervention, and imagine themselves as taking direct action, while entertaining a sense of narcissistic invulnerability.

Gender differences may also influence these sets of appraisals. For example, adolescent boys may feel emasculated by the experience and respond with intense narcissistic rage. When accompanied by a sense of narcissistic invulnerability, this rage places them at risk of taking revenge or engaging in dangerous reenactment behaviors. Whereas, many preteen and adolescent girls may be especially troubled by a sense of their own physical ineffectualness and vulnerability or may be disturbed by their aggressive impulses, and, for example, may show reluctance to explore their fantasies of revenge without proper therapeutic assistance.

Common Misconceptions

Some of the prevalent ideas about children's traumatic experiences have limited childhood trauma theory and approaches to treatment.

Multiple Episodes

There has been a tendency to approach any event as if it were one global experience. Our studies suggest, however, that in remembering life-threatening situations, children's recall is not organized as a single episode. In fact, working-through requires attention to the multiple traumatic episodes within a single event.

Children's organization of memory and strategy of recall differs as they focus on different anchor points, such as life threat, worry about another, cues of distress, sight of victims, injury, or blood, the attributes and movements of an assailant, the efforts to reach safety or be rescued, their own physiological responses, worst moments, location and actions of adults, reunion with parent, parental reactions, guilt, grief, or reminders of past life experience. Spatial and temporal registration, affective and cognitive responses, sets of perceptions, intervention fantasies and psychodynamic attributions differ for each moment or memory anchor point. For example, previous life experience will influence children to emphasize certain details, attribute special meaning to aspects of the trauma, and to be preoccupied with certain psychodynamically relevant internal dangers (Pynoos & Nader, 1989a).

These findings underscore three points: (1) these anchor points, or memory markers, are important clues to pertinent clinical issues; (2) there may be separate sets of reminders for each traumatic moment; and (3) the manner in which they are initially interviewed may be of critical clinical importance because interviewing provides children with a strategy of recall.

Mental Modification

The symptoms of PTSD in children and adolescents have sometimes been represented as if they embodied simple replications or depictions of the traumatic event without the children's own mental modifications or activity. For example, intrusive images, reenactment behavior, dreams or traumatic play are spoken of as if they represented an exact replay of the traumatic experience. In fact, reexperiencing phenomena often include mental efforts to manage traumatic anxiety or to regulate the associated affect, for example, as depicted in their play, drawings, or behavioral reenactments (Pynoos, 1990).

Because children do not apparently exhibit the degree of amnesia that is sometimes seen in adult trauma victims, and seem, at times, readily able to describe horrifying experiences in detail, it has been suggested that children do not employ denial. Denial, in its original usage, did not mean disavowal of reality; indeed, in Anna Freud's original description (1936), it was a means children, especially, employed to mitigate "objective pain" by use of fantasy or imagined action. Thus, they are able to maintain their appreciation of even the most disturbing realities. Some repetitive images contain within them a denial in fantasy; for example, a child may move away from the injured victims or out of the most immediate zone of danger (Pynoos & Nader, 1989a). Furthermore, children omit portions of their experience from conscious memory (e.g., the blood all over her own shirt; the worst danger within the general danger) or reframe aspects of an experience in order to minimize an internal or external threat (e.g., rationalize that a best friend grabbed her foot as she scrambled to safety as an attempt to save her life).

Traumatic play includes the redramatization in play of episodes of the event or the repetition in play of traumatic themes. Terr (1981) observed that children's traumatic play fails to provide relief, may aggravate rather than soothe the condition. and often ends unsatisfactorily in contrast to normal play. In play, children are not simply repeating an action but manipulating the object as well, sometimes toward a more positive outcome. We have observed that children's traumatic play may either provoke anxiety or provide relief for a child, perhaps related to the degree of perceived control over outcome, to the degree a satisfactory ending is achieved, to the degree there is freedom to express the prohibited affect (e.g., revenge), or to the degree a cognitive reworking is facilitated (Nader & Pynoos, 1990). For example, a boy who attempted to engage his peers in shooting games following a school sniper attack was agitated whenever his friends would not allow him to be the successful good guy. In contrast, a boy from the same school who enacted the successful rescue of several endangered schools by police and firemen and the girl who, as nurse, repaired the injured, felt their play to be rewarding and experienced a temporary sense of relief.

Imagined Actions

There has also been a controversy over the relationship of reality and fantasy in children's retelling of traumatic experiences, primarily expressing concern on how to distinguish truth from confabulation or retelling from elaboration. We suggest a different emphasis. In our study of children's acute traumatic memories (Pynoos & Nader, 1989a), we found, in accord with the laboratory findings of Johnson and Foley (1984), that specific trauma-related imagined actions are incorporated into their memory representations of the event.

"Denial in fantasy" (A. Freud, 1966), "inner plans of action" (Lifton, 1979), and "intrapalliative strategies" (Lazarus, 1966) each describe mental efforts to contend with a loss or injurious outcome by employing fantasized or imagined actions to answer the internal or external danger, or both. Those who witness cues of distress (e.g., a dying child calling for help or a wounded parent bleeding) search intensely for effective means of assisting (Pynoos & Nader, 1989a). For example, in her initial recall, one 11-year-old girl described standing over her fatally wounded classmate saying, "I love you," before she died. In fact, no one could get near the dying child because of the continued rapid gunfire. Another classmate stated that someone had moved the fatally injured girl into a protected area where she could have received help when the paramedics arrived. Both children admitted in their more detailed descriptions of the event that they had only wished these moments had occurred.

Intervention Fantasies and Identification

Ongoing intervention fantasies are integral to children's continued reprocessing of traumatic events (Table 46.1). These fantasies involve conscious and unconscious efforts to discover "what could have been done," what might diminish the resulting pain, or what can counter a continued sense of threat. The accessibility and richness of children's conscious fantasy is often underestimated. Revenge fantasies are one overlooked source of understanding how children address their traumatic helplessness after the fact. An overreliance on the term, "identification with the aggressor" (A. Freud, 1936) has limited appreciation of the complexity and psychic economy of these special mental efforts, of their multidetermined identificatory content, and of the interdigitation of mental components to rid the child of the external danger while definitively resolving the internal threat.

Dissociative Phenomena

Dissociative phenomena in children after trauma are also described as if they reflected simply an altered state of mind, rather than a complex developmentally influenced mental effort. When there are dangers to physical integrity (e.g., being penetrated during a molestation or being burned by a cigarette during physical abuse), the child's attention may move away from monitoring the assailant or imagining outside intervention and toward fears of internal damage including frighten-

ing fantasies of physical or psychological harm. The content of the dissociation may be a direct effort actively to offset these fears and to escape from the physical coercion (e.g., by imagining having reached a safe haven or shrunken to an imperceivable dot). In this latter fantasy, a child attempted both to make herself an impossible to find sexual target while, in reducing her own significance, she hoped to diminish her narcissistic importance to an incestuous father.

Guilt and Repression

Sandler (1967) discussed how guilt instigates repression following trauma:

> The motive for the repression stems, not from the traumatic experience proper, but from fear of punishment, which is reflected in internal feelings of guilt, shame and humiliation. (See Ruben, 1974, p. 374.)

Guilt, itself, often incorporates fantasies of ineffectual intervention or interpretation of actions or inaction as endangering themselves or others. We found that guilt significantly increases posttraumatic distress in children (Pynoos *et al.*, 1987).

In summary, because these intervention fantasies become inextricably associated in children's memory with the event, treatment approaches must include specific developmental means to explore these mental activities. The principal underlying treatment is that the mind of a child remains extremely active in processing a traumatic experience; acutely, and over time, children's minds attribute meaning to the details of the event and reprocess different aspects of the experience and its aftermath.

Play and Drawing in the Assessment and Treatment of Trauma

The role of play and drawing in the assessment and treatment of traumatic stress goes beyond the general discussion of play and drawing in psychotherapy or the simple idea that drawing permits an easy access to children who might otherwise find it difficult to speak about their experiences. Drawing and play have a special place in the linking of the internal and external domains. According to Piaget and Inhelder (1969), "drawing should be considered as halfway between symbolic play and the mental image" (p. 54). Winnicot (1971) described play as an interface between a child's intrapsychic reality and the outer world in which a child is attempting to control or manipulate outer objects.

In the specialized treatment of traumatized children, drawing is more than a doorway to the child's mental representation of traumatic material. A more complex model proposes that the visual and other perceptual experiences of the event become embedded and transformed in a child's play and drawings (Nader & Pynoos, 1990). Thus, play and drawings serve as an ongoing indicator of both the child's processing and her or his resolution of traumatic elements. Within the context of the specialized interview, drawings help to identi-

Table 46.1. Intervention Fantasies

To alter the precipitating events
To interrupt the traumatic action
To reverse the lethal or injurious consequences
To gain safe retaliation—fantasies of revenge
To prevent future trauma

fy anchor points and to identify the spatial and temporal misrepresentations that allow the child to contend with anxiety or fear. They permit depiction of the series of actions that occurred and help to understand the circumstances of the child's life into which the trauma intrudes. They also may reveal details imbued with special traumatic meaning to a child (A. Freud, 1966) (e.g., two-pronged buildings or abstract images drawn by a boy who saw his mother killed with a two-pronged pitchfork or the depiction of a special dress borrowed from the daughter the morning that the mother was killed).

Because play can always be redone (Solnit, 1987), it provides opportunities, for example, to reexamine and give new meaning to aspects of the event or to reexperience and rework the memory and emotions. These techniques may assist in identifying intrusive phenomena and ongoing issues of self-blame or of loss of self-esteem. Using play and art in the assessment and resolution of, for example, inner plans of action is not only a method of turning passive into active but, in addition, permits a completion of the desired or fantasied act within a safe therapeutic setting.

Strategies of Intervention

Successful intervention requires triaging and screening for children at risk, reducing stress-induced disturbances in children undergoing normative reactions, and preventing the onset of disorders or reducing their duration and progression. Attention to traumatic experiences in childhood provides the opportunity to implement the principles of preventive psychiatry in outreach intervention strategies. These strategies focus on strengthening individual and family-coping capacities, as well as decreasing adverse influences on recovery. They include fostering the continued adaptation of resilient children, as well as assisting those with severe stress reactions (Pynoos & Nader, 1989b).

In working with families and children at risk for psychiatric morbidity, prevention goals include (1) ameliorating traumatic stress reactions and facilitating grief work, (2) preventing interferences with child development and the resulting maladjustments, and (3) promoting competence in effectively adapting to the crisis situation. Successful preventive intervention requires access to children who are identifiably at risk, treatment of populations undergoing normative reactions to extreme stress and prevention of the onset of disorders, or reduction of their duration and progression.

In the following section, we discuss aspects of four phases of posttrauma treatment: (1) Psychological First Aid and Therapeutic Consultation in Classrooms, (2) Initial Assessment, (3) Brief Therapy, and (4) Long-Term Therapy.

Psychological First Aid and Therapeutic Consultation in Classrooms

The goal of psychological first aid is to provide important initial emotional relief through immediate psychological services. Since many disasters or incidents of community violence or trauma affect large numbers of children and adolescents, we have previously proposed the school setting as an optimum site for any organized intervention program. We have described a detailed day-by-day plan that can be implemented in schools to meet the immediate and long-term needs of those directly and indirectly affected (Pynoos & Nader, 1988a). In this discussion, we will underscore some of the salient features of this work and address some of the misapplications that commonly occur.

First, the first-aid techniques must be developmentally sound both in identifying specific age-related reactions and in providing age-appropriate interventions. We have summarized our current understanding of these issues in Table 46.2. Certain age considerations, for example, the potentially dangerous reenactment behavior of adolescents, can make intervention a psychiatric emergency. Relaxation methods are often recommended for adults and children in the acute aftermath, and may, acutely, give immediate or periodic relief from anxiety. Care must be taken because relaxation exercises may actually permit increased vividness of traumatic imagery (Rachman, 1980) and is most appropriately used in the context of therapeutic *in vitro* flooding techniques that address the accompanying anxiety (Saigh, 1986).

Second, the goals must be appropriate for the school setting. Lacking a clearly delineated overall strategy of intervention, many current programs attempt to do more than is possible or recommended; it is an ideal site for certain interventions, and the wrong setting for others. The school classroom is an optimum setting to identify children at risk for posttrauma stress reactions, to minimize the fear of recurrence and its continued interference with everyday activities or tasks, and to normalize the recovery process.

In the context of a classroom discussion, we use a drawing-and-story-telling technique (Nader & Pynoos, 1990) that allows us to identify traumatic imagery and avoidance and to introduce discussion of the spectrum of children's individual traumatic experiences. Children's spontaneous pictures vary from direct depictions of the traumatic event to peaceful scenes or abstract designs (e.g., a flower, balloons). Their stories often verify their sense of engagement with details of the event, their efforts at avoidance or omission, or their natural independence from what went on (Nader & Pynoos, 1990).

The classroom is also an excellent site for addressing issues of dying and loss (Pynoos & Nader, 1988a). In the classroom, we discuss death in age-appropriate themes and reinforce the physical reality of death through specific group enactment, drawing, or story-telling. As Furman (1973) suggested, grieving requires, even in the youngest children, an understanding of the physical reality of that particular death. The goal is, then, to provide concrete and symbolic representations of the finality of death. Playing out the funeral may be especially effective when the body is not recovered after a traumatic loss (e.g., after a plane crash into the ocean) or when children did not have the opportunity to attend. This exercise also permits the further identification of children's grief reactions. Children may reveal, for example, their disbelief, reunion fantasies, anger, emotional pain,

Table 46.2. Preventive Intervention Strategies

Symptomatic response/issue	First aid
Preschool through Grade 2	
1. Helplessness and passivity	1. Support, rest, comfort
2. Generalized fear	2. Protective shield
3. Cognitive confusion	3. Repeated clarifications
4. Difficulty identifying feelings	4. Emotional labels
5. Lack of verbalization	5. Help to verbalize
6. Reminders become magical	6. Demystification of reminders
7. Sleep disturbance	7. Telling parents/teachers
8. Anxious attachment	8. Consistent caretaking
9. Regressive symptoms	9. Time-limited regression
10. Anxieties about death	10. Explanations of death
Grades 3–5	
1. Responsibility and guilt	1. Expression of imaginings
2. Reminders trigger fears	2. Identification of reminders
3. Traumatic play and retelling	3. Listening with understanding
4. Fear of feelings	4. Supported expression
5. Concentration/learning	5. Telling adults
6. Sleep disturbance	6. Help to understand
7. Safety concerns	7. Realistic information
8. Changes in behavior	8. Challenge to impulse control
9. Somatic complaints	9. Link between sensations and event
10. Monitoring parents anxieties	10. Expression of concerns
11. Concern for others	11. Constructive activities
12. Disturbed by grief responses	12. Positive memories
Adolescents (Grades 6 and up)	
1. Detachment, shame, guilt	1. Discussion: Event, feelings, limitations
2. Self-consciousness	2. Adult nature of responses
3. Posttraumatic acting out	3. Link: Behavior and event
4. Life-threatening reenactment	4. Address: Impulse to recklessness
5. Abrupt shift in relationships	5. Understanding expectable strain
6. Desire for revenge	6. Address: Plans/consequences
7. Radical changes in attitude	7. Link: Changes and event
8. Premature entrance to adulthood	8. Postponing radical decisions

sadness, depression, restlessness, and/or separation anxiety (Pynoos & Nader, 1988a).

However, it is inappropriate to delve into certain highly emotionally charged issues in the classroom exercise. For example, children may illustrate in their picture a horrifying experience of mutilation or a grotesque death. Whereas in individual work, we would explore further these intrusive phenomena, in the classroom we would identify the child who needs individual attention, and then allow the child to draw a more pleasant second or third picture to bring proper closure in the classroom to this renewed anxiety or distress. Also, we do not engage children in their revenge fantasies in this group setting. There is neither the opportunity nor the privacy in which to explore the challenge to the child's own impulse control such fantasies evoke or their private meaning.

Third, in the current enthusiasm to engage children in classroom exercises after disasters or trauma, basic principles of trauma treatment are overlooked. For example, after the October, 1989, earthquake in Northern California, nearly every school engaged children in drawing or dramatizing the force of the earthquake, and, perhaps, their own fears. However, there is sound scientific research to suggest this is an inadequate step, at times, only renewing anxiety, without employing a second constructive, therapeutic step. In the Galente and Foa (1986) study of school interventions in the aftermath of an Italian earthquake, fear of recurrence and other anxieties did not diminish until the children, after demonstrating the destructive force of the earthquake, were then engaged in play to rebuild their villages and provide safer housing. After visualizing or drawing the damage, after a disaster or violence, the opportunity to depict repair is a necessary therapeutic step. Children have been visibly relieved, for example, after restoring in their drawings the physical integrity of an injured person.

Above all, classroom interventions are not a substitute for needed individual or family interventions. All too often, we have observed newly formed school psychological crisis teams carry out extensive on-site initial classroom exercises, offering global assistance to the whole school population, while the most severely affected children remain without further proper treatment. There is a recent interest in the vicarious anxiety experienced by less exposed children, but we hope this trend will not be at the expense of the difficult work of identifying the most exposed and at-risk children and providing them with the fullest attention.

In conducting initial parent's meetings, we have found it most productive first to elicit the parent's own reactions to the event, their own continued concerns and worries, and then to use their responses as a bridge to understanding the responses of their children. This process can also help to identify parents who have had previous traumatic or violent experiences, sometimes in their own childhood. These previous experiences may require special attention before the parents can be helpful to their own children.

Initial Assessment

Children who have been severely exposed to a life threat or who have witnessed injury or death may require individual intervention to avert serious psychiatric morbidity. Only preliminary investigations have been made regarding appropriate therapeutic techniques for children. In the acute aftermath, school-aged children and adolescents have participated in the same kind of clinical debriefing that has been a hallmark of adult trauma work. For adults or children, almost all therapeutic approaches to PTSD incorporate some review and reprocessing of the traumatic events. The emotional meaning, as well as the personal impact, is imbedded in the details of the experience and the therapist must be prepared to hear everything, however horrifying or sad. Special interview techniques may be necessary to assist children to explore thoroughly their subjective experiences and to help them understand the meaning of their responses (Pynoos & Eth, 1986). Encouraging children's expression through drawing, play, dramatization, and metaphor, the therapist attempts to understand the traumatic links and looks for ways to recruit children's fantasy and play actively into communication about their experience. The memory of young children may be especially improved when the original physical context is reinstated, so that going through the scene in drawing, dramatization, or even by *in vivo* return to the actual physical site can sometimes elicit important additional memories.

One treatment goal is to bolster children's observing ego and reality testing functions, thereby dispelling cognitive confusions and encouraging active coping. Children are assisted in identifying traumatic reminders that elicit intrusive imagery, intense affective responses, and psychophysiological reactions. A second goal is to help children to anticipate, understand, and manage everyday reminders, so that the intensity of these reminders and their ability to disrupt daily functioning recede over time. Enabling children to share these reminders with their parents increases the likelihood that they will receive essential parental support and understanding. Another goal is to assist the child in making distinctions among current trauma, ongoing life stresses and previous trauma, and to decrease the impact of the recent trauma on present experience. Helping children recover from the most immediate posttraumatic reactions may directly increase their ability to address the posttrauma changes in their lives.

It is expected and understandable that posttraumatic stress reactions will result from traumatic exposure. By using their authority, primary care professionals can legitimize children's feelings and reactions, and assist them in maintaining self-esteem. Children can also be prepared to anticipate and cope with the transient return of unresolved feelings over time. We will underscore several principles that are important in undertaking this kind of consultation. First, early access is imperative. As with investigators of adult posttraumatic stress disorders, we have found that the optimal time for intervention is in the acute period when intrusive phenomena and incident-specific traumatic reminders are most identifiable, and the associated affect is most available.

Second, the trauma consultation interview differs from the usual child psychotherapy session or initial interview in a number of ways. It has a stated focus. It takes longer than the usual time permitted for a single session; once begun, the therapist must permit sufficient time to explore thoroughly the child's experience. The therapist must remain alert to the tendency not to address central issues, for example, images of the mutilation or revenge fantasies; inadequate therapeutic attention often leads to observable limitations in affective recovery. Care must be taken to bring proper closure to the consultation interviews or the child may be left with renewed anxiety and an unnecessary traumatic avoidance of the therapeutic situation itself. Above all, the clinician must recognize that, in addition to providing immediate therapeutic intervention, he or she is also providing the child with a strategy of recall that may remain with the child. When assisted to go over the event in slow motion, children are able to fill in gaps, to correctly sequence events, to add details, to explore their emotional responses and their intervention fantasies (Pynoos & Nader, 1989a).

The following example is taken from a 90-minute initial interview with a child after a tornado hit her school, causing serious destruction, multiple injuries, and many deaths. It illustrates both the complexity of the child's traumatic experience and the intricacies of conducting even the first consultation interview.

She had been at the site of heaviest damage, and had her front tooth knocked out by a flying table. At first, she did not recall seeing the table coming toward her nor the moment when the table hit her face. In recreating the scene with toys, she initially focused on being trapped by debris and screaming for someone to free her and omitted any mention of her profuse bleeding. However, in her slow motion replaying of the scene, assisted by the clinician, she recalled seeing the legs of the table coming toward her, her ineffective attempt to duck, and, finally, the impact and the subsequent pain. In her drawing, she then placed the trajectile table many more feet away than it had been when first sighted. When the therapist commented on how much she must have wished it had been that far away so that she would have time safely to duck, the child strongly agreed, looked relieved, and became more animated. At the end of her consultation, she picked up this picture excitedly to show her mother, telling her how much she had wished the table had been that far away. The girl used the drawing to convey to her mother the terror of her experience and the subsequent relief provided by the consultation.

The child began by focusing on a true moment of fear—the desperate need for someone to rescue her, to remove her to safety away from any further life threat or injury. At first, she used this moment to screen her memory from the most horrifying moment of being hit by the table legs and the resulting profuse bleeding. After achieving this rescue in her imagination, thereby reaching a safe place in her mind, she then could approach the earlier moment of traumatic helplessness and injury. The therapist recognized the child's efforts to use denial in fantasy by spatially misrepresenting the event, and chose to address the child's superego condemnation for not being able to do more to protect herself (Grinker & Spiegel, 1943). The child visibly showed relief, more directly appreciated her own life threat, and, without less need to minimize the threat, expressed how strongly she wished it had not happened.

Her initial focus on the need to be rescued was also understood to refer to the consultation situation. The child demonstrated a fear of being affectively overwhelmed if she returned in her mind to the most terrifying moments. She wished the clinician would augment her traumatic avoidance by helping her to move her mind away from intrusive preoccupations. The therapist was able to communicate that she was available as an auxiliary ego to help the child approach the most threatening moments, and, suggested by her interventions, that working-through her subjective experience offered more emotional relief than did continued traumatic avoidance.

Brief Therapy

Although trauma debriefing and consultation will prove adequate for some children, many severely exposed and other at-risk children will require extended therapeutic interventions. The use of brief, focal, individual psychotherapy with traumatized children has several therapeutic goals: to counteract traumatic hindrances to normal functioning and development; to identify the child's ongoing processing of traumatic aspects of the event and its aftermath and to rework specific moments of the event; to address ongoing issues of helplessness, self-blame, and passivity; to enhance mastery of traumatic intrusive phenomena; to monitor reactions to anticipated and unexpected traumatic reminders; to address the disregulation of aggression; to explore the interaction between select existing intrapsychic conflicts or the emerging personality and specific features of the trauma; to restore the capacity for normal play; and to address secondary stresses subsequent to the trauma.

Because a traumatic experience may involve many complex traumatic moments, even within a short period of time, brief treatment often requires several months and may extend beyond the first anniversary of the event. Brief therapy allows the exploration of changes in emphasis or in meaning of the multiple significant moments of the event. It permits a contextual understanding of the trauma within the life situation and culture of the child and the family. The clinician must attend to the impact on the child's phase-specific narcissistic vulnerabilities, psychosexual issues, and cognitive maturity in monitoring disturbances in the child's normal developmental progression.

Traumatic experiences often lead to a cascade of changes in the child's life situation, thereby making additional demands on the child's inner resources. Injured children must contend with the stress of medical hospitalization or procedures, and reintegration into their classroom and peer group. Often there are changes in life circumstances, such as relocation, school changes, loss of peers, separation, new responsibilities that are due to death, changes in the intrafamilial matrix that are due to grief, traumatic anxiety in other family members, resultant changes in parenting, change in guardianship, and involvement in ongoing criminal procedures. Furthermore, there are changes related to traumatic symptoms, such as disturbances in peer relationships, school performance, and self-esteem. The clinician must remain attentive to all these subsequent changes and their appearance in the child's mental activity, to continue to be active with family, school, medical, and judicial systems, and to be prepared to assist children and their families constructively to improvise in their practical responses.

Close communication with the family permits an ongoing awareness of the frequency, content, and reaction to traumatic reminders. With therapeutic assistance, children, too, become less afraid to register these reactions and their source, and, over the course of treatment, gain an understanding that allows them to manage even unexpected future reminders. Attention to these reminders may elicit cognitive and affective associations to previously unprocessed portions of the experience.

During brief therapy, a child may continue a particular aspect of the trauma in play until further resolution or may move to some other aspect and incorporate other relevant issues. At different times, different distressing moments or affects may be emphasized. Repetitions of the same play may occur with slight changes over time to incorporate various aspects of the traumatic event. Another child in the tornado incident described seeing the window blown out, turning to run, being grabbed by her friend, and being pinned with her badly injured foot under a table. In the initial session, she focused on her fear, the horror of her own injury and, most importantly, on seeing her friend covered with blood and struggling to breathe. She minimized her reactions to her friend's having held her from running from the scene. In a later session, she approached her conflict over her friend's action, including anger toward her friend and a wish still to have her as a best friend. At first, the child had been irritable and angry with her mother, perhaps as a safe displacement, but after this session, the aggression toward her mother dissipated and the girl seemed more at ease with herself.

At times, the clinician will notice that certain details are omitted repeatedly. Omitted details often represent a child's most disturbing appraisals of a life threat. After a natural disaster, for example, many children continued in their play not to use the siren when an ambulance took injured children to the hospital. The siren had remained a distressing traumatic reminder, and many of them had had subsequent exaggerated startles to loud noises, especially sirens. But more than that, hearing the sirens had indicated to these school-aged children the seriousness and medical urgency of what happened, and, they were afraid to be overwhelmed affectively once more by their fear, helplessness, and terror if they recreated this sound in their play. We pay special attention to omissions, spatial misrepresentations, and altered focus that indicate a suppression of normal fears. As Rachman (1980) discussed, this affective suppression increases the risk of incomplete emotional processing.

One may also observe a transition from overt intrusive images to their incorporation in play. This may be especially true for vivid images of irreversible damage, for example, of the sight of injury or profuse bleeding, especially since children may assess the seriousness of the damage by the amount of blood (Pynoos & Nader, 1989a). For example, a young boy was preoccupied with the sight of the blood surrounding his murdered father. A few months later, he drew, on a coloring book a depiction of a picnic basket, a catsup bottle that had spilled making a pool of red similar to that surrounding his father. In addition to the continuing intrusiveness of the blood, this image represented the child's wish that it had been fake blood and that his father was still alive.

As the child continues to rework the traumatic experience, there is often a progression toward the most terrifying and irreversibly damaging moments. While standing in his front doorway, a 7-year-old boy was wounded in an exchange of gunfire by gang members. Gun pellets lodged in his brain, chest, abdomen, and legs and he lost vision in one eye. During the hospitalization, he feared the assailants would again attack him, and was wary of unfamiliar hospital personnel. After leaving the hospital, he alternately avoided the front doorway and played in session at opening and closing it. Over time, he began to play at throwing things fast and catching them. When the therapist suggested that this play might be related to the shooting in some way, the boy responded, "Yeah, like catching the bullet." Thus, he began his intervention fantasy with stopping the bullet before it struck him. The therapist replied, "Yes, I bet you wish you could have stopped the bullet; it must have been frightening to be hit by a bullet." This exchange represented a crucial phase in the treatment, a prelude to his addressing the most horrifying moment of being hit by the pellets and a terrifying sense of damage. He then adopted a more active role in fantasy at apprehending the assailants and seeking justice. At one point, he played at disguising himself as a detective in order to go out and find the assailants and inform the police. In addressing his need to provide himself a protective disguise, one could approach his underlying sense of danger, his smallness and sense of ineffectualness, and his visual disability. The clinician also ad-

dressed his ongoing wish to put the threat to rest and to take revenge without fear of retaliation.

In subsequent sessions, the boy addressed more directly his sense of narcissistic injury and the permanent loss of his vision in one eye. In the later phases of treatment, when unusual efforts to be a good boy were therapeutically addressed, the child revealed a hidden thought that only bad people get shot. If he could be a totally good boy, he would never again be hurt. He was interpreting his experience through his own emerging superego, and, secondarily, seeking control over external dangers by providing himself a way to prevent future harm. The boy had initially been withdrawn and afraid of being rejected by his peers. The brief therapy and a tailored classroom intervention enabled him to reestablish his friendships.

Certain moments of the traumatic experience may evoke dominant conflicts related to maternal care and parental protection. A fifth-grade child was taken hostage in her classroom by a woman who then shot herself in front of the children. The extremely nervous woman had agitatedly waved the guns at the children and the teacher. The child described moments of intense crying and worry that the woman would shoot the teacher. Subsequently, she became extremely and persistently clinging to her mother and complained of her mother's neglect. Toward the end of the year-long brief therapy, the therapist, the child, and the mother gained a new understanding of the meaning of this worry and the related behavior. At the age of 6 months, after her father had left the family, she became similarly clinging and frightened in the absence of her mother. As this issue was explored further, the girl began to tell her mother, "I am almost a teenager. I want to spend time with my friends. I don't want to be with you all the time"; she exhibited more normal early teenage behavior. Both mother and child recognized that the vulnerabilities from her early life were not fully resolved, but to a significant degree had been disentangled from her traumatic responses.

Trauma and Grief

If the violence or disaster has resulted in the death of a family member or friend, there is an important interplay between the traumatic and grief reactions. Posttraumatic stress reactions keep the minds of children focused on the circumstances of the death, and, in doing so, interfere with the ego resources and full attention needed to address the loss and to adapt to subsequent life changes. Children seem particularly vulnerable to the dual demands of trauma mastery and grief work. Efforts at relieving traumatic anxiety appear to take psychological priority over mourning. For example, one child found his murdered father's body soon after he was shot. The picture of his bleeding wound remained intrusive and interfered with efforts to elicit more positive memories. In play, he acted out his reparative fantasy of taking his father to the hospital where surgery would save him (the extracted bullet is kept for evidence). In imagining the restored, uninjured image of his father, he expressed intense sadness over the poignant wish that his father could once again hug him.

Extended Treatment and Interpretation

Over the course of extended treatment, we are less likely to encourage specific forms of play or drawing and more likely to look for the deeper themes of children's spontaneous play and communication. The skill or art is judging when, how, and if to interpret some portion of the children's play, behavior, or verbal response in terms of specific aspects of their traumatic experience. Children may simply stop their play or conversation if interpretation occurs before they have finished authoring their fantasy. We suggest placing primary attention on the child's fantasies of intervention as both an expression of wished for action and as a means of mitigating the pain or managing the affect. This therapeutic attention serves as an intermediary step: (1) the child's animated efforts underscore both to the child and therapist the close association between the experienced external and internal dangers; (2) it places emphasis on the operations of intrapsychic defenses rather than their outcome (Horowitz and Kaltreider, 1979); and (3) it reduces the therapeutic tension between directly linking a child's productions to the trauma or interpreting within the metaphor of his play, behavior, and words.

Psychopharmacology and Arousal Behavior

If increased arousal behavior leads to direct functional impairment (e.g., reduced attention and learning because of sleep disturbance), or to altered self-concept and personality (e.g., secondary to hypervigilance and exaggerated startle), then modifying arousal behavior can be an important aspect of an overall treatment plan. Early alleviation of these symptoms may decrease chronicity and the number of secondary consequences of these symptoms, especially in highly exposed children.

We are entering into a new era of psychopharmacology where the pharmacologic agent, dosage, and method of monitoring efficacy will be directed at select, neurophysiological effect. This goal is especially important in the treatment of children and adolescents because the decision to use medications must always be done with caution and concern for the functional consequences of side effects (e.g., sedation) and any secondary impact on other neurophysiological functions, including normal growth and development. Animal laboratory experimentation has elucidated the neurophysiology of the fear-enhanced startle pathway and the pharmacological effects of various agents (Davis, 1986). Whereas different agents, such as tricyclic antidepressants, propranolol, clonidine, and other antianxiolytic agents have been reported to attenuate arousal and other PTSD symptoms in adults, each of these agents actually has different effects on brainstem mechanisms (Krystal et al., 1989). For example, antidepressants do not reduce fear-enhanced startle, whereas the other agents do; however, clonidine also reduces baseline startle and is most potent at eliminating fear-enhanced exaggerated startle. At UCLA, we have preliminary data to suggest clonidine may reduce the persistent arousal behavior in children exposed to gunfire incidents, especially the sleep disturbance and exaggerated startle behavior. A recent report has also described the use of propranolol in treating the arousal symptoms in children who were exposed to sexual assault (Famularo, Kinscherff, & Fenton, 1988).

Family Intervention

The family provides the key site for reinstating a sense of safety and security. Research studies as well as children's self-reports often attribute improvement to the supportive behaviors of family and friends (Lystad, 1984). All family therapy must recognize the evolving interpersonal matrix of the family that includes the current developmental phase of each family member as well as the developmental phase of the family as a whole (Brown, 1980). It has been our observation that the most common overlooked adverse influence on this interpersonal matrix is the variability in psychological agendas among family members. Differences in exposure may create different psychological challenges for each member. The mutual lack of appreciation of these may lead to estrangement or impatience between parent and child, or between siblings. These different psychological demands may require different time courses, leading to disharmonious offers and need of support. In this situation, it is easy for children's special needs to be overlooked. A primary goal of family therapy after trauma is to help family members validate and legitimize each others psychological challenge and working-through, thereby facilitating continued mutual support.

The goals for family intervention to assist the child are: (1) to restore in children a sense of personal security; (2) to validate their affective responses rather than dismiss them; (3) to anticipate and respond to situations in which they will need added emotional support, especially in managing traumatic reminders or in handling feelings of vulnerability; and (4) to assist the family in minimizing secondary stresses and adversities.

Before they can effectively help the children, family members often need support and guidance, and sometimes need therapeutic intervention to reduce their own levels of stress and renewed reactions from other prior experiences. Parenting skills can be enhanced if parents can be educated regarding posttraumatic stress reactions (Nader & Pynoos, 1990), realistic expectations about the course of recovery, differing psychological agendas among family members, and the importance of encouraging open communication with their children, not just in the immediate aftermath, but in the months ahead when anniversary or other traumatic reminders may stimulate recollections.

Group Intervention

The small group can be an important therapeutic agent during the immediate weeks or months after violence or disaster (Yule, 1989). It offers the opportunity to reinforce the normative nature of the children's reactions and recovery, to share mutual concerns and traumatic reminders, to address common fears and avoidant behavior, to increase tolerance for disturbing affects, to provide early attention to depressive reactions, and to aid recovery through age-appropriate and situation-specific problem-solving. Groups may become an especially valuable tool in the treatment of adolescents traumatized in a group setting by permitting the working-through of any temporary disturbance in peer relationships. When there has been a peer death related to the trauma, group therapy can take on an added importance for those close acquaintances. It provides an ongoing setting to normalize grief responses, provides additional emotional support and a reserved time for reworking the loss, permits professionally assisted shared reminiscing, and reinforces efforts toward recovery.

Pulsed Intervention

Before proceeding to the topic of long-term treatment, we offer for consideration an additional intervention strategy. Similar to the Wallerstein (1990) proposed treatment for children of divorce, we suggest that a pulsed intervention model may sometimes be most applicable. In such a strategy, an acute phase of treatment is followed by planned periods of consultation in accord with the time trajectory of trauma recovery and ongoing development. This model rests on the knowledge both of what is psychologically most challenging about the trauma at changing developmental phases and of the maturing capacity for an adaptive response at different intervals over the years. The major preventive goal of this strategy is to maintain normal developmental progress. The clinician would then see the child at certain critical junctures, decided on through ongoing communication with the family and the child, by anticipated reminders and normal developmental challenges.

Long-Term Therapy

As treatment is extended from an initial consultation either to brief or to long-term psychotherapy, there is the opportunity to understand the effects of cognitive, affective, and intrapsychic maturation on the child's reprocessing of the trauma and its impact. It allows for exploring the deeper ramifications of the meaning of the event in the child's ongoing life. As the clinician increases the frequency of sessions, there is more opportunity to explore and interpret the psychodynamic attributions.

Maturation as well as experiential growth often lead, not simply to a reworking, but to new reappraisals and evolving psychological challenges. Revised intrapsychic conflicts and narcissistic accommodations may result. Freud (1939/1968) observed that, over time, traumatic responses may be less visible as symptoms and may silently become embedded in a child's ego functioning, thereby playing a significant role in shaping character. Greenacre (1952) noted that these changes and corresponding defects in the sense of self may then leave children vulnerable to future life stresses. Therefore, there is the added goal in long-term psychotherapy or analysis of exploring traumatic influences on the child's emerging character formation.

Indications

There are a number of indications for extended therapy that may be identified during the initial consultations; others may require careful monitoring of children's ongoing development. The intensity, duration, and personal impact of the trauma may prolong the time needed to reprocess their traumatic experience. This may occur, for example, when there is massive violence, with multiple deaths, injury, and loss of family members

or friends, or multiple assaults on the child within a prolonged episode. If there has been concomitant life threat or injury and loss, the dual demands of trauma and bereavement often require more extended treatment.

There may be child-intrinsic or extrinsic factors that suggest strong adverse influences on recovery. Some of these are generic to child psychiatry; for example, preexisting psychopathology in the child or in the child's parents or guardians, or parental discord. Furthermore, there may be extrinsic factors, secondary to the trauma, that can be anticipated to prolong the course; for example, continued participation in criminal proceedings or further need for medical procedures because of trauma-related injuries. Also, any series of posttrauma adversities increases the risk of depression and reduces the child's available inner resources.

We call special attention to two additional factors. One, if there is a previous history of trauma, including chronic or repetitive trauma, then the likely oscillations between past and present experiences, diminished ego resources, and ongoing vulnerabilities, usually require lengthening the treatment duration. Two, when there is intrafamilial violence, especially murder and suicide, especially if the child has been a witness, long-term treatment is usually indicated. The treatment must address the preexisting relationship with the perpetrator and the deceased or injured, complicated issues of identification, intense conflicts of loyalty, issues related to loss, and, often, preexisting vulnerabilities arising from a chronic impulse-ridden environment.

Select Long-Term Issues

We will address only some of the specific features of long-term treatment with children and adolescents who were exposed to violent trauma and disasters. Many of the techniques and goals do not differ from the principles of child psychotherapy or psychoanalysis (Pearson, 1968; Ruben, 1974). However, recognition that the emotional meaning is often embedded in the details of the traumatic experience remains a constant feature of this therapeutic work.

As ego functions mature, in cognition, language, and affective tolerance, prior action memories may become more understandable (Furman, 1973). A 3-year-old boy had watched as his mother's boyfriend chased and shot her. The boyfriend then held a gun inside the boy's mouth but decided to spare him. For the first year, no one knew what he had experienced, until at age 4 he began running up and down the house (like in a chase) telling what had happened. He had often demonstrated a behavioral sequence where he would first make a pulling motion with his fingers over his head, second, open his mouth widely, and, third, become aggressive with his peers. Over a number of sessions, the clinician observed how the boy would engage in this pulling motion whenever he tried to evoke a good picture of his mother with her "beautiful curly hair." In response to therapeutic attention to this pattern, he detailed how his mother's hair had become matted with blood after the shooting. In his efforts to evoke positive memories of his mother, he strove to restore the image of her physical integrity and to counter her marred internal representation.

The content of intervention fantasies may progress with increasing cognitive maturity. One boy, at five years of age, witnessed the shooting assassination of his father from the passenger seat of their truck. In his reworking of the event in his play, he had at first played at ducking in the truck. He built fortresses in the playroom and, at home, maintained an area of his bedroom where he could quickly take cover. Two years later, when he was responding to an unexpected traumatic reminder, he returned to this theme, but now played at putting playdough on the windows in order to bulletproof them. Further along in the treatment, his case illustrated how changes in play may represent secondary exposures, new information, or additional details of the event. It took nearly 3 years before the assailants were brought to trial. During the trial, it was revealed that the boy's house had been under surveillance and the assailants had originally planned to kill the whole family. He responded in session by playing, for the first time, at fighting off armed invaders who entered his home.

We have treated a number of children who have endured witnessing the murder-suicide of their parents. In every case, the children had been exposed to prior violence or abuse and the erratic behavior of a disturbed parent, for example, who suffered from untreated manic-depressive disorder. Furthermore, after the deaths, they have often had to contend with intrafamilial arguments over guardianship, and radical, sometimes frequent, changes in their life situations and in parenting. We have observed a consistent pattern in their long-term psychotherapy. During the initial months, even years, of psychotherapy, the child may remain focused on the murder and loss of the murdered parent. It is often only much later that the child addresses the deep conflict over the parent's suicidal behavior.

Pruett (1984), who provided a rich psychoanalytically informed longitudinal description of two children's responses to the murder of their mother and attempted suicide by their father, ended his account 3½ years later, when, the clinical vignettes would indicate to us, the boy was beginning to manifest conscious thoughts of and conflicts over identification with his father's suicidal behavior. In this case, as we have also observed, there were renewed symptoms, not only in aggressive behavior but also depression, that prompted renewed psychiatric referral.

In addition, other family members may remain preoccupied with issues of identifying a particular child with the murderous or suicidal parent, by appearance, sex, temperament, or behavior. For example, after a father murdered his spouse and then committed suicide, the grandmother caretaker responded to every aggressive act of her young grandson as a frightening indicator that he might grow up to become a murderer as well. His physical appearance also reminded the grandmother of the now hated son-in-law. Her reactions continued to place the young child under the shadow of his father and impeded his own difficult efforts to address his conflicted memories of his father and to struggle with his own emerging self-concept. Finally, the long-term intrapsychic legacy of a murder-suicide may have relevant gender differences. For example, a sister may evidence ongoing psychosexual disturbances owing to attributions of a mother's sexual behavior as instigating a father's murderous behavior, whereas a brother may manifest an unresolved struggle to avoid identification with the father's aggression and to evade his own fantasized masculine culpability.

We have also followed a number of cases where a child has accidentally shot a family member or friend. For example, a 9-year-old boy accidentally shot his brother while playing with a gun he thought he had previously emptied. The bullet struck an artery, and he could not stop the bleeding. The long-term treatment revealed complicated themes of his aggressive fantasies toward his brother, anger at the mother for not stopping the dangerous play, oscillating with transference wishes to elicit her protection against his own dangerous impulses, continuously revised restitution fantasies both to undo the harm and to ease his pain, ongoing reunion fantasies with his brother, and manifestations of self-inflicted punishment. More than the outward stigma, he struggled to contend with the intrapsychic legacy of killing his brother.

One major area of longitudinal concern is the disregulation of aggression or impaired development of conscience that can accompany the exposure to violent trauma. We have observed that children acutely, after violence, usually exhibit a flexibility in identificatory roles. They may vary, even within a single session, in their identification with the assailant, victim, and rescuer and may involve the therapist in any or all of these roles. Although Williams (1987) suggested that one set of children are totally involved with aggressive revenge fantasies and another set turn the aggression inward, we find that such predominance only occurs over time. In addition, character traits and career interest may also reflect a lifelong preoccupation with rescue or reparative roles. However, we think intrapsychic traces of all three pathways remain, and, indeed, early and extended treatment maintains a flexibility and opportunity for interpretative intervention that can preclude disturbances in aggression from becoming rigid before they can be properly worked-through.

When the trauma is violent and massive, there may be continued risk of life-threatening or violent behavior throughout adolescence. A major goal of therapy is to return the child to a normal developmental path with a maturing conscience, and, as a result, to help alleviate dangerous unconscious reenactment behavior. Unanswered intervention fantasies, especially unresolved revenge fantasies, can lead to marked changes in behavior and personality. A 12-year-old boy with no history of behavior problems was shot in both arms during the violent rampage of a sniper through a crowded fast-food restaurant. In addition, the boy witnessed the horrifying death of his best friend and that boy's mother, viewed horrendous mutilation of others, experienced the frightening storming of the restaurant by the SWAT team, and exited through pools of blood. Whenever someone mentioned his friend, he would close his eyes and gradually sink down, taking the position he had taken underneath the table in the restaurant during the massacre. Several hours, sometimes a day later, he would become aggressive, hitting, slugging, or kicking his mother or friends. He provoked his schoolmates into fights or became aggressive toward them. He took a knife into areas known to be frequented by armed youths. In his earliest fantasies of revenge, he imagined jumping up from under that table, and slugging the sniper senseless. As therapy progressed, his reenactment behavior become more restricted to the sessions, diminishing what had been quite dangerous outside behavior. In the second year in treatment, he took a toy gun out into a wooded area behind the therapy room and played at coming up from behind rocks and shooting men in army fatigues. He placed the therapist at the edge of the embattled territory, as if to temporarily park his more maturing superego off to the side and to employ a neutral observer while he engaged in his dramatization. After he had completed his play, he permitted the therapist to speak and responded with superego relief at understanding his desire to be the one with the gun who surprises the enemy instead of the other way around. He was then able to explore his frightening original assumption that the SWAT team (whose army boots, which were similar to those worn by the assailant, were all that he could see from his prostrated position) were there to complete the massacre, and of his continued distrust of the police and of his own internal policing functions. There were many similar dramatizations in which he worked through multiple moments of his experience and engaged in countless efforts to address his traumatic helplessness. He slowly demonstrated a maturing of his impulse control and adolescent conscience.

The violent experience also stimulated intense and prolonged psychosexual disturbance as the boy entered adolescence. There were pretrauma influences that arose out of his early childhood and parental divorce, however, the current violent trend had origins within his terrible sense of being emasculated by his experience of the massacre. He had witnessed his best friend's mother die from a single bullet wound, while her husband survived multiple gunshots. He had also viewed shotgun mutilation to another woman's breast. The experience of lying helpless on the floor during the rampage took on a vulnerable, repulsive, passive, feminine attribution. During the course of treatment, he gave a female doll his hairstyle and dressed it in a jacket with the name of a punk rock group, "Dead Kennedys," written on the sleeve just as he wore. He then bashed, hung, burned, and beat the doll. Although he attempted repeatedly to reverse his helplessness through identification with the aggressor, this too only increased his sexual conflicts, as "macho" behavior with its sexual characteristics took on a murderous meaning. His revenge fantasies then included firing at the sniper repeatedly, both shooting his eyes out, in retaliation for his own observational insult, and shooting point blank at his genitalia. It required a few years of interpretive work before he consolidated a more unperturbed masculine identity.

His treatment also illustrated that as therapy progresses other life issues may emerge. As his ego reconstituted from the traumatic experience, he began to address the psychological impact of his parents' divorce and his conflicts over their respective remarriages and his new stepparents.

There may also be a direct interplay of traumatic elements and ongoing intrafamilial conflict. On her birthday, a 6-year-old girl's father and a maternal relative became involved in a fight over whose day it was to have the child. She saw her father kicked repeatedly and stabbed in the leg with a knife. This child's course was complicated by the intense custody battle between her parents which had precipitated the knifing by the mother's cousin. Initially, she created only accidents or natural disasters in her therapeutic play. The key transition step occurred when she shifted responsibility to human inflicted injury. The child could then be seen to oscillate between the violent incident, the parental fighting, and her own punitive self-image. At different moments, she used attention to the traumatic details to avoid the chronic conflict and at times vice versa.

In situations of chronic or repetitive trauma, because of physical or sexual abuse, usually there are still singular traumatic incidents that require special attention. These unique experiences may hold such psychological priority in the child's mind that by addressing them in a timely fashion a therapeutic alliance is formed, and the subsequent treatment is facilitated. Furthermore, suicidal, self-mutilating, sexual, or aggressive behavior or play of physically or sexually abused children may incorporate traumatic reenactment, identifications or self-blame, which diminish with proper exploration and interpretation. Addressing isolated traumatic experiences often restores sufficient ego functioning so that children are then able to address the less overt, yet substantial influences of a disturbed environment or parental dysfunction.

The school remains an important source for monitoring the long-term impact. Because childhood trauma may lead to increased concretization, one may observe reduced symbolic usage or precocious trauma-related knowledge. Adolescents, especially, may experience a developmental risk in increasing symbolic usage because the enhanced associative capacity may actually lead to a wider spectrum of traumatic reminders. Symbolic thought may evoke intense traumatic emotion with the renewed fear of being affectively overwhelmed. For example, when asked to assess the court system in civics class, one girl whose father's murderers were on trial had to leave the classroom. One teenager, who was the only survivor after she and her family were kidnapped and robbed, burst into tears when she was asked, in religion class, to discuss a Biblical passage on love. One of the goals of long-term treatment is to repair the ability to symbolize and to enable the use of symbolic expression relatively free of impingement from traumatic meaning. Long-term treatment permits continued exploration of the various meanings of the child's overly concretized mental representations and gives the most opportunity to expand the child's symbolic usage and limit any activities (Ruben, 1974).

Conclusion

Anna Freud (1966) argued that the fate of traumatic anxiety in childhood is determined by the degree that adults induce children of even the tenderest years to devote all their efforts to assimilating the reality, however painful and disagreeable. She warned that the fate of the child's ego lies in the balance. Reworking is a complicated task with children because of their facility for dealing in imagination, play, and fantasy, their evolving development, and the reappraisals that accompany experiential growth and cognitive maturity. If a traumatic experience requires integration into a new inner model of the world (Horowitz & Zilberg, 1983), then the challenge for children is twofold, since their inner model of the world is already under constant revision. We hope that our discussion of select therapeutic issues will enhance the interests of other researchers to continue to investigate this important topic.

References

Bergen, M. (1958). Effect of severe trauma on a 4-year-old child. *Psychoanalytic Study of the Child, 31*, 3–32.

Brown, S. L. (1980). Developmental cycle of family: Clinical implications. *Psychiatric Clinics of North America, 3*, 369–381.

Burt, C. (1943). War neuroses in British children. *Nervous Child, 2*, 324–337.

Davis, M. (1986). Pharmacological and anatomical analysis of fear conditioning using the fear-potentiated startle paradigm. *Behavioral Neuroscience, 100*, 814–824.

Famularo, R., Kinscherff, R., & Fenton, T. (1988). Propranolol treatment for children with acute post-traumatic stress disorder. *American Journal on the Diseases of Children. 142*, 1244–1247.

Freud, A. (1936). *The ego and the mechanisms of defence.* London: Hogarth Press.

Freud, A. (1966). Comments on psychic trauma. In *The writings of Anna Freud* (pp. 221–241). New York: International Universities Press.

Freud, S. (1968). Beyond the pleasure principle. In J. Strachey (Ed. and Trans.), *The standard edition of the complete psychological works of Sigmund Freud* (Vol. 18, pp. 7–64). London: Hogarth Press. (Original work published 1920)

Freud, S. (1968). Inhibitions, symptoms and anxiety. In J. Strachey (Ed. and Trans.), *The standard edition of the complete psychological works of Sigmund Freud* (Vol. 20 ,pp. 77–174). London: Hogarth Press. (Original work published 1926)

Freud, S. (1968). Moses and monotheism. In J. Strachey (Ed. and Trans.), *The standard edition of the complete psychological works of Sigmund Freud* (Vol. 23, pp. 3–137). London: Hogarth Press. (Original work published 1939)

Friedman, P., & Linn, I. (1957). Some psychiatric notes on the Andrea Doria disaster. *American Journal of Psychiatry, 114*, 426–432.

Furman, R. A. (1973). A child's capacity for mourning. In Anthony, E. J., & Koupernik, C. (Eds.). *The child in his family: The impact of disease and death* (pp. 225–231). New York: Wiley.

Galente, R., & Foa, D. (1986). An epidemiological study of psychic trauma and treatment effectiveness for children after a natural disaster. *Journal of the American Academy of Child and Adolescent Psychiatry, 25*, 3357–3363.

Greenacre, P. (1952). *Trauma, growth and personality.* New York: International Universities Press.

Grinker, R. R., & Spiegel, J. P. (1943). *War neuroses in North Africa: The Tunisian campaign.* New York: Josiah Macy, Jr., Foundation.

Hoffman, M. L. (1979). Development of moral thought, feeling, and behavior. *American Psychologist, 34*, 358–388.

Horowitz, M. J., Kaltreider N. B. (1979). Brief therapy of the stress response syndrome. *Psychiatric Clinics of North America 2*(2), 365–377.

Horowitz, M. J., & Zilberg, N. (1983). Regressive alterations of the self concept. *American Journal of Psychiatry, 1940*(3), 284–289.

Johnson, M. K., & Foley, M. A. (1984). Differentiating fact from fantasy: The reliability of children's memory. *Journal of Social Issues, 40*, 33–50.

Krystal, J., Kosten, T., Perry, B., Southwick, S., Mason, J. W., & Giller, E. L. (1989). Neurobiological aspects of PTSD: Review of clinical and preclinical studies. *Behavioral Therapy, 20*(2), 177193.

Lazarus, R. S. (1966). *Psychological stress and the coping process.* New York: McGraw-Hill.

Lifton, R. J. (1979). *The broken connection.* New York: Simon & Schuster.

Lystad, M. (1984). Children's response to disaster: Family implications. *International Journal of Family Psychiatry, 5*, 41–60.

Nader K., & Pynoos, R. S. (1990). Drawing and play in the diagnosis and assessment of childhood post-traumatic stress syndromes. In C. Schaeffer (Ed.), *Play, diagnosis and assessment* (pp. 375–389). New York: Wiley.

Pearson, G. H. (1968). *Handbook of child psychoanalysis.* New York: Basic Books.

Piaget, J., & Inhelder, B. (1969). *The Psychology of the Child.* New York: Basic Books.

Pruett, K. (1984). A chronology of defensive adaptations to severe psychological trauma. *Psychoanalytic Study of the Child, 39*, 591–612.

Pynoos, R. S. (1990). PTSD in children and adolescents. In B. D. Garfinkle, G. A. Carlson, & E. B. Weller (Eds.), *Psychiatric disorders in children and adolescents* (pp. 48–63). New York: W. B. Saunders.

Pynoos, R., & Eth, S. (1986). Witness to violence: The child interview. *Journal of the American Academy of Child Psychiatry, 25*(3), 306–319.

Pynoos, R., Frederick, C., Nader, K., Arroyo, W., Steinberg, A., Eth, S., Nunez, F., & Fairbanks, L. (1987). Life threat and post-traumatic stress in school-age children. *Archives of General Psychiatry, 44*, 1057–1063.

Pynoos, R., & Nader, K. (1988a). Psychological first aid and treatment approach for children exposed to community violence: Research implications. *Journal of Traumatic Stress, 1*, 445473.

Pynoos, R. S., & Nader, K. (1988b). Children who witness the sexual assaults of their mothers. *Journal of the American Academy of Child and Adolescent Psychiatry, 27*, 567572.

Pynoos, R. S., & Nader, K. (1989a). Children's memory and proximity to violence. *Journal of the American Academy of Child and Adolescent Psychiatry, 28*, 236241.

Pynoos, R. S., & Nader, K. (1989b). Prevention of psychiatric morbidity in children after disaster. In D. Shaffer, I. Philips, & N. Enzer (Eds.), *Prevention of mental disorders, alcohol and other drug use in children and adolescents* (225–271) (OSAP Prevention Monograph-2). Rockville, MD: U.S. Department of Health and Human Services.

Rachman, S. (1980). Emotional processing. *Behavior Research and Therapy, 18*, 51–60.

Ruben, M. (1974). Trauma in the light of clinical experience. *Psychoanalytic Study of the Child, 29*, 369–387.

Rutter, M. (1985). Resilience in the face of adversity. *British Journal of Psychiatry, 147*, 598–611.

Saigh, P. A. (1986). In vitro flooding in the treatment of a 6-year-old boy's post-traumatic stress disorder. *Behavioral Research Therapy, 24*(6), 685–688.

Sandler, J. (1967). Trauma, strain, and development. In S. Furst (Ed.), *Psychic Trauma*. New York: Basic Books.

Solnit, A. J. (1987). A psychoanalytic view of play. *Psychoanalytic Study of the Child, 42,* 205–219.

Terr, L. (1979). Children of Chowchilla: Study of psychic trauma. *Psychoanalytic Study of the Child, 34,* 547–623.

Terr, L. (1981). Forbidden games: Post-traumatic child's play. *Journal of the American Academy of Child and Adolescent Psychiatry, 20,* 741–760.

Wallerstein, J. S. (1990). Preventive interventions with divorcing families: A reconceptualization. In S. E. Goldston, J. Yager, C. Heinicke, & R. S. Pynoos (Eds.), *Preventing mental health disturbances in childhood* (pp. 154–174). Washington, DC: American Psychiatric Press.

Williams, W. (1987). Reconstruction of an early seduction and its aftereffects. *Journal of the American Psychoanalytic Association, 35,* 145–163.

Winnicot, D. W. (1971). *Therapeutic consultations in child psychiatry*. New York: Basic Books.

Yule, W. (1989). The effects of disasters on children. *Association for Child Psychiatry and Psychiatry Newsletter, 11*(6), 3–6.

CHAPTER 47

Father Kills Mother

Effects on the Children in the United Kingdom

Dora Black, Tony Kaplan, and Jean Harris Hendriks

Introduction

CASE 1

The night before his seventh birthday, William and his sister Anna, aged three, were put to bed as usual by their mother. Their parents were living apart and their mother was seeking a divorce. On the birthday morning, the children were awakened by their father who told them that their mother had left them and would not be coming back. He took the children to his parents' home for that day and afterward cared for them until he was arrested some days later for the alleged murder of their mother. He had buried her body on wasteland.

The children lived briefly with maternal grandparents who were in poor health and then with distant relatives of their mother. The children, by then in state care, were referred to a department of child psychiatry for an opinion, one year after the murder, as to where they should live and whether they should visit their father in prison.

CASE 2

Thomas, aged 20 months, was found by police crying in his cot, wet, smelly, and hungry. Downstairs was the body of his mother, killed by strangulation. The police had broken into the house at the request of relatives and the estranged father of the child who was charged with the murder of his common-law wife. It is not known whether this child was placed in the cot by his mother or by his father after the killing, nor is it known what he saw or heard. It was calculated that he had been alone for 10 hours after the mother's death. He was referred for as-

sessment of a persistent disorder of conduct at the age of 3 years, having been placed with relatives of his father. The arrangement was being challenged by the mother's relatives.

Children whose fathers kill their mothers are orphaned by this act. Not only are they deprived of their mother by the catastrophe of her death, but their father is now suddenly absent, locked up in jail or in a mental hospital, on "the run," or dead by his own hand. These children are the children of women who die a violent death and they are the children of the killer.

For child psychiatric teams, these are difficult cases. For individual workers, there will be little experience of dealing with such children, their families, and their networks.

Prevalence of Homicide among Marital Partners

In England and Wales, although there are likely to be 40 to 50 families each year where the father kills the mother, there is no direct way of calculating this figure, since there are no formal records kept on the children. What records do exist are not coded in a way that enables identification retrospectively. The prison service, the probation service, and the Department of Health do not keep records of the children of convicted killers. Death records of individuals contain no information about their children. The figure of 40 to 50 families affected per year was calculated on the basis that, in England and Wales alone, there are on average 500 to 600 cases of homicide per year, and of these 20% will be of a man killing his wife or cohabitee; 40% of these women will be in their child-bearing years (Home Office, 1984). In the United States, the homicide rate and the propor-

Dora Black, Tony Kaplan, and Jean Harris Hendriks • Department of Child and Adolescent Psychiatry, Royal Free Hospital, Pond Street, London NW3, England.

tion of homicides that are "wife murder" are both higher than in the United Kingdom (Pynoos & Eth, 1985), and even in the United States information is scarce. In reviewing the literature, other than our 1988 paper (Black & Kaplan, 1988), we could find only three English-language papers that dealt specifically with this subject. These papers are case studies in relation to one or two cases only (Isaacs & Hickman, 1987; Pruett, 1979; Schetky, 1978). Pynoos (Pynoos & Eth, 1985) and Malmquist (1986) have written on their work with children who have witnessed extreme violence which includes children who have seen their father kill their mother.

Sample for the Present Study

Since we made known our interest and in response to a pilot questionnaire we developed, we now have information on 46 such cases involving 95 children. Some of these children we have seen personally; on others we have information from the questionnaire only. The sample consists of 49 girls and 46 boys, who were between 8 months and 15 years in age at the time of the killing. The time of referral after the death ranges from within 24 hours to 19 years. Twenty-one children (10 cases) were referred to a child psychiatrist within 1 month, 41 children (25 cases) were referred later than 1 year, and 33 children (11 cases) form an intermediate group referred between 1 month and 1 year. This range reflects the differing reasons for referral, some being referred for crisis intervention, bereavement counseling, or psychotherapy, and some being referred for advice on placement, custody, and access issues. Some requests were for the formal preparation of expert evidence to be presented in civil legal proceedings.

Limitations to the Method

Clearly, this sample is a heterogeneous group. There are children with different backgrounds, histories, and circumstances surrounding the killing of their mother by their father. Limitations in the questionnaire emerged: The questionnaire was completed in some cases by the referrer and in some cases by the assessing clinician, and completed at different intervals after the killing. Some symptom categories are bound to be noticed earlier (e.g., posttraumatic stress disorder [PTSD]), some may emerge only later (e.g., conduct disorder). Some were referred after interventions and some before them. In most cases, we have no data on the children from before the killing of their mother, so it is not possible to say with any degree of certainty which problems emerged as a result of the killing nor how preexisting problems may have been influenced. Standardization and definitions of terms in the questionnaire are inadequate. However, our experience has left us with strong impressions about the particular difficulties for these children, their caretakers, and the involved professionals, impressions which we are able to consolidate in some cases with data from the questionnaire survey. Thus, in organizing the clinical data, the chapter is structured in three parts: (1)

the framework for assessment, (2) identifying psychiatric disorder, and (3) principles for practice.

Framework for Assessment

Posttraumatic Stress Disorder and Crisis Intervention

CASE 1

David, aged 3, was seen at the home of his maternal aunt two days after his father had shot his mother and then turned the gun on himself. David was now 200 miles from his home. He was continually drowsy by day, reluctant to be roused. At night he screamed, refusing to go to bed.

Given the violence these children witness, it is likely that many will develop posttraumatic stress disorder (American Psychiatric Association, 1987). In our sample, 44% of the children had witnessed the killing or had heard it taking place. Posttraumatic stress disorder was only diagnosed in 25% of all cases. This percentage is likely to be *underestimated* because (1) there were many late referrals, and PTSD was not recorded in any of these; and (2) in all cases evaluated by nonpsychiatrists PTSD was not diagnosed, a fact which probably reflects lack of familiarity with the diagnostic category.

Among the most comprehensive and systematic descriptions of PTSD in children is that of Pynoos (Pynoos, Frederick, & Nader, 1987) in relation to exposure to violence (see Chapter 46, in this volume, for a review). There have been two subsequent reviews of PTSD in children in disasters (Lyons, 1987; Sugar, 1989).

The experience of Pynoos and his colleagues (Pynoos, 1986; Pynoos & Eth, 1986) and Ayalon (1983) is that crisis intervention limits the severity of posttraumatic stress symptoms. In essence, this approach depends on helping the child to recount the traumatic events and his or her feelings and integrate them as fully as possible. Pynoos (1986) developed a semistructured interview technique for intervention. He emphasized the need to intervene rapidly since memories of the events are progressively lost to recall and maladaptive responses may become entrenched. This brief intensive form of intervention does not preclude the possibility, in the longer term, of bereavement counseling and psychotherapy. In the present study, crisis intervention had been made (or was to be made) in only 21% of our sample.

Bereavement-Related Problems

Children have an increased rate of pathological grief reactions when compared to adults (Bowlby, 1980; Raphael, 1983). When father kills mother, the children's losses are particularly difficult to cope with, being sudden, simultaneous, and multiple, including the loss of both parents, their familiar home environment, and, in some cases, even friends, school, and neighborhood. In those children suffering from a PTSD, normal grieving may be inhibited (Pynoos & Nader, 1988). Other factors may inhibit the development of normal mourning. The child may feel compelled to remain silent because of shame or because he or she may wish to protect others from the intense feelings of horror, rage, sadness, and powerlessness which the story may provoke. This suppression is particularly likely if the carers are kin, since they will be more emotionally affected by the child's harrowing account.

They may say, as did the relatives of Thomas (Case 2), that the child was too young to be affected by his mother's death and that it was kinder not to tell him that his father was in prison. Relatives of older children, whose tragedies may have been local causes célèbres will insist, in the teeth of probability, that the children know nothing. Children usually know more than adults think they do.

CASE 4

Six-year-old Harry was referred with his two older siblings by social services for advice about access to his father. Harry was invited to draw a picture (see Figure 47.1). We were told by his uncle and aunt, with whom he had lived since his mother was killed, that Harry did not know how his mother had died or where his father was located. Harry's picture indicated that he knew (and maybe witnessed) that his father had hit his mother with a hatchet, and that his father was in prison. It shows his reluctance to leave his own house for his uncle's (he

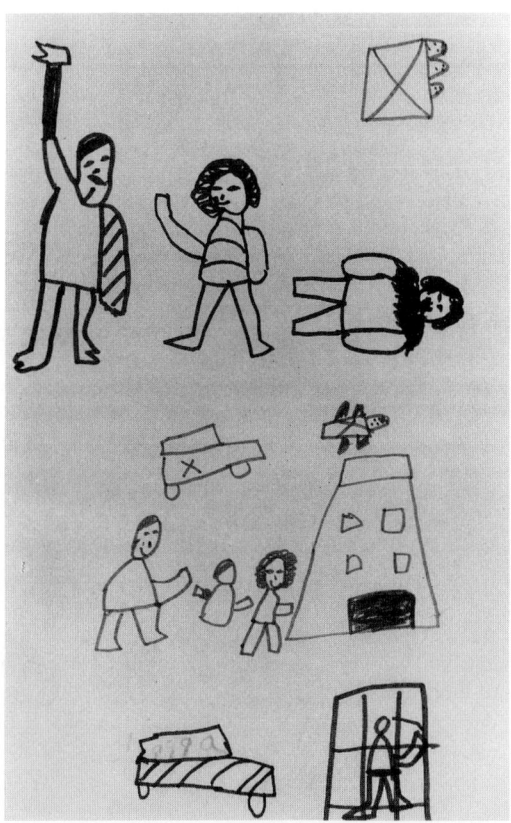

Figure 47.1. Projections of trauma in children's drawings.

has no legs and no face in the drawing of his going to his uncle's house with its coffin-shaped door), and it indicates that he would like to visit his father in jail.

Children then collude with this silence, absorbing the message that this subject is not to be talked about, so that no one can estimate their knowledge. Relatives (as opposed to nonrelated carers) will decide more often not to tell the children of the true nature of their mother's death, or disguise or distort the truth. Of the children who were not told, 70% were living with kin. Without this knowledge, the children will have difficulty in making sense of their changed circumstances and the reactions of those around them and may not be able to mourn their losses effectively.

What to tell the children and how to tell them will depend on their age and understanding. Our practice is to help the carers find the right way for them to tell the children, to make this matter an open one for discussion in the home so that they become more available to support the child.

Inquiry should be made about religious and secular ceremonies subsequent to the death and as to whether the children were included. Did they see their mother's body, attend the funeral, or visit her grave? (If a body is not released for burial, different additional traumas may ensue.) Information should be sought regarding counseling that was made available to children and caretakers at the time of the tragedy. The family's financial status should also be investigated. Also, there may be serious disputes about religious ceremonies and about possessions, money and the disposal of the family home. These conflicts exacerbate the children's difficulties and may contribute to placement breakdown. Such children, behaving as though a storm is raging over their heads, may show prolongation of the detachment and constriction of affect characteristic of PTSD. The children's "goodness" and compliance bring relief to caretakers who may reinforce such responses.

Another complication contributing to difficulty in mourning may be that, with their mother dead and their father in jail, in hospital, or dead, the children may be the only source of information regarding their history, their family, and their social network. They may be too young or too shocked, especially early on, to give a useful account. This may amplify their sense of dislocation. Construction of a "life-story book" (Ryan & Walker, 1985) and visits to home and neighborhood have proved useful in relieving the sense of rootlessness and alienation, and inquiries about these concrete ways of helping the child cope with bereavement should form part of the assessment, especially in cases referred late.

Identifying Psychiatric Disorder

Our questionnaire responders were asked to record whether the children had other problems to be categorized, such as conduct problems, emotional problems, learning problems, difficulties in relating to peers and/or adults, and psychosexual problems. It must be stressed that these represent descriptive categories only. Even with PTSD excluded, half of the children were recorded as positive on 3 or more of the 7 problem categories with only 1 in 10 recorded as having no symptoms at all (see Table 47.1). The children who seemed to have been least disturbed were girls placed with mother's kin where mother and father had previously separated and father had infrequent contact with the child.

Emotional Problems

Of the children who were recorded, 70% were rated as having emotional problems (see Table 47.2). Boys aged 6 to 11, who were placed with other than kin, who missed their fathers or were ambivalent about access, and who had been exposed to previous violence, were the children most likely to develop emotional problems.

Behavioral Problems

Of the children who were rated, 44% had behavioral problems and of these, 70% were boys (see Table 47.3). Age did not appear to be a significant determinant. Also, 87% had witnessed previous violence in the home, although 54% of those who had been exposed to previous violence were not rated as having a behavioral problem. Thus, if they were rated as having a behavioral problem, they were likely to have been exposed to violence, but such exposure by itself did not predict behavioral problems. Of the children with behavioral problems, 70% were not living with kin. Thus, boys not staying with kin, who were exposed to previous violence, are the children most likely to be rated as having a behavioral problem.

Placement

Half the sample had been placed with kin, half with nonrelatives, and, where the referrer cited placement problems, placement in either category was equally likely. The advantages and disadvantages of such placements (already discussed) ought to be, but usually are not, weighed up at the time of crisis.

There may be a presumption that because of their familiarity, relatives are best able to support children at this time. However, bereaved relatives are preoccupied with their own emotional turmoil, and may be emotionally unavailable to the children. A mother's relatives may wish to discourage access of the children to their father, and indeed, 83% of children placed with the mother's relatives were said not to want access and, in most cases, had not seen their fathers since the killing. Conversely, children staying with paternal relatives were said to want access in 100% of the cases. Thus, the relationship that children can have with their father after the killing of their mother is much influenced by placement. Brinich (1989) showed that when relatives become parents by default, because of the death of a parent, usually by violence (as in murder, manslaughter, and suicide), the dynamics of the relationship are often different from voluntary assumption of parenthood. Parents by default both overprotect and subtly reject their foster child and we, too, have found this a common pattern in our studies.

A father's relatives may seek to justify his action and may do so at the expense of the children's mother (e.g., she may be blamed for provoking the father's assault). We found this to be common. If the father receives a short sentence (and most of these men were found guilty of manslaughter rather than murder), his relatives, if they have custody of the children, may have in mind to keep the children only until the father can resume custody. Such children may not be encouraged to form any reliable attachments to caretakers, yet the disadvantages of open-ended, uncertain, unplanned, substitute care are well documented (Harris, 1985).

CASE 5

Charles, aged 12, full of guilt at his mother's death, which he felt he could have prevented had he only awakened at the right time, lived briefly with a recently married sister and then with short-term foster parents. No permanent plans were made for him. Charles lost contact with his mother's relatives when they disapproved of his frequent visits to his father. The father, now released from prison, wished to resume care of Charles, who had developed a severe tic. Having avoided all discussion of his mother's death, he now began to blame her for provoking it and to justify his father's action in killing her.

Although children placed with kin were often less symptomatic than children not so placed, our impression was that where problems did arise, relatives were more resistant to change and to recognition of distress. Many of the children placed with nonrelatives were there because, as with Charles, a placement with kin had failed.

Custody

Data recorded prior to 1988 indicate that most referred children had no formal arrangements, remained in the custody of their father, or were subject to care orders of the local authority. Usually, recent referrals have been wards of the court (see the section on Legal Issues).

Access

Of the total sample of the children, 71% had seen their father after the killing but in only 43% of the cases was access regular. The group was subdivided into those

Table 47.1. Problem Category at Referral ($N = 50$)[a]

Problem	Percentage of referrals
PTSD	26
Bereavement problems	48
Emotional problems	70
Conduct problems	44
Learning difficulties	48
Difficulties in relating to peers	38
Difficulties in relating to adults	38
Psychosexual difficulties	14

[a]Most children had more than one problem.

Table 47.2. Emotional Problems (Rated More Than 6 Months after Death of Mother)[a]

	Percentage with emotional problems	Percentage of sample overall
Witnessed previous violence	78 ($N = 19$)	60
Witnessed killing of mother	39 ($N = 18$)	38
Placed with kin	42 ($N = 19$)	47
Sex		
Boys	58 ($N = 19$)	48
Girls	42 ($N = 19$)	52
Age		
0–5	32	44
6–11	58	46
12 or over	10	10

[a]Most children had more than one problem.

requesting and those refusing access. Of those refusing access, 77% had been exposed to previous violence and 64% had witnessed the death of their mother (a significantly larger percentage than in the group as a whole). Of those wanting access, more than half (56%) had not seen their father killing their mother. Two thirds (67%) *had* witnessed previous violence in their homes but at least half of those children were living with their father's kin, and encouragement and support from relatives for them to visit their father in prison may have counteracted the off-putting effect of previous exposure to violence seen in the group not wanting access.

Many referrers asked for an opinion about the access of children to their fathers. Our principle was that access was a right of the child and that the issue was most clear-cut when children refused access, had a clear understanding of their mother's death, and could explain their refusal. Such wishes should be respected but where, for example, younger children lacked linguistic skills, we considered the same principle should also apply. Children who wished to see their parent should be enabled to do so. In some circumstances, we recommended planned and supervised access with careful preparation. For example, where children feared that their father was dead or regarded him as a vengeful or terrifying figure, access might help them to perceive him as a comprehensible human being. Access may be of particular importance where the father has been the primary caretaker.

We were asked to comment on the frequency of access. This must be related to such practical issues as

distance from the prison or hospital, the views of caretakers, and the availability of social workers as well as to the wishes of the children and the purpose of the meetings.

CASE 6

John (6) and Andrew (5) were referred by social services for advice about whether they should attend their mother's funeral and visit their father in prison. Their father had killed his wife and dismembered her. The children were now living with relatives who believed they were unaware of the dismemberment. At our first consultation, however, John drew a "ghost" which consisted of a disembodied leg and two eyes, perhaps letting us know that he had seen his mother's mutilated body, which we knew had been recovered except for one leg.

Following a visit to their father in prison, John asked one of us (Dora Black) to draw an outline around his body when he lay down on a large piece of paper, following which he tore it in half. He had spoken about the visit and how he had the same name as his father. It seemed that he was showing us the conflict he felt about his identity—the father half and the mother half were unable to be united because of the father's action. After the visit, John was able to talk for the first time about his father. The father had apologized for depriving them of their mother. He had been helped to do so by his probation officer. Andrew had said, "What's the use of apologizing—she's dead." He had dared to face his father and repudiate him instead of fearing him. Further-

Table 47.3. Exposure to Violence and Killing in the Home

	Percentage of children with behavioral problems	Percentage of children in sample as a whole
Witnessed previous violence in home	87 ($N = 23$)	60
Witnessed killing of mother	32 ($N = 22$)	38
Living with kin	30 ($N = 23$)	47
Sex		
Boys	70 ($N = 38$)	48
Girls	30 ($N = 38$)	52

more, these children, too, were violent and difficult to contain in their therapy session, so much so that the therapist was in actual danger.

Legal Issues

In the United Kingdom, children may become wards of court (a modern version of *parens patriae*): All matters relating to their welfare, such as where they live, whom they may visit, and how they are educated, must be reviewed by a judge of the High Court, and the children's interests are paramount. Their financial affairs may be managed by an officer of the court. Where children are unable to live with relatives, care may be shared between caretakers and the state. Some children in the sample were in foster care, while custody remained with the father.

If a parent or guardian is considered to be abusing or neglecting a boy, for example, placing him at risk or failing to plan for him, the boy may be made subject to a Care Order in a lower court or in the course of the matrimonial proceedings his custody may pass to a designated local authority. The balance of probabilities must be that, unless such an order be made, the boy will not receive the care and control of which he is in need. Foster parents do not have the legal rights of guardians, since custody remains with the natural parent, a court, or a local authority. Only after adoption do substitute parents acquire full parental rights with respect to a child.

Thus, legal arrangements made on behalf of a child have a considerable effect on his well-being. Only if he is a ward of court, or if care proceedings are in process but incomplete, does he have a right to personal legal representation and the opportunity for a court official to make independent enquiry into his best interests.

Children as Witnesses

In our experience, it is unusual for children who have witnessed homicide to be asked to give evidence in a criminal trial for homicide. The capacity of children to give truthful evidence has been discussed in relation to sexual abuse rather than to homicide (see Jones & McQuiston, 1989, for a review of this issue) but the principles apply to other presentation of evidence by legal minors. Pynoos (1984; Pynoos & Nader, 1988) review this issue in detail.

Long-Term Psychiatric Sequelae: Prolonged Factors

It is likely that untreated PTSD results in long-term problems. We have clinical examples of placements in which compliant children with constricted affect have been greeted with relief by troubled caretakers, a situation likely to lead to psychiatric disorders at a later time.

As expected, behavioral problems are more common in boys and have a poorer outcome (Robins, 1966).

They may be exacerbated and prolonged where boys identify or are identified with the violent father (see a similar discussion in Chapter 53, in this volume).

Depression in later life may be a sequel to this form of parental loss since Harris, Brown, and Bifulco (1986) found that the death of the mother was more often associated with poor subsequent child care, and this was the main predictor of adult depressive disorder.

We have encountered vengeful, murderous fantasies in both boys and girls and these, in general, are not communicated to caretakers or teachers. We do not know whether such fantasies lead to acting out in later life, but they are common themes in PTSD (Horowitz, 1986). In our experience, these children often have difficulty in establishing and sustaining reliable substitute affectional bonds, even when, as is not commonly the case, they are rapidly and securely available to them.

We have met sibling groups who are closely mutually attached, to the point of enmeshment, but lack affectional bonds with adult caretakers. These children demand attention yet remain distant, polite, and uninvolved with the adults closest to them.

In summary, we postulate increased risk for depressive illness and personality disorders in adult life. Longitudinal follow-up will be highly difficult given the understandable wish for privacy of many children and their families.

Direct Work with Children: Therapeutic Considerations

These traumatized children have lost their caretakers, not because of a shared fate (a plane crash, for example, might be seen as uniting lost parents in death) but because one has destroyed the other. Children may cope by regarding one parent as good, the other as bad. Sometimes there is a split within a sibship, with further family breakdown (Case 5).

Individual or group therapy is a demanding task, resources are limited, and criteria for selection are insufficiently defined. Therapeutic intervention, however, may be economical and effective.

Rebecca, aged 3 years, had seen her father cut her mother's throat. The child's clothes and bare legs were bloodstained. An older child ran for help and did not witness the killing. The younger described feeling paralyzed and unable to leave the house in her bare feet. She developed asthma which disappeared subsequent to interventions by her psychotherapist who began therapy 1 year after the killing. For example, a drawing of a woman whose face and nose, painted in red, smeared and ran over the figure's dress, was accompanied by comments on "dirty water" and marked wheezing. The therapist linked the drawing and the wheezing with the child's experience of her mother's death (the noise of the intake of air through the blood of a cut throat sounding like the wheezing of asthma). These issues are represented in Figure 47.2. Following intervention, Rebecca ceased wheezing.

Having worked through the fear and excitement of his father's coming out of prison, James's therapist noted: "James, aged 6, painted half a rainbow and showed it to me saying 'It's just half, the other half is

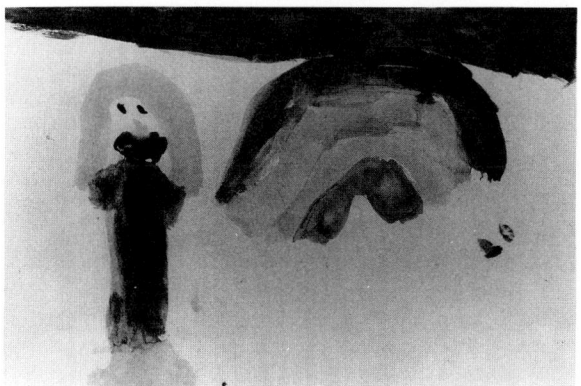

Figure 47.2. A child's depiction of the mother covered in blood.

here,' and he gestured to the imaginary half of the rainbow which would join up to his. I said, 'This is like you; the lovely other half of you is missing.' He said, 'I see Mummy's face very clearly. I can see her.' I said I thought he might see his mother's face in his mind often. He said, 'I do.'"

A sibship of four children, alienated from both families of origin and from their caretakers, were seen as a sibling group. They joined forces to attack their male and female therapists, but split by gender themselves, with the older girls terrorizing and bullying the younger boys. All four children behaved in a destructive and manically angry manner.

Therapy in this case was handicapped by the children's perception that it was offered in a hospital unit where a psychiatrist had written a court report expressing concerns about their foster home (an emergency arrangement that had drifted into being a long-term arrangement, although the foster parents were overburdened and their own children's needs underestimated). The foster children had been immensely powerful in their neediness and their demand to stay where they were and resented the hospital report on the disadvantages of the arrangement. Thus, therapy was offered in what to them was a hostile environment.

Then, though this difficulty was addressed in therapy, the foster parents requested its termination. The children at home and at school were so compliant that no further difficulties were envisaged by their caretakers. The children themselves appeared terrified by their rage, which was demonstrated only in therapy, and also asked not to keep further appointments.

Work with Carers

When caretakers hear the stories of what children have seen and experienced, it is not surprising that they have difficulty in hearing the children, let alone encouraging them to talk. We take the view that it is of fundamental importance to help carers support these children who are disclosing terrible events and being encouraged to open up in therapy. Therefore, a necessary part of psychotherapy is to work in parallel with carers. This includes helping carers to get a sense of the manic rep-

aration they may wish to make, to understand the projections they may experience from the children, especially revenge fantasies which may make the children feel implacably hostile to the father and perhaps to parents in general, yet impotent and inadequate (children may suffer from the feeling that they did not take the right action to save their mother).

Therapy may range from crisis intervention related to PTSD, primary prevention of psychiatric disorder (e.g., by offering bereavement counseling, advice to caretakers, family therapy) to secondary interventions which may include as appropriate the full range of treatments relevant to psychiatric disorder in childhood and adolescence.

Principles for Practice

Immediate Care

1. The children require a *safe place*, preferably with friends or family well known to them, but emergency state provision may be necessary. Caretakers will need immediate advice and support.

2. The children *require emergency decisions about legal custody* and may require independent legal representation and advocacy. Preferably, the state should act as parent to the children while plans are made for them.

3. Primary health care services should be alerted about the children and *early consultations sought from child mental health services* with particular reference to assessment of PTSD and the need for crisis intervention or other treatment. Expert advice should be sought regarding the planning of access to key relatives.

Planning for the Future

1. Such planning should not be delayed pending the outcome of criminal proceedings concerning the father. The emergency placements should not become permanent by default. Children should be freed for adoption (Adcock & White, 1984) if they would be grown by the time father is released or if they are too young to have a memory or any relationship with the father or for other reasons such as his likely incapacity to care for them after release, or their continuing hostility toward him.

2. With regard to access to the father and other key relatives, the guiding principle should be that this is the right of the child.

3. Therapeutic help should be offered as needed by child mental health services that are convenient to the child in his family setting.

Research Implications for the Future

1. There is need for cross-sectional population studies of all cases arising *de novo* within defined communities. Routine immediate referral to child mental health services will allow more focused assessment of PTSD and sustained, systematic assessment of the need for forensic and therapeutic interventions.

2. Longitudinal studies will present great difficulties but are necessary for the testing of hypotheses regarding risk of psychiatric sequelae in adult life.

3. There are ethical and practical difficulties with regard to the evaluation of therapeutic interventions (see Anthony, 1986, for a discussion of these issues). Controlled studies are not achievable for such events as violent murder which are rare, sudden, and unpredictable. Families in crisis require whatever help is available and may not readily or ethically be allocated randomly to alternative treatments.

4. These crises require, as do other emergencies concerning children, a coherent body of law, a flexible, readily available system of judicial hearings, and a recording of decisions in such a way that they may be subjected to rigorous retrospective evaluation.

Summary and Conclusions

Children whose fathers kill their mothers are likely to suffer from PTSD, particularly if they witness the killing. They need urgent crisis intervention with skilled help to uncover what they experienced in order to minimize the risk of disorder in the future. Grieving cannot begin until this work is done, and they may also need bereavement counseling. Their status must be safeguarded by wardship or care proceedings. Careful consideration should be given to where they should live, bearing in mind the difficulties in the role of parents by default. Since it is likely that the children will benefit by psychotherapy, and relatives on the whole find it more difficult to support therapy than unrelated foster parents, children should not drift into unsuitable long-term relationships in the absence of proper planning. Visiting father, at least once, in prison may "cut him down to size" and reduce fear.

In therapy, psychosomatic symptoms may relate to traumatic experiences and they may be resolved when these are linked by the therapist. To be the son of a killer makes for male *identity problems*, which need patient and prolonged exploration. Violent behavior in the therapy room can be difficult to contain and presumably represents an identification with the killer and the acting out of revenge fantasies (Miller, personal communication). We advise that if siblings are to be treated as a group, that there are always be two therapists working together. Miller points out in her work with similar sibling groups, the importance of not getting caught up in punitive zeal and manic reparation which may prevent the therapist from exercising sensitivity to the children's communications. Our impression is that few of the 95 children we studied have had the opportunity of receiving any therapeutic intervention. The awesome horror inspired in professionals and caretakers by the suffering of the children provokes a defensive denial that there could be a problem needing treatment. Our recommendation is that all children, where a parent dies at the hand of the other, should receive an immediate and skilled evaluation by an experienced consultant child psychiatrist or psychologist who can make recommendations about the child care and protection issues, the crisis intervention, the bereavement counseling and

therapy needs, and who can arrange for the necessary treatment, for supervision and support of the therapists and social workers, and appear in court as an expert witness as necessary (Black, Wolkind, & Harris Hendriks, 1991).

ACKNOWLEDGMENTS

The therapists who contributed case material are Ricky Emanuel, Judith Bevan, and Anita Colloms (Department of Child and Adolescent Psychiatry, Royal Free Hospital, London). We are also grateful to the *British Journal of Psychiatry* for permission to quote from our paper (Black & Kaplan, 1988).

References

Adcock, M., & White, R. (1984). Freeing for adoption. *Adoption and Fostering, 8*(2), 11–17.

American Psychiatric Association. (1987). *Diagnostic and statistical manual of mental disorders* (3rd ed., rev.). Washington DC: Author.

Anthony, E. J. (1986). Children's reactions to severe stress. *Journal of the American Academy of Child Psychiatry, 25*(3), 299–305.

Ayalon, O. (1983). Coping with terrorism. In D. Meichenbaum & M. Jaremko (Eds.), *Stress reduction and prevention* (pp. 293–339). New York: Plenum Press.

Black, D., & Kaplan, T. (1988). Father kills mother. *British Journal of Psychiatry, 153,* 624–630.

Black, D., & Urbanowicz, M. A. (1984). Bereaved children: Family Intervention. In J. E. Stevenson (Ed.), *Recent research in developmental psychopathology* (pp. 179–187). Oxford, England: Pergamon Press.

Black, D., Wolkind, S., & Harris Hendriks, J. (Eds.). (1991, 2d ed.). *Child psychiatry and the law.* London: Royal College of Psychiatrists, Gaskell Press.

Bowlby, J. (1980). *Attachment and loss, Vol. 3. Loss: Sadness and depression.* London: Hogarth Press.

Brinich, P. M. (1989). Love and anger in relatives who 'adopt' orphaned children: Parents by default. *Bereavement Care, 8*(2), 14–16.

Harris, J. (1985). *The outcome of adoption in taking a stand.* London: British Agencies for Adoption and Fostering.

Harris, J., Brown, G. W., & Bifulco, A. (1986). Loss of parent in childhood and adult psychiatric disorder: The role of lack of adequate parental care. *Psychological Medicine, 6*(84), 641–659.

Home Office. (1984). *Criminal statistics, England and Wales.* London: Her Majesty's Stationary Office.

Horowitz, M. J. (1986). *Stress response syndromes.* Northvale, NJ: Jason Aronson.

Isaacs, S., & Hickman, S. (1987, April). Double loss. *Community Care, 16,* 22–24.

Jones, D., & McQuiston, M. (1989). *Interviewing the sexually abused child.* London: Royal College of Psychiatrists, Gaskell Press.

Lyons, J. A. (1987). Post-traumatic stress disorder in children and adolescents: A review of the literature. *Journal of Development and Behavioral Pediatrics, 8*(6), 349–356.

Malmquist, C. (1986). Children who witness parental murder: Post-traumatic aspects. *Journal of the American Academy of Child Psychiatry, 25*(3), 320–325.

Miller, S. (1989, March). Personal communication.

Pruett, D. (1979). Home treatment of two infants who witnessed their mother's murder. *Journal of the American Academy of Child Psychiatry*, 647–657.

Pynoos, R. S. (1984). The child as witness to homicide. *Journal of Social Issues*, 40(2), 87–108.

Pynoos, R. S. (1986). Witness to violence: The child interview. *Journal of American Academy of Child Psychiatry*, 25(3), 306–319.

Pynoos, R. S., & Eth, S. (1985). Children traumatized by witnessing acts of personal violence. In S. Eth & R. S. Pynoos (Eds.), *Post traumatic stress disorder in children* (pp. 19–43). New York: American Psychiatric Press.

Pynoos, R. S., & Eth, S. (1986). Witnessing violence: Special interventions with children. In M. Lystad (Ed.), *The violent home* (pp. 193–216). New York: Brunner/Mazel.

Pynoos, R. S., Frederick, C., & Nader, K. (1987). Life threat and post-traumatic stress in school age children. *Archives of General Psychiatry*, 44, 1057–1063.

Pynoos, R. S., & Nader, K. (1988). Psychological first aid and treatment approaches to children exposed to community violence: Research implications. *Journal of Traumatic Stress*, 1(4), 445–473.

Raphael, B. (1983). *The anatomy of bereavement*. New York: Basic Books.

Robins, L. (1966). *Deviant child grown up*. Baltimore: Williams & Wilkins.

Ryan, T., & Walker, R. (1985). *Making life story books*. London: British Agencies for Adoption and Fostering.

Schetky, D. H. (1978). Preschoolers' response to murder of their mothers by their fathers: A study of four cases. *Bulletin of the American Academy of Psychiatry and the Law*, 6, 45–47.

Sugar, M. (1989). Children in disaster: An overview. *Child Psychiatry and Development*, 19(3), 163–179.

CHAPTER 48

Responses of Children and Adolescents to Disaster

Rob Gordon and Ruth Wraith

Introduction

The amnesia of childhood and even adolescence is such a veil that adults must resort to clinical experience and research to reconstruct the impact of trauma in early life. But both child and adolescent lack the perspective to follow the intricate repercussions of trauma as it unfolds in their being. After 7 years of clinical work with families in natural and man-made disasters, preceded by a further 7 years of hospital work, it is time to present our observations of responses to trauma.

Over 100 disaster-affected families have been seen in short- and long-term contexts, including bushfire, massacre, hostage, and plane crash disasters, as well as individual traumata involving murder, physical and sexual abuse, and transport accidents. Although aspects of this work have been reported elsewhere (Gordon, 1986, 1987, 1989a,b; Gordon & Wraith, 1987, 1988, 1991; Wraith, 1987, 1988a,b; Wraith & Gordon, 1987a,b), detailed findings on the nature of children's and adolescents' responses have not been reported. In this chapter, the term *children* also covers adolescents for the sake of brevity.

The Literature

Children's responses to disaster have only been reported in detail in the last 10 years, and the literature is sparse compared to that for adults. Ahearn and Cohen (1983) cited 25 child references out of 297 entries in their disasters and mental health bibliography. Yet the importance of children is indicated by the fact that in one Ash Wednesday (1983) bushfire-affected municipality in Australia, two thirds of the population were either children, parents, grandparents, or other caretakers concerned in their recovery.

Early work reported responses in the first weeks or months of the recovery period (Bloch, Silber, & Perry, 1956; Burke, Borus, Millstein, & Beasley, 1982; Farberow & Gordon, 1981). Longer term reactions were reported in case studies (Newman, 1976; Terr, 1979). Recent reviews (Anthony, 1986; Pynoos, 1989; Raphael, 1986; Terr, 1985, 1987), describe increasing interest in children and unique characteristics of their posttraumatic responses in relation to development. A body of knowledge now exists describing their reaction to disaster, and popular myths are being identified (Terr, 1987; Wraith & Gordon, 1987b).

Myths

Contrary to common opinion, children are not more flexible than adults because of their age and do not easily "forget" bad experiences (Terr, 1983a), although they cease to speak about them in deference to the wishes and expectations of adults (Kinzie, Sack, Angell, Manson, & Rath, 1986). If they do not show disturbance in the immediate posttrauma period, they may still demonstrate later problems (McFarlane, 1987; Terr, 1979); they do not get over trauma quickly though they may resume aspects of normal functioning; nor do they "grow out" of problems. Talking about traumata and reactions does not create problems where there were none (Galante & Foa, 1986). These misconceptions have been encountered in disaster-affected communities, disaster managers, health, education and welfare workers, and even adult- and child-trained mental health professionals.

Rob Gordon • Department of Psychology, Royal Children's Hospital, Melbourne, Parkville, Victoria 3052, Australia.
Ruth Wraith • Department of Child Psychotherapy, Royal Children's Hospital, Melbourne, Parkville, Victoria 3052, Australia.
International Handbook of Traumatic Stress Syndromes, edited by John P. Wilson and Beverley Raphael. Plenum Press, New York, 1993.

Our experience coincides with Gubrich-Simitis (1981), Burke *et al.* (1982), Rosenheck (1986), Kinzie *et al.* (1986), Handford *et al.* (1986), and Earls, Smith, Reich, and Jung (1988) that children often suffer much more than parents and other adults think, and, if anything, collude with adults' wishes to minimize needs rather than exaggerate them (Titchener & Kapp, 1976). We also observed children who were indirectly involved, such as siblings, school fellows, or neighbors, developing post-traumatic disorders. Terr (1987) mentioned this as "vicarious trauma" and Anthony (1986) referred to it as a process of "contagion."

Prevalence

Large-scale epidemiological studies are few (see Galante & Foa, 1986), but available evidence supports our observation that posttraumatic sequelae are prevalent among affected children when a long-term perspective is taken. All 25 children involved in a school-bus kidnapping exhibited symptoms 4 years after the event (Terr, 1983a). Fifty percent of 40 Cambodian adolescent refugees suffered posttraumatic stress disorder (PTSD) 4 years after leaving their country (Kinzie *et al.*, 1986). Twenty-six percent of 35 children affected by the Three Mile Island nuclear accident exhibited personality change one and a half years later (Handford *et al.*, 1986). Because the traumata and degrees of exposure are so varied, generalizing from such data is more hazardous than in other areas of mental health; however, it can be safely said many traumatized children suffer some sort of disorder in the long-term.

Vulnerability

Trauma breaches the psychic stimulus barrier (Freud, 1920/1968; Raphael, 1986; Terr, 1985) by overwhelming quantities of unorganized affect, perceptions, and cognitive demands. High physiological arousal may persist for long periods (Anthony, 1986; Pynoos, 1989; Wilson, 1989). Degrees of traumatization may involve differing mechanisms (Terr, 1983b). There are differences in the symptom patterns presented by children from adults (Terr, 1983a). Reactions are influenced by prior vulnerabilities or special needs (Burke *et al.*, 1982; McFarlane, 1987; Terr, 1983a), separation from family (Kinzie *et al.*, 1986), developmental level (Newman, 1976), reactions of parents and family members (Newman, 1976; Terr, 1987), extent of threat to one's own or loved one's life (Pynoos, 1989), meaning of the trauma in the child's life (Pynoos, 1989), gender with boys more vulnerable (Burke *et al.*, 1982), extent of exposure to trauma (Newman, 1976, though this was not found by Earls *et al.*, 1988, nor by Galante & Foa, 1986), preexisting family pathology (Terr, 1983a), and the degree of community bonding or disorganization (Galante & Foa, 1986; Milne, 1977; Terr, 1983a).

Yet it is unprofitable to account for posttraumatic sufferings of children in terms of predisposing or preexisting factors. As Raphael (1989) noted, it is quite clear that whatever the contribution to variance made by pre-

morbid variables, both clinically and empirically, it is the reaction to the severe trauma itself and its integration that are the most important factors. Terr (1987) was also uncompromising: "If the event they experience is sufficiently shocking and intense, no children can escape psychic trauma." Although family mental health influences the severity of the posttraumatic condition, she said "it will not make the qualitative determination as to whether symptoms will arise."

Symptoms

Symptoms reported are varied (Malmquist, 1986) and span the perceptual, affective, fantasy, cognitive, behavioral, and social life of the child. There is increasing evidence of long-term consequences of these phenomena (Raphael, 1986), evident 4 years after an event (Terr, 1983a), creating vulnerability to future stresses (Newman, 1976), and producing transgenerational effects (Bergman & Jucovy, 1982; Danieli, 1985; Rosenheck, 1986). Our observations concur with Handford *et al.* (1986) and Earls *et al.* (1988) on the disconnection between long-term sequelae and the original trauma. Of particular importance is the 6-month posttrauma period which we have found crucial for the presentation of difficulties as have Terr (1979), Sugar (1988), and McFarlane (1987). The understanding that disasters affect the communities in which they occur (Gordon, 1989a; Raphael, 1986) suggests effects may be wider than just to those directly exposed. There is also little information on how young children recover from trauma.

Resilience

Children's resilience needs to be acknowledged against this picture of vulnerability and long-term difficulty. Malmquist (1986) related recovery to the comforting role of internalized objects and successful resolution of past losses. Community bonds (Terr, 1983a), family support, early reestablishment of daily routines, and opportunities for structured group discussion of experiences (Galante & Foa, 1986) all aid recovery.

Characteristics of Psychic Trauma

Although a trauma is usually discrete, what traumatizes the child in the experience may not be obvious. If the responses are not related to the varied characteristics of psychic trauma, posttraumatic phenomena are misunderstood as preexisting problems, normal developmental issues, or unrelated difficulties. Experience shows trauma has a pervasive effect on the past, present, and future life of those it touches. Unless it is recognized and integrated, simple difficulties are compounded and complex disorders fail to respond. At least eight characteristics can be identified.

A trauma is *beyond normal experience*. It falls so far outside normal expectations that even if the subject responded appropriately in the moment, afterward past experience and problem-solving skills do not apply and accustomed boundaries between fact and fantasy are no longer reliable. A *massive quantity of emotion is generated*, including somatic responses that may be quite unfamiliar. Psychophysiological affects are a trauma in themselves if they have shocked or overwhelmed the child and altered perception, physiological functioning, and personal relationships. They must be contained before cognitive processing is commenced.

Trauma *violates normal psychological assumptions*. Norms, customs, values, habits, and regularities derived from experience ensure predictability and reduce the stress of moment-by-moment processing of experience enabling higher order processing to occur. They are especially important to give young children control over their environment. In violating these assumptions, trauma negates safety and security imposing the need to process all experience, leaving nothing to chance (compare the combat veteran's response to a slamming door). This restricts capacities for dealing with trauma sequelae. Trauma *ruptures expectations about the future*. Not only are they defied by the experience, but ruptured in the sense that any expectation is thrown into question and only reestablished by rehabilitation. This leads to profound uncertainty.

Children establish adaptations to the demands of life in most areas of normal functioning. There are compromise solutions to conflicts, personal deficits, and mismatches with the environment. Trauma *ruptures preexisting adaptations*, throwing them into question. It evokes issues for which no defenses are established (e.g., the homicidal rage of a child against the murderer of his stepfather), that disorganize and destabilize functioning with far-reaching consequences, demanding that earlier solutions be reworked. Trauma also *ruptures meaning*. The inherent drive to meaning in human nature (Bettelheim, 1979; Frankl, 1962, 1977, 1978) creates a fabric of knowledge, understanding, and relations as important for children as for adults, but children use more fantasy to construct it. Trauma violates the preexisting pattern, creates meaninglessness, and undermines the basis for integrating further experience.

The traumatic experience is *placed outside time, constantly repeated in the present*. It is not processed or integrated with other experiences, nor is it placed in a time context. Its traces are not fully consigned to memory and infiltrate current functioning. This leads to attempts at mastery by repeated dreams, recollections, play, imaginative reconstructions, and intrusive thought and imagery. As long as this occurs, trauma does not dim with time, and may reappear later with similar intensity to the original.

Finally, there is an *existential dimension* to the experience. Trauma poses questions about life, existence, and values which have only been faced in a theoretical way, if at all. Everything takes on new significance. Children's perspectives on life, the future, relationships, and themselves change and can become out of step with those around them. Family and peer relations have to be reevaluated, and the difficulty of communicating such experiences may lead to a profound sense of isolation. These characteristics of psychic trauma are the basis for understanding the complex repercussions that clinical observation reveals in the lives of children.

Life Continuum and Mediation of Trauma

Trauma usually has its impact on the process of the child's life at a discrete time. The concept of the *life continuum* has been developed as a framework for tracing its evolution. The life continuum is the result of the individual's activity which generates meaning and predictability, combined with the expression of wishes, needs, and hopes in interaction with those around him or her. Past experience is progressively and continuously integrated with present demands, future goals, and expectations providing coherence and a sense of identity. But the child's integrative functioning is sustained by systems of interactions and relationships without which it is ineffective or breaks down. These systems, therefore, are mediating factors determining the extent to which the child's life is affected.

A trauma is not an objective event, but a construct whose features are soon indistinguishable from its repercussions and whose impact is assessed in relation to these mediating factors within and beyond the individual. Disruption is reduced by those aspects of the child's life-supporting normal experience, but if this support is not available, the effect is compounded or exaggerated.

The first mediating factor is the specific physical detail of the event, or *what is actually traumatic in the experience*. The event is always embedded in a constellation of ancillary incidents which gives it a particular interpretation. It is also situated within a life context and earlier incidents retrospectively change their significance or give personal meaning to some aspect of the experience. The child actively interacts with the event, trying to make sense of it. What traumatizes cannot be taken for granted, but must be carefully established. Perceptions, thoughts, feelings, and circumstantial details accumulate whose significance is estimated by careful reconstruction of the individual's moment-by-moment objective and subjective experience. For example, the most disturbing element of one adolescent's bushfire experience was the abusive language and threatening attitude of police who were sent to evacuate his family; the fire itself was less of a threat standing with his family and their animals in a large dam as it swept past. Individuals' experiences vary widely within a situation and physical details give the trauma its character. For example, two children reacted differently after nearly losing their lives trapped in a car in a bushfire. The elder saw the world on fire out the window (and developed short-term problems), the younger could not and experienced near-suffocation on the floor in the back (and developed long-term problems).

The child's *cognitive capacity and temperament* govern the style and complexity of understanding of the trauma and the particular issues around which it is achieved. Children's understanding of traumatic incidents is invariably *embellished with fantasy* altering the character of the experience and providing the basis for evaluating it. Children rarely communicate fantasies, since they are unclear about what they think or assume everyone sees the situation as they do. Their reactions may be based on unrealistic interpretations never made explicit. For example, a 10-year-old boy thought one third of his peers evacuated from his school following a bushfire had been killed in it and only discovered his mistake weeks later when they began to return. For that time, he lived with a greater catastrophe than the rest of his family.

The significance of the trauma also depends on the child's *developmental stage*, governing cognitive grasp, horizon of understandings, emotional state, and relationship context. Development is a rhythmic process with discontinuities, relationship crises, and sudden increments in awareness and capability alternating with periods of consolidation of skills, stable relationships, and more secure personal identity. Impact is mediated by comprehension of the event, emotional stability, and life issues that are prominent at the time. For example, a 5-year-old boy in a rebellious stage of relationship with his father was separated from him during a bushfire evacuation; he developed phobic symptoms and would not relate to him afterward. Treatment revealed guilt engendered by the possibility of his father's death, which threatened to realize the hostile wish he felt in the midst of his prefire tantrums. His older brother's lack of problem shows what is traumatic at one stage is not at another.

The weight children give to traumatic experiences is influenced by the *reactions of parents and significant others*, such as grandparents, siblings, teachers, and caretakers. Parenting style, confidence, availability, and understanding of children mediate the extent of the crisis, determining whether the trauma is dealt with in its own right or is submerged in multiple repercussions and displacements which are part of children's posttraumatic responses. Family relationships provide the immediate psychological environment for processing much of the experience. Readiness to help understand the events, and sensitivity and responsiveness to unexpected needs in the recovery period provide containment and safety that limit the trauma's extent. Families with poor communication skills, rigid expectations, and preexisting conflicts leave the child to cope with the incident alone, which is itself a serious trauma. Emotional closeness, communication, good past experiences, capacity for enjoyment, mutual support and problem-solving constitute the *fabric of family* life which determines whether the trauma is carried by a mutually supportive family unit, or as an isolating factor by individuals. The incident may be compounded by other issues and start a deterioration in previously manageable family life. For example, parents who narrowly escaped death in a city massacre reacted punitively to their 5-year-old's behavioral problems. She became increasingly difficult until they were helped to understand how she also had been disturbed by the event.

Children evaluate crucial aspects of their experience within *peer and sibling relationships* and may prefer their authority to that of their parents. For example, a fear-inspiring rumor from a high-prestige 4-year-old far outweighed reassuring platitudes of parents after a kindergarten siege until the source was discredited. But some issues children discuss only with peers. Peer relationships reconstruct good experiences, overcome family isolation, and provide support, empathy, and understanding not obtainable in other relationships. Without them, children have more trouble placing events into context and cannot clarify the trauma's effect on age-appropriate identity. Successful peer relations compensate for family inadequacy. For example, the mother of a large family who lost their home in a bushfire complained that her children were always fighting and she had lost her adolescent son and daughter to their peer group. In the stress of rebuilding, the parents had become rigid, insensitive, and demanding on the children who sought support from the peer group. The younger two placated the parents at the expense of their own needs. In treatment, the siblings were rapidly reconstituted as a support group and peer affiliations became more balanced.

Children are in a close rapport with their *community and environment*, and daily activities bring regular contact with the world beyond the family. Although taken for granted, routines, personalities, and landmarks are concrete props for their sense of security, predictability, and confidence in the continuity of life (Gordon, 1989a). Even minor alterations in the environment or familiar people involve a degree of mourning, for adolescents as well as for younger children. Maintenance of normal routine is a support, but if other community members do not acknowledge the trauma or are not involved (as in the case of the local community in a kindergarten siege), it reinforces a sense of unreality making it harder to come to terms with what has happened. If the environment is extensively damaged (as in a bushfire), it symbolizes the destructiveness of life for children, justifying attitudes of pessimism (Terr, 1983a). Community events powerfully mediate the traumatic event, irrespective of the meaning adults may give it. For example, after a ceremony awarding kindergarten teachers for bravery 6 months after a siege, many children had recurrences of earlier disturbances or developed new anxiety symptoms. But it also allowed them to talk about it among themselves for the first time. After a street theater group played the killing of a fire dragon in a bushfire community's festival, children's emotional state improved significantly.

Model of Trauma and Disaster Impact

Support systems promote children's integration of experience by their stability, predictability, attunement to individual needs, availability for communication, age-appropriate expectations, and opportunities for enjoyment and recreation. Their breakdown impairs integrative functioning. Moment-by-moment linking of past and future is sustained in a psychological space formed by these systems that operate as protective sheaths, like the myelin sheath forms a space protecting the synapse for the transmission of nerve impulses, without which consciousness as we know it is inconceivable. The resulting life continuum is modeled as shown in Figure 48.1.

The stream of experience is shown as a discontinuous line broken in the present. The line representing the past emerges from the individual's history as a string of events twining round the line of the future as a string of expectations and goals. In a protected space, they are linked by a third line representing the individual's integrative activity. Three protective layers form a sheath around this "psychical synaptic space." The first, form-

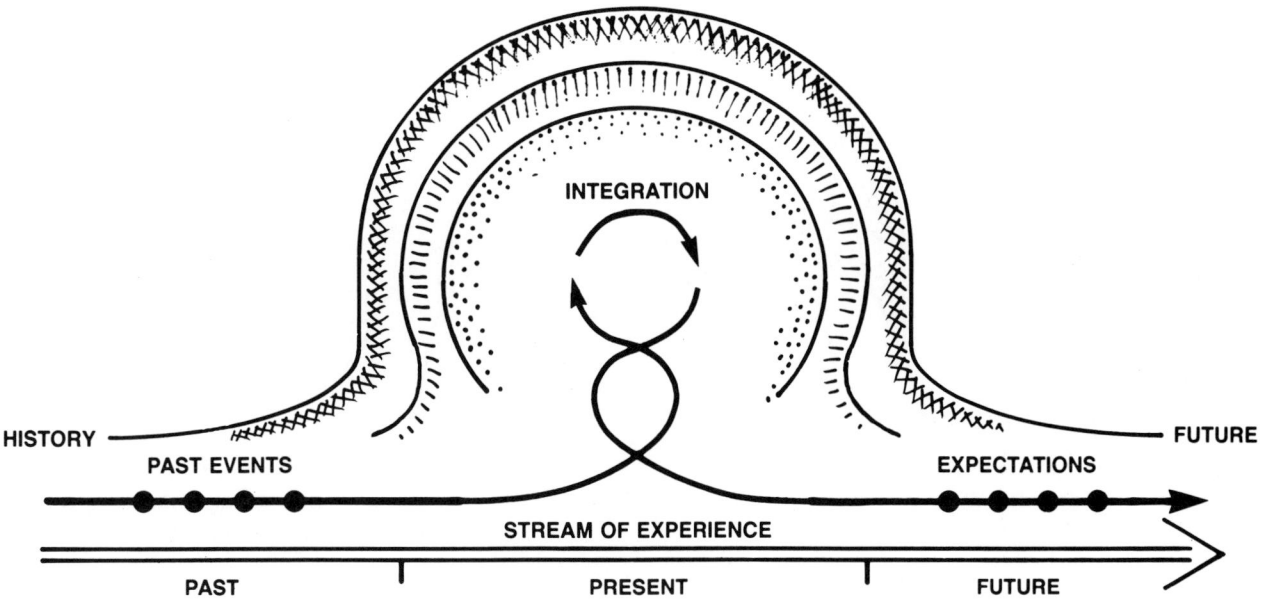

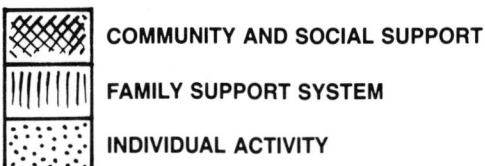

COMMUNITY AND SOCIAL SUPPORT

FAMILY SUPPORT SYSTEM

INDIVIDUAL ACTIVITY

Figure 48.1. The life continuum—normal integration of experience.

ed by the individual's own activity, includes cognitive, emotional, and personality capabilities. This is protected by the second layer, comprising support of family relationships and interactions. A third, more far-reaching layer is formed by community and social relationships constituting the psychosocial environment. (This simplified diagram makes no attempt to map all systems and processes.)

Trauma disrupts this continuum, and posttraumatic reactions can be understood in this light. The psychical apparatus is overwhelmed by the impinging of trauma and the delicate, intertwining linkage of past and future uncouples, as is illustrated in Figure 48.2.

The trauma severs past and future streams of experience which then turn back on themselves. The line of the past curves back to recent and remote events, expressed as preoccupation with the past or regressed behavior. The line of the future tries to link to near and remote goals and expectations, expressed as achievement anxiety or despondency about long-term attainments (see Terr, 1983a). Between the two, tentative, ineffectual attempts are made to bridge the gap in continuity. The individual, family, and community sheaths are ruptured by the sudden drive to reach out to past and future, impairing the containment and support necessary to rework past and future and reestablish the continuum. This is expressed in children's novel, abnormal, or unexpected reactions, which others do not understand or cannot fit into their expectations. The indi-

vidual, family, and others in the community and social system are stressed in attempting to assist children recuperate from trauma, because previous assumptions do not explain what happens.

In disasters, trauma occurs as a simultaneous impact on a significant number of people, or community, as modeled in Figure 48.3.

It shows the same intrusion of trauma in the life of the individual uncoupling past and future. But an added dimension of disruption is created by others also being affected, including the family system and community sheath. Parents, siblings, peers, teachers, and others are coping with traumatic experiences and cannot attend to children's needs. Social and community structures are disorganized and disrupted, and life becomes a series of unusual demands overshadowing normal life, perhaps for years. This is shown as simultaneous disaster impacts throughout the protective sheaths, causing pervasive disruption. In disaster, many phenomena can be understood on the basis that the very structures and systems required for recovery from traumatic experiences are themselves compromised (Gordon & Wraith, 1991).

Constituents of the Life Continuum

The life-continuum model integrates characteristics of psychic trauma and factors mediating its impact along

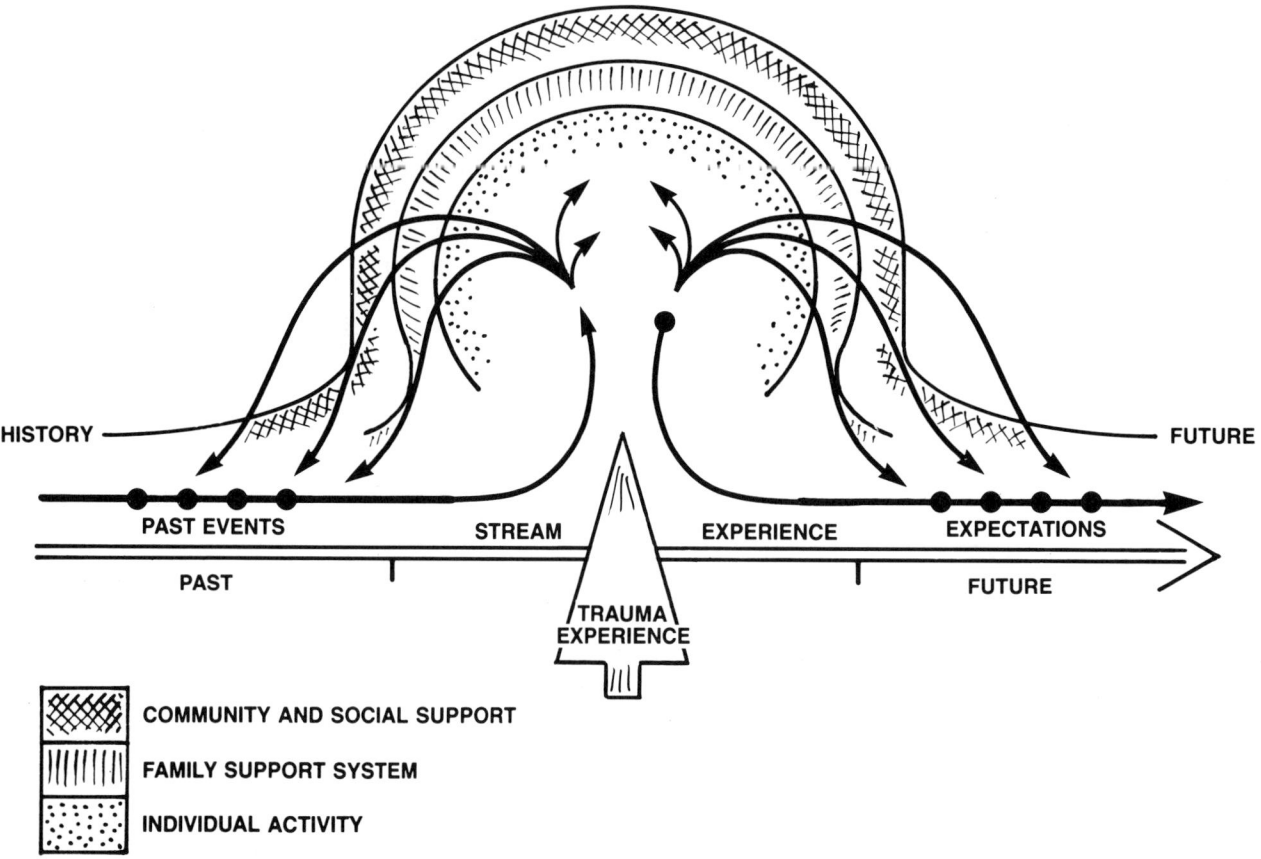

Figure 48.2. Disruption of integration on impact of trauma.

several key dimensions which, like the strands of a rope, contribute to the formation and maintenance of the continuum. Failure or disturbance on any dimension jeopardizes its integrity. The first dimension of continuity is the *developmental process* as an interplay of factors creating a field of experience where play, work, exploration, and learning occur. It is supported by teaching and modeling from adults, imitation and identification with peers. The child's temperament sets the pace and style of the activity, and biologically determined changes form a timetable of new experiences including increases in cognitive skills, emotional repertoire, and instinctual impulses to be mastered. Developmental lines (Anna Freud, 1973) determine the attainment of successive goals in relatively independent areas; for example, bodily autonomy, impulse control, motor skill, social facility, and language competence.

A second dimension of the life continuum is *communication*, comprising verbal interaction, the field of language, and paralinguistic signs (including "body language") by which the conscious representation of psychic experience is attained (Freud, 1923/1968; Lacan, 1977). Traumatic experiences are characterized by failure of adequate psychical representation, only remedied through effective communication about them. This forms an intricate fabric of mutual understanding which renders the body and actions of self and others a trans-

parent expression of their mind and being (Mearleau-Ponty, 1962, 1964). Without this, individuals are isolated in their own experience, neither understanding nor understood by others, unable to establish meaning as a precondition of continuity.

Relationships are a third field of experience where developmental achievements gain their significance. Family and peer relationships are complementary sets of interactions, like longitude and latitude, enabling children to locate themselves as functioning individuals. Dysfunction on either dimension interferes with development.

Fourth, the formation of *identity* as representation of the self to itself is essential to embrace the multiplicity of experiences and interactions of daily life. It is the nucleus for integration of these impressions, and upon it hangs the sense of continuity of the self, as a central strand to the life continuum. It involves a balance between the capacity to be alone and the maintenance of successful relationships with others (Gordon, 1991).

Finally, a dimension of *psychodynamic constitution* comprises relations between the influences and agencies of the child's psyche, including drives, wishes, reality demands, ideals, conscience, and defense mechanisms. It represents compromises and solutions to the dynamic problems set by conflicts. The psychodynamic constitution gives a unique character to the way each child main-

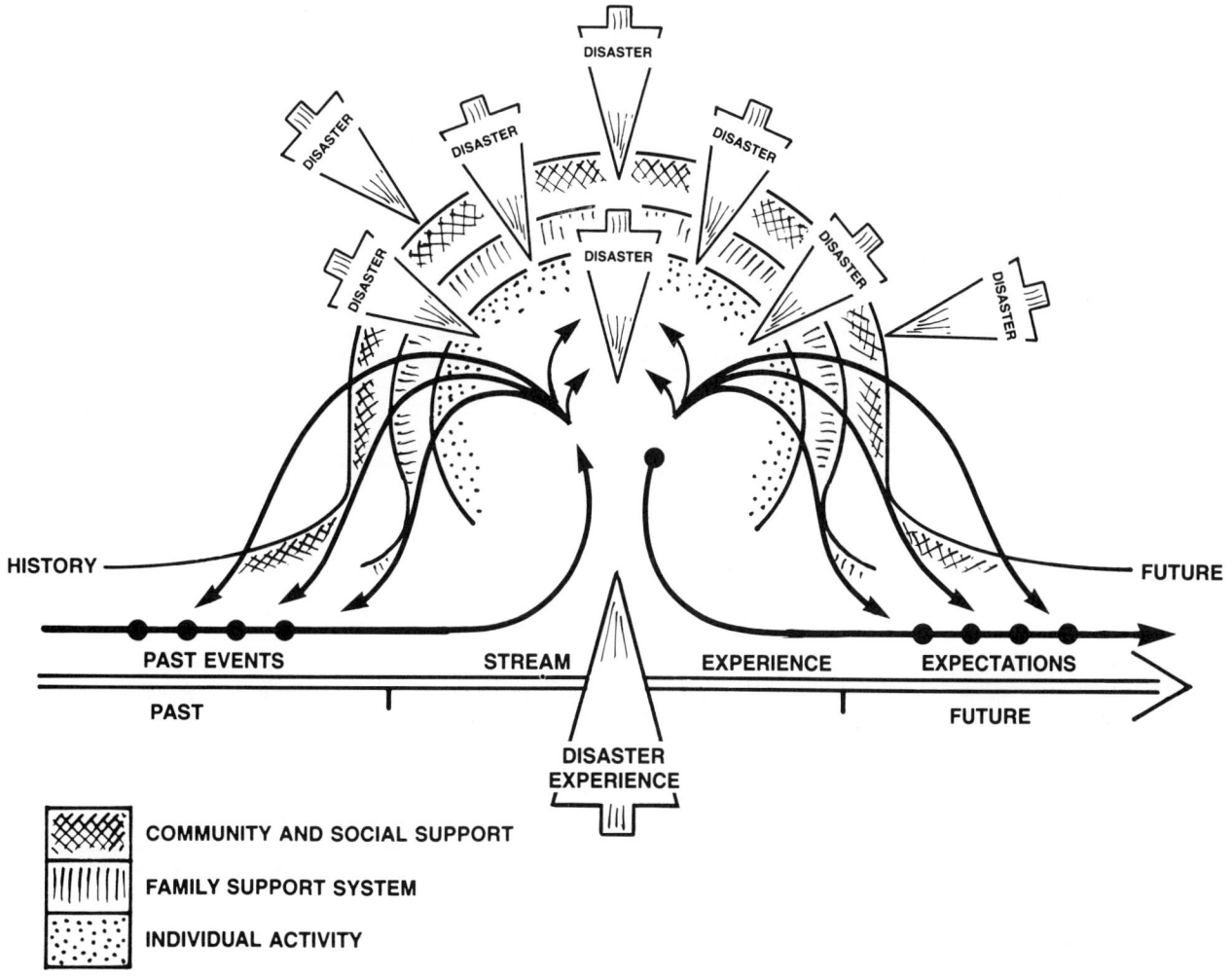

Figure 48.3. Disruption of integration on impact of disaster.

tains psychic stability and achieves continuity. It en-twines him or her intimately with family members from whom many features derive.

Responses to Trauma and Disaster

The model differentiates observed posttraumatic re-actions of children and adolescents into three main groups broadly corresponding to the time intervals fol-lowing trauma. Some responses are transient, others in-dicate ongoing difficulties. Reactions differ depending on the stage of the recovery process and the dimensions of experience or strands of the continuum affected. They can be grouped according to when they are most likely to be found, in the short-, medium-, and long-term. The observed responses are a map of possible reactions to assist in ordering observations and are not intended as definitive. Each child follows its own path, and anyone may have circumstances which interrupt the process or produce variations. Experience also emphasizes these

responses are as likely in children indirectly involved in the trauma, not just the primary "victims."

Short-Term Responses (First Weeks)

Short-term responses include the immediate reac-tion to the experience and the first few weeks. They are devoted mainly to absorbing the impact and dealing with perceptual disruption and emotional impressions. The first task is to reestablish the stimulus barrier so that processing of experience can commence. The most cru-cial dimensions are the developmental process setting the basic repertoire of responses available to express dis-tress, communication as a means of gaining information and clarifying the experience, and relationships as a re-source for comfort and support. They fall into several groups:

Many initial responses can be called *repetition phe-nomena* reproducing elements of the experience in vari-ous modalities. Repetitions may be literal attempts at mastery of perceptual or emotional impressions too intense for assimilation. Examples are compulsive talk of the event, questions about it, dreams and nightmares, hypnogogic confusional states, sleepwalking, imagining the trauma actually happening again, acting out incidents in play, and portraying it in pictures. Usually, these representations are fragmentary, only grasping certain aspects of events. Symbolic repetition phenomena also occur in dreams and nightmares representing the trauma in terms specific to the child. Play and other activities may lack direct reference to the trauma, but express its themes. If they are not accompanied by emotion, discharge can often be detected in other areas of functioning. Although evidence of the repetition compulsion (Freud, 1920/1968), they also serve as vital communication about more of the child's being than can ever be put into words.

Fear and insecurity are common, usually centering on the trauma, but may concern other demanding, frightening, or unusual situations. Innocuous stimuli can become fearful when fantasy elements have been incorporated into the experience. Earlier normal fears may be reawakened. Their effect is to bring relationships into the foreground of the child's experience, thus compensating personal disruption by interaction with trusted others.

Emotional reactions include withdrawal, sadness, anger, difficult or "bad" moods, demanding behavior, fixations, displacing conflicts onto small everyday incidents, excitement, and excessive high spirits. They usually indicate unexpressed ideas or emotions temporarily overwhelming the child and unable to be communicated; or perhaps parents are being protected or mistrusted.

Regressed and disorganized behavior with loss of previously attained habits, motor and cognitive skills, interests, comfort patterns, speech, play, or exploratory activity usually occurs. Separation problems, reduced independence, loss of autonomy, confidence, and initiative are common if the intensity of the traumatic impressions has overtaxed current skills and those of earlier, more established developmental levels are resorted to.

Heightened arousal produces vigilance, alertness, exaggerated startle responses, sensory hyperacuity, sleep difficulties, and restlessness. Although based in physiological states, reactions are expressed in key relationships and in the family fabric, indicating a need for additional support to contain excess arousal. Thus, physiological responses have a social framework.

Precocious awareness of and preoccupation with trauma-related issues may be expressed in questions, comments, interests, social relations, feelings of responsibility, and protection of parents or others in more mature forms than the child's normal style. It indicates a burden of awareness within primary relationships not placed in appropriate perspective. It is often misunderstood as a good adaptation and welcomed, but can lead to later problems.

Confusion and disorientation create a constant need for explanation and reassurance even about the familiar, difficulty organizing, planning, or following instructions. Assistance is required from adults as "auxiliary egos" to undertake these activities necessary to give coherence to their world, but adults easily misinterpret this as "attention seeking."

Short-term effects can be mild or severe and disabling, but usually subside quickly, since the child and others are highly motivated to reestablish stability and continuity. They generally have a clear relationship to the trauma, if only by temporal proximity. Usually, parents and caretakers understand and tolerate them as posttraumatic effects, but if support is not available, or vulnerabilities exist, they may not resolve. Their resolution indicates reestablishment of the continuum and the start of the integration process.

CASE EXAMPLE

Malcolm, a boisterous 4-year-old, was involved in a kindergarten siege. A gunman locked the children in the kitchen for about 20 minutes before they escaped. Four children remained hostage for the remainder of the day, but he was not among them. In the following week, he was fearful, overactive, unwilling to leave his mother, had nightmares, and slept in his mother's bed, was afraid of his father, and refused to go to him for weekend access.

When seen, Malcolm was unwilling to enter the room and refused to interact. Both parents described their uncertainty about how to treat him. The mother adopted a strict, punitive approach for "attention-seeking" behavior, though understood it was somehow related to the trauma. The father was hurt by his son's rejection when wanting to help. Malcolm was invited to paint while the clinician explained his posttraumatic responses and advised the parents about his behavior, including a plan reintroducing weekend visits to the father.

During the discussion, Malcolm did the paintings illustrated in Figures 48.4, 48.5, and 48.6. The first (Figure 48.4) is a chaos of lines and spots of color, showing his initial confusion. The second (Figure 48.5) begins to resolve into a pattern of

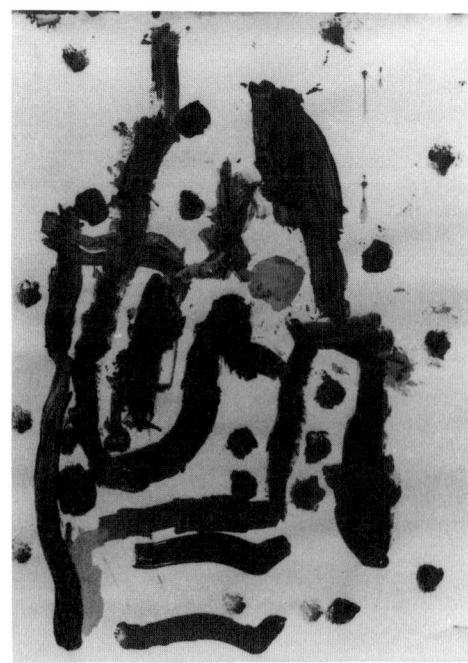

Figure 48.4. Chaotic lines and spots that reflect Malcolm's initial confusion.

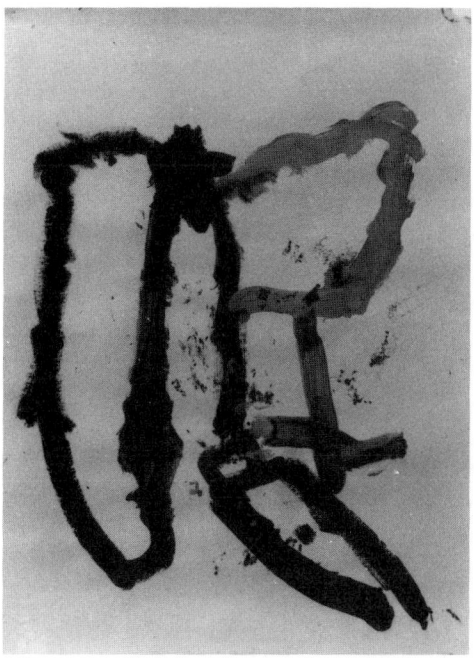

Figure 48.5. Patterns now emerge in Malcolm's painting.

lines. The last picture (Figure 48.6) is clearly representational. When asked, Malcolm said, "That's the sun, the sand, and a shark in the sea" pointing to the triangular fin emerging from the water, which was blue in the original painting. The sequence indicates the first stage in resolving the confused impressions of the trauma into a representation of a malevolent

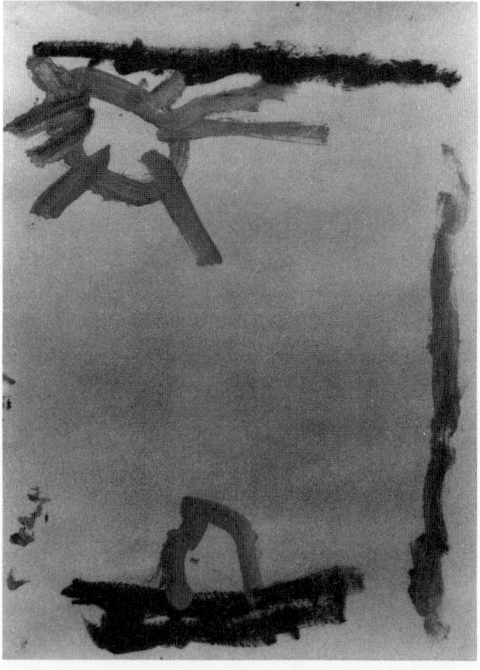

Figure 48.6. Malcolm's initial attempts to resolve the trauma by depicting it as a shark coming out of the sea into the sunlight.

shark. Although a fantasy, the shark enabled him to begin coming to terms with his encounter with death. The pictures demonstrate children's need to develop a representation of the trauma over time before it can be integrated. As this was explained, Malcolm glowed with pride at being recognized, entered the conversation for the first time, and made comments about the incident and his parents' behavior.

The following week when visiting his child care center, Malcolm engaged the clinician in a game by shutting himself in a room when it was time to leave. His mother became angry and authoritarian, provoking him to lean against the door shutting her out, until the clinician pointed out to his mother and Malcolm that he was playing a game as when the nasty man came to the kindergarten, except this time *he* was in control. Malcolm gleefully agreed, invited the clinician and mother into the room, telling them to wait. He then came in by another door and said "boo." After some similar play he was happy to go home.

Most of Malcolm's problem behavior resolved almost immediately. He was soon back to pretrauma relations with his father. However, his high arousal persisted for months and included aggressive incidents toward peers.

Recognizing and giving time to such play is an essential mode of integration of trauma in young children. Unfortunately, without advice or education, many parents react punitively or in a misguided way thereby impeding integration.

Medium-Term Effects (First Weeks to 1 Year)

From several weeks to about a year, effects of persisting arousal states accumulate. The trauma experience interacts as one element with other factors in the child's life forming complex structures sustained by ongoing relationships and issues. Short-term responses may subside and difficulties reappear in different forms indicating persisting underlying processes. Six months to a year is a long time in a young child's life, if it spans a developmental spurt for an adolescent it means coming to terms with cognitive and emotional changes as well as integrating the trauma. The framework shifts when stability is needed most and the trauma is fused and confused with the developmental process. If communication has been impeded by short-term responses, and relationships have suffered, defense mechanisms become prominent in containing posttraumatic affects. As time passes, the implications of ongoing changes affect the child's identity. Medium-term reactions indicate the growing interaction of the trauma and life continuum as integration proceeds in a more or less healthy form.

Short-term effects persist. Where children are not given adequate support or where other stresses exist, the normal recovery process leading to rapid resolution of acute effects is interrupted and they persist unchanged or reappear. Once this has occurred, there is no limit to the time they can continue to be evident because it indicates the continuum is still uncoupled and integration has not begun.

General stress signs, such as poor health, psychosomatic complaints, sleeplessness, emotional instability, and reduced concentration, begin to indicate the continuing struggle to master the trauma. They suggest that the child is not receiving or using enough support from parents and others or is struggling alone.

Relationship, mood, and attitude changes may lead to irritability, chronic dissatisfaction, withdrawal from adults, lack of communication, solitariness, and antisocial or delinquent behavior in some children. Others show such emotional changes as sadness, listlessness, depressed mood, and anxiety. Overconcern for others may displace the child's own needs, giving adults a false sense of their recovery. Although some children make increased demands on relationships and communication, others withdraw from it; both usually reflect the pattern of family interaction.

Discharge behavior expresses the release of tension, emotion, or fear in outbursts, negativism, tantrums, destructive behavior, and conflict. This is evidence of unresolved issues continuing to generate affects. Fantasies, guilt, fear of recurrence or misunderstandings about the events, and the lead-up or aftermath of the trauma are often at the basis. Children take them as accepted by all and they are only revealed upon careful examination.

Pseudoneurotic symptoms may appear as an alternative to discharge of affects in the form of phobias, obsessional preoccupations, superstitious ideas, and anxiety states triggered by symbols or elements of the trauma experience. That these are not genuine neurotic phenomena is indicated by their rapid resolution when the trauma is integrated. If untreated, however, they may form the basis for long-lasting defensive adaptations.

Loss of developmental pathway begins to manifest if the sequence of closely tied experiences necessary for proper development is interrupted. Unusual demands in the recovery period can displace normal developmental requirements. This is especially liable to happen when important milestones fall in the period. For instance, a boy who commenced school some months after a bushfire was failing badly 2 years later because he had been unable to establish himself in the new environment. Problems with developmental lines (A. Freud, 1973) may occur, such as the achievement of bodily independence, separation-individuation, attainment of cooperation, and mastery of emotional impulses if the child remains fixated at the pretrauma stage.

Challenges and new experiences may be avoided because of added stress dealing with problems initiated by the trauma. More serious consequences like avoiding exploration or failing to learn from experience represent a form of deprivation often evident after trauma that can seriously disrupt development if not recognized. Defense mechanisms may be instituted to deny or obscure the inhibitions expressed in this behavior and can become entrenched in the psychodynamic constitution.

Changes in peer relations may occur. Older children and adolescents may become overinvolved to compensate for lack of understanding at home. Peer relations then cause conflict between child and parents, with parents inevitably the losers. Peers may be avoided because of anxiety about normal challenges, or to support the family after the disaster. In either case, the balance between peer and family relations that is necessary to form a healthy identity is upset and the basis for more serious long-term problems is established.

School and performance problems appear as children are expected to return to normal while still preoccupied with the events (often in the privacy of their own minds). Stress impairs educational and social skills; some children may overachieve as a refuge from the trauma, only to encounter longer term problems. Sometimes, misguided teachers pressure children to help them "get back to normal" or "put it out of their minds." Many children are only capable of limited academic application when dealing with posttraumatic responses. Additional pressure compounds problems with school failure, loss of motivation, or conflict with teachers.

Medium-term responses are more complex and represent the interaction of direct effects with further experiences. They are harder for parents and caretakers to understand and often do not overtly demonstrate the link with the trauma, though it is usually evident on examination. Parents and teachers often feel deskilled at this stage and uncertain whether to understand and risk "spoiling" the child or reestablish normal demands. It is always important to give top priority to the reestablishment of the life continuum and integration of the trauma at the individual child's own rate since it is a natural process whose pace cannot be forced. The first year after the trauma should be oriented around recovery needs to keep them in the foreground and ensure that they are not integrated in a maladaptive way.

CASE EXAMPLE

A single mother sought help for Ben, her 9-year-old son, a year after a bushfire had surrounded their town. Their house was untouched, but she had to leave him and his older sister for a short time to evacuate an invalid neighbor. Ben was frightened by the wall of smoke and flame in the distance and for a while thought his mother had been caught in it. She soon returned and they went to safety. For the next couple of weeks he showed the same short-term responses as many other children in the town.

Then an incident altered his perspective. One evening, during a visit from his aunt and cousins, a cousin asked the meaning of "nuclear war" in response to a television program. The aunt replied, "That's when the whole world is on fire and men come round with guns, killing everybody." Ben then began to have regular nightmares of the world on fire and men coming to kill him and his mother. He developed acute anxiety symptoms including enuresis, fear of separation, sleeping in his mother's bed, reluctance to go to school, and behavior problems, becoming disobedient, demanding, and throwing frequent tantrums when he could not get his own way.

The mother was a deprived woman doing her best to understand Ben. In the initial interview, the link between his aunt's words, the fire, and his dreams was identified and he was helped to understand how his fantasy had constructed a worse trauma out of the ingredients. Ben's nightmares stopped, but his behavior problems persisted. After several sessions, his mother came in tears saying she was a bad mother and she should give up her children to save Ben from turning bad. A story emerged of her upbringing in orphanages, her marriage to an aggressive man whom she left, and her one aim in life which was to give her children what she lacked. Her fear of Ben's deterioration derived from a violent paternal uncle who was wanted by the police and who had threatened to kill his parents. Her parents-in-law had said that Ben was another "bad seed, and would turn out just like Uncle Jim."

When it was demonstrated that Ben lacked even early

stages of personality disorder and his willingness to communicate and understand himself indicated he had nothing in common with his uncle, the mother was relieved and was able to accept advice on his management and resume her parenting responsibility. Ben responded positively when he understood the fears that his mother carried on his behalf.

This case demonstrates how posttrauma events can make the objective incident into a different subjective trauma. The resultant responses take on a new meaning quite apart from the trauma when they are maladaptively integrated with other family problems. Ben and his family were at risk for serious and long-term disruption from the bushfire. Although Ben was not an easy child, there was no evidence that this degree of difficulty had been evident before the fire.

Long-Term Responses (Second Year and Beyond)

After 12 months or more, life adds further complexity to the pattern of responses. If difficulties persist into the second year or beyond, the life continuum has been disordered for a considerable time and responses include problems traceable to the trauma and others related to the dysfunction of the continuum and to maladaptive integration. Continuity may be reestablished in some dimensions while others remain impaired. Many children presenting long-term responses have compromised their needs with the demands around them. The further away from the trauma, the more the developmental process becomes a key factor as dysfunctional patterns and symptoms are integrated into the behavioral repertoire. Communication that breaks down in the short or medium term may not be reestablished, and a changed fabric of family life distances the child and family from each other. These situations provide information from which children draw conclusions about their identity, and defense mechanisms and neurotic systems are used to deal with conflict and pressures of life. Sometimes clinical experience allows the reconstruction of very long-term effects from many traumata of years ago. In principle, there is no limit to the time trauma can continue to disrupt children's lives.

Short- and medium-term responses persist or appear for the first time. Acute responses, such as nightmares, fears, and emotional upheaval, can continue 2 years or more after the event even in children who are not directly involved. For example, the son of a policeman sent to a bushfire far from his town continued to have nightmares, fears, and regressed behavior 2 years later. Delayed short- or medium-term responses can present, and children sometimes postpone their own response until other family issues are resolved, such as rebuilding, or the posttraumatic problems of parents. In this case, a pseudocontinuum of limited life has been constructed in the short term, only to uncouple later.

Developmental deviations occur if developmental issues persist into the long-term and continue to compromise the child's experience. Preoccupation with trauma or posttraumatic responses for months or years prevents children from getting on with their lives and critical experiences are missed. Deviant patterns may require considerable effort to rectify; for instance, continued fears create a dependent, passive stance that is inherently frustrating and breeds discontent and conflict for the child. Cognitive development suffers as a child's time is preoccupied by the trauma and interest in other activities is lost.

School failure and poor performance can become chronic if short- and medium-term problems lead to lack of success, bad experiences with teachers, and loss of self-esteem. Learning is displaced by survival-oriented behavior or rumination about trauma-related issues, or education is undermined by pessimism and lack of sense of the future.

Personality changes follow if continued conflict and misunderstanding lead to chronic disillusionment, withdrawal from family contact, acting out of frustrations, and other patterns not evident before the trauma. Chronic anger, depression, distrust, bitterness, and pessimism follow failure to resolve earlier emotional reactions. Relations with parents and others deteriorate, and the child adjusts to being alone. Some children say they have not felt understood by anyone since the trauma. A dysfunctional self-sufficiency develops, and attempts to communicate are rejected as too late. Another outcome is the chronically anxious, timid personality where the trauma-based anxiety is generalized to life in general.

Postponing life issues may occur as children struggle to manage daily life. They remain fixated at the pretrauma stage and avoid confrontation with current challenges and tasks. Loss of family and other support systems leaves them unable to attempt anything but the familiar. Some children function adequately by maintaining a narrow existence.

Chronic peer problems can develop. Adolescents can form support systems almost entirely from peers if the family no longer provides their needs. But usually they are only partially effective and are often based on distrust and opposition to adults. Such individuals are often lonely, wanting contact but are unable to take responsibility. This may culminate in adolescents prematurely leaving home or school a year or more after the trauma. Younger children who make their gang the focus for their life become vulnerable to antisocial activity. The peer group can also become the object of fear and unhappiness displaced from family misunderstanding. Chronic conflict then develops and peer support is lost. Peers are also responsible by teasing and deriding a child's fears and posttraumatic responses that are out of step with them.

Poor physical health can follow the chronic stress of the long-term recovery process, with increased vulnerability to infection and a general run-down state. Risk of accidents is also increased.

Preoccupation with other traumas may occur, leading to constant repetition by fixation on news reports of death, danger, and suffering of others. Trauma becomes an ever present likelihood. Earlier traumata of their own may also be reactivated leading to confusion and disorientation. For example, one adolescent's father died a year before a bushfire nearby. He presented a year later with a delayed grief reaction based on seeing the distant mountainside a mass of smoke and flame at night. In treatment, he revealed this conjured up a vision of hell as taught in his religious denomination, and he was plagued with the thought this was what his father was suffering.

Identity changes occur as children live with changes in themselves, their relationships, and their capacities. They may label themselves cowards, weak, bad, guilty and blame themselves for emotional or behavior problems. They lose confidence in themselves and in the future, and suicidal ideation occurs even in quite young children if their despair is not noticed. One senior emergency services officer confided that, in adolescence, he experienced normal traumatic responses during a bushfire. Family members had called him a coward; he believed them and lived his life and brought up his sons to believe it too.

Philosophical views emerge that generalize from the trauma to form a dismal worldview. Although this may express depression, it can become an entrenched attitude to life. The following piece was written by a 12-year-old boy, who was caught in a bushfire, and whose elder brother a few months later suffered brain damage in a motorcycle accident. When visiting his brother in the hospital, the boy was caught in an elevator with a deranged man who threatened to kill him with a knife and who slashed his clothes.

THE WORLD—Chapter 1

G'day my name is Richie. I'll explain the world to you in my own words from my mind. Well first I think the world to me is having lots of troubles. First there is Wars then Bushfires and Earthquakes. Plus sport, I really like football. Aussie rules of course. But there is fights, the world is spinning and spinning. We don't know when it's gonna stop or whatever. That is the world to me in a couple of words. Goodbye.

Children rarely confide inner feelings and conclusions about the world and life unless encouraged and understood, but then they reveal surprisingly elaborate or sophisticated deductions based on their experiences. Often the act of communication is enough to place them in a perspective that opens them to change. At the same time, children may develop strong altruism and optimism from the experience of suffering. Such philosophical views are often revealed in school essays.

Long-term reactions to trauma can be protracted and severe, and can present in the guise of a wide range of psychopathology, family or social problems. They represent the breakdown of the life continuum and dysfunctional integration. Trauma mediation and life continuum dimensions provide an intricate background. Children and adolescents need assistance and guidance as the various levels of the recovery process interact. The consequences of these experiences can be formative and decisively alter the course of development. However, help to identify and treat the relationship to trauma can produce rapid change.

Helping Children with Trauma

Recovery from trauma involves reestablishing systems that support processing the experience to integrate it into the life continuum. These systems involve structures and networks of children's normal world, and the first priority is to ensure they are properly constructed, informed, and resourced to undertake the task and prevent complications. Effective strategies promote normal recovery by identifying vulnerabilities and interference from relationships or other areas of life and assist the child and the family to take control of them. Attention to the detail of their experiences, fantasies, and confusions by communication within stable relationships assists this process. Successful integration of trauma can be fostered by all people in the child's life.

The first task of a helper is to *discover what is traumatic about the trauma* for the child and not make assumptions. Often the child is unclear about the significance or incorporates fantasy elements into various aspects of the experience, and comes to a better understanding in the course of such an investigation. Adolescents tend to misinterpret events rather than add fantasy. Since a defining characteristic of trauma is *the lack of adequate psychical representation of the experience*, integration cannot occur until this has been achieved. A clear idea of what happened is the first step. Although the child seems to know the facts after the event, crucial elements are usually missing and, as time passes, they become more confused. An additional step is for the child to represent the incident to him- or herself so that the *personal psychological reality* is understood even when the facts are remembered. This takes time and is the most crucial factor for successful recovery. When achieved, the child can do much of the work as his or her normal integrative processes take over.

It is also essential to *promote integration through meaning*. Traumatic incidents undermine or defy established meaning. It is achieved by inserting the trauma representation into a network of other relationships enabling the experience to become part of a set. Free communication promotes this integration by allowing the child to relate the full range of implications of the event for his or her life. Treatment can focus on the details of this and pursue unconscious issues later.

Emotions must be bound by being received in the relationships that surround the child. The high charge of emotion aroused by trauma is a major source of problems. Support systems provide a safe place for their expression, or become the object of displaced emotions. Where the emotions are received, binding can be undertaken by the child. Often it is not necessary to do more than acknowledge emotions and avoid personalizing them to begin this process. *A forum for expression and working-through* of the elements of the experience needs to be created. Action and emotion are repeated many times in the process of working-through. The same theme may be played in several different games, or discussed repeatedly. This is done only where self-expression is freely accepted. Normal relationships and environment provide the basis where the child can do much of the integrative work.

Integration follows the line of association and fantasy, not logic. Caretakers and parents need to allow the child to approach the experience in a piecemeal fashion and to play with it in his or her communication. Adult logic and order are only effective after the child has explored it in his or her own way. Recovery works best when based on the child's terms and preconceived notions of what the issues are or how resolution is achieved are not imposed. The more children follow their own meandering path through the associations of their fantasy about the event, the faster the progress. Improvement often follows the unexpected.

Strategies for Treatment

Space does not permit a detailed discussion of treatment of posttraumatic responses in children and adolescents, but a number of principles are outlined in which strategies can be based. Assuming pretrauma normal functioning and emphasizing strengths and capacities for independent activity maximizes the sense of control which counters traumatic helplessness. Where pathology predates the trauma, it is advisable to promote integration of the experience within the current mode of functioning and only negotiate a shift of emphasis toward dealing with broader issues once this is established. Embarking on general psychological treatment initially is a further traumatization since it was not invited and issues are either unconscious or subject to defenses which it is unwise to dismantle until integration has commenced. Such intrusion can have long-term adverse effects on recovery. For example, a family burnt out in a bushfire were immediately referred for treatment by their lawyer to strengthen their case for compensation. The clinician lacked knowledge of trauma work and, to their surprise, explored family issues and personal histories, and suggested nothing was wrong with them. When the parents anxiously asked how to assist their distressed 8-year-old, they were told it was like loss and should be treated the same way. They felt intruded upon, not helped and did not return. Two years later, they were seen after friends had been successfully helped. Their disabling long-term family problems quickly resolved and could have been prevented by appropriate assistance in the early recovery period.

Therapeutic work with children after trauma can be confusing for clinicians, who may not know what to expect and be uncertain whether something special should be done to meet their needs. The issues that we outlined give the necessary openness to support recovery most effectively. Where clinical treatment is required, the following strategies have been found to be reliable guidelines for traumatized children.

1. *Don't expect what to hear; listen and pick up opportunities.* Crucial messages are often transmitted incidentally and unexpectedly. The pace cannot be forced, and not everything has to be dealt with explicitly. Children may need help with obscure aspects of their experience they cannot articulate for themselves; once this is done, they can make sense of the rest. It is best to wait and work with opportunities offered by the child and deal carefully with whatever is presented, even if it seems irrelevant. Where preexisting problems become fused into a single mass with those provoked by the trauma, they need to be dealt with as aspects of the trauma and not independent problems.

2. *Identify and deal with fantasies and give information; reality is always easier than fantasy.* Children build fantasies around fears and uncertainties. Fantasy is an essential part of integration, but fantasies constructed on uncertainty produce false facts and interrupt the process. Ensuring that the facts are clear and fantasy elements are articulated for the child if he cannot do so himself makes the unreality obvious. A painful reality is the basis for a new future, but a fantasy only leads to another fantasy.

3. *Keep the time perspective; don't rush integration.* It takes years rather than months to integrate traumatic experiences. Usually, treatment need not do more than initiate the process in the right way. But if the appropriate time scale is understood, it takes pressure off those supporting the child's recovery; children then take their time instead of responding to adults' need for them to be recovered.

4. *Create a network with a common understanding of the child.* If those persons who are involved with the child—parents, relatives, and teachers—have a common understanding and shared expectations, they may feel contained in a supportive network which compensates for the violation of expectations and assumptions caused by the trauma. This reforms the protective sheath necessary to reestablish the life continuum. Energy expended in creating and maintaining such a network is well repaid since it represents in external form the very integration of experience that the recovery process is pursuing.

5. *Take a preventive approach.* Often minor problems develop into serious ones in the long-term. A preventive approach highlights the problem in its context and provides parents with information on what to expect, how to respond, when and where to seek help. Intervention should not depend on the presence of significant pathology, since only in the medium and long term do more serious consequences become evident. The earlier the intervention, the more important the preventive component, since resolution of short-term problems does not necessarily prevent long-term ones from developing.

6. *Maintain the normal perspective, but do not ignore signs of disturbance.* After trauma, it is easy to lose the perspective of normal developmental processes, both beneficial and problematic. It is important to maintain normal expectations without missing real manifestations of disturbance where trauma effects are assimilated into developmental issues. Differentiating and relating these is therapeutic in itself. Clinicians often need to supply this balance, because families, teachers, and primary care workers usually feel themselves to be in an unprecedented situation after the trauma and do not know if they can trust their previous knowledge and judgment.

7. *Support normal routines, networks, and relationships.* These provide the structure which facilitates working-through. Social support is a decisive factor determining the degree of posttraumatic disturbance. Children are dependent on these external props to sustain their functioning. Considerable effort may be needed to re-create them in the confusion of the aftermath, and consultation is one of the most efficient modes of service delivery.

8. *Promote meaning through symbols and ritual.* Every human being has a need for symbols and rituals. Children supply this for themselves by fantasy and imaginative play. However, religious, artistic, or other cultural events allow them to place the events in a larger social context in a unique way. Plays and services have a deep

and lasting effect, marking the phases of the recovery process.

Children and adolescents react strongly to the events in their lives, but their resilience and capacity for growth are equal to their vulnerability provided their needs are understood and respected. Assistance is often needed, if not sooner then perhaps later. But information, education, and support always benefit. Usually, children do not feel themselves to be "patients" and respond quickly to being helped to understand what is happening in their lives and commence what is often the first effective communication about the events. Usually, treatment is a matter of helping them conduct their own recovery and attuning other adults to their own special way of doing it. It must also be remembered that they will carry the experience or its imprint through their lives and it has the possibility to provide them with unique gifts if properly integrated.

References

Ahearn, F. L., & Cohen, R. E. (1983). *Disasters and mental health: An annotated bibliography.* Rockville, MD: National Institute of Mental Health.

Anthony, E. J. (1986). The response to overwhelming stress: Some introductory comments. *Journal of the American Academy of Child Psychiatry, 25*(3), 299–305.

Bergman, M. S., & Jucovy, M. C. (1982). *Generations of the Holocaust.* New York: Basic Books.

Bettelheim, B. (1979). *Surviving and other essays.* London: Thames & Hudson.

Bloch, D. A., Silber, E., & Perry, S. E. (1956). Some factors in the emotional reaction of children to disaster. *American Journal of Psychiatry, 113,* 416–422.

Blom, G. E. (1986). A school disaster: Intervention and research aspects. *Journal of the American Academy of Child Psychiatry, 25*(3), 336–345.

Burke, J. D., Borus, J. F., Burns, B. J., Millstein, K. H., & Beasley, M. C. (1982). Changes in childrens' behaviour after a natural disaster. *American Journal of Psychiatry, 139*(8), 1010–1014.

Danieli, Y. (1985). The treatment and prevention of long-term and inter-generational transmission of victimization: A lesson from Holocaust survivors and their children. In C. R. Figley (Ed.), *Trauma and its wake.* New York: Brunner/Mazel.

Earls, F., Smith, E., Reich, W., & Jung, K. G. (1988). Investigating psychopathological consequences of a disaster in children: A pilot study incorporating a structured diagnostic interview. *Journal of the American Academy of Child Psychiatry, 27*(1), 90–95.

Erikson, K. (1976). *Everything in its path.* New York: Simon & Schuster.

Farberow, N. L., & Gordon, N. S. (1981). *Manual for child health workers in major disasters.* Rockville, MD: National Institute of Mental Health.

Frankl, V. E. (1962). *The doctor and the soul: An introduction to logotherapy.* New York: Alfred A. Knopf.

Frankl, V. E. (1977). *Man's search for meaning.* New York: Pocket Books.

Frankl, V. E. (1978). *Psychotherapy and existentialism.* Harmondsworth, England: Penguin Books.

Freud, A. (1973). *Normality and pathology in childhood.* London: Hogarth Press.

Freud, S. (1968). Beyond the pleasure principle. In J. Strachey (Ed. and Trans.), *The standard edition of the complete psychological works of Sigmund Freud* (Vol. 18, pp. 3–64). London: Hogarth Press. (Original work published 1920)

Freud, S. (1968). *The ego and the id.* In J. Strachey (Ed. and Trans.), *The standard edition of the complete psychological works of Sigmund Freud* (Vol. 18, pp. 3–66). London: Hogarth Press. (Original work published 1923)

Galante, R., & Foa, D. (1986). An epidemiological study of psychic trauma and treatment effectiveness for children after a natural disaster. *Journal of the American Academy of Child Psychiatry, 25*(3), 357–363.

Gordon, R. (1986). *Stress in disaster workers and their families.* Paper presented at the International Conference on Stress in Emergency Services, Melbourne, Australia. November.

Gordon, R. (1987). *Longer term personal and family responses following disaster.* Paper presented at the National Hazards Workshop, Boulder, Colorado. July.

Gordon, R. (1989a). Community process and personal responses in disaster. In C. A. Ackehurst, D. Beggs, R. Gordon, J. Isherwood, M. B. O'Connell, & G. D. Smith (Eds.), *Engineering aspects of disaster recovery* (pp. 11–17). (Australian Counter Disaster College Manual No. 1). Mt. Macedon: Australian Counter Disaster College.

Gordon, R. (1989b). *Children and adolescents' responses to disaster and trauma.* Paper presented at the Australian Psychological Society Conference, Hobart, Australia. September.

Gordon, R. (1991). Intersubjectivity and the efficacy of group psychotherapy. *Group Analysis, 24*(1), 41–51.

Gordon, R., & Wraith, R. (1987). Personal and family responses to disaster: The long term perspective. *Australian Child and Family Welfare, 12*(3), 15–17.

Gordon, R., & Wraith, R. (1988). Debriefing after disaster work. *National Emergency Response, 3*(3), 31–41.

Gordon, R., & Wraith, R. (1991). The human response to disaster. In *The Mt. Macedon digest: The Australian newsletter of disaster management: 1986–1988* Mt. Macedon: Australian Counter Disaster College. Reprinted.

Gubrich-Simitis, I. (1981). Extreme traumatization as cumulative trauma: Psychoanalytic investigations of the effects of concentration camp experiences on survivors and their children. *Psychoanalytic Study of the Child, 36,* 415–450.

Handford, H. A., Mayes, S. D., Matterson, R. E., Humphrey, F. J., Bagnato, S., Bixler, E. O., & Kales, J. K. (1986). Child and parent reaction to the Three Mile Island nuclear accident. *Journal of the American Academy of Child Psychiatry, 25*(3), 346–356.

Kinzie, D., Sack, W. H., Angell, R. H., Manson, S., & Rath, B. (1986). The psychiatric effects of massive trauma on Cambodian children: I. The children. *Journal of the American Academy of Child Psychiatry, 25*(3), 370–376.

Lacan, J. (1977). The function and field of speech and language in psychoanalysis. In J. Lacan (A. Sheridan, Trans.), *Ecrits: A selection.* New York: W. W. Norton.

Malmquist, C. P. (1986). Children who witness parental murder: Posttraumatic aspects. *Journal of the American Academy of Child Psychiatry, 25*(3), 320–325.

McFarlane, A. C. (1987). Posttraumatic phenomena in a longitudinal study of children following a natural disaster. *Journal of the American Academy of Child and Adolescent Psychiatry, 26*(5), 794–796.

McFarlane, A. C. (1989). Recent life events and psychiatric disorder in children: The interaction with preceding extreme adversity. *Journal of Child Psychology and Psychiatry, and Allied Disciplines, 29*(5), 677–690.

Mearleau-Ponty, M. (1962). *The phenomenology of perception.* London: Routledge & Kegan Paul.

Mearleau-Ponty, M. (1964). The child's relations with others. In M. Mearleau-Ponty (Ed.), *The primacy of perception and other essays* (pp. 96–155). Evanston: Northwestern University Press.

Milne, G. (1977). Cyclone Tracey II: The effects on Darwin children. *Australian Psychologist, 12,* 55–62.

Newman, C. J. (1976). Children of disaster: Clinical observations at Buffalo Creek. *American Journal of Psychiatry, 133*(3), 306–312.

Pynoos, R. S. (1989). Post-traumatic stress disorder in children. In B. Garfinkel, G. Carlson, & E. Weller (Eds.), *The medical basis of child and adolescent psychiatry* (pp. 48–63). Philadelphia: W. B. Saunders.

Raphael, B. (1986). The young, the old, and the family. In *When Disaster Strikes* (ch. 7, pp. 149–175). New York: Basic Books.

Raphael, B. (1989). Foreword. In J. P. Wilson (Ed.), *Trauma, transformation and healing: An integrative approach to theory, research and post-traumatic therapy* (pp. vii–viii). New York: Brunner/Mazel.

Rosenheck, R. (1986). Impact of post-traumatic stress disorder of World War II on the next generation. *Journal of Nervous & Mental Disease, 174*(6), 319–327.

Sugar, M. (1988). A preschooler in disaster. *American Journal of Psychotherapy, 42,* 619–629.

Terr, L. C. (1979). Children of Chowchilla: A study of psychic trauma. *Psychoanalytic Study of the Child, 34,* 547–621.

Terr, L. C. (1983a). Chowchilla revisited: The effects of psychic trauma four years after a school bus kidnapping. *American Journal of Psychiatry, 140*(2), 1543–1550.

Terr, L. C. (1983b). Life attitudes, dreams, and psychic trauma in a group of "normal" children. *Journal of the American Academy of Child Psychiatry, 22*(3), 221–230.

Terr, L. C. (1985). Psychic trauma in children and adolescents. *Psychiatric Clinics of North America, 8*(4), 815–835.

Terr, L. C. (1987). Childhood psychic trauma. In J. D. Noshpitz (Ed.), *Basic handbook of child psychiatry* (Vol. 2, pp. 262–272). New York: Basic Books.

Titchener, J. L., & Kapp, F. T. (1976). Family and character change at Buffalo Creek. *American Journal of Psychiatry, 133,* 295–299.

Wilson, John P. (1989). *Trauma, transformation and healing: An integrative approach to theory, research, and post-traumatic therapy.* New York: Brunner/Mazel.

Wraith, R. (1987). Children and families in disaster. In *Proceedings of the Inaugural State Conference of the Australian Early Childhood Association, Victoria Branch,* Melbourne, Australia. July.

Wraith, R. (1988a). *Experiencing disaster as a child.* Paper presented at the Annual Conference of the Royal Australian and New Zealand College of Psychiatrists, Cairns, Australia. September.

Wraith, R. (1988b). *Experiences of children of emergency services workers in disaster.* Paper presented at the International Conference on Stress in Emergency Services, Melbourne, Australia. November.

Wraith, R., & Gordon, R. (1987a). The response to disaster of individuals and families within their community. *Australian Child and Family Welfare, 12*(3), 2–10.

Wraith, R., & Gordon, R. (1987b). The myths of response to disaster by people and communities. *Australian Child and Family Welfare, 12*(3), 26–28.

CHAPTER 49

Childhood Sexual and Physical Abuse

Arthur Green

Introduction

The high incidence of physical and sexual abuse in the United States and in other parts of the world and the increased recognition of a history of these forms of victimization in the childhood of adults afflicted with a wide variety of psychiatric disorders make it imperative to document the harmful consequences maltreatment leaves on the child victims and to trace the process of traumatization as it extends into adulthood. The ultimate goal of this chapter is to develop a theoretical framework to help us understand the nature of the trauma associated with the physical and sexual abuse of children and its relationship to posttraumatic stress disorder (PTSD).

Prevalence of Maltreatment

The prevalence of physical and sexual abuse of children is quite alarming. According to Light (1973), approximately a million and a half cases of child maltreatment occur each year, including severe neglect and sexual abuse. According to the findings of the National Incidence Study of Child Abuse and Neglect carried out in 1986 (National Center on Child Abuse and Neglect [NCCAN], 1988) almost two million children were found to be maltreated. Finkelhor and Hotaling (1984) projected the annual number of new sexual abuse cases to be 150,000 to 200,000.

Retrospective studies of women estimate a higher prevalence of sexual abuse during their childhood. Russell (1983) reported that 38% of a community population

of randomly selected women had experienced sexual contact during childhood, whereas Wyatt (1985) discovered that 45% of a community sample of white and Afro-American women in Los Angeles had unwanted sexual contact during childhood. The prevalence of sexual abuse in males is lower than in women. Lewis (1985) found that 16% of males interviewed in a community sample had been sexually victimized during childhood; Miller (1976) found that a sample of adolescents yielded an 8% molestation rate for males.

Comparison between Physical and Sexual Abuse

Physical and sexual abuse are similar in that they both involve the intentional exploitation of a child by a parent or caretaker in the context of a pathological family environment. Both types of maltreatment often result in immediate and long-term sequelae, including stigmatization, scapegoating, and impaired psychological and cognitive functioning. Both physical and sexual abuse are treated as offenses by the family court or juvenile court and must be reported by physicians and other child-care professionals to designated child abuse registries.

Physical and sexual abuse differ in that physical abuse is committed almost equally by mothers and fathers or father surrogates on boys and girls in equal numbers, whereas sexual abuse is primarily inflicted by fathers or father-surrogates on female children.

Impact of Physical and Sexual Abuse on Children

The traumatic impact of physical and sexual abuse on child victims has produced a variety of anxiety disorders, disturbances in affect, and impaired impulse con-

Arthur Green • Department of Psychiatry, Columbia-Presbyterian Hospital, New York, New York 10032.
International Handbook of Traumatic Stress Syndromes, edited by John P. Wilson and Beverley Raphael. Plenum Press, New York, 1993.

trol. In addition, physical abuse has been associated with cognitive and language impairment and central nervous system (CNS) dysfunction. In these key areas of psychopathology, the immediate and short-term effects of childhood victimization will be compared with the long-term sequelae encountered in adult survivors of physical and sexual abuse.

Child Abuse and Anxiety

Frequently, fearfulness and anxiety-related symptoms have been described as immediate and long-term sequelae of physical and sexual abuse. Green (1985) described anxiety states, sleep disturbances, nightmares, and psychosomatic complaints in physically abused children as immediate results of the physical assault. Kempe (1976) observed that abused children were hypervigilant, anxious, and fearful in relating to adults and that they expected punishment and criticism. Visual avoidance, hypervigilance, and extreme wariness in the presence of a caretaker have been described in infants and toddlers by George and Main (1979). Ounstead, Oppenheimer, and Lindsay (1974) reported a hypervigilant attitude, "frozen watchfulness," in otherwise passive infants and toddlers who had been physically abused. Similar fearfulness and anxiety-related symptoms have been observed in sexually abused children by Lewis and Sarrell (1969), Sgroi (1982), and R. Kempe and C. H. Kempe (1978). Sgroi (1982) observed fear reactions in sexually abused children extending to a phobic avoidance of all males. Many of these anxiety-ridden children satisfied the DSM-III-R (American Psychiatric Association [APA], 1987) criteria for PTSD. Kiser, Ackerman, Brown, and Edwards (1988) documented PTSD in 9 of 10 children between the ages of 2 and 6 who were molested in a day-care setting. The most frequently observed symptoms were acting as if the traumatic event were reoccurring (attributable to environmental stimuli), avoiding activities reminiscent of the traumatic event, and intensification of symptoms on exposure to events resembling the molestation. Other symptoms were visualizing the trauma (in neutral situations), nightmares related to the molestation, and sexual acting out.

McLeer et al. (1988) diagnosed PTSD in 48% of sexually abused children who were evaluated at a child psychiatry outpatient clinic based on DSM-III-R criteria. The symptoms included reexperiencing phenomena, avoidance behavior, and autonomic hyperarousal. Seventy-five percent of children abused by a natural father, 67% abused by strangers, and 25% abused by trusted adults met PTSD criteria as opposed to none of the children abused by an older child.

Goodwin (1985) adapted Kardiner's (1959) descriptions of shell-shocked combat veterans to child sexual abuse victims (i.e., they displayed symptoms of fear, startle reactions and anxiety, repetition and reenactment, sleep disturbance and depressive phenomena, ego constriction and regression, and explosive expressions of anger). Goodwin also compared child sexual abuse victims with rape victims suffering from fear, sleep and eating disturbances, guilt, decreased functioning, sexual problems, and irritability. However, Goodwin reasoned that sexually abused children display more severe and long-lasting symptoms than do adult rape victims because the children experience more frequent sexual assaults over a more prolonged period.

Allen, Gaines, and Green (1991) reported that 61% of a cohort of physically abused and sexually abused children fulfilled the DSM-III-R criteria for PTSD using the Columbia Clinical Interview and the PTSD Stress Reaction Index (Pynoos, Frederick, Nader, Arroyo, Steinberg, Eth, Nunez, & Fairbanks, 1987). The majority of the children reported intrusive symptoms and anxiety symptoms in a consistent and reliable manner, whereas the reports of blunting and numbing were inconsistent. These children also manifested high rates of enuresis, phobias, and aggressive behavior.

Thus far, the studies cited have documented contrasting adaptive responses to the stressful experience of physical or sexual abuse: fearfulness and phobic avoidance existing side by side with reenactments and repetitions. The avoidant responses may be interpreted as a defense against the intrusive and repetitive traumatic imagery, as suggested by Horowitz (1976) who described the alternation of intrusive and avoidant numbing responses as the essential feature of PTSD.

Dissociation

Dissociation, or an alteration in consciousness resulting in an impairment of memory or identity, has also been observed in children traumatized by physical and sexual abuse (Kluft, 1985; Putnam, 1984). Signs of early dissociation in children are forgetfulness with periods of amnesia, excessive fantasizing and daydreaming, trancelike states, somnambulism, the presence of an imaginary companion, sleepwalking, and blackouts. Multiple personality disorder (MPD), the most extreme form of dissociation, has been observed in severely sexually and physically abused children (Braun & Sachs, 1985; Kluft, 1985). According to Braun and Sachs (1985), the two major predisposing factors for MPD are a natural inborn capacity to dissociate and exposure to severe overwhelming trauma. Sexual abuse and physical abuse are the most frequent background factors in the etiology of MPD in adults. There appears to be a close relationship between dissociation and PTSD. Coons, Bowman, Pellow, and Schneider (1989) demonstrated significant dissociation in adults suffering from PTSD based on the Dissociative Experiences Scale (Bernstein & Putnam, 1986). Braun (1988) conceptualized a continuum of dissociation from dissociative episodes to PTSD to atypical dissociative disorder to MPD.

Briere and Runtz (1985) reported that adult female survivors of child sexual abuse seeking treatment at a crisis center scored higher on a dissociation scale than their peers without a history of sexual abuse. Liner (1989) found that physically and sexually abused children referred for outpatient treatment exhibited significantly more dissociation than a comparison group of nonabused children who attended a child psychiatry outpatient clinic.

Hysterical symptoms appear to be closely related to dissociation. In his early paper, "The Etiology of Hysteria," Freud (1896/1968) described the importance of childhood seduction and sexual abuse in causing hysterical symptoms in adult life. According to Freud, victims of childhood sexual abuse repressed their memories of these traumatic events, but the memories emerge from the unconscious in the form of hysterical symptoms, which were provoked by situations linked in some way to the original trauma. In the modern literature, Gross (1979) reported hysterical seizures in four incest victims, whereas Goodwin, Cheeves, and Connell (1989) described six cases of hysterical seizures in adolescents who had experienced incest. The hysterical symptoms were interpreted as the child's attempt to "wall off" traumatic impressions of the incest through primitive defenses of denial, isolation of affect, and splitting.

In reviewing the anxiety-related behaviors of abused children, there appears to be a continuum of defensive reactions, beginning with hypervigilance to protect against retraumatization, phobic avoidance as a conscious response to trauma, hysterical symptoms highlighting repression and isolation of affect, and dissociative states involving alterations in memory and identity, the last two defenses operating on an unconscious level. In PTSD, the avoidant and dissociative defenses buttressed by a constricted affect fail to prevent a breakthrough of intrusive recollections of the traumatic event accompanied by autonomic hyperarousal.

Child Abuse and Depression

Depression is one of the most common sequelae of child maltreatment. There is mounting evidence linking physical and sexual abuse to subsequent depression in the victims. This depression is often accompanied by low self-esteem, self-destructive behavior, apathy, and runaway behavior.

Gaensbauer and Sands (1979) studied a group of 48 physically abused and neglected infants between 6 and 36 months of age. Compared to normals, these infants exhibited a variety of distorted affective communications which interfered with mutual engagement and elicited negative responses in caretakers. These consisted of social and affective withdrawal, a failure to respond to or initiate pleasurable responses with others, unpredictable affective communication, shallowness and ambiguity of affect, and a preponderance of such negative affects as distress, anger, and sadness. In a later study, Gaensbauer (1982) indicated that abused and neglected infants displayed less pleasure, less interest in toys, and higher ratings for sadness than did normal infants.

Depressive symptoms and suicidal or self-destructive behavior have been described in physically abused preschool children (P. A. Rosenthal & S. Rosenthal, 1984) and school age children (Allen & Tarnowski, 1989; Green, 1978b). According to Green (1978a,b), the physically abused child's sense of worthlessness, badness, and self-hatred as a consequence of parental assault, rejection, and scapegoating formed the nucleus for subsequent self-destructive behavior.

Depressive symptoms have also been widely observed in sexually abused children (R. Kempe & C. H. Kempe, 1978; MacVicar, 1979; Nakashima & Zakins, 1977).

Sgroi (1982) described depression, guilt, and low self-esteem, along with a sensation of permanent physical damage or "damaged goods syndrome" as pivotal issues facing victims of child sexual abuse. Two studies of sexually abused adolescents admitted to psychiatric inpatient facilities (Cavaiola & Schiff, 1989; Sansonnet-Hayden, Haley, Marriage, & Fine, 1987) reported that the victims of sexual abuse demonstrated a greater severity of depressive symptoms and more suicide attempts than did nonabused inpatients. Livingston (1987) evaluated 13 sexually abused children who were psychiatric inpatients and reported that 10 of them manifested major depressive disorder with psychotic features.

Although the literature clearly documents the presence of depression, alterations in affect, and suicidal behavior in maltreated children, the nature of the link between physical or sexual abuse and depression has not been precisely defined. Green (1981) theorized that the physically abusive parent not only fails to soothe and protect the child from abnormal levels of stimulation, but adds physical assault, scapegoating, and rejection that contribute to a core affective disturbance which forms the nucleus for subsequent depression and a negative self-image. Green (1978b) also posited that the abused child's feelings of badness and self-hatred, which are derived from the parental assault and scapegoating, lead to depression and self-destructive behavior. Green attributed the depressive and self-destructive behavior manifested by physically abused children to primitive learned behavior patterns originating in the earliest painful encounters with hostile caretakers rather than to self-punishment out of a sense of guilt. Self-hatred and self-destructive behavior might also represent the abused child's compliance with the rejecting and destructive parental attitudes directed toward him or her.

Finkelhor and Browne (1986) maintained that the depression in sexually abused children is caused by the betrayal by the parent resulting in the loss of this trusted figure, feelings of powerlessness and exploitation, and stigmatization which produces feelings of badness, shame, and guilt which become incorporated in the child's self-image.

Child Abuse and Impaired Impulse Control

Impaired impulse control is characteristic of physically and sexually abused children. Victims of physical abuse are typically unable to control aggression, while sexually abused children have difficulty containing and modulating sexual impulses.

Green (1978a) described the aggressive and destructive behavior in physically abused children which occurred at home or in school. A controlled study by George and Main (1979) reported hyperaggressive behavior in physically abused infants and toddlers from 1 to 3 years of age. They assaulted their peers in a day-care setting twice as often as did the nonabused controls. Fraiberg (1982) cited "fighting" in toddlers as an early defense against the helplessness and self-dissolution accompanying extreme danger. Livingston (1987) documented a diagnosis of conduct disorder in 87% of a population of abused children who were inpatients in a psychiatric hospital.

Retrospective studies of murderers (Duncan, 1958; Satten, Menninger, Rosen, & Mayman, 1960) and delinquents (Alfaro, 1977) reported that many of these individuals had been physically abused during childhood. Lewis, Shanok, Pincas, and Glaser. (1979) demonstrated that juvenile delinquents with a history of child abuse were more likely to commit assaultive crimes than their nonabused peers.

According to Green (1978a), the loss of control over aggressive impulses is largely determined by the child's basic identification with violent parents, associated with the use of "identification with the aggressor" as a major defense against feelings of anxiety and helplessness. Aggressive behavior associated with the victimization of others also represents an attempt to achieve mastery by turning a passive humiliating experience into an active attempt to control a feared object. The impulsive, hyperaggressive behavior may also be regarded as an intrusion or reenactment of the original traumatic event, which breaches the child's defenses. Whether the aggression is regarded as a learned defensive operation or a breakthrough of uncontrolled impulse, its link to the original abuse is clear. Thus the uncontrolled aggression may ultimately be understood as a posttraumatic symptom. The loss of impulse control is further enhanced by the presence of CNS dysfunction.

Sexually abused children characteristically exhibit defects in controlling and integrating sexual impulses. Yates (1982) described the eroticization of preschool children by incest. These young children were orgastic and maintained a high level of sexual arousal. They failed to differentiate affectionate from sexual relationships and became aroused by routine physical and affectionate closeness. Friedrich and Reams (1987) cited the high level of sexual play by sexually abused children as a major issue in their treatment. MacVicar described compulsive masturbation in sexually abused girls of latency age and reported promiscuity as a common feature of adolescent victims. Browning and Boatman (1977) and Sloane and Karpinski (1942) theorized that the promiscuity in incest victims represented the acting out of conflicts in lieu of developing neurotic symptoms. Brant and Tisza (1977) maintained that these incest victims provoked further sexual contact as a means of obtaining pleasure and need satisfaction and as a technique for mastering the original trauma.

The study of sexual offenders provides another perspective on the link between sexual victimization and dyscontrol of sexual impulses. Several investigators (Abel, Becker, Cunningham-Rathner, Rouleau, Kaplan, & Reich, 1984; Groth & Burgess, 1979; Langevin, Handy, Hook, Day & Russon, 1985) reported a high incidence of childhood molestation in the backgrounds of adult male sexual offenders. Becker and Kaplan (1988) also found a frequent history of childhood sexual victimization in adolescent male sexual offenders. Although fewer women are involved in the sexual abuse of children, studies of these female perpetrators also reveal a high frequency of sexual abuse during their childhood (Marvasti, 1986; McCarty, 1986). McQuire, Carlisle, and Young (1965) suggested that learning is established by the process of fantasizing the initial deviant sexual experience and pairing these fantasies with orgasm, which reinforces the offending behavior.

Van der Kolk (1989) regarded the proneness of physically and sexually abused children to eventually victimize others, or to place themselves at risk for further victimization as a behavioral reenactment of the trauma based on hyperarousal on a neuroendocrine and psychobiological level. The hyperarousal is associated with dysregulation of noradrenergic and serotonergic activity. According to van der Kolk, the abuse victim may become "addicted" to the trauma on the basis of increased endogenous opioid responses which may produce dependence and withdrawal similar to that observed in individuals who are addicted to exogenous opioids. Van der Kolk used the animal model of inescapable shock to buttress his theory concerning human traumatization and the compulsion to repeat the trauma, in that animals that are unable to avoid the shock manifest similar pathological alterations in the levels of neurotransmitters and endogenous opioids.

Although the biological substrate of the dyscontrol of sexual and aggressive impulses needs further study, the psychological dimensions appear to be overdetermined and related to hyperarousal, early identifications and modeling, a need for mastery over helplessness through repetition, and a relative weakness of higher level psychological defenses against the trauma, such as repression, sublimation, and intellectualization. Insofar as the original elements of the physical and sexual assaults are repeated and reenacted and poorly controlled, they should be regarded as evidence of a genuine posttraumatic stress response.

Cognitive Impairment Associated with Physical Abuse

Physically abused children frequently display cognitive and intellectual impairment associated with delayed development on standardized IQ and developmental tests (Elmer & Gregg, 1967; Morse, Sahler, & Friedman, 1970; Smith, 1975). Martin (1972) documented mental retardation in one third of a sample of abused children. Thirty-eight percent of these children exhibited delayed language development. Oates (1986) and Sandgrund, Gaines, and Green (1974) reported depressed IQ scores in abused children compared with nonabused controls. Although some physically abused children sustain cognitive damage as a result of their abuse, in some cases this impairment might have preceded the maltreatment or even provoked it. Speech and language impairment in abused children might be caused by an inhibition of these functions if the child is frequently beaten while crying or vocalizing, on the basis of a conditioned emotional response.

Central Nervous System Impairment Associated with Physical Abuse

Neurological impairment has been documented in several retrospective studies of abused children (Baron, Bejar, & Sheaff, 1970; Smith & Hanson, 1974) but the etiology of this impairment is unclear. Martin, Beezly, Conway, and Kemp (1974) reported that many abused children with skull fractures and subdural hematomas were neurologically intact, but many abused children without head injury exhibited neurological deficits. Green, Voeller, Gaines, and Kubil (1981) reported that 52% of abused children without head injury demonstrated neurological impairment compared with 14% of the nonabused controls. However, the abused sample was not significantly more damaged than a neglected, nonabused comparison group, suggesting that the adverse physical and psychological environment associated with maltreatment, such as inadequate prenatal care, perinatal trauma, poor infant care, inadequate nutrition, and abnormal extremes of sensory stimulation may be more damaging to the CNS than the physical assault itself.

The cognitive and CNS impairment associated with physical abuse/neglect may contribute to the further traumatization of the child victims in that (1) their verbal and language impairment favors behavioral reenactment and direct motor discharge of affects and attitudes concerning the victimization, (2) defenses against aggressive impulses and intolerable affects are weakened, and (3) their deviancy in social and academic areas may lead to further scapegoating and abuse.

Adult Survivors of Child Maltreatment

The study of adult survivors of childhood physical and sexual abuse offers a longitudinal perspective to the traumatization process and the long-range coping of the victims. Many of the symptoms and psychiatric disorders of the survivors are similar to those displayed by the children, but there are also significant differences in the victim's adaptation one generation later. Some of these are caused by the apparent disruption of the linkage between the current symptoms in the adult and the childhood trauma, in some cases, at least, on a conscious level.

Anxiety

Anxiety attacks and anxiety-related symptoms, such as tension, sleep disturbance, nightmares, and somatic preoccupations, have been reported to be more frequent in former sexual abuse victims than in nonabused comparison groups (Briere, 1984; Briere & Runtz, 1985; Sedney & Brooks, 1984). These manifestations of anxiety may be chronic and relatively independent of the original trauma, or might be exacerbated by exposure to events resembling the sexual abuse. Lindberg and Distad (1985) described sleep disturbance, guilt, intrusive imagery of the incest, and feelings of detachment or constricted affect and sexual dysfunction in formerly molested women who were exposed to reminders of the incest. Lindberg and Distad regarded these symptoms as a manifestation of delayed or chronic PTSD. Gelinas (1983) attributed the persistent long-term negative effects of incest, which included symptoms of denial alternating with repetitive intrusions of the traumatic experience, such as nightmares, hallucinations, behavioral reenactments, dissociation, depression, and impulsivity to a chronic traumatic neurosis.

Former sexual abuse victims also report a higher frequency of symptoms of dissociation and "out-of-body experiences" than nonabused comparison groups (Briere, 1984). Briere and Runtz (1985) maintained that the dissociation originally used to escape the unpleasant sensations of the sexual molestation later becomes an autonomous symptom.

Although some of the symptoms of anxiety appear to be chronic and more generalized, the unconscious link to the trauma is clearly visible in the cases of chronic or delayed PTSD, in which symptoms of anxiety and intrusions of the trauma are elicited by exposure to events evoking the victimization.

Depression, Low Self-Esteem, and Suicidal Behavior

According to Finkelhor (1986), depression is the most commonly reported symptom reported among adults who were molested as children. Depressive symptoms have been described by Bagley and Ramsay (1986), Sedney and Brooks (1984), and Peters (1985). Briere and Runtz (1985) reported that formerly sexually abused subjects had more depressive symptoms than nonabused controls as determined by a modified Hopkins Symptom Checklist. There is also widespread evidence of low self-esteem among adult survivors of child sexual abuse (Bagley & Ramsay, 1986; Courtois, 1979; Herman, 1981). These authors describe feelings of alienation, isolation, stigmatization and a negative self-image which is often associated with depressive symptoms.

Suicidal and self-destructive behavior have also been frequently observed in adults with a history of child sexual abuse. Briere (1984) reported that 51% of adult sexual abuse victims had a history of suicide attempts compared with 34% of nonabused patients, whereas Sedney and Brooks (1984) found that 39% of sexually victimized college students described suicidal ideation compared to 16% of a control group. Additional observations of suicidal sequelae in adult survivors of sexual abuse have been made by Herman (1981) and Bagley and McDonald (1984).

Substance Abuse

Drug and alcohol abuse have been frequently documented as long-term sequelae of sexual abuse, and first appear during adolescence or early adulthood. Briere (1984) reported that 27% and 21% of sexual abuse victims had a history of alcohol and drug abuse, respectively. Herman (1981) found that 35% of female incest victims abused drugs or alcohol, whereas Goodwin, Cheeves, and Connell (1990) found that 80% of women attending a psychotherapy group for incest survivors, who had been former psychiatric inpatients, had abused drugs or alcohol. Clinical experience with adolescents and young adults with a history of sexual abuse reveals that these substances help to blot out the painful memories and affects associated with the victimization.

Eating Disorders

There has been increasing evidence of the relationship between victimization experiences and eating disorders. Oppenheimer, Howells, Palmer, and Chandler (1985) found that two thirds of their sample of 78 eating disordered patients with anorexia and bulimia reported a history of sexual abuse. Kearney-Cooke (1988) reported that 58% of 75 bulimic patients had been sexually abused during childhood. Sloan and Leighner (1986) documented a history of sexual abuse in 5 of 6 inpatients on an eating disorders unit. Root and Fallon (1988) reported a high incidence of various types of victimization in a sample of 172 bulimic women. Twenty-nine percent of these women were sexually molested, 23% were raped, 29% were physically abused, and 23% were battered by their spouses. Goodwin *et al.* (1989) hypothesized a relationship between habitual vomiting in patients with eating disorders and conflicts regarding oral sex.

Eating disorders often begin during adolescence, and usually reflect underlying problems in self and body image and in sexual identity. The rigid, obsessional, and avoidant anorexic survivor of child sexual abuse is likely to be defending against sexual impulses and an adult sexual identity in attempting to avoid or postpone physical and psychological evidence of female sexuality.

The bulimic, on the other hand, has a more hysterical and impulsive personality organization in which binging and purging might represent the displacement and reenactment of unconscious incestuous sexual conflicts.

Impaired Impulse Control

Aggressive and Assaultive Behavior

The physically abused child's inability to control impulses is frequently perpetuated throughout adolescence and adult life. They often remain aggressive and violence prone, and often engage in delinquency and antisocial behavior during adolescence and early adulthood. Retrospective studies of murderers (Duncan, 1958; Satten *et al.*, 1960) reported that many of these individuals had been physically abused during childhood. Alfaro (1977) documented a high incidence of delinquent and criminal activity in an adult population who were reported abused or neglected as children in the previous generation. Ressler and Burgess (1985) found that 42% of 31 sexual murderers reported childhood physical abuse, 39% reported child sexual abuse, and 74% were victims of psychological abuse. Lewis *et al.* (1979) demonstrated that juvenile delinquents with a history of physical abuse were more likely to commit assaultive crimes than their nonabused peers. Geller and Ford-Somma (1984) found that two thirds of a population of incarcerated juvenile offenders reported being beaten with a belt or extension cord.

Frequently, physically abused children become abusive parents in the next generation. According to Steele (1983), "with few exceptions, parents and other caretakers who maltreat babies were themselves neglected and abused in their own childhood." Steele maintained that the infant tends to reproduce the affect and behavior of the caretaker and hypothesized a specific kind of identification with a parent aggressor against a child

victim. Retrospective studies indicate that physically abusing parents report a high rate of physical and emotional maltreatment during their own childhood (Steele & Pollock, 1968; Green, Gaines, & Sandgrund, 1974). Egeland, Jacobvitz, and Papatola (1987) followed the child-care practices of women who had been abused in childhood for a period of 3 years. Seventy percent of these mothers either maltreated or provided borderline care for their children, whereas all but one of a comparison group of nonabused mothers with a history of good parenting provided adequate care for her child.

There is considerable evidence that the abused child is at risk for reenacting the original violent interaction with his parents in subsequent relationships with peers and offspring, supporting a theory of intergenerational transmission of violence.

Disorders of Sexual Behavior

Many clinical studies describe sexual problems in adult survivors of child sexual abuse ranging from inhibition and diminished sexual activity because of guilt, anxiety, and dissatisfaction to promiscuity and a compulsive increase in sexual activity (Goodwin *et al.*, 1989; Herman, 1981; Langmade, 1983; Meiselman, 1979). Courtois (1979) found that 80% of former incest victims reported either an avoidance or inability to enjoy sexual activity or a compulsive desire for sex. James and Meyerding (1977) and Silbert and Pines (1981) observed that 55% and 60% of their respective samples of prostitutes had been sexually abused as children.

It appears that the extremes of sexual hyperarousal and sexual avoidance typical of the sexually abused child may be continued into adult life, as a reflection of the original, posttraumatic vacillations between intrusive reenactment and avoidance, corresponding to an inadequate or excessive control over sexual impulses, respectively.

Revictimization

Russell (1986) found that between 33% and 68% of the sexually abused victims (depending on the seriousness of the abuse they suffered) were subsequently raped, compared to an incidence of rape in 17% of nonabused women. Miller Moeller, Kaufman, Divasto, Fitzsimmons, Pather, and Christy (1978) found that 18% of repeat rape victims had incest histories, compared to 4% of first-time victims. In addition to rape, victims of child sexual abuse also seem more likely to be physically abused by a husband or partner (Briere, 1984; Russell, 1986). Green (1980) described the tendency of some women physically abused as girls to reenact their "victim" status by ultimately choosing physically abusive mates. This proneness towards revictimization may be regarded as evidence of the victim's compulsion to reenact the trauma.

Borderline Personality Disorder

The development of borderline personality disorder is a common finding in adult incest survivors, especially females. Stone (1981) and Stone, Unwin, Beacham, and Swenson (1988) documented histories of childhood incest in 36% and 41% of recently hospitalized female patients who had been diagnosed with borderline personality disorder in New York and Brisbane, Australia respectively. Bryer, Nelson, Miller, and Krol (1987) found that 86% of 14 hospitalized borderline patients had a history of sexual abuse before age 16, whereas sexual abuse was reported by only 21% of the entire inpatient population. Herman, Perry, and van der Kolk (1989) reported that 71% of outpatients diagnosed as borderline personality disorder had a childhood history of physical abuse, whereas 68% had a history of child sexual abuse. Herman and van der Kolk (1987) attribute the higher incidence of borderline personality disorder in women to the more widespread sexual victimization of girls. Herman *et al.* (1989) regarded borderline personality disorder as a complicated posttraumatic syndrome in which the subjects fail to perceive a connection between their current symptoms and their abusive childhood experiences. These authors maintained that the memories of abuse become integrated in the total personality organization and become ego-syntonic. Perusal of the DSM-III-R (APA, 1987) criteria for borderline personality disorder highlight the symptoms of impulsivity associated with intense anger or suicidal, self-mutilating behavior, and affective instability with depression, both of which are typical behaviors in maltreated children and in adult survivors of child abuse.

Multiple Personality Disorder

Multiple personality disorder, a chronic and extreme dissociative reaction, usually has its origins in childhood. The primary etiological factor in the genesis of this disorder is childhood trauma, particularly sexual and/or physical abuse (Putnam, 1985; Wilbur, 1984). Using hypnosis, Bliss (1980) documented the role of sexual and physical abuse in the formation of alter personalities in patients with multiple personality disorder. Horevitz and Braun (1984) described the similarity between patients with multiple personality disorder and borderlines. They found that 70% of patients with a diagnosis of multiple personality disorder also fulfilled the DSM-III criteria for borderline personality disorder. Like borderline patients, the patients with multiple personality disorder reacted in an extreme manner to mild environmental stimuli because they were unable to connect their current anxiety with repressed traumatic events. These authors observed that borderlines also exhibit self-fragmentation and dissociation, but to a lesser degree than do patients with multiple personality.

Additional Posttraumatic Syndromes

Frequently, adult survivors of incest and physical abuse engage in self-mutilation (Green, 1978b; Stone, 1989) and exhibit somatization disorder, (Goodwin *et al.*, 1989; Stone, 1989) and histrionic and avoidant personality disorders (Stone, 1989). According to Goodwin *et al.* (1989), suicidality and somatization appear together in about one quarter of adult incest victims. Morrison (1989) reported that 55% of a sample of women with somatization disorder had been molested during childhood.

Comparison of Child Victims and Adult Survivors

The child victims and adult survivors of abuse are alike in that they exhibit similar core symptoms of anxiety, depression, and impulsivity, which cause psychological impairment and suffering. They differ in that the survivors are less consciously preoccupied with the traumatic event because of the passage of time and the absence of the original abuser and the wider variety of defenses at their disposal. The defenses often coalesce into personality traits, attitudes, and identifications which become ego-syntonic and appear to be unrelated to the trauma. Combinations of defenses, identifications, and symptoms form personality disorders which often give rise to disturbances in object relationships. Since the adults are less immersed in the original trauma, they are less likely to experience typical symptoms of PTSD, but a delayed PTSD can be elicited by events resembling the original traumatization. However, the persistence of childhood symptoms, and the deployment of maladaptive defenses and personality traits derived from the original victimization suggest that the adult survivors experience posttraumatic stress reactions in a broader sense. In these situations, the new symptom or defense replaces the original anxiety (i.e., addictive behavior, conversion reaction, self-mutilation, etc.).

The Traumatization Process in Child Abuse

The nature of the traumatic process in cases of physical and sexual abuse of children is different from traditional types of trauma associated with PTSD (i.e., accidents, catastrophes, combat stress, and exposure to single and discrete overwhelming episodes). First of all, the parents are the instruments of trauma in child abuse, whereas parents are usually protective and supportive in extrafamilial traumatic situations. The painful reality of victimization by a parent from whom nurturance and protection is expected and needed cannot be readily assimilated by the child, who may rely on splitting and dissociative defenses as a means of survival. Second, the traumatic events are recurrent and of long duration. Physical and sexual abuse often go on for years before disclosure, so that the dread of retraumatization is ever present. In most other forms of PTSD, there is usually one major catastrophic event which is unlikely to be repeated. The ongoing nature of the trauma in cases of abuse is more likely to result in pathological changes in character structure and personality. Finally, the traumatic elements in a child-abuse situation are numerous and would appear to have a cumulative effect on the victim. Instead of the trauma acting as a single independent variable, the victim must deal with the physical or sexual assault, the lack of protection by the nonoffending parent, frequent rejection and scapegoating associated with the abuse, a deviant and pathological family, and family disruption in the aftermath of disclosure. Another way of conceptualizing the dimensions of trauma in child abuse is to consider the sexual or physical assault as the acute traumatic event which is inflicted upon a background of chronic punitive or inappropriate parenting, scapegoating, and rejection. In cases of physical abuse, CNS dysfunction may be superimposed.

Acute Physical or Sexual Assault

The actual or threatened physical or sexual assault may create a sense of helplessness, fear, and disorganization in the child. The sense of betrayal by the parent paired with coercive threats can also lead to fears of abandonment. A painful affective state often ensues, and the child's defensive organization is unable to process the traumatic stimulation. This traumatic situation is consistent with Freud's concept of traumatic neurosis and the breaching of the stimulus barrier (1920/1968). Freud (1926/1968) subsequently defined the traumatic situation as the experience of helplessness on the part of the ego in the face of an accumulation of excitation, whether of external or internal origin. Boyer (1956) stressed the parent's role as a supplementary stimulus barrier, but in case of abuse, the parent not only fails to buttress the stimulus barrier, but adds to the trauma. When the barrier is breached, the child's receptive, defensive, and integrative ego functions are overwhelmed, rendering the child helpless. The core symptoms of anxiety, depression, and impulsivity begin to emerge. The abused child initiates primitive defenses to deal with the traumatic overstimulation that repression fails to control. Avoidance and distancing behavior, consisting of hypervigilance, gaze aversion, and the raising of sensory thresholds are attempts to control the noxious stimulation. Defenses of denial, projection, and splitting allow the child to maintain the fantasy of having a "good" parent, whereas the parent's malevolence is displaced onto some other person or himself.

These defenses often fail to bind the anxiety generated by the abuse, and the traumatic imagery derived from the physical or sexual assault invades the dreams, fantasies, play, and object relationships of the child victims. The children begin to repeat and reenact traumatic themes to cope with their helplessness and feelings of being overwhelmed. Whether the reenactments involve victimization of others in play or fantasy, actual sexual or physical assaults on peers, or provocative behavior designed to elicit abuse or punishment from the environment, they represent a "fixation" on the trauma as described by Freud (1939/1968).

CASE ILLUSTRATION

Sarah, a 6-year-old girl, had been physically abused by her mother since she was an infant. Her mother beat her severely for letting a bathroom sink overflow when she was four, resulting in a fractured femur. During her first evaluation in the child psychiatry clinic, Sarah responded to the presentation of a hitting scene in a doll family with the comment, "The mother hits the baby for playing with water." During the psychiatric interview a short time later, Sarah appeared quite anxious upon returning from the bathroom. She told the doctor that she was afraid he would punish her for spilling water from the sink onto the floor.

Repetition of the trauma may be regarded as another primitive defense mechanism, in which the traumatic elements are reenacted in a relatively unmodified form in an attempt to achieve active mastery over a passively experienced danger. The child tries to recreate, master, and control painful affects and anxiety engendered during the traumatic assault.

Severe episodes of physical and sexual abuse may produce a PTSD response, with typical symptoms of anxiety, alternating intrusions and avoidance of traumatic stimuli, and evidence of hyperarousal, roughly corresponding to other types of discrete catastrophic events causing PTSD in children. These short "one shot" traumata have been described as "Type I" trauma by Terr (1987).

Long-Term Traumatic Elements in Physical and Sexual Abuse

The chronic parental dysfunction that occurs in abusive families exerts a cumulative, undermining impact on the child's ego functioning and development. The ongoing deficits in parenting constitute "cumulative" trauma, a concept described by Khan (1963) which is caused by the parent's failure to function as a protective shield for the child; these deficits may alternatively be regarded as a form of "strain" trauma (Kris, 1956) which refers to the traumatic effects of long-lasting stressors. These long-standing multiple traumas are also consistent with the Terr (1987) concept of "Type II" trauma.

Harsh and Punitive Child Rearing

Prolonged exposure to a harsh, punitive physically abusing parent or to a coercive sexually deviant parent promotes a primary identification with the aggressive parent. "Identification with the aggressor" is used as a major defense mechanism in situations of anxiety provoked by fears of attack, helplessness, and humiliation. While using this defense, the child's fears of helplessness are replaced by feelings of power, control, and omnipotence.

CASE ILLUSTRATION

Juan, an 11-year-old boy, was referred to a child psychiatry clinic after he forced his 3-year-old half-brother to drink lye. Juan had returned to live with his mother and her boyfriend one year prior to this incident after having spent the previous 7 years with his father and stepmother in Puerto Rico. Juan had been subjected to chronic and severe physical abuse by his father during this period, which consisted of beatings on the head and burns on his body inflicted with a hot iron. Since returning to his mother, Juan became hyperactive and aggressive at home and in school and exhibited extreme jealousy toward his two half-brothers whom he encountered for the first time and whom he hit frequently. He confided in his therapist that he enjoyed catching mice, placing them in boiling water, and smashing their heads with a hammer, after which he would flush them down the toilet. When asked to explain this cruel behavior, Juan pointed to the scars and ridges on his scalp and the burn marks on his shoulder exclaiming, "This is what my father did to me."

"Identification with the aggressor" appears to be embedded in the child's compulsion to repeat and re-enact the trauma. This trauma-induced defense permits the child to displace some of his original rage towards the abusive parent onto a substitute, and may also serve as a tension-relieving device and as a pathologic form of self-esteem regulation. Children such as Juan often display an inordinate degree of excitement during their aggressive outbursts, possibly reflecting an associated autonomic hyperarousal and a loss of impulse control.

Exposure to a sexually aggressive parent may induce a similar type of "identification with the aggressor" but in these cases the aggression is expressed in a driven, hypersexual fashion.

CASE ILLUSTRATION

Sharon, a 6-year-old girl, was referred for a psychiatric evaluation when her precocious sexual behavior at school alarmed the teachers and her classmates, whom she seduced by taking them into the bathroom and fondling their genitals. This seductive school behavior launched the investigation which disclosed that Sharon had been sexually abused by her father and other gays and lesbians at homosexual orgies. During her therapy, Sharon repeatedly tried to apply "makeup" on herself and her male therapist by using crayons and magic markers. She tried to seduce the therapist by attempting to sit on his lap. Further exploration by the therapist revealed that Sharon's father used to dress her up in women's clothing and helped her apply lipstick and makeup as a prelude to their sexual activity.

Like their physically abused counterparts, sexually victimized children reduce their anxiety by identifying with the sexual aggressor, which provides them with a means of actively controlling a passively endured trauma.

Scapegoating and Stigmatization

Severe physical abuse and sexual abuse are usually limited to one child in a family. Often, the abused child is scapegoated and blamed for the inadequacy of the parents and other family members. This child is most closely identified with the abusing parent, who projects his or her own deficiencies onto the child, who assumes that he or she is to blame and is deserving of the punishment. This increases the child's self-hatred, low self-esteem, and depressive affect, which become the nucleus for subsequent masochistic and self-destructive behavior.

CASE ILLUSTRATION

Victor, a small 12-year-old boy, was referred for psychiatric treatment because of poor conduct and academic problems at school and chronic depression. Victor's parents divorced when he was 8 after a stormy relationship in which his mother was frequently battered by his father. His mother resented being pregnant with Victor and tried to abort him by pushing on her stomach. After Victor's premature birth after a 7-month gestation, his mother rarely visited him in the premature nursery and confessed that she had hoped he would die. The mother perceived Victor as a sickly, emaciated, and unresponsive baby who reminded her more and more of her despised husband.

During his initial psychotherapy sessions, Victor referred to himself as a "goofy" kid, and he described being teased by his classmates for being too small and afraid to fight. In his play, he depicted himself as a "sad baby monster" who was destroyed by battleships because he was "different." He was jealous of his three younger sisters and his "tall" older brother who were closer to his mother.

This pervasive sense of badness, shame, and guilt occurs in sexually abused children. Finkelhor (1986) referred to stigmatization of the sexually abused child in which the stigma is induced by the pressure for secrecy by the offender or by the child's awareness that the incest is considered deviant, or if the child is blamed for the sexual activity. Keeping the incest a secret increases the stigma as it reinforces the sense of being different.

Maternal Deprivation, Abandonment, and Family Disorganization

Physical abuse of children, especially if it occurs in multiproblem, impoverished families, is often accompanied by other types of parental dysfunction, such as neglect, multiple caretaking, maternal deprivation, and substandard physical care. These deficiencies in parenting are compounded by a stressful environment and lack of support systems. Therefore, the specific sequelae of physical abuse will be superimposed on the detrimental effects of neglect and deprivation, such as affect hunger, cognitive impairment, impaired attachment, and lack of object constancy. The threat of parental rejection and object loss occurs during beatings which are interpreted by the child as the parent's wish to be rid of him.

Sexually abused children are faced with threats of parental loss and abandonment from a different source, namely threats of harm or imprisonment to themselves or their parents if secrecy about their molestation is breached. When the sexual abuse is disclosed, the marriage is often dissolved and the offending parent, usually the father, is forced to leave home. An additional source of anxiety for the sexually abused child stems from the frequent emotional unavailability of the mothers in incest families. Needless to say, separation anxiety and other attachment disorders in both physically and sexually abused children will be augmented if they are placed in institutional or foster care as a result of their maltreatment. Their vulnerability to separation has been frequently observed in their therapy sessions, where they often exhibit extreme separation anxiety in response to missed appointments and vacations of their therapists.

Central Nervous System Impairment

CNS impairment, as a result of brain trauma or "shaking injury" inflicted during physical abuse, or as a preexisting factor provoking the abuse, will render the child more vulnerable to the traumatic impact of physical abuse. The CNS impairment will further undermine the cognitive, adaptive, and defensive functions of the ego during their response to trauma, and facilitate the acting out of impulses.

Finkelhor and Browne (1986) identified four trauma-causing or "traumagenic" factors in sexual abuse: (1) Traumatic sexualization, occurring through the sexual stimulation and reinforcement of the child's sexual responses so that the child learns to use sexual behavior to gratify numerous nonsexual needs. This leads to inappropriate and premature sexual activity and deviant sexual arousal. (2) Powerlessness, which is derived from the helplessness during the sexual assault, leads to fear and anxiety. (3) Stigmatization, which describes the child's sense of being damaged and blamed for the molestation, leads to shame, guilt, and low self-esteem. (4) Betrayal, which refers to the child's disillusionment at being sexually exploited by a trusted parent or caretaker, may lead to a generalized mistrust of others.

While the traumagenic dynamics conceptualized by Finkelhor and Browne (1986) are comprehensive and helpful in isolating specific traumatic elements and their sequelae, they lack a temporal perspective to account for the occurrence of immediate and long-term symptoms.

Traumatic Process, Choice of Symptoms, and Diagnostic Considerations

The acute, overwhelming physical and sexual assaults, which render the child fearful and helpless, produce anxiety-related symptoms such as sleep disturbance, nightmares, autonomic hyperarousal, intrusive imagery, and reenactments, as well as the avoidant, numbing, and dissociative defenses against the painful experience. This will often produce a clinical picture of PTSD. Sexual and physical abuse of less severe proportions may only satisfy partial criteria for PTSD, or produce signs of overanxious disorder, separation anxiety disorder, or avoidant disorder of childhood or adolescence.

The long-term continuous parental dysfunction is more likely to result in personality disorders, in which the initial anxiety is gradually transformed into distorted personality traits, attitudes, identifications, and self-image, which, in turn, give rise to chronic depressive symptoms and cause difficulties in object relationships. For example, the victims of harsh, punitive parenting who primarily identify with the aggressive aspects of their abusers will be likely to exhibit symptoms of a conduct disorder, other impulse disorders, or antisocial personality disorder as they reenact the original abuser–victim relationship with new objects. Children identifying with sexually abusive parents and who experienced long-standing traumatic sexualization are prone to confusion about their sexual identity, sexually aggressive

behavior, promiscuity, prostitution, and various forms of sexual dysfunction involving extremes of sexual hyperarousal and sexual inhibition.

Children exposed to scapegoating and stigmatization display guilt, shame, low self-esteem and often feel responsible for their victimization. They are vulnerable to major depressive disorder, suicidal behavior, and self-mutilation. Some of these victims of scapegoating exhibit substance abuse, eating disorders, or somatization disorders, which may be regarded as depressive equivalents or as defenses against depressive affect.

Physically or sexually abused children experiencing actual or threatened abandonment during or as an aftermath of their maltreatment, multiple caretakers, or neglect might be vulnerable to depression, apathy, poor self-care, accident proneness, and disorders of attachment, such as separation anxiety disorder and reactive attachment disorder.

Physically abused children with CNS impairment may develop specific learning disabilities and language disorders, hyperactivity, poor impulse control, and seizure disorders.

The choice of personality disorder will ultimately be shaped by the relative concentrations of impulsivity, depression, and dissociation, as well as constitutional factors. For example, high levels of impulsivity and dissociation might produce a histrionic personality disorder, whereas a mixture of impulsivity, dissociation, and depression could lead to a borderline personality disorder. Organicity is another factor that has been etiologically linked to borderline personality disorder (Bemporad, Smith, Hanson, & Cicchetti, 1982). On the other hand, if dissociation is the primary defense, the victim would display dissociative states or multiple personality disorder. The presence of depression with a strong presence of stigmatization and compromised self-image and body integrity might result in an eating disorder or somatization disorder.

The severity of both the acute and long-term sequelae of child maltreatment depends on the following variables: (1) age and developmental level of the child; (2) the child's preexisting personality; (3) onset, duration, and frequency of the abuse; (4) severity of the physical or sexual abuse; (5) the relationship between the child and the perpetrator; (6) the family's response to disclosure; (7) the institutional response (i.e., the nature of evaluations by protective service caseworkers, police investigators, court testimony, hospitalization, placement out of the home, etc.); and (8) the availability and quality of therapeutic intervention.

Traumatic Impact of Physical and Sexual Abuse

The following case histories are presented in order to illustrate the interplay between immediate and long-term traumatic elements that are associated with child maltreatment, their impact on the child's coping strategies over time, and the vulnerability of the children to retraumatization.

CASE HISTORY—PHYSICAL ABUSE

Charles, a 16-year-old boy, was referred for psychiatric evaluation after his second arrest for a weapons violation. At the age of 12, Charles was placed on probation after shooting his junior high school teacher with a pellet gun. This incident occurred after he was reprimanded by the teacher for fighting with another boy in the classroom. After the teacher hit him in front of the class for failing to stop the fighting, Charles announced that he would return with a gun and take revenge. He carried out his threat and proceeded to shoot the teacher in the leg. He was living with his maternal grandfather in Florida at this time. After being placed on probation, Charles returned to his mother in New York, where he continued to exhibit behavior problems in school. He was also abusive to his younger brother and was involved in stealing. During the current shooting episode, Charles shot a gun into a crowd of youths who taunted him and several of his friends with racial epithets. Luckily no one was hit, and Charles was arrested on the spot. Charles had stolen the gun from his friend's father and carried it with him in anticipation of an attack. He explained his actions by stating that he feared the youths would attack him and his friends.

Charles was born when his mother, Sally, was 13. Sally had been living with a female cousin and her husband when Charles was conceived. She had been beaten by her cousin and sexually abused by the husband since she was sent to live with them at the age of 4 when her mother died. When Charles was born, Sally had moved, and lived alone in a small room with insufficient money to feed and clothe her infant. Sally initially reared the baby as "unreal, like a doll" and expected that he would make her happy. However, when he cried out of hunger, she beat him severely, "so he would shut up and go to sleep." "I beat him so long he'd scream until he was exhausted," Sally confessed. "I hit him with a belt, extension cord, and anything I could get my hands on."

Charles lived with his mother until he was 4, and was then sent to live with his maternal aunt for 2 years, where he was also physically abused. After this, he was shifted back and forth between his mother, aunt, and maternal grandfather. Charles successfully repressed any memory of the beatings by his mother, but he did remember beatings with switches at the hands of his aunt, and subsequent beatings by a female teacher. He referred to these beatings as "unreal," and admitted that they terrified him.

Charles seemed unperturbed when confronted with the possibility that he might have killed someone. His principal interests are guns and vicious watchdogs, such as rottweilers, Doberman pinschers, and bullterriers because they can be trained to keep potential attackers at bay and kill them if necessary. In a recurrent fantasy, his bullterrier carries out his command to kill an intruder. When Charles becomes 18, he plans to join the army and become a "ranger" to receive training in special gun tactics. He would like to be a sniper so he can stalk the enemy at a distance and then shoot them. Charles experiences violent nightmares, the most recent one depicting a friend trying to kill him.

Case Discussion

Charles responded to his experiences of long-standing harsh and punitive childrearing and maternal deprivation by forming a basic identification with his violent caretakers, which promoted the use of "identification with the aggressor" as a major defense against feelings of anxiety and helplessness. His hypervigilance and paranoid style of relating to others could be traced to early overwhelming perceptions of beatings which are largely repressed. Fixation to the trauma is reflected by the persistent reenactment his victimization in fantasy and actual behavior. His fixation on guns and vicious watchdogs serves a dual purpose of protection from and destruction of the original and potential abusers. Charles's lack of control over aggressive impulses is probably derived from the impulsivity and disorganization associated with the acute posttraumatic anxiety states and the more chronic identifications with violent caretakers. Although the psychiatric evaluation emphasized the conduct disorder and antisocial personality diagnoses, the recurrent outbursts of violent and potentially lethal behavior in response to actual or imagined physical attack reminiscent of the original abuse may be regarded as an example of delayed or chronic PTSD.

CASE HISTORY—SEXUAL ABUSE

Tina was referred for psychiatric evaluation at the age of 8 by her guidance counselor because of disruptive, aggressive behavior in school. Several months earlier, Tina revealed that she and her 10-year-old sister had been sexually molested by her father for the past 2 years. The disclosure was made after Tina was admitted to the hospital with vaginal bleeding and a discharge. A diagnosis of vaginal warts (condyloma acuminatum) was made and the vaginal culture was positive for gonorrhea. Tina described how her father came into their bedroom regularly at night and had vaginal intercourse with her and occasionally with her sister. Tina was so frightened that she would close her eyes and feign sleep during the molestation. The father threatened both girls with beatings if they were to divulge the secret so that they were afraid to tell anyone. When Tina finally told her mother, she was reprimanded for "making up stories." The mother later admitted that she was afraid of confronting her husband with the sexual abuse because she feared his murderous rage, as she had been frequently battered by him.

After the disclosure of the incest, Tina and her sister were temporarily placed with their maternal grandmother, the father was jailed, and the mother was cited for neglect. The children were returned home after the mother agreed to psychiatric evaluation and treatment for the family.

Psychiatric evaluation of Tina revealed a sad, emotionally constricted child who manifested sleep disturbances with nightmares about her father coming into her room. She exhibited a tarnished self-image as she believed that her classmates in school disliked her because of the incest. Yet she discussed her molestation with everyone in a compulsive manner. At home, she fought with her sibling and felt rejected by her mother. In the treatment setting, Tina acted frightened and needy, and tended to cling to her female therapist. She expressed yearnings for nurturance and safety by caring for doll babies and stuffed animals. At home, she began to overeat and steal money from her mother's purse. A constant theme was that her father would return and sexually attack her. She became involved with a repetitive traumatic story which she reenacted with her sister, called "Runaway Haunted House Island." In the story, two sisters run away from their mother after she cooks bad food. They sneak out in the middle of the night to a castle on the island, open the door, and encounter a witchlike lady who gives them a poison potion. The girls fall asleep and wake up and try to escape, but the witch and a dog chase them. They see a scary devil with horns and red hair who joins in the chase. They run back to their own house and their mother becomes good. In a minor variation of the story, they say, "I feel sleepy but I've got to stay awake" after the witch gives them poison. The story ends when the witch was still there, and they find themselves on the floor, having fallen out of bed.

Case Discussion

The runaway haunted house story, which was repetitively acted out by the sisters, symbolized the need of these children to escape their rejecting, unprotective mother and their "devillike" incestuous and brutal father. However, the would-be rescuers turn into the original abusers, so that these reenactments are often unsuccessful in neutralizing the traumatic anxiety. The traumatic impact of the incest experience was also expressed in Tina's spontaneous drawings of sinister devils with phallic horns and children frightened by snakes. A typical snake drawing included small children who were being threatened by large snakes. The children wear eye masks, and squirrels are hiding in the hollow of a tree. These defensive maneuvers of avoidance reflect Tina's "possumlike" behavior during the nightly sexual encounters with her father in her bed.

Tina's feelings of stigmatization and bodily damage were undoubtedly increased by the actual genital damage. She confided in her therapist that she was afraid to go to summer camp because the girls would notice the bleeding of the vaginal warts, which would identify her as an incest victim. When surgical removal of Tina's vaginal warts was planned two years after the onset of her psychotherapy, she reacted with predictable anxiety and the exacerbation of the posttraumatic symptoms. She perceived the operation as a repetition of the violation of her body by her father and began to reexperience sleep difficulties and nightmares. She insisted on having a female surgeon, which fortunately could be arranged. She was afraid of the anesthesia, and being "put to sleep," since the father's assaults occurred at this time. One can predict additional exacerbations of posttraumatic anxiety in the future as Tina anticipates her menstrual period, and during her first sexual relationships when her original feelings of stigmatization and genital damage associated with the incest would be expected to surface. Tina's shame and guilt were also expressed in her fear that she would be sent to jail when she testified in court, because she had "done something wrong."

Implications for Treatment

A conceptual framework which recognizes the difference between acute and long-term traumatic processes operating in maltreated children, and the tendency of trauma victims to rapidly repress or dissociate from terrifying memories will be helpful in designing intervention strategies. Far too often, children are not referred for treatment after the initial posttraumatic anxiety symptoms subside. The victim's psychopathology and suffering might be underestimated if sexual or aggressive acting out is minimal, and depressive symptoms are not prominent. Parents, or even professionals, are often reluctant to recommend treatment after the child has been protected from further abuse, owing to concern over inflicting additional suffering by confronting the victim with the original frightening memories. If the child's phobic, avoidant defenses and constricted affect predominate, the evaluator might be lulled into a false sense of security and regard the child's response to the abuse as an adjustment disorder which will dissipate over time. In other cases, the initial symptoms of anxiety might be overlooked or absent so that the child is felt to be relatively unaffected by the abuse.

Increasing familiarity with the long latency period between the traumatization and the emergence of symptoms in adult survivors of childhood physical and sexual abuse, which often reflect an unrecognized chronic or delayed PTSD, suggests that these individuals would have benefitted from timely intervention during childhood. Therefore, in some cases, mental health intervention with abused children not only alleviates their current symptoms and personality distortions, but will prevent the development of psychiatric disorders in the next generation. It is therefore recommended that each abused child receive a thorough psychiatric evaluation to identify the acute and long-term sequelae of his or her victimization and to design the most effective treatment strategy.

A wide range of psychotherapeutic and educational techniques has proven successful in alleviating the symptoms and distress experienced by the abused children. Individual psychoanalytically oriented play therapy and psychotherapy have been used effectively with abused youngsters, as well as group therapy, whereas family treatment modalities have been used with some dysfunctional abusive families. Psychoeducational intervention can be employed to deal with learning difficulties based upon cognitive and attentional deficits and CNS impairment.

Core symptoms of anxiety, depression, and impulsivity may be alleviated by modifying the abusive environment and providing an accepting and supportive therapeutic milieu, in which the child may express anxiety and painful affects in words or in play. In cases of severe anxiety or depression, anxiolytics or antidepressant medications may be useful. Impulsivity in physically and sexually aggressive children requires structuring, strict limit setting, and interpretations to help them understand their use of "Identification with the aggressor" as a primary defense. Shame and guilt in the stigmatized or scapegoated child may be alleviated by stressing that the perpetrator and not the child is responsible for the abuse. These children require reassurance that they are not permanently damaged. The therapist should be prepared to gratify some of the dependency needs of the deprived abused youngsters. Strengthening of ego functions becomes a major focus, with an emphasis on reality testing, increasing frustration tolerance, and encouraging verbalization as an alternative to the repetitive reenactment of traumatic events. Higher-level defenses, such as repression and sublimation, are strengthened in order to replace primitive mechanisms of denial, projection, splitting, dissociation, and identification with the aggressor. Ultimately, the therapist must convey to the child that his pathological defenses, personality traits, and distorted object relations—designed to master the abusive experience and to control or ward off further assault—are distinctly maladaptive in nontraumatic environments. This can only be accomplished when the therapist helps the child to link these anxiety-related symptoms and defenses back to the original traumatic experiences which are uncovered, remembered, and "worked through" in the safety of the therapeutic setting.

Summary

This chapter describes the major traumatic components inherent in the physical and sexual abuse of children, and explores their role in the development of symptoms, maladaptive defenses and personality traits, and cognitive impairment which may persist throughout adulthood. The child-abuse syndrome consists of two main categories of trauma: the acute physical or sexual assault generating anxiety, helplessness, and disorganization which is superimposed upon long-term traumatic elements inherent in chronic abnormal parenting, such as harsh, punitive, or sexually coercive caretaking styles, scapegoating, rejection, and maternal deprivation and/or parental loss.

It is hypothesized that the acute trauma creates terrifying memories and affects, which cannot be processed in an effective manner, and that result in cycles of intrusions and avoidance of traumatic imagery and increased arousal, which approximate the clinical diagnosis of PTSD. The pathological impact of the long-term traumatic events are most likely exerted on the child's self-concept, identifications, defensive style, and personality traits which lead to pathological object relationships and the development of persisting trauma-related symptoms and personality disorders. Cognitive and CNS impairment, which are frequently associated with physical abuse, may be regarded as additional chronic sequelae which may potentiate the pathological impact of the acute and long-term components of the abusive environment.

Although many cases of physical and sexual abuse fail to generate severe symptoms of anxiety necessary for a diagnosis of PTSD, the appearance of trauma-related symptoms and sequelae upon exposure to events linked to the original victimization many years later suggests that these sequelae of child abuse are "posttraumatic" in the general sense. The importance of providing timely therapeutic intervention for the abused child is emphasized. If the child is helped to remember and work-through the original traumatic experiences, he or she will be less likely to be adversely affected by them in later life.

References

Abel, G., Becker, J., Cunningham-Rathner, J., Rouleau, J., Kaplan, M., & Reich, J. (1984). *The treatment of child molesters.* New York: SBC-TM (722 West 168th Street, Box 17, New York, NY 10032).

Alfaro, J. D. (1977). *Report on the relationship between child abuse and neglect and later socially deviant behavior.* New York State Assembly Select Committee on Child Abuse, New York, NY.

Allen, R., Gaines, R., & Green, A. (1991). *Post-traumatic stress disorder in abused children.* Unpublished manuscript.

Allen, D. M., & Tarnowski, K. J. (1989). Depressive characteristics of physically abused children. *Journal of Abnormal Child Psychology, 17,* 1–11.

American Psychiatric Association. (1987). *Diagnostic and statistical manual of mental disorders* (3rd ed., rev.). Washington, DC: Author.

Bagley, C., & McDonald, M. (1984). Adult mental health sequelae of child sexual abuse, physical abuse, and neglect in maternally separated children. *Canadian Journal of Community Mental Health, 3,* 15–26.

Bagley, C., & Ramsay, R. (1986). Sexual abuse in childhood: Psychosocial outcomes and implications for social work practice. *Journal of Social Work and Human Sexuality, 4,* 33–47.

Baron, M., Bejar, R., & Sheaff, P. (1970). Neurological manifestations of the battered child syndrome. *Pediatrics, 45,* 1003–1007.

Becker, J. V., & Kaplan, M. S. (1988). Assessment and treatment of the male sexual offender. In D. H. Schetky & A. H. Green (Ed.), *Child sexual abuse: A handbook for health care and legal professionals* (pp. 136–149). New York: Brunner/Mazel.

Bemporad, J. R., Smith, H. F., Hanson, G., & Cicchetti, D. (1982). Borderline syndromes in childhood: Criteria for diagnosis. *American Journal of Psychiatry, 139,* 596–601.

Bernstein, M. A., & Putnam, F. W. (1986). Development, reliability, and validity of a dissociation scale. *Journal of Nervous and Mental Disease, 174,* 727–735.

Bliss, E. L. (1980). Multiple personalities: A report of 14 cases with implications for schizophrenia and hysteria. *Archives of General Psychiatry, 37,* 1388–1397.

Boyer, L. B. (1956). On maternal overstimulation and ego defects. *Psychoanalytic Study of the Child, 11,* 236–256.

Brant, R., & Tisza, V. (1977). The sexually misused child. *American Journal of Orthopsychiatry, 47,* 80–90.

Braun, B. G. (1988). BASK model of dissociation. *Dissociation, 1,* 4–23.

Braun, B. G., & Sachs, R. G. (1985). The development of multiple personality disorder: Predisposing, precipitating, and perpetuating factors. In R. P. Kluft (Ed.), *Childhood antecedents of multiple personality* (pp. 38–64). Washington, DC: American Psychiatric Press.

Briere, J. (1984). *The long-term effects of childhood sexual abuse: Defining a post-sexual abuse syndrome.* Paper presented at the Third National Conference on Sexual Victimization of Children, Washington, DC.

Briere, J., & Runtz, M. (1985, August). *Symptomatology associated with prior sexual abuse in a non-clinical sample.* Paper presented at the annual meeting of the American Psychological Association, Los Angeles.

Browning, D., & Boatman, B. (1977). Incest: Children at risk. *American Journal of Psychiatry, 134,* 69–72.

Bryer, J. B., Nelson, B. A., Miller, J. B., & Krol, P. A. (1987). Childhood physical and sexual abuse as factors in adult psychiatric illness. *American Journal of Psychiatry, 144,* 1426–1430.

Cavaiola, A., & Schiff, M. (1988). Behavioral sequelae of physical and/or sexual abuse in adolescents. *Child Abuse and Neglect, 12,* 181–188.

Coons, P. M., Bowman, E. S., Pellow, T. A., & Schneider, P. (1989). Post-traumatic aspects of the treatment of victims of sexual abuse and incest. *Psychiatric Clinics of North America, 12,* 325–335.

Courtois, C. (1979). The incest experience and its aftermath. *Victimology: An International Journal, 4,* 337–347.

Duncan, G. M. (1958). Etiological factors in first degree murder. *Journal of the American Medical Association, 168,* 1755–1758.

Egeland, B., Jacobvitz, D., & Papatola, K. (1987). Intergenerational continuity of parental abuse. In J. Lancaster & R. Gelles (Eds.), *Biosocial aspects of child abuse* (pp. 255–276). San Francisco: Jossey-Bass.

Elmer, E., & Gregg, C. S. (1967). Developmental characteristics of abused children. *Pediatrics, 40,* 596–602.

Finkelhor, D. (1986). *A sourcebook on child sexual abuse.* Beverly Hills: Sage Publications.

Finkelhor, D., & Browne, A. (1986). Initial and long-term effects: A conceptual framework. In D. Finkelhor (Ed.), *A sourcebook on child sexual abuse* (pp. 180–198). Beverly Hills: Sage Publications.

Finkelhor, D., & Hotaling, G. (1984). Sexual abuse in the national incidence study of child abuse and neglect. *Child Abuse and Neglect, 8,* 22–32.

Fraiberg, S. (1982). Pathological defenses in infancy. *Psychoanalytic Quarterly, 51,* 612–635.

Freud, S. (1896). The aetiology of hysteria. In J. Strachey (Ed. and Trans.), *The standard edition of the complete psychological works of Sigmund Freud* (Vol. 3, pp. 179–221). London: Hogarth Press. (Original work published 1896)

Freud, S. (1968). Beyond the pleasure principle. In J. Strachey (Ed. and Trans.), *The standard edition of the complete psychological works of Sigmund Freud* (Vol. 18, pp. 7–64). London: Hogarth Press. (Original work published 1920)

Freud, S. (1968). Inhibitions, symptoms, and anxiety. In J. Strachey (Ed. and Trans.), *The standard edition of the complete psychological works of Sigmund Freud* (Vol. 20, pp. 77–175). London: Hogarth Press.

Freud, S. (1939). Moses and monotheism. In J. Strachey (Ed. and Trans.), *The standard edition of the complete psychological works of Sigmund Freud* (Vol. 23, pp. 77–175). London: Hogarth Press.

Friedrich, W., & Reams, R. (1987). Course of psychological symptoms in sexually abused young children. *Psychotherapy, 24,* 160–171.

Gaensbauer, T. (1982). Regulation of emotional expression in infants from two contrasting environments. *Journal of the American Academy of Child Psychiatry, 21,* 167–171.

Gaensbauer, T., & Sands, K. (1979). Distorted communications in abused/neglected infants and their parents and their potential impact on caretakers. *Journal of the American Academy of Child Psychiatry, 18,* 236–250.

Gelinas, D. (1983). The persisting negative effects of incest. *Psychiatry, 46,* 312–332.

Geller, M., & Ford-Somma, L. (1984). *Violent homes, violent children.* A study of violence in the families of juvenile offenders. (New Jersey State Department of Corrections, Trenton. Division of Juvenile Services) Report prepared for the National Center on Child Abuse and Neglect, Department of Health and Human Services, Washington, DC.

George, C., & Main, M. (1979). Social interactions and young abused children: Approach, avoidance, and aggression. *Child Development, 50,* 306–319.

Goodwin, J. (1985). Post-traumatic symptoms in incest victims. In S. Eth & R. S. Pynoos (Eds.), *Post-traumatic stress disorder in children* (pp. 157–168). Washington, DC: American Psychiatric Press.

Goodwin, J., Cheeves, K., & Connell, V. (1989). Defining a syndrome of severe symptoms in survivors of extreme incestuous abuse. In J. Goodwin (Ed.), *Sexual abuse: Incest victims and their families* (pp. 196–204). Chicago: Year Book Medical Publishers.

Goodwin, J., Cheeves, K., & Connell, V. (1990). Psychotherapy and psychological trauma in borderline personality disorder. *Psychiatric Annals, 20,* 33–43.

Green, A. (1978a). Psychopathology of abused children. *Journal of the American Academy of Child Psychiatry, 17,* 92–103.

Green, A. (1978b). Self-destructive behavior in battered children. *American Journal of Psychiatry, 135,* 579–586.

Green, A. (1980). *Child maltreatment: A handbook for mental health and child care professionals.* New York: Jason Aronson.

Green, A. (1981). Core affective disturbance in abused children. *Journal of the American Academy of Psychoanalysis, 9,* 435–446.

Green, A. (1985). Children traumatized by physical abuse. In S. Eth & R. S. Pynoos (Eds.), *Post-traumatic stress disorder in children* (pp. 135–154). Washington, DC: American Psychiatric Press.

Green, A., Gaines, R. W., & Sandgrund, A. (1974). Child abuse: Pathological syndrome of family interaction. *American Journal of Psychiatry, 131,* 882–886.

Green, A., Voeller, K.,, Gaines., R. W., & Kubie, J., (1981). Neurological impairment in battered children. *Child Abuse and Neglect, 5,* 129–134.

Gross, M. (1979). Incestuous rape: A cause for hysterical seizures in four adolescent girls. *American Journal of Orthopsychiatry, 49,* 704–708.

Groth, A. N., & Burgess, A. (1979). Sexual trauma in the life histories of rapists and child molesters. *Victimology: An International Journal, 4,* 10–16.

Herman, J. (1981). *Father–daughter incest.* Cambridge: Harvard University Press.

Herman, J., Perry, J. C., & van der Kolk, B. (1989). Childhood trauma in borderline personality disorder. *American Journal of Psychiatry, 146,* 490–495.

Herman, J., & van der Kolk, B. (1987). Traumatic antecedents of borderline personality disorder. In B. van der Kolk (Ed.), *Psychological trauma* (pp. 111–126). Washington, DC: American Psychiatric Press.

Horevitz, R. P., & Braun, B. G. (1884). Are multiple personalities borderline? *Psychiatric Clinics of North America, 7,* 69–88.

Horowitz, M. (1976). *Stress-response syndromes.* New York: Jason Aronson.

James, J., & Meyerding, J. (1977). Early sexual experiences as a factor in prostitution. *American Journal of Psychiatry, 134,* 1381–1385.

Kardiner, A. (1959). The traumatic neuroses of war. In S. Arieti (Ed.), *American handbook of psychiatry* (Vol. 1, pp. 245–257). New York: Basic Books.

Kearney-Cooke, A. (1988). Group treatment of sexual abuse among women with eating disorders. *Women and Therapy, 7,* 5–22.

Kempe, R. (1976). Arresting or freezing the developmental process. In R. E. Helfer & C. H. Kempe (Eds.), *Child abuse and neglect: The family and community* (pp. 64–73). Cambridge: Ballinger.

Kempe, R., & Kempe, C. H. (1978). *Child abuse.* Cambridge: Harvard University Press.

Khan, M. (1963). The concept of cumulative trauma. *The Psychoanalytic Study of the Child, 18,* 286–306.

Kiser, L. J., Ackerman, B. J., Brown, E., & Edwards, N. B. (1988). Post-traumatic stress disorder in young children: A reaction to purported sexual abuse. *Journal of the American Academy of Child and Adolescent Psychiatry, 27,* 645–649.

Kluft, R. (1985). *Childhood antecedents of multiple personality*. Washington, DC: American Psychiatric Press.

Kris, E. (1956). The recovery of childhood memories. *The Psychoanalytic Study of the Child, 11,* 54–88.

Langevin, R., Handy, L., Hook, H., Day, D., and Russon, A. (1985). Are incestuous fathers pedophilic and aggressive? In R. Langevin (Ed.), *Erotic preference, gender identity, and aggression*. New York: Erlbaum.

Langmade, C. J. (1983). The impact of pre-and postpubertal onset of incest experiences in adult women as measured by sex anxiety, sex guilt, sexual satisfaction and sexual behavior. *Dissertation Abstracts International, 44,* 917B. (University Microfilms No. 3592)

Lewis, D., Shanok, S., Pincus, J., & Glaser, F. (1979). Violent juvenile delinquents: Psychiatric, neurological, psychological, and abuse factors. *Journal of The American Academy of Child Psychiatry, 18,* 307–319.

Lewis, I. A. (1985). *Los Angeles Times* Poll #98. Unpublished raw data.

Lewis, M., & Sarrell, P. (1969). Some psychological aspects of seduction, incest and rape in childhood. *Journal of the American Academy of Child Psychiatry, 8,* 606–619.

Light, R. (1973). Abused and neglected children in America: A study of alternative policies. *Harvard Educational Review, 43,* 556–598.

Lindberg, F., & Distad, L. (1985). Post-traumatic stress disorders in women who experienced childhood incest. *Child Abuse and Neglect, 9,* 329–334.

Liner, D. (1989). *Dissociation in sexually abused children*. Unpublished doctoral dissertation, Georgia State University, Atlanta.

Livingston, R. (1987). Sexually and physically abused children. *Journal of the American Academy of Child Psychiatry, 26,* 413–415.

MacVicar, K. (1979). Psychotherapy of sexually abused girls. *Journal of the American Academy of Child Psychiatry, 18,* 342–353.

Martin, H. P. (1972). The child and his development. In C. H. Kempe & R. E. Helfer (Eds.), *Helping the battered child and his family* (pp. 93–104). Philadelphia: J. B. Lipincott.

Martin, H. P., Beezly, P., Conway, E. F., & Kempe, C. H. (1974). The development of abused children. *Advances in Pediatrics, 21,* 439–447.

Marvasti, J. (1986). Incestuous mothers. *American Journal of Forensic Psychiatry, 7,* 63–68.

McCarty, L. (1986). Mother–child incest: Characteristics of the offender. *Child Welfare, 65,* 447–458.

McLeer, S., Deblinger, E., Atkins, M., Foa, E., and Ralphe, D. (1985). Post-traumatic stress disorder in sexually abused children. *Journal of the American Academy of Child and Adolescent Psychiatry, 27,* 650–654.

McQuire, R., Carlisle, J., & Young, B. (1965). Sexual deviations as conditioned behavior: A hypothesis. *Behavioral Research and Therapy, 2,* 185–190.

Meiselman, K. (1979). *Incest: A psychological study of causes and effects with treatment recommendations*. San Francisco: Jossey-Bass.

Miller, P. (1976). Blaming the victim of child molestation: An empirical analysis. *Dissertation Abstracts International*, Vol. 37. (University Microfilms No. 77–10069).

Miller, J., Moeller, D., Kaufman, A., Divasto, P., Fitzsimmons, P., Pother, D., & Christy, J. (1978). Recidivism among sexual assault victims. *American Journal of Psychiatry, 135,* 1103–1104.

Morrison, J. (1989). Childhood sexual histories of women with somatization disorder. *American Journal of Psychiatry, 146,* 239–241.

Morse, W., Sahler, O., & Friedman, S. (1970). A 3-year follow-up study of abused and neglected children. *American Journal of Diseases of Children, 120,* 439–446.

Nakashima, I., & Zakins, G. (1977). Incest: Review and clinical experience. *Pediatrics, 60,* 696–701.

National Center on Child Abuse and Neglect (NCCAN). (1988). *Study findings: National study of incidence and severity of child abuse and neglect*. Washington, DC: Department of Health, Education and Welfare.

Oates, K. (1986). *Child abuse and neglect: What happens eventually?* New York: Brunner/Mazel.

Oppenheimer, R., Howells, K., Palmer, L., and Chandler, D. (1985). Adverse sexual experiences in childhood and clinical eating disorders: A preliminary description. *Journal of Psychosomatic Reserach, 19,* 157–161.

Ounstead, C., Oppenheimer, R., & Lindsay, J. (1974). Aspects of bonding failure: The psychotherapeutic treatment of families of battered children. *Developmental Medicine and Child Neurology, 16,* 446–456.

Peters, S. D. (1985, August). *Child sexual abuse and later psychological problems*. Paper presented at the meeting of the American Psychological Association, Los Angeles.

Putnam, F. (1984). The psychophysiologic investigation of multiple personality disorder. *Psychiatric Clinics of North America, 7,* 31–40.

Putnam, F. (1985). Dissociation as a response to extreme trauma. In R. P. Kluft (Ed.), *Childhood antecedents of multiple personality* (pp. 66–97). Washington, DC: American Psychiatric Press.

Pynoos, R. S., Frederick, C., Nader, K., Arroyo, W., Steinberg, A., Eth, S., Nunez, F., & Fairbanks, L. (1987). Life threat and posttraumatic stress in school-age children. *Archives of General Psychiatry, 44,* 1057–1063.

Ressler, R. K., & Burgess, A. W. (1985). The men who murdered. *FBI Law Enforcement Bulletin, 54,* 2–6.

Root, M. P., & Fallon, P. (1988). The incidence of victimization experiences in a bulimic sample. *Journal of Interpersonal Violence, 3,* 161–173.

Rosenthal, P. A., & Rosenthal, S. (1984). Suicidal behavior by preschool children. *American Journal of Psychiatry, 141,* 520–525.

Russell, D. (1983). Incidence and prevalence of intrafamilial and extrafamilial sexual abuse of female children. *Child Abuse and Neglect, 7,* 133–146.

Russell, D. (1986). *The secret trauma: Incest in the lives of girls and women*. New York: Basic Books.

Sandgrund, A., Gaines, R. W., & Green, A. H. (1974). Child abuse and mental retardation: A problem of cause and effect. *American Journal of Mental Deficiency, 79,* 327–330.

Sansonnet-Hayden, H., Haley, G., Marriage, K., & Fine, S. (1987). Sexual abuse and psychopathology in hospitalized adolescents. *Journal of the Academy of Child and Adolescent Psychiatry, 26,* 753–757.

Satten, J., Menninger, K., Rosen, I., & Mayman, M. (1960). Murder without apparent motive: A study in personality diagnosis. *American Journal of Psychiatry, 117,* 48–53.

Sedney, M. A., & Brooks, B. (1984). Factors associated with a history of childhood sexual experience in a nonclinical female population. *Journal of the American Academy of Child Psychiatry, 23,* 215–218.

Sgroi, S. (1982). *Handbook of clinical intervention in child sexual abuse*. Lexington, MA: Lexington Books.

Silbert, M. H., & Pines, A. M. (1981). Sexual child abuse as antecedent to prostitution. *Child Abuse and Neglect, 5,* 407–411.

Sloan, G., & Leighner, P. (1986). Is there a relationship between sexual abuse or incest and eating disorders? *Canadian Journal of Psychiatry, 31,* 656–660.

Sloane, P., & Karpinski, E. (1942). Effects of incest on the participants. *American Journal of Orthopsychiatry, 12,* 666–673.

Smith, S. M. (1975). *The battered child syndrome.* London: Butterworths.

Smith, S. M., & Hanson, R. (1974). 134 battered children: A medical and psychological study. *British Medical Journal, 14,* 666–670.

Steele, B. F. (1983). The effect of abuse and neglect on psychological development. In J. D. Call, E. Galenson, & R. L. Tyson (Eds.), *Frontiers of infant psychiatry* (pp. 235–244). New York: Basic Books.

Steele, B. F., & Pollock, C. A. (1968). A psychiatric study of parents who abuse infants and small children. In R. E. Helfer & C. H. Kempe (Eds.), *The battered child.* Chicago: University of Chicago Press.

Stone, M. (1981). Borderline syndromes: A consideration of subtypes and an overview—Directions for research. *Psychiatric Clinics of North America, 4,* 3–13.

Stone, M. (1989). Individual psychotherapy with victims of incest. *Psychiatric Clinics of North America, 12,* 237–255.

Stone, M., Unwin, A., Beacham, B., & Swenson, C. (1988). Incest in female borderlines: Its frequency and impact. *International Journal of Family Psychiatry, 9,* 277–293.

Terr, L. (1987, May). *The trauma and extreme stress disorders: An outline and overview.* Paper presented at the Samuel G. Hibbs Lecture, American Psychiatric Association Annual Meeting, Chicago, Illinois.

van der Kolk, B. A. (1989). The compulsion to repeat the trauma: Re-enactment, revictimization, and masochism. *Psychiatric Clinics of North America, 12,* 389–411.

Wilbur, C. B. (1984). Treatment of multiple personality. *Psychiatric Annals, 14,* 27–31.

Wyatt, G. E. (1985). The sexual abuse of Afro-American and white American women in childhood. *Child Abuse and Neglect, 9,* 507–519.

Yates, A. (1982). Children eroticized by incest. *American Journal of Psychiatry, 139,* 482–485.

CHAPTER 50

Father–Daughter Incest

Judith Lewis Herman

Introduction

In the past two decades, as the result of feminist consciousness-raising, sexual abuse of children has been recognized in North America and Western Europe as a serious social problem. The testimony of victims, first in consciousness-raising groups, then in public speakouts, and finally in formal survey research, has documented the high prevalence of sexual exploitation of children. The best available data, drawn from large-scale surveys of nonclinical populations, indicate that the risk of victimization may be as high as 1 in 10 for boys (Finkelhor, 1979), and greater than 1 in 3 for girls (Russell, 1984). Whether the child victim is male or female, the perpetrator is usually male. Most perpetrators are not strangers but are well known to their child victims; often they are in a position of trust or authority that affords them access and power.

Although boys are more commonly abused by extrafamilial perpetrators, girls appear to be particularly vulnerable to sexual abuse by family members; in a probability survey of over 900 women in California, Russell (1986) found that 16% had been sexually abused by a relative, and 4.5% reported sexual abuse by a father or stepfather before age 18. A recent nationwide study of over 1,000 women in the Netherlands yielded almost identical findings: 15.6% of the sample reported sexual abuse by a relative in childhood (Draijer, 1988). Preliminary reports from similar surveys in the Scandinavian countries have also yielded comparable results (Leth, 1989). The vast majority of incest cases are undisclosed and undetected. In the American community survey cited above, only 2% of the intrafamilial sexual abuse cases were reported to the police. Although poor and disorganized families are heavily overrepresented

among reported cases, the actual prevalence of incest varies very little with social class, race, ethnicity, or religion.

Incestuous Family Constellation

Incestuous families are not easily recognizable because of their conventional appearance (Herman, 1981, 1983). Incestuous fathers are frequently described as "good providers," or even "pillars of the community." Although they assiduously maintain a social facade of respectability, within the privacy of their families they often establish a pattern of intimidation and coercive control. This abuse of paternal authority is generally unrecognized, since it simply represents an exaggeration of accepted norms of patriarchal dominance. Incestuous fathers often attempt to isolate their families, restricting the mobility and social contacts of both their wives and their daughters. It is not unusual for survivors to report that their fathers discouraged their mothers from working outside the home, socializing, or even driving a car, that the family never had visitors in the home, or that the children were not allowed to participate in normal peer activities because of their fathers' jealousy and suspiciousness.

Incestuous fathers also frequently enforce their dominance in the family through violence. Numerous studies have now confirmed the strong association between wife-beating and sexual abuse of children (Bowker, Arbitel, & McFerron, 1988). In my own clinical study of 40 survivors of father–daughter incest, half reported that they witnessed their fathers beating their mothers or other children (Herman, 1981). The daughter singled out for the sexual relationship is sometimes spared the beatings; however, the dire consequences of incurring her father's displeasure are only too apparent to her.

For these reasons, incestuous fathers are often described as family tyrants (Maisch, 1972; Summit & Kryso, 1978). However, once the incest has been de-

Judith Lewis Herman • 61 Roseland Street, Somerville, Massachusetts 02143.

International Handbook of Traumatic Stress Syndromes, edited by John P. Wilson and Beverley Raphael. Plenum Press, New York, 1993.

tected, these men are unlikely to present themselves in this manner in a clinical interview. On the contrary, they commonly appear as pathetic, meek, bewildered, and ingratiating. Because they are exquisitely sensitive to the realities of power, they rarely attempt to intimidate anyone of equal or greater social status, such as an adult professional or an officer of the law. Rather, they commonly seek to evoke sympathy and to deny, minimize, or rationalize their abusive behavior. Naive observers may incorrectly conclude that the incestuous father is a relatively powerless figure in the family and may even describe the family system as "mother-dominated."

Most mothers in incestuous families, however, are not in any position to dominate their husbands; often they can barely take care of themselves or their children. One of the most consistent findings in the literature is the unusually high rate of serious illness or disability in the mothers of sexually abused daughters (Finkelhor, 1979; Herman & Hirschman, 1981). These mothers are often further disempowered by domestic battering, or by the inability to take control of their reproductive lives. Economically dependent, socially isolated, battered, ill, or encumbered with the care of many small children, mothers in incestuous families are generally not in a position to consider independent survival, and must therefore preserve their marriages at all costs, even if the cost includes the conscious or unconscious sacrifice of a daughter.

Incestuous fathers do not assume maternal caretaking functions when their wives are ill or disabled; rather, they expect to continue to receive female nurturance. The oldest daughter is often deputized to take on a "parentified" role, assuming major responsibility for housework or child care (Herman & Hirschman, 1981; Justice & Justice, 1979). The daughter's sexual relationship with the father may evolve almost as an extension of her other caretaking duties.

Sexual estrangement of the marital couple is frequently cited as a factor in the genesis of father–daughter incest. However, careful interviewing indicates that most incestuous fathers continue to have sex on demand with their wives as well as with their daughters; those who confine their sexual activities to their children do so by choice (Groth, 1979). A significant proportion of incestuous fathers also commit other sex offenses against both adults and children outside the home (Abel, Mittelman, Becker, *et al.*, 1983). Like other sex crimes, incest may be seen as the compulsive, sexualized expression of a wish for power and dominance.

Diagnostically, it has been difficult to characterize incestuous fathers, other than to note that the great majority do not suffer from psychiatric conditions (psychotic disorders or mental retardation) that might be invoked to diminish criminal responsibility. In fact, on careful evaluation, the majority of offenders in community studies do not qualify for *any* psychiatric diagnosis (Abel, Rouleau, & Cunningham-Rathner, 1985). Even though alcoholism is common in incestuous fathers, it has not been shown to be any more common than in the general male population. The role of alcohol can probably best be understood as a facilitating one, helping to overcome inhibitions and provide socially acceptable excuses for men who are already predisposed to commit sexual offenses. Careful evaluation reveals that the com-

pelling sexual fantasy is present whether the offender is drunk or sober, and the sexual assault is not impulsive but rather carefully planned (Groth, 1979).

The incestuous father's attitude of entitlement to female service, and his willingness to use coercion to obtain it, reflect a kind of circumscribed sociopathy, limited to the domain of private life, and not ordinarily displayed in other social situations. Because paternal domination of the family is socially accepted and condoned, we lack a diagnostic category which recognizes extreme paternal dominance as a form of pathology. Sociopathic, paranoid, and narcissistic personality disorders are frequently described in clinical studies of incest offenders, although there are no controlled studies to indicate that they are any more common in this group than in the general male population. All these disorders involve a preoccupation with one's own fantasies, wishes, and needs, a lack of empathy for others, and a desire to control and dominate others rather than to engage in mutual relationships. In addition, the incestuous behavior, once established, has repetitive and compulsive aspects which liken it to an addiction (Herman, 1988).

Incest History

Incestuous abuse commonly begins when the child is between the ages of 6 and 12, though cases involving younger children, including infants, have been reported (Russell, 1984). The sexual contact typically begins with fondling and gradually proceeds to masturbation and oral penetration. Vaginal intercourse may or may not be attempted before the child reaches puberty. The sexual act itself is not necessarily violent; the overwhelming authority of the parent is usually sufficient to gain the child's compliance.

Secrecy Principle

Secrecy becomes the dominant principle of family life, imposed by the father's need to preserve sexual access to his daughter. The sexual contact is rarely a single event, rather it is repeated over a period of months or years, ending only when the child finds the resources to escape. The child victim keeps the secret, fearing that if she tells she will not be believed, she will be punished, or she will cause the destruction of the family. The consequences of breaking secrecy may be represented to the child as a loss of a parent ("Your mother will have a nervous breakdown"; "I'll be sent to jail"), or expulsion from the family ("You'll be sent away"). These prospects are terrifying to any child. In addition, positive inducements are offered in some cases. The child may be singled out for special attention, privileges, or gifts, and may in the process be alienated from mother and siblings, who become jealous of the "special" father–daughter relationship without knowing of the overt sexual involvement. Usually, the father employs some combination of violence, threats, isolation of the child, and positive inducements to preserve secrecy.

Frequently, clinicians suspect that the mother is aware of and complicit in the incestuous relationship (R. Kempe & C. Kempe, 1978). Although this is undeniably true in some cases, the majority of survivors indicate that they never disclosed the incest to their mothers while it was occurring. Rather, they gave vague and indirect indications of distress, and felt betrayed and disappointed when their mothers failed to recognize the problem. Distress symptoms frequently displayed by incestuously abused children include insomnia, nightmares, bedwetting, fearfulness, social withdrawal or misbehavior, and somatic complaints. A few children may attempt to reenact the sexual encounters with younger playmates. Although in the aggregate these symptoms comprise a classic posttraumatic picture, the symptom picture in individual children is often quite vague and nonspecific (Adams-Tucker, 1982; Burgess, Groth, Holmstrom, et al., 1978; Gomes-Schwartz, Horowitz, & Sauzier, 1984; Goodwin, 1985; Lusk & Waterman, 1986). (A fuller clinical description of sexually abused children may be found in Chapter 49, in this volume.)

As the child victim reaches adolescence, distress symptoms may heighten for several reasons. First, the father may increase his sexual demands, attempting intercourse for the first time. This added intrusion, as well as the risk of pregnancy, makes continuation of the sexual relationship increasingly intolerable. In addition, the normal course of the girl's maturation, which now includes increased social involvement with peers and greater awareness of sexual norms, inevitably represents a threat to the father's monopoly of power. The father may respond with jealousy verging upon paranoia, and may attempt to place severe restrictions on his daughter's social contacts. The result is an increase in family conflict and escalating symptoms of distress. Runaway attempts, suicide attempts, self-injury, drug and alcohol abuse, hysterical conversion symptoms and other somatic complaints, indiscriminate sexual activity, and early pregnancy are frequently seen in teenage incest victims (Goodwin, 1982; Herman & Hirschman, 1981).

As the oldest daughter becomes more resistant and threatens to escape entirely, the father may turn his attention sequentially to younger siblings. Repetition of the incest with more than one daughter or with other children outside the immediate family has been a common finding of numerous clinical reports. On the other hand, there are virtually no reports of cases in which an incestuous relationship was spontaneously ended by the perpetrator's initiative and choice. It seems reasonable to conclude that once an incestuous relationship has begun, the father will seek to perpetuate it, either with his first victim or with another, for as long as he can, until external controls are placed on his behavior.

Father–daughter incest should be suspected in any family that includes a violent or domineering father, a battered, chronically ill, or disabled mother, or a daughter who appears to have assumed major household responsibilities inappropriate for her age. Although the oldest daughter is particularly vulnerable, once incest has been reported with one child, all other children to whom the perpetrator has intimate access should be considered at risk. Incest should also be suspected as a precipitant in the behavior of adolescent girls who present as runaways, sexual delinquents, or drug and alcohol abusers, as well as those who inflict deliberate injuries upon themselves or make suicide attempts.

Principles of Intervention

Effective intervention in incestuous families begins with identification of the problem. Given the prevalence of incest and other forms of child sexual abuse, questions about abuse should be included in a routine clinical evaluation. The main obstacle to obtaining a history is the clinician's failure to ask specific and direct questions. As in the case of other stigmatized or taboo subjects, most patients are not unduly upset by calm, matter-of-fact questioning. When abuse is suspected in young children, a full evaluation may require specialized projective interviewing techniques, such as the use of drawings and anatomically correct dolls. When proper assessment procedures are followed, even very young children are able to give accurate descriptions of what happened to them, though they cannot locate their experiences accurately in time or give a coherent, sequential verbal narrative. False complaints of incest are rare (under 5% of all complaints); on the other hand, it is common for a child to retract a true allegation under pressure from the family (Goodwin, 1982).

Discovery of Incest

The discovery of incest represents a major family crisis, requiring rapid and decisive intervention (Sgroi, 1982). Usually, by the time of disclosure, the incest has been going on for years, and the family has become organized around the preservation of the incest secret. Disclosure represents a serious threat to the survival of the family. The father faces loss of the sexual activity which has become compulsive. He also faces possible loss of his wife and family, social stigmatization, and even criminal sanctions, though in practice these are very rarely applied. The mother faces possible loss of her husband, social stigma, and the terrifying prospect of raising her family alone, a task for which she is ill-prepared.

In this situation, the father usually steadfastly denies the allegations. He insists that the child is lying and directs his efforts to persuading others that he is innocent. The mother finds herself torn between her husband and her daughter. Although she may initially believe the child and attempt to take protective action, unless she receives rapid and effective support, she will usually rally to her husband's side within a short time. If she persists in believing her child, she has a great deal to lose and very little to gain. The daughter, therefore, may find herself discredited, shamed, punished for bringing trouble on the family, and still unprotected from continued sexual abuse. Suicide and runaway attempts are particularly common at this time. Without effective intervention, the child victim may be scapegoated and virtually driven out of the family.

Focus of Crisis Intervention

The initial focus of crisis intervention should be on establishing a safe environment for the child within the family. Reporting to the mandated state authorities should be done promptly, preferably in the presence of the child and her mother. Although some clinicians are reluctant to report for fear of alienating the family, failure to report is a violation of the law, and represents collusion with the perpetrator. No therapeutic alliance can possibly be established on the basis of preserving secrecy.

In order to minimize the reprisals and intimidation that can follow upon disclosure, it is often desirable to have the father leave the home for a brief period during the crisis. Although child protective agencies do not have the legal authority to compel this course of action, the same result can often be achieved either by persuasion or through use of civil protection laws. A court order may be obtained by the mother, requiring the father to vacate the home temporarily and to provide child support. Conditions for supervised visitation and for mandated treatment may also be established by the court. Clinicians working with incestuous families must be thoroughly familiar with these legal procedures, and willing to offer active, concrete guidance to their clients, who are generally terrified at the prospect of involvement in the legal system. For example, following the disclosure, it is often useful to have a knowledgeable person (caseworker, victim witness advocate, or peer counselor) accompany the mother to court to obtain the temporary restraining order.

This form of temporary separation during the crisis period is far preferable to the more traditional intervention, the removal of the child victim from the home. Removal of the child makes her feel as though she is the one at fault, and that she is being punished by banishment from her family. Removal of the child also reinforces the tendency of the parental couple to bond against the disclosing child, and it does nothing to protect the other children at risk. Moreover, it is often difficult to find an appropriate placement for a child victim; the offender, by contrast, does not need a "placement" to leave home temporarily—a nearby motel room will do in a crisis. For all of these reasons, removal of the child should be undertaken only as a last resort, when no other practical means of ensuring safety can be found.

During the crisis period, all family members are in great distress and need intensive support. The child needs to be assured that protective and responsible adults believe her story and will not allow her to be further exploited. The mother needs help believing her daughter and resisting the tendency to side with her husband against her child. If the couple separates, the mother also needs help with practical issues of survival. Previously untreated health and mental health problems should also receive prompt attention. The father needs help facing the fact that secrecy has been irrevocably broken, and that he must now admit to and give up the sexual relationship with his daughter if there is to be any possibility of restoring the family.

The crisis period is resolved at the point that the family is under the supervision of the mandated agency and a coordinated safety plan is in place. Cooperation between all professionals working with the family facilitates quick and effective crisis intervention and greatly improves the prospects for treatment. Some states now mandate interagency cooperation between law enforcement, child protective services, and mental health services on cases of child sexual abuse.

Following disclosure, the family is generally so divided and fragmented that family treatment is not the modality of choice. Experienced practitioners who have begun programs with a family therapy orientation have almost uniformly abandoned this method except in late stages of treatment (Giarretto, 1982). If the father is violent or intimidating toward other family members, family treatment is *contraindicated*.

Group treatment for mothers, fathers, and child victims appears to be a far more promising approach. In some cases, individual or couple therapy, or family meetings with the mother and children may be recommended in addition to group. For all family members, the issues of stigma, isolation, and shame are especially amenable to group treatment. For fathers, group treatment is also effective in breaking through denial and the rationalization of criminal behavior. Many group programs for offenders follow a highly structured model similar to programs for the treatment of alcoholism and other addictions. In early stages of treatment, the offender acknowledges that he has lost control of his behavior and must submit to external control. Progression through the treatment program involves increasing acceptance of responsibility for present behavior and restitution to others for past abuses (Herman, 1988). Opinion is divided on whether incest offenders can be motivated to remain in treatment without a credible threat of legal sanctions for failure to comply. To date, the most highly developed programs have been those which rely on a court mandate.

In addition to group and individual treatment, many programs incorporate a self-help component. Self-help activities may supplement more formal therapeutic work in a number of ways. During the crisis period, the family's intense need for support may be partially met by frequent peer contact. In the postcrisis period, families beginning treatment may benefit from the experience of those further along, while "advanced" group members may gain self-esteem from being in a helping role. Finally, after formal treatment is terminated, self-help groups provide a continued source of support and community.

Restoration of the incestuous family centers on the mother–daughter relationship. On this point, there seems to be wide consensus among experienced practitioners, even those most committed to reuniting the parental couple (e.g., Giarretto, 1982). Safety for the child is not established by improving the sexual or marital relationship of the parents; it is established only when the mother feels strong enough to protect herself and her children, and when the daughter feels sure that she can turn to her mother for protection.

The father may be judged ready to return to his family when he has admitted and taken full responsibility for the incest, and apologized to his victim in the presence of all family members, and taken steps to ensure that he will not offend again. When the father is ready to return to the family, the family may or may not be ready to receive him. This choice properly rests with the mother, once the mother–daughter bond has been restored, and once neither mother nor daughter feels intimidated. A decision for divorce may be as valid as a decision to rebuild the marriage; certainly the preservation of the parent's marriage should not be considered the criterion of therapeutic success. Probably the best gauge of successful treatment is the child victim's subjective feeling of safety and well-being, the disappearance of her distress symptoms, and the resumption of her interrupted normal development.

Given the present state of therapeutic knowledge, no one can claim to "cure" incest; rather, the offender's behavior may be brought under control, first, by outside intervention, second, by empowering the mother as a protective agent within the family system, and, finally, by restoring the alliance between mother and daughter. The father's internal controls should never be considered sufficient to ensure safety; if the family decides to reunite, mother and daughter should be explicitly prepared for an attempt to resume the incestuous relationship (Groth, 1979). Some degree of outside supervision should probably be maintained as long as children remain in the home.

Further investigation is needed to continue the development of effective treatment for all family members. Controlled, long-term follow-up studies of treated and untreated families, and comparative studies of differing approaches to treatment are necessary in order to refine what is at present largely an oral culture of front-line clinical experience.

Long-Term Effects of Incestuous Abuse

Community studies of incest survivors indicate that the long-range effects of childhood incest may be highly variable. In Russell's (1986) community study of adult incest survivors, for example, virtually all the women stated that they were upset by their experiences at the time of occurrence, but half judged themselves to be either entirely or mostly recovered from the trauma they had suffered. These estimates, however, should be considered optimistic, first, because women who were so impaired that they could not function independently in the community were not included in the survey, and second, because these estimates are based only upon self-report. Thus, they measure only the long-term consequences recognized by relatively healthy informants.

Prognosis for Recovery

The likelihood of a good recovery appears to be highly related to the nature of the traumatic experience. Sexual contacts that were not forceful, that did not involve intrusive physical violation, that occurred only once or infrequently, and that involved relatives who were not part of the child's household are the least likely to result in lasting harm. With the more severe degrees of sexual abuse, however, few women are able to escape without long-term sequelae. Survivors who have experi-

enced forceful or repeated, prolonged abuse, or severe physical violation, and those abused by much older men, especially fathers or stepfathers, are very likely to report persistent difficulties in their adult lives. It appears that violent, prolonged, or intrusive abuse, or abuse by a primary caretaker, represent stressors that are beyond the adaptive capacities of all but the most exceptional children, and will regularly produce a long-lasting traumatic syndrome (Herman, Russell, & Trocki, 1986).

The long-term effects that survivors most commonly attribute to incest are injuries to the self in relation to others: distrust and fear of men, lowered self-esteem, and fear of sex. Indeed, when compared with women who have not been incestuously abused, incest victims do not fare well in their sexual and intimate relationships. Abused women are significantly more likely to experience early pregnancy, marital separation and divorce, and repeated sexual victimization. Perhaps in response to their repeated experiences of the world as an unsafe place and other human beings as untrustworthy, incest victims are also much more likely than others to lose their faith in God, and to defect from the religion in which they were raised (Herman, 1981; Herman et al., 1986).

Clinical studies of incest survivors in the general population indicate persistent high levels of distress. Draijer's (1988) comprehensive study of women in the Netherlands found that survivors of incest had much higher levels of psychosomatic and psychiatric symptoms than their counterparts who had not been abused. Significantly elevated symptoms included nightmares, sleep disturbances, eating disorders, generalized anxiety, depression, self-destructive behavior including self-mutilation and suicide attempts, and sexual and relational problems. Very few, however (under 10%), had sought psychiatric treatment for their problems. Similar studies conducted in the United States indicate that incest survivors report generally high levels of distress, with a wide array of symptoms and a good deal of variability in symptoms, both among individuals and in any one individual over time. There is no one symptom profile for incest survivors (Browne & Finkelhor, 1986).

Although most survivors never seek psychiatric treatment, adult women with a history of incest are frequently found among psychiatric patients (Carmen, Rieker, & Mills, 1984; Herman, 1986; Jacobson & Richardson, 1987). In some series, such histories are found in over half of female inpatients (Briere & Runtz, 1987; Bryer, Nelson, Miller, & Krol, 1987). A history of severe childhood sexual abuse, most commonly incest, has been etiologically linked to the development of certain specific psychiatric syndromes such as multiple personality disorder (Putnam, Post, Guroff, Silberman, et al., 1986), and has been documented in the majority of patients with borderline personality disorder (Herman, Perry, & van der Kolk, 1989).

Clinical descriptions of adult patients with a history of childhood sexual abuse are consistent with a formulation of posttraumatic stress disorder that has become chronic and integrated into the victim's personality structure (Gelinas, 1983). Memory of the original stressor may be partially or severely repressed, but fear and hypervigilance usually persist, and the trauma may be reexperienced in intrusive nightmares, flashbacks (often triggered by attempts at sexual intimacy), and dissociated states. Patients are chronically anxious or fearful, and often have chronic sleep disturbances or insomnia. Patients may have become so accustomed to their intrusive posttraumatic symptoms that they no longer complain of them, but rather organize their lives to accommodate them; on careful questioning patients may report, for example, that they always sleep fully clothed, or with a light on. A need for vigilance at night may have become integrated in to the patient's character structure and adaptively expressed in a choice of occupation (night-shift nurse, for example, or security guard).

Constrictive features of the posttraumatic syndrome are most noticeable in the survivor's persistent deficits in self-care and self-protection, and sometimes also in social withdrawal or isolation. Additionally, many patients complain of emotional numbing and chronic dysphoria and describe themselves as "in a fog" or "behind a glass wall." Memory deficits for childhood experiences may become apparent (Herman & Schatzow, 1987). When questioned, patients will often describe conscious or involuntary induction of dissociative states, originating in their childhood attempts to cope with overwhelming trauma. Patients frequently complain of chronic depression, anhedonia, and inner deadness, and may be driven periodically to seek relief in drug and alcohol abuse, self-mutilation, and suicide attempts. Comprehensive reviews of the literature on clinical symptomatology in incest survivors can be found in two recent publications (Briere, 1989; Courtois, 1988).

Characterological adaptation to a childhood environment of severely disrupted caretaking also results in persistent impairments in self-esteem, self-protection, identity formation, and the capacity for intimate relationships. Valued only for her capacity to service the sexual needs of her father, the survivor has great difficulty valuing herself. Scapegoated and blamed for the incestuous relationship, the survivor is frequently left with a heavy burden of shame and a highly stigmatized identity. Exploited and neglected in childhood, the survivor is often extremely fearful and mistrustful in adult relationships. She may attempt to protect herself by avoiding sexual or intimate relationships; such periods of withdrawal may alternate with intense and desperate searching for a special relationship with an idealized rescuing figure (Herman, 1981).

Almost inevitably, the survivor will have difficulty protecting herself in the context of intimate relationships. Her longing for the unconditional care and nurturance which she did not receive in childhood, her well-learned habits of submission and obedience to authority, and her dissociative defensive style, all make it difficult for her to assess danger accurately or to assert herself effectively in an intimate relationship. For all of these reasons, survivors of incest are at unusually high risk for repeated victimization. Incest survivors are highly vulnerable to rape, domestic battery, sexual harassment, and exploitation in pornography and prostitution (James & Meyerding, 1977; Russell, 1986).

The phenomenon of repeated victimization calls for great care in interpretation. For too long the clinical literature has simply reflected the crude social judgment that victims get what they ask for. Traditional concepts of masochism, and more recent formulations of "addiction to trauma," imply that victims actively seek or derive gratification from abuse. Although some victims do seek eroticized reenactments of early sexual trauma, the majority do not; rather they experience their revictimization as the dreaded but unavoidable price of being in an intimate relationship.

Because of the increased risk that survivors will marry an abusive spouse, their children may in turn be at increased risk for physical or sexual abuse (Goodwin, 1982). Clinical observations of abused women who were subsequently unable to protect their children from abuse suggest that victims who have recovered poorly from their own trauma may have particular difficulty protecting their children. It should be noted, however, that the great majority of adult survivors, even those with very severe abuse histories, neither abuse nor neglect their children (Coons, 1985; Kaufman & Zigler, 1987). A second potential mechanism of "generational transmission" may be traced through the sons of incestuous fathers, who may develop abusive behavior in identification with their fathers. Anecdotal reports of such behavior are common, but no controlled studies have as yet been done to document this phenomenon.

Treatment of Adult Survivors

Successful treatment of the patient with a history of childhood abuse begins with obtaining a history. The willingness of the victim to disclose her history is entirely dependent on the clinician's willingness to hear, respect, and validate her experiences and to bear the intense emotions that are inevitably aroused. With increasing tolerance, the clinician can expect to hear an increasing number of histories that include atrocities. The limits of the clinician's own affect tolerance are constantly challenged. Any clinician who works with victims must be assured of dependable access to supportive peers, in order to cope with the contagion of posttraumatic stress disorder that affects caregivers.

Countertransference Issues in Treatment

Male and female therapists often differ in their countertransference responses to victims of sexual assault. These differences may result in staff splitting along gender lines in institutional settings, and to different but equally common therapeutic mistakes in individual practice. Female therapists may tend to overidentify with the victim, becoming overwhelmed by feelings of helplessness and despair or with rage against the offender that the victim may not share. They may tend to shy away from exploring the actual details of the sexual encounters. Male therapists, on the other hand, may tend to identify with the offender. They may focus on aspects of the victim's behavior that might have been interpreted as provocative and may have difficulty supporting the victim's anger against the offender. Male therapists may also find incest victims sexually arousing.

This may lead to inappropriate behaviors ranging from intrusive questioning about the details of the sexual encounter to actual seduction attempts. Since an estimated 5 to 10% of male therapists seduce their patients (Holroyd & Brodsky, 1977; Gartrell, Hermann, Olarte, Feldstein, & Localio, 1986), and since incest victims appear to be particularly vulnerable to repeated exploitation, the risk for revictimization by a therapist is considerable. It is perhaps unnecessary to state that any violation of the boundaries of therapy, however rationalized, represents a repeated trauma to the victim.

Establishment of trust in the context of a therapeutic alliance is the initial task of treatment. Early and explicit clarification of this issue is essential. The patient should be told that, regardless of her behavior, the fact that she had an incest experience means that she was not properly cared for. Her difficulties in establishing trusting relationships and her own lack of entitlement to self-care should be explained as predictable consequences of abuse. Posttraumatic symptoms and defensive strategies should also be explicitly identified. Repeated testing of the therapist's trustworthiness should be anticipated and clarified with the patient. A prolonged time period may be required before a secure trusting relationship is formed.

Once a therapeutic alliance has been established, the patient is able to review and construct new meaning in the incest history. Grieving for both parents and for the lost childhood should be expected. Patients may experience a period of existential despair as they give up their belief that their own intrinsic badness was responsible for their victimization and the hope that their own efforts to be good will eventually create the longed-for good parent. Suicidal, self-destructive, or regressive episodes may occur during this process. However, at the same time, the beginnings of new, more adaptive behavior may also be discerned. As the patient works through her rage and grief, she gives up her stigmatized identity. Self-esteem, self-protection, and peer relationships begin to improve.

Because the trauma of incest is profoundly social, so is the recovery process. A full resolution of the trauma involves the restoration of social bonds and a renegotiation of the patient's relationship with her family of origin. Group treatment and self-help are particularly useful in the recovery process, either in addition to individual psychotherapy, or as a sole treatment modality. In a peer group, survivors find a protected environment in which they can unburden the shame and stigma of victimization, and come to a new understanding of their isolated experience based upon the shared knowledge of other survivors. Mature defenses such as anticipation, altruism, and humor are mobilized as survivors discover their capacity to help others. For patients with memory deficits, group treatment provides a powerful stimulus for the recovery of memories. Disclosures, limit-setting, and confrontations with family members are also more likely to be successful if carefully planned in a group setting and carried out with group support. A fuller discussion of group treatment for incest victims may be found elsewhere (Herman & Schatzow, 1984).

The critical importance of supportive relationships, including but not limited to the therapeutic relationship,

is repeatedly cited in the testimony of survivors who have recovered well. For example, in one community study, survivors who felt they had escaped without serious permanent harm attributed their recovery to helpful intervention from other people. Most frequently cited were supportive friends and family members, who assured these women that they were not at fault, and patient lovers, who helped them reclaim their sexuality (Tsai, Feldman-Summers, & Edgar, 1979). In another controlled study, survivors who had recovered well, as evidenced by greater marital satisfaction and capacity to protect their children, were those who in childhood had told others about the abuse and received a supportive response (Straus, 1981). Although therapeutic intervention at the time of the abuse is clearly the most desirable, even long-belated therapy and social support appear to be beneficial to many survivors.

Furthermore, systematic investigation is needed to identify those environmental factors both in childhood and in adult life that promote long-term recovery for victims. Today's adult survivors endured their abuse at a time when public awareness of the problem was minimal, detection extremely unusual, and societal intervention, if it occurred at all, was often destructive to the child victim. It is our hope that as a result of increased reporting and early detection of child sexual abuse, fewer children will suffer their victimization in silence, more children will benefit from supportive intervention, and fewer survivors will reach adult life still bearing their secrets alone.

References

Abel, G., Mittelman, M. S., Becker, J., Cunningham-Rathner, J., and Lucas, L. (1983). *The characteristics of men who molest young children.* Paper presented at the World Congress of Behavior Therapy, Washington, DC.

Abel, G., Rouleau, J., & Cunningham-Rathner, J. (1985). Sexually aggressive behavior. In A. L. McGarry & S. A. Shah (Eds.), *Modern legal psychiatry and psychology.* Philadelphia: Davis.

Adams-Tucker, C. (1982). Proximate effects of sexual abuse in childhood: A report on 28 children. *American Journal of Psychiatry, 139,* 1252–1256.

Bowker, L. H., Arbitel, M., & McFerron, R. (1988). On the relationship between wife-beating and child abuse. In K. Yllo & M. Bograd (Eds.), *Feminist perspectives on wife abuse* (pp. 158–174). Beverly Hills: Sage Publications.

Briere, J. (1989). *Therapy for adults molested as children: Beyond survival.* New York: Springer Publications.

Briere, J., & Runtz, M. (1987). Post sexual abuse trauma: Data and implications for clinical practice. *Journal of Interpersonal Violence, 2,* 367–379.

Browne, A., & Finkelhor, D. (1986). Impact of child sexual abuse: A review of the literature. *Psychological Bulletin, 99,* 66–77.

Bryer, J. B., Nelson, B. A., Miller, J. B., & Krol, P. A. (1987). Childhood sexual and physical abuse as factors in adult psychiatric illness. *American Journal of Psychiatry, 144,* 1426–1430.

Burgess, A. W., Groth, A. N., Holmstrom, L. L., & Sqroi, S. M. (1978). *Sexual assault of children and adolescents.* Lexington, MA: D. C. Heath.

Carmen, E., Rieker, P. P., & Mills, T. (1984). Victims of violence and psychiatric illness. *American Journal of Psychiatry, 141,* 378–383.

Coons, P. (1985). Children of parents with multiple personality disorder. In R. P. Kluft (Ed.), *Childhood antecedents of multiple personality disorder* (pp. 151–166). Washington, DC: American Psychiatric Press.

Courtois, C. (1988). *Healing the incest wound: Adult survivors in therapy.* New York: W. W. Norton.

Draijer, N. (1988). *Sexksueel misbruik van meisjes door verwanten.* Den Haag: Ministerie van Sociale Zaken en Werkgelegenheid.

Finkelhor, D. (1979). *Sexually victimized children.* New York: Free Press.

Gartrell, N., Herman, J. L., Olarte, S., Feldstein, M., & Localio, R. (1986). Psychiatrist–patient sexual contact: Results of a national survey. *American Journal of Psychiatry, 143,* 1126–1131.

Gelinas, D. (1983). The persisting negative effects of incest. *Psychiatry, 46,* 312–332.

Giarretto, H. (1982). *Integrated treatment of child sexual abuse: A treatment and training manual.* Palo Alto, CA: Science and Behavior Books.

Gomes-Schwartz, B., Horowitz, J., & Sauzier, M. (1984). *Sexually exploited children: Service and Research Project.* Washington, DC: U.S. Office of Juvenile Justice and Delinquency Prevention.

Goodwin, J. (1982). *Sexual abuse: Incest victims and their families.* Boston, MA: John Wright.

Goodwin, J. (1985). Post-traumatic symptoms in incest victims. In R. Pynoos & S. Eth (Eds.), *Post-traumatic syndromes in children.* Washington, DC: American Psychiatric Press.

Groth, N. (1979). *Men who rape: The psychology of the offender.* New York: Plenum Press.

Herman, J. L. (1981). *Father–daughter incest.* Cambridge, MA: Harvard University Press.

Herman, J. L. (1983). Recognition and treatment of incestuous families. *International Journal of Family Therapy, 5,* 81–91.

Herman, J. L. (1986). Histories of violence in an outpatient population. *American Journal of Orthopsychiatry, 56,* 137–141.

Herman, J. L. (1988). Considering sex offenders: A model of addiction sign. *Journal of Women in Culture and Society, 13,* 695–724.

Herman, J. L., & Hirschman, L. (1981). Families at risk for father–daughter incest. *American Journal of Psychiatry, 138,* 967–970.

Herman, J. L., & Schatzow, E. (1984). Time-limited group therapy for women with a history of incest. *International Journal of Group Psychotherapy, 34,* 605–616.

Herman, J. L., & Schatzow, E. (1987). Recovery and verification of memories of childhood sexual abuse. *Psychoanalytic Psychology, 4,* 1–14.

Herman, J. L., Russell, D. E. H., & Trocki, K. (1986). Long-term effects of incestuous abuse in childhood. *American Journal of Psychiatry, 143,* 1293–1296.

Herman, J. L., Perry, J. C., & van der Kolk, B. A. (1989). Childhood trauma in borderline personality disorder. *American Journal of Psychiatry, 146,* 490–495.

Holroyd, J., & Brodsky, A. (1977). Psychologists' attitudes and practices regarding erotic and nonerotic physical contact with patients. *American Psychologist, 32,* 843–849.

Jacobson, A., & Richardson, B. (1987). Assault experiences of 100 psychiatric patients: Evidence of the need for routine inquiry. *American Journal of Psychiatry, 144,* 908–913.

James, J., & Meyerding, J. (1977). Early sexual experience and prostitution. *American Journal of Psychiatry, 134,* 1381–1385.

Justice, B., & Justice, R. (1979). *The broken taboo.* New York: Human Sciences Press.

Kaufman, J., & Zigler, E. (1987). Do abused children become abusive parents? *American Journal of Orthopsychiatry, 57,* 186–192.

Kempe, R., & Kempe, C. (1978). *Child abuse.* Cambridge, MA: Harvard University Press.

Leth, I. (1989). *Sexual abuse of children and adolescents: Results from a Scandinavian research concerning the extent and character of sexual abuse.* Copenhagen, Denmark: University of Copenhagen. Unpublished manuscript.

Lusk, R., & Waterman, J. (1986). Effects of sexual abuse on children. In K. MacFarlane & J. Waterman (Eds.), *Sexual abuse of young children: Evaluation and treatment* (pp. 101–120). New York: Guilford Press.

Maisch, H. (1972). *Incest.* New York: Stein & Day.

Putnam, F. W., Guroff, J. J., Silberman, E. K., Barban, L., & Post, R. M. (1986). The clinical phenomenology of multiple personality disorder: Review of 100 recent cases. *Journal of Clinical Psychiatry, 47,* 285–293.

Russell, D. E. H. (1984). *Sexual exploitation: Rape, child sexual abuse, and sexual harassment.* Beverly Hills, CA: Sage Publications.

Russell, D. E. H. (1986). *The secret trauma: Incest in the lives of girls and women.* New York: Basic Books.

Sgroi, S. (1982). *Handbook of clinical intervention in child sexual abuse.* Lexington, MA: D. C. Heath.

Straus, P. (1981). *A study of the recurrence of father–daughter incest across generations.* Unpublished doctoral dissertation, California School of Professional Psychology, Berkeley, CA.

Summit, R., & Kryso, J. (1978). Sexual abuse of children: A clinical spectrum. *American Journal of Orthopsychiatry, 48,* 237–250.

Tsai, M., Feldman-Summers, S., & Edgar, M. (1979). Childhood molestation: Variables related to differential impacts on psychological functioning in adult women. *Journal of Abnormal Psychology, 88,* 407–417.

CHAPTER 51

Bitter Waters

Effects on Children of the Stresses of Unrest and Oppression

Michael A. Simpson

> When young lips have drunk deep of the bitter waters of
> Hate, Suspicion and Despair, all the love in the world will not
> take away that knowledge.
> —RUDYARD KIPLING, *Baa, Baa, Black Sheep*

In this chapter, I will explore the effects of political repression, chronic unrest, and structural violence on children, adolescents, and families, reviewing the world literature, and using the specific example of local experience in South Africa, a chronically repressive society. The text is based on presentations to the conference "Bårn i Krig," held in Bergen, Norway, in May, 1988 (Simpson, 1988b; Simpson *et al.*, 1988).

I wish to argue the need for a broader and more holistic view of posttrauma reactions. While focussing on responses of children and adolescents, I want to bring to attention a number of usually neglected aspects of trauma and its results such as the matter of community trauma and communal responses to trauma; the nature and effects of continuing and recursive violence; the necessity to recognize the political context of trauma and its effects; the interplay between multiple traumata; and the fact that structural violence, such as that inherent in oppressive systems, has potentially severe and continuing posttraumatic effects.

I will illustrate neglected themes, such as the fact that child abuse is not simply a one-on-one tragedy occurring within faulty families, but that it may be institutionalized in the form of societal child abuse and bu-

reaucratically designed and organized trauma within a country where political and social systems are perverted by a devotion to principles requiring that groups (as defined racially) must be treated differently and, in all senses of that word, with prejudice. The hundred-thousand blows of oppression constitute trauma with the potential for influencing the lives of many individuals and for damaging not only those individuals but also their communities and a whole society.

There has been an excessive emphasis on seeing psychic trauma as a sequel to sudden, unexpected and intense stress, referring to single, short, sharp events, and ignoring stress which is gradual in onset, or recurrent, expected (indeed, dreaded), and of varying intensity. There is no rational basis whatsoever for the oddly elitist view—even, surprisingly, repeated in Terr (1985)—that sees horrible chronic stress as "somewhat removed from the more purely 'traumatized' group because of the chronicity and lack of surprise." She acknowledges that experiences like child abuse, for example, may be similar to trauma, "but they are not, strictly speaking, the same as trauma." We are told (Terr, 1985) that "the idea of repeated, expected dread is no longer a recognized facet in the concept of trauma." If so, then most of the real world was excluded from the ivory tower in which this absurdity was adopted, and there is an urgent need to revise that concept so that it no longer excludes the obvious.

Part of the problem is the extraordinarily sloppy phenomenology of many American workers in this field, who fail to elicit sufficiently detailed accounts from the

Michael A. Simpson • Intermedica, P.O. Box 51, Pretoria, South Africa. Chapter submitted 1990.

International Handbook of Traumatic Stress Syndromes, edited by John P. Wilson and Beverley Raphael. Plenum Press, New York, 1993.

victims, of the manifold components of their traumatization. Many, if not most, of the supposedly "single" traumatic events are single only in the researcher's notepad: they are of significant duration, and their impact is a compound of a grisly variety of stressful components.

This is the "Boo!" fallacy, and unjustifiable bosh. By what logical contortion do we consider that incidents of trauma cease to be trauma merely by repetition? That a single act of rape or assault is more "purely traumatizing" than years of abuse, one day of disaster more so than a year of horrors? Must one discount the Holocaust as trauma, because it lasted longer than an afternoon? Or did it cease to be traumatic to those who knew and dreaded its brutal effects, only traumatizing the odd innocent who wandered into it by mistake?

There is not the slightest logical or research basis for defining trauma by only some of its more puny characteristics. There is no convincing evidence that "surprise" or a single, short, sharp stress are essential elements in producing psychic damage; and mounds of evidence and experience to the contrary. This Halloween fantasy is a typical product of smugly assured communities who experience trauma, if at all, only as brief intrusions into comfortable and ordered life.

Psychic trauma results from stress that overwhelms, and there are many ways of overwhelming someone, none of them pure. The formula is very simple: if the psychic demands of the situation are sufficient (in length, breadth, or depth, in whatever dimensions or combination of characteristics) so as to substantially overwhelm the individual's capacity to cope or defend, psychic trauma will result.

Relevance of Politics

Value-free research is not possible and does not occur. Research may be most perniciously biased by the attitudes of the researcher when these attitudes are hidden from the reader or even from the researcher's own perception. Value-free research is not possible, but value-explicit research is more honest research in which scientists express and clarify their value system. Physicians and other health professionals are never so intensely political, in the worst possible way, as when they consider themselves as apolitical. In an inescapable sense, much or all of human life is political, dealing with or influenced by public affairs and societal governance. Therapy, research, and education are inescapably political activities, whereas health is a necessarily political field. Although a scientist or health professional has no business meddling in party politics, other than as a private citizen, our comprehension of the human situation will always be stunted if we ignore the political context of our patients and their problems.

Biomedical and behavioral texts are *always* political in what the authors choose to include, in what they choose to ignore, in what they do not realize they are including, and in what they do not realize they are excluding (Simpson, 1987). Apparently neutral texts have, in fact, taken a highly political stance by choosing to accept a particular political situation and avoiding overt comment on it. Considering how many stress disorders arise from political causes (warfare, torture, terrorism, concentration camps) the absence of informed recognition of political aspects of the conditions is notable. Certainly, political factors have played a substantial part in the delayed recognition of traumatic stress disorders in many situations and have shaped societal and therapeutic responses to them, including the neglect of victims, which has been so tragically common in so many settings. Young (1980) criticized the extent to which stress research ignores the role of social forces in a way which can individualize and emphasize the naturalness of the reaction, rather than the unnaturalness of the cause.

The matter is even more acute when one is working in relation to topics like oppression and torture. It is not bias to be opposed to cruelty and the planned damage of human beings: it is bias *not* to be opposed to such circumstances. Ethically, one cannot avoid such a position, though one may avoid partisan participation in the underlying disputes. A physician is not "biased" in opposing cancer, but a physician who felt obliged to act in favor of cancer is hard to imagine. Not to be opposed to evil is to participate in it.

Readers living in stable democracies can enjoy the luxury (it is expensive, even though it is usually others who pay the price) of living what they believe to be an apolitical life, that is, one in which they are unaware of all the political matters they take for granted. Especially within a repressive society, whatever you do or do not do is political: politics is inevitable and inescapable. Those who live among acts and policies of deliberate harm to human beings and ignore it, are not being "objective" or "scientific" or "neutral": they are being morally and intellectually blind.

When I worked in a South African university hospital, my black students were not allowed to examine white patients; their father might die of a heart attack because an ambulance could not take him to the white hospital even though it had vacancies in its intensive care unit; my teaching, my research, and my clinical work were expected to be shaped by the "racial group" to which someone was considered to belong; and I was subjected to consistent and ultimately damaging pressures to avoid ethical and practical involvement in critical health problems for political reasons.

How does one work "neutrally" with the grief of a young black or Indian mother mourning her dead child, who says, "Professor, they told me his leukemia could be cured. But then in the black hospital, there were three children in one cot, and just when his resistance to infection was lowest, he had to share the cot with a child with typhoid and another with gastroenteritis, or sleep on the floor with the others; so he died of an unnecessary infection, not of the disease." How does one teach black medical students the meanings of "normal" and "healthy" when in nearby communities 60% of black schoolchildren (and 0% of white children) have blood in their urine, because of schistosomiasis, yet where one is not supposed to discuss all the reasons for such glaring epidemiological discrepancies? How should one ethically participate in the faculty of a university which paid tearful lip service to concepts of equality and justice, but where needy black students were refused admission to the pleasant dormitories on campus and were required to stay miles away, in a segregated and grimy hostel surrounded by an oil refinery?

Children of Southern Africa

South Africa is a very psychologically sick society. The divorce rate, the coronary disease rate, the number of motor vehicle accidents, of suicides, and personal violence (Lester, 1989), and the rates of alcoholism and drug abuse are among the highest anywhere. The "Family Wipe-out syndrome" (Simpson, 1986/1987), in which entire families are killed in a murder–suicide by one of the parents, has been notable. Yet there are only some 2,000 clinical psychologists and psychiatrists in the country, serving some 30 million people. Only a tiny fraction of these mental health professionals are black. Mental health services for the black population are primitive, whereas those for the white population are not greatly better.

Majeke (1952) and Cuthbertson (1987) summarized the nineteenth-century legacy of the violence against the individual from proselytization and predatory missions, the structural violence of British imperialism, and the physical violence of colonial warfare. Boesak and Brews (1987) referred to the recent experience of violence: that between 1960 and 1983 more than 3.5 million people were victims of forced removals, with a further 1.8 million disrupted and under threat (see also Platzky & Walker, 1985); that from the introduction of detention-without-trial in 1963 until June, 1985, at least 72 people died in or as a direct result of detention under such legislation; that during the 1985 state of emergency, an estimated 11,500 people were detained without trial, including more than 2,000 children under the age of 16; and that a further 25,000 people were arrested and charged with "public violence," though only a negligible number ever came to trial, let alone reached a conviction.

Swartz and Levett (1989) referred to collated official figures showing that, between 1984 and 1986 alone, 300 children were killed by the police, 1,000 wounded, 11,000 detained without trial, 18,000 arrested on charges related to protest, and 173,000 were held awaiting trial in police cells. Then there was the violence of pass laws, inferior education, influx control, discriminating labor legislation: but that has been the "normal," endemic violence, all too often taken for granted (see also Jupp, 1986).

For decades, South Africa has been a violent society in the very structure of governmental policy. It is violent to move people forcibly from their place of birth and to dump them in strange places, just to satisfy someone else's racist obsessions. It is violence to separate family members by policy or by designed economic hardship and necessity. It is violence to classify people by race in order to deny privileges to some and to heap privileges on others. It is violence to systematically deny the most basic human rights in the service of such a system. The obvious physical violence that reaches wide attention is the merest tip of the iceberg of such ignored, routinized, structural violence.

The book, *Thula Baba* (Anonymous, 1987a), expresses acutely some of the tragedy of South Africa's children, typifying the manner in which political structures can enforce child neglect. It was written by a group of black women domestic workers, who work in white households, on minimal wages, looking after white children, so as to try to be able to afford to provide even minimal care for their own children, to be able to feed them and send them to school. Many employers do not allow the domestic worker to have her own children live with her, since she has to live in small rooms at the back of the garden, or on the roofs of apartment blocks, while her own children live in the "homelands," those abstract creations of busybody bureaucrats—rural wastelands in which unwanted people are filed.

The incidence and distribution of malnutrition and other social ills is not by act of God alone, but related clearly to apartheid policies. The carefully and deliberately created migrant labor system, and the influx control system (controlling the movement of black people), combined with the Group Areas Act (controlling where people are allowed to live) has been greatly effective in breaking up intact families. De Beer (1984) cataloged some of the routine miseries, such as black hospitals normally well over 100% full. There are massive disparities in infant, child, and maternal mortality rates (see also Hammond & Gear, 1986a,b). The traumatized children who concern us have been discriminated against since before their birth (maternal malnutrition and stress can have left its mark).

The children may be thrust into confrontations with adult responsibilities early in life. In 1986, in the time of the "Comrades," children were active in setting up "alternative" systems in the townships. They set up "people's courts," "people's education," and attempted to organize social and medical services. Although sometimes harsh in judgment and punishment, such enterprises often also showed a strong sense of moral concern with such issues as drunkenness, promiscuity, and violence in the family. Comrades I have interviewed have shown a notable, at times almost prissy, concern with such matters, and a highly idealized image of the sort of idyllic home lives they wanted to create, including materialistic dreams of carefully selected furnishings and consumer goods. In one area, the Comrades ordered *shebeens* (informal drinking houses) to close at 6 P.M. with a resultant drop in alcohol-related crimes being reported.

Such young people showed a high degree of politicization. Although the state repeatedly blamed "political agitators," the state itself was the most omnipresent and effective political agitator: a noisome political system that oppresses and frustrates children at every point will readily cause political sensitization. Dawes and de Villiers (1987), working with adolescents who were preparing for prison, noted that a central copy style involved the use of their political beliefs, striving to control their anxiety in the cause of the "struggle for liberation," though still, commonly, showing anxiety. Some have suggested that children with a coherent ideology may be more stress-resistant than children who are more isolated and apolitical.

The problems of children detained under security

legislation are discussed later. But the fate of the black child detained for "normal" criminal charges has also been highly unsatisfactory. Most juveniles are convicted of typical crimes of poverty, not of viciousness (Arndt, Burgin, Gutknecht, Haesler, Kronsucker, & Schmid, 1989). They are not automatically legally represented under the South African legal system and the court is not obliged to inform the child of its rights to a lawyer. Whipping is one of the commonest sentences, and a child may receive 2 to 4 sentences of whipping before a probation officer is involved. Corporal punishment is commonplace in reformatories, "Places of Safety," and children's homes—the law only takes care to ensure that white girls are excluded from it! Within prisons, gang systems are very powerful, very violent, and compete over food, clothes, money, drugs, and sex.

Problems of Research in Repressive Settings

Curran (1988) reviewed some of the many methodological problems that arise in studying the psychological effects of terrorist violence, but the problems are even more extensive within a repressive society. If we look for clear evidence on the issue of whether the turbulence and stresses of apartheid and its attendant unrest are causing damage to children, we find a great many assertions and few facts; much rhetoric and little data. Partly, this is due to failures of funding (there are few funding sources other than the government, which does not support quality studies of such matters) and partly to the preference for irrelevant research, by Third-World academics who would rather follow (far, far behind) European and American fashions, than meet local needs or use unique local opportunities.

But problems also arise because of the effects of government policy, both in the intrusive effects of extensive restrictions, harassment, and censorship, and in the effects of the alienation, resentment, and suspicion which repression causes. There are very substantial problems imposed by harassment and interference with researchers, emergency and media regulations that interfere with the reporting of findings and which may even prevent intelligent critical discussion of important issues. Any form of research that involves asking questions is interfered with by the existence of secret police actions, informers, and similar mechanics of repression; and results may be distorted either by fearful responders who say what they believe you want to hear, or by responses that are tailored to achieving a politically desired result.

One has to be aware of potential political uses and abuses of research findings. What one writes may be deliberately and cynically selectively misquoted by defenders of the system in trials, for instance, and what one writes about torture will with certainty be attentively read and applied by torturers. There is the possibility, for example, as Gibson (1989) also mentioned, that whatever other valid interpretations might be compelling, a result that demonstrated no psychological damage caused by morally repulsive actions could be misused to imply that such actions were defensible, even justifiable.

Then there can be intense politicization which can distort such studies at many points, rendering both subjects and researchers self-conscious about the potential political interpretations, meanings, uses, and abuses of the findings. They can come to be too concerned about what *should* be, to be able to clearly see what *is*.

Some of the risks are illustrated by Gibson (1989) and especially by Swartz and Levett (1989). Gibson (1989), for example, referred to "the need for this research to be useful to the victims of political violence, either directly or ideologically useful in the broad struggle against apartheid"; a phrase which potentially suggests something that could go beyond the ethical imperative not to harm subjects, or even to produce findings of social benefit, or to choose relevant topics for research (all of which are noble ideas), but that raises the possibility of choosing topics and designing methodologies in order to produce ideologically required results, an inappropriate sense of political predetermination of what findings are acceptable.

Gibson referred to the conflicting value of research as opposed to action in situations of crisis. Indeed, this is a potential problem, where research occupies scarce health professionals also needed by the community as care providers; but action unguided by relevant research, especially where it fails to include the assessment of the effects of such action, has been more potential to be damaging and wasteful of scarce resources. The right sort of relevant research can be an essential part of action and of aid.

Swartz and Levett (1989) referred perceptively to the problem of conceiving of oneself as a "neutral mediator, say, between parents wanting to keep their children indoors and children wanting to go to political rallies which are potential targets for state violence," in the situation where "adults want to 'save' children who do not want to be saved." However, they also illustrate the problems that arise when political ideology distorts scientific argument. While accepting some uses for identifying that some of repression's victims suffer from PTSD, they add that, however,

> progressive professionals are not generally interested in reproducing the elitist and alienating excesses of a mental health industry which is based on assumptions of the type that people respond to hardship with psychopathology, which, in turn, needs to be treated by experts.

This attitude (crammed with untested assumptions driven by fierce ideological positions) they describe as a "value position" which would require us to "refuse to label unhappiness and misery in the face of abuse as pseudo-diseases." That these are *pseudodiseases* is assumed without question, as are the assumptions that such description of human misery is harmful, inevitably prevents communities from caring for the children themselves, is elitist and causes alienation. Such nihilistic gloom is not helpful.

Unrest and Its Effects on Children

What has "ordinary" life been like for the child in the townships? Some children wrote about this during the 1985 state of emergency, in the moving book *Two Dogs and Freedom* (Anonymous, 1986). The children wrote recurrently of wanting freedom and equal rights, of boycotts and pressures to join "the struggle," of bad and neglected schools, and of needing good education ("We cannot be illiterate leaders"). Bothale, aged 12, wrote, "Life in nowadays is like a sick butterfly./ To many of us it is not worth living/ when it is like this."

These children grapple with complex issues. Bathandwa (aged 15) wrote that "the situation in our townships is so disgusting that you sometimes ask yourself a question which has got no answer and that is 'Why did God create a human being?' . . . We are guarded by troops every day as if we are criminals which are life sentenced. We can no longer walk as free men in our own land."

The youngest of the group was Moagi, aged 8, who wrote of the future: "When I am old I would like to have a wife and [two] children, a boy and a girl, and a big house and [two] dogs and freedom. My friends and I would like to meat [sic] together and [talk]."

There has been a breakdown of the traditional intergenerational leadership patterns. In the traditional African family, the young show deference and respect for their elders. Where the parents are seen as having allowed the repression to occur, and/or having failed to vanquish it, their leadership competence and worthiness for respect have been rejected by the children, who have been thrust into forming their own normative structures. In such fearful communities, there is a feeling that no one can or will look after you, that everyone is already or potentially against you. Children feel there is no one to turn to, and that they can only rely on their own norms: their parents' norms are obviously unable to respond to the situation.

Black children, since the 1970s, showed that they were not prepared to passively accept, as they believed their parents had done, an unjust society. It was the children's rejection of the Afrikaner hegemony in the form of the imposition of Afrikaans-medium instruction in schools that drove the 1976 uprising. There was intergenerational conflict, where parents did not support the children, and were perceived to be a generation who had been suppressed and cowed by the preceding repression (Chikane, 1986).

Children are unlikely to learn a respect for authority —*any* external authority—when growing up in a society in which *all* authorities are seen to be associated with a system which so comprehensively oppresses them.

Mpumlwana (1987) referred to force and violence as a means whereby, in Tillich's phrase (1982), "being actualises itself over against the threat of non-being," and comments, "Anyone who has seen young people at a funeral and throw stones at an armoured vehicle spitting live bullets will understand this description of defensive violence as an act of desperation."

In his analysis of violence, May (1972) wrote of "absentee violence" or "instrumental violence," what Mpumlwana calls "the indirect violence of those who claim innocence despite the fact that they live in and benefit from a system that perpetrates violence."

Not all stresses have the same impact. Straker and the Sanctuaries Team (1987) interviewed black children who were subjected to continuing traumatic stress and

high levels of violence, and reported that they were very stressed on witnessing violence against colleagues, less so with violence against strangers. They felt more stress on seeing violence between groups of black people, but much less stress when the victim of violence was seen as "part of the system."

Township mothers have voiced fears for the effects of the unrest on their children (Richman, 1986), as have such clinicians as Swartz, Dowdall, and Swartz (1986), and Straker *et al.* (1987). Straker is, however, significantly mistaken in referring to a "continuous traumatic stress syndrome" and suggesting that posttraumatic stress disorder (PTSD) is a misnomer for what is seen as a sequela to it. No valid research has established any suggestion that any such different syndrome exists with different pathology or features; the more justifiable suggestion is simply to have emphasized that one must recognize some differences in formulation, in situations in which the originating or causative traumata are continuing rather than completed. This is not a distinct condition, though a differing context, which may need variant approaches in diagnosis and therapy.

South Africa provides other stressors. What is the effect on the development of the black child who regularly sees her parents humiliated and degraded by South Africa's peculiarly condescending paternalism, in which grown black men and women are called "boy" and "girl." The children discover that their parents have few of the normal social rights, and no real power over the course of their lives. Disconnected from their roots, dislocated from their past, having a severely constricted present, and facing an uncertain future, there seems little to lose from accepting immediate gratification from sex or aggression. There is little to live for, so the risks of such conduct seem of little account.

The extent of disruption of family structure has led to an increasing number of "twilight children," homeless black urchins living feral lives in city streets. Where the home has not disintegrated around them, they have often run away from home because of family violence and drunkenness. Some are left abandoned, without shelter or protection, after their parents have been forcibly removed and deported; or when they return from a scavenging expedition to the squatter camp in which they lived, to find that it has been bulldozed by the authorities. Some babies are born in the bushes, because their parents did not dare to put up even a flimsy shelter for fear of detection by the authorities.

They sleep in streets and sewers and live by begging, stealing, and fighting. They tend to grow up with no close human relationships at all, with, at best, temporary alliances in the immediate interests of survival. They can become aggressive and isolated adults, with no real interpersonal contacts, low self-esteem, and significant suicidal impulses. At an early age, they may become unloved and unloving mothers who do not know how to care for their babies, as they have never been cared for, and unfathered sons who can become uncaring, deserting fathers. Alternatively, they can become especially concerned parents, determined to ensure that their children are not similarly deprived.

Even where the family has not wholly broken down, the requirements of life under apartheid damages child development. One man complained that his children did not know him because he was only able to be with them for 3 weeks in every year. Political detainees are released to meet a child several years old, who was fathered before their sudden arrest, but whom they may never have seen (Skinner & Swartz, 1989). Other children have been left, perforce in the care of reluctant guardians who may beat them, or with old grandparents who are too exhausted to be able to cope with them.

Severe malnutrition is common, and children may be intellectually stunted by this (Harbison, 1983; Simpson, 1963). Some experts believe that if the child is severely malnourished in the first 2 years of life, it may never fully recover from the effects. In some "homelands" areas, three quarters of the children are stunted physically by chronic poor diet.

Chikane (1986) wrote of children "socialized to find violence completely acceptable and human life cheap" (p. 344), saying that "the experiences and exposure of township children to violence will undoubtedly result in the maiming of children in every sphere of their development" (p. 337). He wrote of the extreme violence of the world of the township child:

> It is a world made up of teargas, bullets, whippings, detention and death in the streets. It is an experience of military operations and night raids, of road-blocks and body searches. It is a world, where parents and friends get carried away in the night. It is a world where people simply disappear where parents are assassinated and homes petrol-bombed. (pp. 342–343)

It is a world encompassing faction-fights, rival anti-apartheid groups, rumors of police death-squads, and right wing vigilantes.

Faction-fighting and long-standing vendettas between rival political factions, such as occurs in Natal, may lead to serial tragedies. Gqubule (1990) wrote about such communities. As one murdered youth is buried, his menfolk pledge revenge, and his sisters sing: "Ingane zethu udkula kwesiba" . . . [Our children are food for the gun]. A popular township song says that if you are black and live in a Natal township, your chances of reaching the age of 30 are slim. David Dlamini, aged 17, died after being tortured by a rival gang, accused of painting an anti-Inkatha slogan (relating to one political grouping) on a road. He told his mother: "Mama, I would rather die for something I am guilty of." He was called from his home one night and shot. After an armed attack by one local gang, students at one school demanded the right to carry arms to school. The principal who refused, saying that "Guns will never become part of the school uniform," was found dead in the streets a few days later. At a funeral, a crowd of 200 men danced and chanted "Ukufa kuyise" [death has no sting; death is nothing].

As repressive police action across the decades skimmed off almost everyone in the black communities who showed leadership abilities, there were less possibilities for the communities to control their angry youth. Among those more purely concerned about liberation are the "tsotsi comrades" or gangster activists, who straddle the line between political protest and sheer wanton violence, and can use a political vocabulary and justifications for frankly criminal activity. They have not contributed toward producing desired societal changes (indeed, they have retarded them), and appear, especially in some areas, to have moved beyond any kind of political or social control or discipline. The risk, as has been so tragically demonstrated in Belfast, Beirut, and elsewhere, is the production of an ungoverned and ungovernable community of self-perpetuating violence.

The militarization of children in such circumstances is seen in the example of the children who functioned as armed guards in "defence units" to protect their home area, in township wars. Mostly aged around 15 to 16, and armed with pangas (knives like machetes), clubs, spears, and knives (mainly homemade), they would stay awake all night to protect their houses. One said, "I do this so my parents and other brothers who have to work do not have to stay up all night."

One 14-year-old was reported to have a "comrade" name which translates as "Kill 'em all and come back alive." He was second in command of "The Scorpions," a "People's Defence Unit," and was also called "Ethiopia" because his colleagues thought he looked like a malnourished Ethiopian child. He claimed there were 3,000 local youths under his command and reported that a 15-year-old friend of his was fatally shot in a riot; another was hacked to death by a rival group (Bekker, 1987, for example). Yet these boys could also be like boy's gangs in other communities: girls were dismissed as "sissies" and were not allowed to join the struggle. "You can't trust the ladies," one explained, "they tell our secrets. Also, they are not strong enough to be with us."

The Report of the Lawyers' Committee for Human Rights (Lock, 1986) pointed out that children are growing up without any perception or understanding of the parameters of acceptable behavior and warned that this could do great damage to the future cohesion of the country, adding that "it is difficult to see what rehabilitative processes, if any, will be effective in undoing all the damage." The report asked, "What is to be done with children who use hand grenades or dance around the dying bodies of people they have set alight? What is to be done when authority has lost all credibility, and respect for the law has been destroyed by the very people trying to implement it?" The committee complained that "when security forces are granted indemnity, then whatever they do appears to show so little respect for the law that they are prepared to abuse their powers to the extent that they do, their victims cannot be expected to respect the law either."

After episodes of publicized complaints of police violence in breaking up demonstrations by schoolchildren, a doctor quoted a man whom he had seen, whose son was hospitalized after the father had severely beaten the child. Unashamed, the father said: "How can the government tell me not to beat my child, when they employ people to sjambok [whip] strangers' children in the streets?"

In a major report, Wilson and Ramphele (1987) emphasized not only the obvious effects of the brutalization of those caught in the violence of the townships among blacks but stated that

> white youngsters are conscripted into the Army after finishing school, and sent into the townships, often into the black schools themselves, [and] become part of the

machinery of oppression maintaining a social, political and economic order which is profoundly corrupting of human well-being and decency.

Vergnani (1986) reported that some white children were so disturbed by ANC bombings that they believed they would end up barricaded behind sandbags in their suburban homes. For a time we saw children around 6 or 7 years of age, suffering from school phobia, aggravated by bomb drills and the fear that they might come to harm at school. Older children showed more depression and anxiety. Black children attempt to deal with the experience in the form of games like Casspir-Casspir (named after the common armored vehicle used by police and army), and Witdoek against Comrades (named after two vigilante fighting factions) can replace cops and robbers. Another popular game was "Funerals."

Much regressive behavior, including bedwetting, has been noted in township children, and some were referred for assistance with anxiety and uncontrolled crying spells. They may show a generalized fear of people in uniform (especially in the colors of the police and the army uniforms); some show an even more generalized fear of white people. The case is quoted of a young black child who screamed in terror when she saw her mother's white friend, crying, "She's going to kill me!"

A great deal of relevant and useful psychosocial research needs to be done. The most relevant of the slim body of potentially relevant international research findings are existing studies of "minority groups": groups identified racially or otherwise, who are prejudicially treated in other societies. South Africa has been notable in contriving to turn the vast majority of its population into a "minority group."

The theory of learned helplessness (Seligman, 1975; Abramson, Seligman, & Teasdale, 1978) has considerable value in understanding the sequelae of traumatic stress. Animal models of inescapable shock are relevant (van der Kolk, Greenberg, Boyd, & Krystal, 1985), and the development of helplessness responses is related to the individual's attributional or explanatory style in regard to life events. Notable among these is *locus of control* (the extent to which individuals feel able to control their own destiny). People with an *internal* locus of control believe they can control their sociopolitical environment and life situations; with an *external* locus, they feel they have no control over what happens to them. Members of minority or disadvantaged groups tend to perceive their locus of control as external (Battle & Rotter, 1963; Gore & Rotter, 1963; Meyter & Raphaely, 1978). In "doll-choice" studies, minority group children tend to identify with dolls representing the dominating group, even when they can cognitively tell the difference. Gregor and McPherson (1966) reported that black children in South Africa also identified with white dolls. When they compared white and so-called colored school children, they found the two groups similar as regards a measure of self-acceptance, but the "colored" children were more external in locus of control.

Significant relations between learned helplessness attributional styles and various measures of PTSD have been demonstrated (McCormick, Taber, & Kruedelbach, 1989), and a relationship between disaster response and locus of control has been shown (Anderson, 1977; Gibbs, 1989; Thurber, 1977).

On the other hand, Garmezy (1985) proposed a sort of reverse of the learned helplessness model, like Rachman's idea of "required helpfulness" (1979), that the act of helping others, in a stressful situation, can empower a person and strengthen their resistance to the stress. Such possibilities need far more study and resemble Simpson's earlier emphasis (Simpson, 1979) on the benefits for the dying patient of retaining usefulness and being able to aid others. It has been argued that prior exposure to trauma (depending on how it was experienced) could enhance the ability to cope. Liu and Cheung (1985), for example, reported that those refugees who had experienced the 1954 Dien Bien Phu evacuation adjusted much better after the 1975 Saigon evacuation than those who had not experienced it.

The Oppressors

A much neglected area of study is the effects of repression on the oppressors themselves. Kelman (1973) examined the dehumanizing effects of violence on the perpetrators as well as the victims. The overprivileged can be traumatized as well as the underprivileged (though the trauma may be far more comfortable). The Afrikaner people of South Africa have been shaped by powerfully warping influences, having been treated with special favoritism by a state devoted purely to their sectional needs, yet without ever having to earn any of their privileges through any personal or group endeavor, such care being guaranteed as an entitlement to anyone with white skin and membership of the Afrikaner tribal system (see van der Spuy, 1978; van der Spuy & Shamley, 1978, on the psychology of apartheid).

Orpen (1970) and others found the Afrikaner to be extremely authoritarian. In fact, the description by Klineberg (1964) of the authoritarian person fits the typical Afrikaner upbringing with uncanny closeness. He

> tends to be a supreme conformist, he sees the world as menacing and unfriendly . . . he is rigid and shows limited imagination; he is hard-minded, exalting his own group and disliking many out-groups. . . . Often these individuals are on the surface, poised, self-confident and well-adjusted, but fundamentally anxious and insecure. . . . They blame others for their faults and imperfections.

They have been a paranoid people, feeling nationally persecuted while they have been the persecutors; and convinced that a massive and co-ordinated "onslaught" seeks to destroy them. Similarly, Miller (1987) argued that where obedience is an undisputed, supreme principle of child-rearing and religious education, this leads to a type of personal development inclined to manipulation and control by propaganda and to violent conduct.

There is also a strong sense of "divine purpose," of being a chosen people with a unique relationship with a Deity who, if He (He must surely be both male and white) condones their actions in recent decades, can bear little resemblance to the Deities recognized by anyone else. Yet they are endlessly pious, with a passion for the Bible from which they have extracted justifications for their determinedly ungodly actions, in the name of that ghastly experiment in social engineering—*apartheid*.

their determinedly ungodly actions, in the name of that ghastly experiment in social engineering—*apartheid*.

Ironically, it was in South Africa that the British invented the concentration camp, during the Anglo-Boer War in the late nineteenth century (De Vitt, 1941; van Rensburg, 1980). Those camps, in which death rates from infectious disease were very high, specifically interned Boer women and children. In those days, there was no counseling for survivors, and no one looked for PTSD. No one has adequately studied the impact of those experiences on the people who shaped Afrikaner society in this century—and on the policies which they later developed.

Van der Spuy (1978; van der Spuy & Shamley, 1978) reported that South African students scored high on neuroticism (compared to other national groups), and showed a high level of anxiety. One means of coping with this has been the awesome obsessionality of petty apartheid. What a feeble ego it is that can find no single other thread of which to weave a sense of self than the hollow and essentially meaningless claim: "But I am white!" If that is all you are, what are you?

The children often show no developing capacity for deferred gratification: If the very existence of a future is seriously in doubt, why work for goals that may never be allowed to happen? There is a tragic irony. Black children can show such effects, from the underprivileged lives apartheid forces upon them, in which life is treated as if cheap and transient; whereas white children show similar effects from their overprivileged experience, knowing at some level within themselves that they do not deserve the materialistically lavish lives they lead, and expecting the whole fragile system that supports them to burst like a bubble, while dreading a retributive black backlash which they fear they have earned.

B. Angus (personal communication, 1988) observed a decline in the mode of moral behavior of white schoolboys; a belief that any conduct is acceptable, so long as nobody finds out; that things you do only become wrong when you are caught. Although a dilettante fashion has emerged among trendy lawyers, to offer "street law" courses to schools, these are meaningless in the absence of a developed sense of morality, except as classes in how not to get caught. It is hard for children to invent a moral system, but easy to invent rebellion against one. It is not easy for them, in the absence of a coherent and obvious, demonstrable, and shared public morality, to devise an organized ethical code for themselves.

Young children can often distinguish between violence for a just cause and violence in the service of injustice. It is a commonplace observation in routine life that children display great indignation and fury over real or exaggerated experiences of injustice: "It isn't *fair!*" is such a common complaint and is felt by them to be a very substantial objection to any action or proposal. Such a sensitivity is not limited to the petty frustrations of regular living. Such aspects of the development of moral sensitivities have not yet been fully explored.

The effort required to live in a system which requires one to ignore the monstrous immorality of an oppressive system like apartheid has a significant effect on stunting moral growth. If we look at Kohlberg's model of the stages of moral development (Kohlberg, 1963), which Turiel (1966, 1973) has shown to develop similarly

in widely different cultural settings, children between 7 and 16 show a sharp rise in the proportion at Level II (Conventional) and a moderate rise in those at Level III (Autonomous or Principled). Our experience in South Africa would suggest that far more children remain at the most basic level (I, the Proconventional level), often at Stage I, the punishment/obedience orientation, even in adulthood, and that few reach Level III. Abu Nasr, Vriesendorp, Lorfing, and Khalifeh (1981) studied the moral judgment of Lebanese children in times of war, but far more such work on the potential impact of trauma on moral development is needed.

Lasting Impact of Unrest on Children

The major single review of the research literature on this issue is that by Dyregrov and Raundalen (1987), and in the book by Dodge and Raundalen (1987). There have been numerous studies of children's responses to warfare (Baider & Rosenfeld, 1974; Bodman, 1944; Boothby, 1986; Brander, 1943; Burbury, 1941; and Burt, 1943). Specific settings have been studied, such as the children of the Lebanese civil strife (Bryce, 1986; Bryce & Armenian, 1986; Day, 1984, 1986; Day & Sadek, 1982; Hourani, Armenian, Zurayk, & Afifi, 1986; Saigh, 1985, 1986); Palestinian and Israeli children (Punamaki, 1982, 1983; Ziv, Kruglanski, & Shulman, 1974); children in the Spanish Civil War (Coromina, 1943); children in Chile (Schirmer, 1986); Southeast Asian refugee children (Carlin, 1979); children from Cambodia (Kinzie, Sack, Angell, Manson, & Rath, 1986); child soldiers in Uganda (Dodge, 1986; Dodge & Raundalen, 1987); and those affected by Central American warfare (Arroyo & Eth, 1984).

It is an unsatisfactory literature—so little research has been done, and so little of this is well done, or useful, or justifies the weight of the conclusions that may be based on it. Most of the literature on disasters, war, and posttraumatic disorders simply ignores children and adolescents. If they look at children at all, many of the studies examine the impact of a single horrible event (such as an earthquake), and few study the effect of the sort of chronic, suppurating violence and unrest that afflict many parts of the world. Most of the emphasis is on short-term effects; very few studies try to look for lasting effects. Except for some studies of Holocaust survivors, there has been little attention to the effects in adult life of exposure to horrors as a child.

Initially, Raphael (1984) was oddly dismissive of "smaller-scale disasters . . . such as civilian violence, riots and terrorism" which "cannot match" war. However, in her excellent work on disasters (Raphael, 1986), in the section "Civilian violence as disaster," she recognized that

> the predictability of disaster, by contributing to psychological preparedness, may lessen shock effects. Thus, the morbidity found with regular flooding may be substantially less than that associated with a highly traumatic and unexpected man-made disaster . . . or with the uncertainty and terror of civilian violence.

There is loss and grief, antipathy, hatred, vendettas, and dislocation. The challenge is *not* simply to survive a single catastrophe and then repair and heal and resume routine life, but to adjust to ongoing stress with episodic occurrences of acute threat, while trying to maintain everyday existence.

The fact that the great bulk of recent research and development work in regard to traumatic stress disorders has focussed on American Vietnam veterans has, to an extent not fully realized by the researchers, biased the findings and misshaped our concept of these conditions in ways not always helpful to our understanding of such problems in other peoples, following other tragedies. Similarly, too much of the recent literature on traumatic stress and children has consisted of repetitive publication of rather limited studies, of highly publicized and peculiar events, such as American sniper incidents. There is a strangely flat and monotonous quality to the bland portrayals of children's apparently essentially similar responses to trauma as portrayed by such authors as Pynoos and Furman. It is not so tidy in the real world or in the Third World, and such models do not deal realistically with continuing or recursive trauma.

It is very important to understand the effects of traumatic, and especially chronic, stressors on children. In adult life, serious late effects may cripple national development in the decades after the resolution of disasters or conflicts. In chronic conflicts, such effects may be a major part of the reason for their chronic awfulness and persistent unsolvability. Just as it has been recognized that the abused child may grow up to become an abusing parent, so traumatized societies may either become chronically traumatic because of internecine violence, or may themselves become traumatizers in internal or international affairs. It is also important because we need a better understanding of the nature of the problems caused, so as to be able to plan relief, aid, and continuing support effectively. When planning to assist children involved in catastrophes, mere survival is not enough.

In World War II, for example, the British policy of evacuating children from heavily bombed areas was due in part to exaggerated fears of the effects air raids would have on the psychological health of civilian populations. In fact, it is likely that far more harm was caused by the enforced separation from parents and familiar environment in the evacuees, than would have been caused had the children remained in the sturdy and healthy communities that were being bombed (see Wolfenstein, 1957, for instance).

The analytic literature is especially given to disguising the extent to which it is speculating. Universal conclusions may be based on studies of a very small number (sometimes one or two) seriously disturbed children, atypical in many ways, including their ability to afford extensive psychotherapy. It is impossible to know how representative or idiosyncratic are their reactions. Even when larger samples of traumatized children are studied, there is rarely a control group. In conducting and evaluating such studies, there are two risks: that we will exaggerate the extent of damage caused, and that we will underestimate it.

Even where it would be perfectly possible to do so, remarkably few studies actually ask the children about their responses. Some ask exclusively the parents or teachers (although it has been well shown that these sources under- or overestimate the child's experience). Some studies rely only on drawings, sometimes interpreted so personally by the researcher (rather than the child) that they seem to serve, like Rorschach's inkblots, more a form of projective test revealing the researcher's psychopathology rather than the child's.

Where there are studies of the long-term effects of childhood trauma, these are almost inevitably retrospective. Rarely are there controls, but there is heavy reliance on the patient's memories; the likely effects of intervening life events are usually ignored; and the subjects are usually exclusively those who are unwell, ignoring both those who survived unscathed, and those so severely affected as not to have survived until the time of the study. There have been few prospective studies; usually they also lack controls; assessment of the children is often indirect or superficial and there is only very brief follow-up. Although other factors, such as culture, religion, and the meanings the individuals apply to life events are clearly significant, these are usually ignored.

Reports of the effects of disaster on children are relevant to our theme. Studies of the effects of bombing during World War II found that children showed acute disturbance—worst in the 8- to 12-year-old age group, in those with previous psychological disorders, and in those from unstable homes. Common major effects were anxiety and fear (especially fear of being separated from parents, a result often thoughtfully arranged by their "caregivers"), restlessness and irritability, dependent and demanding behavior, disturbance of body functions, and difficulty concentrating (Edwards, 1976). Our experience has been that the effects are partly related to broad developmental stages. More regressive modes of coping are seen more in preschool children; elements of political identification and more defiant coping styles emerge in middle childhood and consolidate in adolescence. Boys seem more vulnerable in early childhood, the balance reversing in adolescence, as differing gender expectations become more prominent.

Early in the aftermath of disaster, children show what some researchers call *compulsive behavior patterns*, and what I consider to be attempts in play to rehearse, control, and master events. After the Skopje earthquake, Popovic and Petrovic (1964) described how the favorite play of children was based on earthquakes and burying bodies. As already mentioned, we have seen similar responses in South Africa.

Lyons (1979) described a range of potential reactions. Those who had experienced bombing showed affective problems, or phobias, with some developing agoraphobia. Children often showed separation anxiety. Depression was seen in 29% of the cases, as well as severe irritability, anxiety, sleep disturbances, and startle responses. Sixty-five percent showed posttraumatic anxiety states. The symptoms of the children and teenagers were seen in relation to those of the parents. They also tend to show excitement, and often identify with, and act out violence, and show conduct disorders. In Belfast, the older children and teenagers mostly belonged to paramilitary gangs, and group antisocial behavior was common.

Significantly, Lyons (1979) noted the difference between wars, when a community can be united against an external aggressor, and terrorism or civil war, where a community can be divided, and violence can come from anywhere. Tan and Simons (1973) described similar features as effects of riots in Malaysia. Frazer (1974) agreed that there are major effects on child development and behavior. Abu Nasr, Makhoreli, and Lorfing (1986) found that the population withstood the Lebanese Civil War surprisingly well, because of a strong family system and group cohesion, but reported an increase in psychiatric referrals, including commonly posttraumatic and depressive symptoms, and increased drug addiction and alcoholism. Kinzie *et al.* (1986), studying 40 Cambodian children who had experienced massive trauma, reported that 50% developed PTSD and 85% also had some depressive disorder.

Raphael (1986) summarized other studies of morbidity in children and adolescents. Crawshaw (1963) observed that adolescents have reactions between those of children and those of adults, and may be simultaneously excited by, and fearful of, disasters—the same reaction we see in the face of unrest.

The idea that unrest could engender positive reactions is unfamiliar. But Fogelson (1970), for instance, commenting on the 1960s riots, noted:

> the outpourings of fellow feeling, of mutual respect and common concern . . . camaraderie . . . carnival spirit . . . exhilaration so intense as to border on jubilation . . . a sense of pride, purpose and accomplishment . . . their common predicament revealed in the rioting, blacks looked again at one another and saw only brothers.

He emphasized such positive responses to riots, not to suggest that they are advisable and beneficial, but that there are sufficient psychosocial benefits to help to explain their continuation and acceptance by communities. The sense of common purpose, and of joint outrage against a common enemy, are notable here.

Children seem able to be psychologically quite resilient—if they stay with parents who themselves can cope and can allow their children to express their fears. Rutter (1986) emphasized the extent to which one of the main determinants of a child's reactions to a stresslike hospitalization is the *parent's* level of anxiety. Across a number of studies, it appears that children who remain with their families have less problems than those who are separated from them. As we have seen, in South Africa, apartheid often separates children from parents, but there is often a very supportive larger community, and good sibling and peer relations. It is the younger children who suffer most from the separation effects (see also Skinner & Swartz, 1989).

In studies of bereaved children, Rutter (1986) found that discord and multiple shifts of home are more likely to be factors that influence outcome rather than the bereavement itself. The better the support from the family and community, the less the ill-effects. In South Africa, the black family and community structure have often remained strong, despite the grave damage caused by apartheid.

The relation between the extent of the ill-effects suffered by the child, and the degree of upset and emotional expressiveness of the parents, needs to be studied. One cannot effectively study the child without studying the parents. There may be a grisly interaction. A case is

reported in South Africa where the mother hid her child when another faction of youths wanted to catch and execute him. The father, terrified lest they burn down their humble house he had struggled to attain, fought her off and called out to the gang: "Here he is—take my son, leave my house alone."

Dawes, Tredoux, and Feinstein (1989) provided unusual two-generation data in their study of the effects on children of the Crossroads tragedy, where four squatter communities in South Africa were deliberately burnt to the ground, 53 people were killed, many injured, and 70,000 were left homeless, in a brutal "forced removal." They described an incidence of PTSD of 63.1% in adult women, 32% in adult men, 52.5% in single women, and 69.1% in married women. In the children, the overall incidence of PTSD was 9.2%; 32.4% showed stress symptoms though not PTSD; 58.4% showed no symptoms. Fearfulness, often very specifically triggered, was the commonest type of problem. In the youngest age group, boys showed more stress symptoms than girls; in midchildhood, both sexes were similarly affected; and in adolescence, more girls than boys were symptomatic, and more had PTSD.

Some studies suggest a potentially grim long-term outlook for some severe stressors. Lidz is quoted by Hocking (1965) as finding that all survivors of the Guadalcanal evacuation developed neurotic symptoms in civilian life. Archibald, Long, Miller, and Tuddenham (1963) reported that 15 years after combat trauma, 70% of the survivors suffered from a chronic traumatic neurosis, one third were unemployed, and another one third were only in unstable employment. Bulhan (1985) remarked: "Violence breeds more violence . . . and a community of victims, unaware of its history and unable to control its destiny, engages in much autodestructive behavior."

Accounts of the experiences of Nazi concentration camp survivors, such as those reviewed by Kinston and Rosser (1974), are highly relevant. One should note those studies of the children and families of survivors of the Nazi Holocaust which suggest that psychological effects of such traumatic events may persist so as to affect the next generations (Bergmann & Jucovy, 1982; Epstein, 1979), even where they have had no direct experience of the horrors. Shatan (1975) described World War II "war babies" who experienced the absence of their fathers and the withdrawal/depression of their mothers.

Rosenheck (1985a,b) described special problems faced by Vietnam combat veterans who were sons of World War II combat soldiers. In some cases, they developed what he called a malignant form of PTSD, with "a general valence for aggressive or physically assertive behavior and an episodic loss of impulse control in response to frustration or threat." Rosenheck and Nathan (1985) described the effects that some Vietnam veterans with severe PTSD had on their own children; and in a clinical survey, Rosenheck (1986) described long-term transgenerational effects in the offspring of World War II combat veterans.

The sinister potential for intergenerational transmission of violence (Krugman, 1987) is a cause for real concern. This could add significantly to the potential for prolonged cycles of violence, especially when combined with the potential, such as Kardiner (1941) described, for victims to subsequently seek, voluntarily, reenactment or reexposure to similar trauma, even to the extent that Horowitz (1976) called "traumatophilia."

Where longer follow-up has been attempted, the results are worrying. Higgins and Schinckel (1985) found that the degree of disorder in children 2 years after a disaster was greater than that after 2 or 8 months. The children showed still more morbidity when there was other family dysfunction or posttrauma symptoms in the parents. Up to 13% were affected, and the problems were not minor. Harmful effects seemed to be lessened where there were continuing supportive relationships, and where parents gave children information, answered their questions, and encouraged them to share their feelings about events.

A year after the Ash Wednesday bushfires in South Australia, Clayer (1984; Clayer, Bookless-Pratz, & Harris, 1985) found increased family and marital problems, and problems with the children; and Milne (1977) described similar findings after the Darwin cyclone. Newman (1976) found continuing responses to the Buffalo Creek disaster in children 2 years later, even in children who had been as young as 26 months during the events. The very few studies that looked at the impact on family functioning found an increased incidence of family disorders, which, in turn, affect children, who are thus secondary as well as primary victims of trauma.

Apart from the fearfulness of the events themselves, there is likely to be an increased need for nurturing and caring; at the very time when the family and community are least able to provide it. In a short-interlude disaster that intervenes in the midst of a secure life-style, positive influences may be most noticeable, such as a sense of adventure, the reassuring discovery of one's competence, the pleasure of disrupted routine, and others.

Fragmentary comments in many reports confirm our experience that a common response is the development either of a generalized fearfulness (as if the universe has become so untrustworthy that anything might happen at any time); or with specific fears that are triggered by reminders of primary aspects of the trauma, often with a strong startle response. Children surviving Aberfan (Lacey, 1972) for instance, showed fear of heavy rain and other bad weather such as that which preceded the disaster.

Fearfulness continues even in children who are judged by others to have recovered or to have been unaffected. Troubled sleep and nightmares can be long-lasting, either with replicas of the events, or partly or wholly disguised symbols. In South Africa, Gibson (1987) gave the telling example of the child of 3 or 4 years whose home had been raided by the police, who, in the therapist's office, began systematically emptying desk drawers and bookshelves. These games may be hard for parents to tolerate. Attempts at mastery, they can represent an action replay of the trauma, but with this essential difference: this time around, you can win. Drawings, if allowed, often depict the traumatic events, often with hopeful elements, or magical means of controlling the damaging elements. With more chronic exposure to trauma, these hopeful or control elements may fade out. The games and drawings, like the dreams in adult PTSD, show typical forms. Some are sterile, monotonously repetitive, and produce no sense of relief whatsoever. Where there are elements of empowerment, such as elements of potential mastery or escape, there is more an indication of the tentative development of coping. The first type reenacts central elements of the trauma, whether or not symbolically elaborated, without progress toward resolution. Indeed, each reprise replenishes the anxiety. Progressive, healthy play or depiction of the trauma does not need so much repetition before a useful degree of mastery can be achieved by it.

Incidentally, the therapeutic uselessness of these flashbacks and the sterile variety of traumatic dreams and play demonstrate the fallacy of those pop therapists who market, so expensively, means to achieve rapid intensive affect arousal, as if that, in itself, was therapeutic. It is not. Without a working-through, and the slower fabrication of meaning, it is useless. None of the therapeutic quacks arouses his damp audiences as competently as do these reverberations of trauma, or with less benefit.

General research has shown that "undesirable life events" can have a causal association with the onset of psychiatric disorder in children and adolescents (Goodyer, Kolvin, & Gatzanis, 1985, 1987). The "undesirable" events in such studies are usually very minor compared with those experienced by the children of conflict. Also relevant to assessing the potential damage the children might experience is work like that of Brown and Harris (1978), who showed that the ill-effects of multiple unrelated events have an additive impact. It is not yet quite clear to what extent this effect is quantitative. Much work remains to be done as regards how children personally construe stresses and risks.

Some of the literature has been construed as suggesting that social turmoil and unrest might not have any substantial impact on mental health, but this interpretation is not truly convincing. A major problem is that such studies so often use convenient but unreliable indirect measures of psychopathology (which, it is well known from other studies, do *not* accurately reflect actual rates or types of psychopathology). Many of them use assessments made in nonstandard ways, using undisclosed criteria, variable methods and sensitivities, and, largely, untrained assessors. For example, after the Tower of London bomb explosion, a study (Tucker & Lettin, 1975) reported that 11% of the victims had psychological symptoms, as assessed by orthopedic surgeons!

In a better study (Hadden, Rutherford, & Merrett, 1978) of 1,532 consecutive victims of similar bombings, 50% were found to be psychologically disturbed. In a sensible study of drug-prescription rates in Belfast during the major 1969 riots, Fraser (1971) showed major increases in rates of prescription of tranquilizers, varying from 26% in one general practice, to 135% in another. Also, such studies did not look for the varieties of stress disorders now recognized.

Also, one must distinguish (and such research has not adequately done this) between having symptoms and having access to clinical services; the sensitivity, skills, and knowledge of the clinician seen; successfully and accurately communicating the quality of one's distress; receiving a diagnosis; the accuracy and comprehensiveness of that diagnosis; receiving treatment at the primary, secondary, or tertiary level; and admission to the hospital.

Some studies of specific disasters and conflicts are also relevant to our theme. Terr (1979, 1981, 1983) studied 23 children who survived kidnapping in a schoolbus, and found all suffered significant posttraumatic effects with cognitive disturbance, fear of further trauma, disturbed dreams, and reexperiencing the trauma. They no longer felt able to trust the world, and had multiple fears.

Kaffman and Elizur (1979, 1983) found that around 40% of normal preadolescent Israeli kibbutz children, who lost a father during the 1973 Yom Kippur war, still showed severe maladaptive behavior over 3 years later, including social, volitional, and learning problems. With the poor standard of black education in South Africa, such an impact on learning would be harder to assess. When they compared similarly bereaved kibbutz and urban children, Kaffman and Elizur found persistent signs of "pathological grief" in 48% of kibbutz children and in 52% of urban children, showing little protective effect from the social supports of the kibbutz. In these studies, unfortunately, the data are derived from interviews with the parents and not with the children.

Punamaki (1983) found "outbursts of anger and aggression" common in Israeli and Palestinian children, and Abu Nasr *et al.* (1986) wrote of children becoming "pupils of war." In their work in Uganda, Dyregrov and Raundalen (1987) described a relatively low incidence of aggression and revenge in the children they worked with, whereas 80% of the children were rated as depressed. Psychic numbing and avoidance of painful memories seem to have been common in the Ugandan and Cambodian children described.

Fields (1987) described unique research on children, 6 to 16 years old, in Northern Ireland, Lebanon, the West Bank, Israel, and South Africa, with fascinating results. On the Tapp-Kohlberg measures of legal socialization, she found that Palestinian and Northern Irish children showed truncated development at an early stage of retributive justice or vendetta. The children feel helpless and powerless, feel their parents are unable to protect them, and that violence and destruction are inevitable and inescapable. She reported that, in the Irish sample, "those who became activists in organizations that advocate terror tactics, had usually suffered physical and psychological pain and humiliation at the hands of the authorities." Her work also suggests that exposure to prolonged violent trauma limits the personality development to the egocentric, narcissistic level, and that terrorized children are likely to become terrorists (see also Fields, 1973, 1976).

Fields also raised an important and often overlooked point. She wrote of how Palestinian youths with no personal direct experience of violence identified so strongly with the victims of the Sabra/Shatila massacre that they had nightmares and fantasies of personal victimization, or danger to their parents or sibs. She commented, sagely, that "a child can be traumatised vicariously through his or her identification with a victimized group."

The findings of Yacoubian and Hacker (1989) also illustrate this point, in their description of the reactions of Armenian-American adolescents in Los Angeles to the Soviet Armenian earthquake. They showed intense identification and grief reactions; and also the response of enhanced nationalism and cultural cohesion. They also described "a sort of envious resentment about being excluded from a unique and rallying experience, a longing at least for participation" as well as a variety of survivor guilt. I share, however, the skepticism of Terr (1985) about claims that children's concerns about nuclear war constitute true vicarious traumatization. These other examples are far more real.

Macksoud (1988) studied 2,220 children in Beirut, aged 4 to 16 (average, 9), who were rather different to those seen in South Africa and other troubled lands. About 95% had both parents alive, instead of the predominant single-parent families, and a high percentage had fathers who were employed, many of them in good jobs. The study used a questionnaire completed by the parents. Macksoud showed that one of the traumas for children was watching coverage of violent events on TV. Trauma was ubiquitous, 96% of the children had been exposed to at least one trauma, on average, to 5 or 6, and thus multiple, interacting trauma; a very small portion of the children (perhaps, in part, determined by the method of the study) had personally suffered direct violence.

The chronic horrors of Northern Ireland have resulted in disappointingly few studies. Lyons (1971, 1972) reported temporary "normal fear and anxiety responses" related to the troubles, but no increase in psychotic illness. In the areas of greatest aggression, there seemed to be a decrease in depression, which might be related to an externalization of aggression. Frazer (1974, 1983) found, in contrast, that psychological disorders increased during the 1968 violence in Belfast. He described immediate reactions as hysterical (some children could not stop crying). Common responses included insomnia, enuresis, and nervousness, with persistent abnormal fears. Jahoda and Harrison (1975) compared children in Belfast with children in peaceful Edinburgh. They found high ethnocentrism from an early age, with the Irish children taught to deprive the enemy of identity, a dehumanization effect very powerful by the age of 6. Fields (1973, 1976) found that the stories told by Belfast children were full of helplessness, death, and destruction.

The relationship between actual war stressors and anxiety is not clear (R. M. Milgram & N. A. Milgram, 1976; Saigh, 1985, 1986; Ziv & Israeli, 1973); though the children surveyed in these studies had in fact had limited exposure to the worst of the violence. Where Middle East and Irish data showed no substantial increase in anxiety, and a matter-of-fact, seeming acceptance of menacing events, this is sometimes taken as representing adaptation to, and coping with, the situation. In some ways, such an approach may limit the impact of emotional trauma. But we still need a more thoughtful approach to the issue of what constitutes good and appropriate coping in such highly abnormal circumstances.

Skinner (1986) conducted a most detailed study of the responses of 19 South African preschool children to the detention of a parent. More than half had no contact at all with the detainee during the period of detention. There had been regular or constant presence of security forces near the home in 74% of cases, and harassment of

613

Table 51.1. Responses of Preschool Children to the Political Detention of a Parent

Problem	During detention (%)	Short-term (%)	Long-term (6 months+) (%)
Overdependence, clinging	79	53	36
Will not sleep alone	68	40	27
Fear and phobias			
Of police	63	60	55
Of loud noises	37	40	9
Of being followed	16	20	18
Sleep disturbance	68	27	0
Wakes up crying	32	13	0
Crying by day	79	40	27
Irritable	63	33	9
Tantrums	53	7	9
Depressed	47	20	0
Overactivity	26	13	9
Anger at police, officials	53	33	45
Hate for	37	27	18
Desire to kill or maim	47	40	45
Physical symptoms	79	40	9
Enuresis	42	20	9
Regression	37	13	9
Taking adult role	16	20	9
Learning problems	32	7	0
Nightmares	26	27	0
Reliving trauma	16	13	0

Source: Adapted from Skinner, 1968, and Skinner & Swartz, 1989.

the family by such forces in 42%. In 13% of cases, the parent was subsequently re-detained, and in 47% had to go on the run, after release, as a result of harassment. Problems encountered in the children, during the parent's detention, within weeks of the parent's release, and 6 months later, are shown in Table 51.1 (which was adapted from Skinner, 1986). Although numbers are too small to be sure, there was a suggestion that the children who had fantasized during the detention that their parent was dead showed more short- and long-term problems.

Traumatic Effects of Prejudice

Suffering which falls to our lot in the course of nature, or by chance, or fate, does not seem so painful as suffering which is inflicted on us by the arbitrary will of another.
—SCHOPENHAUER

The great majority of us are required to live a life of constant, systematic duplicity. Your health is bound to be affected if, day after day, you say the opposite of what you feel, if you grovel before what you dislike and rejoice at what brings you nothing but misfortune . . . our soul . . . is inside us, like teeth in our mouth. It can't be forever violated with impunity.
—BORIS PASTERNAK, *Doctor Zhivago*

Allport (1958) reviewed what he called "traits due to victimization," effects of prolonged exposure to prejudicial attitudes. He felt that there were inevitable character effects. He spoke of the child "who finds himself rejected and attacked on all sides" as "not likely to develop dignity and poise as his outstanding traits." Yet my experience in South Africa suggests that very significant numbers of black children develop just such traits from just such a bitter background of experience. Allport wrote of the child being like a dwarf in a world of menacing giants with whom he cannot fight on equal terms, and reviewed what ego defenses are available to such an individual. Such a "dwarf-child" can withdraw and keep to himself, "speaking little to the giants and never honestly"; he can band with a group of similarly afflicted, for comfort and self-respect; "He may try to cheat the giants when he can and thus have a taste of sweet revenge. He may in desperation occasionally push some giant off the sidewalk or throw a rock at him when it is safe to do so"; or he may come to act as the giant expects, and to share his master's prejudiced view of dwarfs.

Other traits can include clowning, aggression against one's own group, prejudice against other outgroups, sympathy with other victims, striving for symbolic status, and fighting back with militancy. As Spinoza wrote, "He who conceives himself hated by another, and believes that he has given him no cause for hatred, will hate that other in return." As Allport commented: "His natural self-love may, under the persistent blows of contempt, turn his spirit to cringing and self-hate"; and also refers to the "obsessive concern" with which the victim wonders whether and when he will be insulted and humiliated.

Allport gave some telling examples of the dawning of race consciousness, and how prejudice affects the "Negro" child. Six-year-old Janet runs home and asks, "Mother, what is the name of the children I am supposed to hate?" A little boy whose mother was warning him never to play with niggers, replied, "No, mother, I never play with niggers. I only play with white and black children."

In a neglected and overlooked section relevant to our studies of traumatic stress symptoms, Allport also referred to "conditioning" following trauma or shock, with the example of the girl, sexually abused by a Filipino houseboy who "now actually shudders when [she is] in the presence of an oriental." He considered that traumatic learning leads to overgeneralization, equivalent to the "total rejection" phase of his model of prejudice. But he cautioned that trauma may merely intensify or accelerate a process already under way; and that people tend to look for simple childhood traumatic experiences to explain their attitudes.

Gross sociopsychological deprivation can result from being politically dominated and exploited (Fanon, 1967; Freire, 1968; Herskovits, 1971). Burke (1984, 1985) described racism-related disorders in blacks as grieflike in kind, resulting from a basic sense of loss and fear of further loss (see also Mannoni, 1964; and Pillay, 1984).

In the past, racially blinkered authors have gone so far as to assert that black people would not be affected by trauma. Green (1914), for instance, argued that the Negro had "a simple nature which gives little thought to the future," so that "depression is rarely encountered even under circumstances in which a white person would be overwhelmed by it." Levy-Bruhl (1910) stated that blacks lacked an individual mind or sense of being a person, sharing some sort of tribal or communal mind, and making little difference between himself and the outside world.

Early research showed that black children in Britain and in the United States had low self-esteem, a negative self-image, and an insecure sense of identity, suggesting, as Coopersmith (1975) implied, that social devaluation of a race or culture can be incorporated within the individual with these results. More recent work has intimated that black children have potentially other sources of self-pride to draw on in building their self-esteem, and that they do not necessarily introject white society's negative valuation of themselves.

Posttraumatic Stress Disorders and Childhood Detentions

In South Africa, the legal definition of a child is a person of 18 or younger, but such definitions were overridden by the Emergency Regulations, and detained children were not protected by welfare legislation. A compilation of figures provided by the authorities (Arndt *et al.*, 1989) shows a total of 8,828 (see Table 51.2).

In addition, other youngsters were in prison awaiting trial on various charges. For example, on February 24, 1988, the Minister of Law and Order told Parliament that, at that date, 63,360 persons under 18 were being held in police cells awaiting trial for "ordinary crimes." In March, 1988, he said that a total of 1,338 youths aged 17 or under had been detained under Emergency Regulations in 1987. The Detainees' Parents' Support Committee (DPSC) estimated that of the 28,471 detained in 1986, 40% were under 18.

One source of criticism has been the fact that a very high proportion of those detained are eventually released without any charges being laid. Of the tiny minority brought to trial, relatively few are convicted. Where the Black Sash (1986) monitored the public violence cases of 226 juveniles, only 22% were convicted, the rest were acquitted, or had charges withdrawn. In 1984, for example, less than 4% of detainees were charged criminally, and less than 3% were convicted of an offense (South African Institute of Race Relations, 1984). In the last half of 1985, 1,045 aged under 20 were arrested on charges of public violence—167 were found guilty. Yet they may all spend months in detention, with many postponements of the cases, prolonged anxiety, loss of schooling and chances of further schooling, or loss of salary and job—and receive no compensation.

Allegations of assaults on detained children were dismissed as "unsubstantiated" by the Minister of Law and Order, who refused to comment on allegations presented to him in a memorandum from a delegation (Collinge, 1986). This report by the Committee of Concern for Children alleged that detainees, aged 11 to 18, had been physically abused and intimidated. Of 40 exdetainees, 24 claimed they had been assaulted with kicks, slaps, fists, canes, and sjamboks (whips). About 20% said they had been forced to exercise and had been assaulted when they tried to rest. One said he was picked up by his arms and legs and dropped repeatedly; a 15-year-old was said to have had a rope put around his neck and to have been suspended, screaming. Two alleged electric shock torture. Others claimed to have been threatened with death, prolonged detention, "necklacing" (being burnt to death with a burning car tire filled with petrol around the neck), or other burning. The group claimed that "an analysis of the statements [of the detainees] does not indicate isolated incidents where one policeman oversteps the mark, but rather a consistent pattern that is occurring countrywide."

The minister said that the allegations lacked detail: "It is yet another example of how untested, unsubstantiated and one-sided allegations are made in public in an obvious bid to discredit the police, not only locally, but also abroad" (Collinge, 1986). Such a comment is naive or cynical. It is not clear how a child, held incommunicado by people who need not identify themselves to him, could possibly provide tested, substantiated, and two-sided allegations, even if the complaints were perfectly true.

In a highly polarized political conflict, it is obviously true that some detainees and their supporters, opposing the regime, might indeed be tempted to invent or exaggerate allegations of mistreatment. But the South African Government has persistently refused to protect itself against such a problem in obvious ways. By refusing independent and objective inquiries, by maintaining deep secrecy about conditions of detention, by imposing strict press censorship, by holding detainees incommunicado and specifically excluding them from the normal protections of law, by routinely denying all allegations, and by specifically providing excessive protection and immunity from prosecution for its agents, the inescapable question is: Why is all this necessary, if none but criminals are detained, and if their interrogation and detention are managed with impeccable care?

Numerous examples have been reported in detail in the press, but there has never been any independent or objective inquiry into such matters. Eleven-year-old William Modibedi alleged that he spent over 2 months in detention. He had been accused of taking part in the burning of cars and shops. On release, he had lost two front teeth. He said one had been knocked out by the police, one by other prisoners. He said he had been forced to stand for long periods, staring at a bright light. He said, "they put a dummy [infant pacifier] into my mouth and the dummy had wires connected to it. The

Table 51.2. Summary of Detained Children

Period	Number of detentions
July 21, 1985 to March 7, 1986	212 under 14, 2,711 aged 14 to 18
June 12, 1986 to June 11, 1987	308 under 14, 4,674 aged 14 to 18
June 11, 1987 to June 10, 1988	18 under 14, 472 aged 14 to 18
June 10, 1988 to January 24, 1989	3 under 14, 430 aged 14 to 18

wires were connected to a socket in the wall, and when a policeman turned on the switch, I experienced a jarring effect. I also felt excruciating pains in my head." He said he was taken to a mortuary and shown corpses.

There are so many such stories (Anonymous, 1987b; Beresford, 1986). A 12-year-old youth left home to buy something at the shop—and came home 9 months later, having been held under Emergency Regulations by mistake. His parents were not notified of his detention; he was released without being charged. A teenage detainee told a court (Kuzwayo, 1987) that the security police had pulled off bits of his hair and forced him to eat them, that he had received electric shocks to his testicles, that he had been assaulted, throttled, kneed in the groin, among other assaults. He had to be admitted to hospital with painful, swollen testes and needed a surgical operation.

Yet South Africa is a signatory of the United Nations Charter on the Rights of Children. A Black Sash report (Black Sash, 1986) on the consequences of such detentions describes a profound sense of helplessness, a sense of the meaninglessness of life, lack of hope for the future, a poor self-image, an all-pervasive alienation from life. "A 15-year-old describes his life as worthless to the police, his parents, his friends, his enemies, himself."

There are reports of anxiety, listlessness, an inability to interact with others, excessive feelings of fear, anger, and suspicion, even directed to friends and family. The Detainees' Parents' Support Committee and others have described how they seem to have lost their childhood, so that often young persons of between 10 and 14 years of age seem to have the seriousness and inflexibility of a 50-year-old.

No formal study has been published that properly assesses such sequelae. One doctor has estimated that 70% of such children suffer from PTSD. Certainly, we are seeing obvious cases of PTSD according to DSM-III and DSM-III-R criteria. Brett, Spitzer, and Williams (1987) observed that the adult criteria usually apply to children, with some modifications, and this finding matches our experience. They also refer to "Omen formation," the false belief in an ability to prophesy future untoward events.

It is essential to recognize that while classic PTSD may be seen, there are also a wide range of other post-traumatic stress sequelae and victimization syndromes, not yet formally recognized in official nomenclatures. There may be nonspecific physiological symptoms, generalized fearfulness, separation anxiety, while diminished interest/constriction of affect is difficult for the child to report, but may be recognized by parents and teachers (Eth & Pynoos, 1985; Frederick, 1984; Pruett, 1984). Quite often, there can be muteness or reluctance to discuss the trauma or its results, which the naive or biased observer or assessor can mistake for a lack of symptoms and, thus, a lack of damage.

It is believed that detention can permanently distort and deform the child's personality development, damaging the capacity to trust others, leaving a legacy of bitterness, resentment, and, at times, an overwhelming desire for revenge. The children can experience difficulties controlling their feelings and behavior and may act out in antisocial ways.

This recalls Rosenheck's (1985b) description of ma-lignant PTSD, where he reported his patients came to "feel most alive when they are in a situation of intense conflict or potential danger," and feel bored or depressed in the absence of such stimulation. Many were anxious or even paranoid in crowds or public places, and could get irritated and argumentative in such situations. He described a severe self-loathing and self-hatred; sometimes "a manifest embracing of their negative identity, a boastful and exhibitionistic pride in being loathsome." Such responses create a horrid potential for self-perpetuating spirals of violence and counterviolence. Such responses are seen in some of the gangs of politicized and gangsterized youngsters in some areas; and some parts of Natal in South Africa are already showing, in the so-called faction-fighting, the typical endemic violence patterns of Beirut and Belfast.

There have been few relevant studies in the world literature to help us understand these events. Cohn, Holzer, Koch, and Severin (1980) reported a study of 75 Chilean children seen in Denmark 2 to 6 years after their parents had been released from prison. The children and/or their parents had been subjected to physical and/or mental torture. Thirty-eight percent were anxious and sensitive to noise; 35% had difficulty falling asleep and had nightmares of police, soldiers, murder, and death. Many walked in their sleep. Twenty-three percent had secondary difficulty with relationships with other children of their own age, whereas 17% showed aggressiveness, 12% were troubled by anorexia, 6% by impaired memory, 8% had psychogenic stomachaches, and 6% had constipation.

There are many problems with this study. There were no controls, the children were seen quite a time after the events and were geographically distant from them, because they had suffered the additional stresses of refugee relocation. They showed a wide range of ages (1 to 21 years); and if they were seen, as the paper states, 2 to 6 years after the events, one child must have been traumatized at least 1 year before birth, which is somewhat odd.

If we consider the factors which have been shown to favor violence (Kastenbaum & Aisenberg, 1976), we see to what extent situations like that in South African can breed the danger of continued violence:

1. *Anything may physically or psychologically separate the potential killer from the victim,* such as when the victim is perceived as fundamentally different from oneself. The entire South African system is based on a profound and unnatural concentration on the differences, rather than similarities, between people; on group membership and identity, specifically in distinction and in opposition to many other groups. The extraordinarily fragile sense of identity of the Afrikaners seems most clearly defined, by themselves, by what they are *not*, than by what they are; and especially by their separateness.

2. *Anything may permit the killer to define murder as something else.* Where the violence and killing can be redefined, and seen as something else—"preserving democracy," "frustrating the terrorist onslaught," or whatever—it becomes far easier to carry out.

3. *Anything may foster the perception of people as objects or as less than human.* This is a very potent catalyst for violence. Apartheid, of course, is based on the proposi-

tion that some people are objects, cogs in a machine of social engineering, and less than human. Earlier, these foundations were very explicitly stated; more recently, they are implicit even when denied. When people are seen not as individuals but as "blacks" or "whites" (or even more insulting epithets), they more readily become targets. Also, where the violence is indirect, as in the actions of a bomber, or in killing by the carefully planned neglect of others' welfare, the victims may be multiple, but usually distant in place and time from the agent responsible. Within a riotous crowd, there is dilution of personal responsibility, and a sense of community support for group actions.

4. *Anything may permit one to escape responsibility by blaming someone else*, as in the classic invalid excuse: "I was only carrying out orders." Violence has been institutionalized within South Africa to an alarming extent, with official violence being given special indemnity—whatever may be done by a very wide range of officials (police, soldiers, etc.) was formally declared to be free from any negative consequences when done in "good faith" (which is presumed to be present)! Lifton (1986) wrote of "genocidal bureaucracy," which facilitates the sequence leading to genocide, rendering it unreal, deamplified, using euphemisms to disguise ugly realities. Within the underclass, actions believed to be on behalf of "liberation" or "the struggle," may be seen as sanctioned by the broad community.

5. *Anything may encourage seeing oneself as debased or worthless*. "If I'm treated like a rat, I might as well act as one. What have I got to lose?" So many people in South Africa have little or nothing to lose. Deliberately and systematically degraded by the system of apartheid, their self-worth is hard to establish or maintain. Unwilling students of brutality may learn to exercise those gruesome skills.

6. *Anything may reduce self-control*, or is believed to have that effect, including alcohol, psychoactive drugs, crowd and mob effects.

7. *Anything may force a hasty decision*, or may not permit time for "cooling off," as occurs in many of the confrontations in which violence erupts.

8. *Anything may encourage a person to feel above or outside the law*. The notion is that one's rank, position, or whatever, makes it possible for one to "get away with murder." For some officials in South Africa, this has seemed, at times, to be literally true; and only long after the events, did the authorities even begin to investigate the police "Hit Squads," and Army murder units. On the other hand, the laws of petty apartheid have been so many and so difficult for any normal person to adhere to, that many, especially within the black community, who would be wholly law-abiding within any normal society, have been made into "law-breakers" by absurd and immoral laws. Where, as under apartheid, laws do not serve to protect morality, but rather to require immorality, the individual is placed in a very difficulty position.

Considering how many of these catalysts to violence are active within South Africa, it is a tribute to the cultural stability and maturity of the African communities that there has been so little violence. The horrific episodes of savage violence that have occurred are appalling and are not excusable. Within their context,

though, they are comprehensible; and they are rare indeed in comparison to the enormous number of invitations to violence which those communities face.

In some major trials of those accused of such violence, Edward Diener of Illinois (in one instance) and myself (in others, e.g., Simpson, 1987, 1988a,b, 1989) have interviewed the accused in depth, so as to prepare reports for the Supreme Court in consideration of mitigation. We have seen the extent of the effects of crowd and mob psychology in stirring mob violence. Diener and I have described the effects of community anger, suggestibility, hyperarousal, conformity, imitation, deindividuation, modeling, and related factors in impelling individuals who would not normally act violently, toward impulsive viciousness toward scapegoat targets who have come to be seen as epitomizing the hated system.

Children's Encounters with Death

The human race is the only one that knows it must die, and it knows this only through its experience. A child brought up alone and transported to a desert island would have no more idea of death than a cat or a plant.

—Voltaire

Generally, we don't recall when we lost our immortality (unlike the loss of our virginity, although that's a far less significant change). It is a more profound loss of innocence, though it more commonly occurs gradually. (Simpson, 1979)

We must address the matter of the child's relationship with death, because one of the central components of potentially damaging trauma and the causation of PTSD and traumatic stress problems is the exposure to undeniable evidence of the mortality of oneself and loved ones. McCarthy (1980) said that "when anxiety is experienced by a child in accomplishing developmental tasks, it may activate the fear of death, and, conversely, the arousal of death anxiety interferes with the mastery of developmental tasks."

In infancy and very early childhood, death is sensed by the child in nonverbal, noncognitive terms. I believe that the very few psychologists and psychoanalysts who have bothered to try to look at the situation have overinterpreted, overliterally, and then overgeneralized. I am far from sure, for instance, that the "oral wishes and fears" they describe are what children are talking about—rather than overformalized approximations, heavily shaped by the inquirer's expectations and conceptual schemata, of those rough approximations which are the closest such a young child can get to describing its broader and more complex, but not verbal, concerns. Terr (1988), referring to psychic trauma before approximately 28 to 36 months of age, similarly recognized that this may leave behavioral rather than verbal memories.

Such infantile metaphors, approximate descriptions of inchoate concepts, need to be heard for what they are. They should not serve as behavioral projective tests into which analysts read shapes more revealing of themselves than their subjects. Whenever we need to speak of concepts as immense and vague as death, we have to use metaphors to depict some of its resemblances. We shape our metaphors, and, in turn, are shaped by them.

Death anxiety was attributed in classical psychoanalytic theory to anal events, castration anxiety, and the lack of object constancy. I attribute it to death anxiety and to death.

As one begins to recognize one's helplessness and complete dependency, recognizing how fiercely one needs care, and that the world is not automatically and uniformly nurturing, fear that one's vital needs might not be met can readily arise: of the possibility that one might lose nurturance. As one begins to develop any concept of life and living, a counterconcept of death and dying must develop. Neither makes sense without the other. No child can begin to distinguish "me" from "not-me" (an essential task, both immunologically and psychologically, and for similar reasons) without recognizing the shadow of nonbeing that defines those edges.

"Children's fears of death begin as formless, undifferentiated anxiety and later take on specific dimensions [such] as the fear of the dark, monsters, ghosts and burglars," wrote McCarthy (1980). For our children of Africa and other settings of chronic unrest, this rather theoretical lack of specificity is often replaced by menaces with all too realistic shapes and names.

I have grave doubts about the validity of much of the rather primitive work that has been done in this field so far. Studies have almost always been of *dominant* culture groups; of children who lead rather privileged lives and who have had relatively little experience of death and loss. Such research has usually failed to pay attention to cultural, ethnic, and life-experience issues, though it is obvious that these will affect children's attitudes. Other studies have shown how much mothers underestimate their own children's concerns about death—yet researchers so often rely on these opinions. Nagy (1948) and Anthony (1940) conducted their studies in the 1940s, and this work has been too uncritically accepted, without appreciation of how heavily it was influenced by its cultural and historical context.

Young children may not be able to verbally define death, as naive psychologists have asked them to do—but they know about it, are scared of it and by it, curious about it, and form lasting images of it, while building special defenses against its fearfulness. There have been very clear examples of children as young as 18 months, and 2 years old, obviously grappling with the idea of death. Rather than the task being an unfortunate intrusion into the child's world, trying to comprehend death is a major and essential developmental task. Yalom (1980) would seem to agree with this view; and Jean Piaget considered the subject of death instrumental in the child's development of mature concepts of causality (without fully exploring this important question). Klein (1948) also recognized the importance of that early relationship with death. Anna Freud (1960; Freud & Burlingame, 1943) from her work with children in the 1940s wrote:

It can be safely said that all the children who were over two years at the time of the London Blitz realized the

house will fall down when bombed, and that people are often killed or get hurt in falling houses.

Sigmund Freud, himself profoundly disturbed about death, misled many. He focussed on the child's curiousity about where he comes from, so as to be able to avoid and largely ignore the far more interesting issue of where one is going to. Yalom (1980) said of Freud that "in the area of death he had a persistent blind spot which obscured for him some patently obvious aspects of man's inner world." He pointed out that it is absurd that Freud insisted that there can be no representation of death in the unconscious, because we have had no experience of death. How did Freud imagine we achieved castration anxiety (a far more complex concept) with no experience of castration? Feebly, Freud suggested that weaning, or the daily loss of feces, is a sufficiently analogous loss. That does not say much about castration, but it says an awful lot about Freud's attitude to feces.

In night terrors, a child is literally frightened of nothing. Children play with being versus non-being even when throwing toys out of sight and having someone recover them. They cannot achieve concepts of object permanence without entertaining the hypothesis of object impermanence. Toilet training is *not* about "anal eroticism" but about possessiveness and loss. Maybe children escape into an interest in sex to avoid the fear of death, as Freud himself did.

The "golden age of latency" is in part about death anxiety, a time when one unlearns what one has discovered, until the denial system breaks down in adolescence, and these matters have to be relearned. Latency is when you learn expertise in *denial*, the skill of being consistently and effectively dishonest with yourself.

Such developmental aspects of dealing with death under normal circumstances are usually achieved with little or no direct confrontation with its grisly realities. The children of unrest do not have the luxury of handling such matters purely theoretically. When one considers the enormous impact that analysts ascribe to such comparatively trivial events as toilet training, a new sibling, or school attendance, what scale of effects should one expect in children who watch their house burnt down or bulldozed flat, or who see human beings burnt to death, parents killed violently, or tortured? If such massive and primal traumata do not have substantial and enduring effects, can the tiny traumata that the classic analyst deals with in comparatively rich and pampered people really have the full and exclusive impact traditionally ascribed to them?

There is also an interaction between external events and a child's own natural aggressive impulses and fears of the effects of the anger and aggression of others, fears of punishment for actions and impulses, and fear of abandonment. When external reality matches the fantasy, to what extent is the impact magnified? When the mother with whom the child is engaged in the normal creative conflict is suddenly lost to detention, or the father against whom aggressive fantasies exist dies horribly in the child's sight, what are the effects?

Summarizing existing research on children's responses to loss and grief, one may say that major early losses contribute to disturbances in self-image and object-relations, and to adult depression. Furman (1974) considered that three major factors influence the child's ability to cope with traumatic loss: (1) the child's maturational level and cognitive ability to comprehend it, (2) the child's previous experience of loss, and (3) the support given by the surviving parent. Hilgard, Newman, and Fisk (1960) found evidence that children could achieve successful mourning—where the home stayed stable, where there was a support network outside the home, and where relationships before the death were stable. Yet the unrest situation may often deny all these healing factors to the very children most exposed to experiences of overwhelming loss.

Some aspects of the situation these children are in are similar to those that Pine (1986) placed centrally in his model of the development of the "borderline-child-to-be," including early experiences of being overwhelmed by major traumatic stress. Similar possibilities were explored in my early studies of self-mutilators (Simpson, 1975, 1977) and by Herman and van der Kolk (1987). This possible outcome needs formal evaluation.

I return to my earlier question of what constitutes normal "coping" or adaptation in very abnormal circumstances. People may accommodate to a maimed world by lowering their expectations of normal social life. But such accommodation may in itself become as pathogenic as the trauma to which it brings some relief. Although doubt has more recently been cast on the Turnbull (1972) account of the Ik, which was discussed by Kaplan (1978), this potential scenario is surely possible. According to Turnbull, the Ik responded to dislocation and existence on the edge of starvation, horribly:

> The Ik abandoned all hope, all belief in the mutualities of love and family. They came together solely for self-interest. Their sexual, marital and group associations became temporary and acrimonious. There was no longer any way for affection or trust to flourish.

If later anthropologists do not consider this an accurate description of the Ik, there can be no doubt that it does represent accurately a way of life that occurs in some people, within chronic unrest situations, and inner-city ghettoes. "He who remains passive when overwhelmed with grief loses his best chance of recovering elasticity of mind" (Darwin, 1872).

Terror and trauma have the potential for profound as well as subtle effects in the child, impacting on a nervous system not yet matured in its cognitive and other functions. Van der Kolk (1987) provided a most valuable review of a wide range of the factors and effects involved. Some have suggested that children are especially susceptible to long-term effects of trauma (Green, 1983), and that the impact may be related to the level of cognitive development (Garmezy & Rutter, 1983). Among the disturbing potential consequences are: progression to a victimizer, learning disabilities, and more basic central nervous system responses—hyperarousal, kindling, and behavioral sensitization (van der Kolk & Greenberg, 1987).

In the important work of Fish-Murray and others (Fish-Murray, Koby, & van der Kolk, 1987) the "strongest finding" was "the inflexibility of organized schematas and structures in all domains." They commented that "function and structure were frozen so that dynamic change could not take place," and noted marked impairment in the capacity to accommodate, to self-correct, as well as verbal impairment, attention deficit disorders, and the like.

Kobasa, Maddi, and Pucetti (1982) and others discussed *hardiness* as a personality style positively resistant to debilitation by stressful life events. Hardy people combine commitment, control, and challenge, show curiosity, and find interest and meaning in their experiences of life; they believe they can influence events (an external locus of control), anticipate change, and tend to optimism. To the extent that detainees and other victims of political repression are political activists or even community leaders, they may be more hardy, which is their resistance to accepting repression that attracts such unwelcome attention. In Kobasa's research, the highly stressed people who showed a low incidence of symptoms of illness were high in hardiness; and variations in such characteristics as hardiness may also explain the variation in community and group responses to severe trauma.

There are other vital issues here, within fields of great importance that rarely receive adequate study. How do children learn love and compassion in such circumstances? An old black woman said of the children in South African townships, "I don't know them. Perhaps they love us, but they don't respect what we know. They are left loose here, and we cannot help them. We had fathers, but our children, oh our children go but they don't believe. Even the little ones. They say 'Your people lied to you.' *They dream the dreams we never had—* because we could look at our land and touch it and we knew, there it was, and it was ours. But the children, they don't look at the future like we did."

What Needs to Be Done

In all the areas of knowledge and controversy I have reviewed in this chapter, so very much more work is needed. Maybe it is part of the denial needed by societies to cope comfortably with such troubles that these issues are not studied. In his book, *Death in Life* Lifton (1982) pointed out that 17 years after Hiroshima, no Japanese individual or group had made a proper study of its general psychological or social effects. Psychic numbing seems to extend to the sciences and to the professions.

We need, urgently and collaboratively, to draw up a research agenda of matters that need to be studied and to make formal arrangements to share data, instruments, and methods. We need governments to recognize the importance of such work, and to facilitate it rather than obstruct it. Within such research (and the development and evaluation of means of helping) we need to understand far more about which components of traumatic stresses are pathoplastic, and how the qualitative as well as quantitative aspects of traumata interact with the personality and other characteristics of the victim. We need to clarify potential modes of prevention, intervention, and postvention. How can we help individuals, families, and communities to avoid damaging situations, to minimize the damage when these occur, and to repair the immediate and lasting damage caused?

One problem is that psychosocially skilled personnel are so rare in Third-World countries, and in this field especially it is essential that intervention be conducted by someone acceptable to the community, who knows its beliefs and practices and is able to speak the vernacular. Mzinyathi (1987) pointed out that "there are less than 10 registered black psychologists to serve the population of more than 20 million blacks" in South Africa, for instance, and that the majority of these psychologists were in teaching posts and were not providing a direct clinical service.

We must not assume that any specific type of trained health professional is the only possible source of aid; and we need to learn both how to use such very scarce resources optimally, and how to reach people tactfully, so that our advice is acceptable and usable. Lindy (1985) pointed out that "from the survivor's vantage point, professionals interested in treating or studying PTSD threaten to disturb a fragile equilibrium. Fear of affect overload makes the survivor wary."

The mode of intervention is very important. In his review of world psychiatric services, Cohen (1988) made this clear. In Israel, for instance, several local psychiatrists told him that they had learned not to intervene too much; to be available, but not to "swamp the place with outside experts." They criticized "foreign volunteers who liked to drop in on a crisis to assuage their guilt" (or gain material for a publication?), saying that "they get in the way. Raise all kinds of expectations and then disappear." They found that "the local people didn't know who the hell we were and were not too keen on discussing their feelings with perfect strangers."

Thus, in events like the Ma'alot disaster (when children were held hostage by guerrillas, and 22 of them were killed) care was provided by a local team including teachers who spoke to parents and relatives, and regional experts intervened only where there was obvious illness and served rather as back-up and support to the local team. Benyamini told Cohen that in times of tension and war, since 1967, it has been found best to help the teachers to handle as much as they could, to support them, and to interfere only as a last resort. Community care should be nurtured slowly and in times of peace (or during lulls in the conflict) rather than instantly demanded or improvised during a crisis.

Cohen (1988) also cited the experiences of the hostages of the South Moluccans in Holland between 1975 and 1978 (having traced their subsequent lives). Many ex-hostages complained fiercely of their treatment by psychologists and psychiatrists after their rescue, of being forced to go to hospital against their wishes, being treated with the assumption that they must become unhinged by the experiences, being pressed with unsolicited help, and dismissed as "disturbed" when they complained about this.

In situations like South Africa, there is no effective funding for much needed intervention, which is done almost entirely by volunteers. Resources are grossly inadequate to meet the needs; research is impractical, though it could be so valuable for so many. There are large numbers of small groups and individuals, with little chance for proper coordination of their efforts or results, and they are tragically vulnerable to suppression, intimidation, and obstruction.

What is needed, with the support of appropriate national and international agencies, is to develop valid international programs to include guided and sponsored carefully planned research and evaluation of intervention methods; to pool and share results and methods; to study how individuals and communities heal themselves; to devise means of providing international training and back-up for local caregivers, and ways to assist in emergencies, acute disasters, and in the chronic disaster areas; and to find ways to assist those on the scene and in the affected communities to work effectively.

In our international responses to the disasters and tragedies children face, we have worried too much about helping children just to stay alive. *Alive is not enough.* There is some concern if they are physically maimed or handicapped. But when the survivors live, mentally, emotionally, and psychologically maimed, to grow into stunted adults, who may well harm future generations of children and produce deformed societies of festering misery, there is little or no concern. The psychological damage may be less immediately obvious but is more infectious than physical damage, and is able to be transmitted across generations.

We do not know enough about child development in so many areas that matter. Researchers, as ever, have measured mostly whatever is easy to measure, preferring the exact measurement of the barely interesting to the less perfect measurement of the highly relevant. What do we really know of the development of affection, love, respect, ideologies, coping skills, and of kindness and compassion—all those components that give quality rather than mere quantity to life?

There are other important issues for which there has not been space to discuss. I believe that PTSD, in children and in adults, reflects a turbulent response to a very primal loss of innocence after one has been faced with the irreversibility of some kinds of knowledge. We tend to ignore, as Marin (1981) emphasized, the problems of living in moral pain. How do we live with the knowledge that mankind is capable of committing acts with such terrible consequences; with the realization of our own capacity for committing as well as suffering terror? We seem to have lost whatever shared ways we once may have had for dealing with such moral pain and guilt. Some events and actions irreversibly change one's life. Oedipus saw, and was blinded; in Marin's words, "he suffered not so much because of what he had done, but because of what he learned he had done" (1981).

Although psychologically we can render many things explicable and understandable, we are uneasy about admitting to our categories the possibility that some actions, some people, are not sick, not immature, not temporarily goaded and provoked into uncharacteristic cruelty; but are simply bad, and evil, in nature and intent. We have not really tried to understand and manage evil. Yet we see among many adults so little guilt, so little shame, so much moral smugness. We have seen in many countries, in Germany in the 1930s and 1940s, in South America and South Africa in the 1960s, 1970s and 1980s, professional people, including doctors, who have been content to see and examine the damaged victims of evil acts, and to remain silent, or help to keep it hidden. How should we relate to them?

Albert Camus, in his acceptance speech for the No-bel Prize (1958, 1961), said:

> We had to fashion for ourselves an art of living in times of catastrophe in order to be reborn before fighting openly against the death instinct at work in our history. Probably every generation sees itself as charged with remaking the world. But its task is perhaps much greater, for it consists in keeping the world from destroying itself.

The effects of the tragedies we have been consider-ing cannot be expressed entirely in scientific prose. Con-sider also the words of a short poem John Bowlby (1980) quoted in his book, *Loss: Sadness and Depression*, which I quote with his permission. It is by a girl of 11, who was separated from her parents for some years:

> The beauty of love has not found me
> Its hands have not gripped me so tight
> For the darkness of hate is upon me
> I see day, not as day, but as night.
>
> I yearn for the dear love to find me
> With my heart and my soul and my might
> For darkness has closed in upon me
> I see day, not as day, but as night
>
> The children are playing and laughing
> But I cannot find love in delight
> There is an iron fence around me
> I see day, not as day, but as night.

I conclude with the words of Alan Paton, writing of just these tragedies in South Africa, in his classic book, *Cry, the Beloved Country* (1958):

> Cry, the beloved country, for the unborn child that is the inheritor of our fear. Let him not love the earth too deeply. Let him not laugh too gladly when the water runs though his fingers, nor stand too silent when the setting sun makes red the veld with fire. Let him not be too moved when the birds of his land are singing, nor give too much of his heart to a mountain or a valley. For fear will rob him of all if he gives too much.

Postscript

Apart from the scientific references, I recommend that readers genuinely interested in the themes that I developed also read artistic works that record such expe-riences more vividly. Regarding the South African scene, these would include books like the great classic *Cry, the Beloved Country* by Alan Paton (Penguin Books and other editions); and poetry such as Oswald Mtshali's *Sounds of a Cowhide Drum* (Johannesburg, Renoster Books, 1971); James Matthews's *Cry Rage!* (Johannesburg, Sprocas-Ravan, 1972); Mongane Wally Serote's *Yakhal'inkomo* (Jo-hannesburg, Renoster Books, 1972); Jeremy Cronin's *Inside* (Johannesburg, Ravan Press, 1983); and the an-thology of black poetry, *To Whom It May Concern* (Johan-nesburg, Ad Donker, 1973).

References

Abramson, L. Y., Seligman, M. E., & Teasdale, J. (1978). Learned helplessness in humans: Critique and reformulation. *Journal of Abnormal Psychology, 87,* 49–74.

Abu Nasr, J., Vriesendorp, S., Lorfing, I., & Khalifeh, I. (1981). *Moral judgement of Lebanese children after the war.* (Monograph of the Institute for Women's Studies in the Arab World). Beirut: Beirut University College.

Abu Nasr, J., Makhoreli, M., & Lorfing, I. (1986). *The develop-ment of three- to six-year-old Lebanese children and their environ-ment.* (Monograph No. 3, Institute for Women's Studies in the Arab World). Beirut: Beirut University College.

Allport, G. W. (1958). *The nature of prejudice.* New York: Double-day Anchor.

Anderson, C. (1977). Locus of control, coping behaviors, and performance in a stress setting: A longitudinal study. *Journal of Applied Psychology, 62,* 446–451.

Anonymous. (1986). *Two dogs and freedom.* Johannesburg: Ravan Press.

Anonymous. (1987a). *Thula Baba.* Johannesburg: Ravan Press.

Anonymous. (1987b, October 16–22). The terror of a detained child . . . the anguish of the parents. *Weekly Mail* (Johannes-burg, South Africa), p. 12.

Anthony, S. (1940). *The discovery of death in childhood.* London: Routledge & Kegan Paul.

Archibald, H. C. D., Long, D. M., Miller, C., & Tuddenham, R. D. (1963). Gross stress reactions in combat. *American Journal of Psychiatry, 119,* 317–322.

Arndt, H., Burgin, D., Gutknecht, K., Haesler, W. T., Kron-sucker, H., & Schmid, S. (1989). *Children and juveniles in the prisons of South Africa: Report of an interdisciplinary group from Switzerland and Germany.* Heidelberg: Druckerei Gebhard.

Arroyo, W., & Eth, S. (1984). Children traumatized by Central American warfare. In S. Eth & R. Pynoos (Eds.), *Post-traumatic stress disorder in children* (pp. 101–120). Washington, DC: American Psychiatric Press.

Baider, L., & Rosenfeld, E. (1974). Effect of parental fears on children in wartime. *Social Casework, 55,* 497–503.

Battle, E. S., & Rotter, J. N. (1963). Children's feelings of person-al control as related to social class and ethnic group. *Journal of Personality, 31*(4), 482–490.

Bekker, J. A. (1987, October 16–22). Children of violence. *Weekly Mail* (Johannesburg, South Africa), p. 14.

Beresford, D. (1986, December 7). South African brutality to-wards children in detention. *Manchester Guardian,* p. 9.

Bergmann, M. S., & Jucovy, M. (Eds.). (1982). *Generations of the Holocaust.* New York: Basic Books.

Black Sash. (1986). *Memorandum on the suffering of children in South Africa.* Johannesburg, South Africa: Author.

Bodman, F. M. (1944). Child psychiatry in war-time Britain. *Journal of Educational Psychology, 35,* 293–301.

Boesak, A., & Brews, A. (1987). The black struggle for libera-tion: A reluctant road to liberation. In C. Villa-Vicencio (Ed.), *Theology and violence: The South African debate* (pp. 51–68). Grand Rapids, MI: Wm. B. Eerdmans.

Boothby, N. (1986). Children and war. *Cultural Survival Quar-terly, 10*(4), 28–30.

Bowlby, J. (1980). *Loss: Sadness and depression.* New York: Basic Books.

Brander, T. (1943). Psychiatric observations among Finnish chil-dren during the Russo-Finnish war of 1939–1940. *Nervous Child, 2,* 313–319.

Brett, E. R., Spitzer, R. L., & Williams, J. B. W. (1987, October

23–26). *The DSM-III diagnostic criteria for post-traumatic stress disorder*. Paper presented at the 3rd annual meeting of the Society for Traumatic Stress Studies, Baltimore, MD.

Brown, G., & Harris, T. (1978). *Social origins of depression*. London: Tavistock Press.

Bryce, J., & Armenian, H. (1986). In wartime: The state of children in Lebanon. In J. Bryce & H. Armenian (Eds.), *In wartime: The state of children in Lebanon* (pp. 155–159). Syracuse, NY: Syracuse University Press.

Bryce, J. W. (1986). *Cries of children in Lebanon as voiced by their mothers*. Cairo: UNICEF, Regional Office for the Middle East and North Africa.

Bulhan, H. A. (1985). *Frantz Fanon and the psychology of oppression*. New York: Plenum Press.

Burbury, W. M. (1941). Effects of evacuation and air raids on children. *British Medical Journal, 2*, 486–488.

Burke, A. W. (1984). Is racism a causative factor in mental illness? An introduction. *International Journal of Social Psychiatry, 30*, 1–3.

Burke, A. W. (1985). Mental health and apartheid. (World Psychiatric Association conference report). *International Journal of Social Psychiatry, 31*(2), 145–148.

Burt, C. (1943). War neuroses in British children. *Nervous Child, 2*, 324–337.

Camus, A. (1958). Nobel Prize acceptance speech. *Atlantic, 101*, 34.

Camus, A. (1961). *Resistance, rebellion, and death*. London: Hamish Hamilton.

Carlin, J. E. (1979). The catastrophically up-rooted child: Southeast Asian refugee children. In J. D. Call, J. D. Noshpitz, R. L. Cohen, & I. N. Berlin (Eds.), *Basic handbook for childhood psychiatry* (Vol. 1, pp. 290–300). New York: Basic Books.

Chikane, F. (1986). Children in turmoil: The effects of unrest on township children. In S. Burman & P. Reynolds (Eds.), *Growing up in a divided society*. Johannesburg: Ravan Press.

Clayer, J. R. (1984). *Evaluation of the outcome of disaster*. Adelaide, Australia: Health Commission of South Australia.

Clayer, J. R., Bookless-Pratz, C., & Harris, R. L. (1985). Some health consequences of a natural disaster. *Medical Journal of Australia, 143*, 182–184.

Cohen, D. (1988). *Forgotten millions: The treatment of the mentally ill—a global perspective*. London: Paladin.

Cohn, J., Holzer, K., Koch, L., & Severin, B. (1980). Children and torture. *Danish Medical Bulletin, 27*(5), 238–239.

Collinge, J.-A. (1986, March 25). Police abuse of minors rejected. *The Star* (Johannesburg, South Africa), p. 4.

Coopersmith, S. (1975). Self-concept, race and education. In H. K. Verna & C. Bagley (Eds.), *Race and education across cultures* (pp. 145–167). London: Heineman.

Coromina, J. (1943). Repercussions of the war on children as observed during the Spanish Civil War. *Nervous Child, 2*, 324–337.

Crawshaw, R. (1963). Reactions to a disaster. *Archives of General Psychiatry, 9*(2), 157–162.

Curran, P. S. (1988). Psychiatric aspects of terrorist violence: Northern Ireland 1969–1987. *British Journal of Psychiatry, 153*, 470–475.

Cuthbertson, G. (1987). The English-speaking churches and colonialism. In C. Villa-Vicencio (Ed.), *Theology and violence: The South African debate* (pp. 15–30). Grand Rapids, MI: Wm. B. Eerdmans.

Darwin, C. (1872). *The expression of the emotions in man and animals*. London: Murray.

Dawes, A., & de Villiers, C. (1987). Preparing children and

parents for prison: The Wynberg Seven. In *Mental health in transition* (Proceedings of the 2nd OASSA National Conference). Cape Town: Organization for Appropriate Social Services in S.A., Western Cape.

Dawes, A., Tredoux, C., & Feinstein, A. (1989). Political violence in South Africa: Some effects on children of the violent destruction of their community. *International Journal of Mental Health, 18*(2), 16–43.

Day, R. C. (1984). The effect of television-mediated aggression and real-life aggression on the anxiety levels of Lebanese children under stress. *Journal of Experimental Child Psychology, 34*, 350–356.

Day, R. C. (1986). A psychological profile of children in Lebanon. In J. Bryce & H. Armenian (Eds.), *In wartime: The state of children in Lebanon* (pp. 155–159). Syracuse, NY: Syracuse University Press.

Day, R. C., & Sadek, S. (1982). The effect of Benson's relaxation response on the anxiety levels of Lebanese children under stress. *Journal of Experimental Child Psychology, 34*, 350–356.

De Beer, C. (1984). *The South African disease: Apartheid health and health services*. Johannesburg: Southern African Research Service.

De Vitt, N. (1941). *The concentration camp in South Africa during the Anglo-Boer war of 1899–1902*. Pietermaritzburg, South Africa: Shuter & Shooter.

Dodge, C. P. (1986). Child soldiers of Uganda—What does the future hold? *Cultural Survival Quarterly, 10*(4), 31–33.

Dodge, C. P., & Raundalen, M. (Eds.). (1987). *War, violence and children in Uganda*. Oslo: Norwegian University Press.

Dyregrov, A., & Raundalen, M. (1987). Children and the stresses of war—A review of the literature. In C. Dodge & M. Raundalen (Eds.), *War, violence and children in Uganda* (Chapter 4, pp. 109–131). Oslo: Norwegian University Press.

Edwards, J. G. (1976). Psychiatric aspects of civilian disasters. *British Medical Journal, 1*, 944–947.

Epstein, H. (1979). *Children of the Holocaust*. New York: Putnam's.

Eth, S., & Pynoos, R. S. (1985). Developmental perspective in psychic trauma in childhood. In C. R. Figley (Ed.), *Trauma and its wake* (pp. 36–52). New York: Brunner/Mazel.

Fanon, F. (1967). *The wretched of the earth*. Harmondsworth, England: Penguin Books.

Fields, R. (1973). *Society on the run*. Harmondsworth, England: Penguin Books.

Fields, R. (1976). *Society under siege*. Philadelphia: Temple University Press.

Fields, R. M. (1987, October 23–26). *Terrorized into terrorist: Sequelae of PTSD in young victims*. Paper presented at the 3rd annual meeting of the Society for Traumatic Stress Studies, Baltimore, MD.

Fish-Murray, C. C., Koby, E. V., & van der Kolk, B. A. (1987). Evolving ideas: The effect of abuse on children's thought. In B. A. van der Kolk (Ed.), *Psychological trauma* (pp. 89–110). Washington, DC: American Psychiatric Press.

Fogelson, R. M. (1970). Violence and grievances: Reflections on the 1960's riots. *Journal of Social Issues, 26*, 141–143.

Fraser, R. M. (1971). The cost of commotion: An analysis of the psychiatric sequelae of the 1969 Belfast riots. *British Journal of Psychiatry, 118*, 257–264.

Frazer, M. (1974). *Children in conflict*. Harmondsworth, England: Pelican Books.

Frazer, M. (1983). Childhood and war in Northern Ireland: A therapeutic response. In M. Kahnert, D. Pitt, & I. Taipale (Eds.), *Children and war: Proceedings of the symposium at the*

Siuntio Baths, Finland. Helsinki, Finland: GIPRI, IPB, Peace Union of Finland.

Frederick, C. J. (1984). Children traumatized by catastrophic situations. In R. S. Pynoos & S. Eth (Eds.), *Post-traumatic stress disorders in children.* Washington, DC: American Psychiatric Press.

Freire, P. (1968). *The pedagogy of the oppressed.* New York: Seabury Press.

Freud, A. (1960). Discussion of John Bowlby's paper. *Psychoanalytic Study of the Child, 15,* 53–62.

Freud, A., & Burlingame, D. (1943). *War and children.* New York: Medical War Books.

Furman, E. (1974). *A child's parent dies.* New Haven: Yale University Press.

Garmezy, N. (1985). Stress-resistant children: The search for protective factors. In J. Stevenson (Ed.), *Recent research in developmental psychology. (Journal of Child Psychology and Psychiatry,* Book Supplement No. 4). Oxford: Pergamon Press.

Garmezy, N., & Rutter, M. (Eds.). (1983). *Stress, coping and development in children.* New York: McGraw-Hill.

Gibbs, M. S. (1989). Factors in the victim that mediate between disaster and psychopathology: A review. *Journal of Traumatic Stress, 2*(4), 489–514.

Gibson, K. (1987). Civil conflict, stress and children. *Psychology in Society, 8,* 4–26.

Gibson, K. (1989). Children in political violence. *Social Science and Medicine, 28*(7), 659–667.

Goodyer, I., Kolvin, I., & Gatzanis, S. (1985). Recent stressful life events in psychiatric disorders of childhood and adolescence. *British Journal of Psychiatry, 147,* 517–524.

Goodyer, I., Kolvin, I., & Gatzanis, S. (1987). The impact of recent undesirable life events on psychiatric disorders in childhood and adolescence. *British Journal of Psychiatry, 151,* 179–184.

Gore, P. M., & Rotter, J. B. (1963). A personality correlate of social action. *Journal of Personality, 31*(1), 58–64.

Gqubule, T. (1990, January 19–25). The children who are food for the guns. *Weekly Mail* (Johannesburg, South Africa), 1, 6, 11–12.

Green, A. H. (1983). Dimensions of psychological trauma in abused children. *Journal of the American Association for Child Psychiatry, 22,* 231–237.

Green, E. M. (1914). Psychoses among negroes—A comparative study. *Journal of Nervous and Mental Disease, 41,* 697–708.

Gregor, A. J., & McPherson, D. A. (1966). Racial preference and ego identity among white and bantu children in the republic of South Africa. *Genetic Psychology Monographs, 73*(2), 217–253.

Hadden, W. A., Rutherford, W. H., & Merrett, J. D. (1978). The injuries of terrorist bombing: A study of 1,532 consecutive victims. *British Journal of Surgery, 65,* 525–531.

Hammond, M., & Gear, J. (1986a). *Workbook I: Measuring community health: Workbooks in community health.* Cape Town: Oxford University Press.

Hammond, M., & Gear, J. (1986b). *Workbook II: Health, human services, and society: Workbooks in community health.* Cape Town: Oxford University Press.

Harbison, J. I. (Ed.). (1983). *Children of the troubles.* Belfast, Northern Ireland: Stranmillis College Learning Resources Unit.

Herman, J. L., & van der Kolk, B. A. (1987). Traumatic antecedents of borderline personality disorder. In B. A. van der Kolk (Ed.), *Psychological trauma* (pp. 111–126). Washington, DC: American Psychiatric Press.

Herskovits, M. J. (1971). *Life in a Haitian valley.* New York: Anchor Books/Doubleday.

Higgins, M., & Schinckel, H. (1985). Psychiatric disorder in primary school children following a natural disaster: A follow-up study. Adelaide, Australia: Flinders University, Department of Psychiatry.

Hilgard, G., Newman, M., & Fisk, F. (1960). Strength of adult ego following childhood bereavement. *American Journal of Orthopsychiatry, 30,* 788–798.

Hocking, F. (1965). Human reactions to extreme environmental stress. *Medical Journal of Australia, 2,* 477–483.

Horowitz, M. J. (1976). *Stress response syndromes.* New York: Jason Aronson.

Hourani, L., Armenian, H., Zurayk, H., & Afifi, L. (1986). A population-based survey of loss and psychological distress during the war. *Social Science and Medicine, 23*(3), 269–275.

Jahoda, G., & Harrison, S. (1975). Belfast children: Some effects of a conflict environment. *Irish Journal of Psychology, 3,* 1–9.

Jupp, M. (1986). Apartheid: Violence against children. *Cultural Survival Quarterly, 10*(4), 34–37.

Kaffman, M., & Elizur, E. (1979). Children's bereavement reactions following the death of the father. *International Journal of Family Therapy, 1,* 203–231.

Kaffman, M., & Elizur, E. (1983). Bereavement responses of kibbutz and non-kibbutz children following the death of the father. *Journal of Child Psychology and Psychiatry, 24,* 435–442.

Kaplan, L. J. (1978). *Oneness and separateness: From infant to individual.* New York: Touchstone/Simon & Schuster.

Kardiner A. (1941). *The traumatic neuroses of war.* New York: Paul B. Hoeber.

Kastenbaum, R., & Aisenberg, R. (1976). *The psychology of death.* (concise ed.). New York: Springer Publications.

Kelman, H. C. (1973). Violence without moral restraint: Reflections on the dehumanization of victims and victimizers. *Journal of Social Issues, 29,* 25–61.

Kinston, W., & Rosser, R. (1974). Disaster: Effects on mental and physical state. *Journal of Psychosomatic Research, 18,* 437–456.

Kinzie, J. D., Sack, W. H., Angell, R. H., Manson, R., & Rath, B. (1986). The psychiatric effects of massive trauma on Cambodian children: I. The children. *Journal of the American Academy of Child Psychiatry, 25,* 370–376.

Klein, M. (1948). A contribution to the therapy of anxiety and guilt. *International Journal of Psychoanalysis, 29,* 114–123.

Klineberg, O. (1964). *The human dimension in international relations.* New York: Holt, Rinehart & Winston.

Kobasa, S. C., Maddi, S. R., & Pucetti, N. C. (1982). Personality and exercise as buffers in the stress-illness relationship. *Journal of Behavioral Medicine, 5*(4), 391–404.

Kohlberg, L. (1963). The development of children's orientation toward a moral order: I. Sequence in the development of moral thought. *Vita Humana, 6,* 11–33.

Krugman, S. (1987). Trauma in the family: Perspectives. In B. A. van der Kolk (Ed.), *Psychological trauma* (pp. 127–151). Washington, DC: American Psychiatric Press.

Kuzwayo, P. (1987, February 15). Doctor tells judge of detainee's operation. *Sunday Tribune* (Durban, South Africa), p. 6.

Lacey, G. N. (1972). Observations in Abervan. *Journal of Psychosomatic Research, 16,* 257–260.

Lester, D. (1989). Personal violence (suicide and homicide) in South Africa. *Acta Psychiatrica Scandinavica, 79*(Suppl. 3), 235–237.

Levy-Bruhl, L. (1910). *Les fonctions mentales dans les sociétés inférieures.* Paris: Alcan.

Lifton, R. J. (1968). *Death in life.* New York: Random House.

Lifton, R. J. (1986). *The Nazi doctors: Medical killing and the psychology of genocide.* New York: Basic Books.

Lindy, J. (1985). The trauma membrane and other clinical concepts derived from psychotherapeutic work with survivors of natural disasters. *Psychiatric Annals*, *15*(3), 153–160.

Liu, W., & Cheung, F. (1985). Research concerns associated with the study of Southeast Asian refugees. In T. C. Owan (Ed.), *Southeast Asian mental health: Treatment, prevention, services, training and research*. Washington, DC: U.S. Government Printing Office.

Lock, H. (1986). *The war against children: Apartheid's youngest victims*. Washington, DC: Lawyer's Committee for Human Rights.

Lyons, H. A. (1971). Psychiatric sequelae of the Belfast riots. *British Journal of Psychiatry*, *118*, 265–273.

Lyons, H. A. (1972). Depressive illness in Belfast. *British Medical Journal*, *1*, 342–344.

Lyons, H. A. (1979). Civil violence—The psychological aspects. *Journal of Psychosomatic Research*, *23*, 373–393.

Macksoud, M. (1988, August 30–September 2). *The types of war related traumas experienced by Lebanese children*. Paper presented to the First European Conference on Traumatic Stress Studies, Lincoln, England.

Majeke, N. (1952). *The role of missionaries in conquest*. Johannesburg: Ravan Press.

Mannoni, D. (1964). *Prospero and Caliban: The psychology of colonization*. New York: Praeger.

Marin, P. (1981, November). Living in moral pain. *Psychology Today*, pp. 68–80.

May, R. (1972). *Power and innocence: A search for the sources of violence*. New York: W. W. Norton.

McCarthy, J. B. (1980). *Death anxiety: The loss of self*. New York: Gardner Press.

McCormick, R. A., Taber, J. I., & Kruedelbach, N. (1989). The relationship between attributional style and post-traumatic stress disorder in addicted patients. *Journal of Traumatic Stress*, *2*(4), 477–488.

Meyter, C., & Raphaely, C. (1978). The effect of minority group membership on the perceived locus of control and self-acceptance of South African school-children. In H. I. J. Van der Spuy & D. A. F. Shamley (Eds.), *The psychology of apartheid: A psychosocial perspective on South Africa*. Lanham, MD: University Press of America.

Milgram, R. M., & Milgram, N. A. (1976). The effect of the Yom Kippur war on anxiety levels in Israeli children. *Journal of Psychology*, *94*, 107–113.

Miller, A. (1987). *For your own good: The roots of violence in childhood*. London: Virago Press.

Milne, G. G. (1977). Cyclone Tracy: II. The effects on Darwin children. *Australian Psychologist*, *12*, 55–62.

Mpumlwana, M. (1987). legitimacy and struggle. In C. Villa-Vicencio (Ed.), *Theology and violence: The South African debate* (pp. 89–99). Grand Rapids, MI: Wm. B. Eerdmans.

Mzinyathi, M. (1987). Mental health care in South Africa: A personal psychological perspective. In A. B. Zwi & L. D. Saunders (Eds.), *Towards health care for all*. (NAMDA Conference 1985). Johannesburg: NAMDA.

Nagy, M. (1948). The child's theories concerning death. *Journal of Genetic Psychology*, *73*, 3–27.

Newman, C. J. (1976). Children of disaster: Clinical observations at Buffalo Creek. *American Journal of Psychiatry*, *133*, 306–312.

Orpen, C. (1970). Authoritarianism in an authoritarian culture: The case of Afrikaans-speaking South Africa. *Journal of Social Psychology*, *81*, 119–120.

Paton, A. (1958). *Cry, the beloved country*. Harmondsworth, England: Penguin Books.

Pillay, H. M. (1984). The concepts "racism," "causation," and "mental illness." *International Journal of Social Psychiatry*, *30*, 29–39.

Pine, F. (1986). On the development of the "borderline-child-to-be." *American Journal of Orthopsychiatry*, *56*(3), 450–459.

Platzky, L., & Walker, C. (1985). *The surplus people*. Johannesburg: Ravan Press.

Popovic, M., & Petrovic, D. (1964). After the earthquake. *Lancet*, *2*, 1169–1171.

Pruett, K. D. (1984). A chronology of defensive adaptations to severe psychological trauma. *Psychoanalytic Study of the Child*, *39*, 591–612.

Punamaki, R.-L. (1982). Childhood in the shadow of war: A psychological study of attitudes and emotional life of Israeli and Palestinian children. *Current Research on Peace and Violence*, *5*, 26–41.

Punamaki, R.-L. (1983). Psychological reactions of Palestinian and Israeli children to war and violence. In M. Kahnert, D. Pitt, & I. Taipale (Eds.), *Children and war: Proceedings of the symposium at the Siuntio Baths, Finland* (pp. 24.3–27.2). Helsinki, Finland: GIPRI, IPB, Peace Union of Finland.

Rachman, S. J. (1979). The concept of required helpfulness. *Behaviour Research and Therapy*, *17*, 1–6.

Raphael, B. (1984). *The anatomy of bereavement*. London: Hutchinson.

Raphael, B. (1986). *When disaster strikes: How individuals and communities cope with catastrophe*. New York: Basic Books.

Richman, S. (1986). *Stress and stress coping mechanisms employed by pre-school teachers in the black townships of Cape Town in relation to the South African crisis*. Unpublished thesis, University of Cape Town, South Africa.

Rosenheck, R. (1985a). Father–son relationships in malignant post-Vietnam stress syndrome. *American Journal of Social Psychiatry*, *5*, 19–23.

Rosenheck, R. (1985b). The malignant post-Vietnam stress syndrome. *American Journal of Orthopsychiatry*, *55*(2), 166–176.

Rosenheck, R. (1986). Impact of post-traumatic stress disorder of World War II on the next generation. *Journal of Nervous and Mental Disease*, *174*(6), 319–332.

Rosenheck, R., & Nathan, P. (1985). Secondary traumatization in children of Vietnam veterans. *Hospital and Community Psychiatry*, *36*(5), 538–539.

Rutter, M. (1986). Bereaved children. In M. Rutter (Ed.), *Children of sick parents* (Maudsley Monographs, Vol. 16, pp. 66–75). London: Oxford University Press.

Sack, W. H., Angell, R. H., Kinzie, J. D., & Rath, B. (1986). The psychiatric effects of massive trauma on Cambodian children: II. The family, the home, and the school. *Journal of the American Academy of Child Psychiatry*, *25*, 377–383.

Saigh, P. (1986). Three measures of childhood psychopathology in Lebanon. In J. Bryce & H. Armenian (Eds.), *In wartime: The state of children in Lebanon* (pp. 155–159). Syracuse, NY: Syracuse University Press.

Saigh, P. A. (1985). An experimental analysis of chronic post-traumatic stress among adolescents. *Journal of Genetic Psychology*, *146*(1), 125–131.

Schirmer, J. (1986). Chile: The loss of childhood. *Cultural Survival Quarterly*, *10*(4), 40–42.

Seligman, M. P. (1975). *Helplessness: On depression, development and death*. San Francisco: W. H. Freeman.

Shatan, C. (1975). "War babies": Delayed impact of war-making, persecution and disaster on children. *American Journal of Orthopsychiatry*, *45*, 289–290.

Simpson, M. A. (1963, October). *Malnutrition and mental develop-*

ment. Paper presented to the Physical Society, Guy's Hospital, London, England.

Simpson, M. A. (1975). The phenomenology of self-mutilation in a general hospital setting. *Canadian Psychiatric Association Journal, 20*(6), 429–434.

Simpson, M. A. (1977). *Self-mutilation and the borderline syndrome.* Dynamische Psychiatrie (Berlin), *1,* 42–48.

Simpson, M. A. (1979). *The facts of death.* Englewood Cliffs, NJ: Prentice-Hall.

Simpson, M. A. (1986/1987). Wiping out families: Stress in South Africa. *Psychology News* (London), *2*(2), 4–6.

Simpson, M. A. (1987, November). *Psychological findings in eight accused of murder by "common purpose" in the course of a township riot.* (Report to the Court in the case of the State versus M. Ncaphayi, V. Jack, B. Sonamzi, S. Booysen, E. Nelani, M. Sgoko, R. Yebe, and N. Madolo). Supreme Court of South Africa (Eastern Cape Division), Grahamstown.

Simpson, M. A. (1988a, June). *Psychological and psychiatric findings in three men accused of terrorist bombings.* [Report to the Court in the case of the State versus Nthunzi Tshika, Theminkosi Nkosi, and Zwellinjani Mathe). Supreme Court of South Africa, Pietermaritzburg.

Simpson, M. A. (1988b, May). *Bitter waters: The problems of children and adolescents in repression and unrest.* Keynote address delivered at the Barn i Krig conference, University of Bergen, Bergen, Norway.

Simpson, M. A. (1989, July). *Physical and psychological findings in a patient alleging beatings and electrical torture.* (Report to the Court in the case of Doris Dlamini versus the Minister of Law and Order). Supreme Court of South Africa, Durban.

Simpson, M. A. Palme, L., Dodge, C., Hundiede, K., Raundalen, M., Dyregrov, A., & Fields, R. (1988, May). *Children under extreme life situations: How to protect children in times of war and crisis.* Panel discussion at the Barn i Krig conference, University of Bergen, Bergen, Norway.

Skinner, D. (1986). The consequences for the pre-school child of a parent's being detained: A study from the Western Cape. Unpublished Honours thesis. University of Cape Town.

Skinner, D., & Swartz, L. (1989). The consequences for pre-school children of a parent's detention: A preliminary South African clinical study of caregivers' reports. *Journal of Child Psychology and Psychiatry, 30*(2), 243–260.

South African Institute of Race Relations (S.A.I.R.R.). (1984). *Survey of race relations in South Africa.* Johannesburg: Author.

Straker, G., & the Sanctuaries Team (1987). The continuous traumatic stress syndrome: The single therapeutic interview. *Psychology and Sociology, 8,* 48–56.

Swartz, L., & Levett, A. (1989). Political repression and children in South Africa: The social construction of damaging effects. *Social Science and Medicine, 28*(7), 741–750.

Swartz, S., Dowdall, T., & Swartz, L. (1986). Clinical psychology and the 1985 crisis in Cape Town. *Psychology and Sociology, 5,* 131–137.

Tan, E.-S., & Simons, R. C. (1973). Psychiatric sequelae to a civil disturbance. *British Journal of Psychiatry, 122,* 57–63.

Terr, L. C. (1979). Children of Chowchilla: A study of psychic terror. *Psychoanalytic Study of the Child, 34,* 547–623.

Terr, L. C. (1981). Psychic trauma in children: Observations following the Chowchilla school-bus kidnapping. *American Journal of Psychiatry, 138,* 14–19.

Terr, L. C. (1983). Chowchilla revisited: The effects of psychic trauma four years after a school-bus kidnapping. *American Journal of Psychiatry, 140,* 1543–1550.

Terr, L. C. (1985). Psychic trauma in children and adolescents. *Psychiatric Clinics of North America, 8*(4), 815–835.

Terr, L. C. (1988). What happens to early memories of trauma? A study of 20 children under age 5 at the time of documented traumatic events. *Journal of the American Academy of Child Psychiatry, 27,* 96–104.

Thurber, S. (1977). Natural disaster and the dimensionality of the I-E scale. *Journal of Social Psychology, 103,* 159–160.

Tillich, P. (1962). *Love, power and justice.* New York: Oxford University Press.

Tucker, K., & Lettin, A. (1975). The Tower of London explosions. *British Medical Journal, 3,* 287–289.

Turiel, E. (1966). An experimental test of the sequentiality of developmental stages in the child's moral judgements. *Journal of Personality and Social Psychology, 3,* 611–618.

Turiel, E. (1973). Stage transition in moral development. In R. M. W. Travers (Ed.), *Second handbook of research on teaching* (pp. 732–758). Chicago: Rand McNally.

Turnbull, C. M. (1972). *The mountain people.* New York: Simon & Schuster/Touchstone.

van der Kolk, B. A. (Ed.). (1987). *Psychological trauma.* Washington, DC: American Psychiatric Press.

van der Kolk, B. A., & Greenberg, M. S. (1987). The psychobiology of the trauma response: Hyperarousal, constriction and addiction to traumatic re-exposure. In B. A. van der Kolk (Ed.), *Psychological trauma* (pp. 63–87). Washington, DC: American Psychiatric Press.

van der Kolk, B. A., Greenberg, M., Boyd, H., & Krystal, J. (1985). Inescapable shock, neurotransmitters, and addiction to trauma: Toward a psychobiology of post-traumatic stress. *Biological Psychiatry, 20,* 314–325.

Van der Spuy, H. I. J. (1978). The psychology of apartheid: I. The psychodynamics of apartheid. In H. I. J. Van der Spuy & D. A. F. Shamley (Eds.), *The psychology of apartheid: A psychosocial perspective on South Africa* (pp. 1–17). Lanham, MD: University Press of America.

Van der Spuy, H. I. J., & Shamley, D. A. F. (Eds.). (1978). *The psychology of apartheid: A psychosocial perspective on South Africa.* Lanham, MD: University Press of America.

Van Rensburg, T. (1980). *Camp diary of Henrietta Armstrong.* Pretoria, South Africa: Human Sciences Research Council.

Vergnani, L. (1986, October 12). The kids under seige. *Sunday Tribune* (Durban, South Africa), p. 3.

Wilson, F., & Ramphele, M. (1987). *Children on the frontline: The impact of apartheid, destabilization and warfare on children in Southern and South Africa.* New York: UNICEF.

Wolfenstein, M. (1957). *Disaster: A psychological essay.* New York: Free Press/Macmillan.

Yacoubian, V. V., & Hacker, F. J. (1989). Reactions to disaster at a distance: The first week after the earthquake in Soviet Armenia. *Bulletin of the Menninger Clinic, 53,* 331–339.

Yalom, I. D. (1980). *Existential psychotherapy.* New York: Basic Books.

Young, A. (1980). The discourse on stress and the reproduction of correctional knowledge. *Social Sciences and Medicine, 14,* 133–146.

Ziv, A., & Israeli, R. (1973). Effects of bombardment on the manifest anxiety level of children living in kibbutzim. *Journal of Counseling and Clinical Psychology, 40,* 287–291.

Ziv, A., Kruglanski, A. W., & Shulman, S. (1974). Children's psychological reactions to wartime stress. *Journal of Personality and Social Psychology, 30,* 24–30.

CHAPTER 52

Traumatic War Experiences and Their Effects on Children

Mona S. Macksoud, Atle Dyregrov, and Magne Raundalen

Introduction

With the growing number of countries involved nowadays in armed conflict, more children have come to suffer the atrocities of war. Displacement, witnessing violent acts, bearing arms, being victims of direct hostilities are some of the traumatic experiences children face growing up in war-torn countries. There is no question that such overwhelming experiences have an impact on the development of children, their attitudes toward society, their relationships with others, and their outlook on life in general. In this chapter, we will examine the nature of childhood war traumata and their potential deleterious effects on children. Based on our own experiences, and drawing from the literature on traumatic stress, this chapter also outlines different treatment approaches to childhood posttraumatic stress disorder (PTSD) and discusses the implementation of such approaches in countries involved in armed conflict.

Childhood Trauma

There has been a recent intensification of interest in defining what constitutes a traumatic experience during childhood (Eth & Pynoos, 1985; Terr, 1984). In the analytical literature, a widely agreed upon definition of trauma refers to an external event (as opposed to an internal stimulation) that is intense, sudden, and that over-

whelms the child's capacity to cope or master the trauma at the time (A. Freud, 1967; S. Freud, 1920/1968; Furman, 1986; see also Chapter 5, in this volume, for a review). In its definition of posttraumatic stress disorder, the DSM-III states that the traumatic stressor must be "outside the range of usual human experience" and must be of sufficient intensity to "invoke symptoms of distress in most people" (American Psychiatric Association, 1987, p. 247).

Two important factors emerge from the above definitions. First, the traumatic event is differentiated from a stressful event in that, because of its intensity and nature, it will be likely to produce distress in all children exposed to it, regardless of the child's prior vulnerabilities or coping resources (Hocking, 1970; Lifton & Olson, 1976; Terr, 1984). An emphasis is thus placed on the *intensity* of the environmental event itself as opposed to differences in the child's predisposing factors toward stress. Secondly, the reaction to a traumatic experience is seen as inevitable and universal among children. Although the symptom presentation and the content of the reaction may vary according to age, the nature of the trauma, and its meaning to the child (Eth & Pynoos, 1985; Furman, 1986), the general features of the posttraumatic reaction are the same. In brief, childhood trauma is thus defined as a function of specific types of environmental experiences and of a person's response pattern to them (Keane, 1986).

Childhood War Traumata

An important challenge in the study of the effects of war on children, is the identification of the specific war experiences that are traumatic to children. However, from the above discussion, it becomes evident that one is looking for unusual war-related experiences that are linked to posttraumatic stress symptomatology in children.

An extensive review of the literature on the experi-

Mona S. Macksoud • Project on Children and War, Center for the Study of Human Rights, Columbia University, New York, New York 10027. Atle Dyregrov • Center for Crisis Psychology, Fabrikkgt 5, 5037 Solheimsvik, Norway. Magne Raundalen • Asligrenda 8, 5095 Ulset, Norway.
International Handbook of Traumatic Stress Syndromes, edited by John P. Wilson and Beverley Raphael. Plenum Press, New York, 1993.

ences of children during World War II, and during more recent wars, indicate that several war-related experiences trigger posttraumatic stress reactions in children (see Arroyo & Eth, 1984; Dyregrov & Raundalen, 1987). The diagnostic entity of what is now termed *posttraumatic stress disorder* (PTSD) did not exist during the prior four decades. However, earlier studies have documented very similar psychiatric symptoms to those of PTSD in children who were exposed to war traumata (Arroyo & Eth, 1984). Among the traumatic experiences children face during wartime are the following:

1. *Violent death of a parent.* The violent death of a parent brought about severe stress reactions for a sample of bereaved Israeli children (Kaffman & Elizur, 1984).

2. *Witnessing the killing of close family members.* Ugandan children who had witnessed the killing of a family member showed severe grief and posttraumatic symptoms following the event (Raundalen, Lwanga, Magisha, & Dyregrov, 1987). Several authors also document the posttraumatic reactions of children who have witnessed such violent acts as the torture, brutal arrest or execution of parents or relatives (Allodi, 1980; Cohn, Kisten, & Koch, 1980; Lebovici, 1974; Malmquist, 1986; Schirmer, 1986; see also Chapter 26, in this volume, for a discussion).

3. *Separation and displacement.* Forced separation from parents and displacement from home, as a result of war conditions, were shown to be related to mental health problems in children during World War II (Bodman, 1944; Burbury, 1941; Coromina, 1943; A. Freud & Burlingham, 1943). The effects on children of separation from their fathers during the latter's involvement in conflict needs also to be considered. More recently, displacement, forced immigration, and refugee status are linked to traumatic stress reactions in Asian children and adolescents (Carlin, 1979; Kinzie, Sack, Angell, Manson, & Rath, 1986; Ressler, Boothby, & Steinbock, 1988).

4. *Terror attacks, kidnapping, and life threat.* Ayalon (1983) showed how children exposed to terror through guerrilla attacks suffer symptoms indicative of posttraumatic stress reactions. The work of Terr (1979, 1983) on the impact of the Chowchilla kidnapping showed the presence of severe long-term effects in most children following the event. Although this was a single event taking place in a relatively peaceful community, the kidnapping of children during wartime would expose children to a threatening situation that goes far beyond the Chowchilla experience. In addition, Pynoos *et al.* (1987) have shown how violent life threats, such as a sniper attack, can trigger posttraumatic stress reactions in children exposed to them.

5. *Participation in violent acts.* Boothby (1986) presented several cases of children and adolescents who were perpetuators of abusive violence and who exhibited stress reactions similar to PTSD. Little is known yet about the effects of training children as child-soldiers and of forcing them to commit atrocities toward their own communities and families. From our own preliminary interaction with child-soldiers in Mozambique, it became clear that they were suffering from PTSD following the violent acts they were forced to commit.

6. *Bombardment and shelling.* Several authors suggested that bombardment and evacuation under shelling are stressors frequently resulting in posttraumatic stress reactions in children (Brander, 1943; Carey-Trefzer, 1949; Dunsdon, 1941; Janis, 1951). Lebanese children exposed to repetitive shelling and combat conditions were shown to exhibit high levels of psychological distress (Day & Sadek, 1982; Hourani, Armenian, & Afifi, 1986).

7. *Witnessing parental fear reactions.* Burt (1943) and later Baider and Rosenfeld (1974) described several cases of war neurosis in children who witnessed parental panic reactions or extreme fear reactions. Parental reactions to violence are a strong predictor of how the children will react to a traumatic event.

It is known that parental post traumatic stress reaction has a significant impact on both childhood development and the creation of psychopathology with the family system.

8. *Physical injuries and handicaps.* Moreover, although no studies document specifically the effects of war injuries on children, several articles describe posttraumatic stress reactions in children who had to cope with amputations (Schechter & Holter, 1979), burns (Galdston, 1972), and mutilating surgeries (Earle, 1979).

9. *Extreme poverty and starvation.* Finally, several researchers in Northern Ireland stress the importance of considering the impact of extreme poverty and deprivation on children as potentially traumatic, although the evidence remains inconclusive (Harbison, 1983).

On the other hand, Kinzie *et al.* (1986, 1988) presented several cases of Cambodian children who had endured starvation, among other traumas, and who developed posttraumatic stress disorders and prolonged depressive symptoms.

The above studies suggest a variety of childhood war traumas that are common experiences during wartime. Because each country has its own type of war, the kinds of traumatic experiences that children face are therefore quite variable from country to country. The development, therefore, of a national childhood trauma profile for a given country allows for the identification of that country's specific types of war traumas. In Lebanon, for example, the distribution of a representative sample of Lebanese children by types of war traumata experienced showed that the most common war experiences were shelling or combat, extreme poverty, displacement, witnessing violent acts, and bereavement (Macksoud, 1988). Once the traumata are defined, their impact on the development of children can then be studied.

What becomes clear from studies investigating the effects of war on children is that war traumata are diverse and multiple and can occur repeatedly over a long period of time (Arroyo & Eth, 1984; Bryce, 1986). On average, a Lebanese child, for example, experiences five to six different types of traumatic events during lifetime (Macksoud, 1988). Thus, the effect of a single trauma cannot be studied in isolation because most traumatic events and their effects are difficult to disentangle. In addition, the repetitive nature of most war traumata (such as shelling or witnessing violent acts) adds another dimension to the assessment of trauma effect, namely, the cumulative effect of trauma exposure.

In summary, the types of war traumata, the magnitude of trauma exposure (i.e., how many traumata), and the extent of exposure (i.e., how often and for how long), are all crucial factors to assess while investigating the effects of war traumata on the development of children.

Short-Term Effects of Trauma on Children

Whether originating in bereavement, displacement, or shelling, children's initial reactions to traumatic events have a great deal in common, although there are some distinctive aspects that relate to particular traumata. For example, with bereavement, feelings of loss and grief dominate the picture. With displacement, homesickness and feelings of anger and alienation toward the new environment predominate (Anthony, 1986). However, the general features of children's reactions to traumatic events are more or less universal (Benedek, 1985) and cluster together to form the diagnostic category of PTSD.

Posttraumatic Stress Disorder in Children

The general criteria for the diagnosis of PTSD in children are the following (see American Psychiatric Association, 1987; Benedek, 1985; Pynoos & Nader, 1988):

1. The identification of a distressing experience in the life of the child that is outside the range of usual human experiences.
2. A persistent reexperiencing of the trauma in a variety of ways, namely, through disturbing intrusions of a specific image or sound related to the actual trauma; traumatic dreams of the actual trauma or of the recurrence of another type of trauma; and traumatic play incorporating different aspects of the trauma.
3. A reduced responsiveness and involvement with the environment, namely, through diminished interest in enjoyable activities, emotional detachment from parents or friends, and reduced tolerance and avoidance of intense feelings.
4. The presence of new trauma-related symptoms and behaviors such as an increased state of alertness, including nervousness, exaggerated startle responses, and sleep disturbances; avoidant behaviors and recurrent anxiety to specific concrete reminders of the trauma; and difficulty in concentrating over school work.

In addition to the above general features of PTSD in children, several studies (Dyregrov, 1985; Pynoos & Nader, 1988; Terr, 1979) reported the presence of other symptoms that seem specific to children's reactions to trauma. These include (1) an increase in attachment behavior toward parents or siblings; (2) the presence of separation anxiety symptoms; (3) loss of recently acquired developmental skills, especially among younger children; (4) fear of the recurrence of the trauma; and (5) feelings of guilt over surviving the traumatic event, especially among older children.

PTSD and Development Stages

Although the general features of PTSD are the same for all children, the symptom presentation and content of the disorder seem to vary according to the age of the child. The developmental achievements specific to each age, whether in the area of cognition, emotions, or social relationships, will influence the child's reaction to a trauma. Eth and Pynoos (1985) proposed age-specific posttraumatic stress reactions for preschool children, school-aged children, and adolescents.

Preschool Children

Preschool children (0–6 years) are dependent on adults for their nurture and safety. They are helpless and passive when confronted with a threatening situation and thus require the assistance of adults to feel secure and to ward off the threatening situation. As younger children do not have the ability to imagine ways they can prevent or alter the trauma, they often feel defenseless. They may go to sleep, but usually there is no way they can escape or avoid a stressful situation. Following a trauma, young children may appear mute and withdrawn. There are several accounts of children staying at the side of their dead parent(s) unable to speak, eat, or play.

The silence does not mean that the event is forgotten. Young children will often give full details of the traumatic event to a trusted person, at a later point in time. On the other hand, some elements of the traumatic event may show up in the child's play activities. Reenactments and play involving some aspects of the trauma are common events with traumatized young children. A 7-year-old Mosambikan boy, for example, who had been forced to light a fire to his own hut and to witness his parents' death, spontaneously acted out a game of setting fire to huts.

Children under 4 years of age often react to a trauma with anxious attachment behavior in the form of separation and stranger anxiety. Thus, they frequently cling to parents, fear going to sleep, and have temper tantrums when left alone. Other regressive behaviors also emerge with young children, namely, a return to former transitional objects.

Because of the pressure in processing the trauma while awake or during sleep, nightmares and sleep disturbances are common occurrences among young children. Somnambulism, sleep talking, and night terrors are the most frequent sleep disturbances among this age group.

The young child has a limited tolerance for sadness and may thus use various forms of denial to ease the pain. In the case of the death of a parent, for example, the mourning process is complicated by the child's need to work through the traumatic death before being able to grieve the loss.

School-Aged Children

School-aged children (6–12 years) can utilize a broader repertoire of cognitive, emotional, and behavioral responses to deal with the trauma. In the cognitive domain, school-aged children will experience difficulties concentrating, and thus their school performance often declines. The child's decreased ability to concentrate is often caused by the intrusions of the traumatic memories, or by the influence of a depressed affect on the child's mental processes. In either cases, the child is distracted from school work. Thus, learning disorders and the associated conduct disturbances are very common among this age group.

School-aged children will often actively deal with the traumatic event in fantasy. They can, for example, fantasize having rescued their parents or tricked the assailant. Play activity and reenactments become more elaborate with this age group. Inner plans of action are devised in order to help the child change the outcome of the trauma. In fantasy, they can undo what had taken place and imagine a happy ending to the traumatic event. The ability to deal with the trauma in fantasy gives the child a way to counteract feelings of helplessness. This cognitive maturity of devising "inner plans of actions," also makes the child more prone to feelings of guilt and self-reproach. For when children imagine ways that could have prevented the traumatic event, they will also blame themselves for not having done enough.

In the event of a death, school-aged children understand the concept of a death in a more advanced manner. They know that death is irreversible and final. Unlike younger children, they do not expect the dead person to return.

Frequently, school-aged children become either more passive and unspontaneous or more aggressive and demanding. Both behavioral changes may interfere with their peer relationships and lead to social isolation.

Finally, this age group is particularly susceptible to the development of such psychosomatic complaints as headaches, stomachaches, and other physical problems.

Adolescents

Adolescents may be forced to assume a premature adult role following a trauma. The abrupt loss of a parent or the witnessing of violence may precipitate a premature identity formation or identity diffusions among adolescents. Having the cognitive maturity for deductive reasoning and the ability to understand the far-reaching consequences of a traumatic event, adolescents are in many ways more vulnerable to trauma exposure than are school-aged children. Although they may be too old to use fantasy as a denial mechanism, they typically do not use play activity and reenactments as coping strategies. Instead, adolescents use self-destructive behaviors as a way to distract themselves from the anxiety of the traumatic memories. A serious consequence of being traumatized in adolescence is the risk of becoming more rebellious and more prone to partake in antisocial acts. Adolescents may embark on a period of acting-out behaviors that are characterized by school truancy, precocious sexual activity, substance abuse, and delinquency.

Unlike school-aged children, adolescents are able to identify how their own behavior may or may not have contributed to the outcome of a traumatic event. However, adolescents may still experience strong feelings of guilt following a traumatic event.

For adolescents, the peer group is very important. A trauma may cause shame and isolation. Fearing that they may be stigmatized, adolescents dread the reaction of their peer group, and they may try to keep the information from reaching friends and fellow students.

Adolescents have the capacity to fully understand how a trauma may affect their lives and they do not conceive of themselves as invulnerable. Following a traumatic event, they may go around expecting a new trauma, or that something bad may happen. At this age, they are apt to experience a lack of future preparedness or a pessimism about the future. Basic assumptions about life, themselves, and others can be thoroughly shaken.

Long-Term Effects of War Traumata on Children

The full-blown picture of PTSD can resolve itself, without treatment, within 6 to 8 months but this is by no means the common outcome. Some children may exhibit symptoms of PTSD chronically following a traumatic exposure. For instance, in her follow-up study of kidnapped children, Terr (1983) found that *every* child still exhibited posttraumatic effects 4 years after the single traumatizing event. Among the long-term effects were recurrent dreams of the trauma, repetitive relating of the trauma, pessimism about the future, fear of further traumata, the development of myths and omens, and personality changes.

Under war conditions children may suffer from the aftermath of distinctive traumata, and exhibit long-term psychological effects in the form of PTSD. The warfare, however, has other more far-reaching, long-term effects on the psychosocial development of children, which may take several forms.

Moral Development

During civil wars, the armed forces commit many atrocities toward the civilian population (see Boothby, 1986; Bryce, 1986; Dodge & Raundalen, 1987; Jupp, 1986). Children often witness the looting, torturing or killing that is carried out by political leaders or army personnel. As a result of identifying with "the aggressor," children's sense of right and wrong may become blurred. They will gradually accept that looting, for example, is different from stealing, or that killing for political reasons is different from murdering. In other words, these children will slowly convince themselves that certain violent acts are morally permissible or acceptable.

In the context of sexual abuse, Finkelhor and Browne (1985) described the feeling of betrayal that children experience when they discover that someone on whom they were vitally dependent had caused them harm. During wartime, children experience a betrayal of another order. The authority figures, whether parents, local leaders, or army personnel, those role models they have learned to trust and respect, have repeatedly breached the expected moral standards of behavior. This deep sense of betrayal may, in turn, affect the moral development of these children.

A Survivor's Identity

Some children who are immunized by their own family's moral standards identify with the helping pro-social forces of their country rather than with the armed forces. Children may want to become doctors or teachers and help to change their country's situation. Most Ugandan children, for example, want to become medical professionals (Dodge & Raundalen, 1987). Such a role seems to fill an important psychological function for these children, namely, a way to obtain control over and even conquer death and disease: "When I get to be a doctor, I will do my best to save peoples' lives. It is very important to save lives" (so said a Ugandan girl who was 9 years old).

Regardless of the type of occupation these children chose, all voiced the wish to acquire material goods. They wanted to become rich and to own a house, a car, a farm, and other such luxuries. This craving for material goods seems to depict a deep feeling of deprivation.

Interestingly, child survivors of the Holocaust often voiced the need to be compensated for the hell they had endured during the war. This might be displayed by an obsessive need for food, clothing, and other material objects (Klein, 1974). Having "lost" their childhood, war children may grow up wanting to actively compensate for that loss, not only on the material level but also on the personal level. The long-term effect of material and psychological deprivation is expected to have a profound effect on the personality formation of these children (E. Kahana, B. Kahana, Harel, & Rosner, 1988).

For instance, Ayalon (1982) referred to a "survivor's identity" as a major transformation of the self-image. Survivors of war traumata either developed a resentment bordering on a paranoid suspicion of others, or an altruistic self-sacrificing attitude. The first attitude is explained as part of a syndrome of unspent aggressiveness projected onto others, whereas the second seems to be activated by a need to reverse the image of a "victim" into that of a "rescuer," conveying a sense of mastery and control over the trauma. Both attitudes influence the child's later occupational choice in specific as well as his or her relationship to others in general.

Pupils of War

In war situations, children become pupils of war and are often recruited as soldiers or militia fighters. The recruitment of these children is often associated with heavy indoctrination programs that glorify violence. Thus, feelings of revenge and aggression come to dominate these children's minds. In addition, during their training, some children are compelled to commit brutal acts toward civilians as "rites of passage" (Boothby, 1986; Dodge & Raundalen, 1987). When such violent aggression is displayed and encouraged by a government, children suffer the consequences. It is well known, for example, that there is an increase in antisocial behavior

and in hostile and aggressive feelings among adolescents during wartimes (Jahoda & Harrison, 1975; Punamaki, 1982, 1983).

Lack of Trust, Feelings of Vulnerability

The constant unpredictability of a war situation can alter children's sense of security and trust in others. During wartime, parents are often unable to protect their children from harm. The fear and anxiety that children feel when their parents are unable to control noxious events can be intensive. If such an insecurity is experienced in the early years of life when "basic trust" is formed, children's attachment behavior will be affected and they will become anxious and over-dependent (Solnit, 1982). Similarly, Ayalon (1982) found that traumatic events, such as terrorist activities, can inhibit children's capacity in trusting themselves and others and in enjoying life in general. Trauma victims of all ages report difficulty reestablishing trust after the traumatic event. However, children appear to be especially vulnerable to the collapse of basic trust under traumatic conditions (Lyons, 1987).

Pessimism about the Future

The exposure to war events on a "daily" basis, coupled with a constant feeling of insecurity, may leave children uncertain about their future. Although this aspect has not been thoroughly studied among children in war situations, the Ugandan study showed that around one fourth of the children who were interviewed made remarks that conveyed their uncertainty about the future (Dyregrov & Raundalen, 1987): "If I am not a bunch of bones in my grave, I will be a businessman." "If I reach 2000 and I am still alive. . . ." "So if God wishes and all goes well, I should like to become a lawyer."

In her follow-up study of children who were exposed to terrorist attacks, Ayalon (1982) noted how some children may live for years harboring catastrophic expectations of the future, while others live with the conviction of being "protected for life" by some supernatural forces.

Data on the consequences of war traumata on children's view of themselves in the future and on their ability to make plans for their lives are still very limited. However, anecdotal data on children in Uganda and in Lebanon seem to indicate that most children in these war-torn countries have a rather pessimistic view of their future.

School Performance

Little is known about the long-term effect of war on school performance. In many war-afflicted societies, it is difficult to keep the schools functioning, and it is even more difficult to evaluate the children's school performances. It is interesting to note that schools, as institutions, are among the few relatively safe places that children could turn to during wartime. Schools also offer a sense of continuity in the children's daily lives. In addition, through cultural activities, schools allow for the symbolic expression of some of the children's experiences. Data, however, on how warfare affects school performance remain scarce.

Kinzie *et al.* (1986) described a study of Cambodian children who survived extreme suffering under the Pol Pot regime. They were studied after escaping and settling in the United States. In school, these children presented as behaviorally deviant (25%) rather than academically deviant (15%). Despite their past history, they performed well academically. However, their classroom behavior suffered; they become withdrawn in class and did not participate in class discussions. They also spent a lot of time daydreaming.

Kinzie *et al.* (1986) argued that cultural values must be taken into consideration when investigating the effects of war traumata on school performance. The effects of war may be channelized in different ways in different societies. Traditionally, Asians, for example, have a deep commitment to learning and hold a deep respect for the teacher as an authority figure. This attitude might have acted as a buffer against more disruptive behavior in school (see Chapter 25, in this volume, for a discussion of these issues).

Arroyo and Eth (1984) found that latency-aged children who had escaped Central American warfare were primarily referred to a psychiatric service because of school difficulties and conduct disorders. The school performance of these children was impaired by the intrusion of past traumatic memories, and of more recent stresses associated with parental separation and immigration.

Intervention

Short-Term Interventions

The aims of the short-term interventions are to restore the traumatized child to a pretrauma level of functioning, and to alleviate the fears and anxieties of the child's families. Several treatment approaches (behavioral, psychoanalytical, crisis-intervention) and treatment modalities (child, parents, teachers) have been described by researchers working with children during the acute phase of posttrauma reactions. In the following section, we offer a brief summary of those therapeutic efforts.

Pynoos and Eth (1985) described a one-to-one interview format that aims at offering immediate relief for the child and at buffering further distress. Both authors use drawings and storytelling to help the child gain some control over the traumatic event. In the case of mass trauma (in this instance an earthquake), Galante and Foa (1986) and Frederick (1985) discussed the advantages of group sessions with children who had shared common traumas. Again, drawings and play sessions involving storytelling and role-playing were used to encourage the free expression of fears and to facilitate trauma resolution.

The working through of fears, whether individually or in a group can be handled by trained parents and would not necessarily require trained professionals (Galante & Foa, 1986; Rigamer, 1986). This is deemed necessary in order to reach a larger number of children.

There is some evidence suggesting that the well-being of children living in dangerous environments depends on the capacity of the parents to sustain a strong attachment to their children, maintain a positive sense of self, and establish stable routine care-giving arrangements following a trauma (Garbarino, 1988). Using a crisis intervention model with families of traumatized children, parents are initially assisted in understanding the dynamics of unusual behaviors (such as PTSD symptomatology) on the part of the affected child (Nir, 1985). A next step entails training the parents to attend to their children's needs and to provide a structured opportunity to discuss and work-through their children's fears and experiences (Galante & Foa, 1986). Finally, parents are advised to reestablish a daily routine as soon as possible following a trauma, such as having the child resume school attendance.

Several authors stress the importance of establishing outreach programs that extend intervention from the child and family to community members (such as teachers) (Blom, 1986; Frederick, 1985; Rigamer, 1986). The community intervention programs include didactic expositions of studies on PTSD in children, recommendations for action, and discussion groups for the community members to share their experiences and problems (Frederick, 1985; Rigamer, 1986). As with parents, community members are thus trained to attend to the special needs of children who are exposed to trauma.

Although little effort was made to evaluate the effectiveness of such short-term therapeutic efforts, the rapid therapeutic gains that are accomplished during the time-limited period following a crisis have long been proven (Caplan, 1964). By intervening during the acute phase of posttrauma reaction, the child is assisted in the stress recovery process and in trauma resolution.

Long-Term Interventions

Interventions that address the long-term effects of war traumata are, of course, more complex than in acute treatments. The effects of war traumata, involve not only PTSD but also the associated problems that have developed over time, in part as a result of unresolved PTSD, but mainly as a result of the child's struggle to cope with the overpowering consequences of war. Long-term interventions on behalf of children caught up in war are often based on the following premises:

1. Violence breeds violence, that is, the children of today's wars are to become the terrorists and warriors of the future.
2. The chronic exposure to destabilization has deleterious effects on the psychological development of children.
3. Children escape unscathed by wars if they have access to parental protection.

Our experience with children living under war conditions has lead us to challenge this rather dark picture of the effects of war and to introduce new premises for long-term interventions.

The Violent Child

Are the children of today's wars the easy recruits of terror? When we analyzed the stories written on war and violence by a sample of children from Uganda and Mozambique, we came to realize that the war created two groups of victims. The "passive recipients of war," those children who are unexpectedly caught in the firing line with their families, and "the pupils of war," those children that actively participate in the fighting.

It was interesting to note that children who were the passive recipients of war wrote stories that did not portray any feelings of hate, violence, or revenge. Most of these children did not identify any specific enemy. Rather, they saw the "war" as the enemy. A minority wanted to punish the assailants, but relied on the "authorities" and on "God" to administer the punishment. The majority of these children had identified with the "good-doers" and wanted to become doctors or relief workers in order to help others.

Children who were the pupils of war, on the other hand, had stories portraying more aggressive themes. They were more vindictive, brutal, and less hesitant about using violence. They had been recruited and trained to commit violent acts. For many of these children, violence had become a way of life, a "drug" to cure feelings of grief and hopelessness.

These two groups of children represent, of course, two extremes on a continuum. Children vary in their assimilation of violence depending on the types of experiences they face during wartime. Thus, war does not automatically create violent children.

For children who were not involved directly with violence, intervention programs include working-through the traumatic experiences and treating the depression and the grief that stem from the loss of significant others. For those children who were trained to commit violent acts, the intervention package includes a school program aimed at gradually reducing aggressive and violent behaviors. In Zimbabwe, for example, such a school program was organized by the army. Teachers were replaced by army personnel, and the children were gradually rehabilitated to a normal nonviolent existence.

The Child Politician

A 12-year-old boy from Mozambique related the following statement after he was released from a 16-month captivity:

> Renamo destroys our schools, our hospitals. They force the farmers to be refugees, they destroy the nation and our future. We ask the whole world to help fight the bandits. We want you to know that we suffer. Children are kidnapped and forced to kill, even their own families. I have seen it myself and I want the world to know.

This youth's political appraisal of his experience of war was typical of how Mozambican children tackled the psychological impact of destabilization and violence.

Teachers in several war-torn countries have shared with us the importance of informing children about the political background of a war and of teaching them the important role they play in rebuilding their nation. With such a "political-cognitive" frame of reference, children are better able to process the atrocities of a war situation.

The aims of the political-cognitive method are three-fold: (1) to allow children to experience their world as rational, relatively predictable, and thus understandable; (2) to give children the opportunity to involve themselves intellectually—and sometimes practically—in putting an end to the war in a constructive way. Youths could, for example, appeal to world opinion to put pressure on the war makers, or take part in demonstrations, or discuss the political situation at school or at home; and (3) to prepare the young for the future by helping them build realistic hopes and expectations about their future.

The Child Refugee

Should relief workers by all means reunite children with their families? Do all parents want their children back? The argument that all children should stay with their parents during wartime is supported by studies that took place during World War II. Evidence then showed that parents acted as "protective shields" against the taxing demands of war (Coromina, 1943; A. Freud & Burlingham, 1943). Similarly, more recent studies suggest that children are better off remaining with their families even though by doing so they may witness destruction and deprivation (Ressler *et al.*, 1988). It is worth noting that the "buffering effect" of parents is strongest the younger the child and the more resourceful the parents (Garbarino, 1988).

Although we definitely agree with family reunification during times of war, anecdotal data from Lebanon and Sudan led us to question the move to reunite children with their families regardless of the circumstances surrounding the separation. Some young adolescents in Sudan, for example, had willingly fled their war-torn region and settled in another region of the country. For them, staying with their families would have meant death. They were described by relief workers as resilient and resourceful in adapting to their new status of refugees.

In another situation, some parents had urged their children to leave and seek better opportunities elsewhere. Children were given money and placed on the first bus or train leaving the war-torn region.

It is difficult to assess the significance of these anecdotal observations. However, while planning intervention programs for refugee children (especially those above 10 years of age) the circumstances around and after the separation should be carefully assessed and weighted. If reunification is considered, a program should then be set up to help the child work-through the traumatic experience of separation and the associated feelings of loss, anger, and helplessness. Anxieties about the possible recurrence of a separation should be addressed, and the child should gradually be assisted in his "reentry" to his family.

In the event that refugee children cannot be reunited with their families, alternative placements should be arranged. Again, children should be helped to process their traumatic experiences and feelings of loss. As new attachments with other adults are formed and educational and social activities are resumed, refugee children will begin slowly to adjust to their new status.

Conclusion

In this chapter, we have identified the types of problems that children face growing up in war-torn countries. Children are the innocent victims of wars. Their lives are affected by the violence and the atrocities they experience on a daily basis. We have seen how war traumata can post a significant and persistent burden on the development of children. Some of the short-term effects of war can be addressed through simple intervention programs. However, the state of the art in the study of the long-term effects of war is still novel. Many questions remain unanswered.

Since wars will not vanish, we need to know what are the mitigating circumstances during wartime that may buffer the long-term effects of war. Some children come through the experience of war surprisingly less damaged than others. A good deal seems to depend on the availability of the parents and on the solidarity of the community (Anthony, 1986; Garbarino, 1988). The identification of such other protective factors becomes crucial.

We also need to know whether stress-inoculation techniques, such as those applied in Israel (Ayalon, 1979), steel children and prepare them for future traumata, or whether they produce unnecessary anxiety and unwarranted fears.

It is only through long-term studies in war countries that the answers for these questions and others may become possible. Meanwhile, urgent action is needed on a larger scale to resolve ongoing political conflicts and to prevent the occurrence of new wars. For as yet, we do not really know what happens to a generation of vulnerable children who have lost their sense of safety, who have acquired a high tolerance for violence, who are haunted by terrifying memories, mistrusting and cautious of others, and who hold a pessimistic view of the future.

References

Allodi, F. (1980). The psychiatric effects in children and families of victims of political persecution and torture. *Danish Medical Bulletin, 27,* 229–332.

American Psychiatric Association (1987). *Diagnostic and statistical manual of mental disorders* (3rd ed.). Washington, DC: Author.

Anthony, E. (1986). Children's reactions to severe stress: Some introductory comments. *Journal of the American Academy of Child Psychiatry, 25*(3), 299–305.

Arroyo, W., & Eth, S. (1984). Children traumatized by central American warfare. In S. Eth and R. Pynoos (Eds.), *Post-traumatic stress disorder in children* (pp.101–120). Washington DC: American Psychiatric Press.

Ayalon, O. (1979). Community oriented preparation for emergency: COPE. *Death Education, 3,* (pp. 227–244).

Ayalon, O. (1982). Children as hostages. *Practitioner, 226,* 1773–1781.

Ayalon, O. (1983). Coping with terrorism: The Israeli case. In D. Meichenbaum & M. Jaremko (Eds.), *Stress reduction and prevention* (pp. 293–340). New York: Plenum Press.

Baider, L., & Rosenfeld, E. (1974). Effect of parental fears on children in wartime. *Social Casework, 55,* 497–503.

Benedek, F. (1985). Children and psychic trauma: A brief review of contemporary thinking. In S. Eth & R. Pynoos (Eds.), *Post-traumatic stress disorder in children* (pp. 1–16). Washington DC: American Psychiatric Press.

Blom, G. E. (1986). A school disaster—Intervention and research aspects. *Journal of the American Academy of Child Psychiatry, 25,* 333–345.

Bodman, F. M. (1944). Child psychiatry in war-time Britain. *Journal of Educational Psychology, 35,* 293–301.

Boothby, N. (1986). Children and war. *Cultural Survival Quarterly, 10*(4), 28–30.

Brander, T. (1943). Psychiatric observations among Finnish children during the Russo-Finnish war of 1939–1940. *Nervous Child, 2,* 313–319.

Bryce, J. W. (1986). *Cries of children in Lebanon as voiced by their mothers.* UNICEF: Regional Office for the Middle East and North Africa.

Burbury, W. M. (1941). Effects of evacuation and air raids on children. *British Medical Journal, 2,* 486–488.

Burt, C. (1943). War neuroses in British children. *Nervous Child, 2,* 324–337.

Caplan, G. (1964). *Principles of preventive psychiatry.* New York: Basic Books.

Carey-Trefzer, C. (1949). The results of a clinical study of war-damaged children who attend the child guidance clinic, the Hospital of Sick Children, Great Ormond Street, London. *Journal of Mental Science, 95,* 535–559.

Carlin, J. E. (1979). The catastrophically up-rooted child: Southeast Asian refugee children. In J. D. Call, J. D. Noshpitz, R. L. Cohen, & I. N. Berlin (Eds.), *Basic handbook for childhood psychiatry* (Vol. 1, pp. 290–300). New York: Basic Books.

Cohn, J., Kisten, I. M. H., & Koch, L. (1980). Children and torture. *Danish Medical Bulletin, 27,* 238–239.

Coromina J. (1943). Repercussions of war on children as observed during the Spanish civil war. *Nervous Child, 2,* 324–337.

Day, R. C., & Sadek, S. (1982). The effect of Benson's relaxation response on the anxiety levels of Lebanese children under stress. *Journal of Experimental Child Psychology, 34,* 350–356.

Dodge, C. P., & Raundalen, M. (1987). *War, violence and children in Uganda.* Oslo: Norwegian University Press.

Dunsdon, M. I. (1941). A psychologist's contribution to air raid problems. *Mental Health, 2*(2), 36–41.

Dyregrov, A. (1985, November). Children in crisis: What will happen if emotional wounds are not treated? *Journal of Emergency Services,* 39–43.

Dyregrov, A., & Raundalen, M. (1987). Children and the stresses of war: A review of the literature. In C. P. Dodge & M. Raundalen (Eds.), *War, violence and children in Uganda* (pp. 109–132). Oslo: Norwegian University Press.

Earle, E. (1979). The psychological effects of mutilating surgery in children and adolescents. *Psychoanalytical Study of the Child, 34,* 527–546.

Eth, S., & Pynoos, R. (1985). Developmental perspective on psychic trauma in childhood. In C. R. Figley (Ed.), *Trauma and its wake* (Vol. 1, pp. 36–52). New York: Brunner/Mazel.

Finkelhor, D., & Browne, A. (1985). The traumatic impact of child sexual abuse: A conceptualization. *American Journal of Orthopsychiatry, 55*(4), 530–541.

Frederick, C. J. (1985). Children traumatized by catastrophic situations. In S. Eth & R. Pynoos (Eds.), *Post-traumatic stress disorder in children* (pp. 71–100). Washington, DC: American Psychiatric Press.

Freud, A. (1967). Comments on trauma. In S. Furst (Ed.), *Psychic trauma*. New York: Basic Books.

Freud, A., & Burlingham, D. T. (1943). *War and children*. New York: Medical War Books.

Freud, S. (1968). Beyond the pleasure principle. In J. Strachey (Ed. and Trans.), *The standard edition of the complete psychological works of Sigmund Freud* (Vol. 18, pp. 7–64). London: Hogarth Press. (Original work published 1920)

Furman, E. (1986). On trauma: When is the death of a parent traumatic? *Psychoanalytic Study of the Child, 41*, 191–208.

Galante, R., & Foa, D. (1986). An epidemiological study of psychic trauma and treatment effectiveness for children after a natural disaster. *Journal of the American Academy of Child Psychiatry, 25*, 357–363.

Galdston, R. (1972). The burning and healing of children. *Psychiatry, 35*, 57–66.

Garbarino, J. (1988). *A note on children and youth in dangerous environments: The Palestinian situation as a case study*. Unpublished manuscript, Erikson Institute for Advanced Study in Child Development, Chicago.

Harbison, J. I. (1983). Children in a society in turmoil. In J. I. Harbison (Ed.), *Children of the troubles* (pp. 1–11). Belfast: Stranmillis College, Learning Resources Unit.

Hocking, F. (1970). Extreme environmental stress and its significance for psychopathology. *American Journal of Psychotherapy, 24*, 4–26.

Hourani, L., Armenian, H., & Affifi, L. (1986). A population-based survey of loss and psychological distress during war. *Social Science Medicine, 23*(3), 269–275.

Jahoda, G., & Harrison, S. (1975). Belfast children: Some effects of a conflict environment. *Irish Journal of Psychology, 3*, 1–19.

Janis, I. (1951). *Air war and emotional stress*. New York: McGraw-Hill.

Jupp, M. (1986). Apartheid: Violence against children. *Cultural Survival Quarterly, 10*(4), 34–37.

Kaffman, M., & Elizur, E. (1984). Children's bereavement reactions following death of the father. Special issue: Family psychiatry in the kibbutz. *International Journal of Family Therapy, 6*(4), 259–283.

Kahana, E., Kahana, B., Harel, Z., & Rosner, T. (1988). Coping with extreme trauma. In J. P. Wilson, Z. Harel, & B. Kahana (Eds.), *Human adaptation to extreme stress: From the Holocaust to Vietnam* (pp. 55–76). New York: Plenum Press.

Keane, T. (1986). Defining traumatic stress: Some comments on the current terminological confusion. *Behavior Therapy, 16*, 419–423.

Kinzie, J.D., Leone, P., Bui, A., Ben., R., et al. (1988). Group therapy with Southeast Asian refugees. *Community Mental Health Journal, 24*, 157–166.

Kinzie, D., Sack, W., Angell, R., Manson, S., & Rath, B. (1986). The psychiatric effects of massive trauma on Cambodian children. *Journal of the American Academy of Child Psychiatry, 25*(3), 370–376.

Klein, H. (1974). Child victims of the Holocaust. *Child Psychology, 3*, 44–47.

Lebovici, S. (1974). Observations on children who have witnessed the violent death of one of their parents: A contribution to the study of traumatization. *International Review of Psycho-Analysis, 1*(102), 117–123.

Lifton, R. J., & Olson, E. (1976). The human meaning of total disaster: The Buffalo Creek experience. *Psychiatry, 39*, 1–18.

Lyons, J. A. (1987). Posttraumatic stress disorder in children and adolescents: A review of the literature. *Developmental and Behavioral Pediatrics, 8*, 349–356.

Macksoud, M. (1988, September). *The war traumas of Lebanese children*. Paper presented at the First European Conference on Traumatic Stress, Lincoln, England.

Malmquist, C. (1986). Children who witness parental murder: Posttraumatic aspects. *Journal of the American Academy of Child Psychiatry, 25*(3), 320–325.

Nir, Y. (1985). Posttraumatic stress disorder in children with cancer. In S. Eth & R. Pynoos (Eds.), *Post-traumatic stress disorder in children* (pp. 121–132). Washington, DC: American Psychiatric Press.

Punamaki, R-L. (1982). Childhood in the shadow of war: A psychological study on attitudes and emotional life of Israeli and Palestinian children. *Current Research on Peace and Violence, 5*, 26–41.

Punamaki, R-L. (1983). Psychological reactions of Palestinian and Israeli children to war and violence. In M. Kahnert, D. Pitt, & I. Taipale (Eds.), *Children and war: Proceedings of the symposium at the Siuntio Baths, Finland* (pp. 24.3–27.2). Helsinki, Finland: GIPRI, IPB, Peace Union of Finland.

Pynoos, R., & Eth, S. (1985). Children traumatized by witnessing acts of personal violence: Homicide, rape, or suicide behavior. In S. Eth & R. Pynoos (Eds.), *Post-traumatic stress disorder in children* (pp. 17–44). Washington, DC: American Psychiatric Press.

Pynoos, R., & Nader, K. (1988). Psychological first aid and treatment approach to children exposed to community violence: Research implications. *Journal of Traumatic Stress, 1*(4), 445–474.

Pynoos, R., Frederick, C., Nader, K., Arroyo, W., Steinberg, A., Eth, S., Nuez, F., & Fairbanks, L. (1987). Life threat and posttraumatic stress in school age children. *Archives of General Psychiatry, 44*, 1057–1063.

Raundalen, M., Lwanga, J., Magisha, C., & Dyregrov, A. (1987). Four investigations on stress among children in Uganda. In C.P. Dodge & M. Raundalen (Eds.), *War, violence and children in Uganda* (pp. 83–108). Oslo: Norwegian University Press.

Ressler, E., Boothby, N., & Steinbock, D. (1988). *Unaccompanied children: Care and protection in wars, natural disasters, and refugee movements*. New York: Oxford University Press.

Rigamer, E. (1986). Psychological management of children in a national crisis. *Journal of the American Academy of Child Psychiatry, 25*, 364–369.

Schechter, M., & Holter, F. (1979). The child amputee. In J. Noshpitz (Ed.), *The basic handbook of child psychiatry* (Vol. 1, pp. 427–432). New York: Basic Books.

Shirmer, J. (1986). Chile: The loss of childhood. *Cultural Survival Quarterly, 10*(4), 40–42.

Solnit, A. J. (1982). Developmental perspective of self and object constancy. *Psychoanalytic Study of the Child, 37*, 201–218.

Terr, L. C. (1979). Children of Chowchilla. *Psychoanalytic Study of the Child, 34*, 532–623.

Terr, L. C. (1983). Chowchilla revisited: The effects of psychic trauma four years after a school-bus kidnapping. *American Journal of Psychiatry, 140*, 1543–1550.

Terr, L. (1984). Children at acute risk: Psychic trauma. In L. Grinspoon (Ed.), *Psychiatry update* (Vol. 3, pp. 104–120). Washington, DC: American Psychiatric Press.

CHAPTER 53

Transgenerational Transmission of War-Related Trauma

Laurie Leydic Harkness

Introduction

Awareness of transmitted intergenerational processes will inhibit the transmission of pathology to succeeding generations.
—Yael Danieli, 1982

I became tight-lipped and resentful. I got on with my life. I married and had children. But the rules of survival I mastered in Vietnam made parenting difficult. I can't forget those rules . . . they are there like a broken record: "Kill or be killed," "Don't grieve," "Survive at all costs," "Be unpredictable—it's safer," "Shut off feelings."

—39-year-old Vietnam veteran

Traumatic events affect individuals, families, and society in many different direct and indirect ways. In this chapter, I examine specific aspects of the *intergenerational transmission* of combat-related trauma by assessing the impact of a father's combat-related posttraumatic stress disorder (PTSD) on family life. What, if any, are the transgenerational effects of having a parent whose combat experiences have led to PTSD? In the United States, it is estimated that 30 million people (Lipsky *et al.*, 1976), 13% of the total population has served in the Armed Forces and 50% percent have a first degree relative who is a veteran. Many of these veterans are combat soldiers who served in World War II, Korea, or the Vietnam War and may have combat-related PTSD. Investigation and understanding of intergenerational transmission are essential to comprehend the long-term outcome for the combat veteran with PTSD and his or her family.

Laurie Leydic Harkness • Yale University, Community Support Program and Psychiatric Rehabilitation Program, Veterans Administration Medical Center, West Haven, Connecticut 06516.

International Handbook of Traumatic Stress Syndromes, edited by John P. Wilson and Beverley Raphael. Plenum Press, New York, 1993.

The symptoms of PTSD, particularly the numbing of responsiveness and social withdrawal, have profound implications for interpersonal and family life. Studies of children of Holocaust survivors (Freyberg, 1980; Kestenberg, y1980; Krystal, 1968; Rakoff, Sigal, & Epstein, 1965; Sigal, Silver, & Rakoff, 1973) and children of psychiatrically disturbed parents (Beardslee, Bemporad, Keller, & Klerman, 1983; Rolf & Garmezy, 1974; Sameroff & Seifer, 1980; Weissman, Leckman, Gammon, & Prusoff, 1984) found that these children have considerable impairment in their cognitive-intellectual functioning, social-interpersonal functioning, and affective functioning. McFarlane, Blumbergs, Policansky, and Irwin (1985) have shown in disaster studies that ongoing parental PTSD is one of the most significant variables leading to disaster related morbidity in the child. These studies have clearly shown that the psychological reverberations of traumatic events can affect other family members. In other words, if massive trauma has produced psychopathology in a generation of parents, many of their offspring may also suffer from emotional disturbances and psychiatric symptoms. These symptoms may be the result of genetic predisposition or from the child's identification with the parents and/or dysfunctional family structure.

In particular, Vietnam veterans with PTSD have been found to experience a high incidence of divorce, marital discord, and domestic violence. They also experience high unemployment, drug and alcohol abuse, and suicide. Until recently, relatively little has been done to investigate the characteristics and problems of the families these veterans have formed in the postwar period.

After presenting a conceptual overview of family systems theory, I will review the various ways PTSD can affect family life from a systems perspective as well as extending to the impact of PTSD on daily family life. The results of a descriptive research study which examined the various ways a father's combat-related PTSD affected his children's social competence and behavior patterns will then be reviewed. A discussion of this study and its clinical implications, including several clinical vignettes, will follow.

PTSD and the Family

Most of the relevant family literature relies on "family systems theory" for its theoretical foundation. For the purposes of this chapter, three basic tenets of family systems theory will be identified and reviewed.

The first tenet is that the family is a highly complex system which consists of a number of interlocking parts engaged in patterned interaction. The family must be viewed as a whole unit and cannot be reduced to the properties or characteristics of its individual members. The second tenet is that individuals influence each other through their interaction. This influence can either increase or decrease the frequency or intensity of certain behavior. In other words, what affects one part of the system (family) is felt by others in that system. A corollary is that concerns need not be openly shared in order to be deeply felt. The third tenet of systems theory is that interactions are hierarchically organized. Each generation in the family plays a different role with respect to the others. Thus, the interactive patterns between parents are, or should be, quite different from those between parents and children.

Several researchers have suggested, and family systems theorists tend to agree, that, in general, the impact of a father's PTSD on the second generation depends to a significant extent on how the family "handles the matter." Therefore, when the effects of a parent's combat-related PTSD on the family are examined, it is important to differentiate the various ways PTSD affects family functioning both at the systems level and at the daily interactive level.

Patterns of Family Structure and Interaction

At the systems level, three patterns of family structure and interaction emerge. Two of these patterns follow the Minuchin concepts of *enmeshment* and *disengagement* (Minuchin, 1974), and a third is characterized by *impulsivity* and *violence*.

Disengagement

The tendency of Vietnam veterans to have disengaged relationships with their spouses and families is most often reported. These families show a relative absence of structure, order, and authority. Ties between family members are weak or nonexistent. Excessive distance between members is seen, with very little communication or protection available. These families tend not to respond to stress; members receive little or no support from each other, and they have few problem-solving abilities. In these families, it is not unusual to find a child elevated to a parental-functioning role.

Enmeshment

A second and quite different family pattern is characterized by *undifferentiated role boundaries* and *enmeshed relationships*. Husbands continue and wives collude in the perpetuation of the soldier–protector role; the family becomes a closed unit and isolated from the outside world. The world is seen as unsafe, uncaring, and treacherous. The family feels the need to band together in order to survive. Family members often see themselves solely in relation to the veteran father and his problems. These enmeshed relationships are an attempt to avoid reexperiencing the anxieties and vulnerabilities of the war. In these families, there is little tolerance for disagreement. Familial interactions are rigid because family members fear that any change would lead to more pain. Self-protection is learned through emotional constriction and avoidance of emotionally intense issues. Krugman (1987) wrote that these families are organized on the *reparative fantasy* that a "family in which nobody ever leaves or develops autonomous strivings and competing loyalties will provide safety that at one point in time was not there for a family member." These families are uncomfortable with personal growth in individual members because change threatens the family's static but "safe" boundaries. One effect of this on the children is difficulty in separation and individuation; their individuation may be regarded as a challenge to authority or as another loss.

Impulsivity and Parental Violence

A third family pattern occurs as a result of the veteran father's inability to control his impulsive behavior, which leads to chaos within the family. Krugman (1987) observed that these families are highly reactive to both their environment and to disagreements among their members. There is little or no capacity for affect modulation. These families are constantly in turmoil and crisis. Family members tend to be anxious and uptight, always waiting for the explosion to occur. Children from these families grow up in homes where there is little sustained closeness, where anger may explode without apparent provocation or explanation, and where the child is likely to become a pawn in parental conflict.

For each of these patterns, the most profound impact of PTSD on family life centers around the emotional inaccessibility of the father. His need to be disengaged, if successful, protects him from discomfort but also keeps him removed from other family members. Wives often try to reach these husbands but fail. As parents become enmeshed in their own pain, there is little time or energy to devote to the child(ren).

It is important to note that in all these family patterns differences may be related to the veteran's combat-related PTSD being superimposed over varying levels of preexisting character pathology. The combat experiences may also interact with existing dysfunctional family patterns that have developed over time. In addition, many of the veterans and their spouses that I have evaluated come from dysfunctional families of origin and lack individuation. They choose their marriage partners based on what is familiar or have the wish to rescue or save the partner. Therefore, couples frequently develop a complementary process which only perpetuates dysfunction.

Effect of Combat-Related PTSD on Children

Some of the problems observed in children of Vietnam veterans with PTSD include impaired self-esteem, poor reality testing, hyperactivity, and aggressive behavior. Many children express a need to identify with their father's suffering in order to understand him better and to feel more intimate with him. Others report difficulty in communicating with him about the war for fear of upsetting him or causing him pain. And still others report problems coping with their own feelings, especially with their own fears, rage, guilt, and mistrust. Most children struggle with their fantasies of what really happened in Vietnam. One child stated he was relieved finally to know some details because he knew then that he was not just imagining things.

Vicarious Traumatization: The Overidentified Child

Children raised in any of these families generally fall into one of three categories. The most destructive child pattern is that of the overidentified or secondarily traumatized child. Through a process Rosenheck (1986) has termed *secondary traumatization*, other family members come to experience an emotional disequilibrium not unlike that of the originally traumatized member. Their reciprocal reactivity and distress may further compound a dysfunctional family interaction. These children become their fathers' closest companions; often they relive their fathers' trauma and share the flashbacks and nightmares. But they pay a high price for this special relationship. They have few friends; their whole world revolves around their fathers. In school, they often have difficulty with concentration because they are frequently concerned with how their fathers are doing.

Role Reversal: Children as Nurturing Rescuers

A second pattern is for some children to become *rescuers*, frequently taking on parental roles and responsibilities. They blame themselves or feel guilty when there is trouble at home. They assume if they are good that homelife will go well. They often lose their spontaneity and find little joy in life. As with the children of alcoholics, these children are at risk of continuing this role into adult life. They believe it is their responsibility to keep people happy and to ensure that nothing goes wrong.

The Emotionally Isolated Child

A third pattern centers around those children who are not triangulated into the family pathology but who receive little support from their parents. These children know about their fathers' war experiences and are not caught up in the dysfunctional patterns of the family, but seem, rather, emotionally uninvolved in family life. To gain acceptance, they do well in school but go through life with their feelings repressed. They build a wall or *protective shield* around themselves. This can be highly adaptive in childhood but may cause problems in adulthood in forming close, intimate relationships.

Overt and Subtle Exposure to Parental PTSD

The effects of trauma on the second generation can occur in many ways, both subtle and overt. A child can experience the impact of a parent's traumatic symptoms of anxiety, depression, withdrawal, or anger; hear repeatedly about the father's war experiences; observe how other people treat the father; become overprotected; adopt the parent's reactive attitudes of bitterness or suspicion; and feel pressure to compensate for his or her parents' deprivation and suffering. However, research with some groups of trauma survivors (e.g., Holocaust survivors) has shown that the consequences are not always pathologic (Krell, 1982). Some children can shelter themselves from the negative impact of the environmental and familial sequelae of a traumatic experience. They seem surprisingly resilient. They have the capacity to elicit positive responses from parents, friends, and teachers. The risks associated with parental PTSD can also be buffered by constitutional characteristics of the child.

These perspectives on the impact of a family member's PTSD on the family are primarily based on reports of experienced clinicians. In order to quantitatively measure some aspects of the impact of a father's PTSD on family and child function, I studied 40 families in which the father had combat-related PTSD.

Methodology

The primary purpose of my study was to examine the relationship between the severity of a father's Vietnam War combat-related PTSD and his child(ren)'s social competencies and behavior patterns. The specific hypothesis was that in families with similar levels of family functioning, the severity of the father's PTSD symptoms would be positively correlated with the child(ren)'s increased difficulties in social competence and abnormal behavior patterns.

Sample and Measures

Eighty-six children from 40 families participated in the study. The father in each family was a Vietnam war veteran who was diagnosed with PTSD. The fathers had been extensively interviewed about their war experiences and current symptoms using a number of standardized instruments including the Schedule of Affective Disorders and Schizophrenia (Endicott & Spitzer, 1978), the Structured Clinical Interview (SCID) for PTSD (Spitzer & Williams, 1985), the Jackson Interview (Keane, Fairbank, Caddell, Zimering, & Bender, 1985), the Figley Structured Interview for PTSD (Figley, 1978), the Impact of Events Scale (Horowitz, Wilner, & Alvarez, 1979), and the Vietnam Stress Inventory Scale (Wilson & Krauss, 1980, 1982) to establish their diagnoses. Each veteran also completed a demographic questionnaire which included questions about psychosocial adjustment since the war. Each family member then completed the Family Adaptability and Cohesion Scale (Olson, Sprenkle, & Russell, 1979, 1983) and the Parent/Child Communication Questionnaire (Olson, McCubbin, Barnes, Larsen, Muxen, & Wilson, 1982); these scales were used to assess the level of family functioning. To assess the child's functioning, the Achenbach Child Behavior Checklist (CBCL) and the Teacher's Child Behavior Checklist (TBCL) were used (Achenbach & Edelbrock, 1983). Both self-administered questionnaires are designed to record in a standardized format the social competencies and behavioral problems of children aged 4 to 16, as reported by their parents or teacher. The 9 behavior scales derived from the 118 behavioral problem items are: schizoid or anxious, depressed, uncommunicative, somatic complaints, obsessive-compulsive, social withdrawal, hyperactive, aggressiveness, and delinquent. Derived from these are two more general factors called *internalizing* and *externalizing* behaviors. Data are presented in one of two ways. Raw mean CBCL subscale scores are used to report specific sex/age group scores and to compare them to those of a normative group of agemates as well as with the mean scores of a clinic-seeking group of agemates. Second, when CBCL scores are used to examine the group as a whole or subgroups within other than age (i.e., severity of PTSD), scores are reported using *T* scores, which allow for comparison across age and sex groups. The CBCL and TBCL have been standardized and results were compared to values obtained for both nonclinic- and clinic-seeking samples.

Results

Symptom Clusters in Children

In general, parents saw their children as depressed, anxious, somatized, schizoid, uncommunicative, hyperactive, aggressive, and delinquent, with boys being perceived as having slightly more problems. These children resembled a clinic-patient population on many problematic behavior scales, and were, therefore, identifiable as a group of children at risk of experiencing significant functional disruption. Within this "high-risk" group, a lower level of family functioning, father's past combat experience, and current violent behavior in the father were found to be significantly associated with the behavior problems of the children. It is important to note that teachers saw a subgroup of 55 of these 86 children as significantly less behaviorally problematic than did the children's parents; they rated these 55 children as more similar to a normative sample. This may reflect that when the child is in the family environment he or she is

triangulated into a dysfunctional family role, but outside the family the same child, without role expectations, may behave very differently. Because child behavior scores are based on the perceptions of these parents, the scores may reflect parental distortions based on the parents' clinical state and poor self esteem. Families of Vietnam veterans can often consist of at least two people with low self-esteem who experience great despair from years of dealing with failure and frustration. The wives of Vietnam veterans often feel a reciprocal lack of self-esteem and loss of identity. They report loneliness, social isolation, and self-blame for their husbands' depression, rage reactions, and/or wide fluctuations in mood (Jurich, 1983; Krugman, 1987). Rosenheck (1986) described many of these wives as secondarily traumatized by the experience of living with someone with PTSD. In addition, many of the children in these families have been exposed to frequent marital tensions, rigid family boundaries, poor intrafamilial communication, and poor models of adult interaction. It is not surprising that these children may be experiencing difficulties, and that these are more frequently expressed at home where there are fewer limits and less communication between parents.

Child Behavior Problems in Relation to Father's Violence Potential

Many of the child behaviors reported by the parents resembled behaviors exhibited by the father (e.g., depression, anxiety, low frustration tolerance, and outbursts of anger). These behaviors might be the children's attempt to identify with their fathers or to understand their fathers' behavior—or these children might be secondarily traumatized by having a father with PTSD. In working with these children, clinicians need to be sensitive to the presence of these behaviors in the fathers as they diagnose and treat the children.

A major finding of the present study was that children with a violent father were significantly more likely to have more behavior problems, poorer school performance, and less social competence than children with a nonviolent father (see Table 53.1). Girls aged 6 to 11 years with violent fathers were more frequently per-

Table 53.1. Summary of Child Behavior Checklist Scores

Scale	Nonviolent fathers (N = 102) M ± SD	Violent fathers (N = 70) M ± SD	t	p
Behavior				
Internalizing	59.2 ± 7.9	67.1 ± 9.5	5.73	.0001
Externalizing	58.7 ± 9.1	66.0 ± 10.5	4.76	.0001
Social competence				
Activity	41.5 ± 12.0	39.4 ± 10.2	1.28	.201
Social	44.6 ± 9.2	41.5 ± 14.0	1.59	.114
School	46.8 ± 12.7	42.2 ± 13.9	2.16	.032
Total competency	43.3 ± 14.5	37.9 ± 12.7	2.59	.011

639

Table 53.2. Summary of Behavior Scale Values for Boys 12 to 16

Behavior	Nonviolent fathers (N = 28)		Violent fathers (N = 16)		Clinical sample[b]		Nonclinical sample[b]	
	M	SD	M	SD[a]	M	SD	M	SD
Somatic complaints	3.0 ± 2.8		7.4 ± 5.6		4.5 ± 4.6		1.4 ± 2.0	
Schizoid/anxious	2.2 ± 2.0		4.6 ± 2.9		3.0 ± 2.8		1.1 ± 1.5	
Uncommunicative	6.0 ± 3.6		12.1 ± 5.5		9.1 ± 5.5		3.2 ± 3.6	
Immature	1.0 ± 1.2		3.5 ± 3.1		3.1 ± 2.6		0.9 ± 1.3	
Obsessive/compulsive	1.9 ± 1.5		4.5 ± 3.7		4.4 ± 3.1		1.7 ± 1.9	
Hostile/withdrawn	2.6 ± 3.0		8.1 ± 6.7		8.0 ± 5.1		1.8 ± 2.5	
Delinquent	1.7 ± 2.8		6.6 ± 5.7		6.6 ± 4.6		1.2 ± 2.0	
Aggressive	8.1 ± 6.1		17.4 ± 9.8		16.1 ± 8.9		5.7 ± 5.9	
Hyperactive	4.3 ± 3.0		8.1 ± 4.4		9.0 ± 4.1		3.0 ± 2.9	

[a]Ratings comparable to a clinical sample reported by Achenbach and Edelbrock (1983).
[b]All N = 250.

ceived as socially withdrawn and delinquent. Girls aged 12 to 16 from families with a violent father resembled the clinic treatment-seeking population, with the externalizing behavior aggressive scale score and all internalizing behavior scores (anxious/obsessive, schizoid, depressed/withdrawn, and immature/hyperactive) significantly higher than for those girls with nonviolent fathers.

For boys aged 6 to 11 with a violent father, it was the externalizing behavior scores that were significantly higher. Of special concern is the fact that boys aged 12 to 16 years old with a violent father and boys aged 12 to 16 years old with a nonviolent father were compared, *all* behavior scale scores were significantly higher ($p \leq .012$) for those with a violent father. In addition, those scores were not just higher than the nonclinical range, but frequently higher than the clinic range (see Table 53.2). Teacher-reported scores also found a significant difference between children from families with violent and nonviolent fathers. They reported the children with violent fathers as demonstrating poorer academic performance, not learning as much, not behaving as appropriately, and less happy than their peers (see Table 53.3). They also reported them as being anxious, socially withdrawn, unpopular, inattentive, immature, self-destructive, and aggressive (see Table 53.4).

Table 53.3. Social Competency Scale Scores for Children

Behavior	Nonviolent fathers (N = 33)		Violent fathers (N = 22)		t	p
	M	SD	M	SD		
Academic performance	3.5 ±	.8	2.7 ±	.7	3.70	.0001
Hard working	4.4 ±	1.7	3.7 ±	1.8	1.33	.190
Behaving appropriately	4.5 ±	1.6	3.6 ±	1.6	1.88	.066
Learn much	4.8 ±	1.4	3.8 ±	1.7	2.25	.029
Happy	4.6 ±	1.3	3.8 ±	1.6	1.98	.058

Violent behavior has a powerfully destructive effect on children and appears to be more influential than either the father's PTSD or the level of family functioning. Children do not know how to cope with violent behavior by one of their parents and become fearful and helpless. Some younger children fill the void of not knowing with a sense of primitive guilt or responsibility for the outburst: "If only I were better" or "If only I had not done that." They turn their fear and pain inward, often somatizing and becoming hyperactive and/or depressed. Some engage in self-destructive activity or attempt to provoke attack from others, including siblings and authority figures. Other children, especially older ones, seem to externalize the behavior, that is, exhibit more aggressive, cruel, and delinquent behavior. These behaviors can be seen as an attempt to not only defend against the anxiety but also as a way to emulate and identify with their fathers and thereby feel closer. This identification permits the child's fears of helplessness and annihilation to be replaced by feelings of power and omnipotence.

Social and family factors have been found to explain as much as 90% of the variance in family violence (Steele & Pollock, 1968; Straus, Gelles, & Steinmetz, 1980). Among the identified factors are: (1) the intergenerational transmission of violence (i.e., if you have been abused as a child it is more likely you will abuse as an adult); (2) lower socioeconomic status; (3) social and structural stress such as unemployment, larger family size, and illness in a family member; (4) social isolation with little involvement in the community; and (5) family structures where there is little shared decision-making and/or a cold emotional atmosphere. Many Vietnam veterans and their families suffer from at least several, if not all, of these factors. In the present study, I found that violence was most strongly related to a lower level of family functioning (families with lower cohesion and adaptability), lower socioeconomic status, larger family size, and unemployment or underemployment. In addition, prominent among symptoms of PTSD are the social isolation and alienation which comprise another social/family factor that increases the likelihood of family violence. The presence of these factors places the individual children

Table 53.4. Summary of Tacher's Child Behavior Checklist Scores

Behavior scale	Nonviolent fathers (N = 33)		Violent fathers (N = 22)		t	p
	M	SD	M	SD		
Anxious	56.9 ±	3.3	59.9 ±	5.5	2.31	.025
Social withdrawal	57.4 ±	4.2	60.9 ±	8.3	1.84	.072
Unpopular	57.4 ±	4.8	62.5 ±	8.9	2.47	.017
Obsessive/compulsive	59.0 ±	6.8	62.8 ±	9.0	1.15	.262
Inattentive	56.9 ±	3.7	60.8 ±	7.8	2.17	.035
Immature	56.6 ±	2.7	62.7 ±	7.6	1.90	.070
Self-destructive	59.3 ±	5.2	62.8 ±	7.1	1.97	.054
Aggressive	57.0 ±	4.4	62.5 ±	10.1	2.42	.019
Nervous	60.6 ±	10.2	61.6 ±	7.6	.31	.760

in these families at risk of violence, as well as the family system at risk for extreme dysfunction.

Premorbid characteristics are possible predisposing vulnerability factors in the development and perpetuation of violence. Those individuals and families without preexisting pathology seem to adapt better and develop healthier patterns. Families where pathology existed before the combat trauma often lack basic skills which make them more vulnerable to stress and to the development of maladaptive behaviors. In a recent survey of the wives who participated in treatment at the Vietnam Veteran Readjustment Counselling Centers, Matsakis (1988) estimated that one fourth of the 15,000 Vietnam veteran wives could be considered battered women (i.e., they had endured at least two severe beatings by their husbands) and that their lives had become organized around avoiding or trying to control their husband's anger. These veterans and their wives need to take responsibility for this destructive behavior and be taught to resolve their conflicts by other means. Consequently, clinical interventions may be more effective at the character and learned-generational structure level than at the level of the neurosis.

Clinical Implications

Children of Vietnam veterans with PTSD, especially those whose fathers are violent, are identifiable as high-risk children. In addition, many of these families have problems in family functioning, including communication patterns, expressions of intimacy (cohesion), and problem-solving abilities (adaptability).

Parental perceptions can influence children's behavior; if parents see their child as problematic, the likelihood of the child behaving that way is increased. In the present study, very few differences were found between father's and mother's perceptions of child behaviors and social competencies: Both parents saw their children similarly. The similarity in parental perceptions could also be due to a more general characteristic of these families. Figley and Sprenkle (1978) found that many of the PTSD symptoms (i.e., intrusive memories, impaired

self-concept, depression, etc.) have a severe, ongoing and disruptive effect on marital and family life. In the present study sample, there was an overrepresentation of families in the low range of functioning, that is, in the rigid/disengaged range. In addition, the families with fathers who had severe PTSD were significantly more likely to be in the low range of functioning, mainly because of their low cohesion scores, which reflect their inability to feel close and connected to each other. Both groups of families, however, described their familial interactions as controlled with little spontaneity and flexibility. These findings support the works of Figley and Sprenkle (1978), Haley (1974), Rosenheck (1986), and others who have hypothesized that this difficulty was related to the guerrilla nature of the Vietnam War, where anyone could be the enemy, even women and children. Thus, closeness to women and children or the responsibility of family life may, in some veterans, activate a stress response and a fear and distrust of those they most want to love. They both desire and avoid closeness and intimacy. One veteran told me, "I feel committed to my family but not close. I'll never let myself feel that vulnerable again." Many veterans reported wanting relationships but expressed a strong need to be in control so as not to feel the helplessness or painful sense of loss they experienced in Vietnam. In addition, because traumatized individuals and dysfunctional families tend to have static defenses and perceive change as threat, they have difficulty lowering interpersonal boundaries and in developing intimate relationships.

DeFazio and Pascucci (1984), Haley (1974), and others have written that a man's war experiences may affect his ability to function as a husband and/or father, especially in the expression of affect and behavioral impulsivity. For example, veterans in Vietnam learned to suppress emotions as a defense against overwhelming loss, pain, and anger. When they returned home, this constricted and often hypervigilant attitude persisted and continued to plague their intimate and family relationships. In general, fathers tend to be both overprotective toward and distant from their children. For example, when his child is ill, a father will pull away even though he can feel very loving toward the child. This seems to reflect either his emotional numbing and/or an inability to grieve. One veteran reported that when he goes to the park with his young child, he does not look for ways to have fun together but worries about ways his child can get hurt. Some fathers turn to alcohol and/or drugs to help them forget or manage the pain, but sometimes it only serves to intensify the rage. Figley (1978) and Wilson and Krauss (1982) found that the extent of combat played an important role in the coping ability of the veteran to handle everyday problems. When activities, responsibilities, or interactions with family members did not go smoothly, the veteran was quick to respond angrily or to withdraw emotionally. In my present study, extent of combat exposure was significantly related to severity of PTSD, general level of family functioning, and receiving a service-connected disability pension (financial compensation for either a medical or psychiatric disability which was determined to be related to time in military duty). Subjects receiving a service-connected disability pension were more likely to be unemployed and violent.

For many veterans, their wives and children are what give meaning and purpose to their lives. Many feel it is their children who keep them alive, keep them from running away, or from committing suicide. Yet family life is also a significant source of stress for these veteran fathers. As the family unit progresses through the various stages of development, the family has to change in order to adapt to new demands (Minuchin, 1974). Pressure for these changes comes from internal and external sources and must be responded to at the individual and the systems levels. These changes can be extremely stressful for the veteran father who has only rigid, structured patterns of interaction to control his environment. The family must respond to these stresses or develop dysfunctional patterns (Stanton & Figley, 1978).

PTSD and the Family Life Cycle

The family life cycle is also characterized by the making and breaking of emotional bonds. For the veteran father, these emotional bonds are often painful triggers of anger, guilt, and grief that are connected to combat memories. Therefore, fatherhood and the process of raising children may for many reasons be an inordinately difficult task for combat veterans to tolerate. Haley (1985) observed that child-rearing seemed to interfere with the veterans' working-through their transition from the "reflex" of combat aggressiveness to adaptive, nondestructive aggression in their current lives. For example, the obstinacy of the "terrible twos" seemed to reawaken the painful affects of combat aggression and sadism in veteran fathers. Many fathers reported feeling helplessness or a fear of losing control when their children had temper tantrums or stubbornly refused to obey orders. Another example of a potentially stressful life-change is a child's entry into adolescence. This is a time when a child needs the psychological space to explore the outside world and needs to test the family's beliefs and authority in the process of his or her own search for identity. Many parents have difficulty tolerating their adolescents' rebellion, but Rosenheck (1986) and others have suggested that this may be particularly difficult for

Vietnam veterans. The adolescent's push to differentiate often leads to conflict in the family complicated by the feelings of betrayal, loss, and/or abandonment in the family. In addition, these children are nearing the age when their fathers were called to war, which may raise unresolved issues of their own adolescence. The study found that adolescent children, especially those who have violent fathers, were perceived to have more difficulties during this stage of development.

Rakoff *et al.* (1965) examined issues of *parental control* in the families of Holocaust survivors. They found limit setting to be overly rigid, ineffectual, or consisting of a combination of pampering with inconsistent discipline because of unresolved guilt and/or overcompensated aggression. This may also be true for the Vietnam veteran and his family, who tend to have more rigid family interaction patterns. The veteran has experienced or seen unleashed aggression at an age when sadomasochistic fantasies were rampant, and made attempts to inhibit and control his feelings. Thus, even though familial interactions are characterized by this rigidity and distance, it may be the fear of "losing it" or unleashing aggression, not disinterest or self-centeredness, which keeps these fathers from being more involved in disciplining their children.

Effective intervention and treatment begins with identifying these families as high risk and making an early comprehensive assessment targeting specific problem areas. The assessment needs to focus on individual and family dynamics, including addressing the issue of violence. A family-of-origin history for each spouse often facilitates knowledge of what resources and liabilities the individual brought to the marriage, as well as to the traumatic experience. Individual, couple, and family therapy may all be necessary, depending on the individual and family circumstances. Clearly, treatment issues will vary depending on the focus of treatment.

Family Dysfunction and Homeostasis

Frequently identified problems for these families include difficulties in communication, intimacy, and problem-solving abilities, as well as the presence of substance abuse and/or violence. It is important to remember that although these families look (and many are) dysfunctional, they have found the roles and patterns that maintain their homeostasis just as any other family does. Therefore, it is important not to disrupt this homeostasis until there is something to put in its place. In general, these families do require standard family therapy interventions, but this treatment is more effective after specific trauma issues have been addressed and after some improvement in self-image is achieved. In his article on the disjointed/conjointed model of family therapy, Rosenheck (1986) described this process and stated that the "disarming of the war experiences facilitates discussion of developmental issues, family problem-solving, and task performance."

Treatment Considerations

For all families, the therapist needs to provide the system with a "safe environment" first and then begin to intervene at all necessary levels to allow movement. It is important to be aware, especially in the early stages of treatment, of the tolerance of the family (and its individual members) for affect expression, because they will flee from experiences that reproduce the experience of being out of control. Establishing and enforcing ground rules, such as no violence, can be one way to accomplish this. Teaching new ways of relating and dealing with problems enables them to collaborate in producing a reinforcing environment and to keep motivation for change high.

Although for the veteran father the war can never be completely forgotten or erased (nor should it be), he must learn to put it in its proper place, dealing with war issues when necessary, and get on with improving the current quality of life. The veteran's family can provide a present life-experience focus to help motivate these changes.

Couples therapy with veterans and their wives must address their individual needs, their strengths and weaknesses as a couple, and help them develop more effective parenting skills and a stronger, more cohesive parental dyad.

The strengthening of ego functions should be a major focus of treatment with these children, with an emphasis on reality testing, increased frustration tolerance, and encouragement of verbalization as an alternative to reenactment. These children need to recognize their separateness from their fathers and to discover that being different from their fathers would be what would make them most proud. They need to become aware that they are not responsible for their parents' behavior and pain and do not have to feel guilty about it. Thus, they can gain needed distance from the intensity of family interactions and begin to address more appropriately their own developmental issues.

The role of the family in the psychosocial generational transmission of trauma should be further studied. During development, a child is subject to an array of factors which include the quality of the parents' interaction with each other and with the child, the mother's personality and her reactions to the father's PTSD, the influence the father's symptoms have on the family life, the family dynamics, the child's constitution, and other life circumstances. These factors may aggravate or ameliorate particular potential problems. It is important to continue to identify those factors which make the children in these families high risk, and to continue to expand the data base which will guide clinicians toward more optimum interventions in the future.

Conclusion

To date, the relationship between violent behavior, PTSD, and child development has not been a focus of significant professional attention. This study represents the first empirical work to examine the transgenerational effects of combat-related PTSD on the family system, especially on children's social competence and behavior patterns. The findings of this study support the need for preventive programs for children of combat veterans with PTSD, particularly those from lower functioning families and/or violent families. Longitudinal follow-up studies are needed which assess further the risks in the different age groups and examine what happens to these families and children without treatment. It is important for clinicians to think about the multiple social and family factors that influence the outcome of combat-related PTSD. If lack of social supports, poor familial communication, and early childhood abuse are important contextual variables, then treatment strategies should aim at addressing these problems. Strategies should be developed which will identify and begin to treat those families that are at high risk for developing problems from combat-related PTSD so that succeeding generations will be spared their pathology.

References

Achenbach, T., & Edelbrock, C. (1983). *Manual for the Child Behavior Checklist and Revised Child Behavior Profile*. Burlington, VT: Queen City Printers.

Beardslee, W. R., Bemporad, J., Keller, M. J., & Klerman, G. (1983). Children of parents with major affective disorder: A review. *American Journal of Psychiatry, 140*(7), 825–832.

Danieli, Y. (1982). Families of survivors of the Nazi Holocaust: Some short- and long-term effects. *Series in Clinical and Community Psychology: Vol. 8. Stress and Anxiety* (pp. 405–421).

DeFazio, V. J., & Pascucci, N. J. (1984). Return to Ithaca: A perspective on marriage and love in post traumatic stress disorder. *Journal of Contemporary Psychotherapy, 14*, 76–89.

Endicott, J., & Spitzer, R. L. (1978). A diagnostic interview: The Schedule for Affective Disorders and Schizophrenia. *Archives of General Psychiatry, 35*, 837–844.

Figley, C. R. (Ed.). (1978). *Stress disorders among Vietnam veterans: Theory, research, and treatment*. New York: Brunner/Mazel.

Figley, C. R., & Sprenkle, D. H. (1978). Delayed stress response syndrome: Family therapy indications. *Journal of Marital and Family Therapy, 4*, 53–60.

Freyberg, J. (1980). Difficulties in separation-individuation as experienced by offspring of Nazi Holocaust survivors. *American Journal of Orthopsychiatry, 41*, 101–116.

Haley, S. (1974). When the patient reports atrocities. *Archives of General Psychiatry, 30*, 191–196.

Haley, S. (1985). Some of my best friends are dead: Treatment of the PTSD patient and his family. In W. Kelly (Ed.), *Post-traumatic stress disorder and the war veteran patient* (pp. 54–70). New York: Brunner/Mazel.

Horowitz, M. J., Wilner, N., & Alvarez, W. (1979). Impact of Events Scale: A measure of subjective distress. *Psychosomatic Medicine, 41*, 209–218.

Jurich, A. P. (1983). The Saigon of the family's mind: Family therapy with families of Vietnam veterans. *Journal of Marital and Family Therapy, 9*, 355–363.

Keane, T. A., Fairbank, J. A., Caddell, J. M., Zimering, R. T., & Bender, M. E. (1985). A behavioral approach to assessing and treating post-traumatic stress disorder in Vietnam veterans. In C. R. Figley (Ed.), *Trauma and its wake: The study and treatment of post-traumatic stress disorder* (pp. 257–294). New York: Brunner/Mazel.

Kestenberg, J. (1980). Psychoanalyses of children of survivors from the Holocaust: Case presentations and assessment. *Journal of the American Psychoanalytic Association, 28*, 775–804.

Krell, R. (1982). Family therapy with children of concentration camp survivors. *American Journal of Orthopsychiatry, 36,* 513–522.

Krugman, R. (1987). The assessment process of a child protection team. In R. E. Kempe & R. S. Kempe (Eds.), *The battered child* (4th ed., rev. & exp., pp. 127–136). Chicago: University of Chicago Press.

Krystal, H. (Ed.). (1968). *Massive psychic trauma.* New York: International Universities Press.

Lipsky, *et al.* (1976).

Matsakis, A. (1988). *Vietnam wives: Women and children surviving life with veterans suffering posttraumatic stress disorder.* Kensington, MD: Woodbine House.

McFarlane, A. C., Blumbergs, V., Policansky, S. K., & Irwin, C. (1985). A longitudinal study of psychological morbidity in children due to a natural disaster. Unpublished manuscript. Department of Psychiatry, Flinders University of South Australia, Beford Park, South Australia.

Minuchin, S. (1974). *Families and family therapy.* Cambridge: Harvard University Press.

Olson, D., McCubbin, H., Barnes, H., Larsen, A., Muxen, M., & Wilson, M. (1982). *Family inventories.* Beverly Hills, CA: Sage Publications.

Olson, D., Sprenkle, D., & Russell, C. (1979). Circumplex model of marital and family systems: Cohesion and adaptability dimensions, family types, and clinical applications. *Family Process, 18,* 3–15.

Olson, D., Sprenkle, D., & Russell, C. (1983). Circumplex model of marital and family systems: VI. Theoretical update. *Family Process, 22,* 69–83.

Rakoff, V., Sigal, J., & Epstein, N. (1965). Children and families of concentration camp survivors. *Canada's Mental Health, 14,* 24–26.

Rolf, J. E., & Garmezy, N. (1974). The school performance of children vulnerable to behavior pathology. In D. F. Ricks, A.

Thomas, & M. Roff (Eds.), *Life history research in psychopathology* (Vol. 3). Minneapolis: University of Minnesota Press.

Rosenheck, R. (1986). Impact of post-traumatic stress disorder of World War II on the next generation. *Journal of Nervous and Mental Disease, 174*(6), 319–327.

Sameroff, A. J., & Seifer, R. (1980). The transmission of incompetence: The offspring of mentally ill women. In M. Lewis & L. A. Rosenbaum (Eds.), *The uncommon child.* New York: Plenum Press.

Sigal, J., Silver, D., & Rakoff, F. (1973). Some second generation effects of survival of the Nazi persecution. *American Journal of Orthopsychiatry, 43,* 320–327.

Spitzer, R. L., & Williams, J. B. (1985). *Instruction manual for the Structured Clinical Interview for DSM-III (SCID).* New York: Biometrics Research Department, New York State Psychiatric Institute.

Stanton, D., & Figley, C. R. (1978). Treating the Vietnam veteran within the family system. In C. R. Figley (Ed.), *Stress disorders among Vietnam veterans: Theory, research, and treatment* (pp. 281–289). New York: Brunner/Mazel.

Steele, B. F., & Pollock, C. A. (1968). A psychiatric study of parents who abuse infants and small children. In R. E. Helfer & C. H. Kempe (Eds.), *The battered child.* Chicago: University of Chicago Press.

Straus, M., Gelles, R., & Steinmetz, S. K. (1980). *Behind closed doors: A survey of family violence in America.* New York: Doubleday.

Weissman, M. M., Leckman, J. K., Gammon, D. G., & Prusoff, B. (1984). Depression and anxiety disorders in parents and children. *Archives of General Psychiatry, 41,* 845–852.

Wilson, J. P., & Krauss, G. E. (1980). *Vietnam Era Stress Inventory.* Cleveland, OH: Cleveland State University.

Wilson, J. P., & Krauss, G. E. (1982). *Vietnam Era Stress Inventory.* Cleveland, OH: Cleveland State University.

CHAPTER 54

Apartheid

Disastrous Effects of a Community in Conflict

Derrick Silove and Robert Schweitzer

Introduction

Primo Levi, the prolific Italian-Jewish author, who committed much of his life to documenting his experiences as one of the Holocaust survivors of Auschwitz, was plagued by two persisting fears (Cameron, 1988). His first concern was whether he, as a writer, was capable of expressing the enormity of the disaster he had lived through. How does one record immeasurable suffering or attempt to explain the inexplicable? His second fear was that the information that he was able to record would not be understood or believed by a new generation which lacked firsthand experience of the concentration camps. He questioned whether the contemporary human mind, so conditioned by the influences of normal society, is capable of understanding that, under certain circumstances, mass human behavior can become fundamentally deviant and perverted. For these reasons, he feared that the Holocaust of World War II would fade into a collective community amnesia or be so sanitized that the essence of its lessons would be lost.

His predictions have been at least partly correct. As part of a strong revisionist movement in German academia, some reputed historians have claimed that the historical importance of the Holocaust has been exaggerated, giving substance to the fear that increasing tem-

poral distance from the event may increase the likelihood of its importance being minimized.

Those who have confronted the enormity of the human-engineered disaster in South Africa can understand in small measure Primo Levi's fears. South Africa is undergoing a period of rapid social and political change, with its leaders claiming to be committed to the dismantling of the system of apartheid. As such promises of change assuage international criticism, there is a risk that the psychosocial consequences of decades of apartheid will lose currency as an issue for concern.

Both authors of this chapter grew up in South Africa, and yet we still have to remind ourselves that apartheid is not simply an aberration of our imaginations, not some elaborate form of delusion that has stricken us. Indeed, it is a commonly held maxim among anti-apartheid workers that to explain South African society convincingly to the outside world, one has to dilute the truth to make it plausible—the reality is so improbable that incredulity quickly takes over. It is very difficult to comprehend that, in the modern world, a culture which claims to form part of the western tradition has, nevertheless, carefully designed a political system which bases its viability on the exclusion and degradation of the majority of its citizens. The outcome of the rapid political transition period that South Africa is undergoing at present remains unknown. This chapter will deal with the period of apartheid prior to these changes and will focus particularly on the youth-led rebellion of the 1980s and its psychosocial consequences.

To understand the stark reality of the apartheid system, it is useful to suspend the rationalizations of the adult mind and to attempt to view reality through the eyes of the children of South Africa. Children and adolescents have not yet developed inflexible adult defenses, motivations, and cognitions, and they tend to have simple notions of morality: good is good and bad is

Derrick Silove • Academic Mental Health Unit, University of New South Wales, Liverpool Hospital, New South Wales 2170, Australia. Robert Schweitzer • Department of Psychology, University of Queensland, St. Lucia, Brisbane, Queensland 4067, Australia.

International Handbook of Traumatic Stress Syndromes, edited by John P. Wilson and Beverley Raphael. Plenum Press, New York, 1993.

bad. Although they are certainly capable of acting deviantly, children do not, as a rule, rise up against the authority of the state unless there is good cause. In many respects then, we would suggest that the ideas, behavior and psychological health of the youth of a country provide a barometer against which the social well-being of that society may be judged.

Children of Apartheid

Unlike their white counterparts, who are energetically shielded from the truth, the black children of South Africa have been direct witnesses of the apartheid system. In contrast to their parents, black children are more able to penetrate white areas if only as newspaper sellers, beggars, and car washers. At times, they are allowed to visit their mothers who work as maids in the white-owned houses—a privilege that is denied their fathers. While walking through white suburbs, black children have ample opportunities to observe the white schools, hospitals, and recreational facilities from which, until recently, they have been excluded. They have experienced at the most fundamental level the reality of the two worlds into which apartheid has split South Africa— the privileged world of the white person and the deprived world of black people.

The extent to which the South African state has differentially neglected black children in every aspect of their lives has been amply documented. In the area of health, according to a report from the Department of Paediatrics at the University of Natal (Moosa, 1984), rates of severe malnutrition in the forms of marasmus, kwashiorkor, and pellagra reach as high as 66% in many regions. The infant mortality rate is 11 times that found in the white population (South African Institute of Race Relations, 1988), and most of these deaths are from preventable nutritional and infective diseases. The paradox is that South Africa has been a rich supplier of food to other countries. UNICEF has noted this exceptional disproportion between the wealth of South Africa and the poor state of health of its black children—which can only be explained by a willful misallocation of resources according to racial criteria (Seedat, 1984).

Few black children have escaped the ravages of serious illnesses, such as kwashiorkor, marasmus, tuberculosis, malaria, or gastroenteritis, and most families have experienced the trauma of one or more of their children dying at home while other family members look on helplessly. While the first author was working in an understaffed, overcrowded clinic in Kwazakhele in Port Elizabeth, he had to send many dying children home knowing full well that they would not survive until the next appointment. They had exhausted their right to a 2-week supply of protein-enriched food supplement, and the local hospital could not admit them because it was full.

The woeful state of mental health services in South Africa, and especially the inadequate services for children, recently drew a sharp comment from Chris Allwood, the Director of Psychiatry at the University of Witwatersrand (South African Institute of Race Relations, 1988):

I think it is true to say that in the white population and other population groups psychiatric facilities are fair. But when it comes to caring for African mentally ill patients, we find that just about anything which is provided is grossly oversubscribed, understaffed and overloaded.

Social Effects of Apartheid

In the wider social sphere, black children have experienced the full impact of the extreme social disintegration that has been caused by apartheid. They have witnessed the separation of members of their families by official racial reclassification, they have seen bulldozers flattening their shacks, and they have experienced forcible removals to remote "resettlement" areas where the means to sustain life are barely available (Silove, 1988). Few children have escaped the effects of apartheid on family life: the prolonged separation from parents and the destruction of family cohesion caused by the ubiquitous migrant labor system, the high death rate of fathers who work in the mines, and the ravages of alcoholism and lawlessness which are an inevitable consequence when established communities have been dislocated and destroyed by forced removals.

The implementation of "grand apartheid" has affected millions of families. Between 1950 and 1981, over 120,000 families were forcibly moved in accordance with the Group Areas Act, and as recently as 1986, 64,000 people were resettled in rural areas (Apartheid Barometer, 1987).

Education under Apartheid

In the past, black children were constantly reminded that their educational system was specifically designed to ensure that they were destined, according to an Afrikaner nationalist maxim, to be "hewers of wood and drawers of water." Young children were turned away from school because of lack of space, and those who returned the next year often found themselves sitting on the floor in overcrowded classrooms with inadequate staffing, few materials, and little hope of being able to afford textbooks. Per capita expenditure on the education of white children was six times more than on their black counterparts and only a minute proportion of black students were able to surmount all the obstacles to complete their matriculation (South African Institute of Race Relations, 1985).

Effects of Apartheid on Morale

Possibly more damaging than all these material deprivations, and an experience that the child was unable to escape, was the indignity and humiliation of being treated as an *untermensch* (an unworthy being), and the effects that these insults have had on relationships in the family and the community as a whole. The young boy watched with confusion as his respected father, who himself was called "boy," stood subserviently with bowed head and shoulder, while being instructed in surly tones by the white "boss." The young girl wondered why she hardly ever saw her mother who cared for the white "madam's" children while she, the daughter, was left to fend for herself in the township. South Africa is a rich source of tragic anecdotes which illustrate these repeated assaults on the self-esteem of children. A tale which we have recently been told involved an adolescent of "colored" (mixed-race) descent, who, just prior to emigrating to Australia, scrubbed her knees to the point of severe excoriation to try to remove the areas which were most obviously pigmented. By so doing, she hoped that no one would notice her "colored" status on arrival in the new country.

Children are very sensitive to the prevailing value system of the society, and, during the years of apartheid in South Africa, virtually every experience invoked in the black child a sense of being different and of being excluded. Although the violence and the overt conflict which now beleaguer South Africa are tragedies in their own right, the divisive effects of apartheid on human relationships have been arguably more destructive. The creation of the apartheid society has sown deep-seated suspicion, mutual misunderstanding, and loss of genuine human contact among the diverse communities within the country. It is this psychological, spiritual, and cultural polarization which will be the most difficult task to reconcile once the formal structures of apartheid are dismantled.

Uniqueness of Apartheid in the Modern World

To make sense of the political system in South Africa, many individuals will understandably try to compare the deprivations suffered by its black people with situations of prejudice and hardship in other countries—and certainly there are many states where oppression, poverty, and social dislocation are prevalent. What can be overlooked in these comparisons, however, and what underpins the uniqueness of apartheid are that the system is an expression of a deliberately designed government program whose raison d'etre was quintessentially racist. In essence, according to the ideology of apartheid which was promulgated in its most developed form in the late 1940s and early 1950s, the laws of the land completely controlled the destiny of each person according to one criterion only, his or her skin color. No other contemporary political system, certainly not one subscribing to a Western philosophy of morality and culture as does South African white society, uses race as the sole criterion for controlling every aspect of the citizen's life. Such a "total" system as apartheid cannot by its very nature be reformed or tinkered with to make it more palatable. For this reason, the seeming reluctance of white South Africans to overturn completely the principles underlying apartheid continues to be a source of conflict within the country.

Protest by Black Children

Evidence that the black youth of South Africa understand this fundamental issue—that their deprivations

and humiliations are not just the result of a generally poor economy or incompetent government—was made clear by the spontaneous protests of 1976 which began in Soweto. Significantly, the protests were provoked by a directive from the government to introduce Afrikaans as the medium of instruction in schools. This imposition symbolized to the black youth the final invasion of their dignity—being forced to learn the language of the oppressor who excluded them from participation in the wider society. The 1976 uprising started as a peaceful protest and created a watershed in the history of South Africa. The authorities responded swiftly and brutally: children were shot by the police, many in the back while running away, many at funerals where they were burying their dead. The face of the oppressor was visible as never before, and the collective psyche of the youth changed in a way which is likely to be irreversible. The experience allowed the youth to develop a sense of their own empowerment and their own dignity as effective human beings, even though their rejection of the passivity of the older generations caused great strain within traditional family structures. The psychological revolution had occurred, and the mythology of white superiority was eradicated from the minds of the youths who emerged as leaders in the community. They developed organizational skills by mustering large and effective student bodies and voiced their deep ideological commitment to a genuine progressive transformation of South African society.

Recent Uprising

By 1984, when a combination of factors sparked the recent and most widespread rebellion in South Africa's history, the black youths were ready to take the vanguard. At the height of the struggle, the authorities were expelled from large areas in the townships which were declared liberated zones. Youths were instrumental in creating street committees which attended to civic matters and took over legal and administrative functions. Justice was often a crude business, governed by overriding fears of collaboration and treachery within the community. When the authorities retaliated with unrestrained force, invading the townships with armored cars, guns, and teargas, the anger of the youths was displaced onto symbols of the apartheid system, such as black counselors, government clinics and schools which were easier targets than were the armored vehicles. In the state of chaos which overtook the townships, the cycle of police action and community reaction became very complex so that the source of the violence sometimes was difficult to ascertain. Those who defend the South African government would claim that the violent insurrection preceded the widespread arrest, incarceration, and torture of young people which followed.

Tracing the history of protests in South Africa to that time, supports the view that such protests had always been provoked by substantive issues—opposition to pass laws, unfair changes in education, or crushing increases in the cost of rent—and that initial protests had generally started in an orderly and peaceful way until the intrusion of the police. In any event, detention without trial and torture of detainees in South Africa long antedated the 1984 uprising, and, as has been documented by the Department of Criminology at the University of Cape Town, children have never been spared the harshest of treatments by the police (McLachlan, 1984).

Political Abuse of Children

The first author has documented elsewhere (Silove, 1988) allegations that the South African police have subjected black children (some as young as 12 years old) to beatings, interrogation, and torture. A reputable monitoring group, the Detainees' Parents' Support Committee (1986) has claimed that since 1984, over 10,000 children were detained during the period of rebellion (Apartheid Barometer, 1986). Other organizations which have substantiated these claims are *inter alia* the Black Sash (1986), which is a women's organization aimed at defending civil rights, academics from the University of Cape Town (Foster, Davis, & Sandler, 1987), organizations of concerned medical practitioners, psychologists, and social workers (Detainees' Parents' Support Committee, 1986), and a number of international organizations, such as Amnesty International. Reports prepared by these organizations reveal a consistent pattern of intimidation against the youths who were involved in challenging the system. Police or soldiers repeatedly raided township homes in the middle of the night, smashing down doors, assaulting parents, and setting police dogs on family members. Police also apprehended children on the street and subjected them to beatings in police vehicles or police stations. Some of these children were detained for longer periods in jail where they were allegedly intimidated, interrogated, and tortured (Black Sash, 1986; Detainees' Parents' Support Committee, 1986). No automatic legal right of access to lawyers or family existed, and the police subsequently charged only a minority of detained children with substantive crimes.

Released children complained about the inadequacy of the diet that was provided in jail and their lack of access to medical care. Children were denied writing and reading materials, and facilities for washing and exercise were rudimentary. One of the most serious allegations was that young adolescents were incarcerated in large cells with adult prisoners, many of whom were hardened criminals, so that the risks of exploitation and sexual abuse were high.

Many families faced the predicament of not knowing whether a child who had disappeared was in a jail, on the run, injured, or dead. Under the arbitrarily declared Emergency Regulations, the authorities were not obliged to inform anyone about the fate of those who had been apprehended, and the government had persistently refused to release a full list of detainees.

Evidence of Torture of Children

A comprehensive study from the University of Cape Town (Foster *et al.*, 1987) has detailed the experiences of 176 victims of torture, of whom 58 were below the age of 20 years. Although few very young adolescents were included in this study, the data suggest that adolescents were not spared the harshest treatments, including torture. To the contrary, detainees under the age of 20 years reported more experiences of physical torture than did any other age group.

The Black Sash (1986) and the Detainees' Parents' Support Committee (1986) compiled numerous case descriptions of children who were subjected to torture. We record the experiences of one adolescent whose testimony was documented by the DPSC.

A youth of 18 years described his experiences:

> I was taken to the police station and the police then assaulted me with sjamboks [leather hide whips] on my back, arms, thighs, buttocks, legs, and on my head and face. They also choked me until I could hardly breathe. . . . They also poured some liquid which smelled like paraffin (kerosene) over my body after they had assaulted me. They also put a tire from a van around my neck—they threatened to necklace me [the practice of putting a petrol-soaked tire around the neck of a victim and setting it alight] unless I pointed my leader out. I was taken to the toilet where I was blindfolded and given electric shocks on my back and on the small finger of my right hand.
>
> Later I was taken to another police station. Here they handcuffed me and two hoods were put over my head. Something like a ring was put on the small finger of my left hand and on my left cheek. I felt shocks all over my body. They kept asking me who my leader was.

The detainee's ordeal did not always end following release from prison. Many children reported being threatened that they would be re-detained if there was "any trouble in the township" (Detainees' Parents' Support Committee, 1986), leaving them with a residue of fear and foreboding.

Released detainees and their families were often harassed by the security police or unknown confederates of the authorities who intimidated and assaulted family members and fire-bombed homes. As a consequence, many released detainees fled into permanent hiding as "internal refugees," thereby swelling the ranks of the growing number of homeless children in South Africa. A father interviewed by the Detainees' Parents' Support Committee (1986) remarked:

> There are so many of these children (on the run). We do not know where our own children are. Therefore we must help any child that we find and try to give them some of the things that they can no longer get from their parents. We must give them food, shelter and love. Maybe in another place it will be my child that is getting this, so I must give to those I find. We all must.

Consequences of the Torture on Children

A small group of concerned social workers, psychologists, and doctors in South Africa have attempted to record the effects of torture they have observed in children released from detention. In addition to manifesting severe symptoms of the posttraumatic stress disorder, released children frequently expressed feelings of helplessness and powerlessness and seemed to have lost a sense of control over their inner psychic worlds, suggesting that intensive interrogation can threaten, at the most fundamental level, the ontological security of the child. Many tortured children were avolitional and tended to obey orders in a catatonic manner. On the other hand, repressed anger was expressed in unpredictable and purposeless ways, and suspicion of all adults was intense and remorseless. Loss of self-esteem, self-hatred, suicidal urges, and a numbed, wooden unresponsiveness to the world were all phenomena frequently noted by those professionals who have tried to help these children.

Effects on the Community

The ramifications of the widespread political abuse of children on the community are manifold. Many children fled their homes after detention, partly to protect their families from further intimidation, but also because of the fears generated by intrusive memories of being apprehended at home. These children joined the ranks of the growing bands of internal refugees, fugitives who wandered from place to place trying to avoid contact with the authorities. Those who returned home often rejected traditional patterns of authority within the family because of the perceived impotence of parents in offering protection to the child against unjust treatment. Township children who were fortunate enough to escape the detention dragnet were nevertheless constantly exposed to the daily chaos and violence of township life. The overriding sense within the community was one of loss and dread (Detainees' Parents' Support Committee, 1986): loss of the dead, loss of limbs, loss of children, and dread of more trauma in the future.

Discussion

A number of important issues arise from the catastrophic events that have befallen black children in South Africa—events that can only be seen as the inevitable outcome of a system whose very conception sowed the seeds of violence and destruction. We need to consider the allegation that the arrest and brutalization of children has, in the past, formed part of a deliberate and planned government policy. It is well recognized that in the modern world, torture is no longer used primarily to extract information or confessions, but rather to act as a potent form of intimidation aimed at deterring the victim and the wider community from engaging in political opposition to the ruling regime. The torture of children by the South African regime in the mid-1980s would have served a number of purposes: to break the important nexus of power held by the students, to intimidate the community by targeting its most vulnerable members, and most seriously, to break the spirit of self-assertion, political initiative, and psychological liberation which has emerged among the youth in that decade.

Although it is not possible to penetrate the inner workings of the apartheid system, a number of observations lend support to this theory. The disproportionate number of children detained, the random manner in which children were apprehended, the fact that many

detained children have not had any organizational links (Detainees' Parents' Support Committee, 1986), and the extent of the wanton brutality against these children, all suggest that policies governing detention were not simply made at the battlefront. It does not take long for even inexperienced policemen and soldiers to learn that no useful information will be obtained from young adolescents after they have been subjected to sustained and prolonged torture.

The long-term outlook for the mental health and social functioning of children exposed to detention in South Africa is a cause for great concern. Some children, as they grow into young adulthood, bear their experiences in detention as a badge of heroism and commitment, and the restitutive effects of this identification with a common community purpose should not be underestimated. On the other hand, we know from recent evidence that the posttraumatic stress disorder is not necessarily self-limiting and can become chronic (MacFarlane, 1988). Also, we know from the studies of adult torture victims that the majority are still severely symptomatic many years later (Petersen, Abilgaard, Jess, Marcussen, & Wallach, 1985).

A psychiatrist who treated traumatized refugee youths in exile in Southern African "frontline" states observed that those children were so fundamentally disturbed that the term posttraumatic stress disorder was inadequate to describe fully the psychological problems they suffered (Reddy, 1988). He suggested that the term *existential paranoia* more adequately captures the tortured child's experience of a fundamental mistrust of adults and loss of faith that the world can be a safe, nurturing, and benign place. So fearful and resentful were some of these children that their suspiciousness frequently spilled over into frankly delusional thinking. Such symptoms isolated them from each other and particularly from adults whom many of the children mistrusted completely. Their social and psychological development were fundamentally disrupted by their traumatic experiences. Although Reddy (1988) reported that, from his own experiences, these children responded gradually to psychotherapy, he also expressed doubt as to whether full psychological recovery was possible.

Conclusion

The reactions to torture do raise one last issue. The development of the posttraumatic stress disorder category has had valuable consequences in so far as it has focused attention on the regular and predictable cluster of symptoms that are experienced by human beings when they are confronted with overwhelming stress. There is, however, a risk that more complex response patterns may be obscured by assigning all major trauma victims to this blanket category, although it may be equally unsatisfactory to encourage a proliferation of terms, such as the "Concentration Camp Syndrome" (Thygesen, 1980) or the "War Sailors Syndrome" (Askevolde, 1980). Nevertheless, it is possible that in comparison to natural disasters, human-engineered disasters like apartheid may have singularly damaging effects on the individual's long-term sense of social integration and feelings of fundamental trust, and that these effects may be particularly marked in the child. Because the aim of torture is explicitly to disintegrate and alienate the personality of the victim—an aim which is directly antithetical to that of psychiatric treatment—psychiatrists have a responsibility to demand effective action to prevent such atrocities. South Africa demands particular attention because it not only stands accused of the widespread torture of children, but this degradation has occurred against a background policy of deliberate humiliation and deprivations based on racist principles.

References

Apartheid Barometer. (1986, October 17–23). *Weekly Mail*, p. 4.

Apartheid Barometer. (1987, March 27-April 2). *Weekly Mail*, p. 4.

Askevolde, F. (1980). The war sailor syndrome. *Danish Medical Bulletin, 27*, 220–223.

Black Sash. (1986). *Memorandum on the suffering of children in South Africa*. Johannesburg, South Africa: Author.

Cameron, J. M. (1988, March 17). The lie in the soul. *New York Review of Books, 25*, 3–6.

Detainees' Parents' Support Committee. (1986). *A memorandum on children under repression*. Johannesburg, South Africa: Author.

Foster, D., Davis, D., & Sandler, D. (1987). *Detention and torture in South Africa*. Cape Town: David Phillip.

McFarlane, B. (1988). The phenomenology of post-traumatic stress disorder following a natural disaster. *Journal of Nervous and Mental Disease, 176*, 22–29.

McLachlan, F. (1984). Children in prison in South Africa. *Institute of Criminology, University of Cape Town, 5-16u*, 21–39.

Moosa, A. (1984). The health of children in South Africa: Some food for thought. *Lancet, 1*, 779–782.

Petersen, H. D., Abilgaard, G. D., Jess, P., Marcussen, H., & Wallach, M. (1985). Psychological and physical long-term effects of torture. *Scandinavian Journal of Social Medicine, 13*, 89–93.

Reddy, F. (1988, May). *Health for all by the year 2000: An idle dream for South Africa*. Paper presented at the meeting of the World Psychiatric Association Regional Symposium, Sydney, Australia.

Seedat, A. (1984). *Crippling a nation: Health in apartheid South Africa* (pp. 16–29). London: Internation Defence and Aid Fund for South Africa.

Silove, D. (1988). Children of apartheid: A generation at risk. *Medical Journal of Australia, 148*, 346–353.

South African Institute of Race Relations (S.A.I.R.R.). (1985). *Survey of race relations in South Africa*. Johannesburg, South Africa: Author.

South African Institute of Race Relations (S.A.I.R.R.). (1988, April 15). *News*. Johannesburg, South Africa: Author.

Thygesen, P. (1980). The concentration camp syndrome. *Danish Medical Bulletin, 27*, 224–228.

CHAPTER 55

Psychotherapy with Young Adult Political Refugees

A Developmental Approach

Guus van der Veer

Introduction

In this chapter, I will discuss some aspects of psychotherapy with *political refugees*. The exposition will be limited to political refugees who have had serious traumatic experiences, such as on the battlefield or physical and psychological torture during imprisonment. Moreover, only work with *young adult political refugees* will be discussed. The term young adult refers to persons who were between 16 and 26 years old at the time they asked for assistance, and who became traumatized during adolescence. Their traumatic experiences occurred during a period which is critical for personality development, and *before* the developmental tasks of adolescence had been sufficiently completed. In their initial presentation, they make a very adult impression—and this applies to the youngest among them—but sometimes they also behave as adolescents—and this also applies to the older ones.

My goal in this chapter is to present some of the possibilities which developmental theories of adolescence provide for understanding the problems of young adult political refugees and to show that this approach also provides a point of departure for intervention and therapy.

In particular, I will discuss two of the issues which are relevant for psychotherapy with these young adults in some detail: (1) the so-called testimony method and (2) the analysis and use of dream material. I will attempt to show how both methods are aimed at the *assimilation* of *traumatic experiences* on the one hand, and at the *stimulation* of normal adolescent development on the other hand.

Important aspects of psychotherapy with young adult political refugees, especially other psychotherapeutic methods which can be useful, and many of the important questions related to diagnosis, have been discussed elsewhere (van der Veer, 1992) and will not be considered here.

Traumatization and Adolescence

An obvious point of departure for building a theory of adolescent traumatization seems to be the fact that there may be an interaction between traumatization and the normal process of development in the adolescent period. Traumatic experiences and the mental consequences of these experiences can affect cognitive development, moral development, psychosexual development, the development of social cognition, the separation-individuation process, the process of identity formation, and more. Furthermore, interference can occur with the problems which, according to psychoanalytic theory, result from the reactivation of unsolved conflicts from previous phases of life (see Chapter 5, in this volume, for a discussion).

As far as we know, there is little literature based on scientific research from a developmental perspective on the long-term consequences of traumatization during adolescence. Knowledge gained from experience with this phenomenon has only seldomly been made explicit in the light of the psychology of adolescence. The work of Glover (1984) and the research of Wilson (1988) on Vietnam War veterans are exceptions.

Based on my own experience, I will present *five*

Guus van der Veer • Social Psychiatric Centre for Refugees, Cornelis Schuystraat 17, 1071 JD Amsterdam, Netherlands.

International Handbook of Traumatic Stress Syndromes, edited by John P. Wilson and Beverley Raphael. Plenum Press, New York, 1993.

themes which illustrate how traumatization can interfere with the normal process of development during adolescence: (1) loyalty, (2) future orientation, (3) the need for recognition, (4) changing motivation, and (5) mistrust.

Loyalty

The first important theme when giving assistance to traumatized adolescents is the relationship with their parents. This is obvious when the parents are directly involved in the process of traumatization, such as in cases of maltreatment or sexual abuse within the family. When adolescents have been traumatized in a family context, the process of overcoming the trauma can be complicated by feelings of loyalty toward the parents, and the process of separation from the parents can be complicated by the fact that the adolescent has not come to grips with his traumatic experiences. Experience has now shown that the same interweaving of emotionally loaded themes is present in young refugees (see Chapter 26, in this volume), and that the process of coping with the trauma can be better understood if it is considered within the context of the process of emotional separation from the parents. Moreover, separation from the parents is further complicated by the fact that the adolescents in question were forced to leave their parents at a time when the separation-individuation process of adolescence had not yet been completed.

It seems that these young refugees still need the strong emotional support of their parents. Moreover, they are often very worried about their parents and feel that they have failed in their responsibility toward them. In some cases, individuals have left their parents behind in perilous situations, and, in a few cases, this was partly the result of the political activities of the refugee himself. In other instances, the young refugees have made promises to their parents before fleeing (e.g., that they will complete their studies) which they now realize they cannot honor. For these adolescents, contact with their parents is very important, but because of circumstances, it is also often difficult, if not impossible.

If these young refugees can maintain contact with their parents, they may be afraid to express openly their everyday worries for a variety of reasons. The refugees find themselves in an alien culture governed by different rules and norms. If they conform to the customs of the country of exile, then their behavior may deviate from that which is considered normal and desirable in their own culture. Thus, the adolescent refugees have reason to fear that their parents will not understand their behavior and the problems which they encounter, and as a result, of their traditional culturally bound ideas, they will disapprove of their attempts to adapt to their new culture.

The feelings which young refugees have toward their parents are also complicated by other factors, such as the political views of their parents. In some instances, their political activities were the result of a *first independent choice*, or a *first act of rebellion* against their parents. But if the first independent step has such a disastrous or traumatic consequence it may not be easy to take a second one on account of fear, anxiety, and uncertainty.

Furthermore, if their parents have political sympathies with those who use torture as a political instrument, then this may profoundly influence their attitude toward their parents.

In yet other cases, adolescent refugees carry out their political activities with the approval of their parents and later reproach them for not having provided adequate protection (though they are not initially aware of such negative feelings). Thus, a traumatic experience during adolescence affects existing loyalties to persons and institutions. As a consequence, the image which the traumatized person has of his parents or those who are important to him can be severely shaken. This is one reason why traumatic experiences are so painful and difficult to overcome.

Future Orientation

A second theme which is central in helping young refugees is their attempt to build a future orientation or perspective for themselves. This is to be expected, given their stage of epigenetic development. According to Erikson (1968), the process of restructuring during adolescence is only possible in the light of an anticipated future (de Wit & van der Veer, 1987). Owing to traumatic episodes, it is not easy for young refugees to develop plans for the future. Traumatization may lead to disillusionment about the perspective to the self in the future; thus, the development of a new future perspective is more than just a developmental task for them; it is also an aspect of dealing with the trauma. The refugees have to learn to live with the fact that some of the possibilities of which they dreamed are temporarily or permanently closed because the political situation in the country of exile is not suitable for their realization and the current alternatives may not be available or clear in terms of achievement. Moreover, as long as the refugees are still awaiting the outcome of their request for asylum, they are not even certain that they will have a future in the country of exile. However, when this does become clear, the adolescents will have to once again reorient themselves to a future perspective.

The parents of young refugees usually have made very great financial sacrifices to make the flight of their son or daughter possible. Often, in such cases, the parents have given instructions to their child to "achieve something" (see also Bruers, 1985; Lin, Masuda, & Tazuma, 1982). These adolescents internalize the need to fulfil this obligation to their parents. Ambivalent feelings toward their parents can combine with ambivalent feelings about their vocational pursuits. Language problems, teaching methods which are different from those in the country of origin, and concentration problems which result from posttraumatic stress syndromes all contribute to problems of education. These types of problems may be experienced as a failure to live up to the parents' expectations, a situation which they in turn, may find difficult to comprehend. As an inadvertent consequence then, the parents may complicate an already difficult situation. On the basis of my practical experience with young refugees, I can state that the development of a future perspective is facilitated if there is a sense of security (e.g., when the refugee has been granted asylum) and at least some of the traumatic experiences and related emotions have been discussed in therapeutic interviews. A discussion of the future perspective which the adolescent had before his traumatic experiences, and of his parents' expectations, can shed light on problems which occur in the search for a new future perspective.

Need for Recognition

A third theme in the provision of assistance to young adult political refugees can be referred to by the word recognition. The security and safety which are conditions for the development of a future perspective are also related to the granting of asylum to the refugee. The recognition of his or her status as a political refugee provides this safety and security and it grants a sense of certainty that he or she will not be sent back to the country in which the trauma occurred. But official recognition does not only have practical consequences,it also has a psychological meaning.

With the concept of recognition, I am once again making use of the terminology of the Erikson (1968) theory of identity development. Erikson stated that it is very important for the adolescent to have the feeling that that which he considers essential for himself is also recognized and respected as such by others (1968, p. 50).

Political refugees in general, and those requesting asylum in particular, often have the experience that people do not believe what they have endured or been subjected to in the trauma. It is also common for people either to minimize or deny the reality of the traumatic experience. The fact that a therapist takes the time to listen, takes the *content* of their story seriously (i.e., the trauma story), and sympathizes with the fact that they are still haunted by their traumatic experiences is usually their first episode of recognition. In the technique of the "testimony method" of the Chilean psychologist Elizabeth Lira (which will be discussed below) recognition and respect are fundamental points of departure.

Changing Motivation

In working with traumatized adolescents, the therapist is, as far as motivation for psychotherapy is concerned, confronted with the same kind of problems as occur in work with adolescents in general. Adolescents often have an ambivalent attitude toward the therapist: asking for and accepting assistance does, after all, conflict with the need which adolescents usually feel to be independent and to arrange their own affairs (de Wit & van der Veer, 1987). Additionally, traumatization often results in ambivalence toward assistance. When assistance is aimed at the assimilation of traumata, the client will be confronted with experiences which would rather be forgotten. The ambivalent attitude toward the therapist becomes apparent, especially in the case of the youngest refugees, from the way they inconsistently attend the appointments which have been made. More-

over, in the case of older refugees, ambivalence is expressed more in terms of changes of attitude within the therapeutic situation. These fluctuations in motivation demand a flexible and accommodating approach on the part of the therapist since there is a complex set of interactions between posttraumatic adaptation, developmental processes, and transference reactions that occur simultaneously within the therapeutic context.

Mistrust

People who have been traumatized during adolescence are often very mistrustful of social workers and therapists. According to Glover (1984), this distrust can often be explained by the fact that before they underwent the traumatic experiences these people put their full trust in an adult person whom they respected, who did not protect them, or who may have abandoned them during the traumatic experiences. Glover's conclusion is in agreement with the more general hypothesis that the results of traumatization can be understood better if they are seen in the light of existing or former loyalties, persons of trust, security and stability, and likely transference phenomena.

Basic Assumptions in Psychotherapy with Political Refugees

In the present political climate in many European countries, political refugees experience the feeling that they are not welcome and that people do not believe their traumatic stories. Thus, one basic condition in psychotherapy with political refugees is that refugees feel welcome and respected, and that their description of their traumatic experiences be taken seriously. It is not only the attitude of the therapist which gives the refugee the feeling of being welcome: Other factors, such as reading matter in his native language in the waiting room, presence of a dictionary, a map of his country of origin, and the like, all contribute to the feeling of being welcome.

Moreover, as is the case in psychotherapy with adolescents, a flexible and accommodating attitude is also a basic condition. This is important not only because of the client's changing motivation and mistrust but because he or she is occupied with so many different problems: (1) coming to grips with a traumatic past; (2) the terrible uncertainty as to whether asylum will be granted; (3) fitting into a new cultural situation; (4) separation from parents; (5) experimenting with new social roles; (6) establishing intimate relationships; and (7) sometimes the assimilation of childhood conflicts. The therapist will have to respond to these factors in a flexible and open-minded manner. In order to be purposefully flexible, the psychotherapist needs to be aware of the various techniques which can be employed.

In psychotherapeutic work with political refugees, I prefer two approaches: (1) the so-called testimony method and (2) the discussion of dreams, particularly nightmares.

Testimony Method of Posttraumatic Therapy

It is unfortunate that in the various writings on psychotherapy with political refugees or other victims of political violence, little reference is made to the kind of therapeutic methods which were used. The work of Cienfuegos and Monelli (1983), E. Lira (personal communication, November 10, 1986), and Ochberg (see Chapter 65, in this volume, for a discussion) are exceptions. The testimony method was developed in Chile, as a result of experiences with victims of the military dictatorship there. Of course, the method is closely bound to the Chilean situation, but certain aspects have been found to be applicable in other countries.

In the testimony method, a client is encouraged to describe his or her traumatic experiences in as much detail as possible, as if he or she were making a testimony. The client is encouraged to express emotions which are related to his or her experiences. The life history and the reasons for becoming politically active are also discussed. In addition, the strong aspects of the client's personality and the way in which he or she coped with difficult situations are also discussed. What the client says is recorded and transcribed by the therapist, and this text is discussed with him or her. According to Cienfuegos and Monelli (1983), this approach is effective because it provides the possibility of constructively channeling aggression in the form of a charge or indictment. Moreover, it gives the client a better total picture of what has happened to him or her: fragmentary experiences become integrated in the life history. Since the client's experience of suffering has been symbolized in a different form (in a written testimony), and the importance of that experience has been recognized by the therapist, the need to express that suffering through somatic complaints often disappears or lessens in frequency.

The success of the testimony method is largely dependent on the motivation of the client. It is particularly effective in the case of people who know exactly what they want to talk about and realize that it is important to talk about it. The client's coping skills are also important. In Chile, the method has produced good results with farmers and mine workers, or, to put it more generally, with those who have had little education and are not accustomed to talk about themselves and their emotions. The method is less useful in the case of the highly educated, who are able to write down their stories themselves (E. Lira, personal communication, November 10, 1986). Moreover, the testimony method is not suitable for all victims of political violence, but it is most effective in the case of victims of torture. It does not produce satisfying results when applied to the relatives of political detainees who have disappeared: In their case, mourning and grief reactions have to be specifically dealt with (Cienfuegos & Monelli, 1983).

On the basis of limited personal experience with the testimony method, it can be said that it is useful with clients who are used to talking about themselves and their emotions, but who were psychologically isolated in a situation where there was no one whom they could trust with their recollections. The method seems to be especially effective in the case of those who still experience oppression as a reality in their present situation, such as those who live with the fear of being sent back to the country from which they have fled. These individuals feel that they have some support during the process of application for asylum because their stories have been translated into the language of the country of exile and transcribed in a comprehensive account. During therapy, they often describe essential details that they did not mention during the interrogation by an official from the Ministry of Justice because they did not trust the official or the interpreter. So the testimony becomes an instrument which can be used in the active defense of their request for asylum. The compilation of the testimony breaks through the feeling of extreme helplessness which is often experienced by these clients.

The reexperiencing of the past may be directly utilized in the construction of a new future. The discussion of life history, political views, and the nature of their personality traits (as these were manifested during traumatization) contribute to the formation of a balanced self-image and a strengthening of personal identity.

The testimony method is aimed specifically at the experiences in relation to which clients feel lonely and unacknowledged, but which are central to their self-image. When in contact with the therapist, the loneliness in these patients is reduced and they receive acknowledgment, respect, and appreciation, even if matters or emotions of which they are ashamed are discussed. For these reasons, the method is very supportive for the development of a personal identity. Furthermore, the method helps to make traumatic experiences easier to discuss without being overwhelming. Finally, it contributes to making memories of pleasant moments which occurred during the period in which the traumatic experiences were undergone more accessible.

In the application of the testimony method, I do not make use of a tape recorder but rather take notes which are worked out after the session. I try to get the refugees to relate their narrative chronologically, but remain flexible if they digress. At the beginning of each session, I give the client the chance to discuss other matters which may be important at that moment. I may inquire: "How are you?" or "Is there something that you particularly want to discuss today?" or I may ask about specific complaints: "How have you slept during the last week?" This then leads on to topics, such as recent developments in the client's country of origin; news of friends and relatives; contacts with immigration officials which were experienced as offensive; problems in connection with his request for political asylum; experiences of discrimination or lack of understanding of his cultural background; incidents which seem to stem from his lack of understanding of the customs in the country of exile; language problems; housing problems; somatic complaints; and so forth. This means that it is not always possible to follow the testimony method exactly, and, after such deviations, the thread has to be reestablished. In other cases, it is easy to make the transition to a discussion of the past since those events are reported in the testimony (see also Chapter 57, in this volume).

Nightmares

Many young adult refugees complain about nightmares. The discussion of nightmares is therefore directly related to their motivation to seek assistance and is an

655

important psychotherapeutic point of departure. The most important theme in the nightmares of young adult political refugees is a feeling of extreme helplessness. Many of the dreams of political refugees with mental problems can be seen as posttraumatic nightmares. They differ from normal nightmares to the extent that they contain elements from memory rather than fantasy and are repetitive.

Posttraumatic nightmares follow from such experiences as the death (often in gruesome circumstances) of someone who was important for the person in question, having been in a life-threatening situation, or in conditions of extreme helplessness and powerlessness. These traumatic experiences are reexperienced in dreams (Hartmann, 1984).

Some authors, particularly those who have studied the posttraumatic nightmares of Vietnam War veterans, explain the occurrence of chronic nightmares by the fact that those involved were traumatized during adolescence—and this point of view also applies to young adult refugees who suffer from nightmares. Hartmann (1984) proceeds from the Piagetian idea that the way in which adolescents think about reality, and the emotions which are related to it, are strongly determined by *absolute* contrasts, such as those between good and bad, dependent and independent, active and passive, love and hate. They therefore experienced the feeling of helplessness during the traumatic occurrences as absolute. That feeling is apparently so frightening that it is radically warded-off. In practice, this means that the person in question does not speak of or think about his or her experiences during that traumatic event, and generally tries to suppress memories which are related to it. This means that these memories cannot be transformed by thought processes; so the achievements of further cognitive development, which make relativizing possible, cannot be applied.

In nightmares, these memories are reexperienced. The nightmare is a reexperiencing of the almost unbearable feeling of absolute powerlessness, partially stimulated by occurrences during the day which remind the dreamer of the traumatic experiences and feelings related to them. Moreover, young refugees sometimes undergo traumatic experiences as a result of decisions which they made without the knowledge of their parents, or against their parents' wishes. These traumatic occurrences may form the catastrophic result of their first independent experiment, and this is damaging to their self-confidence and reduces their self-image. These themes may also be symbolized in nightmares.

In summary, nightmares are based on traumatic experiences. The self-image of the refugees and their attitude toward other people are also represented in the content of the nightmare. Discussing nightmares therefore not only provides the possibility of giving support in dealing with the trauma, but also of stimulating (1) cognitive development, (2) identity development, and (3) identity integration (see Erikson, 1968).

Discussing Nightmares

Some authors (e.g., Schwartz, 1984) see nightmares as dreams which have gone wrong, that is, dreams in which there is a failure or partial failure to integrate distressing experiences and emotions related to them in the light of previous experiences.

The integration process can be facilitated during psychotherapy by discussing with refugees the feelings, memories, and actual events which are associated with their nightmares. Also, their self-image and their attitude toward other people can be discussed, and this makes the discussion of the nightmares more future-oriented.

As a result of this process, the nightmares may become less frequent, less frightening, or may disappear altogether. In this connection, it is useful to mention that, at the start of therapy, the nightmares are often about being persecuted or taken prisoner, with the refugees' waking up at the moment when they dream that they are so helpless that they will not be able to escape and will be killed. Those who have requested asylum often dream that they have been arrested by the police in the country of exile and are sent back to their country of origin, where they are persecuted, and so forth.

The dreams of some of those who have requested asylum end when the dreamer witnesses a friend commit suicide, or gets into a hopeless situation and is on the point of taking his or her own life. When this situation occurs, it is a sign of an increased suicide risk (van der Veer, 1992).

The content of the dreams often changes with time, as the refugees build up more self-confidence, feel less helpless, and get confirmation that they will be granted asylum. The patients may then dream that they can escape or can help others to escape to a safer place.

Mr. X., a refugee from an Asian country, had participated in political activities against the wishes of his father. He was arrested when he was 18 years old and spent 3 months in a torture center.

One of the methods which the police used to torture him was to throw a boa constrictor into his cell. The snake coiled itself around his body and he fainted, totally helpless. When he regained consciousness the snake had disappeared. Mr. X. has a recurring nightmare in which he is attacked by a dangerous animal—an aggressive dog or a poisonous snake. He tries to escape but whichever way he runs he is stopped by other snakes or dogs. It appears to the therapist that Mr. X. experiences absolute powerlessness in his nightmares. That feeling is associated with traumatic experiences which occurred 4 years previously, when Mr. X. was 18. But there is also a more actual aspect: This refugee has good reason to feel helpless because he has been waiting for a decision on his request for asylum for more than 3 years.

In his relationship with Mr. X., the therapist has the impression that Mr. X. places him on a pedestal. For example, when the therapist hands him his coat at the end of a session, Mr. X. exclaims: "Why do you do that? . . . You're higher than me?"

This last remark can be explained by Mr. X.'s cultural background. But one could also conclude that Mr. X. feels more inferior than would be expected from a political idealist who is struggling for the equality of all people, that his self-image has been devalued. This led the therapist to decide on the following supportive intervention:

"I think that you have this dream because you feel small and helpless and powerless and unimportant, and also because you feel all alone" (the therapist thinks of as many synonyms as possible and looks them up in a dictionary of Mr. X.'s language. He repeats them until he has found a few to which Mr. X. nods in agreement). "When you were tortured, you were also really helpless and alone. You weren't treated like a human being but like a piece of rubbish. It's just as if you still feel like that, even though you are now in a very different situation. If the Ministry of Justice turns down your request for asylum, then you can still appeal. You can still defend yourself. You are not alone anymore, because you have a very experienced lawyer who wants to help you. And there are other people who want to help you with other things. You've already done a lot yourself; you've managed to learn the language, for example. You don't speak it perfectly, but its good enough for us to be able to converse. In spite of your nightmares and your worries, you've managed to learn a lot of the language. That's a great achievement, it means that you've got the power and the will to succeed."

Five Pragmatic Points in Nightmare Therapy

1. The nightmares of political refugees can, of course, also be related to unassimilated emotions from much earlier periods. This is why knowledge of the total life history of the refugee is desirable.

2. Even when refugees have confronted their own traumatic experiences, the nightmares may still return as a result of actual circumstances which evoke a feeling of helplessness; for example, the arrival of bad news from their country of origin. It is therefore useful for refugees to learn to think about their nightmares and to relate them to actual events (Genefke, 1984).

3. In psychotherapy with young adult political refugees, pharmacological support is not an unnecessary luxury. But it must be remembered that some refugees have an aversion to psychiatric medication. This aversion can often be seen as a healthy distrust which is based on experience; for example, with doctors who "treated" them so that the torturers could continue their work, or who tortured them directly by administering psychiatric or other drugs by force (Vladar Rivero, 1988).

4. It is not self-evident that people are willing and motivated to discuss their dreams. Cultural factors can play an important role here. In some cultures, it is not customary to speak about dreams. Cultures also differ in the value which they attach to the content of dreams; for example, a dream can be seen as a prediction—which makes nightmares all the more frightening—or the result of an evil spirit, which is no more reassuring.

In some cultures fear is itself considered to be an emotion which suggests inferiority, so that a taboo has to be overcome before it is possible to discuss nightmares. When therapists are able to explain why it is useful to discuss dreams, and how they propose to try to discover their meaning, refugees will be more willing to discuss their dreams with them. Working with refugees is a long series of language problems and cultural misunderstandings, and this does not make psychotherapy any easier (van der Veer, 1992). Language problems are all the more bothersome when it comes to discussing dreams.

5. Refugees often experience nightmares as a new calamity in the face of which they feel helpless. During psychotherapy, the therapists can try to bring about a more active attitude toward the nightmares on the part of their clients. This can be done, for example, by letting them write down (in their own language) what they have dreamt as soon as they wake up, or by prescribing certain kinds of behavior after the nightmare, such as active breathing exercises. This may help to relativize the absolute feeling of helplessness which they have experienced during the nightmare.

Conclusion

The therapist who works with adolescent victims who are political refugees needs to be aware that traumatic experiences can intensify epigenetic developmental processes that are normative during adolescence, and that they may have an impact especially on the processes relevant to (1) identity formation, (2) separation-individuation, (3) future goals and values, (4) intimate relations, (5) parental relations, and (6) current motivational states. During adolescent years, traumatization often leads to factors that may become the focus of treatment: (1) loyalty, (2) future perspective, (3) need for recognition, (4) changing motivations, and (5) mistrust. Based on my own experiences, I discussed two major techniques of therapy—the testimony method and the discussion of nightmares. Both approaches have been valuable in treating the posttraumatic sequelae of victimization.

References

Bruers, J. J. M. (1985). *Vervreemding, geborgenheid en integratie* [Alienation, security and integration]. Psychiatrisch Ziekenhuis, Wolfheze.

Cienfuegos, A. J., & Monelli, C. (1983). The testimony of political repression as a therapeutic instrument. *American Journal of Orthopsychiatry, 53,* 43–51.

de Wit, J., & van der Veer, G. (1987). *Psychologie van de adolescentie* [The psychology of adolescence]. Nijkerk: Uitgeverij Intro.

Erikson, E. H. (1968). *Childhood and society.* New York: W. W. Norton.

Genefke, I. K. (1984). *Rehabilitation of torture victims.* Copenhagen: International Rehabilitation and Research Center for Torture Victims.

Glover, H. (1984). Themes of mistrust and the posttraumatic stress disorder in Vietnam veterans. *American Journal of Psychotherapy, 38*(3), 445–452.

Hartmann, E. (1984). *The nightmare: The psychology and biology of terrifying dreams.* New York: Basic Books.

Lin, K. M., Masuda, M., & Tazuma, L. (1982). Problems of Vietnamese refugees in the United States. In R. C. Nann (Ed.), *Uprooting and surviving* (pp. 11–24). Dordrecht, Netherlands: D. Reidel.

Lira, E. (November 10, 1986). Personal communication with author.

Schwartz, H. J. (1984). Introduction: An overview of the psychoanalytic approach to the war neurosis. In H. J. Schwartz (Ed.), *Psychotherapy of the combat veteran* (pp. xi–xxviii). Lancaster, England: MTP Press, Falcon House.

van der Veer, G. (1992). *Counseling and therapy with refugees:*

Psychological problems of victims of war, torture and repression. New York: Wiley.

Vladar Rivero, V. (1988). *Het gebruik van psychofarmaca bij de hulpverlening aan politieke vluchtelingen, Psychische problemen en de gevolgen van onderdrukking en ballingschap* [Political refugees: Psychological problems and the consequences of repression and exile]. Nijkerk: Uitgeverij Intro.

Wilson, J. P. (1988). Treating the Vietnam veteran. In F. Ochberg (Ed.), *Post-traumatic therapy and victims of violence* (pp. 278–295). New York: Brunner/Mazel.

PART VI

Trauma Related to Torture, Detention, and Internment

Part VI contains nine chapters concerned with the traumatic consequences of torture, detention, and coercive internment. By its nature, the various forms of torture and detention are political acts of oppression of freedom and attempts to subjugate the will of the victim to the ideological views and the pathological needs of the perpetrator. The chapters in this Part cover the domain of what is currently known about the effects of torture and detention on the psyche and include the psychosexual trauma of torture; physical and somatic manifestations in behavior; and medical, psychotherapeutic, and group-oriented approaches to treatment.

In Chapter 56, Michael A. Simpson presents an overview of the effects of torture and coercive interrogation on the victims of apartheid in South Africa. He begins by placing the use of torture in a historical context and notes that from the days of the Spanish Inquisition, through witch hunts, to modern times torture has been a tool of oppression designed to produce psychological disorder and the diminution of will. However, Simpson argues that advances in the psychological sciences have changed the methods of torture employed to inflict traumatic scars to the deepest levels of the self and states:

> In the old days, prisoners were treated with elaborate apparatus, a technology of torture that owed most to a perverted talent for structural engineering, and reflecting the peak of the technological progress of their times. They were stretched on racks, had their fingers crushed with thumbscrews, or were dipped in boiling oil. In more recent years, it is clear that the avant garde of awfulness has learned more from the behavioral sciences, in an unethical application of knowledge of how brain and mind can be pressured into dysfunction. This has improved the ease and efficiency with which suffering can be carefully tailored so as to break down an individual detainee, to bruise his soul and render him cooperative against his will. We are now capable of far more sophisticated sadism. Physical brutality is not really necessary anymore, though it quite easily occurs when interrogators get carried away by their own power and indemnity from repercussions.

At the core of torture techniques are a number of key elements that are used to render the victim helpless and vulnerable to the manipulations of the perpetrator. These include (1) psychological isolation in an environment or institution totally controlled by the captors, (2) unpredictability as to fate, (3) loss of time scale as to outcome or release, and (4) loss of normal relationships with others and their replacement with an abnormal or perverted relationship with the perpetrator. Once these elements are in place, threats, sleep deprivation, and physical torture can be applied to the victim according to the purposes created by the captor. Simpson cites case examples throughout the chapter from the South African experience, such as this one, which is regarded as typical, if not commonplace:

> He ordered me to remove my shoes . . . then he stamped on my toes with the heels of his shoes for several times . . . he banged my head against the wall at least four times. My nose began to bleed heavily . . . they covered my face with a tight rubber tube like a balaclava, so that I couldn't breathe, but pulled it off while I was struggling, then put it back. . . . I was then tied, lying on my back, to what felt like a table (I was blindfolded, so I couldn't see what they were doing). My limbs were tied down with damp cloths. Then I experienced excruciating pain, like when you accidentally contact a live wire. I then realized I was being electrocuted. I tried to scream, but the pain was too severe. This took place at intervals of about 10 minutes, for about 3 hours. Then I was taken back to my cell.

It is not unexpected that as a consequence of these types of experiences, victims manifest PTSD, depression, exhaustion, poor concentration, and sleep disturbance, among other psychological symptoms. Simpson carefully reviews the literature on the psychiatric sequelae of torture for the victims in South Africa. Based on the knowledge of the unique effects torture creates for the survivor, various therapeutic considerations are discussed. Problems are also noted with the DSM-III-R stressor Criterion A, since it is nearly impossible to objectively verify the torture event. This thought-provoking chapter ends with a call for more flexible and creative approaches to the clinical treatment of torture victims so that the "soul that was bruised" will eventually heal to restore a sense of wholeness.

In Chapter 57, Inger Agger and Søren Buus Jensen present a discussion of the psychosexual trauma of torture which, according to Amnesty International in 1984, is practiced in one third of the world's countries. In their work in Denmark, the authors have treated refugees seeking asylum from countries in which they were the victims of political oppression and, in many cases, torture. Indeed, 75% of the refugee referrals at one hospital reported having been tortured.

Similar to the analysis presented by Simpson in Chapter 56, Agger and Jensen have identified the central elements of the torture experience. They state that

> the aim of *psychological* torture is to break down and shatter the victim's psychological defense mechanisms and sense of will by causing psychic pain. Among the frequently used methods are long-term isolation, extensive and exhausting interrogation, sensory and sleep deprivation, threats, mock executions, witnessing the torture of others, and other forms of humiliating treatment, such as nakedness and *sexual torture*.

The purpose of sexual torture, like all torture, is to break the will of the victim and to destroy ego-identity. The methods of sexual torture that are discussed by the authors include (1) homo- or heterosexual rape, (2) the rape of women by trained dogs, usually Alsatians, (3) electrical stimulation of the sexual organs, (4) mechanical stimulation of the erogenous zones, (5) manual stimulation of the erogenous zones, (6) the insertion of overly large penis-shaped objects (which can be electrified) into body openings, (7) the forced witnessing of perverse sexual acts, (8) forced masturbation (by self or others), (9) fellatio and oral coitus, and (10) exposure to lewd and humiliating aggressive remarks by the captors. Additionally, subjugation and belittlement of the victim are attempted by the heterosexual rape of women and the homosexual rape of men.

Among the many traumatic consequences of sexual torture are the loss of sexual pleasure, gender identity confusion, emotional detachment, and PTSD. It is, of course, the goal of the sadistic perpetrator to cause as much damage as possible to the victim. The authors state that

> in sexual torture, the interchange between the victim and the torturer is characterized by an ambiguity consisting of both aggressive and libidinal elements. The victim's as well as the torturer's sexual structures are involved in the psychodynamics of this interaction, and the victim experiences the torture as directed against his or her sexual body image and identity with the aim to destroy it.

To illustrate the nature of sexual torture, Agger and Jensen present four case illustrations that involve a Latin American woman, a torturer from the Middle East, a Kurdish man, and a Latin American couple. In each case, the nature of the traumatic experience is explored as is the process of treatment and psychotherapy. The authors clearly indicate that powerful countertransference reactions occur in their work with victims of torture. The trauma story is often so laden with depictions of violence, brutality, cruelty, and degradation that it is difficult to believe what actually happened. Yet the emotional turmoil of the patient forces the therapist to confront the reality of what must have happened to that person. Finally, the authors discuss posttraumatic therapy and note that in work with the victims of torture

> review of the trauma story was not necessarily therapeutic. Often, it could stimulate further intrusive thoughts which intensified existing symptoms. . . . it [is] especially important that the memory of the painful events get reframed. . . . The therapist should not try to break through the resistance to get to "the feelings." . . . A provocation of this kind may lead to an increase of the "private" pain of the person at the expense of the "political" pain, and the therapist might be identified with the torturer in the transference situation.

In Chapter 58, Stuart W. Turner and Caroline Gorst-Unsworth discuss the psychological sequelae of torture, based on their work at the Medical Foundation for the Care of Victims of Torture in London, England. They begin their chapter with an overview of the psychological effects of torture and, consistent with the other authors in Part VI, consider it to be an attempt to break the will of the victim through physical and psychological means.

In discussing the psychological sequelae of torture, Turner and Gorst-Unsworth indicate that the victims manifest a common set of symptoms which include impaired memory and concentration, headaches, anxiety, depression, sleeplessness with nightmares and other intrusive phenomena, emotional numbing, sexual disturbances, rage, social withdrawal, lack of energy, apathy, and helplessness. Establishing these symptoms within the context of PTSD, the authors then discuss each cluster of reactions in depth, illustrating their relationship to the stressors experienced during the torture period. Furthermore, based on a sample of the first 20 torture victims who were treated in the medical facility in London, a list of at least 20 methods of torture were identified, which included beatings, kicking, slapping; striking with heavy cables or belts; electric shock; *falaka* (beating the soles of the feet); hooding and blindfolding; mock executions; burns to the body; *telefono* (violent boxing of the ears); suspension by ropes or chains; *submarino* (cold water immersion); sexual molestation; handcuffing; removal of fingers; pins under thumbnails; and the like.

The chapter concludes with a discussion of treatment strategies. In working with torture victims, the authors suggest that clinicians need to be sensitive to patterns of symptomatology present and state that

> incomplete emotional and cognitive processing with intrusive, avoidance, and hyperarousal symptoms is common, although it may be atypical with the development of unusual defensive mechanisms, including chronic hyperventilation disorder. On theoretical grounds, it may also be predicted that successful avoidance behavior would be disrupted by the method of torture and that intrusive features would predominate. . . .
> For each individual, the predominant reaction is likely to guide the choice of treatment.

In Chapter 59, Tony Jaffa discusses methods of therapy with families who have experienced torture. As noted by Harkness in Chapter 53, families are systems which have defined roles, responsibilities, and affective relationships among their members. Thus, a trauma to one or more members of the system is very likely to upset the stasis of the system and cause disequilibrium. As Jaffa states:

> I see a healthy family as an interacting evolving system which operates for the mutual benefit of its members. This involves ideas of continuity and also of adaptability. The family influ-

ences and is influenced by changes in its members and in its environment. My goal is to help the families come closer to this state.

How does the psychotherapist work with families whose members have experienced torture? Jaffa believes that following an initial assessment and identification of the problem areas that have developed in the system, it is necessary to establish a mutually agreed upon agenda. In terms of his work with families at the Medical Foundation for the Care of Victims of Torture in London, England, the author has identified family coping patterns with victims of torture which include these thematic elements: (1) the need to *preserve* the myth of the competence of the husband and father, (2) attempts to *rescue* the fallen (traumatized) husband and father, (3) attempts to *replace* the absent husband and father by a "parent-child" who engages in *role reversal* by "filling the father's shoes," and (4) the development of symptoms in children as an indirect attempt to maintain or restore family cohesion.

Since torture is such a powerful and abusive experience, the issue of trust emerges early in the treatment process. As a result, the therapist may be tested severely by the family in an attempt to establish the boundaries of his or her trustworthiness. Once the therapeutic alliance is established, a number of concrete steps may be taken to assist the distressed family. These therapeutic activities include (1) practical aid, such as writing reports to support asylum or lining up resources to help with securing housing, jobs, or medical care; (2) addressing manageable problems first in order to overcome feelings of hopelessness and despair that might exist; (3) addressing openly the unspoken and latent fears that might exist among family members; and (4) facilitating and empowering a sense of personal control over life-events and decisions to controvert states of helplessness and depression.

Clinical work with families who have experienced torture is not easy and inevitably blocks to progress occur. Through his own experiences, Jaffa notes that this includes a reluctance of family members to attend sessions, the need for interpreters to translate foreign languages, countertransference reactions in the therapist, and a lack of funding support to carry out long-term counseling. In his conclusion and summary, the author states:

> Even when there is no clinical intervention, when no skill and no technique come to mind, there is still the *person* of the therapist who can be there for the client at the moments of deepest despair. To remain there and not run, deny, panic, or hide in a professional role may be the most important thing the therapist has to offer.

In Chapter 60, Stuart W. Turner and Alexandra Hough discuss one of the more powerful psychosomatic reactions to torture: the hyperventilation syndrome (HVS). The authors note that the relationship between breathing and emotion is well established as in, for example, "a *sigh* of sadness or a *gasp* of surprise." However, HVS is often difficult to diagnose precisely because it may be associated with other psychiatric conditions, such as a panic disorder. In terms of reactions to traumatic stressors, the activation of the autonomic nervous system and levels of hyperarousability may be causally associated with overbreathing and HVS.

The authors studied 10 survivors of various torture practices, which included falaka, telefono, beatings, burns, electric shock, suspension, mock executions, and the witnessing of torture and executions. About one half of the subjects developed HVS during torture and imprisonment, whereas the onset was uncertain for the others. In torture victims, HVS may be part of a complex psychobiological response which includes dissociative states. Thus, it is possible that hyperventilation during torture may be one of several physiological pathways to dissociative states. This phenomenon is illustrated in a case vignette provided by Turner and Hough, who describe a 32-year-old man who was imprisoned for three years:

> The falaka was continued for periods lasting from 1 to 2 hours and, despite the development of swelling and infection, was repeated frequently. The pain was described as "appalling." Early in the torture, he was repeatedly hit on the head and remembers losing consciousness several times. After several weeks, he found that, after only 20 to 30 minutes of torture, he would lose consciousness without head trauma. This was preceded by subjective anxiety with autonomic accompaniments. He also remembers that his hands and his body would shake before he passed out.

To treat HVS in the victims of torture, Turner and Hough suggest a holistic approach which incorporates education about HVS and PTSD, physiotherapy in breathing retraining, relaxation training, and emotional support. Where co-diagnoses exist, such as PTSD, a multiprofessional, multimodal approach to therapy is recommended.

In Chapter 61, Richard Douglas Blackwell extends the discussion of how to help victims of torture and detention at various levels of therapeutic response. He observes that torture not only injures the psyche of the victim but destroys family systems and entire communities. Thus, the reconstitution of the family and community is an important task for the survivors. But this is not an easy thing to accomplish, and no therapist can magically restore what was torn apart by the torture experience. However, as Zev Harel, Boaz Kahana, and Eva Kahana found in their study of Holocaust survivors (as reported in Chapter 20), the reestablishment of social support systems and networks within a meaningful community is important to recovery and mental health. In a similar observation, Blackwell writes that "reconstitution of systems, families, networks, and communities can be done only by the exiled survivors themselves. It is their existential project and not something that we can take over and manage for them."

The fact that the victim of torture has the personal responsibility to reconnect to others in a community which is psychologically valuable does not mean that therapeutic interventions cannot assist in the recovery process. The author, a member of the Medical Foundation of the Care of Victims of Torture in London, England, discusses some of the ways in which the Foundation attempts to facilitate a process that enables reconstitution of families and communities.

First, the Foundation is regarded as a community in itself which can provide a "bridge for an individual to move from isolation to contact with others; a place in which network relationships can develop and in which families can find support in reestablishing themselves."

Second, there are levels of therapeutic intervention which includes support for asylum, medical care, social work services, a therapeutic milieu, the testimony method, and individual and group psychotherapy. The potential benefit from this multilevel approach to intervention is that it creates a healing environment of care. In his conclusion, Blackwell states:

> In our work with torture survivors we focus not just on the torture and its impact on these individuals, but also consider how their relationships have been changed and how they understand themselves now as members of a community.

In Chapter 62, Lars Weisaeth chronicles the posttraumatic aftermath of a Norwegian ship's crew that was tortured in May of 1984 by Libyan captors who thought that the journey of the ship from London to Libya was part of an international coup to overthrow their government. The crew was detained for 67 days and during that time was subjected to torture, interrogation, beatings, false confessions, mock executions, threats of violence, and exposure to a fellow sailor who had been beaten to death. Upon their return to Norway, the crew was interviewed at two points in time and administered psychological questionnaires, which included the General Health Questionnaire (GHQ), the Impact of Events Scale, and measures of anxiety and PTSD.

The results of the study revealed that 46% of the crew met the DSM-III criteria for PTSD. However, at the 6-month follow-up, 54% of the men suffered from PTSD and none of them was able to return to work at sea. The GHQ scores revealed a caseness prevalence of 83%, suggesting that there were severe psychiatric disturbances among the crew members. A similar result was also obtained on an Amnesty International Scale for victims of torture, which showed high levels of startle reaction, bodily tension, repetitive nightmares, reduced performance capacity, reduced affect modulation, increased alcohol consumption, exhaustion, depression, and emotional lability. The scores on the Impact of Events Scale were consistent and similar to those of persons suffering from PTSD. Thus, the configuration of findings in this study provides additional evidence with regard to the deleterious and prolonged effects of torture on individuals' psychological well-being and adaptive behavior.

In Chapter 63, Margaret Cunningham and Derrick Silove present an overview of their work with refugees and victims of torture who have immigrated to Australia. They observe that there are at least six phases of transition for refugees as they leave behind their previous culture and assimilate the new one. These six phases include (1) living in the home culture in which war, violence, and torture exist; (2) torture, detainment, and imprisonment; (3) exile out of the home country; (4) initial adaptation to the new country; (5) transition between cultures; and (6) resettlement in the country of asylum.

Based on their work at the Service for the Treatment and Rehabilitation of Torture and Trauma Survivors in Sydney, Australia, the authors discuss the organizational development and philosophy of treatment approaches in working with torture victims and traumatized refugees. They note, for example, that

> conditions in camps vary, but refugees who manage to resettle in Western countries frequently recount traumatic experiences associated with this phase, including illness, overcrowding, poor sanitation, malnutrition, domestic violence, rape, bribery, and extortion. Regional and global political factors greatly influence attitudes toward refugees and hence their treatment. Host governments in countries of first asylum often have a policy of "deterrence" which militates against camp authorities who provide more than a subsistence level of survival. . . . It is important to note that over 70% of those living in refugee camps are women and children who are most vulnerable to neglect, abuse, and exploitation.

The authors proceed to discuss the many complex issues that face the specialist working with refugees and victims of torture. They state that having a bilingual staff is important to bridge the gap between cultures. So, too, is it important to have staff that is knowledgeable and sensitive to cross-cultural differences so that they can be

> cultural brokers . . . to translate the issues of torture to the dominant culture, to assist the immigrant community in demystifying the norms and mores of the dominant culture, and to develop a *modus operandi* which allows access to and participation in the new society without devaluing their own traditional cultures.

Like the other contributors to Part VI, Cunningham and Silove recommend a flexible and creative approach to treating victims of torture. Among the principles they have identified are (1) the need to reempower survivors of torture; (2) the need for awareness of torture as a political issue; (3) the need for pragmatic assistance to aid refugees in meeting basic security needs for housing, food, and medical care; (4) respect for religion and cultural rituals for healing and recovery; (5) creating resource manuals for the clients; and (6) networking with other agencies that can provide services which are needed by the torture survivors or refugee immigrants. The authors conclude their chapter with a discussion of specific treatment principles and a set of recommendations with regard to staff selection and note that "it is as important for staff to focus on organizational and service development as it is to develop effective approaches to clinical assessment and treatment."

Part VI concludes with Chapter 64, by Marrianne Juhler, who concisely discusses the diagnosis and medical treatment of torture survivors. Based on her work at the Rehabilitation Centre for Torture Victims in Copenhagen, Denmark, Juhler outlines the steps of a medical examination. Although a medical evaluation is rather routine for the nontraumatized individual, it may be threatening and may reactivate aspects of torture among those victimized. Thus, Juhler states that it is important, if not imperative, for the physician to have "knowledge of torture in general and of specific torture methods [which] . . . facilitate both questioning and interpretation of the information obtained." For example, the application of EKG electrodes to monitor cardiovascular functioning may precipitate a flashback (reliving) of electrical torture and intensify sympathetic nervous system functioning, thereby providing a false measurement of cardiac function. For this reason, Juhler recommendes that "it is unwise to subject patients to diagnostic procedures, if the same information can be obtained in a way which is simpler and less straining for the patient." However, should the medical examination result in the need to hospitalize the patient, Juhler recommends that it only occur in a setting where the staff have a "special interest and knowledge in dealing with torture survivors," in order to avoid aggravating the symptoms of PTSD or other psychiatric conditions associated with the torture experience.

In a most useful way, Juhler specifies the most common somatic and psychological symptoms that torture victims manifest. These include pseudodementia, headaches, muscle and joint aches, lower back problems, heart palpitations, dyspnea, peptic ulcers, gastritis, visual disorders, chronic fatigue, gynecological complaints, and abdominal or pelvic pains. These and other symptoms can usually be linked to the events that happened in the torture experience or as a somatic component of PTSD.

CHAPTER 56

Traumatic Stress and the Bruising of the Soul

The Effects of Torture and Coercive Interrogation

Michael A. Simpson

> He who has been tortured remains tortured. . . . He who has suffered torment can no longer find his place in the world. Faith in humanity—cracked by the first slap across the face, then demolished by torture—can never be recovered.
> —JEAN AMERY, cited in Levi (1987)

> To live is to suffer, to survive is to find meaning in the suffering.
> —GORDON ALLPORT

In the struggle to exert power over the minds of others (for whatever political, philosophical, religious, or other aims) one may gain the agreement and cooperation of others by free discussion, debate, exchange of opinions, and the attempt to convince the other person by the quality of one's facts and logic. But throughout history some have chosen, instead, to force others to agree by using war and fearful conflict, captivity, pain, degradation, and fear; indeed, by the deliberate creation of traumatic stress and its sequelae.

"The politico-religious struggle for the mind of man may well be won by whoever becomes most conversant with the normal and abnormal functions of the brain, and is readiest to make use of the knowledge gained." Thus wrote my pioneering colleague William Sargant in his classic book *Battle for the Mind* back in 1957. Over 30

years later, it has become clear that a great many governments and other political groups have become deeply conversant with the means to induce peculiarities of brain function, and are very ready to use whatever techniques are potentially effective.

There is an awful similarity, ultimately, between the stresses (and their consequences) that result from all varieties of conflict. We see post-traumatic stress disorders (PTSD) arising after natural disasters, those conflicts between mankind and the inexorable realities of nature. But what of the consequences of man-made cruelties, the unnatural disasters? It is a recurrent propensity of mankind (or man-unkind) to deliberately generate overwhelming horror for other humans not as an occasional, freakish, accidental occurrence, but, rather, as an expectable and regular feature of human intercourse.

More disturbing in their universality than the results of flood and earthquake are the disorders we see following the deliberate and carefully orchestrated cruelty of captivity and interrogation. Much of the recent literature on posttraumatic stress has concentrated on the unplanned and unintended consequences of conflict. But we also see PTSD as a deliberate and carefully nurtured

Michael A. Simpson • Intermedica, P.O. Box 51, Pretoria, South Africa. Manuscript submitted May, 1990.

International Handbook of Traumatic Stress Syndromes, edited by John P. Wilson and Beverley Raphael. Plenum Press, New York, 1993.

product of malicious skills; an evil bloom, occasionally visible in the open air and light of society, with its roots deep in the spiritual manure of secret interrogation chambers.

There have been numerous published studies of the victims of torture and interrogation. Like botanists classifying the varieties of beetle, most authors have been content to solemnly tabulate torture techniques and to summarize survivors' symptoms, without drawing any particularly useful conclusions. We have relatively little more to learn from such simplistic catalogs of cruelty. There are other problems (see Engdahl & Eberly, 1990, for a useful literature review and research critique). Usually, those studied are not typical. Survivors with few or no problems will not seek help; those severely afflicted may never reach the treatment center; those who did not survive long enough to reach evaluation are omitted. Overall, there are well-recognized ranges of horrid methods, used with minor variations in every country where torture and coercive interrogations are used.

In this chapter, I have omitted any detailed review of the literature, whose monotony and lack of conceptual vigor and methodological rigor make it so disappointingly unhelpful. These studies are often sloppy (considering the comparative luxury of the facilities available to those assessing refugees, far from the torture site). Corroborating tests and measurements are often not done or not recorded. The simple and repetitive collating of cases blurs the essential individual details into tidy piles. Enough! The obvious facts have been established: torture is bad for one's health; the worse the torture, the worse the results; and a little torture can cause a lot of suffering and damage. But what else do we need to know and do? The really important thing is what the individual victims suffered, and how they were affected by this activity.

Therefore, instead of this, and based on such documentation and particularly my own experiences as victim and in working with victims and on our experiences in the chronic tragedy of South Africa, I will explore some neglected aspects of this field. One of the challenges in traumatic stress research is the constraint that it is ethically and practically impossible to create experimentally most of the conditions whose effects we study. We must rely on natural experiments, on naturally occurring tragedies and disasters. Often, we study the effects of war and disasters, situations in which an enormous number of factors (most of them ignored by researchers) impinge on the individual; in which the stress experience is a complex compound of noxious and irrelevant stimuli.

Coercive interrogation and torture, in contrast, are in fact perverted experiments, in which the interrogator/torturer uses a grisly expertise to deliberately induce traumatic stress problems in his subjects. Usually, the intention is to produce disorder, and the modern torturer inherits an ancient expertise, developed with malignant care over the centuries; tested in the witch hunts (Kramer & Sprenger, 1971), the Spanish Inquisition, the Czarist police, the Stalinist purges (Lermolo, 1955), North Korean and Chinese "brain-washing" (Biderman & Zimmer, 1961), and the brutal beastliness of numerous countries in recent decades.

In the old days, prisoners were treated with elaborate apparatus, a technology of torture that owed most to a perverted talent for structural engineering, and reflecting the peak of the technological progress of their times. They were stretched on racks, had their fingers crushed with thumbscrews, or were dipped in boiling oil. In more recent years, it is clear that the avant garde of awfulness has learned more from the behavioral sciences, in an unethical application of knowledge of how brain and mind can be pressured into dysfunction. This has improved the ease and efficiency with which suffering can be carefully tailored so as to break down an individual detainee, to bruise his soul and render him cooperative against his will. We are now capable of far more sophisticated sadism. Physical brutality is not really necessary anymore, though it quite easily occurs when interrogators get carried away by their own power and indemnity from repercussions.

Generally, the torturers have realized that more subtle but no less cruel pressures can break the human spirit more efficiently, and with far less risk of leaving behind tell-tale marks. Scars on the psyche and searing of the soul are harder for the victim to demonstrate to the press or to the courts, should any opportunity arise. If someone gets carried away and inflicts visible physical damage, release from detention can usually be delayed until the marks have faded.

Enthusiasm for electrical shock torture is based in part on its capacity to provide closely calibrated cruelty, varying the severity with finesse; and partly because it was believed to be impossible to prove afterward that it had taken place. When it was shown that microscopic skin changes could reveal the placement of electrodes, there was a trend toward supplying the current through wet cloths instead, to avoid leaving unwanted traces. My discovery of chemical tests which can show traces of such torture after the events (e.g., Simpson, 1989a,b) seems also to have restrained some of those who favored this method. Similarly, our understanding of the stress disorders can provide a delineation of psychic bruises and scars, which, by helping to reveal these sequelae of maltreatment, may also inhibit the torturer.

In order to know how to assist the victim, we must understand what has been done to them, and how and why it has affected them. We can formulate therapeutic interventions based on an understanding of the ways in which damage has been caused.

From the point of view of our scientific need to understand the nature of traumatic stress itself, and the means by which it induces pathological effects, I believe that our work with torture victims can shed unique light in such issues (Simpson, 1987).

For some people, *torture* is such an emotive word that they hesitate to use it for what so frequently happens to political detainees in so many countries. Torture is any systematically applied unpleasantness used to make a prisoner psychologically pliable, to get information or a confession that would not freely be given, to change behavior and opinion, and/or to deter opposition.

Significant components of the torture process include: (1) taking someone into a totally controlling situation or institution with an unknown time-scale and unpredictability regarding his or her fate; (2) providing threats and menaces of unpleasant things that might happen; and (3) reducing or preventing normal human interactions with sustaining others. These elements are noticeably similar to those features of the combat or disaster situation that I believe constitute the formula for inducing PTSD: being in an uncontrollable situation and at high-risk of death or of horrible events occurring to oneself or to others whom one cares about, and with impaired access to sustainment.

South African Experience

Before I discuss the main themes of this chapter, I would like to examine some of the findings reported in South African studies that are not widely known. Increasingly, between 1960 and 1990, the South African government developed a wide variety of laws that ignored the basic principles of human rights, under which any person might be detained, effectively indefinitely, if in the opinion of a remarkably wide range of law-enforcement officials (even quite junior) they posed in any one of a large range of vaguely defined ways, a risk to the state. They could be interrogated at great length, while generally being held incommunicado, often with no access to lawyers, the courts or their family. Eventually, under the regulations of the long-running State of Emergency, it was a possibly serious offense even to announce or remark that someone else was in detention or to seek their release. Doctors and scientists were legally advised that it was potentially an offense to publish any article about detainees or their conditions or problems, or to give a public lecture on the subject.

After their release, or when they eventually reached a court, numerous detainees have alleged that they had been tortured, usually in order to produce a confession. Usually, the courts have preferred to believe the police disavowals of such conduct, though the detainees have told harrowing, consistent, and credible stories. When held incommunicado, of course, there is little chance for the detainee to prove subsequently what happened, even when there has been notable corroborating evidence. The organized medical profession has almost entirely ignored these matters (Rayner, 1987).

Typical of accounts given by detainees is the story of STN:

He ordered me to remove my shoes . . . then he stamped on my toes with the heels of his shoes for several times . . . he banged my head against the wall at least four times. My nose began to bleed heavily . . . they covered my face with a tight rubber tube like a balaclava, so that I couldn't breathe, but pulled it off while I was struggling, then put it back. . . . I was then tied, lying on my back, to what felt like a table (I was blindfolded, so I couldn't see what they were doing). My limbs were tied down with damp cloths. Then I experienced excruciating pain, like when you accidentally contact a live wire. I then realized I was being electrocuted. I tried to scream, but the pain was too severe. This took place at intervals of about 10 minutes, for about 3 hours, Then I was taken back to my cell.

It must be realized how extraordinarily difficult it has been for us to study these problems in South Africa.

Individual clinicians may see individual cases after detention, but are normally denied any access to detainees during their detention. In unique cases, I have seen people during their detention, when examining them to provide expert evidence for human rights court cases. Formal study is extremely hard to achieve: obviously, the authorities will not cooperate, and ex-detainees are understandably suspicious of any attention they receive.

One of the few studies reported was by Paul Davis (1986) who reviewed his experience of 21 ex-detainees seen over the previous 2 years. The length of their detention ranged from 2 weeks to 4 years, and four had been detained more than once. All of them alleged that they had received mental and physical abuse, usually early in their detention, including beatings to body and head, using hands, fists, truncheons, sticks, planks, and booted feet; electric shocks to ears, nipples, neck, and scrotum; abuse of sexual organs; and near-suffocation manually, with belts or wet canvas bags.

All detainees gave a history of being in solitary confinement for periods of 13 days to 4 months; 18 reported deliberate deprivation of sleep and food, and 14 described major variation of routine and time disorientation. Periods of uninterrupted interrogation of up to 10 hours were reported, often combined with the use of extremely uncomfortable positions, such as prolonged standing, crouching, or being naked and shackled.

All cases examined by Davis were diagnosed as suffering from PTSD. All had such sleep disturbance as insomnia, nightmares, night sweats, or early morning wakening; 18 had significant disturbance of previously good relations with wives, friends, parents, and children; 18 had sexual dysfunctions, including impotence, premature ejaculation, and anorgasmia. Five (23.8%) showed "moderately severe depression" after release.

Davis also experienced the sort of persecution that illustrates the dangers experienced in attempting such research. He was subpoenaed and brought to court on bizarre grounds. It was said that, because some of the patients described in his paper had alleged that they had been assaulted while in detention, the police required him to provide them with the names and addresses of all the detainees he had seen and treated, claiming that they wished to investigate the allegations (the only occasion on which they had made any such attempt, despite many other allegations). For more than a year, despite his explanation that he could not recall such names and addresses, and had not recorded them, he faced the threat of detention, for failing to disclose to the Security Police the patient details they wanted. This episode was a transparent attempt to intimidate all those who were providing counseling and assistance to ex-detainees; and to dissuade ex-detainees from seeking assistance. In the whole ethically obscene episode, the South African Medical and Dental Council, which has persistently failed to apply basic ethical principles in political matters, made no attempt to defend those principles.

Friedlander (1988) reported on his findings in 28 former detainees. The commonest symptoms were poor concentration (96%), disturbed sleep (88%), intrusive fearful thoughts about the future (73%), depressed mood (69%), irritability (65%), and tension headaches (62%); guilt was evident in 42%. His diagnoses were major depressive disorder with PTSD in 29%, major depressive episode in 18%, and PTSD alone in 14%. Taking into account those cases with double diagnoses, there were thus 47% with depression, and 43% with PTSD. Of his subjects, 80% claimed to have been beaten, 8% claimed to have received electric shock. They were seen soon after release, 86% within a month of release.

The most detailed study in this field is that of Foster, Davis, and Sandler (1987) documented in their book *Detention and Torture in South Africa*. The South African authorities have worked hard to discredit this work, using very minor and politically biased academics at government universities to make unrealistic and naive criticisms of it in legal cases where it has been cited. It is based on interviews with 158 ex-detainees, describing 176 episodes of detention. Eighty-three percent reported instances of physical torture, 75% reported beatings, 50% forced standing, 34% being forced to maintain an abnormal and uncomfortable body posture, 28% described forced exercises, 25% having to wear a bag over the head, 25% reported electric shock, and 18% strangulation among other methods.

All 158 ex-detainees reported instances of psychological torture, including 79% who experienced solitary confinement, 71% verbal abuse, 64% threatened violence, 41% threats of execution of self or family, and 27% being forced to undress. This study was not conducted by assessors competent to make diagnoses, but they did collect data on symptoms experienced after release from detention. Only 3% of the ex-detainees complained of no symptoms. Common symptoms included fatiguability (46%), problems relating to friends (39%), problems relating to family (34%), difficulty getting to sleep (34%), nightmares in 33%, irritability in 31%, depression in 24%, and problems in concentrating in 24%.

In one of my studies of political detainees, who were seen and assessed during their detention at the request of their lawyers, I compared 11 who made no allegations of torture or intensive interrogation, with 12 who did make such allegations. Of the 11 making no allegations of mistreatment, none merited any psychiatric diagnosis, and none complained of substantial symptoms. Of the 12 who did allege maltreatment, 5 (41.6%) had posttraumatic stress disorder (PTSD) (according to DSM-III criteria), and one (8.4%) had PTSD and major depression; giving a total incidence of PTSD of 50%. Three (25%) showed significant symptoms of depression and of PTSD, but without meeting all the diagnostic criteria. Three (25%) showed no significant current symptoms. Although the numbers in this series are small, this unique study provides the only comparative data available on psychiatric assessments during such detention.

The situation has posed significant ethical dilemmas for those few doctors who have not carefully hidden from and avoided the problems of detainees. Ethically, one cannot refuse to see a detainee who needs medical advice, because one cannot refuse to help someone in need. But once one is treating such a patient, one may be in the position of resuscitating the victim to help restore him to a condition in which he will be fit for further abuse. One can be officially asked to declare the victim fit to return to the situation which harmed him. My approach to the dilemma has been to refuse to do so, on the grounds that no one is ever fit to be subjected to or

returned to a harmful process, just as no one is ever fit to be thrown off a cliff or fit to be run over by a bus.

Similarly, one may be faced with the difficulty of trying to treat someone in an entirely inappropriate prison setting; or, if one insists that the patient be transferred to a hospital, the authorities may insist that he be isolated, manacled to the bed, and closely guarded at all times. One may have to struggle to insist that proper medical advice is followed.

At first, one is inclined to see PTSD as an unfortunate and unwanted side effect of the processes of interrogation and detention. But I suspect that it is at times a deliberate and desired effect. In situations in which large numbers of restive and socially active individuals are placed in custody, more may be wanted than simply removing them from circulation for a time. The induction of PTSD may serve to ensure that after release, they may be continuously less active and less effective members of any opposition.

It is not only political detainees who developed PTSD and related stress symptoms in relation to the political unrest. Young white men conscripted into compulsory military service were involved in highly politicized conflicts, including service on the Namibian/Angolan border, and in the townships. Like the American Vietnam veterans, they faced guerrilla warfare, for ambiguous and unpopular goals, against an ambiguous enemy. Unlike Vietnam, the fighting was almost entirely unpublicized (indeed, news coverage was banned) so that few outside the military comprehended what they had experienced, or even believed that they had actually met any of the horrors they encountered.

Many of these men describe absolutely classical features of PTSD. There are also some unique horrors. One of these men, who was serving in the townships during the riots, saw someone being necklaced by a mob and commented: "When they're burning, all men are the same colour; there's no skin left, just this thing on the ground moving and burning, like lamb on a spit . . . those eyes staring at me; he couldn't blink, there were no eyelids." He began to have nightmares that hordes of small animals were eating him. Later, in conflict on the border, he escaped physical injury, but his friends were killed and blinded. He showed classical PTSD.

The Nature of the Stressors

"One might describe an interrogator as a man who tries to obtain information from another man who may or may not possess it, and who is not necessarily motivated to give the information if he does" (Hinkle, 1961). The interrogator would like to get the information rapidly, accurately, completely, and without irrelevant or untrue additions. In such a situation, there are many ways (to be discussed below) in which a detainee's free will, resistance, and ability to make independent, freely voluntary decisions (such as whether to make a statement and what to say in it) may be impaired or influenced These factors have the effects of inducing suggestibility, compliance with external instructions, malleability, and plasticity, and, thus, an impaired capacity to freely exercize a voluntary and informed choice of decision and

671

action. If sufficiently severe, such factors will produce stress disorders.

Factors Affecting Subjects of Interrogation

The factors that influence those who experience torture and coercive interrogation are multiple and include those that are now outlined separately.

Fears

Examples

Menaces and threats are conveyed by deed and word of death and suffering, of endless isolation, of never getting home, of awful things happening to one's family and friends, of betrayal, of disgracing oneself, of indefinite continuation of isolation, interrogation, and incarceration. Threats are made and there are fears of death, of torture, of pain, of indefinite continuation of isolation, of interrogation, and of incarceration. Unorthodox practices may imply that captors are not subject to normal controls. Vague threats are often the most effective, allowing individuals to project their deepest secret fears into the menace.

Effects

There is anxiety, dread, despair, and an increasing willingness to sacrifice long-term interests for relief from these fears.

Isolation

Examples

There can be physical isolation, social isolation (separation from sustaining others), isolation in small groups, hooding, and solitary confinement. There is also the practice of alternating intense stimulation with isolation (each amplifying the other's impact).

Effects

Isolation forces a dependence on the interrogator, deprives the subject of social and emotional support, fosters intense concern with self and the immediate predicament, impairs coping, and amplifies the effects of other factors. The detainee is more open to suggestion and has increased susceptibility to pressures to conform. Deterioration of complex thinking and higher functions are seen and there is a drive for companionship and a desire to talk.

Exhaustion

Examples

Debility can be induced with poor food, exposure to heat or cold, prolonged constraint, prolonged standing or awkward postures (self-inflicted pain being most effective) lack of exercise, sleep disturbance, prolonged interrogations, and sustained tension.

Effects

These deprivations result in weakness, tiredness, exhaustion, decreased physical and mental ability to resist, and impairment of higher functions.

Helplessness/Hopelessness/Powerlessness

Examples

The interrogator demonstrates omniscience and omnipotence; he demonstrates his power and the subject's impotence. The interrogator may enforce trivial commands, forced writing, hooding, and "Yes" questions.

Effects

These actions convince the subject of the futility and impossibility of resistance. The captor develops a habit of compliance.

Manipulation of Hope and Motivation

Examples

Promises may be given directly or by hint and implication to the detainee of better treatment, rewards, or even simply the withdrawal of threats and the prospect of enhanced safety. There may be occasional indulgences and small rewards for partial compliance that influence the subject's assessment of likely outcomes of his choices (e.g., that minimize the crime or the likely sentence).

Effects

Such manipulation gives positive motivation for compliance, makes the benefits of compliance seem greater than the benefits of silence or resistance, and gives an unrealistic impression of the consequences of compliance.

Unpredictability

Examples

There may be unpredictable responses to a subject's behavior: unexpected kindness or cruelty of an indefinite duration, or relocation to an unfamiliar environment. The interrogator may display severe anger, *not* closely related to the subject's actions, which only enhances confusion, uncertainty, and ambiguity.

Effects

Unpredictability impairs adjustment, may prevent coping, fosters a sense of unreality, and impairs higher functions and decision-making.

Monotony

Examples

Monotony is induced by deprivation of environmental stimulation or a barren environment, no books or recreation, monotonous food, restricted movement, hooding, and the absence of normal varying stimuli.

Effects

The effects of monotony include cognitive disturbances, disorientation, difficulty concentrating, and memory disturbances. An intense focus of attention by the subject on his immediate predicament fosters introspection, eliminates the benefits of distraction, and damages coping capacity.

Humiliation

Examples

Manipulation of self-esteem, interference with personal hygiene, dirty surroundings, demeaning acts, being stripped naked, along with insults, taunts, and the denial of privacy result in humiliation.

Effects

Humiliation damages the captor's self-esteem, makes continued resistance seem more threatening to his self-esteem than noncompliance, exaggerates status difference by amplifying effectiveness of persuasion. It focuses the captor's attention on "animal" values and needs and impairs his higher-order decision-making.

Questioning Forms and Methods

Examples

In the simulation of omniscience, the interrogator asks questions to which the subject cannot know the answers, then switches to relevant questions; he is a hard man/soft man and discourages the subject from expressing his own attitudes. Silence is interpreted as incriminating ("It must mean you have something to hide"). Silence can also be interpreted as confirmation or assent; he may pretend others have betrayed the subject, seeking to alienate the subject from his allies, supporters, or cause. "Have you stopped beating your wife? Answer yes or no" are a favored type of question.

Effects

Such questioning fosters the concept that cooperation by the detainee is inevitable; it is a psychological entrapment that induces suggestibility.

This model is based on the early studies of the Group for the Advancement of Psychiatry (1956, 1957), modified in the light of more recent research and experience.

Relationship between Torturer and Victim

As Ignatieff (1985) wrote: "It is the most intimate of all relations between strangers: eye to eye, hand to hand, breath on breath, torturer and victim are as close as lovers"; and "the more inhuman the screaming, the more bestial the torment, the less human . . . the victim can seem." Once the torturer has begun, the victim's responses can be dehumanizing in effect, thus making it easier for the torturer to continue. Inadvertently, the victim becomes easier to victimize.

Of course, the torturer degrades and dehumanizes himself, by his actions, but this is rarely appreciated. Although some torturers may be brutes, they are generally technologists, often sophisticated. Few are unaffected, once they begin to learn to inflict pain on the victim, by the heady exercise of such unlimited power. He may strive to avoid producing lasting marks (just as any other criminal tries not to leave fingerprints). Yet, while his actions may produce no visible signs of damage, the victim's pain may remain unreal to the perpetrator, and will not serve to inhibit his actions (see also Scarry, 1985). Sartre (1958) wrote: "the victim must disgrace himself by his screams and his submissions, like a human animal. In the eyes of everybody and in his own eyes, he who yields under torture is not only to be made to talk, but is also to be marked as sub-human."

The victim's very existence may be subsumed by pain, the suffering being an amalgam of the pain that preceded this, the present pain, and the dreaded future pain. "It takes over all that is inside and outside . . . it exhausts and displaces all else until it seems to become the single broad and omnipresent fact of existence" (Scarry, 1985). Coping and maintaining one's integrity are very difficult; as defenses, coping skills and morale are eroded rapidly.

Pain is incorporated; your body hurts you; your own body, in pain, causes a sense of self-betrayal; your own body, the battleground, can become the ultimate weapon they can use against you.

Pain is a great biological solvent; everything dissolves in it. First, the outside world, then the world of captivity, the room, the body itself, until only the pain remains. Once the torture has begun, the interrogator may feel he has to continue, until some shred of evidence can be extracted, to vindicate the decision to use torture. Once he has taken that step, the interrogator may feel committed, by whatever means, to get such evidence, whether the subject is guilty or innocent.

The torturer and his support system have become paranoid, too, building a grand conspiracy theory to justify themselves; and then are frightened by their own creation. And they have seductive elitist benefits: within such a brutal system, they may fear that they, too, may receive what they have given to others, if they disobey orders.

Aspects of the Pathology of Traumatic Stress

The torture experience usually starts precipitately. Timerman (1982) described the entry phase in which

> a man is shunted so quickly from one world to another that he's unable to tap a reserve of energy so as to confront this unbridled violence. That is the first phase of torture: to take a man by surprise, without allowing him any reflex defense, even psychological.

E. Kahana, B. Kahana, Harel, and Rosner (1988) spoke of the effect of there being "no predictable end to the experience," and no opportunity to remove the stress or influence it, except by cooperating. Total life experience is disrupted, the total fabric of normal life is replaced with an unfamiliar, unreal reality; a hostile, threatening, dangerous environment. Coping attempts may include identification with the aggressor, depersonalization, focus on purpose of survival, regression, and denial. Critical is the significance of overwhelming experiences with complete helplessness, when, as Op den Velde (personal communication) said "the immunity of the inner self snaps."

Guilt, where it is appropriate, arises "in the gap between what I am and what I could have been" said David Roy (personal communication). I see it more in the gap between what I have done and what I might otherwise have done; or between what I did not do, and what I could have done—in the unfulfilled potential. It is not apt in victims, for whatever they did (or did not do), however awful, was the best they could have done under the circumstances. A moral *realpolitik* is needed. To expect of oneself the best of which one is capable is reasonable. But to expect to function better than that best, for failing to be more than superhuman, is unrealistic self-blame. It is in how one faces the horror that one has the opportunity for greatness; in bearing the awful, in surviving. Much of the heroism that wins medals and acclaim is simply stupidity: lack of capacity (permanent or in a temporary high) to realize the extent of the risk. Far greater courage is seen in the survivor who has no such option for ostentatious bravery.

Psychic numbing, as a defense against overwhelming emotions and as a preemptive strike to remove one's vulnerability to further sources of loss and grief, has long been recognized. In the Albert Camus play *Cross Purpose*, a character who has killed her own brother says to his wife: "Pray God to harden you to stone. It's the happiness He has assigned to Himself, and the one true happiness. Do as He does, be deaf to all appeals, and turn your heart to stone while there is still time." Wilfred Owen (1985), the great English poet of World War I, himself a victim of PTSD who recovered and returned to the battlefront only to be killed just before the armistice ended the war, wrote brilliantly of PTSD in his poem "Insensibility":

> Happy are men who yet before they are killed
> Can let their veins run cold
> When no compassion fleers
> Or makes their feet
> Sore on the alleys cobbled with their brothers.
> . . . .
> And some cease feeling
> Even themselves or for themselves
> Dullness best solves
> The tease and doubt of shelling.

Some authors have raised a bizarre concern about the diagnosis of PTSD, saying, like Engdahl and Eberly (1990), that "it is curious that in a diagnostic manual that purports to eschew etiologic considerations (on grounds of insufficient knowledge) PTSD is the lone companion of the organic mental disorders in having a pinpointed causal sequence." Why on earth should the failure to be able to determine the etiology of *other* psychiatric disorders make anyone feel squeamish about defining it when we can? No one feels timid about describing alcoholism as related to alcohol consumption: how could we contemplate an alcohol-free definition of alcoholism? No one has qualms about diagnosing posttraumatic leg fractures in relation to the "purported" causative trauma. We need feel no overwhelming obligation to overlook the obvious, in the service of some abstract and artificial sense of diagnostic purity. By all means let us eschew (one should always eschew carefully, before swallowing such a proposition) classifications based on unproven etiologies. But which of us is seeing PTSD that does *not* follow a trauma, and a trauma whose grimy fingerprints lie all over the symptomatology?

If one has to face unpleasant events, both animals and humans prefer predictable to unpredictable aversive events (Badia, Harsh, & Abbott 1979; Pervin, 1963). Petersen and Seligman (1983) offer a cognitive theory for the experience of victimization and focus on the uncontrollability of the onset and end of the experience, as this combination bedevils coping. One cannot cope with a danger of unknown content, risk, course, and duration.

Misfortune that is perceived (by the recipient) as a random accident is potentially less damaging than grief caused deliberately by a specific agency. Most damaging of all may be the perception that misery is in the nature of things, in the very warp and weft of the weave of life. The level of generality of the causal hypothesis shapes the extent of the generality and pervasiveness of the symptoms and of the triggers which can elicit them. The degree of generalization determines the extent of the loss and of the subsequent vulnerability.

Where the female victim attributes the cause of events to herself, symptoms are more likely to be more pervasive across situations, because she herself will be a common factor, present in every situation she encounters; whereas any other enemy or source of danger is likely to be absent from at least some settings, actual or potential.

As with predictability, so it is with control. Controllable noise is experienced as less aversive than uncontrollable noise (e.g., Glass & Singer, 1972). Other work, reviewed by B. Melamed, J. L. Melamed, and Bouhoutsos (1990), showed that the autonomic impact and behavioral consequences of uncontrollable events are greater.

Previous experiences have a variable effect. Where one has successfully handled similar stressors, there may be enhanced coping skills and confidence (the "stress innoculation" theory). But when such a confident/competent person, facing extreme trauma, finds himself unable to cope, the impact may be much worse. Where the individual has previously failed to cope, reexposure may be far more disasterous in its impact.

Research has shown that people under stress have an enhanced need for support from others (e.g., Schachter, 1959). Many studies have shown that cohesive social support can lessen the effects of strife and aid healing. But, while increasing the potential or actual number of sources of support, it also increases the number of opportunities for loss, and the vulnerability to vicarious trauma. (Anyone you love is a hostage to potential loss; griefs are the wages of love.)

Denial is a psychic lubricant that mediates between the external, shared reality and the internal reality of the worldview. Relatively minor challenges to the worldview can be ignored, and the damaging impact of major threats to it can be delayed or limited, where it is practical to effectively use *denial*, that splendid existential ointment. Denial is a most valuable skill (Simpson, 1979, 1982); and the common "denial of denial" (Simpson, 1982), by professionals, is unhelpful. It helps to resist any tendency to change too radically in response to the challenge of trauma. As Kuhn (1962) pointed out, "As in manufacture, so in science—retooling is an extravagence to be reserved for the occasion that demands it."

Janoff-Bulman and Frieze (1983), Janoff-Bulman and Timko (1987), and Lazarus (1983) are among the few other authors who have respectfully recognized the value of denial.

Denial is *not* a sign of serious psychopathology, as some have claimed. Absence of denial is more likely to be pathological. It is not routinely maladaptive, but usually adaptive. It does not inevitably interfere with the accurate perception of reality: in fact, like sunglasses, by avoiding dazzle, it can aid such perception. Usually, it has been studied only in seriously disturbed individuals; hence its valuable role in normal individuals facing trauma has often been overlooked.

The torture victim confronts the world's loneliness, mercilessness, and nothingness. These events horrify us because they are *evil*. (What else is horror but a response to evil?) As Yalom wrote (1980), they

> stun us because they inform us that nothing is as we have always thought it to be, that contingency reigns, that everything could be otherwise than it is; that everything we consider fixed, precious, good, can suddenly vanish; that there is no solid ground; that we are "not-at-home" here or there or anywhere in the world.

Locus of control is relevant to the existential issue of responsibility and freedom. (Lefcourt, 1976; Phares, 1976; Rotter, 1966; Seligman, 1975). There is some evidence that early family environment is important in the formation of internality versus externality; and that an inconsistent, unpredictable milieu favors the development of a sense of individual helplessness and an external locus of control.

The right to privacy (the right to be left alone) is an essential feature of liberty. Another simple but potent aspect of torture and interrogation is the aggressive invasion of privacy, of being forced into a "total institution," such as Goffman (1961) described, where "these territories of the self are violated, the boundary that the individual places between his being and the environment is invaded and the embodiment of self profaned."

Privacy is the state of being secure from unwanted access by others—whether physical access, access to personal information, or to unwelcome attention. People naturally protect the privacy of their personal space, their names, their thoughts, their hopes and fears. Ironically, the detention and torture experience may contrive both to provide the stress of isolation from sustaining others, and the stress of invasion of privacy by unwelcome others (Bok, 1984; Laufer & Wolfe, 1977; Margoulis, 1977).

Another aspect of the trauma is being forced to disclose secrets. To gain the power to remain silent is an early and significant part of realizing control over events; and its loss is a central experience of powerlessness. Piaget (1959) saw the young child as "unable to keep a single secret," "incapable of keeping to himself the thoughts which enter his head. He says everything. He has no verbal continence." It is in playing with "secrets" that children learn about loyalty and betrayal. Although Piaget underestimated the complexity of the issue, the achievement of verbal continence, of the capacity to keep secrets, is an important developmental target. Adults forced to lose this can feel as shamed and regressed as if losing anal continence (this relation is analogous, not symbolic). Jung (1963), too, emphasized the significance of having and keeping a secret:

> No one could discover my secret and destroy it. I felt safe, and the tormenting sense of being at odds with myself was gone. . . . This possession of a secret had a very powerful formative influence on my character; I consider it the essential fact of my boyhood.

Confessions, even in the most benign setting and with the most wholesome of mutual motives, are highly delicate matters, even in religious or therapeutic settings. When occurring at a time and place selected for the benefit of the individual who has chosen to confess, to whom to confess, and what to confess, they can be most beneficial. But interrogation and torture, as acts of communicational rape, can subsequently interfere with needed, desired, wholesome confession.

America's noisy rediscovery of death has so often illustrated denial by acceptance and ignores, in almost its entire literature, the fact that psychology and history are both primarily about humanity's attempts to deal with (literally, for there is dealing to be done, deals to be made) several archetypal horrors of life (not just one). Death, the fact that life ends, and always will, is just one pain. The fact that it hurts, and always will, is another. Cruelty and evil, the fact that they will hurt you because someone else *wants* you to suffer, are other pains. Meaninglessness, the fact that it might be all for nothing, all nonsense, all worthless, is one more.

Many people have wrestled with the death problem. Victor Frankl and others have dealt with the problem of meaninglessness. Frankl, the meta-Pollyanna, avoids the very real possibility that the truth may be that there is, indeed no meaning whatsoever, except what we invent in order to console ourselves; metaphysical comforters to suck on when times get hard. It is not just denial of death that occurs but denial of meaninglessness. Why *should* life have meaning? I would like it to but there is no inescapable need for life to oblige me. One could, instead, consider Sartre's merciless view: "All existing things are born for no reason, continue through weakness and die by accident . . . It is meaningless that we are born; it is meaningless that we die" (Sartre, 1965). Frankl's writings, in an oddly elitist and uncaring way, are very literally careless about those who cannot emulate his noble discovery of meaningfulness in the dirt of life: if they cannot manage his mode of denial, then he seems to deny their grief.

That people can discover transcendent meanings in terrible circumstances is undeniable and ancient knowledge. Frankl's work is stubbornly flawed: the texts shamelessly play to the emotions (oddly undignified for a philosopher); they are extraordinarily repetitive (I have never read a new Frankl book without wondering why it felt as if I had read it before), contain proclamations rather than developed arguments, and a poorly developed therapy that does *not* connect to his themes. Although claiming to be secular, they are actually very religiose. They are so tirelessly self-aggrandizing, boastful, so busy name-dropping, filled with incessant self-citation, so carefully reminding us of all the places he has lectured, his titles, his applause. He shows a curiously powerful need to do this, for a man who can claim what he claims.

My main objection, in relation to working with victims of traumatic stress, is that Frankl is so very authoritarian. He gives the patient his own meaning, like a blood transfusion, when the real challenge is to enable the patient to find his or her own true meaning. But he is right in one essential: it is not the pleasure principle that is primal, but the *meaning* principle. Pleasure does not give meaning, though meaning gives pleasure. Yet, in therapy, I prefer to explore *purpose*, rather than meaning. Purpose implies at least some sense of an agenda for activity, rather than the more passive and contemplative demand for meaning.

Far fewer authors in the clinical sciences have ever grappled with the problems of pain and cruelty and evil. But the torture victim is forced to confront them all: definitively cruel and evil, meaningless pain at risk of death. The victim has to find an immediate way to survive in the face of undeniable evidence of the rotten core of life; to discover during the experience of torture, some workable and acute accommodation with central problems of existence which the world's sages, working at leisure and in comfort, over the centuries, have failed to handle.

The view that Sigmund Freud and others have propagated, that man cannot imagine his own death, is nonsense and is the product of a very stunted vision. Ludwig Wittgenstein understood these matters far better than Freud. I can envision my own death: surely many of us can. Yes, I cannot be certain exactly how it will occur: nevertheless, growing experience of life has taught me more and more examples of how it might occur. Yes, I cannot imagine what being dead will feel like: not through any failure to attain any achievable vision of that, but because being dead will be like nothing, and not like anything: it is not a human failure, but a logical trick. Whatever I might imagine, would be something—and that, failing to be nothing, would not be like death at all.

I believe American writers have greatly exaggerated the universality of survivor guilt. Undoubtedly, it is frequent and miserable; but it is not universal. It is absent in very many traumatized survivors. Sometimes this is because the circumstances of the trauma did not encourage it. Where, for example, an innocent is picked up mistakenly, and tortured to reveal information that he or she does not have, there may not be material to form a realistic basis of survivor guilt; and there may not be enough neurotic grounds for forming inappropriate guilt. Also, the formulation of *survivor guilt* may depend significantly on the individual's worldview and cultural philosophy. If one considers all events, good and bad, as intended by God or Fate, and meant to be our lot in a fatalist sense, then survival may be seen as equally intended, and no grounds whatever for guilt. I wonder whether the American ethos, which avoids intellectual dialectic in favor of a highly activist physical dialectic with life, expecting an active struggling with life, and wresting a good result out of any circumstances, may not be more at risk for survivor guilt for failing to overcome the bad buys, for failing to save one's buddies. If one does not necessarily expect to vanquish the forces of evil, or to be able to save everyone, there is far less opportunity for guilt.

And it is survivor guilt we talk of, related to a perceived failure to meet inner expectations, not survivor shame, which would relate to a perceived failure to meet community and societal expectations. This, too, is a possible outcome, but one that has so far been ignored.

Guilt may be a most unpleasant experience, but it may be preferable to the feeling of powerlessness, of being unable to influence events at all. It can represent an attempt to regain perceived controllability, because it requires the postulate that one could have acted otherwise, that one could by one's own effort have produced a different outcome. I made a similar point in my earlier work (Simpson, 1979, p. 244) on grief and the malignant chorus of "if only's": "If only I had . . ."; "If only I hadn't. . . ."

Sometimes the survivors feel called upon to show bravado and devotion to the struggle, but not fear or signs of damage: there may not be social support for those natural responses. Guilt may be seen while in custody as being unable to care for the family—separation guilt, a companion to *separation anxiety*.

Traumatic stresses shake multiple relationships, rarely comprehensively explored in the literature or in therapy with the victim: one's relationship with oneself, with one's closest relationships, with one's community, with society at large, and with God and the universe. The encounter with torture shows us that some things can be just too big to mourn. There is not just self-blame, but God-blame, or universe-blame.

Anger can be a common reaction, and a more healthy one than the numbness and withdrawal, one more easily converted into constructive engagement in a continuing future existence. While I am angry, I am not dead. On the other hand, captivity provides such a vivid experience of impotence that sexual problems are quite common, especially impotence and premature ejaculation.

There may be a very well-based mistrust of others. This attitude can be based on one's experience of how deceptively cruel others can be; but also on a realistic assessment of the true motivations of some of the eager helpers. In the old phrase, the need of the cow to give suck may be greater than that of the calf to drink. Many helpers are primarily driven by their own agendas; and this may be more obvious to the survivor who has had to learn to be more acute in assessing others than to colleagues.

Lifton (1976, 1983) has written of how survivors of the Hiroshima atomic bomb could find fulfillment in working for peace, and some Holocaust survivors, in working for the formation of the State of Israel. An alternative response is the *disinvestment* policy: never trust anyone again, never care about anything. This is not merely psychic numbing, which it is often mistaken for; it can be a logical damage-control, damage-limitation policy. After severely traumatic experiences, investing in loving relationships and caring about anything make oneself once again a hostage to horror, again vulnerable to traumatic breach of these relationships. Choosing to maintain a minimal and autonomous internal psychic economy may reduce vulnerability. The cost of that strategy, of course, is that it may effectively protect one against the loss of love in the future, by imposing an absence of love in the present; it may protect one against a future loss of faith in communal values by choosing not to share any common values forever. As Paul Tillich (1952) said of neurosis, this can be "the way of avoiding non-being by avoiding being."

It is not just the survivor's own numbing and denial that cause problems. As one sees on a smaller scale in the griefs of normal bereavement, if no one will truly listen and hear what one tells of one's awful experience, one cannot let it rest. One must keep it alive until it has been recognized by others. If others deny it and ignore it, then the survivor may feel far more compelled to keep the embers burning. One factor that may have made traumatic stresses more damaging in this century has been the loss, to a very significant degree, of shared ceremonies that symbolize the social recognition and acknowledgment of what has happened and of its importance for society; of continuity of values, of defiance of wickedness rather than compliance with evil. Modern society babbles with inane statements, in word and symbol, perpetuating the trivial; while it has become strangely inarticulate, verbally and symbolically, and unable to signify the significant.

For the tortured and the victims of state repression, of course, there can be the added factor that there will be no monuments, no commemoration. A cunning refinement of evil that has become common has been the explicit methods for rendering this impossible: repressors now take very great care to ban the symbols and to make the remembrance as difficult as possible. With the "dis-appeared," there is, deliberately, no certainty as to their fate, no body to bury, no specific place to commemorate them. Governments which fear ideas, often from an instinctive realization of the extremity of the poverty of their own imaginations, take great care not just to physically remove dissidents, but to ban their words and ideas from public availability. The South African Government, for example, even gave itself the power to "ban" someone beyond death: forbidding the publication of any of a dissident's words, or the possession of any publication containing those words; it could not only lock up important leaders, but ban even the printing of pictures or likenesses of them. Such forms of psychological and social repression can significantly impair the ability of individuals and communities to recover from traumatic losses. However, they can also render those very banned symbols more powerful icons of comfort and inspiration in all contacts that escape the bannings.

Some individuals may be diminished by the attempt to live safely in a malicious world. There is a serial amputation of human potentials; cut off this, cut off that, hedge oneself in with safeties and precautions, a sort of spiritual shrinkage. As they get more limited, the fear grows, for it is fear of the unknown. And when you avoid personal growth, the unknown grows. Freedom will be of little help to them, for when it comes, they may have forgotten what to do with it.

There has been a shift in the technology of torture, from the torture chamber with awful, specialized instruments to the abusive use of simple daily objects: a broomstick, a pencil, water, a knitted hat, a motor tire inner tube, a plastic bucket or soda bottle, car battery jump leads, and wet cloths. Now, common daily objects have been treacherous, with much scope for generalization of cues for fear. With malignant creativity, the South African government devised "house arrest," a sort of privatization of repression, in which the individual was placed, within very severe restrictions, forcing the detainee and his family to be his jailers.

Traumatic experiences also shatter some of life's protective delusions. For example, Perloff (1983, 1987) and others (Langer, 1975; Schlenker, 1987; Snyder & Ford, 1987) have written of the illusion of unique invulnerability which nonvictims hold, believing themselves to be far less likely to be the victims of unfortunate events than others, and greatly underestimating the actual risks of such occurrences. These illusions may increase a sense of safety and comfort, but can be dangerous in that they enhance a tendency to ignore appropriate and needed protective and preventive behavior. As Perloff's review (1987) showed, people underestimate the probability of natural disasters, the frequency of mortal diseases and their own risks of contracting them, their chances of being involved in automobile accidents, or to be victims of crime. It is not just that they underestimate the menaces of life, but that people see themselves, personally, as less likely to suffer such misfortunes than other people. Similarly, there is an "illusion of control" over random events, or an exaggerated belief in one's ability to control chance outcomes (e.g., Langer, 1975). Such beliefs contribute to the unjust blaming of innocent victims for their misfortune.

Lerner (1980; Lerner & Miller, 1978) posited the *just world theory*, according to which, people believe in a fair and orderly world in which people get what they deserve, and deserve what they get; a world in which bad things do not happen to good people. Trauma and torture seriously damaged these comforting beliefs.

Yalom (1980) illustrated this when he wrote of his own experience after a head-on automobile collision.

> The world seemed precarious. It had lost, for me, its hominess: danger seemed everywhere. The nature of reality shifted, as I experienced what Heidegger called "uncanniness" (*Unheimlich*)—the experience of "not being at home in the world" which he considered (and to which I can attest) a typical consequence of death awareness.

See also Heidegger (1962).

Problems with DSM-III-R in Relation to Torture Victims

One problem has arisen several times when torture victims have attempted to establish the nature of their psychiatric injuries in South African courts. Some people, mistakenly, assume that in diagnosing PTSD, one must assess the severity of the stressor as an abstract concept, and in relation to the assessor's guess as to how severely it would affect the mythical "average person" absolutely ignoring any aspect relating to the vulnerabilities of the individual involved. This is nonsense and should not be required by any criteria. The confusion may arise in regard to the introductory section on the use of the DSM-III-R (American Psychiatric Association, 1987), which discusses the severity of psychosocial stressors for Axis IV. This is not in reference to diagnosing PTSD but causes problems when it is read in that context.

The DSM-III-R is surely in error, however, where it says that even "though a specific stressor may have a greater impact on a person who is especially vulnerable . . . the rating should be based on the severity of the stressor itself, not on the person's vulnerability to the particular stressor." Presumably, the intention in proposing such a rating method for this particular axis is to attempt to make an abstract and general, mock-"objective" measure of the overall extent of stresses the individual faced, temporarily ignoring the interaction between these and the individual, so as to subsequently consider this specific relation.

It is inevitably an artificial and false exercise, however. It pretends to a degree of objectivity that cannot be achieved. It is believable that a clinician can, with useful accuracy, assess how a particular person experienced particular stressors, and how severe such stressors were for that individual. But, realistically, what actually happens if we try to apply the Axis IV guidelines? The assessor elicits how this particular person experienced a specific stressful occasion, an account inevitably and inescapably shaped by that individual's experience and vulnerability; then tries to extract from it an allowance for that person's vulnerabilities and personal characteristics; then tries to imagine how severely some fantasized "average person" would be affected; and derives an idea of how severe the stressor was. No one ever assesses an

"average person": we only, ever, assess specific individuals. What is pretending to be an objective assessment becomes a projective test for the assessor. The more assessors try to ignore the person before them, and to invent this average person, the more likely it is that the result will represent the imagination and fantasy of the assessor.

There are other large objections to this phoney exercise. Bizarrely, the DSM-III-R asks us to rate the stress that would be felt by this "average person" in similar circumstances and with similar sociocultural values. Thus, while trying to ignore the actual person's vulnerability, one should attend to the "circumstances" and "sociocultural values" of that person. This is simply silly.

Above all, stressors simply do not, ever, exist in the abstract. The events might exist independently, but not as a stressor. If, for example, a rocket goes out of control and explodes in the middle of the desert, it might cause a massive explosion. But it would not be a stressor (except perhaps for some passing lizards, such as rarely consult psychiatrists). If no one was stressed, it was not a stressor. If suitable instrumentation was at hand, the severity of the event could be measured in many ways: the loudness of the bang could be measured in decibels; one could measure the earth movement caused, in centimeters of displacement, or in kilograms of earth; the brightness of the flash as so many candela, and so on. But the only instrument capable of assessing its severity as a stressor would be a human being, with vulnerabilities, and warts, and all, and in terms of stress we can consider how the event affected the affected person: the litmus paper of psychological stress. Trying to remove the real, genuine people, in their totality, from the stress assessment is like removing the litmus from the paper. What the DSM-III-R proposes in this specific regard is Zen exercise, like measuring the noise of one hand clapping, or the sound of a tree falling in an uninhabited forest.

This is obviously relevant to PTSD, and the context in which we are considering it in this chapter. As Curran (1988) pointed out, with reference to a terrorist bombing: "a vulnerable person at home five miles away, hearing the same explosion or even watching it on television news, might react more adversely psychologically than some 18-year-old male who thoroughly enjoys the excitement." There is no pathology in which an external stressor is the sole determinant of outcome, regardless of the strengths and weaknesses of its recipient.

The most disgusting way in which the DSM-III-R can be abused is seen when, as in the Cele case (Simpson, 1989a) a person was detained without trial, held in solitary confinement for months, interrogated for lengthy periods, and eventually produced a confession. When in court facing the resultant charges, he repudiated the confession, saying that he had been tortured. There was some supporting evidence supporting his story. On careful clinical examination, he had all the features of PTSD, and met the DSM-III-R criteria, and the defense psychiatrist made that diagnosis. A psychiatrist working for the South African State insisted that it was impossible to make the diagnosis: because, he argued, one cannot ever diagnose PTSD unless there is "objective, collateral proof" of the existence of the stressor (a requirement invented by him, and so very convenient to hide the effects of torture). This cynical and false proposition would mean that PTSD could only be diagnosed in victims of torture and rape, with the consent and assistance of the torturer and the rapist. He also argued, abusing the criteria with regard to the stressor, that solitary confinement and incommunicado detention of indefinite duration were not severe enough to meet Criterion A.

The DSM-III-R definitions of the characteristics of the stressor are empty hypotheses with insufficient data to support them, and are based on too little experience of too limited a range of trauma. As regards the attempt to ignore vulnerability, no other mental or physical insult to the human being is assessed thus. Is someone's leg any the less broken because a fall from the same height would not have broken the leg of *most* average people, and, thus, was not "outside the range" of human falls?

The apparent distinction between the so-called objective definition of trauma that concentrates on the characteristics of the event alone, as artificially opposed to the "subjective" definition that encompasses predisposing and other factors is phony. The so-called objective measure is merely disguised subjectivity. Are we to measure the likely psychopathological impact of an earthquake on a human being by using the Richter scale?

Third-Order Premises

Watzlawick, Beavin, and Jackson (1968) made a usable distinction between First-Order knowledge (direct sense experience), Second-Order knowledge (meta-knowledge about objects), and Third-Order knowledge, which is of still higher abstraction, dealing with the attribution of levels of meaning to the environment. One of the essential tasks of development is to evolve third-order premises about existence and the characteristics of the universe in which one exists. Damage to these third-order premises, violations of the sense of meaning of the world one has adopted, can be profoundly disruptive. This is what Friedrich Nietzsche meant when he said that he who has a *why* of living will endure almost any *how*. To go further than Nietzsche, one must add that if one loses the *why* of living, almost any *how* can be overwhelming.

Human beings have great difficulty surviving psychologically in a world that does not behave as their third-order premises predict, a world which now seems senseless; a world such as that in which one experiences torture.

Gollwitzer (1956) showed, as reflected in final messages and letters, that prisoners condemned by the Nazis for various political crimes varied in their responses. Those who were able to feel that their actions had served to help to defeat the evil regime, managed to face death with some calm and even serenity. The most desperate anguish was seen in those who had received the death sentence for such pathetic offenses as listening to an Allied radio broadcast, or making some improper comment about Hitler. As Watzlawick *et al.* (1968) commented: "Their deaths were apparently a violation of a significant third-order premise: that one's death should

be meaningful and not petty." The torture victim faces just such a ridiculous, absurd death; just such a rape of third-order premises.

A Kuhnian Model: The Maimed Paradigm

We each have a personal theory of the construction of reality; an internal model of reality, its structure and conduct; a cohesive set of assumptions and expectations about who we are and how the world works, which influences our planning and behavior, as it shapes our decisions as to how we will act, and how we expect the world to respond. Generally speaking, such a set of assumptions are shaped by our experiences (as well as shaping them). People vary as to how stable, how resistant or susceptible to change this is. Parkes (1971, 1975) called this one's "assumptive world"; Marris (1975), similarly, spoke of "structures of meaning"; and Bowlby (1969) of "world models." Horowitz (1983) has provided a somewhat similar model, though its terminology is rather clumsy.

It is illuminating to apply to the field of traumatic stress a model analogous to Kuhn's model of the nature and progress of science (Kuhn, 1962). In "normal life" (analogous to "normal science" in his model) the regular daily conduct of life is based on the internal paradigm, the set of primal postulates, which the individual accepts (some consciously, some unconsciously) as a basis for continuing life. These define the legitimate problems and methods, as in Kuhn's model. But, unlike Kuhn's model, these are ultimately individual and internal, though many elements of them may be shared by a community, like those discussed above. They are regularly and routinely tested and confirmed in social exchanges with others, which is why the social isolation of solitary confinement can be so disturbing: just when the individual faces unusual challenges and stresses, he is denied access to the community with whom he shares paradigms. Who then could assist in the fabrication of an amended model to enable the individual to cope with this new and strenuous challenge?

Such a model can be fractured by trauma, which requires, insists upon, major revisions of most such models. Predictions (and their underlying assumptions) that prove alarmingly wrong are abandoned or modified in the light of the results. Minor adjustments are common; a major paradigm shift is rarer. Indeed, it is a valid definition of traumatic stress to view it as stress severe enough for the individual to require very major revision of this internal belief set, such as cannot be rapidly achieved. This drastic revision leaves a pile of *paradigms lost*.

These models are mental maps, ways of seeing, organizing principles, very like Kuhn's (1962) paradigms. Developing such a paradigm is unavoidable. In fact, the process is highly analogous to Kuhn's model of how science functions. Within our set of paradigms, we can conduct the "normal science" of normal life, and it works; and we can tolerate a fair number or degree of failures or contradictions. When the cumulative weight of these becomes burdensome, or when the challenge is too overwhelming to be managed in the regular way (following an awful lot of little awfulnesses, or one massively nasty event), the system must change rapidly and radically. In this psychic equivalent to a Kuhnian scientific "revolution" a radical revision is forced on us.

Most of us can (and must) tolerate living with a worldview that contains inconsistencies, even contradictory elements, so long as we refrain from examining the model too closely, and while circumstances do not require us to try to rely on incompatible elements at the same time. Kuhn writes of "anomalies," which "call into question explicit and fundamental generalizations of the paradigm." These can lead to crises (trauma is the crisis), which lead to revolutions, and then to a new paradigm. PTSD represents an unresolved revolution, in which no new paradigm has been found. Such a model, I submit, is more useful than the rather pneumatic simplified "stress" and analytic models.

Trauma leads to a disruption and instability of the paradigm. We are rarely directly aware of the assumptions of the model: they are like the lenses in my spectacles. They let me see the world much more clearly, though I cannot be directly aware of how they affect what I see. Crisis is induced by events that do not and cannot fit, yet which cannot be ignored or denied, and which demand accommodation. Trauma shatters the illusory assumptions, the functional illusions, of individual invulnerability, of a basically benign universe, of meaningfulness, and of self-worth, as discussed above.

Attempting very large-scale change of one's paradigm needs to be relatively slow and gradual. The challenge is similar to that of managing major structural changes to a hospital, while maintaining its usual services. While core revisions are being made, one must maintain a structural capacity for continuing normal functions, and retain an ability to handle new traumata while work is in progress. As Janoff-Bulman and Frieze (1983) said, denial "provides for the proper pacing in the revision and rebuilding" of one's basic theories and assumptions. The challenge is to maintain balance; to allow access to enough of the task to allow timeous and efficient completion of it, but in installments that are not so large as to encompass overwhelming anxiety.

Hope is an intermediate, postulated new model. Usually highly favorable, pleasant, and unrealistic, this postulate is not usually achievable in any detail, but it does not need to be, for it serves as a most valuable navigation aid in charting a course from the ruins to the future. It is a template for a new, functional paradigm, setting the direction of desired positive outcomes. "Hope is the search for a future good of some kind, and depends on the knowledge and belief that there is an alternative, preferable, reachable situation or state" (Simpson, 1982).

Trauma is uncomfortable but can be fruitful. Crises may be a necessary precondition for the emergence of novel and creative models. One is, as a result, genuinely sadder but wiser. The change we are discussing here is truly revolutionary. Just as political revolutions, in Kuhn's words (1962), "aim to change political institutions in ways that those institutions themselves prohibit," after normal politics has failed to resolve the crisis; so massive psychological trauma changes our view of the world in ways which that worldview prohibits.

Such paradigm change causes us to see the world differently: we see things we have not seen before, both by looking in new places, in new ways, and by seeing things newly even where one had looked before. Once one has achieved this major shift, there is an enormous amount of work to do, a great many revisions to be made to the previous schemata, and a large amount of necessary discovery of new implications of the new formulation.

It is ironical that even if there were any validity in the criticisms mounted in works like Lakatos and Musgrave (1970), Kuhn's concepts may apply more effectively in our field than in his own!

Aspects of Therapy with Torture Victims

The torture victim has learned three awful things: about themselves (Such things can happen to me); about other people (They can do such things to me); and about the world (It can let such things happen: no one cares enough to stop it). Torture is like being a murder victim, but being murdered slowly, while you watch and wait.

Therapy needs to be a sort of antitorture, or countercoercion. In planning a therapeutic approach for the torture victim, one should recognize the forms of stressors and coercion which were used to damage them, and plan interventions so as to reverse the damaging effects that were so deliberately created. The torture victim is not simply showing generic responses to generic stress, special perhaps only in its extent. Although there are notable similarities in responses, both in the form of PTSD and of other traumatic stress disorders, there are also relevant particularities in the relation between the type of deliberate stresses used and the individual's vulnerabilities.

Damage was caused in the horridly intimate relationship between torturer and victim, in the closely calibrated cruelty which matched the person's weaknesses, fears, and sensitivities. From the victim's account of the methods used, one can better understand what psychic wounds are likely to need care. If one considers some of the coercive and damaging forces listed above, matching therapeutic issues are apparent. For example, several of the pressures are designed to induce a habit of compliance with the captor. Subsequently, the patient may be unreliable about keeping appointments and obligations, and may need help to develop independence and a creative capacity for noncompliance. This requires the freedom to be compliant when it is functional, because if one is automatically, reflexly, noncompliant with regard to others' wishes, one is just as totally controlled by others as when one is wholly, automatically compliant. Freedom lies in the independence that allows you to make the best choice for yourself, whether or not it is what someone else wants.

Those characteristics of the experience that forced the individual to view resistance as futile can be profoundly convincing lessons in *learned helplessness*. In therapy, this needs to be worked with to help the victim reexperience personal efficacy and empowerment. Victims often need assistance in rediscovering motivations other than pure survival, and in regaining normal hopefulness. Threats, fears, and the infliction of physical pain often leave the individual, even those who do not show all the features of PTSD, with acute psychological and even physiological reactivity to situations which directly, partly, or symbolically recall the original traumata. Many aspects of the usual processes of assessment, investigation, hospitalization, and therapy may stir highly disturbing reexperiencing of earlier terror. Patients may be highly sensitive to small rooms, mysterious equipment, people in uniforms, and to being questioned. I find it important to be flexible and open to novel settings for assessment and counseling; working on the beach, at a hotel, in a park, or in settings free of interfering connotations.

The degradation and humiliation inflicted on the victim may have severely impaired self-esteem, and particular care must be taken to assist in the rebuilding of the damaged self-image. Physical exhaustion and debility may require medical attention, or simply rest. Those especially affected by the unpredictability of the traumatic experience may need help regarding tolerance of ambiguity, and realistic management of their need for clarity. Quite apart from the emotional numbing which may be induced by such experiences, victims who have spent extended periods in situations in which any expression of their true emotions may endanger them or attract fresh torment may have derived the lesson: "Try not to bleed, but if you must, bleed internally"—and may show a persistent inhibition of the expression of emotions and responses, which can need assistance.

It is important to clarify that whatever the victim did was a normal response to a highly abnormal situation. Validate the victim's views not merely by one's own expertise, but by the victim's unique expertise. I find it useful to use an element of *paradoxical intention*, by drawing attention to the fact that the goals of torture were to induce precisely the sort of symptoms from which the victim is suffering. Framing the symptoms as being desired by the torturer recruits resistance to the symptoms. It is important to form a shared purpose to gain control over the symptoms as a means of gaining a lasting victory over those who sought to damage us. Otherwise, there is a significant risk of the adoption of a new life role as victim, as weak and damaged goods, deserving special handling in perpetuity. One sees, after many different varieties of traumatic stress, people who adopt a life career as supervictim, a role which can seriously maim the individual's remaining experience of life.

Dreams are relevant, not jut as potential symbols of other matters, but as valid reflections of the objective or subjective reality of the traumatic experiences. Dream management and rescripting, with the mutual drafting of new endings to the nightmares, providing either ridiculous endings (which remove the power of the images) or endings that exemplify positive coping, is remarkably effective.

Survival work is like grief work; it is essential, sustaining, and reoperative work that needs to be done urgently and at a time when one's personal resources are minimal. One should adapt the principles of *grief counseling* as follows:

1. Help the survivor actualize the experience, realize how much and how little it means, and to bear witness to what happened.

2. Help the survivor to identify and express feelings and fantasies related to what happened.
3. Assist the survivor to live *despite* what has happened.
4. Facilitate decathexis and withdrawal of emotional centering on the events, and reinvestment in life.
5. Provide time and space for grief work and healing.
6. Interpret the survivor's normal behavior and responses as normal.
7. Allow for individual differences, and do not require the survivor to follow some specific model or sequence of recovery.
8. Provide continuing support, as and when required.
9. Identify and enhance the survivor's coping styles.
10. Recognize substantial pathology when it occurs and refer appropriately.

Note the form of the words used in the above. I am concerned by the impression given in some of the very scanty literature on the treatment of torture victims (perhaps because of a faulty translation) of authoritarian forcefulness in therapy. For example, I became uneasy when Ortmann, Genefke, Jakobsen, and Lunde (1987) wrote: "We seek to make the client recall and describe all the details"; and, later "his resistance must be broken down." Similarly, Somnier and Genefke (1986) said: "The victim must describe precisely what he experienced," must fully understand and accept," and "humiliations must be discussed point for point." This sounds so much like what the interrogator was demanding! One absolutely must not imitate the methods of the interrogator, however pure we believe our motives to be. Some of the resistance to talking to the therapist is because it is so similar to what the interrogator or torturer demanded. The therapist must not reassault the victim. Victims in therapy must not be "musted": they are suffering from the "musts" of others.

Adaptation requires a reevaluation of the traumatic experience, placing it in perspective. It will not be forgotten, but needs to be detoxified. As Somnier and Genefke (1986) effectively expressed it: "Forgetting is not the answer; nor is atonement through obsessive remembering." In the related phenomenon of pathological grief reactions (Simpson, 1979), one encounters people who preserve the room and belongings of the dead individual as a shrine, in a type of social embalming which has been called "mummification." Similarly, there is a risk that the torture victim may be left preoccupied with unproductive cyclic recall of the events.

Apart from specific techniques and interventions, in a very acute sense, the relationship is the therapy. It is so important for the victim of deliberate cruelty to be able to have a benign relationship with someone strong enough to accept the burden of hearing about the awful events. Once the trauma of torture has impressed upon you the tragic truths that there are no powerful rescuers who can protect you, and that there is no safe place, externally or internally, where you can hide from horror, the formation of a therapeutic alliance can be complicated by alternation between unrealistic pessimism and difficulty in trusting another, and by unrealistic expectations. The therapist needs to provide empathy and sympathy but not sentimentality.

There have been relatively few published accounts of specific therapies for torture victims. Larsen (1988) (and Larsen & Pagadian-Lopez, 1987) wrote of using muscle relaxation for the relief of physical and psychological symptoms that had a prompt effect still apparent 3 months later. Lyons and Keane (1989) described "implosive therapy," exposing the patient to trauma-related cues until there is a reduction in the associated anxiety. Although I have not called it implosive therapy, I first used that technique in 1977, in similar cases. I used deconditioning, systematic desensitization, and abreaction with imaginal flooding. There are studies suggesting the value of such techniques, but with extremely small numbers of subjects; far more data are needed. Jacobsen and Vesti (1989) described interdisciplinary treatment (an impractical luxury in many situations, but ideal), including psychotherapy (they overemphasize guilt), physiotherapy, somatic treatment, social counseling, work with spouses and children, and nursing care.

Lister (1982) reviewed the implications of the victim's forced silence about the event, where some explicit or implicit threats prohibit such communication. This can leave the individual unable to discuss or work through the pain; both conscious and subliminal recall of it may be rendered unshareable, unacknowledged. Where the victim has internalized the image of the torturer, he may be left with a twisted sense of obligation, binding him to his tormentor, with a fear that the real trauma may return if he betrays the confidential obligation of his betrayal.

There is often a strongly felt need to prove what happened. It is awful to be the victim of a secret Apocalypse, which no one else will believe was real. Cienfuegos and Morelli (1983) emphasized the concept of testimony so as to provide a detailed account for others to know of what happened. There is also the need to prove it, to convince others that it happened, to bear witness to what happened to those who cannot tell of it (being dead or still detained). Cienfuegos and Monelli (1983) used a formal technique, in which the testimony of a patient's account of experiences is taperecorded and turned into a jointly written document. We use that too, without the tape phase, to help someone to speak the unspeakable, and to bear witness for those who did not survive. Where there can be a trial, testifying may also be therapeutic. This testimony is the confession the torturer did not want, a denunciation rather than a betrayal, as Cienfuegos and Monelli pointed out.

When reviewing the experience, there can be difficulties with the mereness of words; the experience of torture drives one back, regressively, beyond language. Some clients find it easier to depict the experience in art, or to write about it: though not necessarily so, where the interrogator used "forced writing," the technique whereby the victim is required to write lengthy confessions and accounts of his life story, which are then abused and torn up, and he is instructed to start again.

The victims are often resistant to follow-up. This may be for reasons of personal safety. In South Africa, for instance, the Security Police have shown much unwholesome interest in the identity of ex-detainees who receive assistance. They may not be able to afford to travel to appointments. They may be re-detained. This has led to a need for single-session approaches. For many reasons, rapport is not always easy to achieve. Understandably there are suspicions and the reality of police informers and harassment which may mean that both therapist and client may be at risk and may have realistic difficulties in trusting each other that are not purely psychodynamic in origin. This additional, poorly studied range of factors I call "under-the-counter transference." One can hardly be value-free in the face of repression. If you attempt it, you are seen as yet another part of the repression or an ignorant fool. Talking cures are unfamiliar to many victims and need careful explanation.

Countertransference problems have been largely ignored in the literature on torture, though two papers are especially relevant. Haley (1974) in a classic study of Vietnam veterans wrote of cases in which a patient reports atrocities, and where the patient can frighten or repulse the therapist, and arouse retaliatory impulses. Danieli (1984) wrote of the complexities of countertransference in treating Holocaust victims, including such issues as "bystander's guilt" in which the therapist feels guilt for having escaped such experiences and views the survivor as a hero. The therapist's impulse is to be a liberator or savior, with a feeling of privileged voyeurism at access to such stories, and rage against the perpetrators of such suffering.

In some circumstances, there is an additional complication in that the therapist or counselor may be personally at risk simply for providing aid to the torture victim. The realistic possibility that one might be subjected to similar maltreatment because one is conducting therapy with the patient is an element that needs exploration.

Racial issues are usually not difficult to deal with in the South African setting (except where the therapist is racist) because the sincere and predominant attitude among the majority of the people is nonracial. Also, though the system responsible for their misery is "white," the state has generally used paired white and black police in handling detainees, so that a white therapist does not necessarily arouse unpleasant echoes of those responsible for the patient's grief.

Whereas various authors have described the situation of the older victim of the Holocaust, and the secondary effects on the younger generation, I see the reverse. In the South African situation, the younger generation has been, preponderantly, the victims; and it is the older, parental generation that shows the secondary effects. Not infrequently, the effect of the martyrdom or victimization of the child has been a radicalization of the parents (often very conservative people originally) and a move toward the parents' sharing their child's ideals and joining the struggle. This deserves more study.

Finally, I must emphasize the need for more imaginative and creative responses to comprehending and assisting those of our fellows who have suffered what Martin Buber called a "wound in the order of Being." It is the arts, rather than the sciences, that have made the most acute comments.

We must remember, and require our societies to remember, that while any nation may wish to maintain law and order, this is done not for its own sterile sake but so as to preserve the liberty and freedom of the individual. And the laws of humanity are the very first of those which must be upheld, to preserve order, above all, between the human ears and within our soul. If ever, in the pursuit of justice and security, we promote injustice and insecurity, we defeat our own ends. If to defend ourselves against what we see as an enemy, we adopt the methods of an enemy, we damage our own society and become our own enemy.

Those of us who have been privileged to work with torture victims have learned of the freedom that men can seize from their captors. As Epictetus wrote:

I must die. I must be imprisoned. I must suffer exile. But must I die groaning? Must I whine as well? Can anyone hinder me from going into exile with a smile? The master threatens to chain me: but what say you? Chain Me? My leg you will chain—yes, but not my will—no, not even Zeus can conquer that.

We have also learned, some of us from personal experience, of how much can be created from the encounter with destruction. As Elie Wiesel wrote: "I know the paths of the soul, overgrown, often know only the night, a very vast, very barren night, without landscapes. And yet I tell you: we'll get out. The most glorious works of man are born of that night."

We must learn to blend the tools of scientific inquiry with the compassion of a fellow victim. As Wilfred Owen (1985), the poet who knew PTSD so intimately, wrote, we must not let ourselves be immune:

To Pity and whatever moans in man
Before the last sea and the hapless starts;
Whatever mourns when many leave these shores;
Whatever shares
The eternal reciprocity of tears.

References

Allodi, F., & Cowgill, G. (1982). Ethical and psychiatric aspects of torture: A Canadian study. *Canadian Journal of Psychiatry*, 27, 98–102.

American Psychiatric Association. (1987). *Diagnostic and statistical manual of mental disorders* (3rd ed., rev.). Washington, DC: Author.

Arendt, H. (1978). *Willing—the life of the mind: Vol. 2*. New York: Harcourt, Brace Jovanovich.

Astrom, C., Lunde, I., Ortmann, J., Boysen, G., & Trojaberg, W. (1989). Sleep disturbances in torture survivors. *Archives of Neurology of Scandinavia*, 79, 150–154.

Badia, P., Harsh, J., & Abbott, B. (1979). Choosing between predictable and unpredictable shock conditions: Data and theory. *Psychological Bulletin*, 86, 1107–1131.

Biderman, A. D., & Zimmer, H. (Eds.). (1961). *The manipulation of human behavior*. New York: Wiley.

Bok, S. (1984). *Secrets: On the ethics of concealment and revelation*. Oxford, England: Oxford University Press.

Bowlby, J. (1969). *Attachment and loss (Vol. 1): Attachment*. London: Hogarth Press.

Charlesworth, M. (1975). *The existentialists and Jean-Paul Sartre*. Brisbane, Australia: University of Queensland Press.

Cienfuegos, A. J., & Morelli, C. (1983). The testimony of political repression as a therapeutic instrument. *American Journal of Orthopsychiatry*, 53, 43–51.

Curran, P. S. (1988). Psychiatric aspects of terrorist violence: Northern Ireland, 1969–1987. *British Journal of Psychiatry*, 153, 470–475.

Danieli, Y. (1984). Psychotherapists' participation in the conspiracy of silence about the Holocaust. *Psychoanalytic Psychology*, 1(1), 23–42.

Davis, P. (1986). Medical problems of detainees: A review of 21 ex-detainees seen in the past two years in Johannesburg. In A. B. Zwi & L. D. Saunders (Eds.), *Towards health care for all: NAMDA Conference 1985* (pp. 15–18). Johannesburg, South Africa: National Medical and Dental Association.

DPSC, DESCOM. (1988). *A woman's place is in the struggle. Not behind bars*. Johannesburg: Federation of Transvaal Women.

Engdahl, B. H., & Eberly, R. E. (1990). The effects of torture and other captivity maltreatment: Implications for psychology. In P. Suedfeld (Ed.), *Psychology and torture*. Washington, DC: Hemisphere Publishing.

Faraone, S. V. (1990). Psychology's role in the campaign to abolish torture: Can individuals and organizations make a difference? In P. Suedfeld (Ed.), *Psychology and torture*. Washington, DC: Hemisphere Publishing.

Foster, D., Davis, D., & Sandler, D. (1987). *Detention and torture in South Africa: Psychological, legal and historical studies*. Capetown, South Africa: David Phillip.

Friedlander, R. I. (1988). Stress in detention. In *Stress: The modern scourge*. Johannesburg, South Africa.

Glass, D. C., & Singer, J. E. (1972). *Urban stress: Experiments on noise and social stressors*. New York: Academic Press.

Goffman, E. (1961). *Asylums: Essays on the social institution of mental patients and other inmates*. Chicago: Aldine.

Gollwitzer, H. (1956). *Dying we live: The final messages and records of the Resistance*. New York: Pantheon.

Group for the Advancement of Psychiatry. (1956). *Factors used to increase the susceptibility of individuals to forceful interrogation: Observations and experiments* (GAP Symposium No. 3). New York: GAP Publications Office.

Group for the Advancement of Psychiatry. (1957). *Methods of forceful indoctrination: Observations and interviews* (GAP Symposium No. 4). New York: GAP Publications Office.

Haley, S. A. (1974). When the patient reports atrocities: Specific treatment considerations of the Vietnam veteran. *Archives of General Psychiatry*, 30, 191–196.

Heidegger, M. (1962). *Being and time*. New York: Harper & Row.

Hepburn, R. (1965). Questions about the meaning of life. *Religious Studies*, 1, 125–140.

Hinkle, L. E. (1961). The physiological state of the interrogation subject as it affects brain function. In A. D. Biderman & H. Zimmer (Eds.), *The manipulation of human behavior* (pp. 19–50). New York: Wiley.

Horowitz, M. J. (1983). Psychological response to serious life events. In S. Breznitz (Ed.), *The denial of stress*. New York: International Universities Press.

Ignatieff, M. (1985, September 20). Torture's dead simplicity. *New Statesman*, pp. 24–26.

Jacobsen, L., & Vesti, P. (1989). Treatment of torture survivors and their families: The nurse's function. *International Nursing Review*, 36(3), 75–80.

Janoff-Bulman, R., & Frieze, I. H. (1983). A theoretical perspective for understanding reactions to victimization. *Journal of Social Issues, 39*, 1–17.

Janoff-Bulman, R., & Timko, C. (1987). Coping with traumatic life events: The role of denial in light of people's assumptive worlds. In C. R. Snyder & C. E. Ford (Eds.), *Coping with negative life events: Clinical and social psychological perspectives* (pp. 135–160). New York: Plenum Press.

Jung, C. G. (1963). *Memories, dreams, reflections.* London: Routledge & Kegan Paul.

Kahana, E., Kahana, B., Harel, Z., & Rosner, T. (1988). Coping with extreme trauma. In J. P. Wilson, Z. Harel, & B. Kahana (Eds.), *Human adaptation to extreme stress: From the Holocaust to Vietnam* (pp. 55–80). New York: Plenum Press.

Kinzie, J. D., & Boehnlein, J. J. (1989). Posttraumatic psychosis among Cambodian refugees. *Journal of Traumatic Stress, 2(2),* 185–198.

Kramer, H., & Sprenger, J. (1971). In M. Summers (Ed. and Trans.), *The Malleus Maleficarum of Heinrich Kramer and James Sprenger.* New York: Dover Publications. (Original work published 1486)

Kuhn, T. (1962). *The structure of scientific revolutions.* Chicago: University of Chicago Press.

Lakatos, I., & Musgrave, A. (Eds.). (1970). *Criticism and the growth of knowledge.* London, England: Cambridge University Press.

Langer, E. (1975). The illusion of control. *Journal of Personality and Social Psychology, 32,* 311–328.

Larsen, H. (1988). Stress-tension reduction program for torture victims. *International Newsletter on Treatment and Rehabilitation of Torture Victims, 1(1),* 4–5.

Larsen, H., & Pagadian-Lopez, J. (1987). Stress-tension reduction treatment of sexually tortured women: An exploratory study. *Journal of Sexual and Marital Therapy, 13,* 210–214.

Laufer, R. L., & Wolfe, M. (1977). Privacy as a concept and a social issue: A multidimensional developmental theory. *Journal of Social Issues, 33,* 29–36.

Lazarus, R. S. (1983). The costs and benefits of denial. In S. Breznitz (Ed.), *The denial of stress* (pp. 1–30). New York: International Universities Press.

Lefcourt, H. (1976). *Locus of control.* Hillsdale, N.J.: Lawrence Erlbaum.

Lermolo, E. (1955). *Face of a victim.* New York: Harper & Brothers.

Lerner, M. J. (1980). *The belief in a just world: A fundamental delusion.* New York: Plenum Press.

Lerner, M. J., & Miller, D. T. (1978). Just world research and the attribution process: Looking back and ahead. *Psychological Bulletin, 85,* 1030–1051.

Levi, P. (1987). *The doomed and the saved.* New York: Summit Books.

Lifton, R. J. (1976). *Death in life: The survivors of Hiroshima.* New York: Touchstone Books.

Lifton, R. J. (1983). *The broken connection: On death and the continuity of life.* New York: Basic Books.

Lister, E. D. (1982). Forced silence: A neglected dimension of trauma. *American Journal of Psychiatry, 139(7),* 872–876.

Lyons, J. A., & Keane, T. M. (1989). Implosive therapy for the treatment of combat-related PTSD. *Journal of Traumatic Stress, 2(2),* 137–152.

Margoulis, S. T. (Ed.). (1977). Privacy as a behavioral phenomenon. *Journal of Social Issues, 33,* 5–21.

Marris, P. (1975). *Loss and change.* Garden City, NY: Anchor Doubleday.

Melamed, B., Melamed, J. L., & Bouhoutsos, J. (1990). Psychological consequences of torture: A need to formulate new strategies of research. In P. Suedfeld (Ed.), *Psychology and torture.* Washington, DC: Hemisphere Publishing.

Ortmann, J., Genefke, I. K., Jakobsen, L., & Lunde, I. (1987). Rehabilitation of torture victims: An interdisciplinary treatment model. *American Journal of Social Psychiatry, 8(3),* 161–167.

Owen, W. (1985). *The poems of Wilfred Owen* (J. Stallworthy, Ed.). London: Hogarth Press.

Parkes, C. M. (1971). Psychosocial transitions: A field for study. *Social Science and Medicine, 5,* 101–115.

Parkes, C. M. (1975). What becomes of redundant world models? A contribution to the study of adaptation to change. *British Journal of Medical Psychology, 48,* 131–137.

Perloff, L. S. (1983). Perceptions of vulnerability to victimization. *Journal of Social Issues, 39,* 41–61.

Perloff, L. S. (1987). Social comparison and illusions of invulnerability to negative life events. In C. R. Snyder & C. E. Ford (Eds.), *Coping with negative life events: Clinical and social psychological perspectives* (pp. 217–242). New York: Plenum Press.

Pervin, L. A. (1963). The need to predict and control under conditions of threat. *Journal of Experimental Psychology, 31,* 570–585.

Petersen, C., & Seligman, M. E. P. (1983). Learned helplessness and victimization. *Journal of Social Sciences, 2,* 103–116.

Phares, J. (1976). *Locus of control in personality.* Morristown, NJ: General Learning Press.

Piaget, J. (1959). *The language and thought of the child.* London: Routledge & Kegan Paul.

Rasmussen, O. V., & Lunde, I. (1980). Evaluations of investigation of 200 torture victims. *Danish Medical Bulletin, 27,* 241–243.

Rayner, M. (1987). *Turning a blind eye? Medical accountability and the prevention of torture in South Africa.* Washington, DC: Committee on Scientific Freedom and Responsibility, American Association for the Advancement of Science.

Rotter, J. (1966). Generalized expectancies for internal vs. external control of reinforcement. *Psychological Monographs, 80(1,* Whole No. 609).

Sargant, W. (1957). *Battle for the mind.* London: William Heinemann.

Sartre, J. P. (1958). Introduction. In H. Alley, *The question.* New York: John Calder.

Scarry, E. (1985). *The body in pain: The making and unmaking of the world.* New York: Oxford University Press.

Schachter, S. (1959). *The psychology of affiliation: Experimental studies of the sources of gregariousness.* Stanford, CA: Stanford University Press.

Schlenker, B. R. (1987). Threats to identity: Self-identification and social stress. In C. R. Snyder & C. E. Ford (Eds.), *Coping with negative life events: Clinical and social psychological perspectives* (pp. 273–321). New York: Plenum Press.

Seligman, M. (1975). *Helplessness: On depression, development and death.* San Francisco: W. H. Freeman.

Simpson, M. A. (1979). *The facts of death.* Englewood Cliffs, NJ: Prentice-Hall.

Simpson, M. A. (1982). The therapeutic uses of truth. In E. Wilkes (Ed.), *The dying patient: The medical management of incurable and terminal illness.* Lancaster, England: MTP Press.

Simpson, M. A. (1987, October). *Traumatic stress and the bruising of the soul.* Plenary address to the Annual Meeting of the Society for Traumatic Stress Studies, Baltimore, MD.

Simpson, M. A. (1989a). *Physical and psychiatric findings in a patient alleging beatings and electrical torture* (Report to the Court in the case of *Doris Damiani* v. the *Minister of Law and Order*). Durban: Supreme Court of South Africa.

Simpson, M. A. (1989b). *Physical and psychiatric findings in a patient alleging beatings and electrical torture* (Report to the Court in the case of the *State* v. *Mandla Cele*). Newcastle: Regional Court, Natal Region, South Africa.

Snyder, C. R., & Ford, C. E. (Eds.). (1987). *Coping with negative life events: Clinical and social psychological perspectives.* New York: Plenum Press.

Somnier, F. E., & Genefke, I. K. (1986). Psychotherapy for victims of torture. *British Journal of Psychiatry, 149,* 323–329.

Tillich, P. (1952). *The courage to be.* New Haven: Yale University Press.

Timerman, J. (1982). *Prisoner without a name, cell without a number.* Harmondsworth, England. Penguin Books.

Watzlawick, P., Beavin, J. H., & Jackson, D. D. (1968). *Pragmatics of human communication.* London: Faber & Faber.

Yalom, I. D. (1980). *Existential psychotherapy.* New York: Basic Books.

CHAPTER 57

The Psychosexual Trauma of Torture

Inger Agger and Søren Buus Jensen

Introduction

In accordance with the view of many political refugees, we regard the exile of victims as part of the political repression of the country of origin. The activities in the home country against individuals who have individually or collectively resisted social and economic exploitation have been met by dictatorial or other forms of authoritarian persecution which results in imprisonment and torture, and—as the last step—coercion to leave the country. In this way, political regimes rid themselves of troublesome individuals they have abused without physically killing them.

Many political refugees have suffered psychosexual trauma under imprisonment and torture. Although deliberate and systematic attempts at breaking down political opponents physically and psychologically are known to be practiced in one third of the world's countries (Amnesty International, 1984), little is known about the psychosexual traumatization inherent in torture. According to Bustos (1988), Chilean ex-prisoners have begun to break "the conspiracy of silence" surrounding sexual trauma in prisons, and this also appears to have been the case for some Iranian exile groups, but we still know little about sequelae and appropriate interventions in a Western exile setting (Mollica & Lavelle, 1988).

The United Nations High Commissioner for Refugees (UNHCR) (1988) estimates that there are about 12 million political refugees in the world. Of these, four

million are in exile in Western countries (Australia, North America, and Western Europe). We do not have any data on how many of these have suffered torture trauma, but an investigation from the Danish Red Cross shows that, of 3,200 refugees who applied for asylum in Denmark in 1986, 20% had been exposed to torture and had severe psychological and physical problems (Kjersem, 1987). This figure is based on interviews made at arrival at the Danish refugee camp. In this situation, many refugees feel too insecure to reveal facts about torture, so this figure probably only expresses a bare minimum. What we might infer from this investigation is that *at least* 20% of the political refugees in the Western countries have suffered torture trauma, as there is no reason to believe that the 3,200 refugees who have sought asylum in Denmark differ substantially from refugees in other Western countries.

In Denmark, there are about 25,000 refugees, with 54% from the Middle East, 30% from Asian countries, 13% from Eastern Europe, and 3% from Latin America (Agger, 1988a). If the refugees are permitted to cross the Danish border and apply for asylum (and this has become increasingly difficult), they are first placed in a camp under the auspices of the Danish Red Cross while their asylum application is under consideration. If asylum is granted, they leave the camps and become the responsibility of the Danish Refugee Council during an 18-month integration period at which time suitable accommodation is sought for the refugees. During this period, language school is started and plans for a future occupation are made. Following this period of time, the refugees become the responsibility of the municipal authorities in which they live.

The waiting period in the refugee camps, often protracted, with no knowledge of whether asylum will be granted or not, adds to the expectable stress experienced during prison, torture, and flight. Clearly, this means that exile in itself can be considered as a traumatic event, in addition to other traumas that often occur in such

Inger Agger • Department of Social Studies and Organization, Aalborg University, DK-9220 Aalborg, Denmark. **Søren Buus Jensen** • Center for Psychosocial and Traumatic Stress, Aalborg Psychiatric Hospital, Mølleparkvej 10, Aalborg, Denmark.

International Handbook of Traumatic Stress Syndromes, edited by John P. Wilson and Beverley Raphael. Plenum Press, New York, 1993.

situations of political violence, coercion, and purposeful manipulation.

It is important to recognize that a significant number of refugees waiting for asylum are referred for psychiatric treatment. In an investigation carried out at Hillerød Central Hospital, 73% of the refugees who were seen at the ward were asylum applicants. In the same investigation, it was found that the 75% of the refugee referrals who were questioned about this had suffered the trauma of torture. Moreover, the fact that the ward staff had not asked all referrals for this information reveals something about the professional reticence connected with the subject of torture (Jensen, Schaumburg, Leroy, Larsen, & Thorup, 1989).

Investigations carried out, both in exile and in one of the countries where torture is performed (El Salvador), show that about three fourths of the political prisoners who have been tortured have also suffered psychosexual trauma (Agger, 1989; Agger & Jensen, 1987).

Sexual Torture

We shall now focus initially on the general aspects of torture before going into a more detailed description of sexual torture and its psychological sequelae.

In a simplistic sense, the methods of torture are classified as either physical or psychological. The primary aim of *physical* torture is to inflict upon the victim varying degrees of physical pain by use of blows, kicks, suspension, electric or water torture, and/or many other forms of physical violence.

The aim of *psychological* torture is to break down and shatter the victim's psychological defense mechanisms and sense of will by causing psychic pain. Among the frequently used methods are long-term isolation, extensive and exhausting interrogation, sensory and sleep deprivation, threats, mock executions, witnessing the torture of others, and other forms of humiliating treatment, such as nakedness and *sexual torture*.

The victims often described the *psychological methods* of torture and degradation as being the most difficult to defend themselves against and survive. The torturers "break down" and humiliate the victims through manipulation of a complex lattice of common human feelings. And afterward, typically in exile, the victim often comes to a situation where the reality of his or her suffering may be met with mistrust, doubt, and disbelief. It is so difficult, for those of us who have not experienced it, to understand the knowledge of the torturers' bestialities, that we—in order to protect ourselves—may deny, avoid, or mistrust what we are told: Is it really true? Can it be proved? Who will supply proof, and what would it consist of? Thus, it is an integral part of the torturers' choice of torture methods and thought reform to ensure that, if the story is told, no one would believe it. Therefore, it is often hopeless to count on various agencies of authority to give confirmation. On the contrary, many prisoners are forced to sign a declaration before they are released in which they testify or affirm that they have not been subjected to torture (Sveaass, 1987). Clearly,

freedom exacts a price psychologically which contributes to further victimization and exploitation.

It is not surprising, therefore, that the use of sexual torture is so widespread. Sexual torture is deeply traumatic, but at the same time often leaves no evident or discernable external physical traces. However, as the physical and psychological methods are often interchangeable, it may seem artificial to segregate them. Nevertheless, it is important for psychotherapy that the psychological and "sexological" aspects of torture, because they have severe and traumatic effects, are more closely and exactly defined and understood.

The Aim of Torture

Lira and Weinstein (1986), Chilean psychologists, have described, on the basis of wide experience with treatment of torture victims, the aim of sexual torture. They define sexual torture as "the use of any form of sexual activity with the purpose of manifesting aggression and of causing physical and psychological damage" (p. 1). It is stressed that the goal of sexual torture is to destroy the prisoner's identity, but that it also is directed at the prisoner's sexuality, seeking to disturb future sexual function.

The aim of these pernicious methods of behavioral change is not primarily to force the victims to confess or to give information. Rather, it must be seen as the authorities' attempt to deprive victims of both personal and political identity with the aim of neutralizing individuals without killing them. In addition, there are the more general aims of terrorizing the population and preventive punishment of "subversive" elements.

Hence torture seeks deliberately to change the psychoformative processes and bring about those changes which are generally described in posttraumatic theory as the sequelae of extreme stress: changes in the self structure of the individual which include an experience of disintegration and a changed view of the world (Wilson, 1989). The extreme stress of sexual torture, therefore, may fulfil the aim of torture as it can bring about "a loss of self-continuity and self-sameness; a loss of a coherent and cohesive sense of self; feelings of narcissistic injury and a fragmentation of the ego and identity processes" (Wilson, 1989). The changed view of the world that results from this process, can, of course, also affect the political identity of the prisoner.

Methods of Torture and Dehumanization

According to Lira and Weinstein (1986), the systematized "breaking down" process is primarily carried out in two ways: by forcing the prisoner to take part in humiliating ("perverse") sexual relations, and by inflicting physical pain to the genitals, which brings the prisoner to associate pain and/or panic with sexuality. The sexual methods of torture can consist of:

(1) Either hetero- or homosexual rape; the rape of women by the use of specially trained dogs; the use of electric

currents upon the sexual organs; *mechanical* stimulation of the erogenous zones; *manual* stimulation of the erogenous zones; the insertion of penis-shaped objects into the body openings (these can be made of metal or other materials to which an electrical current is later connected, are often grotesquely large and cause subsequent physical damage, and are used on both male and female victims); (2) the forced witnessing of "unnatural" sexual relations; forced masturbation or to be masturbated by others; fellatio and oral coitus; and (3) finally, the general atmosphere of sexual aggression which arises from being molested, from the nakedness, and from the lewd and lecherous remarks and threats of sexual aggression made to the prisoner and his or her family and threats of the loss of ability of reproduction and enjoyment in the future. (pp. 2–3)

Thus, some sexual torture methods are directed at women, others at men, and some are directed at both genders. *Heterosexual rape* has a dominant position in the torture of women, whereas *homosexual rape* is the dominating element in the sexual torture of men. As a consequence of these experiences, future sexual functioning is threatened in both genders.

Psychodynamic Definition of Sexual Torture

On the basis of the above-mentioned and other sources (Agger, 1987, 1988b, 1989, 1992; Agger & Jensen, 1990), the following psychodynamic definition will be proposed: In sexual torture, the interchange between the victim and the torturer is characterized by an ambiguity consisting of both aggressive and libidinal elements. The victim's as well as the torturer's sexual structures are involved in the psychodynamics of this interaction, and the victim experiences the torture as directed against his or her sexual body image and identity with the aim to destroy it.

Thus, the essential part of sexual torture's traumatic and identity-damaging effect is the feeling of being an accomplice in an ambiguous situation which contains both aggressive and libidinal elements of a confusing nature.

The individual experiences himself (or herself) as a partaker in homo- (or hetero-) sexual relations and is overwhelmed by a feeling of being a party to the act, with an intensity which is much greater than the feelings experienced in connection with other forms of torture. (Lira & Weinstein, 1986, p. 6)

Because of the nature of the torture situation, a great degree of moral conflict and complexity is involved in the trauma of sexual torture. Pathological outcome of trauma is, as noted by Wilson (1989), in general directly proportional to the magnitude of moral conflict and complexity.

Clinical Interventions

In clinical work with political refugees in a Western exile setting, we consider the following issues to be especially important: (1) ideological and political issues, (2) transcultural issues, and (3) issues of posttraumatic therapy.

Ideological and Political Issues

As stated in the Geneva Convention, a refugee is a person who is outside of his or her home country because of well-founded fear of persecution on account of race, religion, nationality, membership in a special group, or political opinion. Therefore, ideology plays a crucial role for the refugee both by virtue of its presence or its absence. The degree of identity loss which the refugee experiences after the separation from life in the home country will be strongly influenced by the extent to which he or she is able to perceive the persecution as part of the ideology of those in power, instead of seeing it as individually directed persecution. Therefore, ideological and political consciousness influences both the outcome of treatment and life in exile. We believe that previous refugee research has not sufficiently taken this factor into account.

Since ideological issues are important for the refugee, the therapist is often asked about his or her ideological convictions. Experience shows that a "neutral" position seldom has a convincing effect—especially if the refugee has maintained his or her ideological consciousness. On the contrary, our experience suggests that it has a positive effect to concede the fact of *not* being directly involved in the individual refugee's struggle; but rather engaged on a more general level in the struggle against injustice, abuse of power, and suppression of democratic rights. On a theoretical level, the discussion about the concept of neutrality can raise many questions, but, in practice, it has not been difficult to administrate.

Thus, the loss of personal and ideological consciousness can be seen as a major part of the refugee's psychological problems. Erikson (1968) stressed in his life-span epigenetic model that the development of identity moves in the direction of a state which can be characterized by many qualities ranging from trust to despair. "Ideological engagement" plays a major role in the experience of integrity, whereas the state of despair is sometimes marked by value confusion. Among refugees who come to the attention of the mental health system, we often see reflected the negative dimension of the process described by Erikson: identity confusion, isolation, stagnation, and despair. Therefore, the ideological consciousness of both therapist and refugee will play an important role in the treatment, which aims at reinforcing the experience of integrity and identity (Wilson, 1980, 1989).

Even after approval of the therapist by the refugee, the working alliance will often be marked by continuous distrust and hopelessness. In this situation, the therapist can use ideological consciousness and education as a starting point. First, explain the aim of those in power—explain why they use torture—explain that the aim is to make the pain private to a degree where the political prisoner is made impotent as an opponent. Second, place the torture and its sequelae into a meaningful context which might be more relevant than employing a traditional psychotherapeutic approach. For the refugees who have individualized their pain, this perspective may be the first step in a process of deindividualization within a *reframing process* (Agger, 1992).

Transcultural Issues

In anthropology, discussions have been raging for years between the proponents of *universalism*, who emphasized the similarities underlying human cultures (e.g., Kiev, 1964), and proponents of *cultural relativism*, who emphasized the untranslatable differences between cultures (e.g., Kleinman, 1988). It is not our intention to try to solve this dispute but only to point out the dangers of falling either into the universalist or the relativist trap. In some immigrant and refugee research, there has been a tendency to explain social and political problems by "cultural differences" (Schwartz, 1985a,b). But "culture . . . is not a list of traditions but a tool kit of resources and skills . . . culture is also transformation, renovation . . . culture is in constant development" (Schwartz, 1985a, p. 36).

As therapists, we do not want to exert an attitude of cultural imperialism; but if we fall into the trap of cultural relativism, we might find it impossible to deal with the treatment of refugees, since we neither have a thorough knowledge of the refugee's cultural background nor do we belong to the refugee's own culture. In effect, this would limit the individual therapist's possibilities for working with different refugee groups, and thereby contribute to an extreme exaggeration of cultural determinism.

As noted by Wilson (1989), we still know too little about the various ways cultural differences affect the perception, interpretation, and assimilation of traumatic events. Nor do we know to what extent we can apply Western concepts and classification schemes to the symptoms presented by the refugees. But studies of Indochinese refugees suggest that many refugee patients suffer from both depressive and trauma-related symptoms (Mollica & Lavelle, 1988).

The anthropologist Clifford Geertz (1973, 1984) takes the stand of an "anti-antirelativist" focusing on the *meeting* between representatives of two cultures in which something new and different is created: a "third culture" in which no one takes on the other's values and patterns (see also Bloch, 1977).

In the meeting between therapist and refugee, culture-sensitive questions and informative elements can become part of the formation of therapeutic contact and alliance. The refugee is already confronting a foreign culture. In the field of sexuality, for example, there might be great differences between homeland and exile country, but not so great as to prevent a recognition of similar traits; for example, we are also familiar with discrimination of homosexuals although homosexuality is not forbidden by law.

Therefore, in the clinical treatment of the torture victim, an exchange is introduced: "It is like this in our society," and the refugee tells how it is in his or her country. This may be a challenge to the refugee but it might be an even greater challenge to the therapist who may see some of his or her ingrown values called into question or directly challenged by differences in value orientations.

Issues of Posttraumatic Therapy

Wilson (1989) and Ochberg (see Chapter 65, in this volume) have written on the unique nature of post-traumatic therapy (PTT). How to handle the *trauma story* (Wilson, 1986, 1988, 1989) is a crucial issue in therapy with torture victims. This refers to both the refugee's and the therapist's reactions (see Danieli, 1988, and Wilson, 1989, for a discussion of countertransference reactions).

From experience with Indochinese refugees, Mollica and Lavelle (1988) found that a review of the trauma story was not necessarily therapeutic. Often, it could stimulate further intrusive thoughts which intensified existing symptoms. This has also been our experience and for these reasons we find it especially important that the memory of the painful events get reframed. Through reframing, the reliving of the trauma is not only a repetition of the pain, it is also experienced and understood in a new and more meaningful manner (Lindy, 1986). "It helps the patient give meaning to their questions, 'Why did this happen to me? How can human beings be so cruel?' " (Mollica & Lavelle, 1988, p. 290). Therefore, the therapist should not try to break through the resistance to get to "the feelings." A provocation of this kind may lead to an increase of the "private" pain of the person at the expense of the "political" pain, and the therapist might be identified with the torturer in the transference situation.

As noted by Mollica (1988, p. 304), "the psychotherapy of torture survivors is in its infancy. . . . Except for a few outcome studies, there is almost a total lack of literature in this area." Therefore, we will extend our discussion of clinical interventions by presenting four detailed case examples of psychotherapies in which different aspects of the psychosexual trauma of torture are seen. In these case presentations, we have attempted to illustrate the central ideological, transcultural, and clinical issues as well as the all important *countertransference reactions* on the part of the therapist who is confronted with this kind of material.

We will present the cases of a Latin American woman, a torturer from the Middle East, a Kurdish man, and a Latin American couple. Confidentiality has been maintained by changing identities and other information to ensure anonymity.

Case One: Silvia

The following case history is not a clear-cut story of an ordinary person who suddenly experiences "an event that is generally outside the range of human experience"

689

(American Psychiatric Association [APA], 1987). The woman who is depicted here has a background of a difficult childhood which has left her especially vulnerable to further trauma. The case is chosen because it shows the mechanisms of psychosexual trauma in a very vivid way.

Silvia is a woman whose psychological defenses are frail. She was able to describe at a deep level how she reacted and still reacts to the trauma she was subjected to and how it is constantly intertwined with previous and later life events. She shows a whole array of stress response symptoms normally associated with post-traumatic stress disorder (PTSD): hypervigilance, memory and concentration impairment, illusions, distressing intrusive thoughts, nightmares, hallucinations, flashbacks, shame, self-hatred, avoidance of situations that activate recall of torture, daze, numbness, sense of unreality, withdrawal, self-medication with alcohol, and excessive sleeping.

As the trauma story gradually unfolds, the therapist's reactions are also analyzed in order to attempt to demonstrate the powerful countertransference reactions which this kind of material can elicit in the clinician. The treatment, which was supervised throughout its course, lasted for 1 year.

THE STORY OF SILVIA

Silvia is a political refugee from Chile, and she has been in exile in Denmark for 8 years. She is 30 years old, divorced, and lives with her son in an apartment in a major city. She is unemployed and does not participate in any form of educational activity. Because of memory and concentration difficulties, she has only been able to learn very little Danish in spite of the duration of her stay in the country. The therapy is therefore conducted in Spanish without an interpreter present in the room.

The first impression of Silvia is that of a nice looking, slender woman with a shy smile. She wears somewhat dull clothes in comparison with other Latin American women. The therapeutic alliance is established easily, perhaps because the Danish female therapist is able to communicate with Silvia in her native language. She reveals a traumatic childhood with a sadistic mother who beat her and forced her to work hard in the house and to take care of her two younger sisters. Silvia's parents were divorced before adolescence. She was very attached to her father, who continued to visit the house after the divorce. According to Silvia, he wanted to lead a free life with other women. Silvia's home was in a large city in Argentina, and her family was from the lower middle class. She joined a socialist party during her teenage years, but she did not hold a prominent office. Silvia stated that the events of imprisonment and torture occurred when she was 20 years old. She cries when she tells her story of imprisonment. She complains of lying in bed all day and sleeping while her son is at school, of anxiety-ridden nights, and of difficulties establishing a relationship to a man. She says that she feels abnormal.

Silvia starts the next session by talking about her abusive mother. She feels that her childhood, and especially her mother, is the reason why she today cannot establish any permanent relationship to a man. Her mother had a very restrictive view of sexuality. She also treated Silvia poorly and said that she should never have been born, and had no abilities and would be a failure in life. She was frequently beaten and blamed for her

sisters' wrongdoings. Silvia discloses her story of childhood abuse without any sign of anger. When this is pointed out to her by the therapist, she replies: "You cannot be angry towards the person who gave you life."

She continues the subject of motherhood in the following session by disclosing that she herself is a good mother to her son, and does not parent like her mother did. She adds that the only person who gave her love during her childhood was her grandmother with whom she spent three months every summer. Silvia cries as she remembers her grandmother who died when she was 16. After her death, she felt that her grandmother was still with her but this religious belief could not be reconciled with the ideology of the socialist party. When the therapist comments that her grandmother can exist inside her as something good which she also can use in her relationship with her son, it is evident that Silvia feels relieved of her ambivalence of contradictory beliefs. To the therapist, the central themes now seem to be the evil mother, the good mother, and the anger which cannot be expressed. In the background looms the story of the torture trauma, of what happened to Silvia in prison, but the therapist decides not to press Silvia on this subject; she decides instead to continue with the themes Silvia feels impelled to talk about. There is something very fragile and anxious about her which brings the therapist to feel protective towards her. A "good mother" transference is being built up, but also, in the countertransference, a feeling of danger, of permeable boundaries, and the feeling that both she and Silvia could go to pieces if these issues are not handled carefully in therapy.

In the next session the therapist is surprised, when Silvia begins to approach the difficult subject of torture by telling how nervous she is today. She had awakened several times during the night and had dreams, but she cannot remember their content. On this morning she sweated and her hands trembled. Silvia evades going further into the subject by asking the therapist what she wants her to talk about. Perhaps she is actually asking the therapist to help her talk about the dangerous subject. The therapist does not direct her attention and Silvia tells that she felt relief after having talked about her grandmother at the last session. It seemed as though Silvia wants to hold on to the "good" before moving into the "evil." She goes on to talk about a lover she had when she was 17 to 19 years old and states that her mother was very opposed to the relationship and once beat her with a stick which resulted in two bumps in the back of her head. On another occasion the mother locked her in the house for an entire week in order to prevent her from seeing her boyfriend. All this led Silvia to run away with her boyfriend with whom she had her first sexual experience, a fact mentioned in passing. They escaped to Valledoza where she broke off the relationship. Silvia felt that she did not really love the man but had used him to get security and affection and get away from home. After this, she had a happy and harmonious period in Valledoza, where she felt herself to be a completely new and different person. However, this period of moratorium in development was interrupted by her arrest and imprisonment. She states that she experienced the prison as being a better place than her mother's home, because she knew why she was being mistreated and made attempts to defend herself. She reflects that maybe she acted out her anger toward her mother by attacking the torturers and soldiers, and eventually this may have made them believe that she was insane. She indicated that she did not care if she died and hit, bit, kicked, and pulled her torturers' hair until she was beaten unconscious.

Silvia ended the session by disclosing that there are long passages of the time in prison that she cannot remember and that this frightens her. She leaves the session saying that there are many stories to tell from the prison. Apparently, Silvia has to approach the trauma story by focusing on the good part of it. It is as if she is gaining confidence in herself and in the good relationship which is being built up in the therapy room before taking the dive into the prison experiences, "which she cannot remember" but which might be revealed as "many stories."

At the start of the next session, the therapist feels anxious. She believes that the disclosure of the trauma story is getting closer and that she must face it together with Silvia. She also observes her countertransference reactions in the reversal of roles. Last time, it was Silvia who started out by being anxious; this time it is the therapist. The therapist tries to take control of the situation by asking Silvia if she has thought about what happened during the last session. Silvia goes back to the time before imprisonment when she was still living with her mother. At that time, she had seen movies about the Nazi era and horror movies about torture. She had also heard about torture from comrades in the party who had been in prison. She had, however, always experienced all this as something unreal—only as stories. Her own stay in the prison had the same unreal depersonalized character. She then describes her arrest and what followed. She was taken to the barracks where they took her handbag, watch, and papers. She was put in line with other prisoners in a dimly lit corridor. A hood was placed over her head. It was morning and Silvia could glimpse under the hood and, as the light changed, get an impression of the passage of time. While she was standing in this corridor, she was convinced that she would soon be released again, that the whole thing was a misunderstanding. She kept on saying that she had to leave because she had to start work at 12:30. However, she was not released but during the afternoon was instead taken out to the courtyard where she was forced to stand in *planton*; that is, she must stand with her legs spread apart and her arms behind her head. A piece of cardboard with her name on was hung on her. At nightfall, when it became cold, her sweater was taken off her so that she was only wearing a chemise and jeans. She stood there the whole night and when she fell down, she was kicked or beaten onto her feet again. At one point, they pushed a chair between her legs to keep them apart. Later, a large Alsatian (German Shepherd) dog was placed between her legs. If she moved the dog bit her. Silvia recalls in detail about these first days when she was taken inside during the day and outside during the night. Once, when she went to the toilet, she was able to make a small hole in the hood with a safety pin she had in her jeans. In this way, she could catch a small glimpse of what was happening around her. She fought with a soldier who tightened her hood around her neck so much that she almost could not breathe. She bit his hand and pulled his hair. He twisted her arm and beat her so hard that she lost consciousness and woke up in a dark isolation cell. She continues by describing a scene in the torture chamber, where she was brought to a large torturer who pulled the hood off her. In her own words she said: "I see that there is blood on the walls and on his arms. He asks me if I want to go for a swim. I answer no, and I say that it looks as if they have slaughtered chickens in here. He pulls me up and down a couple of times and hits me on both ears at the same time (*teléfono*). He hits me other places on my head and he puts my head under water three or four times (*submarino*). Then, he asks me if I have been to bed with my lover. I am completely confused—the situation is incomprehensible. At last, he kicks me out of the room with such force

that I crash into the wall of the corridor outside. I don't remember more until I wake up in the isolation cell. One time, I am confronted with my cousin who says that I should tell everything. But I don't have anything to tell. I sign a paper. Another time, I also meet my other cousin who is only 13 and who has not been able to eat anything for many days because she was so scared." When Silvia tells this, she starts crying. She says at the end of the session that it felt awful to tell all this—"It was just like being back there again." The therapist answers that it is good for her to go back to all this because it will help her get rid of it. The therapist, herself, feels shaken and upset by hearing Silvia's story.

At the beginning of the next session, the therapist doubts whether it really had been beneficial for Silvia to go back to the past because Silvia apparently was in a dissociative state for a while after the session. She says that she does not want to tell more about what happened in the prison because she felt so strange after the last session. While going home, she felt as if she were in another world and upon arrival, stood in the window and looked at her son's school as if he no longer existed. She states that if one of her girlfriends had not reminded her that she should go get her son she might not have done it. For the rest of the day and the evening she says that she was not herself. She said that she did the housework automatically and that her girlfriend told her that she looked strange. Silvia is frightened by this slip in her connection to reality and she is afraid of going "mad." During the night, she had many dreams but does not remember their content. When she awakes, she is herself again. She says that her mother and the torturers said she was "mad." To this, the therapist comments that she does not think Silvia is mad. Silvia answers that the other Argentineans also think she is crazy. She then starts to cry and says she does not have normal relations with anyone except her son. She adds that there is another reason why she will not talk more about the prison and it is because she saw things so horrible that she cannot tell about them. The recollections of these things pursue her, both while she is awake and while she is asleep. Sometimes she thinks that she hears dogs howl and the sounds of beatings and screams. She can, however, connect these sounds to noises in the surroundings. The therapist tells her that she will feel better if she tells about these memories—as it is impossible for her to forget them. But she must do it at her own pace. Silvia accepts this explanation. Apparently, the trauma story is very close to the surface and manifests itself in intrusive thoughts, flashbacks, and dreams. The therapist now sees it as her task to keep Silvia in contact with reality and be supportive of her ego. Since the recollections of the trauma seem to have an immense force, it also seems valid to slow up the process of working through the distressing material. The therapist wonders about the kinds of difficulties Silvia has in her relationships to men.

Silvia cancels the next appointment because she has an opportunity to take a short trip to Sweden without her son. She looks brilliant when she arrives for the following session. She has put on makeup and attractive clothes. She starts by saying that she does not remember anything about what happened during the last session. She is silent for a long time and at last the therapist becomes impatient. She feels the need to help both Silvia and herself and asks Silvia if she truly cannot remember one single thing. Silvia then gives a short summary containing all the main issues—but leaves out her present problems with heterosexual relationships. The therapist repeats the agreement from the last session about going into the experiences in prison even though she had actually decided to slow up the process. This is her reaction to Silvia's repeating her complaints about problems with sleep disturbances. Silvia continues this topic and tells that she had an especially bad evening and night after coming home from the trip, which she enjoyed. She sensed that someone was trying to come in through the front door with a key, and at one point, she also heard a loud noise as if something fell. She got out of bed to check these things but did not find anything wrong. After that, she went to sleep with all the lights in the apartment illuminated. The therapist tries to connect to reality by saying that Silvia actually lives in an apartment building with a lot of different noises during the night and that these noises can very well be connected to her fantasy and her anxiety. Silvia tells that she was not afraid of the dark before being in prison. The therapist points out that her torture was performed during the night, and Silvia adds that arrests were also made at night. The therapist comments that it is understandable that she is particularly anxious at night. Silvia asks how she can get over this anxiety and the therapist replies that Silvia should tell more about what happened in prison so that she can be better at distinguishing what happened *then* and what happens *now*. Silvia then speaks about the night when the leading members of the party were arrested and brought to the prison. Silvia and the other prisoners were awakened and ordered to put on their hoods and go out into the courtyard without shoes. There, they had to stand in *planton*. The children present were crying. Now, Silvia is also crying in the session. Somehow, she had caught a glimpse of some of her comrades hanging down from a wall. They were in a terrible physical condition. She heard the soldiers saying that they would shoot them all and she heard the sound of the safety catches of the rifles being released and the shots. She also heard the sound of someone beside her falling and felt a blow on her head. She woke up in a completely dark isolation cell and thought that she was dead. She thought she was in a casket and buried. When they came to get her, she asked where she was and they said with a grin that she was in Hell. She was taken in for interrogation. In the room was the commandant and the large man who had tortured her. They said that she should tell where the weapons were; otherwise she would be taken to torture again. She began saying a lot of crazy things and talked at cross-purposes. They then took her to another room where they tied her to a table with rope around her wrists, ankles, and neck. Silvia begins to sob violently and the therapist goes to get her a cup of coffee. The fact that the therapist, in this situation, leaves Silvia alone can probably be interpreted as a result of her own anxiety and a feeling of not being able to contain more horror. When she comes back with the coffee, Silvia is quiet for a while and then continues her story. They gave her an injection, she says, which was supposed to make her tell the truth. She does not remember more before she again awoke in the isolation cell. The therapist asks why this was especially painful for her to tell and Silvia answers that the pain comes from not knowing what actually went on. She did not really know where she was. Anything could have happened to her. She could have said something she should not have revealed. Silvia changes to the present time and tells again of how scared she is of going to sleep; scared of waking and not knowing where she is; of waking and being dead; and of being abducted. At the end of the session, Silvia again talks about her terror of darkness. The therapist had the distinct impression that Silvia has *not* told everything which happened while she was strapped to the table; that Silvia was in fact raped there and that Silvia's fear of being abducted is actually a fear of being abducted *and* raped. Silvia probably refrained from telling the whole story because

she sensed from the therapist's act of leaving the room that the therapist was not able to tolerate more of the trauma story at that time.

At the beginning of the next session, the therapist feels tense and anxious. She has a feeling that Silvia has not told the worst and fears that she will not be able to listen to it. Silvia is silent for a long time. Then she says that she never knows how to begin. She sits for a long time and turns her ring around nervously. At last, she says that it was now the period when she was in the barracks of Calla. Then she is again silent, and at last the therapist repeats "the barracks of Calla?" Actually, Silvia had not said that the events she described at the previous session had taken place in another prison. Then Silvia says: "Yes, I don't know how long I was in Calla. I don't have any perception of the passage of time there. But from Calla, they brought us back to Valledoza with our hands tied behind our backs. Maybe it was after 5 months, and they took the hoods off us and I was put in a large cell together with many other comrades. I was in this cell for 3 months. They were very well organized and they helped me a lot. After Calla, I only wanted to sleep. While I had the hood on, I slept as much as possible under the hood, but when they took it off, I couldn't sleep so much. I had to keep my eyes open. I was like an automaton. They had to lead me everywhere. If I was sat down, I stayed sitting until they stood me up again. I didn't utter a word. At last, I was released because they said that I was 'mad.'" There is a long pause.

"What happened in Calla?" the therapist asks. Silvia becomes very nervous. "There were so many things that happened. I don't know in which order they happened." "It doesn't matter with the order," the therapist replied. There is again a long pause. Silvia says: "One evening they took us to the pigsty and said we should stay there for the rest of the night. Besides the pigsty there was a cage with Alsatians (dogs) and they barked all through the night. We did not sleep at all. The next morning they took us out and we washed ourselves in cold water. Then my cousin and I were led into a room and they told us to confess. I did not say anything and they beat me. They took my cousin into the next room and I heard screams, the barking of dogs, and loud music. The guards in my room told me what they were doing to my cousin. Afterwards, they took me into the same room. I can't tell it." "What did they do to you?" the therapist asks. "I will tell what they did to my cousin—they did the same to me. There was an Alsatian which was held by a guard in a chain. My cousin was naked and someone was holding her arms. And the dog was over her and bit her. She had blood all over. And they made it lick her everywhere and they also made it rape her. They said that now there was going to be a ball. They were many and there was very loud music. They told us to dance with the dog. They said that we were animals and that they didn't feel inclined to rape us. Afterwards, they did the same to me. Ever since, it has been very difficult for me to be together with a man. When I was pregnant with my son, I dreamt that I would give birth to a beast. I am scared of seeing films like 'The Wolfman' and of being near big dogs." Silvia is shaking all over and the therapist tries to de-privatize the situation by saying that this is a common torture method; that they have done this to many. Silvia says that she has never told this to anyone. She seems overwhelmed by shame and the therapist feels a painful shame seep into her as well. Silvia wants to talk about ordinary things now and does so for the last 15 minutes of the session. When the therapist later tells her supervisor about this session, she reexperiences the shame. Not only shame, but also guilt pervades her. She feels like a voyeur; as if she had witnessed something which should never have been seen by anyone. In this confusing mixture of feelings, there is also an element of being a party to the torture; that is, the therapist is identified with Silvia and the torturer at the same time.

In the next session, the therapist wants to start talking about ordinary things, again reversing roles with Silvia in order to avoid the distress associated with the trauma story. Then she asks Silvia how she has been. Silvia says she has not felt well. She says she feels as if she were in an empty void. When she came home, she went to get her son because she wanted to be together with someone with whom she felt secure. Silvia is anxious that someone will learn about her state of anxiety. The therapist answers that what Silvia has experienced, other have experienced as well; that she should try *not* to see it as something directed at her personally. This attempt at reframing calms Silvia a bit. She goes on with her story and tells that after her release she could not allow any man to approach her in any way. When she met her son's father, it took a very long time before she dared let him touch her. It was as if sexuality had become something bestial. After a long pause, Silvia says that there is something else that she needs to tell. After another long pause, she tells that she had to get drunk to have intercourse with her husband and that it is still so. She thinks that everything which has to do with sex is very complicated. The therapist comments that it does not seem so complicated to her; that there must evidently be a relation between her experiences in Calla and her feelings about sex now; that alcohol helps her reduce anxiety and that her mother's attitude toward sex might also influence the situation. Silvia denies that her mother could have influenced her so profoundly in this matter. She had a rewarding sex life during the two years before she went to prison. But after prison, she feared that her lovers would find out about what had happened to her. The therapist tries to hold Silvia to reality by telling her that this is a fantasy; that no one can ever find out about it, and that she does not need to tell it. It is important, however, that Silvia talks about it in therapy so that she can liberate herself from this fantasy and its negative effects on her well-being. Silvia then goes on to tell about a man she met during her recent trip to Sweden. She indicated that she had a nice time with him and they went to bed together but, as usual, Silvia was drunk in order to have sexual relations. Moreover she said that this man wants to see her again and calls her every day, but she does not know if she wants to see him again. She is afraid of having a man in her house, especially in her bed. The therapist supports the part of Silvia which wants to see him again and tells her that this could be an opportunity for her to work with her anxiety and get rid of it. She also encourages Silvia to gradually reduce the amount of alcohol intake before intercourse. Silvia apparently likes this proposal. She says that she would never have gone on this trip if she had not been in therapy. It has given her more confidence in herself. The atmosphere in this session is light and positive.

In the next session Silvia begins by saying that she never knows where to start talking. The therapist senses that Silvia wants to talk more about the trauma, and she chooses to be quiet and await Silvia's opening. After a long pause, Silvia says that the therapist has told her to come out with everything which happened in Calla. She then continues the story. After the episode with the dogs, the three women were put in a dog cage outside the house. There was barbed wire around it. Silvia makes a drawing of it. They were held there for the next 12–14 days. It was cold and stormy and they only wore jeans and a shirt—it was a gray prison uniform. They did not have any

shoes to wear. Silvia adds that this is maybe why she is always so afraid when it storms. They were treated like animals and their food was placed on the earth as if they were dogs. At intervals, they were taken for interrogation. Afterwards, they were taken back to Valledoza. She was put in a cell with other women prisoners and they also had female guards and this felt a little better. The therapist senses that Silvia has gone very quickly past the rest of her stay in Calla and asks Silvia to explain a little more about the way in which they were treated as animals. The therapist is unsure whether she is right in doing this, but also feels that she is at the core of the trauma and that she must help Silvia get it out. Silvia is again overwhelmed by shame, a shame which the therapist can also feel and which again makes her doubt whether she should have gone further into the subject. Silvia says: "It was as if they did it for fun and not to get information. They came and beat the cage with sticks, as you would if you wanted to tease dogs. Sometimes we were trained as if we were dogs: We had to walk on four legs in a collar and we were beaten with a dog whip. Food was served in a bowl for animals—not on plates—and it was not real food, but leftovers from the kitchen. We barely talked together but took turns being on watch so that we could wake the others if the soldiers came." It is very difficult for Silvia to tell this, and the therapist tries to reframe it by talking about the general aim of torture: to humiliate and break down the identity of the prisoner. It is therefore that such humiliating methods are chosen. This seems to give relief to Silvia. She then makes a jump to the period after her release and tells that she had to go to the barracks once a week for a while, and thereafter once every two weeks. At last it was once every month. Sometimes they kept her for 24 hours. Once, they made her stand in *planton* for 20 hours. Finally, this was too much for Silvia and she decided to flee the country.

As usual, at the beginning of a session, Silvia doesn't know where to start, and the therapist decides to give her a lead by making a short summary of the last session. Somehow it feels necessary to establish continuity and get the rest of the story in order to provide a structure out of the chaos which threatens both the therapist and Silvia. From Silvia's remarks at the end of last session it also seemed that the trauma story was about finished. It provided some sort of relief for the therapist, perhaps, to establish how it ended, and give the horrors a conclusion. How was it when she came out, the therapist asks? Silvia tells that a relative came to fetch her from the prison and they went together to her house. Here, Silvia isolated herself in her room and she stayed there completely secluded for the next 10 days. She only talked with her relative about the most necessary ordinary things. The relative asked her a few times what had happened in the prison and every time Silvia passed it off. The relative also asked her about her cousin and Silvia said that she was well. During these 10 days of numbness, Silvia tried to block the period in prison out of her consciousness. Little by little, she began going out with her younger cousins, but mostly she kept to herself and walked in the most quiet streets. Silvia heard about a theatrical group in which former prisoners participated and she asked to join this group. She wanted to show that she had conquered the torturers and that what had happened in prison and what she had done had only been a grotesque theatrical play in which she had taken part. She wanted to show that she was not mad. Silvia participated in this group for a year and liked it but continued to keep to herself and she always left the conversation if someone mentioned the prison. She had to check in at the barracks every Monday and Saturday, and afterwards on these days, she always went home to bed and stayed in her room for the rest of the day without eating or drinking or talking to anyone. At the theater, she met her husband, and after a year, she became pregnant and they moved to another town. During the pregnancy, Silvia was haunted by fantasies of giving birth to a monster or to a deformed child and she regretted that she had become pregnant. She decided that she would kill the baby by smashing its head against the floor if something was wrong with it. She studied books about newborn babies and the first thing she did after her son was born, was to inspect him closely and examine his reflexes. She then realized that the baby was normal. She did not want to give birth to "a fruit of the torture," as Silvia put it. During a pregnancy many years later, she had the same fantasies and anxieties. She was later sterilized because she did not want to experience these feelings any more. Also in this session, Silvia is convinced that there is a risk that she could give birth to something ugly because of the torture. It seems that Silvia feels that the evil has so penetrated her that it could destroy her children.

The therapy continues another 6 months until Silvia wants to stop and instead join a women's group composed of other exiled Latin Americans. During the rest of the therapy, the dominating issues were all related to her sense of identity: (1) her concepts of herself as a woman, (2) as a mother and as a lover, and (3) she feels physically damaged and believes that her genitals are deformed and that her body is not really feminine. She wonders if the evil is inside of her, and if anyone can "see" what has happened to her. She feels that she must not cry and be a perfect mother to her son. Ultimately, she has a fear of falling into an empty void and being strangulated. Clearly, this suggests the level of her state of identity diffusion at this point in therapy.

During the last sessions, the focus is primarily on here-and-now issues: problems in Silvia's relationships with other people. When she decides to terminate the therapy, it seems as if her symptoms have lessened, but there is still much unresolved work to do in the future. The therapist's reaction to Silvia's termination is one of relief, tinged with an uneasy feeling that she has been through something horrible together with Silvia and that she felt powerless against it.

As Wilson (1988, 1989) noted, the question generally arises in the minds of both the victim and the witness, be it a therapist or other listeners: How can human beings be so cruel? How can anyone become a torturer? The following case story of a torturer is presented in an attempt to show some of the mechanisms which can bring a human being to take this position. It also depicts some of the ethical and clinical issues involved in the encounter with extreme human cruelty.

Case Two: Ahmed, a Torturer

There do not exist many testimonies of torturers. It is dangerous to leave the job, let alone to tell anything about it. This torturer felt disturbed by his job and decided to leave it. He was caught and tortured himself; he was also exposed to combat and war stress. Thus, he had suffered multiple stressor events in the stage of transition into early adulthood. Such a history can be expected to have severe impact on personality propensities and ego identity (Wilson, 1980, 1988).

He was seen at a psychiatric ward for 5 days, during

which time he had two long sessions of 3 hours each with a Danish male psychiatrist and a female interpreter from his own country. During these two sessions, he willingly told his story in great detail. His rational reason for doing so was a belief that it would help him obtain asylum (this proved to be correct), and on a less rational level, it could have been a search for atonement. From a clinical viewpoint, he might be seen as a person "entrapped within his trauma story" (Wilson, 1985, 1986, 1989) in his obsessive wish for telling the story over and over again.

At his dismissal from the ward, he was diagnosed as suffering from a personality disorder and PTSD. These diagnoses, however, both have transcultural and clinical implications which should be taken into consideration. The torturer came from a small village in a country with a very different culture than the middle-class Danish culture to which the therapist belonged. Since we know very little about the transcultural applicability of Western diagnostic concepts, the diagnoses could be an expression of ethnocentrism (Kleinman, 1988; Mollica & Lavelle, 1988). Moreover, on the clinical level, symptoms of personality disorder are often seen to overlap with PTSD symptoms. Thus, the "appearance of being cold and unemotional" (Wilson, 1988, p. 248) could be an effect of emotional numbness, one of the symptoms of PTSD.

The most profound issues raised in this case, however, are ideological and ethical. In the meeting between the torturer and the therapist, a powerful negative countertransference was rapidly built-up and traditional concepts of neutrality in the therapist were challenged.

THE STORY OF AHMED

Ahmed comes from a country in the Middle East and is 21 years old. After his arrival in Denmark, when he applied for refugee status, he was referred from a refugee camp for psychiatric evaluation, suspected of being psychotic. He arrives to the session well-groomed, dressed in black shirt and black trousers, and is accompanied by an interpreter, an elegant woman, who is old enough to be his mother. He says hello formally and continues a minor argument with the interpreter about cigarettes and some belongings which he did not bring with him. His behavior is commanding.

From the beginning, the therapist feels uncomfortable, senses that Ahmed has an aura of power about him, and that it is not a psychotic but a well-structured person that confronts him. The therapist had been called by the staff of the refugee camp because they did not know what to do with Ahmed. He had told the interpreter that he had been a torturer and that he wanted to see blood. He had also said that he felt as if he were two persons, and wanted to be isolated for security reasons. The interpreter had been shaken, and the refugee camp dared not keep him. They suspected that Ahmed was psychotic and asked that he be admitted to the ward for diagnostic evaluation.

During the entire course of the first 3-hour session, there was no eye contact between Ahmed and the therapist, but there was some during the following and last session. In these two encounters, Ahmed told his story readily without any signs of emotion, remorse, or guilt.

"I grew up in a poor family and I only went to school for a few years before I started to work to support my family. My parents supported the dictatorship in the country, and one day my father suggested that I should join the army for the sake of my parents and our religion. My father said that it was my duty to fight for our religion, and besides that, the wages were also good in the army. I therefore reported to the army headquarters in our town. I was then 17 years old.

"I started military training, which also included religious training. I was sent to the Kurdish territory where our task was to destroy the Kurdish villages. We shot with bazookas and we threw grenades into the village houses. Once, I remember we drove through a village and threw bombs into all of the houses. Afterwards, I saw a woman sitting in one of the houses I had bombed. She sat as if she tried to protect her child, but both of them were dead. We also trained in the mountains, but after a while, I could not endure it any longer and fled back to my home town.

"When I came back, I discovered that my family thought that I was dead. They had already received a large compensation check. They were, however, glad to see me again and my father tore the check into pieces. But I did not dare do anything else than report again to the army headquarters. They enlisted me again, and together with some others, I was commanded to go out onto a large square and stand in the position of attention. We could not see anyone but were given orders through loud-speakers. We were ordered to stare upwards and it was forbidden to look at any of the others. After that, I sensed that some-one was walking around us. There was also someone who stopped in front of me and hit me and tried to push me out of the position I was in, at the same time threatening me and ordering me to stay in the position of attention and keep a straight face. I was pulled aside and I thought I should be punished but instead I was told that I had been selected for training in the Capital City. I was put on an airplane together with some others and about 35 of us were selected to start at the torture school.

"We were all put in the same class, and it was apparent that none of us had much education. But this did not matter because we should not read but learn practical tasks. Usually, the teacher entered without presenting himself and gave us different assignments which we were trained to solve. People say that those who go to that school are all brainwashed, but I don't think this happened to me. The teacher might say that we should imagine that we had arrested a socialist who insists that he is just an occasional visitor. The task is then to make him confess. They taught us that we should start by putting them in a dark cell in the prison for 4 weeks. This also meant that their nails would grow so that it was easier to get hold of them with a pair of tongs. I learned that during interrogation you should pull one or two nails off each time, because if you pulled more off, the hand or the foot would become anesthetized so that it wouldn't do any good. Some prisoners knew that you could avoid this by biting your nails, but then you could always start with the toes, especially the big toe. Other times, we practiced in a special way on dolls which were made for that purpose. We also learned to plait 'horses' tails' which consisted in plaiting a few strands of horsehair of a length of 10 to 12cm. This was meant for inserting in the urethra of men, whereafter the 'horses' tail' was pulled out very quickly. This resulted in bleeding, pain, infection, and difficulties with urinating. I was at this school for about 3 months with theory, practical training, and demonstrations."

For the sake of observing Ahmed in the most neutral way, the staff of the ward had only been told that he was a refugee and should be observed for psychosis. A nurse who was a member of Amnesty International sat in at the sessions, and

she started listening to Ahmed's story with a great deal of sympathy, but when she realized that he was more of a torturer than a victim, an uneasiness was clearly felt in the room and her goodwill froze to ice. From then on, the nurse sat with her arms folded in front of her and her eyes wide at the horror of having met evil personified.

The interpreter was also clearly affected by the situation. Several times she lost the thread, and later it was discovered that she identified Ahmed with her own son of the same age, and that she felt pity for Ahmed. When the story became too incriminating, she translated unprecisely. For example, "the horses' tails" became "I don't really understand it—I think it is something dirty." After the therapist insisted, the interpreter could only translate correctly after several attempts.

On the conscious level the therapist was absorbed in the task of getting to know the story of a torturer, in order to gain a deeper understanding of the experiences of the victims—of the survivors of torture. He therefore insisted on getting the whole story, even when the interpreter and Ahmed hesitated. On the emotional level, the therapist in the beginning had a feeling of unreality, of hearing a "tale," with intermediate flashbacks to torture victims he had treated. He felt a growing anger, however, as it became more and more difficult to deny the reality of the story: It fit too well the accounts he had heard from the victims that had been treated. The possibility that the story could be pure invention did not completely disappear, but the defense of denial was hard to maintain in the face of Ahmed's consistent and logical speech which poured out in a way typical for a person in crisis who needs to tell his story. It was not the speech of a psychotic. Ahmed kept direct eye contact with the interpreter who was clearly the only person who felt sympathy for him.

"I was sent for further training in another town. In the beginning, I learned to tap telephones and try to intercept code messages. When we decided that someone talked in code, we went out and got hold of the people, blindfolded them and drove them around in the town in such a way that they would not know where they were. After that, we delivered them to the torture people. Later on, I was sent to do duty in the prison itself. Here, I received further training in the performance of torture. My first task was to participate in the interrogation of two persons that had been arrested at the border. I was to learn how you interrogate. Besides using the methods with the nails, they also used whips, and I saw how they were whipped until their backs were completely bloody. Thereafter, I was ordered to go into them and continue whipping them; but when I came in, I couldn't do it. I went out again and told my teachers that their backs could not take more whipping, but they answered that in that case, they would be forced to whip me. When I had tried that for a while, I was willing to go in and try again. The two prisoners screamed and moaned. I tried to close my eyes and give more gentle blows, but my teachers insisted that I should strike harder and faster. I then did that, and I must confess that after a while I enjoyed it. I also learned to use the ironbed where we gave electric shocks and to give blows with a baton. I learned how to use the horses' tails that they had taught us about at the school. If you didn't feel like doing the things that they ordered you to do, you were threatened with being punished yourself.

"After a while, I liked my job. I passed the final examination one day in which I was ordered to shoot the two persons whom I had earlier whipped. They had been condemned to death for the sake of our religion. They were just like small children when a sack was put over their heads. I was given a piece of firearm, but my hands were shaking so much that I missed the first shot. My teachers shouted and insisted that I should keep my eyes open. After several shots, the prisoners collapsed and my colleagues tapped my shoulders and said that now I was one of them. As I said before, I came to like my work little by little. It became a job like any other job, although I gradually had greater and greater difficulties sleeping at night and had nightmares."

He began telling about the nightmares he had in the ward. In these dreams, he alternated between being a torturer and a victim. He presented evident symptoms of PTSD and pleaded for sleeping tablets. He was also given the tablets even though the therapist felt, in countertransference, a desire to refuse: Ahmed deserved to suffer himself.

Ahmed very quickly started participating in the social life of the ward. He moved in, made himself comfortable, and watched TV. He reacted to a program about the war in Afghanistan by bragging, with his few English words, about his own merits in war and of how he had shot with a bazooka, and he gave a convincing representation of shooting in a somewhat teasing and provoking manner to his fellow patients. A senile woman patient reacted to this by giving him a slap in the face, which he found ridiculously funny. He had continuous discussions about cigarettes and minor privileges with the staff.

"I began to doubt if I was a human being or an animal and when I was off work I went to see my uncle. He told me to get away from the job, but he asked me to notice, until he could help me get away, what I saw in the prison; where they buried the dead and how they tortured and executed. In return, he would help me to flee. I did the physical torture. The psychological part required more training. It was the most experienced who stood for that. It wasn't the army but the people from the secret police. I only performed sexual torture against men. This consisted in inserting a bottle or egg into the rectum. To your question about homosexual rape or threat of rape I can only answer that I don't consider that to be torture.

"My uncle got me out of the country and I fled to another country where I was arrested in the airport and put in prison. There, I wasn't submitted to torture but the stay in prison was nearly worse than the torture I knew about. All the prisoners carried heavy iron chains on both arms and legs, and during the night, the prisoners were chained together. We lived in darkness, cramped together under miserable circumstances, and we were seldom given food, and if so, only poor food. Nor were we able to wash.

"After 5 months, I was sent back to my country. They had suspected me of being a spy. When I arrived in my own country I was put in prison again.

"They took me to my home village and I was myself tortured. First, they put me in an isolation cell which was in ground area 1 meter × 0.8 meter, which means that it is impossible to lie down. There was a hole in the middle of the floor which served the function of a toilet and there was a bottle of water. The floor in the cell was nearly always covered with water, and when I tried to sleep I had to push as much of the water as possible into the hole in the middle. Water ran down the walls, and above the cell, there was nearly always noise. Sometimes I was awakened by strange noises, as if someone called for help or was being tortured. They moved me to another cell and I received beatings under my feet, *falaka*, and I was also submitted to psychological torture, a kind of brainwashing where they tried to make me forget everything that I knew from before. Among other things, they used electric shocks for this purpose. I was in this prison for many months

until at last my family got me out on condition that I reported to the army headquarters at intervals.

"When I came out, I felt very lonely and I found out that I missed my former job in the prison. My only friends were in the prison. It is strange, but I found out that I missed the sight of blood. Therefore, I went back to them and asked if I could have a job there again. They almost laughed at me and instead of sending me to the prison, they sent me to the front."

The therapist was very attentive to Ahmed's theme of "missing the sight of blood." In a way, he wished that something psychotic would surface around this theme: a flaw in the connection to reality, a loss of control. But Ahmed remained well structured when telling about this, with an aura interpreted by the therapist as being sadistic rather than psychotic. The therapist sensed the impulses of a murderer rather than of a psychotic. Actually, Ahmed's desire for seeing blood could be interpreted as a wish for symbolic and actual reenactment of the trauma—a symptom seen in severe cases of PTSD (Wilson, 1988). In dissociated states, Ahmed would cut himself and carry out actual reenactments, as he related later in the story. The therapist, however, reacted to this with a feeling of discomfort and disgust rather than "empathy."

"At the front we were on duty every second night. One night when I was on duty, my friend was shot and I saw him lying in the dark in front of me with his cerebral matter and blood running out of him. He had been hit by a grenade."

This was presented with so much detail that the therapist felt that "now it could bloody well be enough."

Ahmed continues: "I felt very strange and suddenly I fired all my bullets into the air, completely desperate. The enemy must have found out from which direction the shots came and they started launching rockets at us. I remember that I watched the first and the second rocket arrive, and from the time when the third rocket came, I don't remember any more before I woke up in hospital. I don't know how many of my comrades from the platoon were killed in that attack.

"I was in hospital for some weeks and my mother was allowed to visit me. During one of her visits, I was able to escape and from then on I was hiding until I succeeded in fleeing to another country. When I first arrived at the capital, I lived in a hotel; but after a while, I did not have any more money and I lived for several months in the parks. Here, I met some Christians from my own country who went to the parks and gave the homeless food. I became friends with some of them and they took me into their house. I didn't think that my own religion had done me any good so I decided to become a Christian. They taught me to confess my sins and that, if I did so, I would be forgiven. While I was with them, I sometimes felt strange during the night. I could not sleep or I did not dare go to sleep. I found out that I again had the desire to see blood and sometimes I cut myself in the arm with a knife and smeared blood all over my face. After that, I could come back to myself and rather quickly I could feel normal again. At last, they asked me to leave and my brother sent me some money so that I could travel to Denmark by air with false papers.

"When I arrived in the Danish refugee camp I also had difficulties sleeping. I was afraid and felt insecure among the others. I was scared that they would find out who I was. I asked to be isolated but after some days I told my story to an interpreter from my country. She told it to the nurse and after that I was referred to the psychiatric ward."

As Ahmed ends his story, the therapist realizes how his attitude has changed during the two sessions. He started out as the *clinician* who wanted to make a correct diagnostic evaluation; he discovered that the patient is not psychotic, that he was a torturer and that this is undeniable and real. The therapist knows that Denmark has signed the United Nations Convention against Torture (Sørensen, 1988) and that this might oblige the therapist to inform against Ahmed so that he can be punished. However, was it he who should take the first step?

At the conclusion of the last session, the therapist informed Ahmed in a sharp manner that he would either be returned to his own country or put in prison in Denmark. As he said this, the therapist had the feeling of being a torturer himself. The events which followed showed that the therapist judged Ahmed more severely than the Danish authorities, who, in the name of humanitarianism, granted Ahmed asylum within a few days and concealed his past from the refugee organization which took over his case.

The therapist was left feeling anger toward a system which grants quick asylum to murderers while many victims of torture have to wait in insecurity for long periods of time. Other considerations were also raised: Should Ahmed be offered treatment? Or are there certain categories of patients we will not treat? The therapist was also concerned with his credibility among the survivors: If he treated torturers, where then was his solidarity?

Issues of trust and mistrust are, then, an essential determining factor for whether a treatment process can be established at all for victims of extreme man-made stress such as torture (Wilson, 1989). The experiences they have had might naturally lead to a loss of belief in humanity. Moreover, it is an integral element in psychosexual torture that a person is submitted to acts which are so bizarre that others who hear about it will easily feel mistrust. The therapist may experience doubt: For example, is he telling the truth? This mistrust contributes to the victim's feeling of isolation and to his or her mistrust of the surroundings.

In the following anecdote, a course of treatment is shown where the mistrust is overcome by a reframing process which later makes it possible to use testimony as a psychotherapeutic tool (Agger & Jensen, 1991a,b; Jensen & Agger, 1988). During the process of bearing testimony, symptoms are gradually reduced, and there is a marked improvement in the patient's general level of adaption.

Case Three: Mehmet, a Torture Victim

Mehmet is a Kurd and he is 37 years old. He has been in Denmark for almost 3 years waiting for asylum to be granted. His application has been refused twice because his statement has been questioned and he has not been able to deliver convincing proofs. The authorities in his home country have declared that Mehmet will not run any risks by returning.

He has the status of a leader among his fellow countrymen in Denmark, and he has, therefore, felt too proud to ask for help. However, after thinking it over for several months, he has accepted an offer of help at a psychiatric ward as an outpatient.

The referral symptoms are nightmares in which events from prison and torture are reexperienced, intrusive phenomena during the daytime which manifest themselves as flashbacks accompanied by aggressive outbursts toward other asylum applicants—an unusual behavior for this otherwise quiet and deliberate man. He keeps to himself, avoids talking to anyone, cannot concentrate, and believes that his memory has been damaged. Politically, he is disillusioned. He feels that the struggle he believed in which would lead to an independent Kurdistan has been lost. He does not have the energy to commit himself any longer to political causes. At the same time, he feels guilty because he has saved himself by fleeing the country while several members of his family have been killed, and women and children suffered for the sake of "his" cause. He questions what it all has been worth. During most of the day Mehmet sits dark and scowling in a corner without contact with anyone.

THE STORY OF MEHMET: USE OF THE TESTIMONY METHOD

At the first session, Mehmet verifies the referral symptoms. His mood is still depressed and he is angry. At the same time he has a bearing of affected politeness.

He is openly skeptical toward the therapist before the therapist has even uttered a word and he is angry toward the Danish system, which mistrusts him. He believes that his referral to a psychiatric ward is an expression of racism. He believes he will not be taken seriously as he must obviously be considered insane. He knows the interpreter and accepts him immediately, although there is a minor argument about whether communication should be Turkish or Kurdish.

The spontaneous countertransference reaction of the *therapist* is a feeling of injustice. He has taken on this task because of his commitment to and interest in the refugee cause. He does not like to be mistrusted and he likes even less to be seen as a racist. He feels that it will be a tough job to establish a solid contact and working alliance and get to work. However, he tries to get through to Mehmet by delivering a series of statements in which he attempts to reframe the symptoms. He tells Mehmet that what he is experiencing is not strange or special but is universally found in people who have suffered traumatic events, and that these symptoms have a name: PTSD. He emphasizes that this is a reaction which anyone would have if they experienced extreme trauma. He exchanges "cultural information" by telling Mehmet that in Denmark people who treat refugees in that particular referral area are staff of the psychiatric ward and that it is an expression of this particular staff's interest in helping refugees who need it. It is therefore not because they think Mehmet is insane. On the contrary, the staff basically sees Mehmet as a "sane person who has been submitted to an insane situation." The therapist asks if the psychiatric system is different in Mehmet's homeland, which he affirms in the positive. Finally, the therapist emphasizes that he has no power of decision in his asylum case.

Mehmet reacts with some confusion; he apparently feels insecure but also curious. A certain degree of contact is established with Mehmet for the first time making direct eye contact with a hint of friendliness in it.

The therapist asks Mehmet what he believes is wrong with him, and he answers that he thinks the torture has "crushed" him and that there is no longer any hope. He does not think that anyone can help him and appears to have given up striving.

The therapist reacts to this by telling Mehmet that the authorities have used torture to change the *political pain* to private pain; that they have used a strategy of destruction which has the aim of forcing the victim to be so preoccupied with his own symptoms and so unsure of his own identity that he becomes harmless as an opponent. However, it is explained that the aim of therapy is the opposite: to change the private pain to political dignity. Briefly, he mentions the *testimony method* as an example of how to accomplish this change.

At the end of the first session, there is a certain relief in the atmosphere. There is more friendliness and more eye contact. The therapist is satisfied with the course of this first intervention and, in the talk afterward with the interpreter, he instructs him in the use of the testimony method. He also goes through the basic rules for interpretation in therapy.

At the beginning of the next session Mehmet conducts himself exactly as he did at the beginning of the first session. His mood is depressed, he is hopeless, mistrustful, and angry at the Danish system. He emphasizes that the long period of waiting in the camp reminds him of the insecurity in prison: That is, you never knew when something terrible would happen. He experiences the interrogation of lawyers and police in his asylum case as a repetition of the interrogations in prison, and on these occasions his symptoms are intensified. He thinks that this makes the Danish authorities even more mistrustful of him because his anxiety in these situations is expressed as bursts of anger.

Mehmet then directs his mistrust toward the interpreter. Why is he in Denmark? What is his political stand? Does he support the Kurdish cause? The interpreter is a friendly immigrant who has lived in Denmark for many years. He is taken by surprise at this sudden mistrust and becomes confused and insecure. The therapist, therefore, uses a considerable amount of time to clear up the relation between the interpreter and Mehmet, until Mehmet finally approves of him. When the atmosphere between these two has become more relaxed, the mistrust is again directed toward the therapist. How is *his* stand in the Kurdish cause? Will information given in the sessions come out? Once again, time must be used to establish a secure atmosphere. The reframing of the symptoms begun during the last session must be repeated as if it were for the first time. On his own initiative, the interpreter points out that Mehmet had complained of memory problems. The therapist, thus, chooses to repeat his statements from the last time with the same conviction—and with the same effect. He ends up by introducing the testimony method once more, and asks Mehmet to consider until they meet next time, whether he wants to work with this method. At the end of the session, the atmosphere is again more relaxed.

At the third session, a few minutes are spent on reviving the issues of the last time, whereafter Mehmet suddenly declares himself ready to bear testimony.

In practical terms, the process is started by the therapist who asks Mehmet to tell about his background, and they then move swiftly up to the time shortly before the first imprisonment torture and flight. The story is continually translated by the interpreter who talks into a dictaphone while the therapist gets Mehmet to elaborate the trauma story. The account of *what* happened is the cognitive lead, while the therapist works at getting Mehmet to realize *how* he reacted to the traumatic events—especially at the emotional level. The therapist also encourages Mehmet's understanding of *why* it happened by emphasizing the political context of the torture. In this way, the therapist tries to resolve some of the fundamental questions of "(1) What happened? (2) Why did it happen? (3) Why did I and others act as we did, then and since then? And (4) If something like this happens again, will I be able to cope more effectively?" (Figley, 1988, p. 87).

Between the weekly sessions, a secretary transcribes the dictation and at the beginning of the following session the interpreter translates the statement from the last session back to Mehmet who, in turn, corrects errors and approves of it before the testimony is continued.

Mehmet starts the testimony by telling that he is 37 years old and born into a poor family with many children. He does not have any formal education but has worked in many different fields. He committed himself politically by joining a democratic party which worked for an independent Kurdistan. He tells about the family, his general background, and then comes to his first experiences of torture.

Between sessions Mehmet is asked to do homework. He records his dreams and sometimes he makes a drawing of a dream or of a certain event (he is very good at drawing). An abbreviated account of Mehmet's story of the torture trauma is as follows:

"We were around 30 people and we were put one or two together in each cell. They were in a corridor. There were about 20 cells along the corridor. On the walls of the corridor were hanging different kinds of torture instruments so that we could constantly be reminded about it.

"We were first ordered to take off our clothes, were blindfolded, and led into a room. I was pushed so I fell and an *automobile tire* was pulled down over me so that I was lying squeezed into it.

"Later, we talked about how we were lying there like turtles: Either we could, completely helpless, be turned so we were lying on our backs—or we could be turned the other way and be raped from behind. They were all the time shouting impudent remarks and insinuated that we were homosexual. It all went on in one room so that you could constantly hear how they tortured the others. You could hear the sounds of beatings and the screams. We also heard voices of women and children. Maybe it was from a tape recorder. They tried to make us believe that they were torturing and raping someone from our families. While I was lying there, I felt completely helpless even though I would not confess anything. They tried to make me confess something I had not done. On my drawing I have 'forgotten' to make myself naked (see Figure 57.1).

"The automobile tire is one of the first things they use. After that comes *falaka*—especially if they think that you are a powerful person in the organization. In *falaka*, the man who sits on top of you shakes your head and beats you while he at the same time hinders you from banging your head onto the ce-

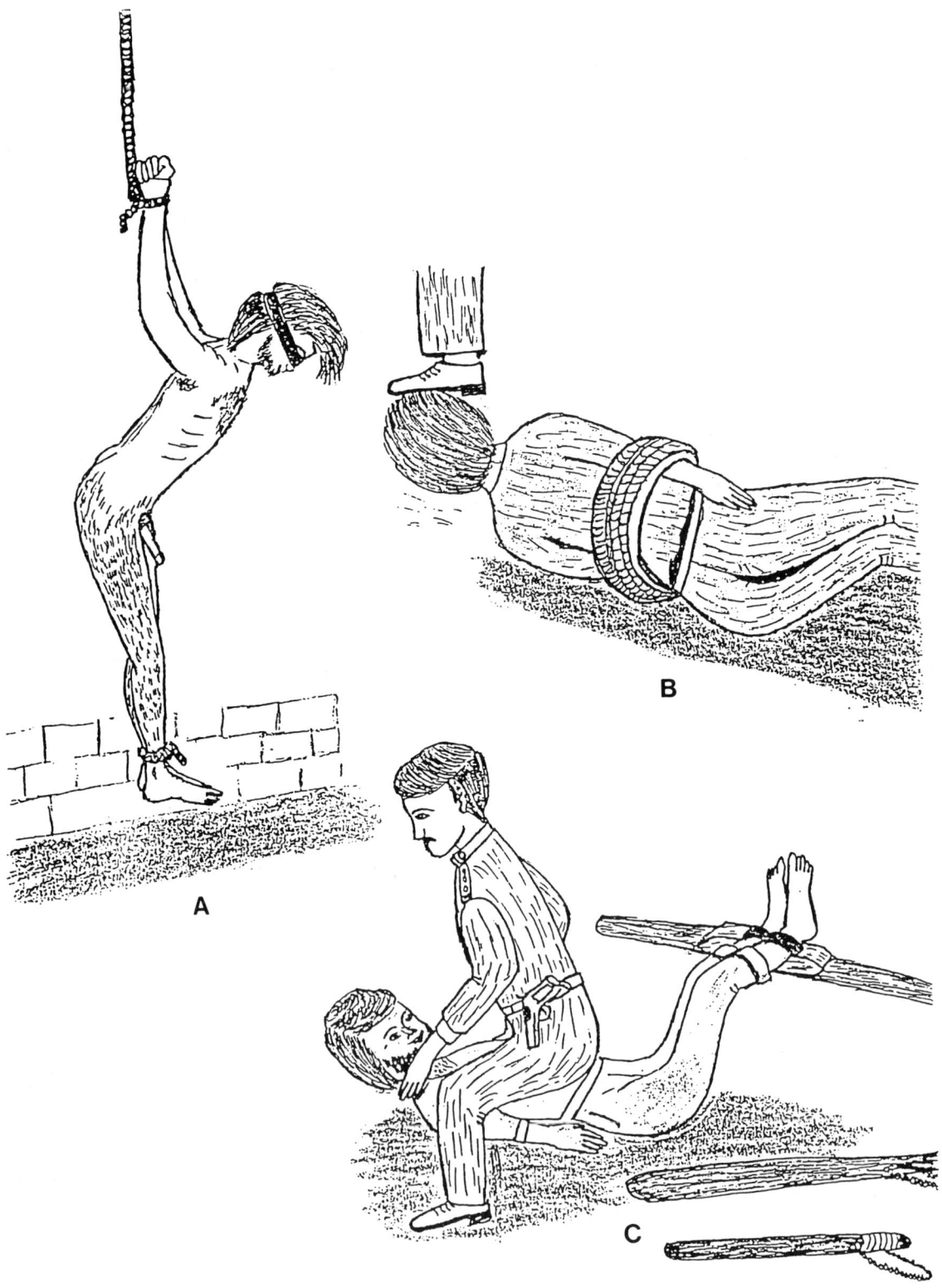

Figure 57.1. Common torture techniques: (A) *Filistin askisi*, (B) the automobile tire, (C) *falaka*.

ment floor, for in that way to make yourself unconscious. In between, they beat you under the footsoles, and later I had to walk around in the room where they had strewn salt on the floor. They said it was to make the swellings go away and to avoid that anyone could afterward see that you had been tortured. They said that no one would believe me if I told it. I felt mostly pain, but I also felt anger in the middle of my powerlessness.

"The next step was *filistin askisi*, Palestinian suspension. Here, you are hung up naked as is shown on the drawing (see Figure 57.1). They came past and shouted dirty words at me. While I was hanging there, they gave me electrical currents on my genitals. They told me that from now on I would be impotent for the rest of my life and that I would not be able to have any children. At that time I did not know if it was true. They also inserted a baton in my rectum while they laughed and shouted dirty things. At last you faint from mere exhaustion and maybe also from shame. Another time they told me to masturbate and when I refused one of the guards began touching me and tried to give me an erection. I cursed him but he continued and when nothing happened he said that I could see for myself that now I was impotent. Every time I have been together with a woman later on I have had this fear inside of me. They could be right! I know now that it is not true but I still avoid sexual contact."

Mehmet works himself through his story during subsequent sessions while his symptoms diminish. He is very keen on telling the whole story and corrects details when the account from the last session is read aloud. He wants the document to be reliable. The therapist senses that Mehmet is sometimes "back there in the past" (i.e., reliving the torture) when he tells about the traumatic events. Sometimes it is difficult to get him diverted from his flashbacks but it helps when the therapist makes interventions about the general aspects of the situation: "We know that they use this method in many countries—and the aim is usually to . . . ," etc.

Later on, Mehmet describes daily life in the prison as illustrated by his drawing (see Figure 57.2), with special emphasis on the unequal treatment based on social differences among the prisoners.

At the end of his story, he is visibly better. The story is worked through once more. It is stated more exactly and shortened in some parts, and finally signed by Mehmet, the interpreter, and the therapist. It is then read aloud one more time and symbolically handed over to Mehmet. His pain has now become a document which is in his power. He may use it for his own cause if he chooses to.

Mehmet wants to use it as a support for his asylum case and he also wants it to be used for teaching therapists who work with political refugees. He is granted asylum a few

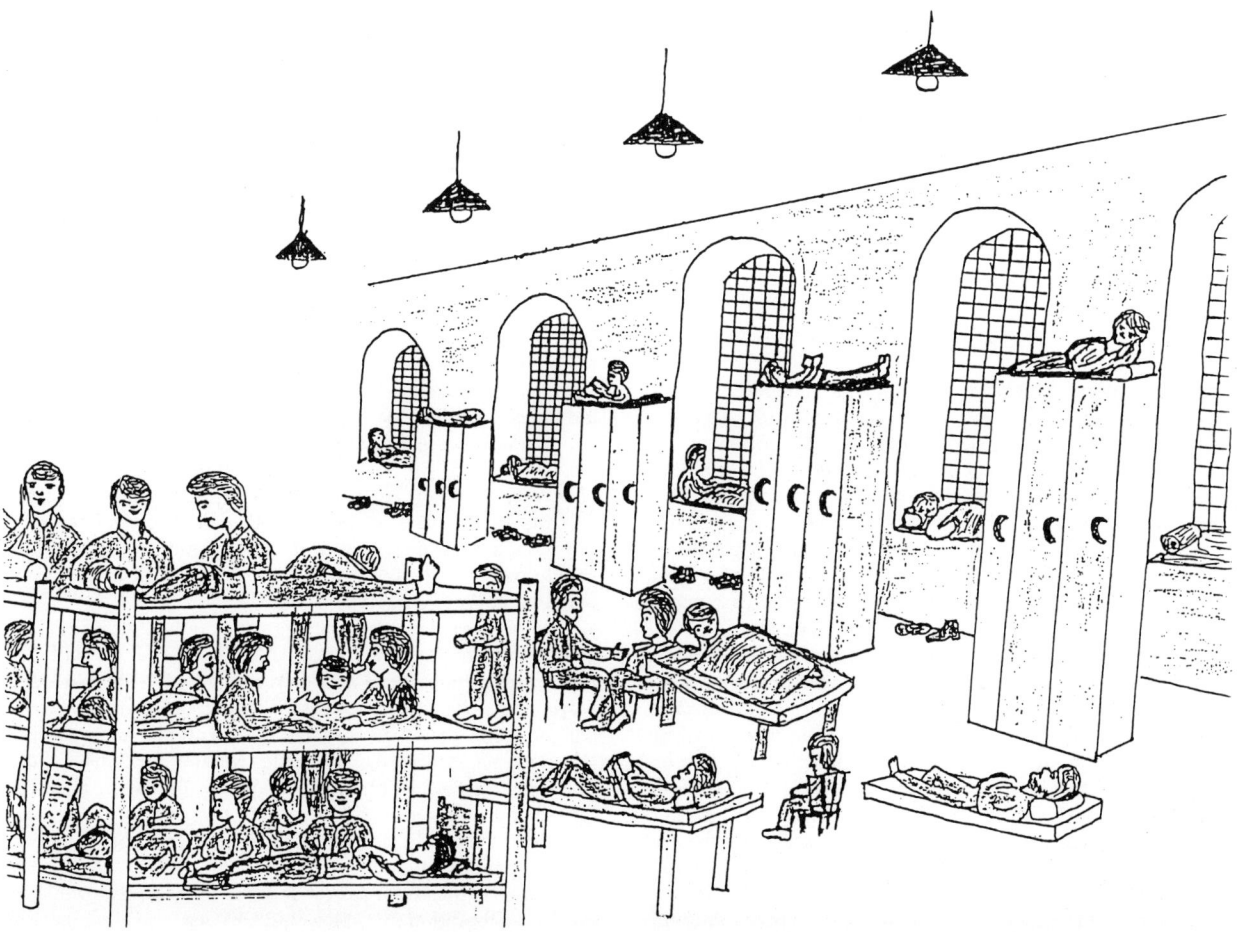

Figure 57.2. The prison compound.

months later, and at that time, there is a revival of his symptoms whereafter they fade out again. He can still have symptoms in situations which have a similarity to traumatic events in the past, but his ideological commitment has awakened again and helps him in these situations. His anger against the Danish system has been converted to a commitment to the Kurdish cause and to a fight for better conditions for applicants for asylum including the right to psychiatric assistance. The treatment process is terminated by Mehmet himself when he feels that he does not need any more assistance. He offers to participate in educational activities if needed, and he intercedes for one of his friends also receiving treatment.

Mehmet's PTSD symptoms have gone into remission following treatment. The therapist contemplates his initial diagnosis since there were also evident depressive elements. Mehmet contacts the ward 2 years later because of sexual problems in his newly established relationship to a Danish woman. One session seems to be sufficient to clear up Mehmet's unrealistic anxiety about impotency. He is invited to bring his partner if he feels the need of additional assistance.

Partners of victims of psychosexual trauma and families in which one or more members have undergone torture are naturally greatly affected. The stress of exile is also a factor which affects both the individual and the family system. As "each person experiencing traumatic stress must be viewed within a social network of supporters, including family members" (Figley, 1988, p. 83), it will be important in the work with exiled couples and families to include both family members *and* relations to the exile group from the refugee's particular country (Agger & Jensen, 1989). In the following and last case example, we look more closely at this aspect of torture and exile.

Case Four: Carlos and Maria—Political Conflict in a Marriage

This Latin American couple was referred for psychotherapeutic treatment because of marital troubles. They had already consulted the social worker of the Danish Refugee Council about divorce and had been asked if they were interested in seeing a therapist before they went further in the procedure. They had accepted this on the condition that a certain woman interpreter, who has followed them throughout their stay in Denmark, could participate. Although the therapist spoke Spanish quite well, she accepted this, and, in fact, was able to make a good team with the interpreter, who was very experienced in the field. An arrangement was made in which the interpreter was "the voice" of the therapist, which meant that she only translated the interventions of the therapist since it was most difficult for the Danish therapist to express herself accurately in Spanish. In effect, the interpreter became a valuable co-therapist, as the couple felt very secure with her and trusted the words coming from her mouth more than if they had come directly from the therapist. Before and after the sessions, the interpreter could supply the therapist with valuable information about the couple, and when the

couple saw that the interpreter supported what was going on in the therapy, they were encouraged to go more fully into the process.

THE STORY OF CARLOS AND MARIA

Carlos and Maria had arrived three years ago. Carlos was in his late twenties and Maria was around 20 years old. They had a 2-year-old daughter. Carlos had been politically active in Chile, had been imprisoned a couple of times, but "had not been severely tortured," as he put it. After being released from prison, he had been continuously followed by the police and he decided to leave the country as he feared renewed imprisonment. Just before flight, he married Maria, whom he had been dating for a while, in order that she could follow him in exile.

Maria had never been involved in political activities. On the contrary, she had kept out of everything "political." Both were from a big city and were skilled laborers.

After arriving in exile, they had a long stressful stay in a Red Cross camp while their asylum application was under consideration. During this period, Maria became pregnant.

At last, they were granted asylum, got an apartment, and started language school. During the stay in the camp, Carlos had already established connection to the Chilean exile group and he was very busy attending meetings and activities. He was so busy that he was nearly never at home.

Maria stayed at home with the child and refused to participate in any of the group's activities. She was called by several women of the group who tried to persuade her to attend the meetings of the women's group. She felt very hostile toward these women, wondering if any of them had a sexual relationship with her husband.

At the same time, she refused to have sex with Carlos, complaining of fatigue and a lack of desire. When they occasionally had intercourse, she felt very good about it and she did not have any problems reaching orgasm.

Every time Carlos went to a meeting, he and Maria had arguments. She tried to prevent him from going and he stayed away—sometimes overnight—refusing to give her any time for his return. There was also continuous quarreling over the upbringing of the child—Carlos complained that Maria was spoiling the child, while Maria felt that Carlos was too demanding.

Maria was consumed by loneliness and a strong longing for her country and especially for her mother, to whom she had been very attached. Further, because of the incessant quarrels and the lack of sex life, they considered divorce. They felt, however, a great deal of warmth toward each other and they sought couple's therapy in an attempt to solve the sexual problem and stop the quarrels.

In therapy, Maria revealed a great amount of anger toward Carlos for bringing her into exile. Also, she was angry with her mother for urging her to marry Carlos and follow him in exile. Maria had never before expressed this anger openly. Instead, she punished Carlos by not having sex with him and by refusing to have anything to do with the central issue in his life, the political struggle. He, in return, responded by staying away for longer and longer periods. It seemed that both of them were escalating the conflict in order to force some kind of solution to end the painful situation.

Carlos expressed a strong desire to stay together with her but on the condition that she would have sex with him regularly and accept his political activities. Maria felt very attached to him and she was willing to stay on the condition that he spend more time at home and with the child. With respect to the sexual problem, they were both willing to participate in a sensate focus exercise program which in the beginning consisted in caressing each other with intercourse being forbidden.

During these exercises, Maria felt it quite easy to caress Carlos, and she also enjoyed it, while she felt it very uncomfortable to be passive and let him caress her. Her unwillingness to give in to him was interpreted by the therapist as a refusal to give up her anger toward him (and her mother). However, little by little, the couple saw this dynamic and recognized the sexual symptom as part of the power struggle between them. Around the political issue, they also saw the dynamics as part of this power struggle; her sexual withholding in contrast to his incessant political activities.

At last, a working alliance between them was established. She started accompanying him to some meetings, and Carlos set time limits to his involvement. Eventually, they started having intercourse at intervals which they could both accept.

An important factor in the therapy was for them to see how they expressed their mutual anger, and how they turned the difficult personal and political situation of exile against one another. In this way, they developed a "healing theory" (Figley, 1988) which helped them toward finding a new equilibrium in their family system.

At the end of the couple therapy, the therapist suggested to Carlos that he might one day feel prepared to come back and talk about his imprisonment. Carlos declared that he did not think it was necessary but that he would think it over.

Conclusion

What we have been examining here are different expressions of person-inflicted *organized violence*. This concept was adopted by a WHO working group in 1986 (Ministry of Welfare, Health and Cultural Affairs, 1987). Organized violence is here defined as

> the interhuman infliction of significant, avoidable pain and suffering by an organized group according to a declared or implied strategy and/or system of ideas and attitudes. It comprises any violent action which is unacceptable by general human standards and relates to the victim's feelings. (p. 9)

To this definition the Dutch Deputy Chief Medical Officer of Health adds that

> The violence which occurs in these situations as a direct consequence of repression is of a structural nature and can only disappear when human and social relationships are profoundly changed. This practically always means a fundamental change in the imbalance of powers. (van Geuns, 1987, p. 8)

As therapists, we can work at helping the psychic consequences of trauma to heal. We can also attempt to make our small contribution to the change of that imbalance of power, which causes organized violence, by aiding the process of transforming private, individualized shame to political identity and dignity. We can, for example, testify to what we see and hear from our clients.

In the complex and confusing stress of psychosexual trauma, we see the traumatic fusion of sexuality and political aggression. We see how victims' feelings of complicity can aid those in power in crushing their identity, including the political identity, of their opponents, as was illustrated in the story of Silvia.

Therapy for political refugees, therefore, is permeated with politics. Maybe we want to take a "neutral" stand, but, of course, in doing so we are also taking a stand; namely, for those in power who instigated the organized violence. Some of these ethical questions were seen in the story of the torturer, Ahmed.

As therapists in Western culture meeting people from other parts of the world, we might mistake social and political problems for cultural differences, since, in fact, there also exists a common purpose which is innately human: the struggle against injustice. In this process we need not fall into the traps of cultural universalism or relativism. As in the story of Mehmet, the meeting can take place within the setting of a testimony, which serves both as a psychotherapeutic tool for reframing *and* a political document supplying evidence against the repressive system. Moreover, this method has proved to be transculturally applicable in a Western exile setting for people who do not see the blessings of the kinds of therapy we usually subscribe to.

In the story of Carlos and Maria, we saw how the couple turned the political pain of exile against each other so that it manifested itself as private symptoms. This reframing helped the couple to develop a healing theory by giving them answers to the important question of "Why has this happened?" We also saw that Carlos was not ready to tell his story from the prison and that the therapist chose not to provoke him into disclosing the trauma story until he felt ready for it.

In the stories of both Silvia and of the torturer, we recognized the powerful countertransference reactions elicited in the therapists through confrontation with such dimensions of human evil. We saw emotional reactions of fear, anger, guilt, shame, and distress in the therapists. In the testimony of Mehmet, we could have foreboding of a prosocial, positive, overcommitted countertransference (Wilson, 1989).

These reactions indicate that close supervision of therapies with victims of torture trauma is necessary both on the individual level and also on the institutional level (Jensen, 1991). Otherwise, specialized institutions working with torture victims could become infected with the trauma and symbolically reenact in their internal dynamics the repression and organized violence which their clients have been subjected to (Bustos, 1991).

Most political refugees wish to return to their home countries as soon as it is safe to do so, and we, as therapists who meet them in their exile, might be able to establish relations with therapists working in the human rights movement of the countries of origin. Repatriation is, as many Uruguayan, Chilean, and Argentinean refugees have already discovered, a difficult process which can revive symptoms. By establishing contact and alliance, professionals in both exile and home countries can contribute to the common cause of opposing organized violence and restoring human dignity.

References

Agger, I. (1987, June). *The female political prisoner: A victim of sexual torture*. Paper presented at the 8th World Congress of Sexology, Heidelberg, Germany.

Agger, I. (1988a) *Flygtningekvinder i Danmark* [Refugee women in Denmark]. Repro-Serie, 10, University of Copenhagen, Institute of Cultural Sociology.

Agger, I. (1988b). Die politische Gefangene als opfer sexueller Folter [Female political prisoners as victims of sexual torture]. *Zeitschrift für Sexualforschung, 1,* 231–241.

Agger, I. (1989). Sexual torture of political prisoners: An overview. *Journal of Traumatic Stress, 2*(3), 305–318.

Agger, I. (1992). *Det blå værelse: Kvindeligt vidnesbyrd fra exilet* [The blue room: Feminine testimony from exile]. Copenhagen: Hans Reitzels Forlag. Spanish edition: *La pieza azul: Testimonio femenino del exilio.* Santiago de Chile: Cuarto Propio, 1993.

Agger, I., & Jensen, S. B. (1990). *La potencia humillada. Tortora sexual de presos politicos de sexo masculino* [The humiliated potency. Sexual torture of male political prisoners]. In H. Riquelme (ed.), *Era de nieblas.* Caracas: Editorial Nueva Sociedad.

Agger, I., & Jensen, S. B. (1989). Couples in exile: Political consciousness as an element in the psycho-sexual dynamics of a Latin American refugee couple. *Sexual and Marital Therapy, 4*(1), 101–108.

Agger, I., & Jensen, S. B. (1990). Testimony as ritual and evidence in psychotherapy for political refugees. *Journal of Traumatic Stress, 3*(1), 115–130.

American Psychiatric Association. (1987). *Diagnostic and statistical manual of mental disorders* (3rd ed., rev.). Washington, DC: Author.

Amnesty International. (1984). *Torture in the eighties.* London: Martin Robertson.

Bloch, M. (1977). The past and the present in the present. *Man (N.S.), 12,* 278–292.

Bustos, E. (1988). Sexualitet och exil hos traumatiserade flyktingar. En psykodynamisk förståelse [Sexuality and exile in traumatized refugees. A psychodynamic understanding]. *Nordisk Sexologi, 6,* 25–30.

Bustos, E. (1991). Dealing with the unbearable: Reactions of therapists and therapeutic institutions working with survivors of torture. In P. Suedfeld (Ed.), *Psychology and torture.* Washington, DC: Hemisphere Publishing.

Erikson, E. H. (1968). *Identity, youth and crisis.* New York: W. W. Norton.

Figley, C. R. (1988). Post-traumatic family therapy. In F. M. Ochberg (Ed.), *Post-traumatic therapy and victims of violence.* New York: Brunner/Mazel.

Geertz, C. (1973). *The interpretation of cultures.* New York: Basic Books.

Geertz, C. (1984). Distinguished lecture: Anti-relativism. *American Anthropologist, 86,* 263–278.

Jensen, S. B. (1991). Traumatized refugees meet psychiatry: Comparative studies of refugees exposed to organized violence. *Proceedings of the WHO Advisory Group on the Health Situation of Refugees and Victims of Organized Violence, August 26–27, 1988.* Gothenburg, Sweeden: The Nordic School of Public Health.

Jensen, S. B., Schaumburg, E., Leroy, B., Larsen, B. Ö., & Thorup, M. (1989). Refugees exposed to organized violence meet psychiatry: A comparative study of refugees and immigrants in a Danish county. *Acta Psychiatrica Scandinavica, 80*(2), 125–131.

Kiev, A. (1964). *Magic, faith, and healing.* New York: Free Press.

Kjersem, H. (1987). *Erfaringer fra arbejdet for asylsogere* [Experience from the work for applicants for asylum]. Copenhagen: The Danish Red Cross.

Kleinman, A. (1988). *Rethinking psychiatry: From cultural category to personal experience.* New York: Free Press.

Lindy, J. D. (1986). An outline for the psychoanalytic psychotherapy of post-traumatic stress disorder. In C. R. Figley (Ed.), *Trauma and its wake* (pp. 195–212). New York: Brunner/Mazel.

Lira, E., & Weinstein, E. (1986, May). *La tortura sexual* [Sexual torture]. Paper presented at the Seminario Internacional: Consecuencias de la represion en el Cono Sur. Sus efectos medicos, psicologicos y sociales, Montevideo, Uruguay.

Ministry of Welfare, Health and Cultural Affairs (Eds.). (1987). *Health hazards of organized violence.* The Hague: Center of Government Publications (DOP).

Mollica, R. F. (1988). The trauma story: The psychiatric care of refugee survivors of violence and torture. In F. M. Ochberg (Ed.), *Post-traumatic therapy and victims of violence* (pp. 295–314). New York: Brunner/Mazel.

Mollica, R. F., & Lavelle, J. P. (1988). Southeast Asian refugees. In L. Comas-Diaz & E. E. H. Griffith (Eds.), *Clinical guidelines in cross-cultural mental health* (pp. 262–305). New York: Wiley.

Schwartz, J. M. (1985a). From "social conditions" to "cultural collisions": A review of migration research in Danish social science, 1970–1984. In Center for Comparative Cultural Research (Eds.), *Integration.* University of Copenhagen.

Schwartz, J. M. (1985b). *Reluctant hosts: Denmark's reception of guest workers.* Copenhagen: Akademisk Forlag.

Sveaass, N. (1987). Intervju med psykologerne Elizabeth Lira og Juana Kovalsky [Interview with the psychologists Elizabeth Lira and Juana Kovalsky]. *Tidsskrift for Norsk Psykologforening, 24,* 102–105.

Sørensen, B. (1988, August). *United Nations Convention against Torture.* Paper presented at the meeting of the WHO Advisory Group on the Health Situation of Refugees and Victims of Organized Violence, Gothenburg, Sweden.

United Nations High Commissioner for Refugees. (1988). *Refugees* (Special Issue). New York: United Nations Publishing.

van Geuns, H. A. (1987). The concept of organized violence. In Ministry of Welfare, Health and Cultural Affairs (Eds.), *Health hazards of organized violence.* The Hague: Center of Government Publications (DOP).

Wilson, J. P. (1980). Conflict, stress, and growth: The effects of war on psyhcosocial development among Vietnam veterans. In C. R. Figley & S. Leventman (Eds.), *Strangers at home: Vietnam veterans since the war* (pp. 123–165). New York: Brunner/Mazel.

Wilson, J. P. (1986). Post-traumatic stress disorder and the disposition to criminal behavior. In C. R. Figley (Ed.), *Trauma and its wake: Vol. 2. Traumatic stress theory, research, and intervention* (pp. 305–322). New York: Brunner/Mazel.

Wilson, J. P. (1988). Understanding the Vietnam veteran. In F. M. Ochberg (Ed.), *Post-traumatic therapy and victims of violence* (pp. 227–253). New York: Brunner/Mazel.

Wilson, J. P. (1989). *Trauma, transformation and healing.* New York: Brunner/Mazel.

CHAPTER 58

Psychological Sequelae of Torture

Stuart W. Turner and Caroline Gorst-Unsworth

Introduction

Although much has been written about the history and methods of torture, and moving testimonies have been produced by individuals and groups of survivors, there have been few attempts to produce an explanatory model which systematically deals with the common physical and psychosocial sequelae. Never has this been more important (Pilisuk & Ober, 1976). Torture is prohibited by the *United Nations Universal Declaration of Human Rights* (United Nations [UN], 1948) and the *Convention against Torture* (UN, 1984), yet it is widely used by state authorities throughout the world as an instrument of interrogation and systematic repression (British Medical Association, 1986). Amnesty International (1987a) has reported the use of "brutal torture and ill-treatment" in over 90 countries in the 1980s.

Developments in the social and clinical sciences during this century have provided the opportunity for advancement in our understanding of the long-term reactions to torture. In this chapter, one approach is outlined. It is based on our personal experience of working in a London-based center, the Medical Foundation for the Care of Victims of Torture (Turner, 1989) and in an academic traumatic stress clinic.

Torture is not a new phenomenon. It has been mentioned in ancient Greek and Roman law. In the thirteenth century, at the beginning of its resurgence in Europe, torture was defined as the "inquiry after truth by

means of torment." Confession was seen as the most important of the proofs of guilt and in the presence of other indicators, torture was perceived as a legitimate means of obtaining confession (Peters, 1985).

Changes in legal practice and philosophy have reduced the central importance of personal confessions in the legal process. Similarly, advances in forensic sciences and in the techniques of investigating crime have provided powerful alternative ways of obtaining evidence. Peters (1985) asserts that the increasing dependence on torture in the twentieth century is a result of changing concepts of political crime during this period. Usually, the current use of torture appears to be part of a process of systematic repression of dissent by a regime acting within its own country (Martin-Baro, 1988).

So torture has been defined in broader terms, as for example, "the deliberate infliction of pain by one person on another in an attempt to break down the will of the victim" (Stover & Nightingale, 1985). Similarly, the World Medical Association (1975) has defined torture as the

deliberate, systematic or wanton infliction of physical or mental suffering by one or more persons acting alone or on the orders of any authority to force another person to yield information, to make a confession, *or for any other purpose.*

Finally, under the terms of a recent UN convention (UN, 1984), the position is made clear: Torture is always carried out "by or at the instigation of or with the consent or acquiescence of a public official or other person acting in an official capacity." It is in its nature, therefore, an action of a state against an individual, and moreover an action usually outside the normal process of criminal investigation and punishment.

Of course, states have other means at their disposal to impose political change on groups of people or even on whole communities. The concept of organized state violence has recently been introduced to include other forms of persecution in addition to torture. Derived in part from the *Universal Declaration of Human Rights* (UN, 1948), it includes imprisonment without trial, mock ex-

Stuart W. Turner • Department of Psychiatry, University College and Middlesex School of Medicine, Wolfson Building, Middlesex Hospital, London W1N 8AA, England. **Caroline Gorst-Unsworth** • The Medical Foundation for the Care of Victims of Torture, 96–98 Grafton Road, London NW5 3EJ, England.

International Handbook of Traumatic Stress Syndromes, edited by John P. Wilson and Beverley Raphael. Plenum Press, New York, 1993.

ecutions, hostage taking, or any other form of violent deprivation of liberty carried out for political or repressive purposes (Van Geuns, 1987).

It is our contention that torture, in common with many other forms of organized violence, is an activity with particularly complex social, psychological, and physical sequelae. The man, or woman, or child who survives torture has not merely been the victim of physical injury or threat of death, such as occur in a natural disaster (and these are disturbing enough), but has also received the focused attention of an adversary who is determined to cause the maximal psychological change. This perversion of an intimate relationship (Ritterman, 1987; Schlapobersky & Bamber, 1988) will often include the deliberate intention to disrupt the normal healing process and leave the survivor condemned to a life of misery.

However, it is not just the individual who suffers. For every person tortured there are mothers and fathers, wives and children, and friends and relatives who wait in uncertainty and fear (Cohn et al., 1985).

Unlike other forms of trauma, the primary aim of torture is to effect a specific psychological change in each person. The desired effect will vary for different people in different situations. Although subjugation of the will of the victim to that of the torturer is the common theme, for some it will be one aspect of interrogation, for others it will be punishment, and for many it will form part of the process of political or religious repression. It would be naive to assume that torturers do not achieve some of their aims. Indeed, one way of approaching an understanding of the types of reaction to this form of extreme trauma is to consider what it was that the torturer was attempting to achieve and on whom.

Psychological responses described in survivors of torture are protean. They include impaired memory and concentration, headache, anxiety, depression, sleeplessness with nightmares and other intrusive phenomena, emotional numbing, sexual disturbances, rage, social withdrawal, lack of energy, apathy, and helplessness (e.g., Abildgaard et al., 1984; Allodi & Cowgill, 1982; Cathcart, Berger, & Knazan, 1979; Rasmussen & Lunde, 1980). In a recent review, Goldfeld, Mollica, Pesavento, and Faraone (1988) have attempted to introduce some order by breaking down these symptoms into three categories: cognitive, psychological, and neurovegetative (Table 58.1). Although this approach is useful in describing common elements of the reactions to torture, it lacks a theoretical basis and has little heuristic value. The range of symptoms listed is very wide, includes features of many of the common psychiatric conditions, and is hard to interpret as representing a single disorder.

Many torture victims continue to have physical and psychological symptoms for long periods (Petersen et al., 1985). Some will have developed ways of responding to torture (e.g., the induction of altered states of consciousness during torture by hyperventilation) which persist as maladaptive behaviors following release; these may come to dominate these individuals' symptom profiles. In addition, there may be differences in the capacity to resist the torturer between those who were actively engaged in resistance prior to torture and those who were picked up at random or by mistake, or between people

Table 58.1. The Psychological Symptoms Commonly Reported Following Torture[a]

Cognitive symptoms
  Confusion/disorientation
  Memory disturbance
  Impaired reading
  Poor concentration
Psychological symptoms
  Anxiety
  Depression
  Irritability/aggressiveness
  Emotional lability
  Self-isolation/social withdrawal
Neurovegetative symptoms
  Lack of energy
  Insomnia
  Nightmares
  Sexual dysfunction

Note: Adapted from "The Physical and Psychological Sequelae of Torture" by A. E. Goldfeld, R. F. Mollica, B. H. Pesavento, and S. V. Faraone, 1988, *Journal of the American Medical Association, 259*, p. 2727. [a]Goldfeld et al. list the relative frequencies of these symptoms in the main published clinical surveys (*n* = 294).

of different cultures (Kinzie, 1985). Any systematic account must allow for these and other variables.

We therefore reject the notion of a single "torture syndrome" (Allodi & Cowgill, 1982; Basoglu & Marks, 1988). Not only are individual reactions more complex—it must be acknowledged that torture has effects on communities and on whole societies.

We believe that it is more helpful to conceptualize the common sequelae of torture under four distinct headings that form dimensions of the torture reaction. As will be discussed later, they are not only of heuristic value, they also stand to have important implications for treatment.

Direct (Individual) Responses to Torture

Incomplete Emotional and Cognitive Processing

The conceptual development of the posttraumatic neuroses in different settings has been reviewed comprehensively (Wilson, 1989; Horowitz, 1976; Kinston & Rosser, 1974; Raphael, 1986; Raphael & Middleton, 1988; Trimble, 1981; Wilson, 1989). The evidence obtained from all these sources points to the conclusion that similar stress response syndromes are found as sequelae to a wide range of traumatic events. It also became evident that, although premorbid personality was not necessarily unimportant (McFarlane, 1987), these reactions may occur in any one who is exposed to sufficient stress (Wilson, 1988a). Some have reported a dose-related effect to trauma (e.g., Shore, Tatum, & Vollmer, 1986, following the Mount St. Helens volcano eruption). Horowitz (1976) points out that the phrase "everyone has his breaking point" is derived from experience with reactions to combat. Lifton and Olson (1976) were able to write of the Buffalo Creek flood disaster that the psychological impact had been so extensive that no one in Buffalo Creek was unaffected.

The two central features of the specific traumatic stress response syndrome are (1) the compulsive tendency toward repetition of some aspect of the disturbing experience (as thoughts of the original event, as feelings associated with the experience or as behavioral reenactments), and (2) the avoidance of internal or external representations which recall or resemble the traumatic episode (Horowitz, 1976). There are several differing theoretical explanations for these phenomena (Basoglu & Marks, 1988; Brett & Ostroff, 1985; Wilson, 1989; Wirtz & Harrell, 1987).

Horowitz (1976) preferred a cognitive and emotional processing model. He suggested that painful experiences need to be processed in the mind, in the same way as any other formative experience. In this view, he is supported by Rachman (1980), who wrote of emotional processing as a normal way of dealing with affective material; sometimes this processing may be arrested or incomplete and it is then a source of continuing distress for the individual. Horowitz suggested that there are natural (protective) limits to the rate of cognitive and emotional processing. He wrote of "massive ideational denial and emotional numbing" as being the opposite phenomena to intrusive repetitiousness. Material which threatens to overwhelm the person leads to the invocation of these defensive mechanisms. In his theoretical and descriptive work, Horowitz pointed to a cyclical process in which the individual shifts between avoidance and a state of emotional distress associated with these intrusions into consciousness. In extreme cases, a state of denial and even patchy amnesia for the traumatic event may be induced.

To move on from this condition and complete the task of processing requires the intrusion of manageable chunks ("doses") of this material into consciousness. In this way, successful processing is accompanied by a phasic process of intrusion that alternates with denial. Of course, the traumatic event may be brought into consciousness not just by internal systems but also by external stimuli which resemble the circumstances of the traumatic episode; there may be frank avoidance of such stimuli.

Subsequently, the criteria for posttraumatic stress disorder (PTSD) have been modified in the revised edition of the Diagnostic and Statistical Manual (DSM-III-R) (American Psychiatric Association [APA], 1987). They are now based more closely on this etiological model.

Those elements central to PTSD, the intrusions, the avoidance, and the hyperarousal phenomena, undoubtedly occur in people who have been subjected to torture (Mollica, Wyshak, & Lavelle, 1987b). In torture, where the infliction of physical and psychological pain can continue over many months, the reactions may be particularly severe. The deliberate application of pain at a time which suits the torturer and which is intended to have the maximum impact on the victim makes it much more difficult for the victim to mount any satisfactory defense. It may be predicted that survivors of torture are less able to control their later intrusive recollections than others who have experienced major trauma.

Indeed, it is likely to be the aim of the torturer to overwhelm the normal cognitive and emotional processing mechanisms. Factors which stand to impede emotional processing have been described (Rachman, 1980) and several of these are common in torture. The induction of high arousal levels, fatigue, sleeplessness, and the irregularity of presentation of dangerous, intense, uncontrollable traumata are all said to militate against successful processing. Many of these factors appear to be manipulated deliberately by torturers to achieve this effect. Some survivors have learned (often by chance) alternative methods of reducing the pain of torture. These behaviors may include hyperventilation as a way of dissociating from the impact of the violence (see Chapter 60, in this volume).

The impact of prolonged exposure to painful stimuli, and the ever-present threat of a recurrence of attack, also lead to a state of chronic anxiety during detention. Following release, survivors are often vulnerable to repeated arrests, and even if they escape the country where torture took place, they may equally be subject to detention and forcible repatriation. It is the fear of further persecution and torture which drives people into exile and refuge. They may deal with these chronic anxiety symptoms by using the increasingly maladaptive responses that were learned during the torture. These avoidance behaviors appear to differ from those seen in war veterans, who may more commonly resort to the use of excessive drugs and alcohol (Yager, Laufer, & Gallops, 1984). Differences between combat and torture survivors may include not only the degree of access to these chemical agents during the traumatic process, but also cultural and philosophical factors. For example, those tortured because of their political beliefs may have a strength of personal commitment to a cause which is lacking in many combat troops.

Depressive Reactions and Life Events

Even in other fields of work with survivors of trauma, PTSD has been recognized to be an insufficient diagnosis to explain all the reactions reported. For example, Shore et al. (1986), in the study of the Mount St. Helens volcano disaster, reported increased rates of generalized anxiety and major depression as well as PTSD. McFarlane (1984) found that the two common disorders following the Australian bushfires were PTSD and major depression.

Intimately involved in the experience of torture are many emotionally charged processes chiefly concerned with loss. The survivors of torture may have lost body parts (e.g., a limb or an eye), a normal bodily function, or bodily health. They are likely to have lost work, status, family, and credibility. Even if they succeed in resisting torture, their colleagues are likely to be suspicious of them. If they stay in the same region, they know that there is the continuing threat of repeated detention and torture. They know that there is a similar threat to their families and friends. If they leave the region to seek asylum elsewhere, the losses are compounded (Miserez, 1988; UN, 1951). Torture, therefore, must be seen not only as a very important life event in its own right, but also as the cause of many others.

In the context of torture, the depressive reaction is a common sequel and is almost certainly related to these loss events (Brown & Harris, 1978). This is particularly likely when the individual is examined as an asylum seeker or refugee (Kinzie, Fredrickson, Ben, Fleck, & Karls, 1984). In a recent series of 52 Southeast Asian refugees reported by Mollica et al. (1987b), only one had PTSD alone; the remaining 25 individuals with PTSD also had another diagnosis, usually major affective disorder. Major depression was the single most common diagnosis, being present in 37 of the 52 subjects. Those Cambodian widows who had experienced at least two of the three traumata of rape, loss of spouse, or loss of children had the highest levels of depressive symptoms. They perceived themselves as socially isolated and living in a hostile social world.

Somatic Symptoms

Symptoms suggestive of physical illness and the signs of cognitive impairment are common following torture (Cathcart et al., 1979; Rasmussen & Lunde, 1980; Rasmussen & Marcussen, 1982). The physical sequelae are often the obvious and direct consequences of torture (Goldfeld et al., 1988). One example is the pain on walking experienced by someone who has been subjected to falaka, in which the soles of the feet are beaten repeatedly with a light cane or whip. It has been demonstrated that certain physical signs are specific to certain physical tortures and could not have been caused in any other way (Goldfeld et al., 1988; Gordon & Mant, 1984; see also Chapter 64, in this volume). These are of particular importance in the medical documentation and verification of the survivor's torture story.

However, in a person whose body has been tortured as a way of gaining control over his or her mind, somatic symptoms may have a multitude of meanings. Not infrequently they appear to be intimately related to a disturbed emotional state. It is important not to dismiss them lightly. A thoughtful clinical assessment is needed which does not rely too heavily on physical investigation. For example, in a person who has survived electrical torture, special care is required before advocating even a simple investigation such as an electrocardiograph (EKG).

Hyperventilation is not uncommon in survivors of torture and may be an important mechanism involved in the production of physical symptoms (see Chapter 60, in this volume). Similarly, sexual dysfunction is often reported in survivors of torture but so far the etiological mechanisms are unclear (Lunde, Rasmussen, Lindholm, & Wagner, 1980). Although sexual violence is a common form of torture especially in women and female adolescents (Goldfeld et al., 1988), dysfunction may also occur in those victims who have not experienced sexual torture. It is likely that the symptom has a complex etiology, with psychological processes being more important than organic factors.

Similarly, the etiology of cognitive impairment following torture is unknown. Thygesen (1980) believed

the symptoms experienced by the concentration camp survivors (Table 58.2) to be an expression of an organic damage which affected the brain. Physical and mental symptoms were reported in over 50% of cases with a significant disability assessment. The risk factors for the "dementia" which he believed to be present were older age, greater weight loss during detention, and lower social class.

It was the surprising resemblance between the psychological syndromes affecting war sailors and concentration camp survivors which challenged this view (Askevold, 1980). War sailors had been exposed to psychological stress but had not endured the physical privation of the concentration camp; they had been well fed and well looked after although they had frequently faced threats of death in action. Of particular importance was the finding that even apparently "organic" sequelae, such as memory impairment and reduced concentration, were obvious in people with the "war sailor" syndrome (95.8% and 89.1%, respectively). This suggested that it was not the physical hardship of the concentration camp, but the psychological impact of living under continued threat of death and personal disaster which was the crucial factor.

Thus, cognitive impairment (especially associated with PTSD) is likely to be a consequence of two processes. There are often changes in the person's emotional state which stand to affect concentration and the processing of cognitive information. There may also be organic brain damage from direct injury, electrical torture, malnutrition, or chronic illness. In survivors of torture, there is often a history of multiple head injuries (Goldfeld et al., 1988). The relative importance of the emotional and organic factors is unknown.

Existential Dilemma

The existential dilemma may be the most important and enduring of the psychological reactions to torture, although the most difficult to conceptualize in medical terms. With torture, as with some other forms of ex-

Table 58.2. Main Symptoms of Concentration Camp Syndrome

Physical
  Weight loss
  Pathological fatigue
  Periodic or constant diarrhea
  Dizziness
  Headache
  Hot flushes, nightly sweating
  Sleep disturbances
  Reduced sexual potency
Mental
  Depression/moodiness
  Lability
  Nightmares/other fear phenomena
  Reduction in memory and/or ability to concentrate

Note: Adapted from "The Concentration Camp Syndrome" by P. Thygesen, 1980, Danish Medical Bulletin, 27, pp. 226–227.

treme trauma, it is impossible to ignore the broader social and political dimensions. People are tortured for a purpose. Often it is not that the individual has important information or that a confession is required. If a regime is acting outside the usual rules of law, there are other simpler ways of investigation and people may be punished or killed ("disappeared") without proof being required. It seems that torture is used for a combination of reasons, but chief among these are punishment and systematic repression of whole communities. Membership of a political, social, tribal, or religious group may be sufficient reason in itself for a person to be detained and tortured (Stover & Nightingale, 1985).

Torture is a "catastrophic existential event" (Bendfeldt-Zachrisson, 1985). Survivors of torture face the double dilemma both of coming to terms with the full reality of torture in their world and also of surviving unchanged the insidious pressure of the torturer to change, to act or react in relation to the torturer's wishes.

The need to live in a world of such unremitting cruelty is the material of testimony and autobiography (e.g., Levi, 1987). The purpose of existence itself is challenged by the fact of torture.

It is probably in this area that early experiences and political or religious cultures are likely to have the strongest effects. Individual differences in reactions to other forms of severe trauma have been reported. For example, there appears to be increased emotional disturbance in black rather than in white soldiers who took part in the atrocities in Vietnam (Yager et al., 1984). This finding was interpreted (with some additional anecdotal evidence) as indicating that those who were more able to dehumanize their victims (to identify less well with them) were less severely affected themselves.

Similarly, in surviving torture, those who are able to retain some of their human values may have the best outcome. One man recalled how, when he himself was in prison and was being severely tortured, he comforted another victim whose torture he had witnessed with these words: "Old man, I cannot defend you now. But whilst we are here in prison I shall teach you to read and write and that will be our victory" (Schlapobersky & Bamber, 1988).

The trauma of torture may have important unconscious meanings. Ullman and Brothers (1988) argued that, in some cases, before the traumatic event, an individual may maintain fragile narcissistic fantasies of omnipotence which are completely shattered by the traumatic experience. This is seen in the fragmentation and disintegration of the self (and has been postulated as an explanation for the dissociative elements of the traumatic stress reaction). Frequently, for whatever reason, survivors of torture seen in the United Kingdom report that one of the most difficult tasks in the recovery process is not the control of evident symptoms but the rebuilding of their shattered sense of self.

Survival may bring its own guilt. A man who persisted in asking where his brother was being detained under one repressive regime was later detained himself and killed. He went to the security forces to ask about his brother once too often and never came back; his brother survived and is now alive and living in the United Kingdom, living with the guilt of his brother's death.

Following release, those who are able to obtain sufficient peer support or who are able to return to active religious or political groups may be able to overcome or suppress some of the broader aspects of torture in their internal lives. Those who are affected by torture and who have to seek asylum elsewhere may find themselves in a joyless world in which they can find little personal meaning or fulfillment. To some extent, they must come to reconcile the "new self" with the "new reality" of the external world.

The survivors may have to face victimization. They may have the experience of being blamed for their own condition. Similar processes have happened in the past. In World War I, for example, physical explanations for symptoms of "daze, fear, trembling, nightmares, and inability to function" were preferred; psychological mechanisms were seen to resemble weakness and cowardice (Horowitz, 1976). Shell shock was attributed to a combination of concussion and cerebrovascular damage, which was brought on by proximity to loud explosions. Some of the attempted "cures" of traumatic stress reactions, based on this understanding of the reaction as a combination of physical damage and psychological inferiority, were barbaric. Showalter (1987) reported the use of coercive treatments. Lewis Yealland, for example, is said to have described, with "complacent pride," his clinic in London. One young man, a veteran of Mons, Marne, Ypres, Hill 60, Neuve Chapelle, Loos, and Armentières had collapsed and subsequently had been mute. For 9 months he had resisted all efforts at "cure": including "hypnotism, electric shocks to his neck and throat, hot plates in his mouth, and cigarette burns on the tip of his tongue." Yealland, by a process of electric shocks of increasing intensity and the use of military discipline, managed to return this man's speech (Yealland, 1918, quoted in Showalter, 1987).

Following World War II, the survivors of concentration camps and the Holocaust had their own shattering histories to recount (Eitinger, 1980). However, even after the survivors had been seen and interviewed, there was debate about the validity of offering compensation based on disturbed psychological states. Many survivors were assessed only on the basis of physical handicaps. The early views of Sigmund Freud had indicated that stress reactions in adult life were often merely the reactivation of some childhood conflict or trauma which had not been dealt with completely at the time (Horowitz, 1976). If this was the case, how could their adult experiences of life in a camp be seen as causal of neurosis? It was argued that those who developed neuroses did so because of a prior constitutional deficiency. The medicolegal council eventually made a ruling (with important political and financial consequences) that "there cannot, in our opinion, be any doubt that the distress described here must be regarded as illness in the normal medical meaning of the word" (quoted by Thygessen, 1980).

It has been said that these existential aspects of the posttorture condition are a form of "bondage" through which the torturer ensures that his interventions will persist. Seen in this way, the work of rehabilitation is centered on the task of "freeing" survivors from these existential chains (Schlapobersky & Bamber, 1988).

Survivors of torture may gain the greatest support

from each other. Another survivor has described the members of a self-help group he attended in this way:

> This is a chain, one link and then another. It will be a great chain. When we eventually shake this chain it will be like thunder. You will hear thunder. The world will stop to listen, humanity will come to its senses and there will be no more torture. (Schlapobersky & Bamber, 1988)

In making this assertion, he is trying to reclaim for himself and his colleagues personal meanings, to find their ways out of the existential despair he and others had experienced and to stake his claims on the future he would like to see.

Indirect (Social) Responses to Torture

The problems arising in the survivor's community cannot be ignored and may be construed under some of the same dimensions as for the individual (Table 58.3). For example, close relatives of a man or woman undergoing torture have their own psychological reactions to deal with. These include incomplete emotional processing, depression, and the existential dilemma.

Young children of victims of torture have been reported to show social withdrawal, chronic fear, depressive moods, clinging and overdependent behavior, sleep disorders, somatic complaints, and an arrest or regression in social habits or school performance (Allodi, 1980). In another series of Chilean children who were being treated in Denmark, common symptoms included anxiety, oversensitivity to noise, sleep disturbance and nightmares, secondary nocturnal enuresis, anorexia, somatic symptoms, depression, and difficulty in social relationships (Cohn, Holzer, Koch, & Severin, 1980; Cohn et al., 1985). Others have reported symptoms of PTSD in school-aged children following a fatal sniper attack on the elementary school playground (Pynoos et al., 1987) and in adolescent survivors of the Pol Pot regime in Cambodia (Sack, Angell, Kinzie, & Rath, 1986).

Torture thus has important effects not just on the individual victim but on others who were not directly traumatized. There are also profound existential changes, described by some children of Holocaust survivors, and by many who have seen people close to them suffer torture and persecution.

In Argentina, a group of relatives (Argentina's National Commission on Disappeared People, 1986) provides a tragic example of people who were unable to discover the fate of the "disappeared." Were the disappeared people really dead? Were they being tortured? Were they still living in secret camps? How could these relatives begin to work through their feelings of grief when they could not know the reality?

In countries subject to repression and torture on a very large scale, whole communities may be affected. Torture and killing of individuals may have a striking effect on the social and political life of a country or region (Martin-Baro, 1988). This is certain to be one of the primary aims of the regime responsible for the violence, including torture, against its citizens.

The often arbitrary nature of the process is another destabilizing factor. In Cambodia, under Pol Pot, there was mass genocide. Amnesty International (1983) reported that intellectuals "were singled out for particularly harsh treatment and in many regions of the country were summarily executed." The same report indicated that intellectuals were "often crudely identified as those that wore spectacles."

In countries which practice torture, there is often no real democratic option for change, and nonviolent political dissent is sufficient reason for individuals to be detained and tortured. To be effective as a social control, it has to be widely known that behavior perceived as difficult or subversive to the authority of the regime is likely to lead to this sort of extreme response.

In one example of torture affecting a doctor, the reason was explained. The doctor, working in a poor district, was shot and wounded, then arrested. He was told that his wife and two daughters had already been captured and "disappeared." He was hooded and taken to a torture center.

> Then I heard another voice. This one said he was the "Colonel." He told me they knew I was not involved with terrorism or the guerrillas, but that they were going to torture me because I opposed the regime, because: "I hadn't understood that in Argentina there was no room for any opposition to the process of National Reorganization." He then added: "You're going to pay dearly for it . . . the poor won't have any goody-goodies to look after them any more!" (Argentina's National Commission on Disappeared People, 1986)

Table 58.3. The Dimensions of the Torture Reaction

Psychological reactions	Personal sequelae	Immediate social network	Broader political effects
Incomplete emotional and cognitive processing	++	+	−
Depressive reactions	++	++	+
Somatic symptoms	++	−	−
Existential dilemma	++	++	++

++ Very likely; + Likely; − Unlikely.

A Personal Series

Scrutinizing the detailed case notes of the first 20 people who were subjected to torture and referred to a psychiatrist (Stuart W. Turner) at the Medical Foundation revealed a long list of tortures (Table 58.4). Nine subjects were from Iran, and the remainder came originally from Iraq, Ghana, Peru, Angola, Chile, Uganda, and South Africa. Only one had a history of psychiatric treatment prior to torture. The mean age was 34 and the sex ratio was 18 men to 2 women.

Eighteen (90%) had evidence of PTSD, 14 (70%) met the criteria for major depression, and four (20%) had clinical evidence of a chronic hyperventilation disorder (confirmed by reproducing symptoms on voluntary over-breathing). Two (10%) were frankly psychotic: One had a manic illness and the other had a paranoid psychosis. It has to be said that all were referred to a psychiatrist; the sample was therefore highly selected. However, it does illustrate the complexity of the reactions, with most people having multiple diagnoses.

The case histories that follow illustrate some of the psychological reactions.

INCOMPLETE EMOTIONAL AND COGNITIVE PROCESSING

A 35-year-old man described his detention and torture in Iran. He reported nightmares which disturbed his sleep. Dur-ing the day, he tried to avoid things which reminded him of his torture. One of the worst experiences for him had been being forced to witness the torture of children. Now, whenever he saw an adult showing anger or hitting a child, he was reminded of his detention and felt extremely distressed. He described anxiety symptoms including a marked startle response.

MAJOR DEPRESSION

A 31-year-old survivor of torture, in fear for his life, described a crisis he had experienced. He developed hypochondriacal delusions. His concentration was impaired. He had almost no interests and no enjoyment. He appeared miserable. He had thought of killing himself. He had sleep disturbance with both early morning wakening and latency. He had lost his appetite and about 20 kilograms in weight. He made a very good symptomatic response to a tricyclic antidepressive drug.

SOMATIC SYMPTOMS

A 30-year-old man had survived severe torture including frequent beatings and electrical torture. He remained extremely troubled by his experiences, with disturbed sleep, nightmares, anxiety symptoms, and irritability. However, he also found that he could be quite forgetful. For example, he often forgot names and addresses that he would previously have remembered easily. On assessment, his concentration was impaired, and he

Table 58.4. Methods of Torture in a Retrospective Case Note Survey (n = 20)

Torture	Incidence	Percentage
Beating, slapping, kicking, punching	16	80
Striking with heavy cables or belts	9	45
Electric shocks	5	25
Falaka[a]	5	25
Hood or blindfold	5	25
Striking with rifle butts	4	20
Mock executions	4	20
Food withheld or restricted	4	20
Burns (cigarettes, hot liquid, or chemical)	3	15
Suspension	3	15
Cold water showers	3	15
Sexual molestation	3	15
Bad or rancid food	3	15
Sleep deprivation	2	10
Telefono[b]	1	5
Tear gas in cell	1	5
Walking on thorns	1	5
Pins under thumbnails	1	5
Handcuffed to post, arms twisted behind back	1	5
Finger chopped off	1	5

[a]In falaka, the soles of the feet are beaten with a cane or flexible whip over long periods. One man gave a typical description of this. He said that he would usually be strapped prone to a bench and have the soles of his feet beaten with a cane. After these sessions, his feet would be swollen and eventually became blackened. The pain was described as appalling. His feet became infected. Even now, some years later, he has painful feet which limit his ability to walk long distances.
[b]In telefono, there is violent boxing of the ears, which often leads to permanent hearing impairment.

made several errors in tests of memory including only being able to recall two out of three objects at 3 minutes on a cued recall test. There were both physical and psychological explanations, either of which could explain his pattern of poor concentration and impaired memory. All of these symptoms may well be a direct manifestation of PTSD.

EXISTENTIAL DILEMMA

Another survivor of torture had been forced to give information which led to the detention of some colleagues in his political group. As a refugee in the UK, he reported symptoms of PTSD, but more than anything else, he gave a sense of utter hopelessness and loss of direction in his life. For him the world would never, could never be the same again. His purpose in living had been destroyed.

Choices Facing Health Professionals

Eight (40%) of these survivors reported seeing a doctor *during* their period of detention. Some were transferred to hospital and later were returned to the detention center. Others were seen by doctors in prison. One said "the doctor took no notice of the wounds people presented with following beating or other ill treatments." One woman required surgery; this was carried out at the local hospital but, although she accepts that it was the right thing to do, she said that at no point was she asked to give consent. Many more victims saw doctors following their release; it is hard to see how torture on any scale can be carried out without the medical and allied professions having some concrete evidence of this.

An example of how forensic examiners can inhibit the abuse of detainees is said to have taken place in Northern Ireland between 1977 and 1979 (Stover & Nightingale, 1985). Here the Forensic Medical Officers Association made confidential reports, then public statements, finally leading to threats of resignation. This action led to important changes in practice and a marked reduction in allegations of assault.

Of course, speaking out under certain regimes may be fraught with considerable personal danger. Doctors themselves have been subject to torture or state killing. Several doctors who were tortured have been seen at the foundation. Recently, there have been reports of detentions of doctors in Iran, protesting about changes to the organization and autonomy of their professional body (Amnesty International, 1987b).

Thus, health professionals and others who work in countries where torture is practiced may become involved and implicated in the procedure. They have their own existential dilemmas.

Rational Approach to Treatment of the Individual Survivor

As noted sensitively in Chapter 65, in this volume, the principles of posttraumatic therapy (PTT) must include the initial establishment of trust in order for therapy to proceed. It is only in such a context that the treatment outlined below can be undertaken.

Approaches designed to have an effect only on intrusive and avoidance phenomena are rare in practice. Perhaps the nearest analogies are guided mourning in bereavement (Ramsay, 1975) and exposure-based treatments in the anxiety-based disorders (Basoglu & Marks, 1988; Wirtz & Harrell, 1987). These behavioral approaches have yet to be tested adequately in survivors of torture and thus warrant great caution. Although it may be predicted that some measures such as these are of value in the specific features of the reaction (especially on any phobic avoidance), they are unlikely to prove popular as the only method of treatment. They involve planned reexposure to memories and memorabilia of torture. Without an adequate therapeutic alliance, in which many of the more general aspects of the person's situation can be examined, this would be impossible. However, as an adjunctive therapy, in certain people, they may prove to be very useful.

It is hardly surprising to report that antidepressive medication has been successfully used in some patients with posttraumatic neuroses (arising from torture and other causes). Boehnlein, Kinzie, Ben, and Fleck (1985) reported on a group of 12 Cambodian concentration camp survivors who met the DSM-III (APA, 1980) criteria for PTSD. They found that tricyclic antidepressants were helpful in treating the "depression" as well as the PTSD symptoms of nightmares, startle reactions, and intrusive thoughts. Avoidance symptoms responded much less well. Imipramine has been successfully used for night terrors associated with the posttraumatic syndrome (Marshall, 1975). A monoamine oxidase inhibitor (phenelzine) has been successfully used in combat PTSD (Hogben & Cornfield, 1981; Levenson, Lanman, & Rankin, 1982), again probably having the greatest effect on anxiety symptoms (including panic attacks) and sleep disturbance. However, in a group of 25 Israelis, benefit appeared to be marginal (Lerer *et al.*, 1987). It appeared that those who responded best were patients with additional diagnoses of mood disorder or panic disorder. The common coexistence of more than one diagnostic category must be considered in the design of further research in this field (see Chapter 66, in this volume).

The use of testimony has developed as a common intervention in survivors of torture (see Chapter 55, in this volume, for a discussion). It is a way of systematically reordering the survivor's view of what has happened. It is aimed at helping the person to assimilate the experience of torture and to work toward a restoration of self-esteem. The process of healing requires that the individual be able to see him- or herself once again as (to some degree) in charge of his or her destiny. This involves making that person's previous history (in terms of political commitment, work, and personal relationships) meaningful again. This formal use of testimony is said to act by restoring affective ties, by orienting aggression in a constructive manner, and by integrating fragmented experiences. In this way, the possibilities for personal growth are reopened (Cienfuegos & Monelli, 1983).

Similar methods have been applied successfully in other countries. In Denmark, for example, one group is using what is essentially a cognitive approach. They regard torture as having the aim of converting "political pain into private pain." The purpose of their treatment, which is based on the testimony method, is to "focus on reverting the private pain into political pain with a relief in symptoms and a reestablishment in ideological consciousness." This is done through a process of "reframing," which is akin to cognitive restructuring (Jensen & Agger, 1988). Similar approaches have been successful in survivors of sexual torture (Agger, 1988). Work at the Indochinese psychiatric clinic in Massachusetts also confirms the central importance of looking at the "trauma story" in therapy (Mollica & Lavelle, 1986; Mollica et al., 1987b). At the International Center for Rehabilitation of Torture Victims (RCT) in Copenhagen, a psychotherapeutic approach is used which includes the recounting of the torture story in detail (Somnier & Genefke, 1986). This is said to lead to a transformation away from the role of victim and toward the greater expression of creativity.

All these authors describe the effects of the testimony in terms of changes in personal outlook. After experiencing torture, people need to regain a sense of direction in their lives, and they often need to relearn their personal scale of values. In many cases, not only have survivors suffered frank barbarity, they have also witnessed others being tortured and often killed and for many the worst aspect is that they have been forced to give information or to stand helplessly and watch the rape or torture of those they love. Inevitably, these events have profound effects on personal philosophies. Making a testimony statement may be the first step in asserting a right to recovery. It may help to set in context the meaning of their own actions within a broad social and political framework.

However, it is also possible that describing the events in detail is beneficial for other reasons. Writing about traumatic events has been shown to reduce medical consultations by students (Pennebaker & Beall, 1986), possibly by facilitating emotional processing. It may have a direct effect on intrusive memories and experiences, and the associated need to avoid recall.

Therapy may be best carried out in family units or in other social groups. Children often come from families in which others may also show signs of PTSD and depression (Sack et al., 1986) and are probably best treated in family units (Allodi, 1980; Svendsen, 1985). All involved will have to come to terms with a world in which torture is not only theoretically possible, but is also a stark reality in their own lives.

Similarly, treatment must take into account the effects of the cultural base both of individuals and groups. Questionnaires have been translated for use in other languages (e.g., Kinzie et al., 1982; Mollica, Wyshak, & Lavelle, 1987a). There may be striking differences in the use of words to describe emotions, in cross-cultural diagnostic patterns, and in interpreting common cultural belief systems between people of different ethnic and cultural backgrounds (Westermeyer, 1985). The common need to use an interpreter may present its own difficulties (Marcos, 1979). The formal training of community workers may be a better approach where the numbers of people from one or more cultures are sufficiently large.

In the early work of the Medical Foundation, an emphasis on group work emerged in which survivors of torture would help each other through a process of self-help and mutual support. Political factors had to be taken into account. Generally, no more than one person from any single country could be included in a group for reasons of personal safety. Paradoxically, this meeting of people from different cultures and backgrounds was often extremely powerful. The person best able to talk to the condition of a survivor of torture may be another survivor.

Conclusion

In this attempt at a synthesis, it is suggested that the type and severity of individual reactions to torture can be conceptualized under four main headings. Incomplete emotional and cognitive processing with intrusive, avoidance, and hyperarousal symptoms is common, although it may be atypical with the development of unusual defensive mechanisms, including chronic hyperventilation disorder. On theoretical grounds, it may also be predicted that successful avoidance behavior would be disrupted by the method of torture and that intrusive features would predominate. Depressive reactions constitute another characteristic reaction, particularly in people who seek asylum in other countries. There are somatic symptoms, including the apparently "organic" signs of cognitive impairment. These somatic features are likely to have many causes. For example, they may be the direct consequence of the physical method of torture; they may be related to a maladaptive response following torture, such as the chronic hyperventilation syndrome; they may be intimately associated with a person's emotional condition, or they may be part of a dissociative phenomenon. Finally, the existential dilemma of the survivor may be the dominant feature and may be the most difficult for the person to overcome. It requires a broadly political perspective, and some clinicians have found success using a method based on personal testimony.

There are implications for treatment in the many different treatment approaches that have been attempted with survivors of torture. For each individual, the predominant reaction is likely to guide the choice of initial treatment. If the social, political, and existential changes dominate, then a longer and more difficult process of healing and readaptation is required. During this time, the knowledge that others are in the same position and are struggling to reach their own understandings may be essential, and the group therapeutic approach over substantial periods of time may be the ideal way of dealing with these problems.

Also, it must be acknowledged that the individual does not exist in isolation. The consequences of torture will affect others; specifically, this includes children and other family members, local networks, and even whole communities. The survivor may view others differently, for example, being unable to trust. There may also be changes in the way the person is perceived by friends and relatives.

It is hoped that this extensive review will act as a stimulus to urgently needed public research directed at understanding reactions to torture and at identifying the most appropriate ways of intervening. There is a risk that publishing material about the sequelae of torture will better inform the people who order or perpetrate these acts of violence. We believe that it would be naive to assume that the more sophisticated torture schools do not themselves engage in research designed to evaluate their own activities. The greater risk, therefore, is the perpetuation of ignorance in the general public and in those who are called to help survivors of torture either in their own countries, or, commonly, as refugees.

Medical and other health professionals can no longer pretend or turn a blind eye on the problem of torture (Best, 1986). It is impossible to imagine a setting in which torture could take place without health care personnel being informed (Stover & Nightingale, 1985). Even if they are not involved at the time of torture, they will be asked to help people following their detention. There is, therefore, a particular professional duty in safe countries to define good methods of practice and to support colleagues who are practicing defiantly in more dangerous parts of the world.

References

Abildgaard, U., Daugaard, G., Marcussen, H., Jess, P., Petersen, H. D., & Wallach, M. (1984). Chronic organic psychosyndrome in Greek torture victims. *Danish Medical Bulletin*, 31, 239–242.

Agger, I. (1988, August). *Psychological aspects of torture with special emphasis on sexual torture: Sequels and treatment perspectives*. Paper presented at the WHO Advisory Group on the Health Situation of Refugees and Victims of Organized Violence, Gothenburg, Sweden.

Allodi, F. (1980). The psychiatric effects in children and families of victims of political persecution and torture. *Danish Medical Bulletin*, 27, 229–232.

Allodi, F., & Cowgill, G. (1982). Ethical and psychiatric aspects of torture. *Canadian Journal of Psychiatry*, 27, 98–102.

American Psychiatric Association. (1980). *Diagnostic and statistical manual of mental disorders* (3rd ed.). Washington, DC: Author.

American Psychiatric Association. (1987). *Diagnostic and statistical manual of mental disorders* (3rd ed., rev.). Washington, DC: Author.

Amnesty International. (1983). *Political killings by governments*. London: Amnesty International Publications.

Amnesty International. (1987a). *Amnesty International Report 1987*. London: Amnesty International Publications.

Amnesty International. (1987b). *Iran violations of human rights*. London: Amnesty International Publications.

Argentina's National Commission on Disappeared People. (1986). *Nunca mas* [Never again]. London: Faber & Faber.

Askevold, F. (1980). The war sailor syndrome. *Danish Medical Bulletin*, 27, 220–223.

Basoglu, M., & Marks, I. (1988). Torture: Research needed into how to help those who have been tortured. *British Medical Journal*, 297, 1423–1424.

Bendfeldt-Zachrisson, F. (1985). State (political) torture: Some general, psychological, and particular aspects. *International Journal of Health Services*, 15, 339–349.

Best, J. (1986). Torture—The cancer of democracy. *Medical Journal of Australia*, 145, 416–417.

Boehnlein, J. K., Kinzie, J. D., Ben, R., & Fleck, J. (1985). One-year follow-up study of post-traumatic stress disorder among survivors of Cambodian concentration camps. *American Journal of Psychiatry*, 142, 956–959.

Brett, E. A., & Ostroff, R. (1985). Imagery and post-traumatic stress disorder: An overview. *American Journal of Psychiatry*, 142, 417–424.

British Medical Association. (1986). *The Torture Report*. London: Author.

Brown, G. W., & Harris, T. (1978). Social origins of depression: A reply. *Psychological Medicine*, 8(4), 577–588.

Cathcart, L. M., Berger, P., & Knazan, B. (1979). Medical examination of torture victims applying for refugee status. *Canadian Medical Association Journal*, 121, 179–184.

Cienfuegos, A. J., & Monelli, C. (1983). The testimony of political repression as a therapeutic instrument. *American Journal of Orthopsychiatry*, 53, 43–51.

Cohn, J., Danielsen, L., Holzer, K. I. M., Koch, L., Severin, B., Thogersen, S., & Aalund, O. (1985). A study of Chilean refugee children in Denmark. *Lancet*, ii, 437–438.

Cohn, J., Holzer, K. I. M., Koch, L., & Severin, B. (1980). Children and torture. *Danish Medical Bulletin*, 27, 238–239.

Eitinger, L. (1980). The concentration camp syndrome and its late sequelae. In J. E. Dimsdale (Ed.), *Survivors, victims, and perpetrators: Essays on the Nazi Holocaust*. New York: Hemisphere.

Goldfeld, A. E., Mollica, R. F., Pesavento, B. H., & Faraone, S. V. (1988). The physical and psychological sequelae of torture. *Journal of the American Medical Association*, 259, 2725–2729.

Gordon, E., & Mant, A. M. (1984). Examination of a teacher from El Salvador. *Lancet*, i, 213–214.

Hogben, G. L., & Cornfield, R. B. (1981). Treatment of traumatic war neurosis with phenelzine. *Archives of General Psychiatry*, 38, 440–445.

Horowitz, M. J. (1976). *Stress response syndromes*. New York: Jason Aronson.

Jensen, S. B., & Agger, I. (1988, August/September). *The testimony method: The use of testimony as a psychotherapeutic tool in the treatment of traumatized refugees in Denmark*. Paper presented to the First European Conference on Traumatic Stress Studies (Lincoln, England).

Kinston, W., & Rosser, R. (1974). Disaster: Effects on mental and physical state. *Journal of Psychosomatic Research*, 18, 437–456.

Kinzie, J. D. (1985). Cultural aspects of psychiatric treatment with Indochinese refugees. *American Journal of Social Psychiatry*, 5, 47–53.

Kinzie, J. D., Fredrickson, R. H., Ben, R., Fleck, J., & Karls, W. (1984). Post-traumatic stress disorder among survivors of Cambodian concentration camps. *American Journal of Psychiatry*, 141, 645–650.

Kinzie, J. D., Manson, S. M., Vinh, D. T., Tolan, N. T., Anh, B., & Pho, T. N. (1982). Development and validation of a Vietnamese-language depression rating scale. *American Journal of Psychiatry*, 139, 1276–1281.

Lerer, B., Bleich, A., Kotler, M., Garb, R., Hertzberg, M., & Levin, B. (1987). Post-traumatic stress disorder in Israeli combat veterans. *Archives of General Psychiatry*, 44, 976–981.

Levenson, H., Lanman, R., & Rankin, M. (1982). Traumatic war neurosis and phenelzine. *Archives of General Psychiatry*, 39, 1345.

Levi, P. (1987). *If this is a man: The truce*. London: Penguin Books.

Lifton, R. J., & Olson, E. (1976). The human meaning of total disaster. *Psychiatry*, 39, 1–18.

Lunde, I., Rasmussen, O .V., Lindholm, J., & Wagner, G. (1980). Gonadal and sexual functions in tortured Greek men. *Danish Medical Bulletin, 27,* 243–245.

Marcos, L. R. (1979). Effects of interpreters on the evaluation of psychopathology in non-English-speaking patients. *American Journal of Psychiatry, 136,* 171–174.

Marshall, J. R. (1975). The treatment of night terrors associated with the post-traumatic syndrome. *American Journal of Psychiatry, 132,* 293–295.

Martin-Baro, I. (1988). From dirty war to psychological war: The case of El Salvador. In A. Aron (Ed.), *Flight, exile, and return: Mental health and the refugee.* San Francisco: Committee for Health Rights in Central America.

McFarlane, A. C. (1984). The Ash Wednesday bushfires in South Australia. *Medical Journal of Australia, 141,* 286–291.

McFarlane, A. C. (1987). Life events and psychiatric disorder: The role of a natural disaster. *British Journal of Psychiatry, 151,* 362–367.

Miserez, D. (1988). *Refugees—The trauma of exile.* Dordrecht, Netherlands: Martinus Nijhoff Publishers.

Mollica, R. F., & Lavelle, J. P. (1986). The trauma of mass violence and torture: An overview of the psychiatric care of the southeast Asian refugee. In L. Comas-Diaz & E. H. Griffith (Eds.), *Clinical practice in cross-cultural mental health* (pp. 262–305). New York: Wiley.

Mollica, R. F., Wyshak, G., & Lavelle, J. (1987a). Indochinese versions of the Hopkins Symptom Checklist-25: A screening instrument for the psychiatric care of refugees. *American Journal of Psychiatry, 144,* 497–500.

Mollica, R. F., Wyshak, G., & Lavelle, J. (1987b). The psychosocial impact of war trauma and torture on southeast Asian refugees. *American Journal of Psychiatry, 144,* 1567–1572.

Pennebaker, J. W., & Beall, S. K. (1986). Confronting a traumatic event: Toward an understanding of inhibition and disease. *Journal of Abnormal Psychology, 95,* 274–281.

Peters, E. (1985). *Torture.* Oxford, England: Blackwell.

Petersen, H. D., Abildgaard, U., Daugaard, G., Jess, P., Marcussen, H., & Wallach, M. (1985). Psychological and physical long-term effects of torture. *Scandinavian Journal of Social Medicine, 13,* 89–93.

Pilisuk, M., & Ober, L. (1976). Torture and genocide as public health problems. *American Journal of Orthopsychiatry, 46,* 388–392.

Pynoos, R. S. Frederick, C., Nader, K., Arroyo, W., Steinberg, A., Eth, S., Nunez, F., & Fairbanks, L. (1987). Life threat and post-traumatic stress in school-age children. *Archives of General Psychiatry, 44,* 1057–1063.

Rachman, S. (1980). Emotional processing. *Behavior Research and Therapy, 18,* 51–60.

Ramsay, R. (1975). Behavior therapy and bereavement. In J. Brengelman (Ed.), *Progress in behavior therapy.* Berlin: Springer.

Raphael, B. (1986). *When disaster strikes.* New York: Basic Books.

Raphael, B., & Middleton, W. (1988). After the horror. *British Medical Journal, 296,* 1142–1143.

Rasmussen, O. V., & Lunde, I. (1980). Evaluation of investigation of 200 torture victims. *Danish Medical Bulletin, 27,* 241–243.

Rasmussen, O. V., & Marcussen, H. (1982). *The somatic sequelae to torture.* Copenhagen: International Center for Rehabilitation of Torture Victims (RCT).

Ritterman, M. (1987, January/February). Torture, the countertherapy of the state. *Networker,* pp. 43–47.

Sack, W. H., Angell, R. H., Kinzie, J. D., & Rath, B. (1986). The psychiatric effects of massive trauma on Cambodian children: II. The family, the home and the school. *Journal of the American Academy of Child Psychiatry, 25,* 377–383.

Schlapobersky, J., & Bamber, H. (1988, February 14). *Rehabilitation and therapy with the victims of torture and organized violence.* Paper presented to the annual meeting of the American Association for the Advancement of Science.

Shore, J. H., Tatum, E. L., & Vollmer, W. M. (1986). Psychiatric reactions to disaster: The Mount St. Helens experience. *American Journal of Psychiatry, 143,* 590–595.

Showalter, E. (1987). *The female malady.* London: Virago Press.

Somnier, F. E., & Genefke, I. K. (1986). Psychotherapy for victims of torture. *British Journal of Psychiatry, 149,* 323–329.

Stover, E., & Nightingale, E. O. (1985). *The breaking of bodies and minds.* New York: W. H. Freeman.

Svendsen, G. (1985). *When dealing with torture victims social work involves the entire family.* Copenhagen: International Rehabilitation Center for Torture Victims (RCT).

Thygesen, P. (1980). The concentration camp syndrome. *Danish Medical Bulletin, 27,* 224–228.

Trimble, M. R. (1981). *Post-traumatic neurosis: From railway spine to the whiplash.* Chichester, England: Wiley.

Turner, S. W. (1989). Working with survivors: The Medical Foundation for the Care of Victims of Torture. *Psychiatric Bulletin, 13,* 173–176.

Ullman, R., & Brothers, D. (1988). *The shattered self: A psychoanalytic study of trauma.* London: Analytic Press.

United Nations. (1948). *Universal Declaration of Human Rights.* Office of Public Information. New York: United Nations.

United Nations. (1951). *Convention relating to the status of refugees.* Office of Public Information. New York: United Nations.

United Nations. (1984). *Convention against torture and other cruel, inhuman or degrading treatment or punishment.* Office of Public Information. New York: United Nations.

Van Geuns, H. (1987). The concept of organized violence. In O. Aalund, P. Riss, P-G. Svensson, P. Thorvaldsen, & H. Van Geuns (Eds.), *Health hazards of organized violence.* The Hague, Netherlands: Distribution Center of Government Publications, Ministry of Welfare, Health and Cultural Affairs.

Westermeyer, J. (1985). Psychiatric diagnosis across cultural boundaries. *American Journal of Psychiatry, 142,* 798–805.

Wilson, J. P. (1988a). Understanding the Vietnam veteran. In F. M. Ochberg (Ed.), *Post-traumatic therapy and victims of violence* (pp. 227–253). New York: Brunner/Mazel.

Wilson, J. P. (1988b). Treating the Vietnam veteran. In F. M. Ochberg (Ed.), *Post-traumatic therapy and victims of violence* (pp. 254–277). New York: Brunner/Mazel.

Wilson, J. P. (1989). *Trauma, transformation, and healing.* New York: Brunner/Mazel.

Wirtz, P. W., & Harrell, A. V. (1987). Effects of post-assault exposure to attack-similar stimuli on long-term recovery of victims. *Journal of Consulting and Clinical Psychology, 55,* 10–16.

World Medical Association. (1975). *Declaration of Tokyo.* Ferney-Voltaire, France: Author.

Yager, T., Laufer, R., & Gallops, M. (1984). Some problems associated with war experience in men of the Vietnam generation. *Archives of General Psychiatry, 41,* 327–333.

CHAPTER 59

Therapy with Families Who Have Experienced Torture

Tony Jaffa

Introduction

I have not been tortured. Being tortured and its after-effects are largely beyond my imagination. I do know the devastation of the lives of those who have been tortured and those around them. I also understand some of the difficulties in the struggle to restore meaning and purpose to those who have been tortured. Sometimes that struggle seems hopeless and futile. It is not.

Working with families who have experienced torture is difficult. At times the anxiety levels of the family and the therapist seem unbearable. It is difficult to hear the trauma story (Wilson, 1989). The resources of the therapist and patient are often stretched to their limits. What is achievable varies greatly from case to case and is difficult to predict. Therapists, aware of the enormity of the problems remaining for the torture victim, will find it difficult to appreciate the value of the work and progress already accomplished. Therapists who are not prepared to work under these conditions or who are not knowledgeable in posttraumatic therapy (see Chapter 65, in this volume, for a review) should not attempt to treat these families.

Torture and Torture Survivors

Most of those who have been systematically tortured are dead. In describing work with those who are alive, it is fitting to talk not of torture victims but of *torture survivors*.

Tony Jaffa • The Medical Foundation for the Care of Victims of Torture, London, and The Adolescent Community Team, 32b York Road, Battersea, London SW11, England.

International Handbook of Traumatic Stress Syndromes, edited by John P. Wilson and Beverley Raphael. Plenum Press, New York, 1993.

It has been estimated that torture occurs in approximately one third of the countries of the world (Amnesty International, 1987). There are a number of definitions of torture; one of the more commonly cited is that of the World Medical Association (1975). The following features are emphasized:

1. It is the deliberate inflicting of suffering.
2. This may take physical or psychological forms. Most commonly there are elements of both.
3. It is carried out by or on behalf of authorities.
4. It has a purpose. This may be the extraction of information or a confession. More important may be the suppression, of individuals, families, and communities, as part of a political struggle.

Effects of Torture on Levels of Functioning

The Individual

The torture survivor may be rendered unable to function effectively. Trust and, therefore, the maintenance of cooperative relationships typically become difficult or impossible. The suffering of some may be understood in terms of posttraumatic stress disorder (PTSD) (American Psychiatric Association [APA], 1980, 1987), or of bereavement syndromes (Raphael, 1983). There may be disabling physical sequelae, such as the pain of walking following repeated beatings to the soles of the feet known as *falaka* (see also Chapter 57, in this volume, for a description of common torture methods).

The Family

Relationships within a family are formed on the basis of shared expectations of the roles individuals will assume as well as what sort of future the family might have together. If there are children, they, too, are incorporated into this system of beliefs and expectations. Family members know what they can reasonably expect of each other and what is expected of them. This balance in the family system may be destroyed by the imprisonment, torture, and the return of the survivor who is inevitably a changed person. It must be remembered that one goal of torture is to break the "will" of the victim. Through subjugation and helplessness the individual becomes defiled and diminished in ego-vitality (Ochberg, 1988).

The Community

Widespread, seemingly arbitrary imprisonment and torture are part of a pattern of fear and political intimidation. Those who are being tortured and those who flee the country are missing and may never return. Those who have been tortured and those who fear torture may withdraw and isolate themselves in a more private world. It is common for there to be an increase in alcohol or drug abuse. The structures that hold the fabric of society together may be weakened or broken, resulting in a situation of secondary traumatization (Erikson, 1976).

This chapter focuses on the family. How does one think about the psychological effects of torture on the family? How can therapists usefully intervene?

The Therapist

The decision to engage in therapy with families who have experienced torture and the ways that this therapy can be approached are intimately linked to the personality of the therapist. I relate my decision to enter this field to my guilt concerning my affluence and privilege, and, as a Jew born in the 1950s, to my childhood conversations about persecution and injustice. The way that I behave in therapy is part of who I am: a male, in my thirties, and a child psychiatrist from London, England. The undertaking of posttraumatic therapy requires consideration of such factors. How does what I bring to therapy affect my relationship with client families? Am I a healer, a colonialist, a physician, a rescuer, or all or none of these? How do my clients "see" me in my role, then? Clearly, our personalities and potential for powerful countertransference reactions must be acknowledged and addressed in posttraumatic therapy (Wilson, 1989).

It may be that there are things about the therapist which he or she feels are contraindications to working with particular clients. For example, my continuing confusion and internal conflict over the situation in the Middle East has led me to the decision that, for the time being, I should not attempt to do therapy with traumatized Palestinians. For other therapists, such ideological, political, moral, or religious views may profoundly affect how effectively they can work with victims of torture and their families.

Work with Torture Victims in a Time and Place Context

I am a child psychiatrist who spends a few hours a week on a voluntary basis at the Medical Foundation for the Care of Victims of Torture in London. This independent charity works with refugees and asylum seekers from many parts of the world (Turner, 1989). All clients are assessed initially by caseworkers and are then referred to the appropriate medical, psychological, social, and legal agencies. Although most clients are alone, there are a number who are with part of their family in the United Kingdom. It is with these cases that I become involved. Over the past few years, I have worked with families from Latin America, Africa, and Asia. All have included one family member who has been imprisoned, harshly treated, and, in most cases, tortured.

Pynoos and Eth (1986) described a model of therapeutic work with traumatized children. Intervention occurs in the children's hometown, and relatively soon after the trauma; the trauma is the focus of the therapy. Similarly, Straker (1989) described the single therapeutic interview in work with ex-detainees in South Africa where the client is at risk of further detention and of further physical and psychological assault. There are major differences between my working context and those of Pynoos and Eth and Straker. I work with families who are hundreds, if not thousands, of miles away from their homes. In all cases, there has been a period of at least 6 months between the end of the imprisonment and torture and my contact with the families. Generally, I see them once every two weeks typically for 6 to 12 months and sometimes longer. The focus of my work is not the torture *per se* or even the experience of torture. It is the family system and its members. The content of the sessions is usually whatever is most anxiety provoking for them at the time.

In broad terms, I see a healthy family as an interacting evolving system which operates for the mutual benefit of its members. This involves ideas of continuity and also of adaptability. The family influences and is influenced by changes in its members and in its environment. My goal is to help the families come closer to this state. This may involve a number of types of intervention: some supportive, some challenging, some directed to present concerns, and some to past trauma.

My work stems from a clear personal moral conviction that torture is wrong. In the struggle between torturer and tortured, I am on the side of the tortured. However, regarding a client's struggle for political change in his or her country of origin, my position is somewhat different. I have political views on a number of ruling regimes and am free to give my support to a number of national and international organizations. However, in my role as a therapist, I am involved in a personal, rather than in a political, struggle to help the victim to well-being. This enables me to work with clients with widely differing views and even those who might see each other as political opponents. My position is different from that of a therapist who is working within a community, in one's own and one's clients' country of origin. Such a therapist would be likely to have twin goals of facilitating the psychological well-being of clients and furthering the cause of the political struggle in which they are both involved.

Assessment

Family Needs

In a very short time sitting with a family including a victim of torture, I am sometimes overwhelmed by the number and severity of the problems confronting them. It is not uncommon for a family to be faced with the stresses associated with most or all of the following: (1) the physical and psychological effects of torture, (2) death of family or friends, (3) uncertainty about the fate of family or friends, (4) the loss of all that is familiar in the country of origin, (5) life in a strange place with different language, culture, and climate, (6) economic hardships, (7) life as asylum seekers with limited rights and an uncertain future, and (8) having work skills and training which are not recognized or needed.

As a therapist, I am very aware of the risk that, in a state of high anxiety, I might decide what needs the family has, as well as what their priorities and problems are, without listening properly to what they have to say. Not only is this patronizing but it also makes a *therapeutic alliance* unlikely if not impossible. It is important to explore the concerns of all family members. Neither extremes of age, inability to speak the English language, nor the presence or absence of obvious psychological disturbance give a person any less right to have his or her voice heard. Effective therapeutic work must be a collaborative effort with an agenda agreed upon between therapist and family. This agenda is not necessarily fixed, but evolves in time with the changing relationships within the therapeutic setting.

Family Functioning

Families which have experienced torture vary widely in their level of adaptive functioning. The grouping of them as a class of families is somewhat arbitrary and implies, probably mistakenly, that their torture experience is the most important thing about them. As I see more families of torture victims, however, I have begun to construct patterns of their functioning. I claim no objective validity for these patterns and recognize that they are not mutually exclusive. They are, however, a useful reflection of my current thinking.

In many of the families I see, the husband and father has been a prominent member of the community— for example, a trade union official—who has been imprisoned and tortured. Previously, this man has been the authority figure in the family with a younger, sometimes submissive wife. These families attempt to cope with the changes in their lives in a number of ways. The broad themes of these are listed below.

Family Coping Patterns with Victims of Torture

1. *Preserving the Competence, or the Myth of the Competence, of the Husband and Father.* How can this be done when the man is physically and psychologically damaged, especially when he has lost that which gave him his status in society, and when he is unable to provide for his family? The man may become more irritable, tense, unreasonable, and distant. Although inflexible and somewhat of a caricature of his previous self, he is often feared and yet does retain at least some of his authority within the family. In response to the changes evident in the behavior and personality of the victim, the woman and children may become depressed, anxious, or develop other symptoms, responses which may provide the man with the opportunity to take on a nurturing role if he is capable of doing so.

2. *Attempts to Rescue a Fallen Husband and Father.* In this situation the man is a shadow of his former self— changed, diminished, and ineffective. He becomes increasingly withdrawn and irritable; he believes that he cannot be part of the family, as he must think of other things, which may include intrusive imagery of torture. Often his wife feels unsupported and becomes frustrated, depressed, and angry. She may attack her husband for not fulfilling his obligations as a husband and father. In many cases, she hopes her action will provoke him into a response, even if an angry one, which will increase his involvement in the relationship and the family. She may be partly successful in reducing his isolation, but there will be a price for this. Her husband may become more irritable, trying harder to withdraw and isolate himself. Typically, one of the children, seeing that the mother has attacked the father while he is vulnerable, intervenes on the father's behalf. The child's attack on the mother is intended to rescue the father and to show him that it is possible for him to be more assertive. However, the father may become increasingly aggravated by the noise, argument, and conflict. He may, in turn, explode with anger at the child. At this point, the wife either colludes, by joining in the attack on the child, or tries to protect the child from the excessive force of the attack.

3. *Attempts to Replace an Absent Father and Husband: The Parental Child.* In this situation, the husband (and father) is dead, imprisoned, has left the family, or is present but ineffectual and psychologically debilitated. A child, usually a son, attempts to fill the place vacated by his father. As a result, he attempts to parent his or her siblings and may try to be a partner to his mother, resenting intrusions by other adults. These attempts are limited in their success by the child's inability to truly carry out the functions of an adult and by the ambivalence of the mother regarding this behavior. The tendency of children to take up an authoritative pseudoadult position (role-reversal) is increased by their greater ability to adapt to the new culture and to learn a new language.

4. *Development of Symptoms in a Child as an Attempt to Maintain Family Cohesion.* Hoffman (1981) described a pattern in single-parent families in which the develop-

ment of symptoms in a child focuses the attention of the parent onto the family. I see a similar pattern in some of the families who have experienced torture, both in single- and in two-parent families. The parents are often physically or psychologically wounded and are struggling to cope with the hardships and uncertainties of life as asylum seekers. Family members may be in conflict or withdrawing from each other and drifting apart. Distressed or disturbed behavior in a child *diverts attention* to parenting and away from these other issues. If anxieties lessen—for instance, when the family is granted refugee status—the child may cease acting out. If anxieties rise, for instance, when a relative is arrested in the country of origin, or if family conflict or fragmentation increase, the child's disturbance typically increases as well. This sounds like a simple reflection of family stress in one of its members, but actually it is more complex. The child and the symptoms are serving a function for the family and for its continued survival. A "problem child," as described here, may coexist in the same family with a "parental child." The parental child provides extra nurturance for the problem child, who, in turn, ensures a degree of assistance for the parental child by the real parents. Thus, in a traumatically stressed family there may be established a form of symbolistic dependency in order to meet the complex needs of the family unit.

Previous or Background Family Functioning

An excessive narrowness of vision may lead the therapist to relate all problems directly to the effects of trauma. In 1941, Anna Freud made a useful observation in this regard when she noted that the fears of children concerning bombing in World War II were more related to parental anxieties than to actual experience of bombing (A. Freud, 1974). It is easy to see the overpowering effect of the trauma experience as overshadowing many normally occurring psychosocial events and crises in a family system.

For example, I saw a couple who had presented at the Medical Foundation for help with their asylum applications, but whose degree of conflict had worried the worker they initially saw. At first, I attributed their difficulties to their situation and to their trauma. However, on further questioning, I discovered that their relationship had been poor for many years. They were a badly matched couple from very different backgrounds with little in common. Their relationship difficulties, while exacerbated by their traumatic experiences and by their isolated, insecure existence in the United Kingdom, certainly predated both of these.

Key Events in the Family's History

It may seem unnecessary to emphasize that the therapist needs to explore events in the family's history and the way family members make sense of these experiences. There is a fascination and horror concerning

torture which coexists in the mind of the therapist who empathically seeks to understand what has happened to the victim. As a result, this may lead to an avoidance of, or alternatively an endless preoccupation with, torture in the therapeutic sessions. Excessive preoccupation with the torture may prematurely force a reliving of the trauma. A sensitive exploration of the trauma story explores the torture events as well as other events in the family history which may have equal or even greater significance.

A Developmental Perspective

The ability to employ a life-cycle, epigenetic-developmental framework helps the therapist to see a family as an *evolving system* which has become arrested and impeded rather than as a unit of pathology. I believe it is important to understand the stage of development at which the family has become fixated. Issues include, for example, the development of a secure marital relationship, the adjustment of the couple to relating to a child as well as to each other, and the negotiation of gradual increasing independence of the adolescent children (Haley, 1973). To facilitate helping the family, it is useful to ask how they would be progressing if they were not fixated or preoccupied with the traumatic event. Among the very basic questions are (1) What is preventing the family from doing this now? and (2) How can they be helped to move in this direction?

Family's Cultural Context

A proper assessment requires an understanding of culture and history (Parson, 1985). Barot (1988) pointed out that "cultures of minorities, far from being static, are dynamic and respond to social conditions in which groups and individuals find themselves." The culture that is bound up with family life is not the same for a refugee family in London as it is for their relatives in their country of origin. Relevant questions are not so much "What is this family's cultural tradition?" as "What are the conflicting demands of old and new cultures?" and "How is the family managing this period of transition?" The most useful answers are often those given by the family members themselves.

Intervention

Trust

The importance of trust in a therapeutic relationship has long been recognized (Truax & Carkhuff, 1967); this is imperative in posttraumatic therapy (Chapter 65, in this volume; Wilson, 1989). Torture is an abuse of the body and mind occurring within the context of the intimate relationship between torturer and victim. It is such a perversion of this intimate relationship that the survivors usually find it impossible subsequently to develop or rediscover intimacy and trust with family and friends. This may be exacerbated by the infiltration of refugee groups by hostile or mistrusted agencies. Therapy involves the creation of a secure environment within which the torture survivor and family may explore and develop trusting relationships once more. This is, in itself, a goal of therapy as well as a prerequisite for other cooperative work. It is not as straightforward as it may appear. The therapist's trustworthiness and commitment will be *severely* tested by the family (see Figley, 1988; Wilson, 1989). This may be manifested in their missing of appointments or their assessing the therapist's reaction to a part of their story before they decide it is safe to further disclose personal concerns. It is not encouraging to the family for the therapist to be either unmoved or overwhelmed by emotion (see Wilson, 1989, for a discussion of countertransference in posttraumatic therapy).

Practical Aid: Concrete Steps Which Facilitate Therapy

There are many practical things the therapist can do in the course of posttraumatic therapy. For example, this may involve writing a report in support of an asylum application. If the family is preoccupied with a problem that I cannot help them with, such as physical ill health or housing, then facilitating an alliance with other people and agents not only facilitates work on this problem, but also makes it more likely that they will trust me. Such concrete actions and useful, pragmatic advice seem to strengthen the therapeutic alliance.

Facing the Unfaceable in Small Steps

In the course of posttraumatic therapy with victims of torture, the resources of the family and of the therapist are often limited. Current economic and practical difficulties, fears for the future, and rage and distress over the past events seem overwhelming for many families. I find it helpful to acknowledge feelings of hopelessness and despair. This allows me to model an ability to express and cope with these feelings and to continue the work of therapy.

In my view, the therapist should start with a relatively manageable issue. In order for the family to remain in therapy, they must value the process as important. Thus, the establishment of trust is central to posttraumatic therapy. Therefore, I start by establishing with the family what might be a small, meaningful, and achievable goal. From my perspective, the experience of therapy as a joint venture helps me to avoid seeing myself as the rescuer of the family. Given the profundity and complexity of the various issues (Figley, 1988), "knights in shining armor" do not survive long in this particular struggle.

Giving a Nudge: Saying the Unsayable

There will be occasions when it is appropriate to actively encourage the family to face anxiety-provoking issues in treatment. In my experience, this often involves being quite directive, sometimes saying the things which I feel the family is too anxious to say, or to hold in mind.

For example, I worked for some time with a 70-year-old torture survivor, his 60-year-old wife, and their 33-year-old youngest daughter. At a time when the father was imprisoned and the mother was struggling to cope with the situation, the previously well-adjusted daughter, then aged 18, became progressively more disturbed. Over the years, she was variously diagnosed as epileptic, schizophrenic, and mentally retarded. Because of her decompensation, the mother's attention focused more on her and on her care. Eventually, it was the severity of the daughter's condition which enabled the family and the father to leave for the United Kingdom. Once there, the daughter remained dependent and immature and continued to suffer occasional "falling" episodes. She was clearly the center of family life.

In view of the family dynamics, I felt it was important for her to develop as an autonomous individual. My individual therapy with her is described in a later section. It was clear to me that whatever desire for growth might be mobilized in the daughter, success in this endeavor required the support and assistance of her parents. The parents agreed with this view, but there still did not seem to be a great energy for change. I hypothesized that there was a fear of change because this would activate issues involving loss. Hence, the daughter would lose her neurotically based security. The parents feared that if they "lost" their daughter as the central stabilizing focus of their lives, they would be faced with other issues, some of which I knew about, and some I would identify later in treatment. However, continued stability of the current pattern of family functioning was not a realistic possibility, and I could only help the family by holding this in mind. I reminded the family that the parents would not be able to care for their daughter indefinitely. Eventually, they would become infirm, continue aging, and die. The parents nodded in agreement and repeated my words several times to their daughter. In turn, she looked frightened. I asked the parents what they would want for their daughter. They insisted that she must become more independent. With her parents' help and encouragement, the daughter became involved in a program of graded exposure to achieve greater independence.

Control and Meaning

Torture survivors describe a number of strategies to maintain a sense of personal control and the ability to make decisions, even during periods of imprisonment and torture. An example is the decision of when to drop to the floor during a beating: if too soon, the beating continues; if too late, there is additional suffering.

Torture is designed to deprive the victim of a sense of meaning or of control. Victims are made to believe that there is a course of action which will stop the torture. The victim tries to make sense of the experience in a way which will provide a solution and stop the torture, but, in reality, the problem is insoluble and the torture continues. In the face of this inability to influence the environment (the torture), the victim may become withdrawn and passive, relinquishing the struggle to maintain autonomy. Often, a degree of passivity is still evident when clients present for help months or years later. This phenomenon has been called *learned helplessness* (Seligman & Weiss, 1980; Garber & Seligman, 1980). It may be somewhat less likely to happen in the case of the activist who understands torture and imprisonment in terms of a political struggle. Those who are imprisoned and tortured at random may be more vulnerable.

The concepts of *meaning* and of *control* are crucial to posttraumatic therapy with these families. Sometimes families seem very cooperative. They agree with what I say and do what I suggest. For a time, I may believe that the therapy is going very well. Then I realize we are actually getting nowhere, because I am encouraging them to remain passive and dependent. Together we are maintaining our shared myth that I can somehow take care of them, a common countertransference theme (Wilson, 1989).

Effective therapy makes demands on the clients. It challenges them to make decisions and to think about meaning. How does one give meaning to a life which is so different and, in many ways, so much more limited than that which was anticipated?

For some, the answer lies in the telling of the stories of the many who have not survived, giving them a voice even after their death. The very act of survival against all odds may be seen as an act of defiance that gives meaning and value to life (see the "testimony" method in Chapter 55, in this volume).

Others withdraw their energy from past traumata and focus more on developing a new existence and life in the host culture. As a therapist, I am still struggling to accept that not only can I not influence the meaning people give to their lives, but I also do not know what is best for them. The way I can be of use is to help them in whatever journey *they choose* to embark on.

Dysfunctional Interactional Patterns

As described earlier in this chapter, the stresses of torture and of other traumata commonly cause disruption of the previous family functioning. When parents find it difficult to work together, they may become conflicted; one or both may draw the child or children into the marital conflict. In working with these problems, I have found the model of family therapy described by Minuchin (Minuchin, 1974; Minuchin & Fishman, 1981) most helpful.

The therapist works in an active directive manner to reinforce the authority of the parents and to free the children from becoming involved in parental issues. I have found it useful to suggest that a couple who are in conflict on most things actually negotiate and make a joint decision on a specific issue, such as the bedtime of their child. I block the repeated attempts of the child to take an adult parental role in the discussion and state that this is a matter of parental responsibility and is not for children.

The parents are likely to need help, not only in finding a joint solution, but also in implementing it. This work required great persistence, but once the parents realize they can effectively cooperate on one issue, they are likely to repeat the process with another one. Thus, it is often possible to help strengthen the parental unit and to help the children behave in age-appropriate roles rather than as allies for one or the other parent. Freed from this interference, the parents may then be able to work more effectively on their problems.

Therapy When Only One Family Member Will Attend

It may be that only one member of a family that has experienced torture will come for help. This may not be the person that has directly experienced the torture. Supporting this individual is likely to have some value. However, it may be more useful to attempt to change the family functioning through this individual and his or her interactions within the family (Fisch, Weakland, & Segal, 1982).

A Latin American woman in her late thirties had been attending the Medical Foundation for some years. Her complaints remained the same. Her husband had been a powerful union leader in his country of origin before being arrested and tortured. Subsequently, he had become a shadow of his former self, managing only a menial job and participating little in family life. He worked long hours; in his free time, he watched television and ate meals provided for him.

Their 16-year-old son was becoming increasingly violent; he was fighting other local youths and had begun carrying a knife around with him, threatening that he would kill someone. At home, he was uncooperative, refusing his mother's demands that he be in on time, clean his room, and perform other chores.

The mother had gained much support from a church which she attended regularly. She had also seen a number of therapists, each of whom had attempted unsuccessfully to get the family into treatment, and had then offered support to the mother alone. Several times, she had realized that this was not bringing about a significant change and she left treatment; later, she would ask to be seen by somebody else.

She was referred to me. I, too, attempted and failed to convene the family. I reviewed what I knew of them, suspecting that the son used his behavior to keep his mother's attention focused on himself rather than on her unsatisfactory relationship with her husband. The son provided considerable excitement for the family and attempted to take the strong authoritative role that had been vacated by his father. This could not continue as he would be likely to attack someone or end up severely injured or, perhaps, incarcerated.

I gave the mother a choice. I said that I could continue to support her until she was fed up with me, as had happened with the other therapists, or we could work together to produce some change in the family. Taken aback by my statement, she agreed to consider her position and let me know the outcome. Some weeks later, she requested that we work for change.

I knew that I could not work directly with the son but could try to influence the mother. I assumed that her behavior, though intended to resolve the problem, was actually contributing to it. Her worrying, pleading, reasoning, and demanding, and her son's risk-taking, resistance, and violence were the two halves of an out-of-control escalation. The principle of my intervention would be to interrupt her half of the cycle. The most effective way of doing this would be not to suggest that she stop her behavior—this, in practice, can be almost impossible—but rather to suggest that she do something else instead.

We agreed to start with a relatively trivial problem; the son's refusal to make his bed in the mornings and her pattern of trying to deal with this by repeated demands. Instead of this, she was to make the bed dutifully each morning, but to fill it with toast crumbs (compare *paradoxical intent*). After some discussion, she consented to do this. When he complained about the crumbs, rather than saying that he should make his own bed, she apologized profusely and said she would try not to make a mess next time. She explained that she was so short of time that she was having to eat her breakfast while doing her domestic chores. Of course, she continued to put crumbs in his bed, and continued to apologize when challenged. After a few days, he began to make his bed himself.

Similar interventions were devised for a number of fairly trivial behaviors with mixed success. It was clear that she was enjoying herself. She became *creative* in the planning of interventions and seemed much less of a downtrodden victim. After five sessions, she discontinued therapy without explanation. Later, I heard that she had returned to her country of origin, perhaps for an extended holiday or longer. Although I would like to have done much more, and to know more about the outcome, my hope is that by interrupting the pathological cycle of interactions, I helped them to avoid the seemingly inevitable disaster. The family members were given an opportunity to find other ways of behaving; although their problems were certainly not over, this was perhaps a start in their working toward a new solution.

Competence

Much of posttraumatic therapy is oriented towards the working-through of traumatic material. Given the nature of the trauma experienced by these clients, this may be a recipe for never-ending therapy. It is arguable as to whether this approach is desirable, or whether it maintains people in an incompetent client role indefinitely.

There is a further problem in the application of this "damage-repair" approach to clients who have suffered such severe trauma. The effects of the trauma may be so deep and pervasive that the clients do not have a sufficiently competent undamaged part of themselves which can think about, make sense of, and find a language system to communicate about the torture experience. These clients may be better served by being helped to develop nontraumatized aspects of their functioning, which may be in the area of relationships, or may start with very basic acts of self-care and self-determination (see Alvarez, 1989).

Earlier, I described my involvement with a 70-year-old torture survivor, his wife, and their daughter. While her father was enduring a prolonged and hazardous period of imprisonment, his daughter had become increasingly disturbed; she had been variously diagnosed as mentally retarded, schizophrenic, and epileptic. When I first met this family, the daughter was sharing a bed with her mother, had acquired no English, had not been out of her parents' sight for more than a few minutes in years, and had not gained any work or domestic skills. When I or her parents asked her about worries, thoughts, or feelings, she smiled blankly and sometimes looked slightly anxious. The daughter's disturbance was understandable to me in terms of regression in the face of overwhelming anxiety, and as providing a focus for her parents' concern and activity.

After some questioning, I learned that she could knit a little bit. The subsequent sessions were occupied by my talking about her knitting, encouraging her to do more, to show it to me and my admiring it. After several more sessions, she began attending English classes. She now speaks some English, can cook two dishes, and has been shopping on two occasions. Although this can hardly be described as efficacious or superior functioning, it is a start. It involves acknowledgment that independence and autonomy are issues in working with families who have been victimized. Helping clients increase their competence not only aids self-esteem but enhances organismic vitality.

Thus, sometimes from a small start, clients can develop or strengthen areas of their being which are not contaminated by torture and in which they can function effectively. Some clients use these areas of competent functioning as a base from which to think about and start to repair the trauma damage. Others choose to continue to develop their competencies and to work around and avoid encapsulated areas of traumatic damage.

Limitations of Working in a Family Context

There are times when working within a family context is inappropriate. Most certainly, there are individual as well as interactional components to the problems presented; clients should be able to choose to work on these alone or with their families.

However, there is also often useful work to be done in liaison with other agencies. For example, the torture survivor who has suffered electric shocks is likely to have great anxieties over an electrocardiogram or similar physical examination, for which leads are attached to his chest to measure the electrical activity of his heart. The presence of a familiar therapist, who understands these fears and who can combine understanding and reassurance, may make the procedure bearable.

Use of Interpreters

Therapy can be seen as a conversation between the therapist and the family. When the two parties do not share a common language, conversation is only possible through an interpreter. In my work, when no one in the family speaks English, an interpreter is needed. This is a straightforward if sometimes difficult problem. More problematic is the situation in which one or more family members speak English, but others do not (see Chapter 55, in this volume). Arranging for an interpreter to be present can be difficult; there is always the temptation to manage without one.

In practice, this means that I communicate with the English-speaking member, who then interprets for the rest of the family. I am drawn into an alliance with this family member, and hear a particular version of the family's story. My words may be modified in translation according to this family member's view. Treating a family with non-English-speaking members without the use of an interpreter may be expedient, but it is not conducive to good therapy.

What is being interpreted is not just language but also culture and cultural differences. How the interpreter is able to carry out these functions will depend on his or her own background and abilities, especially knowledge in posttraumatic stress disorder. Is the interpreter fluent in both languages? Does the interpreter share the culture of the therapist, that of the family, or neither? If the family and the interpreter are from the same country, there may be problems in their relationship that are due to differences in political views or status in the society. The family and the interpreter will be aware of such factors; the therapist who does not take the trouble to find out may be working at a severe disadvantage. A helpful account of these and other issues in working with an interpreter is that of Baker and Briggs (1975).

In the therapy session, the therapist should generally make eye contact with family members rather than with the interpreter. Even without a common language, family and therapist will communicate nonverbally and will develop a working relationship. A balance must be found between the extremes of a literal word-for-word translation which loses meaning, and a brief summary which omits important detail. If a point seems unclear or a translation of a particular idea seems difficult, the account should be repeated or approached from a different angle. The therapist may need to turn to the interpreter for advice. Of course, working with an interpreter is time consuming and difficult, but is essential in order to uncover the trauma story.

Where possible, the interpreter should have an association or contract with the institution which provides the therapy, rather than being a friend of the family. He or she should be treated as part of the therapeutic team. There should be an opportunity before and after each session to clarify the interpreter's role in relationship to the therapy, and also to provide the interpreter with support and an opportunity to share his or her feelings about what has been said.

Support, Supervision, and Training

These three important issues are often grouped together. However, they are different; failure to consider them as such may mean that none of them are carried out adequately. All three are very important in the process of posttraumatic therapy (see Chapter 65, in this volume). They all require that institutional resources be allocated to therapists. Although allocating resources to therapists may mean funding for fewer clients, the alternative is high staff turnover, a high burn-out rate, and poorer quality therapy; understanding countertransference reactions is the cornerstone of good posttraumatic therapy (Danieli, 1988; Wilson, 1989; see also Chapter 65, in this volume).

Support

Working with individuals who have been tortured can be traumatic, as noted by Raphael (1986). An unsupported staff team tends to fragment; workers isolate from one another to seal off their collective pain. Effective support enables therapists to share their feelings about working with torture victims. It makes therapists feel valued and accepted in their work and able to continue it. Support may be effectively and economically provided in a peer-group setting (see also Chapter 76, in this volume, for a discussion of debriefing).

Supervision

Supervision occurs in the context of a supervisor–supervisee relationship, or these roles may be taken alternately, with two or more therapists supervising each other. An advantage of the latter arrangement is that it helps get away from the idea, never far away in work with torture survivors, that somewhere there is an expert who can provide all the answers and repair all the wounds.

Given that this is a field which attracts therapists with a range of approaches to therapy, it is worth stating the obvious: Supervision should be consistent with models used by the therapist in the work with clients. It is also imperative that the supervisor be knowledgeable in PTSD and countertransference issues in order to assist effectively in the treatment protocol (see Chapter 65, in this volume).

Training

Therapists working in this field often feel inadequate. At times, it seems as though nothing one can do is enough. Self-doubt is common; there is a nagging feeling that this is a reflection of lack of therapeutic skills. Given encouragement, all therapists who have been working in this field for some time will have skills and insights to pass on to colleagues (Figley, 1988; Ochberg, 1988; Wilson, 1989).

A formalized program of training should be incorporated into the functioning of any institution working in this field as well as ongoing workshops and annual conferences. Such a program should be varied and flexible, covering such areas as trauma dynamics, bereavement, ethnicity and culture, posttraumatic stress disorder, countertransference reactions, and working with interpreters. Even if there are no acknowledged experts available in these areas, much can be gained from shared experience and from reviews of relevant literature.

Conclusion

I have tried to present a broad view of my experience and thoughts concerning my work with families who have experienced torture. It is a truism that this work is difficult; one can never achieve all that one would wish. Even when there is no clinical intervention, when no skill and no technique come to mind, there is still the *person* of the therapist who can be there for the client at the moments of deepest despair. To remain there and not run, deny, panic, or hide in a professional role may be the most important thing the therapist has to offer. Trust, honesty, empathy, and a willingness to *hear* the trauma story and its impact in the lives of individuals and families are the core of healing and recovery from torture.

References

Alvarez, A. (1989, February). *Child sexual abuse: The need to remember and the need to forget.* Paper presented at the Association of Child Psychology and Psychiatry study day, London. Summary published in *Newsletter of the Association for Child Psychology and Psychiatry, 11*(3), 28.

American Psychiatric Association. (1980). *Diagnostic and statistical manual of mental disorders* (3rd ed.). Washington, DC: Author.

American Psychiatric Association. (1987). *Diagnostic and statistical manual of mental disorders* (3rd ed., rev.). Washington, DC: Author.

Amnesty International. (1987). *Amnesty International Report 1987.* London: Amnesty International Publications.

Baker, R., & Briggs, J. (1975). Working with interpreters in social work practice. *Australian Social Work, 18*(4), 31–37.

Barot, R. (1988). Ethnicity and family therapy. *Journal of Family Therapy, 10*(3), 271–282.

Danieli, Y. (1988). Confronting the unimaginable: Psychotherapists' reactions to victims of the Nazi Holocaust. In J. P. Wilson, Z. Harel, & B. Kahana (Eds.), *Human adaptation to extreme stress: From the Holocaust to Vietnam* (pp. 219–238). New York: Plenum Press.

Erikson, K. (1976). *Everything in its path.* New York: Simon and Schuster.

Figley, C. (1988). *Post-traumatic family therapy.* In F. M. Ochberg (Ed.), *Post-traumatic therapy and victims of violence* (pp. 83–109). New York: Brunner/Mazel.

Fisch, R., Weakland, J., & Segal, L. (1982). *The tactics of change: Doing therapy briefly.* San Francisco: Jossey-Bass.

Freud, A. (1974). *Infants without families and reports on the Hampstead nurseries 1939–45.* London: Hogarth Press.

Garber, J., & Seligman, M. (Eds.). (1980). *Human helplessness.* New York: Academic Press.

Haley, J. (1973). *Uncommon therapy: The psychiatric techniques of Milton H. Erickson, M.D.* New York: W. W. Norton.

Hoffman, L. (1981). *Foundations of family therapy.* New York: Basic Books.

Minuchin, S. (1974). *Families and family therapy.* Cambridge: Harvard University Press.

Minuchin, S., & Fishman, H. (1981). *Family therapy techniques.* Cambridge: Harvard University Press.

Ochberg, F. M. (Ed.). (1988). *Post-traumatic therapy and victims of violence.* New York: Brunner/Mazel.

Parson, E. R. (1985). The black Vietnam veteran: His representational world in post-traumatic stress disorders. In W. Kelly (Ed.), *Post-traumatic stress disorder and the war veteran patient* (pp. 170–192). New York: Brunner/Mazel.

Pynoos, R., & Eth, S. (1986). Witness to violence: The child interview. *American Journal of Child Psychiatry, 25*, 306–319.

Raphael, B. (1983). *Anatomy of bereavement.* New York: Basic Books.

Raphael, B. (1986). *When disaster strikes: How individuals and communities cope with catastrophe.* New York: Basic Books.

Seligman, M., & Weiss, J. (1980). Coping behavior: Learned helplessness, physiological activity, and learned inactivity. *Behaviour Research and Therapy, 18*, 459–512.

Straker, G. (1989). Child abuse, counselling and apartheid: The work of the Sanctuary counselling team. *Free Associations, 11*, 7–38.

Truax, C., & Carkhuff, R. (1967). *Toward effective counselling and psychotherapy: Training and practice.* Chicago: Aldine.

Turner, S. (1989). Working with survivors. *Psychiatric Bulletin of the Royal College of Psychiatrists, 13*(4), 173–176.

Wilson, J. P. (1989). *Trauma, transformation and healing: An integrative approach to theory, research and post-traumatic therapy.* New York: Brunner/Mazel.

World Medical Association. (1975). Declaration of Tokyo. *World Medical Journal, 20*, 87–88.

CHAPTER 60

Hyperventilation as a Reaction to Torture

Stuart W. Turner and Alexandra Hough

Introduction

A relationship between exposure to psychological stressors and a syndrome variously titled "soldier's heart" or "effort syndrome" has long been recognized (Margarion, 1982; Wood, 1941). Now acknowledged to be a consequence of overbreathing (Bass & Gardner, 1985b; Kerr, Dalton, & Gliebe, 1937), common symptoms include breathlessness or sighing breathing at rest, chest wall pain, giddiness, fatigue, numbness and tingling of the hands, blurred vision, and syncope (Bass, 1981). That these symptoms occur in survivors of organized violence including torture is hardly surprising. There is an association between breathing and emotion that is recognized by the gasp of surprise, the sigh of sadness, and the altered breathing patterns of laughing and crying. Often, torture is a devastating event for the individual to survive. For those who do, their problems may be compounded by the stresses of flight to a new country, loss of society and status, uncertainties over refugee status, and separation from family.

The severity of the handicaps resulting from hyperventilation syndrome (HVS), the delay in recognizing the nature of the disorder and the good outcome with appropriate treatment are all good reasons for further study (Evans & Lum, 1977). Of equal importance, however, may be the insight that the experiences reported by survivors of torture offer into the pathophysiological mechanisms of the hyperventilation syndrome.

Chronic Hyperventilation Syndrome

Hyperventilation may be defined as breathing in excess of metabolic requirements (Bass & Gardner, 1985a). The chronic hyperventilation syndrome (HVS) is more difficult to define, but diagnosis should usually rest upon the presence of typical symptoms and characteristic abnormalities in breathing patterns, either at rest or in provocation tests (Gardner, Meah, & Bass, 1986). Although HVS may occur in people with no demonstrable psychological or respiratory abnormalities (Bass & Gardner, 1985b), it is usually associated with anxiety, panic, and phobic symptoms and provides an illustration of the often complex relationships between physiological and psychological processes. The common signs and symptoms are listed in Table 60.1 (Margarion, 1982).

Physiological and Psychological Processes

Under conditions of psychological stress, with sympathetic nervous system overactivity, a number of adaptive physiological responses occur. These include increased heart and respiratory rates and increased tidal volume (Grossman, 1983). It has been suggested that many, if not all, people may react to stress and anxiety by overbreathing (Hibbert, 1984). An altered psychological state may therefore be seen as the primary abnormality in the etiology of this condition. On the other hand, Lum (1983) has persistently argued that habitual overbreathing is usually the fundamental cause of both the physical and the psychological symptoms of HVS; anxiety symptoms are secondary to the breathing habit and may be exacerbated by the failure of doctors to recognize

Stuart W. Turner • Department of Psychiatry, University College and Middlesex School of Medicine, Wolfson Building, Middlesex Hospital, London W1N 8AA, England. **Alexandra Hough** • St. Thomas' Hospital, London, and The Medical Foundation for the Care of Victims of Torture, 96–98 Grafton Road, London NW5 3EJ, England.

International Handbook of Traumatic Stress Syndromes, edited by John P. Wilson and Beverley Raphael. Plenum Press, New York, 1993.

Table 60.1. Signs and Symptoms of Hyperventilation Syndrome[a]

General
Chronic and easy fatigue, weakness, sleep disturbances, headache, excessive sweating, sensation of feeling cold, poor concentration and performance of tasks

Neurologic
Numbness and tingling, especially of distal extremities, giddiness, syncope, blurring or tunneling of vision, and impaired thinking

Respiratory
Sensation of breathlessness or inability to take a deep enough breath with sighing, yawning, and excessive use of upper chest and accessory muscles of respiration, nocturnal dyspnea superficially mimicking paroxysmal nocturnal dyspnoea of cardiovascular origin, and nonproductive cough with frequent clearing of throat

Cardiovascular
Chest pains often mimicking angina, palpitations, and tachycardia

Gastrointestinal
Aerophagia resulting in full/bloated sensation, belching, flatus, esophageal reflux and heartburn, sharp lower chest pain, dry mouth, and sensation of lump in throat

Musculoskeletal
Myalgias, increased muscle tone with muscular tightness (stiffness), cramps with occasional carpopedal spasms and rarely a more generalized tetany

Psychiatric
Anxious, irritable, and tense though may superficially appear calm (suppression of emotional release), depersonalization or a feeling of being far away, phobias, and panic attacks

[a]From Margarion (1982).

and treat the disorder. In the established condition, a positive feedback loop commonly exists by which overbreathing may produce such physical symptoms as chest pain, leading to increased apprehension and hence to increased overbreathing (Lum, 1983).

In their review, Bass and Gardner (1985a) considered the relative merits of theories which were based upon a psychological predisposition in people with trait anxiety or neuroticism, or a physiological abnormality with undue reactivity of the respiratory center. Both extremes are likely to be insufficient. Although it has been demonstrated that normal volunteers with high neuroticism scores are more likely to show affective symptoms on hyperventilating (Clark & Hemsley, 1982), Bass and Gardner (1985b) have demonstrated that some people with HVS have no demonstrable psychological or respiratory disorders.

Anticipation of an electrical shock (Suess, Alexander, Smith, Sweeney, & Marion, 1980) during a perceptual task has been demonstrated to produce overbreathing with lowered end-tidal $paCO_2$ levels (a noninvasive measure of alveolar and hence arterial $paCO_2$ levels). This result is not easy to interpret. It appears to suggest that traumatic stress may be directly responsible for hyperventilation. However, none of these subjects went on to develop HVS. This has been taken to indicate that abnormal psychological condition alone may be insufficient to explain the etiology of HVS.

Lum (1983) appeared to accept that overbreathing is a normal response to stress, but believes that habitual overbreathing is of fundamental importance in the etiology of HVS. In experiments on healthy young men, he cited evidence that by manipulating inhaled CO_2 levels, it is possible to demonstrate low-resting $paCO_2$ levels and abnormally sensitive respiratory function in about 12% of subjects (Lambertsen, 1960). In established HVS, there is evidence in favor of relatively stable, abnormal respiratory control (Gardner et al., 1986) and there are characteristic abnormalities in breathing behavior, including sighing, irregular, and thoracic respiration (Lum, 1983).

The clinical situation is probably more complex, because whatever the primary abnormality, there are usually both psychological and physiological disturbances which require treatment. Bass and Gardner (1985a) also pointed out that the process by which people become "patients" is complex and partly determined by extraneous factors, such as complaint threshold and symptom attribution. In the absence of large-scale longitudinal investigations, theories of primary causation of HVS are in their nature speculative.

Even the mechanisms by which HVS produces symptoms are not always clear, although the lowered $paCO_2$ levels and increased pH appear to play an important part (Lum, 1983). Thus, a fall in $paCO_2$ produces cerebral arterial vasoconstriction and may lead to cerebral hypoxia, with consequent neurological and psychological symptomatology (Lum, 1983; Pincus, 1978). Other biochemical processes may also be important, including the Bohr effect by which lowering the arterial $paCO_2$ levels leads to a reduction in the bioavailability of the circulating oxygen (Margarion, 1982). However, these simple mechanisms may not be sufficient to explain all the symptoms of HVS. Hyperventilation can also lead to transient cardiac changes associated with abnormal EKG recordings, and, if associated with air swallowing, it can lead to gastrointestinal symptoms (Pincus, 1978). There have been recent attempts, for example, to understand the detailed mechanisms behind the etiology of chest pain (Freeman & Nixon, 1985a,b) and unilateral neurological symptoms (O'Sullivan, Harvey, Bass, Sheehy, Toone, & Turner, personal communication).

Survivors of Organized Violence

Survivors of torture and other forms of organized violence often have a multitude of problems. They may present with physical symptoms following torture; they may have a depressive reaction; they may share with other survivors of extreme trauma the features of posttraumatic stress disorder (PTSD) (American Psychiatric Association [APA], 1987); and they may have had the meaning systems in their life shaken or destroyed (see Chapter 58, in this volume).

A proportion also have HVS and they may offer a unique insight into the way that HVS develops. A series of 10 survivors of organized violence, all with HVS and seen by one or both of us at the Medical Foundation for the Care of Victims of Torture (Turner, 1989), is reported here (Table 60.2).

Table 60.2. Summary of the Ten Survivors of Organized Violence[a]

	Age	Sex	Previous psychiatric history	Organized violence	HVS onset	Symptoms	PTSD	Depression
A	25	F	None	Political detainee for 3 months, tortured, deprived of food, severely burned, falaka	During torture	Pseudoseizures, headache, shortness of breath	Y	Y
B	32	M	None	Political detainee for 3 years, tortured, falaka, beaten, heard friends' torture and death	During torture	Pseudoseizures, chest pain, paresthesiae	Y	Y
C	34	M	None	Political detainee for 31 months, tortured, falaka, suspension, beaten, mock executions, required surgery, made to witness torture	During torture	Headaches, anxiety symptoms, chest pain, unilateral neurological symptoms	Y	Y
D	34	F	None	Political forced deportee to country at war, victim of organized persecution there	During persecution	Shortness of breath, palpitations, weakness, unilateral neurological symptoms	Y	Y
E	31	F	None	Political detainee, harassed and forced to witness husband being beaten	Uncertain	Fatigue, anxiety, lightheadedness, chest pain, neurological symptoms, emotional outbursts	Y	Y
F	37	M	None	Political detainee subjected to severe torture	Uncertain	Insomnia, anxiety, chest and arm pain	Y	N
G	42	M	None	Political detainee for 24 hours, tortured, electric shocks to arm and genitals, teléfono	On release	Headaches, tension, dizziness, anxiety, shortness of breath	Y	Y
H	32	M	None	Political detainee for 1 month, tortured, beaten, burns, forced standing, soiled food	On release	Chest pain, palpitations, headaches, shortness of breath	Y	N
I	40	F	None	Politically active, friend detained 1 year, lived in fear friend would give her name	During time of fear	Burning sensations, anxiety symptoms	Y	Y
J	31	M	None	Political detainee, tortured, beaten, burned, denied food	On release	Insomnia, cramps, peripheral paresthesiae	Y	N

[a]Based on a retrospective case note survey.

The study group comprised six men and four women with a mean age of 34 years. Most but not all had been tortured. All had been victims of organized violence under repressive regimes. Eight were from the Middle East, one was African, and the other South American. All had clinical evidence of HVS and all improved with relaxation and breathing retraining.

Perhaps the most interesting finding is that although none had any history of psychiatric disturbance before their traumatic experiences, four reported the onset of symptoms during exposure to organized violence, three first experienced symptoms shortly after release from detention, and another developed HVS when she lived in fear that a friend, who had been detained and was being tortured, would give her name to the authorities. Two of these cases illustrate the way that the traumatic procedure is closely implicated in the onset of HVS.

Localization of the Onset of HVS

A 25-year-old woman (Mrs. A.) reported how she had been tortured in her own country by being beaten, burned with cigarettes, and subjected to *falaka* (a form of torture in which the soles of the feet are beaten using a cane or whip). One day, after several months of detention, she was standing in the interrogation room, hooded and tied to a post, when she suddenly experienced an agonizing pain as very hot or corrosive liquid was poured over her legs. At this point she lost consciousness and woke up in the "sick bay" of the torture center. She was later transferred to the local hospital, an event which led to her eventual release. Her legs were very badly damaged and subsequently she spent several months in the hospital. Within a few days of this assault, she had the first of many pseudoepileptic seizures. She has a markedly reduced breath-holding time (1–2 seconds) and 10 seconds of voluntary overbreathing produced symptoms identical to those which precede a typical attack. An EEG was normal.

Another Example of Onset of HVS

A 32-year-old man (Mr. B.) gave a similar history of imprisonment for 3 years in his native country. In addition to frequent kicking, punching, and beating during his detention, he was also subjected to falaka. The falaka was continued for periods lasting from 1 to 2 hours and, despite the development of swelling and infection, was repeated frequently. The pain was described as "appalling." Early in the torture, he was repeatedly hit on the head and remembers losing consciousness several times. After several weeks, he found that, after only 20 to 30 minutes of torture, he would lose consciousness without head trauma. This was preceded by subjective anxiety with autonomic accompaniments. He also remembers that his hands and his body would shake before he passed out. At this point, the torturers would stop and he was usually transferred to a local hospital. In the United Kingdom, where he is now a refugee, he experienced similar attacks, usually worst at times of high distress. They were precisely reproducible by voluntary hyperventilation. He also had evidence of a depressive illness.

An EKG, EEG, and CT scan revealed no significant abnormalities.

These cases may be taken as illustrations of two processes. First, the severity of the stressor is greater, by many orders of magnitude, than that in any ethical scientific experiment. In torture it is common, and may be the rule, for survivors to develop psychological reactions even in the absence of any pretorture psychological disturbance (see Chapter 58, in this volume). The severity of the stressor is so great that probably everyone is affected in some way. A similar process may occur in relation to HVS. The infliction of uncontrollable, severe, and prolonged pain and deprivation may be sufficient, in the absence of any individual predisposition, to lead to the development of a sustained breathing abnormality in a way that the experiments of Suess *et al.* (1980) could not demonstrate.

Second, they illustrate how, at first, overbreathing may be adaptive by inducing lightheadedness, by reducing pain perception, by terminating torture, and sometimes by leading to transfer into a less harsh environment. However, following release and asylum in another country, this breathing habit may be persistent and maladaptive. The same responses occur but in a nonspecific and maladaptive way. Particularly for those with PTSD (APA, 1987), who have persisting intrusive phenomena and hyperarousal, it is easy to see how HVS may persist and how symptoms may be made worse at times of intrusive recall of the trauma which first led to the syndrome. Because of this potential relationship between intrusive phenomena and symptoms, there may be differences between posttorture HVS and the HVS seen more commonly in psychiatric practice. Gardner *et al.* (1986) report normalization of $paCO_2$ levels during sleep. In those especially troubled by nightmares following torture, this may not be the case.

Nocturnal Hyperventilation

A 34-year-old man (Mr. C.) complained of severe headaches. He had survived torture including beating and falaka. For him the worst part of his experience was witnessing the torture of children. The typical pattern was that the headaches, when they occurred, would commence on awakening. On these days, his girlfriend later told him, he would have had a very restless sleep, muttering and looking very distressed. He told me that his hands would be clenched into fists; the marks of his fingernails would be deeply scored into his palms. Interestingly, during the day, he had developed a series of coping strategies to reduce the impact of intrusive thoughts. Usually, the headache persisted for 12 to 24 hours. There was evidence of a major depressive disorder. Voluntary overbreathing reproduced his symptoms, and HVS was confirmed by measuring end-tidal $paCO_2$ levels at rest and on provocation.

It is likely that for this man, the intrusive recall was worse during sleep and that the hyperventilation mirrored this process.

Severity of the Handicaps Associated with HVS

HVS can be frankly disabling both in relation to the symptoms of the disorder, for example, pseudoepileptic seizures, and as a result of the meaning ascribed to the symptoms.

The Severity of the Symptoms of HVS

Mr. C., a man with severe and intractable headaches, reported that the pain was so severe that he had tried banging his head against a wall in an attempt to gain relief and had seriously contemplated suicide. He had been extensively investigated in two neurological centers but no diagnosis had been established. Successful treatment has allowed him to take up a job for the first time in this country.

The Ascription of Meaning to Symptoms

Mrs. D., aged 34, reported persistent pain and numbness affecting the right side of her body. She had not herself been tortured but had been subject to state persecution over several years. She had been told by a doctor that she would never be able to use her right hand again. These symptoms were associated with the development of PTSD and in 2 months of treatment, including breathing retraining, she had lost all her right-sided symptoms and also showed a significant improvement in her psychological state.

Of the sample of 10 clients reported earlier, it is worth pointing out that none had been correctly diagnosed elsewhere and for some the symptoms were both chronic and very severe. In addition to the two cases described above, several had hospital admissions and investigations and another had been confined to bed.

Diagnosis of HVS

HVS is common yet often undiagnosed in medical practice (Margarion, 1982). Reasons for this may include inadequate education and poor communication skills in doctors who approach patients looking for textbook stereotypes (Bass, 1981; Rice, 1950). HVS may coexist with established organic respiratory disease such as asthma or multiple pulmonary emboli (Bass & Gardner, 1985b). There is often a failure to recognize that the overbreathing may not be visibly obvious (Margarion, 1982). Patients may suffer from early labeling by professionals as "neurotic" or in survivors of torture as having the "torture syndrome" (e.g., Abildgaard, Daugaard, Marcussen, Jess, Petersen, & Wallach, 1984): an overinclusive attempt to produce a single syndromal diagnosis to describe what is inevitably a complex psychological reaction (Goldfeld, Mollica, Pesavento, & Faraone, 1988).

Clinical diagnosis rests on the history and a provocation test (Hibbert, 1984; Margarion, 1982) which can include breath-holding as well as voluntary overbreathing. The overbreathing is usually at a rate of 30 to 40 deep breaths per minute and should be continued for 4 to 5 minutes or until the client complains of dizziness. If chest pain has been part of the history, the test should be carried out under EKG control. After the provocation test, rebreathing in and out of a brown paper bag held loosely over the mouth and nose, which has the effect of raising $paCO_2$ levels, can be demonstrated to terminate symptoms (Margarion, 1982). If the provocation test reproduces the symptoms precisely, the diagnosis of HVS becomes very likely. Indeed, many researchers have argued that this clinical test should be regarded as diagnostic (Blau, Wiles, & Solomon, 1983; Margarion, 1982). However, there are several pitfalls. First, organic respiratory disease may be associated with HVS, and where the two coexist, the physical pathology may be missed by this approach. Second, overbreathing may lower the threshold for other disorders, the obvious example being reduced seizure threshold; in other words, overbreathing may provoke a genuine epileptic seizure in some predisposed people. Finally, the clinical provocation test may be negative in the presence of HVS, possibly because of low levels of perceived threat in the clinical environment.

Therefore, the best method of making the diagnosis, where the equipment and expertise are available, may be to measure $paCO_2$ levels under several different conditions. This may be particularly important in people who fail to show a good initial response to treatment. Overbreathing is reflected by lowering of $paCO_2$ as this is eliminated through the lungs. The measurement is most conveniently carried out using nasal catheters and a system which measures end-tidal pCO_2 levels as these closely approximate to arterial $paCO_2$ levels. Where it is demonstrated that a person is breathing in excess of requirements in different situations and for prolonged periods after different provocations, the diagnosis is fairly secure (Bass & Gardner, 1985a).

Management of HVS in Survivors of Torture

In treating survivors of torture, who have endured some of the worst imaginable physical injuries and psychological distress, it is particularly important to look, first of all, at the therapeutic relationship.

Whether psychiatrist, psychologist, psychotherapist, or physiotherapist, the worker must be prepared to listen to the trauma story, and to offer a "whole person response." In torture, where the body is abused for psychological effect, it is impossible not to look at each symptom as having a range of physical and psychological meanings. Usually, survivors need to know that their pain can be acknowledged even if it is beyond the range of experiences that most of us can understand.

Torture often takes place within a personal, perverted relationship. In other words, the victim of torture received the focused attention of an adversary determined to break down the will to resist, and hence to achieve psychological change. Therapeutic work must take place in a different psychological environment, one in which a degree of trust has been fostered and in which survivors can be encouraged to regain their self-confidence and esteem. They must feel welcome and know that their problem is being taken seriously. They need space, time, privacy, and an attentive ear.

HVS is a good example of a mechanism with, at least in the established condition, interacting psychological and physiological processes. It demands a holistic approach.

One of the first and most important steps is to listen to the client's own understanding of the symptoms. Very often, people will have been given incorrect diagnoses in the past or will have made erroneous assumptions about their state. The clinical provocation test is a useful therapeutic as well as diagnostic maneuver. By demonstrating that symptoms can be provoked by such simple maneuvers as breath-holding or voluntary over-breathing, clients can start to learn something about the nature of their condition. Moreover, they may start to appreciate that they are, at least to a very limited degree, in control.

Time should be spent informing clients about HVS. This is often reassuring to those clients who may start to realize that other symptoms which they had not mentioned or which have now disappeared are also understandable in relation to overbreathing. Not only does this reassure survivors about their symptoms, it also provides some additional reassurance that the diagnosis is correct. It can be quite puzzling to learn that symptoms affecting so many different parts of the body, and associated with so many feelings, can be produced by a breathing disorder. There may be myths which need to be abolished, such as the common belief that breathing deeply will enhance relaxation. Education is not a single step in treatment; it needs to be continued as long as it is needed.

Coexisting psychiatric disorders require treatment. For example, a sedative antidepressant drug may be useful in people with mixed anxiety and depressive symptoms. The broader psychological meanings must not be overlooked either and many people will require a psychotherapeutic approach (see Chapter 58, in this volume). However, these must be coupled with a program of relaxation and breathing retraining (Bonn, Readhead, & Timmons, 1984; Hough, 1991) and it is this which will be considered in more detail in the rest of this chapter.

During breathing retraining, the client has to experience the discomfort of air hunger and learn to resist the drive to overbreathe. This is necessary if there is to be readjustment of the respiratory control center. This procedure has to be accompanied by reassurance and relaxation, and must have been explained and accepted in advance.

A typical program would start with the client's being asked to lie in a comfortable position on a couch, perhaps with a pillow under the knees for support. Awareness of breathing is encouraged by asking the client to imagine the air going into his or her lungs, as if the air is passing down a tube and filling a balloon every time a breath is taken. Different breathing maneuvers, such as breathing in, breathing out, and breath-holding (for a short time) can be rehearsed, asking the client to concentrate on each of these automatic experiences. Ask-

ing the client to put one hand on the upper chest and another on the abdomen is useful in learning awareness of thoracic and abdominal breathing. One of the aims of treatment is to encourage people to use abdominal rather than thoracic breathing.

Usually, treatment will include relaxation training. It is very difficult, if not impossible, to learn new methods of breathing in the presence of high levels of arousal or tension. Relaxation training will take one of the standard forms, although the one used in our practice is a simple relaxation program described by Mitchell (1977).

Sometimes, a combination of education, learning abdominal breathing, and relaxation training is sufficient, and breathing patterns return to normal. If not, time should be spent teaching the client to use slower, and if necessary, more shallow breaths. To do this, the first step is to take a baseline measurement of respiratory rate and then ask the client to breathe in time with words or numbers. For example, the therapist could initially repeat aloud "in-and-out" or "in-and-out-two-three," pacing these words to a steady rhythm, resulting in slight slowing of the client's breathing (Innocenti, 1987). Care must be taken to watch for any evidence of increasing depth of breathing, a return to thoracic breathing, or increasing tension. Although some discomfort is inevitable as breathing is slowed, this should not reach the point of creating tension.

As this slowing is practiced, there should be occasional breaks for feedback and discussion. Clients may be reassured that slight discomfort is usual and indicates success. This is necessary for there to be resetting of the breathing control mechanisms.

From time to time, repeat measurements of resting respiratory rates should be made to monitor progress. However, although this is useful, the final evidence of success is loss of symptoms and these provide a much better outcome indicator. Nonetheless, if the rate can be reduced to six to eight breaths a minute in the resting state, this is a good result, likely to be associated with loss of symptoms.

The exercise is then transferred from a couch to a sitting position in a chair, and from there to more normal situations, such as walking and talking. This may take several sessions. Eventually, breathing control is practiced while hurrying, on stairs, and even while jogging (Lum, 1983). Because of the nature of the complaint, these should not be hurried and an undisturbed hour should be set each time. Between sessions, the client should be encouraged to practice alone. These practice sessions should be short but frequent. Clients should also be encouraged to set aside 20 minutes each day for relaxation. Only by carrying the treatment techniques into everyday life, can ultimate success be achieved. Part of each formal treatment session should be spent reviewing progress in this "homework" and discussing any difficulties experienced.

Advice may be offered about dealing with difficult situations. For example, swallowing is a way of suppressing the urge to take a deep breath or if a deep breath has been taken, it may be useful to follow with a compensatory breath-hold to reduce the physiological effects. Similarly, for those who experience real difficulties in transferring their practice into their everyday life, it may be helpful to look again at some of the situations which seem to trigger symptoms and see if other ways can be found to deal with them.

The Beneficial Role of Education

Mrs. E. was a qualified nurse who had suffered harassment, loss of her home, and a traumatic flight from her country. She presented with fatigue, insomnia, lightheadedness, paresthesia in her hands, air hunger, and feelings of a weight on her chest and of her breath being "cut short." Her breathing was punctuated with sighs and her conversation with outbursts of uncontrolled laughter, followed by embarrassed apologies. The whole of the first treatment session with a physiotherapist was spent in listening and explaining the purpose of the treatment and in teaching relaxed abdominal breathing. She found the relationship between her symptoms and hyperventilation hard to accept at first. However, once convinced, she was an enthusiastic and highly motivated client. She managed to slow her respiratory rate with counting, but when practicing deeper relaxation she began to experience feelings of fear. Once again, she had to be reassured that expression of feeling in a physiotherapy session is not only permissible but is often therapeutic. Offering a strategically placed box of tissues was a useful nonverbal communication. At first, the treatment was slow and she found air hunger particularly difficult to control but the final outcome was good.

A Whole-Person Approach

Mr. F. had arrived in the United Kingdom 6 years before his presentation for treatment. He had suffered severe torture and in the United Kingdom, had been continuously unemployed, disturbed by symptoms of insomnia, anxiety, and chest and arm pain. The first treatment session with a physiotherapist was again spent listening, and in explanation and reassurance. Relaxation was readily achieved, but many weeks passed before breathing became controlled. During his treatment, as he started to regain control and learn to trust, he started talking about his feelings. After some time, he felt able to take up the suggestion of participating in group therapy, where he found that his ability to support others was a major step in his own path to recovery (see Chapter 65, in this volume, for an explanation of the principles of posttraumatic therapy).

In the series of 10, there was a good outcome in all cases. Sometimes, the beneficial effects of treatment were dramatic with a rapid and total loss of all HVS symptoms.

Conclusions

HVS is common in survivors of torture. The etiology of HVS remains a matter for debate, but, in torture, important elements may be the severity of the traumatic event and the adaptive functions of overbreathing as the trauma continues. Following release from detention, the syndrome of HVS may be a disabling result. It may lead people to contemplate suicide or to believe that they have a very serious physical illness. Usually, the treatment is multiprofessional and is often very successful. Indeed, the outcome may be better for survivors of torture than for others with HVS, because, in their release from detention, the maintaining factors for HVS may be reduced. An important element of treatment is breathing retraining and this procedure has been presented in some detail.

References

Abildgaard, U., Daugaard, G., Marcussen, H., Jess, P., Petersen, H. D., & Wallach, M. (1984). Chronic organic psychosyndrome in Greek torture victims. *Danish Medical Bulletin, 31*, 239–242.

American Psychiatric Association. (1987). *Diagnostic and statistical manual of mental disorders* (3rd ed. rev.). Washington, DC: Author.

Bass, C. (1981). Diagnosis and treatment of breathlessness. *Lancet, i*, 220.

Bass, C., & Gardner, W. N. (1985a). Emotional influences on breathing and breathlessness. *Journal of Psychosomatic Research, 29*, 599–609.

Bass, C., & Gardner, W. N. (1985b). Respiratory and psychiatric abnormalities in chronic symptomatic hyperventilation. *British Medical Journal, 290*, 1387–1390.

Blau, J. N., Wiles, C. M., & Solomon, F. S. (1983). Unilateral somatic symptoms due to hyperventilation. *British Medical Journal, 286*, 1108.

Bonn, J. A., Readhead, C. P. A., & Timmons, B. H. (1984). Enhanced adaptive behavioural response in agoraphobic patients pretreated with breathing retraining. *Lancet, ii*, 665–669.

Clark, D. M., & Hemsley, D. R. (1982). The effects of hyperventilation: Individual variability and its relation to personality. *Journal of Behavior Therapy and Experimental Psychiatry, 13*(1), 41–47.

Evans, D. W., & Lum, L. C. (1977). Hyperventilation: An important cause of pseudoangina. *Lancet, i*, 155–157.

Freeman, L. J., & Nixon, P. G. F. (1985a). Are coronary artery spasm and progressive damage to the heart associated with the hyperventilation syndrome? *British Medical Journal, 291*, 851–852.

Freeman, L. J., & Nixon, P. G. F. (1985b). Chest pain and the hyperventilation syndrome—Some etiological considerations. *Postgraduate Medical Journal, 61*, 957–961.

Gardner, W. N., Meah, M. S., & Bass, C. (1986). Controlled study of respiratory responses during prolonged measurements in patients with chronic hyperventilation. *Lancet, ii*, 826–830.

Goldfeld, A. E., Mollica, R. F., Pesavento, B. H., & Faraone, S. V. (1988). The physical and psychological sequelae of torture. *Journal of the American Medical Association, 259*, 2725–2729.

Grossman, P. (1983). Respiration, stress, and cardiovascular function. *Psychophysiology, 20*, 284–300.

Hibbert, G. A. (1984). Hyperventilation as a cause of panic attacks. *British Medical Journal, 288*, 263–264.

Hough, A. (1991). *Physiotherapy in respiratory care: A problem solving approach.* London, England: Chapman & Hall.

Innocenti, D. M. (1987). Chronic hyperventilation syndrome. In P. A. Downie (Ed.), *Cash's textbook of chest, heart and vascular disorders for physiotherapists* (4th ed.). London, England: Faber & Faber.

Kerr, W. J., Dalton, J. W., & Gliebe, P. A. (1937). Some physical phenomena associated with anxiety states and their relation to hyperventilation. *Annals of Internal Medicine, 11,* 961–992.

Lambertsen, C. J. (1960). Carbon dioxide and respiration in acid-base homeostasis. *Anaesthesiology, 21,* 642–651.

Lum, L. C. (1983). Physiological considerations in the treatment of hyperventilation syndromes. *Journal of Drug Research, 8,* 1867–1872.

Margarion, G. J. (1982). Hyperventilation syndromes: Infrequently recognized common expressions of anxiety and stress. *Medicine, 61,* 219–236.

Mitchell, L. (1977). *Simple relaxation.* Bath: Pitman Press.

O'Sullivan, G., Harvey, I., Bass, C., Sheehy, M., Toone, B. K., & Turner, S. W. (1990). Personal communication.

Pincus, J. H. (1978). Disorders of conscious awareness: Hyperventilation syndrome. *British Journal of Hospital Medicine,* 312–313.

Rice, R. L. (1950). Symptom patterns of the hyperventilation syndrome. *American Journal of Medicine, 107,* 691–700.

Suess, W. M., Alexander, A. B., Smith, D. D., Sweeney, H. W., & Marion, R. J. (1980). The effects of psychological stress on respiration: A preliminary study of anxiety and the hyperventilation syndrome. *Psychophysiology, 17,* 535–540.

Turner, S. W. (1989). Working with survivors: The Medical Foundation for the Care of Victims of Torture. *Psychiatric Bulletin, 13,* 173–176.

Wood, P. (1941). DaCosta's syndrome (or effort syndrome). *British Medical Journal, i,* 767.

CHAPTER 61

Disruption and Reconstitution of Family, Network, and Community Systems Following Torture, Organized Violence, and Exile

Richard Douglas Blackwell

Introduction

The process of arrest, torture, release, flight, and exile involves trauma at many levels. Insofar as humans are social beings, this trauma can be understood, not only as an assault on the individual person, but also an assault on the links and connections between people and the patterns of relationships through which people define themselves and give meaning to their lives.[1]

In this chapter, I am concerned not so much with specific techniques and models of treatment, but rather with presenting an orientation to work with torture survivors, specifically those in exile. It is an orientation that was adopted by the Medical Foundation for the Care of Victims of Torture in London, which works mainly with people who have suffered persecution in other countries and who have fled to the United Kingdom from many different parts of the world.

[1]Although this chapter focuses on the relationships between people and the importance of social context, I do not wish to obscure the violence done to individual persons and the assault on individuality and personal integrity constituted by torture and organized violence. Rather, I wish to establish the extent to which the individual's uniqueness is an emergent property of a context of social relationships, and to emphasize the impossibility of separating the violation of individuals from the violation of their significant relationships with others.

Richard Douglas Blackwell • Medical Foundation for the Care of Victims of Torture, 96–98 Grafton Road, London NW5 3EJ, England.

International Handbook of Traumatic Stress Syndromes, edited by John P. Wilson and Beverley Raphael. Plenum Press, New York, 1993.

In this setting, our concern at the foundation is to move beyond a medical model, which sees the individual as a damaged organism to be repaired by the efforts of professional staff; this type of a model tends to render the patient a passive recipient of professional help. We regard such a model as particularly inappropriate for patients who have already suffered the attempts of oppressors to render them passive and helpless. Instead, we seek an existential approach which pays attention to the subjective experience of the survivor and develops a dialogue between survivors and professionals in such a way that each learns from the other. For us as professionals, it is our clients who teach us how to help them.

This active client role is particularly important for clients whose countries have already been colonized by foreign powers which have imposed their own cultures and ideologies on the indigenous population. It is of further special significance when the new host country (in this case Great Britain) has been the colonizer or when colonialism is perceived as having come from white, European, or English-speaking nations. It is all too easy to repeat the colonizing process by imposing a therapeutic ideology that is rooted in the culture of the host community, giving meaning to the survivor's experience in the language and symbols of that host community and its professionals, and failing to recognize the rich sources of meaning and symbolism available to the survivor from his or her own culture. This does not mean that we feel bound to accept or go along with whatever the survivors think or say; it does mean, however, that in cases of disagreement we must always be aware that differences between the survivor's view and ours is just as likely to be rooted in the differences between our cultures as it is in the survivor's symptomatology. Such disagreements can then be respected as part of a dialectic within which there are new creative possibilities, and not interpreted as the survivor's resistance to our efforts to help.

In paying attention to the survivor's existential status and subjective experience, it is necessary to take account of the social nature of human existence and to recognize that a person's sense of self is rooted in his or her relationships with others. Our focus, therefore, shifts from the "individual" *per se* to the "individual in relationship to others." Thus, we regard torture and organized violence as an assault, not on an individual alone, but on the family and the community to which that individual belongs. It is on these social units that we focus when we think in terms of rehabilitation.

Indeed, when we look at the overall nature of organized violence, we see that it is rarely directed against individuals as such. Usually, its purpose is the control and repression of whole groups of people. It is directed against political movements or populations which provide the seed bed for such movements: against villages, or tribes, or communities, or religious and ethnic minorities whose very existence is seen as a threat. It is used to induce a state of fear, apathy, or compliance in whole populations and to discourage any thoughts or speech against the dominant power. Vinar (1989), in Uruguay, and Kordon *et al.* (1988), in Argentina, described how people became afraid to speak, even among themselves, about the repression and the disappearances. A rule of silence became operative in whole populations, and people would rather not think of what was happening because it could not be spoken of; to think it, without being able even to speak of it, was painful and seemed pointless. Argentina's National Commission on Disappeared People (1986) includes the testimony of a doctor who was arrested and told by his torturers that they knew he was not involved with terrorism or with guerrillas but that he would be tortured because he opposed the regime. They told him, "You're going to pay dearly for it . . . the poor won't have any goody goodies to look after them any more!" Kordon *et al.* described how members of a family in which someone had disappeared would be encouraged by others, including psychotherapists, to give up the hope of seeing that person again. They were encouraged to mourn that person as lost, or even to deny the existence of that person, and get on with their own lives. It was the great achievement of the mothers of the Plaza de Mayo that they refused to submit to this pressure, made known the disappearances of their children and demanded to know what had happened to them.

Thus, we can see how organized violence is aimed at severing the connections between people, controlling their ways of being together and relating to each other, and destroying the possibility of free dialogue and thought.

Theoretical Framework

Theoretically, we can consider three levels of social life which can provide a focus for our rehabilitative work: *families*, *networks*, and *communities*. We can under-

stand these as dimensions of systemic interaction in which individuals participate and through which they generate meaning and purpose in their lives.

Family Systems

The term *system* has been applied within family therapy to denote a definable group of people, usually a family, engaged in habitual patterns of interaction which can be said to have rules that determine these observable patterns. According to Watzlawick, Beavin, and Jackson (1967), all behavior is communicative, so that these interactions can be understood to be communication at the verbal and nonverbal levels.

From these patterned, rule-governed communications, participants derive and construct meaning. The meaning of themselves as persons, their sense of self, identity, and purpose are thus derived from their patterned interaction and communications with other participants in the "system."

The basis for the individual's understanding and interpretation of the world in which he or she lives is similarly derived from such systems of interaction. Thus, an individual who grows up in a family inherits and internalizes a range of meanings and habitual patterns of behavior through which he or she relates to others to give meaning to the experience of the world. Individuals internalize rules for relating, experiencing, and creating meaning.

In psychoanalytic theory, the term *transference* is used to describe the way in which a person repeats habitual patterns of interaction with significant others (usually parents) which have begun their formation in infancy. Also, the metaphor of *internal objects* is used to describe the way in which rules of relating to others are represented and patterned in an individual's mind. Subsequently, I shall speak of internalized rules for relating and making sense of the world (i.e., giving meaning to experience) as an internal meaning system.

Networks

Individuals who have grown beyond the stage of infancy relate to many other individuals outside their families: friends, neighbors, colleagues, comrades, enemies, bosses, subordinates, and the like. Insofar as these relationships have a sort of regularity and continuity of pattern over time, they can be called *networks* in which the individual participates. Through these networks of relationships, the individual develops further patterns of interaction and communication and thereby elaborates his or her meaning system, whose basis is first formed in the family system. Thus, an individual may learn artistic appreciation (rules for experiencing art) or a political ideology (rules for giving meaning to social process) through relationships with fellow students or friends, even though such things are beyond the repertoire of the family of origin. Also, as in the family system, these rules form part of the individual's sense of identity: who the person is and where the person belongs in the world.

Community

Both the family and the network exist within the context of a larger group of people with a shared language, a shared system of meanings, shared pattern of, and rules for, interactions and communication, and shared symbols, values, and concepts of individuality, relationships, and society. This is called a *community*. The rules and meanings of an individual's family and network are variations on an overall theme derived from the community. Thus, strangers from the same community have an immediate basis for establishing interaction and communication and for correcting misunderstandings, based on their shared membership in the same community. They bring to a new relationship the differences derived from their participation in different networks and their origin in different families, but have a common basis for understanding these differences.

By way of illustration we may take a rather simplistic analogy from football. A man becomes a footballer by joining a team in which he learns the formal rules of the game. He also learns a language (the terminology of football) and a range of patterns of play. He learns skills and how to fit those skills to the skills of others so that he can participate in the team's tactical and strategic plays. He learns to recognize patterns of play so that he can anticipate what might happen next and position himself accordingly—in football language he learns to "read the game." In this way he acquires the identity of being a "footballer."

In addition to being a member of his own team, he will have contact with other teams against whom he plays in a particular league. He may talk to players from other teams and, through this encounter, learn other skills and patterns not familiar to his own team. If we see the team in which he starts as analogous to a family, we can see the additional contact with other teams and players as a network. All this takes place within an overall context of the game of football which has many teams and players who never meet but who have in common the rules of the game and a certain terminology and body of skills and understandings, styles and fashions, rules and meanings. This can be seen as analogous to the community. Thus, in the same way that a person becomes a footballer through participation with others in a team, and through contact with other players in other teams, all within the overall framework of the game of football, so individuals become persons through their participation with others, in a family, through their contact with others in wider networks, all within the framework of a community.

S. H. Foukes, who founded Group Analysis as a mode of group psychotherapy, used the term *matrix* to describe the connections between members of a psychotherapy group. He distinguished two levels: the *foundation* matrix and the *dynamic* matrix. The former matrix referred to the common basis of shared understanding with which all the members began—their common membership of some sort of community. This might be no more than their all being members of the human community. Or it might be that they also had a common language, or a common experience of being soldiers, or of being patients in the same hospital, or of having a common problem, such as alcoholism. The subsequent web of communication and understanding which developed between them through their interaction and communication within the group he called the *dynamic matrix*. It was through their participation in this dynamic matrix that they could redefine themselves and their relationships, thereby developing new internal meaning systems.

Impact of Torture, Organized Violence, and Exile

Approximately fifteen years ago, there was a film called *Rollerball*. It depicted a fictitious sport of the future whose administrators began to change the rules to increase the spectator appeal. The rule changes allowed and encouraged increasing levels of violence in the game to the point where killing opponents was permitted. The object of the game ceased to be pursuit of the ball and scoring of goals; it became killing and surviving. If one can imagine football players being encouraged to kill each other in the course of a football game and doing so on a regular basis, then one can see that the relationships between players would be dramatically changed and the definition of being a footballer would be so transformed as to be virtually meaningless in terms of how we currently understand it.

Players, loyal to the original terms of the game and the original definition of what it meant to be a football player, might flee to a country where football was not played. In such a country, it would be exceedingly difficult if not impossible to maintain their identity as football players. Transformation of the original football game would have been so great that its original rules and meanings would be only history. Furthermore, anyone announcing himself as a fellow football player might be a friend of the old sort or a killer of the new sort. Recollection of the original team would carry unbearably painful recollections of its disintegration under the onslaught of violence.

The analogy is admittedly crude and simplistic but reflects many similarities to the crisis of identity of the exiled torture survivor. The normal rules and expectations of everyday life have been changed. The historically predictable conduct of social life has been replaced by violence, terror, and the consequently pervasive sense of insecurity.

In its description of posttraumatic stress disorder (PTSD), the revised third edition of the *Diagnostic and Statistical Manual of Mental Disorders* (DSM-III-R) of the American Psychiatric Association (APA) (1987) refers to exposure to an event outside the range of usual human experience. Frequently, torture and organized violence constitute events so far outside the range of usual experience that the individual's internal meaning system—his or her rules for making sense of experience—is nullified. The established patterns of communication and interaction within families, networks, and communities through which that internal meaning system is maintained are shattered, and the individual faces a crises of discontinuity. Often alone in an alien environment, he or she must attempt to reestablish relationships with others through which rules for relating, communicating, understanding, and giving meaning to life can be reconstructed. The only available resource is a sense of identity rooted in a past which is extremely painful to remember. The following stories of survivors illustrate some of these traumatic disruptions.

Example 1—John. John grew up in an African village. In his family, he was the eldest son and therefore had a particularly close relationship with his father and a particular set of family responsibilities. The bond between father and son in his culture appears to be greater than that between husband and wife. When John grew up and went to the university, both he and his father were members of the political party that was in power at the time. John's community was not politically sophisticated or pluralistic. Everyone in the village supported the same party with a largely uncritical loyalty.

Following the overthrow of the government, John's village became a target for the new army. One day they went to the village looking for John and his father. John was away, but they killed his father and his brother whom they mistook for him. John returned home to bury his father and brother. In the middle of the funeral service, soldiers arrived and arrested him.

In prison, he lost hope and wished his torturers would kill him, but they were clever enough to keep him alive. Meanwhile, army and bandit attacks on his village destroyed the cattle on which the village economy was based and killed many of the leaders of the village. John eventually escaped to England, but his suffering continues. His father returns to him in his dreams, seeking the completion of his burial and the continuation of the family traditions. He is haunted by the feeling that his brother died in his place. He is worried about the safety and well-being of his remaining brothers and sisters and of his wife and child. A letter arrives from his home telling him that his uncle has been killed and that his sister may have to give up her studies because she has no money and nowhere to live. John cannot discharge his responsibilities as the eldest son. He has no work and no money in England. He cannot send instructions back home for some cattle to be sold to finance his sister's education because the cattle are all gone. He cannot hope that other members of the extended family or friends in the village will help because they are struggling to survive themselves. There is no longer a village community, and John feels that even if it were safe for him to return, there is no longer anything to return to.

In England, he lives in a single room, one of five bedsitting rooms occupied by fellow countrymen. He receives a small welfare allowance, so small that his fares to come to the Medical Foundation have to be paid by us. Because he has only temporary admission, he is not allowed to work until 6 months after lodging his application for asylum. He has no job, no money, and no friends. He finds it unbearably depressing to talk to his fellow countrymen, who live in the same building, because all they can talk about is what is happening back home and how bad it all is.

He cannot arrange for his wife and child to come to England because he has no money to pay the fare. He cannot understand English society: No one talks to each other on buses or on the underground, and he does not know the people who live on the same street. (One of his fellow countrymen once told me, "If you came to my village, in a week you would know everyone. You could go anywhere without me, and you would be greeted.") He spends much of his time alone in his room. When he meets with me and I ask about his family, his friends, and his community—the relationships and structures which have given his life its meaning—it is almost too painful for him to talk about it.

Example 2—Michael. Michael grew up in the Middle East. He was and still is an idealistic man with humor, compassion, and hope for a more just and fair society. He was arrested because of his membership in a political party and his role in an officially legal workers council which had incurred the government's displeasure.

He survived torture from which he still limps. He was forced to witness the torture of others and face mock executions in which others standing alongside him were killed and he was spared. In the prison, he made friends who were subsequently killed. His wife and child were brought to the prison in an attempt to put further psychological pressure on him.

When he was released, he was kept under observation by the security police. His friends and associates had all gone into hiding, and he was afraid to try and find them in case he unwittingly led the police to them. Eventually, he went into hiding himself, fearing that he would be rearrested. He had to live in a separate town from his wife and children, and when the town in which they lived was under military attack, he was unable to be with them to look after them, and so he suffered acute anxiety about their safety.

Finally, with the help of a relative, he and his family got together and fled the country. Clear of its borders, they felt, at last, that they were safe. At the second country in which they stopped, they were rearrested and told they would probably be sent back. After an agonizing period of waiting in fear, they were allowed to continue to England. Unlike many other such refugees arriving in England, they were not again arrested by the immigration department and threatened with being sent back. Instead, Michael was granted exceptional leave to remain in England. This is renewable on an annual basis. So he watched closely the diplomatic relations between the United Kingdom and his home country, always fearing that a minor increase in friendliness between the two governments might lead to his exceptional leave's being revoked.

He and his family had to live in one room for nearly a year. None of them could speak English. They were wary of contact with others from their own country because of the possibility of spies, and further betrayal, hostility, or violence. When they eventually found a house, it was in an area where everyone else was English and white.

Michael's physical and mental distress resulting from his torture made it hard for him to relate easily to his wife and children. He would frequently become acutely depressed and cut off, or suddenly and unpredictably angry. News coverage of accidental disasters in England, such as a fire at a railway station, reactivated his anxiety from the death and destruction to which he had been so close at home. His wife, struggling to care for him and their children, desperately missed the support of her own relatives and friends. He blamed himself for being the cause of his family's having to live in this alien environment where they could find no support. He blamed himself for not being able to support them. Unable to speak English, he blamed himself for being unable to help his children with their schoolwork. Each time he received news of the deteriorating situation in his own country, he blamed himself for having left and for being in a position where he could now do nothing to help. Letters would arrive from home asking what he was doing to generate help and support in England for the people back home. These left him feeling helpless, hopeless, and alienated from a political movement and a collective hope for a better future for which he had risked his life and for which he continues to suffer.

Impact on Family Systems

Gregory Bateson (1979) described engaging himself in some experiments with optical illusions such that when he walked out into the street, he could no longer trust his perception and was unable to cross the road. His rules for making sense of what he saw were no longer reliable.

Schlapobersky and Bamber (1987) described torture as a perverted form of intimacy. The victim is forced into a position of helplessness and vulnerability and is violated. The previously established patterns of relating to another person, the sense of meaning as to what it is to be a person in relation to another, which is derived from those patterns, are fundamentally violated in an attempt to nullify them. Mock executions attack the meaning of life and death. In such circumstances, the torture victim may seek to preserve his sense of meaning through relationships with other prisoners; these relationships are then further violated by the torture and death of those others.

Thus, when the survivor returns to his or her family, the meaning of intimate relationships has been perverted for that person.[2] Even if no other member of the family has been harmed, their patterns of relationship have been transformed by the shock of the sudden removal and violation of one member. The problem of reestablishing meaningful relationships in such a family are considerable. In worse cases, where other members of the family have been killed, it may feel to the survivor that there is no longer a family within which a meaningful system of communication can be reestablished.

Impact on Networks

Like families, networks may be largely wiped out. Where members of networks—friends, colleagues, com-

[2]It is worth noting that torturers and perpetrators of violence suffer similar difficulties. The acts they have committed transform for them, too, the meaning of relationships with others and the identity of being human with other human beings.

rades, and so forth—have survived, they have often been driven into hiding or their relationships have become permeated by suspicion and mistrust so that they can no longer function as they did before. The released prisoner may also be fearful of contacting friends and associates in case he is being watched and would endanger anyone with whom he were seen to be connected. He may also have been told convincingly by his torturers that members of his network have betrayed him, so that the meaning of friendship and comradeship has been undermined and subverted. Again, as in the family, the reestablishment of meaningful patterns of interactions through which the survivor might begin to reconstruct meaning and purpose are not only severely damaged, but extremely difficult to begin to recover.

Impact on Communities

The destruction of the community, within which the family and network have existed and from which they have derived their most fundamental values and systems of meaning, is one of the most demoralizing experiences for survivors. (How can one be a footballer, if football itself no longer exists?) When a whole village has been decimated by the killing of many or most of its members, or where the economic basis of the community's life has been destroyed through the destruction of crops or animals, or where all its values and laws have been perverted through terror and the rule of violence, it is likely that the survivor will experience the whole meaning of his life's being called into question. Even if there is contact with family and network members, it takes place in a vacuum, like a meeting between two trees that have both been uprooted and no longer have any soil from which to draw sustenance.

Impact of Exile

All the problems described above are enormously exacerbated by the process of flight and subsequent exile in an alien society.

If the family escapes together, they are likely to share an experience of flight during which they feel in constant danger of rearrest and enforced return to their own country, probably to face further violence. Sometimes they are, in fact, arrested in the countries through which they pass.

Such arrests, often involving separation of family members, tend to constitute repeats of their original ordeal. Even if there is no actual violence, the experience is sufficiently similar to reactivate all the anxieties and fears associated with the original arrest. Often they are detained again on arrival at their destination, in this case the United Kingdom. This arrest comes at the point at which they believe they are clear of danger and have arrived in a place of safety. Again, they may be separated; again, they may face the questions: Will we be sent back? Will some of us be allowed to stay and others sent back? Will we ever find anywhere to be safe and attempt to recover something of our past family life? Thus, the meaning system on which they had previously built their lives is further undermined. It is replaced by a meaning system which is permanently mistrustful and uncertain, unable to take anything for granted in terms of trust and predictability; the family can no longer be assumed to be a secure unit with predictable patterns of behavior but is constantly under threat. If the family is granted leave to remain in the country but not full refugee status, then they achieve temporary safety but with a continued threat that, at some point in the future, they may still be sent back.

After all this, the meaning systems of uncertainty and of helplessness in the face of large threatening institutions, the sense of constant threat, and the sense of prior systems of meaning being no longer applicable or trustworthy tend to persist, even when, and if, refugee status is actually granted. An example of this is a man who had been arrested and tortured as a result of his political activities and who escaped to the United Kingdom with his family. Even after they had lived there in safety for some time, his mother, who had not been politically involved nor threatened in any way in their home country, would become anxious whenever he went out. Although not conscious of it, she continued to live with the anxiety that his arrest and torture could happen again. Those who have to leave their families behind must endure the hazards of flight and the struggle to obtain asylum alone. They then find themselves cut off from their families, unable to begin the work of restoring meaningful patterns of relationships of trust and intimacy. They are left with only the anxiety and uncertainty about what has happened to their families, and a sense of guilt at having left them behind and possibly of having placed them in a dangerous position by prior political activity, or merely by the act of escaping from the country. Where communication with the family in the home country is possible, the news received may be about the arrest or death of other family members. Or there may be requests for the exiled family member to perform his traditional role perhaps by organizing or financing a funeral or the education or accommodation of children. Already cut off from his family, the survivor's inability to fulfill these traditional roles further confirms the breakdown of the whole system of meaning, tradition, and history through which he has a personal identity.

Networks are even less likely to remain intact than families. Often, the exiled members' only contact with networks in their own country is the receipt of bad news about further arrests or deaths or the deteriorating overall situation. This may be worsened by the network members in the home country who expect the exiled members to be able to campaign or raise money or engage in other effective activities on their behalf. They may convey a message along the lines of "Things are very bad here, but you are free and safe and in England (often perceived as a center of influence), what are you doing for us?" Thus, the only role or identity offered to the survivor by his erstwhile network is that of someone who has saved himself but is not doing enough for the others, a surviving failure from a network (and community) which is all failing.

In the host country, the exiled survivor will face great difficulties in trying to establish himself in new networks, whether these be with members of the host community or with members of the exiled community. In the host community, the ways of relating and the systems of meaning are so radically different that it is hard to find enough common understanding to begin to establish friendship or membership. Even the meaning of such terms as *friendship* or *membership* or *neighbor* will be different. Many Africans find it amazing that they cannot immediately get to know all their neighbors and that people do not greet each other in the street or talk to each other on buses.

Attempts to gain employment are frequently frustrated because the qualifications the exile brings from his home country (as, for example, a doctor or accountant) are not recognized in the host society. Thus, the exile faces the choice of long-term retraining or completely giving up his professional identity and the concomitant relationships with professional colleagues. Additionally, of course, for many exiled survivors, all this takes place within the context of having to learn an entirely new language. So network relationships with members of the host community offer little possibility of a sense of continuity and far more potential for discontinuity and a split between the past and the present. As one exile put it, "In my country I am a man, I have friends who know me, from the past. Here, no one knows me. I am not trusted; I have to keep proving myself, trying to show I am O.K. Here, who I am, I am not!"

The networks available within the exile community present other problems. Even where the survivor can make contact with people he knew in his home country or who are from the same village or are part of the same extended family, they meet in a completely different context which imbues their meeting with different meanings from those of the past. Because of the many problems of integrating into the host community (language, culture, racism, etc.), exile communities are, to various degrees, "ghettoized." To the extent to which they are turned in on themselves, their problems tend to become magnified. If, for example, there are few jobs available within the Kurdish community, then competition between members of that community for those jobs will be intensified by the lack of opportunities for Kurds to find jobs outside that community.

The problems of the home country are also reproduced. The fear, mistrust, anxiety, and sense of defeat generated by the organized violence from which they have fled continue to be dimensions of the community's life. A child with little memory of the oppression from which her family fled and who managed to adapt well to the cultural change, remembers most vividly her mother's instructions about whom she should and should not talk to and make friends with within the exile community. One exile stated bluntly about his community, "We are here because we lost." What has been lost is not only a political struggle but a collective vision of hope for the future of their country. Thus, network relationships can be permeated by a sense of loss and failure which is further fueled by news from the home country of further deterioration—waves of arrests, executions, and the like. Another exile said that in spite of having no friends or associates except for his fellow countrymen with whom he shared accommodation, it was depressing for him to spend much time talking with them, because all they had to discuss was how bad things were back home.

Returning to our theoretical view of there needing to be a foundation matrix, a set of shared values, beliefs, meanings, and symbols, for people to build their specific dynamic matrices of family and network relationships, we can see that for exiled torture survivors, their foundation matrix, insofar as it exists at all, is permeated by experiences of suffering, mistrust, danger, and pessimism. Terms, symbols, and relationships which previously carried positive meanings of hope, loyalty, and trust have been destroyed or subverted to take on new negative meanings. The individual is constantly threatened with fragmentation and discontinuity. In such a situation, it is hardly surprising that many individuals withdraw into isolation, finding the pain of trying to relate to others too much to manage.

Therapeutic Response

From the point of view outlined above, it makes little sense to us to think in terms of trying to treat or cure individuals according to a conventional medical paradigm. Conversely, it is tempting to become either excessively ambitious, trying to influence an enormous range of circumstances—trying to provide everything— or overwhelmed by the enormity of the problems and do too little. It is necessary, therefore, to try to locate ourselves *within* the process of reconstitution.

Reconstitution of systems, families, networks, and communities can be done only by the exiled survivors themselves. It is their existential project and not something that we can take over and manage for them. But this does not mean that it is something from which we must stand back, leaving them entirely to get on with it and contributing nothing more than a little professional and medical expertise at the periphery. It is a process within which we can struggle to find for ourselves a meaningful role through a dialogue with those individuals, families, and communities with whom we work.

One of the central concepts of the Medical Foundation is to see ourselves as a community. We have a paid core staff of less than 10, approximately 50 professionals working voluntarily, over 1,000 new clients per year, and a number of interpreters who interpret not just language but also culture, and who provide a link between our organization and exile communities. We regard this as a community which can provide a bridge for an individual to move from isolation to contact with others, a place in which network relationships can develop and in which families can find support in reestablishing themselves. It is also a community which is connected with other communities, both exile communities and the host community.

Levels of Therapeutic Intervention

The Process of Asylum

Our work is carried out at a number of different levels. First, we are concerned with the process of obtaining asylum, which establishes the individual's right to stay in the United Kingdom. Thus, many initial medical examinations and testimonies (which involve the survivor's recounting what has happened to him or her) take place within the context of establishing that the survivor has indeed been tortured and has a well-founded fear of persecution in the home country. This initial contact is an important opportunity for Medical Foundation staff to convey warmth, friendliness, and concern at the very basic level of examining an abused body and of inquiring about horrifying experiences with particular sensitivity and respect. Where the survivors approach the foundation after their right to stay has been established, the initial examination and taking of testimony can proceed under less pressure while still providing the important first contact.

Medical Care

Subsequent medical care, which can include massage, physiotherapy, osteopathy, and dentistry, is an important way of communicating care and respect for the survivor's body, and of reestablishing the meaning of intimate physical contact as an expression of concern.

Social Work Services

The expression of caring is extended through practical social work help in obtaining accommodation, social security payments, and, at later stages, career counseling and assistance in obtaining employment. Psychiatric assessment and treatment, counseling, psychotherapy on individual, family, and group basis, child psychotherapy, and art therapy are all available.

Although clients normally attend the foundation on an appointment basis, it is not uncommon for them simply to turn up or to telephone and talk to whoever is available. The waiting room and kitchen (to which clients have full access) are often the site of much activity, conversation between clients, games of chess, making coffee together, and sometimes sharing food. A deliberate attempt is made to create an atmosphere of informality so that clients can regard the foundation less as a medical facility and more as a safe place, a place in which they can feel a sense of belonging. Sometimes, a family will formally arrange to bring a meal to the foundation and invite staff members to share it with them. Some clients have contributed to the foundation by decorating, repairing furniture, providing refreshments at meetings, and contributing their own personal and professional expertise to seminars and to publicizing the foundation's work through the media.

Therapeutic Milieu

In this way, we attempt to create a setting where survivors can experience themselves as significant persons rather than as victims or supplicants. For so many of them, their reason for coming to the foundation, the violence and destruction they have suffered and survived, is all they have in common. Their potential foundation matrix, their basis for relating to others, is the damage done to their internal meaning system, their families, networks, and communities.

The Medical Foundation tries to provide a larger foundation matrix, helping to establish common ground with others in which they can experience a common personhood and humanity, and recover and build upon their sense of history and continuity. Our approaches to testimony taking, group therapy, and individual therapy give some illustration of this.

Testimony Method and Process

Testimonies involve the survivor telling her or his story. We regard it as important to begin with birth and go right through the survivor's personal history and that of the person's family. In this way, the traumatic experience is not only approached slowly, but is also set within a larger story of an individual in a family, a network, and a community. The violence and torture are then events within a story—terrible events to be sure, and events which threaten to fracture the story completely—but they are not the whole story or the only story.

Individual and Group Psychotherapy

Similarly, in individual counseling and psychotherapy, we regard it as important not to focus excessively or exclusively on the trauma, but to talk about the survivor's past, beliefs, interests, communities, and politics. This includes not only the past but also the current situation in the home country, in the family, and in relation to friends.

In my own experience of doing psychotherapy, it is not possible for me to understand the meaning of a survivor's current difficulties in English society without that person's explaining to me much of the background of his or her own society and customs. It was in the course of such a discussion that one client explained that, in his mind, he still lived in his home country. He looked forward to a day when he could return and felt unable to commit himself to any course of action in England because his future was not there. Within this context, many of his difficulties took on a different significance.

Another client seemed glum and uninterested in our conversation until I asked a question about the president who had been overthrown during the coup in which the client had been tortured and from which he had fled. At the mention of the name, his face brightened, his posture changed, and he said with conviction, "He was *my* president." He then began to tell me, in a much more engaged way, about *his* president and about his own beliefs and feelings.

In group therapy in the past, we have avoided placing two people from the same country in a group together. Apart from the possibility of their being from opposing factions within the country, many survivors feel suspicious about informers or fearful that things they have said will be talked about elsewhere and will get back to their own country. However, one group discovered that they were all Africans. (They had not been consciously assembled as such.) They quickly began to relate on this basis, discussing the history of Africa and the place of their own countries within it. When the therapist observed that no reference had been made to the persecution they had all suffered, he was told by a member

that they had to get to know each other first and become a group before they could deal with the bitterness.

Nationalistic and Regionalistic Commonalities

Their sharing and mutual support in terms of their common identity as Africans seemed an important part of this process. We are now thinking more about the value of continent-based groups and have a Latin American group running at present. There has also been a successful women's group. This seems to suggest a value in having a common basis, whether rooted in culture, gender, or some dimension other than the common basis of having been tortured. This can provide a holding connection between people at the time when one of them begins to talk about his or her torture, thereby reminding the others of their own experience and putting the cohesion of the whole group under considerable stress. It is at this point that absenteeism and fragmentation of the therapy group are most likely to occur.

Conclusion

At the beginning of this chapter, it was stated that little is being offered in the way of models, techniques, and strategies. Instead, what has been presented is an orientation toward understanding the individual within the contexts of family, social network, and community. It is through relationships in these contexts that individuals establish and maintain a sense of identity and a sense of meaning and purpose in their lives.

Torture and organized violence radically transform and sometimes destroy these contexts of family, network, and community and the patterns of relationships within them. The transformation or loss of these patterns of relationship drastically undermines the individual's sense of purpose and meaning in life. It is, therefore, extremely difficult to retain a sense of continuity and to reassert a sense of identity, purpose, and meaning. These problems are greatly compounded by the process of flight and exile in an alien society. The individual is not only physically cut off from these contexts but is faced with a new culture whose systems of meaning are radically different from those of the survivor's original culture.

In our work with torture survivors, we focus not just on the torture and its impact on these individuals, but also consider how their relationships have been changed and how they understand themselves now as a members of a community. We are aware that it is their relationships which need to be reconstituted. Our therapeutic task, therefore, is to provide a context in which previous systems of meaning can be recovered and new ones can be developed. For any population of clients, this involves (1) addressing the history of the individual survivors, their networks and community, and often the politics of their society; (2) addressing the disparity between the culture of their society and that of ours and the consequent difficulties of living in our society and relating to us, including the disadvantage and discrimination that are encountered in our society; and (3) providing new relationships in which trust and empathy can be reestablished, new meanings can be generated to make sense of their experience, and purpose and continuity can be reclaimed.

We are further aware, not only of the value of scientific theories, generalized categories, and conceptual frameworks, but also of their *limitations*. We see our role not so much as directors and organizers of the reconstitutive process, but as participants in it. This calls for us to engage in the process not only at a professional level, but also at a human level; to be prepared to subordinate our scientific theories and professional defenses to the dialectic of an encounter between fellow human beings who are cooperatively engaged in a struggle for human rights and human values. We are mindful of the words of Max Horkheimer: "The hope that earthly horror does not possess the last word is, to be sure, a nonscientific wish."

ACKNOWLEDGMENTS

I am indebted to Perico Rodriguez and Erol Yesilyurt, my colleagues at the Medical Foundation, for contributing their experience and understanding of the processes described above. Without them, this chapter could not have been written. I am also grateful to Antonia Hunt and Rachel Tribe for their critical reading of the manuscript. Like all our work at the Medical Foundation, this chapter represents the efforts of a team and not just the work of one individual.

References

American Psychiatric Association. (1987). *Diagnostic and statistical manual of mental disorders* (3rd ed., rev.). Washington, DC: Author.

Argentina's National Commission on Disappeared People. (1986). *Nunca mas (Never again)*. London, England: Faber & Faber.

Bateson, G. (1979). *Mind and nature: A necessary unity*. New York: Wildwood House.

Horkheimer. Foreword. In Martin Jay, *The dialectical imagination: A history of the Frankfurt School and Institute of Social Research, 1923–1950*. Canada: Little, Brown & Co.

Kordon, D., Edelman, L. D., Nicoletti, E., Bozzolo, R., Siaky, D., Hoste, M., Bonano, O., & Kersner, D. (1988). *The psychological effects of political repression*. Buenos Aires: Sudamericana Planeta Publishing.

Schlapobersky, J., & Bamber, H. (1987). Rehabilitation work with victims of torture. In D. Miserez (Ed.), *Refugees—The trauma of exile*. London, England: Martinus Nijhoff Publishers.

Vinar, M. (1989). Pedro or the demolition: A psychoanalytic look at torture. *British Journal of Psychotherapy, 5*, 353–362.

Watzlawick, P., Beavin, J., & Jackson, D. D. (1967). *Pragmatics of human communication*. New York: W. W. Norton.

CHAPTER 62

Torture of a Norwegian Ship's Crew

Stress Reactions, Coping, and Psychiatric Aftereffects

Lars Weisæth

Introduction

Medical reports on torture sequelae are usually based upon examinations of previous prisoners of war (Eitinger & Strøm, 1973; Ursano, Boydstun, & Wheatley, 1981) or exiled persons. Expatriated victims in particular have been subject to medical and psychological research during the last 10 to 20 years, especially in Canada (Allodi & Cowgill, 1982), Norway (Fossum, Hauff, Malt, & Eitinger, 1982), and in Denmark (Rasmussen & Nielsen, 1980; Somnier & Genefke, 1986) where the International Rehabilitation Center for Torture Victims opened in 1984 in Copenhagen. For obvious reasons, it has been difficult to perform systematic studies in the country where the torture and violence took place. Refugees make up a selected group of torture victims, and the additional stress of expatriation may produce adverse health effects that are difficult to separate from the torture effects (Thorvaldsen, 1987; see also Chapter 55, in this volume, for a discussion).

Although the classical aim of torture is to make the victim yield information or to destroy his or her personality, victims of terrorism and political hostage incidents are threatened or killed mainly as a way of exerting pressure upon a third party, often a government. Also, long-term psychiatric sequelae have been reported in such victims (Støfsel, 1980; Terr, 1984).

Dutch researchers found that one third of ex-hostages reported continuing negative psychological effects 6 to 9 years after the incident, and 12% were still in need of professional treatment (Ploeg & Kleijn, 1989).

The subjects in this study were in a different position from other victims of torture, terrorism, or hostage taking. Their Libyan captors wrongly believed that the sailors were secret agents who possessed valuable information. Thus, the torture was without any meaning whatsoever to the victims who had no information to confess nor any involvement in a political cause. Neither were the sailors exploited as hostages in the usual sense of the term. They were accidental victims to torture and terror and exposed to what is probably a uniquely stressful experience.

The Norwegian government's Directorate for Seamen asked our department to examine and evaluate all the sailors immediately upon their return to Norway. The purpose was (1) to determine whether they were suffering from somatic or psychosocial problems as a result of the imprisonment/torture, and (2) to provide adequate treatment and help them achieve the best possible restitution.

My purpose in this chapter is to describe the nature of the stress experience, the reactions to the stress during the arrest and torture, the acute posttraumatic stress disorder (PTSD), and the incidence of PTSD 1 month and 6 months after the release of the sailors. Clinical interviews are compared to various psychiatric rating instruments when it comes to identifying the PTSD cases. The purpose of using several tests was to examine the specificity and sensitivity of these instruments in identifying and assessing PTSD. My discussion also focuses on torture as a risk factor for development of PTSD and on some clinical characteristics of the psychopathological sequelae.

Lars Weisæth • Division of Disaster Psychiatry, Department of Psychiatry, University of Oslo, Oslo 3, Norway.

International Handbook of Traumatic Stress Syndromes, edited by John P. Wilson and Beverley Raphael. Plenum Press, New York, 1993.

As part of the ongoing studies of risk factors for the development of PTSD, I also want to categorize the severity of the stress exposure, to investigate premorbid functioning, and to record immediate responses to the stress and coping mechanisms. In fact, having a maritime occupational background had appeared as a particularly valuable coping factor in my previous studies of disaster behavior and subsequent PTSD (Weisæth, 1985, 1989) so one could hypothesize that the crew would be rather resistant toward the severe stress and traumatization.

Material

The study included all 13 seamen who returned from Libya. Their ages ranged from 24 to 64 years, averaging 42 years old. They were all experienced sailors who had worked at sea for several years. Eight were married, some had small children, one lived steadily with a female partner.

None had suffered from any severe mental disorder or from PTSD earlier. Four of the men had a history with a period of prior emotional instability, of whom only one had needed sick leave for a time.

Methodology

The main approach that I used was semistructured personal clinical interviews at two points in time supplemented with psychological test instruments following the second interview. In several of the interviews and therapeutic sessions, Leo Eitinger, who is a very experienced researcher and clinician in the sequelae of torture (Eitinger & Strøm, 1973) took part in the evaluations. The first interview was carried out as soon as possible after the crew had sailed the ship from Libya to Norway. The range from the start of the imprisonment to the first examination was 93 to 114 days, with an average of 106 days. Family members took part in about half of the interviews, which provided, among other things, an opportunity to obtain comparative information.

At the first interview, an extensive precoded rating form developed by a group of psychiatrists at the Medical Faculty of the University of Oslo (Fossum et al., 1982) was used. This form has been used by this research group in work with victims of torture for Amnesty International. The precoded forms made it possible to carry out a detailed categorization of the various torture techniques that had been applied. By means of this instrument, data could also be coded on background and sociodemographic factors, on previous somatic and mental health, on stress reactions and coping attempts during the torture experience, and on acute and prolonged effects of a somatic, psychosomatic, and psychological nature. In this particular study, the 36 posttraumatic stress symptoms listed in the amnesty form (see Table 62.3), which were considered typical for aftereffects of torture, have been converted into an index score that was termed the *Amnesty Score*, by giving one point to

each symptom present. The Amnesty Score thus had a possible range from zero to 36 points.

A second interview was carried out after 6 months, supplemented with standardized paper-and-pencil tests: the State Anxiety Scale from the State-Trait Anxiety Inventory (STAI) (Spielberger, Gorsuch, & Lushene, 1970), and the 20-question version of the General Health Questionnaire (GHQ) (Goldberg, 1978). A posttraumatic stress scale (PTSS-10) developed by Holen, Sund, and Weisæth (1983) was found to be effective in screening out psychiatric risk cases among disaster survivors, along with the Impact of Event Scale (IES) (Horowitz, 1982; Malt, 1988), with its two subscales. The intrusion subscale (range 0–35) measures the intensity of involuntary reexperiences of the trauma. The avoidance subscale (range 0–40) yields a measure of how strongly the person tries to avoid being reminded of the trauma.

Although the State Anxiety Scale measures general anxiety and the GHQ measures psychological distress and psychiatric impairment, the PTSS-10 and IES are designed to record the presence and intensity of specific posttraumatic stress symptoms. The Amnesty Score does the same but even more specifically for posttorture sequelae.

Seizure of the Norwegian Ship

Since the seizure event is not internationally well-known, in order to be able to discuss the severity of the stress as a mental health risk factor, it is necessary to describe the ordeal and the torture in some detail. On May 13, 1984, a Norwegian merchant ship arrived in Libya after a voyage from London. Immediately upon arrival, the entire crew and the ship were taken in arrest. The Norwegian authorities were not informed of this action, and it took weeks to find out what had happened to the crew. When arrested, all the seamen were told that they were accused of participating in a coup against the Libyan state and that country's leader and that "they should understand what the consequences would be." Clearly, this statement implied the death penalty to the crew members. The accusation, which was never formally written, said that the seamen were either undercover British or Israeli secret agents. When torture was applied immediately after the arrest, it was because Libya wanted information about a secret operation which they suspected. It was obvious that the Libyan captors and the officials in charge were themselves convinced that the ship's voyage to Libya was a covert operation as part of a scheme to overthrow the government. The crew on this particular vessel probably became the targets and victims because the ship had left London for Libya just after the siege of the Libyan embassy in London, and Libya presumably expected reprisals for the killing of an English police officer during the London incident.

After an unknown period of time, the Libyans must have begun to doubt, and gradually to acknowledge, their mistake. The terror continued, but from then on, the aim was probably to force false confessions about an agent operation so that those responsible for the death and maltreatment of the sailors could go free.

Torture

For the captured seamen, the first days were the worst of their entire incarceration period. One seaman was beaten to death. Before he died, he was taken to the ship so that his comrades could see him. Another had been abducted and was believed to be dead. The third man had sustained head and brain injuries after blows to his head. The seamen were also subjected to psychological torture which included death threats, interrogations with threats of physical torture, and listening to their fellow crew member being beaten to death. Some of the crew still believed, however, that the sailor's death by beating had not been planned by the captors but that it resulted from their lack of expertise and control in the use of violence. Moreover, the seamen were also exposed to raids and searches and were confronted with false information about weapons found on the ship and with "confessions" made by other crew members. Threats of violence against their families in Norway were also expressed. These kinds of threats were quite credible to the sailors who knew of Libyan "hit actions" abroad, and who were told that "Libya has eyes and ears everywhere." Toward the end of their 67 days of arrest, the seamen were also threatened with reprisals wherever they were in case they talked critically about their experiences in Libya. The crew was kept totally isolated from the outside world during the first month.

The seamen were kept in arrest on board ship but were allowed to stay together as a group while the interrogations were held at a nearby police station to which they were brought in cars. On board the ship, they could watch Libyan TV, which aired trials of these "enemies of the Libyan state," in which the accused confessed their guilt and then were publicly executed. The young guards were often intoxicated, probably drugged, and were very hostile and sometimes sadistic but also very fearful of their "dangerous captives." Every day the seamen were targets for these unbalanced youths who aimed at them with loaded, unsecured guns.

Several episodes approaching mock executions occurred. The situation was characterized by total unpredictability and was absolutely uncontrollable, and, in this respect, the seamen were all equally exposed. To the crew it was apparent that the man killed became the victim just because he happened to be on deck duty when the ship entered the Tripoli harbor.

Physical stressors other than violence were also present but did not measure up to the terror and included extreme heat, entrapment, infectious diarrhea, and the lack of medical treatment. Of the 13 men, 9 suffered weight losses of from 5 to 15 kilograms (about 11 to 35 pounds).

In spite of similarities in their stress exposure, a scaling of the severity of the stress may be justified. Only 3 levels of exposure severity are distinguished: *extreme*, *severe*, and *strong*. The last category consisted of the 4 sailors who never were taken to the interrogation center. The majority, 7 in all, qualified for the *severe* exposure category. They were all interrogated at the place where their comrade was killed, and 6 of them heard him scream when being beaten to death. As a rule, they had been brought in several times and had to wait for

hours in uncertainty before the interrogation was canceled or until it actually took place. The interrogators would tell about their ability to extract "the truth" and demonstrate their methods, like pulling out nails, without actually doing any physical harm. Of the two sailors who can be put in the *extreme* stress exposure category was the one who was physically beaten and the other who was abducted to a prison and maltreated.

Results

Stress Reactions and Coping Mechanisms during Arrest and Torture

Although 5 of the 13 seamen reported that they had been apprehensive when approaching Libya, none of them were prepared for what was to come. As a result, surprise and disbelief were common to all; numbing and depersonalization, as seen in Table 62.1, occurred in a number.

Common themes in the repetitive nightmares were flight, fight, and torture. These intrusions constituted constant preoccupations. In spite of these substantial anxieties, none of the seamen suffered panic attacks. No hallucinations, confusional states, or other psychotic symptoms developed. Less than half experienced severe anger, but fear of their own anger and loss of control were more of a problem. Although only three seamen seem to have suffered a reduction in self-esteem, there were widespread ruminations about whether they could have done more to prevent the death of their comrade. Because of their total isolation, many of the sailors felt that they were let down by their own government.

Of the symptoms that may have been psychosomatic in nature, diarrhea developed in five and gastrointestinal bleeding, probably from peptic ulcers, developed in two sailors.

Asked to select the three most stressing experiences of the entire captivity, 12 out of the 13 sailors listed uncertainty. The two other stressors noted as particularly

Table 62.1. Stress Reactions Reported to Occur for a Shorter or Longer Period during Imprisonment ($N = 13$)

Reaction	n^a	Percentage
Sleep disturbance	11	85
Fear of dying	11	85
Anxiety	9	69
Depersonalization	6	46
Repetitive nightmares	5	38
Severe hopelessness	5	38
Severe anger	5	38
Tremor	4	31
Fear of madness	4	31
Amnesia	4	31
Numbing	4	31
Reduced self-esteem	3	23

$^a n$ = number of sailors who reported the symptom.

painful were hearing the screams from their comrade being tortured and to witness his torture.

Not one of the sailors gave in to the pressure of admitting to something they had not committed. From the start, at least eight were unable to see any meaning in the situation; as the time passed, it seemed as if *not to yield* to pressure and to maintain the truth of whatever happened became *a meaning* and *goals* in themselves. The meaninglessness of having to sacrifice one's life for a cause that really did not exist constituted a problem. As one of the sailors said: "If there had been something to die for, it would have been easier."

The following appeared to have been important coping mechanisms: trust in leadership, increase in group cohesion, search for deeper meaning, psychological reduction of the terrorists, strengthening of personal identity and values, information search, religious faith, activity as a distraction from reality, and use of daydreams and fantasy. As many as four wrote diaries, at high risk because they were searched repeatedly. The main motive for writing was to have some evidence of their history and fate in case none survived to tell it.

Some of these coping responses were engaged rather directly in attempts to master specific stressors: The psychological reduction of the torturers protected one's own self-esteem and may be related to the fact that so few suffered a reduction in self-esteem and virtually no one developed general feelings of guilt or shame.

Acute Posttraumatic Stress Disorder

Based upon the first clinical interview, six sailors, or 46% of the crew, satisfied the DSM-III criteria of a posttraumatic stress disorder (American Psychiatric Association, 1980). If an attempt is made to grade the *clinical severity* of the PTSD conditions, two of the disorders can be labeled *severe*, implying total loss of function and intense and continuous subjective suffering, two were *marked*, and two of *moderate* degree. Both severe conditions had developed in the two men who had been subjected to the extreme stress exposure. Generally, the PTSD represented the continuation of the stress symptoms that were evoked already during the stress exposure. The PTSD cases seemed to have had the more pronounced stress reactions already at that time as compared to those who did not suffer from PTSD.

Amnesty Scores and PTSD

As seen from Table 62.2, the Amnesty Score differentiated between the PTSD and the non-PTSD with scores in the 6 clinical cases ranging from 20 to 32 points, while the 7 non-ill subjects had scores from zero to 3 points.

The number of sailors who suffered from a variety of the 36 posttraumatic stress symptoms, as clinically rated on the Amnesty rating scale, appears in Table 62.3.

Although symptoms of cerebral concussion could still be demonstrated in the seaman who had sustained head injuries, no other severe physical ailments were found. At least two seamen who were classified as PTSD cases had started to drink heavily.

Table 62.2. Amnesty Scores Approximately 1 Month after Release (N = 13)

Points	Points
PTSD cases (*n* = 6)	Non-PTSD cases (*n* = 7)
32	3
27	2
27	2
23	2
22	1
21	0
20	0
	0
Mean 24.2	*Mean* 1.1
SD 4.5	*SD* 1.2

Two months after their release, one crew member developed PTSD. On his way to the sailors' office, where he was to inquire about a new job at sea, he suffered a severe anxiety attack which was the start of a disorder of moderate intensity.

One of the 7 PTSD cases, the man who had been abducted and maltreated, suffered a paranoid breakdown in the form of a brief reactive psychosis when he attempted to go back to sea again after about 5 months. The psychotic symptoms disappeared but he went ashore, while his PTSD symptoms persisted.

Six-Month Follow-Up

Six months after their release, the same seven men (54%) of the crew still suffered from PTSD, although there were no new cases. In spite of considerable improvements, not one of the seamen who had a PTSD had been able to go back to sailing in international waters during these 6 months.

During the 6-month observation period, one man, not suffering from PTSD, developed a drinking problem. It seemed that his drinking was not related to the recent stress experience, but this is difficult to rule out.

Table 62.4 shows the 13 sailors' scores on the 5 mental state-rating instruments at the 6-month follow-up interview. The 7 PTSD cases are subjects 1 through 7 in the table.

Some of the test instruments differed in their accuracy in distinguishing between subjects with and without PTSD. The Amnesty Score, PTSS-10, and the IES intrusion subscale that typically yield specific measures of posttraumatic stress symptoms had all a higher sensitivity, specificity, and positive predictive power than the more general instruments (the GHQ and the State Anxiety Scale). The IES avoidance subscale was less accurate than the other posttraumatic stress scales (see Table 62.5). The relationship between severity of stress exposure and ensuing PTSD fails to reach significant statistical correlation (see Table 62.6).

Table 62.3. Frequency of Posttraumatic Stress Symptoms Rated on the Amnesty Scale Approximately 1 Month after Release (N = 13)

Symptom	n	Percentage	Symptom	n	Percentage
Startle reactions	7	54	Insecure	4	31
Bodily tension	7	54	Hyperactivity	3	23
Repetitive nightmares	7	54	Depression	3	23
Repetition experiences	6	46	Headache	3	23
Restlessness	6	46	Loss of initiative	3	23
Reduced performance capacity	6	46	Memory problems	3	23
Concentration problems	6	46	Feelings of insufficiency	3	23
Anxiety	6	46	Sexual impotence	2	15
Traumatophobia	6	46	Conversion symptoms	2	15
Ruminating about event	6	46	Dysphoria caused by insufficiency	2	15
Psychological withdrawal	5	38	Dyspepsia	1	08
Reduced affect control	5	38	Vertigo	1	08
Alcohol or drug use	5	38	Dyspnea	1	08
"Nightmares" when awake	5	38	Guilt	1	08
Social withdrawal	4	31	Short-term memory problem	1	08
Diffuse bodily pain	4	31	Shame	0	0
Emotional lability	4	31	Psychotic symptoms	0	0
Easily tired	4	31	Concrete thinking	0	0

Discussion

The results show quite convincingly that the 67 days of arrest and torture brought forth significant symptoms of stress *during* the stress experience, in the *immediate* aftermath, as well as *6 months later*. Although nearly all the crew members had some significant symptoms during the captivity, about half the group suffered from psychopathological sequelae after the release, as well as 6

months later. Judged from the Amnesty score, there was a tendency in the early aftermath to suffer from either a broad range of posttraumatic stress symptoms or from none at all. Being free of symptoms then, did not mean that the risk of developing a PTSD was absent. In the one case, with a somewhat delayed PTSD onset, only some motoric restlessness was noticeable and no subjective complaints were registered at the first examination. In this case, the delayed onset seemed to result from

Table 62.4. Scores on Five Psychiatric Rating Scales 6 Months after Release (N = 13)

Subject number	GHQ	State Anxiety Scale	Amnesty Score	PTSS-10	IES Intrusion[a]	IES Avoidance[b]
			PTSD			
1	17	77	19	10	30	35
2	20	70	22	9	35	29
3	20	57	18	8	22	25
4	17	69	9	10	25	22
5	16	59	15	8	26	27
6	14	45	29	9	25	12
7	7	38	9	7	21	18
			Non-PTSD			
8	6	38	4	4	9	15
9	2	38	0	4	2	30
10	1	27	0	0	0	10
11	1	24	7	1	10	14
12	0	27	0	0	0	13
13	0	21	0	0	2	12

[a]PTSD cases: IES Intrusion *Mean* 26.3, *SD* 4.8; non-PTSD cases: IES Intrusion *Mean* 3.8, *SD* 4.5.
[b]PTSD cases: IES Avoidance *Mean* 24.0, *SD* 7.5; non-PTSD cases: IES Avoidance *Mean* 15.7, *SD* 7.2.

Table 62.5. Diagnostic Summary of PTSD

Rating scale	Cutoff point	Sensitivity	Specificity	Positive predictive power
GHQ (20 items)	4	1.00	0.83	0.88
State Anxiety Scale	38	1.00	0.66	0.77
Amnesty Score	8	1.00	1.00	1.00
PTSS	6	1.00	1.00	1.00
IES Intrusion subscale	20	1.00	1.00	1.00
IES Avoidance subscale	20	0.71	0.83	0.83

reactivation and followed a latency period that was symptom free.

The treatments that were provided probably attenuated the degree of the disorders, and it cannot be excluded that the preventive and therapeutic measures that were taken may have prevented the development of more cases of PTSD. The findings show a high level of psychopathology, considering that the men had been well functioning before the stress exposure. Their extensive maritime expertise in handling severe danger situations could not be put to use in this uncontrollable situation for which they were completely unprepared, which resulted in experiences of helplessness and, also, for some, severe hopelessness. The short-term incidence of psychopathology in this study readily compares with the high incidence of chronic long-term psychiatric sequelae found in other populations who were exposed to severe violence (Allodi & Cowgill, 1982; Eitinger & Strøm, 1973; Støfsel, 1980; Ursano et al., 1981).

From a methodological point of view, the usual considerations of retrospective influence upon memory and report must be made. Some tendency to a stereotypical response set was noted in the filling out of self-report questionnaires and had to be countered. Anger against Libya contributed to aggravation in one case. The main limitation in this study is the small number of subjects. However, considering these small numbers, it is not surprising that the relation between stress exposure and PTSD failed to reach statistical significance. On the basis of clinical judgment, it appeared that premorbid *vulnerability* played a role: All four sailors who previously in their lives had suffered from some kind of psychological problems developed PTSD, compared to only three of the other nine sailors who had an unremarkable premorbid function. The predisposing vulnerabilities in the four

men were: (1) sequelae of previous head injury, (2) two of the men had earlier in life experienced neurotic anxiety symptoms, and (3) passive-dependent personality. In the study of the captured crew of the USS *Pueblo* (Ford & Spaulding, 1973), passive-dependent personality was the predominant diagnosis in the group with lower coping ability during the captivity. The psychiatric morbidity in the *Pueblo* crew had not been reported in follow-up studies.

The analysis of stress as the etiological factor is also complicated by the fact that those of the crew who had been most badly treated, the deck crew, also had fewer coping possibilities than the engine staff and the catering personnel. Although the latter two groups were allowed, after some time, some degree of routine work on board the ship, the deck crew got few possibilities to engage in activities that were reported as very helpful in coping with the stressful situation. Considering that the majority of crew members did develop PTSD afterward, perhaps the better question is why did not every one?

Clinically, the PTSD symptoms directly reflected the many hardships the men experienced. Compared to the PTSDs in survivors of a technological industrial disaster (Weisæth, 1985), perceived as accidental, two striking differences appeared in the contents of the clinical symptoms of the posttorture PTSD. First, it was always one or more persons who made up the threatening element in the recurring experiences of the traumatic situation. This seemed to reflect the constant state of *death threat* created by the captors and interrogators, in contrast to the material/technological dangers that dominated the PTSD symptoms after the industrial disaster. Second, the aggression in the sailors was a direct reaction to the violence they had suffered. In the technological disaster, angry feelings developed only after some time and then as a neurasthenic irritability secondary to longstanding anxiety and sleep deprivation. This difference in development and content of aggression symptoms may be a distinguishing clinical feature between man-made and accidental causation of PTSD.

The torture experience also seems to produce a higher incidence of PTSD than civilian disasters and accidents (Malt, 1988; Weisæth, 1985). Since the subjects in the study of the industrial disaster (Weisæth, 1989) and in the present study were healthy, reasonably well-functioning, fully employed at the time of the exposure, and were offered comprehensive preventive and therapeutic programs soon afterward, the difference in resulting psychopathology probably can be ascribed to the duration, severity, nature, and intensity of the stress.

Table 62.6. Distribution of PTSD Diagnoses at 6-Month Follow-Up

Intensity of stress exposure	PTSD		Total
	Yes	No	
Extreme	2	0	2
Severe	4	3	7
Moderate	1	3	4
Total	7	6	13
$p = .22$			

Luchterhand (1971) postulated that man-made disasters are psychologically more harmful than non-man-made. The captivity stress was also dominated by low predictability and control, and it was completely meaningless and difficult to comprehend, in contrast to the industrial workers who were exposed to the factory explosion. In this last respect, the crew differed also from the military crew on the USS *Pueblo* which was captured by North Korea in 1968 and whose crew went through a somewhat similar captivity and torture in North Korea for about a year (Ford & Spaulding, 1973).

Compared to a diagnosis of PTSD which is based upon a clinical interview, the PTSS-10 and intrusion subscale of the IES had a very high sensitivity and specificity in discriminating between cases and non-cases. This is not surprising considering the consistency of the core symptoms of the PTSD and the absence of other psychiatric sequelae in this material. It remains to be seen, however, if the instruments have the same predictive validity when used separately without a simultaneous psychiatric interview. The GHQ is regarded as a reliable measure of nonpsychotic psychiatric impairment. In a study of Australian firefighters who were exposed to a natural disaster, McFarlane (1986) found that the 12-item GHQ had a 90% specificity, a 78% sensitivity, and a misclassification rate of 12% for detecting PTSD. In our study, the 20-item GHQ discriminated even better, producing only one false positive. In view of the overall findings, the GHQ and the State Anxiety Scale should probably be supplemented with one of the specific posttraumatic rating scales when traumatized people are to be assessed. Although the IES was constructed to serve as a measure of distress, the present findings indicate that the IES intrusion subscale is also a valid case-finding instrument. All the PTSD cases had intrusion scores higher than 20. This accords well with the findings of Horowitz, Wilner, and Alvarez (1979) regarding male patients at a stress clinic who averaged a score of 21.2.

After 6 months, 54% of the sailors still had high scores, compared to 15% of the rescuers 9 months after an oil rig disaster (Ersland, Weisæth, & Sund, 1989), to 77% of the raped women in the acute phase as described by Dahl (1989), and only 5% in accidentally injured patients in the acute phase, respectively, after the 28-month follow-up (Malt, 1988). The fact that high IES intrusion scores related more closely to psychopathology than high avoidance scores was also in accordance with findings in the study of disaster rescue workers (Ersland, Weisæth, & Sund, 1989).

Conclusion

The strong validity of the psychological test instruments in discriminating between cases and noncases of PTSD is a finding of considerable interest when the task is to screen large numbers of stress-exposed subjects in order to identify the psychiatric at-risk cases. The Amnesty Score appears to have been a good discriminator of these subjects who were clinically felt to have had PTSD and should be further studied as a clinical and research instrument in the examination of victims of torture.

ACKNOWLEDGMENTS

I am grateful for the cooperation that was given by the Directorate of Seamen, particularly their consulting social worker Mr. Jan Frydenlund. I also appreciate the stimulating exchanges with fellow psychiatrists who have treated PTSD patients. I wish to thank Leo Eitinger for sharing with me his unique clinical and research experience with torture victims. Richard J. Sokol and Robert L. Ursano provided valuable comments to this chapter.

References

Allodi, F., & Cowgill, G. (1982). Ethical and psychiatric aspects of torture. *Canadian Journal of Psychiatry, 27*, 98–102.

American Psychiatric Association. (1980). *Diagnostic and statistical manual of mental disorders* (3rd ed.). Washington, DC: Author.

Dahl, S. (1989). Acute responses to rape—A PTSD variant. *Acta Psychiatrica Scandinavica, 80* (Suppl. 355), 56–62.

Eitinger, L., & Strøm, A. (1973). Mortality and morbidity after excessive stress: A follow-up investigation of Norwegian concentration camp survivors. Oslo: Universitets-forlaget.

Ersland, S., Weisæth, L., & Sund, A. (1989). The stress upon rescuers involved in an oil rig disaster. *Acta Psychiatrica Scandinavica, 80* (Suppl. 355), 38–49.

Ford, C. V., & Spaulding, R. C. (1973). The Pueblo incident: A comparison of factors related to coping with extreme stress. *Archives of General Psychiatry, 29*, 340–343.

Fossum, A., Hauff, E., Malt, U., & Eitinger, L. (1982). Psykiske og sosiale følger av tortur [Psychosocial consequences of torture]. *Tidsskrift for den Norske Lægeforen, 102*, 613–616.

Goldberg, D. (1978). *Manual of the General Health Questionnaire.* Windsor, England: NFER Publishing.

Holen, A., Sund, A., & Weisæth, L. (1983). *Questionnaire for screening disaster victims, in the* Alexander Kielland *disaster March 27, 1980: Psychological reactions among the survivors.* Oslo University, Division of Disaster Psychiatry. (In Norwegian)

Horowitz, M. J. (1982). Stress response syndromes. In L. Goldberger & S. Breznitz (Eds.), *Handbook of stress* (pp. 711–732). New York: The Free Press.

Horowitz, M. J., Wilner, N., & Alvarez, W. (1979). Impact of Event Scale: A measure of subjective stress. *Psychosomatic Medicine, 41*(3), 209–218.

Luchterhand, E. G. (1971). Sociological approaches to massive stress in natural and man-made disasters. In H. Krystal, & W. G. Niederland, Psychiatric traumatization: Aftereffects in individuals and communities. Boston: Little, Brown.

Malt, U. (1988). The long-term psychiatric consequences of accidental injury: A longitudinal study of 107 adults. *British Journal of Psychiatry, 153*, 810–818.

McFarlane, A. C. (1986). Chronic post-traumatic morbidity: Implications for disaster planners and emergency services. *Medical Journal of Australia, 145*, 561–563.

Ploeg, H. M., & Klein, W. C. (1989). Being held hostage in the Netherlands: A study of long-term after-effects. *Journal of Traumatic Stress, 2*(2), 153–169.

Rasmussen, O. V., & Nielsen, I. L. (1980). Evaluation of investigation of 200 torture victims. *Danish Medical Bulletin, 27*, 241–243.

Somnier, F. E., & Genefke, I. K. (1986). Psychotherapy for victims of torture. *British Journal of Psychiatry, 149*, 323–329.

Spielberger, C. D., Gorsuch, R. L., & Lushene, R. E. (1970). *STAI manual for the State-Trait Anxiety Inventory* (p. 24). Palo Alto: Consulting Psychologist Press.

Støfsel, W. (1980). Psychological sequelae in hostages and the aftercare. *Danish Medical Bulletin, 27,* 239–241.

Terr, L. C. (1984). Chowchilla revisited: The effects of psychic trauma four years after a school bus kidnapping. *Annual Progress in Psychiatry and Child Development,* 300–317.

Thorvaldsen, P. (1987). *Health hazards of organizational violence* (pp. 18–49). Ministry of Welfare, Health and Cultural Affairs, The Hague.

Ursano, R. L., Boydstun, J. A., & Wheatley, R. D. (1981). Psychiatric illness in U.S. Air Force Vietnam prisoners of war: A five-year follow-up. *American Journal of Psychiatry, 138,* 310–314.

Weisæth, L. (1985). Post-traumatic stress disorder after an industrial disaster. In P. Pichot, P. Berner, R. Wolf, & K. Thau (Eds.), *Psychiatry—The state of the art,* vol. 6 (pp. 299–307). New York: Plenum Press.

Weisæth, L. (1989). A study of behavioural responses to an industrial disaster. *Acta Psychiatrica Scandinavica, 80* (Suppl. 355), 13–24.

CHAPTER 63

Principles of Treatment and Service Development for Torture and Trauma Survivors

Margaret Cunningham and Derrick Silove

Undoubtedly, torture is one of the most traumatic threats to psychic integrity that any human being can undergo. Systematic assaults on the integrity of the personality are used by repressive regimes to incapacitate the individual in order to intimidate the family and the wider community. Torture aims to destroy the victim's sense of identity and to engender feelings of "debilitation, dependency, and dread" (British Medical Association, 1986). The wider goal of this process is to render political leaders and social militants powerless, to prevent further political opposition to the ruling regime, and to act as a strong deterrent to potential opponents in the community (Ugalde & Ziwi, 1989). Techniques which deliberately induce a sense of helplessness in conjunction with feelings of guilt and shame combine with physical, sexual, and psychological violence to paralyze the psyche and dissipate opposition to the status quo.

The challenge for therapists who work in this field is to reverse the effects of these experiences and to help survivors restore a sense of hope, dignity, and empowerment, while allowing them to reestablish their capacity to trust fellow human beings. Torture and trauma services therefore need to develop organizational structures and models for relating to affected immigrant communities which are congruent with these aims and which support appropriate clinical practices and treatment modalities.

Services for Survivors

There are now a variety of services and models for the treatment of survivors of torture and refugee trauma within repressive countries themselves, in countries of asylum, and in countries of resettlement. In determining principles of practice and priorities for these services, it is critical to acknowledge that survivors suffer a sequence of traumata so that a continuum of services is needed. Increasing awareness that service priorities vary substantially at sequential points on this continuum of trauma will facilitate a more rational and coherent international response to the needs of survivors.

Examples of Services

Currently, services exist at various points on this continuum of torture and refugee trauma. The Medical Action Group in Chile and the Sanctuary Project in South Africa are examples of services that provide crucial treatment in countries of repression. In countries of asylum, informal services exist as well as programs supported by international and humanitarian agencies in refugee camps in Pakistan, Thailand, and elsewhere. Services have proliferated in countries of resettlement, examples being the Medical Foundation for Victims of Torture in England, R.C.T. and Oasis in Denmark, the Canadian Centre for Victims of Torture in Canada, and the Service for the Treatment and Rehabilitation of Torture and Trauma Survivors (STARTTS) and the Victorian Foundation for Survivors of Torture, both in Australia.

Margaret Cunningham • Service for the Treatment and Rehabilitation of Torture and Trauma Survivors, 28 Nelson Street, Fairfield, New South Wales 2165, Australia.   Derrick Silove • South West Sydney Area Health Service, Liverpool Hospital, Liverpool, New South Wales 2170, Australia.

International Handbook of Traumatic Stress Syndromes, edited by John P. Wilson and Beverley Raphael. Plenum Press, New York, 1993.

By understanding the sequence of traumata and social stresses suffered by refugees, it becomes easier to
consider the need for differing treatment priorities on
the continuum of refugee trauma, and the ways in
which services need to relate to each other to provide a
coherent and comprehensive response to this global
problem.

Sequence of Refugee Trauma: Six Phases of Transition

The refugee experience involves a number of
phases. Phase 1 involves living in a home country that is
at war or in the midst of widespread violence and social
upheaval which result in the progressive disruption of
educational, health, and other social facilities. Militants
and their families, and to a variable extent many other
citizens, experience a sense of constant threat accentuated by the breakdown of law and order. Phase 2 which
is common but not suffered by all refugees, involves
attacks, torture, imprisonment, and/or the disappearance of individuals and family members. Detainees may
be forced to carry out slave labor or are incarcerated in
degrading conditions in detention centers, concentration or "re-education" camps. The mass detention of
children is particularly traumatic to families and a potent
weapon of intimidation against the community in general (Goldfeld, Mollica, & Pesavento, 1988).

In Phase 3, ex-detainees, fearing further reprisals
against themselves or their families, become fugitives or
internal exiles in their own countries. Families then
struggle to trace lost family members while attempting
to cope with grief, uncertainty, and ongoing fear. Phase
4 involves family members who flee the country in hazardous circumstances, such as the Vietnamese boat people who risked being attacked by pirates or dying from
drowning, dehydration, and starvation on the voyage,
or the Afghan refugees who treacherously trekked
through the desert while risking starvation and attack
from militant groups. In Phase 5, the refugee gains entry
to a country of first asylum. For many individuals and
families, this involves living in refugee camps, or border
camps where the individual suffers many deprivations,
isolation, and uncertainties about the future. Individuals
may have little or no knowledge of the whereabouts or
safety of family members and often are subjected to
crowded, unsanitary, and unstimulating circumstances
in a milieu that is often hostile to the refugee's presence.
Phase 6 supervenes when refugees receive permission to
enter a host country for resettlement, where they often
experience problems concerning residency status, racial
prejudice, and socioeconomic, educational, occupational, and linguistic obstacles. Many of the stresses of previous phases may be ongoing, such as concern about
family/friends and the situation of strife at home, ambivalence and grief about fleeing from their country, and
coping with disturbing, traumatic memories and the
other physical and psychological sequelae of torture and
related trauma (Goldfeld *et al.*, 1988). The refugee's
sense of isolation and helplessness may be accentuated
by factionalism within the refugee communities in the
host country, and ongoing fears of reprisal by external
agents of repressive regimes. For all these reasons, it is

important to recognize that, even in "safe" host countries, refugees are often in a state of "continuous" stress
because of unresolved political and family calamities in
the home country which are superimposed on the difficulties they have in adapting to their new and often alien
environments (Collins, 1988; Littlewood & Lipsedge,
1982; Raphael, 1986).

Service Provision

In 1989, we contacted a number of torture and trauma services throughout the world to inquire about aspects of their organizational development and preferred-
treatment modalities. We solicited comments about their
service priorities and the obstacles and pitfalls which
individual organizations had encountered. Although the
information that was collated is somewhat selective, it
provides a broad range of viewpoints and experiences.
We will draw on this material as we attempt to trace the
needs and priorities of torture services at consecutive
points on the continuum of trauma that survivors suffer.
We will then report on approaches we have implemented to counter some of the problems which appear
to be common to most torture and trauma services in
establishing treatment principles, management of staff,
training and education, initiating preventive programs,
and the development of relationships with affected ethnic communities.

Countries of Repression

Services established in such countries as Chile, El
Salvador, the Philippines, and South Africa have developed in direct response to the political turmoil endemic
in these states. These services tend to focus on two
broad areas; first, a broad-based emphasis on providing
health care to disrupted families of victims of persecution, and second, a wide range of psychological, social,
and educational strategies which enable the individual
and the family to survive the experience of repression
while maintaining their integrity and commitment to
their struggle. It is important to remember that one of
the strategies used by repressive regimes against people
is to label dissidents and their families and thus exclude
them from mainstream public services which are available to other sectors of the population. Services are available to anyone identified as being victimized by repressive forces and extend to all family members. They
include the provision of practical assistance, such as the
provision of food and milk programs for children, along
with legal advice, medical assistance, and special educational programs.

There are risks for all workers who are involved in
these programs, since the very act of providing such
services signifies solidarity with the forces opposing the
repressive regime. Inevitably, staff find themselves providing medical treatment and psychological support
within the context of shared solidarity in the political
struggle and with consequent personal risk which is
shared not only with the client but also with the worker's
colleagues and family. Psychotherapy used by these services is often modified to provide psychological support

which enables targeted individuals to cope with repression, to face the possibility that torture may occur again, to deal with grief for tortured, dead, or "disappeared" comrades or family, and to utilize social and political action as a means of dealing with anger (Straker, 1988). The provision of educational programs for children of victims is an example of the preventive work which is a major focus of these services.

Usually, staffing of these services depends on volunteer professionals who may also have close associations with human rights organizations. Training programs are often directed at establishing a network of lay health workers who are drawn from the client group, who provide basic medical care, first aid, and crisis intervention as well as assist in the identification of people in the community who require more specialized services. Health professionals in these services, and in the community at large, need to be guided not only about the medical and psychiatric consequences of torture and political repression, but also in the ethical responsibilities and the risks in collaborating with repressive authorities (British Medical Association, 1986). Services in Chile, the Philippines, and elsewhere have developed detailed guidelines for health professionals concerning appropriate conduct in a variety of challenging situations (e.g., where a doctor is confronted by someone arriving at the doorstep in the middle of the night with gunshot wounds). The funding of these services is usually minimal and, consequently, resources are often scarce with a reliance on international funding bodies for support and ongoing education.

Countries of First Asylum

Countries such as Thailand, Pakistan, and Iraq have provided emergency domicile for the mass immigration of people from neighboring states which are beset by revolution, social upheaval, or war, adding an enormous strain to these "countries of first asylum," which are themselves Third World countries that are struggling to provide for their own population and to manage major economic problems. The establishment of refugee holding camps near the borders in these countries is one means that has been adopted to manage the huge influx of people from neighboring countries. With six million Afghans living outside Afghanistan, mostly in Pakistan and Iran, and with refugee camps in Thailand and Hong Kong housing thousands of Vietnamese and Cambodian refugees, the task for countries of first asylum to cope beyond the provision of basic shelter and nutrition for these refugees is arduous.

Conditions in camps vary, but refugees who manage to resettle in Western countries frequently recount traumatic experiences associated with this phase, including illness, overcrowding, poor sanitation, malnutrition, domestic violence, rape, bribery, and extortion. Regional and global political factors greatly influence attitudes toward refugees and hence their treatment. Host governments in countries of first asylum often have a policy of "deterrence" which militates against camp authorities who provide more than a subsistence level of survival (Mollica & Jalbert, 1989). It is important to note that over 70% of those living in refugee camps

are women and children who are most vulnerable to neglect, abuse, and exploitation (United Nations, 1989). The multiple factors which threaten the mental health of refugees who live in camps include the effects of previous trauma, such as torture and direct danger, for example, ongoing shelling around the campsite, lack of effective law enforcement and internal security systems to prevent intimidation, increased levels of domestic violence, chronic malnutrition, overcrowding, and poverty which leads to feelings of demoralization, powerlessness, hopelessness, and despair (Mollica & Jalbert, 1989). Many people face the prospect of being confined in refugee camps for 2 to 15 years, with the only option being to return to their own country to face persecution and possible death. Mollica and Jalbert (1989) have observed that the combination of military confinement and ongoing humanitarian assistance to interned refugees has generated pathological dependency, low self-esteem, and lack of initiative.

Staff members who work in refugee camps are plagued by inadequate training and support, few well-established organizational structures, and actual physical threat. They are often drawn from camp occupants as well as a wide range of sponsoring organizations and countries, with the employing organization having the responsibility for staff training and orientation. Staff may be employed according to specific skills they possess and not necessarily for any particular aptitude for working in a cross-cultural setting. Many staff members have no access to orientation programs, as they often request employment in the refugee camp while traveling overseas.

The task for staff in refugee camps—to provide meaningful services within the resources available and within the philosophy of their employing authority—is overwhelming. Usually, services focus on physical health, welfare, and education. Mental health programs are often poorly coordinated and underresourced.

Mollica and Jalbert (1989), in their report on the Site 2 camp in Thailand, emphasized that all agencies with personnel working in refugee camps need to develop strict guidelines for staff support and training, and that structures should be established to monitor compliance with these requirements. These guidelines need to cover clinical supervision and program support, as well as opportunities for personal development, debriefing for staff, and recreation. Involvement of traditional healers and religious leaders in treatment programs is essential, as is recruitment and training of bicultural counselors from camp occupants. Work training and education are essential to limit pathological dependency and ongoing social disability after relocation in a country of settlement.

The task of providing psychological services in a setting where people's lives are arduous and often threatened, and their future is uncertain, is difficult and demanding. Clearly, international cooperation in resolving the conflicts underlying the need for refugee camps is of paramount importance. In the meantime, if refugee camps are recognized as one point on the continuum of trauma suffered by displaced people, then early intervention and preventive programs could be designed in collaboration with staff in countries of repression and resettlement. This cooperation across countries would allow services to initiate integrated training programs with continuity of treatment as refugees progress through different phases. It would also allow interested agencies and services to make more comprehensive and coherent recommendations concerning amelioration or even prevention of refugee trauma.

Countries of Resettlement

Services in countries of resettlement fall into two categories: services addressing the broad range of welfare and medical needs faced by refugees, and services which specifically focus on the psychological needs of people who have been tortured.

There is a reciprocal relationship between these two types of services. The capacity of specialized services to focus on the specific needs of torture survivors in countries of resettlement depends on the strength and coherence of the wider service(s) which are available to meet the more general health and welfare needs of refugees.

Three main specialized service models for survivors of torture and refugee trauma have developed. At one extreme are services which are based primarily on highly trained clinical staff with an emphasis on psychotherapy and medical treatment, whereas at the other, are some centers which are organized to provide assessment, coordinating, and referral functions with clients who are referred to a network of volunteer professionals who provide definitive treatment on a continuing basis. A third and intermediate model encompasses a mixture of the previous two, with clinical staff employed by the center providing assessment, treatment, and coordination of clinical services, while volunteers provide social assistance and support.

The issues for staff training vary enormously depending on the service model used and the availability of resources for training. Services which use volunteer professionals as staff members experience ongoing difficulty with arranging training programs for volunteer professionals who have a high level of commitment to other professional roles while providing the primary treatment for torture and trauma survivors. Usually, staff who work in torture and trauma services have a high commitment to human rights, and service providers find client demands often take precedence over their own need for continued training, supervision, and support.

In countries where there is a well-coordinated program to manage all the resettlement needs of refugees, torture and trauma centers are able to provide a highly specific and specialized treatment service for clearly defined groups. This facilitates research into assessment and treatment and aids in promoting the training of outside staff and in providing expert consultancy roles to assist the development of new services. However, in countries which lack a broad-based, well-coordinated program for the resettlement needs of refugees, the staff of torture and trauma services are at risk of being overwhelmed by social welfare and legal issues such as the demands for expert reports to support asylum applications. This role quickly becomes an overriding function of the center as clients' urgent demands to support their

residency applications, and requests from government departments who request expert medical assessments to validate refugees claims of torture take precedence. This function can place the torture and trauma service in an invidious position of ambiguity where its role as part of the decision making process concerning the refugee's residency status may conflict with attempts to create a therapeutic milieu independent of external influences.

Staffing, Treatment Principles, and Service Development

In the discussion which follows we address some specific issues concerning staff selection, treatment of survivors, and service development in countries of resettlement.

Role of Biocultural Staff

The model we have developed at STARTTS is similar to that of the Boston Indochinese Psychiatry Clinic (Kalucy, 1988), where bilingual workers are not simply interpreters but participate actively as "specialized mental health clinicians" in counseling and therapy. For this reason, and to emphasize their bridging role between the two cultures, the bilingual staff preferred the appellation of "bicultural worker" to their original designation of "bilingual counselor." Some workers were employed with little formal training or experience in counseling but have brought to the position the invaluable assets of linguistic skills, shared experiences with clients' culture and recent history, and the capacity to educate Anglo-Australian health professionals in developing a deeper understanding of the experiences of refugees (Reid, Silove, & Tarn, 1989).

The principles of professionalism are difficult to teach by formal instruction in a short period of time, so our major emphasis in the training of bicultural workers was to develop their learning by direct experience. Each bicultural worker works closely with an experienced senior therapist who aims to develop a trusting and mutually enhancing co-therapist partnership. Respect for the special areas of expertise and knowledge of each partner is emphasized, with the professional therapist providing a modelling experience in the principles of diagnosis and counseling, and facilitating the processes used to enable the bicultural worker and client to talk together. The bicultural worker contributes linguistic skills, cultural interpretations, and a more intimate awareness of the nuances of the client's mental state. Staff members aim to maintain an ethos of mutual respect and consideration; for example, discussions in English between co-therapists are always immediately translated to the client to avoid any sense of exclusion. Clarification between co-therapists focuses on the interpretations of psychodynamic and interpersonal meaning, rather than on simple translation of language. Although initially it was feared that this elaborate model of therapy would be cumbersome and slow, therapists have found that the process allows a closer examination of client's nonverbal cues and the precise meanings which they are attempting to convey—aspects which paradoxically may be lost in conventional therapies where assumptions about the commonality of language may obscure highly individual and personalized experiences. These therapeutic partnerships have also facilitated the development of trust between co-workers as they confront together the importance and meaning of therapeutic processes utilized with clients and develop a closer sharing of cultural perspectives.

Because the bicultural workers are members of their clients' communities, they are confronted by the daunting task of separating their professional roles in which confidentiality and privacy are paramount, and their community roles as leaders, friends, or social activists. Some bicultural workers hold strong opinions about the regimes they have fled (or were loyal to), and these beliefs may be at variance with those of clients from opposing factions. Similarly, some refugee communities are politically divided, so that if a worker is perceived as having sectarian affiliations, needy members of antagonistic groupings may avoid consulting the service. There is always the potential for conflict in a service where individual staff members have suffered victimization by regimes that profess diametrically opposite ideologies. Although often difficult to implement, an important role for the professionally trained staff is to discourage sectarianism and to emphasize the humanitarian and nonpartisan commitment of the service.

Bicultural workers are often untrained and need an intensive period of initial training to prepare them for their counseling roles. Occasional symposia and case management meetings, while necessary, are not sufficient to meet the needs of ongoing training and supervision. Each service needs to develop comprehensive policies and strategies for staff training and development, and it will be helpful to newly developed services if these strategies are recorded in writing and made freely available. Consideration must also be given to the career structures of bicultural workers and the formal certification of acquired skills so that their professional status can be enhanced and their own resettlement facilitated.

Staff Selection

Questions are often raised about the type of staff members who work in trauma services and whether therapists from the dominant culture who have never experienced political persecution can ever really effectively work satisfactorily in this area.

It is our belief that culture need not be an intimidating obstacle to becoming an effective therapist for refugee survivors. Our bicultural workers are able to be "cultural brokers" while the role of Western therapists is, in part, to translate the issues of torture to the dominant culture, to assist the immigrant community in demystifying the norms and mores of the dominant culture, and to develop a modus operandi which allows access to and participation in the new society without devaluing their own traditional cultures. In this way, therapists from the mainstream culture can help to build bridges between the dominant culture and the traumatized ethnic communities. Many clients find it too shameful to speak of their experiences to people from

their own culture, and it can be especially therapeutic for such clients to convey the horror of their experience to someone outside their cultural group. To use incest as an analogy, the capacity of the survivor to be able to tell someone outside her normal network provides a method for breaking the silence at a more universal level. The partnership of bicultural counselor with the professional therapist who is usually drawn from the country of resettlement provides a balanced approach which seems to meet the needs of most refugees. For the reasons outlined above, selection of staff members also needs to be made as much on criteria of commitment to human rights and personal flexibility, as on specific skills needed by the service.

Terminology

Terminology varies across services, yet the language used reflects important underlying concepts and models for treatment. The majority of services use the term victims of torture in the titles of their services and in publicity material. This emphasis may inadvertently encourage the notion of victims as passive recipients of persecution who are permanently disabled. Usually, these services focus primarily on medical assessment and treatment aspects of their work, apparently with little time being given to networking with affected ethnic communities in the host country, developing volunteer services or group programs, or providing preventive programs. Services which focus on people as "survivors" share concepts developed by practitioners who work in other areas of posttraumatic stress, such as those who work with incest survivors (Bass & Davis, 1988). From this perspective, clients are regarded as people who have resources and assets which have allowed them to survive their victimization, and the aim of treatment therefore, is to enhance their reempowerment. Perhaps there is less emphasis on the use of intensive psychotherapy and more concern with ensuring symptom reduction, providing assistance with social difficulties, and devoting time to networking with other community organizations within the mainstream society and within ethnic communities. The rationale for this approach is that if survivors are provided with enough support and relief from immediate symptoms and anxieties, they will be able to mobilize natural inherent capacities for healing and coping.

Treatment Principles

When torture and trauma services were established initially, there was a pressing need to document fully accounts of torture in order to publicize its widespread use and its deleterious effects on psychological functioning. Although this work needs to continue, it is equally important to consider what principles of treatment can be derived from the growing fund of experience that is accrued by health professionals in torture and trauma services across the world. Possibly as a result of the alacrity of the development of services, some of the formulations in the earlier literature concerning the treatment of survivors of torture seem somewhat simplistic. For example, there is reason to be concerned by the assertion of some influential therapists that survivors who present for treatment need to disclose the full details of their torture experiences for therapy to be successful (Silove, Tarn, Bowles, & Reid, 1989). An excessive emphasis on eliciting the "trauma story" may lead overly zealous therapists to be intrusive or directive inadvertently. Therapists are inevitably regarded as authority figures, and an excessively interrogatory interview can, even when sensitively undertaken, evoke strong memories of the torture experience in the survivor. People who have been tortured commonly suffer a devastating loss of control over their physical, psychological, and moral integrity, so that pressure by a therapist to reveal these painful memories may be experienced as persecutory and, on occasion, lead to regression, retreat from therapy, and additional loss of self-esteem.

Although the process of catharsis and cognitive reappraisal is undoubtedly beneficial for many survivors, we concur with Kalucy (1988) that a broader consideration of the torture experience is necessary to formulate appropriate treatment. Working-through traumatic experiences is an integral component of therapy for many survivors, but, for some patients, detailed self-disclosure may be premature, unnecessary, ineffective, or, if used as the only strategy, potentially harmful. In view of the sequential traumata that refugees experience, successful therapy for survivors often requires the therapist to subordinate the examination of intrapsychic material to a more fundamental need of patients to regain a sense of empowerment in their struggle for survival in the country of resettlement.

Dealing with Emotions in Therapy

In the memory of many survivors, the nadir of their torture experiences was their devastating loss of control over their inner emotional, moral, and psychic worlds which was often attended by dehumanized pleading, regression, and inability to contain primitive emotions. These responses, together with survivors' direct experiences of deliberately planned brutality at the hands of fellow humans, tend to leave them with an intense residual fear of expressing such strong emotions as anxiety and anger, which become inextricably identified with destructiveness and humiliation.

Like survivors of other major disasters (Raphael, 1986), victims of ongoing persecution often employ strong defenses of denial and dissociation, so that they may seem outwardly blunted and lacking in feeling. However, this emotional repression may be adaptive at the time of persecution, because it allows the person to attend exclusively to the immediate needs of survival (Raphael, 1986). Emotions may remain repressed for many years but may erupt as posttraumatic stress symptoms, such as the intrusion of unbidden images from the traumatic past into the survivor's waking hours and nightmares overwhelming their inner worlds at night. Dynamically, survivors face persisting difficulties in modulating their conflicting needs for "calming reassurance" to maintain ego-function on the one hand, and the pressure to maintain extreme vigilance against the intrusion of inner memories or outside threats on the

other (Rundell, Ursano, & Holloway, 1989). The learned helplessness model (Abrahamson, Alloy, & Metalsky, 1989) seems particularly pertinent to the posttraumatic dynamic of victims of torture who experience such a profound loss of control over their inner psychic worlds that it is difficult for them to reclaim their identity or a sense of self-efficacy and purpose on release.

Many survivors experience major difficulties in adapting their defenses to the more flexible demands of the "normal" world on release and for some, such defenses as projections, denial, or dissociation may remain rigid. One of the characteristics of people who employ such defenses is that they have difficulty modulating strong emotions, especially anger and irritability, and this may result in domestic and other forms of violence. Some survivors may also respond in resentful, hostile, and frankly paranoid ways when confronted by insensitive or ignorant officials in bureaucracies and in places of work. The risk of these reactions to authority figures is magnified by the linguistic and cultural obstacles which refugees face in dealing with officialdom in the host country.

Facilitative Self-Mastery: The Need for Flexibility in Counseling

We propose that the aims of therapy for survivors of torture should be to promote a sense of self-mastery over their turbulent inner psychic worlds and a feeling of social reempowerment and identity. Usually, this requires a flexible two-pronged approach which allows the therapist to give equal attention to the intrapsychic residue of the torture experience, as well as to strategies which will aid survivors to develop a sense of agency in dealing with their new and often alien environment.

The therapist's willingness to be involved actively in the process of providing practical assistance helps to cement the therapeutic alliance and often facilitates later disclosures of the survivors past trauma. Therapists' familiarity with their clients' current difficulties aids the hermeneutic process of psychotherapy in which attempts are made to integrate the raw experience of torture into the meanings and symbols of the survivors' current reality.

One strategy which therapists can use to enhance the survivors' sense of personal mastery is to offer initial counseling for the family at home. Survivors can then assume greater control over the transaction by ordering the environment according to their needs and by offering the therapist hospitality in the tradition of their culture. It also provides the opportunity for the survivor to reveal positive aspects of his or her past experience; for example, by showing the therapists a photograph album or artifact from the home country. Symbolically, the therapist's role of "respectful guest" is appropriate to the aid of treatment, which is to generate a greater sense of identity, autonomy, and efficacy in the client. The home environment also allows the natural inclusion of other family members in the therapy, and their presence can mitigate the therapist's fears about leaving the survivor in a state of severe distress at the end of the sessions. However, the home can be an inappropriate setting for individual psychotherapy where confidentiality and privacy are essential.

On the other hand, therapists need to remain clear that their aim is to reempower the survivors and their families, and that there are boundaries to the friendship which is developed in therapy. These limits often need to be explained to clients who are unfamiliar with the procedures and goals of Western therapy.

The Political Dimension

During the process of reempowering survivors of torture, the therapist also needs to be sensitive to existential and ideological issues, because some torture survivors are political militants who need to understand their experiences as part of a broad social framework. These refugees hold strong political and moral views and tend to judge themselves and others according to stringent ethical and social codes of behavior.

The importance of the political dimension raises many important issues concerning the appropriateness of orthodox models of psychotherapy in the treatment of torture survivors. It can be argued that "conventional" therapies provided in countries of resettlement are limited in their scope since they are excessively individualistic and tend to be administered by professionals who are raised in stable Western countries who lack the experiential background to relate fully to the survivors' beliefs and concerns. A particular concern is that health professionals may "medicalize" the problem of torture, thereby invalidating the existential meaning of the experience for survivors. There is therefore, a need for all mental health workers in this field to have at least a minimum knowledge of the social and historical context in which torture occurs so that they are able to understand the possible political meanings of the experience to the survivor. The therapist also needs to understand the relationship of the survivor and his or her political allegiances to the rest of the ethnic community in the host country.

Practical issues flow from these considerations; for example, the need for services to pay special attention to matching clients and therapists, to the choice of interpreters according to known political affiliations, and to the special need for confidentiality of any information that is divulged. The use of psychodynamic interpretations in therapy also needs to be widened to include not only the examination of defenses and unconscious material, but also such issues as the pain of exile and feelings of frustration and loss which arise out of the survivor's altered political identity.

Cultural and Religious Factors

Knowledge about and respect for cultural and religious issues is of paramount importance for therapists to be successful in treating refugees. In some groups, there may be strong cultural prohibitions against showing emotions, particularly for men who may fear breaking down in front of other family members or female therapists. Similarly, cultural factors may accentuate the natural inhibition that women may have in disclosing to male therapists experiences of rape, which is a common form of political violence against women (Goldfeld *et al.*, 1988). Self-disclosure to a counselor is foreign to some cultural groups (e.g., the Indochinese), so that this consideration is another reason for therapists to be cautious in expecting rapid revelation of personal and sensitive information by these clients in therapy.

However, cultural barriers to psychotherapy are not rigid. Where whole societies have experienced mass social traumatization and cultural upheaval (such as has occurred in Cambodia), refugees have already endured rapid social changes so that they may no longer adhere as firmly to traditional cultural constraints, for example, to concealing private feelings. In these circumstances, clients' notions about healing can undergo complex transformations allowing them to accept diverse therapeutic interventions from both traditional and Western medicine. It is important that therapists not only keep pace with the client's changing views, but that they be willing to integrate into Western-based therapies both culturally based attributions concerning the cause of symptoms, whether these are based on mythical, religious, magical, or superstitious beliefs, and shamanistic approaches to treating them.

Creating Resource Manuals: Culture-Specific Techniques

For these reasons, in our service we have encouraged bicultural staff members to prepare resource manuals on their respective communities to assist the professional staff. The manuals aim at detailing the common ways people from the relevant cultures express anger, joy, loneliness, sadness, and grief. They also detail healing customs that are relevant to the various communities, which helps to inform other staff of the processes involved, the purpose of the custom, the symbolism expressed, the conditions under which this custom could be practiced, and whether its application is restricted to a designated healer within the culture. This inventory of cultural and religious customs has greatly enhanced the breadth of psychotherapeutic interventions we are able to provide. Through sharing of knowledge about these customs, we have also been able to identify similarities in practices across different cultures, and this has facilitated our understanding of the ways to help people from little-known ethnic groups. The presentation of some of these customs as well-timed interventions in the therapeutic process has served to heighten clients' feelings of affiliation with the service and has ensured that our therapeutic practices are acknowledged as being culturally appropriate.

Many of our clients are deeply religious people who need to understand their experiences not only in a sociopolitical but also in a spiritual framework. For example, a 29-year-old woman who was a political activist from a Middle Eastern country interpreted most of her torture experiences in terms of her relationship with Allah and the idea of a just Islamic society. One method she initiated to regain a sense of empowerment has been to meditate every night while wearing the traditional Muslim sackcloth to purify herself. She has shown interest in developing an active group of compatriots who will try to integrate an understanding of their shared persecution within a religious framework.

One of the advantages in establishing specialized services for the treatment of survivors of torture is that a database of information can be developed along with a resource network which supports the therapist in understanding the intricate sociopolitical and cultural issues which are important for effective therapy with patients from diverse backgrounds.

Treatment Guidelines

In summary, we offer a brief list of treatment guidelines for the provision of a service in countries of resettlement for refugees who have suffered severe torture or multiple traumata. Some of these principles, which have been outlined by Reid and Strong (1988) and Kinzie and Fleck (1987) include:

1. The provision of a nonthreatening milieu for therapy
2. The willingness of therapists to engage clients in a trusting, patient, and long-term relationship in which the latter may feel at ease to return to the service in times of crisis
3. A willingness to respond to clients' expressed needs even if these seem only distantly related to their trauma
4. The careful judgment of the client's readiness to disclose details of his or her past trauma
5. The ability of the therapist to judge the extent of catharsis that the client can tolerate at various points in therapy
6. The provision of an explicitly multimodal approach to therapy in which target symptoms and disabilities which most trouble the client will receive primary attention
7. An understanding of the historical, political, cultural, and religious context in which the refugee tries to reconstruct his or her reality
8. An advocacy role in which the therapist actively assists (albeit within the limitations of resources) with social, family, medical, legal, and residency issues which will all help to empower the survivor to overcome distrust of the new society and cope more effectively with resettlement.

Confidentiality

An important aspect of work in torture and trauma services is the need for developing recording processes which are secure and confidential, yet able to be utilized for the educational development of staff and members of other organizations who require training. Some services have reported infiltration of spies who report the attendance of survivors to political regimes in the country of origin. Clients and ethnic communities need to feel involved in designing methods which ensure that the center is able to maintain confidentiality and impartiality in service provision.

Service Development

It is as important for staff to focus on organizational and service development as it is to develop effective approaches to clinical assessment and treatment. These two activities are closely interlinked and mutually enhancing. In the following discussion, we will identify areas which were of prime importance in the first two years of establishing STARTTS in Sydney, Australia, and which have been cited by other services as important issues in their development.

Service Autonomy versus Government Sponsorship

The experiences of refugee communities of the misuse of government power by repressive regimes has often led to a heightened collective fear of government bureaucracies so that the communities are often concerned that torture and trauma services be removed from the possibility of government interference, even in countries of resettlement. Where refugee services are funded primarily by government, there is a legitimate concern that the service may be used to foster, directly or indirectly, the government's policies. For example, service provision may be restricted to those who are accepted for asylum or who are granted residency status. This often means that large numbers of refugees who are awaiting change of status or who are "illegal" residents may be restricted in their access to urgently needed treatment. Government policies may also preclude staff of services from publicizing or criticizing government practices which, even in countries of resettlement, may be experienced by refugee communities as violations of human rights. For example, conditions within detention centers for illegal refugees may fall far short of providing an adequate milieu for detainees who have suffered extreme trauma.

An alternative model which helps to retain service independence and autonomy is for centers to be private foundations. The advantage of a foundation is that, given an adequate funding base, creativity can be enhanced through the range of independent initiatives which can be implemented. In practice, funds are usually provided by a combination of government grants and/or private benefactors. The precariousness of funding and the difficulty in establishing ongoing and continuing financial support can absorb staff in concerns about organizational survival, often inhibiting the growth of services to meet the demands of increasing refugee numbers. For this reason, an emphasis on the early development of a diverse funding base from a multiplicity of agencies and sources is valuable both in the time and effort spent, because it provides stability and security for the organization which ensures ongoing service development and independence.

Service Management

Dilemmas also arise concerning representation on management committees or boards which oversee torture and trauma services. If these committees comprise mainly members from refugee communities, problems of equity arise in that there are often large numbers of different ethnic communities who legitimately warrant representation. In addition, many leaders of refugee communities are relatively recent arrivals who have yet to develop strong enough political links within the mainstream culture which are necessary to ensure the continued success and survival of the program. At the same time, it is understandable that ethnic communities find it unacceptable for management committees to be dominated by representatives of the mainstream culture. We have found that a heterogeneous membership, some members with strong human rights affiliations or holding positions in human rights organizations, some with appropriate professional backgrounds, and some representing the needs of the major refugee groups, helps to create a management committee which is sensitive to the broad range of services needed and which has access to appropriate sources of policy-making and funding.

On a wider front, it is time for services to focus on the task of organizing structures which are aimed at promoting international cooperation in dealing with the problems of torture and refugee trauma. In this task, trauma services may benefit from examining models established by environmental groups, women's organizations, and international human rights groups. International linking of services is essential to establish a coherent continuum of services which are responsive to the sequence of traumata that are suffered by refugees. The informal exchange of information which currently occurs at the international level is the first step in disseminating and comparing organizational methodologies and approaches to practice, as well as contributing to combating the spread of torture by raising consciousness concerning human rights abuse and violations.

Flexible Therapeutic Models

The diversity of models and practices in the torture and trauma field highlight the creativity which has developed in this complex area of service delivery.

Some services utilize multidisciplinary teams in a way which emphasizes professionally proscribed roles (e.g., the social worker sees the family, the doctor manages the team and performs medical assessments, and the psychologist provides testing and counseling). Our application of a multidisciplinary model involves making use of all skills each staff member possesses, both personal and professional. This provides substantial flexibility in that most staff member, irrespective of their qualifications, can accept case-management responsibility, have access to clinical supervision and personal support on a regular basis, and may share leadership roles and organizational functions.

It has also been useful to include somapractitioners and Feldenkrais therapists (Hanna, 1988) as part of the physical services, because these practitioners have particular expertise in understanding the somatization of clients. The physical exercises which are used for pain relief focus on giving clients a sense of control over the therapeutic process and assists them in understanding their body functions which have often been distorted by the torture experience. Self-management programs are often developed and monitored by the somapractitioner. The availability of this alternative therapy has meant that our physiotherapist has been able to provide a specialist treatment role as well as a training and supervision role in establishing the range of physical therapies.

Since a large majority of our clients are drawn from the Indochinese community, we have needed to con-

sider ways in which to integrate practitioners of Chinese medicine into our Western treatment modalities. The use of such modalities as therapeutic massage can often bridge the gap between concepts of healing ("laying on of hands") in traditional culture and Western medical practices. The intercultural transposition of therapies has been detailed by Wilson (1989), who has shown the value of using Native American Indian Sweat Lodge rituals with Vietnam veterans who were suffering posttraumatic stress disorder. Similarly, Peseschkian (1986) in Germany has developed a model of "positive psychotherapy" using Oriental stories as a major tool in the treatment of Middle Eastern refugees.

The use of groups for oral history, writing, art, and drama all provide the potential for creative and therapeutic experiences which can empower survivors by assisting them to focus on ways of expressing their feelings, either directly or through creative symbols, and thus to construct meaning from their experiences. This helps survivors overcome their feelings of helplessness and impotence in expressing rage, guilt, and shame which defy verbal expression. We have noted, too, that little use is made in refugee trauma services of the skills and knowledge offered by occupational therapists and medical anthropologists (one of whom was instrumental in developing STARTTS) in devising appropriate therapeutic interventions.

A broader use of recent concepts developed in social psychology with its research formulations based on attribution theory (Abrahamson, Garber, & Seligman, 1980) and self-control strategies (Taylor, 1986) may assist services in developing more effective assessment and evaluation tools. The treatment modalities developed by therapists who were working with incest and domestic violence survivors (Bass & Davis, 1988) provide an array of creative and flexible therapeutic methods which may, in modified form, be applied to survivors of torture and their families.

Prevention through Community Development and Group Work

Currently, these two areas are underdeveloped in torture and trauma services in countries of resettlement, although in repressive countries they are a primary component of services. Many staff members who are working in countries of resettlement express concern at the lack of involvement in service policy-making and development of some of the refugee communities for which services are provided. We have found that focusing on community development and group work provides a useful way of enhancing the commitment of refugee communities to the work of our service.

Initially, we established one staff position to have primary responsibility for community development for our center. This worker has access to a third of the time of every other staff member in our center in order to develop projects and group programs. Meetings are arranged with representatives from affected ethnic communities on an annual basis to promote dialogue with each community about the provision of the service and its implications for their community. We then provide feedback to the people of these communities about how we have implemented their ideas and concerns into our practice. This process of ongoing dialogue and commitment has provided feedback to community leaders who are able to assist in engaging the ethnic community as a whole in our work. Consequently, this has allowed us to establish a process of rapid self-referral to our agency by members of communities who are familiar with our work, thereby helping to overcome some of the resistances to presentation (e.g., by men) which are described by many other agencies. The community development process has also assisted us to be aware of the difficulties of smaller refugee communities who, as yet, have not developed effective infrastructures within the dominant culture and may therefore be overlooked. Our community orientation has assisted us to link more effectively with appropriate mainstream services which provide specific services for immigrant communities. For example, in a community consultation conducted for the Tamil community, we became aware that residency status issues were a major source of concern for this group. We facilitated a meeting between community leaders and senior officials of the Department of Immigration to attempt to clarify procedures for gaining formal residency approval. On another occasion a consultation with the Lao community provided information about the arrival of a large group of Lao men who had recently been released from labor camps. This news allowed us to respond rapidly by establishing a group program for these men which was conducted by our bicultural worker, the community development worker, and Lao workers from other relevant community organizations. This group is ongoing and reports to date from participants indicate that this intervention has had a preventive function in reducing the stress of resettlement and in facilitating the reentry of these men into their families.

Need for Networking: Links to Other Agencies

The success of community development programs depends on effective *networking* with ethnic organizations and communities, developing supportive media coverage, and employing concepts of volunteerism which we believe should be based on principles of *exchange* rather than of *rescue*. To give an example of this idea, our agency assisted a group of Latin American artists with funding applications and a venue to meet, and, in return, these artists are assisting with the development of art programs for our clients. Often volunteerism based on notions of "rescuing" people leads to inappropriate choices of volunteers, with the attending risk of perpetuating paternalistic and colonial attitudes. If volunteers are selected carefully and receive appropriate briefing and education, then they can be invaluable in helping services promote attitudes of quality and respect. By recruiting volunteers with specific skills, it is possible to promote creative projects, such as using writers from the host community to assist survivors in writing their stories for publication, or in enlisting members of an embroiderers' guild to assist women refugees to record their traditional work, the wider aim being to validate and give recognition to the culture and personal histories of clients.

Preventive programs can utilize staff and facilities from other agencies that are involved in multicultural work. With the assistance of staff and accommodation at an adolescent service, we have conducted effective multicultural camps during school holidays for 10 to 16-year-old children whose parents have been tortured. This provides staff at STARTTS with a unique opportunity to train other workers in dealing with the psychological difficulties faced by the children of refugees, enables children to meet their peers who have experienced similar traumatic histories, and promotes an understanding of multiculturalism among these people. Working with the children of survivors can involve after-school programs and can be extended to camp programs which include adults and wider family groups.

All torture and trauma services recognize the responsibility they have in raising consciousness about torture and in providing training for the wider community and especially for staff of government and voluntary organizations. One approach we have utilized is to combine clients and professionals in one training group. For example, we were invited by teachers to an English as a Second Language (ESL) class to talk to potential clients about the services we provided. We presented information concerning the rationale for our service, described some of the experiences our clients had suffered, and outlined some of the repercussions of torture for individuals and families. Our aim was to present this material in an informal yet thought-provoking manner, using an approach which demonstrated to these potential clients the manner in which professional therapists and bicultural staff work together. Students responded by discussing the way they felt their past torture affected their present functioning. This not only validated the information we had provided, but also was the first time teachers, who chose to attend the session, had heard of any of these experiences of their students. The affected students went on to talk about some of the difficulties they had experienced in class when confronted by certain behaviors of their teachers (e.g., teachers unintentionally causing them distress by the interrogatory nature and style of their questioning). The outcome of this process was that students were able to identify the relevance of our services to them, while simultaneously raising the consciousness of teachers in an explicit and direct way. It was necessary, however, for STARTTS staff to spend considerable time debriefing the teachers who expressed guilt and distress concerning their own lack of knowledge and sensitivity to their students' previous experiences. The outcome was that staff members reviewed their classroom management practices, and further recognition was given to the need to educate adult migrant education teachers on the availability of torture and trauma services. The preventative potential of this exercise has had widespread implications for consciousness raising and the implementation of changes to services in countries of resettlement.

Media Relationships

In using the media for raising community consciousness on torture, we have established policies which have discouraged the use of individual refugee histories as a means of gaining publicity for the service. This has often made it difficult to promote ongoing publicity, but we have found that this firm policy of discouraging media sensationalism has won the support of ethnic communities through our respectful treatment of refugees and their problems. We believe that it is important that the public image of torture and trauma services be as credible and professional as the private context of our treatment milieu.

Staff Management and Training

Staff of torture and trauma services are working not only in multidisciplinary contexts but also in multicultural contexts. It is important that the various services develop an identifiable culture and unifying ethos which can be shared by staff as well as clients. It is important for staff to meet together to discuss the organization's philosophy and its mission, so that all members can identify goals which are meaningful to them. At STARTTS, staff members focused on such questions as: What is the culture of our service? and How do we communicate it to clients as the way of dealing with issues of philosophy and mission in a staff group with diverse educational and cultural backgrounds?

Management of torture and trauma services requires ongoing planning of support strategies to facilitate team building as well as to ensure that staff members are able to evaluate their work and receive feedback with the aim of maintaining the quality of work while reducing the ever-present risk of staff burnout. Many services have policies in place which provide for a portion of staff time to be allocated to nonintensive clinical work. This is in recognition of the high degree of stress involved in constantly being exposed as a therapist to the horror of torture experiences. Usually, this time is used to raise consciousness in the dominant culture concerning refugees, as well as to participate in research, community development, teaching, and training.

Senior staff members need to maintain a high degree of awareness that all workers experience some emotional upheaval when listening to clients recount their "trauma stories." For the bilingual counselor, there is the added stress associated with listening to experiences of the client which resonate with (and amplify) his or her own memories, pain, and despair. Added risks to staff are overidentification with and excessive protection of our clients, as well as the possibility of falling prey to other distortions, such as using the work to displace personal sources of anger, or developing a vicarious fascination with the intricacies of the sadistic behaviors or torturers. We have therefore established a system of external supervision implemented so that each worker can undergo weekly debriefing while, at the same time, receiving additional clinical training. This external supervision program was deliberately designed to involve senior clinicians outside the service, which provides a moderating influence, mitigating any feelings of service isolation or the development of doctrinaire views within a small and highly cohesive team.

In addition, we have found it useful to involve staff members in writing their own antiburnout strategy as part of their own work management. This strategy aims to promote the recognition that we each have a responsibility to support ourselves and our colleagues from burnout. The staff group has implemented this policy by developing a peer-monitoring system to ensure that all staff members maintain their own antiburnout strategies, which include a broad range of personal activities that enrich their work and leisure time. For bicultural staff, the emphasis on recognizing their own needs has enabled them to establish boundaries between their work life, their own survival experiences, and their ongoing resettlement needs.

Conclusion

We now provide a synopsis of guidelines that are derived from our own experiences and those of colleagues who responded to our survey concerning priorities for service development in the treatment of torture survivors. These insights may provide both working guidelines and a stimulus for future research.

- Carefully screen volunteers for particular skills and personal resources needed to work in the area.
- Indicate clearly the limitations of the service, proceed slowly and carefully in development, and be cautious in publicizing services so that the center is not swamped by demand.
- Plan service growth in a coherent manner.
- Ensure that the guiding principle of the service is humanitarian and not political.
- Minimize staff burnout through their involvement in project work and training work, and institute appropriate self-monitoring strategies.
- Recognize that treatment services are likely to reflect both positive and negative aspects of the society in which it is located. In particular, avoid paternalism and dominance of the mainstream culture within the service.
- Establish realistic aims and implementation priorities.
- Establish affiliations with universities and other educational institutions.
- Strengthen international cooperation among treatment services.
- Develop research instruments and evaluation tools which facilitate the assessment of innovative interventions.
- Assist the development of refugee mental health programs in countries of first asylum.
- Aim in therapy to empower the survivor and to avoid colonial and oppressive attitudes. Base treatment firmly within a context that recognizes the realities faced by refugees in countries of resettlement.
- Develop holistic and interdisciplinary approaches.
- Attend to the need for marital and family therapy to address relationship disturbances, and to assist the refugee family to resettle in their adoptive culture.
- Encourage a broad perspective acknowledging that torture is not only a medical problem but needs to be understood within a social and political context.

In conclusion, it is worthwhile to remember that refugees, as a group, are neither heroes nor victims. The victims of torture are dead, or have permanently disappeared; the survivors are those who are seen. In the words of Rigoberto Menchu, a Guatemalan Indian woman, "all of us who are alive can be the voice of the dead."

We would encourage torture and trauma services to reflect on the principles which were developed in 1987 at the World Health Organization's conference on Healthy Public Policy that was held in Adelaide, South Australia: (1) to create supportive environments, (2) to strengthen community action, and (3) to develop personal skills.

Torture and trauma centers will only be able to meet these aims if there is adequate international coordination so that services are able to respond appropriately to the sequential needs of survivors on the continuum of refugee trauma.

ACKNOWLEDGMENTS

Special gratitude is expressed to all the staff members at STARTTS for their commitment to developing the model and their creative implementation of these principles and practices.

References

Abrahamson, L., Alloy, L. B., & Metalsky, G. I. (1989). Hopelessness depression: A theory-based subtype of depression. *Psychological Review*, 96(2), 358–372.

Abrahamson, L., Garber, J., & Seligman, M. E. P. (1980). Learned helplessness in humans: An attributional analysis. In J. Garber & M. E. P. Seligman (Eds.), *Human helplessness*. New York: Academic Press.

Bass, E., & Davis, L. (1988). *The courage to heal*. New York: Harper & Row.

British Medical Association. (1986). *The torture report*. London, England: Chamelon Press.

Collins, J. (1988). *Migrant hands in a distant land*. Sydney: Pluto Press.

Goldfeld, A. E., Mollica, R. F., & Pesavento, B. H. (1988). The physical and psychological sequelae of torture. *Journal of the American Medical Association*, 259, 2725–2729.

Hanna, T. (1988). *Somatics*. Reading, MA: Addison-Wesley.

Kalucy, R. S. (1988). The health needs of victims of torture. *Medical Journal of Australia*, 148, 321–323.

Kinzie, D. J., & Fleck, J. (1987). Psychotherapy with severely traumatized refugees. *American Journal of Psychotherapy*, 42, 82–94.

Littlewood, R., & Lipsedge, M. (1982). *Aliens and alienists*. Harmondsworth, England: Penguin Books.

Mollica, R. F., & Jalbert, R. R. (1989). *Community of confinement: The mental health crisis in Site Two* (Report for the Committee on Refugees and Migrants). World Federation of Mental Health.

Peseschkian, N. (1986). *Oriental stories as tools in psychotherapy*. Berlin: Springer-Verlag.

Raphael, B. (1986). *When disorder strikes*. Sydney, Australia: Century Hutchison.

Reid, J. C., Silove, D., & Tarn, R. (1989). *The development of the New South Wales Service for the treatment and rehabilitation of torture and trauma survivors (STARTTS): The first year*. Unpublished manuscript.

Reid, J. C., & Strong, T. (1988). Rehabilitation of refugee victims of torture and trauma: Principles and service provision in NSW. *Medical Journal of Australia*, 148, 340–346.

Rundell, J. R., Ursano, R. J., & Holloway, H. C. (1989). Psychiatric responses to trauma. *Journal of Hospital and Community Psychiatry*, 40(1), 68–74.

Silove, D., Tarn, R., Bowles, R., & Reid, J. (1989). *Psychosocial needs of torture survivors*. Unpublished manuscript.

Straker, G. (1988). Post traumatic stress disorder: A reaction to state-supported child abuse and neglect. *Journal of Child Abuse and Neglect*, 12, 383–395.

Taylor, S. E. (1986). *Health psychology*. New York: Random House.

Ugalde, A., & Ziwi, A. (1989). Towards an epidemiology of political violence in the Third World. *Journal of Social Science and Medicine*, 28, 633–642.

United Nations House Committee on Refugees (UNHCR). (1989). *Report on refugees*. New York: United Nations Publishing Services.

Wilson, J. (1989). *Trauma, transformation and healing*. New York: Brunner/Mazel.

CHAPTER 64

Medical Diagnosis and Treatment of Torture Survivors

Marianne Juhler

Introduction

In this chapter I will focus on the diagnosis and treatment of the somatic sequelae of torture. Summarily, these can be divided into (1) a general stress-related condition which is found to some extent in most untreated survivors, irrespective of the type of torture; and (2) the symptoms and findings related to specific torture methods and to body parts and organ systems directly affected by the torture.

Medical History

As in all other therapist–patient contacts, the medical history is of crucial importance. A precise knowledge of the type of torture to which the patient has been subjected, his or her present complaints, and the diseases or trauma prior to torture provide the necessary guidelines for focusing on certain items in the general medical exam, for ordering additional paraclinical tests, and for specialist referral. Furthermore, this is the only way to obtain a holistic view of the patient's problem and to avoid futile diagnostic testing and medical therapy for isolated organ complaints, which often make sense only when brought into the broader context of torture survival (Juhler & Vesti, 1989).

The medical interview provides information on the presence and severity of elements from the general stress picture, as well as specific organ-related complaints. Knowledge of torture in general and of specific torture methods in particular facilitate both questioning

Marianne Juhler • Rehabilitation and Research Center for Torture Victims, Juliane Mariesvej 34, 2100 Copenhagen 0, Denmark.

International Handbook of Traumatic Stress Syndromes, edited by John P. Wilson and Beverley Raphael. Plenum Press, New York, 1993.

and interpretation of the information obtained. Thus, the medical approach to torture survivors becomes—if not a task for specialists—at least a task for doctors with a particular interest.

In addition to the diagnostic information, the individual torture history calls attention to special considerations which must be taken when subjecting the patient to various medical tests. Diagnostic procedures and treatment methods, which are easily accepted in the general, nontortured patient population, may remind the torture survivor directly or indirectly of the torture. Thereby uncontrollable anxiety may be provoked leading to an irreparable loss of confidence in the therapist. Only thorough attention to the history ensures that the risk of such situations is minimized (Stover & Nightingale, 1985).

Purpose of the Medical Examination

It is often mentioned (and rightly so) that psychological mechanisms are the major matter in posttorture symptoms. However, only a minority of the survivors perceive their problem to be mainly or entirely of a psychological nature. The majority experience and present their situation as somatic disease. It is important to understand that the somatic complaint picture, irrespective of any organic basis or not, is an important (and perhaps the only) access for initial treatment. The torture survivor has a right to have his or her situation taken seriously, and a somatic complaint which is listened to and which results in a normal medical examination may be the gateway to confidence without which later psychotherapy is impossible. Starting out with a psychological approach to a problem classified by the therapist as purely psychosomatic, with little or no organic substrata, may thus be a bad idea, if the survivor/patient experiences it differently. Naturally, it is not the task of doctors to confirm or invent organic disease if it is not present. On the contrary, they must, on the basis of his professional knowledge, reassure the torture survivor that he is not suffering from disease or chronically progressing ill health, as they have been led to believe by deliberately erroneous information from the torturers concerning the connection between torture and chronic disease.

In case of actual somatic disease—whether traceable to torture or not—the torture survivor has a right to medical examination and relevant treatment. In other words, it may be dangerous to assign all symptoms to psychological and social sequelae of torture without a closer look to determine whether this is actually the case. As is the case with all other patients, psychosomatic disease is a diagnosis of exclusion. Torture survivors should not be at a disadvantage just because their torture history immediately offers itself as a plausible explanation of all complaints.

Special Considerations Concerning Diagnosis and Treatment

Prior to any diagnostic procedure, it should be considered whether it is really necessary to carry out the contemplated examination. In general, it is unwise to subject patients to diagnostic procedures, if the same information can be obtained in a way which is simpler and less straining for the patient. In particular, this applies to torture survivors who because of their torture experience may suffer from pronounced fear of procedures and medical equipment. For the same reason, it is important to "institutionalize" examination and treatment as little as possible. It promotes trust and thereby cooperation and diagnostic yield of examinations, if examinations can take place in an atmosphere and in surroundings which are as nontechnical as possible (Danish Medical Association and The International Rehabilitation and Research Centre for Torture Victims, 1987).

In cases requiring examination or instrumentation with special equipment (possibly in a hospital environment), it is necessary to prepare the torture survivor thoroughly for this in order to minimize the psychological trauma of the procedure.

The preparation consists of giving the patient an understanding of the purpose of the examination, the technical procedure, the equipment that will be used, and the expected aftereffects. When the result of the examination is ready, it is important to immediately inform the patient of this and any consequences thereof. Also when the outcome of an examination is completely normal, it is important that the doctor inform the patient, as the fear of suffering from disease may thereby be removed.

It is obvious that painful and unpleasant examinations should be completely avoided (e.g., electromyography or nerve conduction velocity studies). These tests might seem reasonable to perform because of frequent complaints of paresthesia in hands and feet from torture survivors, who have been exposed to torture methods involving suspension or the tying of hands and feet. However, a thorough clinical neurological examination is sufficient to disprove the presence of the suspected polyneuropathy, as is spontaneous subsidence of symptoms along with the patient's mental improvement through psychotherapy. Generally speaking, problems which remain after significant mental improvement should be reconsidered medically. Once again, it is preferable if the diagnosis can be reached by relatively untraumatic methods (i.e., blood or urine tests, noninvasive radiology, etc.).

Also, routine procedures which are hardly stressful at all to the general patient population may be extremely traumatizing to torture survivors, if they are even remotely reminiscent of torture. Examples include electrocardiography resembling electric torture, taking blood samples resembling torture with needles, and dental treatment resembling torture to the oral cavity and teeth.

Major and thus more stressful diagnostic procedures may be necessary to perform under general anesthesia to protect against discomfort, anxiety, and pain. However, general anesthesia also requires special considerations toward the torture survivor. The fear of losing consciousness and thereby control of oneself may be overwhelming, probably because it recalls the fear of dying during torture. Therefore, the anesthetist should take enough time in talking to the patient and in establishing a relationship of trust. It is preferable if the patient can be accompanied to the examination by nursing staff or another person whom he or she already knows and trusts. That person should stay with the patient during induction of anesthesia until the patient is asleep and intubated. The same person should also be present during the recovery from anesthesia.

Naturally, the same precautions apply to any kind of surgery under local or general anesthesia. The postoperative period requires efficient analgesic treatment, considerate nursing care, and time to talk the experience over with the patient.

Framework for Examination and Treatment

The first systematic examination of a group of torture survivors was carried out during the early 1980s on an inpatient basis at the University Hospital in Copenhagen (Rigshospitalet). The project included examination of all organ systems clinically as well as paraclinically, including an extended blood test screening, radiological and neuroradiological evaluation, EKG, EEG, neuropsychological examination, tests of endocrine function, and the like. The examinations were performed on approximately 30 torture survivors who had all given their acceptance to the purpose of obtaining knowledge about the sequelae of torture possibly leading to cure and prevention. The results form the basis of outpatient examination and treatment at the Rehabilitation Centre for Torture Victims (RCT) in Copenhagen, as it turned out that almost all examined persons had normal test results, and that symptoms requiring hospital treatment or sophisticated diagnostic procedures constituted a small minority. It was decided, therefore, that the routine program for all referrals to the RCT should include a general medical examination, examination of joints and muscles by a rheumatologist, eye and ear examinations, EKG and a chemical screening which required limited technical resources that could be carried out in an outpatient structure. Specialist consultants, additional paraclinical tests, and hospitalization are used only when warranted by the patient's symptoms.

This structure has the advantage that the treatment and responsibility rest with a small number of persons, all of whom the client gets to know; and that the client goes through a minimum number of examinations without danger of misdiagnosis. Geographic separation from a hospital or other large institutions, which is desirable for the previously mentioned reasons, is also obtained by creating a small outpatient nucleus dedicated to the one task of rehabilitation of torture victims.

Apart from the permanent medical staff, a number of other specialist consultants are called upon when necessary. These specialists are chosen on the basis of their particular interest in torture survivors. On the first visit, the torture survivor is accompanied to and from the specialist treatment by a person whom he or she already knows and trusts.

If hospitalization becomes necessary, it should take place in only one department where the staff have special interest and knowledge in dealing with torture survivors. The responsibility for the hospital course should rest with or at least be supervised by the admitting doctor, because a single person should have the responsibility for coordinating the various specialist examinations and treatments thereby observing the principles outlined above, so that the physical and psychological strain on the patient is as negligible as possible. It is also the responsibility of the same doctor to discuss with the patient the contemplated procedures, and, subsequently, to explain the test result and its consequences to the patient. If these rules are not observed, the patient may pass through the hands of many different doctors, some of them perhaps only once or twice. This procedure makes the patient confused, and at worst the examination and treatment are unsuccessful. An irreparable loss of trust in the therapist may also arise making both diagnosis/treatment of somatic disease and psychotherapy impossible.

General Complaints of Torture Survivors: Diagnosis and Treatment

The most frequent complaints of torture survivors relate to the central nervous system (85%), the motor system (90%), the heart (75%), and the gastrointestinal tract (70%). They are often related to general stress rather than to exposure to specific torture methods.

Complaints from the *central nervous system* are dominated by headache. The headache is of a psychomyogenic type and is often significantly relieved or disappears completely along with a mental improvement through psychotherapy. Almost as frequent are complaints which at first glance suggest dementia, such as difficulties in concentrating and learning, poor memory, adaptation problems, irritability, and sleep disorders. The general clinical impression is often that of a "pseudodementia" caused by another underlying psychological cause. This impression can be confirmed by neuro-

psychological examination. The complaints are related to psychodynamic disorders as a consequence of the torture, for example, posttraumatic stress disorder (PTSD). The psychodynamic disturbances are the target of well-directed psychotherapy. Again, it is characteristic that the complaints decline as successful psychotherapy progresses.

Symptoms from the *motor system* fall mainly into two categories: (1) joint symptoms from overstretching, for example, by tight confinement or suspension, and (2) muscular pain related to tension by general stress. Low back pain is a common symptom. During imprisonment, many torture survivors have been subjected to beating on the back or forced to perform heavy labor. Both may lead to back problems. A large minority of torture survivors with back problems have symptoms which indicate lumbar root compression. The objective examination sometimes produces findings which support that suspicion (reflex differences, minor sensory changes, pain-related reduction of muscle power). "Hard findings" consistent with intervertebral disk herniation (actual paresis, dermatomic sensory changes) are rare. If radiological studies (myelography and/or CT scanning) are performed, they show mostly normal conditions or minor changes which do not suggest that improvement should be sought surgically. Back problems with or without radicular symptoms will, in most cases, be fully amenable to physiotherapy or other conservative treatment, perhaps supported by medication therapy for a short period.

Heart symptoms typically involve complaints of palpitation, stabbing in the heart region, and dyspnea. Many torture survivors are convinced that they suffer from heart disease, especially if they have been subjected to electric torture on the thorax. General clinical examination, EKG, and chest X rays are often sufficient to determine that this is not the case. *Hypertension-arterialis* is described as part of the concentration camp syndrome, and its presence should also be considered in torture survivors (Eitinger, 1973). The population of torture survivors who were examined at the RCT is composed of young people (typically 25–35 years), and the observation period is a few years at most. This could explain why high blood pressure has been only rarely encountered among the treated torture survivors.

Symptoms from the *gastrointestinal tract* are often suggestive of peptic ulcer or gastritis. In these cases, X rays or gastroscopy will show the expected changes, with gastritis being more frequent than peptic ulcers. In the mild cases of gastritis, antacids and nutritional guidance are fully sufficient; severe cases and ulcer patients benefit well from H_2 antagonists. Complaints of bloating, nausea, diarrhea, constipation, loathing of food, and consequent uniform diet and possible weight loss may well coexist with typical ulcer complaints. Sometimes these problems are explained as irritable colon, but the pathoanatomical basis is significantly less tangible than in ulcer/gastritis patients. Treatment consists of nutritional guidance and eating in calm surroundings. There is no specific treatment and the problems disappear with the mental improvement in the patient.

The above-mentioned complaints are present in almost all untreated torture survivors (Rasmussen & Marcussen, 1982). From a number of other organ systems, there are complaints which are frequent, but do not show up with the same regularity. (1) *Symptoms from the eyes* are most frequently uncharacteristic visual disorders (previously called cerebral asthenopia). Furthermore, there may be visual disorders which are often related to severe headache. (2) *Pulmonary complaints* involving dry cough are occasional complaints. Thorough stethoscopy and chest X ray should be performed; on simultaneous presence of lymphadenopathy, fever, chronic fatigue, and perhaps anemia, the search should be intensified for pulmonary disease or chronic infection. Many torture survivors have experienced deplorable sanitary conditions, bad cells without protection against climatic changes, and a poor-quality diet. On occurrence of relevant symptoms, these patients should thus be examined for tuberculosis or other endemic infectious diseases from their area of origin. (3) *Gynecological complaints* can result because chronic stress often produces disorders in the menstrual cycle, most often oligomenorrhea or perhaps amenorrhea. Abdominal or pelvic pain is often complained of by female torture survivors. Many of them have been subjected to sexual violations, electric torture, or other kinds of instrumental torture to the genitalia. This in itself indicates the necessity of a gynecological exam (e.g., to exclude chronic pelvic inflammation).

Specific Symptoms Related to Torture Methods

Apart from the diffuse stress reaction and psychological suffering which torture inflicts on the victim, there may be acute as well as chronic symptoms and findings from the organs at which the torture was directed.

Many torture survivors have been exposed to situations which are potentially brain damaging, such as (1) direct cranial trauma, with or without subsequent unconsciousness; (2) anoxic episodes caused by submersion or airway obstruction until the stage of fainting; and (3) electric torture with convulsions and consequently insufficient respiration. It was mentioned above that the neuropsychological examination rarely confirms suspicion of organic brain damage. Clinical/neurological examination, CT scan of the brain, and EEG are almost always normal.

Uncharacteristic visual disorders are mentioned above. However, there are also symptoms from the eyes which are specifically related to torture methods; for example, chronic irritation and conjunctivitis following submersion in contaminated water, direct eye lesions, and cataract which, in some cases, must be suspected to be traumatically induced.

Symptoms from ears/hearing are almost always directly related to the torture method. Repeated beatings on the ears result in damage to the middle ear with subsequent conduction disorders. Labyrinth damage and all degrees of nerve deafness are also seen as direct sequelae of head trauma.

Corresponding to the infectious/irritative condition in the eyes following "submarino," there are similar otologic sequelae of submarino; such as otitis externa/eczema of the auditory canal, chronic otitis media, and sequelae from previous untreated acute otitides. Owing to the social disablement which potentially lies in impaired hearing (especially in the torture survivor, who besides having to overcome the sequelae of torture, also has to handle the exile situation and learn a completely new language), it is important to diagnose even minor hearing impairment and to establish contact to an otologist for a correct diagnosis and treatment, being, for example, reconstructive middle ear surgery or a hearing aid recommendation.

Many torture survivors have marks on their skin after the torture to which they have been subjected. The legal validity of such evidence is obvious. In most cases, the scars warrant no treatment, but if they are disfiguring or in any other way a problem (e.g., because of contractures) they will often be amenable to surgical correction. Examples are facial scars, disfiguring scars in other places, scars close to joints with consequent contractures, and secreting sinus connected in depth to, for example, chronic osteomyelitis.

Fractures can be diagnosed by X ray. Like skin changes, they may have important legal validity. Although infrequently encountered, there are a number of conditions after fracture which may require corrective treatment (e.g., malalignment, pseudoarthroses, or chronic osteomyelitis).

Conclusion

In the above text, I explained how the physician has a significant role in treatment and rehabilitation of torture survivors. In most cases, the physician can exclude any somatic disease which either the present symptoms or the torture history might suggest. In these cases, it is fully sufficient to perform a general medical examination together with the short screening program mentioned. This can be done by one or two consultations and, after this, the emphasis is on psychotherapy.

In some cases, physical torture sequelae require further medical diagnosis and treatment, and perhaps hospitalization. The special considerations and caveats in dealing with torture survivors should be conscientiously observed by the involved medical and paramedical staff.

References

Danish Medical Association and The International Rehabilitation and Research Centre for Torture Victims. (1987). Doctors, ethics and torture (Proceedings of an International Meeting, Copenhagen). *Danish Medical Bulletin, 34,* 185–216.

Eitinger, L. (1973). Late effects of imprisonment in concentration camps during World War II. In *Physical and mental consequences of imprisonment and torture* (pp. 89–113). London: Amnesty International.

Juhler, M., & Vesti, P. (1989). Torture: Diagnosis and rehabilitation *Medicine and War, 5,* 69–79.

Rasmussen, O. V., & Marcussen, H. (1982). The somatic sequelae of torture. *Maanedsskrift for Praktisk Laegegerning, 3,* 124–140.

Stover, E., & Nightingale, E. O. (Eds.). (1985). *The breaking of bodies and minds.* New York: W. H. Freeman.

Intervention, Clinical Treatment, and Psychotherapy
Approaches to Recovery and Treatment

Part VII contains 11 chapters on the clinical treatment of traumatic stress syndromes. These chapters present different approaches to aiding persons who are suffering from posttraumatic stress disorder and associated conditions, such as depression, substance abuse, and personality alterations. This section includes discussion of pharmacological considerations, focal psychoanalytic techniques, neurocognitive stress deconditioning procedures, group psychotherapy, inpatient specialty programs for PTSD, and 12-step self-help programs.

In Chapter 65, Frank M. Ochberg discusses posttraumatic therapy (PTT), a specific approach to treatment that has arisen out of the author's extensive psychiatric work with victimized persons. Ochberg begins by defining the fundamental principles of PTT: (1) PTSD is a normal reaction to extremely stressful life events; (2) to overcome phases of reexperiencing and negative affect, the client must be empowered through a collaborative relationship with the therapist; and (3) each individual has a unique pathway to recovery. With these fundamental concepts established as the core orientation in PTT, Ochberg proceeds to elaborate the techniques of the therapeutic approach, which is both holistic and eclectic in nature. The result is a clearly written set of guidelines to assist clinicians in working with the intricacies of PTSD, especially for professionals with little experience in treating victims of massive trauma.

In Chapter 66, Matthew J. Friedman discusses the psychobiological and pharmacological approaches to the treatment of PTSD. Friedman's chapter integrates well with van der Kolk and Saporta's explication of PTSD in Chapter 2. However, Friedman focuses on the various psychobiological strategies for intervention with medication to regulate brain functioning, especially in terms of the hyperarousal condition inherent in PTSD. He states that

> Neuropharmacological and neuroendocrinological observations in PTSD patients suggest that exposure to trauma can evoke persistent biological abnormalities. Some, but not all, research findings to date indicate that PTSD may be associated with a hyperadrenergic state, hypofunctioning of the hypothalamic-pituitary-adrenocortical (HPA) axis and dysregulation of the endogenous opioid system.

Friedman then reviews the research literature on the brain-behavior relationship in PTSD and discusses how pharmacological approaches (e.g., tricyclic antidepressants) are showing success in symptom reduction and aiding the process of deconditioning the hyperaroused state in the HPA axis. Moreover, the relationship between PTSD and substance abuse, especially alcohol dependence, is explained within the psycho biological framework:

> The adrenergic hyperarousal and opioid dysregulation associated with PTSD may make affected individuals particularly susceptible to chemical abuse/dependency. . . . The implications for treatment are clear. When PTSD and chemical dependency occur simultaneously, they must be treated simultaneously. Unfortunately, most (especially inpatient) treatment approaches attempt to treat the two disorders sequentially rather than simultaneously. . . . Such an approach is doomed to failure because it fails to acknowledge programmatically that the complex self-sustaining interrelationships between intrapsychic, behavioral, and biological aspects of PTSD and concurrent chemical abuse/dependency demand a comprehensive approach.

In Chapter 67, George S. Everly, Jr., continues a discussion of the neurophysiological considerations in the treatment of PTSD. Everly considers PTSD as a disorder of arousal and that the "phenomenological epicenter of PTSD resides in a functional neurologic hypersensitivity within the anatomical boundaries of the limbic system." Thus, consistent with the research of van der Kolk and Saporta in Chapter 2 and that of Friedman in Chapter 66, Everly proposes that PTSD be treated as a disorder of arousal. The goal of treatment, then, is to effect neurological desensitization—a shift from ergotropic functioning to a trophotropic one—to reduce arousal at both the central and peripheral levels.

Based on his review of the experimental research on the HPA axis, Everly discusses a number of clinical techniques that can be employed to achieve neurological desensitization. These include the induction of the relaxation response, hypnosis, and cognitive behavioral therapy designed to facilitate a restructuring of the distressing, intrusive recollections of the trauma.

In Chapter 68, Jacob D. Lindy presents a discussion of the use of focal psychoanalytic psychotherapy of PTSD. He begins by noting that focal psychoanalysis

> distinguishes itself from other treatment modalities in that its focus is on the meaning of trauma-related symptoms and behaviors and on the meaning of catastrophic life events to the person as a whole. The analytically oriented therapist is also curious about the ways in which a person's psyche and soma fend off, experience, cope, and adapt to extreme stress.

Lindy suggests that the process of focal psychoanalysis for PTSD can be divided into three phases: opening, middle, and terminal. Each phase has its own focus and purpose, such as establishing the therapeutic alliance and discovering the "meaning configuration" of the trauma for the client. Lindy notes that this is not always an easy thing to accomplish because of the difficulty for the victim to fully disclose, remember, and make sense of what happened in the traumatic event and the powerful nature of countertransference reactions in working with PTSD. The successful management of these reactions through a stance of genuine empathy allows the therapeutic process to unfold. In the last phase, however, Lindy notes that

> even after the survivor achieves considerable mastery over the trauma, separating from the therapist is often difficult. It requires attending to the newly formed continuity between the pre- and posttraumatic self, and often it must acknowledge the incompleteness of the recovery. Setting a final date sets off unworked-through grief and mourning that are connected with the traumatic memories. Increased energy, altruism, and sublimation of trauma are often rewarding consequences to the survivor and to the therapist.

In Chapter 69, Noach Milgram discusses principles of traumatic stress prevention in Israel. Milgram notes that the State of Israel has been subject to many threats and stressors because of its conflicted relationship with Palestine and other Arab states in the region. These various stressor events (e.g., war, terrorist attacks, high potential of threat, etc.) have been continuous in nature and are experienced by large segments of the population. Given the history of a substantial potential for reoccurrences, the question naturally centers on how people cope with such adversity. Milgram states that "there are certain peculiar features of life in Israel today that appear to have buffered many citizens against the deleterious effects of war-related stressful events. These features may be conceptualized as principles of traumatic stress prevention or management."

The author reviews three major approaches to stress prevention and management: (1) stress inoculation, (2) indoctrination (i.e., ideological conviction), and (3) implosion techniques of desensitization and incongruity reduction. In his conclusion, Milgram draws an analogy between a state and a therapist:

> Societies function like therapists for the potential and real stress reactions and disorders of their members. . . . Applying the stress and coping paradigm to an entire society may help social and behavioral scientists and practitioners better assess the strengths and weaknesses of the society and facilitate professional planning for large-scale primary and secondary stress intervention.

In Chapter 70, Erwin Randolph Parson presents an analysis of posttraumatic narcissism (a form of self-disorder) which affects some victims of trauma with PTSD. In order to treat posttraumatic narcissism, Parson argues that group psychotherapy is the method of choice for effective intervention. In particular, the author discusses the use of group therapy in the treatment of Vietnam veterans.

Many specialists who work with PTSD have noted that narcissistic scarring to the self is common and may be expressed in lowered self-esteem, identity changes, states of rage and aggression, as well as a grandiose sense of entitlement and exploitative interpersonal relationships. Parson reviews the clinical literature on narcissistic states and explains their relationship to trauma and victimization. With this perspective established, he next proceeds to outline a model of group psychotherapy which is closed-ended and time-limited for about eight members. Parson suggests that there are six phases to group psychotherapy: "(1) effectance, (2) uncertitude (fragmented sense of power), (3) essential trust and dependency, (4) autonomy and interdependence, (5) initiative and responsibility, and (6) self-cohesion."

In each of the six phases, the process of therapy is discussed with a focus on the emergent themes and symptoms which are manifest as part of the restorative attempt at healing the narcissistic injury produced to the self-structure by the traumatic event. In his conclusion, Parson states:

> Treating posttraumatic narcissistic disorders in Vietnam veterans and in other survivors is a complicated matter, requiring a multiplicity of conceptual bases and the application of a number of techniques. The Curvilinear Regressive-Progressive Group (CuRePro) model was applied to demonstrate the complexities of unconscious developmental motivations of the group. . . . Most chronic traumatic states have often caused significant character alterations, which become embedded and structuralized into the self-system. Long-term treatment as suggested by the CuRePro model would be appropriate in these instances.

In Chapter 71, Henry Krystal discusses therapeutic considerations in PTSD based on his extensive experience in working with Holocaust survivors. After a general review of theoretical and clinical perspectives of PTSD, Krystal lays out his paradigm of adult catastrophic trauma:

> When an individual concludes that the impending danger is not avoidable, and that the situation is hopeless, and when that individual surrenders to it, then the affective response changes to a catatonic-like reaction. . . . When we study posttraumatic states retrospectively, we find that remaining in the traumatic situation for a significant period of time, the catatonic-like reaction initiates or continues into a traumatic state. When individuals judge themselves to be totally helpless in the face of overwhelming danger and surrender to it, an evolution-determined pattern is initiated, which is common to all animals, and since it may end in a purely psychogenic death . . . it may be said that individuals carry their self-destruct outfit at all times.

In Krystal's view, traumatic events dramatically affect hedonic regulation, cognition processes, and the capacity for bonding and intimacy.

When the motivational system of hedonic regulation is adversely affected by trauma, the victim may manifest anhedonia and alexithymia, or, alternately, unmodulated affect which is painful and unbearable. The configuration and structure of a trauma within a person may vary depending on its developmental onset. Krystal notes that there are at least three trauma patterns which he labels as infantile, child, and adult trauma patterns. Thus, depending on the severity of the traumatic experience, the consequence is likely to include impairment in the capacity for basic trust, alexithymia and anhedonia, as well as the quality of ego identity.

The narcissistic scar to the self-structure presents a challenge to the therapist. According to Krystal: "The therapeutic orientation must address itself to the major injury: the fragmentation of the self-representation, and the repression of the 'opposite side' in victim/perpetrator duality by erecting powerful defenses against reintegration of it." Thus, in order for psychotherapy to be fully successful, it is necessary for the traumatized patient to form a therapeutic alliance in order to rebond in a trusting relationship characterized by empathy. However, one of the difficulties in treatment is that the presence of anhedonia and alexithymia may prevent the patient from identifying and confronting feelings which were defensively numbed for purposes of survival. Furthermore, the layers of defense associated with affect regulation may be so strong that the victim fears that by letting-go of them, he or she will be rendered vulnerable again and regress back to a catatonic-like state approximating death itself. When this is the case, there is often little transference that would permit systematic interpretation and the working-through of the traumatic material.

In Chapter 72, Ofra Ayalon discusses posttraumatic stress recovery of terrorist survivors. Specifically, she analyzes the effects of three terrorist attacks on families who were living in villages in Israel between the years 1974 to 1980. The attacks involved murder, kidnapping, and abusive violence. Additionally, the author lists the stressors which typify terrorist activities: (1) fear of death, (2) arbitrariness, (3) uncertainty, (4) frustration, (5) exposure to cruelty, (6) confrontation with violence, and (7) ambivalent attachment to the aggressor. The initial emotional reactions to such experiences included anxiety and fear reactions, depressive reactions, paranoid reactions, and perceptual distortion (e.g., time deceleration).

In a manner similar to stress prevention as discussed by Milgram in Chapter 69, Ayalon describes a multilevel set of strategies for intervention and treatment of the survivors. First, she underscores the need for "circles of support" since "insufficient support and its danger of secondary victimization on the part of society increase the importance of community intervention." Second, techniques of stress inoculation and psychological immunization are reviewed and considered important in terms of limiting the severity of emotional damage that might be produced by future terrorists' acts. Third, brief psychotherapy and critical incident stress debriefing are techniques for addressing acute psychological reactions in the wake of a terrorist attack.

The chapter concludes with nine recommendations that summarize "the similarities and differences between short-term therapy for terrorist victims and short-term therapy for victims of other crises."

In Chapter 73, Joel Osler Brende outlines a 12-step recovery program for victims of traumatic events. Twelve-step programs have been widely used to treat addictions, such as alcoholism, and have evolved throughout the years as paradigms of self-help groups. Brende adapts the model program of Alcoholics Anonymous (AA) to a recovery program for persons suffering from PTSD and notes seven general principles of treatment which are similar to those proposed by Ochberg in Chapter 65 for posttraumatic therapy. Among the core principles are those of the admission of helplessness and surrender, the willingness to acknowledge that PTSD has become destructive in their lives, the need for intragroup support, education about the disorder, and the trust in a higher power for spiritual strength.

In Chapter 74, Raymond M. Scurfield discusses an in-patient program to treat PTSD among Vietnam veterans. This rich chapter chronicles the evolution and development of a unique program at the American Lake Veterans Administration medical facility in Tacoma, Washington, which is one of several programs specially designed for the treatment of PTSD.

Following a theoretical and conceptual overview of the central objectives of the in-patient program, 11 principles of treatment are presented. These 11 principles overlap with the others discussed in the chapters in Part VII and clearly show the convergence in the accumulating body of knowledge in terms of approaches to psychotherapy. For example, Scurfield discusses the establishment of the therapeutic alliance; educational programs about PTSD; the facilitation of reliving traumatic events; exposure to symptom-producing stimuli; the use of medication; placing the trauma in a whole-life perspective; and out-patient aftercare.

Similar to the arguments put forth by Parson in Chapter 70, Scurfield discusses the advantages and disadvantages of peer-group treatment. When a person has been screened and deemed appropriate for treatment, a set of guidelines and rules is established regarding the small group therapy process. These rules (e.g., no violence, weapons, or substance abuse; insured confidentiality) help to establish boundaries and limits which focus the painful work of self-disclosure and the cognitive restructuring of the traumatic experiences.

Moreover, as the treatment progresses, there appears to be a natural progression of themes which emerge among the group members. By the end of the peer-group treatment, the focus has shifted away from war experiences onto current life choices and situations. Noteworthy, too, in this chapter is the discussion and suggestion on the management of countertransference reactions among staff members. Since powerful countertransference reactions are expectable, if not unavoidable reactions in the treatment of PTSD, it is important to design ways programmatically to facilitate their resolution in order to avoid burnout or ineffective therapeutic responses to the patients.

In Chapter 75, the last chapter in Part VII, Yael Danieli discusses the treatment of Holocaust survivors and their children. It is clear from the accumulating body of scientific evidence that internment in the Nazi concentration camps or being a partisan in hiding or in resistance against enemy forces was a profoundly stressful experience that left an emotional legacy for those who survived it. It is also the case, as noted by Harel and his colleagues in Chapter 20, that many Holocaust survivors have been able to reconstruct social networks and live normal lives. Yet, for those who have sought out professional care, the adverse effects of the Holocaust have had prolonged effects in their lives and within their families.

As the director of the Group Project for Holocaust Survivors and Their Children in New York City, Danieli brings a wealth of experience to the understanding of posttraumatic reactions to the victims of the Nazi Holocaust. This chapter summarizes many clinical insights into the difficulties in working with this population, such as powerful countertransference reactions among psychotherapists. Unique to this chapter is the use and illustration of the "Family Tree" to describe intergenerational effects of the Holocaust experience. This technique is simultaneously creative, heuristic, and informative because it distills a great amount of information into a graphic form which can lead to new clinical insights into psychodynamic functioning.

CHAPTER 65

Posttraumatic Therapy

Frank M. Ochberg

Introduction

Most victims of violence never seek professional therapy to deal with the emotional impact of traumatic events. If they did, they would be sorely disappointed. There are not enough therapists in the world to treat the millions of men, women, and children who have been assaulted, abused, and violated as a result of war, tyranny, crime, disaster, and family violence. When people do seek help, suffering with posttraumatic symptoms, they may find therapists who are ill equipped to provide assistance. The credentialed clinicians in psychiatry, psychology, nursing, social work, and the allied professions are only recently learning to catalog, evaluate, and refine a therapeutic armamentarium to serve traumatized clients. The ambitious collection of chapters in this volume is one such arsenal. The prodigious efforts of Charles Figley, co-founder of the Society for Traumatic Stress, and organizer of the Psychosocial Stress book series (Brunner/Mazel) and the Stress and Coping Series (Plenum Press), are important resources for professionals concerned with traumatic stress reactions. A cadre of clinicians have also shared insights and approaches, face-to-face, and through written works, defining principles and techniques that address the worldwide problem of posttraumatic readjustment. Recently, I assembled a sampling of those clinical insights (Ochberg, 1988) and attempted to define the commonalities in assumptions and approaches to therapy. The common ground is the foundation of posttraumatic therapy (PTT). The individual distinctions that separate clinicians who share this common ground are the inevitable differences of creative minds.

Frank M. Ochberg • Department of Psychiatry, Michigan State University, East Lansing, Michigan 48824. The material addressed in this chapter was previously published, in a slightly different format, in *Psychotherapy*, Volume 28, No. 1, Spring, 1991.

International Handbook of Traumatic Stress Syndromes, edited by John P. Wilson and Beverley Raphael. Plenum Press, New York, 1993.

My purpose in this chapter is to enlarge upon the foundation of PTT and clarify some of the clinical techniques that stand upon this foundation.

Foundation of Posttraumatic Therapy

Fundamental Principles

Several principles are fundamental to posttraumatic therapy, and discussing these at the outset of therapy is usually advisable. Since traumatized and victimized individuals are, by definition, reacting to abnormally stressful events, they may confuse the abnormality of the trauma with abnormality of themselves.

The first principle of PTT is, therefore, *the normalization principle*: There is a general pattern of posttraumatic adjustment and the thoughts and feelings that comprise this pattern are normal, although they may be painful and perplexing, and perhaps not well-understood by individuals and professionals not familiar with such expectable reactions. The word normal can mean many things. Offer and Sabshin (1966) described, among other connotations, the use of the term normal to designate health, an ideal, and a statistical mode. When a doctor says, "This is a normal reaction," any or all of those three possibilities could be implied. For example, after breaking a bone, a patient has the fracture examined and set. A few days later there is pain and swelling, some itching under the cast, but good circulation and no sign of infection or nerve damage. The doctor has seen this pattern many times before, knows the physiological reasons for discomfort, and the danger signals of disease. The doctor's reassurance, "This is normal," means that a healthy healing process is underway. Further explanation of the healing pattern allows the patient to participate actively in the recovery process, understanding the reasons for symptoms, the time course of reequilibration, and the signs of abnormal interference, such as a wound infection.

The emotional healing process often includes *reexperiencing, avoidance, sensitivity,* and *self-blame*. These symptoms are easily described, explained, and "set" in a context of adaptation and eventual mastery. By sharing such information, the second principle of PTT, the *collaborative* and *empowering principle*, is recognized: The therapeutic relationship must be collaborative, leading to empowerment of one who has been diminished in dignity and security. This principle is particularly important in work with victims of violent crime. The exposure to human cruelty, the feeling of dehumanization, and the experience of powerlessness create a diminished sense of self. This diminution is normal when it is proportional to the victimization. Survivors of natural disasters experience powerlessness, too, although they are not subjected to cruelty and subjugation. They benefit greatly from a therapeutic alliance that is experienced as collegial and empowering.

A third principle is the *individuality* principle: Every individual has a unique pathway to recovery after traumatic stress. Cannon (1939) and Selye (1956) may have identified common physiological and psychological reactions in states of extreme stress, but Weybrew (1967) and others noted the complexity of the human stress response and the fact that one's pattern is as singular as a fingerprint. This principle suggests that a unique pathway of posttraumatic adjustment is to be anticipated and valued, and not to be feared or disparaged. Therapist and client will walk the path together, aware of a general direction, of predictable pitfalls, but ready to discover new truths at every turn.

These three principles can be expressed in various ways and supplemented with other important tenets. For example, an appreciation of coping skills rather than personality limitations allows therapy to proceed without undue emphasis on negative characteristics, and the devastating implication that victimization is deserved (Wilson, 1988). PTT begins with the assumption that a normal individual encountered an abnormal event. To ameliorate the painful consequences, one must mobilize coping mechanisms. How dramatically different this is from the hypothesis that posttraumatic stress disorder and victimization symptoms are products of personality flaws and neurotic defenses that must be identified and treated according to traditional paradigms! Furthermore, an interdisciplinary approach, recognizing the contributions of biology, psychology, and social dynamics, stimulates clinician and client to see beyond any singular explanation for posttraumatic suffering and to search for remedies in many different fields. The contributions of pharmacology, education, nutrition, social work, law, and history are recognized and valued. Interventions may include introduction to a self-help network, exposure to inspirational literature, explanation of the victims' rights movement, establishment of an exercise regimen, or prescription of anxiolytics. PTT is interdisciplinary. Practitioners should therefore be aware of community resources that are of potential benefit and be willing to assess the merit of these adjuncts to their direct clinical intervention. Often, this requires personal meetings with colleagues from disparate fields. To some degree it also requires a cognitively flexible attitude as to how best serve the patient suffering from PTSD who may need many special (yet not traditional) therapeutic interventions to facilitate the stress recovery process.

Techniques of Posttraumatic Therapy

Many techniques have been used effectively to help survivors readjust after traumatic events. I have found it useful to classify the various methods into four categories:

1. The first category is educational and includes sharing books and articles, teaching the basic concepts of physiology to allow an appreciation of the stress response, discussing civil and criminal law with new participants in the process, and introducing the fundamentals of holistic health. The educational process is one of mutual exchange (i.e., a "two-way street"). The client may have resources that he or she finds helpful and wants to share with the clinician.

2. The second grouping of techniques falls within the category of holistic health. Although the term *holistic health* has its critics as well as its supporters, I offer it in the spirit of Merwin and Smith-Kurtz (1988), who noted how physical activity, nutrition, spirituality, and humor contribute to the healing of the whole person. The clinician who promotes these aspects of healing serves as a teacher and a coach, offering concepts that might be new to the client, and shaping abilities that may be latent.

3. The third category includes methods that enhance social support and social integration. Family and group therapy could be included here. Exposure to self-help and support groups in the community are other examples. But most important is the sensitive assessment of social skills, the enhancement of these skills, the reduction of irrational fears, and the expert timing of encouragement to risk new relationships. Traditional analytical tools and traditional social work skills are employed to promote healing in supportive human groups.

4. Finally, there are clinical techniques that are best categorized as therapy. These include working through grief, extinguishing the fear response that accompanies traumatic imagery, judicious use of medication for target symptoms, the telling of the trauma story, role play, hypnotherapy, and many individualized methods that are consistent with the principles of PTT.

These four clusters of techniques are not comprehensive. There are innovations that defy categorization, such as the Native American sweat lodge technique (and other techniques of healing and purification) discussed by Wilson (1988) and testimony of political repression, used as a therapeutic instrument (see Chapters 55 and 57, in this volume; Cienfuegos & Monelli, 1983). But it is not my purpose here to prepare an exhaustive catalog of techniques. My intent is to explain those approaches that I have employed, in residential (Ochberg & Fojtik, 1984) and in outpatient settings, with victimized, traumatized clients.

Education

Reading the DSM Together

I will never forget the first time I brought out my green, hardbound copy of the DSM-III (American Psychiatric Association, 1980), moved my chair next to Mrs.

M., and showed her the chapter on PTSD. Mrs. M. is a thin, soft-spoken woman in her thirties who was assaulted and raped in South Lansing, Michigan. She was referred by a colleague and had just finished telling me her symptoms, 8 or 9 weeks after the traumatic event. She was frightened, guarded, perplexed, and sad. She had no basis for trusting me. But after she saw the words in the book, as I read them aloud, she brightened, sat up tall, and said, "You mean, that's me, in that book! I never thought this could be real."

Seldom have I found such a reversal of mood and such a sudden establishment of trust and rapport since Mrs. M., but I have never missed an opportunity to read the criteria list with a client, when it seemed appropriate.

The responses vary, from satisfaction that the symptoms are officially recognized, to surprise that anybody else has a similar syndrome. Some patients take pride in making their own diagnosis, pointing out exactly which symptoms apply. Few show any interest in other sections of the book. Most seem to enjoy hearing my explanation of the trouble we (i.e., the members of the American Psychiatric Association committee on PTSD criteria) had formulating the diagnostic category—how some of us argued for placing the description in the "V Code" section with other "normal" reactions, such as "uncomplicated bereavement," but others prevailed and the practical consequence of placing this normal reaction to abnormal events in the chapter on anxiety is that insurance companies pay their fair share of the bill!

Reading the DSM-III (American Psychiatric Association, 1980) or DSM-III-R (American Psychiatric Association, 1987) together begins the educative and collaborative process. It opens the door to further education about the physiology of stress and the range of human responses to adversity. The DSM-IV is scheduled for production in 1993, and the architects are considering a "Victim Sequelae Disorder," in addition to PTSD (R. L. Spitzer, S. J. Kaplan, & D. Pelcovitz, personal communication, 1989). This should help clinicians and clients, since the list of potential criteria supplements the PTSD symptoms and includes those common features that affect *victimized* rather than *traumatized* individuals. I have long considered the distinction important (Ochberg, 1984, 1986, 1988, 1989) and am delighted to see it considered in the DSM-IV (see Appendixes 1 and 2 at the end of this chapter).

Introducing Civil and Criminal Law

A therapist need not be a lawyer to know about the law. When our clients face the criminal justice system for the first time, understandably they may be concerned, confused, and overwhelmed.

Mr. A. was shot in the abdomen at close range by an intruder and almost killed. After heroic surgery, he awoke to the hubbub of an intensive care unit. Between hallucinations, he learned what occurred, received family visits, and began looking at mug shots. His introduction to the world of detectives, prosecutors and judges was better than most. They appreciated his condition

and worked slowly and sensitively, after realizing the futility of expecting a positive identification. He appreciated their professional responsibilities and their regard for him. Would it were always so!

Victims of violent crime are often treated like pawns in an impersonal bureaucracy (Young, 1988). President Ronald Reagan realized this in commissioning the President's Task Force on Crime Victims (1982), and the U.S. Congress followed suit by passing the Victims of Crime Act of 1984.

Usually, I offer clients who are victims of violent crime several articles and brochures that explain their rights under state law and the role of the victim-witness in the American judicial justice system. In the United States, Michigan is blessed with a model victims' rights law (Ochberg, 1988 Van Regenmorter, 1989), and a Crime Victim's Compensation Board that provides financial aid. Clinicians who counsel victims could easily find resources and references in their own states. I find that many clinicians, even in Michigan, are unaware of these resources, but are pleased to know that a portion of their bills can be paid by the state, if their clients report their victimization within a year of the crime.

A patient who is in the middle of a trial, cooperating fully with the prosecutor, may know nothing of his or her right to sue the assailant, to have a court injunction against harassment, to receive workers compensation, and, in some instances, to receive representation from the *pro bono* committee of the county bar association. Moreover, finding the right lawyer is as difficult as finding the right therapist, so I pay close attention to my patients' experiences with attorneys and maintain an up-to-date referral roster. Sharing information about legal resources is part of the education process.

Discussing Psychobiology

Few clients are interested in reading about autonomic nervous system activation, but some read voraciously. To understand the physiology of mammalian arousal during stress is to begin mobilizing the mind in pursuit of recovery. It is relatively easy to impart a basic understanding of the fight/flight mechanism (Cannon, 1939) and the General Adaptation Syndrome (Selye, 1956). Wilson (1989) and Merwin and Smith-Kurtz (1988) explained the concepts clearly and Roth (1988) and van der Kolk (1988) discuss more complex implications in the same volume (Ochberg, 1988). Without turning therapy into a didactic exercise, without burdening the client with unsolicited instruction, one can convey the fact that lethal threat has a powerful impact on body chemistry; that our adrenal glands are stimulated; that we are prepared to fight or to flee as if we were facing a wild beast, millennia ago; that all this circuitry is out of date and usually destructive when we face threats in modern society; that PTSD is the predictable outcome in general after extraordinary stress; and that everyone's individual pattern is different.

Furthermore, vigorous use of the large muscles is the intended result of adrenal activation, and physical activity is an advisable measure to ameliorate the effects of PTSD. This point leads to the next educational objective.

Reviewing Concepts of Fitness and Holistic Health

In designing the milieu and program of the Dimondale Stress Reduction Center (Ochberg & Fojtik, 1984), I hoped for a blend of a health spa, a community college, and a hospital. For several years, we maintained this balance but eventually the hospital bureaucracy crowded out the other elements. I was disappointed, but not surprised. American medicine, particularly hospital-based medicine, places the patient in a passive role and ignores the power of health promotion. In elementary school, we used to call health promotion "hygiene." Gym teachers, not doctors, got the points across.

Now, in an office-based, part-time practice, I do what I can to educate patients about the benefits of exercise and nutrition. The syllabus is in the Merwin and Smith-Kurtz (1988) chapter of *Post-traumatic Therapy*. My approach includes nagging, begging, and heartfelt approval when interest is shown. Since the general category of holistic health promotion includes this educational goal, let us move there now.

Promoting Holistic Health

Physical Activity

Writing about the development of a healthy fitness routine for PTT clients, Merwin and Smith-Kurtz (1988) observed that

> techniques of physical training have changed in recent years as the maxim "no pain, no gain" has been discarded. Exercising past the pain threshold risks injury to muscles, joints, or tendons. The watchwords today are "balance," "moderation," and "listen to your body."

They go on to describe the three elements of a balanced program: strength, cardiovascular efficiency, and flexibility, and they note the generally accepted activities that provide these elements. Nowadays, I find few clients who are unfamiliar with these principles, but many who lack the motivation to begin or to resume an interrupted routine. Some fear social interaction. Some have injuries that limit activity. Some are generally lacking in initiative, evidencing Criterion C.(4) of PTSD (American Psychiatric Association, 1987), "markedly diminished interest in significant activities." Relatively early in therapy, I will evaluate the client's potential for supervised physical activity. I want to know that a recent medical examination has been performed and there are no limitations or restrictions. If there are limitations, I may still promote allowable activity, but only after consultation with the examining physician.

Often, the client and I develop an exercise plan, with goals and methods listed in the record. Usually, this process occurs after a preliminary discussion of stress physiology and before agreement on overall treatment objectives. (The client may be ready to take daily walks, but not ready to discuss the details of victimization.) Agreeing on an exercise plan and fulfilling the agreement are separate issues.

When there is resistance to exercise, the resistance itself must be confronted. The therapist should not assume to know an individual's underlying motive for avoiding healthy activity. A gentle, collaborative search for the obstacles and the construction of a path around these obstacles comprise an important chapter of PTT. Having said this, I must admit that I find it very difficult to avoid the methods that ultimately motivated me to undertake a fitness routine: the unremitting urging of well-meaning friends.

Therapists are advised to become familiar with supervised, structured fitness programs in their communities. A referral to a specific YMCA, health club, or aerobic instructor can assure that the milieu is appropriate, the regimen is reasonable, and the opportunity for reinforcement is available.

I am delighted when clients adopt a healthy exercise routine, and they know it.

Nutrition

We never learned much about nutrition in medical school (other than infant formulas in pediatrics). I am still baffled by conflicting professional and lay advice on the value of various "healthy" diets. But it makes sense to evaluate a client's eating habits and look for the common mistakes that contribute to anxiety, irritability, and depression. In general, this is part of good clinical work, but particularly important for posttraumatic (Stress Syndrome) patients who are vulnerable to mood swings and who may have neglected their nutrition.

Caffeine Intoxication

The DSM-III-R (American Psychiatric Association, 1987) requires 5 out of 12 signs, plus the presence of recent excessive caffeine ingestion and the absence of other causes, to make the diagnosis of caffeine intoxication (or "caffeinism"). The 12 signs overlap with the hallmarks of panic, generalized anxiety, and aspects of PTSD: restlessness, nervousness, excitement, insomnia, flushed face, diuresis, gastrointestinal disturbance, muscle twitching, rambling flow of thought and speech, tachycardia or cardiac arrhythmia, periods of inexhaustibility, and psychomotor agitation. Clients who experience numbing may consciously or unconsciously increase their coffee consumption. A demoralized indifference to preparing and consuming adequate meals may result in excessive drinking of tea, or coffee, or alcohol. Also, caffeine is found in soft drinks, candy, and certain desserts as well as in coffee and tea. The incidence of true caffeine intoxication is relatively rare, but good clinical practice requires that we rule out the diagnosis when anxiety symptoms are present. Furthermore, a discussion of caffeine effects leads to the broader issues of diet, appetite, and meal rituals.

Meaning of Healthy Eating

Food gathering, preparation, and consumption have ritual significance in most cultures. Full participation in the family or tribe requires the equivalent of "bringing home the bacon" or "fixin' dinner" or "getting to the table on time." Food sharing is a critical aspect of nurturing and of family cohesion. When a traumatic event interferes with one's desire to eat, one's ability to face the ordeal of shopping, and one's participation in shared meals, more than nutrition is at stake. There is disruption of biochemistry, interpersonal relations, self-esteem, and connection to culture. PTT requires attention to all of these issues, agreement on desired objectives in the short-term and long-term future, and a collaborative search for remedies.

Mrs. A. developed agoraphobia in addition to PTSD after being held hostage and surviving a sexual assault. Her therapy was prolonged, involving residential and outpatient treatment. She read every book she could find about coping with stress, and understood the significance of reestablishing her role in her family and community. But a major obstacle was her fear of meeting people who knew about her assault and who felt compelled to make well-intentioned remarks about her recovery. We discussed this situation at length. As she learned to respond to the sympathetic comments of friends and acquaintances without feeling invaded, she overcame her fear of the marketplace. The later phases of PTT were supportive and nondirective. She resumed her functions in the family, and meals became a source of pleasure rather than pain.

Referral to Nutrition Experts

My community has a state-supported university with a department of food science, four hospitals with dietitians, and a professional association of dietitians that holds regular educational conferences. It is relatively easy to identify competent colleagues. Several expressed interest in counseling clients on the fundamentals of food selection and diet. They are experienced in working with eating disorder patients, but not with victims of violence and extreme stress. In those few instances where I made referrals, the outcome was generally good. The clients learned new facts and experienced a feeling of mastery. Those therapists who do not have colleagues close by to assist with nutritional counseling are advised to review the basic facts and the supplementary reference list provided in Ochberg (1988), Chapter 4.

Humor

Following the advice of my colleagues who wrote the section on humor in the chapter just mentioned (Merwin & Smith-Kurtz, 1988), I asked Mrs. R., an adult survivor of incest, to tell me about her ability to laugh. "Do you think my life is funny?" she fumed, casting a look at me that could wither an oak tree. My timing was awful. But usually I can succeed in initiating a discussion about humor, its salutary effect, and ways that we can improve our ability to laugh at ourselves. Smith-Kurtz

cites the remarkable example of Norman Cousins (1979), a genius in marshaling humor as a coping mechanism for critical illness. Furthermore, she provides techniques and references to enhance the therapist's sense of humor.

The goal in adding humor to PTT is not for the therapist to be witty, but for the client to have the capacity to laugh. A clinician can facilitate the recovery and the improvement of a client's sense of humor by setting an example, by searching for instances when the client used humor well, and by providing a good audience when spontaneous humor arises.

A week after Mrs. R. cut me down to size, I told her how clumsy a therapist can feel, trying to uncover humor and failing completely. She laughed. Now we can talk freely about her tendency toward sanctimoniousness and her neglect of humor as a healing art. She is interested in elevating her capacity for laughter, and that is a step in the right direction.

Spirituality

Long before psychology and psychiatry were invented, before medicine was a science, there were healers who treated the sick and the wounded. Sometimes they used remedies with a chemical basis for efficacy, unknown at the time (e.g., belladonna for diarrhea). But, invariably, there was a sacred, ritual dimension to the treatment. The medicine man invoked spiritual assistance. Sacrifices were required to the gods. Prayers were said, individually and collectively. There is abundant evidence that healing was facilitated (see Wilson, 1989, for a review).

The power of prayer in surviving captivity and torture is well known (Fly, 1973; Jackson, 1973), although the mechanism of action is subject to debate.

Although I once felt that religion and spirituality had no place in the clinical sciences, I am now convinced that clinicians must evaluate their clients' spiritual potential. By this I mean their ability to benefit from their own beliefs, particularly a sense of participation in universal, timeless events. For adherents to the major religions, this spiritual dimension may be conceptualized as feeling God's love. For others, spirituality may be described as a transcendent feeling of harmony and communion with humanity or Nature or the unknown reaches of space.

Merwin and Smith-Kurtz (1988) explained that

> spirituality is a state of being fully alive and open to the moment. It includes a sense of belonging and of having a place in the universe. A deep appreciation of the natural world, an openness for surprise, a gratefulness for the gratuity of everything, joy and wonderment are all a part of spirituality. Although spiritual growth is a type of healing from which most of us could benefit, a victim's sense of spirit may be acutely dimmed for a period after the victimization.
>
> Over time, however, as the victim heals in all areas, the potential for spiritual growth may become greater than ever before and greater than for many people who have not faced the reality of their individual death.

Usually, I avoid these issues early in therapy. Many patients have complained to me about clergy who focused on their own method of spiritual healing after a trauma, ignoring the feelings of the victimized individual. On the other hand, many clients have been helped by sensitive pastoral counselors, and continue seeing them while seeing me. My role is not to promote any specific spiritual approach. But after a relationship is established, after some progress has been made, I express interest in the client's experience of spirituality. Often I am surprised by the strength of religious conviction that coexists with pessimism and helplessness. In therapy, the issue then is not creating *de nova* a spiritual capacity, but identifying and overcoming the obstacles to feeling the embrace of one's faith.

An excellent example of personal triumph over childhood sexual assault, and the effects of racism and sexism, can be found in the autobiographical prose and poetry of Maya Angelou (1978). Her faith in her own indomitable spirit inspires others. I have referred her works to clients and students, when the spiritual dimension of overcoming adversity was relevant. Here is a powerful poem of hers (Angelou, 1978) that can reach the right client at the right time:

*And Still I Rise**

You may write me down in history
With your bitter, twisted lies,
You may trod me in the very dirt
But still, like dust, I'll rise.
Does my sassiness upset you?
Why are you beset with gloom?
'Cause I walk like I've got oil wells
Pumping in my living room.
Just like moons and like suns,
With the certainty of tides,
Just like hopes springing high,
Still I'll rise.
Did you want to see me broken?
Bowed head and lowered eyes?
Shoulders falling down like teardrops,
Weakened by my soulful cries.
Does my haughtiness offend you?
Don't you take it awful hard
'Cause I laugh like I've got gold mines
Diggin' in my own backyard.
You may shoot me with your words,
You may cut me with your eyes,
You may kill me with your hatefullness,
But still, like air, I'll rise . . .
Out of the huts of history's shame I rise.
Up from a past that's rooted in pain I rise . . .
Leaving behind night of terror and fear
I rise
Into a daybreak that's wondrously clear
I rise.
Bringing the gifts that my ancestors gave
I am the dream and the hope of the slave.
I rise.
I rise.
I rise.

*From Maya Angelou, *And Still I Rise*. New York: Random House. © 1978 by Maya Angelou. Reprinted with permission.

Holistic health recognizes that the healing process is more than chemical reequilibration. Attention to exercise, nutrition, humor, and spirituality are important elements of the holistic approach. Beyond these elements is the human group, whether it is a family, a support network, or a community. The individual who is victimized cannot recover in isolation. Therefore, the clinician must attend to the demands of social integration.

Social Integration

A supportive family is the ideal social group for healthy posttraumatic healing. Figley (1988) described how such families promote recovery by "(1) detecting traumatic stress; (2) confronting the trauma; (3) urging recapitulation of the catastrophe; and (4) facilitating resolution of the trauma inducing conflicts." After reviewing the first 50 admissions to the Dimondale victims' assistance program, a residential treatment facility with an average stay of 2 weeks, I was surprised to find that less than 10% of the patients had supportive families. My conclusion is that victimized individuals with loving, effective families would rather recover at home than be separated from their primary source of nourishment. However, even the ideal family can be sorely strained after one or more members are seriously traumatized. There is an important role for the posttraumatic therapist in assessing family strengths and weaknesses, and in assisting in the design and implementation of strategies for optimum recovery. Referral to support groups and self-help networks may complement or supplement the healing function of the family.

Posttraumatic Family Therapy

The formula for posttraumatic family therapy includes an assessment phase (Figley, 1988) and four distinct treatment phases. Before summarizing these, I must emphasize that family therapy is not necessarily the best approach, particularly when violation occurs within the family. For example, Herman (1988) cautioned that following the crisis of disclosure, the incestuous family is generally so divided and fragmented that family treatment is not the modality of choice. Experienced practitioners who have begun programs with a family therapy orientation have almost uniformly abandoned this method except in late stages of treatment (H. Giarretto, A. Giarretto, & Sgori, 1978). Stark and Flitcraft (1988) minimized family therapy and emphasized the shelter movement and individual, empowering therapy for battered women: "Assuming that violence has stopped, principal treatment objectives are to overcome the sense of physical and psychological violation and restore a sense of autonomy and separateness."

Family Assessment

Eleven criteria distinguish functional from dysfunctional families, according to McCubbin and Figley (1983): the traumatic stressor is clear, rather than denied; the problem is family-centered rather than assigned completely to the victim; the approach is solution-oriented rather than blame-oriented; there is tolerance; there is commitment to and affection among family members; communication is open; cohesion is high; family roles are flexible rather than rigid; resources outside of the family are utilized; violence is absent; drug use is infrequent. Standardized protocols can supplement clinical judgment, but ultimately the clinician and client together must decide whether family therapy is feasible.

Treatment Phase I: Building Commitment to Therapeutic Objectives. When the clinician and the client agree that family therapy is indicated, the first phase of treatment requires that as many family members as possible disclose their individual ordeals, and the therapist demonstrate recognition of their suffering. Figley (1988) suggested that the therapist's sense of respect for each family member's reaction, coupled with optimism and expertise, promotes trust and commitment to therapy. Highlighting differences in individual responses leads to the next phase.

Treatment Phase II: Framing the Problem. Now each family member is encouraged to tell his or her view of the traumatic event, and to understand how each member was affected. The therapist reinforces discussion that shifts the focus away from the victimized individual, toward the impact on the family as a whole. This is the time to recognize, explore, and overcome feelings of "victim blame." When positive consequences of the ordeal are mentioned (e.g., a greater appreciation of life after a close brush with death), they are duly noted.

Treatment Phase III: Reframing the Problem. After individual experiences, assumptions, and reactions are expressed and understood, the critical work of melding these viewpoints into a coherent whole begins. "The therapist must help the family reframe the various family member experiences and insights to make them compatible in the process of constructing their healing theory," notes Figley (1988), illustrating this principle with an example from his work with Vietnam veterans. A combat veteran felt rejected by his wife who avoided talking with him. She felt like a failure as a spouse because she could not help him overcome PTSD symptoms. In this treatment phase, "he began to reframe his perception of her behavior from a sign of rejection to a sign of love." Eventually, the whole family rallied, seeing obstacles as challenges to be overcome.

Treatment Phase IV: Developing a Healing Theory. The goal of posttraumatic family therapy is consensus regarding what happened in the past, and optimism regarding future capacity to cope. An appraisal that is shared by all family members, that accounts for the reactions of each, and that contributes to a sense of family cohesion is a healing theory. Figley (1988) suggested a fifth phase that builds upon this consummation, emphasizing accomplishment and preparedness. However the therapist chooses to clarify the closure of successful therapy, the family will know that they have fulfilled their potential as a healing, nurturing human group.

Alternatives to Family Therapy

Self-Help Groups

Lieberman, Borman, and their colleagues (1979) described and evaluated self-help groups, noting how effective they are, particularly in those countries and cultures that do not rely upon the extended family for support. Self-help and mutual support groups tend to be specific, rather than generic. It is unusual to find a group for all victims of violent crime, but common to have groups for parents of murdered children, adult survivors of incest, and victims of domestic assault. Groups that endure tend to have extraordinary leaders, compatible members, and an optimum blend of ritual and flexibility. Often, professionals are in the background, available for consultation and referrals, but not intruding upon the autonomy of the group.

Therapists who work with victims of violence should become familiar with community groups that offer opportunities to share experiences, promote normalization, combat victim blame, and provide a nonthreatening social experience. Some groups will complement individual therapy. Some provide unique opportunities to help others, restoring a sense of purpose and potency. But some groups do more harm than good, encouraging premature ventilation, allowing self-styled "experts" to dominate, confusing and demoralizing the new participant.

Dyadic Support

I have found several ex-patients who were willing to meet with current clients to share experiences. Usually, this worked best one-on-one, at the ex-patient's home or at a restaurant. Since I knew both individuals, I could arrange the meeting, giving a bit of background information to each. I would choose the pairs carefully, thinking about compatible personalities, common traumatic events, and timing with respect to each. For example, Mrs. L., a 35-year-old mother of two children, a survivor of rape by a man eventually convicted of serial rape and murder, told me, after therapy, that she would be pleased to help other women with similar terrifying experiences. Mrs. L. was of considerable help to Mrs. A., the woman mentioned earlier who was held hostage and assaulted. Both were mothers, career women, and articulate and assertive. Mrs. A. did not want sympathy from strangers, had difficulty returning to work, feared entering a supermarket, but rallied as therapy and self-help efforts progressed.

Later, Mrs. L. assisted other clients. But when she went through a separation and divorce from an abusive husband, she was not available to help. I therefore recommend that any attempt to promote contact between ex-clients and current clients be made with caution, knowing the current status of each, and protecting confidentiality by withholding names and personal information until each has been consulted, each agrees, and the timing seems appropriate. However, a carefully screened dyadic "support group" can be extremely beneficial, and is well worth the effort on the part of the therapist. Most of my clients tell me they would appreciate an opportunity to assist others, and I believe them.

Support Services for Victims

Social integration refers to the use of sensitive, supportive companions in the course of recovery from traumatic events, and also to the goal of reentering society without fear. Victims of violent crime who participate in the criminal justice system have little choice about the timing of some stressful social experiences. They are questioned, cross-examined, brought to crowded court rooms, and sometimes forced to share a waiting room with the perpetrator. For them, social integration can be sudden and traumatic. Fortunately, efforts are underway in most states to provide specialized services for victims facing these stressful ordeals. Marlene Young, Director of the National Organization for Victim Assistance, describes these efforts and the generic model of ideal victim services in her chapter, "Support Services for Victims" (1988). Young points out the need for advocacy and assistance at every stage of the process, including the precourt appearance, the trial, and the sentencing hearing.

There are victim-witness specialists who are trained to support an individual throughout the criminal justice gauntlet, but caseloads are overcrowded, budgets are tight, and too often, the victim-witness specialist is ignored. I have not hesitated to meet with prosecutors and to attend court hearings when my clients felt it would help. PTT objectives are advanced, particularly the objective of sensitive facilitation of social contact. Moreover, court personnel take more interest in the client, and I learn about the wheels of justice in my hometown. Some colleagues argue that this type of intervention fosters dependency and interferes with the therapeutic relationship. They would be correct if psychoanalysis were the modality. But PTT recognizes the reality of revictimization by busy bureaucrats and officious officials. Partnership between clinician and client in the pursuit of justice is both ethical and professional.

Psychotherapy

When I concluded a dozen years in federal and state government to return to full time practice of psychiatry, Perry Ottenberg congratulated me and said, "It's a great occupation. You've got your tools in your *tuchas* (Yiddish for backside)—right here!" And he pointed to his head. Wherever the tools of the trade are located, most therapists rely on their own stock of intervention methods, sharpened by years of use. Good therapists establish rapport easily, facilitate discussion of painful material gently, and help their clients or patients to make informed choices about critical decisions, such as use of medication. PTT requires and employs these basic skills. There are several additional psychotherapy tools, specialized tools, that deserve mention. These are the timing of the telling of the trauma story, symptom suppression, the search for meaning, and the handling of coexisting problems.

Telling the Trauma Story

PTT is never complete if the client has not told the details of traumatization. This does not mean that a person who has seen several therapists must tell every detail to every clinician. Nor does it mean that one unemotional synopsis will suffice. Persons who suffer PTSD and victimization symptoms are still captured by their trauma histories and often feel "trapped in the trauma" (Wilson, 1985, 1988, 1989). They are unable to recollect without fear of overpowering emotion. And they recollect what they do not want to recollect, recall, or remember, especially when they are least prepared to remember. As a therapist, the purpose of hearing the details of the trauma story is to revisit the scene of terror and horror and, in so doing, remove the grip of terror and horror. The client should *feel* your *presence* at that moment. The purpose is more than *catharsis*. It is *partnership* in survival. It is painful and it is necessary and unavoidable.

There is no sense in exploring these corridors before a bond of mutual trust is established. Usually, I know some details from a referral source before beginning my first session with a client, and I will mention them in a matter-of-fact manner, but I make it clear from the beginning that there will be a time for sharing the details, and that will come later.

I believe that highly charged events are filed in the brain's special filing system according to emotional tone, not chronologically, certainly not alphabetically. My objective with respect to the traumatic memory is to file a memory of the two of us, client and clinician, revisiting the trauma, right next to the original file. The co-location of this experience of controlled, shared recollection, with the original, terrifying event, allows mastery and respect to permeate the experience of lonely dehumanization.

Obviously, a mechanical retelling of events will not produce a memory file that ends up in that "special" drawer reserved for extreme emotion. And an uncontrolled, unanticipated abreaction lacks the healing quality of guided, collegial reexploration. There is an optimal emotional intensity, strong enough to assure association with the original trauma, but not so strong as to obliterate the recognition of mastery and respect.

I have employed hypnosis and guided imagery to facilitate recall of trauma scenes, but always with continual reassurance that we are proceeding together, that safety is assured. With female sexual assault survivors I have always used a female co-therapist during hypnotic revisiting of trauma scenes.

Occasionally, the properly timed telling of the trauma story is the dramatic crux of therapy.

Mrs. M., a 60-year-old woman married to a man with advanced senile dementia, was driving with her lover on a snowy night. There was a crash and he died in her arms. She could not share her horror with her daughters and she had PTSD symptoms for over a year. My colleague Alice Williams, a social case worker, worked with her on an outpatient basis, and I consulted once or twice. Symptoms remained. But after 3 days in a residential unit, we revisited the terrible snowy night together with Mrs. M., who was placed in a light hypnotic trance. She cried and screamed as she narrated the events, then blurted out, "Alice, why didn't I do this before?" then cried some more. But now they were clearly tears of relief. The lonely terror was welded to the reenactment experience with a respected therapist. Symptoms abated completely. Telephone follow-up 2 years later confirmed enduring relief.

More frequently, the telling of the trauma story is not curative. One re-enactment with a trusted clinician is not enough. Aspects of the trauma are still hidden. Implications of victimization are profound. Symptoms remain entrenched. PTT continues, with all applicable tools applied.

Symptom Suppression

Roth (1988) asked the pertinent question in his chapter on the role of medication in posttraumatic therapy: "Is the treatment of a psychological disorder by biological means a short-sighted suppression of symptoms that robs the patient of the motivation and resources to solve his or her true underlying psychological problems?" He then provided an "integrated psychobiological viewpoint" of posttraumatic stress, justifying the temporary suppression of symptoms that interfere with adaptation. Whether medication, biofeedback, or behavior modification are offered to suppress symptoms, the client should have the opportunity to make an informed choice among effective options. Common posttraumatic symptoms that can be suppressed at any stage of PTT include insomnia, panic, and generalized anxiety. Medication can help with each of these, but there are pitfalls and contraindications. Roth (1988) and van der Kolk (1988) discussed these issues well.

I have found that judicious use of sedatives (e.g., triazolam, 0.125 mg every other night) often restores a normal sleep pattern without creating dependency. The dosage may be increased, but the client avoids using medication nightly, and discontinues the drug within a month. Some sleep disorders are very difficult to treat, however, with or without drugs.

Similarly, moderate use of tricyclics for panic and benzodiazepines for anxiety have allowed many of my patients to accelerate recovery, reenter social groups, and restore self-esteem. Both of us know that symptoms are being suppressed to facilitate PTT, not to replace it.

Individualized Search for Meaning

By definition, catastrophic stress shakes one's equilibrium, breaks one's attachments, and removes a sense of security. Inevitably, confrontation with deliberate human cruelty strains one's sense of justice, shatters assumptions of civility, and evokes alien, sometimes bestial, instincts. Those clinicians who describe therapy with Holocaust victims and refugee survivors of violence and torture (Danieli, 1988; Mollica, 1988) recognize these profound effects, often transmitted to a second generation, cast in the shadow of cruelty.

Victor Frankl, the famous Viennese psychiatrist, pondered the profound questions about life's meaning as he endured the Nazi concentration camp and, afterward, as he provided therapy to fellow survivors. "Woe to him who saw no more sense in his life, no aim, no purpose, and therefore no point in carrying on," stated Frankl, recalling the death camp (1959).

> What was really needed was a fundamental change in our attitude toward life. We had to learn ourselves and, furthermore, we had to teach the despairing men, that *it did not really matter what we expected from life, but rather what life expected from us*. We needed to stop asking about the meaning of life, and instead to think of ourselves as those who were being questioned by life—daily and hourly. Life ultimately means taking the responsibility to find the right answer to its problems and to fulfill the tasks it constantly sets for each individual.

It is a rare privilege to work with a client who reaches the philosophic stage of PTT, consciously formulating a new attitude toward life. But when patients are overwhelmed with symptoms, discussion of life's meaning has little relevance. However, as *normalization* restores a sense of dignity, as *empowerment* restores a will to endure, and as *individuality* restores a sense of self, clients do take responsibility to find the "right answer" for themselves. Their behavior demonstrates their fulfillment of Frankl's ideal, even if they lack the ability or inclination to formulate a philosophy of life.

The therapist, however, should have the aptitude to guide a search for meaning, to recognize existential despair, to confront self-pity, to reinforce recognition of one's responsibility for one's own life. A final phase of PTT includes articulation of the meaning of life in terms that are specific to the individual, not general or abstract.

Coexisting Problems

PTSD may mimic personality and anxiety disorders. It may precipitate physical and psychiatric conditions. It may exacerbate preexisting disorders. It may be confounded by coexisting problems, including normal stages of life adjustment (Mowbray, 1988; Wilson, 1988). To illustrate this point, Wilson (1988) cites the remarkable findings of Green, Lindy, and Grace (1984) who found "that only 13% of a treatment seeking population of Vietnam veterans manifest a single diagnosis of PTSD." Therefore, it is important for posttraumatic therapists to recognize coexisting problems and to clarify these in therapy.

Certain coexisting disorders, particularly *borderline personality*, may be impossible for the posttraumatic therapist to manage according to the principles of PTT. Where borderline cases are at issue, for example, *collegiality* may be misinterpreted as intimate friendship, and a *willingness to intervene* with criminal justice officials may lead to insatiable requests for help with personal affairs. Unfortunately, abused children may evidence combinations of borderline personality, multiple personality and PTSD. This presents enormous challenges to the therapist. A treatment strategy must be individualized, and may involve several therapists, concurrently or in sequence.

Recently, I served as a consultant to a therapist who was treating a client with borderline personality disorder and PTSD. I provided educational material to the client and his spouse, and shared my clinical hunches with the therapist. The client made several attempts to enlist my aid in undercutting therapy, calling me at home, complaining that his therapist never saw him after the therapy hour, citing previous papers of mine to "prove" how insensitive his therapist was to the needs of traumatized patients. His therapist confronted him respectfully, maintained appropriate therapeutic boundaries, and continued undeterred. I am grateful for therapists with the maturity and stamina to treat borderline patients, and I am thankful for lessons in the limitations of PTT.

It is not unusual for a traumatized patient to request help with psychological issues that antedate the trauma. Several clients have embarked upon long-term therapy for dysthymia, avoidant personality disorder, or dependent personality disorder, after achieving mastery of PTSD and victimization symptoms. In these cases, I continually clarified the contract and the objectives, to avoid self-blame when working with victimization issues, and to promote self-reliance when treating the preexisting condition. There is no way to untangle completely PTSD and a personality disorder, treating one first and then the other (see Wilson, 1988). But the therapist can maintain the fundamental principles of PTT and use tools in the general armamentarium of techniques, as long as there is no contraindication that is due to coexisting problems.

Conclusion

The clinician and the client have no difficulty realizing when posttraumatic therapy approaches its conclusion. Symptoms subside, although they may be present to some degree. There is an understanding of the causes and significance of autonomic echoes. There is a sense of mastery and control. But most significantly, there is a shift from victim status to survivor status. To clarify this change of self-perception, I wrote the *Survivor Psalm* and use it with clients to gauge progress and to mark termination:

I have been victimized.
I was in a fight that was not a fair fight.
I did not ask for the fight. I lost.
There is no shame in losing such fights, only in winning.
I have reached the stage of survivor and am no longer a
    slave of victim status.
I look back with sadness rather than hate.
I look forward with hope rather than despair.
I may never forget, but I need not constantly remember.
I *was* a victim.
I *am* a survivor.

With every client who travels that painful path from victim to survivor, I feel a surge of hope for all of us who are engaged in the larger struggle for survival.

It is no accident that many of the same principles that guided the community mental health movement in the 1960s are rediscovered in the victims' rights movement of the 1980s. There is a vast, underserved population. There is a need to mobilize help from separate disciplines. There is a crescendo of attention that cuts across ideology. There is a scientific basis for humanitarian aid. There are atavistic approaches that do more harm than good, and that beg for reform. Treating rape victims on the same psychiatric unit as chronic schizophrenics is the modern equivalent of institutionalizing the mentally ill. Removing sexually abused children from their mothers rather than removing the abusive father is reminiscent of persecuting psychotic individuals as demons. And denying that thousands of Vietnam veterans and millions of refugees can benefit from clinical attention is tragically similar to the national myopia

that culminated in President Kennedy's call for *Action for Mental Health* (1963).

Participation in any aspect of the healing arts and sciences is a source of gratification and humility. The rewards are great; the problems are never-ending.

Appendix 1

Proposed Diagnostic Criteria for Victimization Sequelae Disorder

A. The experience, or witnessing, of one or more episodes of physical violence or psychological abuse or of being coerced into sexual activity by another person
B. The development of at least (number to be determined) of the following symptoms (not present before the victimization experiences):
   1. A generalized sense of being ineffective in dealing with one's environment that is not limited to the victimization experience (e.g., generalized passivity, lack of assertiveness, or lack of confidence in one's own judgment)
   2. The belief that one has been permanently damaged by the victimization experience (e.g., a sexually abused child or rape victim believing that he or she will never be attractive to others)
   3. Feeling isolated or unable to trust or to be intimate with others
   4. Overinhibition of anger or excessive expression of anger
   5. Inappropriate minimizing of the injuries that were inflicted
   6. Amnesia for the victimization experiences
   7. Belief that one deserved to be victimized, rather than blaming the perpetrator
   8. Vulnerability to being revictimized
   9. Adopting the distorted beliefs of the perpetrator with regard to interpersonal behavior (e.g., believing that it is OK for parents to have sex with their children, or that it is OK for a husband to beat his wife to keep her obedient)
   10. Inappropriate idealization of the perpetrator
C. Duration of the disturbance of at least one month

Appendix 2

Victimization Symptoms: A Distinct Subcategory of Traumatic Stress

1. *Shame:* Deep embarrassment, often characterized as humiliation or mortification.
2. *Self-blame:* Exaggerated feelings of responsibility for the traumatic event, with guilt and remorse, despite obvious evidence of innocence.
3. *Subjugation:* Feeling belittled, dehumanized, lowered in dominance, and powerless as a direct result of the trauma.
4. *Morbid hatred:* Obsessions of vengeance and preoccupation with hurting or humiliating the perpetrator, with or without outbursts of anger or rage.

5. *Paradoxical gratitude:* Positive feelings toward the victimizer ranging from compassion to romantic love, including attachment but not necessarily identification. The feelings are usually experienced as ironic but profound gratitude for the gift of life from one who has demonstrated the will to kill. (Also known as pathological transference and "Stockholm syndrome.")

6. *Defilement:* Feeling dirty, disgusted, disgusting, tainted, "like spoiled goods," and in extreme cases, rotten and evil.

7. *Sexual inhibition:* Loss of libido, reduced capacity for intimacy, more frequently associated with sexual assault.

8. *Resignation:* A state of broken will or despair, often associated with repetitive victimization or prolonged exploitation, with markedly diminished interest in past or future.

9. *Second injury or second wound:* Revictimization through participation in the criminal justice, health, mental health, and other systems.

10. *Socioeconomic status downward drift:* Reduction of opportunity or life-style, and increased risk of repeat criminal victimization due to psychological, social, and vocational impairment.

Note. From *Post-traumatic Therapy and Victims of Violence* (Chapter 1) by F. M. Ochberg, 1988. New York: Brunner/Mazel. Copyright 1988 by Brunner/Mazel. Reprinted by permission.

References

American Psychiatric Association. (1980). *Diagnostic and statistical manual of mental disorders* (3rd ed.). Washington, DC: Author.

American Psychiatric Association. (1987). *Diagnostic and statistical manual of mental disorders* (3rd ed., rev.). Washington, DC: Author.

Angelou, M. (1978). *And still I rise.* New York: Random House.

Cannon, W. B. (1939). *Wisdom of the body.* New York: W. W. Norton.

Cienfuegos, A. J., & Monelli, C. (1983). The testimony of political repression as a therapeutic instrument. *American Journal of Orthopsychiatry, 53,* 43–51.

Cousins, N. (1979). *Anatomy of an illness.* New York: Norton.

Danieli, Y. (1988). Treating survivors and children of survivors of the Nazi Holocaust. In F. M. Ochberg (Ed.), *Posttraumatic therapy and victims of violence* (pp. 278–294). New York: Brunner/Mazel.

Figley, C. R. (1988). Post-traumatic family therapy. In F. M. Ochberg (Ed.), *Post-traumatic therapy and victims of violence* (pp. 83–109). New York: Brunner/Mazel.

Fly, C. L. (1973). *No hope but God.* New York: Hawthorne Press.

Frankl, V. E. (1959). *Man's search for meaning* (pp. 121–122). New York: Pocket Books.

Giarretto, H., Giarretto, A., & Sgroi, S. (1978). Coordinated community treatment of incest. In A. W. Burgess, A. N. Groth, L. L. Holmstrom, & S. M. Sgroi (Eds.), *Sexual assault of children and adolescents.* Lexington, MA: D. C. Heath.

Green, B., Lindy, J., & Grace, M. D. (1984). *Prediction of delayed stress after Vietnam.* Unpublished manuscript, University of Cincinnati, Cincinnati, Ohio.

Herman, J. L. (1988). Father–daughter incest. In F. M. Ochberg (Ed.), *Post-traumatic therapy and victims of violence* (p. 186). New York: Brunner/Mazel.

Jackson, Sir G. (1973). *Surviving the long night.* New York: Vanguard Press.

Kennedy, J. F. (1963). *Messages from the President of the United States relative to mental health and illness.* 88th Congress, Document House of Representatives No. 58, February, 1963.

Lieberman, M. A., Borman, L. D., & Associates. (1979). *Self-help groups for coping with crisis: Origins, members, processes, and impact.* San Francisco: Jossey-Bass.

McCubbin, H., & Figley, C. R. (1983). Bridging normative and catastrophic family stress. In H. McCubbin and C. R. Figley (Eds.), *Stress and the family: Vol. I: Coping with normative transitions* (pp. 218–228). New York: Brunner/Mazel.

Merwin, M., & Smith-Kurtz, B. (1988). Healing of the whole person. In F. M. Ochberg (Ed.), *Post-traumatic therapy and victims of violence* (pp. 57–82). New York: Brunner/Mazel.

Mollica, R. F. (1988). The trauma story: The psychiatric care of refugee survivors of violence and torture. In F. M. Ochberg (Ed.), *Post-traumatic therapy and victims of violence* (pp. 295–314). New York: Brunner/Mazel.

Mowbray, C. T. (1988). Post-traumatic therapy for children who are victims of violence. In F. M. Ochberg (Ed.), *Post-traumatic therapy and victims of violence* (pp. 196–212). New York: Brunner/Mazel.

Ochberg, F. M. (1986). The victim of violent crime. In L. A. Radelet (Ed.), *Police and the community* (4th ed., pp. 285–300). New York: Macmillan.

Ochberg, F. M. (1988). *Post-traumatic therapy and victims of violence.* New York: Brunner/Mazel.

Ochberg, F. M. (1989). Cruelty, culture and coping. *Journal of Traumatic Stress, 2*(4), 537–541.

Ochberg, F. M., & Fojtik, K. M. (1984). A comprehensive mental health clinical service program for victims: Clinical issues and therapeutic strategies. *American Journal of Social Psychiatry, 4*(3), 12–23.

Offer, D., & Sabshin, M. (1966). *Normality: Theoretical and clinical concepts in mental health.* New York: Basic Books.

President's Task Force on Crime Victims (1982). Final Report. Washington, DC: U.S. Department of Justice.

Roth, W. T. (1988). The role of medication in post-traumatic therapy. In F. M. Ochberg (Ed.), *Post-traumatic therapy and victims of violence* (pp. 39–56). New York: Brunner/Mazel.

Selye, H. (1956). *The stress of life.* New York: McGraw-Hill.

Stark, E., & Flitcraft, A. (1988). Personal power and institutional victimization: Treating the dual trauma of woman battering. In F. M. Ochberg (Ed.), *Post-traumatic therapy and victims of violence* (p. 127). New York: Brunner/Mazel.

van der Kolk, B. A. (1988). The biological response to psychic trauma. In F. M. Ochberg (Ed.), *Post-traumatic therapy and victims of violence* (pp. 25–38). New York: Brunner/Mazel.

Van Regenmorter, W. (1989). *Crime victim's rights act and other victim information.* Room 115, State Capitol, Lansing, MI 48913.

Weybrew, B. (1967). Patterns of response to stress. In M. H. Appley & R. Trumbull (Eds.), *Psychological stress.* New York: Appleton-Century-Crofts.

Wilson, J. P. (1988). Treating the Vietnam veteran. In F. M. Ochberg (Ed.), *Post-traumatic therapy and victims of violence* (pp. 262–268). New York: Brunner/Mazel.

Wilson, J. P. (1989). *Trauma, transformation and healing.* New York: Brunner/Mazel.

Young, M. A. (1988). Support services for victims. In F. M. Ochberg (Ed.), *Post-traumatic therapy and victims of violence* (pp. 330–351). New York: Brunner/Mazel.

CHAPTER 66

Psychobiological and Pharmacological Approaches to Treatment

Matthew J. Friedman

Introduction

Posttraumatic stress disorder appears to be associated with a complex array of abnormalities in several biological systems. Despite the fact that systematic research in this area is at a relatively early stage, robust findings from a number of experimental approaches suggest that PTSD patients exhibit distinctive physiological, neuropharmacological, and neuroendocrinological alterations. In addition, there is a wealth of psychological and neurobiological theory and data that may be directly applicable to our understanding of PTSD. Moreover, unlike most other psychiatric disorders, there are several animal models that may be directly applicable to PTSD, including conditioned fear (Kolb, 1987, 1988), two-factor theory (Keane, Zimering, & Caddell, 1985), learned helplessness to inescapable shock (van der Kolk, Greenberg, Boyd, & Krystal, 1985), and kindling (Friedman, 1988, 1991; van der Kolk, 1987).

In my opinion, psychobiological laboratory techniques designed to elucidate the pathophysiology of this disorder will also lead to the development of clinically useful biological approaches to the diagnosis and treatment of PTSD. Although diagnostic and methodological considerations must be factored into any interpretation of such data, current biological research findings have fostered a growing conviction among many clinicians that pharmacotherapy is sometimes useful in reversing the biological abnormalities associated with PTSD.

In this chapter, I will begin by describing the physiological, neuropharmacological, and neuroendocrine abnormalities that current research suggests are associated with PTSD. This should provide a background for understanding and predicting why certain pharmacological approaches might be more effective than others in treating this disorder. Along the way, I'll point out some methodological problems with these research findings and how such problems limit the generalizability of current data on the pathophysiology of PTSD. I will then move on to clinical pharmacology *per se* and review current research findings on antidepressants, anxiolytics, carbamazepine, lithium, and neuroleptics. Finally, I'll discuss the widespread clinical phenomenon of chemical abuse/dependency among PTSD patients and argue that high co-morbidity rates between PTSD and chemical abuse/dependency may have a neurobiological basis which, in turn, has significant implications for treatment.

Physiological and Neurohumoral/Neuroendocrinological Alterations in PTSD

As shown in Table 66.1, physiological findings with PTSD patients (most of whom so tested are male Vietnam combat veterans) suggest that the homeostat for both the central and the autonomic nervous systems has been set at a level of higher arousal. Pulse rate and blood pressure appear to be elevated in the resting state, and PTSD patients exhibit greater cardiovascular arousal following exposure to either a neutral stimulus (white noise) or to a meaningful traumatomimetic stimulus,

Matthew J. Friedman • National Center for PTSD, Veterans Administration Medical and Regional Office Center, White River Junction, Vermont 05009, and Department of Psychiatry and Pharmacology, Dartmouth Medical School, Hanover, New Hampshire 03755.

International Handbook of Traumatic Stress Syndromes, edited by John P. Wilson and Beverley Raphael. Plenum Press, New York, 1993.

Table 66.1. Physiological Alterations Associated with PTSD

Sympathetic hyperarousal
   Tonic—resetting of the homeostat at a higher level
   Episodic—in response to neutral stimuli
   Episodic—in response to traumatomimetic stimuli
Excessive startle reflex
   Lowered threshold
   Increased amplitude
A reducer pattern of cortical evoked potentials in response to neutral stimuli
Abnormalities in sleep physiology
   ↑ Sleep latency, ↓ sleep time, ↑ movements, ↑ awakenings
   Disturbances in sleep architecture
   Traumatic nightmares differ from other types of nightmares

such as the sounds or images of combat (Blanchard, Kolb, Pallmeyer, & Gerardi, 1982; Kolb, 1987; Malloy, Fairbank, & Keane, 1983; Pitman, Orr, Forgue, de Jong, & Claiborn, 1987). The startle response to neutral stimuli in children and in adults indicates that PTSD patients, in contrast to appropriate controls, exhibit a lower startle threshold as well as a significant enhancement of the startle response itself (Ornitz & Pynoos, 1989; Paige, Reid, Allen, & Newton, 1990).

Paige *et al.* (1990) reported robust differences between PTSD patients and others with respect to the pattern of cortical evoked potentials recorded in response to a stimulus pulse of white noise. PTSD patients showed significant responses to sound intensities that were at or below threshold for most normal subjects. Furthermore, the pattern of cortical evoked potentials elicited by auditory stimuli in PTSD patients showed a reduced rather than an augmented electrical pattern. Interpreting these findings in the context of the augmenting/reducing literature (Buchsbaum, 1976), Paige *et al.* (1990) suggested that PTSD patients are "reducers" in whom inhibitory feedback loops are activated to dampen a tonic state of hyperarousal.

Finally, sleep and dreaming are altered in PTSD. PTSD patients have difficulty initiating and maintaining sleep. Several studies indicate marked disruption of sleep architecture in PTSD exemplified by increased Stage 1, increased Stage 2, decreased Delta sleep, increased rapid eye movement latency, and decreased total REM percentage (Friedman, 1988; Kramer & Kinney, 1985; Lavie, Hefez, Halperin, & Enoch, 1979; Schlossberg & Benjamin, 1978). Other studies have failed to find such abnormalities (Greenberg, Pearlman, & Gampel, 1972; Kauffman, Reist, Djenderedjian, *et al.*, 1987; Ross, Ball, Sullivan, & Caroff, 1989; W. Van Kammen, Christiansen, D. Van Kammen, & Reynolds, 1987) and this controversy may actually reflect failure to distinguish PTSD from depressive sleep pathology (see below). Finally, traumatic nightmares are unique phenomena that differ from classic nightmare/ night terror Stage 4 episodes as well as from the dream anxiety attacks associated with REM sleep (Friedman, 1981; Ross *et al.*, 1989). On the one hand, PTSD dream processes are similar to

REM events. Like typical REM events, they appear to the dreamer like videotape replay sequences. However, since REM sleep is associated with atonia, the nocturnal movements and panic attacks that often accompany traumatic nightmares are more similar to a State 4 nightmare/night terror attack.

In short, most physiological data support the DSM-III-R (American Psychiatric Association, 1987) and indicate that PTSD symptoms include hyperarousal, insomnia, and startle. If replicated, the results showing reduction of cortical evoked potentials may actually represent a pathophysiologic aspect of the avoidant/ numbing behaviors listed among the PTSD Category C symptoms.

Likewise, neuropharmacological and neuroendocrinological observations in PTSD patients suggest that exposure to trauma can evoke persistent biological abnormalities. Some, but not all, research findings to date indicate that PTSD may be associated with a hyperadrenergic state, hypofunctioning of the hypothalamic-pituitary-adrenocortical (HPA) axis and dysregulation of the endogenous opioid system. These findings are summarized in Table 66.2.

Pharmacological evidence for increased catecholamines is, of course, consistent with sympathetic hyperarousal noted in Table 66.1. Twenty-four-hour urinary epinephrine and norepinephrine levels in PTSD patients are significantly higher than those of normals and of patients with most other psychiatric disorders (Mason, Giller, Kosten, & Harkness, 1988; Mason, Giller, Kosten, Ostroff, & Harkness, 1986). Furthermore, PTSD patients have the highest 24-hour urinary norepinephrine/free cortisol ratio of any psychiatric diagnostic group tested to date (Mason, Giller, Kosten, & Harkness, 1988). If, as implied by this research, PTSD is associated with higher levels of circulating catecholamines. such increased adrenergic activity should desensitize or down-regulate adrenergic receptors. Indeed, this appears to be the case since the number of both alpha-2 and beta adrenergic receptor sites is reduced in platelets and lymphocytes of combat veterans with PTSD (Lerer, Garb, Siegel, & Bleich, 1986; Perry, Cella, Falkenberg, & Heidrich, 1987).

Additional evidence for central nervous system adrenergic dysregulation comes from preliminary experiments with yohimbine, an adrenergic alpha-2 antagonist that increases CNS sympathetic arousal by disinhibiting locus coeruleus activity. It is well established, that yohimbine can precipitate panic attacks in panic-

Table 66.2. Neurohumoral/Neuroendocrinological Abnormalities Associated with PTSD

Increased circulating catecholamines
   ↑ Urinary catecholamine levels
   Down-regulation of alpha-2 and beta receptors
Hypothalamic-pituitary-adrenocortical axis abnormalities
   ↓ Urinary-free cortisol levels
   Blunted ACTH response to CRH
Opioid system dysregulation
   ↓ Pain threshold at rest
   Stress-induced analgesia elicited by traumatomimetic stimuli
   ↓ Beta-endorphin levels

disordered patients (Charney, Woods, Goodman, & Henninger, 1987). Preliminary experiments with yohimbine at the National Center for PTSD (Southwick, Krystal, & Charney, 1989) indicate that after Vietnam veterans with PTSD receive this drug, they respond with hyperarousal, anxiety, panic, and intrusive recollections of traumatic combat experiences. In some patients, yohimbine appeared to elicit frank flashback (dissociative) episodes. If these results can be replicated, the fact that such a specific pharmacological probe can precipitate such specific trauma-related symptoms strongly implicates the central adrenergic system in the pathophysiology of PTSD.

HPA abnormalities have also been shown in combat veterans with PTSD. Urinary free cortisol levels are significantly lower among PTSD patients than among other psychiatric diagnostic groups (Mason et al., 1986). Furthermore, PTSD patients exhibit a blunted ACTH (adrenocorticotropin hormone) response to CRH (corticotropin-releasing hormone) in contrast to normal controls (Smith et al., 1989). (CRH is the hypothalamic hormone that stimulates the release of ACTH from the pituitary gland.) Both findings suggest that PTSD is associated with HPA axis hypofunction. Such an interpretation, however, may not do justice to complex HPA axis abnormalities which may include both tonic and episodic components and which may also depend upon the recency of exposure to traumatomimetic stimuli.

Reports of lower pain thresholds (Perry et al., 1987) and increased susceptibility to chronic pain (Benedikt & Kolb, 1986; Rapaport, 1987) among PTSD patients suggest that this disorder is associated with lower available levels of endogenous opioids. Consistent with this possibility is a finding by Hoffman, Burges Watson, Wilson, and Montgomery (1989) who found lower beta-endorphin levels among combat veterans with PTSD. Paradoxically, although opioid levels appear to be reduced in the resting state, the pain threshold may become elevated after exposure to traumatomimetic stimuli. Pitman, van der Kolk, Orr, and Greenberg (1990) exposed Vietnam veterans with PTSD to combat scenes from the movie Platoon. They found that pain thresholds increased significantly after such exposure. This response, which they believe is a clinical example of what psychologists call stress induced analgesia (SIA), results from a sudden increase in opioid levels following exposure to stressful stimulation. Moreover, Pitman and co-workers were able to prevent the development of SIA by pretreatment with naloxone, the narcotic antagonist, indicating that SIA mediated by the endogenous opioid system is dysregulated in PTSD. Such dysregulation of the opioid system in PTSD may, in effect, represent a biological coping strategy. Van der Kolk, Pitman, Orr, and Greenberg (1989) suggested that endogenous opioids are released to attenuate the extreme arousal triggered by traumatomimetic stimuli. To go one step further, these investigators hypothesized that endogenous opioid fluctuations may serve as the biological vehicle for some of the avoidant/numbing symptoms associated with PTSD. They have shown that PTSD patients who are exposed to traumatomimetic stimuli exhibit greater anxiety, anger, guilt, and dysphoria following injection of naloxone, than following a placebo.

Finally, since the adrenergic, HPA, and opioid systems are related to one another through a variety of neuropharmacological feedback loops and since many experimental analogues to PTSD abnormalities can be reproduced in laboratory animals exposed to inescapable shock, there is growing confidence in some circles that the complex puzzle of PTSD's pathophysiology will be solved by further experimentation.

Methodological Considerations

Before progressing from basic biological research to clinical psychopharmacology, it is necessary to sound the cautionary notes that follow:

1. Results are few and far between. Except for sympathetic/adrenergic arousal (and perhaps heightened startle responses) most findings have not been replicated by many investigators. In addition, some findings are controversial; especially with regard to alterations in sleep and in HPA function.

2. Some studies report only baseline (i.e., catecholamine or cortisol) results in PTSD patients. Others obtain their measurements after exposure to neutral (i.e., white noise) stimulation. Others obtain biological measurements after exposing patients to traumatomimetic stimuli. Whereas still others have different combinations of the above procedures in their experimental protocols. Certainly, such findings are interesting snapshots of PTSD physiology but will remain difficult to interpret without more global information on the biological manifestations of PTSD in all three conditions. Future studies should compare baseline conditions with those provoked by physiological, pharmacological, and/or psychological provocation.

3. Research conducted to date has not controlled adequately for different diagnoses associated with PTSD that may seriously confound interpretation of experimental results. For example, depression is often associated with PTSD. Depression is a disorder that is known to be associated with abnormal sleep and HPA function. Therefore, experiments must be designed with adequate control groups in order to clarify whether observed sleep and HPA abnormalities are associated with PTSD alone, with depression alone, or with some biological hybrid when the two disorders occur simultaneously in the same individual. Finally, we must determine whether the depression associated with PTSD is a true major depressive disorder (according to the DSM-III-R) or whether it is (biologically) a qualitatively different type of depression/dysthymia that represents a specific affective subtype of PTSD (Friedman, 1990).

4. Almost all quantitative biological research has been conducted on male Vietnam combat veterans. Studies with female war zone veterans are needed to determine whether current findings are gender-specific. Furthermore, quantitative data are needed on male and female survivors of other types of traumatization before we can extrapolate from the current results to other groups of survivors.

5. We must acknowledge the pessimistic possibility that unraveling the pathophysiology of PTSD may not necessarily help us discover an effective drug for treating this disorder. The complex interrelationships

between the several biological systems affected in PTSD may rule out the possibility of a penicillin, lithium, or other magic bullet for PTSD. For example, our understanding of the vicious cycle of cholinergic subsensitivity and dopaminergic supersensitivity thought to occur in tardive dyskinesia has not led to a specific pharmacological intervention for that disorder.

Pharmacological Treatment for PTSD

From the previous discussion, it would appear that any drug that can dampen physiological hyperactivity, ameliorate the disturbed sleep/dream cycle, attenuate sympathetic hyperarousal, or reduce anxiety should be helpful in PTSD. In this regard, most psychotropic drugs that are effective in other disorders have been used in PTSD. In particular, antidepressants, both tricyclic antidepressants (TCAs) and monoamine oxidase inhibitors (MAOIs), have reportedly ameliorated PTSD symptoms in uncontrolled clinical trials involving many patients. Unfortunately, the few published controlled trials of TCAs and MAOIs have presented mixed and modest results. The same can be said for anxiolytic agents, especially propranolol and clonidine, for which controlled studies are needed to bolster earlier enthusiastic anecdotal reports.

Despite the current paucity of evidence, however, there is growing conviction among many clinicians that pharmacotherapy is useful for PTSD and that it is only a matter of time before an effective pharmacological approach will be demonstrated.

Antidepressants

Antidepressants are a very interesting class of drugs to consider since in addition to their actions on affective disorders, they are effective anxiolytic and antipanic agents that can dampen sympathetic arousal through a variety of mechanisms (Charney, Menkes, & Heninger, 1981; Kahn, McNair, Lipman, et al., 1986; Sheehan, Ballenger, & Jacobsen, 1980).

Antidepressants, especially TCAs, are becoming first-line drugs in PTSD pharmacotherapy. This finding is based on numerous uncontrolled studies and case reports asserting that TCAs and MAOIs reduce specific PTSD symptoms, such as hyperarousal, intrusive recollections, traumatic nightmares, and flashbacks. Associated symptoms, such as depression and anxiety, have also been responsive to antidepressant treatment but PTSD numbing/avoidant symptoms have generally been unaffected by these drugs (Blake, 1986; Boehnlein, Kinzie, Ben, & Fleck, 1985; Burstein, 1982; Davidson, Walker, & Kilts, 1987; Embry & Callahan, 1988; Falcon, Ryan, Chamberlain, & Curtis, 1985; Friedman, 1981, 1988, 1991; Hogben & Cornfield, 1981; Marshall, 1975; Milanes, Mack, & Dennison, 1984; Shen & Park, 1983; van der Kolk, 1987).

To date, there are three published controlled trials of TCAs and two of MAOIs. (There are actually only four separate studies since Frank, Kosten, Giller, and Dan, 1988, compared TCA, MAOI, and placebo in the same study.) Results are mixed and somewhat difficult to in-

terpret. Frank et al. (1988) had the most favorable findings in an 8-week double-blind comparison of imipramine (a TCA), phenelzine (a MAOI), and placebo in 34 Vietnam combat veterans with PTSD who exhibited significant reduction in PTSD intrusion (but not avoidant) symptoms as measured with the Impact of Events (IES) Scale (Horowitz, Wilner, & Alvarez, 1979). Phenelzine was somewhat more potent than imipramine in this regard, but both were significantly superior to placebo. Davidson, Kudler, Smith, and Mahorney (1990), also using the IES to assess PTSD symptomatology, found 8 weeks of treatment with the TCA amitriptyline to be modestly but significantly superior to placebo. They also observed that depressed PTSD patients appeared to show greater remission than nondepressed patients and suggested that such improvement was most likely attributable to amitriptyline's antidepressant and anxiolytic properties rather than to a specific anti-PTSD effect. A third TCA study evaluated desipramine and placebo in a 4-week double-blind comparison and found no difference between the two groups with regard to remission of PTSD symptoms (Reist, Kauffmann, Haier, & Curtis, 1989). Finally, Shestatzky, Greenberg, and Lerer (1988) conducted a 4-week double-blind crossover comparison of phenelzine and placebo. In contrast to the positive results with phenelzine of Frank et al. (1988), this group reported no difference between MAOI and placebo with regard to remission of PTSD symptoms.

Obviously, more research is needed and it is necessary to invoke the usual caveats about research findings in a new field such as the need for larger clinical samples, better attention to dosage, and concern (recently expressed by Kudler, Davidson, Stein, & Erickson, 1989), about the lack of a well-validated observer-rated scale in current PTSD research. Certainly, the lack of significant differences could reflect a lack of statistical power since sample sizes in most of these experiments were small.

Kudler et al. (1989) have also pointed out that the two negative studies (Reist et al., 1989; Shestatzky et al., 1988) only carried out their drug trials for 4 weeks whereas positive results (Davidson et al., 1990; Frank et al., 1988) only emerged after an 8-week trial of imipramine, phenelzine, and amitryptyline, respectively.

A third methodological issue concerns the failure of Shestatzky et al. (1988) to demonstrate phenelzine's superiority over placebo in their 4-week double-blind crossover trial. Examination of their data, however, shows that failure to demonstrate superiority of MAOI over placebo was not because subjects were refractory to phenelzine but rather because they were extremely responsive to placebo.

Finally, failure to separate PTSD patients from PTSD + MDD (Major Depressive Disorder) patients may contribute to differences between the findings of Frank et al. (1988), and those in the other two TCA double-blind trials. Whereas Frank's group excluded patients with MDD from their experimental groups, both Davidson et al. (1987) and Reist et al. (1989) included relatively large numbers of MDD patients in their PTSD group. As argued elsewhere (Friedman, 1988, 1990, 1991), PTSD and MDD have many symptoms in common and patients often meet DSM-III-R criteria for both PTSD and MDD.

One recent report found that 46% of hospitalized PTSD patients also met diagnostic criteria for MDD (Reaves, Hansen, & Whisenand, 1989). Furthermore, as mentioned previously, both PTSD and MDD are associated with alterations in both the sleep cycle and the HPA axis. Thus, much of the current confusion regarding which sleep and/or HPA abnormalities are attributable to PTSD alone or MDD (among PTSD patients) probably is due to failure to control for the presence of MDD among many patients included in the PTSD experimental group. This same argument also applies to interpretation of clinical drug trials. Future research will have to identify separate PTSD-alone and PTSD + MDD subgroups in order to determine whether antidepressant drugs have a specific anti-PTSD action or whether their usefulness in this disorder is due to their antidepressant, anxiolytic, and/or REM-suppressant actions.

In summary, there are many methodological concerns about the few controlled trials of antidepressants in PTSD. Certainly, it is premature to pass judgment about the efficacy or lack thereof of TCAs and MAOIs in PTSD. Furthermore, many psychiatrists remain convinced by their own clinical experience that antidepressants are very effective in some but not all cases of PTSD. Finally, a new report that fluoxetine is extremely effective in PTSD (Shay, 1991) joins the enthusiastic chorus of uncontrolled positive reports on the efficacy of antidepressants suggesting, at the very least, that clinical trials with this serotonin uptake inhibitor must be placed on the agenda for clinical psychopharmacological research on PTSD.

Anxiolytics

PTSD is classified in the DSM-III-R as an anxiety disorder. Although that may change in the forthcoming DSM-IV, the current classification is based on the fact that PTSD patients exhibit symptoms, such as anxiety, fear, autonomic arousal, irritability, and insomnia, that accompany most anxiety disorders. In certain respects, PTSD appears most similar to panic disorder because (1) episodic surges of anxiety (especially following exposure to traumatomimetic stimuli) resemble panic attacks, (2) avoidant behavior may become phenomenologically similar to phobic avoidance or agoraphobic withdrawal, and (3) because PTSD flashbacks meet the DSM-III-R criteria for panic attacks (Mellman & Davis, 1985).

For these reasons, one might expect that anxiolytic/antipanic drugs will prove efficacious in PTSD. Since MAOIs are the most potent antipanic agents, with TCAs close behind, the preceding discussion is certainly applicable in this regard. In other words, the possible effectiveness of MAOIs and TCAs in PTSD may be attributable to their antipanic/anxiolytic properties rather than to their antidepressant actions.

Other anxiolytics with reported efficacy in PTSD are sympatholytic agents, such as propranolol and clonidine, and benzodiazepines, such as diazepam and alprazolam. These drugs reduce sympathetic arousal and anxiety through several different mechanisms of action (Charney, Brier, Jathow, & Heninger, 1986; Ravaris, Friedman, & Hauri, 1986; Sheehan, 1982; Tanna, Penningroth, & Woolson, 1977; Tyrer & Lader, 1974). Given

the sympathetic hyperarousal associated with PTSD (see above) and given the fact that propranolol, clonidine, and alprazolam (but not other benzodiazepines) reduce central and/or peripheral adrenergic activity, one might expect that such sympatholytic agents might prove beneficial in PTSD.

The only published controlled drug trial on any of these drugs is a small study on the efficacy of propranolol for 11 children with acute PTSD who had been physically and/or sexually abused (Famularo, Kinscherff, & Fenton, 1988). The study was an A-B-A design (off-on-off medication) in which propranolol was administered in doses up to 2.5 mg/kg/day. The children exhibited significant reductions in PTSD intrusive and arousal symptoms during the active drug phase of the experiment. Furthermore, when placebo was substituted for propranolol, all symptoms returned with the same intensity as before. In another study, an open trial with 14 Vietnam combat veterans treated with 120 to 160 mg of propranolol daily for 6 months appeared to effectively reduce PTSD symptoms, such as nightmares, intrusive recollections, hypervigilance, insomnia, startle reactions, and angry outbursts (Kolb, Burris, & Griffiths, 1984). Negative results with propranolol have been reported by Kinzie (1989) in a clinical report on treatment of PTSD in traumatized Cambodian refugees. Since published reports indicate that among clinical treatment-seeking patients, 60% to 80% of PTSD patients have a concurrent diagnosis of alcohol or drug abuse/dependency (Branchey, Davis, & Lieber, 1984; Keane et al., 1988), the low abuse potential of beta-blockers such as propranolol will make them an attractive treatment option if their efficacy can be demonstrated conclusively.

There are two favorable reports on the anti-PTSD potency of clonidine, an alpha-2 adrenergic agonist that reduces central sympathetic activity through locus coeruleus inhibition. Both reports are open trials rather than controlled double-blind clinical studies. Kolb et al. (1984) reported that eight combat veterans had a favorable response to 0.2 to 0.4 mg/day of clonidine marked by reduced explosiveness, fewer nightmares, improved sleep, lessened startle, reduced intrusive recollections, and a general reduction in sympathetic arousal. Kinzie (1989) found that clonidine effectively lowered anxiety and autonomic arousal among Cambodian refugees with PTSD, especially when combined with tricyclic antidepressants.

Benzodiazepines are potent anxiolytics that have been prescribed widely for PTSD, despite the lack of any published controlled trials attesting to their clinical efficacy in PTSD. At one VA hospital, 71% of PTSD patients received benzodiazepines either exclusively (36%) or in combination with other drugs (Ciccone, Mazarek, Weisbrot, et al., 1988). Many clinicians are extremely reluctant to offer benzodiazepines to PTSD patients, however, because of the risk of addiction/dependency among patients who already have very high rates of alcoholism and chemical abuse/dependency (Branchey et al., 1984; Keane et al., 1988). These cautionary remarks are especially pertinent to alprazolam (Xanax) which, because of its short half-life, is more likely to produce clinical complications such as rebound anxiety and withdrawal symptoms in addition to more general concerns about benzodiazepine addiction and dependence (Higgitt, Lader, & Fonagy, 1985). Despite all these reservations, benzodiazepines in general are excellent anxiolytics and alprazolam in particular has potent anxiolytic/antipanic actions (Sheehan, 1982). Therefore, these drugs may prove effective in PTSD for carefully selected patients in whom the risk of addiction and dependence is minimal. Furthermore, from a theoretical point of view, the kindling model of PTSD (see below) offers a neurobiological argument for prescribing benzodiazepines for appropriate patients since limbic kindling is associated with increased benzodiazepine receptor binding (McNamara, Bonhaus, Shin, Crain, Gellman, & Giacchino, 1985; Morita, Okamoto, Seki, & Wada, 1985; Tietz, Gomaz, & Berman, 1985). In other words, benzodiazepines and other gamma-aminobutyric acid agonists or synergists may prove particularly useful in PTSD for well-selected patients.

Other Drugs and PTSD

Carbamazepine

Kindling is a process by which neuroanatomic structures, especially those in the limbic system, become increasingly sensitized following repeated exposure to electrical stimulation or stimulant (cocainelike) drugs. Kindling can lead progressively to profound neurophysiological abnormalities, such as grand mal seizures, or to the progressive development of aberrant behavior. Once established, kindling is a relatively stable neurobiological alteration. According to this model, chronic high intensity central sympathetic arousal mediated by the locus coeruleus kindles limbic nuclei thereby producing a stable neurobiological abnormality.

Kindling was first invoked as a neuropsychiatric model to explain lithium-refractory bipolar affective disorder by Post and Kopanda (1976). They suggested that carbamazepine (Tegretol) be prescribed for this disorder because it is an anticonvulsant that effectively counters the neurobiological changes produced by kindling. Likewise, van der Kolk (1987) and Friedman (1988) independently hypothesized that the chronic CNS sympathetic arousal associated with PTSD produces an endogenous state that optimizes the conditions for limbic kindling. Furthermore, a kindling model explains the well-known clinical fact that PTSD is extremely stable—if untreated it can persist for decades (Archibald & Tuddenham, 1965; Kluznik, Speed, van Valkenburg, & Magraw, 1986).

Motivated by such a theoretical perspective, two groups have conducted open clinical trials of carbamazepine in Vietnam combat veterans with chronic PTSD. Lipper, Davidson, Grady, *et al.* (1986) reported reduced intrusive symptoms, such as traumatic nightmares, flashbacks, and intrusive recollections. Wolf, Alavi, and Mosmaim (1988) observed alleviation of impulsivity, irritability, and violent behavior in 10 combat veterans with PTSD. Whereas Lipper's group assessed carbamazepine's effect on PTSD intrusive and avoidant symptoms, Wolf's group did not monitor specific PTSD symptoms; therefore, their positive results could be due to carbamazepine's attenuation of anger and rage (Eichelman, 1988) rather than to an anti-PTSD effect. From a different perspective, however, it is noteworthy that all patients in the Wolf *et al.* (1988) study had normal

EEGs and no evidence of temporal lobe epilepsy. Therefore, since the Wolf *et al.* patients definitely did not suffer from a PTSD-like syndrome caused by complex partial seizures as proposed by others (Greenstein, Kitchner, & Olsen, 1986; Stewart & Bartucci, 1986), the positive results with carbamazepine cannot be attributed to a traditional anticonvulsant effect and may instead reflect specific anti-PTSD potency for this drug.

Lithium

There are uncontrolled clinical reports that lithium is an effective treatment for PTSD, even for patients without a personal or family history of bipolar affective disorder or cyclothymia (Kitchner & Greenstein, 1985; van der Kolk, 1983). Van der Kolk (1987) reported that 14 out of 22 PTSD patients treated with lithium exhibited diminished sympathetic arousal, a decreased tendency to react to stress as if it were a recurrence of their original trauma, and reduced alcohol intake. He has stated that the clinical response to lithium in his PTSD patients was "clinically indistinguishable" from the response to carbamazepine, as was described in the previous paragraph. As with most other reports of pharmacological efficacy in PTSD, there are no published systematic double-blind trials of lithium in PTSD.

Neuroleptics

It is not difficult to understand why neuroleptics were widely prescribed during the 1960s and 1970s for Vietnam war zone veterans who presented clinically with behavioral problems and/or psychotic symptoms. During the pre-DSM-III (American Psychiatric Association, 1980) era, PTSD did not exist as a classifiable psychiatric diagnosis to the average psychiatrist. At that time (what we would now call) unrecognized PTSD sometimes appeared to be a bizarre and explosive psychotic disorder marked by agitation, paranoid thoughts, loss of control, potential for violence, and brief psychotic episodes, which are now called *PTSD flashbacks*. Therefore, neuroleptics frequently were prescribed as the drug of choice for such patients.

Since then, we have learned that adrenergic hyperarousal, intrusive recollections, avoidant/numbing behavior, and reactivity to traumatomimetic stimuli are the primary target symptoms of PTSD rather than psychotic thinking. Currently, antidepressants and anxio-lytic/antipanic agents show the greatest promise as first-line drugs for PTSD. After two decades of misuse and overuse of antipsychotic agents, it is now apparent that neuroleptics have no place in the routine treatment of PTSD.

Although neuroleptics should never be prescribed until other agents have been tried, they do have a role in the treatment of refractory PTSD marked by paranoid behavior, aggressive psychotic symptoms, overwhelming anger, fragmented ego boundaries, self-destructive behavior, and frequent flashback episodes marked by frank auditory and visual hallucinations of traumatic episodes (Atri & Gilliam, 1989; Friedman, 1981, 1991; Walker, 1982). It has been suggested that PTSD patients with auditory hallucinations constitute a distinct subgroup for whom neuroleptics are specifically indicated (Mueser & Butler, 1987). Again, as mentioned above with most other drugs reviewed, there are no published controlled clinical trials of neuroleptic agents on PTSD patients.

Treatment of PTSD and Concurrent Chemical Abuse/Dependency

Alcohol and chemical abuse/dependency are very high among Vietnam veterans with war-zone-related PTSD and presumably among other traumatized groups as well. Epidemiologic data from the National Vietnam Veterans Readjustment Study indicate that among individuals currently suffering from PTSD, current and lifetime prevalence rates for alcoholism are 23% and 75%, respectively, while rates for current and lifetime drug abuse/dependency are 6% and 23% respectively (Kulka et al., 1988). As one might expect, rates for alcohol or drug abuse/dependency are even higher, 60% to 80%, among clinical treatment-seeking cohorts of Vietnam veterans with PTSD (Branchey et al., 1984; Keane et al., 1988). Furthermore, there is a linear correlation between war-zone exposure and chemical abuse/dependency so that Vietnam veterans with higher levels of war-zone stress are more likely to exhibit chemical abuse/dependency than those who experienced lower levels of traumatic exposure (Keane et al., 1988; Kulka et al., 1988).

There may be a neurobiological reason for such high co-morbidity rates between PTSD and chemical abuse/dependency. The adrenergic hyperarousal and opioid dysregulation associated with PTSD may make affected individuals particularly susceptible to chemical abuse/dependency. Suppression of the adrenergic hyperarousal state with alcohol, central depressants, marijuana, or opiates should provide temporary relief to the person suffering from PTSD intrusive and hyperarousal symptoms. Moreover, reversal of the postulated opioid deficiency (Friedman, 1991; Perry et al., 1987; van der Kolk et al., 1985) through self-medication with heroin, methadone, or with other opiates would be expected to ameliorate intolerable PTSD symptomatology.

One may extend this line of reasoning another step and argue that once the vicious addiction-withdrawal cycle is established, PTSD patients may have even more difficulty achieving (and maintaining) abstinence than chemically dependent individuals without PTSD. This is because the rebound hyperarousal experienced by physically dependent PTSD patients undergoing withdrawal may itself trigger a conditioned emotional response associated with PTSD symptoms. Kosten and Krystal (1988), in an elegant review on this subject, proposed that withdrawal-induced hyperarousal will serve as a conditioned stimulus that elicits traumatomimetic PTSD symptoms. In other words, the routine difficulties of treating chemical dependency are multiplied by the complex risk of exacerbating PTSD symptoms during detoxification. This may be an even greater problem with opiate addicts, since heroin-like drugs may replenish a depleted endogenous opioid system in addition to reducing the adrenergic hyperarousal of PTSD.

The implications for treatment are clear. When PTSD and chemical dependency occur simultaneously, they must be treated simultaneously. Unfortunately, most (especially inpatient) treatment approaches attempt to treat the two disorders sequentially rather than simultaneously. Gatekeepers for such programs usually insist that patients undergo chemical detoxification/rehabilitation as a prerequisite for admission to inpatient treatment for their PTSD. Such an approach is doomed to failure because it fails to acknowledge programmatically that the complex self-sustaining interrelationships between intrapsychic, behavioral, and biological aspects of PTSD and concurrent chemical abuse/dependency demand a comprehensive approach. The recent establishment of Dual Diagnosis inpatient programs at several VA hospitals is a hopeful sign that more appropriate treatment alternatives are being introduced for patients with concurrent PTSD and chemical abuse/dependency.

Summary

1. PTSD appears to be associated with a unique pattern of biological abnormalities.

2. Physiological alterations associated with PTSD include hyperarousal of the sympathetic nervous system, an excessive startle reflex, a reducer pattern of cortical evoked potentials, and abnormalities in sleep and dreaming.

3. Neurohumoral and neuroendocrinological alterations in PTSD include increased adrenergic activity, hypothalamic-pituitary-adrenocortical axis abnormalities, and endogenous opioid dysregulation.

4. Methodological concerns about the current status of research on the neurobiology of PTSD include: (a) the small amount of published research findings; (b) lack of standardized protocols—future studies will have to compare baseline conditions with those provoked by physiological, pharmacological, and/or psychological stimulation; (c) failure to control for different diagnoses (e.g., depression, chemical abuse/dependency, etc.) that are frequently associated with PTSD; and (d) almost all quantitative biological research is on male combat veterans; research is needed on females with war-zone-related PTSD and on male and female survivors of other types of trauma.

5. Despite a growing body of open drug trials and clinical anecdotes, there have only been four double-blind trials of TCAs and MAOIs and one controlled trial of propranolol. Results with antidepressants and anxiolytic/antipanic agents are promising but inconclusive at this time.

6. Neurobiological alterations associated with PTSD may make affected individuals more susceptible to alcohol, opiates, and other illicit drug use. Therefore, when PTSD and chemical abuse/dependency occur simultaneously, they must be treated simultaneously.

7. Most open and controlled trials indicate that successful pharmacotherapy for PTSD generally results in attenuation of the DSM-III-R intrusive recollections and arousal symptoms. Avoidant symptoms, impacted grief, guilt, problems with intimacy, and moral pain do not appear to respond to medication. It appears, therefore, that drug treatment alone can never alleviate the

suffering in this disorder. At this time, pharmacotherapy appears to be primarily useful as an adjunct to psychological (intrapsychic and/or behavioral) treatment of PTSD.

References

American Psychiatric Association. (1980). *Diagnostic and statistical manual of mental disorder* (3rd ed.). Washington, DC: Author.

American Psychiatric Association. (1987). *Diagnostic and statistical manual of mental disorder* (3rd ed., rev.). Washington, DC: Author.

Archibald, H. C. & Tuddenham, R. D. (1965). Persistent stress reaction after combat: A 20-year follow-up. *Archives of General Psychiatry, 12,* 475–481.

Atri, P. B., & Gilliam, J. H. (1989). Comments on posttraumatic stress disorder. *American Journal of Psychiatry, 146,* 128.

Benedikt, R. A., & Kolb, L. C. (1986). Preliminary findings on chronic pain and posttraumatic stress disorder. *American Journal of Psychiatry, 143,* 908–910.

Blake, D. J. (1986). Treatment of acute posttraumatic stress disorder with tricyclic antidepressants. *Southern Medical Journal, 79,* 201–204.

Blanchard, E. B., Kolb, L. C., Pallmeyer, T. P., & Gerardi, R. J. (1982). A psychophysiological study of post-traumatic stress disorder in Vietnam veterans. *Psychiatric Quarterly, 54,* 220–229.

Boehnlein, J. K., Kinzie, J. D., Ben, R., & Fleck, J. (1985). One-year follow-up study of posttraumatic stress disorder among survivors of Cambodian concentration camps. *American Journal of Psychiatry, 142,* 956–959.

Branchey, L., Davis, W., and Lieber, C. S. (1984). Alcoholism in Vietnam and Korea veterans: A long-term follow-up. *Alcoholism: Clinical and Experimental Research, 8,* 572–575.

Buchsbaum, M. S. (1976). Self-regulation of stimulus intensity. In G. E. Schwartz & D. Shapiro (Eds.), *Consciousness and self-regulation.* New York: Plenum Press.

Burstein, A. (1984). Treatment of post-traumatic stress disorder with imipramine. *Psychosomatics, 25,* 681–687.

Charney, D. S., Menkes, D. B., & Heninger, G. R. (1981). Receptor sensitivity and the mechanism of action of antidepressant treatment: Implications for the etiology and therapy of depression. *Archives of General Psychiatry, 38,* 1160–1180.

Charney, D. S., Brier A., Jathow P.I., Heninger, G.R. (1986). Behavioral, biochemical and blood pressure responses to alprazolam in healthy subjects: Interactions with yohimbine. *Psychopharmacology, 88,* 133–140.

Charney, D. S., Woods, S. W., Goodman, W. K., & Heninger, G. R. (1987). Neurobiological mechanisms of panic anxiety: Biochemical and behavioral correlates of yohimbine-induced panic attacks. *American Journal of Psychiatry, 144,* 1030–1036.

Ciccone, P. E., Mazarek, A., Weisbrot, M., Greenstein, R. A., Olsen, K., & Zimmerman, J. (1988). Letter. *American Journal of Psychiatry, 145,* 1484–1485.

Davidson, J., Kudler, H., Smith, R., & Mahorney, S. (1990). Treatment of posttraumatic stress disorder with amitriptyline and placebo. *Archives of General Psychiatry, 47,* 259–266.

Davidson, J., Walker, J. I., & Kilts, C. (1987). A pilot study of phenelzine in the treatmentof post-traumatic stress disorder. *British Journal of Psychiatry, 150,* 252–255.

Eichelman, B. (1988). Toward a rational pharmacotherapy for aggressive and violent behavior. *Hospital and Community Psychiatry, 39,* 31–39.

Embry, C. K., & Callahan, B. (1988). Effective pharmacotherapy for post-traumatic stress disorder. *VA Practitioner, 5,* 57–66.

Falcon, S., Ryan, C., Chamberlain, K., & Curtis, G. (1985). Tricyclics: Possible treatment for posttraumatic stress disorder. *Journal of Clinical Psychiatry, 46,* 385–389.

Famularo, R., Kinscherff, R., & Fenton, T. (1988). Propranolol treatment for childhood posttraumatic stress disorder, acute type: A pilot study. *American Journal of Diseases of Children, 142,* 1244–1247.

Frank, J. B., Kosten, T. R., Giller, E. L., & Dan, E. (1988). A randomized clinical trial of phenelzine and imipramine for posttraumatic stress disorder. *American Journal of Psychiatry, 145,* 1289–1291.

Friedman, M. J. (1981). Post-Vietnam syndrome: Recognition and management. *Psychosomatics, 22,* 931–943.

Friedman, M. J. (1988). Toward rational pharmacotherapy for posttraumatic stress disorder. *American Journal of Psychiatry, 145,* 281–285.

Friedman, M. J. (1990). Interrelationships between biological mechanisms and pharmacotherapy of posttraumatic stress disorder. In M. E. Wolf & A. D. Mosnaim (Eds.), *Posttraumatic stress disorder: Etiology, phenomenology, and treatment* (pp. 204–225). Washington, DC: American Psychiatric Press.

Friedman, M. J. (1991). Biological approaches to the diagnosis and treatment of post-traumatic stress disorder. *Journal of Traumatic Stress, 4,* 67–91.

Greenberg, R., Pearlman, C. A., & Gampel, D. (1972). War neuroses and the adaptive function of REM sleep. *British Journal of Medical Psychology, 45,* 27–33.

Greenstein, R. A., Kitchner, I., & Olsen, K. (1986). Posttraumatic stress disorder, partial complex seizures, and alcoholism. *American Journal of Psychiatry, 143,* 1203.

Higgitt, A. C., Lader, M. H., & Fonagy, P. (1985). Clinical management of benzodiazepine dependence. *British Medical Journal, 291,* 688–690.

Hoffman, L., Burges Watson, P., Wilson, G., & Montgomery, J. (1989). Low plasma beta-endorphin in post-traumatic stress disorder. *Australian and New Zealand Journal of Psychiatry, 23,* 269–273.

Hogben, G. L., & Cornfield, R. B. (1981). Treatment of traumatic war neurosis with phenelzine. *Archives of General Psychiatry, 38,* 440–445.

Horowitz, M. J., Wilner, N., & Alvarez, W. (1979). Impact of events scale: A measure of subjective stress. *Psychosomatic Medicine, 41,* 209–218.

Kahn, R. J., McNair, D. M., Lipman, R. S., *et al.* (1986). Imipramine and chlordiazepoxide in depression and anxiety disorders. *Archives of General Psychiatry, 43,* 79–85.

Kauffman, C. D., Reist, C., Djenderedjian, A., Nelson, J. N., & Haier, R. J. (1987). Biological markers of affective disorders and posttraumatic stress disorder: A pilot study with desipramine. *Journal of Clinical Psychiatry, 48,* 366–367.

Keane, T. M., Zimering, R. T., & Caddell, J. M. (1985). A behavioral formulation of posttraumatic stress disorder in Vietnam veterans. *The Behavior Therapist, 8,* 9–12.

Keane, T. M., Gerardi, R. J., Lyons, J. A., & Wolfe, J. (1988). The interrelationship of substance abuse and posttraumatic stress disorder: Epidemiological and clinical considerations. *Recent Developments in Alcoholism, 6,* 27–48.

Kinzie, J. D. (1989). Therapeutic approaches to traumatized Cambodian refugees. *Journal of Traumatic Stress, 2,* 75–91.

Kitchner, I., & Greenstein, R. (1985). Low dose lithium carbonate in the treatment of post traumatic stress disorder: Brief communication. *Military Medicine, 150,* 378–381.

Kluznik, J. C., Speed, N., van Valkenburg, C., & Magraw, R. (1986). Forty-year follow-up of United States prisoners of war. *American Journal of Psychiatry, 143,* 1443–1446.

Kolb, L. C. (1987). A neuropsychological hypothesis explaining posttraumatic stress disorders. *American Journal of Psychiatry, 144,* 989–995.

Kolb, L. C. (1988). A critical survey of hypotheses regarding post-traumatic stress disorders in light of recent findings. *Journal of Traumatic Stress, 1,* 291–304.

Kolb, L. C., Burris, B. C., & Griffiths, S. (1984). Propranolol and clonidine in the treatment of the chronic post-traumatic stress disorders of war. In B. A. van der Kolk (Ed.), *Post-traumatic stress disorder: Psychological and biological sequelae* (pp. 97–105). Washington, DC: American Psychiatric Press.

Kosten, T. R., & Krystal, J. (1988). Biological mechanisms in posttraumatic stress disorder: Relevance for substance abuse. *Recent Developments in Alcoholism, 6,* 49–68.

Kosten, T. R., Mason, J. W., Giller, E. L., Ostroff, R. B., & Harkness, L. (1987). Sustained urinary norepinephrine and epinephrine elevation in post-traumatic stress disorder. *Psychoneuroendocrinology, 12,* 13–20.

Kramer, M., & Kinney, L. (1985). Is sleep a marker of vulnerability to delayed post traumatic stress disorder? *Sleep Research, 14,* 181.

Krystal, J. H., Kosten, T. R., Southwick, S., Mason, J. W., Perry, B. D., & Giller, E. L. (1989). Neurobiological aspects of PTSD: Review of clinical and preclinical studies. *Behavior Therapy, 20,* 177–198.

Kudler, H. S., Davidson, J. R. T., Stein, R., & Erickson, L. (1989). Measuring results of treatment of PTSD (letter). *American Journal of Psychiatry, 146,* 1645–1646.

Kulka, R. A., Schlenger, W. E., Fairbank, J. A., Hough, R. L., Jordan, B. K., Marmar, C. R., & Weiss, D. S., (1990). Trauma and the Vietnam War generation: Report of findings from the National Vietnam Veterans Readjustment Study. New York: Brunnes/Mazel.

Lavie, P., Hefez, A., Halperin, G., & Enoch, D. (1979). Long-term effects of traumatic war-related events on sleep. *American Journal of Psychiatry, 136,* 175–178.

Lerer, B., Garb, R., Siegel, B., & Bleich, A. (1986). PTSD following combat exposure: Clinical features and psychopharmacological treatment. *British Journal of Psychiatry, 149,* 365–369.

Lipper, S., Davidson, J. R. T., Grady, T. A., Edinger, J. D., Hammett, E. B., Mahorney, S. L., & Cavenar, J. O. (1986). Preliminary study of carbamazepine in post-traumatic stress disorder. *Psychosomatics, 27,* 849–854.

Malloy, P. F., Fairbank, J. A., & Keane, T. M. (1983). Validation of a multimethod assessment of posttraumatic stress disorders in Vietnam veterans. *Journal of Consulting and Clinical Psychology, 51,* 488–494.

Marshall, J. R. (1975). The treatment of night terrors associated with the posttraumatic syndrome. *American Journal of Psychiatry, 132,* 293–295.

Mason, J. W., Giller, E. L., Kosten, T. R., Ostroff, R, & Podd, L. (1986). Urinary free-cortisol in posttraumatic stress disorder patients. *Journal of Nervous and Mental Diseases, 174,* 145–149.

Mason, J. W., Giller, E. L., Kosten, T. R., & Harkness, L. (1988). Elevation of urinary-norepinephrine/cortisol ratio in post-traumatic stress disorder. *Journal of Nervous and Mental Disease, 176,* 498–502.

McNamara, J. O., Bonhaus, D. W., Shin, C., Crain, B. J., Gell-

man, R. L. & Giacchino, J. L. (1985). The kindling model of epilepsy: A critical review. *CRC Critical Reviews of Clinical Neurobiology, 1,* 341–391.

Mellman, T. A., & Davis, G. C. (1985). Combat-related flashbacks in posttraumatic stress disorder: Phenomenology and similarity to panic attacks. *Journal of Clinical Psychiatry, 46,* 379–382.

Milanes, F. S., Mack, C. N., Dennison, J., & Slater, V. L. (1984). Phenelzine treatment of post-Vietnam stress syndrome. *VA Practitioner, 1*(6), 40–47.

Morita, K., Okamoto, M., Seki, K., & Wada, J. A. (1985). Suppression of amygdala-kindled seizures in cats by enhanced GABAergic transmission in the substantia innominata. *Experimental Neurology, 89,* 225–236.

Mueser, K. T., & Butler, R. W. (1987). Auditory hallucinations in combat-related chronic posttraumatic stress disorder. *American Journal of Psychiatry, 144,* 299–302.

Ornitz, E. M., & Pynoos, R. S. (1989). Startle modulation in children with posttraumatic stress disorder. *American Journal of Psychiatry, 146,* 866–870.

Paige, S., Reid, G., Allen, M., & Newton, J. (1990). Psychophysiological correlates of PTSD. *Biological Psychiatry, 27,* 419–430.

Perry, S. W., Cella, D. F., Falkenberg, J., Heidrich, G., & Goodwin, C. (1987). Pain perception in burn patients with stress disorders. *Journal of Pain and Symptom Management, 2,* 29–33.

Pitman, R. K., Orr, S. P., Forgue, D. F., de Jong, J. B., & Claiborn, J. M. (1987). Psychophysiologic assessment of posttraumatic stress disorder imagery in Vietnam combat veterans. *Archives of General Psychiatry, 44,* 970–975.

Pitman, R. K., van der Kolk, B. A., Orr, S. P., & Greenberg, M. S. (1990). Naloxone-reversible analgesic response to combat-related stimuli in posttraumatic stress disorder: A pilot study. *Archives of General Psychiatry, 47,* 541–544.

Post, R. M., & Kopanda, R. T. (1976). Cocaine, kindling and psychosis. *American Journal of Psychiatry, 133,* 627–634.

Rapaport, M. H. (1987). Chronic pain and posttraumatic stress disorder. *American Journal of Psychiatry, 144,* 120.

Ravaris, C. L., Friedman, M. J., & Hauri, P. (1986, May). *A controlled study of alprazolam and propranolol in panic disorder and agoraphobic patients.* Paper presented at 139th Annual Meeting of the American Psychiatric Association, Washington, DC.

Reaves, M. E., Hansen, T. E., & Whisenand, J. M. (1989). The psychopharmacology of PTSD. *VA Practitioner, 6*(5), 65–72.

Reist, C., Kauffmann, C. D., Haier, R. J., Sangdahl, C., DeMet, E. M., Chicz-DeMet, A., & Nelson, J. N. (1989). A controlled trial of desipramine in 18 men with posttraumatic stress disorder. *American Journal of Psychiatry, 146,* 513–516.

Ross, R. J., Ball, W. A., Sullivan, K. A., & Caroff, S. N. (1989). Sleep disturbance as the hallmark of posttraumatic stress disorder. *American Journal of Psychiatry, 146,* 697–707.

Schlosberg, A., & Benjamin, M. (1978). Sleep patterns in three acute combat fatigue cases. *Journal of Clinical Psychiatry, 39,* 546–549.

Shay, J. (1991). Fluoxetine reduces explosiveness and elevates mood of Vietnam combat vets with PTSD. *Journal of Traumatic Stress, 5,* 97–101.

Sheehan, D. V. (1982). Current perspectives in the treatment of panic and phobic disorders. *Drug Therapy, 7,* 179–193.

Sheehan, D. V., Ballenger, J., & Jacobsen, G. (1980). Treatment of endogenous anxiety with phobic, hysterical and hypochondriacal symptoms. *Archives of General Psychiatry, 37,* 51–59.

Shen, W. W., & Park, S. (1983). The use of monoamine oxidase inhibitors in the treatment of traumatic war neurosis: Case report. *Military Medicine, 148,* 430–431.

Shestatzky, M., Greenberg, D., & Lerer, B. (1988). A controlled trial of phenelzine in posttraumatic stress disorder. *Psychiatry Research, 24,* 149–155.

Smith, M. A., Davidson, J., Ritchie, J. C., Kudler, H., Lipper, S., Chapell, P., & Nemeroff, C. B. (1989). The corticotropin-releasing hormone test in patients with posttraumatic stress disorder. *Biological Psychiatry, 26,* 349–355.

Southwick, S. M., Krystal, J. H., & Charney, D. S. (1989). Yohimbine effects in PTSD patients. *ACNP Abstracts,* p. 185.

Stewart, J. T., & Bartucci, R. J. (1986). Posttraumatic stress disorder and partial complex seizures. *American Journal of Psychiatry, 143,* 113–114.

Tanna, V. T., Penningroth, R. P., & Woolson, R. F. (1977). Propanolol in the treatment of anxiety neurosis. *Comprehensive Psychiatry, 18,* 319–326.

Tietz, E. I., Gomaz, F., & Berman, R. F. (1985). Amygdala kindled seizure stage is related to altered benzodiazepine binding site density. *Life Sciences, 36,* 183–190.

Tyrer, P. J., & Lader, M. H. (1974). Response to propanolol and diazepam in somatic and psychic anxiety. *British Medical Journal, 2,* 14–16.

van der Kolk, B. A. (1983). Psychopharmacological issues in posttraumatic stress disorder. *Hospital and Community Psychiatry, 34,* 683–691.

van der Kolk, B. A. (1987). The drug treatment of post-traumatic stress disorder. *Journal of Affective Disorders, 13,* 203–213.

van der Kolk, B. A. (1988). The trauma spectrum: The interaction of biological and social events in the genesis of the trauma response. *Journal of Traumatic Stress, 1,* 273–290.

van der Kolk, B. A., Greenberg, M., Boyd, H., & Krystal, J. (1985). Inescapable shock, neurotransmitters, and addiction to trauma: Toward a psychobiology of post traumatic stress. *Biological Psychiatry, 20,* 314–325.

van der Kolk, B. A., Pitman, R. K., Orr, S. P., & Greenberg, M. S. (1989). Endogenous opioids, stress induced analgesia, and posttraumatic stress disorder. *Psychopharmacology Bulletin, 25,* 417–421.

Van Kammen, W. B., Christiansen, C., Van Kammen, D. P., & Reynolds, C. F. (1987). Sleep and the POW experience: 40 years later. *Sleep Research, 16,* 291.

Walker, J. I. (1982). Chemotherapy of traumatic war stress. *Military Medicine, 147,* 1029–1033.

Wolf, M. E., Alavi, A., & Mosnaim, A. D. (1988). Posttraumatic stress disorder in Vietnam veterans clinical and EEG findings: Possible therapeutic effects of carbamazepine. *Biological Psychiatry, 23,* 642–644.

CHAPTER 67

Neurophysiological Considerations in the Treatment of Posttraumatic Stress Disorder

A Neurocognitive Perspective

George S. Everly, Jr.

With the exception of the sudden death phenomenon, posttraumatic stress disorder (PTSD) represents the single most severe and recalcitrant variant of pathogenetic stress arousal known to modern medicine (Everly, 1989). Its symptomatology includes both psychiatric and somatic manifestations (Everly, 1989) which often prove to be enigmatic to traditional treatment approaches. In this chapter, I will offer a reconsideration of the neurophysiology of PTSD wherein PTSD is viewed within the context of the "disorders of arousal" nosological genre as formulated in earlier research (Everly & Benson, 1989). Such a reformulation will give rise to a neurophysiological rationale for the use of therapeutic interventions designed to lower the "state-and-trait" levels of neurophysiological arousal within the PTSD patient. Indeed, it may be argued that successful treatment of the PTSD patient is contingent upon the successful diminution of manifest arousal.

Posttraumatic Stress Disorder

The latest edition of the *Diagnostic and the Statistical Manual of Mental Disorders* (American Psychiatric Association, 1987) categorizes PTSD as an anxiety disorder. Disorders thusly categorized possess as key features psychophysiological arousal and avoidance behaviors.

George S. Everly, Jr. • Health Psychology Laboratory, Loyola College, Baltimore, Maryland, and Psychological Services and Behavioral Medicine, Homewood Hospital Center, The Johns Hopkins Health System, 204 Glenmore Avenue, Catonsville, Maryland 21228.

International Handbook of Traumatic Stress Syndromes, edited by John P. Wilson and Beverley Raphael. Plenum Press, New York, 1993.

As early as 1941, Kardiner (1941) had empirically defined the syndrome that would later come to be called PTSD as possessing five key clinical features: (1) constriction of personality functioning, (2) exaggerated startle reflex, (3) psychic fixation upon a traumatic event, (4) atypical dream experiences, and (5) a tendency for explosive and/or aggressive reactions.

It is now generally agreed that PTSD possesses three phenomenological/symptomatological constituents subsequent to an individual's exposure to some traumatogenic stimulus outside the usual realm of human experiences: (1) recollective ideation relevant to the traumatic event, (2) pathognomonic autonomic nervous system arousal, and (3) withdrawal from usual activities and/or what appears to be a dysphoric numbing to stimulation (see American Psychiatric Association, 1980, 1987).

If one considers the phenomenology of anxiety, the formulations of Kardiner (1941), and the recent attempts at phenomenological convergence regarding PTSD (Everly, 1989, 1990), one is struck by the emergence of the recurrent and homogenizing theme that psychophysiological arousal plays.

Arousal and PTSD

Kardiner (1941) originally considered posttraumatic syndromes as variants on a theme of "physioneurosis." This term is the embodiment of the notion that posttraumatic syndromes reflect exquisite intertwinings of psychosocial and physiological phenomena. It seems clear after reviewing Kardiner's own criteria that the key physiology of the posttrauma syndrome is the physiology of arousal; arousal of the central nervous system (CNS) and the autonomic nervous systems with their numerous and diverse peripheral effector mechanisms (Everly, 1989).

Consistent with the formulations of Kardiner, van der Kolk (1988) viewed PTSD as a pathological manifestation of the inability to modulate arousal.

Investigations by Foy *et al.* (1984) and Horowitz, Wilner, Kaltreider, and Alvarez (1980) revealed that self-reported symptoms of arousal and distress were key features of the posttrauma syndrome and serve as useful diagnostic criteria.

Neuroendocrine research conducted by Mason *et al.* (1986) revealed that patients diagnosed with PTSD exhibited unusually high norepinephrine/cortisol ratios when compared to patients diagnosed as depressed or schizophrenic. Such a profile was interpreted as being consistent with hyperactivity of the sympathetic neuroendocrine axis. These findings and interpretations are in concert with the formulations of Kolb (1987, 1988) and Friedman (1988), who view PTSD as a pathological condition consistent with a syndrome of pathological hyperarousal (see also Wilson, 1989, for a useful review of the physiology of PTSD).

Wilson (1989) insightfully analyzed PTSD and found it to be consistent with the phenomenology of heightened arousal within Gellhorn's construct of "ergotropic tuning" (Gellhorn, 1967). Wilson's analysis is particularly revealing in that it shows the potential linkage within PTSD between heightened arousal of Cannon's "fight or flight" neuroendocrine axis and the hypothalamic-adrenal cortical axis with the release of its constituent glucocorticoid hormones (e.g., cortisol).

Finally, I (Everly, 1989, 1990) first proposed that PTSD be viewed within the phenomenological context of a "disorder of arousal." The disorders of arousal nosological genre was first proposed and formulated by Herbert Benson and myself (Everly & Benson, 1989) and is reflective of the notion that all stress-related disorders are manifestations of and variations on a theme of pathognomonic neurologic hypersensitivity, in effect, a lowered threshold for psychophysiologic excitation within the limbic system and its numerous efferent pathways. Consistent with the formulation, I proposed (Everly, 1990) that the phenomenological epicenter of PTSD resides in a functional neurologic hypersensitivity within the anatomical boundaries of the limbic system. More specifically, I proposed that hypersensitivity and manifest arousal within the septal-hippocampal-amygdalar nuclei, and their efferent projections, stand to define anatomically and physiologically the condition known as *PTSD*. Thus, I concluded (Everly, 1990) that PTSD represents a disorder of arousal and as such represents the antithesis of what Benson (1975) referred to as the "relaxation response" (i.e., a hypometabolic response engendered by a wide and diverse variety of so-called relaxation techniques, such as mantra meditation, yoga, biofeedback, etc.). Interestingly enough, the relaxation response has been shown to be effective in the treatment of a wide array of stress-related disorders of arousal (Everly & Benson, 1989). Indeed, it was Ivan Pavlov himself who said that the strength of the central nervous system resides in its ability to inhibit arousal. According to the present formulation, PTSD represents an extreme pathological manifestation of insufficiently bridled arousal.

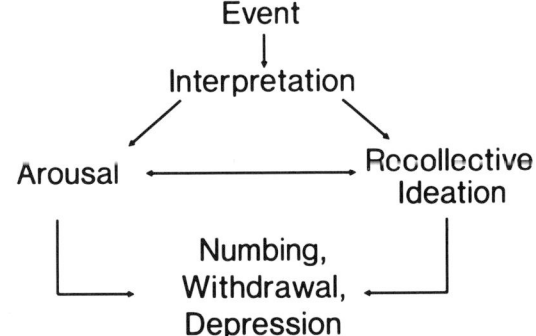

Figure 67.1. A model of PTSD.

Neurophysiological Model of PTSD

The previous section concluded with my assessment (Everly, 1990) that PTSD represents a disorder of arousal and as such possesses neurologic hypersensitivity and hyperexcitation as key phenomenological features. Figure 67.1 represents an effort to show how the major constituencies of PTSD are integrated around the core phenomenological feature of pathognomonic arousal.

Traumatic Events

The current psychiatric nosologies establish as a *sine qua non* of PTSD exposure to some event outside the usual realm of human experience. Such a norm-referenced criterion, while valuable in one sense, could also be potentially confounding to the formal diagnostic process. The notion that a traumatic event must lie outside the usual realm of human experience in order to be truly "traumatic" establishes an excessively restrictive norm-referenced comparison paradigm as the key diagnostic criterion. Phenomenological evidence, however, recognizes the role that religious or cultural variables may play to augment or mitigate the impact of potentially traumatic events upon the individual (Wilson, 1989). Furthermore, psychophenomenologists might argue that an individual's idiosyncratic perception and appraisal of potentially traumatic events exert far more influence upon the pathogenic process than does the mere exposure alone (Ciaranello, 1983; Wilson, 1989).

Cognitive Appraisal-Emotional Integration

In a review of stress-related disorders, I summarized the prevailing opinion that the cognitive appraisal of a given event plays the primary deterministic role in the etiology of pathogenic stress arousal (Everly, 1989). It may be argued, consistent with this perspective, that the wide variety and variability of response patterns to traumatogenic events are largely functions of the cognitive interpretation of the event by the individual's experiencing of that event.

Interestingly, a similar view is reportedly shared by the noted traumatologist Pierre Janet. According to van der Kolk, Brown, and van der Hart (1989), "Janet thought that the victim's state of mental preparation determined the degree of 'vehement emotion' " (p. 375). Furthermore, it was believed that the intensity of "vehement emotion" resulted largely from the cognitive appraisal of the event as opposed to the event itself. Finally, "Janet noted that the traumatizing event itself need not be a dramatic one: it is the intensity of the emotional reaction that determines whether an event precipitates post traumatic psychopathology" (van der Kolk *et al.*, 1989, p. 375). Thus, we see that mere exposure to an unusual event does not necessarily lead to PTSD, rather the key determinants of PTSD reside in the cognitive appraisal and subsequent emotional reaction to the event (Ciaranello, 1983; Everly, 1989; Wilson, 1989). Most basically, trauma represents a contradiction to one's personal worldview (weltanschauung).

Arnold (1984) developed an elegant formulation of the neuroanatomical locus of cognitive appraisal. In her review, she concluded that the prefrontal poles in integration with the cingulum serve as the primary anatomical substrates supporting the process of cognitive appraisal.

Recollective Processes

The diagnostic criteria for PTSD contain direct references to recollective processes associated with the traumatic event. Symptoms, such as flashbacks, intrusive dreams, illusions, intrusive ideation, and repetitive memories associated with the trauma, serve as indicia of pathognomonic recollective processes. These recollective processes should be viewed as one-half of the "core" phenomenological constituency of PTSD.

Speculations into the nature of PTSD leads one to question what role the recollective processes may play in PTSD. It seems likely that an enhanced memory of the traumatic event and conditions associated with the event may serve some self-preservation function. It may be that conditions that are associated with life-threatening circumstances are encoded in such a manner so as to aid in some greater hypervigilance function designed to reduce the likelihood that one will be traumatized again. Simply restated, an enhanced memory of life-threatening experiences serves to increase the likelihood that one would avoid situations in any way related to those which might engender a threat to one's life or well-being. This notion seems to warrant even greater consideration when recollective processes as just described are paired with a status of, or propensity for, hyperarousal.

As an interesting side note, while memories of the trauma are usually enhanced in the PTSD patient (with the notable exception of trauma-related amnestic syndromes which probably serve to protect the ego from recollections that would be in and of themselves traumatizing), there is evidence that the "nonspecific" short-term memory of many PTSD patients may be inhibited. Extreme stress arousal has been shown to suppress neurological functioning in the hippocampus (Sapolsky, Krey, & McEwen, 1984). It is the hippocampus that is well known for being the anatomical locus for short-term memory. Everly and Horton (1989) provided initial documentation of this nonspecific short-term memory suppression effect in PTSD patients.

Thus, it seems as if the memory of the PTSD patient is imprinted with a reiterative, recollective function to serve in combination with a hyperarousal function so as to create a state of hypervigilance and constant readiness. Let us now explore the second of the "core" constituents in PTSD—psychophysiological arousal.

Arousal

The diagnostic criteria for PTSD are replete with evidence of excessive neurologic hypersensitivity for, and a status of, arousal. Sleep disturbance, hyperstartle responses, irritability, and related symptoms are clearly evidence of the neurologic hypersensitivity and hyperarousal constituency with PTSD. Early in this chapter, I argued that PTSD is best understood as a disorder of arousal as formulated by myself and Benson (Everly & Benson, 1989). It is a primary thesis of this chapter that arousal, as a pathognomonic constituent of PTSD in combination with the myriad of recollective processes, represents the phenomenological "core" of PTSD.

The symptoms of arousal within PTSD are largely consistent with arousal of the sympathetic branch of the autonomic nervous system and its effector mechanisms residing within the sympatho-adrenal medullary axis (Everly, 1989). Should the sympatho-adrenal medullary excitation be protracted for excessively chronic periods, or be excessively intense in response magnitude, two potential outcomes are likely to occur: (1) diminution of available catecholamines, and/or (2) increased levels of glucocorticoids, such as cortisol and its tropic hormone adrenocorticotropic hormone (ACTH). Both of the outcomes are associated with behavioral withdrawal, avoidance, and depression (see Everly, 1989, for an integrative review).

The PTSD patient suffers from a pathognomonic hypersensitivity for and status of arousal. This notion, which I applied to PTSD (Everly, 1990), has been extended to virtually all DSM-III-R anxiety disorders (of which PTSD is one) by Barlow and Beck (1984), Carr and Sheehan (1984), and Sheehan (1983). The notion that hyperarousal can play such a central role in disease is by no means new. Such authors as Gellhorn, Weil, and Post have agreed that patients subjected to intense stress arousal can suffer a form of neurologic "sensitization."

Gellhorn's Formulations

Over two decades ago, Gellhorn (1957, 1967; Gellhorn & Loofbourrow, 1963) described the limbically based "ergotropic tuning" process which was thought to serve as the neurophysiological basis of affective lability, anxiety, and stress-related disorders. The term *ergotropic tuning* was used to refer to a neurologic hypersensitivity existing within the mechanisms of the sympathetic branch of the autonomic nervous system. Etiologically, Gellhorn (1965) noted that

in the waking state the erogotropic division of the autonomic is dominant and responds primarily to environmental stimuli. If these stimuli are very strong or follow each other at short intervals, the tone and reactivity of the sympathetic system increases. (pp. 494–495)

Thus, either extremely intense, acute (traumatic) stimulation or chronically repeated, intermittent lower-level stimulation can lead to a state of autonomic nervous system hyperarousal. The causal stimuli, Gellhorn noted in later writings, could be environmentally exogenous or could be endogenously manufactured.

Weil's Formulations

Weil (1974) developed a model similar to that constructed by Gellhorn. In fact, Weil made brief reference to the work of Gellhorn in his construction of a neurophysiological model of emotional behavior. Weil agreed with Gellhorn that the activation thresholds of the limbic system can be altered. More specifically, Weil noted that the neurologic activation thresholds of the limbic system and its efferent mechanisms can be lowered to a point as to render the limbic system hypersensitive. This process he called "charging of the arousal system." Similar to Gellhorn, Weil noted that the arousal system can be charged (i.e., rendered hypersensitive), through high intensity stimulation and/or chronically repetitive stimulation. The behavioral result of a "charged" limbic arousal system, according to Weil, would be affective lability, anxiety-related dysfunction, and stress-related somatic discord.

Post's Formulations

Post proposed that extraordinary stimulation of limbic structures may result in a condition whereby the neurological tissues themselves become hypersensitive to subsequent excitation or arousal (Post & Ballenger, 1981; Post, 1985, 1986). Drawing on the classic experiments of Goddard (Goddard, McIntyre, & Leech, 1969) on "kindling," which demonstrated that intense or protracted stimulation of limbic nuclei could create permanent changes in the structure and function of the limbic system, Post chose the term *behavioral sensitization* to reflect the condition where limbic neurons could become hypersensitive based upon exposure to psychosocially related stimuli. This hypersensitivity, Post noted, is considered to be reversible. He has implicated such a behavioral sensitization phenomenon as being involved in various affective mood disorders and other psychopathological conditions. Doane (1986) implicated the sensitization phenomenon within the limbic system, not only with affective disorders, but also with a host of somatic, psychophysiological disorders. (Readers interested in the morphological bases of sensitization should refer to Delanoy, Tucci, and Gold, 1983, and Fifkova and Van Harreveld, 1977.)

Thus, we see that the PTSD patient is one who is best thought of as neurologically "sensitized." A review of the efforts of Joy (1985), Post and Ballenger (1981), Post and Kopanda (1976), and Nutt (1989) reveal several mechanisms potentially responsible for this neurologic hypersensitivity or sensitization: (1) an augmentation of available excitatory neurotransmitters, (2) a diminution of available inhibitory neurotransmitters, (3) an augmentation of excitatory postsynaptic receptor sites (in both number and area), (4) a diminution of presynaptic inhibitory receptors, and (5) the creation of excitatory rever-

berating feedback loops within the highly plastic limbic circuitry. Recent advances in neurophysiology have lead to a more comprehensive understanding and appreciation of the physiology of high-intensity stimulation, as might be experienced in trauma. It is now well documented that excessively intense stimulation can actually be toxic to neural substrates. This is known as *excitatory toxicity* (E. McGeer & P. McGeer, 1988; Olney, 1978).

The excitotoxic phenomenon was first articulated by Olney and his colleagues. According to E. McGeer and P. McGeer (1988),

> it proposes that a depolarization mechanism underlies the neurotoxic effects. The process is initiated by activation of excitatory receptors . . . the excitotoxin [excitatory neurotransmitters such as glutamate] when present in high concentrations . . . produces a state of pathological depolarization in which the neuronal plasma membrane permeability is increased for extended periods of time. (p. 108)

This depolarization effect is then thought capable of taxing the neuron's energy-producing mechanisms to a point of dysfunction, and even neuronal death. The neurons of the hippocampus and the amygdala appear strikingly vulnerable to excitotoxicity (E. McGeer & P. McGeer, 1988), thus implicating convulsive phenomena within the context of PTSD.

Numbing, Depression, and Withdrawal

Current formulations of PTSD include among their diagnostic criteria symptoms of avoidance, detachment, numbing, and/or depressive symptomatology. The position taken within this chapter is that these symptoms are best understood as "secondary symptoms" in response to the "core" constituencies of PTSD (i.e., the recollective processes in combination with the neurological hypersensitivity and arousal). It will be recalled from an earlier section that under conditions of extreme arousal catecholamine debt and/or increased cortisol release may occur (see Everly, 1989; Wilson, 1989). Both conditions are associated with behavioral withdrawal and depressive affect. Thus, the numbing, depressive, an withdrawal symptoms seem best viewed as residing subsequent to initial excitation and representing symptoms indicative of fatigue, self-preserving withdrawal, and perhaps even depression in response to an event perceived as overpowering, catastrophic, and perhaps inescapable. As noted by Wilson (1989), "Van der Kolk, Krystal, and Greenberg's conceptualization of compensatory responses appears to be a parsimonious explanation for the characteristic avoidance symptoms of PTSD" (p. 32).

Treatment of PTSD via Neurologic Desensitization

Previous sections within this chapter have developed and proposed the notion that PTSD is a *disorder of arousal* (i.e., a disorder which has as its core pathophenomenological constituency a neurologic hypersensitivity residing within the subcortical limbic circuitry). This hypersensitivity is proposed to exist as a lowered functional threshold for depolarization of neurons within the limbic system and its immediate neurologic and neuroendocrine effector mechanisms (e.g., the sympathetic nervous system, the adrenal medullary catecholamine system, and even the adrenal cortical axis). The net result of this functional hypersensitivity is thought to be unusually high levels of excitation within the effector systems. Thus, this excitation serves to create and protract a wide potential variety of psychiatric and somatic symptoms within the overall contruct of PTSD.

As Leonardo da Vinci noted, "First study the science, then practice the art." Thus, the study of pathophenomenology with regard to PTSD should not be seen as an exercise unto itself; rather understanding PTSD as a disorder of arousal should allow us to better practice our therapeutic arts. In this case, cognizance of the neurologic hypersensitivity intrinsic to the PTSD patient allows the emergence of a therapeutic desideratum. Successful treatment of PTSD is based largely upon the neurologic desensitization of the PTSD patient with a resultant diminution in the levels of central and peripheral pathogenic excitation.

Techniques for Neurologic Desensitization

Based upon a review of relevant resources, it is most likely that neurologic desensitization is best achieved through therapeutic technologies which reduce central and/or peripheral arousal (Everly, 1989). Numerous techniques exist which are capable of achieving that end.

I have argued that removing an individual from a set of conditions which engender arousal is a useful first step in promoting a decrement in manifest arousal (Everly, 1989). Similarly, I have noted that simply allowing the individual to talk about circumstances, feeling, reactions, and the like can achieve dramatic decrements in psychophysiological arousal (as long as such cathartic ventilation is guided by a trained professional toward some therapeutic closure).

Wilson (1989) developed an elegant formulation of how the American Indian sweat lodge ritual and its parallels can be of value in achieving a reduction in pathogenic arousal and may then be useful in achieving neurologic desensitization. He noted that such rituals often involve a set of factors known to engender a form of altered state of consciousness. This altered state, as described by Wilson, appears ideally suited to achieve a reduction in hyperarousal and perhaps neurologic desensitization. He noted important therapeutic factors include the elicitation of a positive mood, relaxation, drowsiness, cognitive clarity, and a general sense of well-being. Wilson posited that engendering such factors serves to shift temporarily an individual's status of neurologic functioning from an ergotropic status to a trophotropic one, in effect, achieving neurologic desensitization and a reduction in manifest arousal on both central and peripheral levels.

Benson has written extensively on what he has termed the *relaxation response* (i.e., a hypometabolic response capable of being engendered by wide and diverse variety of relaxation techniques). The relaxation response appears to gain its therapeutic effectiveness from several factors: (1) its ability to reduce catecholaminergic reactivity, (2) its ability to reduce neuromuscular tone, (3) its ability to interrupt cognitive ruminations, and (4) its ability to engender a sense of self-efficacy/self-control (see Everly & Benson, 1989, for a review).

It should be noted that according to Wilson (1989), PTSD has as key elements of its pathological constituency (1) increased catecholaminergic reactivity, (2) increased neuromuscular tension, (3) cognitive ruminations, and (4) a diminished sense of self-control. Thus, we see, at least theoretically, that the use of the relaxation response should prove to be an almost ideal strategy for the treatment of PTSD.

Evidence has failed to demonstrate that there is one best technique to engender the relaxation response, therefore, therapists should employ the techniques that are most likely to be of value on a case-by-case basis. Such techniques as biofeedback may prove of value to individuals who have a high susceptibility to boredom and/or who need to see their therapy "quantified." Imagery and mantra meditation, on the other hand, may be quite useful for patients who are more cognitively flexible (without having schizoidal or psychotic propensities) and can more readily harness their own imagination in a positive manner. I made special note of the value of breathing techniques in reducing ergotropic tone and manifest arousal (Everly, 1989).

Regardless of the relaxation technology employed, Benson (1983) noted that

> the relaxation response results in physiological changes which are thought to characterize an integrated hypothalamic function. These physiological changes are consistent with generalized decreased sympathetic nervous system activity. (p. 282)

Interestingly, Gellhorn and Loufbourrow (1963) noted over a quarter of a century ago, "If it were possible to alter the autonomic reactivity at the hypothalamic level important therapeutic results might be obtained" (p. 90). It now seems clear that such an effect or its approximation is indeed attainable. Furthermore, it is clear that it is attainable on the basis of behavioral interventions. Psychotropic medications, such as benzodiazepines, certain antidepressants, and especially certain anticonvulsants, may achieve a similar end (Everly, 1989). A discussion of those agents is not the focus of this chapter, such a discussion appears elsewhere in this volume. Yet it is worth noting that, for some PTSD patients, psychotropic medication may be less than effective or desirable. Similarly, medication does little to engender a sense of self-efficacy. Thus, it may be that in some cases the use of behavioral interventions which reduce arousal and foster neurologic desensitization can be used to (1) augment the usual course of psychotropic medication or (2) facilitate recovery without the aid of psychotropic medications. Clearly, however, there will be instances where psychotropic medication will be a necessary aspect of the treatment of PTSD.

Neurocognitive Therapy for PTSD

As noted earlier, Wilson (1989) described PTSD as possessing several important constituents: (1) increased catecholaminergic activity, (2) increased neuromuscular tension, (3) ruminative processes, and (4) a diminished sense of self-control. This formulation is consistent with my own (Everly, 1984, 1985, 1989) homogenizing "neurocognitive" construct within which I posit that stress-response syndromes, including PTSD, possess a two-factor dysfunction: (1) pathognomonic arousal and (2) cognitive-affective processes which serve to engender, or otherwise facilitate, arousal. This chapter has similarly portrayed the phenomenology of PTSD as residing within the two-factor neurocognitive construct of pathognomonic arousal (catecholaminergic and neuromuscular) and cognitive-affective facilitation of arousal (recollection of a contradicted worldview, weltanschauung, and a feeling of helpless inefficacy).

From within this two-fact construct may emerge an integrated approach to the treatment of PTSD. This integrated treatment approach has been referred to as *neurocognitive therapy* (Everly, 1984, 1985, 1989). Critical in the neurocognitive approach to the treatment of PTSD is the recognition that PTSD possesses a dual dysfunction expressed in its core constituents: (1) pathognomonic psychophysiological arousal, and (2) ruminative, recollective cognitive and affective processes, which are pathognomonic in and of themselves, and which serve to support and further ignite subsequent cascades of arousal. Neurocognitive therapy entails the creation of an integrated treatment plan and an operationalization of that plan so that *both* core constituent domains receive therapeutic intervention. Therapeutic attention to both constituent domains, in a direct and coordinated manner, is likely to create a condition of reciprocally augmenting and synergistic therapies.

Therapeutic interventions such as rest, light-duty work assignments, training in the relaxation response, biofeedback, and even psychotropic medications have shown their value in reducing pathogenic or pathognomonic arousal (Everly, 1989). These therapies may be seen as directed toward the goals of not only reducing arousal but also achieving the neurologic desensitization as described earlier.

Classic psychotherapeutic strategies may be directed toward the cognitive-affective domain. Techniques ranging from the cognitive-based to the hypnotic-based have all shown some utility in the treatment of PTSD. The work of Bandura (1977, 1982) has unique applicability in the treatment of PTSD from a neurocognitive perspective. Bandura's concepts can be conceptualized in four therapeutic strategies: (1) vicarious learning—wherein one's confidence and coping abilities are increased through learning from others who have had similar problems; (2) enactive attainment—where one learns to cope through confronting anxiogenic people, places, or things; (3) physiological self-regulation—wherein one learns to reduce arousal; and (4) encouragement—wherein one receives support and encouragement from significant others. Bandura's formulations have the potential to contain therapeutic strategies that address virtually all of the pathognomonic constituents of PTSD as

described by Wilson (1989) and myself (Everly, 1989, 1990). Ultimately, however, if trauma represents a contradiction to one's worldview, successful psychotherapy may equate to mending that traumatic contradiction.

In sum, the neurocognitive therapy of PTSD resists the temptation to dictate specific therapeutic strategies; rather, it simply directs therapeutic interventions in an integrated manner toward the core constituents of PTSD: pathognomonic psychophysiological arousal (neurological domain) and the ruminative, recollective cognitive-affective processes which are distressing unto themselves and which serve to fuel further arousal (cognitive-affective domain).

Summary and Conclusions

My intent in this chapter has been to explore the nature of PTSD in search of shedding light on issues of pathophenomenology as well as therapeutic intervention.

PTSD has been presented within this chapter as possessing two *core* constituents: (1) recollective processes and (2) hypersensitivity and excessive psychophysiological arousal. Consistent with this perspective, PTSD has been categorized within the generic formulation of disorders of arousal. The key taxonomic criterion for inclusion in this nosological formulation is neurologic hypersensitivity and pathognomonic arousal. A review of empirical and theoretical evidence found the phenomenology of PTSD to be consistent with the disorders-of-arousal construct. More specifically, it is believed that the biology of PTSD resides in a functional hypersensitivity and ergotropic tonus within the septal-hippocampal and amygdaloid nuclei of the subcortical limbic circuitry.

The conclusion that PTSD represents a disorder of arousal leads directly to implications for therapeutic intervention. It may be argued that successful treatment of PTSD is contingent upon reducing a condition of pathognomonic arousal to a level of excitation which is responsive to homeostatic and autogenic modulation within a range of nonpathogenic functioning. This reduction in manifest excitation can often be achieved by behavioral technologies alone; nevertheless, the use of psychotropic medication to achieve this end may also be considered.

Perhaps the most powerful therapeutic assault on PTSD resides in some form of *neurocognitive therapy*. Neurocognitive therapy is defined as an integrated, coordinated psychotherapeutic effort directed at the psychophysiological arousal (neuro-) and the ruminative recollective cognitions (cognitive) virtually simultaneously. Such an effort reflects an appreciation of the inextricable intertwinings of mind and body, and of the duality of dysfunction intrinsic to PTSD.

Even though much effort was spent in this chapter directed toward a pathophenomenological analysis of PTSD, this analysis derives its greatest value when considered toward the goal of treatment planning. To that end this chapter is dedicated.

References

American Psychiatric Association. (1980). *Diagnostic and statistical manual of mental disorders* (3rd ed.). Washington, DC: Author.

American Psychiatric Association. (1987). *Diagnostic and statistical manual of mental disorders* (3rd ed., rev.). Washington, DC: Author.

Arnold, M. (1984). *Memory and the brain*. Hillsdale, NJ: Lawrence Erlbaum.

Bandura, A. (1977). Self-efficacy. *Psychological Review, 84,* 191–215.

Bandura, A. (1982). Self-efficacy mechanisms in human agency. *American Psychologist, 37,* 122–147.

Barlow, D., & Beck, J. (1984). The psychosocial treatment of anxiety disorders. In J. B. Williams & R. Spitzer (Eds.), *Psychotherapy research* (pp. 29–69). New York: Guilford Press.

Benson, H. (1975). *The relaxation response*. New York: William Morrow.

Benson, H. (1983). The relaxation response. *Trends in Neuroscience, 6,* 281–284.

Carr, D., & Sheehan, D. (1984). Panic anxiety. *Journal of Clinical Psychiatry, 45,* 323–330.

Ciaranello, R. D. (1983). Neurochemical aspects of stress. In N. Garmezy & M. Rutter (Eds.), *Stress, coping, and development in children*. New York: McGraw-Hill.

Delanoy, R., Tucci, D., & Gold, P. (1983). Amphetamine effects on LTP in dendate granule cells. *Pharmacology, Biochemistry, and Behavior, 18,* 137–139.

Doane, B. (1986). Clinical psychiatry and physiodynamics of the limbic system. In B. Doane & K. Livingston (Eds.), *The limbic system* (pp. 285–315). New York: Raven Press.

Everly, G. S. (1984, December). *A neurocognitive analysis of stress response syndromes associated with trauma.* Paper presented to the FEMA/NIMH Conference on Role Conflict and Support for Emergency Workers, Washington, DC.

Everly, G. S. (1985, April). *Neurocognitive therapy and rehabilitation of psychiatric syndromes in response to stress.* Paper presented to the International Conference on Stress and Behavioral Emergencies, Balto.

Everly, G. S. (1989). *A clinical guide to the treatment of the human stress response*. New York: Plenum Press.

Everly, G. S. (1990). Post-traumatic stress disorder as a "disorder of arousal." *Psychology and Health: An International Journal, 4,* 135–145.

Everly, G. S., & Benson, H. (1989). Disorders of arousal. *International Journal of Psychosomatics, 36,* 15–22.

Everly, G. S., & Horton, A. M. (1989). Neuropsychology of posttraumatic stress disorder: A pilot study. *Perceptual and Motor Skills, 68,* 807–810.

Fifkova, E., & Van Harreveld, A. (1977). Long-lasting morphological changes in dendritic spines. *Journal of Neurocytology, 6,* 211–230.

Foy, D., Lund, M., Sipprelle, C., & Strachan, A. (1984). The Combat Exposure Scale: A systematic assessment of trauma in the Vietnam War. *Journal of Clinical Psychology, 40,* 1323–1328.

Friedman, M. (1988). Toward a rational pharmacotherapy for PTSD. *American Journal of Psychiatry, 145,* 281–285.

Gellhorn, E. (1957). *Autonomic imbalance and the hypothalamus.* Minneapolis: University of Minnesota Press.

Gellhorn, E. (1965). Neurophysiological bases of anxiety. *Perspectives in Biology and Medicine, 8,* 488–515.

Gellhorn, E. (1967). *Principles of autonomic-somatic integration.* Minneapolis: University of Minnesota Press.

Gellhorn, E., & Loofbourrow, G. (1963). *Emotions and emotional disorders.* New York: Harper & Row.

Goddard, G., McIntyre, D., & Leech, C. (1969). A permanent change in brain function resulting from daily electrical stimulation. *Experimental Neurology, 25,* 295–330.

Horowitz, M., Wilner, N., Kaltreider, N., & Alvarez, W. (1980). Signs and symptoms of PTSD. *Archives of General Psychiatry, 37,* 85–92.

Joy, R. (1985). The effects of neurotoxicants on kindling and kindled seizures. *Fundamental and Applied Toxicology, 5,* 41–65.

Kardiner, A. (1941). *The traumatic neuroses of war.* New York: Paul B. Hoeber.

Kolb, L. C. (1987). A neuropsychological hypothesis explaining post-traumatic stress disorders. *American Journal of Psychiatry, 144,* 989–995.

Kolb, L. C. (1988). A critical survey of hypotheses regarding PTSD in light of recent research. *Journal of Traumatic Stress, 3,* 291–304.

McGeer, E., & McGeer, P. (1988). Excitotoxins and animal models of disease. In C. Galli, L. Manzo, & P. Spencer (Eds.), *Recent advances in nervous system toxicology* (pp. 107–131). New York: Plenum Press.

Mason, J. W., Giller, E. L., Kosten, T. R., et al. (1986). Urinary free cortisol in PTSD. *Journal of Nervous and Mental Disorders, 174,* 145–149.

Nutt, D. (1989). Altered central a2 adrenoreceptor sensitivity in panic disorder. *Archives of General Psychiatry, 46,* 165–169.

Olney, J. W. (1978). Neurotoxicity of excitatory amino acids. In E. McGeer, J. Olney, & P. McGeer (Eds.), *Kainic acid as a tool in neurobiology* (pp. 95–122). New York: Raven Press.

Post, R. (1985). Stress, sensitization, kindling, and conditioning. *Behavioral and Brain Sciences, 8,* 372–373.

Post, R. (1986). Does limbic system dysfunction play a role in affective illness? In B. Doane & K. Livingston (Eds.), *The limbic system.* New York: Raven Press.

Post, R., & Ballenger, J. (1981). Kindling models for progressive development of psychopathology. In H. Van Pragg (Ed.), *Handbook of biological psychiatry* (pp. 609–651). New York: Marcel Dekker.

Post, R., & Kopanda, R. (1976). Cocaine, kindling, and psychosis. *American Journal of Psychiatry, 133,* 627–634.

Sapolsky, R., Krey, L., & McEwen, B. (1984). Stress downregulates corticosterone receptors in a site specific manner in the brain. *Endocrinology, 114,* 287–292.

Sheehan, D. (1983). *The anxiety disease.* New York: Scribner.

van der Kolk, B. (1988). The trauma spectrum. *Journal of Traumatic Stress, 1,* 273–290.

van der Kolk, B., Brown, P., & van der Hart, O. (1989). Pierre Janet on post-traumatic stress. *Journal of Traumatic Stress, 2,* 365–378.

van der Kolk, B., Greenberg, M., Boyd, H., & Krystal, J. (1985). Inescapable shock, neurotransmitters, and addiction to trauma. *Biological Psychiatry, 20,* 314–325.

Weil, J. (1974). *A neurophysiological model of emotional and intentional behavior.* Springfield, IL: Charles C Thomas.

Wilson, J. P. (1989). *Trauma, transformation, and healing.* New York: Brunner/Mazel.

CHAPTER 68

Focal Psychoanalytic Psychotherapy of Posttraumatic Stress Disorder

Jacob D. Lindy

Introduction

Psychoanalytic psychotherapy of posttraumatic stress disorder (PTSD) distinguishes itself from other treatment modalities in that its focus is on the meaning of trauma-related symptoms and behaviors and on the meaning of catastrophic life events to the person as a whole. The analytically oriented therapist is also curious about the ways in which a person's psyche and soma fend off, experience, cope, and adapt to extreme stress. The analyst is concerned about the dilemmas which the person in the traumatic situation faced, and faces, as a result, in the present. The therapist uses introspection, intuition, and empathy in order to try to comprehend and then verbalize a dilemma which stretches beyond his or her own internal experience. The analytic therapist hopes that insights regarding the meaning of symptoms, both conscious and unconscious, and the consequences of catastrophe can be utilized by the survivor to identify and help master future danger situations and to try to make whole again the fabric of life.

The analytically oriented therapist uses theory to guide this quest, both metapsychological theory and the theory of technique. Psychoanalytic theory of massive psychic trauma presupposes that once the organism's stimulus barrier is overwhelmed, emergency defenses, such as disavowal, dissociation, splitting, identification with the aggressor, and other unconscious mechanisms (often pathological) are put into play. Because energy is continually being drained by the trauma, developmental

arrest, fixation, and regression may occur. Symptoms indicate the ongoing presence of unresolved elements in the trauma and may lead subsequently to altered character formation.

These suppositions as well as the differing views of analytic authors regarding the role of early childhood in subsequent reactions to catastrophic events are developed more fully in the chapter on analytic theory and PTSD (see Chapter 5, in this volume).

In this chapter, I shall focus primarily on principles of analytic theory of technique and discuss the modifications in these principles called for in the focal psychoanalytic psychotherapy of PTSD.

Figure 68.1 helps to identify some of the elements of concern which apply to all psychoanalytically oriented psychotherapies: the course of the working alliance, the development and interpretation of transference phenomena, and the monitoring and therapeutic use of countertransference tendencies.

Analytic Model in the Treatment of PTSD

An extensive literature on these constructs of technique exists and are well summarized by Sterba (1934), Zetzel (1956), Greenson (1967), Gill (1982), and Racker (1968). Figure 68.1 also highlights central therapeutic tasks in each phase of the treatment. These tasks are consistent with the growing literature on time-limited supportive expressive psychoanalytic therapy (Luborsky, 1984a), and brief psychoanalytic psychotherapy (Malan, 1976). They are consistent with tasks involved in understanding a core-conflict relationship theme (Luborsky, 1984b) and the central pathogenic beliefs (Weiss & Sampson, 1986), although the metaphors chosen to describe these tasks have a special reference to the area of trauma.

Jacob D. Lindy • Department of Psychiatry and Traumatic Stress Study Center, University of Cincinnati Medical School, Cincinnati, Ohio 45267–0539.

International Handbook of Traumatic Stress Syndromes, edited by John P. Wilson and Beverley Raphael. Plenum Press, New York, 1993.

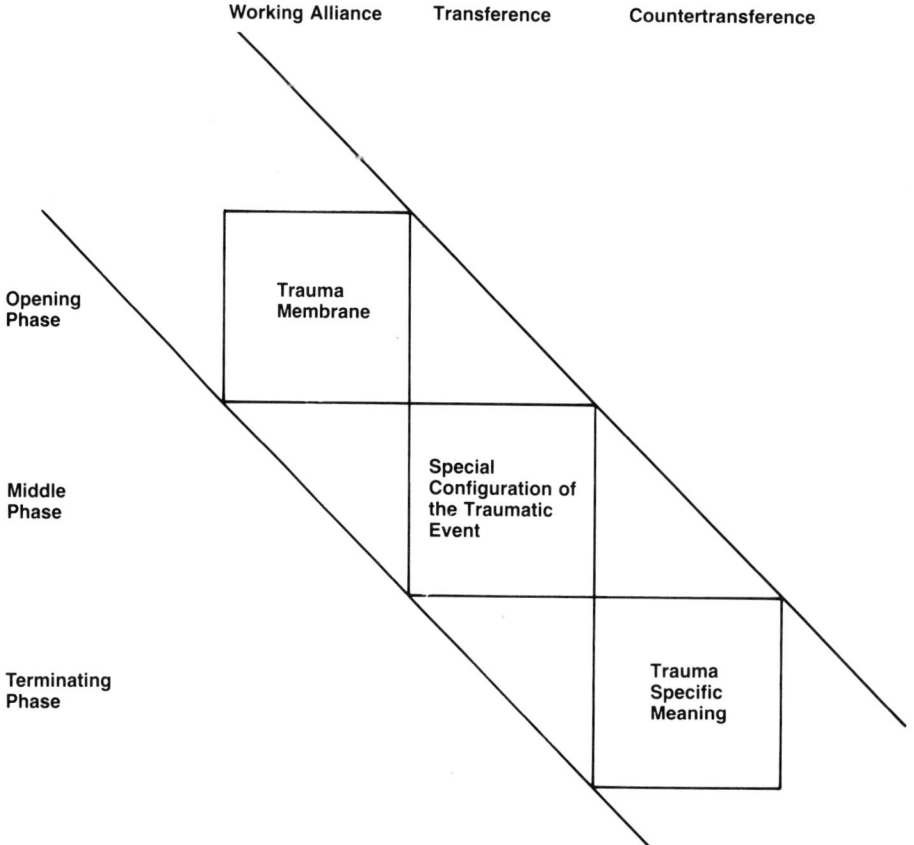

Figure 68.1. Focal psychoanalytic therapy: phases and processes.

The summary presented in Figure 68.1 looks at several traditional elements within psychoanalytic clinical theory as orienting points toward conceptualizing crucial stages of therapeutic activity during the course of the focal psychotherapy of PTSD. Along one axis we have the opening phase, the middle phase, and the terminating phase (perhaps in this case better termed "separating from the therapist"). Along another axis we have the working alliance, transference, and countertransference. Proceeding diagonally, beginning with the quadrant defined by the opening phase and the working alliance, and proceeding to the quadrant defined by separating from the therapist and countertransference, we have two lines; one representing the therapist and the other the survivor. Within each quadrant we have a primary therapeutic task. The first is gaining and maintaining entry beneath the trauma membrane. The task in the middle quadrant is identifying and ultimately metabolizing the special configuration of the traumatic event; and the task in the third quadrant is the acquisition of trauma-specific meaning which permits continuity, sublimation, and mourning.

Biological Metaphors: Analogues to PTSD

Several terms are introduced in this schema: trauma membrane, special configuration of the traumatic event,

metabolizing trauma, and trauma-specific meaning. I begin with definitions and illustrations of these concepts and later follow the fate of each of the new constructs through the course of the treatment. Specific and nonspecific interventions and attitudes relating to the working alliance, transference, and countertransference as they pertain to the special case of the treatment of traumatic stress disorders are discussed next. Last comes a summary of the opening, middle, and terminating phases of the focal treatment of PTSD in light of the above discussion.

Several biological metaphors are used to describe central therapeutic tasks in the treatment of PTSD. They take as their backdrop the structure of the human cell and the nature and function of certain kinds of molecules in it. Central to the model is the differential capacity of the cell, by means of a semipermeable membrane, to take in molecules from components in its adjacent environment which are useful for its ongoing metabolism, and to exclude those elements which might be destructive. Trauma disrupts the semipermeable function of this membrane and indiscriminately allows into the "cell" a wide variety of potentially noxious agents; alternately, the cell closes itself off to all input, becoming impermeable, but thereby being unable to release its own toxic metabolites. In the survivor with PTSD, perception is altered by a disrupted trauma membrane. The overwhelming trauma has not only overcome a "stimulus barrier" (Freud, 1922) but it has left lasting damage at the site of perceptual input to the organism. Thus, trauma has produced an ongoing defect in reality testing. Trigger stimuli, like small toxic molecules, pass through the disrupted membrane and interact directly with traumatic memory traces to which the body responds as though the past is the present. As a construct, the trauma membrane remains important throughout all phases of the treatment. Gradually, the survivors come to position the therapist as functioning on the trauma membrane and acting as the semipermeable discriminator to allow manageable sizes of potentially metabolizable trauma to enter. The therapist directs patients' attention to those aspects of their current life which direct themselves towards those pieces of trauma which conceivably can be worked-through. Later, in the termination process, the survivors reclaim this function. They internalize the therapist's discriminating function and reestablish the viability of this reality-testing function for themselves.

Special Psychic Configuration of Traumatic Events

Here, it is as if the molecular arrangements of a central working segment of a cell, say, for example, the mitochondria, have been realigned and twisted upon each other into a new form. The resultant large configuration or macromolecule functions like a pathogenic enzyme. It is as though the positioning of the molecular fragments attracts and then uses up metabolites and other energy sources in producing reactions which are no longer useful to the organism. The specific form this molecule takes has its origin in the differing disavowed memories (affects, defenses, and object configurations) contained within or surrounding the traumatic events themselves. The trigger stimuli, mentioned earlier, such as the sound of rain in Buffalo Creek, the smell of burning flesh following the Beverly Hills Fire, the sensation of a warm sultry day to a Vietnam veteran, represent sensory warning signals to potential danger situations. Interpersonal configurations, such as potential betrayal or abuse of power, may also set off the special configuration, and special affect states, such as helplessness, rage, guilt, shame, terror, and panic, may also set it off. At the outset of treatment, with an impaired trauma membrane, this large configuration can be set off by a wide number of apparently matching molecular structures: dangerous rules, misplaced objects, the cry of a frightened child, and unidentified object mistaken for a human part. Once the matching molecule sets the macromolecule into action, a whole series of psychic events occur almost simultaneously which usually take the form of a reenactment, a traumatic dream, or an intrusive image. Sometimes this is an unidentifiable complex of overwhelming affect states. The net effect is an overexpenditure of energy on psychic or physical activity which is maladaptive in the current situations. The signs and symptoms of the maladaptation and efforts to avoid it represent the entity of posttraumatic stress disorder.

Meaning Structure of the Special Configuration

The meaning of the special configuration of the traumatic event implies that the whole is greater than the sum of its parts. Thus, the special configuration includes not only the multiplicity of stressors which were active in and around the period of trauma, such as fright, loss, threat of bodily harm, or exposure to grotesqueness; for example, it is more than the multiple interacting affect states of helplessness, rage, guilt, and shame. It is even more than the expectable compensatory fantasies which these states stir up, such as omnipotence or murderous aggression. The meaning of the special configuration of the traumatic event presupposes a uniquely organized, highly integrated percept, action, or fantasy within the trauma which, by virtue of its radical departure from the survivor's preexisting identity, forms a discontinuity between the person and his or her view of self and the world before the events and after them.

Case Illustrations of Special Configuration

Consider the case of Tom and his fellow American prisoners of war, who were being killed by their Vietnamese captors, one per day in random executions. The traumatic memory contained more than a threat to his own life, the fright he experienced, his efforts to cope with that fright as well as the grotesque images of himself observing the mutilations of his comrades and the visual impact of the public executions. The peculiar twist to the configuration meant that for Tom to wish to survive would mean that he would have to wish his comrade's death. Such a self-view was inconsistent with own his sense of personal identity and contributed to his sense of discontinuity as a result of the traumata.

Buddy Lee, Vietnam veteran, having been exposed to a wide variety of combat stressors in Vietnam, including being injured, having his unit overrun, and seeing close friends killed, also witnessed and participated in abusive violence. When he was transferred from a weapons-expert position in a rural village to a new assignment—probably in Operation Phoenix—Buddy Lee left many friends (including children) behind. In his new role, he carried out assigned assassinations on what he supposed to be Vietcong leaders in other rural villages. He came to suspect that, at times, the figures assassinated were actually part of a tactic to stage massacres as though they had been carried out by the Vietcong against United States sympathizers. Eventually, he came to suspect that some of the victims of these assassination squads were actually friendly to the United States. One day, he returned to the village in which he had befriended many people earlier in his tour of duty. He found the village destroyed and discovered the mutilated body of one of the children who had been his friend. He came to believe that this new role as patriot-assassin violated his strongest value, loyalty. Now, loyalty to his task endangered the lives of those whom, paradoxically, he was assigned to protect.

Mrs. K., a married Catholic mother of four, was brutally raped for more than 3 hours in the parking area of an inner-city industrial plant where she worked the night shift. Reasoning that it was better to submit than to risk being murdered by the rapist, she disassociated during much of the assault. When she was late for her menstrual period and believed she was pregnant by the rapist, she came to an inner decision to have an abortion. Although rationally comfortable with her choice, she felt severely guilty and alienated. The rape trauma and its consequences had cut her off from her previous perception of herself as a good Catholic person. The irrational basis of this harsh self-criticism only served to force her to work harder to convince herself that she was, in fact, good, thus worsening her PTSD.

Chip, an air traffic controller and law student, dreamed of a career in air traffic safety. When a severely damaged aircraft was reported in his area, he carefully guided the plane to a relatively successful emergency landing and was viewed as a hero. Nonetheless, the crash landing killed 35 people. Chip recognized that certain errors in the technical landing of the plane may have occurred and were being sidestepped. He blamed himself for failing to speak up loudly enough or soon enough during the subsequent investigation. He felt that he had marred his integrity. Eventually, his life became a grim recrimination, sapping pleasure and ambition from his world. He came to believe that he could no longer trust his own sense of integrity. There was discontinuity in his ideals and expectations of himself. He gave up his career goals and took on atonement-related tasks without relief.

Thus, the special configuration and its meaning depends not only on the complexity of the multiple stressors and reactions, on the accompanying defenses, coping mechanisms, and fantasies, but also on the unique organization of such percepts, actions, and fantasies which tend to disconnect the survivor psychologically from the person before the event.

Three Central Tasks in Focal Analytic Psychotherapy

Focal analytic psychotherapy of PTSD calls for the therapist to address these central tasks: (1) earning the right to gain access beneath the trauma membrane and maintaining that position in the presence of tests to disprove worthiness, thereby clarifying the contours of the special configuration of the traumatic event by linking day residue with traumatic memory; (2) "lysing" trauma into more manageable segments, while comprehending, empathizing, and verbalizing the specific meaning of the trauma as a whole through shared metaphors; and (3) helping the survivor find continuity in self and to disconnect from the therapy.

Therapeutic Posture in PTSD Treatment

Toward these ends, a number of attitudes, behaviors, and interventions are important. Together they describe the *therapeutic posture* of the analytic therapist in dealing with the trauma patient. They differ in pointed ways with some stereotypes of the analyst as rigid, silent, and impassive.

The therapist is invited beneath the *trauma membrane* by the survivor. To take this risk, the survivor weighs heavily the recommendation of other survivors that this person "understands." "Expert" knowledge may be an asset but is clearly secondary to the recommendation of a trusted fellow survivor. In the absence of such facilitating introductions, the survivor is initially wary and must frequently test the therapist in a variety of ways. To some extent, these tests will likely occur somewhere, with or without easy initial access beneath the membrane. How they are responded to will provide the form and durability of the working alliance. They address the central question: Is the therapeutic situation a safe one?

Does the therapist withdraw from the survivor through signs of alarm, fright, or disbelief? Or, on the other hand, does the therapist push counterphobically or voyeuristically too hard for trauma details thus leading to overwhelming affect? Does the therapist push the survivor away with hints of disgust or condemnation? Are the therapist's motives suspect? Is the therapist reliable in behavior and accurate in words? In short, is the therapist concerned, well-paced, nonjudgmental, and ethical? Frequently, the sites around which such tests develop involve the structure of the sessions themselves: the time and frequency of appointments, confidentiality, the relative activity or inactivity of the therapist, the fee, responses to requests to write letters to employers, lawyers, or in regard to disability claims.

Specific responses during the opening phase are of special usefulness in addition to the general attitudes described above. These behaviors and interventions establish, *in toto*, the wisdom of the survivor's judgment to invite the therapist closer to the trauma.

In the initial phase, the therapist makes specific interventions as well. She/he clarifies that certain symptoms, such as hyperalertness, distractibility, and episodes of intrusive images and anxiety are part of a disorder—posttraumatic stress disorder. The syndrome has a natural history and can occur to anyone who is exposed to catastrophic events. Furthermore, the symptoms are set off in the present as a result of reminders of the trauma itself, and that establishing the specifics of these linkages will be the work of both the therapist and the survivor.

In general, continuing to establish specific linkage between derivative current behavior and symptoms and disavowed traumatic memory is the work of the middle phase of treatment and helps to map the contours of the trauma configuration. However, on occasion where intrusive phenomena dangerously dominate the clinical picture early, the therapist may need to assume a link between current acting out and disavowed trauma memory simply to provide a working structure and to get the treatment started.

For example, when Tom broke his hand as he struck the basement wall while writhing as if he were chained down, his therapist assured him that part of his POW experience was likely being played out without his awareness (i.e., he explained the nature of the reenactment), and that the details of this otherwise bizarre behavior will be invaluable in reconstructing Tom's personal experience of traumatic memory.

Current Life Stress and Traumatic Reactions

Alternatively, the linkage between current stress and trauma may need to be massively fended off by numbing. Here, the therapeutic stance is to appreciate the intensity of the need to keep the memory split off; in essence, to appreciate the power of resistance *first*. For example, Abraham, a well-functioning but depressed adult, was *nearly* aware that his bursts of anger at his 14-year-old son were rekindling the memory of a nightlong death vigil he experienced years earlier with a 14-year-old Vietnamese boy whom he had shot. But he was not yet ready to face the enormous guilt and shame he felt over the past event. Literally, if he were to press the linkage between residue (his son) and trauma (the Vietnamese boy) too early, he would risk suicide. Instead, the therapist needed to build an extended alliance patiently and await the veteran's readiness to proceed.

Gradually, in a dosed manner, the therapist and the survivor bring together the many current day situations and feelings which threaten to set off the traumatic memory. The survivor begins to feel that the universe of trigger stimuli is a defined one. The trauma itself now has boundaries and contours with known triggers. One by one, these subelements become clearer and loosened from the trauma as a whole, and the survivor gains some energy to begin to direct in productive, rather than in precautionary, actions.

Here, the therapist encourages a layering of understandings: how bravery and panic, duty and guilt, honor and retaliation rest beside each other in the emotional complexity of traumatic memories. Gradually, each painful emotional state is opened and responded to with acceptance. But grasping the essence of the trauma and responding acceptingly is by no means an easy task. Use of transference formulations becomes an essential guiding principle to the technical work. But first, we must take a step backward. Based on the theoretical importance of the repetition compulsion, analytically oriented therapists are accustomed to search and find—in the here-and-now transactions between patient and therapist—latent references to key relationships in the childhood past of the patient. The analytic therapist draws on these projections to formulate, interpret, and facilitate change. But because of the recurrence and intensity of traumatic intrusive phenomena in the survivor with PTSD, it is more likely that the here-and-now transactions between survivor and therapist will reflect "transference" phenomena from the trauma itself, rather than from the early past.

Clinical Issues in the Three Phases of Treatment

In the initial phase of treatment such transference reactions, which are often negative, may gravely threaten the working alliance. The therapist must link these reactions to the trauma itself in order to build and preserve the working alliance.

For example, in the second session, Spike leaped up from his chair and stuck his finger against the therapist's head: "*You* don't know what it's like to have to blow off the head of a Vietnamese child." Spike had become anxious as the interviewer proceeded and had made reference to the therapist's "interrogating" him. Using his transference understanding, the therapist said, "Someone who was asking about your experience in Vietnam didn't understand but kept *interrogating* you." Spike settled down and recounted his excruciating interrogation by American legal officers upon his return from the troublesome missions in Vietnam. Spike could now distinguish that his doctor in the present was not the legal officer who threatened him many years ago; he could tell what he felt ready to tell, when he felt ready to tell it (i.e., the treatment could proceed).

In the middle phase of treatment, transference reactions many give incisive information about the special configuration of traumatic events which are in the process of being reconstructed.

Jonah, who was always punctual, was 30 minutes late for an appointment; he repeated the phenomenon (to the minute) a second time. The therapist said, "There was a crucial 30-minute lapse in the events we are trying to understand." "Yes, the 30 minutes that I kept radioing in for choppers to get my buddy and . . . (and was abandoned by my commanding officer) . . . (and goes on to describe a most brutal part of the trauma previously disavowed)." Such reactions take many forms and they offer the therapist an opportunity to narrow down the field of trauma to a highly specific one.

Note also that the therapist is using the transference to reconstruct the traumatic past, so as not to bring unnecessary added affect to the here and now, which is already extremely tense. Such centripetal interventions, as "You must be having angry feelings about the treatment because you are 30 minutes late"; or in the case of Spike, "It looks as if you want to kill me because I express interest in you" would be less productive.

As the treatment proceeds toward the termination phase, it is often a transference–countertransference interaction which stirs in the therapist a unique twist to the trauma-specific meaning for the survivor. Buddy Lee's habit of insisting that he pay $10 in cash at each session alerted the therapist to the story of a Vietnamese boy whom Buddy Lee liked and protected and to whom he gave 10 cents of military money, thereby marking each encounter.

Through this transference dimension, the therapist now understood it was in the role of the defenseless child that he, the therapist, was most closely connected to Buddy Lee. When the veteran sensed that the therapist was under attack from the VA, he feared irrationally for the therapist's life. The therapist was able to say, "Something terrible happened to that little boy you tried to protect." "Yes, he was killed by our side; I found him; and it was as though I had done it."

Transference had led the way toward discovering the special meaning of Buddy Lee's trauma: his lifelong goal of protecting the naive and the helpless had been shattered; instead, he would now bring destruction to those who were loyal to him. At *this* point then, it was feasible to return to the debilitating illness of his mother as a child, and to begin to search for the origins of the meaning of loyalty and protection for Buddy Lee. Gradually, the survivor displays in transference reactions to the therapist a *special* configuration of his trauma. Those are the ways in which his memories contain actions, perceptions, and fantasies which alienate himself from his previous sense of self. Empathically, the therapist begins to *feel* this essential twist to the trauma and may even temporarily "fall ill" himself as he struggles with it.

Countertransference precedes the treatment and proceeds simultaneously along with each of the phases (Wilson, 1989). Countertransferences are evoked by stereotypic views which interfere with the uniqueness of the individual's survivor experience and the reactions. Countertransferences occur as the stories of trauma take shape to the objects, drives, and affects contained within these stories. Finally, countertransference occurs in unconscious reenactments within the treatment where the traumatic experience is revived. Monitoring countertransference tendencies is a major activity for a therapist in the treatment of a traumatic neurosis, and, as a consequence, ongoing peer-group support and/or supervision is probably indispensable at any level.

In ways which require more research to explain, the therapist's own internal work at living with knowledge of the trauma, as experienced and related by the survivor, leads to the synthesis of a metaphor—a story or "bridge of words"—which allows the therapist to convey to the survivor that he or she is being understood. Once this occurs, the work can proceed to the final stage: examining with the client the meaning of the trauma with the goal of finding continuity between the survivor's pretrauma sense of self and a current self that incorporates this meaning. Interventions in the termination phase of treatment are directed at integrating the meaning of the trauma with life which preceded it and life which followed it.

Such integration often involves transforming earlier ideals and values in light of a newer, more worldly sense of self. Survivorship may move into a more central positive place in the client's identity, which is connected with a sense of mission to help or to warn others. Altruism and sublimation arise spontaneously. Increasing mastery of managing oneself in the presence of trigger stimuli indicate that time for separation from the therapist is drawing near. Setting the date is difficult and provokes severe reactions; it also sets off mourning for those lost in the trauma and for the years that were lost while absorbed in the trauma's psychic aftermath.

Analytically oriented authors who focus on differing aspects of the therapeutic process find themselves alluding to differing metapsychological systems and points of view. Initial overvaluation of the therapist (viewed here as necessary to enter beneath the trauma membrane) is seen by Ullman and Brothers (1988) as the beginning of an idealizing transference. Pathological defenses that are engendered by the trauma itself are seen and interpreted variously, per therapeutic focus, as splitting (object relations), as traumatic overstimulation and loss of cohesion (self-psychology), or as dissociative states (ego psychology). Termination is viewed by Ullman and Brothers (1988) as a giving up of restorative narcissistic fantasies, whereas from the focal-analytic viewpoint, it is the restitution of epigenetic development by integration and transformation of the specific meaning of the trauma.

The terminology presented here is introduced because it appears to be close to actual work with trauma survivors. Another intention is to stimulate in today's therapist trauma-specific ideas as to how the psyche copes in terms of clinical theory and the theory of technique. In terms of metapsychology, I suggest that "borrowing" concepts derived from transference work with other forms of pathology is not, in the long run, the best way for the field to proceed. Rather it is our job to describe newly and freshly those transference reactions we *do* observe in the trauma patient and to build new theory from these observations.

Conclusion

In summary, the working-through of the impact of traumatic memories in focal analytic psychotherapy involves a series of interactions between survivors and therapist. In the opening phase, the survivors, who are wary of anyone who has not experienced what they have, elect to allow the therapist access to some of their pain, while testing the therapist's concern, commitment, capacity to dose affect, and to remain nonjudgmental. Initially, the therapist listens, conveys empathy, explains the syndrome of PTSD, and points out explicitly how residues of discomfort in day-to-day life relate to specific elements in the traumatic past.

In the middle phase, the survivor and the therapist outline the contours of the trauma by repeating the above process in numerous areas. The therapist appreciates how stressors, affects, and defenses are layered, and listens for ways that the elements of the trauma are repeated in the treatment situation. Often, the unique "twist" to the trauma meaning is gained only after the therapist has also experienced some appreciable countertransference tendency, and, while working internally, has emerged with a metaphor, story, or myth which bridges the world of experience of the survivor and the therapist.

Even after the survivor achieves considerable mastery over the trauma, separating from the therapist is often difficult. The separation process requires attending to the newly formed continuity between the pre- and the posttrauma self, and often it must acknowledge the incompleteness of the recovery. Setting a final date sets off unworked-through grief and mourning that are connected with the traumatic memories. Increased energy, altruism, and sublimation of trauma are often rewarding consequences to the survivor and to the therapist.

References

Freud, S. (1922). Beyond the Pleasure Principle. In J. Strachey (Ed. and Trans.), *The standard edition of the complete psychological works of Sigmund Freud* (Vol. 18, pp.29–30). London: Hogarth Press. (Original work published 1923)

Gill, M. (1982). *Analysis of transference* (Vol. 1, pp. 85–106). New York: International Universities Press.

Greenson, R. (1967). The working alliance. In R. Greenson (Ed.), *The technique and practice of psychoanalysis* (Vol. 1, pp. 190–215). New York: International Universities Press.

Luborsky, L. (Ed.). (1984a). *Principles of psychoanalytic psychotherapy* (pp. 71–141). New York: Basic Books.

Luborsky, L. (1984b). An example of the core conflictual relationship theme method: Its scoring and research supports. In L. Luborsky (Ed.), *Principles of psychoanalytic psychotherapy* (pp. 199–228). New York: Basic Books.

Malan, D. H. (1976). *Toward a validation of dynamic psychotherapy: A replication*. New York: Plenum Press.

Racker, H. (1968). *Transference and countertransference* (pp. 127–173). New York: International Universities Press.

Sterba, R. (1934). The fate of the ego in analytic therapy. *International Journal of Psychoanalysis, 15*, 117–126.

Ullman, R., & Brothers, D. (1988). *The shattered self* (pp. 216–247). Hillsdale, NJ: Analytic Press.

Weiss, J. (1986). Unconscious pathogenic beliefs. In J. Weiss & H. Sampson (Eds.), *The psychoanalytic process* (pp. 68–83). New York: Guilford Press.

Weiss, J., & Sampson, H. (Eds.). (1986). *The psychoanalytic process*. New York: Guilford Press.

Wilson, J. P. (1989). *Trauma, transformation, and healing: An integrative approach to theory, research, and post-traumatic therapy*. New York: Brunner/Mazel.

Zetzel, E. (1956). Current concepts of transference. *International Journal of Psychoanalysis, 37*, 369–376.

CHAPTER 69

War-Related Trauma and Victimization

Principles of Traumatic Stress Prevention in Israel

Noach Milgram

Introduction

The first half of the twentieth century has been characterized as the *age of anxiety*. The major emphasis was on neurotic anxiety arising from intrapsychic conflict and producing reactions in vulnerable people that were, from the point of view of an objective observer, either inappropriate or disproportional to the largely innocuous overt eliciting stimuli. The second half of the century may be aptly called the *age of stress*, with the major emphasis on objectively stressful life events and the adverse reactions they engender in normal people. Such topics as the assessment of stressors and stress reactions, stress inoculation, stress management, and crisis intervention have become major fields of research and practice.

All kinds of stressors have been examined—"normal" stressors associated with schooling, marriage, parenting, occupation, and aging, for example; and "abnormal" or traumatic stressors, such as floods, hurricanes, fires, drought, and famine, on the one hand, and man-made violence (rape, physical attack, terrorism, political torture, and war) on the other (Milgram, 1989). In this chapter, I will deal with the cumulative effects of war-related stressors.

The bulk of research and practice on this topic has centered on the diagnosis and treatment of acute and chronic stress reactions in one category of *primary* victims—soldiers directly exposed to any of the many facets of war. Thomas Salmon's intervention principles—immediacy, proximity, expectancy, and community—have been extensively applied to secondary and tertiary treatment of war-related stress reactions in the military (Milgram & Hobfoll, 1986) and their efficacy has been well documented (Figley, 1978; Figley & Leventman, 1980). Far less attention has been given to the effects of war on civilians in general and on *secondary* victims within an affected society in particular: (1) family and friends of primary victims or of people who are at risk for primary victimization; (2) bystanders caught up in violent acts; and (3) audiences of the mass media that depict the horrors of war (Milgram, 1986).

Still less scientific and professional concern has been given to an analysis of an entire society at war (Hobfoll, Lomranz, Eyal, Bridges, & Tzemach, 1989). The well-known concepts associated with the field of stress and coping—categories of stressor, cognitive appraisals, intrapersonal resources, interpersonal supports, and modes of coping—have not been analyzed for their contribution to our understanding of why some societies endure despite lengthy wars with enormous human costs, while others do not.

This chapter is a modest beginning in this direction. In it, I will attempt to analyze these concepts in Israel, and to derive principles and generalizations applicable to other societies. The reference to Israelis throughout this chapter is to Israeli Jews and not to Israeli Arabs.

Noach Milgram • Department of Psychology, Tel-Aviv University, Ramat-Aviv 69978, Israel.

International Handbook of Traumatic Stress Syndromes, edited by John P. Wilson and Beverley Raphael. Plenum Press, New York, 1993.

Salutogenic versus Pathogenic Orientations to the Stress and Coping Paradigm

Antonovsky (1979) drew a distinction between two major orientations to stress and coping. The most common orientation, the *pathogenic*, investigates the relationship to illness, physical or mental, of adverse stressors, deficient intrapersonal resources, inadequate support systems, and ineffectual coping mechanisms. It investigates those variables that contribute to breakdown in stressful situations. By contrast, the less common orientation, the *salutogenic*, investigates the relationship to physical and mental health of positive features of the stress situations and of the people who are exposed to these situations. It investigates those variables that contribute to sustained, effective functioning and to symptom-free health status, notwithstanding the adverse circumstances to which people are exposed and required to adapt. The salutogenic orientation does not assume that an exposed individual, a group, or a society is necessarily healthy in absolute or relative terms. It determines, however, the focus of investigation and the choice of antecedent and consequent variables. The present analysis draws upon aspects of both orientations and asks what features of Israeli society account for the fact that Israel continues to survive and even appears to prosper, notwithstanding highly adverse war-related stressors that might be expected to bring about severe stress reactions and disorders.

Adverse Stressors Inherent in the Arab-Israeli Conflict

There are a number of adverse stressor parameters that characterize the Arab-Israeli conflict. These parameters include duration, intensity, multiplicity and aperiodic recurrence, palpability, probability, and personal relevance.

Duration

A stressor of lengthy duration has a more deleterious effect than one of short duration (Lazarus & Folkman, 1984). In the present instance, the history of armed conflict between Jews and Arabs in Palestine goes back more than 100 years. Before 1948, the year of the establishment of the State of Israel, there were countless attacks against farmers and city dwellers, with considerable loss of life. Since 1948 a state of hostility has existed between Israel and neighboring Arab countries, resulting in thousands of military and civilian casualties. One might argue that Israelis have adapted to the interminable character of the conflict such that its duration has made it less rather than more stressful. This argument is inconsistent with evidence pointing to (1) an inverse relationship between periods of belligerency and national mood, and (2) a pervasive desire within the society to end the conflict.

Interview data on 11 national Israeli samples be-

tween 1979 and 1984 show an increase in depressed mood as a function of the War in Lebanon (Hobfoll *et al.*, 1989) and surveys of earlier wars show a similar pattern (Guttman & Levi, 1983). There are many popular songs dealing with the theme of peace and none (since 1973, the year of the Yom Kippur War) glorifying the martial spirit or victory in war. There was an enormous outpouring of emotion when Anwar Sadat visited Jerusalem and later when the peace treaty with Egypt was signed. Affirmation of this treaty is still widely maintained despite its falling far short of a "true" peace and amity between the two countries. Many Israelis are willing to make further dangerous territorial concessions for peace (Goldstein, 1989).

Intensity of Threat

A threat to life and limb and to the survival of the society and its people is more stressful than the threat of loss of property, natural resources, territory, or even sovereignty (Milgram, 1986). The national legitimacy of the adversary is not in question, and the survival of its people is not threatened in other Middle East conflicts (e.g., the Iraq-Iran War), or in conflicts elsewhere in the world (e.g., India and Pakistan, or Vietnam and Cambodia). Many, if not most, Israelis believe, however, that the Arab-Israeli conflict differs from other conflicts between nation states in that if Israel loses, the Jewish State will cease to exist.

Impartial examination of the contents of schoolbooks, the preachings of Islamic religious leaders, and the editorials and essays written by intellectuals in all Arab countries today, including Egypt, produces ample support for the thesis that a sovereign Jewish State in the Middle East is perceived by Arabs as an illegitimate entity with no right to exist (Bartov, 1989; Lewis, 1986). Opinions to the contrary are rare and, if made, are almost immediately retracted. Recognition by Arabs of the *fact* of Israel's existence is not reassuring to Israelis since under some future conditions Arabs might come to believe that it is possible to eliminate the Jewish State and take steps to do so. What would be reassuring to the national mood of Israelis is acknowledgment by any Arab leader of the *legitimate right* of Jews to establish and maintain a sovereign Jewish State, but this acknowledgment has not been forthcoming.

Multiplicity and Aperiodic Recurrence of Traumatic Events

The occurrence of a number of traumatic events at the same time or within a short time span and the unpredictable recurrence of stressful events every few years are far more stressful than a single one-time traumatic event or the predictable recurrence of several events over time (Dohrenwend & Dohrenwend, 1974). Many Israeli families have suffered injury or loss of life of loved ones, military and civilian, once every decade or generation—a son dying in one war, a son-in-law wounded in another, a child killed by a terrorist attack in a third.

Threat Palpability and Personal Vulnerability

Threats upon life and limb are far more stressful when they are repeatedly realized and on a large scale than when they rarely if ever occur and only to a small number of people. In Israel, the toll of war affects all: The percentage of Israeli families today who have suffered injury or loss of life of loved ones or who have close relatives or personal friends who have experienced this suffering approaches 100%. The threat is immediate and personal, it has been translated into tragedy on numerous occasions, and it is close to home.

The small size of Israel (smaller than Massachusetts, one of the smaller states in the United States) and the relative size of the Jewish and Arab populations in Israel and of the Arab populations in the neighboring Arab countries do not permit intellectual or emotional detachment about the threat of violent attacks against Jews by Arabs living or working in Israel, of armed incursion against Israeli civilians from outside its borders, or of the full-scale invasion of the state itself. No Israeli citizen lives more than 20 miles from resident Arab populations that are potentially, if not actually, hostile. It is not surprising that a large percentage of Israeli youth (60%) report that terrorist attacks in Israel upset them (Mayseless, 1989) or that many Israelis are uneasy about driving in many sections of Israel today.

Probability of Threat Realization Given the Declared Intentions of the Threatener

Threats with high probability of occurrence and realization are more stressful than threats of low probability. Israelis note the barbaric conduct of conventional war in the Middle East (e.g., the ongoing civil war in Lebanon, the recent Iran-Iraq War, the wholesale murder of local dissidents in Syria) and, most recently, the campaign of terror waged by Palestinian Arabs in 1989 against fellow Palestinians regarded as dissidents or collaborators with Israel. The official description of how these 750 people met their death and the resulting color photographs are not for the squeamish. A partial listing of the manner of killing includes decapitation, bodies burnt beyond recognition, bodies smashed to an unrecognizable pulp, bodies axed and cut to ribbons, and cutting open the stomachs of pregnant women (Kaplan, 1989; Levi, 1989).

Israelis listen to and read Arab declarations of intent to eliminate the Jewish State. Israeli women and children, even preschool children, have been killed by terrorists subsequently regarded as heroes in the Arab press. Consequently, they believe that should Arab armies occupy any part of Israel and capture any portion of its civilian population, they will not return the conquered territories by negotiation or release the people unharmed.

Isolation versus Support

The psychic toll of extended exposure to stressors is strongly affected by perception of the strength and availability of support—moral, economic, technical, and military—from others. The stressors cited above would be more tolerable if Israel commanded the respect and sympathy of most nations. Unfortunately, respect and sympathy for the peculiar and precarious predicament of the Jewish State are far less evident today than in the past. Israelis believe that many United Nations (UN) member nations would accede to Israel's demise. These nations assented to the delegitimization of Israel for 20 years by formally designating Zionism as a form of racism, the latter a patently illegitimate entity, and frequently censure Israel in a one-sided manner. Israel's sense of isolation (Bartal, 1986) is further reinforced by the biased coverage of the world press (Chafetz, 1985).

There are some sources of support that mitigate Israel's isolation. These are the forms of support given by a few foreign countries (chiefly the United States), by Jewish communities in other countries, and by some non-Jewish secular and religious organizations in Western countries. This support is substantial, but it does not outweigh in the minds of many Israelies the animosity or ill will directed toward Israel.

Evidence for Different Hypothesized Models of Coping

Given these stressor parameters, we might well expect to find increased war-associated physical and mental distress and illness in Israeli society—especially in the last 20 years when the toll of casualties has exceeded that of the previous 80—but we do not find evidence to support this hypothesis.

Sociological data on draft evasion, suicide (including suicide during military service), homicide, traffic and work injuries and deaths, family breakdown and divorce, substance abuse and addiction provide no support for the notion of a society under siege or on the verge of collapse (see Fishman, 1983, Landau & Pfeffermann, 1987, and Landau & Raveh, 1987, for confirmation of many of these points). On the contrary, the birthrate has been stable for over a decade, and is rising in some groups within Israeli society. Emigration from Israel has remained stable for the past decade, with only minor variations associated with economic vicissitudes, whereas immigration to Israel exceeded emigration by 50%, and has risen more in recent years than in any other period (Alon, 1989).

Survey data provide little support for various maladaptive response models. There is little evidence, for example, of a reactance response (Brehm, 1966)—a hypervigilant, trigger-happy, jingoist, nationalist, racist society, convinced of its inherent superiority to presumably despised adversaries. In fact, foreign observers are impressed with the degree of self-criticism and restraint shown in Israel. Film exhibitors in Brazil expressed surprise that the major Israeli entry could be highly critical of government policy with regard to the Palestinian uprising and still receive government subsidies for its production (Dishi, 1989). There is also little support for a mindless hedonistic response—"Eat, drink, and be merry because tomorrow we die."

Prevalence rates for adverse stress reactions in children living in vulnerable areas do not tax the mental health services. The northern part of Israel has been the scene of numerous rocket attacks and occasional terrorist incursion with hostage taking and loss of life for the past 20 years. Israeli children living in Judea, Samaria, and Gaza have been stoned in their school buses and family cars for the past 4 years, and some have witnessed loss of life and limb. The few efforts to survey the prevalence of children's acute and chronic stress reactions have not encountered data that would cause apprehension in mental health workers or in parents (Limor & Lessinger, 1989; Milgram, 1982; Raviv & Klingman, 1983). The most exposed groups, 100,000 settlers living in Judea and Samaria and 120,000 Israeli residents of Jerusalem, in areas developed since 1967, have not sold their homes and moved closer to "safer" areas. They are, in fact, being joined by new families (Bar-Yosef, 1989; Horowitz, 1989).

These conclusions do not imply that there are not instances of stressful reactions or even of severe psychopathology. There is a degree of demoralization in a highly visible and vocal group within Israel, the left-wing intellectuals—writers, artists, poets, columnists, and the electorate they represent (Milgram, 1990). These people are by their own admission genuinely distressed by the government's handling of the Palestinian uprising and their own inability to bring the country and the government in line with their views. Dreman (1989) published a 10-year follow-up of two families who were traumatized by terrorist attack. In the first, the father was killed by a booby-trapped refrigerator; in the second, the father was killed and the wife and children narrowly escaped injury in a bus commandeered by terrorists on a suicide mission. The adjustment of the adult children was found to be fair to good in the first family and very poor in the second. Ayalon and Soskis (1986) found that survivors of a large-scale massacre of high school children taken as hostages were functioning reasonably well at work and at home, but reported considerable psychic upset and phobic restrictions of freedom of movement as residuals of the original traumatic episode. One may extrapolate from these instances of chronic maladjustment to the larger population of children and youth. Follow-up research of soldiers who suffered from posttraumatic stress disorder indicates that some soldiers do not regain satisfactory levels of adjustment in military reserve duty, work, marriage, and family life, and that of those who function well in these areas, many report considerable subjective distress and other symptoms (Solomon, 1987, 1989).

Stress-Resistant Factors and Practices before 1948

The magnitude of the war-related stressors on Israeli society is so impressive that it is legitimate to seek salutogenic explanations for its continued vitality and stability. On the whole, why are Israelis functioning so well? Why are Israeli soldiers coping "surprisingly well" (Gal, 1989), despite the difficulties associated with the military response to the Palestinian uprising now entering its fifth year?

When we learn that an individual has coped well in difficult circumstances, we usually ask whether she or he has coped successfully with stressors of this sort in the past, operating on the assumption that past performance is a predictor of present and future performance. In the present context, two historical periods are analyzed briefly in terms of coping style—the exile from the Land of Israel up to the late nineteenth century, and from 1870 to 1948.

Lazarus (1982) identified two kinds of mastery in Jewish history since the destruction of the first and second Jewish Commonwealths (586 B.C.E. and 70 C.E., respectively). External mastery is characterized by efforts to control the external environment, adaptive problem-solving, coping with and accommodating to adverse environmental conditions. By contrast, internal mastery, is characterized by canalization, in Murphy's sense (1947), of energies and resources to achieve culturally and religiously defined goals within a more narrowly defined community, by the exercise of self-control, inhibition of aggression, and emphasizing the satisfactions and security of the inner world. The latter is a more attainable goal than mastery of the external, especially in adverse times. The two forms of mastery are not mutually exclusive and have alternated or co-occurred at different points in time with varying emphases. Both have been instrumental in sustaining Jewish religious, communal, and quasinational life and in promoting important contributions by Jews to the societies and countries in which they lived.

The secularist founders of the modern Jewish State broke with the legacy of internal mastery as well as with religious traditions of the past. They demonstrated active external mastery to the extreme, espoused socialist utopianism to create a new reality, sustained optimism despite discouragement and failure, resolved that "Massada will never fall again," and insisted that Jews rely on themselves and not on the good wishes or intentions of others. This heroic image persisted despite major crises in which the Jewish community of Palestine was threatened with annihilation—first, in the waning days of the Turkish occupation of Palestine during World War I, and later, during World War II, when Rommel's tanks threatened to overrun the entire Middle East. The strong belief by Israelis in the efficacy of efforts to achieve mastery over external conditions has been confirmed in cross-cultural studies, with Israeli university students reporting a more internal locus of control than students from other countries (Parsons & Schneider, 1974).

This feature of national character was challenged and illusions about absolute military security and supremacy were shattered by the outbreak of the Yom Kippur War (October, 1973) when Egyptian and Syrian armies threatened to overrun Israel. Consequently, some groups in Israel today argue for drastic reappraisals of Israel's proper national aspirations, security needs, Palestinian aspirations, and necessary Israeli accommodations. This shift of orientation has created a major rift in Israeli intellectual, political, and psychological thinking. This rift, a major stressor in and of itself, is discussed later in this chapter.

Coping Practices in Israeli Society Today

There are certain peculiar features of life in Israel today that appear to have buffered many citizens against the deleterious effects of war-related stressful events. These features may be conceptualized as principles of traumatic stress prevention or management and are summarized below under four headings: inoculation, indoctrination, implosion, and incongruity reduction. The reader may note that examples cited below for a given principle might well be assigned to another, since a given practice illustrates more than one principle.

Inoculation

Stress inoculation refers to a series of behaviors designed to facilitate the proactive and retroactive mastery of stressful life experiences. These behaviors include the transmission of information about the stressful experience to people at risk for exposure to said stressor. People are informed about stressful situations that have occurred and may recur and how others conducted themselves or should conduct themselves in these kinds of situations (Janis, 1969; Meichenbaum & Jaremko, 1983). This information may be dispensed formally and informally via the mass media, by classroom discussions, workshops, and contacts with mental health or crisis intervention centers.

Inoculation may be offered at the primary, secondary, or tertiary levels of intervention (Caplan, 1974; Ochberg & Soskis, 1982). A number of optimistic assumptions are made about the consequences of intervention at the primary level: Limited, vicarious exposure initiates learning, retention, spontaneous imaging, and rehearsal of the experience and its mastery, with concomitant reduction of the anxiety associated with anticipation or actual confrontation with the feared event. At the secondary level, these developments are not assumed or left to chance: High-risk groups or groups exposed to traumatic events are given specific, graduated instructions to assist them to achieve mastery and symptom alleviation. At the tertiary level, afflicted people are offered a wide variety of behaviorally oriented treatment approaches (e.g., multimodal behavior therapy in Lazarus, 1976).

A great deal of inoculation at the primary and secondary level occurs routinely in Israel, partly because of the open character of the society. Civilians, soldiers, politicians, newspaper reporters, and radio and television commentators freely reveal what they have seen or heard, without regard for instructions to the contrary, official secrets acts, discretion, or even prudence. The Israeli public is informed on countless occasions how family members react when a deputation of military and medical personnel come in person to inform them of the severe injury or death of a family member. It is exposed to articles about bereavement and the management of grief, about posttraumatic stress reactions and disorders in soldiers and in civilian victims of terrorist attack, about the difficulties of families of soldiers missing in action, and the like. The anecdotal illustrations of coping with adversity are believable, because they are not all of

one stripe. Some human interest stories tell of the heroic rebuilding by survivors of shattered lives, others tell of breakdown. Many stories do not have a happy ending (Meiri, 1989; Mualem, 1989).

Inoculation in the Israel Defense Forces (IDF) includes such training activities as hiking for 150 kilometers with full battle gear to running for miles with their buddies on their backs. The first drives home the point that one has reservoirs of physical stamina beyond belief and the second, that if a soldier is wounded, he will not be left behind to the mercies of the enemy. The various branches of military service prepare annual celebrations open to the public displaying their weapons and achievements. Children climb on tanks in army camps or in their own neighborhoods, people witness an aerial formation, a paratroop jump, or visit a naval base. The Civil Guard requires civilians in highly exposed areas to practice air raid drills, that is, the northern part of Israel where there is danger of rocket attack or terrorist incursion from Lebanon, and the settlements along the Jordan River exposed to similar dangers.

Indoctrination

A major personal resource enhancing one's ability to cope for an extended period in highly adverse circumstances is a belief system that provides an explanatory context for why one is exposed to political and military threats to begin with, and an ideological context for why it is worthwhile to persevere in the struggle to achieve one's goals. The context affirms the suffering of the individual or of the group as necessary and even desirable, and thereby enhances the ability to cope (Hobfoll, 1986).

Every society, religion, ethnic group, or nation-state instructs its young people, formally and informally, in the belief systems considered essential for the preservation of the group and the realization of its aspirations. The term indoctrination is typically defined as teaching people to accept a system of thought uncritically. The term is defined here as the transmission of the major belief systems and values of the group, without implying uncritical acceptance. Israel's indoctrination task is complicated by the problem of how to explain to its young people why the Jewish State engenders such hostility and criticism in the Middle East in particular and in the world in general, and why it is worthwhile to live and, if necessary, to die to preserve a democratic Jewish nation-state in a turbulent, undemocratic part of the world.

One might question whether Israel possesses a coherent and persuasive context, given the intense cleavages within Israeli society in religion (orthodox vs. secular), ethnic membership (Western vs. Asian-African ethnic background), and political allegiance (right vs. left). In fact, the majority of Israelis share common views on many issues, especially those associated with Jewish national sovereignty and security, although they may arrive at the same conclusion from different starting points.

Evidence of the existence of this consensus is the widespread acceptance of compulsory military service for young men (3 years) and women (2 years) in the IDF from all walks of life; youth from the extreme orthodox communities comprise the only group who do not serve. This acceptance is expressed in the infrequency of draft evasion, the willingness of young men to volunteer for hazardous military service (e.g., commandos, frogmen) far beyond the numerical needs of these branches, the relatively high rate of combat casualties among commissioned officers, and the low frequency of conscientious objection to military service.

Willingness to accept an onerous burden and to expose oneself to life-threatening events is affected by whether one perceives the burden to be shared equally by all or shouldered primarily by less powerful, disadvantaged groups within the society. A demoralizing factor in the American armed forces serving in Vietnam was the awareness that the burden of combat duty was imposed on the few. By contrast, part of the commitment to service in the IDF stems from the accurate perception that the IDF is an egalitarian citizens' army in which young men and women serve, without regard to social class, ethnic background, or family connections, and in which advancement is based on merit rather than special influence. Recently a pilot, the son of a senior member of the Ministry of Defense, died in a training accident. A newspaper article pointed out that his death was in the egalitarian tradition of a society in which the sons and daughters of the mighty and powerful endanger their lives along with the sons and daughters of the less visible, less powerful families and groups.

In order to maintain high regard and confidence in the IDF, most Israelis draw a sharp distinction between the IDF and the wars it is called upon to fight (Milgram & Hobfoll, 1986). Israelis may differ, even vehemently, about the legitimacy or the advisability of a given war, its goals and its conduct (e.g., the War in Lebanon), but not about the universal high regard with which the IDF is held, higher than that of any other institution in Israeli life.

Implosion

The term *implosion* refers to a form of therapy developed by psychologists working within the cognitive behavior modification tradition (Linden, 1981; Stampfl & Levis, 1967), in which clients are instructed to imagine fearful, threatening scenes for prolonged periods. The rationale is that by producing a highly intense, frightening experience in the absence of reinforcements that maintain the emotionally upsetting response, fear of the particular situation will be lessened rather than heightened. In the present discussion, the term refers to the repeated exposure of individuals and groups to *externally* produced powerful scenes rather than to *internally* produced images. These scenes are public representations, reenactments, and reminiscences of highly stressful events and responses to these events.

The mass media bring into each family's home powerful human dramas: hospital visits to injured persons, funeral processions of mourners; follow-up of the adjustment (successful or unsuccessful) of survivors and the families of survivors and those who did not survive; making public the behavior of afflicted individuals and groups engaged in restitutive acts following tragic, irreversible losses; construction of memorial edifices and landmarks honoring the war dead; annual memorial ceremonies; and periodic assessments of earlier wars and battles. There is an annual recapitulation of the Yom Kippur War on its anniversary.

Special significance is attached to Memorial Day (for fallen soldiers) scheduled the day before Independence Day. Schools are either closed or devote part of the classroom time to honor the dead. Business hours are curtailed. During the morning, a nationwide siren brings all traffic and activity to a standstill throughout the country for a minute of silence. There are solemn ceremonies in military cemeteries throughout the country, and the entire content of radio and television broadcasting is tailored for the solemnity of the day. Personal and family reminiscences depict the depressive reactions and maladjustment of some people and the transcendent solutions of others. The public receives a strong dose of bitter medicine and even people who have not suffered personal loss empathize and weep with those who have. The induced depression in the national mood is relieved by the joyous ceremonies and festivities of Independence Day. Its juxtaposition to Memorial Day makes it clear that national independence is contingent upon the willingness of the society to make periodic sacrifices.

There are entire series of behaviors prescribed by Israeli society without reference to the calendar that reexpose injured and traumatized people to earlier losses. Each family whose son or daughter has died in military service is encouraged to create a book memorializing the deceased person—photographs, printed statements by former comrades, poems and letters by family members eulogizing the deceased, letters and remarks of the deceased himself or herself, and other memorabilia. This book is printed at government expense and is distributed to family and friends. Every city or town has a memorial building that serves as a repository of the memorabilia of each deceased soldier. The building is located in a prominent place, usually in the center of the town, and is seen and visited by all residents at some time or another, since it also serves as a cultural center for the locale. Soldiers who died in military service may also be buried in the national military cemetery on Mount Herzl in Jerusalem or in special military sections of civilian cemeteries throughout the country, by the decision of the family.

Military tombstones possess a silent eloquence. The size and shape of the tombstone for military dead are uniform—a rectangular slab resembling a bed and a smaller stone resembling a pillow or headrest that carries the vital statistics of the dead person: full name and nicknames, rank, serial number, branch of military service, first names of parents, date of birth and death, and name of battle or war in which the soldier died. Visitors to a civilian cemetery invariably pass the gravestones of the military dead, while visitors to the gravesite of a soldier relative pass by the graves of other soldiers from all preceding wars of Israel. All read the vital statistics of some of these headstones and come away impressed with the continuity of sacrifice in war, across the generations and groups that comprise modern Israel. Visits to the cemetery establish death in the defense of one's country as part of the landscape and as the price of statehood that future generations of parents and adult children may be called upon to pay. They also serve to reduce the sense of intolerable loss by emphasizing its group rather than its private character: No soldier is alone in death and no family is alone in its mourning.

Notification of the family that a family member has been injured or has died is always done in Israel by a team consisting of a local military person, a physician, a nurse, and, in some instances, the commanding officer of the deceased. Comrades of the deceased attend the funeral or the unveiling of the stone where possible, often name their newborn children after the deceased soldier, maintain contact thereafter with the bereaved family, and permit contact between the bereaved parents and the namesake child if asked. Each of the branches of the IDF has its own way of remembering its dead and honoring the living. The Air Force provides an annual Bar Mitzvah ceremony for all sons of deceased airforce men when they reach age 13.

Most of these practices are at marked variance with military practice in other countries. The British bury soldiers where they fall, in Europe, or, more recently, in the Falkland Islands. The United States honors its military dead in a low key and with limited appeal and scope on Memorial Day, a day that often passes with most people unaware that anything solemn is taking place. Efforts by the American government to locate the whereabouts or the remains of soldiers missing in action are far less convincing than in Israel (Bar-Zohar, 1991).

The Holocaust, the greatest single atrocity committed in World War II and a traumatic experience by any standard, receives special treatment in Israel. A day is set aside to honor the memory of six million Jews killed merely because they were Jews, and to commemorate the resistance movements, ghetto uprisings, and the struggle to maintain dignity to the very end despite inhuman and degrading circumstances. The ceremonies and associated educational activities are very explicit in their portrayal of the dehumanizing and genocidal behavior of Germans and their collaborators, and are frankly shocking even to those familiar with that bitter period. Many high schools arrange for their students to visit concentration camps and grave sites in Poland. These planned experiences outside of Israel and commemorative events at home are relevant to many Israeli families who lost loved ones in the Holocaust or who include survivors. The trials of Nazi war criminals, both the earlier Eichmann trial and the more recent Demjanjuk trial, received exhaustive coverage in the mass media, evoking once again in many survivors and their children the intolerable images and experiences of that period and exposing these experiences to new, innocent generations.

Incongruity Reduction and Confidence in Leadership

An individual's ability to cope well with stressors is related to high congruity, coherence, or correspondence between different aspects of one's experience. A major source and determinant of experiential congruity is leadership behavior. An individual or an entire society functions better in crisis situations when people in positions of leadership and authority (1) communicate information and their interpretation of the same in a clear and internally consistent manner that does not conflict with other credible sources of information; (2) do not differ markedly from one another in marshaling and summarizing the facts as well as in their interpretations and implications of these facts; (3) practice what they preach, rather than preach one thing and do another; and (4) give true rather than false warnings about the dire consequences of certain actions or lack of action.

Confidence in Leadership

Leadership is a valuable resource that may be squandered or jeopardized when leaders engage in incongruous behaviors that are inconsistent with other behaviors, when they appear to be uncertain, conflicted, unreliable, and unable to shoulder the responsibility of directing the society toward commonly held goals, and when they are, in fact, found to be lacking in integrity and good judgment. Under these circumstances, many adverse consequences follow: confusion in the ranks, a lowering of group morale, and decreased ability to cope effectively with recurring stressors. The situation is no better when leaders do the opposite—pretend to have answers when it is painfully evident that they do not, offer appealing, unrealistic, solutions to pressing problems, or offer false assurances (Peled & Katz, 1975).

Two features of Israeli life have tended to minimize perceived incongruity in the statements and decisions of its leaders. The openness of Israeli society and its capacity for self-criticism have served as a safeguard against excesses of either type of irresponsible leadership. An open, critical stance stripped away discrepancies between preachments and practice, and revealed the vacillation, hypocrisy, and duplicity of leaders. Forewarned, many leaders avoided behaviors that would undermine their credibility and authority.

Second, the unquestioned rule of the country by a single party for nearly 30 years tended to temper the incisiveness of criticism and to encourage an accepting, if not a forgiving, attitude toward observed instances of incongruity. Leadership was competent, decisive, and worthy of trust, or at least was so perceived by the majority of the people, and so portrayed by accommodating members of the mass media. Adverse criticism of the leadership was tempered by the common belief that there was no acceptable alternative to the leadership of the Left-wing Socialist elite who established the state. The opposition Right-wing party headed by Menachem Begin was commonly regarded by opinion makers as fascist, incompetent, and likely to lead the country to economic ruin, moral and cultural bankruptcy, and military disaster. Consequently, the founding elite remained in power for nearly 30 years. During that period, there was a steady deterioration in the trust and regard in which it was held, resulting in a so-called upheaval or earthquake in 1977, when the Right wing came to power. This party had come to represent the ethnic and socioeconomic groups that had been hitherto powerless—the poor, the working classes, the less educated, the children of immigrants from Arab-speaking countries, the new European immigrants—an electorate likely to increase in number and give the Right wing ever greater majorities in future elections.

This dramatic shift of power has not yet been assimilated by the Left, who regard the Right as unworthy and unfit to govern, or by the Right, who are still unfamiliar with the exercise of power. As a consequence, an adversary system has evolved in which rival political leaders equate the good of the country with their acquiring dominant political power, and they behave accordingly. Pressing issues are not examined on their own merits, but rather as a vehicle for attacking and embarrassing the opposition. Political expediency has become the guiding principle to political behavior. This debate has centered primarily on the most explosive and most dangerous issue in Israeli life today, the nature of the political settlement to be achieved with the Arab States in general and with the Palestinian Arabs in particular. Politicians have even enlisted the support of high-ranking military officers to bolster their case, thereby undermining the confidence of the people in the apolitical professionalism of their military leaders as well.

Today, we find two relatively new, interrelated stressors: serious erosion of the people's confidence in the proper motives and sound judgment of their leaders, and a divisive ideological conflict between the Left and the Right. These stressors are especially debilitating because they contribute twice to the stress-outcome equation. First, because they multiply the cumulative stressor index, and, second, because they subtract the positive, buffering effects of confidence in leadership and perceived internal social cohesiveness that had prevailed before 1977. Quality of leadership and group cohesiveness have been found to be the best predictors of the behavior of soldiers during combat and the probability of their experiencing acute and chronic stress reactions afterward (Dasberg, 1982; Milgram, Orenstein, & Zafrir, 1991; Steiner & Neumann, 1982). It is reasonable to assume that these variables will affect the behavior of large groups of people in society as well. The recent return to power of the Labor party (June, 1992) is due in part to public perception that the head of the Labor party is a more decisive, trustworthy leader than his opponent.

Mental Health, Denial, and Hope

This chapter has based its somewhat optimistic appraisal of the coping stamina of Israeli society on the self-report of its more vocal members and on overt behavioral indices. These sources of data may not reflect the underlying psychic cost or vulnerability to breakdown of individuals and of the society as a whole. Denial, the reluctance to acknowledge subjective distress, and other symptoms, and restricted awareness of the "real" state of one's internal reality may lead citizens, leaders, and behavioral researchers to conclude that there is nothing to worry about.

Lazarus (1982) raised this question and applied to it the concept of *middle knowledge*, which was employed by Weisman (1972) in his research with dying patients. These patients constantly struggle to see things as they are, yet maintain hope that they will somehow recover, thereby denying the nature of their plight. The denial process is never complete, however, and doubt alternates with denial. This fluctuating state of affairs is called *middle knowledge*. In using this analogy, Lazarus did not mean to imply that Israel is a dying patient but does not know it yet. He merely pointed out that we may be lulled into a false sense of security about the coping ability of a society when we rely exclusively on surface observation and report.

Breznitz (1983) attacked the issue from another perspective. He asked what are the long-term effects of continuous exposure to a variety of stressors, and answered that two outcomes are possible—immunization or exhaustion, and growing strength or progressive vulnerability. He marshaled theoretical arguments for both possibilities, cited evidence on the adverse transgenerational effects of the Holocaust experience on the children of survivors, and closed with a discussion of realistic hope. By interpreting a situation objectively in a way that is more conducive to hope, individuals can better cope with their difficulties. By perceiving a stressful situation as a challenge, an opportunity to develop new strategies, new creative solutions, we pay less psychic costs than when we interpret the situation as a dire threat mandating fight or flight.

I agree with this analysis and recommend that we attempt to obtain valid estimates of psychic cost and the probability of breakdown. These estimates are never the sole criterion for decision-making or action, however, because psychic costs are not invariably life-threatening, whereas optimistic but unrealistic assessments of the intentions and future behavior of the "enemy" may threaten the present and the future of Israel.

No one should ignore the price that Israelis pay for living in a much-promised land in a contentious part of the world. Some parents commit suicide on the graves of their fallen sons; some soldiers commit suicide during their military service; some people become highly disturbed after a violent, unexpected attack on their persons or property; and some leave the country altogether to seek peace of mind and freedom from Israel's persistent stressors. These incidents are the exception rather than the rule, and I believe that the fabric of Israeli society has not yet come unraveled.

Difficulties in Analyzing Stress and Coping in Israel

Many problems were encountered in undertaking the present analysis: objectivity, comprehensiveness, and generalizability, to cite but a few. With regard to objectivity, it is difficult to analyze any aspect of the Arab-Israeli conflict without appearing to make political or ideological statements. There are diverse, conflicting opinions within Israel itself about the legitimacy of Zionism (the Jewish Nationalist Movement in modern times) and the morality of the means undertaken by the Jewish State to protect its perceived national interests (Goldstein, 1989). These ideological differences affect how mental health workers and researchers in Israel assess the mental health and morale of Israeli society as a whole and the recommendations they make for optimal functioning (Imut, 1989; Staff, 1988). It is difficult for an observer-participant in this conflict, however disciplined, to raise questions and provide answers to these questions without being affected by one's attitudes toward the conflict and its resolution. I have attempted to deal with *factual* events and parsimonious interpretations of these events in an objective manner. *Factual* refers to behavioral events whose occurrence is routinely acknowledged by a majority of Israelis and to interpretations shared by this majority. Following the theoretical distinction Murray (1938) made between alpha press (or stress) and beta press—the former referring to the objective parameters of the stress situations, and the latter referring to subjective, idiosyncratic, or culturally determined perceptions and aperceptions of these situations—I have endeavored to adhere to the former. These distinctions are difficult to maintain in small groups, and are even more problematic in an entire society (Eisenstadt, 1983).

The comprehensiveness and generalizability of the analysis were additional problems. The proper analysis of a society takes into consideration many more features than those required for analyzing an individual. However, the demand for comprehensiveness may be overwhelming—even in the age of the computer—and prevent us from drawing informed conclusions because we have not taken all relevant data into consideration. Consequently, any analysis of a society at war is necessarily incomplete. Furthermore, it is difficult to generalize findings and interpretations from one society to another. Each society is unique, so that generalizations are at best suggestive and not convincing.

This chapter has been restricted to an Israeli perspective. The stress, coping, and suffering of Palestinian Arabs are no less important than those of Israeli Jews. This latter topic awaits a Palestinian researcher with the background and ability to deal with the same difficulties cited above for an Israeli researcher.

The working assumption of this chapter is that societies function like therapists for the potential and real stress reactions and disorders of their members. The difference between society qua therapist and the mental health therapist is that the latter is acutely aware of the mental health implications of what the client is saying and doing and what he or she as a therapist should be saying and doing. Society is not. Applying the stress and coping paradigm to an entire society may help social and behavioral scientists and practitioners better assess the strengths and weaknesses of the society and facilitate professional planning for large-scale primary and secondary stress intervention.

References

Alon, G. (1989, November 9). Peretz: This year more than 20,000 new immigrants will arrive—the largest number in more than ten years. *Haaretz*, p. 9. (In Hebrew)

Antonovsky, A. (1979). *Health, stress and coping*. San Francisco: Jossey-Bass.

Ayalon, O., & Soskis, D. (1986). Survivors of terrorist victimization: A follow-up study. In N. A. Milgram (Ed.), *Stress and coping in time of war: Generalizations from the Israeli experience* (pp. 257–274). New York: Brunner/Mazel.

Bartal, D. (1986). The Masada syndrome: A case of central belief. In N. A. Milgram (Ed.), *Stress and coping in time of war: Generalizations from the Israeli experience* (pp. 32–51). New York: Brunner/Mazel.

Bartov, C. (1989, January 27). Cairo: A cup of coffee I waited 15 years for. *Maariv Weekend Edition*, Section 2, p. 7. (In Hebrew)

Bar-Yosef, A. (1989, September 29). A new kind of settler. *Maariv End of Decade Edition*, pp. 72–73. (In Hebrew)

Bar-Zohar, M. (1991). *The unknown soldier*. Tel-Aviv: Sifriat Maariv. (In Hebrew)

Brehm, J. W. (1966). *A theory of psychological reactance*. New York: Academic Press.

Breznitz, S. (1983). The noble challenge of stress. In S. Breznitz (Ed.), *Stress in Israel* (pp. 265–274). New York: Van Nostrand.

Caplan, G. (1974). *Support systems and community mental health*. New York: Human Sciences Press.

Chafetz, Z. (1985). *Double vision: How the press distorts America's view of the Middle East*. New York: William Morrow.

Dasberg, H. (1982). Belonging and loneliness in relation to mental breakdown. In C. D. Spielberger, I. G. Sarason, & N. A. Milgram (Eds.), *Stress and anxiety* (Vol. 8, pp. 143–150). New York: Hemisphere.

Dishi, S. (1989, December 1). "Green Fields" was viewed for the first time at the film festival Pastreo in Brazil. *Haaretz*, p. 20. (In Hebrew)

Dohrenwend, B. S., & Dohrenwend, B. P. (Eds.). (1974). *Stressful events: Their nature and effects*. New York: Wiley.

Dreman, S. (1989). *Children of victims of terrorism in Israel revisited: Intrapsychic and interpersonal aspects of coping and adjustment*. Unpublished manuscript, Ben Gurion University of the Negev, Israel.

Eisenstadt, S. (1983). Structure, interrelations and solidarity of elites, and reactions to stress. In S. Breznitz (Ed.), *Stress in Israel* (pp. 95–101). New York: Van Nostrand.

Figley, C. R. (1978). *Stress disorders among Vietnam veterans: Theory, research and treatment*. New York: Brunner/Mazel.

Figley, C. R., & Leventman, S. (1980). *Strangers at home: Vietnam veterans since the war*. New York: Praeger.

Fishman, G. (1983). On war and crime. In S. Breznitz (Ed.), *Stress in Israel* (pp. 165–180). New York: Van Nostrand.

Gal, R. (1989, February 7). Psychological and ethical factors in the coping of Israel Defense Force soldiers with the disturbances in the territories. Paper presented at the 22nd Scientific Conference of the Israeli Psychological Association, Haifa University. (In Hebrew)

Goldstein, D. (1989, September 29). Politics. *Maariv End of Decade Edition*, pp. 8–9, 13–14. (In Hebrew)

Guttman, L., & Levi, S. (1983). Dynamics of three varieties of morale: The case of Israel. In S. Breznitz (Ed.), *Stress in Israel* (pp. 102–113). New York: Van Nostrand.

Hobfoll, S. E. (1986). The ecology of stress and social support among women. In S. E. Hobfoll (Ed.), *Stress, social support, and women* (pp. 3–14). New York: McGraw-Hill.

Hobfoll, S. E., Lomranz, J., Eyal, N., Bridges, A., & Tzemach, M. (1989). Pulse of a nation: Depressive mood reactions of Israelis to the Israel-Lebanon War. *Journal of Personality and Social Psychology, 56*, 1002–1012.

Horowitz, D. (1989, December 1). Mood at Ofra confident and defiant. *Jerusalem Post*, pp. 1, 14.

Imut, Mental Health Workers for the Advancement of Peace. (1989, May 15–16). Conference on Psychological Obstacles to Peace, Jerusalem.

Janis, I. (1969). *Stress and frustration*. New York: Harcourt, Brace, & Jovanovich.

Kaplan, K. (1989, December 1). Defence Ministry scraps horror album of "collaborator" victims. *Jerusalem Post*, p. 16.

Landau, S., & Pfeffermann, D. (1987, November). *A time series analysis of violent crime and its relation to economic and security-related stress factors: The Israeli case.* Paper presented at the Annual Meeting of the American Society of Criminology, Montreal, Canada.

Landau, S., & Raveh, A. (1987). Stress factors, social support, and violence in Israeli society: A quantitative analysis. *Aggressive Behavior, 13,* 67–85.

Lazarus, A. A. (1976). *Multimodal behavior therapy: I.* New York: Springer.

Lazarus, R. S. (1982). The psychology of stress and coping. In C. D. Spielberger, I. G. Sarason, & N. A. Milgram (Eds.), *Stress and anxiety* (Vol. 8, pp. 13–36). New York: Hemisphere.

Lazarus, R. S., & Folkman, S. (1984). *Stress, appraisal, and coping.* New York: Springer.

Levi, Y. (1989, December 5). Violence for its own sake. *Jerusalem Post,* Part 4, p. 1.

Lewis, B. (1986). *Semites and anti-Semites.* New York: W. W. Norton.

Limor, B., & Lessinger, T. (1989, February 10). Soon they will not know another reality. *Nekudah, No. 127,* pp. 22–25, 64–65. (In Hebrew)

Linden, W. (1981). Exposure treatments for focal phobias: A review. *Archives of General Psychiatry, 42,* 602–611.

Mayseless, O. (1989). *Perceived stress in Israel due to terrorist acts and war—A national survey of high-school students.* Paper presented at the Fourth International Conference on Psychological Stress and Adjustment in Time of War and Peace, Tel-Aviv. (In Hebrew)

Meichenbaum, D., & Jaremko, M. E. (1983). *Stress reduction and prevention.* New York: Plenum Press.

Meiri, B. (1989, October 27). Please, mother, come back to us. *Maariv Weekend Edition,* pp. 10–12, 20. (In Hebrew)

Milgram, N. A. (1982). The effect of war-related stress on Israeli children and youth. In L. Goldberger & S. Breznitz (Eds.), *Handbook of stress: Theoretical and clinical aspects* (pp. 656–676). New York: Free Press.

Milgram, N. A. (1986). General introduction to the field of war-related stress. In N. A. Milgram (Ed.), *Stress and coping in time of war: Generalizations from the Israeli experience* (pp. xxiii–xxxvi). New York: Brunner/Mazel.

Milgram, N. A. (1989). Children under stress. In T. H. Ollendick & M. Hersen (Eds.), *Handbook of child psychopathology* (pp. 399–415). New York: Plenum Press.

Milgram, N. A. (1990). *Antisemitism and the Israeli Left.* Unpublished paper, Tel-Aviv University, Israel.

Milgram, N. A., & Hobfoll, S. (1986). Generalizations from theory and practice in war-related stress. In N. A. Milgram (Ed.), *Stress and coping in time of war: Generalizations from the Israeli experience* (pp. 316–352). New York: Brunner/Mazel.

Milgram, N. A., Orenstein, R., & Zafrir, O. (1991). Stressors, intrapersonal resources and interpersonal supports in military performance during wartime. *Military Psychology, 1,* 185–200.

Mualem, M. (1989, November 2). Waiting for Ilan to wake up. *Maariv Weekend Edition,* Section 4, p. 1. (In Hebrew)

Murphy, G. (1947). *Personality: A biosocial approach to origins and structure.* New York: Harper & Brothers.

Ochberg, F. M., & Soskis, D. A. (1982). Planning for the future: Means and ends. In F. M. Ochberg & D. A. Soskis (Eds.), *Victims of terrorism* (pp. 275–290). Boulder, CO: Westview Press.

Parsons, O. A., & Schneider, J. M. (1974). Locus of control in University students from Eastern and Western societies. *Journal of Consulting and Clinical Psychology, 42,* 456–461.

Peled, T., & Katz, E. (1975). Media functions in wartime: The Israel home front in October 1973. In J. G. Blumler & E. Katz (Eds.), *The uses of mass communications: Current perspectives on gratifications research* (pp. 49–69). London: Sage Publications.

Raviv, A., & Klingman, A. (1983). Children under stress. In S. Breznitz (Ed.), *Stress in Israel* (pp. 138–162). New York: Van Nostrand.

Solomon, Z. (1987). *Reactivation of combat stress reaction.* Technical Report, Medical Corps, Research Branch, Department of Mental Health, IDF.

Solomon, Z. (1989). *Delayed PTSD: Course and correlations.* Technical Report, Medical Corps, Research Branch, Department of Mental Health, IDF.

Steiner, M., & Neumann, M. (1982). War neuroses and social support. In C. D. Spielberger, I. G. Sarason, & N. A. Milgram (Eds.), *Stress and anxiety* (Vol. 8, pp. 139–142). New York: Hemisphere.

Staff. (1988, December). Jews and Arabs form peace group. *Psychological Monitor,* p. 15.

Stampfl, T. G., & Levis, D. J. (1967). The essentials of implosive therapy: A learning-based-psychodynamic behavioral therapy. *Journal of Abnormal Psychology, 72,* 496–503.

Weisman, A. (1972). *On dying and denying.* New York: Behavioral Publications.

CHAPTER 70

Posttraumatic Narcissism

Healing Traumatic Alterations in the Self through Curvilinear Group Psychotherapy

Erwin Randolph Parson

I supposed if there were any phenomenon of which one could say with some degree of truth "It's all done with mirrors" it would be group . . . the mirrors are there—reflecting not only each other . . . into infinity. . . . Group . . . taught me the use of mirrors—to find self in and through others.
—Garland, cited in Pine (1983), p. 15

Treating Vietnam veterans in groups has been regarded the *sine qua non* of effective intervention (Brende, 1981; Brende & McCann, 1984; Brockway, 1987; Egendorf, 1975; Lifton, 1973; Parson, 1984a,b, 1986, 1988a,b; Walker, 1983). However, most writers on group treatment avoid any mention much less an analysis of the role of narcissistic reactions and disorders in groups with veterans, whose self-organizations are often under persistent threats of narcissistic regression and dissolution. These reactions have great implications for understanding veteran/patient variables, expectational variables, assessment and treatment process variables, as well as outcome variables in psychotherapy.

Intense combat exposure, in essence, traumatically shatters the self and adversely impacts the survivor's capacity for self-regulation and psychic cohesion. Moreover, the veteran's cognitive and drive-affective controls, and the basic regulation of consciousness (so essential to an inner sense of predictability and stability lost in altered states of consciousness), are rendered ineffectual in managing inner states of mind, interpersonal relating,

social and political outlook and connectedness, and economic achievement (Parson, 1989a).

Understanding the role of posttraumatic pathological narcissism (deregulated sense of self) is crucial to successful psychotherapy with Vietnam veterans. Etiologically, the point of view here is that narcissistic vulnerabilities and pathology among help-seeking symptomatic Vietnam veterans originate primarily from a combined "dual traumatic matrix"; that is, psychic trauma in Vietnam ("combat traumatic stress") and psychic trauma at home ("sanctuarial traumatic stress") (Parson, 1988a). Of course, the diagnostician will determine whether and to what extent precombat developmental, familial, social, and economic factors are operative in the constellation of traumatic symptomatology presented by the veteran. Extreme combat trauma produces alterations in the veteran's psychobiological system with related changes in self-identity. Contributing to pervasive narcissistic impairment among these veterans in the aftermath of war was the overwhelming "tearing assunder separation" caused by the death of a self-object "buddy" in the war, combined with the loss of the normal narcissism of the combat-shattered adolescent self.

Clinical experience shows that some veterans' responses and attitudes toward their self, wives, sons, daughters, other relatives, and friends, as well as toward their communities, its institutions, and authority persons are manifestations of a generalized narcissistic

Erwin Randolph Parson • P.O. Box 62, Perry Point, Maryland 21902-0062.

International Handbook of Traumatic Stress Syndromes, edited by John P. Wilson and Beverley Raphael. Plenum Press, New York, 1993.

transference regression tendency. This transference response is observed in pervasive egocentric, nongiving behavior, and in the frequent irrational demandedness and sense of entitlement among some Vietnam veterans, particularly those who served in heavy combat.

Intrapsychic and interpersonal avoidance are related to narcissistic defenses dynamically connected to psychic splitting and numbing, and to dissociation, identity fragmentation, depersonalization, derealization, demoralization, guilt, depression, and manic-mastery defenses (as in "sensation-seeking behavior"; Wilson, 1989). In these veterans, posttraumatic narcissism plays a major role in chronic lifeline dysadaptations (Parson, 1988a)—during their adolescence, young adulthood, and now at middlescence (average age of 44). This narcissistic pathology affects the veteran's capacity to give and receive love; to take normal emotional, interpersonal, social, and behavioral "risks"; to "seek and receive help" (Brende & Parson, 1985), and to achieve and maintain stable economic mainstreaming (Parson, 1985a). Moreover, unresolved narcissism undermines the three basic lifeline challenges at midlife which Wilson (1977), with astute insightfulness, had predicted many years ago. He believed that when Vietnam veterans reached the fourth decade of their lives, they would, by virtue of that developmental achievement, seek resolution to pressing concerns that they had heretofore avoided. These lifeline challenges are: (1) finding meaning, (2) integrating their problems with authority figures as they themselves become authority persons, and (3) examining their war experience and its effects on their lives.

My objectives in this chapter are twofold: (1) to highlight the etiology, dynamics, behavior, and pathology of posttraumatic narcissism, by first briefly discussing the concept of narcissism—its definitions and symptomatology, and identifying various sources of narcissistic traumatic stress to which Vietnam veterans were exposed—from basic training to the homecoming and beyond; and (2) to describe the phases and procedures of a novel group psychotherapy model called the *progressive-regressive curvilinear group model* for working-through narcissistic vulnerabilities, defenses, and problematic behaviors in veterans who are diagnosed with posttraumatic stress disorder (PTSD) (American Psychiatric Association, 1980, 1987). Intrinsic to PTSD, is a narcissistic disorder. As Ulman and Brothers (1988) maintained, PTSD symptomatology is a manifestation of faulty attempts at restoration of narcissistic equilibrium in the individual. It is recognized here that many combat-experienced veterans suffer a number of narcissistic symptoms even in the absence of a diagnosable PTSD.

Narcissism

Cultural myths and legends often extend to us certain universal features about the complexities of human experience and behavior—about individuals' histories, tragedies, and comedies intrinsic to the drama of life.

The Greek prophet Teresias first told the story of a handsome youth, named Narcissus. In response to an inquiry about her son's future, the prophet told the boy's mother that Narcissus would have a long fulfilling life, provided he never looked upon his own reflection. (In ancient Greece there was a superstition that it was unlucky or even fatal to see one's reflection.) Because the youth rejected the love of men and women, this angered the gods and Narcissus subsequently fell in love with his own reflection in the water of a spring.

According to Pausanius' account, Narcissus, after the death of his twin sister (his exact "other self" in appearance), consoled himself by gazing into the spring to recall her image by viewing his own reflection. He was so aflamed by the view of his own image, that he remained fixed gazing upon his reflection and pined away because of self-neglect and abuse. Another and more recent version of this ancient myth is as follows: Narcissus made an agreement with the gods that they allow him to view his own image forever, which was granted to him. To ensure his wish, Narcissus was tied to a fruit tree, but he was too low to reach the fruits and too high to reach the water below. He therefore was dependent for his survival upon the kindness and whims of people passing by (Nicholas, 1983).

From these versions of the legend of Narcissus, one can derive a number of dynamic and behavioral characterizations of narcissistic persons, who often tend to experience tremendous difficulties in giving and receiving love, in forming and maintaining long-term intimate and nonintimate relationships, and in letting go of the fixity with which they dwell upon their own emotional and material needs.

> Behaviorally, narcissistic traits are observed in individuals' need and desire to be admired, loved, and "spoiled" by others, though they themselves are incapable of an empathic realization of others' internal states and needs. To be narcissistically vulnerable means to be extremely sensitive to slights; to be demanding of others' undivided attention; and to be absolutarian in the expectation that every need and wish will be fulfilled to one's own satisfaction and specifications. (Parson, 1987, p. 31)

Contrary to prevailing belief, narcissistic individuals are not people who love their self too much, but rather too little. They have a penchant for drawing attention to themselves to gratify their own needs, but are disinclined to openly and directly let those needs be known to others. Narcissists' self-inflated styles often preclude getting their needs realistically addressed. They tend to be out of sync with other people—either they are too high above everyone else or they perceive the avenues to having these needs met as too far below them.

Normal and Pathological (Disorder) Narcissism

The perspective on narcissism being discussed in this chapter views it as an intrinsic aspect of human life and experience; it is not viewed as something to be overcome as a bad illness, nor as self-seeking moral depravity. Instead, narcissism is viewed as an essential condition of life. It ranges—on a continuum—from normal or healthy to abnormal or pathological, and, from a developmental position, from immature to mature forms

(Kohut, 1971, 1977). Pathological narcissism or narcissistic disorder, such as "posttraumatic narcissism" (being postulated here) is a result of a traumatic disequilibration of the veteran's narcissism or sense of self. Only significant pathogenic influences from unusual events, including problematic parental interactions and internalization, can create the profound upheavals in the central organizing narcissistic core of a person we observe in traumatized individuals.

There are a number of definitions of narcissism. The five most salient applications appearing in the clinical/psychoanalytical literature are identified here: (1) a type of sexual involvement with one's self, (2) a mode of relating to self and to others, (3) a stage of psychological development, (4) a means of regulating self-esteem and a sense of self, and (5) a diagnostic category (Freud, 1912/1968, 1914/1957; Joffe & Sandler, 1967; Kohut, 1971, 1977; Pulver, 1970; Stolorow & Lachmann, 1980; Tolpin, 1971). My discussion of posttraumatic narcissism draws upon applications 2, 4, and 5, which will be elaborated later.

Functional Definition of Narcissism

Let us now focus on a most critical perspective of narcissism that frees us from the need to use "experience-distant" concepts like drives and energies in our descriptions and understanding of human psychic activity and behavior. Stolorow and Lachmann (1980) advanced a specific definition of narcissism which is consistent with my own and other contemporary analysts' position that essentially replaces energic-hydraulic concepts with more "experience-near" conceptualizations. Borrowing from the works of others and their own clinical observations of severely disturbanced patients, these authors advanced a groundbreaking functional definition of narcissism to which I have subscribed for over a decade:

> Mental activity is narcissistic to the degree that its function is to maintain the structural cohesion, temporal stability, and positive affective coloring of the self representation. (Stolorow & Lachmann, 1980, p. 10)

This functional definition of narcissism is instrumental to the understanding of a variety of post-Vietnam attitudes, behaviors, and symptomatologies in veterans with and without a diagnosable PTSD, as well as the posttrauma responses in survivors of other traumatized populations (i.e., rape, incest, earthquake and other natural disasters, aircraft mishaps, technological accidents, etc.). For example, the posttrauma symptoms and reactions of denial-numbing and general avoidance phenomena can be viewed as functional "tools" to assist the veteran in building self-esteem, or as functional "weapons" in the battle to survive environmental threats and assaults to self-esteem. Additionally, these narcissistic maneuvers facilitate the achievement of an inner sense of self through reducing the sense of inner fragmentation, while bolstering identity, and reducing the chances of further insults to self-esteem from an environment that had proven to lack reliability and predictability.

Etiology and "Maintenance Phenomena" in Posttraumatic Narcissistic States

According to my own clinical experience and observations of veterans and other survivor groups, unrecognized narcissistic concerns intensify PTSD and other symptoms, while undermining the veteran's chances of attaining meaningful long-range resolutions to intraself conflicts. In a *Stars and Stripes* article entitled, "Narcissistic Injury in Vietnam Veterans: The Role of Post-Traumatic Stress Disorder, Agent Orange Anxiety, and the Repatriation Experience," I noted (Parsons, 1982) that the adverse impact of war stress and the homecoming was not circumscribed to one or more single, identifiable "parts" of the veterans psychic organization, but in actuality adversely impacted "the self-as-a-whole"—replete with cognitive, affective, physical-biological, experiential, social, cultural, and spiritual aspects (Brende & McDonald, 1989; Parson, 1984, 1985b; Wilson, 1989).

A close examination of etiological factors shows three major sources of narcissistic traumatic stress for Vietnam veterans: (1) traumatic war stress (in Vietnam), (2) negative "honor" traumatic stress (at home), and (3) PTSD-linked narcissistic stress. To these I add two "maintenance factors"; that is, psychological and biological mechanisms that maintain postwar disorders and undermine resolution: (1) "lifeline-wounded masculine narcissism" and (2) the psychobiology of narcissism. These latter factors relate to the veteran's lifeline narcissistic depletions which keep PTSD and allied problems from reaching a state of resolution. Each of these factors is discussed below.

Traumatic Alteration of the Adolescent's Sense of Self

As a consequence of war stress in Vietnam veterans psychic trauma is conceptualized as etiologically emanating from four narcissistically mortifying events: (1) devastation of normal adolescent grandiose fantasies essential for successful negotiation of this developmental period, (2) self-structural alteration through boot camp and military indoctrination, (3) exposure to the mental and biological assault of combat, and (4) the premature and violent "ripping-asunder" experience involving the death of a buddy to whom the veteran was narcissistically ("twin") merged.

Shattered "Rambo Fantasies"

Lifton wrote about the soldier's "warrior identity" which in Vietnam was based on a "violence-prone-super-maleness, and a hyperaggressive, numbed, omnipotent maleness" (Ulman & Brothers, 1988, p. 171). Veterans who served in Vietnam were the youngest group of soldiers to have served in any American war (Brende & Parson, 1985; Wilson, 1977). Still caught up in the developmental throes of normal narcissism (of adolescence), these youthful combatants' normal fantasy systems were marked by a "showing off" attitude (or exhibitionism), and a self-inflated magical grandeur of being uniquely special and even omnipotent.

Boot camp had laid a bolstering foundation: the soldiers had been taught to magnify their normal "Rambohood" to high pinnacles of excited states of mind. They were programmed (involving some principles of brainwashing) to disavow fear and decry weakness in anyone, to include themselves. So "pumped up" were they, as they partook of the "immortalizing grandeur of [the] group" (Lifton, 1973, p. 172), they could do anything. Shatan (1974) wrote about the structural transformation of the young soldier's psyche during Marine Corps training. He noted that the drill instructor (DI) frequently reminded the new trainees that he was both mother and father to them, in an institutionally inspired attempt to replace well-established family-of-origin values with the tactical group values of the Corps.

In many soldiers, a self-developmental arrest occurred as a consequence of both boot camp/military training and the war's psychic and biological impact. As adolescents, these soldiers experienced "invincibility and omnipotent fantasies" in relation to killing (Brende & McCann, 1984, p. 62). These factors undermined the normal evolutionary transformation of soldiers' narcissistic "Rambo prowess" into mature narcissism with attendant ideals and inner guiding values. Such values would contribute to the veterans' transitional and postwar adaptational success in the many spheres of civilian life. As a direct product of this "developmental arrest" (Stolorow & Lachmann, 1980) in narcissistic maturational processes was the intensification of adolescent propensities which Kohut (1971, 1977) in his self-psychological theory attributed to a (narcissistic) structure he called "the grandiose self." For many veterans today, this narcissistic tendency remains deeply structuralized within the self.

Absence of Transformation and the "Narcissistic Vortex"

A very critical point that needs emphasis because of its relevance for group therapy is that the reinforcing of grandiose self tendencies occurred in the absence of a transformation of normal adolescent narcissism into mature narcissism (i.e., the sense of self) so essential to young adulthood and to later adult developmental epochs. This transformation would be critical if the adolescent is to grow beyond infantile grandiose self-inflation (a basic craving for admiration and attention) to attaining matured values, inner guidance, and self-direction in later life. Blos (1962) aptly noted that the adolescent's developmental achievement of "self as an effectively organized entity depends on the relinquishment of infantile megalomania and magic powers" (p. 192).

Ulman and Brothers (1988) made a similar observation when they wrote that "the adolescent combat soldier fighting in Vietnam had no 'psychosocial moratorium,' and, hence no opportunity to develop a cohesive and stable adult sense of self" (p. 160). They went on to state that many soldiers were caught up in

a psychologically devastating "narcissistic vortex" generated by the combination of boot camp and combat. . . . This vortex is created by almost simultaneous yet countervailing intense inflation and then rapid deflation of already unstable and volatile male narcissistic fantasies. (p. 160)

These factors added to the already heightened "narcissistic peril in development" during this developmental period (Ulman & Brothers, 1988; Wolf, Gedo, & Terman, 1972). A goal of group therapy would be to facilitate the transformational process—from adolescent fixations to mature ideals and a stable sense of self, albeit 15 to 20 years after the war.

Central Organizing Fantasies

Ulman and Brothers (1988) offered a very illuminating conceptualization of psychic trauma from the self-psychological perspective. They maintained that traumatic events "shatters the self," and that subsequent symptomatic expressions—as in PTSD—are manifestations of faulty restorative efforts at healing shattered "central organizing fantasies" about the self in relation to the self-object (i.e., persons, situations, institutions, etc.). Self-objects are experienced as extensions of the self and provide essential mirroring. The violence of combat thus shattered young soldiers' grandiose fantasies (i.e., "structures of meaning"; Stolorow & Lachmann, 1985, p. 26) making it difficult, and, for some, virtually impossible, to give up their "infantile megalomania and magic powers." The appropriate healing variable to assist these men and women with this shattering experience would be a cohesive, "containing" postwar environment.

Narcissistic Identification with the Dead

Making matters even worse for many soldiers in Vietnam were the losses of close buddies, with whom they were self-objectally merged. The premature death of such a friend was thus experienced not as the loss of a separate person (with whom they had been close), but as loss of a part of the self (via narcissistic identification). This kind of identification is devoid of memory or representation of the dead friend; it allows the survivor to experience the dead as a live object (or person) as he was once experienced prior to death.

This "identification-in-death," a faulty narcissistic mechanism, is the basis of much of the unresolved pathological mourning among combat veterans today. Clearly, this kind of identification is related to profound feelings of guilt, "impacted grief" (Shatan, 1973), sorrow, and survivor's guilt.

In concert with this view, van der Kolk (1987) mentioned Fox's findings concerning the narcissistic implications of a buddy's death in Vietnam. He thus writes

that soldiers with PTSD had reacted to the death of a friend as a narcissistic injury rather than as an object loss. In other words, they had experienced their friends as extensions of themselves rather than as separate individuals. This resulted in a need to avenge the friend's death, which persisted "despite the passage of time and even after specific acts of revenge had been committed against the enemy." (p. 161)

One of the empirical studies of van der Kolk, Greenberg, and Boyd (1985) also found an association between war stress and buddy-loss, and the development of chronic PTSD. The implications of these observations make group approaches to treatment with traumatized veterans an important modality in the total healing enterprise after Vietnam. Being empowered to give up these pathological identifications with dead friends is another crucial task of psychotherapy in groups with fellow combatants.

Sociopsychic Trauma of the Homecoming

Vietnam veterans' "negative honor" experienced at the homecoming is a narcissistic trauma conceptualized here as "tripartite narcissistic stress" situation involving (1) the failure of the United States to mirror the veteran's need for honor, respect, and a safe place to heal after the war; (2) active vilification; and (3) failure to assist veterans with transitional (from military life) assistance to increase the chances of healthy adaptation to civilian life. My position is that these narcissistic stresses lay at the core of many veterans' "psychological isolation" (Wilson & Krauss, 1985) after coming home. According to Wilson, psychological isolation was a consequence of veterans' inability or lack of opportunity to talk about the war, and that the "lost sense of communality . . . meant that the network of bonding, support and mutuality with the larger corpus of society was no longer functional" (p. 141). Psychological isolation among combat veterans, then, is a massive manifestation of narcissistic stress which is related to being a "stranger at home" (Figley & Leventman, 1980).

There are two kinds of human-mediated destructive acts which lead to psychic trauma in people: acts committed by an individual, and acts perpetrated by a society. In their discussion of the concept of "failed empathy" as the central theme in Holocaust survivors' experience, Laub and Auerhahn (1989) made a similar etiologic classification of trauma. Of societal-induced trauma, they wrote: "When a human being deliberately inflicts pain upon another, the resulting symptomatology in the victim . . . [is] inextricably linked to the . . . traumatic violation." This is especially true when the collective social structure condones the violation (Laub & Auerhahn, 1989, p. 378).

The traumatic violation of the precious covenant between soldier and society has inextricably linked the veteran to societal (sociopsychic) trauma; they are unable to forget it; they are unable to turn the pain off. This is because the pain is narcissistically based: the hurt pervades the veterans' cognitive (perceptual and intellectual), affective, conative capacities and social relationships. Although Nazi death camp survivors' psychic violation is different in many respects from the American society-inspired violation of the Vietnam veteran, there are certain parallels. For example, both experienced a failure of societal empathic self-object functions; and both groups experienced the devastation of those internal structures that connect the individual with the human and nonhuman environment.

The young soldier returns home from Vietnam in a state (narcissistic) of heightened self-vulnerability and a pronounced need for social admiration and fulfillment of shattered grandiose self-expectations. A restorative reentry would have provided the returnees with the opportunity for rebuilding shattered self-other psychic structures. The absence of mirroring and idealizing provisions caused primitive grandiose self-fantsies and structures to "go underground" through repressive and dissociative defenses. Because of exposure to war, these

men and women were now even more in need of mirroring (benevolent person-specific "reflected" pride and admiration) than every before. They craved for a need-mediating environment to replace the inner sense of "falling apart," emptiness, terror, and unneutralized narcissistic rage.

The fear-inducing, noncontaining homecoming experience ruptured the essential structure which provides an inner sense of security and linkage with the human environment. Ideally, as mentioned before, the homecoming could have provided the returnees with opportunities for initiating and maintaining self–self object linkages with the human environment. But this did not occur; instead the event "was a profound insult, a breaking of the covenant between a nation and its soldiers" (Parson quoted in Gelman, 1988, p. 64).

Discussing the work of Cohen on trauma and repression, Laub and Auerhahn (1989) stated

> that representations of need-satisfying interactions with the human environment provide the basis for the link between personal existence and social connectedness. But it may also be the case that satisfying interactions with the nonhuman environment can initiate linkages between self and other. . . . All trauma may well be recognizable not by quantity of impact but rather by its structure-destroying properties. (p. 398)

There is nothing irrational in veterans' expectation of a welcome home reception befitting a hero. Returnees of all wars expect honor and positive recognition: these assist with integration of war-torn self-structures, allowing the veteran to find personal meaning.

Extending beyond intuitive judgment is the now empirically documented finding that the "recovery environment" (Green, Wilson, & Lindy, 1985; Lindy & Grace, 1985; Wilson, 1989) after catastrophic stress has the potential to facilitate or hamper healing and recovery. The force of people's narcissistic needs exists throughout the life cycle (Kohut, 1977); however, owing to intrinsic adolescent vulnerabilities (Haley, 1985; van der Kolk *et al.*, 1985; Wilson, 1977, 1989), the Vietnam veteran probably required greater social mirroring and support than more developmentally mature soldiers of earlier periods (i.e., World War I, Korea, and World War II).

I maintain that veterans' current self-presentations to private and public service delivery systems is often narcissistic. Those who work with veterans over the years, particularly at public-operated systems, describe the Vietnam veteran as demanding, hard-to-please, irritable, angry, and temperamental. Underlying these attitudes are the dynamics of narcissistic aggression, which motivate narcissistic reparative demands. Veterans' demandingness may operate as a self-healing device, "preconsciously and unconsciously motivated to 'repair' insult-induced damage to the self" (Parson, 1984b, p. 31). Observing veterans' help-seeking behavior leads one to sense the presence of "a deeply recorded attitude: "You have deprived me; devastated me; coerced me to do everything you wanted me to do in Vietnam . . . now, you take care of my needs, all of them without question" (Parson, 1980, p. 4).

Rather than professionals' becoming judgmental about this behavior pattern, the group leader needs to understand the unconscious subjective structures of meaning behind the behavior. Too often professionals are "turned off" to such behavior, which then contributes to intensifying the veteran's sense of inner fragmentation or narcissistic mortification. Through being open to experience the veteran on his own terms, Lindy and associates (1988) were able to provide top-rank quality psychotherapy to a cohort of Vietnam veterans. These professionals learned that success in treating traumatized veterans may require divergent strategies in psychotherapy. Traditional approaches were never abandoned fully, but served as a means of monitoring narcissistic defenses.

Being made to feel as strangers is painful enough; but being made targets of hostility and of active vilification and culture-inspired stigmatization (as in "baby killers," "losers," "psychopathic killers," etc.) and institutional neglect, proved very overwhelming to many Vietnam veterans. Triply narcissistically injured (by war, buddy-loss, and at homecoming), they needed a societal response that would make them feel competent and worthy of life and living. The resulting sense of fragmentation, meaninglessness, guilt, and further disintegration of self-structures became an increasing problem in these veteran's postwar lives.

America's Shattered Narcissistic Image: A Parallel Process

From a "collective self-psychological" point of view, and complicating veterans' recovery from the war, was a sense of narcissistic injury to the national self-image. So painful was this shattering for the nation that the United States became possessed by an obsession to reduce its own pain through attempts to outmaneuver its anxieties and despair by "sweeping Vietnam and its veterans under the rug" of indifference, neglect, and stigmatization. These collective defenses made the disavowing of veterans' needs and their very existence psychologically expedient. But as individual veterans know very well, the use of these "defensive maneuvers of convenience," such as denial, projection, suppression, pseudorepression (ineffectual repressive barriers to awareness), and avoidance, do not work. They learned very well that it is impossible to overcome something one is either unwilling to recognize, or fearful of facing—frontally. For these defenses do not offer long-range protection from reality and the truth. Unconsciously, the collective psyche was motivated to repair its damaged self-image by abandoning, rejecting, and villifying its veterans.

In many respects, America's perceptions, attitudes, and patterns of behavior, like those of its own adolescents in Vietnam, were marked by immaturity and lack of awareness. The nation

> was guided by a black and white image of the world that led to a series of disastrous miscalculations during the Vietnam War. . . . The military leaders believed it was infallible, ignoring arguments against its strategy of attrition—[i.e.,] turning back the Viet Cong by killing them until there were no more. . . . The two characteristics of the American people during the period of the Vietnam war were "innocence, in the sense of unawareness, and ignorance, which reinforced that innocence." "We didn't see it because we thought that we Americans were exceptions to history. . . . "We thought that every-

thing we did was right and good because we were Americans." (Neil Sheehan quoted in Beidel, 1989)

With this kind of narcissistic-based blindness, it may be no wonder that it was difficult, if not starkly impossible, for the United States to reach out to veterans who had fought in the first war that the country had lost.

Narcissism, Transitional Stress, and Two Families: "Who Am I, and Where Do I Belong?"

Many people still ask the question: "Why does the negative homecoming have such long-term and devastating consequences on the veteran's lifeline? Why is it that for so many Vietnam veterans a supportive family environment was insufficient to fully compensate for the painful homecoming?" Answers are by no means simple. However, one possible answer is that the issue for many veterans was not so much the uncharitable responses of family members, but rather that their "new, adopted family" (i.e., the American public as "family through military service")—the one that seemed to count the most after war, had been willfully injurious and neglectful. Many veterans found that they could not "go home again" and integrate into their families of origin and their communities as before the war.

In essence, this new family had broken up the recruit's psychic connection to family of origin through intensive military indoctrination and boot camp training to alter their identities (Brende & Parson, 1985) associated with their families of origin. Giving up family values and putting the "superego in uniform" (Redl, 1971) produced "one of the most damaging effects [of the war; namely,] . . . the stripping away of their adolescent illusions and the tarnishing of their ego ideals" (Haley, 1985, p. 60). The narcissistic sense of injustice and injury here is found in the veteran's sense of having been "possessed" or "owned" by the military family, and then, as one veteran put it, "thrown away without a prayer." For though military indoctrination (and "militarized superego") was essential to the "preservation of psychic integrity in the face of catastrophe" (Haley, 1985, p. 61), many veterans felt abandoned by a coherent "moral inner agency" (Parson, 1989d).

PTSD-Linked Narcissistic Stress

As I noted elsewhere (Parson, 1982), the subjective experience of the symptoms of PTSD is a narcissistic injury to many Vietnam veterans. This is because of the veteran's awareness of his basic inability to stave off and control intrusive thoughts, feelings, and behaviors associated with traumatic events in the war. To be convinced that one is unable to even regulate one's own mind, that unbidden inner events come and go at will, is shattering to the masculine sense of control.

Factors Maintaining Posttraumatic Narcissistic Vulnerabilities

Lifeline-Wounded Masculine Narcissism

Freud (1919/1968) believed that symptoms he found in World War I veterans were related to a state he called "wounded self-love." The point of view here is that for many Vietnam veterans the painful discovery of "perennial powerlessness" exists in the absence of confidence that things will ever change. For so many, this proves an ongoing source of narcissistic stress. This stress is based primarily on the survivor's realization that he is incapable of mastering basic challenges of life which are expected of him by life and culture.

This self-wound essentially comes from the narcissistic conviction of personal failure in interpersonal relationships—as husband, or lover, as father, as son, daughter, and friend, as well as in the social, political, and economic areas—involving social isolation and noninvolvement, political alienation, unemployment, and underemployment. A low sense of inner competence (e.g., over intrusions from war and/or PTSD) and external mastery over the environment is an area of importance explored during group therapy as well. Most people have the need to experience the self as competent. In fact, there is a theory advanced by Hendrick (1943) that contrary to the basic Freudian position which indicates that human activity is motivated by sexual and/or aggressive aims, "work is . . . motivated . . . by the need for efficient use of the muscular and intellectual tools." He used the concept of the "work principle" to suggest

> that primary pleasure is sought by efficient use of the central nervous system for the performance of well-integrated ego functions which enable the individual to control or alter his environment. (p. 311)

White (1963) also developed a theory of human competence. He used the term "effectance" to denote "the active tendency to put forth effort to influence the environment, while feeling of efficacy refers to the satisfaction that comes with producing efforts" (p. 85). He goes on to state that "competence is the cumulative result of the history of interactions with the environment," while "sense of competence" refers to the subjective dimensions with these interactions with the environment.

As adolescents, many Vietnam veterans learned very early in life that competence—the ability to impact the environment in Vietnam—was crucial to their identities and sense of self. Now at age 42, many of these veterans have found that former competence is not enough, that competence in the various spheres of their lives is a constant challenge of discovery and rediscovery—an ongoing task of maturing human beings.

The essence of lifeline-wounded masculine narcissism is a pressing concern in the life of persons who prided themselves in the achievement of competence over the environment and over the vicissitudes of powerful and memorable life-and-death events in the war. Many veterans with this narcissistic problem find themselves constantly comparing their "Vietnam self"—a competent and masterful self—with the post-Vietnam or contemporary self," experienced as incompetent men.

Psychobiology of Posttraumatic Narcissism

In Vietnam's guerrilla war, soldiers experienced intense and continuous states of biopsychical arousal in their day-to-day combat actions. This intensity produced some changes in the central nervous system (CNS). Freud's (1916–1917) concept of the "self-preservative in-

stincts," which incorporates significant biological elements, can be understood as fostering self-cohesion and identity. And those who experienced overwhelming events underwent even more changes in their biopsychical organization. Since the "brain is the organ of the mind" (Harris, 1986), its feedback systems organize the complex interactions between biology and phenomenology.

It is quite possible to conceptualize the symptoms of symptoms of PTSD, particularly those involving diminished interest, as having narcissistic motivational underpinnings. For example, survivor's diminished interest, numbing and denial reactions may be understood as a narcissistically-inspired maneuver. This can be best understood when the functional definition of narcissism (Stolorow & Lachmann, 1980) is applied. Survivor's basic inability to regulate physiological arousal after trauma often trigger feelings of "subjective incompetence—the fundamental cause of demoralization (Figueiredo & Frank, 1972). This often results in narcissistic mortification in the veteran, which then leads to defensive maneuvers to "combat" narcissistic stress.

Diminished interest and avoidance as narcissistic defenses against intrusion have their own biological properties connected to changes in the central neurotransmitter systems in veterans with PTSD (Kolb, 1984; van der Kolk et al., 1985). Wilson (1989) discussed the neurophysiological processes related to avoidance phenomena, and his findings are relevant here. He wrote that "in traumatized individuals chronic NE [norepinephrine] due to involvement in the original trauma creates a noradrenergic hyperactivity resulting in decreased tolerance for arousal" (p. 32).

This decreased tolerance of arousal "regulates" psychic and behavioral withdrawal and isolation to avert the occurrence of narcissistic pain and intense fears of losing control. In a sense, we may speak of an "instrumental psychophysiology" that underlies narcissism from the functional perspective. Perhaps the concept of Atwood and Stolorow (1984) of "supraordinate motivational principle" can be applied here. These writers stated that the need to maintain the organization of experience is a central motive in "the patterning of human action." In the present context, the psychobiological substrate in PTSD is centrally involved in the survivor's organization of experience, which means to gain and maintain a sense of self.

Symptoms of Posttraumatic Narcissism

Self Theory

A posttraumatic narcissistic reaction is a pathological narcissism that originates in psychological traumatization. The self is understood to be "a multidimensional psychological construct reflecting the subject's experience of mental being and physical existence" (Ulman & Brothers, 1988, p. 5). The concept of "self," moreover, (in contrast to "personality," a broader concept) "is a more delimited and specific term referring to the structure of a person's experience of himself" (Atwood & Stolorow, 1984, p. 34). More specifically, the self is the center of the human personality—the center of initiative and personal power—and is the supraordinate manager of cognition, affection, and experience, as well as of the various structures and functions that regulate interpersonal, social, cultural, and spiritual dimensions.

In Kohut's (1971, 1977) self-psychological theory, the self is viewed as a "living self" [that] has become the organizing center of the ego's activities" (Kohut, 1971, p. 12), but later (Kohut, 1977) the role of the self was accorded greater salience in the personality, and seen by Kohut "as a supraordinated configuration whose significance transcends that of the sum if its parts" (p. 97).

During the course of development, the infant's nuclear (or core) self is organized to include two archaic structures in need of active nurturing as well as protection from empathic failures by the environment, comprised chiefly of mothering persons in the infant's environment. Kohut maintained that the self is unable to exist in the absence of an empathic self-object, that the self and its self-object together comprise a psychological unit—inseparable, joined together internally to last the entire life cycle of the individual Thus, if the infant's (or older person's) self is to grow and mature, with a balance in narcissism (the spice of psychological life), a self-object is critical, more specifically, an empathic self-object.

Kohut also postulated the existence of two psychic poles (structures) of the self, which he called the "gransiose self" and the "idealized parental image." The former represents the person's need to "show off" his or her skills and have them affirmed, while the latter relates to the need to be psychologically merged with persons of power and strength. But these needs cannot be met without the self-object—a person who is experienced by the infant, or even someone more mature, as an extension of the self. The self-object provides opportunities for "transmuting internalizations"; that is, the bit-by-bit acquisition of psychic structure during development (Ornstein, 1979). Providing the person received sufficient self-object "mirroring" of his or her normal grandiosity, and had opportunities to merge with powerful parental figures, the developmental achievements of ambition and ideals, and the utopian developmental achievement of a cohesive self is then possible. Here self and self-object have differentiated—that is, both independent but also interdependent entities.

Symptoms of the Shattered Self

There are two fundamental ways in which self-pathology develops in the individual: (1) through traumatically unempathic parenting that fails to empathically mirror and provide opportunities for merger contacts with parental figures; and (2) through traumatically shattering (as in war) of the psychological structure "that organizes the experience of the self" (Atwood & Stolorow, 1984, p. 34). This means that the two component polar structures of the self (the grandiose self and the idealized parental image) are severely damaged, fragmented, and destabilized. This state produces a loss of the original self-image involving self in relation to self-object. Zetzel (1973) also found the inability of war-traumatized veterans "to reconstitute their previous self-image. The image had been in effect shattered" (p. 248). Damaged self-structures result in impoverished ambi-

tion, disturbed will and aspirations, and absence of an integrated set of human ideals, goals, and values. Additionally, there is narcissistic vulnerabilities and narcissistic rage; poor social functioning; and an "incapacity to tolerate narcissistic injury" (Zetzel, 1973, p. 263) as well as injury to self love (Ferenczi, 1916–1917), and counterintimacy—a fear of love and sexuality in human relationships.

In general, the Vietnam war and the homecoming experiences have shattered these veterans' subjective world of experience. Because of these deficits, narcissistic pathological defenses are psychically and biologically erected to ensure that the veteran's "disintegration-prone structures of experience" (Atwood & Stolorow, 1984, p. 92; Stolorow & Lachmann, 1980) are restored or maintained, albeit faultily. Such faulty, restorative attempts aim to provide some sense of self; that is, self-continuity, increased self-esteem, and reduced subjective "sense of internal falling apart" (Parson, 1984a). The pervasive symptomatology of posttraumatic stress disorder is evidence that this self-strategy has not worked effectively.

Posttraumatic Group Psychotherapy

Group psychotherapy holds a very important place in the total treatment enterprise of survivors of catastrophic experiences. Because most traumatized individuals feel lonely and distrustful of others (particularly those who did not go through similar traumatic experiences), and have a deep conviction that no one could understand their inner suffering and despair, group approaches to healing can be seen as an important option, or as one modality of intervention within a total treatment plan for the individual survivor. The "therapeutic factors" are of Yalom (1970, 1983) are intrinsic aspects of the group's processes on the way to its achieving its goals and include (1) imparting of information, (2) instillation of hope, (3) universality, (4) altruism, (5) the corrective recapitulation of the primary family group, (6) development of socializing techniques, (7) imitative behavior, (8) interpersonal learning, (9) group cohesiveness, (10) catharsis, and (11) an existential factor.

Pregroup Process

Group therapy with survivors of catastrophic events is very intense therapy, with many complicating factors, replete with indications and contraindications. Careful assessment and diagnostic considerations for each prospective group member is imperative, as well as achieving a good understanding of both conscious and unconscious meanings the trauma contains for the specific individual. Also critical is to determine whether and to what extent the presenting complaint is a "posttraumatic crisis" (PT-Cr), precipitated by a specific instigating event (i.e., elements of trauma in Vietnam, in childhood, or in the post-Vietnam period; Parson, 1988a). Since preservation of the group's healing potential must be guarded, the clinician needs to continually ask a key question and make decisions accordingly: "Is this survivor good for the group?" (Parson, 1984b, 1985c, 1988b).

Specific information pertaining to the veteran's tri-historical background is essential in developing a treatment plan and in understanding the veteran's potential therapeutic response repertoire in the group.

Thus, it is important to explore and understand (1) the veteran/survivor's Vietnam experience in a chronologically ordered and very detailed fashion; (2) early childhood, nature of family organization, school adjustment, and other pre-Vietnam personal experiences to include losses and traumatic events; and (3) homecoming and posthomecoming experiences to include traumatic losses. Identifying and assessing the veteran's "narcissistic stress career" (i.e., insults to the sense of self over time) before, in, and after Vietnam, and attendant "subjective structures of meaning," provide information essential to treatment planning and to group treatment itself.

Assessment is never complete with trauma patients without a clear delineation of the range of present and past strengths and positive personal attributes of the veteran. Once identified, these strengths can be "exploited" to help areas of deficit to mature.

Selection Criteria

The group treatment being discussed in this chapter consists of the formation and use of small "close-ended" groups comprised of six to eight members. I have advanced two reasons for close-ended groups: (1) to forestall the possible increase of narcissistic peril and threat which comes from being "exposed" to "strangers." The impact of these strangers' presence is often experienced by members "as a narcissistic trauma" (Kaplan & Roman, 1963, p. 235), plunging them (the group) into renewed affective embattlements to regain narcissistic equilibrium. (2) To promote the group sense of boundary and identity.

Type and Degree of Psychopathology

Certain prospective members of the group are to be screened out for the group's sake (Parson, 1984b). This is because of the potential undermining, destructive, and anxiety-provoking nature of their personal pathologies to the group's process. Excluded are veterans with (1) severe borderline conditions, with chronic acting-out behavior and strong paranoid-aggressive personality features; (2) severe psychopathic dynamics and behavior; (3) organic brain syndromes; and (4) psychosis.

Homogeneity-Heterogeneity Variables

The group model proposed here (CuRePro) encourages selection criteria to be based on both homogeneous and heterogeneous considerations. In terms of homogeneous variables, group members are to be (1) in-country or theater veterans; (2) at midlife; (3) combat or theater veterans with varying degrees of combat exposure and PTSD (ranging from mild to almost severe), as well as varying degrees of other war-related psychological symptoms (e.g., intimacy problems, difficulties in attaining and maintaining employment, narcissistic injury,

rage, etc.); and (4) a high degree of motivation for change and recovery from the Vietnam experience.

I believe that heterogeneous variables are equally important to the group's success (Parson, 1984b): (1) a range in degree of PTSD and related pathology and psychic structure (i.e., varying degrees of healthy capacity for adaptive functioning in life and in the group), and related to this, (2) a range of exposure to war stress (i.e., low, moderate, and heavy combat, as well as veterans with no combat experience).

Goals of Posttraumatic Group Psychotherapy

In addition to the above issues of selection and composition, the goals of posttraumatic group therapy are: (1) to create and maintain (as much as possible) a climate of security and empathic self-object "holding", and, through this, (2) to promote acceptance among members for each other and for the group and its goals, (3) to promote self-disclosure, (4) to develop group-as-a-whole and individual "healing theories" (the Figley, 1979, 1983, 1988, application of the term to individual and family therapies), (5) to work-through pathological narcissistic defenses, and (6) to find meaning.

Curvilinear Regressive-Progressive Group (CuRePro) Model

Many group developmental theorists have written about the stages or phases the group goes through on its way to filling its mission. In general, the literature highlights three types of group developmental processes: (1) the "linear-progressive" model—the group moving forward toward its goals; (2) the life-cycle model—the group following the life cycle of the individual and ending in psychic and physical decline and death; and (3) the "pendular" model—the group participating in the oscillations, the up and down, and the appearance-disappearance-reappearance sequences of certain issues, themes, and processes. Like other researchers, such as Gibbard, Hartman, and Mann (1974), Kellerman (1981), and Wong (1981), I espouse an integrative model that incorporates these three kinds of group processes.

The CuRePro model's fundamental premise is that, in addition to expected or normative developmental stages, group members are immersed in a multiplicity of unconscious forces which exponentially combine to contribute to the utter complexity of group processes. Identified in the following are transference reactions to group-as-a-whole unconscious currents reverberating within the group. By symbolic analogue, members thus unconsciously experience the group as (1) maternal figure, (2) mirroring self-object, (3) idealizing self-object, and (4) Vietnam tactical fighting group (engaging the enemy). From the individual dynamic point of view, group members may experience each other as maternal, paternal, and sibling figures.

Symbolic analogue processes shape group perceptions of the leader as: (1) an idealizing figure, with nurturant and adaptive aspects (nurturant aspects gratify group members' needs, while the adaptive aspects handle reality within and beyond the group); (2) combat leader (squad, platoon, company); (3) combat peer; and (4) mother to group-as-child.

Writers on group therapy hold that group life progresses from one phase or step to another—from immature levels to mature levels of personal and group integration. For example, Bales and Strodtbeck (1960) noted that "most of the theories about steps or stages in group problem-solving seem to be more or less direct extrapolations of steps or stages assumed to exist in individual mental processes" (p. 629). Appelbaum (1974) thus viewed group development as progressing from oral, to anal, to phallic stages. Along the same basic lines, but using different nomenclature, Kaplan (1967) advanced a tripartite model comprising dependency, power, and intimacy, whereas the duophasic model of Bennis and Shepard (1956) features the authority-dependence and interdependence stages (with a number of subphases).

Gibbard et al. (1974) described a group model they referred to as "linear-progressive," whereas Kellerman (1979) advanced a "linear-regressive model." Kellerman proposed an interesting shift in ordinary conceptualization. He held that group development processes reverse themselves and so begin with the phallic stage, progressing regressively to the anal, and then to the oral stage. The group approach that I advance in this chapter is the "curvilinear regressive-progressive group model." (It integrates linear-progressive, linear-regressive, pendular, and life-cycle models.)

I have discovered that group processes with traumatized populations (veterans and other survivor groups) do not follow the usual developmental path. The developmental sequence incorporates "regressive modes" (e.g., phallic, anal, and oral, or, put in other terms, assertive-narcissistic, power, and dependency), "progressive modes" (i.e., dependency, power, and assertive-narcissistic [phallic]), and a "curve mode"—an intermediary mode which connects both regressive and progressive modes.

The CuRePro model consists of six phases: (1) effectance, (2) uncertitude (fragmented sense of power), (3) essential trust and dependency, (4) autonomy and interdependence, (5) initiative and responsibility, and (6) self-cohesion.

Group Variables

Phase 1: Effectance

Tactical Family Imagery

Typically, Vietnam veterans view the psychotherapy group (with fellow combat veterans) as the most important social institution for them since the war. Second only to their family of origin, the social-affective interactions which characterized the military unit in Vietnam, the group relives together many elements of members' original families, but they especially relive the "tactical family" that originated in Vietnam. Mutual narcissistic elements bonded soldier to soldier ("fellow mirroring"), creating a security-engendering organization, which is now relived in the therapy group. Like the members' original family which provided them the most important pre-Vietnam security-granting institution, the group is experienced as another critical institution in their post-Vietnam lives. This means that group members unconsciously experience the group-as-a-whole as the original tactical military group to which they belonged in Vietnam (Parson, 1984a, 1985c). As it was in the war, members now feel besieged by unseen dangers from within and without.

Narcissistic Fantasy

Associated with the power of fellow mirroring is members' unconscious fantasy system organized around the belief that their peers would never do or say anything that would threaten their fragile sense of self. They believe that people who did not go through Vietnam (or in the case of other survivor groups, go through their specific trauma [or other traumata]) could never understand what they have gone through; and may, therefore, be insensitive and perhaps even condemning and retraumatizing to them. The unconscious belief is that fellow combat veterans with similar experiences can together create a cohesive, safe, and containing climate that would essentially increase mutual mirroring, the beginning of their retrieving a lost sense of self in and after the war.

Mixed groups (veterans and nonveterans) often fail because the veterans need to locate within the group a narcissistic mirror—that is, a person or persons who are able to reflect the self, and the self alone. Veterans often have a deep sense of vulnerability and distrust for "strangers" in the group. They thus experience mixed groups as intrinsically unempathic, with potential for "assaults" against their tenuously organized sense of self. This fear is the basis for the perennial expression among survivors: "If you didn't go through it (i.e., the specific trauma), you can't understand (i.e., empathically reflect) me." Basically, this means that traumatized persons in groups require an "isomorphic configuration of experiences" which comes from interacting with others who have identical needs, feelings, cognitions, and posttrauma patterns of behavior.

Mirroring and Idealizing Group Axes

I have identified two aspects of group process observed in most nonsurvivor groups. Recognition of these are particularly critical with veteran/survivor therapy groups. There are two fundamental dynamic axes: (1) the group-as-a-whole is unconsciously experienced as providing maternal "containing" qualities, such as nurturing; and (2) the unconscious view of the group leader (of both genders) as a paternal figure which provides limits, guidance, and controls. These two types of basic dependency needs can also be conceptualized "as the need for an affirmation of being [the idealized self-object]" (Menaker, 1979). Additionally, from the self-psychological point of view, the group-as-a-whole may be said to provide mirroring for members' grandiose self-omnipotence, while the leader provides opportunities for idealization and power mergers. As expected, these functions overlap for group members.

Transference and Biology

Groups in general have a particular pull toward regressive functioning in members (Bion, 1959; Freud, 1921). Veteran group members partake of two general response tendencies: (1) "state of transference readiness" (Freud, 1912/1968)—mentioned earlier; and (2) tendency to limbic system regression. The former set of responses reactivates archaic grandiose self and idealizing feelings and cognitions. Transference responses will be elaborated later in this chapter.

Lymbic system-level responses are a consequence of the group's capacity to lull members into regressive states of mind. Much of the learning which occurred in the heat of combat is activated in the group. As transference reactivations arise, so do "latent biological programs" originating in Vietnam's behavioral conditioning, especially classical conditioning (Keene, Fairbank, Caddell, Zimmering, & Bender, 1985; Kolb, 1984; Mowrer, 1960; and Pavlov, 1960) "wired into" their neurological systems. The group is thus immersed in both psychologically and biologically mediated experiences and sensations. In their discussion of regressive experiences in combat veterans, Brende and McCann (1984) mentioned a Vietnam veteran who recalled that "When I was in Vietnam, I felt like an animal . . . lived by the law of the jungle . . . I had to kill to survive" (p. 61). They go on to state that

> The experience of "fused" primitive aggression and sexuality, typical of limbic system arousal characterizing phylogenetic regression, was sometimes subjectively experienced as a powerful "high"—even "addicting." As one veteran said, "the 'adrenalin high' I experience in 'Nam was even better than heroin.'" (p. 61)

The above observations give the early group its patent archaic defensive and adaptive organization. Along with these primitive biological systems are the primitive psychological grandiose self and idealized images, sentiment, and behavior which together dominate the early stages of the group. At this stage, members are unable to tolerate honest self-observation. They need to be protected from their own inner feelings of guilt, terror, aggression, and depressive affects, and only good empathic self-objects, which they feel, can achieve this.

Veterans' profound mirror hunger makes them vulnerable to unempathic slights and other narcissistically mortifying behaviors in nonmirroring persons. Members cannot tolerate criticism from anyone, and so find it self-integrating to relate to fellow members whom they believe understand them, and are capable of empathically resonating their fears and anxieties, their deeply felt injustices, their anger, their aspirations, and their hopes.

Archaic Cohesion and Mirroring

In the group's formative period, intense mirror hunger forms a "posttraumatic accelerated cohesion" (p-TAC) (Parson, 1985c). This kind of cohesion occurs very quickly before members have sufficient time to get to know each other. It is based upon a sense of "fantasied familiarity" (Day, 1976), and a "false-self" organization (Winnicott, 1965). Thus, p-TAC contrasts developmentally with more advanced forms of cohesive states (seen in later phases of the group) and exemplified by the terms "in-group consciousness" (Bennis, 1964) and "group spirit" (Coffee *et al.*, 1950). However, p-TAC has intrinsic healing properties which benefit group members and motivate them to remain in the group. Additionally, this cohesion begins "the repairwork" (Parson, 1988a) to fill narcissistic emptiness and deal with the self-affective connection to each other is an important first step in realizing hope, inspiration, and a sense of a safety against internal and external sources of threats to self-esteem.

As positive as p-TAC is for the group, it may have countertherapeutic properties as well, depending on how it is understood and managed, and on the individual and "total group" ego strength represented in the group. As a potentially negative force, p-TAC can undermine individual growth, while stifling development of the group-as-a-whole. For it is well known that "high cohesion . . . is not a universal cultural attribute that should be valued for its intrinsic goodness" (Kellerman, 1981, p. 13).

In contrast to other group formations, the central dynamic operations in survivor groups are to reexperience the original effectance-based power and peer-dominated social system, which group members, as young soldiers, had experienced decades before in Vietnam. Thus, veteran first-phase group members express effectance issues around courage, competence, and surviving while others died, and about guns, machine guns, APCs, tanks, rockets, artillery, securing a hill, gun boats, landmines, pistols, rifles, killings, "firefights," booby-traps, search-and-destroy missions, fighting, surviving, dying, masculine prowess in outsmarting and beating the enemy, and around the ghoulish occurrences on both sides. In this phase, group "consensus" permits some mutual vying for power and dominance among members. Members serving in the most prestigious units, who have the most wounded, or who have "seen the most action," emerge as the most admired, respected, and idealized members of the group (Parson, 1988b). Often, these members because the "group process leaders"—the unofficial leaders who wield much power and influence in the group.

Seductive Nature of Veteran's Complaints

Even the most experienced group leaders can become overly fascinated and "glued" to surface, conscious articulations of group members. They therefore often miss the "subterranean message" and the struggles this message reveals. The leader realizes that though members talk about physical and mental pain and anguish, their guilt, losses, poor social functioning, and their feelings of distance from their wives, children, parents, and friends are important but not the most critical dimension of the group's healing potential. When leaders do not know that first-phase dynamics are phallic-narcissistic (or assertively narcissistic) they may err in guiding the group to dwell prematurely on oral-based conflicts and concerns, and thereby unwillingly remortify (retraumatize) members' sense of phallic narcissism and pride. Oral-based dependency is the antithesis of assertion-based competence.

During this phase, moreover, survivors' fragmented sense of self makes it too frightening to assume the passive role characterized by the oral phase. It portends self-disintegration while it threatens the endangered self of the group with further loss of a sense of control. As one veteran stated in group: "It [dependency] is worse than death!" The tendency to use the "phallic-intrusive mode" (Erikson, 1950) allows members to "combat" unseen dangers and enemies that threaten their sense of self and self-esteem. This tendency also "ensures" safety against intrapsychic fears that come from intrusive threats of the "return of the dissociated" (Parson, 1984b).

Fears of Magical Self–Other Annihilation

A great source of intrapsychic and interpersonal threat in the group is members' fear of losing control over aggressive drive, a cardinal source of posttrauma defensiveness, for many have associated aggressive ideation and behavior with the someone's death. Because of this association, members are less inclined to express anger or other derivatives of the aggressive drive, such as confrontation and expression of disagreement with fellow combatants in the group. The intense fear is that "Were I to express anger or rage toward Bill, I will kill him, and possibly myself, just as it happened in Vietnam when somebody got 'pissed off.'" This fear, referred to as "aggression–annihilation phobia," is the basis in early group phases for members' reluctance to confront each other and express honest evaluation of fellow members' resistances and defenses in the group.

Psychology of Blame

Blaming is central to groups. Kellerman (1981) identified three patterns of managing blame in the group: search for scapegoats, group self-blame, and self-examination. Members' concerns about ineffectual leadership in the war, and in the government of the United States that led to disastrous consequences, are reactivated in the group as well. The "blaming attitude" is fueled by "unconscious identifications with ineffectual leadership in the war enterprise" (Parson, 1988a). The group's first-phase "coziness" and absence of ego-observational capacity leads to externalization of blame, and self-observation is virtually nill. This predisposition results in projections onto the leader in which members question the leader's ability to lead the group on its mission, as members blame the "leaders out there."

Because of this tendency, one of the leader's qualities must be his or her idealizability. This quality represents the leader's ability to attract confidence, admiration, and respect from group members. In part, this comes through the leader's demonstrated competence and experience in working with survivors, his or her intellect, group presence, and ability to connect with the group's processes. Idealizability forestalls the premature projection of hyperaggressiveness and intense paranoid fears onto the leader, which would be overwhelming for the group. When aggression is unmodulated during this phase, the group comes to its demise quite early. Often the leader toward which aggression is directed may be the "unofficial" leader (a group member designated as "leader" from the group process perspective). In either case, premature expression of aggression in the group is destructive.

This proves to be a major challenge to the leader and the leader's success in managing this potential goes a long way to ensuring the group's success in achieving its long-range goals. In terms of veterans' therapy groups, the leader who is perceived as idealizable is one who is either a Vietnam veteran, a veteran of other wars, or a nonveteran with extensive, demonstrated experience and effectiveness with Vietnam veterans. In nonveteran survivor groups, the idealizable leader is one who has either gone through a similar (or related) traumatic event, or is one with great experience whose past interactions with survivors has been competent, sensitive, and successful.

Criticism and Punishment

Being hypersensitive to criticism, members are unable to tolerate criticism from anyone—in or outside the group. Only "ambitendent and attenuated" criticism coming from fellow members can be tolerated without increase in narcissistic stress; however, criticism directed toward a fellow member is rare in the early phase of the group's journey. Criticism, from whatever source, may prove narcissistically disorganizing, particularly if the superego weight of the group is heavy (because of unresolved "moral stress" related to violence in the war). This is one reason the leader's presence and authority are minimized by the group: to avert recognizing the person of the only member of the group who can punish. The leader's potential to mete out punishment for moral-based infractions creates punitive anticipatory anxiety in members, while ambivalence toward the leader prevails. Elsewhere, I recommended that the leader assume a technical stance as the "ghost presence"—a group presence whose perceived absolutarian power is transformed into "senior peer" relating. In ghost presence (Parson, 1985c), the leader's role does not assume a clear demarcation between self and group, but seeks cognitive, affective, and behavioral integration.

Integrating Yalom's "Therapeutic Factors"

The Yalom (1970) therapeutic factors—instillation of hope, imparting of information, and universality—are incorporated in this phase. They promote understanding and heightened mirroring among members. For example, mutual encouragement helps each member see himself in the other, the other having been demoralized in the past, but now feels better and hopeful about life and the future. Information-imparting offers vital knowledge about members' problems and resources within the group and services at community-based organizations, as well as at the Veterans Administration Medical and Regional Centers and Offices (in the case of veterans). Finding that they are not unique in their misery, members share their isolation, traumatic dreams, problems with substance abuse, marital and parental difficulties, as well as problematic careers.

Relating to fellow group members is experienced as integrating: veterans feel they have finally found the empathic self-object mirroring they had always needed since the war but had never found until this group experience. The feeling is that members understand and that they are able to resonate empathically their deepest fears, their sense of humiliation, their narcissistic injuries, and to bolster their self-esteem.

Unseen Dangers

From the perspective of narcissism—or, more appropriately, posttraumatic narcissism (as indicated earlier), the group's theme represents phallic-narcissistic revivals of war-linked (and prewar, in many instances) grandiose self and idealizing mechanisms. Because members unconsciously experience the group-as-a-whole as the original tactical military group to which they belonged in Vietnam, the group is beset by a number of dangers—from both within and without the group self—responded to by paranoid fears which contribute to the phallic-intrusive defensive tendency in the group. However, it is the external forces that are mostly feared and defended against, and they ultiize each others' capacity to provide "soothing mirroring" to help overcome group fears. "It's we against them." The group's "pervasive tactical family imagery" (Parson, 1988b) contributes to binding members together, as mentioned before, in a peer-centered emotional glueing, akin to the concept of "exaggerated perfect unity" (Day, 1976), which might be referred to as a "proveteran/peer group organization."

Phase 2: Uncertitude

The group struggles with the conflict of holding on and letting go of Vietnam, reminiscent of the contradictory tendencies of the retentitive-eliminative mode Erikson (1950). Whereas in the former phase the central dynamic issue was a "sense of self-efficacy versus personal impotence," in this phase the issue is a "sense of power versus a sense of personal defect" undergirded by shame and doubting. As in the first phase, it is marked by "experiential blindspots" (or an inability of members to "see" their cupability and responsibility for their lives). However, as the group moves on, members are no longer so sure that the entities external to the group self are to blame for all problems. Many veterans need to hold onto Vietnam in order to bolster fragile self-esteem and restore positive self-experience.

"The basic attitude for this phase is observed in the Query Constellation as follows: 'Does the government have total power over us? Can it be totally responsible for all our problems.' If the government and others are not fully to blame, then are we to blame for the parts we played in Vietnam and the life unlived within us?" (Parson, 1988b, p. 293). "Maybe society is right: we are mean and depraved." This phase is also marked by group concerns about death, lost buddies, killing, culpability, preguilt (forerunner of true guilt), which are ultimately connected to shame and doubt. The ambitendency of this phase also leads to an increase in splitting defenses resulting in the perception of the group as alternately "all good." This phase marks the beginning of a redirecting of blame toward the group self, as opposed to exter-

nal persons, situations, and institutions. (This does not mean, however, that the group is ready to assume responsibility for itself.)

Whereas in Phase 1 members were caught up in manic other-directed blame, in this phase group members are now prone to self-blame and depression. Phase 1 morphologically mimics the intrusive phase (of PTSD), while Phase 2 resembles numbing, denial, and avoidance. The threat which comes from letting go of pathological omnipotence often results in a sense of narcissistic injury, and to counteract this is the tendency to holding on to remnants of grandiose self images. Autonomy and independence are abandoned within the group, for to be independent means to stand alone, face guilt (from a variety of sources), and become blameworthy. Like the previous phase, the group's dynamics are peer-centered and counterauthoritative in nature, with the beginning of "the development of socializing techniques (Yalom, 1970, 1983).

Phase 3: Essential Trust and Dependency

This phase of the CuRePro model marks the beginning of an authority group organization of the group's structure. Moreover, this phase marks another emerging defensive pattern: dependency. This phase resembles the "basic trust" of Erickson (1950), in which total dependency exists, and mutual regulation occurs between the child and the mothering one. The leader is experienced as all-powerful, omnipotent—"as an archetypal figure of immense authority and power, possessing magical means of healing" (Anthony, 1967, p. 60). The group members' grandiose omnipotence is projected onto the leader. The leader is perceived as both mother and father, as both empathic mirroring and idealizing selfobjects. Group members are now dependent upon the leader, after coming in full awareness of their narcissistic neediness.

This phase is divided into three subphases: immature dependency, confrontative operations, and the beginning of mature dependency. Fear of being "used" as in Vietnam, fear of criticism, ridicule, scorn, rejection, abandonment, and condemnation give the group process a paranoid flavor. Additionally, fears and anticipation of narcissistic injuries at the hand of the leader abound. In Subphase 1, p-TAC dynamics are still quite operative, but anxiety over the leader's power and fear of the outside world are diminished. The group has very little insight into their resistances and narcissistic pathological fixations.

As the leader's position is viewed with less trepidation, the group's self is now bare to the full impact of the treatment experience. In Subphase 2, the group is confronted by the leader who can now explore pathological posttraumatic narcissistic defenses, oral aggression and resistances, paranoid defenses, and deep authority conflicts. Yalom's (1970, 1983) therapeutic factors of "corrective recapitulation of the primary family group" (surfaces pre-Vietnam configurations and homecoming familial-social issues), "imitative behavior," and the beginning of "catharsis" are most evident during this time.

After successful and prolonged working through of pathological identifications with the dead, mourning, and power and control conflicts, a new cohesive group structure evolves. This new organization is based on mutuality and interdependence functioning among and between members. True guilt (as opposed to pre-guilt) is experienced fully during the essential trust phase. (Parson, 1988b, p. 291)

In this phase, the self is vulnerable and least resistant to experiencing the full impact of the therapy. The collective self can now tolerate self-examination, as collective self-blame is manifested in the group process.

Phase 4: Autonomy and Interdependence

As a consequence of working-through pathological identifications, pathological mourning, and pathological grandiose self-images, members are able to now see each other as individuals. Since psychic trauma is the breakdown of self-structure which secondarily leads to self-protective avoidance (of the recognition of people's separateness), only structural development and integration (relative) can give group members the strength to come to terms with being separate individuals, without untoward levels of fragmenting, annihilating anxiety. With this increased capacity in members for ego boundary regulation and control, the members' mirroring and ideal needs and feelings have achieved greater maturational development and concomitant development of individual group-as-a-whole intrapsychic structures.

During this phase, veterans feel centered and more grounded in the real world; they have developed "a larger personal perspective on the traumatic event . . . and think more about the future and . . . [are] less fixed on the past" (Brende & Parson, 1985, p. 186). Concerns of individual self-identity emerge along with concerns about relationships with spouse, son, daughter, father, mother, siblings, and friends in terms of intimacy and autonomous relating and, in general, are important dynamic issues during this phase. This phase relates to the "autonomy versus shame and doubt" of Erikson (1950). Blame is managed through confronting the group and individual self and in seeking new standards to which to aspire.

This phase marks the first time during the treatment in which members feel fully capable of confronting each other and do. In Phases 1 and 2 members need to protect their peers against criticism; narcissistic injury has virtually disappeared in the group. In contrast to a purely narcissistic mirror (which reflects no one but the self) is the social mirror achieved within the group. "The social mirror [is] based on the reflected appraisals of others [in the group and later in society]. This move from the narcissistic mirror to the social mirror is reflected in George Herbert's phrase 'the best mirror is a good friend'" (Pine, 1983). Interpersonal learning and feelings of altruism are salient at this milestone of the group's journey (Yalom, 1970, 1983).

Phase 5: Initiative and Responsibility

Facing one's life as an individual who is separate but related to others, with a self that has private and public aspects, permits one in the group to take responsibility for one's self. The blaming attitude is replaced by initia-

tive, and shame and guilt give way to inner freedom and responsibility. "Gaining cognitive and emotional independence from Vietnam" (Parson, 1988b, p. 295) increases the sense of self. Group members are now able (for the first time during the course of treatment) to truly face their guilt—progressing into "self-lacerating guilt" through to a state of inner peace of self-integrity. Here the guilt stems from violence meted out against the enemy, particularly in terms of "abusive violence" (Frey-Wouters & Laufer, 1986) and "self-violence" in terms of destructive behavioral patterns directed against self, spouse, son, daughter, and others in one's life. Additionally, this "guilting review" at this phase takes in the highly personalized form of guilt—"the transgression against oneself," the failure to live one's life to its fullest (the wasted portions of one's life).

This is a form of "existential guilt" (Yalom, 1980, p. 147), and other "existential factors" (Yalom, 1970, 1983) relating to ultimate concerns about human isolation, meaninglessness, freedom, and death, as well as the "middlessence review." This review includes group members' sense of work and competence, reflection upon the positive or salutogenic aspects of service in Vietnam (Parson, 1989a), and the midlife concerns outlined by Opp (1987): one's death, confidence, demonic (one's selfishness, hedonism, and cruelty), change in sex role, the aspiration-achievement gap, sexual potency, affiliative needs, marriage relationship, one's identity, future goals, and generativity (pp. 177–178). In many respects, this phase is akin to the "initiative versus guilt" of Erikson (1950).

Phase 6: Self-Cohesion

The final phase of the curvilinear group model marks the cohesiveness of the sense of self, which is achieved through "structural replacement" of parts missing because of trauma. Thus, the survivors' former "absence of structure and representable experience in a region of the self" (Cohen, 1985, p. 178) is now replaced by an inner representation and capacity for symbolization. Posttraumatic narcissism has been transformed from a state of unmirrored, isolated pain and suffering to a state of "pretertraumatic narcissism"—a "beyond," matured form of narcissism marked by differentiation and integration of trauma elements and the self in relation to the self-object. Independence from both Vietnam and from self-sustaining/infantilizing, symbiotic relationships, and interdependence, inner freedom, awareness, and self-understanding are achieved. The various strands of the trauma have become integrated into a tapestry of personal meaning. The retrieval of dormant skills learned in the war are activated in earlier phases but especially during this phase. The salutogenic (positive, facilitating) areas of maturity and growth secondary to service in Vietnam are highlighted, reinternalized, and integrated. These are in relation to personal strengths, special skills, talents, leadership abilities, teamwork, tough mindedness, resiliency, and the competencies learned in the war (and still available to the enlightened, aware self). Additionally, group members find meaning in being a survivor and in acknowledging that Vietnam was not all pain, but also had value in terms of surviving where others died, of experiencing the unusual lessons of the dialectic between life and death, of heightened sensitivity, compassion, and caring for other people, and of bringing home vital talents and latent ambitions to be actualized now in their lives. As part of this "Vietnam personal rediscovery" process, members become aware of having learned how to function under extreme external and internal stresses in the war (and possibly even before the war), and they construct a new foundation upon which new ideals, ambitions, initiatives, and values are established.

Having worked-through dread, resistance, and the unconscious meaning of trauma, group members, during this phase, are like Egendorf's (1982) subjects, who have matured "beyond avoidance, blame, self-pity, and self-punishment" (p. 905). Knowing and being known are key achievements. Knowing one's self through honest self-observation (of early childhood experiences, Vietnam traumata, homecoming narcissistic trauma, and the sense of failure since the war) is a noteworthy attainment during this phase. Moreover, knowing others as never before, feeling close to them in unthreatening and nondefensive relating, feeling safe with another, as well as finding one's place in the world of work and people are also salient indices of a cohesive sense of self. Blaming, paranoid projections, denial, disavowal, and other defensive maneuvers are now integrated and understood by group members as "faulty attempts at self-cure" (Ulman & Brothers, 1988; Simmel, 1944). The group is now in an emotional and psychic position to adapt to history—of competence and self-esteem in Vietnam—(and other past experiences) in exchange for the narcissistically injurious adaptation to the social categories that once defined and distorted their humanity, competence, and identity.

Leader Variables

Phase 1

Intrinsic to the CuRePro model is the assumption that leader variables are very important to the group's success. Thus, the leader's skill, technique, knowledge of trauma, PTSD, and allied disturbances, as well as the belief in survivors' intrinsic potential for growth, interact with group members' problems and needs.

Idealizability

As indicated earlier, idealizability is a key requirement for being a leader of a survivor group. The nonidealizable leader often stirs up group unconscious fury against authority persons (i.e., "responsible" for the trauma) prematurely, thus bringing the group to an early demise. However, being idealizable does not automatically mean absolute trust, but relative trust. Most survivors entering a group are ideal hungry; that is, they tend to seek protection by merging with powerful persons and institutions (the leader being unconsciously perceived as "all-powerful"). An important feature of idealizability is a perceptible demarcation separating the leader from the "traumatizing agent" (person or institution viewed as responsible by survivors). For survivors

of Vietnam in the first group phase, leaders must demonstrate that their philosophies and theories about the war, its veterans, and about healing differ significantly to the narcissistically injurious attitudes of others in our society (government, politicians, and family).

Process Manager

The leader is "process manager" (Parson, 1984b, 1988b); which means that he or she "plans, organizes, and coordinates the business of the group. To do this successfully, however, the leader must be aware (and remain aware) of the emerging unspoken (often unspeakable) thoughts, needs, affects, impulses, and defenses of the [trauma] group" (Parson, 1988b). Moreover, the leader must understand group process, and the query constellation around "Who is in charge?" "What is the mission?" "How will the mission be evaluated, and by whom?" "How will I fare in this evaluation?" and the like. These questions are loaded with dread: they require responses that are direct, honest, and sensitive. Genuine, informed, steadfast, and compassionate interaction with the group is critical in all phases.

The leader monitors the group in every phase to ensure manageability of toxicity related to group reliving (intrusive) experiences. The leader is also aware that rigid, traditional approaches may limit effectiveness, as they threaten an increase in group sense of mortal danger (Hurvich, 1989). This then often results in some members' leaving or premature termination from the group. For there are times when the leader will find that "often an emotional response, small gift, taking a stance, or a prescription . . . [are] necessary to capture a sense of empathic presence in the transference" (Laub & Auerhahn, 1989, p. 395).

Technical Presence

The peer-dominated deep social structure of the group requires the leader to assume the "ghost presence" as indicated earlier. This means that the leader is fully present (a participant-observer), and, for the sake of the group, becomes a part of the group's horizontal relationships (peers as opposed to authority). The leader is warm and emotionally available to the group. Critical treatment concerns, such as confidentiality, trust, and exploitation, will arise in the group and must be addressed by the leader. And the leader must always be ready to accept that he or she is the symbolic (transference) platoon leader or some other authority person and as such is a potential target for affect-laden projections.

Preparation for the Work and Need for a Transtheoretical Orientation

Leaders' preparation for work with traumatized individuals begins with (1) self-understanding in terms of motivations for wanting to work with the specific population (i.e., veterans, Holocaust survivors, rape victims, incest survivors, etc.), and (2) specific training in traumatic stress, replete with supervision and/or peer supervision. In terms of the first requirement, the prospective leader explores the following questions: "Is he or she a survivor? If the answer is yes, then what does this mean?" "If it is no, is there someone else in their history that was catastrophically overwhelmed by an extraordinarily toxic life-event?" In any event, leaders need to know how to increase their awareness of self: working with survivors is often much more difficult and demanding (particularly in the early phases of the treatment) than with nonsurvivor populations, owing to pervasive loss of the sense of self and constant threats posed by annihilation anxieties.

Additionally, preparation to treat veterans of the Vietnam war requires that therapists be convinced that veteran survivors are not helpless, nor social victims without hope. When therapists begin with this bias, the group intuits it. Therapists often need to be mindful of the many ways they may unwittingly contribute to stereotyping and villification of veterans (Parson, 1989a, 1989c). Improving the public image of the veteran, first in his or her mind and then in society at large, is integral to treating traumatized veterans (Parson, 1989c, 1989e, 1989f). Veterans' bad public image as "people having posttraumatic stress disorder" (in the absence of strengths) is a narcissistic injury professionals unwittingly perpetrate against the Vietnam war veteran in many instances. The leader is aware of, and able to sensitively and appropriately apply, a medley of techniques, from a number of schools of psychotherapy; for example, behavioral, cognitive, psychodynamic, and existential approaches to healing in the aftermath of psychic trauma.

Countertransference Reactions

The leader's feelings about the social and political forces surrounding the particular trauma must be very clear in his or her mind, and highly charged emotional reactions need to be monitored so as to not interfere with the group's goals; that is, of achieving integration and healing for each member. I identified (Parson, 1988a) at least three problematic countertransference reactions in groups: (1) leaders' envy of members "unit cohesion" and of feeling excluded; (2) members' ability to express murderous wishes and actual aggression in the war in comfortable manner; and (3) sense of masculine impotence of overidentification with members' phallic-centered character resistances. Many reactions can be very helpful if appropriately monitored and incorporated to enhance the treatment process. I have discussed in detail other sources of countertransference responses (see Parson, 1988a).

Phase 2

Personal Stability

Stability is obviously a requirement for each successive phase of the treatment. The leader's personality integration and personal awareness is very important in the group. Being fully anchored psychologically and being self-assured assist the group when issues around blame, doubt, shame, depression, and suicidal behavior arise, as well as when members use the leader as "screen" for group projections.

Phase 3

The leader addresses the group's oral-based impulses, conflicts, and defenses to enhance structural growth and development. According to Parson (1988b), "narcissistic aggression-borne transferences involving the VA, the government, specific hateful Vietnam objects (i.e., officers), and now the leader, are worked through aided by the predictable, stable person of the leader, combined with the sense of group safety, and the systematic use of interpretation, confrontation, clarification, and modeling." I have reviewed other interventions found useful in the group (Parson, 1984a, 1984b), which are to be employed at the leader's discretion based upon a psychodynamic understanding of the group's process. These are: (1) self-instructional training (Meichenbaum, 1977), (2) cognitive restructuring (Beck, 1976; Ellis, 1974), (3) relaxation training (Borkovec & Sides, 1979), and (4) psychoanalytic therapy (DeFazio & Pascucci, 1984; Lindy, 1988; Parson, 1984a, 1984b, 1988a).

Many psychoanalytically oriented professionals may have some misgivings about the intermingling of nondynamic techniques with more traditional approaches. Behavioral and cognitive therapists may feel the same. However, when the survivor's needs dictate the treatment strategies, no one approach will do the job (Crump, 1984). Because it is clear by now that no one school of psychotherapy can systematically address the self-devastating symptoms and reactions of the traumatic syndrome, it appears prudent (in behalf of the patient) to do what needs to be done.

The broad spectrum of needs presented by survivors should dictate what procedures are used—not vested interest procedures determining patients' needs. Undoubtedly, therapists who are unable or unwilling to "bend" the ground rules of their particular technical school will fail to be successful with trauma survivors, particularly those whose narcissistic pathology are in the advanced (chronic) states of posttraumatic breakdown. These and other techniques can be used throughout the six phases of the group treatment. However, in terms of specific techniques or approaches, it is here recommended that the objective is to begin with highly structured approaches (mostly cognitive and behavioral), and end with relatively unstructured, dynamic procedures and techniques.

Phase 4 through Phase 6

During these latter phases, the leader assumes a less active stance, shifting his or her technical "gear" into psychodynamic approaches. This is now possible because group members' self-structures are presumably more integrated and cohesive and so are able to handle anxiety better than before as well as to regulate self-esteem. The leader's interpreting, clarifying, and confronting of members' wishes to remain symbiotically tied to "Vietnam's unit," and the leader's own stability and independence modeled in the group offer reassurance. A major leadership challenge is to assist members to resolve guilt by confronting it rather than by expiating or externalizing it. Intense feelings about Agent Orange-related guilt (pertaining to offspring and a condensation of other "guilts" from the war) contribute to the sense of "inner mortal dangers" at this time (Parson, 1989e; Parson, 1990).

In these phases, the leader explores issues of guilt and responsibility, the interactive effects of which Smith (1982) has written. He notes that "guilt rises exponentially" (p. 1023) in veterans who assume responsibility for the death of others. Dealing with guilt, in its many forms, emerges as an important issue particularly in this phase.

Through employing more openness, therapeutic activity, and advocacy (as appropriate), the leader thus assists survivors with posttraumatic narcissistic pathology by facilitating the working-through of narcissistic injury and rage (Kohut, 1972), fragmentation, denial, numbing, depression, grief states, and suicidal proclivities (and other self-destructive behaviors) and to achieve an integrated sense of self as partly evidenced by members newly acquired ability "to find a home, to care about . . . individuals, . . . ideas or projects, to search, to create, to build—these and other forms of engagement are . . . rewarding . . . intrinsically enriching" (Yalom, 1980, p. 482).

Conclusion

Treating posttraumatic narcissistic disorders in Vietnam veterans and in other survivors is a complicated matter, requiring a multiplicity of conceptual bases and the application of a number of techniques. The Curvilinear Regressive-Progressive Group (CuRePro) model was applied to demonstrate the complexities of unconscious developmental motivations of the group. These motivations shape the enterprise and the various phases the group goes through on its way to realizing its objectives. The phasic-developmental approach upon which the model is based acknowledges the need to address the unfolding and changing needs of members in the group over time (Brende & Parson, 1987; Parson, 1984b). This model acknowledges the fact that survivors having multifaceted problems "defy wholesale remedy by any one theory" (Crump, 1984). It thus employs a "menu of techniques" (Parson, 1988a), referred to in recent years as "psychotherapy integration" (Beutler, 1983; Lazarus, 1981; Norcross, 1986; Parson, 1984a, 1988a; Prochaska & DiClemente, 1984; Stricker, personal communication, 1986; Wachtel, 1977), believed to be the new paradigmatic shift in psychotherapy.

The model recognizes that traumatic changes in group members' personalities cannot be remedied by most short-term methods (Ulman & Brothers, 1988). Short-term methods seem to work best with acute traumatic syndrome cases when the survivor possesses a cohesive self with adequate defensive and adaptive capacities. Most chronic traumatic states have often caused significant character alterations, which become imbedded and structuralized into the self-system. Long-term treatment as suggested by the CuRePro model would be appropriate in these instances.

The vicissitudes of posttraumatic narcissism in the group also require a working-through of social and political issues associated with intraself disturbances (Parson, 1988a; Shapiro, 1978), and attention to the social and internalized (from the society at large of the "drug-crazed psychopathic baby killer" and/or the more recent image of the "sick, disordered, helpless vet") negative self-image of the Vietnam war veteran (Parson, 1989d).

The group in this model meets two to three times per week, for $2^{1}/_{2}$ to 3 hours per session during Phases 1 through 3; and for the same number of hours on a twice per week basis for Phases 4 through 6. The group treatment approach espoused here takes at least $2^{1}/_{2}$ to 3 years to complete, depending on a number of group factors, such as degree of PTSD-related numbing and denial, pathological unconscious guilt, and the severity of posttraumatic narcissistic pathology (i.e., degree of traumatic loss of the sense of self).

My focus in this chapter has been on veterans of the Vietnam war who are suffering from posttraumatic narcissism stemming from combat-linked shattering of subjective structures of experience, and from homecoming narcissistic trauma in being strangers at home and feeling rejected and neglected by a whole society. The pervasive self-damage to the personality of the survivor cautions therapists against allowing empathy to become lost in the transference. As I have written elsewhere (Parson, 1984b, 1988a), during the first phases of the group, the leader may have to meet survivor's concrete needs by direct action (e.g., making a phone call for a veteran who is seeking housing facilities or disability compensation from the VA; contacting the victim's bureau for a terrified rap victim, etc.). Abstractions and symbolizations are not integratable (or utilizable) by the shattered self. This is because the traumatic event cannot be represented internally owing to the disjuncture of self–self-object relations, which contributes to the sense of depersonalization, derealization, and demoralization. Concrete interventions are experienced as real (as "experience-impacting"), filling concretely inner emptiness and narcissistic needs in direct fashion. Such sensitivity to need goes beyond narrowly prescribed theoretical procedures; it expands to envelope the shattered self as the leader's "adaptation to need" (Winnicott, 1975) promotes the reparation of the self.

References

American Psychiatric Association. (1980). *Diagnostic and statistical manual of mental disorders* (3rd ed.). Washington, DC: Author.

American Psychiatric Association. (1987). *Diagnostic and statistical manual of mental disorders* (3rd ed., rev.). Washington, DC: Author.

Atwood, G., & Stolorow, R. (1984). *Structures of subjectivity.* Hillsdale, NJ: Analytic Press.

Bales, R., & Stodtbeck, F. (1953). Phases of group problem-solving. In D. Cartwright & A. Zander (Ed.), *Group dynamics* (pp. 386–400). New York: Row, Peterson.

Beck, A. T. (1976). *Cognitive therapy and emotional disorders.* New York: International Universities Press.

Beidel, T. (1989, November 30). Author discusses Vietnam: Sheehan faults U.S. perceptions. *The Times Union.*

Bennis, W., & Shepard, H. (1956). A theory of group development. *Human Relations, 9,* 415–437.

Bennis, W. G., Shepard, H. (1964). *Interpersonal dynamics: Essays and readings on human interaction.* Homewood, IL: Dorsey Press.

Beutler, L. (1983). *Eclectic psychotherapy: A systematic approach.* New York: Pergamon Press.

Bion, W. (1959). *Experiences in groups.* New York: Basic Books.

Borkovec, T., & Sides, J. (1979). Critical procedural variables related to the physiological effects of progressive relaxation. *Behaviour Research and Therapy, 17,* 119–125.

Blos, P. (1962). *On adolescence.* New York: Free Press of Glencoe.

Brende, J. O., & Parson, E. R. (1985). *Vietnam veterans: The road to recovery.* New York: Plenum Press.

Brende, J. O., & Parson, E. R. (1987). Multiphasic treatment of Vietnam veterans. *Psychotherapy in Private Practice, 5,* 51–62).

Brende, J. O., & McCann, L. (1984). Regressive experiences in Vietnam veterans: Their relationship to war, post-traumatic symptoms and recovery. *Journal of Contemporary Psychotherapy, 14,* 57–75.

Brockway, S. (1987). Group treatment of combat nightmares in post-traumatic stress disorder. *Journal of Contemporary Psychotherapy, 17,* 270–287.

Cohen, J. (1985). Trauma and repression. *Psychoanalytic Inquiry, 5,* 164–189.

Crump, L. (1984). Gestalt therapy in the treatment of Vietnam veterans experiencing PTSD symptomatology. *Journal of Contemporary Psychotherapy, 14,* 90–98.

Day, M. (1976). The natural history of training groups. In M. Kissen (Ed.), *From group dynamics to group psychoanalysis* (pp. 135–144). Washington, DC: Hemisphere Publishing.

DeFazio, V., & Pascucci, N. (1984). Return to Ithaca: A perspective on marriage and love in post-traumatic stress disorder. *Journal of Contemporary Psychotherapy, 14,* 76–89.

Egendorf, A. (1975). Vietnam veterans rap groups and themes of war life. *Journal of Social Issues, 31,* 111–124.

Egendorf, A. (1982). The post-war healing of Vietnam veterans: Recent research. *Hospital and Community Psychology, 33*(11), 901–908.

Ellis, A. (1974). *Humanistic psychotherapy.* New York: McGraw-Hill.

Ferenczi, S. (1916–1917). Two types of war neuroses. In *Further contributions to the theory and technique of psychoanalysis.* New York: Basic Books.

Figley, C. R. (1979, May 14). *Combat as disaster: Treating combat veterans as survivors.* Paper presented at the annual meeting of the American Psychiatric Association, Chicago.

Figley, C. R. (1988). A five-phase treatment of post-traumatic stress disorders in families. *Journal of Traumatic Stress, 1*(1), 127–141.

Figley, C. R., & Leventman, S. (1980). *Strangers at home.* New York: Praeger.

Figley, C. R. (1983). Catastrophes: An overview of family reactions. In C. R. Figley & H. I. McCubbin (Eds.), *Stress and the family: Vol. II. Coping with catastrophe* (pp. 3–20). New York: Brunner/Mazel.

Freud, S. (1968). The dynamics of transference. In J. Strachey (Ed. and Trans.), *The Standard edition of the complete psychological works of Sigmund Freud* (Vol. 12, pp. 99–108). London: Hogarth Press. (Original work published 1912)

Freud, S. (1957). On narcissism: An introduction. In J. Strachey (Ed. and Trans.), *The standard edition of the complete psychological works of Sigmund Freud* (Vol. 14, pp. 69–102). London: Hogarth Press. (Original work published 1914)

Freud, S. (1968). Introduction to psycho-analysis and the war neuroses. In J. Strachey (Ed. and Trans.), *The standard edition of the complete psychological works of Sigmund Freud* (Vol. 17, pp. 207–215). London: Hogarth Press. (Original work published 1919)

Frey-Wouters, E., & Laufer, R. (1986). *Legacies of a war.* New York: Sharpe.

Gelman, D. (1988, August 29). Treating war's psychic wounds. *Newsweek,* pp. 62–64.

Gibbard, G., Hartman, J., & Mann, R. (1974). *Analysis of group.* San Francisco: Jossey-Bass.

Green, B., Wilson, J., & Lindy, J. (1985). Conceptualizing post-traumatic stress disorder: A psychosocial framework. In C. R. Figley (Ed.). *Trauma and its wake: The study and treatment of post-traumatic stress disorder* (pp. 53–69). New York: Brunner/Mazel.

Haley, S. (1985). Some of my best friends are dead: Treatment of the PTSD patient and his family. In W. Kelly (Ed.), *Post-traumatic stress disorder and the veteran patient* (pp. 54–71). New York: Brunner/Mazel.

Hendrick, I. (1943). *Facts and theories of psychoanalysis.* New York: Knopf.

Hurvich, M. S. (1989). Traumatic moment, basic dangers, and annihilation anxiety. *Psychoanalytic Psychology, 6*(3), 309–323.

Kaplan, S. (1967). Therapy groups and training groups: Similarities and differences. *International Journal of Group Psychotherapy, 17,* 473–504.

Kaplan, S., & Roman, M. (1963). Phases of development in an adult therapy group. *International Journal of Group Psychotherapy, 13,* 10–26.

Keene, T., Fairbank, J., Caddell, J., Zimmering, R., & Bender, M. (1985). In C. R. Figley (Ed.), *Trauma and its wake: The study and treatment of post-traumatic stress disorder* (pp. 257–294). New York: Brunner/Mazel.

Kellerman, H. (1979). *Group psychotherapy and personality: Intersecting structures.* New York: Grune & Stratton.

Kellerman, H. (1981). *Group cohesion.* New York: Grune & Stratton.

Kohut, H. (1971). *The analysis of the self.* New York: International Universities Press.

Kohut, H. (1972). Thoughts on narcissism and narcissistic rage. *Psychoanalytic Study of the Child, 27,* 360–400.

Kohut, H. (1977). *The restoration of the self.* New York: International Universities Press.

Kolb, L. (1984). The post-traumatic stress disorder of combat: A subgroup with a conditioned emotional response. *Military Medicine, 149,* 237–243.

Laub, D., & Auerhahn, N. (1989). Failed empathy—A central theme in the survivor's Holocaust experience. *Psychoanalytic Psychology, 6,* 377–400.

Lazarus, A. (1981). *The practice of multimodal therapy.* New York: McGraw-Hill.

Lifton, R. J. (1973). *Home from the war: Vietnam veterans: Neither victims nor executioners.* New York: Simon & Schuster.

Lindy, J., & Grace, M. (1985). The recovery environment: Continuing stressors versus the healing psychosocial space. In B. J. Sowder (Ed.), *Disaster and mental health: Selected contemporary perspectives* (pp. 137–149) (DHHS Publication No. (ADM) 85-1421.) Washington, DC: U.S. Government Printing Office.

Lindy, J. (1988). *Vietnam: A casebook.* New York: Brunner/Mazel.

Meichembaum, D. (1977). *Cognitive-behavior modification.* New York: Plenum Press.

Menaker, T. (1979). Passive dependency and overidealization. In L. Saretsky, G. Goldman, & D. Milman (Eds.), *Integrating ego psychology and object relations theory: Psychoanalytic perspectives on psychopathology* (pp. 65–79). Dubuque, IA: Kendal/Hunt.

Mowrer, O. H. (1960). *Learning theory and behavior.* New York: Wiley.

Nicholas, J. (1983). The narcissistic personality in group psychotherapy. *Group 7*(4), 27–32.

Norcross, J. (1986). *Handbook of eclectic psychotherapy.* New York: Brunner/Mazel.

Opp, R. (1987). Normative mid-life concerns among Vietnam veterans with post-traumatic stress disorders: Some preliminary empirical findings. *Journal of Contemporary Psychotherapy, 17,* 174–194.

Ornstein, P. (1979). The psychology of the self. *Issues in Ego Psychology, 2*(2), 17–19.

Parson, E. R. (1980, September). *The CMHC-based treatment of Vietnam combat veterans: An alternate psychotherapy model.* Paper presented at the 32nd Institute on Hospital and Community Psychiatry, Boston, MA.

Parson, E. R. (1981, April). *Veterans Administration Medical Center as transference object: Implications for the treatment of Vietnam veterans.* Paper presented at the Continuing Education Symposium, Northport, NY.

Parson, E. R. (1982, November 18). Narcissistic injury in Vietnam vets: The role of post-traumatic stress disorder, agent orange anxiety, and the repatriation experience. *Stars and Stripes.*

Parson, E. R. (1984a). The reparation of the self: Clinical and theoretical dimensions in the treatment of Vietnam combat veterans. *Journal of Contemporary Psychotherapy, 14,* 4–56.

Parson, E. R. (1984b). The role of psychodynamic group therapy in the treatment of the combat veteran. In H. J. Schwartz (Ed.), *Psychotherapy of the combat veteran* (pp. 153–220). New York: Spectrum Medical and Scientific Books.

Parson, E. R. (1985a). *Unconscious guilt and fear of authority dominance as psychological impediments to economic mainstreaming in Vietnam veterans.* Paper presented at the Medical Continuing Educational Conference at the VA Medical Center, Montrose, NY.

Parson, E. R. (1985b). Ethnicity and traumatic stress: The intersecting point in psychotherapy. In C. R. Figley (Ed.), *Trauma and its wake: The study and treatment of post-traumatic stress disorder* (pp. 314–337). New York: Brunner/Mazel.

Parson, E. R. (1985c). Post-traumatic accelerated cohesion: Its recognition and management in group treatment of Vietnam veterans, *Group, 9,* 10–23.

Parson, E. R. (1986). Life after death: Vietnam veterans' struggle for meaning and recovery. *Death Studies, 10,* 11–26.

Parson, E. R. (1987). Reparation of the self—II. In W. Quaytman (Ed.), *Studies in post-traumatic stress disorders* (pp. 6–57). New York: Human Sciences Press.

Parson, E. R. (1988a). Post-traumatic self disorders (PTsfD): Theoretical and practical considerations in psychotherapy of Vietnam war veterans. In J. Wilson, Z. Harel, & B. Kahana (Eds.), *Human adaptation to extreme stress: From the Holocaust to Vietnam* (pp. 245–383). New York: Plenum Press.

Parson, E. R. (1988b). The unconscious history of Vietnam in the group: An innovative multiphasic model for working through authority transferences in guilt-driven veterans. *International Journal of Group Psychotherapy, 38,* 275–301.

Parson, E. R. (1989a, April). Economic recovery, stabilization, and integration for Vietnam veterans. Paper presented at the Second Annual Boston Council President's Conference on the Concerns of Vietnam Veterans, Boston, MA.

Parson, E. R. (1989b). Vietnam traumatic war stress: Considerations in the psychological treatment of veterans. *New York State Psychologist, 40,* 10–12.

Parson, E. R. (1989c). *Image 2001: Economic recovery and future public image of Vietnam veterans.* Testimony presented before the Congress of the United States. The 101st Congress, Subcommittee on Oversight and Investigations, Cannon House Offices Building, Washington, DC, May 3, 1989.

Parson, E. R. (1989d, May 16). *The Media and Veterans: Transforming public images of Vietnam veterans.* Paper presented at the Conference on Vietnam: The War and Its Legacy, at Bentley College, Waltham, MA.

Parson, E. R. (1989e, June). *Post-traumatic moral stress.* Paper presented at the William Joiner Center Conference, University of Massachusetts, Boston, MA.

Parson, E. R. (1989f, May). Future looks good: Vietnam veterans find hope in past. *Joiner Center Newsletter, 3,* 3, 7.

Parson, E. R. (1990). Agent Orange stress response syndrome: Recognition and management. In P. Atwood (Ed.), *Agent Orange: Medical, legal, political, and psychological issues.* Boston: William Joiner Center.

Parson, E. R. (in press). The endangered self: Managing inner mortal dangers in psychotherapy. *American Journal of Psychoanalysis.*

Pavlov, I. P. (1960). *Conditioned reflexes: An investigation of the physiological activity of the cerebral cortex.* New York: Dover Books.

Pine, M. (1983). On mirroring in group psychotherapy. *Group,* 3–17.

Prochaska, J., & DiClemente, C. (1984). *The transtheoretical approach: Crossing traditional boundaries of therapy.* Homewood, IL: Dow Jones/Irwin.

Pulver, D. (1970). Narcissism: The term and the concept. *Journal of the American Psychoanalytic Association, 18,* 319–341.

Shatan, C. F. (1973). The grief of soldiers: Vietnam combat veterans self-help movement. *Journal of Orthopsychiatry, 43,* 640–653.

Shatan, C. F. (1974). Through the membrane of reality: Impacted grief and perceptual dissonance in Vietnam combat veterans. *Psychiatric Opinion, 11,* 6–15.

Simmel, E. (1944). War neuroses. In S. Lorand (Ed.), *Psychoanalysis today* (pp. 227–248). New York: International Universities Press.

Stolorow, R., & Lachmann, F. (1980). *Psychoanalysis and developmental arrests: Theory and treatment.* New York: International Universities Press.

Stolorow, R., & Lachmann, F. (1985). Transference: The future of an illusion. *Annual of Psychoanalysis, 10,* 205–220.

Ulman, R., & Brothers, D. (1988). *The shattered self: A psychoanalytic study of trauma.* Hillsdale, NJ: Analytic Press.

van der Kolk, B. A. (1987). *Psychological trauma.* Washington, DC: American Psychiatric Press.

van der Kolk, B. A., Greenberg, M. S., & Boyd, H. (1985). Inescapable shock, neurotransmitters and addiction to trauma: Towards a psychobiology of post-traumatic stress. *Biological Psychiatry, 20,* 314–325.

Wachtel, P. (1977). *Psychoanalysis and behavior therapy: Toward an integration.* New York: Basic Books.

Walker, J. I. (1983). Comparison of "rap" groups with traditional group therapy in the treatment of Vietnam combat veterans. *Group, 7*(2), 48–57.

White, R. (1963). Ego and reality in psychoanalytic theory: A proposal regarding the independent ego energies. *Psychological Issues Monograph,* Vol. 11. New York: International Universities Press.

Wilson, J. P. (1977). *Identity, ideology, and crisis: The Vietnam veteran in transition, Part I.* Paper presented at the Disabled American Veterans Association, Forgotten Warriors Project. Cleveland State University, Cleveland, OH.

Wilson, J. P., & Krauss, G. E. (1985). Predicting post-traumatic stress disorder among Vietnam veterans. In W. Kelly (Ed.), *Post-traumatic stress disorder and the war veteran patient* (pp. 102–147). New York: Brunner/Mazel.

Wilson, J. P. (1989). *Trauma, transformation and healing: An integrative approach to theory, research, and post-traumatic therapy.* New York: Brunner/Mazel.

Winnicott, D. W. (1965). *The maturational processes and the facilitating environment.* New York: International Universities Press.

Winnicott, D. W. (1975). *Through paediatrics to psychoanalysis.* New York: Basic Books.

Wolf, E. S., Gedo, J. E., & Terman, D. M. (1972). On the adolescent process as a transformation of self. *Journal of Youth and Adolescence, 1*(3), 257–272.

Wong, N. (1981). The application of object-relations theory to an understanding of group cohesion. In H. Kellerman (Ed.), *Group cohesion.* New York: Wiley.

Yalom, I. (1970). *The theory and practice of group psychotherapy.* New York: Basic Books.

Yalom, I. (1980). *Existential psychotherapy.* New York: Basic Books.

Yalom, I. (1983). *Inpatient group psychotherapy.* New York: Basic Books.

CHAPTER 71

Beyond the DSM-III-R

Therapeutic Considerations in Posttraumatic Stress Disorder

Henry Krystal

Introduction

The diagnostic criteria of the DSM-III-R (American Psychiatric Association [APA], 1987), which have already been discussed in various parts of this book, represent a spirit of compromise to reduce our criteria to the lowest common denominator. By limiting our criteria to the descriptive ones exclusively, we created a simple enough picture, so that we communicate about certain conspicuous essentials common to virtually all posttraumatic states. These criteria reflect the essential, but not all, points made by the leading contributors in this field. The most explicit statement which summarized the psychoanalytic experiences, as well as his own, was the work of Kardiner (1941). Among Kardiner's classic findings were: (1) a fixation on the trauma altering the perception of the whole world, (2) a typical dream life, (3) a contraction of the general level of functioning, (4) increased irritability, and (5) a proclivity to aggressive action.

Kardiner also stressed (using Freud's old classification) that trauma was apt to produce a *physioneurosis* rather than a *psychoneurosis*. Although the DSM-III (APA, 1980) eliminated both of those terms, it is important to note that Kardiner knew that the damages from long-term trauma were apt to produce problems related more to psychosomatic diseases than to neuroses.

In my review of the subject, I felt that, in regard to "massively traumatized individuals," it was essential to add or reemphasize relative retrograde amnesia (life begins with trauma), regressive behavior, compulsive repe-

tition of trauma in life, and massive somatization (Krystal, 1968, p. 24).

Of course, even though we are still in the descriptive mode, already we are outside the words permissible in the DSM-III. We have to leave those rules in order to talk about regression of any kind, which we must do. Also, we have to add that the "compulsive repetitions" are often part of specific character types. Since the DSM-III recognizes only eleven "Personality Disturbances," leading us to conclude that the rest of mankind, which does not fit those 11 categories is normal, we will just have to mention frequent characterological problems that we see in posttraumatic states as "unofficial" problems.

Among the early observations, which made me realize that the problems of the Holocaust survivors did not fit the descriptions of "traumatic neuroses" nor the classical psychoanalytic formulations of trauma were their *object relations*. Krystal and Niederland (1968) noted that the general impression in this group was of greatly impoverished object relations, with great ambivalence. General rigidity, withdrawal, infantile relationships, and even schizoid withdrawal were observed. Survivors showed a high incidence of abnormal object relations which could be arbitrarily classified as follows: (1) 21% of the patients related some disturbance of affectivity, (2) 18% stated that they could not relate warmly to anyone, (3) 13% had few friends, (4) 18% had no friends, and (5) 9% could be considered isolates (p. 334).

After their liberation, survivors entered into many marriages hastily in order to restore families, and were hostile stalemates plagued with constant fears that some terrible tragedy would befall their children.

In my subsequent work (Krystal, 1971), I felt that some Holocaust survivors showed such pervasive and all-encompassing distrust and suspicion that only the destruction of their capacity for basic trust could account

Henry Krystal • Michigan Psychoanalytic Institute, 26011 Evergreen Road, Suite 206, Southfield, Michigan 48076.

International Handbook of Traumatic Stress Syndromes, edited by John P. Wilson and Beverley Raphael. Plenum Press, New York, 1993.

for such desolation (p. 24). Of course, the horror of this picture is exceeded by those Vietnam veterans who had to escape the proximity of all their love objects and seek solitary refuge in the wilderness.

Posttraumatic Reactions

There is a wide range and variety of characterological traits and problems that we have learned to recognize as "posttraumatic" or "persecution-related." I think that there is a deep wisdom in the Japanese appellation of survivors and other people whose life was significantly influenced by the dropping of the atom bomb as "Hibakusha" (i.e., "explosion-affected person") (Lifton, 1968b). The variety of survivors' problems runs the gamut from reactive aggression, some aptly described by Hoppe (1968, 1970) as "hate addicted," to such severe masochism, inhibitions, reactive dependence, and "broken lifeline" (Venzlaff, 1967) that their inability to be assertive at home. Such behavior has often provoked a protective response on the part of their children. This spectrum of characterological problems, related to the handling of aggression, is but one of the variety of sequelae of traumatization which illustrate that the net effect of the DSM III-R is obfuscation. Of the literally countless attempts to delineate various posttraumatic character problems, I will mention just a few. But first, a historical note.

When Freud was reviewing his life experience with trauma (1939/1968, pp. 75–76), he expected that the long-range effect could be anticipated to be "negative reactions" involving everything that could prevent the return of the trauma or its conscious recall; this would include "avoidances," phobias, inhibitions, and characterological traits based on hypervigilance, avoidance, and inhibitions. On the other hand, to the extent that the memories of the trauma are successfully and "safely" repressed, then they can be acted out in a variety of symptomatic or character distortions. Thus, a Holocaust survivor may require a wife, a boss, or a partner who is the representation of the oppressor or the victim.

In Michigan, a couple who had a mixed marriage (he was an Eastern European Holocaust survivor and she an uprooted "Volks" German) were operating a farm, using mostly family members who felt oppressed and left as soon as they could. The couple then acquired a couple of mentally retarded men who worked for them for years. Eventually, the case came to the attention of the Michigan Attorney General who prosecuted the couple for engaging in slavery.

It will not come as a surprise that the most serious characterological problems turned up in connection with our beginning to gain an appreciation with the discovery that the catastrophic trauma process may end in psychogenic death.

Through his repeated submersion in the traumatic experiences of the Korean War and Chinese "brainwashing," Lifton (1961), through the atomic bombing (Lifton, 1968a), sharing in our work with Holocaust survivors (Lifton, 1968b), became convinced that a "new psychology" was needed, and should be based on the paradigm of "death and the continuity of life" (Lifton, 1968a, p. 29). With the added stimulation of dealing with Vietnam

veterans, Lifton came to the conclusion that for an understanding of the consequences of the universal confrontation with death, he had to start to elaborate a psychology which encompassed a theory of symbolic immortality, and which involved death imagery.

In returning to our attempt to follow sequelae of trauma, for which there is no room in the DSM-III-R, we must underline that all this is necessary in order to understand the psychological equivalents of death which were recognized in so many forms in posttraumatic states. We used to call them the "walking dead," the "shuffling dead," and the "Musulmans." The work of Lifton (1968a) gave structure to the idea of "death in life," a loss of vitality of feeling which was the very state which he called "psychic numbing" (p. 19).

The conception of "psychic numbing" (Lifton, 1968) represents a form of desensitization; it refers to an incapacity to feel or to confront certain kinds of experience because of "the blocking or absence of inner forms of imagery that connect with such experience" (Lifton, 1968, p. 27). By discarding the customary psychoanalytic terms, Lifton put suddenly and unpreparedly in front of perhaps the most difficult dilemma concerning posttraumatic patients the whole question of "primary repression."

With a bow of admiration to Lifton, I shall leave his amazing insight for later. Lifton felt that not only did traumatized individuals but all of us in this nuclear age combine the imagery of extinction and dislocation with the result that we cannot maintain the tradition, religions, myths, and visions of eternality to maintain the denial of death (see Chapter 1, in this volume, for a discussion).

Lifton sees the normal process of conceptualized imagery or symbolic representation of inner imagery of death evolving along three subparadigms of (1) connection versus separation, (2) integrity versus disintegration, and (3) movement versus stasis. Thus, connection is illustrated by the child's attachment to the mothering parent. Manifestations of impaired imagery of death and continuity of life are: death anxiety, psychic numbing, and suspicion of counterfeit nurturance. This last idea, probably the most original of Lifton's concepts, involves a profound reproach from each generation upon the discovery of the transience of their own legacy on a private and global level. In addition to these, Lifton has given a couple of very useful conceptual tools: *centering* and *grounding*. The major aspect of centering that pertains to our therapeutic interests involves "making discriminations and, therefore, more peripheral" (Lifton, 1973, p. 71). Lifton feels that there are a number of core areas of one's self on which our lives would be centered. They would include: sexuality and personal bonds; learning, working, and making; death, play, and transcendence; home and place; relationship to society and environment; and nurturance and growth. He commented "that though these core areas can be conceptualized somewhat differently, they could not, within a formative perspective, be reduced to the single Freudian 'nuclear (Oedipus) complex'" (Lifton, 1979, p. 72).

Grounding is easier to define: It is the relationship of the self to its own history, individual and collective, as well as to its biology. The beauty of Lifton's work in my present endeavor of demonstrating what aspects of posttraumatic stress disorder (PTSD) are missing in the DSM-III-R is that having defined his terms, Lifton can tell us right off five psychological patterns which are bound to identify a survivor. First, the survivor has an indelible "death imprint" consisting of a death image and death anxiety. This means that the survivor loses the ability to mobilize the sense of momentary omnipotence and invulnerability. Second, the pattern is survivor guilt (recently eliminated from the DSM-III-R). Third, survivors are apt to show desensitization, diminished capacity to feel, or what Lifton calls "psychic numbing"—the breakdown of symbolic connectedness with their environment. Fourth, survivors show a "death taint" associated with a "morbid contamination" and the result is an aura of suspicion that always surrounds the survivor. And, lastly, a pattern which Lifton considers fundamental to all survivor psychology and encompassing the other four: It is "the struggle toward inner form or formulation, the quest for significance in one's death encounter and remaining life experience" (Lifton, 1979, pp. 114–115).

In his elaboration of the consequences of the confrontation with the actual danger of death and disintegration, Lifton (1979) stressed that the survivor "actually undergoes a radical but temporary diminution in his sense of actuality" (p. 173), which he chose to explain teleologically (i.e., the individual chooses to accept death in a temporary and symbolic way and thus escapes death). This point of view is open to some questions, particularly in relation to therapeutic approaches. The very "heart of the matter" in the view of Cohen and Kinston (1984) is that a traumatic situation is one which is so overwhelming, that it cannot be integrated and has to be handled by primary repression. This development radically changes the therapeutic prospects, in the opinion of these authors. But it is worth noting that in his work on the paradigm and survival, Lifton (1979) was led to the conclusion that not only confrontation with death, but, as Pierre Janet also found, fear may "narrow the field of consciousness" (p. 180). Anxiety of "the possibility of anxiety" can bring on an inertia, can cause psychic numbing: "Rather than experience anxiety, the mind constricts. The symbolizing process, or at least elements of it, shut down" (p. 130).

Ullman and Brothers (1987) stressed the self-psychological consequences of the kind of traumatic event which shatters unconscious archaic narcissistic fantasies on which (they find, retrospectively) the entire operation of an individual rested. They also found, as so many of us have, that the traumatic experience caused severe and disabling intrapsychic splitting, which contributes to the impossibility of restoring the grandiose self-representation. The symptomatology of PTSD results from various affective responses to the overwhelming event and the subsequent helplessness and narcissistic mortification. But the therapist focuses his or her attention on patients' discovering the unrealistic nature of their previous predominant self-views. The therapist is empathetic with the patient's predicament and promotes the construction of a realistic self-image through transmuting internalization of workable self-views and objectives.

Recently, a prominent psychoanalytic scholar and theoretician (Wurmser, 1989) made the point that the widespread denial following severe trauma seems at first to serve the mastery, but it turns out that it has a more urgent and profound motivation than just getting around the terror. He claimed to have discovered that the danger of uncovering the grudge and the resentment is much worse, for the resentment hides the buried "complex" of revenge, destructiveness, and bitterness directed to punish all those related to the original abuse and harm.

This brings me to the point that I can make an important generalization, although I started my reflections on the sequelae of traumata that have no way of getting into the DSM-III by virtue of being unacceptable characterological problems. With the work of Wurmser, we are alerted to the possibility that, posttraumatically, certain affect and moods may become the secret major motivators and determinants of an individual's life-style. Wurmser (1989) has stressed the importance of resentment and shame (Wurmser, 1981) as well as the consequence of narcissistic mortification on affect regression and the setting up of a vicious cycle which included substance addiction (Wurmser, 1978). Hoppe (1962, 1968, 1969) has long worked on the problems of reactive hate addiction. He found that the problem of hate has to be understood in the context of the superego problems in both participants of an atrocity of abuse (Hoppe, 1965).

Paradigm of Adult Catastrophic Trauma

The well-known emotions of fear and anxiety are, amazingly, poorly understood. They are both the affects which signal impending *avoidable* danger. In order to facilitate the escape or prevention of the danger or its potential ill-effect, they are both endowed with the ability to initiate arousal of the entire organism and mobilization of a variety of evolutionarily determined physical and mental responses. When an individual concludes that the impending danger is not avoidable, and that the situation is hopeless, and when that individual surrenders to it, then the affective response changes to a *catatanoid reaction* (Stern, 1951, 1953).[1]

When we study posttraumatic states retrospectively, we find that remaining in the traumatic situation for a significant period of time, the catatanoid reaction initiates or continues into a traumatic state. When individuals judge themselves to be totally helpless in the face of overwhelming danger and surrender to it, an evolution-determined pattern is initiated, which is common to all animals, and since it may end in a purely psychogenic death—with the heart stopping in diastole—it may be said that individuals carry their self-destruct outfit at all times. The surrender is based on one's psychic reality; in other words, the determination is based on the subjective evaluation of the situation and one's self.

Thus, the evaluation of a danger situation is subject to all the vicissitudes and vagaries of the information-processing functions, including the nature of one's capacity for attention and perception, its processing

---

[1]Catatonic-like.

(which involves associations and thereby defenses), registration, evaluation by cognition (which also involves the nature of one's consciousness, the influence of one's superego, and the availability of benign introjects, the question of inhibitions, and unconscious impulses and identifications), and, finally, the range of one's affect tolerance, and the availability of mature affect signals which favor evaluation of a situation according to one's best judgment and the selection of the most adaptive response out of a big "menu" of possible actions. In other words, people vary greatly in regard to their ability to cope with a given challenge of danger. Nonetheless, as Freud noted back in 1893, once the individual surrenders to the danger helplessly, the trauma process is "on," and it makes no difference whether the victim was "right," or whether his evaluation was correct or not.

The traumatic process then starts with submission, which means that the victims are going to obey orders, and just like hypnotized persons (or animals), the more they obey orders, the more they submit or we may say the deeper they go into a traumatic or hypnotic trance. Eventually, persons can be brought to a state of automatic obedience, ready to cooperate even in their own execution.

The next development in the continuing trauma process is the blocking of affective experiencing, in particular, in regard to the hedonic aspect of affects and proprioception. In effect, the point here is the achievement of total numbness. Our impressions to the contrary, it probably does not hurt the rabbit to be devoured by a predator.

Since ancient times, there have been many observations that wild animals go into trances when apprehended and, if held in restraint long enough, will die. Meerloo (1959) and Seligman (1975) reviewed the recorded evidence and concluded that the cataleptic surrender pattern was common to the entire animal kingdom. In my follow-up studies of concentration camp survivors, I found that although the "affective anesthesia" (Minkowski, 1946) was most conspicuous, the complexity of the posttraumatic problems with emotional and physical pain, on the one side, and alexithymia and anhedonia on the other created such an extraordinary therapeutic problem, that many of the classical conceptions simply did not fit. Eventually, I came to the conclusion that in order to be able to understand the phenomenology, it was necessary to consider the hedonic element of emotions as having developed separately (actually becoming functional earlier and serving as the sole available affect forerunner, a signal in the attachment to the mother), and only later becoming an integral part of the affect experience. But in order to be able to study, we have to include knowledge derived in part through hypnotic research (Hilgard, 1970). We must consider pleasure as separate from gratification, pain as different and separate from suffering, and all for being related to appetitive or gratificatory experiences separately and registered along several spectra of consciousness.

We urgently need a revision of the concepts of the *hedonic regulation* of the organism. The persistence of residues of drive theory is producing the persistence of "discharge of drives" as the explanation of the experience of pleasure. This ancient model based on energy transformation theories, has much popular appeal, and

the use of it is particularly confusing when therapists think that the anxiety and aggression can be relieved by riddance of the excess affects. Of course, no affect can ever be eliminated, although we still sometimes call the physiological arousal attending some affects their "expressive" component. This is an antiquated residue of Freud's idea that drives which could not be discharged to the "outside" were discharged into the body via the affects. Since we now know that there are anatomically identifiable centers which particularly and sensitively register pain or pleasure, it is time to bring the whole concept of the hedonic aspects of emotions for review. In order to be able to understand the posttraumatic disturbance in pleasure regulation, we have to start out by differentiating pleasure from gratification, and pain from suffering. All the points made in the above paragraph are essential to provide tools for helping with the disturbance in the hedonic regulation which is the rule in all posttraumatic states.

The next development in the continuing traumatic process is the constriction of cognition. In certain ways, this reaction is very familiar to us and in other ways still awesome and mysterious. It is virtually common knowledge, in the management of typical man-made and natural disasters, that as soon as the local population exhausts their physical and emotional resources in trying to maintain and restore the usual (normal) state of affairs, they find that resources are not adequate to meet the challenge, even if the noxious agent has stopped (e.g., when we deal with the aftereffects of a tornado, we have to send in outside help because the local population is in a daze, sitting and staring into space, or pacing, sometimes around the ravages, expressing their incredulity and inability to imagine or to register what happened). Actually, besides their conspicuous disturbance in consciousness, their temporary loss of the ability to take care of themselves (the usual Red Cross coffee, sandwiches, and blankets not only shelter them from overexposure but from "ordinary" stress conditions), some people develop an impairment of temperature and other self-regulatory functions, a remarkable regression which confirms our conceptions. But tough as it is, the ideal of everyone is to maintain self-control (Wolfenstein, 1977). At this point, psychological testing shows a progressive impairment in problem-solving ability to evaluate one's resources as related to the demands of the emergency, a general deterioration of conation, accuracy of perception, and progressive diminution of conscious registration, judgment, recall, symbolization, abstraction, and, most of all, integration.

When we deal with the victims of massive catastrophic traumatization, one of their common painful experiences is that "nobody wants to listen." Their complaint has some elements of truth, because their urgency is to master the traumatic past while the host's urgent agenda is to master the potentially traumatic present of receiving their impaired loved and to deal as quickly as possible with their mostly unconscious reactions to the returnee, so as to be able hopefully to reestablish affectionate bonds with this changed person. But in the hypothetical situation, if we could provide recently traumatized persons with the perfect audience they would discover, to their chagrin, that recollection of what happened is spotty and irregular.

From the days of World War I, when a small group of psychoanalysts in German and Austrian armies were trying to cure "traumatic neuroses" by "abreaction," through to World War II, certain psychiatrists like the American Roy Grinker came all equipped to restore most emotional casualties not just with hypnotherapy but aided by a sophisticated pharmacopoeia (Grinker & Spiegel, 1945). It was proven repeatedly that the memory of the traumatic event was registered outside of consciousness and in a greatly impoverished form. What there was could not be taken "straight" because it was already changed, "worked over," as we would say, according to the dictates of the rule of the unconscious mind, thus introducing the subject's necessary conflict defenses and the life-long accumulation of theories about everything built up and remaining unrevised from childhood.

But this was not the big surprise. What surprised me was that when I hired a librarian and a doctoral candidate in literature to find me all the survivor accounts of the subjective recollection of the thoughts and feelings during the traumatic experience, I got nothing but the "facts." The onset of cognitive constriction in traumatic states is a very subtle and gradual process. Like many of these processes which are of evolutionary derivation, they set in, mercifully sparing the victims' conscious recognition of their condition. It is likely to come on when survival becomes barely possible, and what thought can be generated is essential to live at that instant. If someone was available to observe that person, the observer might report that the individual shows no interest in the past or future. Greenson (1949) observed American POWs in Japanese captivity and, 4 years later, reflected on their apathy. He described quite sensitively and accurately that in "combat fatigue," anxiety gives way to apathy, and that in prisoners, once they realized that they were in an inescapable situation, the early attempts to surrender to various fantasies eventually gave way to deeper apathy, restriction, and diminution.

Actually, once the traumatic process has reached the point of cognitive constriction, it may progress to death very rapidly, or may be arrested at any point, depending on a number of subjective and external factors. In concentration camps, there were two waves of deaths among the inmates. One was soon after arrival, within a week or less; the other one set in for individuals at a point when they exhausted their physical and emotional resources (reached what we call the "Musulman" state). This was sometimes ushered in by an outburst of randomly directed aggression, followed by the collapse. One of the factors that might arrest the regression and the cognitive constriction was any kind of group support.

This is the reason why military captives do better if they can remain with their unit, particularly with their officers. But in the absence of such supports, which help to preserve as much as possible the previous realistic self-representation (and secretly also the ideal self), the mental functions are lost one after the other, to the point before psychogenic death sets in, when only minimal self-observing functions are preserved.

As the traumatic state continues, there is a rapid deterioration of the individual's chance to survive, even if he or she should be rescued at this point. The mortality continues to be high in the wake of extreme traumatic situations: for instance, in rescuing survivors who were shipwrecked. In retrospective studies in concentration camp survivors, I found a surprising number of histories of postliberation transient psychosis, most which involved an inability to believe or imagine that the ordeal which came to be accepted as the "ultimate reality" was over. Many starved people died when food became available. Some just seemed to have lost the vitality or motivation to start life all over again. But by far, the most important development related to the endstage of the traumatic state, which had to do with the confrontation with death. I believe that the above-mentioned work of Lifton has not become adequately incorporated into the fabric of psychiatric knowledge, and certainly it has not been noted in the DSM-III. The individuals dealing with the episode during which the denial of death was temporarily or irreparably broken frequently had serious consequences, albeit they may have been silent or unnoticed for a long time.

The mind being incredibly complicated, it may not be possible to discover unconscious identification with death, with the dead, or with the incorporation of some private explanation of the trauma which may surface as "destiny neurosis" or even as sudden death. Lifton (1968a,b,c, 1973, 1976, 1979) presented convincing evidence that some paranoid schizophrenics can be best understood as being identified with death. Lifton spoke for himself in Chapter 1 of this volume, so in connection with the ideal of identification, I would like to mention that, in my opinion, the one universal reaction to mass holocausts or individual misfortunes is the creation in the minds of a warring and irreconcilable "victim" and "oppressor" the walled-off parasitic object representations which are the more powerfully absorbing, and which intrude themselves within the survivor's consciousness the more the posttraumatic conflicts are raging. Among such conflicts in survivors are the unconscious yearnings for revenge, sometimes notable in psychotherapy in forms of "role reversal," in which the victim gets a turn at being the oppressor.

Anyone who has doubt about such needs has only to refresh his memory of the great revolutions which have preoccupied mankind for three centuries. The common outcome of tyranny is that it is generally replaced by another tyranny.

But, for the most part, survivors are busy fighting off conscious recognition with the "other side," a need which is reinforced by survivor guilt: the need to build memorials as well as permanent commemorations of the evil of the oppression, and, if possible, protective laws such as the still not fully ratified United Nations convention against genocide, as an example.

The oppressors get a choice of (mostly symbolic) judgment, a gesture of punishment followed by "rehabilitation." But, if at all possible, they prefer to escape the purification and conversion rites and to cling to the original ideology that motivated their action. In this way, they preserved their original paranoid position, avoided any conscious guilt, and kept refreshing their original view of the world, according to which things were terribly bad and unfair, and, therefore, all the martial and destructive things they did were their own sacrificial and heroic acts intended to rid mankind or their nation of evil.

Amos Oz's novella, "The Crusade" (1978), is a perfect illustration of the relationship of the build-up of paranoid ideas in preparation for unbridled aggression and how, once frustrated, the aggression may become self-destructive. Adolf Hitler's paranoid "Four-Year Plan" could not be changed or abandoned by him despite the urging of all his advisers; and, instead, the true core of his psychosis was revealed: If the Germans could not live up to the warrior stance with contempt for the weak and imperfect, then they should all die supporting his "heroic" vision (Hilberg, 1961).

Three Kinds of Trauma and Their Aftereffects

In my previous reviews of the history of the psychoanalytic approaches to trauma, I pointed out that Freud started out by proposing two different models on the same page (Krystal, 1978a, referring to Freud, 1893–1895, p. 122). A third model was proposed primarily by Joseph Breuer; namely, a key factor in causation, and later understanding of trauma was the phenomenon of hypnoid states. In first mentioning it, Breuer and Freud acknowledged that in using this concept they "concurred with Binet and the two Janets" (1893, p. 12). By the time Breuer was given the task of writing the theoretical chapter, Freud (1905/1953) was increasingly skeptical about the importance of "hypnoid states" which he eventually disclaimed. Breuer, on the other hand, found an even earlier support to the idea in the 1898 work of Paul Julius Moebius. The reason for my recalling the hypnoid model of the reaction to trauma on the one hand and the causation of conversion reaction on the other is to emphasize that although Freud and Breuer were studying the kind of trauma which causes neuroses, they did describe three models of it which are still valid.[2]

In addition to the kind of trauma which causes neuroses, we now commonly recognize certain patterns of *childhood trauma* which produce posttraumatic states similar to PTSD, with enough differences to keep brilliant researchers busy.

However, I have to add that if we define trauma as an overwhelming experience which is followed by obligatory psychopathology, then conceivably other patterns of trauma will be described. I have identified three trauma patterns. The adult catastrophic trauma pattern is clearly recognizable. In addition, the infantile trauma

[2]The modern application of the idea of "hypnoid" states is with regard to trances. Trances are recognized as startlingly common in posttraumatic states, and often are part of the traumatic experience. The reason for our reverting to the term *trance* instead of *disassociation reaction* is because besides the defensive role of trances related to splitting of consciousness, there is another aspect which is vital to our present inquiry: In trances people sometimes become able to exercise functions for which they have the potential and the capacity, but from which they are commonly blocked by inhibitions. These involve a wide spectrum of self-caring and self-soothing activities, from the ability to relax and go to sleep to the ability to lower their blood pressure.

pattern is different from childhood trauma. It takes place in the earliest life, most commonly in the first 2 years of life, but, occasionally, with regression, it may take place later. This type of trauma is caused by the relatively slow process of affect development. The early affect precursors are only minimally differentiated and remain mostly somatic (the infant is the "complete" psychosomatic individual). The intensity of the "expressive" element of the emotions is not yet mollified by specific vocalization and verbalization. Since the infant has not developed any affect tolerance, it depends on affective attunement of a mothering parent to respond speedily to its needs correctly. If the parent fails to stop the distress, the baby rapidly becomes frantic. Depending on the child's temperament, the baby may become agitated in a "geometric progression" so as to become inconsolable. If such trauma is frequent or severe enough, it may lead to a failure to thrive and related syndromes. The aftereffects may include impairment of the capacity for basic trust, alexithymia, and anhedonia. The history of this disaster frequently becomes a family secret, and sometimes it is accepted as "natural fussiness." In some cultures, including ours in the past, it was long considered desirable to "break the child's spirit" to make it more docile or to prevent the later development of the "sin of pride." Infantile trauma of this kind should be suspected, and may even be assumed in many cases of psychosomatic disease, substance dependence, eating or sleeping disturbances, and masochistic characters. Besides this identifiable form of infantile trauma, there is another which thus far is recognizable only by the effect or the traces it leaves.

I became aware of it when I tried to get alexithymic patients to verbalize their emotions and fantasies (1982–1983). I had repeated experiences with alexithymic psychosomatic patients who were getting biofeedback training at the same time we were also trying to do psychoanalytic psychotherapy. I discovered that although the patients were learning to relax and control voluntarily some visceral functions, they could do it only in the laboratory in the presence of the trainer. When they tried to practice the same skills at home, even using tapes prepared for them by the psychologist, they developed incredible "resistances," in effect, making any progress impossible. In psychotherapy, we discovered that they were experiencing terrible fears. Eventually, I realized that the meaning of their fears was that if they "took over" the control of their affective and vital functions, they would be committing an unforgivable sin punishable by a "fate worse than death" (Krystal, 1978b).

Finally, I was able to decode the meaning of those fears which had plagued those patients all of their lives: that their viscera were part of their maternal transferences; in other words, only mother or her surrogates were allowed to soothe and regulate them. If they tried openly and directly to take over this power reserved for mother, the punishment would be the return of the infantile trauma state. The best, if not the only adult representation of the infantile trauma state can be found in the religiously detailed description of *Hell*. There it is complete with the infantile expectation of every kind of torture, and the infantile timelessness promising that suffering will go on "forever and ever." Inhibitions to exercise conscious voluntary control over vital and affective functions are universal and include difficulties in relaxation and sleeping.

Despite the fact that the infant is able to recognize its mother by hearing and smell practically from birth, yet the illusion of symbiosis seems to be necessary for the harmonious development of the baby. We have repeated and convincing evidence that, in the normal course of development, the child experiences all the mother's care as its own thriving self, and the normal course of development has no impedance to exercising the "normal" amount of self-caring, self-soothing, and self-regulation. But a traumatic event is any experience that prematurely interrupts the illusion of symbiosis and confronts the baby with its own helplessness and the inability to control the "external" object. Such a traumatic event leaves as a trace the predisposition to severe inhibition in the capacity for self-caring, the kind we see in psychosomatic patients, substance dependent patients, substance dependent individuals and alexithymic people (Khantzian, 1978; Khantzian & Mack, 1983; Krystal, 1978a,b).

Sequelae of Adult Catastrophic Trauma Affecting Psychotherapy

Every one of the component reactions of catastrophic psychic trauma leaves traceable and recognizable residuals. But to save space, I will not review those aftereffects which have been described by Kardiner (1941), Niederland (1961, 1964, 1968), or in our joint work (Krystal & Niederland, 1968, 1971). The DSM-III-R has received enough attention in this volume, and I will only mention that the symptoms listed there fall into three groups: (1) those related to the old idea of "traumatic neurosis" with repetitiveness of intrusive thoughts and predominantly anxious (but actually differentiated, therefore, mixed "waves" of affects), flashbacks, hypermnesias, recurrent dreams, and other manifestations of "reliving" the traumatic experience; (2) the "avoidance" group of symptoms, which, however, also contain an admixture of symptoms which really are a continuation of cognitive constriction, notably amnesias, inability to resume professional and parental functions, withdrawal from social (actually all human) contacts, and, we may add, severe distrust, weariness to the point that all contacts, even desired ones with special, safe fellow survivors are extremely draining (exhausting); and (3) an intimation of the continuation of affective blocking, which is referred to in terms no more sophisticated than Minkowski used in 1946 (in fact, less insightfully described).

Moreover, in the words of the DSM-III, such as "feeling of detachment or estrangement from others" and "restricted range of affects" (309.89, C5 and C6), we must question whether we are not referring to alexithymic patients without having described or defined them. The problems created by the tunnel vision of descriptive criteria as our sole tool is illustrated in the very next category: persistent symptoms of increased arousal. Among those we find "outbursts of anger." The problem is that among alexithymic patients, including posttraumatic ones, scrutiny reveals that some rages are ex-

perienced by the patients as "crazy intrusions on their minds" while other patients in therapy reveal that they got into the habit of throwing fits "for show," claiming that sometimes they feel "nothing" (Nemiah et al., 1976).

Of course, the problem is that the DSM-III shuns any knowledge derived from psychotherapy and strives to avoid mentioning anything useful in psychotherapy. So we will take the opposite stance: We will concentrate on those direct aftereffects and residuals of trauma that are relevant to psychoanalytic psychotherapy. In order to make this text most useful for the psychotherapist, I will renounce by own inclination to list the aftereffects in the order in which they appear in the traumatic state, and, instead, will present them in the order that they should be considered by the therapist.

Is This Patient Alexithymic?

Since alexithymic patients are not able to use psychoanalysis or psychoanalytic psychotherapy, and, in the coincidence with psychosomatic disease of addictive problems, psychotherapy may be dangerous and contraindicated, we should consider this possibility early. Ideally, the intake interview should give the examiner enough clues to at least suspect the problem. We should expect to find this state in many posttraumatic states (Krystal, 1978a), and in a significant number of acute PTSDs. Most conspicuous is their inability to recognize or name their feelings while bitterly complaining of the physiological components of the painful affects, particularly the symptoms of anxiety and depression, along with a variety of physical symptoms suggestive of malaise, exhaustion, and requests for relieving medication. Patients' urgency to get medication which will produce dreamless sleep is motivated in part by their recognition that they are not able to describe to the examiner the nature of their distress.

We are dealing with the affective disturbance of alexithymia, but the patients are not able to name their feelings. Should we now administer to them one of the tests of alexithymia, we would discover that they show an operative type of thinking. If questioned how they would feel if they were to be assaulted or accursed unfairly, they have given us action responses. Even when they manage to name an emotion, they cannot localize it in their bodies. Although we already have a significant number of tests of alexithymia (J. H. Krystal, 1988), it is helpful to learn to recognize the clinical picture by an interview.

Frequently, affective impairment is revealed spontaneously by patients who may volunteer the observation that they are "action people" not given to using their feelings to make choices in life, but rather tending to reason their problems. We may notice that such statements are euphemisms; when pressed, these patients will admit that they really can not tell "about those things," that they really could not say if they have ever been in love, or, for that matter, whether anyone had ever loved them. If we pursue this line of questioning, we find that many difficulties in their lives could be understood as resulting from their having little or no empathy with the people around them, and that, in point of fact, they treat themselves as machines, too.

In alexithymia, the affective problem makes the emotions less useful in the process of conscious problem-solving, and even less effective as signals in information-processing. The result is that some people learn to ignore their feelings. They become stoical, ignore all danger signals from their minds and bodies, and develop rigid postures and wooden faces: They are the psychosomatic patients. The other group develops a dread of the physiological components of the affects and strives to block them by every possible means; this becomes a predisposition to addictive mechanisms including substance dependence.

If we now turn our attention to their cognitive style, we find severe inhibitions in their ability to use symbols and particularly a severe blocking of the capacity for wish-fulfillment fantasy. They can not ever understand what in the world "free association" could mean and whoever in the world could think of such wasteful absurdity? But those who are motivated to try (usually the psychosomatic and not the addictive patients) give a sterile recitation of all the trivia that happened since last we chronologically presented. This last convention turns out to be a device by which they deny their responsibility in organizing and authoring their narrative.

Since they are not able to have wish-fulfillment fantasies or conflicts about them, they cannot form neuroses, and, in the same fashion, they do not form neurotic-type transferences; and naturally, they also do not have transference neuroses. So what do we talk about with them? We could use the widely prevalent difficulties in getting along with people as an opening gambit. In other words, we can start working on their characterological problems as long as we are prepared to look for the actual object relations, even object conceptions and distortions in self-representations. As mentioned before, we can expect a variety of characterological problems—as long as we do not expect to encounter the eleven DSM-III "Personality Disturbances." Forever though, the object relations tend to be of an exploitative and controlling type. A great deal of work has to be done on them; otherwise, because of their daytime soap-opera nature, they tend to produce such difficult and complicated interpersonal crises and emergencies that any attempt at treatment becomes sabotaged. In desperation, therapists try to expand the sphere of influence and go through attempts at family therapy, but may not be able to control the mass uprisings or general despair that has been building up during the period when the posttraumatic survivor was trying to "normalize" his or her life while trying to deny, disavow, suppress and keep out of consciousness his or her walled-off traumatic "abscess."

But this period may be considered the symptom-free time, and even dreams and projective psychological testing may show a false calmness and a spurious conclusion may be reached that everything is under control (van der Kolk & Ducey, 1987).

Finding alexithymia accompanied by anhedonia suggests a traumatic origin of the alexithymia. Finding alexithymia without anhedonia in the absence of the history of adult catastrophic trauma suggests that we are dealing with residues of infantile trauma. Confirmatory findings are lifelong severe fears and panics the object of

which the patient cannot describe. They have a "doomsday orientation": Their profound belief is no matter how well things are going, doomsday is on the way and with it a fate worse than death—the return of the infantile trauma.

Because infantile psychic trauma was intrapsychically entirely experienced as the (total) arousal of every affect, pain, and everything else that was excitable, there is a lifelong expectation of the return of that doomsday state when the punishment starts for all one's known and unknown, conscious and unconscious transgressions. Also, because the child and the toddler must each have an omniscient, omnipotent, and benevolent mother, therefore, they must assume the guilt for everything the mothering parent has done "bad" or "evil" to them. Since affects ushered in the infantile trauma the first time, the person with the frequently secret history of infantile trauma is apt to have a lifelong dread of emotions in general.

In the aftereffects of adult catastrophic trauma there is a valiant attempt to maintain a superficial latent period as long as possible. Physiologically, they are hyperactive, and it takes little effort to demonstrate their hypervigilance and hyperactive startle responses. They are, in fact, in the process of developing chronic physiologic aftereffects of the trauma (van der Kolk, Boyd, Krystal, & Greenberg, 1984). So they, too, have very good reasons to have a variety of misconceptions of their emotions, which brings us now to the issue of affect tolerance.

Affect Tolerance

The reason we are switching to talking about *affect tolerance* without having talked about any therapeutic considerations of alexithymia is because before we can even speak to individuals about their alexithymia, we must find out what these persons think of their emotions, and how they react to "having them." Actually, this question is exceedingly important in every case of affective disturbance. All of them come to us at the end of a vicious cycle of maladaptive responses to a particular affect which causes this affect to "snowball" to a point that it becomes a clinical problem. Many of our colleagues have a propensity when they see such a patient to forget that depression or anxiety are emotions and prefer to think of them as "diseases." The patient has been "into that" for some time, so we see a perfect agreement for the blind to bravely undertake to lead the blind.

To put this discourse back onto a more proper positive track, every normal person has the task to keep his or her emotions in tolerable intensity, to constantly monitor these emotions, to periodically inspect them, so to say, and to make sure that they are still reflecting appropriate responses to the current life situation. Every once in a while we discover that the current developments in our lives have strong associative links to some powerfully exciting (usually unresolved) similar experience from the past. If that happens, then the affect intensity becomes reintensified. Such unwarranted hedonic and activating responses in our bodies may interfere with the proper information-processing of the situation.

Normally, the affects do not attract too much attention to themselves, and we can concentrate on the cognitive aspects of the operation: What happened? What does it mean? and, What is the most appropriate, that is, the most adaptive response selected from the wide repertoire of possible responses? Normally, it is so self-evident that once the situation is solved, the affect is itself self-limited in duration, as our attention turns to the next item at hand.

But when things start going wrong with affects, operations work out rather differently. If persons are not comfortable and familiar with their affects and familiar with the signal function of affects, they usually are also not used to keeping their emotions in "sotto voce" range, and things tend to get messed up. Some people retain their infantile habits of using the intensity of their emotions to control their significant objects. Particularly when they are angry, they are especially impressed with the cognitive element. The meaning of anger is that something bad had been done by a bad person, and, therefore, they are entitled to hate and punish that person and/or the evil people while they are at it. So frequently when they are provoked, they work themselves into the most intense rage they can have. The outcome is that they are not going to be able to deal with the situation on the basis of their best judgment but rather with a knee-jerk response. Needless to say, it can get them into all sorts of trouble right there. But there are many problems to follow. Working up one's rage to a very high intensity may terrify the subjects. They may become frightened of the fantasized destructive power of their wishes; they may become scared of the observations that the intensity of rage was overwhelming and disorganizing to their own mental and general functioning. And once convinced of the righteousness of their grievance and the limitation of the powers to adequately punish the offender, how and when will they ever be able to stop the powerful rage?

Dealing with problems of affect tolerance is going to be part of all psychotherapeutic work. Now that we understand the nature of our reactions to having the affect as an important part of one's attentive, perceptive, and cognitive style, there is no excuse to ignore it in attempting psychotherapy. In fact, the emotions we are talking about, that is, the affects which are intense enough to come to our conscious attention, are by far the least important part of the affective function. On a subliminal level, affects are the "switches" that operate all of our information-processing operations. Just to try to list them would fill this book.

But to return to our alexithymic patients, we need to acquaint them with the nature of their problem, just as we must explain to color-blind persons the details of the nature of their deficit, and how shrewdly and creatively they have been getting around (covering up) their deficit, doing pretty well, considering the nature of their handicap. Usually, the patients are much relieved to finally receive a rational explanation of something that they have long dimly perceived. Sometimes they say: "I always thought there was something so dreadfully wrong. I am glad I am not crazy!" But next we face the big question: "How are we going to help them with their problem?"

Therapeutic Considerations in Posttraumatic States

Early on, I made an assumption that greatly influenced my thinking and experiences in treating patients who showed what I understood to be residuals of infantile psychic trauma or adult catastrophic trauma. I assumed that if they showed alexithymia, they could not work in a psychoanalytic relationship successfully. Many of them are quite willing to come as frequently as advised and proceed to talk about random material as they can. Years pass, and with the luxury of private practice, the patient continues to keep coming and talking. Sometimes they show some improvement, which pleases the patient and the therapist.

One of my patients, who had a history of having had infantile colic, followed by severe eczema for which his arms had to be restrained on boards during his early childhood, followed by asthma, noted in the course of his treatment that his asthma had disappeared. He had a sadomasochistic relationship with his wife; he divorced her and married a much warmer, younger woman, whom he treated much better, although once in a while, maybe twice a year, he would become unreasonably mean to her, but after a few days he would apologize to her and treat her extra nice for quite a while. He made improvements in handling his employees (he learned that it was smarter in his profession to give them a chance to become partners eventually, because he had a bad experience with a couple whom he treated exploitatively). He never developed a workable transference but always had a friendly and trusting relationship with the therapist so that, after his termination, he would call me and come and talk over problems of almost any kind, most of which I could claim no expertise; but that was OK, because after talking things over, he'd make his own decision. He used the therapist in a manner similar to what Bartemeyer once called "a professional friend." He was never able to truly associate, and although he did report a few dreams over the years, he never could associate to them either. Not "officially," that is, because his dreams, like all of his communications, were matters of practical everyday concern, we ended up talking about the same kinds of things, in the same manner, whether he started with a dream or not. He did not produce any fantasies, but he took pride in being a keen observer, and so he always pointed out whenever anything was changed in my office, the smaller and less significant the better. One year he reported with pride that he discovered that in that year the car licenses contained three letters but the middle one was never a vowel. He never noticed if I was not well, or out of sorts, or if I feel asleep during his session. On one occasion a number of years after his treatment was over, I learned something interesting about him from a person close to him—that he didn't like going to movies because in the theater he was so preoccupied with what was going on in the audience (he was not going to miss anything), that he usually did not follow the story of the film.

As can be inferred from the general tone, we never recovered any repressed memories, and nobody minded that, least of all the patient who was fully satisfied with his treatment, and has become a fine source of referrals. We did spend a lot of time and effort trying to get a "feel" for what it must have been for him as a child going through his private hell, and the realistic problems which also plagued his early life. There was never any significant change in his alexithymia, but since he was such an excellent student in regard to powers of observation, he learned to pick up clues as to the affective state (especially of other people—hardly any in himself), and he learned to use them in his work, becoming very successful financially.

A few years after the treatment was over, he developed rheumaticlike pains of a moderate degree. I referred him for biofeedback training because there was some question whether he had a true myositis or whether tenseness was a major part of it. He did very well in the training, but after a while he stopped practicing relaxation. When I saw him on later occasions, he would sometimes mention that he was having some pains, and that he should resume practicing biofeedback; he never used the expression "practicing relaxation" and to this day has actually never gone back to any formal way of relaxing, but he is in good health and does a number of sports.

The assumption about alexithymic patients to which I referred above, was indeed borne out in this case; it was, to recapitulate briefly, that these patient had severe limitations in their ability to develop a neurotic type of transference, and that this was a manifestation of any special problem not found in "normal" neurotics. In my opinion, alexithymia is the most important and most common cause of failure of psychoanalytic psychotherapy. In order that potential therapists be alerted to this phenomenon, it must be included in any worthwhile delineation of posttraumatic sequelae. The joker in the deck is that it can be done on purely descriptive criteria, because alexithymia varies in intensity from person to person, and within an individual, according to a multitude of factors (e.g., the state of the corpus callosum [Hoppe, 1988]). But, if someone were to ask me, "What is the single most important thing that anyone who deals with posttraumatic alexithymic individuals needs to know?" I would answer without a moment's hesitation, "Whatever the potential helpers' orientation or means of intervention, they need to be aware that these patients have severe inhibitions in regard to exercising self-caring, self-soothing, self-regulating functions." They can be absolutely counted on, when instructed to carry out any therapeutic or self-improvement measure, to sabotage it in every way conceivable. Little wonder that they behave that way; as I explained before, they see all vital and affective parts of themselves to be reserved for mother (or God), and any attempt or even wish on their part as equal to Satan's rebellion, *the* most terrible sin, punishable by a fate worse than death.

This penalty, which can also be stated as "being condemned to Hell forever," translates nearly into our language as "the threat of return of the infantile traumatic state." Anyone who is averse to dynamic formulation can equally and conveniently describe the problem as follows: In posttraumatic states, especially in the wake of infantile trauma, people develop a "doomsday orientation." No matter how well things go for them, no mat-

ter how secure their lives actually are, no matter how long their success or good fortune has lasted, they expect that any minute their good situation will collapse like a house of cards, and they will "go to Hell in a hurry." But, if they defy the most powerful prohibition in the world, it will happen to them instantly.

The updated view of PTSD depends in an important measure on the relinquishing of the topographic view of repression. Psychoanalysis has been remiss in establishing the view of repression. It has also been remiss in establishing the view that mental material can be repressed by a lack of recognition of it as part of one's own self-representation, the lingering older model resulting in "relapses" of entire rehabilitation centers to the traumatic neurosis model with resumption of treatment methods based on the idea that bringing the memory of trauma into consciousness is the proper and adequate cure.

The therapeutic orientation must address itself to the major injury: the fragmentation of the self-representation, and the repression of the "opposite side" in victim/perpetrator duality by erecting powerful defenses against reintegration of it. All the hypervigilant, anxiety-depressive (regressed) affects signal the struggle against what we might call (using a somewhat dated term) the *evil* and *poisonous introject*. As we review our lives, whether it is in psychoanalytic psychotherapy or in the ordinary life review necessary in old age, whenever we encounter any mental element related to those repressed memories, we experience pain. The pain may manifest itself as any painful affect, which in alexithymia is a mixture of the physiological components of painful affects as well as physical pain. The pathognomonic sign of this repressed material is that it has the capacity to "intrude itself upon the mind." Actually, this process shows that the wish to rid one's self of bad memories is forever frustrated. We cannot destroy a memory; we can only deny its self-same nature temporarily. Repression is based on an illusion.

So what is there to be done with these repressed, unbearably painful memories? Psychoanalytic psychotherapy consists of three parts: (1) We slowly help patients to renounce their defenses under the influence of the positive transference, and bring whatever material that lends itself to it into the conscious mind and verbalize it. (2) We review the material with the patients to reinterpret attached infantile interpretations and magical thinking and present the purified memory to the patients as their own mental material which needs to be integrated. (3) If the patients agree, then they proceed to work on the process of integration through mourning. This part is sometimes called "working-through." To the extent that the patients are successful, at the end of this travail they can call their souls their own by having accomplished the creation of the most comprehensive self-representation possible for them. The ability to grieve effectively involves the capacity for affect tolerance because mourners have to be able to monitor themselves in order not to overwhelm themselves with painful affects, but rather to use a variety of resources to terminate the activity. Just as in bereavement or in the process of mastery of an acute very disturbing event, the noxious memory of self-recognition may be denied and removed from conscious awareness or temporarily shrouded by self-distraction, consciousness modification, or a (manic) defense against the affect. After a respite, the idea intrudes itself on the mind again, and/or the person experiences a "wave" of painful affects signaling the resumption of the self-integration work (Freud, 1914; Lindemann, 1944; Horowitz & Becker, 1976). Neither acceptance of a loss nor a negative self-discovery can take place without an inner battle, involving protest, bargaining, and compromise (Bowlby, 1981), which is carried with conscious recognition of the self-sameness of all the "agencies" involved, or else requires the involvement of divine authority. To the extent that most people operate under their "franchise" of various transferences (i.e., without conscious recognition of significant parts of themselves), they may require help of various people who provide the liaison to those alienated divine and mother-attributed powers.

The problem is that in the process of integration of alienated parts of the self-representations, fears are mobilized that one will become evil, unlovable, or lose one's identity and ideal self. For this reason, one important approach to posttraumatic states is by addressing oneself to the shattered grandiose fantasies and helping to restore a realistic self-view. Ullman and Brothers (1987) report good results in PTSD and rape victims through self-psychology models. In essence, the empathic acceptance of the patient's needs for mirroring and idealizing transference permits the development of realistic self-views. There remains the question of the problem with alexithymia: namely that the patient's affects are being regressed (i.e., redifferentiated or resomatized), thus making it impossible for the patient to grieve effectively. When we engage in the process of helping patients to recognize the situations in which emotional responses are called for and they develop the physiological component of affects in the form of psychosomatic symptoms, we also can demonstrate to them their lack of empathy with significant objects and even with themselves.

We have gone over countless times, just as we do with a child—in fact much more than with a normal child—that it is necessary for the patient to take better care of himself, and stop treating himself and his significant objects as robots. In trying to animate the world, we encounter again and again the patient's inhibition of imagination and symbolic representation, but particularly severe blocking of the ability to form wish-fulfillment fantasy.

For instance, one patient who for almost 20 years had the driven need to pick up streetwalker-type prostitutes, when questioned repeatedly about his thoughts from the time he became aware of the urges through the particular details of the activity, could only say that he experienced excitement in connection with the idea that it would be a *new* woman.

When we engage in these efforts to obtain or promote fantasy elaboration, we may become aware that the patient becomes uneasy when pressed to violate his inhibitions, and, on occasion, the transference becomes manifest by the worsening of the inhibition. Edgecumbe (1984) reported the case of a woman in which the analyst (being accustomed to working with children) after some years helped the patient to verbalize her emotions and supported her in taking care of herself. The patient was "unable to distinguish between nausea and most other physical or mental feelings." She also suffered severe abdominal distress for which the gynecologist could find no cause, and partly due to these and other physical problems, she developed an "intense dependent transference" (pp. 1 and 3). When she was away from the analyst, the patient felt herself to be "useless," and she was trembling, felt cold, and her heart was pounding. When the analyst ventured that this picture sounded to her like fear, the patient was surprised, expecting that because of contact with the therapist everything should be all right. At this point, Mrs. Edgecumbe was looking back on "seven years of analysis" and the following development:

> She gradually told me how she never took the initiative in conversations, always waited to be asked questions. The most she could ever manage was a brief mention of events that were important to her. She then left it to the other person to pursue the topic or not. She was often miserably angry. (p. 3)

When the analyst or the husband did not take over the directing of the conversation, they organized it for her by asking appropriate questions. Only in this manner could she relate the story. The analyst reported that finally

> one transference comment made a lot of sense to her . . . that she seemed to feel incomplete at times when she was apart from me, since I had to be the part of her which did the thinking and feeling. (p. 4)

Here, then, we have a perfect example of the concurrence of the maternal transference and inhibitions of self-caring functions which demonstrates that, in that state, part of one's own self-regulatory functions are experienced as being part of the object representation. But it is a golden opportunity to see that some people have such severe inhibition in self-caring and self-regulating that they cannot even openly admit that they are organizing their thoughts! Perhaps this is the reason why alexithymic patients usually recant the trivial details of the interval since we have seen them—chronologically organized—so they pretend that time, the order which things happened, is responsible for the organizing of their thoughts, and escape recognizing their responsibility for self-regulation.

The early maternal transferences contain 2 or 3 years' "worth" of affective memories which are devoid of the usual verbal or symbolic components. The transference is a repetition of the affective attunement which develops after 7 months of age when the infant has established essential self-representation and several "senses" of self-hood, particularly the affective and "historical" sense of the self in terms of a continuity of experience. There follows the practicing of the experiencing of "being with" the primal object and, at a rapid rate, in attachment based on the pure hedonic function, with a participation of melody (prosody) which is more closely linked to affects than to words (D. N. Stern, 1983, 1985). Aprosodia is, of course, a frequent component of alexithymia giving us another "archeological" marker of the timing of the origin of the problems, or the depth of regression. Now the alexithymic patients who have "no imagination at all" are really a confusing paradox. Many of them are distinguished for their imaginative and creative work in technical, mathematical, and financial areas. The rest of them are capable of "borrowing" fantasies.

One of my patients was an alcoholic anhedonic who was unable to make up a story either about a vacation she would like to take nor could she elaborate upon any story on the TAT cards, but was an ardent reader of spy mysteries. She watched television in all her spare time, but she never could tell me a story about either. This blocking of fantasy is a fascinating paradox. These patients are just like musicians who can play any kind of tune but require a composer to organize it for them. They can follow him and the director, but not be *autonomous* musicians. The above-mentioned case of the "woman who could not think for herself" by Mrs. Edgcumbe is a perfect example. Recently (H. Krystal, 1988), I postulated that this defect was another aspect of the sequelae of infantile psychic trauma: namely, the interference with the freedom to utilize transitional object precursors and to transform them into increasingly more abstract forms. This is a similar influence to the forces pushing the child toward autistic objects (Tustin, 1980). But I feel that it is also related to the problems of primary repression.

This brings us to the two subjects I saved for the end because they are the hardest to deal with. They are *holes* and *trances*. There are areas, sometimes large areas of the traumatic past, that are blocked in extraordinary ways so that they cannot be brought back into consciousness the way usual repressed neurotic memories can be.

Recently, I had an opportunity to work with a "juvenile" concentration camp survivor who was fortunate in having had a course of psychoanalytic treatment back in the 1960s. He felt quite satisfied with the progress he had made at the time. He came to see me at this time because of acute panic reactions. I noticed that he did have alexithymic characteristics, and that a few years ago his oppressor/partner got greedy and allowed the patient to buy him out. Not too long afterward, the patient became convinced that he could succeed on his own and he developed severe anxiety mixed with depression and other physiological aspects of emotions. He responded well to a small dose of imipramine, and we spent some time talking about his affect tolerance and health maintenance problems. He related that as a public service, he was giving talks to high school students about the Holocaust. He finally brought himself to confess to me that he had still, untouched by his analysis or with me, a total amnesia for the events of 1942–1945, although by talking to fellow survivors, reading, and other sources, he has reconstructed the story which he still cannot recall directly.

McDougall (1974) was the first researcher to spell out clearly that in analysis with psychosomatic-alexithymic patients, one finds oneself searching for something that is not there. She felt that the future psychosomatic managed early to "decathect" parts of his object representation, and even self-representation, and replaced it with nothing at all. This question brings back the issue of the relation of trauma and primary repression. As mentioned, I am inclined to think of it as a residual of the cognitive constriction which occurs in the traumatic states. However, I find much merit in the work of Cohen and Kinston (1984) and Kinston and

Cohen (1986), who hold that the traumatic memories which have been subjected to primary repression require special considerations. First, it challenges our imagination and all the familiar models of the mind to consider that in posttraumatic states a hole is created in the associative network of our functionally accessible mind. The fear of discovery of this hole is intuitively guarded against (we seem to have a hard-wired reaction as automatic as the reaction to a physical wound), and therefore we tend to develop what Cohen and Kinston (1984) call "object narcissistic" rather than neurotic defensive structures around it. The therapeutic process proceeds along what the therapist can see as the problems that surface and/or need attention and are related to present life problems and resistances. The analysis of the resistances reveals that they are miniature examples of the patient's predominant characterological traits. Although I have been emphasizing the special preparatory work relating to alexithymia, I assume that all other principles of psychotherapy are kept in mind, particularly the following point made by Cohen (1980). He reminds us that Kardiner (1941) pointed out that trauma results in the destruction of adaptive capacity, and the availability of effectively functioning signal anxiety:

> Some portion of the integrated ego is either destroyed or inhibited, a portion which normally enables them to carry out certain functions automatically on the basis of innumerable successes in the past. . . . Being deprived of these protective devices, their psychic representatives, the subject feels deserted and obliged to face a hostile world because he has no longer any defenses against it, or at least has lost command of the more highly integrated forms of defenses against it. (p. 210)

Even though we thus conduct our psychotherapy cautiously and empathically, we also pass a multitude of tests which the patients set for us with various degrees of consciousness. Thus we arrive at a point when the patient may spontaneously go into a trance and relive a traumatic experience. The tendency to develop trances is greatly increased in posttraumatic states.[3]

Disassociative states frequently set in during the traumatic state in children (Eth & Pynoos, 1985; Terr, 1983, 1985). My reason to emphasize the occurrence of trances in treatment is twofold. First, I feel that there are important connections between the onset and aftereffects of psychic trauma and the phylogenetically derived cataleptic responses. We know that the traumatic pattern is the return of essential evolutionary-derived lifesaving and also life-terminating patterns. Second, I feel that one cannot really work effectively with the early preverbal, presymbolic transferences unless patients on their own go into a trancelike state. In particular, I am certain that with it is not possible to relive the traumatic state and together with the patient to work with the patient in creating, for the first time, the psychic contents of the "dead zone," and, at the same time to reclaim the patient's soul unless he or she is in a state very much like a trance. The most profound aspect of self-

---

[3]A related significant study showed that the subjects of repetitive dreams were originally experienced in a depersonalized state (Warren, 1985).

853

healing and self-integration is to reclaim the part of one's self which was mistakenly attributed to the primal love object. Only in this way is the inhibition against self-caring finally lifted.

To paraphrase Cohen and Kinston (1984) and Winnicott (1971), to whom this conception owes much: When object narcissistic defenses are renounced, and a primal relation is established, then primal repression can be repaired by the patient's freely exercising his or her creativity. The patients will do it as they used to in that potential (nonexisting) space between themselves and their mother. The missing remnants and functions will be created anew, and the capacities and potentials that lay fallow will at last germinate and resume their growth and development.

It is now becoming clear that third-party payers and the government agencies acting as third-party payers are increasingly refusing to pay for any psychotherapeutic procedures, or for any medical or surgical procedure which is not included in definitions in diagnostic and statistical manuals. Therefore, in the interest of future patients, it is essential to press for the consideration and recognition of the problems listed in this chapter. Otherwise, our patients and ourselves will be outside the health care coverage and, in effect, outside the law.

References

American Psychiatric Association. (1980). *Diagnostic and statistical manual of mental disorders* (3rd ed.). Washington, DC: Author.

American Psychiatric Association. (1987). *Diagnostic and statistical manual of mental disorders* (3rd ed., rev.). Washington, DC: Author.

Bowlby, J. (1981). Loss: Sadness and depression. In *Attachment and loss* (Vol. 3). New York: Basic Books.

Caplan, G. (1981). Mastery of stress: Psychosocial aspects. *American Journal of Psychiatry, 138,* 413–420.

Cohen, J. (1980). Structural consequences of psychic trauma: A new look at beyond the pleasure principle. *International Journal of Psychoanalysis, 61,* 421–454.

Cohen, J., & Kinston, W. (1984). Repression theory: A new look at the cornerstone. *International Journal of Psychoanalysis, 65,* 411–422.

Edgcumbe, R. (1984). On learning to talk to oneself. *Bulletin of the British Psychoanalytic Society 5,* 1–13.

Eth, S., & Pynoos, R. S. (Eds.). (1985). *Post traumatic stress disorders in children* (pp. 47–70). Washington: American Psychoanalytic Association.

Freud, S. (1953). Fragments of an analysis of a case of hysteria. In J. Strachey (Ed. and Trans.), *The standard edition of the complete psychological works of Sigmund Freud* (Vol. 7, pp. 3–124). London: Hogarth Press. (Original work published 1905)

Freud, S. (1957). On the history of a psycho-analytic movement. In J. Strachey (Ed. and Trans.), *The standard edition of the complete psychological works of Sigmund Freud* (Vol. 14, pp. 7–66). London: Hogarth Press. (Original work published 1914)

Freud, S. (1957). Mourning and melancholia. In J. Strachey (Ed. and Trans.), *The standard edition of the complete psychological works of Sigmund Freud* (Vol. 14, pp. 237–258). London: Hogarth Press. (Original work published 1939)

Freud, S. (1968). Moses and monotheism. In J. Strachey (Ed. and Trans.), *The standard edition of the complete psychological works of Sigmund Freud* (Vol. 23, pp. 3–137). London: Hogarth Press. (Original work published 1939)

Greenson, R. R. (1949). The psychology of apathy. *Psychoanalytic Quarterly, 18,* 290–302.

Grinker, R. R., & Spiegel, J. P. (1945). *Men under stress.* Philadelphia: Blakiston.

Hilberg, R. (1961). *The destruction of European Jews.* Chicago: Quadrangle Books.

Hilgard, J. R. (1970). *Personality and hypnosis.* Chicago: University of Chicago Press.

Hoppe, K. (1962). Persecution, depression and aggression. *Bulletin of the Menninger Clinic, 26,* 195–203.

Hoppe, K. (1965). Persecution and conscience. *The Psychoanalytic Review, 52,* 106–116.

Hoppe, K. (1968). The psychotherapy with concentration camp survivors. In H. Krystal (Ed.), *Massive psychic trauma* (pp. 204–219). New York: International Universities Press.

Hoppe, K. (1969). Reactions of psychiatrists to examination of survivors of Nazi persecution. *Psychoanalytic Forum, 3,* 182–211.

Hoppe, K. (1970). *Image formation and cognition.* New York: Appleton-Century-Crofts.

Hoppe, K. (1971). The aftermath of Nazi persecutions reflected in recent psychiatric literature. In H. Krystal & W. G. Niederland (Eds.), *Psychic traumatization.* Boston: Little, Brown.

Hoppe, K. (Ed.). (1988). Hemispheric specialization. In *The psychiatric clinic of North America* (Vols. 2 & 3). Philadelphia: W. B. Saunders.

Horowitz, M. J., & Becker, S. S. (1976). *Stress response syndrome.* New York: Jason Aronson.

Kardiner, A. (1941). *The traumatic neuroses of war.* New York: Hoeber.

Khantzian, E. (1978). The ego, the self and opiate addiction. *International Journal of Psychoanalysis, 5,* 189–198.

Khantzian, E., & Mack, J. E. (1983). Self-preservation and the case of the self. *Psychoanalytic Study of the Child, 38,* 209–232.

Kinston, W., & Cohen, J. (1986). Primal repression: Clinical and theoretical aspects. *International Journal of Psychoanalysis, 67*(3), 337–356.

Krystal, H. (1968). *Massive psychic trauma.* New York: International Universities Press.

Krystal, H. (1971). Trauma: Consideration of its intensity and chronicity. In H. Krystal & W. G. Niederland (Eds.), *Psychic traumatization* (pp. 11–28). Boston: Little, Brown.

Krystal, H. (1978a). Trauma and affect. *Psychoanalytic Study of the Child, 33,* 81–116.

Krystal, H. (1978b). Self-representation and the capacity for self-care. *Annual of Psychoanalysis, 6,* 209–247.

Krystal, H. (1988). *Integration and self-healing: Affect, trauma, and alexithymia.* Hillsdale, NJ: Analytic Press.

Krystal, H., & Niederland, W. G. (1968). Clinical observations of the survivor syndrome. In H. Krystal (Ed.), *Massive psychic trauma* (pp. 327–348). New York: International Universities Press.

Krystal, H., & Niederland, W. G. (1971). *Psychic traumatization.* Boston: Little, Brown.

Krystal, J. (1988). Assessing alexithymia. In H. Krystal (Ed.), *Integration and self-healing* (pp. 286–310). Hillsdale, NJ: Analytic Press.

Krystal, J. (1989). On some roots of creativity. In K. Hoppe (Ed.), *Hemispheric specialization: Psychiatric clinics of North America, Vol. 11* (pp. 475–492). Philadelphia: W. B. Saunders.

Lifton, R. J. (1968a). *Death in life: Survivors of Hiroshima.* New York: Random House.

Lifton, R. J. (1968b). Observations on Hiroshima survivors. In H. Krystal (Ed.), *Massive psychic trauma*. New York: International Universities Press.

Lifton, R. J. (1973). *Home from the war*. New York: Simon & Schuster.

Lifton, R. J. (1976). *The life of the self*. New York: Simon & Schuster.

Lifton, R. J. (1979). *The broken connection*. New York: Simon & Schuster.

Lindemann, E. (1944). Symptomatology and management of acute grief. *American Journal of Psychiatry, 101*, 141–148.

McDougall, J. (1974). The psychosoma and psychoanalytic process. *International Review of Psychoanalysis, 1*, 437–454.

Meerloo, J. A. M. (1959). Shock, catalepsy and psychogenic death. *International Rec. Medicine, 172*, 384–393.

Minkowski, E. (1946). L'anesthesie affective. *Annual of Medicopsychology, 104*, 8–13.

Nemiah, J. H., Freyberger, H., & Sifneos, P. E. (1976). Alexithymia: A view of the psychosomatic process. In Hill (Ed.), *Recent advances in psychosomatic medicine, vol. 2* (pp. 26–34). London: Butterworth.

Niederland, W. G. (1961). The problem of the survivor. *Journal of the Hillside Hospital, 10*, 233–247.

Niederland, W. G. (1964). Psychiatric disorders among persecution victims—A contribution to the understanding of concentration camp pathology and its aftereffects. *Journal of Nervous and Mental Disease, 139*, 458–474.

Niederland, W. G. (1968). Clinical observations of the "survivor syndrome." *International Journal of Psychoanalysis, 49*, 313–315.

Oz, A. (1978). The crusade. In *Unto death*. San Diego: Harcourt Brace Jovanovich.

Seligman, M. E. P. (1975). *Helplessness: On depression, development and death*. San Francisco: W. H. Freeman.

Stern, D. N. (1985). *The interpersonal world of the infant*. New York: Basic Books.

Stern, M. M. (1951). Anxiety trauma and shock. *Psychoanalytic Quarterly, 20*, 179–203.

Stern, M. M. (1953). Trauma and symptom formation. *International Journal of Psycho-Analysis, 34*, 202–218.

Terr, L. C. (1983). Chowchilla revisited: Affects of psychic trauma four years after school bus kidnapping. *American Journal of Psychiatry, 140*, 1543–1530.

Terr, L.C. (1985). Posttraumatic disorder in children. *American Journal of Psychiatry*.

Tustin, F. (1980). Autistic objects. *International Review of Psychoanalysis, 7*, 30–38.

Ullman, R. B., & Brothers, D. (1987). *The shattered self*. Hillsdale, NJ: Analytic Press.

van der Kolk, B. A., Boyd, Krystal, H., & Greenberg, M. (1984). Post traumatic stress disorder: Psychological and biological sequence. In B. A. van der Kolk (Ed.), *Post traumatic stress disorder* (pp. 123–134). Washington DC: American Psychiatric Press.

van der Kolk, B. A., & Ducey, C. (1987). Clinical implications of research in PTSD. In B. A. van der Kolk (Ed.), *Psychological trauma* (pp. 30, 42). Washington, DC: American Psychiatric Press.

Venzlaff. (1967). Mental disorders resulting from racial persecution. *International Journal of Social Psychiatry, 10*, 177–183.

Warren, J. C. H. (1985). *Dissociation and the traumatic dream in Vietnam veterans*. Unpublished doctoral dissertation, University of Michigan, Ann Arbor.

Winnicott, D. W. (1971). *Playing and reality*. New York: Basic Books.

Wolfenstein, M. (1977). *Disaster: A psychological essay*. New York: Arno Press.

Wurmser, L. (1978). *The hidden dimension*. New York: Jason Aronson.

Wurmser, L. (1981). *The mask of shame*. Baltimore: Johns Hopkins Press.

Wurmser, L. (1989). *Die zerbrochene Wirklichkeit*. Berlin: Springer.

CHAPTER 72

Posttraumatic Stress Recovery of Terrorist Survivors

Ofra Ayalon

Face to Face

The nature of terrorist activity is such that it calculatedly and systematically fosters fear in the defenseless civilian population. Terrorists use noncombatant persons as targets and as a means of intensification of psychological demoralization in order to demonstrate their ability to strike at any place and at any time. The victim is not the real target, but the means toward a goal (Shreiber, 1978); he is used as a form of blackmail and as a demonstration of destructive power. The arbitrary choice of victims means that almost anyone can become a target. In this way, terror transforms whole groups of the population into potential victims. The direct and indirect threats create a "traumatic situation" (Figley, 1978, 1985) necessitating therapeutic intervention to minimize the psychological damage done to the survivors.

In this chapter, I concentrate on the therapeutic and diagnostic aspects of the injury in 3 out of 15 terrorist attacks which involved kidnapping and face-to-face killing of Israeli civilians in the years 1974 to 1980 (see Ayalon, 1983a,b). I also deal with the psychological harm caused by personal, communal, and societal trauma and examine the means of therapeutic intervention.

Circles of Vulnerability

In the examination of activities of sabotage, kidnapping, and murder, one recognizes three target groups which differ from each other in the proximity to the event, the intensity of the threat, and the reality of the loss:

1. Direct victims of kidnapping taken as hostages who are harmed themselves and/or are witness to the murder of family and friends.

2. Members of the family exposed for the duration of the attack or siege to a sense of helpless anxiety about the wellbeing of their loved ones, and afterward must bear the burden of loss and mourning.

3. Those miraculously saved from being hurt (near-miss) and those who were threatened by their geographical proximity to the event or were witnesses to the catastrophe. Also included in this group are those who have certain characteristics in common with the victims, such as age, sex, profession, nationality, and so forth (Janis, 1971).

The civilian population living in the area of the attacks is under pressure and in danger of psychological burn-out. The anxiety stems from a lack of certainty and feelings of helplessness and passivity which are intensified by lack of preparation and forewarning.

Sources of Trauma in Hostages

It is important to discern between damage caused from bombardment and explosion of hidden bombs and that caused by terrorists infiltrating a settlement, attacking civilians, and taking hostages. The hidden or long-distance attacks have immediate results, and most of the damage is caused during the event itself. Assistance arrives the moment the event is over: aiding the injured, controlling the panic, and taking safety measures after the fact. As in natural catastrophes, the destructive force here is perceived as an anonymous and formless element.

The direct, face-to-face confrontation with terrorists is quite different. Until recently, the process of socialization did not prepare us for this kind of confrontation in times of peace, despite the dramatic media exposure to real and fictional violent terror. Even those who experience violence in their daily lives rarely encounter murderous acts perpetrated in cold blood and out of a complete disregard for the victims as human beings. A face-to-face encounter with someone whose intention is to

Ofra Ayalon • School of Education, University of Haifa, Haifa 31999, Israel.

International Handbook of Traumatic Stress Syndromes, edited by John P. Wilson and Beverley Raphael. Plenum Press, New York, 1993.

kill, wherein the victim is totally unable to protect himself or others, involves many elements which are conducive to prolonged trauma on the part of the survivors.

Stressors in Terrorist Activities

The trauma, which involves a total disruption of the daily habits of the individual (Dasberg, 1985), stems from a combination of physical and mental suffering created by the following elements:

Fear of Death

Direct threat to life shatters the illusion of invulnerability, which accompanies every person as a shield against overwhelming anxiety (Krystal, 1984).

Arbitrariness

This element intensifies the fear of the victim. He is degraded to a subhuman level, and his sense of personal identity is badly shaken (Shreiber, 1978).

Uncertainty

Uncertainty about the duration and seriousness of the situation and the chances of being rescued has a destructive influence (Freud, 1950). This increases one's anxiety and diminishes one's ability to adjust to stressful conditions.

Frustration

The sudden impairment of the ability to defend oneself and the barring of routes of escape cause increasing frustration. This frustration breeds aggression, which has no way of being diffused, and is consequently directed inward and turned into desperation (Seligman, 1975).

Exposure to Cruelty

The prolonged proximity to an attacker who seems to enjoy causing suffering destroys the victim's basic comprehension of what is acceptable human behavior.

Confrontation with Violence

Identification with the aggressor (Bettelheim, 1979) undermines the victim's psychological balance between repressed aggressive urges and various defense mechanisms developed through socialization. The victim seems to take on the violent urges, yet is unable to give them expression. The feeling is one of "destruction of the boundaries of the ego" and the infiltration of the alien aggression in the personality.

Ambivalent Attachment to the Aggressor

The victim is totally dominated by the circumstances, and is totally dependent upon the attacker for the most basic and private daily functions, such as mobility, speech, nourishment, toilet functions, and the like. Out of this dependency there slowly develops between the attacker and his victim a feeling of shared fate, which explains the complex phenomenon of the attachment to the kidnapper (the Stockholm Syndrome). This attachment acts as a double-edged sword: It might save the life of the victims, yet after their rescue, the victims might suffer fear and guilt which could interfere in the process of their rehabilitation (Strenz, 1982).

The comprehension of the traumatic elements is essential for the processes of therapy and recuperation, as will become clear in the discussion of the development of appropriate therapeutic systems.

Victims

Face-to-face attacks planned as a means of blackmail and extortion have befallen the Israeli civilian population with some frequency between 1974 and 1980. In some cases, the victims were murdered at the onset of the attack; in others, they were held as hostages until their liberation by force through a military operation. The victims vary in age (babies, children, teenagers, and adults) and in kinship. In certain cases, the attacks were directed toward an entire family, and in others the victims were captured in the company of peers, friends, or strangers. Many of them were wounded, and almost all were eyewitnesses to murders.

The severity of the trauma is measured, among other factors, by the duration of the event, which varied from a few moments to a number of days, and by the death toll. Table 72.1 shows the dramatic and extraordinary circumstances of the damage, which calls for an unconventional approach to the treatment of the victims-survivors.

In prior research, we surveyed the circumstances and results of the attacks at length (Ayalon, 1983a,b). Each of the groups attacked was characterized by its size, form of organization, previous level of functioning within the population, and the presence or lack of support systems. These elements of social environment greatly influence the coping behavior of the individual and the group, for both the short-term and the long-term duration. It became evident that a small united group with reliable leadership having an efficient division of roles and a high degree of interpersonal communication was able to contribute much to the power of their individuals to cope with stress both at the time of the attack and during the period of rehabilitation. Cognitive factors such as faith and a sense of social responsibility are also conducive to coping with the situation of stress (Soskis & Ayalon, 1985), and social support systems are essential for rehabilitation (Caplan, 1974).

Immediate Reactions during Attack

The range of reactions reflects the whirlpool of drives, fears, attitudes, and norms of behavior, wherein every possible solution seems to lead to an even greater catastrophe. A deeper comprehension of the extraordinary conflict faced by those involved, which leaves an indelible mark on their personalities, can contribute to their therapy and rehabilitation. Survivors of terrorist

Table 72.1. Terrorist Attacks in Israel

Date	Place	Duration (hours)	Killed	Injured
April 11, 1974	Kiriat Shmona	5	18	16
May 15, 1974	Ma'alot	0.10	4	1
	Malalot-Safed	16	22[a]	56
June 13, 1974	Kibbutz Shamir	0.20	3	—
June 25, 1974	Nahariya	2	3	—
November 7, 1974	Beit Shean	2.5	4	21
December 1, 1974	Reihanya	1	1	1
December 6, 1974	Kibbutz Rosh Hanikra	0.10	—	—
March 6, 1975	Savoy Hotel	6	7	11
June 15, 1975	Kfar Yuval	2	2	—
November 20, 1975	Ramat Magshimim	0.5	3	2
July 4–11, 1976	Entebbe	168	5	
March 11, 1978	Egged bus	5	38	25
March 3, 1979	Ma'alot	1.15	1	1
April 23, 1979	Nahariya	1.5	4	—
April 4, 1980	Kibbutz Misgav Am	8	2	7

[a]Number of children killed.

attacks have reported (Ayalon & Soskis, 1986) being overwhelmed by a variety of conflicting reactions characteristic of extreme stress, ranging from counterattack, escape, and petrification to palliative thought patterns and to coping by taking active initiative.

Attack

In most of the cases, a counterattack was virtually impossible. However, one heroic attempt in which a hostage succeeded to overpower the terrorists and kill them, thus saving the lives of many of the hostages or potential victims, levied a heavy toll on its initiator—the death of his wife and daughters, and his own grave injury. In another case, hostages' plans for a counterattack met firm opposition on the part of their fellow hostages.

Escape

The decision to escape must be made on the spur of the moment. It involves a high degree of risk-taking and assuming responsibility for one's own life and the lives of others. Escape raises questions that can hardly be answered: Can one desert one's family? Should one attempt to rescue others? Whom? Is the escape attempt more dangerous than staying?

The psychological outcomes of escape are later complicated by consequent feelings of guilt and regret toward those remaining in captivity and by the possible criticism and denouncement by relatives of other victims.

Petrification and Panic

The shock of the first moments cause total panic: running wildly, screaming and crying, and losing control of bodily functions, as well as reactions of petrifica-

tion: temporary loss of mobility and speech and the numbing of emotion, thought, and ability to feel pain. At a later stage, the conflict between the impossible dilemmas causes both physical and spiritual paralysis. These reactions may recur later on in the victims' life, long after the termination of the affliction.

Palliative Thoughts

When the attacks occurred, some individuals attempted to relieve their anxiety through apathy, sleeping, flight into daydreams about hearth and home, fantasizing about a beloved person, childhood memories, magical thinking, taking vows, and bargaining with fate ("If I survive, I will always be good"). Some found consolation in prayer and religious rituals. Faith in God or in rescue seemed to permeate most thinking.

Initiative

The capacity to be active was found in only a few instances. Whenever it happened, it illustrated the fact that stress can activate unexpected personal power. This activity took the form of accepting responsibility, calling for help, taking care of the wounded, and mediating between terrorists and rescuers, each activity carried out at considerable personal risk.

Another form of activity was communicating with the terrorists. There is much evidence showing that these ties might influence the terrorists and make it difficult for them to go through with their murderous intentions (see "The Stockholm Syndrome," Ochberg, 1978; Ayalon & Lahad, 1990). Yet, in retrospect, such activity might damage the survivor's self-image to such a degree as to make therapeutic intervention necessary. As an example, we refer to the report of a girl, held hostage for many hours together with her schoolmates, who shared her bread with one of the terrorists. After her rescue from the bloody attack, in which many others were killed, she developed an aversive reaction to the eating of bread, which for her became contaminated and repulsive (Ayalon, 1983).

In Entebbe, communication with the captors seems to have saved life: when the Israelis and Jews were separated from the rest of the hostages, one of the Jewish passengers exposed the number which had been tattooed on his arm in a German concentration camp in the Holocaust, accusing the German terrorist of being a Nazi. Later, the same terrorist, during the rescue operation by the Israeli Army, hesitated to shoot him and the man was saved (Schreiber, 1978). In this case, communication with the captor seemed a heroic stance and helped rehabilitation of the survivor from his traumatic experience.

Survivor Syndrome

Four kinds of threat influence the perceptions of the event and state of stress, and all of them are activated together in the event of a terrorist attack: threat to life, threat to physical integrity, injury and loss of loved ones, and threat to self-image and values. These threats, which are also common to states of war, genocide, and natural calamities (Lazarus, 1966), are liable to damage the physical and mental reactive systems, either temporarily or chronically. However, there is no way to discern between the various threats or connect them with specific symptoms which are revealed later. One can compare the intensity of the mental harm suffered by the victims of terror with the syndrome of "massive psychic traumatization" of survivors of concentration camps (Eitinger, 1983; Krystal, 1968), that is reported by survivors of plane hijacking (Jacobson, 1973) and hostages who had been liberated (Fields, 1980; Ochberg, 1982; Zafrir, 1982; Terr, 1983).

In order to requisition this posttraumatic state from the realm of psychopathology and underline the universality of reactions to stress that might appear in any person in similar circumstances, a new diagnostic classification has recently been determined. It is based on the statistical profile of the most frequent symptoms: posttraumatic stress disorder (PTSD). This syndrome is described in detail in the DSM-III (American Psychiatric Association, 1980) the first to recognize states of stress (stressors) as activators or exacerbators of specific mental reactions (see sections 308.30, 309.81, p. 236, in the DSM-III).

The first condition for the diagnosis of PTSD is the objective identification of an incident of extreme stress in the life of the victim. The syndrome is diagnosed according to symptoms not present before the event, which belong to the following categories: increase in sensitivity, dulling of sensations, and disturbance in the performance of daily functions. Horowitz (1986) suggested a dichotomic division into two reactive poles: disturbances based on recollection and reliving of the traumatic incident, and disturbances based on denial and disavowal.

Without changing the description of the essential elements of the syndrome, the division into three reactive groups as follows might facilitate the focusing of the therapeutic treatment:

1. *Anxiety and fear reactions*: Reliving the catastrophe through fantasy, hallucinations, sleep disturbances, or nightmares; avoidance of objects which cause recollection of the event, oversensitivity to noises (startle reaction), and nervousness.

2. *Depressive reactions*: Numbing of sensations (psychic numbing); regression and withdrawal; depersonalization, a loss or break in the sense of personal, sexual, or professional identity; memory disturbances; problems of concentration.

3. *Paranoid reactions*: Feelings of persecution; preparedness for catastrophes—expectation of the recurrence of the event; search for prophetic signs (omens and portents); regret and guilt toward the victims who had not been saved; total blame of society and its institutions; suspicion and alienation ("A stranger could never understand it").

Further essential changes in outlook are expressed in the distortion of the sense of time ("The clock seems to have stopped") and loss of immunity ("Fate is chasing me") or the contrary, the feeling of invincibility ("Nothing bad could ever happen to me").

Professional recognition of the stress syndrome of terror survivors presents psychiatry with a new challenge (similar to the acknowledgment of combat reaction syndrome). Although it enables us to differentiate between the mental suffering caused by exposure to situations of extreme stress and the clinical diagnosis of neurotic or psychotic disturbance, it recommends special methods of psychotherapy for relief of this suffering. The universal acknowledgment of reactions to stress must support the right of the survivor to receive psychological help, yet simultaneously to liberate him or her from the sense of failure and the stigma of pathology. Therapy is necessary in two respects: (1) in order to relieve immediately the suffering and to facilitate quick rehabilitation and return to normal living, (2) in order to prevent the development of long-term symptoms and functional disturbances.

Of course, as in any new area, care must be taken that lack of familiarity with the posttraumatic syndrome does not lead to a mistaken diagnosis and inappropriate treatment (Krystal, 1984).

Although the classification of the DSM-III-R (American Psychiatric Association, 1987) frees the victims of terror from the definitions of psychopathology, it does not indicate which factors might contribute to their normal coping. The planning of therapeutic intervention depends on the definition of the behaviors and attitudes which strengthen the survivor, in contrast to those which endanger his or her mental balance. An attempt to find a key to the solution of this problem can be found in the phenomenological approach, which bases itself on the victims' own evaluations of their reactions.

Phenomenological Approach to the Evaluation of Coping

Integration of Diagnosis and Treatment

Rather than relying on external criteria to diagnose normal or pathological coping, Ayalon and Soskis (1986)

Table 72.2. Dimensions of the Coping Self

Helpful	Disruptive
Short-term	
Sleep	Paralysis
Denial	Fear
Compulsive eating	Confusion
Fantasy of rescue	Guilt toward parents
Childhood memories	Blaming guards' failures
Talking to captors	
Helping others	
Prayer to God	
Vows	
Hope for rescue	
Long-term	
Having a slight injury	Severe injury
Writing a diary	Excessive dependence
Talking about the event	Shame over contact with captors
Trying to forget	Loss of faith in people
Helping other survivors	Guilt toward dead friends
Altruistic behavior	Fear of dangerous places
Observing religious rites	Fear of noises
Self-improvement learning	Haunted by memories
	Expecting disaster

applied an original approach by using the survivors' evaluation of themselves as indicators of the degree of harm or benefit caused by their reactions—both during and after the event. This method is based on an attempt to comprehend the idiosyncratic reactions of persons caught in a situation of extreme stress and their choice of unique defense mechanisms necessary for the preservation of their identity. Our approach to the survivor as a partner might also assist us in our effort to understand the "experience" which lies beyond both the range of normal human experience (Trimble, 1985) and the concept of clinical perception. The diagnostic process which turns the survivors into active partners becomes the first step of therapy. It fulfills patients' needs to "regain" themselves—whether in symbolic or tangible fashion and enables them to view the event in a new light, not only as helpless victims, but also as individuals capable of choosing and shaping their own fate.

I will now show how, with the active participation of the victims, it is possible to analyze what has happened to them (see Table 72.2). Those interviewed were asked to classify their behavior according to the following criteria: What feelings, thoughts, and actions at the time of the event and afterward were helpful or disruptive to you?

Circles of Support

Insufficient support and the danger of secondary victimization on the part of society increase the importance of community intervention. This intervention takes place on two levels: intervention of the community itself for the sake of the injured individuals and intervention of therapeutic agents within the affected community as a whole.

Community intervention supplies a support system which is vital for the recuperation of the survivors. "Support-systems are groups which maintain longstanding ties which protect the physical and mental integrity of the person in need" (Caplan, 1974). The more familiar and more similar the supporters are to the supportee, the smaller the gap between them. In contrast, professional services have certain advantages stemming from their knowledge and expertise in various areas of mental health. Since victims of terrorism need both kinds of assistance, it is worthwhile to differentiate between them. The advantage of informal support systems is that they free the victims from the stigmatization of mental illness, while giving legitimate psychological assistance.

Objectives of Psychological Support

Support is given with three objectives in mind: (1) to provide opportunities of sharing the emotional burden by listening and accepting, (2) to actively participate in the solving of problems, and (3) to contribute additional resources, whether they be material resources or new knowledge, which improves the capacity of the victims to make use of their own existing resources.

We can identify two distinct circles of support. The first is spontaneous and is composed of family members, friends, neighbors, and colleagues at work or school. The second, intentionally initiated, is comprised of groups of others who share the same fate in which the giving and receiving of support takes place on an equal basis, with the tacit agreement that "only someone who has gone through what I have can understand my suffering." The brothers of "shared fate" use others' personal examples of coping at various stages of the crisis in order to prepare themselves for future coping. The effectiveness of this support is not only in teaching how to cope with the difficulty, but also in strengthening the individual by means of group identification (Wilson, 1980).

In the following examples, I shall describe two events that differ greatly in the support systems that were mobilized and in the resultant degrees of effectiveness.

Community Support Systems during a Tragedy

An example of the organization of a community support system can be found in the activity of the "Egged" Transportation Cooperative following the terrorist attack on a bus conducting family tours on the coastal road in 1978. The bus was highjacked and bombed. Out of the 36 people who were killed, 18 were Egged employees or family members; many others were seriously wounded.

Egged took full responsibility for the care of the victims and immediately and thoroughly organized support through their chief psychologist (Zafrir, 1982).

The full and voluntary involvement resulted from the cooperative's own description of itself as "one big family." In this sense, the community system reflected two circles of support at the same time: the spontaneous informal one and the professional one. The activities of the support system expressed the special needs of the survivors: (1) stabilizing shaken feelings by emphasizing the validity and regularity of the contact; (2) legitimizing all forms of expression and behavior, thus relieving the victims from the stigma of social failure and/or mental illness; and (3) improving the damaged self-image and reducing the feelings of rejection and alienation, by assuring the survivor's position and reabsorption into the workforce, with special consideration given to his or her limitations.

Volunteers performed a wide range of roles, as required by the size and suddenness of the catastrophe: preparing lists of victims, identifying bodies, notifying the families and helping them through their mourning, sending the wounded to hospitals and subsequently supervising and following their convalescence, mediating between family members and the wounded, and taking care of their immediate financial needs. The volunteers served as a bridge between the survivors and the familial and social system, and later between the survivors and the official agencies of welfare and education.

A combination of professional expertise and human devotion was evident in the care of the affected children. Under the guidance of the psychologist, volunteers filled the role of surrogate parents for those whose parents had been killed or wounded. In this role, they helped to work—through the period of mourning, offering support and affection, and fostering feelings of stability by spending time with the child, celebrating a birthday, and so forth. This behavior helped the children to accept anger and pain, enabling them to dissipate the trauma of the experience by means of play, storytelling, and forms of artistic expression. The volunteers also served to bridge the gap between the children and their families and the social and educational environments created by distance, time, and the bitter experience itself. Their success can be measured by the extent to which they were able to help the children to resume the regular pattern of their lives despite their considerable losses.

It is worthwhile to note the methods of care for those whose injuries were not physically apparent ("invisible wounds"), a group most frequently neglected among trauma victims. Their therapeutic care was not based on a psychiatric diagnosis, thus emphasizing the idea that the justification for receiving help lies in the suffering itself, rather than mental instability or failure. The therapy concentrated on dissipating the survivors' excessive guilt (a sensation of guilt which troubles the survivors over the fact that they remained alive) (Krystal, 1968; Lifton, 1967), on acceptance of regressive behavior and increased dependency, and on rechanneling excessive aggression and anger.

Egged's therapeutic team expanded its scope of activities in an attempt to assist other social-therapeutic agents (doctors and teachers) to understand the "survivor syndrome," which defines the "narcissistic wound," the damage to personal, sexual, or professional identity, and strange or irregular behavior. As a result, the danger of judgment and rejection was avoided, as was the danger of secondary victimization, which threatens victims of human tragedies (Eitinger, 1983; Symonds, 1980).

The Egged group can be classified in the "near-miss" category of the "circles of vulnerability," owing to the high degree of similarity and proximity between the victims and the rest of the members of the cooperative. The feeling that "it could have happened to me" was the key to the level of vulnerability of the members. The support which they provided to the victims of the tragedy reflected their effort to overcome this latent threat.

The preceding description of Egged as a cohesive system shows how, out of a capacity for organization and identification, a complete system of support was geared to cope effectively with the anxiety and pain of the victims and those close to them. In this process of strengthening, the system also increased its own cohesiveness and resourcefulness (see "The Snowball Effect" in Ayalon, 1983b).

Crisis without Aid

In light of this example of total support and acceptance of full social responsibility for the victims of terror, the lack of social organizations and public programs for the efficient treatment of terror victims following other terrorist attacks is especially evident. The failure of society to provide psychological first aid for victims and their families increases the risk of the attack's aftereffects on both individual and communal levels. In such cases, not only is the community incapable of aiding the victims, it goes into a state of crisis itself and is in danger of breaking down.

The failure of the community's ability to cope is often caused by the accumulation of stress and problems, both in the collective and personal past. The elements of erosion which are characteristic of troubled communities are: forced immigration, imposed cultural changes, loss of traditional values, educational deprivation, poverty, low levels of professionalism, inferior living conditions, and multiproblem families (Marx, 1970; Samooha & Peres, 1974; Zuckerman-Bareli, 1979). Prolonged economic, cultural, and social deprivation generates the characteristic traits of underprivileged communities: lack of leadership and cohesion, insufficient communication within the group and with outside government agencies, and lack of autonomy in the approach to problem-solving.

Indeed, such weak social systems have undergone severe crisis as a result of terrorist attacks; and their resources for coping—insufficient from the outset—were almost completely depleted, according to the principle of the "snowball effect." I refer here to two highly vulnerable communities which were the targets of one terrorist attack: Ma'alot and Safed. Four residents of Ma'alot and 22 high school students from Safed were killed in the attack, with dozens of others injured after being held hostage for 16 hours.

Both communities reacted severely. The immediate reactions of the inhabitants were shock, confusion, feelings of helplessness, search for a scapegoat, rage and violence. Over time, persistent fears and a decrease in the level of health were evident (Ayalon, 1983). Community services also broke down; not only did they fail to organize support for the victims, but they also stood in the way of outside attempts at assistance.

The "snowball effect," first and foremost, caused damage to the survivors themselves. Group therapy, which the Social Security agency tried to organize by means of outside social workers, was met with hostility on the part of local education and welfare authorities and was never allowed to develop (Social Security, 1974). This unsuccessful attempt at therapy only intensified the sense of frustration and alienation of the victims. They had no one to turn to but their families, who were themselves paralyzed by anxiety and worry.

The education system also failed after the attack. It did not provide its students with counseling services, which would have helped those who were "near-misses" as well (i.e., the whole student population of the school). A harsh policy was adopted toward the survivors: they were suspected of taking advantage of their weakness in order to avoid study and discipline requirements. A number of girls were sent home because they broke the religious dress code and wore trousers in order to hide their wounds, thus adding secondary victimization to the primary traumatic damage.

The students and their families lost their faith in the school, and expressed great anger toward those teachers who escaped from the siege, leaving their students in the hands of the terrorists.

Evidence of the lack of cohesion among those students who were held hostage is that no organization of "brothers in fate" was formed (Gal, 1980). Instead, an opposite and painful process began: growing alienation and both latent and overt competition over resources and compensation.

Hostility on the part of families of those who were killed only intensified the guilt feelings. The alienation of the establishment intensified their suffering. Those who had been lightly wounded were the luckiest, because their wounds entitled them to attention and care and also served as some measure of "guilt atonement."

In the follow-up study (Ayalon & Soskis, 1986), the survivors described society's attitude toward them in the 8 years since the attack, largely expressing disappointment in the behavior of others.

Stress Inoculation: Preventive Care

As is evident in the two preceding examples, victims of terror are in need of therapeutic care. Although such therapy has no capacity to free them from the pain of the loss, it decreases the risk of additional problems. One can call such therapeutic intervention, which is intended to diminish the damage caused by the original trauma, "psychological immunization." According to Caplan (1964), there are three levels of preventive care:

1. Preparation for excessive stress is conducted in times of minimal or normal stress (and sometimes as a reaction to a crisis in another place), with the goal of increasing the participants' consciousness of various kinds of stressful situations and making them aware of alternative modes of reaction. Stress inoculation is, in fact, "primary prevention." It aims to understand the development of a stressful situation, to stimulate the

feelings accompanying such a situation, and to practice appropriate modes of reaction. Even when it is impossible to foresee the particulars of an event, one can prepare programs for stress inoculation in advance by developing generic coping skills (Meichenbaum, 1977):

- In the cognitive realm, by supplying information and knowledge of the situation
- In the emotional realm, by giving expression to oppressive feelings (catharsis), while giving and receiving support
- In the behavioral realm, by providing activity, initiative, playing a known and clearly defined role, giving a feeling of control, and offering various strategies for problem-solving

2. When the crisis is at its peak, there is need for "secondary prevention." Its purpose is to identify the reactions to stress and to treat them while they are still forming, in order to minimize the danger of fixation on traumatic stress and to stop it from becoming a chronic state. The critical period for this intervention is within 6 weeks of the initial stress. The principles of this approach are immediacy, concentration on problems of "here and now," and orientation of activity. The function of activity is to divert attention and to instill hope. An example of this approach can be found in the treatment of victims of terror in Ireland (Fraser, 1977).

3. "Tertiary intervention," a rehabilitative intervention, treats posttraumatic syndrome and reactions of delayed mourning with a wide range of therapeutic methods. The duration of the treatment depends on the depth of the disturbance, the personality of the individual, and the therapeutic ideology.

A plan for therapeutic intervention in emergencies designed according to these principles at the University of Haifa (Ayalon, 1978) was accepted for application throughout the education system by the Israeli Ministry of Education. The program, based on a systematic approach, is intended to enable educators and mental health workers to support children in times of crisis. It provides a wide variety of tools that are oriented to the development of coping skills in emotionally expressive, cognitive, and behavioral areas, by means of work in groups, bibliotherapy, creative expression through writing and play, simulated situations, drama, and guided imagination exercises that are suitable for all ages.

Primary intervention has proven its effectiveness in a controlled experiment, and in such events as sabotage and mortar bombardment (Lahad, 1981, 1984). As for face-to-face attacks, no study has yet been conducted, although use has been made of the principles of secondary prevention during field work (Ahronstam & Wolf, 1975; Ayalon, 1988; Ben-Eli & Sella, 1980; Ophir, 1980).

The principles contained in *Rescue! An Emergency Handbook* were taught intensively to psychologists and educational advisors in the northern border areas of Israel (Ayalon, 1977; Klingman & Ayalon, 1980). This program has also been used by those therapists who treat near-miss groups for short durations, as well as in other forms of therapeutic intervention.

Brief Group Therapy for a Near-Miss Population

During a terrorist attack in Nahariya, a policeman and another man and two of his daughters were killed, and a sense of terror spread throughout the neighborhood. A crisis intervention was called to abate the panic and reduce posttraumatic stress disorders in the community. The intervention was planned at the following levels: (1) for all pupils in school and kindergarten, an explanation and working-through of mourning processes (an intervention that was not fully carried out awing to parents' and teachers' objections); (2) for "high risk" students, those who were close to the event itself and children who had recently suffered the loss of family members; and (3) for families of students who showed signs of stress.

The crisis intervention was conducted in the schools themselves by a therapeutic team consisting of psychological and educational professionals who had volunteered for this purpose. Approximately 60 children received therapy in order to cope with various symptoms of anxiety: fear of noises and the dark, inability to concentrate, difficulties with eating and sleeping, stomachaches, headaches, bedwetting, and tantrums. The therapeutic framework was composed of peer groups of six to eight participants. The group setting was intended to serve as mutual support and assistance systems.

Eclectic methods were used, combining various dynamic behavioral and cognitive techniques: encouraging catharsis, bringing the experience to a conscious level, channeling fear and anger toward problem-solving, extinction of startle responses by means of relaxation therapy, overcoming phobic reactions to places contaminated by the disaster (such as the beach where the killings took place), cognitive working-through of the experience, and, finally, practicing various alternative behaviors in case of another attack.

Therapeutic meetings were held on 5 consecutive days, accompanied by follow-up meetings of a lesser frequency for 2 weeks, while parents received counseling as well. In only one case was there any need of further individual therapy. In a follow-up study conducted approximately 1 year later (Ben-Eli & Sella, 1980) no signs of morbidity were found, except a lingering startle reaction to noises. These findings validated the benefit, drawn from a prompt crisis intervention program, to reduce traumatic aftereffects.

Mass Media and Treatment

An act of terrorism is a media event which brings the victims into the headlines. The concern expressed by the public may reflect society's shared mourning process, and as such may offer some consolation to the survivors. Yet the exposure of the victim's plight in the media can encourage public meddling in the private life of the victim, often motivated by curiosity and sensation seeking. The public and the media take the liberty to criticize and judge the victim's behavior during and after the event. In one extremely tragic case, some newspapers went as far as to insinuate that the sole survivor from the massacre of her whole family was better off committing suicide! Thus the media becomes the perpetrator of a secondary victimization of the already afflicted victims (Frederick, 1987).

Sometimes politicians attempt to transform the victim into a national symbol or to use victims for political advantage. This is, in fact, a continuation of the process begun by the terrorists: the abuse of random victims as pawns in a power game not of their own.

Another aspect of this publicity that may reflect positively on the audience occurs when victims present a model for coping behaviors under extreme situations. Their example helps to assuage anxiety in other high-risk social groups. This observation is especially valid in cases of survivors' self-reports of their captivity and rescue, which highlight the coping aspects of the event (e.g., the case of Vaders, who was held hostage by terrorists in Holland: Vaders, 1976; Ochberg, 1982). However, this publicity may also cause new problems for the survivors and may jeopardize their recuperation. Survivors who become "famous" may be trapped in their newly formed public image and feel coerced to hold onto this image. Such pressures interfere with the therapeutic intervention and may postpone the necessary working-through of the mourning process.

In such cases, the therapist is faced with additional difficulties, such as a possible bias toward the survivor and an overidentification, enhanced by the disaster and its tragic or heroic circumstances. To some extent, the therapy itself is also subject to public scrutiny. Ethical problems arise when the exposure of the victims' identity causes a breach of professional secrecy.

The attraction of publicity causes competition between the appointed therapists and other social agencies, which puts additional stress on the therapeutic process and causes real damage to the patient (Raphael, 1986). The following is an example of one of the most publicized cases of bereavement following a terrorist attack in recent years in Israel (Ayalon, 1992).

Individual Therapy for Media-Publicized Bereavement

The first therapeutic contact was formed following an emergency call to administer psychological first aid to a young woman who had just lost her husband and two small daughters in a terrorist attack. While the husband and their 5-year-old daughter were dragged from their home by the terrorists and brutally killed on the beach, the mother with her 2-year-old daughter was hiding in the attic. In trying to stop the baby from crying while the armed terrorist was searching the apartment, the mother put her hand over the girl's mouth and eventually caused her death by suffocation.

The details of this gory event unfolded in the media, revealing the tragic scenario, and causing a surge of public emotional reaction that vacillated between strong compassion for the bereaved survivor and appalling resentment of her actions.

Typical to interventions in emergency, the beginning of the therapy in this case was marked by a lack of structure and a flexible setting of location and duration of the therapeutic encounter. The initial stage was marked by a certain confusion between the personal feelings and professional attitudes of the therapist. The major task facing the therapist was to penetrate beyond the confusion and shock in order to form an initial contact and win the patient's trust. The patient, herself a second-generation Holocaust survivor, perceived her plight as a repetition of the Holocaust experience. This perception, which she presented on national television, stirred up a host of contradictory emotions nationwide. It also raised special problems in the relations between the therapist and the patient, creating confusion between the national and the private spheres.

The therapist oscillated among an expression of compassionate support, step-by-step directing of the daily activities, and trying to deal with the terrible conflict and guilt which had beleaguered the patient since the event. The enmeshment of boundaries between the therapist's personal involvement and professional responsibilities exacerbated the problems of transference and counter transference. There was hardly any role model for such extraordinary therapeutic practice.

Despite external pressures and personal difficulties, the therapist was able to establish boundaries and rules for a proper brief therapy in an emergency: immediacy, proximity, variety in intervention methods, short-term duration, and clear definition of goals.

In conjunction with the individual intervention, the therapist carried out network interventions, involving a large number of family members and representatives of State Welfare agencies that are responsible for caring for victims of terrorism. The aim of these meetings was to reach some measure of coordination among the diverse attitudes, and hold at bay attempts to "flood" the patient with contradicting rehabilitative practices. Relatives and friends were instructed in methods of support and assistance.

The therapy terminated gradually, with special care not to add further loss (of the therapeutic contact) to the previous traumatic losses. Follow-up was maintained for a year after the event (Ben-Eli, 1986).

From Getting Help to Giving Help: A Role Change

Short-term therapy was found appropriate for tertiary intervention, as the following case history shows:

A survivor of a terrorist attack applied for therapy 6 years after the event. It should be pointed out that this treatment took place in a phase in the survivor's life cycle which was different from the phase of the trauma, when she had been a teenage schoolgirl. When she requested therapy, she was already married, was a mother, and had developed a successful teaching career.

The patient survived, badly wounded, after having been held hostage for 16 hours by three armed Palestinian terrorists. From the 105 classmates abducted as hostages on a school ground, 17 escaped at the onset of the attack, 22 were killed, and 56 were wounded prior to the military rescue raid. The patient endured hospitalization and surgery from which she emerged with many scars and a limited use of her right hand. Shortly after the attack, she took part in an abortive attempt at group therapy, which apparently was too short and diffused. It

left her even more frustrated and reluctant to seek help for a long time. As part of the search to give meaning to her experience and her rescue, she joined a class on Stress and Trauma at a university, where she found the courage to apply for therapy.

The principles of short-term therapy were applied. The treatment concentrated on the present, and examined the effect of the trauma on the patient's various roles at her present phase of life.

The main complaints were the patient's persistent fear of a recurring terrorist attack (catastrophic expectation), a fear of noises (startle reaction), avoidance of dangerous places (phobia), and a deep worry of passing her fears on to her son. These difficulties had persisted ever since she had been wounded in the terrorist attack that killed and wounded dozens of her fellow students. Despite the disability caused by her injury, and despite the posttraumatic reaction, she coped with developmental tasks with considerable success. Nonetheless, an increasing feeling of distress, along with a growing rift between her social image as a "good coper" and her mounting internal stress, caused her to seek help. Ambivalent feelings, particularly shame and fear of being stigmatized as "emotionally disturbed," accompanied this decision.

The therapist examined the various areas of home activity, her relationship with her spouse, and her professional and maternal performance. The therapy was conducted according to a strategic approach of problem-solving. It concentrated on two major issues: overcoming phobias by means of cognitive desensitization, and ventilation of pent-up anger using the Gestalt method and guided fantasy. Working-through the traumatic events, the therapy provided a corrective experience, building an internal image of strength and courage. In order to introduce greater flexibility into her present behavioral patterns, the patient was given behavioral tasks for coping with fear and anger in her everyday encounters with her husband, her child, and society.

The therapy, which was terminated by the patient, was defined by her as "a chance to learn some common sense and ways to solve problems." This definition expresses the struggle for rehabilitation of her self-image, which had been severely damaged by the traumatic event. In her attempt to regain the shattered feeling of control, she identified with the role of the "healer." Consequently, she decided to study psychology and make use of the therapeutic techniques, which she had experienced firsthand, as a means of assisting children in distress.

Strategic Method of Short-Term Family Therapy

The tragic conflicts in the aftermath of traumatic experiences affect the entire family. The following case history is an example of the treatment of a family that ceased to function because of acute anxiety and phobic reactions after narrowly escaping a terrorist attack.

A couple and their two daughters became separated in the course of a nocturnal escape from a murderous band of terrorists. Each sought separate hiding, regarding all others as dead. Reunited after the ordeal, they all suffered acute posttraumatic reactions, despite the fact that none had suffered any physical injury.

The regular daily functioning of the family broke down. At night, they fortified themselves in their home behind huge barricades of furniture, standing guard against further attack. The father developed a depression accompanied by feelings of guilt and helplessness; the mother's reaction was complete dependency on her husband; the daughters developed phobic reactions toward their bedroom; and all evinced excessive sensitivity to noise and sleeping difficulties. A prolonged family encounter with a therapist did not bring any relief, because of mutual reinforcement of the maladjusted behaviors.

The therapist suggested a new contract for the family therapy, according to which the girls were chosen as the focus of treatment. A multimodal strategy was then successfully employed, using the following elements: (1) development of control by means of activity; (2) use of humor for dissipating tension; (3) gradual desensitization of fears and oversensitivity to noises and voices; (4) reenactment of fear-producing situations through play; (5) acquiring skills for mutual support; and (6) paradoxical instructions.

Examples of the therapeutic suggestions given to the girls may clarify the multimodal strategy: writing a "fear diary"; "grading fear" in each room of the house; developing a protective attitude toward "scared" dolls.

The therapy combined cognitive and magical elements; the redefinition of fear as a necessary reaction, using a method of relaxation in which a "magic word" was repeated to diminish fear. All these various strategies were applied simultaneously.

The girls' condition stabilized after two therapeutic sessions. Further problems of the parents that were not directly related to the event required additional treatment (Alon, 1980).

Discussion and Recommendations

We have attempted to clarify the similarities and differences between short-term therapy for terrorist victims and short-term therapy for victims of other crises:

1. The crises occurring regularly in the life cycle, such as death, divorce, unemployment or immigration, tend to be considered the personal domain of the individual and/or family, who remain anonymous and must themselves contact the appropriate therapeutic agencies. In contrast, a terrorist attack is of social interest, with public ramifications and direct and indirect responsibility resting on the state. The victims lodge complaints with the state, as well as claims for material and psychological compensation. I have illuminated some of the problems and therapeutic solutions to this specific situation. Scrutinizing the available information, I found a dire need for governmental organization for the provision of psychological aid to the victims.

2. All therapeutic intervention in extreme situations of stress must be immediate in both time and focus, geared to treat the victim as a well person reacting to stressful circumstances and aiming to return that person

to normal functioning as quickly as possible. This intervention makes eclectic use of various therapeutic methods—dynamic, behavioral, and cognitive—in order to achieve catharsis, relieve tension, and teach methods of problem-solving. It emphasizes "support systems" as a major therapeutic agent and recommends cooperation between professional therapists and lay volunteers.

3. The target of terrorist attacks is the community at large, so the "community-intervention" approach is highly appropriate in the treatment of its victims. It is necessary to raise the awareness of those who provided the services, so that they will be able to start treatment on site immediately after the attack, in order to prevent the development of a morbid stress syndrome. Because of media and political aspects, a great deal of attention is given to the terrorists. (Note the number of publications dealing with the psychology of terrorists compared with the prominent lack of research of the victims—Ayalon, 1987; Fields, 1982.) There is a tendency in many cases to neglect the victims or to "sacrifice" them on the altar of political interests or prejudice. Note that only a handful of the 15 face-to-face attacks reported in this study, along with many other terrorist attacks that have taken place in Israel over the last decade, were followed by planned therapeutic interventions—all of them as a result of local initiative. The assumption is that there were other sources of treatment, especially within the kibbutz society, and it is appropriate for them to be brought to the attention of the profession and the public. A national clearinghouse of data is badly needed, in order to help develop professional skills for dealing with this sensitive subject.

4. For most of the individual and community situations of stress, whether in times of peace or war, it is recommended to make use of primary preparation and stress inoculation. Such stress inoculation programs have recently been developed at Haifa University and at the Community Stress Prevention Center in Kiriat Shmona: "Coping with Death" (Ayalon, 1979a, 1979b, 1980; Klingman, 1980); "Coping with Divorce" (Ayalon & Flasher, 1993); "Coping with Disability" (Ayalon & Levi Segev, 1985); "On the Border" (Ayalon, 1978; Ayalon & Lahad, 1990; Lahad, 1982, 1986). The question then arises: "How can people be effectively inoculated against terrorist attacks?" Any answer must go beyond the realm of psychology toward that of ethics and politics. In various countries, special briefings have been developed for public persons and their families at risk of kidnapping (Jenkins, 1978). Yet in Israel, there are still great reservations about the application of inoculation programs such as those mentioned above to a wide segment of the population. The psychological price for primary preparation seems too high—and thus "stress inoculation" is prevented from being applied to the entire population at risk. The damage that could be caused by this neglect must be considered.

5. The available information about the psychological injury which victims of terror suffer, and about their therapeutic requirements, is mainly derived from research on captivity (Segal, 1974) and on victimology (see publications of the National American Council for Aid to Victims; NOVA, 1983). We learn that the danger common to all victims of human violence is damage to their self-

image (Tinklenberg, 1982). Feelings of humiliation, degradation, loss of dignity and identity are all part of the high price which the victim must pay—and the therapy must take this into account. One of the methods of rehabilitation used in a small number of countries is the involvement of the survivors in advisory teams for fighting terror and caring for the victims, which contributes greatly to the fostering of the victims' feelings of self-worth. In Holland, a therapeutic team for treating victims of train hijacking was selected from those who had themselves been victims of similar incidents in the past (Bastians, 1982). It would be worthwhile to develop such an approach in Israel as well, and to investigate its effect on the rehabilitation of both the assisting and the assisted victims.

6. The "hidden victims," whom most therapeutic approaches still disregard, are the victims' family members. They suffer anxiety and bereavement and their lives are disrupted as a result of the injury to their loved one; yet they do not even receive the minimal degree of support given to the survivors themselves (Bastians, 1982).

7. There are also a number of positive implications to my research. It seems that the human spirit is strong and capable of withstanding the vicissitudes of fate with great initiative. The hostages' accounts reveal various ways of helping themselves to cope with captivity, of preserving sanity and a feeling of self-worth and, in some cases, of actual rescue. A young woman, while being held hostage at the Savoy Hotel in Tel-Aviv, managed, through unexpected initiative, to become the mediator between the terrorists and the army (Golan, 1979); a boy found a way to free himself and kidnapped friends who had been buried in a pit in the ground (Terr, 1983); the Dutch journalist Vaders recorded his impressions inside the hijacked train (Ochberg, 1982); the psychologist, Jacobson, observed and documented the behavior of her kidnapped friends in a plane in the Jordan desert for an entire week (Jacobson, 1973); a South African psychologist, held hostage for more than 24 hours under degrading conditions, applied her therapeutic skills when dealing with her kidnapper. She thus prevented herself from being thrown into panic, preserved her sense of self-worth, and even managed eventually to obtain her release (M. Freidman, personal communication, 1985). These unexpected activities, which exceed the immediate resources available to the prisoner, indicate that a situation of stress can become a challenge for growth and creativity.

8. In conclusion, I shall touch upon the issue of the burn—out of those psychologists who are called upon to provide assistance for the victims of terror. The therapeutic community is also in a quandary. The common fate of victims, survivors, and therapists in a society which is constantly exposed to terror puts an extra stress on the professionals. As a near-miss group, they too suffer anxiety and guilt. Overidentification can impede their functioning. They must be prepared to absorb the fear and guilt of those whom they wish to help. They must be familiar with survivors' reactions, and also know when to back off and allow natural support systems to aid in the process of recuperation. This issue of the erosion of the therapist, the helper who also shares the fate of the victim, is worthy of further investigation.

9. In these areas of assisting the victims of terror, the unknown supersedes the known. There is need for research, courage, and creativity in the development of appropriate forms of intervention. A start in the right direction can be seen in the activities of the Community Stress Prevention Center, which has recently opened in Kiriat Shmona (Lahad, 1986), preparing guidelines for doctors, psychologists, social workers, and educators, who will work as a multiprofessional team in times of crisis, and enhancing public vigilance.

References

Alon, N. (1980). *Treatment of a family with phobic reaction*. Paper presented at the meeting of the International Congress of Behavior Therapy, Jerusalem.

American Psychiatric Association. (1980). *Diagnostic and statistical manual of mental disorders* (3rd ed.). Washington, DC: Author.

American Psychiatric Association. (1987). *Diagnostic and statistical manual of mental disorders* (3rd ed., rev.). Washington, DC: Author.

Ahronstam, S., & Wolf, O. (1975). Kiryat Shmone project. *Journal of Psychology, Counselling and Guidance in Education*.

Ayalon, O. (1977). Preparing the school-system for coping with stress in emergency situations. *Studies in Education, 15*, 149–166. (In Hebrew)

Ayalon, O. (1978). *Rescue! An emergency handbook*. Haifa: University of Haifa Press. (In Hebrew)

Ayalon, O. (1979a). C.O.P.E. *Journal of Death Education, 3*(4), 222–244.

Ayalon, O. (1979b). Is death a proper subject for the classroom? *International Journal of Social Psychiatry, 25*, 252–257.

Ayalon, O. (1980). Death as a subject in the curriculum. In A. Raviv, A. Klingman, & M. Horowitz (Eds.), *Children under stress and in crisis* (pp. 251–259). Tel-Aviv: Ozar Hamroreh.

Ayalon, O. (1983a). Coping with terrorism: The Israeli case. In D. Meichenbaum & M. Jaremko (Eds.), *Stress reduction and prevention* (pp. 293–339). New York: Plenum Press.

Ayalon, O. (1983b). Face to face with terrorists. In A. Cohen (Ed.), *Education as encounter* (pp. 81–102). Haifa: University of Haifa Press. (In Hebrew)

Ayalon, O. (1987). Living in dangerous environments. In B. Germain, M. Brassard, & S. Hart (Eds.), *Psychological maltreatment of children and youth*. New York: Pergamon Press.

Ayalon, O. (1988). *Rescue! Community oriented preventive education*. Haifa: Nord Publications.

Ayalon, O. (1992). A community from crisis to change. *Community Stress Prevention, 2*.

Ayalon, O., & Levi Segev, R. (1986). *Hand in hand* (3rd ed.). Haifa: Nord Publications. (In Hebrew)

Ayalon, O., & Soskis, D. (1986). Survivors of terrorism: A follow-up. In N. Milgram (Ed.), *Stress and coping in time of war*. New York: Brunner/Mazel.

Ayalon, O., & Lahad, M. (1990). *Life on the edge*. (In Hebrew)

Ayalon, O., & Flasher, A. (1993). *Chain reaction—Children and divorce*. London: Jessica Kingsley Publishers.

Bastians, J. (1982). Consequences of modern terrorism. In L. Goldberg & S. Breznitz (Eds.), *Handbook of stress*. New York: Free Press.

Ben-Eli, Z., & Sella, M. (1980). Terrorists in Nahariya. *Journal of Psychology and Counselling in Education, 13*, 94–101. (In Hebrew)

Bettelheim, B. (1979). *Surviving and other essays*. New York: Knopf.

Caplan, G. (1964). *Principles of preventive psychiatry*. New York: Basic Books.

Caplan, G. (1974). *Support system and community mental health*. New York: Behavioral Publications.

Dasberg, J. (1985). *Trauma in Israel*. Paper presented to the Sinai Center Symposium on Trauma and Society, Amersfoort.

Eitinger, L. (1983). Jewish concentration-camp survivors. In A. Ayalon, L. Eitinger, J. Lansen, A. Sunier, *et al.* (Eds.), *The Holocaust and its perseverance*. Netherlands: Van Gorcum.

Fields, R. (1980). Victims of terrorism: The effects of prolonged stress. *Evaluation and Change*, pp. 76–83.

Fields, R. (1982). Research on the victims of terrorism. In F. Ochberg, D. Soskis (Eds.), *Victims of terrorism* (pp. 137–171). Boulder: Westview.

Figley, C. (Ed.). (1978). *Stress disorders among Vietnam veterans*. New York: Brunner/Mazel.

Figley, C. (Ed.). (1985). *Trauma and its wake* (Vol. 1). New York: Brunner/Mazel.

Fraser, M. (1977). *Children in conflict*. New York: Basic Books.

Frederick, C. J. (1987). Psychic trauma in victims of crime and terrorism. In G. T. VandenBos & B. K. Bryant (Eds.), *Cataclysm, crises and catastrophes* (pp. 59–108). New York: American Psychological Association.

Freud, S. (1950). One problem of anxiety. In *Collected papers* (Vol. 5). London: Hogarth Press.

Gal, P. (1980). *Psychic trauma and support systems*. Unpublished masters thesis, Tel-Aviv University.

Golan, A. (1979). *The hostage city*. Tel Aviv: ZBM. (In Hebrew)

Horowitz, M. J. (1986). *Stress response syndromes* (2nd ed.). New York: Jason Aronson.

Jacobson, S. (1973). Individual and group responses to confinement in a sky-jacked plane. *American Journal of Orthopsychiatry, 43*, 459–469.

Janis, I. (1971). *Stress and frustration*. New York: Harcourt, Brace, Jovanovich.

Jenkins, B. (1978). Rand research on terrorism. *Terrorism, 1*, 85–95.

Klingman, A. (1980). Discussing death in the classroom through literature. eds. In A. Raviv, A. Klingman, & M. Horowitz (Eds.), *Children under stress and in crisis* (pp. 260–263). Tel Aviv: Otzar Hamoreh. (In Hebrew)

Klingman, A., & Ayalon, O. (1980). Primary intervention: A model for coping with stress in the school-system. In A. Raviv, A. Klingman, & M. Horowitz (Eds.), *Children under stress and in crisis* (pp. 192–211). Tel Aviv: Otzar Hamoreh. (In Hebrew)

Krystal, H. (Ed.). (1968). *Massive psychic trauma*. New York: International Universities Press.

Krystal, H. (1984). Psychoanalytical views on human emotional damages. In B. van der Kolk (Ed.), *Posttraumatic stress disorders: Psychological and biological sequelae*. Washington: American Psychiatric Press.

Lahad, S. (1981). *The preparation of teachers and pupils for coping with stress situations*. Unpublished masters thesis, Jerusalem, Hebrew University. (In Hebrew)

Lahad, S. (1982). *Nobody is alone*. Kiryat-Shmona: Center for Emergency Situations. (In Hebrew)

Lahad, S. (1984). *Evaluation of a multi-modal program to strengthen the coping of children and teachers under stress of shelling*. Unpublished doctoral thesis, Columbia Pacific University.

Lahad, S. (1986). *Newsletter*. Kiryat-Shmona: Center for Emergency Situations. (In Hebrew)

Lazarus, R. (1966). *Psychological stress and the coping process*. New York: McGraw-Hill.

Lifton, R. J. (1967). *Death in life*. New York: Random House.

Marx, E. (1970). Violence of individuals in development towns. *Megamot, 17*(1), 61–67. (In Hebrew)

Meichenbaum, D. (1977). *Cognitive-behavior modification*. New York: Plenum Press.

NOVA. (1983). *Victim rights and services*. Washington DC: National Organization for Victim Assistance.

Ochberg, F. (1978). The victim of terrorism: Psychiatric consideration. *Terrorism: An International Journal, 1*(2), 147–167.

Ochberg, F. (1982). A case study: Gerard Vaders. In F. Ochberg & D. Soskis (Eds.), *Victims of terrorism* (pp. 9–38). Boulder: Westview.

Ophir, M. (1980). Simulation games as treatment of situational anxiety. In A. Raviv, A. Klingman, & M. Horowitz (Eds.), *Children under stress and in crisis*. Tel Aviv: Otzar-Hamoreh. (In Hebrew)

Raphael, B. (1986). *When disaster strikes*. London: Hutchinson.

Segal, J. (1974). *Long-term psychological and physical effects of the POW rxperience*. (Report 74–2). Washington, DC: Bureau of Medicine and Surgery, Department of the Navy.

Seligman, M. (1975). *Helplessness: On depression, development and death*. San Francisco: W. H. Freeman.

Shreiber, J. (1978). *The ultimate weapon*. New York: William Morrow.

Samooha, S., & Peres, Y. (1974). Ethnic inequality in Israel. *Megamot, 20*, 4–42. (In Hebrew)

Social Security (1974). *Report on treatment of Ma'alot children*. Jerusalem: Welfare Ministry. (In Hebrew)

Soskis, D., & Ayalon, O. (1985). A six-year follow-up of hostage victims. *Terrorism: An International Journal, 7*(4), 411–415.

Speck, R., & Atteneave, C. (1974). *Family networks*. New York: Basic Books.

Strenz, T. (1982). The Stockholm Syndrome. In F. Ochberg & D. Soskis (Eds.), *Victims of terrorism* (pp. 149–164). Boulder: Westview.

Symonds, M. (1980). The second injury to victims of violent crimes. *Educational and change*, pp. 36–38.

Terr, L. (1983). Chowchilla revisited: The effects of psychic trauma four years after a school-bus kidnapping. *American Journal of Psychology, 140*, 1543–1550.

Tinklenberg, J. (1982). Coping with terrorist victimization. In F. Ochberg & D. Soskis (Eds.), *Victims of terrorism* (pp. 59–72). Boulder: Westview Press.

Trimble, M. (1985). Posttraumatic stress disorder: History of a concept. In C. R. Figley (Ed.), *Trauma and its wake*. New York: Brunner/Mazel.

Vaders, G. (1976). *Strangers on a train: The diary of a hostage*. Netherlands.

Wilson, J. (1980). Conflict, stress and growth. In C. R. Figley & S. Leventman (Eds.), *Strangers at home*. New York: Brunner/Mazel.

Zafrir, A. (1982). Community therapeutic intervention in the treatment of civilian victims after a major terrorist attack. In C. Spielberger, I. Sarason, & N. Milgram (Eds.), *Stress and anxiety* (pp. 303–315). Washington: Hemisphere.

Zuckerman-Bareli, H. (1979). Effects of border tensions on residents of an Israeli town. *Journal of Human Stress, 9*, 29–40.

CHAPTER 73

A 12-Step Recovery Program for Victims of Traumatic Events

Joel Osler Brende

Introduction

On June 9, 1985, a twin-engine airplane crash-landed on a small airport runway 20 miles short of the Dallas-Fort Worth airport. The nine passengers were staff members and wives from the First Baptist Church of Indian Rocks in Largo, Florida, and were enroute to a church convention. The pilot, also a member of the same church, was an experienced commercial pilot. Ten minutes before their nonstop flight was scheduled to land, it became apparent to the pilot and passengers that they would run out of fuel.

Within a few minutes, they did, shortly after the pilot made radio contact with a small nearby airport and was cleared to make an emergency landing. As the two engines abruptly stopped running 3 minutes short of the landing strip, all passengers sat in eerie silence, praying intensely, some silently, some softly. The passengers who dared to look could see the onrush of treetops rising toward them below. The pilot, gliding the plane without power, was able to land on the runway but unable to lower the hydraulically operated landing gear.

With a sudden jarring impact and sparks flying, the plane skidded and bounced on concrete and stopped on the grassy downslope on the runway's far end. The first man out of the small rear door was the church minister who was the last man to board the plane 5 hours earlier while he jokingly remarked, "This door is impossible to open. I hope you won't ever expect me to open it." Later

he reported no recollection of how he got the door open so quickly. None of the passengers nor the pilot were injured as they followed him out and quickly ran for safety from the stricken aircraft which neither burned nor exploded.

Observers within the control tower told them later that they had expected a much worse outcome since this was the first crash landing at that airport without fatalities.

Following 4 days of attending their church conference, the 9 passengers and the pilot all flew back to Florida together by commercial jet. One of them had posttraumatic phobic symptoms about flying and found it difficult to fly for at least a year. One year later, the pilot continued to have guilt feelings about running short of fuel, although he had been exonerated several months after the accident when FAA officials discovered an error in the operating manual's description of fuel consumption.

In spite of the fact that these 10 individuals experienced "a stressful event outside of the range of usual human experience" (DSM-III-R) they did not suffer from posttraumatic disorder as defined in the diagnostic manual of the American Psychiatric Association: (1) persistent reexperiencing of the traumatic event in thought, imagery, and behavior; (2) persistent avoidance of stimuli linked concretely or symbolically with the trauma or numbing of general emotional reactivity; (3) symptoms of increased arousal, hypervigilance, startle reactions, and the like (American Psychiatric Association, 1987).

The absence of symptoms in these 10 survivors can be ascribed to such factors as: there were no fatalities and no survival guilt. All the survivors provided mutual support as they shared their feelings with each other. Clearly, they shared a common religious belief system and sense of purpose.

Other nontraditional factors that were important included the survivors' common belief in God, their capacity to surrender to His purpose, their belief in His

Joel Osler Brende • Martin Army Community Hospital, Fort Benning, Georgia 31905; Adult Outpatient Services, The Bradley Center, Inc., Columbus, Georgia 31907; and Department of Psychiatry, Mercer School of Medicine, Macon, Georgia 31206.

International Handbook of Traumatic Stress Syndromes, edited by John P. Wilson and Beverley Raphael. Plenum Press, New York, 1993.

protection, and their communication with Him in prayer.

The survivors of the airplane crash described the reasons they responded so positively and rapidly from its effects, summarized as follows:

1. *Power and protection*. The survivors all believed in and prayed to a personal God. Since they were Christians, their belief also included a sense of ongoing prayerful contact with Jesus Christ and a belief that He had power to intervene in their lives.

2. *Meaning*: The survivors each had a strong sense that there was a meaning why the accident occurred, which provided a foundation for greater emotional and spiritual strength following the accident.

3. *Trust*: The survivors shared a common belief that they could trust God and surrender themselves to His guidance and protection.

4. *Sharing*: The survivors were able to share openly their feelings, thoughts, and reactions to the accident together and with other members of the church community immediately after the accident and on many occasions in the future. There was no secretiveness or shame.

5. *Anger*: Some of the survivors felt angry at the pilot for running out of fuel; however, these feelings were only short-lived as the passengers were very supportive of him later.

6. *Fear*: Their belief in the protective power of God enabled them to be free of any persistent fear, although one survivor developed phobic symptoms of flying which lasted about a year.

7. *Guilt*: Only the pilot experienced guilt, and he found relief by talking with the other passengers and by praying.

8. *Grief*: There were no lives lost and no grief.

9. *Self-destructive wishes*: There were no persistent negative emotions and no depressive or self-destructive symptoms.

10. *Bitterness*: All survivors believed strongly in forgiveness and there was no bitterness or hatred.

11. *Purpose*: The shared survival experience provided a foundation for a greater sense of purpose in their work.

12. *Relationships*: The shared survival experience enhanced their relationships with each other and provided a basis for more empathy and understanding for others who had suffered traumatic experiences.

These 12 themes coincided with my 12 theme and step recovery program that was developed for combat veterans (Brende & McDonald, 1988, 1989; Sorenson, 1985) and later expanded to include 12 groups of posttraumatic symptoms.

These 12 themes also provided a model from which I have built a nontraditional recovery program for survivors of posttraumatic stress disorder (PTSD), to be described later in this chapter. This 12-step program of stress recovery builds on the tradition of self-help support groups and can be readily applied by individuals who may not be able to access traditional mental health systems or who would prefer such an alternative approach to alleviating the painful symptoms associated with traumatic stress syndrome.

Posttraumatic Symptoms, Recovery, and Religious Beliefs

The survivors of this accident did not require or seek professional help. Nor would they have likely to have sought help from professionals who did not strongly adhere to Christian teachings similar to their own. Yet other trauma survivors with differing religious beliefs or cultures may seek mental health care from professionals who do not understand or believe as they do. Health care professionals and "healers" attempting to aid patients whose cultural or religious beliefs are different from their own should learn the importance of understanding other religious and cultural backgrounds.

Cross-Cultural and Pantheistic Views of Stress Recovery

Some medical professionals working with the Asian population in California have learned to incorporate indigenous healing practices into their treatment practices (including providing acupuncture along with psychotherapy and medication) for Asians with emotional problems (Kinzie, 1989; Lee & Lu, 1989, p. 111).

The religious belief system of Native Americans has been incorporated successfully into a healing program for PTSD. Their healing ritual has been found to be helpful for Vietnam combat veterans: it has been called the *Sweat Lodge Ceremony*, which is led by the tribal medicine man, and is essentially a purification rite where all of the participants feel that they "grow stronger by praying and overcoming pain and suffering together" (Silver & Wilson, 1988; Wilson, 1989).

When individuals believe that spirits can cause symptoms, they will seek "healers" who have awareness and power over these supernatural spirits. In their study of folk beliefs in Laos, Westermeyer and Wintrob (1979) found that those who suffered from emotional and mental disorders believed such disorders were caused by supernatural or spiritual events.

Similarly, a number of Christians believe that demonic spirit possession is responsible for mental illness and will seek the help of a minister or healer who also believes and has the power to exorcise these spirits.

Refugees from Asian countries may prefer to visit their own native folk healers who believe, as they do, that their problems could have been caused by an offense against deities or spirits (Lee & Lu, 1989). Cambodian and other Asian refugees who left behind their Buddhist monks and religious rituals, feel that they have lost power over or cooperation with the unseen spirits they previously communicated with in their native land. This may be one reason that Southeast Asian refugees, after losing touch with their religious heritage, have more difficulty coping with grief and loss (Kinzie, 1989).

Within the eastern religions there is a belief that one's existence does not cease upon physical death and follows the principle of Karma (Mollica, 1988). Consequently, those who expect that their Karmic future will result in a more positive outcome are not likely to fear death. Within the theory of transmigration, for example, the Hindu soul is believed to pass through a series of births. Thus the Hindu's existence is only one manifestation of universal animation. As a result, Hindus are likely to "surrender" themselves to the inevitabilities of life, including death.

Many Asians, particularly those who follow Buddhist teachings, are often able to deal with stress quite well. But many Westerners who are unfamiliar with the concept of "accepting fate" will find it hard to understand these Buddhist teachings

> that catastrophe and suffering are a normal part of existence . . . and that [Cambodian survivors] accept and deal with terrible events as gracefully as possible and try to find meaning in them. The Chinese proverb "the best plan is made in heaven," the Japanese expression called Gaman ("just patiently enduring it") and Shikatajanai ("it can't be helped, nothing can be done about it") sum up a philosophy of life which has helped survivors to accept adversity willingly. (Lee & Lu, 1989, p. 101)

Since Asians often believe that personal misfortune is inevitable, and that suffering may be caused by misdeeds from a previous life, they hope that their death and reincarnation will provide them with a better outcome in the future.

Cambodian refugees, frequently Buddhists, have been seen to suffer from the "dark side" of this philosophy. They believe that

> the atrocities [committed in Cambodia are] a national shame. . . . [They believe that they] must have done something very bad in the past to deserve this kind of punishment. The group shame and the traditional acceptance of life as it is have made it difficult for refugees to speak of events in Cambodia. (Kinzie, 1989, p. 77)

Many Cambodian survivors believe that the civil war was perhaps the result of previous dishonorable events in Cambodian history and therefore Cambodians must experience shame and suffering on behalf of the whole nation (Kinzie *et al.*, 1989).

Upon reading the "holy books" of major religions, the reader will find numerous accounts of human suffering and subsequent attempts of find meaning and purpose from traumatic experiences. Trauma is found in the past and current history of the three major religions of Judaism, Islam, and Christianity, all of whom claim to be descendants of Abraham (Juri, 1946). The earliest reported traumatic events began with Adam and Eve's expulsion from a perfect relationship with God in the garden of Eden. They suffered posttraumatic symptoms including meaninglessness, shame, distrust, physical pain, anger, fear, guilt, and grief (Gen. 3:7–19). It is recorded that from that time on, beginning with murder in the next generation and for nine generations, the people suffered major destructive and self-destructive symptoms, becoming "corrupt before God, and the earth was filled with violence" (Gen. 6:11). This led to the single worst natural recorded disaster—a major flood which only Noah and his family survived but with no reports of symptoms (Gen. 7:20).

Principles of Recovery and Religious Belief

In this section an attempt will be made to delineate some of the major principles of recovery that emanate from a study of cross-cultural and theistic views of personal integration and transcendence of unusually stressful life events. Among these time-honored principles are such concepts as surrender, letting-go, strength through acceptance of vulnerability, limits to responsibility, and personal control of actions and choices. Although many examples and illustrations will be cited from Christian principles and beliefs, most, if not all, of the principles of recovery can be found in the other major religions in the world as well.

Faith and Surrender

During Abraham's life, 10 generations after Noah, his nephew Lot survived the destruction of Sodom and Gomorrah (Gen. 19:13–29). Abraham is noted for his faith in God, which was tested when he nearly sacrificed his son in blind obedience to God's request until an angel intervened and brought Abraham an animal to sacrifice instead (Gen. 22:1–13). God honored Abraham's willingness to surrender his son and made a promise to him and his descendants that the future would look better because of it.

> "By Myself I have sworn," says the Lord, "because you have done this thing, and have not withheld your son, your only son, in blessing I will bless you, and in multiplying I will multiply your descendants as the stars of the heaven and as the sand which is on the seashore; and your descendants shall possess the gate of their enemies. In your seed all the nations of the earth shall be blessed, because you have obeyed my voice." (Gen. 23:16–18)

The principle of blind faith and surrender to the will of God is a major teaching within most religions of the world, Muhammad, in A.D. 610 preached a message of submission and surrender to the will of God [Allah] and founded Islam, one of the three religions where the believers, now comprising an approximate one eighth of the world's population, believe in a single God (Juri, 1946).

Christians hold to a similar belief in the importance of surrender to the will of God, the example of total submission unto His death by crucifixion provided by Jesus Christ, the son of God (Luke 24:7). The reported examples in the New Testament include a willingness by believers to surrender to the will of God in the fact of beatings and imprisonment (Acts 16:37; 27:1–32), stoning and death (Acts 7:57–60). This surrender combined with faith can lead to transcendence of the situation at the spiritual level.

Buddhists believe in accepting life as it comes, including traumatic events. They follow the teachings of the prophet Buddha, who found freedom from the bondage of riches and power through surrender to a new life of service to the poor. Thus, by acting prosocially and altruistically, Buddha received enlightenment beyond his origin at birth.

Surrender in Recovery

The Native American Sioux Indian sweat lodge purification ritual is

> a religious event of thanksgiving and forgiveness led by a medicine man . . . [and] regarded as a serious occasion in which spiritual insights, personal growth, and physical healing may take place. The process of purification is physical, symbolic, and metaphysical. (Wilson, 1989, p. 265)

An attitude of surrender is important for those who choose to participate in this ritual. This attitude is manifested from the beginning of the ritual as participants crawl naked into the sweat lodge in an attitude of humility into a womblike tent and follow the spiritual guide's teachings.

> Through the guidance of the medicine man and the process of four rounds of prayer, the members emerge again from the interior of the womb with a profound sense of release, rebirth, and personal renewal of spirit. (Wilson, 1989, pp. 268–269)

The attitude of surrender during the sweat lodge enables the participants to move freely, sharing their feelings, memories, and fears, surrender their destructive thoughts and establish a bond with other participants while "each of the participants offers his or individual prayer, which often begins with the words 'Thank you, Grandfather/Grandmother' and ends with 'all my relations' ('Mitakuye oyasin')" (Wilson, 1989, p. 47).

The ceremony takes place primarily in darkness as the participants develop a strong spiritual and emotional bonding to one another as they share their pain and suffering. Finally, they leave the heat of the sweat lodge and emerge into the light and the cool air with a sense of cleansing and humility, offering prayer and a thank you as they look to the power of the spiritual leader for expectation and hope.

Role of Surrender in Recovery from Addictions

The psychiatrist Harry Tiebout contributed toward an understanding of the role of surrender for those who were recovering from alcohol addiction (Keller, 1985). "Having applied all of his analytic concepts, approaches, and experience to his treatment of alcoholism patients, he completely failed to help them recover" (Keller, 1985, p. 34).

Then Tiebout discovered that one of his alcoholic patients made a basic change in her attitude and behavior somewhat unexpectedly and began to recover. When he asked her what she had done, she said she had "surrendered." Only after she had done this did she discover any hope for herself. Tiebout concluded that what she had surrendered was her sense of *omnipotence* and *egocentricity* which had covered over her emotional pain and inadequacy.

Alcoholics Anonymous (AA) and similar 12-step programs for those addicted to drugs, food, sex, gambling, and the like, have helped hundreds of thousands of individuals. The 12 steps which provide the basis for these programs strongly emphasize the *principle of surrender*. Today, many individuals suffering from a variety of self-destructive patterns and addictions have found hope by gaining freedom from their own unique victimization patterns by following the principles of the 12-step programs.

Twelve-step programs, which began with Alcoholics Anonymous over 50 years ago and have followed a tradition of success since that time, are based on the following seven major principles: (1) recovering is often a life-long process; (2) education about the disorder is important for participants; (3) frequent attendance provides support and stability (sometimes 90 meetings in 90 days); (4) anonymity, intragroup support, and reaching out to others is important to maintain group participation; (5) accepting one's powerlessness and surrendering to a higher power is the first principle for recovery; (6) continued self-inventory is a basis for introspection, change, and personality growth; and (7) the 12 spiritual steps are the core principles for recovery, including surrender to a "higher power" (God as individually understood).

The 12 Steps of Alcoholics Anonymous: Parallels for Stress Recovery

- Step 1: We admitted we were powerless over alcohol—that our lives had become unmanageable.
- Step 2: Came to believe that a Power greater than ourselves could restore us to sanity.
- Step 3: Made a decision to turn our will and our lives over to the care of God as we understood Him.
- Step 4: Made a searching and fearless moral inventory of ourselves.
- Step 5: Admitted to God, to ourselves, and to another human being, the exact nature of our wrongs.
- Step 6: Were entirely ready to have God remove all these defects of character.
- Step 7: Humbly asked Him to remove our shortcomings.
- Step 8: Made a list of all persons we had harmed, and became willing to make amends to all of them.
- Step 9: Made direct amends to such people whenever possible, except when to do so would injure them or others.
- Step 10: Continued to take personal inventory and when we were wrong promptly admitted it.
- Step 11: Sought through prayer and meditation to improve our conscious contact with God as we understood Him, praying only for knowledge of His will for us and the power to carry that out.
- Step 12: Having had a spiritual awakening as the result of these steps, we tried to carry this message to alcoholics, and to practice these principles in all our affairs.

Twelve-Step Recovery Program for Victims of Trauma

Like addicts, trauma victims may suffer repetitive victimization symptoms and/or behavior patterns (van der Kolk, 1987). Frequently, these are manifested by cyclic experiences of powerless victimization alternating with omnipotent defensive behaviors. Like addicts, trauma victims may begin their recovery when they are willing to surrender the omnipotence, denial, and egocentricity which covers their emotional pain and powerlessness.

Recognizing the impact that 12-step recovery programs have had on the lives of alcoholics and addicts, I developed a unique 12-step program in 1985 for Vietnam combat veterans suffering from chronic symptoms of PTSD that were unresponsive to lengthy durations of traditional treatment (Brende & McDonald, 1988). This 12-step program was based on the following 12 themes: (1) Power versus victimization, (2) Seeking meaning, (3) Trust versus shame and doubt, (4) Self-inventory, (5) Anger, (6) Fear, (7) Guilt, (8) Grief, (9) Suicide versus life, (10) Revenge versus forgiveness, (11) Finding purpose, and (12) Love and relationships.

The combat veterans who chose to participate in this program were asked to meet three times a week for 90-minute psychoeducational meetings, focusing on a single theme each week (i.e., for 12 weeks and 54 hours of counseling). During the first meeting, the group leader would initiate the discussion about the posttraumatic symptoms associated with the theme. During the second meeting, the leader would begin discussion about coping techniques for symptoms. The spiritual step was introduced during the third weekly meeting.

Approximately 200 veterans who participated in the psychoeducational discussion groups that were based on these 12 themes gained improvement over their symptoms. For those who were motivated to continue the program over a 9-month period of time, improvement was significant. These men read the theme-related literature, voluntarily repeated the program two additional times, and continued to meet in a separate "Combat Veterans Anonymous" group, using the spiritual steps based on the 12 themes (Sorenson, 1985).

Trauma Survivors Anonymous: A Program for Recovering Survivors

I have since developed a similar program for survivors of a variety of different traumatic experiences. This program is also based to some extent on the 12-step recovery model and emphasizes the principle of surrender.

The 12-step program for survivors, which has been named *Trauma Survivors Anonymous* (TSA), is based on the following principles:

1. Recovery is considered an ongoing, often lifelong, process and participants should be encouraged to take "one day at a time."
2. The spiritual dimension, including recognition of and surrender to a "Good Higher Power" or God, as individually understood, is the core of the program.
3. Self-inventory and acknowledgment of symptoms, shortcomings, and destructive behavior are a basis for personal growth.
4. Group leadership is emphasized, yet should come from the membership of the group. For best re-

sults, leaders should receive training but, as the group continues, leaders can be rotated within the group membership.
5. Education about posttraumatic symptoms is important for all participants. Instruction about one of the 12 posttraumatic recovery themes can be a part of each meeting. Twelve theme and step literature is also available for participants.
6. Anonymity, confidentiality, and sharing are important for the life of the group. Open sharing of experiences with other group members is encouraged, and confidentiality is expected. Yet sharing emotionally painful memories is not expected unless participants have developed adequate trust.
7. There are no restrictions on participants' involvement in traditional therapy or other helpful activities. In fact, these are encouraged.
8. Attendance at frequent group meetings or other kinds of helpful activities are important for survivors to sustain recovery and prevent relapse.
9. Hope is very important. Survivors need help from other participants within the group to believe that they will find relief from emotional pain. Although participants will often share painful traumatic experiences, this must only take place in an atmosphere of protection, caring, and hope. Meetings should be structured so that they end on a positive theme.
10. Some participants may benefit if they focus extra time on certain significant steps that present major problems for them. For example, some survivors may need to give extra time to Step 7: resolution of guilt or to Step 8: Resolution of grief, or to Step 10: Resolution of revengeful thoughts. In these cases, they would benefit from additional counseling or the help of a sponsor.
11. In general, each of the 12 steps is designed to follow the one before it. For best results, participants who feel blocked in their recovery should review earlier steps and build upon a foundation of successful completion of pertinent earlier steps.
12. The "12th-step work" for recovering survivors is very important. Not only should participants help one another during and between meetings, but should also reach out to help other survivors needing help. Experienced group members are encouraged to become sponsors for other participants (of the same sex), to provide emotional support, encouragement, and guide them toward taking action needed to break victimization cycles.

Participants are encouraged to follow the principles described for each of these 12 steps, which will help them to break the victimization cycle, as follows: (1) *Acknowledge* the problem or symptom which is causing victimization; (2) *Seek help*; (3) *Surrender* the problem to God, as individually understood; (4) *Take action*; and (5) *Pray daily*.

Although these 12 steps can be followed without the help of a group, they are most helpful within a group setting. To structure individual meetings, it is suggested that the leader begin by introducing new group members, then give a brief explanation of the 12 themes and steps after which he or she may choose or ask the group to select a specific step to focus on during the meeting. In order to facilitate discussion, different participants may be asked to read aloud from the available step literature, including the four items pertaining to breaking the victimization cycle listed in above. To close the meeting, the participants should read the appropriate daily prayer together as a group.

Twelve Themes and Spiritual Steps: A Practical Guide for Survivors of Traumatic Events

What follows is an outline to be used as a guide to help the stress-recovery program. All the steps are important, but certain ones will apply more specifically than others. If you are a group participant or a group leader, focus on any one of the 12 steps or proceed through the steps in sequential order as your group meets together.

If you have been in other anonymous 12-step programs, these steps are meant to supplement those programs and not replace them. If you are receiving spiritual help, psychotherapy, or counseling, please use the steps as an adjunct to that process. As you take each of the 12 steps, practice breaking the victimization cycle each time, by acknowledging the symptom, seeking help, surrendering the problem to God or a higher being taking action, and praying each day.

Twelve Themes toward Posttraumatic Recovery: Healing

In the sections that follow, twelve themes are present toward recovery from posttraumatic stress problems. These 12 steps have been developed by me during my work in the United States primarily in conjunction with helping Vietnam veterans who were suffering with PTSD. Individuals in different cultures and countries (e.g., non-Western countries) may wish to adapt these themes in more culture-specific ways that are congruent with the experiences of those traumatized in many different ways (e.g., starvation, torture, rape, political persecution, earthquakes, and natural disasters).

Step 1: Power versus Victimization

"We admitted we were powerless over victimization and sought the help of a Good Higher Power (God, as individually understood), to gain power in our lives."

This step focuses on understanding and finding ways to gain power over victimization from our posttraumatic symptoms—meaninglessness, self-doubt and shame, uncontrollable angry outbursts, recurring memories and dreams, frightening dreams, night terrors, panic, violent and suicidal thoughts, and isolation from people; or the use of power in destructive ways, including abusing, defrauding, or victimizing individuals, families, groups, or organizations.

As victims, we recognize that the ways we have attempted to protect or defend ourselves from victimization have often been ineffective or self-destructive, and include isolation, emotional numbing, avoidance, aggressive retaliation, or abuse of others. Unfortunately, these ways merely perpetuate a cycle of victimization. We can begin to break our self-destructive victimization cycle in the following ways:

Acknowledge that we are powerless to control many or all of our posttraumatic symptoms, protect or defend ourselves adequately from abusive or destructive forces that attempt to control our lives, or control our own destructive use of power.

Seek help from a Good Higher Power—individuals, organizations, and God, as individually understood.

Surrender our symptoms and destructive uses of power—to God, as individually understood.

Take action by asking for help from individuals, organizations, and God to intervene in our destructive behaviors and regain power in our lives.

DAILY PRAYER

God, help me to accept that I have little or no power over symptoms of victimization and destructive behaviors. Help me to recognize which of these I can begin to change. Grant me the wisdom to know the difference.

Step 2: Seeking Meaning

"Came to believe that a power greater than ourselves could help us find meaning."

This step is focused on beginning to seek meaning after surviving a traumatic experience or suffering the loss of the lives of others. It is very difficult to imagine that meaning can be found, but to begin the search means sharing our experiences with others, accepting their support and understanding, and listening to those who may have found meaning in their own traumatic experiences. We can begin to seek meaning in the following ways:

Acknowledge that it is difficult, if not impossible, to accept what has happened to us and to find meaning from the traumatic event and in surviving, particularly if others were injured or lost their lives.

Seek support, understanding and direction from God and others to help us begin to find meaning.

Surrender despair, confusion, and meaninglessness to God, as individually understood.

Take action by seeking answers from God, friends, and counselors; listen to the stories of other survivors who have survived in spite of their emotional pain and who have found meaning.

DAILY PRAYER

God, help me to seek for meaning out of tragedy; to seek for understanding why I am alive even though others' lives may have been lost. Grant me the courage to seek clarity rather than remain a prisoner of confusion, despair, and self-pity.

Step 3: Trust versus Shame and Doubt

"Burdened with distrust, shame, and doubt, we made a decision to seek the help of God, as we understood Him, in order to learn to trust."

This step focuses on helping us regain our capacity to trust selected others, those who want to help us, God, and ourselves. As victims, we may have lost our capacity to trust, even to trust those who have wanted to help us. We may have been abandoned or betrayed by those who should have protected us. And we may have trusted out of blind faith. We may continue to seek someone we can trust, even if we were repeatedly abused or misused in the past. And we may not trust anyone but ourselves, and eventually may have found that we cannot even do that. We can begin to break the cycle of shame, doubt, and distrust in the following ways:

Acknowledge that we continue to experience shame, doubt, and distrust in ourselves and others.

Seek to gradually discover we can truly trust God and others who want to help us resolve shame, doubt, and distrust.

Surrender our shame, doubt, and distrust to God.

Take action by putting trust to the test in God, friends, and counselors.

DAILY PRAYER

God, grant me an understanding of the shame and doubt that lies behind my false pride. Teach me how to trust. Grant me the courage to take the risks necessary to trust, gain freedom from shame, and overcome self-doubt.

Step 4: Self-Inventory

"Admitted to ourselves, another human being, and to God, our faults, and sought His help to accept our positive traits and change our negative ones."

As survivors we may have thought of ourselves as unable to survive unless we are able to master frightening situations, save others, or defeat our enemies. As victims of traumatic events, we may repeat patterns that, because of our survival instincts, cause us to repeatedly relive victimization experiences. We may suffer repeated victimization or self-destructive patterns of behavior as a means of self-punishment because of hidden traumatic secrets we would be ashamed to reveal to ourselves or others. A personal inventory can help us discover the truth about ourselves—about hidden destructive or self-destructive life-styles or ways in which we may hurt others, hurt ourselves, or destroy relationships. If we are open to listening, a group feedback session can provide us with more truth about ourselves, enhance trust and self-esteem, and help us to more easily accept our good qualities and change those which are negative. We can begin a self-inventory in the following ways:

Acknowledge that we often do not accept our positive traits and find it difficult to change negative ones; that we are sometimes guilty of doing self-destructive things, hurting others, breaking relationships, punishing ourselves, and keeping shameful secrets.

Seek to be free from self-destructive or destructive behaviors, shameful secrets, and self-condemning attitudes; to be open-minded to positive and constructive criticism.

Surrender our self-destructive behaviors, our shameful secrets, our resistances to receiving help and constructive criticism from others.

Take action by being open to change and ask for feedback from God, friends, and counselors in order that we can learn more about ourselves. Then accept the positive and begin to change the negative.

DAILY PRAYER

God, help me to accept my positive traits, change those traits which continue to hurt myself or others, and make amends to those I have harmed, when possible. Grant me the courage to accept the truth—both positive and negative—about myself in order that I can begin to "grow" toward a more accurate self-understanding.

Step 5: Anger

"Sought God's help to understand anger, control its destructiveness, and channel it in constructive ways."

Anger is a normal emotion for all people as they live life day-to-day. Anger and sometimes homicidal rage are likely to be normal responses to life-threatening events. In fact, for those who have been repeated survivors, anger may be an automatic response to any perceived threat, and anger and fear may have become opposite sides of the same coin. For some, anger has become a habitual response to danger instead of fear. In fact, for some survivors, anger has become a predominant emotion—a substitute, not only for fear but all other emotions, including guilt and grief. These individuals are not just survivors but are victims—of their own destructive and self-destructive anger.

Many of those who have suffered repeated traumatic experiences are now aware that their anger has become dangerously volatile. If we suffer from this, we must face the fact that anger may have become an uncontrollable and unmanageable problem causing frightening, destructive, and self-destructive consequences against property and people.

For those of us who have become afraid of expressing anger, we suffer from another problem, passivity and an inability to be assertive. In fact, we may not even be able to recognize that we are angry until it suddenly explodes destructively. We can begin to break the victimization cycle of anger in the following ways:

Acknowledge that we may be powerless to recognize normal angry emotions, control angry outbursts, or express anger constructively.

Seek help from God and others to control it or express it in constructive ways.

Surrender our destructive and self-destructive anger and the blocks that keep us from perceiving it to God.

Take action. Reduce excessive and pent-up anger by exercising and participating in healthy activities. Learn how to recognize suppressed anger. When anger is out of control, seek help from God, friends, and counselors to keep it from being destructive. Begin to learn to express anger normally, constructively, and directly in a calm manner. Learn to be assertive.

God help me to accept my anger as a normal emotion even though it may be suppressed or may erupt in destructive and self-destructive ways. Help me to control it when it is unmanageable and be more aware of it when it is suppressed from my awareness. Grant me the wisdom to know the difference between destructive and constructive anger.

Step 6: Fear

"Sought God's help to relinquish 'the wall' around our emotions and His protective presence during moments of terror and risk."

This step focuses on helping us understand and cope with fear. Fear is normal, even life-saving. But the terror that we may experience at times—both day and night—can be just as severe as the original trauma. Some of us may have the experience of reliving the terror again and again. Others may only experience the terror and panic but do not know why. Sometimes, this kind of repetitive fear can become so paralyzing that we are no longer able to function normally.

Some survivors who suffered repeated trauma learned to experience fear from an awareness and have come to believe they do not feel fear any longer. If this happened to us, we may have erected a "wall" around our emotions. If so, we suffer the consequences through isolation, distrust, and "numbing" of all our feelings. Yet, because fear remains hidden behind the wall, we can still suffer from phobic or panic attacks in certain situations that are reminders of the original trauma or of a time when we felt abandoned and unprotected.

If we continue to feel emotionally numb, we may seek the "adrenalin rush" that comes from taking dangerous risks in order to feel something. Unfortunately, we are likely to suffer other consequences from such repeated unhealthy risk-taking behavior. We can begin to break the victimization cycle of unresolved or blocked fear and emotions, as follows:

Acknowledge that fear is either excessively in control of our lives or completely suppressed so that we keep a "wall" around our emotions and may take dangerous risks in order to "feel" something.

Seek the help of God and others that we may be able to relinquish the 'wall' around our emotions; to learn to depend on God and others during terrifying emotions, dreams, and memories; and to learn how to take risks—but only in constructive ways.

Surrender the wall around our emotions and the terror and panic which prevents us from doing things we would like to do.

Take action by seeking help, beginning to let down the "wall," and learning that fear can be normal again. Discover that depending on God and others is a healthy thing to do. Begin to take risks, but only in positive ways. Face frightening situations with the help of God and others.

God, help me the fact that fear is a normal emotion but control that excessive fear which has controlled me.

Help me to relinquish the "wall" around my emotions. Grant me the wisdom to know the difference between normal fear and risk-taking and abnormal fear and risk-taking.

Step 7: Guilt

"Sought God's help to face Guilt, to make amends when possible, to accept His forgiveness, and to forgive ourselves."

In this theme, we will focus on understanding our guilt and to begin to find ways to gain relief from its destructive consequences. We may feel guilt but not know why. Guilt feelings can be unbearable if we suffer from repetitive horrifying or guilt-ridden thoughts, dreams, and images; or from persistent depression, physical illness, and suicidal wishes. There are a number of causes for trauma-related guilt. Survivor guilt can be pervasive and self-destructive, particularly when one or more persons were injured or died and we escaped.

Guilt may result from feeling responsible for the deaths, sufferings, or injuries to others, even though there may be different degrees or guilt, depending on whether the others were enemies, lawbreakers, or the innocent; and whether nor not we were directly or indirectly responsible.

Guilt also may result from witnessing violence or trauma. Guilt by association can result from being a party to destructive activities or by having knowledge of a "traumatic secret." Guilt and shame may be associated with having been abandoned or betrayed rather than protected, but not understanding why. Guilt and shame may result if we believe we should have had control over the traumatic event and believe we should be able to control our posttraumatic symptoms or behaviors. Guilt is painful. Automatically, we tend to find ways to keep from feeling it or being aware of it. We tend to prefer to feel numb from the pain or to avoid the price of emotional distress and remorse.

Guilt that remains unresolved, unforgiven, or "pushed underground" causes a deadening of emotional and spiritual sensitivity. If this happens, we may, at best, become calloused about the needs of others. At worst, we can become abusive, perverse, or antisocial. If this is the path we find ourselves on, eventually we will suffer the consequences and become victims of suffering, retaliation, arrest, or incarceration—enslaved by a victimization cycle fueled by unresolved guilt.

Unresolved guilt seeks resolution, either punishment or forgiveness. Our goal is to find resolution through forgiveness so that we can be freed from the burden of continued guilt or the bondage of calloused disregard for others. We can begin to find freedom from the victimization cycle of unresolved and unforgiven guilt as follows:

Acknowledge that excessive and unresolved guilt may cause callousness and disregard for others, victimization, suffering and self-punishment; that if we are caught in this cycle, we need help; that if we have been responsible for the injury, suffering or deaths of others, we seek resolution and forgiveness.

Seek freedom from self-destructive behaviors, guilty secrets, self-condemning attitudes, self-destructive symptoms, and a distorted or absent conscience; forgiveness from guilty acts wherein we have hurt others; and the capacity to forgive ourselves.

Surrender our self-destructive and destructive behaviors and our guilt secrets to God; our resistances to seeking forgiveness from others and from God; and our resistances to forgiving ourselves when we are assured of our forgiveness from God and others.

Take action by asking for help from God, friends, and counselors to find relief from irrational guilt. Accept forgiveness from God, seek the forgiveness of others we have wronged, when appropriate, and forgive ourselves.

DAILY PRAYER

God, forgive me for things I have done or failed to do, particularly if those things have led to the deaths or injury of others. Help me to regain my sensitivity and to make amends to those I have hurt, when possible. Grant me freedom from guilt, self-punishing symptoms, and destructive actions which have kept me in bondage.

Step 8: Grief

"Sought God's help to grieve those we have lost, face our painful memories and emotions, and let our tears heal our sorrows."

In this step, we will focus on being able to complete the grief process. Grieving is a normal response to loss: loss of a friend or loved one through death, loss of a relationship, loss of a job, loss of a pet, loss of health, loss of body parts, loss of country or community, loss of a leader, therapist, or even national figure, loss of values, loss of self-esteem, loss of innocence, loss of dignity, loss of ideals, loss of boundaries, and the sharing of someone else's loss.

As we grieve, we are likely to experience many different emotions or even a numbing of our emotions. We may be angry, depressed, crying, or overwhelmed with intrusive memories which cloud our thinking and block our ability to function normally. All these are normal responses to loss.

If we have not completed the grieving process, we remain victims, not only of our losses but of unresolved emotional pain: emotional numbing, unresolved grief, unresolved anger, unresolved guilt, painful reminders, and depression. We can be obsessed with thoughts about our losses or we can deny our grief. We can withdraw and avoid people and keep our relationships at an emotional distance by never depending on others; or we can become clinging and overpossessive.

It is important for us to understand that we should complete our "grief work," have emotions, say "goodbye" to whatever or whomever we have lost, and let our tears heal our emotional wounds. We can begin to break the victimization cycle of unresolved grief as follows:

Acknowledge that we may be emotionally blocked, unable to resolve feelings of guilt or anger, unable to grieve losses, fearful about being alone, and fearful of establishing close relationships once again.

Seek to be free from painful emotions associated with losses—anger, fear, guilt, grief; *to be free* from the fear of being alone, fear of close relationships, guilt related to the loss, obsessive thoughts about the lost person or parts of ourselves, and persistent unresolved grieving.

Surrender our persistent thoughts, memories, and painful emotions related to losses; our unresolved emotional numbing, anger, fear, guilt, and grief; our fear of relationships; our fear of being alone to God.

Take action by saying "goodbye" to those we have lost; let down the barrier; "feel" anger, guilt, sadness, and tears; take steps to resolve guilt; risk establishing close relationships once again—with help from God, friends, and counselors.

DAILY PRAYER

God help me to become aware of whom and what I have lost, to grieve my losses, change those attitudes and behaviors which keep me from making close relationships. Grant me the courage to learn the difference between "hanging on" from fear of loss and remembering out of reverence and love for whomever or whatever I have lost.

Step 9: Life versus Death

"Revealed to God and someone we trusted all remaining self-destructive wishes and, with His help, made a commitment to life."

This step focuses on helping us gain freedom from our self-destructive wishes and behavior; helping us face the hopelessness, guilt, or self-directed anger which blocks us from embracing life. Fear, guilt, grief, and rage were once normal responses to survival from traumatic events. However, these emotions, as they persist chronically, lead to depression, apathy, suicidal thoughts, suicide, or death from indirect methods. If suicide thoughts begin to provide a source of comfort, the risk of self-destruction is high now or in the future, particularly, if we keep a "suicide plan" in the backs of our minds.

How can we change this? It may not be easy; in fact, facing death may seem easier than facing life, particularly if we believe that we have a "just cause" that is worth dying for.

Remember that if we were to succeed in taking our own lives, we will have made a final decision without a second chance. And those who survive us will live with the guilt and pain of our death for the rest of their lives. Is that the legacy we want to leave them? Breaking the cycle of destructive, self-destructive, and suicidal anger can begin in the following ways:

Acknowledge that we are powerless to control our self-destructive and suicidal thoughts and feelings; that we may be contemplating suicide without full awareness of the pain that would remain for the survivors.

Seek help from God, family, friends, and counselors to resolve self-destructive thoughts and feelings, ways to find life worth living, and courage to make a commitment to life.

Surrender self-destructive and suicidal thoughts, feelings, and plans to God.

Take action by asking for help from God, friends, and counselors and talking about it with someone you trust. Replace your suicidal plans and death wishes with a commitment to life and find positive thoughts, activities, and relationships to focus on.

DAILY PRAYER

God, help me to surrender my self-destructive and suicidal thoughts to You and to make a commitment to life. Grant me the courage to learn the difference between surrendering my life from motives of selflessness and love, and taking my life because of self-centeredness and hatred.

Step 10: Justice versus Revenge

"Sought God's help to pursue the cause of justice, to gain freedom from revengeful wishes and plans, and for a desire to be channels of God's forgiveness to those we once hated."

This step focuses on helping us gain freedom from our destructive wishes for revenge and face the hatred, bitterness, and relentless anger which victimizes us and blocks us from achieving true justice. As victims, our homicidal rage has been a normal reaction to feeling victimized, betrayed, abandoned, or losing the health or lives of our friends or family. And it may seem impossible to forgive those who were responsible, because hating is easier than living in peace and love, particularly if life has no other purpose beyond achieving "vengeance."

There is a difference between achieving justice and revenge. Justice is the basis for love, peace, and freedom—for ourselves and those we live with. Revenge, although bringing temporary relief, ultimately becomes a basis for repetitive hatred, destruction, and war. Revenge feeds upon itself and causes destructive consequences, further victimization, and bondage. If our hatred persists, we can bring our friends, families, and country into bondage with us. Revenge breeds only destructive consequences that can easily get out of control—an enormous price for ourselves, our friends, and family to pay.

If we have violent thoughts, if those thoughts are buried within our minds, if we have a mental "blueprint" to kill someone, if our hatred has become dangerous to others and to ourselves, we need help. Breaking the victimization cycle of bitterness, violence, and revenge can begin in the following ways:

Acknowledge that we are powerless to control our hatred, revengeful thoughts, and bitterness which only victimizes us, our friends, and our family; that bitterness and hatred may lie deep within us, and even though not fully aware, we hurt our friends and families.

Seek help from God and others to be aware of the presence of hatred and understand the reasons for it; help to control destructive thoughts and feelings; help to find avenues to achieve justice rather than revenge.

Surrender our hatred, our destructive and revengeful thoughts, feelings, and plans to God.

Take action by asking for help from God, friends, and counselors. "Let go of" revengeful wishes and plans and replace them with a commitment to seek justice for those who have been wronged. Seek God's forgiveness through us to those we have hated.

DAILY PRAYER

God, help me to surrender my destructive and revengeful thoughts and plans to You and to seek Your justice for those who are abusers or violators. Grant me the courage to know the difference between justice and revenge, and to be a channel for Your forgiveness to those I have once hated.

Step 11: Finding a Purpose

"Sought knowledge and direction from God and surrendered ourselves to His leadership in order to find a renewed purpose for our lives."

This step focuses on helping us find a purpose for our lives. As victims, our lives were once seemed meaningless. But as we have progressed through the first 10 steps, we have begun to discover freedom from the victimization of meaninglessness, distrust, shame, rage, terror, guilt, grief, suicidal desires, hatred, and isolation. Paradoxically, this freedom, results from acknowledging, seeking, surrendering, and taking action to change old self-destructive "baggage" that we have carried with us for years. Now that we have surrendered all of our "baggage," there is nothing else to surrender but ourselves, which is the next step toward finding a purpose for our lives:

Acknowledge that periodically we slip back into the bondage of meaninglessness, victimization patterns, distrust, shame, rage, terror, guilt, grief, suicidal desires, hatred, and isolation; that when this happens we find it difficult to believe there is a purpose for our lives.

Seek to "let go of" the baggage of posttraumatic symptoms and find a new sense of purpose; to find a new relationship to God.

Surrender not only our posttraumatic baggage but also ourselves to God's leadership and purpose for us.

Take action by talking to others who can help us discover ourselves. Daily renew a commitment to seek God's purpose in our lives. Renew our spiritual strength through uplifting words, thoughts, readings, friends, and activities.

DAILY PRAYER

God, renew me as I surrender myself to You and seek Your purpose for my life today. Lead me on a creative and fulfilling path. Grant me the courage to know the difference between my seemingly fulfilling but self-centered way and Your way, a path not easily followed, of selflessness, justice, truth, and love.

Step 12: Love and Relationships

"Sought God's love in our lives, renewed our commitment to friends and family, loved those we found difficult to love, and helped those who have been victims os we once were."

This step focuses on helping us remain free from self-centeredness and tendencies to slip back into meaningless victimization experiences through learning to love and help others.

Having had a spiritual awakening as a result of these first 11 steps, we will find that it is important to practice these principles with others. But we may still have some blocks which prevent us from helping others or accepting and giving love. Thus, it is important to remove any blocks that prevent us from accepting the love of God, friends, and family.

To build a foundation of loving relationships, it is important to understand and open ourselves to God's love; to renew our commitment to those friends and family whose love we have taken for granted; and to renew the vitality of love and friendships which had died from neglect. With this foundation we can be open to building new friendships—practicing what it means to give and receive. With an attitude of love, we can then carry the recovery message to other survivors and victims who are mired in the bondage of their own unique victimization patterns. We can begin to love by following these steps:

Acknowledge that it is often difficult for us to be open to accept the love of others, to accept God's love, to love those whom we had taken for granted in the past, or to love those whom we have found difficult to love.

Seek openness to receive God's love and the love of others in our lives; the capacity to commit ourselves to friends and family; and the willingness to be channels of God's love to those who are difficult to love.

Surrender ourselves to God's love so that it may flow into and through us.

Take action by committing ourselves to learning how to receive God's love and the love of others. Commit ourselves to our friends and family members. Daily seek to be channels of God's love to those we find difficult to love, and help those who are suffering from victimization in their lives.

DAILY PRAYER

God, renew your love in me as I surrender myself to You today. Help me to commit myself to those whose love I have taken for granted and who depend on me. Grant me the courage to love those I have not been able to love and to know the difference between my self-centered attempts to "love" and the selfless love which can flow from You to others.

Summary

Traumatic events occurring worldwide with increasing frequency have left multitudes of survivors from wars, natural disasters, imprisonments, tortures, and the like who are suffering from posttraumatic symptoms. Their recovery is dependent on the love, support, and understanding of those who will listen empathically to their traumatic memories and painful emotions.

However, recovery is difficult when survivors feel abandoned, betrayed, feel persistent fear, guilt, or grief, have no one who will listen, or are not understood because of cultural or religious differences.

Professional counseling and psychotherapy can be very helpful when available, but survivors need to find additional ways to help their recovery, such as time-honored healing principles and religious traditions. Among them are the 12-step spiritually based recovery programs that have helped thousands, perhaps millions, of persons with "addictions."

Using principles that have been found helpful in other 12-step self-help recovery programs, I have developed a similar 12-step model for recovery from posttraumatic symptoms for survivors open to believing in a "Good Higher Power," or God, as individually understood, and the support provided by other survivors seeking similar help.

This 12-step model utilizes five healing principles for each of the steps: acknowledging the problem, seeking a solution, surrendering the problem or symptom, taking action, and praying to God as individually understood.

References

AA. (1989). *Alcoholics Anonymous* (3rd ed.). New York: Author.

American Psychiatric Association. (1987). *Diagnostic and statistical manual of mental disorders* (3rd ed., rev.). Washington, DC: Author.

Boehnlein, J. K., Kinzie, J. D., Ben, R., & Fleck, J. (1985). One year follow-up study of posttraumatic stress disorder among survivors of Cambodian concentration camps. *American Journal of Psychiatry, 142,* 956–960.

Brende, J. O., & McDonald, E. (1988, October). *Spiritual alienation in Vietnam combat veterans with posttraumatic stress disorder.* Paper presentation at the Annual Meeting of the Society for Traumatic Stress Studies, Dallas, Texas.

Brende, J. O., & McDonald, E. (1988, October). *A twelve theme and step program for Vietnam combat veterans with posttraumatic stress disorder.* Paper presented at the Annual Meeting of the Society for Traumatic Stress Studies, Dallas, Texas.

Brende, J. O., & McDonald, E. (1989). *Spiritual alienation in Vietnam combat veterans with posttraumatic stress disorder.* Unpublished manuscript.

Holy Bible. (1984). New King James Version. New York: Thomas Nelson.

Juri, E. J. (1946). *The great religions of the world.* Princeton: Princeton University Press.

Keller, J. E. (1985). *Let go, let God.* Minneapolis: Augsburg Publishing.

Kinzie, D. J. (1989). Therapeutic approaches to traumatized Cambodian refugees. *Journal of Traumatic Stress, 2*(1), 75–91.

Lee, E., & Lu, F. (1989). Assessment and treatment of Asian-American survivors of mass violence. *Journal of Traumatic Stress, 2*(1), 93–120.

Mollica, R. F. (1988). The trauma story: The psychiatric care of refugee survivors of violence and torture. In F. M. Ochberg (Ed.), *Posttraumatic therapy and victims of violence.* New York: Brunner/Mazel.

Silver, S. M., & Wilson, J. P. (1988). Native American healing and purification rituals for war stress. In J. P. Wilson, Z. Harel, & B. Kahana (Eds.), *Human adaptation to extreme stress from the Holocaust to Vietnam* (pp. 337–355). New York: Plenum Press.

Sorenson, G. (1985). Twelve steps to PTSD treatment prove successful. *Vet Center Voice, 6*(1), 10–12.

Westermeyer, J., & Wintrob, R. (1979). Folk explanations of mental illness in rural Laos. *American Journal of Psychiatry, 136*(7), 901–905.

Wilson, J. P. (1989). *Trauma, transformation and healing.* New York: Brunner/Mazel.

CHAPTER 74

Treatment of Posttraumatic Stress Disorder among Vietnam Veterans

Raymond Monsour Scurfield

> When I got back from Nam, the only people who I could relate to were other Vietnam vets—but they were the last people I wanted to be around.
> —Interview with a Vietnam veteran, Brentwood VA Medical Center, Los Angeles, 1981

Introduction

To heal from war requires time and understanding. Today appropriate treatment modalities for posttraumatic stress disorder (PTSD) among Vietnam veterans continue to be debated. Advocating a particular approach is dependent upon clinical and theoretical points of view, therapeutic and diagnostic skills, conceptualizations about posttrauma psychiatric sequelae, therapeutic needs and treatment objectives, and countertransference issues and dynamics about the trauma of the Vietnam war and the personnel who were sent to fight it (Wilson, 1989; Parson, 1988). In this chapter, I will present one perspective about the treatment of PTSD among Vietnam veterans: comprehensive, holistic peer-group approach. The aftermath of the impact of the Persian Gulf War and "Operation Desert Storm" should be a pointed reminder to us all. Most of the dynamics, issues, and strategies discussed in this chapter transcend various eras of war as well as generational and national boundaries; they are applicable to a range of war-related and civilian trauma (Scurfield, 1992; Scurfield & Tice, 1992).

Successful treatment of PTSD must include understanding of the relationship among significant pretrauma, trauma, and posttrauma factors, as well as the dynamics inherent in experiencing one or more of several types of traumatic events (Green, Wilson, & Lindy, 1985). Such understanding provides the underpinning for the 11 PTSD treatment principles that have been developed and implemented at the American Lake VA Medical center PTSD Treatment Program in Tacoma, Washington. There is a discussion of the techniques, themes, structure, and common pitfalls in peer-group treatment of Vietnam veterans, which I advocate as the treatment of choice for war veterans with PTSD. Possible positive outcomes of military and Vietnam war experiences are described and proper attention to positive aspects of trauma experiences is described as a necessary component of the stress recovery process.

Raymond Monsour Scurfield • Pacific Center for PTSD and Other War-Related Disorders, U.S. Department of Veterans Affairs, P.O. Box 50188, Honolulu, Hawaii 96850 (formerly at Northwest Posttraumatic Stress Treatment Program, American Lake VA Medical Center, Tacoma, Washington 98493). The views expressed in this chapter are solely those of the author and do not purport to represent any official viewpoint of the U.S. Department of Veterans Affairs or the Pacific Center for PTSD.

International Handbook of Traumatic Stress Syndromes, edited by John P. Wilson and Beverley Raphael. Plenum Press, New York, 1993.

Trauma within the Life Cycle

Putting PTSD into a comprehensive, whole-life perspective is absolutely critical to an adequate stress recovery process. Most veterans with PTSD either put too much attention on the war ("Vietnam experience"), or they underemphasize Vietnam as a partial or total explanation of persistent postwar problems.

Issues for Consideration in a Life-Course Analysis

There is no way that one can begin to understand the possible impact of a war unless one has a clear sense about the individual personality before, during, and after the exposure to war trauma. The following is an outline to aid ex-servicemen understand the continuities and changes in their life-course trajectory.

Questions for the Ex-Serviceperson (Veteran)

- In what ways have "threads of personality" (i.e., behaviors, attitudes, interests, and traits) been identifiable by you or people around you as descriptive of you *from very early* in childhood?
- Have these continued to be descriptive of you *throughout* your entire life?
- Or have they seemed to stop or disappear during the war and to resurface later?
- Or have the threads never reappeared? Continue this line of thought concerning threads of personality that seemed to begin at later times in your life and may or may not have continued or reappeared during the course of your life to date.
- Have there been other traumata that have occurred, before and/or after the war? For example, physical or mental abuse as a child; losing a parent traumatically; having an alcoholic parent; traumatization by a near-drowning, fire, imprisonment, vehicular accident, rape, shooting, serious illness or disability, suicide, or other unnatural loss of a significant other? If so, what has been and continues to be the impact of the trauma on you?

It is important to understand the interrelationship of several traumata to each other. When a person is traumatized, the dynamics of emergency survival will occur: shock, terror, denial, or suppression of fully experiencing the horror of the trauma, the emergence of painful intrusive recollections and bodily sensations, emotional numbness, and the like. Often, there are significant complications concerning memory following exposure to trauma at different points in the life cycle. One complication is that memories of life before the trauma may have become distorted or idealized, confused or forgotten (Chodoff, 1970). A second complication is that memories at the time of the trauma sometimes are confused, disjointed, or out-of-sequence. There is a tendency for survivors to fill in the missing parts of memory with something because "unexplained gaps in memory" are uncomfortable to live with.

War Traumata and Other Stressful Life Experiences

Most trauma experts would agree that there are at least two general categories of trauma: natural disasters and "human-induced" trauma. Natural disasters are "acts of nature," such as floods, earthquakes, and typhoons. Human-induced trauma include such events as war, rape, assault, industrial accidents, and kidnapping. There appear to be a number of similarities between natural disasters and human-induced trauma, such as the three DSM-III-R (American Psychiatric Association, 1987) categories of PTSD symptoms (intrusive, avoidance, and arousal). In contrast to survivors of human-induced trauma (Frederic, 1980), victims of natural disasters have little or no self-blame for having experienced the event and are rarely rejected by others or humiliated. Human-induced trauma can also be classified into one of at least seven types: (1) bereavement, (2) personal injury (both actual and threat of), (3) exposure to death and dying, (4) agent of harm, (5) self-inflicted harm, (6) bystander witness of trauma, and (7) responsibility-based trauma (see Chapter 6, in this volume, for a discussion). It is important to understand these different categories of trauma since different symptom patterns may develop and require different types of therapeutic work. Within each of the categories of trauma it is not necessary that a survivor will have to work therapeutically on every element or episode of the trauma. Rather, there usually are one or two "prototypical" episodes that occurred that predominate in memory in distressing ways.

PTSD Treatment Principles

The following principles are central to the therapy of war-related PTSD. It is important to note that all of them are provided within the context of an intact, cohesive cohort or peer group setting and therapeutic milieu. I believe that it is critical to the stress recovery process of war veterans for treatment to be primarily embedded in the peer-group modality. The peer group as the treatment of choice is based on the following factors: (1) that war-related trauma occurs within the context of a peer group (e.g., the small, operation-sized military unit); (2) that trauma survivors are inherently suspicious of nontrauma survivors; (3) that peers offer a special role in terms of identification, self-worth, familiarity with the trauma context, and reality-based feedback; (4) that common PTSD symptoms of isolation, withdrawal, numbing of feelings, and denial of the impact of the trauma can be directly confronted by peers; and (5) that sharing of trauma experiences by other veterans provides the other group members with powerful sources of direct therapeutic exposure to common trauma experiences (Scurfield, 1989; Scurfield, Corker, Gongla, & Hough, 1984).

Treatment Principles for Vietnam Veterans with PTSD

The 11 PTSD treatment principles that follow are explained to the veterans in the first person at the American Lake PTSD unit as part of the orientation to the program. For an elaboration of the potent interface of veteran's disability compensation on the stress recovery process and several additional treatment principles (cognitive reframing, determining and resolving "percentages of responsibility," spirituality and religion, leisure/relationship activities and mind–body connectedness, and community education and advocacy), see Scurfield (in press).

1. *Separation of compensation, legal or job status consequences, and treatment.* It is not possible for a patient to have an open and trusting therapeutic relationship with the person who will be deciding disability for compensation benefits or legal consequences. Our program does not have regular contact with the VA's regional adjudication office and does not provide clinical information to that office about a claim pending for a current inpatient. We do provide upon request a hospital discharge summary at the conclusion of the patient's hospitalization.

2. *Establishment of the therapeutic alliance.* Many expert clinicians in PTSD believe that the very establishment of a trusting relationship with a counselor is central to treatment (see Chapter 65, in this volume, for a discussion). The collusion of sanitization and silence about the impact of war cannot be underestimated in terms of its impact on veterans' trust issues and the therapist's ability to engage the veteran survivor in a helpful recovery process (Scurfield, 1992). By developing trust, the person will begin to work on symptoms and dynamics that are primary aspects of PTSD. Furthermore, we purposefully have significant numbers of both war veterans (60%) and nonveterans (40%), and males and females, on our staff. The challenge to the client is to allow some level of trust to develop with these various staff members. We also have a cohort, group-admission policy. Patients go through the program as an intact, closed-membership group in order to facilitate the development of peer-to-peer bonding, cohesion, and trust. Since trust is a paramount issue in the treatment process, we found it necessary to facilitate its development in every facet of the in-patient program.

3. *Education regarding the stress recovery process and PTSD.* We found it important to educate the patients about PTSD and the recovery process. This includes explaining the nature, course, and dynamics of PTSD in the life cycle, the nature of the stress recovery process, and the reductions and changes to be expected in symptom levels with treatment. For example, it is not unusual for trauma survivors to be preoccupied with fear of loss of control over powerful emotions if they let themselves remember and feel the original trauma; and PTSD symptoms almost always will temporarily get worse before they get better once the survivor engages in or begins a deeper phase of trauma treatment.

4. *Symptom management.* We believe that it is both necessary and a responsibility for us to provide the client with symptom management techniques *before* they begin intensive war-focus therapy groups. It is important for them to both believe that they have the ability and actually attain increased ability to control feelings and symptoms that occur in the course of intensive treatment. Anger control, stress management, and sleep disturbance are three of the most critical issues to address.

5. *Facilitation of the cycle of reexperiencing (intrusion) and avoidance (numbing) symptoms.* In the American Lake Program, we facilitate the clients' abilities to consciously permit a reexperience of what happened to them in Vietnam. They learn "dosing" techniques and how to manage the level of reexperiencing versus the need to avoid or modulate distressing recollections (Horowitz, 1976).

6. *Reexperiencing aspects of the trauma.* Most of the accepted ways of treating PTSD that have proven successful have one central commonality: there is a "direct therapeutic exposure to the trauma" (Fairbank & Nich-

olson, 1987), which is accomplished through several approaches: (a) *Simply talking about the trauma.* Sometimes it is therapeutic merely to verbally share one's thoughts, feelings, and memories of a trauma experience. (b) *Reenacting or reliving aspects of the trauma.* This technique elicits not only words about the trauma but one's feelings as well. In the group therapy (war-focus) sessions, most of the therapeutic techniques are designed to facilitate at least a partial reenactment of the words, thoughts, emotions, and actions as they occurred at the time of the original trauma. This is critical to accomplish since most trauma survivors typically have distorted recollections of what actually happened during the event. Various therapy techniques are utilized to facilitate reenactment of the trauma: *here-and-now techniques,* such as having the veteran talk in the first person, present tense, as if the event were occurring (i.e., "Here I am, walking point on a rainy, dark evening and I see . . ."); *verbal confrontation* (i.e., "I don't hear any feelings from you, just words . . ."); and *role-playing* some aspect of the traumatic experience ("talking now to the rest of the group as if they were your unit that set up a night ambush"). (c) *Exposure to symptom-provoking stimuli.* A common PTSD treatment strategy is to utilize audiovisual and other aides that elicit reexperiencing and/or arousal symptoms related to the original trauma (Keane & Kaloupek, 1982; Scrignar, 1988). At American Lake we utilize selected films of: (1) a realistically dramatized combat event; (2) reactions of veterans attending the national dedication of the Vietnam Veterans Memorial in Washington, DC; (3) a Vietnamese woman's sharing of her trauma experience in Vietnam and afterwards; in addition to films, we also utilize (4) *action-oriented experiences* that elicit memories and feelings similar to those experienced during the war that may trigger war-associated memories and feelings, such as a helicopter ride in collaboration with the Washington State Army National Guard (Scurfield, Wong, & Zeerocah, 1992) and a 5-day "Outward Bound" wilderness river rafting and rappelling course; and (5) a visit to the Washington State Vietnam Veteran Memorial. All these experiences are carefully planned to include orientation and briefings prior to the event, participation as an intact peer group, staff participation, and debriefings afterward. It is important to emphasize that the action-oriented activities are carefully designed not only to arouse troubling memories of war trauma but for the promotion of positive recollections as well. This "new" corrective, positive, here-and-now experience in the context of a supportive peer group and staff provides positive associations to coexist alongside historical negative associations. (d) *Journal writing and sharing.* Veterans are required to write daily in their own personal journals about significant feelings, thoughts, and behaviors that occur while in treatment. They also are required to share some of their written entries with the other group members and staff once a week during their "reflective reading" sessions.

7. *Psychiatric medications.* We have found that the psychosocial program components are the primary treatment needed for PTSD and associated problems. However, there are a number of veterans who have severe PTSD and/or coexisting disorders that require selective utilization of medications in order to permit optimal benefit from the psychosocial treatment provided (see Chapter 66, in this volume, for a review of phar-

macological approaches to treatment). Our program is particularly concerned about the impact of benzodiazepine medications as well as their potentially serious withdrawal side effects (Risse, Whitters, Burke, Chen, Scurfield, & Raskind, 1990).

8. *Placing the trauma into a whole-life context.* It is very evident that most trauma survivors tend to over- or underemphasize the role that the trauma has played in their lives and that other life experiences pre- and posttrauma must also be given the appropriate amount of attention if there is to be a successful recovery. It is rare for veterans with chronic and severe PTSD to have "pure" PTSD and no coexisting disorders (e.g., only about 9% of the veterans discharged from the PTSD Program are PTSD positive only) (Scurfield, Kenderdine, & Pollard, 1990). Treatment of PTSD that is coexisting with other disorders requires attention to the whole-life context.

9. *Integration of and coexistence with trauma.* Since the survivor with PTSD is preoccupied with the negative aspects of the trauma experience, other dimensions of the trauma may be suppressed. Integration of both the positive and negative aspects of trauma is a central goal of treatment. Also, since trauma is literally *unforgettable*, it is important to help the veteran *come to a better attitude and relationship with the traumatic memories* (e.g., to learn how to *better coexist* with reexperiencing and memories). This is only possible if and when an integration of all aspects of the experience occurs.

10. *Outpatient aftercare.* A veteran whose PTSD was severe enough to have entered an intensive inpatient treatment program will not be "cured" by the end of the inpatient phase of treatment. The nature of treatment of a longer duration requires a transitional period following hospital discharge. Outpatient follow-up care is necessary in order to continue the gains made during hospitalization and posttraumatic therapy. For some veterans, the inpatient experience makes it more possible for them to fully utilize outpatient treatment because we are able to break through significant denial and avoidance while the veteran is in an intensive inpatient setting for 12 weeks. This may have taken years of outpatient treatment to accomplish.

11. *The role of significant others in the treatment process.* PTSD is a condition that inevitably has a substantial impact on significant others (see Chapter 53, in this volume, for a review). Research of graduates of the PTSD Program indicates that the area of intimate relationships is both of a continuing, central concern *and* shows improvement among a significant proportion of veterans after treatment (Scurfield *et al.*, 1990). Our program attempts to provide some attention to this critical area through a relationships class cofacilitated by male and female staff, family and couple's therapy, as well as once-weekly spouse support groups and biweekly couples' groups. There is not adequate space in this chapter to do justice to a full discussion of the dynamics and issues concerning PTSD impact on the family (see Brown, 1984; Danieli, 1984; Davis & Friedman, 1985; Mason, 1990; Matsakis, 1988; Palmer & Harris, 1983; Williams, 1987). The major areas of impact include: the marital or partner relationship, the parental role with children, the impact on the partner and the partner's self-image and life-functioning even outside of the partner relationship, and the dynamics among the children of veterans with PTSD. Also it is important to note that

there are significant institutional obstacles to the provision of adequate services to significant others of veterans; for example, cost-reimbursement models by the U. S. Department of Veterans Affairs typically are extremely biased toward clinical contacts with veterans versus almost no reimbursement for significant others *per se.*

Interestingly, there is a very sparse body of literature concerning the specific impact of PTSD among Vietnam veterans on their children (see Chapter 53, in this volume, for a discussion; see also Scarano, 1982). I will briefly explicate some important factors that we have learned through another treatment group in which we treat youths between the ages of 11 to 19 who are children of veterans in our program (Scurfield, Neal, & Hoffstetter, 1988).

Similar to treatment approaches to partners of Vietnam veterans with PTSD, children must be provided with accurate and understandable information about stress reactions and combat. This task is two-fold: to optimize a positive relationship between child, veteran, and partner, and to attend to the child's own needs which may include severe reactions to family-related trauma. Typically, such children manifest a number of the following reactions: (1) a sense of guilt "for the problems my dad has"; (2) confusion, anger, and helplessness about the veteran's chronic symptoms; (3) internalized conflict over the dual standard of being punished for behaviors exhibited similar to those of the veteran or both parents (e.g., substance abuse, swearing, authority conflicts); (4) a tendency for the veteran to be extremely protective, significantly lax, or markedly fluctuating in parenting; (5) acting-out the unconscious attitudes of the parents; (6) role reversal where the veteran or partner uses the child to vent to or get advice from; (7) intense sibling rivalry; (8) violence and/or sexual acting-out; (9) conflicts associated with multiple divorces and/or de facto relations; and (10) a paucity of opportunity to "just be kids" and have enjoyments in life that may be taken for granted.

Overall, the children appear to be very lonely with poor self-esteem and a need to talk with a rationally expressive adult. Our peer-group treatment that involves children from several different families has been a profoundly positive experience for many of the same reasons that veteran peer group treatment is helpful: mutual support and clarification, validation of having "normal" feelings and perceptions, realization that one is not necessarily crazy or alone, and the opportunity to talk about and enjoy themselves in a safe and understanding environment. Although such children initially may be more willing and receptive to peer feedback, they yearn for the friendship of both peers and adults. A particularly impactful aspect of our groups is to have veterans with PTSD who are *not* fathers of any of the children present attend and interact with the youths; honest expressions on both sides occur in a way not yet possible with one's own father or with one's own child. Treatment for children can occur only after careful assessment of the family system.

Peer-Group Therapy for PTSD

The salient role that peer-group therapy with Vietnam veterans has played over the years stems from two primary sources. One source is steeped in the profound rage and mistrust that many Vietnam veterans felt toward the United States, the Veterans Administration, and other health care professionals and institutions. Many veterans found themselves deeply troubled by their war experience and unable to "just forget about it," as was frequently advised. Rage was also exacerbated by the "unwelcome home" that many veterans received and the lack of knowledge about and/or denial of the impact of war trauma among many persons and institutions. Consequently, there was a refusal by many veterans to utilize "traditional" mental health services which, in turn, gave birth to the veterans' "self-help movement" in many locations throughout the country. This movement was characterized by groups of veterans initiating and organizing their own discussions, often in community-based storefront locations. Meetings were characterized by sharing the painful aspects of the war and postwar experiences and were similar in function to other self-help groups (e.g., Alcoholics Anonymous). There were proactive mental health professionals, a number of whom were Vietnam veterans themselves, who also participated in and frequently provided a nontraditional clinical leadership to these groups. These groups typically utilized peer-to-peer discussions of Vietnam and postwar experiences and the broader societal and governmental issues related to the war and its aftermath (Egendorf, 1975; Kormos, 1978; Lifton, 1978; Shatan, 1973, 1974; Smith, 1980). It is my experience that peer-group therapy with Vietnam veterans with PTSD is the treatment of choice. This modality may and frequently should be used in conjunction with supportive individual, couple, family, and/or biologic therapy.

Dimensions of Peer-Group Treatment

The importance of peer-group treatment for Vietnam veterans is due to the factors which are listed below. Potential caveats are mentioned as well.

1. War-related trauma occurs within the context of a peer group (e.g., the small, operation-sized military unit). Hence the dynamics and issues of trauma experiences inherently are interwoven with small-group dynamics. The peer-group setting provides the ideal modality for reexamining the war and postwar consequences in the lives of veterans.

2. Trauma survivors inherently are suspicious of nontrauma survivors ("How could you possibly understand . . ."). They feel stigmatized, ashamed, misunderstood, and perhaps mistreated by others. Healthy self-disclosure with fellow survivors facilitates resolution of those feelings.

3. Common PTSD symptoms of isolation, withdrawal, numbing of feelings, and denial of the impact of war stress is directly and impactfully confronted in the healthy supportive environment of a well-run and cohesive peer group.

4. Sharing of trauma experiences by other veteran survivors provides the other group members with very useful sources of direct therapeutic exposure to the trauma—an exposure that appears remarkably efficacious in promoting recall of aspects of repressed traumatic experiences.

Contraindications to Peer-Group Therapy

1. Severe co-morbidity will significantly interfere with and change group process, goals, and objectives, especially psychotic, substance abuse, and personality disorders. Such co-morbidity necessitates a dual-disorder emphasis (see Daniels & Scurfield, in press).

2. An extremely anxious person who is unable to participate in peer-group therapy may require some preparation in individual counseling, For example: (a) The veteran who is "new" to PTSD treatment may be terrified of what may happen by even talking about the trauma. (b) The veteran who has had poor previous experience in peer-group treatment may require special attention. (c) The veteran may have had a traumatic peer-group experience in the war (e.g., was ostracized by the unit and scapegoated). (d) The veteran's traumatic history may be so profound and there is such massive detachment, denial or numbing, or self-denigration that intimate interactions with peers in a group setting simply cannot be tolerated at this point.

3. Some special-population veterans (ethnocultural minorities, women, the physically disabled, ex-POWs) may be particularly resistant to peer-group therapy for specific reasons (see Scurfield, in press).

Group Membership Criteria

Group therapists rely on their clinical judgment regarding criteria for membership in the group. Presented below are a set of practical considerations that are useful when screening individuals for group treatment.

- Axis I disorders must be carefully assessed to determine if the person will be able to tolerate uncovering of traumatic memories and feeling, and/or the intensity of peer-group bonding and intimacy.
- Axis II disorders must be assessed essentially to determine if the veteran is motivated to change and honestly attempt to deal with troubling war-related issues.
- In my clinical experience, the homogeneity and or heterogeneity of traumatic experiences indicates that American war zone veterans of all eras (World War II, Korea, Vietnam, Persian Gulf) and of varying military specialties (combat, direct combat support, and rear echelon) can be successfully combined together in one group. Usually, however, there is significant initial resistance to such an integration. We also have had some success bringing together visiting Soviet "Afgantsi" veterans with U.S. veterans in our program who volunteer to interact together.

Mandatory Group Operating Rules

Although many of the following operating rules may seem obvious and generic to group treatment *per se*, the dynamics of war-related PTSD are such that they must be *explicitly addressed and agreed to by all*. The dynamics surrounding *how* the therapist and group together will process and resolve the establishment and enforcement of rules will actually be a major component of the establishment of therapeutic trust as well as the ongoing treatment effort with war-related PTSD.

1. *Violence and threats of violence.* The group must agree that violence and threats of violence will not be tolerated and will constitute grounds for immediate discharge from the group. In order to provide the members with adequate consequence to deal with their own rage and impulse control issues, an anger-control strategy (e.g., utilization of time-outs) must be laid out, agreed to, and enforced by the entire group and not by the therapist alone.

2. *No weapons.* Many war veterans own and carry personal weapons. A number of veterans with severe PTSD have carried weapons since their war days. Specific questions to each member about personal weapons, their location and types, and strategies and agreements to prevent easy access to such in times of emotional upheaval, *must* be addressed.

3. *Substance abuse.* There must be specific agreement as to the procedures and consequences if someone comes to a group session under the influence of alcohol or drugs. Generally, at a minimum, the veteran is immediately confronted by the group, given a brief amount of time to think about his actions, and is asked to leave. A calm, simple explanation of the rationale for the decision may be explained along with information on PTSD and self-medication. If the group is dual disorder (PTSD and substance-abuse) in emphasis, further rules are necessary, such as both routine and unannounced monitoring through urine analysis and breathalyzer readings (see Daniels & Scurfield, in press).

4. *Issues of confidentiality.* This is a major concern among war veterans with PTSD and concerns rest in three primary areas: (a) Discussion of "secret" or classified military operations and involvement in atrocity-like incidents that might be construed by someone as a "war crime." (b) Concern will exist about the therapist's record-keeping, particularly in regard to classified military activities and atrocity-like incidents. The therapist should consider the strategy of agreeing not to record details of atrocities and of allowing the veteran the opportunity to have access to review what is being recorded about sensitive war-trauma experiences. It is essential to emphasize that such concerns about sensitive war-trauma experiences will almost always be present to some if not a considerable degree whether or not such concerns are actually expressed to the therapist. Hence, a proactive discussion in this area by the therapist is essential. (c) Clarification will be needed of the therapist's legal and professional responsibilities concerning notification of others when there is a clear and present danger to the veteran (e.g., suicide) or to others (e.g., homicide). Clarification about these issues are particularly relevant to Vietnam veterans with severe PTSD for whom there typically are significant issues of trust with therapists, as well as a real risk of suicide or issues of impulse control.

5. *Attendance requirements and expectations.* These, of course, are critical to the group's functioning. Two elements are crucial to consider: (a) the responsibility and authority of the therapist versus the group as a whole versus individual members regarding attendance, punctuality, and notification if unable to attend; (b) telephone exchange and possible establishment of a buddy system.

6. *Number of sessions: specified versus open-ended.* My

experience is that a contract for a limited number of sessions has the advantages of offering and expecting a time commitment that is relatively realistic and promotes the intact peer-group experience. For veterans who are more willing and able to make a longer-term commitment to sustained PTSD-related treatment, a 12 to 16-week series of sessions appears particularly useful. Recontracting for *additional* specified numbers of sessions and with a specific content focus may be offered. Three of the major advantages of such time-contracted therapy with Vietnam veterans with PTSD is that it forces a formal reevaluation and stock-taking, it provides the veteran with the opportunity to "walk out the front door, head held high," having fulfilled his or her commitment to the number of sessions contracted, and is consistent with the cyclical ebb and flow of PTSD symptoms.

7. *Length of sessions.* Depending on the number of participants, a 1½ to 2-hour block of time is required for any *realistic* opportunity for a group to delve into sensitive war-related issues and debrief adequately before the session ends. There will be a number of veterans who will attempt to judge, test, and attack the therapist's commitment by insisting that the sessions have no firm ending time and extend well beyond whatever is the specified time frame. It is also important to note that having intense war focus therapy groups in the evenings has the effect of contributing negatively to sleep disturbance and should be carefully assessed so that adequate debriefings can occur to minimize the impact on sleep disturbance. Finally, there are some war-trauma issues that may require considerably longer than a 1½ to 2-hour block of time, usually because of the complexity of the event, ingrained denial and avoidance, and/or the desirability to have *several* group members do "focus" work (in the same session) who have a similar issue to resolve. Thus, special extended-length sessions may be scheduled as necessary.

8. *Treatment objectives in the peer-group setting.* In many cases, outpatient therapy groups with war veterans with PTSD may be the primary or sole therapeutic intervention of a systematic nature that is accessible. In such situations, the treatment objectives necessarily must cover the exploration, discussion and resolving of both war-specific and current problems in living. With the preceding as a general guideline, there are four specific life time-frames that are appropriate for such a group treatment approach with veterans with PTSD: (a) war-trauma events and experiences; (b) current problems in living; (c) premilitary factors that appear significantly related to the individual veteran's negative and positive war experiences; and (d) interactions between war zone, current life, immediate premilitary, and premorbid factors.

Thematic Patterns Which Emerge with Time in Groups

A seemingly "natural" progression of major themes in outpatient therapy groups for veterans with PTSD was demonstrated in a research assessment of three different such groups over a 1-year period (Scurfield *et al.*, 1984):

1. First four months: There was discussion of PTSD

symptoms, troubling Vietnam experiences, and how they negatively affect current life.

2. Second four months: As the Vietnam experiences were more openly discussed and some resolution began, there was more of an emphasis on current life dynamics and a somewhat lesser emphasis on the link between Vietnam and current life.

3. The last four months: Relatively little discussion of Vietnam *per se* and major emphasis on "moving on" to current life situations and future goals.

A second major approach to thematic structure is to focus primarily on one area in a session. For example, to "alternate" between war-focus issues in one session and current concerns in the next session. The actual number of sessions devoted to either area can be adjusted according to the treatment needs. This approach is particularly important when one group session a week is the *only* therapeutic modality that a veteran is participating in.

A third thematic approach is to "walk each member of the group through" a chronologically progressive series of themes (Mazejko, 1986; Scurfield & Blank, 1985).

Group Themes Common to the Vietnam War Experience

Listed below are themes that are likely to emerge within the discussion context of the war experience:

1. Fear of mental illness and what is "normal" versus "abnormal."
2. Responsibility assignment. There is a tendency for trauma survivors to take extreme positions (e.g., denial to false blame).
3. Stigma and shame over what one did or did not do. (The issue of external versus internal "responsibility" is central to many war-trauma-related issues; for a detailed discussion of the cognitive and experiential technique of "determining percentages of responsibility," see Scurfield, in press.)
4. The role and relationship to professional staff in Vietnam (e.g., clergy, physician, and psychiatrists).
5. Other authority figures, including military officers and civilians, both in and outside of the war zone.
6. Moral, ethical, and spiritual issues.
7. Racial and ethnic issues and conflicts; one common experience was that "there wasn't racism in the bush (combat) but there sure was back in base camp."
8. Attitudes toward Vietnamese and other Asian groups.
9. War injuries, medical evacuation, and disabilities (Scurfield & Tice, 1992; Tice *et al.*, 1988).
10. Combat versus noncombat status.
11. War, sex, violence, and rape.
12. Fear. A number of veterans have profound issues related to their inner experiences of terror and fright in the war zone and denial of the same both then and now.
13. The brutal side of war. Many veterans have struggled for years with guilt, moral pain, fear, and self-condemnation at having crossed over the boundary to what the veteran considers to be evil or bad behaviors and attitudes, such as having gone "kill crazy" against Vietnamese following the death of a comrade.
14. Rest and recreation and issues about having difficulties in enjoying life.
15. The search for meaning and pride. Many veterans with PTSD struggle over the seeming wastefulness of death and wounding in Vietnam and over their own pain suffered both during and since the war.

Analogy of the Small Military Unit

It can be very helpful to the therapeutic process to facilitate the peer-group treatment to consciously draw a parallel when appropriate to the veterans previous experiences while on active duty as members of a small, tactical military unit. For example, that the person "walking point" in the field cannot get too far ahead and the rear guard can not get too far behind ("bringing up the rear"), or else there is a danger to the unit and to the individual. "Keep the group together as a unit," "pull your own weight," and "cover for each other" are all concepts that in the peer-group treatment can actively be utilized in working toward the common objective of stress recovery and promoting equitable participation by all group members.

Attending to Countertransference

I would be remiss not to reemphasize the critical need to pay close attention to the range of powerful cognitions, feelings, and countertransference issues inevitably aroused in the clinician who is providing PTSD treatment to Vietnam veterans. The controversial and divisive nature of the war, the collusion of sanitazation and silence about war's negative and profound psychological and social impact (Scurfield, 1992), the tendency for trauma experiences of all types to elicit powerful reactions in clinicians, and some typical presenting symptoms of Vietnam veterans with PTSD (projected rage, isolation, suspicion, self-destructive, demanding, needy) all contribute to countertransference dynamics (see also Parson, 1988; Newberry, 1985; Wilson, 1989). I would like to delineate on four sources of countertransference dynamics that are inherent in treating Vietnam veterans and that therapists must honestly address within themselves: (1) attitudes toward war and military service (i.e., Is any death or killing in a war zone "justifiable"?); (2) issues of collective and individual responsibility toward the national policy governing the war (i.e., Is it okay that the Selective Service indeed has been *very* selective—of the lesser educated, poor, and ethnic minorities?); (3) specific attitudes toward the Vietnam War and its veterans (i.e., How does the clinician feel about the guerillalike nature of the war and the use of women and children as combatants and booby-traps?); (4) specific reaction to individual veteran's experiences and personality dynamics (i.e., How comfortable are you talking about missing limbs with an amputee?).

It is important to note that one conceptualization of countertransference is that much of it is of a *positive* nature and equally needs to be recognized and appreciated. Our determination to advocate the cause of trauma survivors may occur, or our renewed determination to continue working in this field, or our sense of accomplishment when a trauma survivor is facilitated to "let go" of some of the terrible burdens that have followed him or her for years or decades. For me, reaffirmation of the strengths of human beings to not only withstand but persevere and succeed in the face of adversity is continually refueled through clinical contact with war veterans and their families.

Strategies to Address Countertransference Dynamics

We have instituted several strategies to deal directly with countertransference dynamics that routinely occur among staff. Most importantly, there is an *expressed recognition* that this is very demanding work on the caregivers. There must be a *regular* attention to identification and processing of countertransference dynamics and issues. There is the expectation of the staff to share some of their own countertransference issues. Therefore, we have a "staff support group" every Friday following the last scheduled clinical activity for the week. As the program director I try to set the example by attending and participating regularly. The group is also officially "leaderless," with all participants as peers in this group. Information discussed in this support group is considered confidential (and not material to be used in performance evaluations).

Generally, countertransference dynamics and issues tend to be in three areas: specific triggers and reactions elicited by exposure to the sharing of war trauma or other sensitive clinical material; intrastaff territorial battles and personality disputes; and personal self-disclosures about issues beyond the program that may have a negative or positive impact on work performance. Overlaying all such countertransference dynamics are the individual staff's own possible issues about authority and the degree to which personal disclosures of any type may put one at risk with one's supervisor and/or colleagues. Other strategies to deal with countertransference dynamics and stress reactions include debriefings at the end of each day, co-facilitated groups, limiting work schedules to 40 hours, widespread programmatic involvement by staff in a variety of roles with periodic rotation in and out of activities, and systematic sharing of positive feedback.

Enhancement of Positive Aspects of Trauma and Its Aftermath

In addition to the sensitive uncovering, reexploration, and reflections of troubling and painful aspects of trauma, it also is essential to give appropriate attention to the positive aspects as well. It appears that a majority of both male and female Vietnam veterans report more positive than negative impacts of their war experiences (Card, 1983; Schnaier, 1985). Also, there is a subset of veterans who appear to have transformed their traumatic experiences into positive outcomes (see the discussion of "post-conventional, humanistic orientation" in Wilson, 1989). Finally, as described in this section, *all* trauma experiences contain both troubling and potentially positive aspects; a central strategy, especially in the middle and later stages of stress recovery, *is to facilitate the discovery and appreciation by the trauma survivor of such positives.* These positives often have been embedded beneath negative preoccupations and are overlooked or minimized by the survivor unless a reframing is facilitated to enable self-acknowledgment that the positive aspect also is true. A utilization of "helicopter-ride therapy" has demonstrated a significant ability to promote positive associations with the war (Scurfield *et al.*, 1992).

A listing of some of the common negative preoccupations of war-trauma survivors and coupled also with the valid positive aspects follows:

1. There is a sense of loss, grief, and preoccupation with hurt, versus the comradeship that may have occurred at an extraordinary level and perhaps never attained before or since. The fact that such comradeship occurred at one time means not only that the potential but the actualization of such has been achieved by the war veteran.

2. There are feelings of confusion, of not being clear about what is valued in life, or where one is going versus development of very healthy questioning and/or a reaffirmation of one's values, such as what is important and what is not, and what is really meaningful.

3. Difficulties arise in dealing with "everyday" stresses, versus maintaining a continuing ability to have a sense of integrity and proficiency under very trying circumstances.

4. Very low self-esteem at what one did in the war and one's difficult postwar adjustment may be troublesome versus appreciation of the strength that it took to survive both the war and the continuing reexperiencing of the original trauma in the postwar years.

5. Mistrust and loss of faith in the country's institutions can be disturbing versus a healthy questioning of the motivations and behaviors of those institutions.

6. The veterans may have little tolerance or may act out when confronted by depersonalized and insensitive behaviors of authority and institutions, versus the development of very strong convictions that he or she is entitled to be treated with dignity and respect.

7. Veterans may experience isolation and alienation, feeling that others could not possibly understand their trauma experience, versus rediscovery of the shared bonding among other war veterans, a specialness that would not be possible without having had the Vietnam experience to begin with.

8. Loss of belief in God, religion, or faith in humanity can arise versus marked positive changes in outlook, expansiveness of worldview, and profound insights, perceptions, and quasireligious or religious/spiritual insights.

9. There may be a morbid dwelling on the fact that one should have died or not survived, or resentment over physical pain and loss suffered and endured all these years versus the concept of "bonus time"—to consider it extraordinary that one did survive and to appreciate this bonus time to enjoy and take advantage of (Tice, 1988).

10. There may be terror of taking risks or exposure to danger *or* being an "adrenalin junkie" who is constantly exposed to dangerous and unnecessary risks versus appreciation of the thrilling and peak experiences that did occur in the war and the willingness to promote "healthy and safe" stimulations to enhance one's life today.

11. Continual bemoaning and resentment of one's postwar difficulties and deprivations may be a problem versus a deep appreciation of the value of freedom and one's abilities to persevere in the face of extraordinary and unrelenting pain.

12. There may be pain over remembering repeatedly the troubling aspects of the war experience versus understanding and appreciating that it can be a sign of health *not* to forget war trauma—lessons that should not be forgotten by anybody or by our country (Scurfield, 1992).

13. Accepting total or exaggerated degree of responsibility for trauma that occurred in the war zone can be a problem versus the realization and appreciation that when a nation goes to war, *everyone* in that nation bears some responsibility for all that happens in that war.

The therapeutic discovery is that aspects of *both* negative preoccupation *and* the accompanying positive dialectic are valid and that even the most horrible traumatic experience also can and does contain extraordinary growth possibilities.

Summary and Conclusions

Appropriate treatment of PTSD and associated problems among Vietnam veterans is a most complex, challenging, and rewarding task. The relationship between pretrauma, trauma, and posttrauma factors complicates an accurate assessment, treatment focus, and outcome. Oftentimes it is difficult both for the client and the professional to pay adequate attention to these various factors. It also is challenging to "stay with" deeply painful and disturbing reexperiencing of traumatic events long enough to elicit expression, cover the various issues and pain that are embedded deeply, and attain cognitive and experiential insights.

The treatment approach that has been described in this chapter is an integration of several approaches to treatment of PTSD among Vietnam veterans. I do not think it is possible to emphasize enough the salient role that several factors play in stress recovery: (1) the *right* of the survivor to have a therapeutic trust relationship, which includes the right to experience the clinician as a real person who is willing to share in the stress recovery process; (2) the necessity for the survivor to relive experientially some aspects of the trauma in a controlled, safe therapeutic environment; (3) the necessity to provide behavioral and cognitive tools to assist the client to assume control over painful and powerful emotions and symptoms; (4) judicious utilization of psychiatric medications when necessary as a supplement to the therapeutic process; and (5) helping the veteran and family to integrate both the war and postwar trauma experiences into identity, self-esteem, and relationship with others and with society. To aim to do any less with the survivor of pro-

tracted, massive trauma who is manifesting moderate or severe PTSD is ignorant at best, and not infrequently harmful to a successful stress recovery.

There are three elements of PTSD treatment with Vietnam veterans that seem particularly vital. The first element is the healing power of positive peer relationships, both in the group treatment setting and in the support necessary to permit reintegration with a supportive and enriched social environment. The second element in PTSD treatment is ensuring that systematic and adequate attention is given to "caring for the caregivers"; to pay less than adequate attention to this axiom of PTSD treatment will be destructive to clients and to the staff. The third element comes from military and civilian veterans of war in many countries and periods in history. "For those who have fought for it, freedom has a taste that the protected will never know." Let us join in our efforts to rekindle the latent power inherent in rediscovery of that truth, and in actualizing the joy of freedom—in this case, freedom from the destructive legacies of the trauma of war.

References

American Psychiatric Association. (1987). *Diagnostic and statistical manual of mental disorders* (3rd ed., rev.). Washington, DC: Author.

Brown, D. C. (1984). Legacies of a war: Treatment considerations with Vietnam veterans and their families. *Social Work, 29*(4), 372–379.

Card, J. (1983). *Lives after Vietnam: The personal impact of military service.* Lexington, MA: Lexington Books.

Chodoff, P. (1970). The German concentration camp as a psychological stress. *Archives of General Psychiatry, 22,* 78–87.

Danieli, Y. (1984). Psychotherapists' participation in the conspiracy of silence about the Holocaust. *Psychoanalytic Psychology, 1*(1), 23–42.

Daniels, L. R., & Scurfield, R. M. (in press). War-related PTSD, chemical addictions and non-chemical habituating behaviors. In M. B. Williams and J F. Sommer (Eds.), *Handbook of post-traumatic therapy.* Westport, CT: Greenwood Publishing.

Davis, R. C., & Friedman, L. N. (1985). The emotional aftermath of crime and violence. In C. R. Figley (Ed.), *Trauma and its wake: The study and treatment of post-traumatic stress disorder* (pp. 90–112). New York: Brunner/Mazel.

Egendorf, A. (1975). Vietnam veteran rap groups and themes of postwar life. *Journal of Social Issues, 31*(4), 111–124.

Fairbank, J. A. & Nicholson, R. A. (1987). Theoretical and empirical issues in the treatment of post-traumatic stress disorder in Vietnam veterans. *Journal of Clinical Psychology, 43*(1), 44–66.

Frederic, C. (1980). *Effects of natural vs. human-induced violence upon victims: Evaluation and change.* Minneapolis Medical Research Foundation, Inc./NIMH, Mental Health Services Development Branch. Special Issue: Services for Victims Survivors.

Green, B. L., Wilson, J. P., & Lindy, J. D. (1985). Conceptualizing post-traumatic stress disorder: A psychosocial framework. In C. R. Figley (Ed.), *Trauma and its wake: The study and treatment of post-traumatic stress disorder* (pp. 53–69). New York: Brunner/Mazel.

Horowitz, M. J. (1976). *Stress Response Syndromes.* New York: Jason Aronson.

Keane, T., & Kaloupek, D. (1982). Imaginal flooding in the treatment of post-traumatic disorder. *Journal of Consulting and Clinical Psychology, 50,* 138–140.

Kormos, H. R. (1978). The nature of combat stress. In C. R. Figley (Ed.), *Stress disorders among Vietnam veterans.* New York: Brunner/Mazel.

Lifton, R. J. (1978). Advocacy and corruption in the healing profession. In C. Figley (Ed.), *Stress disorders among Vietnam veterans* (pp. 209–230). New York: Brunner/Mazel.

Mason, P. (1990). *Recovering from the war: A woman's guide to helping your Vietnam vet, your family and yourself.* New York: Penguin Books.

Matsakis, A. (1988). *Vietnam wives.* Kensington, MD: Woodbine House.

Mazejko, W. (1986). "Walk through Vietnam" spells out one approach to group therapy. *Vet Center Voice, 7*(4), 2–7.

Newberry, T. B. (1985). Levels of countertransference toward Vietnam veterans with posttraumatic stress disorder. *Bulletin of the Menninger Clinic, 49*(2), 151–160.

Palmer, S., & Harris, M. (1983). Supportive group therapy for women partners of Vietnam veterans. *The Family Therapist, 4*(2), 3–11.

Parson, E. R. (1988). Post-traumatic self disorders (PTsfD): Theoretical and practical considerations in psychotherapy of Vietnam War veterans. In J. P. Wilson, Z. Harel, & B. Kahana (Eds.), *Human adaptation to extreme stress: From the Holocaust to Vietnam* (pp. 245–283). New York: Plenum Press.

Risse, S. C., Whitters, A., Burke, J., Chen, S., Scurfield, R., & Raskind, M. A. (1990). Severe withdrawal symptoms following discontinuance of alprazolam in combat-induced post-traumatic stress disorder. *Journal of Clinical Psychiatry, 51*(5), 206–209.

Scarano, T. (1982, December). Family therapy: A viable approach for treating women partners of Vietnam veterans. *The Family Therapist, 3*(3), 9–16.

Schnaier, J. (1985). Women veterans. In C. Kubey, D. Addlestone, R. O'Dell, K. Synder, B. Stichman, & Vietnam Veterans of America (Eds.), *The Viet vet survival guide: How to cut through the bureaucracy and get what you need and are entitled to* (pp. 257–268). New York: Ballantine Books.

Scrignar, C. B. (1988). *Post-traumatic stress disorder: Diagnosis, treatment and legal issues* (2nd ed.). New Orleans: Bruno Press.

Scurfield, R. M. (1989). *Techniques of peer group therapy for PTSD in Vietnam veterans.* Paper presented at the American Psychiatric Association Annual Meeting, San Francisco.

Scurfield, R. M. (1992). The collusion of sanitization and silence about war: An aftermath of "Operation Desert Storm." *Journal of Traumatic Stress, 5*(3), 505–512.

Scurfield, R. M. (in press). Treatment of war-related trauma. In M. B. Williams and J. F. Sommer (Eds), *The handbook of post-traumatic therapy.* Westport, CT: Greenwood Publishing.

Scurfield, R. M., & Blank, A. S. (1985). A guide to obtaining a military history from Vietnam veterans. In S. M. Sonnenberg, A. S. Blank, & J. A. Talbott (Eds.), *The trauma of war: Stress and recovery in Vietnam veterans* (pp. 2262–2292). Washington, DC: American Psychiatric Press.

Scurfield, R. M., Corker, T. M. Gongla, P. A., & Hough, R. (1984). Three post-Vietnam "rap/therapy" groups: An analysis. *Group, 8,* 3–21.

Scurfield, R. M., Kenderdine, S. K., & Pollard, R. J. (1990). Inpatient treatment for war-related post-traumatic stress disorder: Initial findings on a longer-term outcome study. *Journal of Traumatic Studies, 3*(2), 1–37.

Scurfield, R. M., & Tice, S. N. (1992). Interventions with medical and psychiatric evacuees and their families: From Vietnam through the Gulf War. *Military Medicine, 157*(2), 88–97.

Scurfield, R. M., Wong, L. E., & Zeerocah, E. B. (1992). Helicopter ride therapy. *Military Medicine, 157*(2), 67–73.

Scurfield, Neal, & Hofstetter. (1988). PTS Treatment Program Handbook, American Lake VA Medical Center, Tacoma, WA (unpublished handbook).

Shatan, C. F. (1973). Through the membrane of reality: "Impacted grief" and perceptual dissonance in Vietnam combat veterans. *Psychiatric Opinion, 11*(6), 6–15.

Shatan, C. F. (1974). The grief of soldiers: Vietnam combat veterans' self-help movement. *American Journal of Orthopsychiatry, 43*(4), 640–653.

Smith, J. (1980). *Rap groups and the stress recovery process.* Unpublished manuscript. Reprints from: Dr. J. Smith, Stress Disorder Program, Brecksville VA Medical Center, Brecksville, OH.

Tice, S. (1988, April). *Physically disabled Vietnam vets: Treatment issues.* Paper presented at the conference on Healing from the Trauma of Vietnam. University of Oregon, Eugene.

Tice, S. N., Hinds, R. Bialobok, E., Carter, H., Cecil, J., Koverman, D., Makowski, N., Pierson, R., & Batres, A. R. (1988). Report of the Working Group on Physically Disabled Vietnam Veterans. Submitted to Readjustment Counseling Service, Department of Veterans Affairs, Washington, D. C. VA monograph.

Wilson, J. P. (1989). *Trauma, transformation, and healing: An integrative approach to theory, research, and post-traumatic therapy.* New York: Brunner/Mazel.

CHAPTER 75

Diagnostic and Therapeutic Use of the Multigenerational Family Tree in Working with Survivors and Children of Survivors of the Nazi Holocaust

Yael Danieli

Introduction

The following was related with agitation during a child survivors' group therapy session of the Group Project for Holocaust Survivors and their Children by a child survivor/psychotherapist, after attending an initial class at a family therapy institute, where she and her fellow students were asked to draw and discuss their geno-grams[1] (Guerin & Pendagast, 1976):

> The contrast was so unbelievable. There was a feeling of shock, both in me and in everybody watching me. I couldn't relate to all their full, big genograms [family trees]. And they looked at me pretty much like somebody from another planet. [In mine] everybody was crossed off, those I remembered, and half I didn't know. There it was. A cemetery up there. The contrast was absolutely unbelievable. It does you in, stares you in the face. You can't see it and not be profoundly affected. Literally no one survived. Its there, all the crosses. The machine gun just went throughout a whole blackboard. I had to call my mother and ask her how many brothers

[1]A *genogram* is a structural diagram of a family's three-generational family relationship system.

Yael Danieli • Group Project for Holocaust Survivors and Their Children, 345 East 80th Street, Apt. 31-J, New York, New York 10021.

International Handbook of Traumatic Stress Syndromes, edited by John P. Wilson and Beverley Raphael. Plenum Press, New York, 1993.

and sisters father had. I also didn't remember mother's sisters.

> Mother is depression. She is always gray, like she is walking through ashes. Compared to most of you [her group members], at least I have some memory of father [She was 11 years old when she last saw him]. We built our lives on nothing. No. We built on a cemetery without graves and full of horrors. That is why this group is so unbelievable to me: the fact of how much life and accomplishments we built on this terror and horror we sustained. I can't comprehend it. We were all children, ages 2 to 16, some went through five or six concentration camps. Imagine! You [another group member] were three years old and you knew not to say that you were Jewish! We came out in the end of it and many had absolutely, literally no one. [Gesturing an embrace, she exclaimed,] This group and our Project are my family and extended family. This is real continuity!

Group Project for Holocaust Survivors and Their Children

The Group Project for Holocaust Survivors and their Children was established to counteract the profound sense of isolation and alienation among Holocaust survivors and their children—the most common consequence of a pervasive *conspiracy of silence* which has existed between survivors, their children, and society since the end of World War II. This silence resulted from negative societal reactions and attitudes, such as indifference, avoidance, repression, and denial of their Holocaust experiences, and victimization histories and sequelae that most survivors encountered after the war. The project also compensated for the neglect by mental health professionals who, for many years, typically participated in this conspiracy as well.

Elsewhere, I have reviewed in detail the literature on the conspiracy of silence (Danieli, 1982a), described its impact on the survivors (Danieli, 1981e, 1989), their families (Danieli, 1981a,c, 1985b), and their psychotherapies (Danieli, 1988a,b), and reported my research on therapists' difficulties in treating survivors of the Nazi Holocaust and their children (Danieli, 1980, 1984, 1988a). There I have identified and systematically examined 49 countertransference reactions and attitudes reported by 61 psychotherapists. My research strongly suggests that the source of these reactions is the Holocaust itself—horrific loss—rather than the actual encounter with its survivors and their offspring. These results, and the pervasive absence of training for professionals working with this as well as other victim/survivor populations (see Danieli & Krystal, 1989) informed the inclusion of a training component in the project in addition to its research and various therapeutic functions.

Central Role of the Group Modality

Since its inception in 1975 in the New York City area, the Group Project has recognized and capitalized on the unique reparative and preventive value of the group modality in meeting the needs of survivors and their offspring (Danieli, 1982b). First, maintaining bonds of loyalty and mutual help proved of utmost importance for survival during and immediately after the war (Davidson, 1984; Des Pres, 1976; Eitinger, 1972; Luchterhand, 1967, 1971; Matussek, 1975; Moskovitz, 1983). Group and community therapeutic modalities serve to counteract their sense of isolation and alienation and affirm the central role of "we-ness" in their identity as victim/survivors and the need for a collective search for meaningful responses to their experiences. This seems true particularly with regard to mourning, the nature of relationships and communication between the generations, issues of Jewish identity after the Holocaust, and the relationship of the survivors and their children with the non-Jewish world. By participating in groups, survivors and offspring who were plagued by mistrust and the feeling that nobody who had not undergone the same experiences would "really understand" them, could at last talk about their memories and experiences. They were also able to explore with each other and comprehend the long-term consequences in their lives of the Holocaust and the conspiracy of silence that followed it, and share their feelings and current concerns.

Group modalities have been particularly helpful in compensating for countertransference reactions. Whereas a therapist alone may feel unable to contain or provide a "holding environment" (Winnicott, 1965) for his or her patient's feelings, the group as a unit is able to. Although any particularly intense interaction invoked by Holocaust memories may prove too overwhelming to some people present, others invariably come forth with a variety of helpful "holding" reactions. Thus, the group functions as an ideal absorptive entity for abreaction and catharsis of emotions, especially negative ones, that are otherwise experienced as uncontainable (Krystal, 1975, 1978; Wilson, 1985). Finally, these modalities also help rebuild a sense of extended family and community, which were lost during the Holocaust (Danieli, 1988d). The Group Project for Holocaust Survivors and their Children provides individual, family, group, and intergenerational community assistance in a variety of noninstitutional settings. Survivors' resistance to institutions—their fear of being stigmatized, labeled crazy (stemming from the Nazi practice of gassing the sick or mentally ill), or considered emotionally damaged by their victimization (thereby granting Adolf Hitler a posthumous victory)—specifically precluded making the project part of a mental health facility.

Some excellent reviews of the psychiatric literature on the long-term effects of the massive traumata experienced by survivors of European Jewry and of their treatment can be found in articles by Krystal (1968), Krystal and Niederland (1971), Chodoff (1975), Rijswijk (1979), Dimsdale (1980), Eitinger and Krell (1985), Dasberg (1987), and Braham (1988), among others. Kestenberg (1989a,b) provided a relatively new focus on child survivors (those who were children during the war).

Literature on the intergenerational transmission and treatment of the psychological effects of the Holocaust on survivors' offspring (children born after the war) began with the article by Rakoff (1966). A review of the literature and an up-to-date bibliography can be found in Danieli (1981c, 1982a), Bergman and Jucovy (1982), Sigal and Weinfeld (1989), and Steinberg (1989). Recently, concern has also been voiced about the transmission of pathological intergenerational processes to the third and succeeding generations (P. A. Rosenthal & S. Rosenthal, 1980; Rubenstein, 1989).

My descriptions (Danieli, 1981a, 1988b), corroborated by the studies of Rich (1982) and Sigal and Weinfeld (1989), and findings by others, such as Klein-Parker (1988) and B. Kahana, Harel, and E. Kahana (1989), of a heterogeneity of adaptation and quality of adjustment to the Holocaust and post-Holocaust life experiences of families of survivors, caution against the simple grouping of individuals as "survivors" who are expected to exhibit the same "survivor syndrome" (Krystal & Niederland, 1968), and the expectation that children of survivors will manifest a singly transmitted "children of survivors syndrome" (Phillips, 1978). Detailed descriptions of the four differing adaptational styles of survivors' families—the *Victim* families, *Fighter* families, *Numb* families, and families of "*Those who made it*"—can be found in Danieli (1981a,c).

The Project's goals, which are preventive as well as reparative, are predicated on two major assumptions: (1) that integration of Holocaust experiences into the *totality* of the survivors' and their children's lives, and awareness of the meaning of post-Holocaust adaptational styles (Danieli, 1981a,c) will liberate them from their traumata and facilitate mental health and self-actualization for both; and (2) that awareness of transmitted intergenerational processes will inhibit transmission of pathology to succeeding generations.

Except for participation in the Intergenerational

Community Meetings (Danieli, 1989), each prospective Project participant is interviewed in order to determine the appropriate therapeutic modality. Many participants choose to combine a variety of modalities (e.g., individual and group therapy). The central therapeutic goal of integrating rupture, discontinuity, and disorientation informed the diagnostic and therapeutic choice of constructing a multigenerational family tree during initial interviews with newcomers to the Project.

Psychological/internal liberation from the trauma of victimization and its effects is the ultimate goal of treatment of survivors and their children. *Integration* is its central and guiding dynamic principle; that is, integration of the trauma into one's life span such that it will become a meaningful part of the survivor's and the survivors' offspring's identity, hierarchy of values, and orientation of living. Such integration can only be achieved through acquiring a full longitudinal perspective of one's life, which will include the victimization experiences and their impact at any point in time. An essential aspect of the establishment of such perspective is that when we speak of integration for severely victimized people we speak of integrating a rupture (Danieli, 1985b, p. 307) and the *extraordinary* into one's life—that is, confronting and incorporating aspects of human experience that are not normally encountered. The massive catastrophe of the Nazi Holocaust not only ruptured continuity but also destroyed all the individual's existing supports. The conspiracy of silence exacerbated the situation by further depriving survivors of *potential* supports.

Use of the Multigenerational Family Tree

Begun as a pragmatic way of trying to systematically collect patients' histories, the use of the family tree emerged not only as an extremely effective diagnostic and therapeutic tool in working with this population, but as an organic context, an orienting guide, a leitmotif in the framework of charting or mapping treatment progress. As one of our participants ironically declared, "This family tree has such visual impact! It's not only for the therapist. This is a therapy tool for the patients!" Indeed, as a metaphor the genogram makes explicit and visually expresses the goals and assumptions of the project—(re)establishing a sense of rootedness, belongingness and continuity with the *totality* of one's life (see also Lifton, 1973, 1979; Krystal, 1988).

Thus, to understand postwar adjustment, when constructing the multigenerational family tree it is critical to explore the pre-Holocaust background. In addition to learning the names of family members, and such factors as the nationality, places of residence, age, birth order, education, occupation, and marital, economic, societal, and communal status and aspirations of the survivors at the onset of the Holocaust, this includes becoming acquainted with the characteristics and dynamics of the survivor's family of origin in the pre-World War II European Jewish cultural and religious life, in its heterogeneity. The latter may prove particularly important when the survivor or offspring needs to discuss the meaning of being a Jew and the belief in God before and after the Holocaust, and the creation of the State of Israel (Danieli, 1981b, 1984; Marcus & Rosenberg, 1989).

The details of the family's war history are of paramount significance to the identities of its survivors and of their offspring, and should be thoroughly explored in their therapies. Children of survivors seem to have consciously and unconsciously absorbed their parents' Holocaust experiences into their lives. Holocaust parents, in the attempt to give children their best, taught them how to survive and in the process transmitted to them the life conditions under which they had survived the war. Thus, one finds children of survivors, who psychologically , and sometimes literally, live in hiding. Others are always ready to escape or continuously run from relationships with people, from commitment to a career, or from one place of residence or country to another. Some keep split or double (fake) identities. Yet others adopt a resigned passivity as their mode of being in the worldcamp. We see tireless manipulators and those who, in whatever they do, are resistance fighters. These modes of being are manifested in their language, behavior, fantasy life, and dreams.

Like their parents, many children of survivors manifest these Holocaust-derived behaviors particularly on the anniversaries of their parents' traumata (Axelrod, Schnipper, & Rau, 1980). Moreover, some survivors' offspring have internalized as parts of their identity the images of those who perished (see also Kestenberg, 1989a) and hence experience themselves as living in different places (Europe and America) and different time zones (1942 and the present) simultaneously.

Working with the Holocaust is always painful, but during the taking of the patient's history nothing else so starkly depicts the abyss as constructing the multigenerational family tree. The impact of the visual image is inescapable. It makes compellingly evident the degree of the loss, the fragmentation, desolation and rupture of the whole constellation of immediate and extended family and community. A child of survivors who came "to learn how to tell" her 11-year-old daughter their family history, abruptly stopped constructing their family tree, insisting that "it's so small. . . . There is nothing there. That is not what I want to know." It also mercilessly demonstrates the potential transgenerational distortions and damage to the concept, myths and sense of family, and time (Lomranz & Shmotkin, 1985). Patient(s) and therapist *see* the *broken* cycle of the generations and ages. "This is like a private Yad Vashem," remarked a survivor at the completion of a rather lengthy process of constructing his richly elaborate family tree, during which he was very engaged in describing the *living*, prewar period. In Elie Wiesel's words (1979) "they have no cemetery; we are their cemetery." Indeed, the commemorative function (Chodoff, 1980, 1981) of "survivor guilt" (Carmelly, 1975; Krystal & Niederland, 1968; Niederland, 1961, 1964); and its functions related to mourning, loneliness, loyalty, a sense of justice, and helplessness (Danieli, 1981d, 1985a, 1988c; Goodman, 1978; Klein, 1968), are easily implied upon examining the survivors' multigenerational family tree. Roskies (1984) reports that ultraorthodox Jews send invitations to their murdered relatives, addressing the cards to the death camps where they perished.

The family tree structurally organizes one's history and makes immediately evident the issues and themes primary to these families (see Figure 75.1). In this chap-

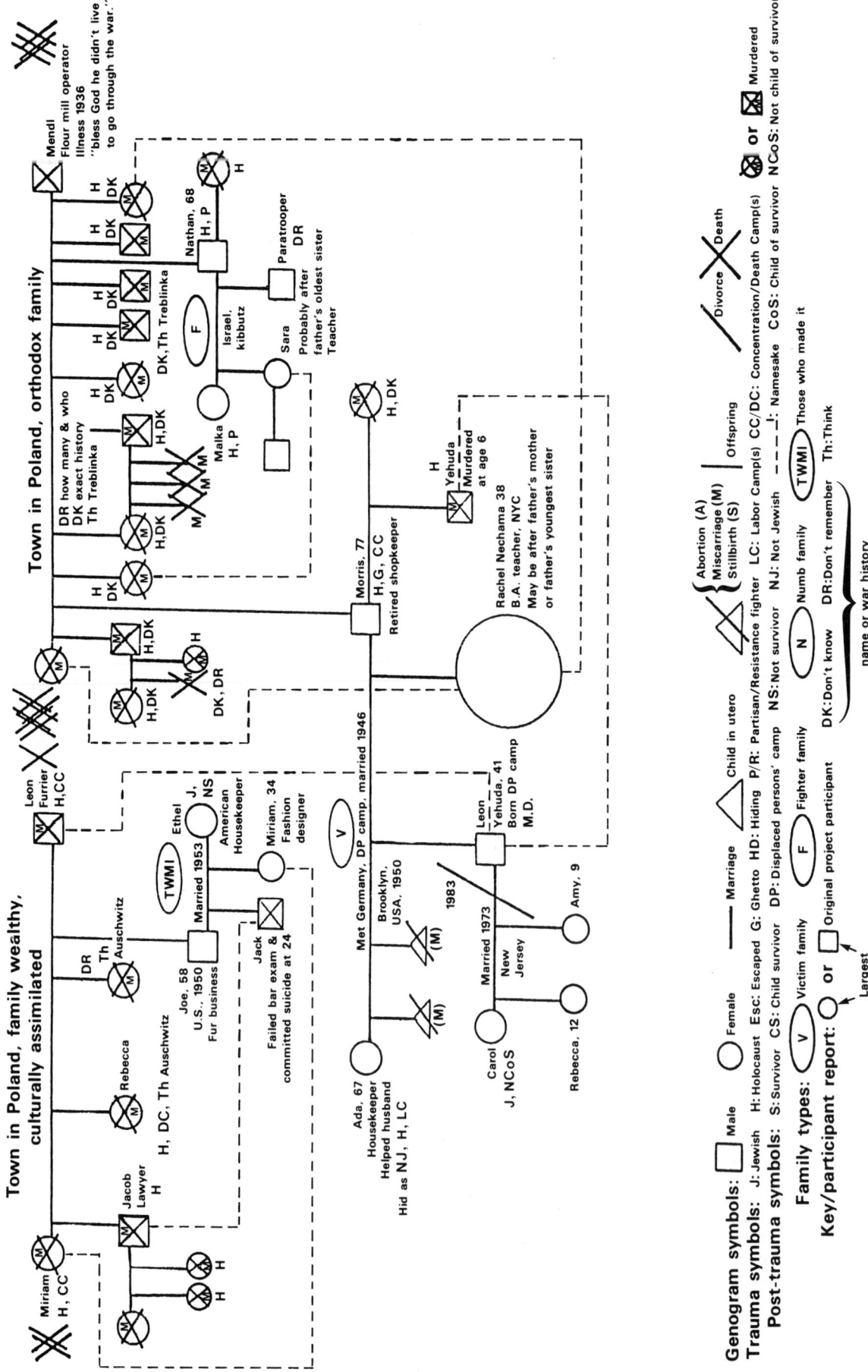

Figure 75.1. Survivors' family tree (structural).

Genogram symbols: ☐ Male   ◯ Female   △ Child in utero   ⎯⎯ Marriage   │ Offspring

Trauma symbols: J: Jewish   H: Holocaust   Esc: Escaped   G: Ghetto   HD: Hiding   P/R: Partisan/Resistance fighter   LC: Labor Camp(s)   CC/DC: Concentration/Death Camp(s)   DP: Displaced persons' camp   NS: Not survivor   NJ: Not Jewish

Post-trauma symbols: S: Survivor   CS: Child survivor   'I: Namesake   CoS: Child of survivor   NCoS: Not child of survivor

Family types: ◯ Victim family   Ⓝ Numb family   Ⓕ Fighter family   (TWMI) Those who made it

Key/participant report: ⓥ Original project participant   DK: Don't know   DR: Don't remember   Th: Think

⊗ or ⊠ Murdered   ╲ Divorce   ✕ Death

A: Abortion (A)   M: Miscarriage (M)   S: Stillbirth (S)

name or war history

ter, I address some of the themes which most directly bear on its diagnostic and therapeutic use. First and foremost is the degree of the loss, murder, and destruction and the consequent shock, disbelief, horror, helplessness, and overwhelming sense of loss of control and vulnerability; rage, outrage, and anger at the desolation, profound sense of (survivor and other) guilt and shame, and excruciating pain and grief. Second, a keen realization of the genuine impossibility of mourning (Danieli, 1981c, 1989; Meerloo, 1963; Sigal, 1971; Terry, 1984; Trautman, 1971), not only the loss of so many (de Wind, 1972; Klein, 1968; Krystal, 1981), but also the absence of dates and "evidence" of their death (Bettelheim, 1984; Leitner, 1985), "transitional objects" from their "past lives" (Bychowski, 1968; Spiegelman, 1986; Wiesel, 1972), and the want of words to describe and express it all.

Not surprisingly, emerging out of such an unprotective history, many survivors and children of survivors feel vulnerable to a return of anything that might signify the Holocaust. Although some of the literature reports good adjustment in survivors' children, Solomon, Kotler, and Milkulincer (1988) demonstrated in them a special vulnerability to traumatic stress. The family tree clearly illustrates a potential vulnerability to further separations and losses, to life's changes, fear of trusting "outsiders" (including psychotherapists), while maintaining mutual overprotectiveness within the family, as mentioned in the above literature (see also Freyberg, 1989) and as described in the case material below.

The tree further demonstrates how very small survivors' remnant families are and how this fact alone suggests possible psychological limitations (Eitinger, 1980). For example, the burden on the marital unit to meet unconscious restorative expectations were bound to fail, especially in the context of *marriages of despair* (Danieli, 1981c, 1988b; Davidson, 1984). Also, the size of the family partly explains the intensity of affect, of activity, of frozenness and silence that pervades many survivors' households. Frankle (1978) described the effects on the nature of *parenting* of the absence of the survivors' parents to provide help and support and serve as realistic, rather than ideal(ized), parental models at appropriate stages of their children's development. One emerging hypothesis in need of further testing is that the survival of the mother/child unit of continuity should predict better adaptation. Many child survivors include the families that rescued them during the war in their family tree. Ornstein (1981) viewed grandparenting and the creation of postwar "adoptive" extended families as highly adaptive and healing, especially for aging survivors.

The multigenerational family tree also illustrates the sense of burden the children may experience (H. Barocas & C. B. Barocas, 1979) at choosing, out of a deep loving mission to undo the Holocaust for their parents and for themselves, to become both the "carriers" and replacement of the family tree, and its future "resurrectors." It suggests their longing and their determination to have a large family again, their envy and estrangement when visiting such "clans," their tendency to seek and "adopt" others as "relatives," or to construct a family in fantasy. Some become "family addicts," whose overwhelming need to transform every situation into a romanticized,

often extremely idealized, rigidly pure and moralistic family situation may lead to inappropriate work and social expectations and behaviors.

An essential aspect of the diagnostic use of the family tree is to evaluate the survivor's and or offspring's general cognitive approach (see Shafir, Hirsch, & Shepps, 1975; Dor-Shav, 1978; also see discussions of the "posttraumatic constellations," notably alexithymia and anhedonia, in Krystal, 1981; for the availability and ability to use fantasy in the offspring, see Auerhahn, 1980, and Kleinplatz, 1980). The quantity and quality of memory and remembering vary in these families. Some children of survivors do not know the names of their grandparents, uncles, and aunts, how many they may have had, their ages, or who they are named after. Most children of survivors remember their family's and war history *"only in bits and pieces,"* and experience the *healing of the narrative* as most integrative and therapeutic (Auerhahn & Laub, 1984). The activity of rebridging is often experienced as healing the family wound, which may free one to go on with life more fully. Survivors and children of survivors who have distinct memory gaps may identify with absence and death and, as a result, transferentially relate to their therapists and others as absent or dead. Thus, one's sense of coherent identity, place, and comfort in the world, and one's definition of where and when he or she begins (i.e., in Biblical times or after the Holocaust) and his or her sources of growth and strength are intimately related to *(re)claiming* or *owning* one's family tree and the totality of its history (Danieli, 1981b).

Families differ in their styles of communication and in the permitted quantity and quality of sharing. Some parents decided to forget their Holocaust experiences for fear that the memories would corrode their and their children's lives. Some children will not ask questions to protect their parents and themselves against the hurt of remembering, reliving, and knowing. Some want to know all the details, who, what, why, where, read everything they can, go on pilgrimages to their parents old hometowns, visit notorious camps with their parents or alone, and retrace and integrate their Holocaust "journey"—"trying to make it real." In the case of children whose survivor parents have died, doing their "homework" to complete their family tree can cause an additional "horrible sense of loss, of missed opportunities" when "it's too late for oral history . . . I am so frightened and lost. With their death I also lost my whole history, forever." The healing significance of a stable narrative is evident in the story of a survivor who always believed that his grandmother died in Auschwitz, and who found out, during a visit to a Holocaust museum, that she had actually died in Treblinka. He remarked:

> Not that it changes anything. But such elementary things of where a person died gave me a jolt 30 years later, and told me yet another thing I don't know for sure. . . . To my mind there I was, fooling myself. Having been to Auschwitz, somehow I knew the place and understood a little more. Fortunately, I have never been to Treblinka, but I have read a lot. It hurt all over again, and as much.

Similarly, a child of survivors who learned that his grandfather had actually died just 2 days before liberation, rather than much earlier, experienced anew his sense of helplessness, hurt, and outrage. When, after 3 years in therapy, a survivor's daughter discovered that her mother had an additional sister she did not know about [making the mothers family consist of *three* sisters and four brothers] she experienced a simultaneous gain and loss, and felt that her *"whole world has to be re-arranged."*

Survivor families also differ in their tolerance for affect and fantasy. Thus, some survivors tell their stories in great detail, but without any affect. Others become overwhelmed by intense emotions and are unable to contain the details. Concrete and discrete thinking are rather common.

> Everything is either/or, totally one way or the other, with nothing in between. Its all like life or death. Words don't really make it. We take things literally because things *really* happened.

However, as Bettelheim (1984) commented, "what cannot be talked about can also not be put to rest; and if it is not, the wounds continue to fester from generation to generation" (p. 166). Indeed, Cahn (1987) demonstrated that the more able and willing the parents were to acknowledge and openly share their experiences, the less likely were their children to experience depression and separation-individuation difficulties. In the context of the use of the multigenerational family tree, she[2] noted the importance of articulating their experiences, and commented that the tree

> gives specificity to the general sense of loss and instead of nebulous emptiness you begin to feel pain associated with real loss. . . . [By conjuring up the images] You get in touch with the objects you carry around, you describe accurately and identify with *real* people, not vague, idealized, impossible to identify with, martyred figures.

She also commented on the immediate therapeutic value of seeing the context of many of one's core issues of living, of "seeing connections regardless of the degree of sophistication" and likened the shared activity of building the family tree to "sitting with a grandparent who reminisces with you, which most children of survivors don't have."

Constructing the family tree *together* also has a containing therapeutic effect and underlines again the importance of the full psychological availability of the listener.

The family tree as a metaphor has a restorative impact as well. It focuses on what was destroyed rather than on the consequences of the destruction alone. Although it triggers an acute sense of pain and loss, it reaffirms the importance of continuity and belongingness. One child of survivors commented:

> There is loss and connection at the same time. I have a family tree like every other family. There *are* roots. After the war, third cousins became first cousins and you adopt relatives. They are sort of there in my personality and they serve a purpose. They are here, and they are a part of me. My parents talked a lot about their families. Some families don't and that is so tragic. It is bad enough

that people are gone, but it's awful when their existence is denied. We are mourning them, but they existed. The pain I feel is because I have to deal with the loss, but it also brings people into life.

Another child of survivors commented, "My mother's mother has been transformed into *my* grandmother. My life has been enriched with a totally new, and real, dimension."

One invaluable yield of exploring the family tree is that it opens communication within families and between generations and makes it possible to work through toxic family secrets. Breaking the silence about the Holocaust and pre-Holocaust experiences within the family is generally helpful in (family) therapy, but it is particularly crucial for aging survivors and their offspring (Danieli, 1981e).[3]

The family tree also helps to develop one's ability for fantasy, which has been damaged in survivors and in their children by their family's traumata. Its development then allows them to also "fill the vacuum with creative responses." Indeed, members of the Project have been very active in searching for symbolic expressions for their own and their family's experiences in the creative arts. Again, this underscores the therapeutic value of the group modality, in that it offers a multiplicity of options for expressing, naming, verbalizing, and modulating feelings. It provides a safe place for exploring fantasies, for imagining, "inviting," and taking on the roles of murdered relatives or victimizers, and for examining their significance in the identity of group members. The group encourages and demonstrates mutual caring, which also draws on comforting memories, and ultimately enhances self-care in survivors and their families.

As stated at the beginning of this chapter, the Group Project for Holocaust Survivors and their Children offers a variety of therapeutic modalities, and most participants choose to combine more than one. However, regardless of the therapeutic modality used, individuals and families are viewed within the context of their multigenerational family tree, with its unique dynamics, history, and culture (E. F. Wachtel & P. L. Wachtel, 1986).

Transitions and Continuity

It is particularly during times of transition in people's lives that they tend to conjure up their family tree, to reexamine its relation to their changing life, and consequently remap their role in it.

Upon deciding to get married and have children, JR, a child of survivors, went through a period of "hallucinations breakdown" wherein she, feeling excruciating pain and fear, experienced her murdered relatives emerging out of her bleeding fingertips. She couldn't stop it. They had "an exodus out of [her] body." She had "to evacuate and free [her] inner spaces for new full loves and commitments to begin a future family." She no longer could "serve as a cemetery for people who had none, to

---

[2]A. Cahn (personal communication, May, 1988).

[3]For issues and concerns particular to aging survivors, see Blau and Kahana (1981).

house their souls because their bodies were gassed and burnt." The "bleeding" meant to her that she was in labor, somehow giving birth to them. At the same time, she felt overwhelming guilt for letting them go. Her ruptured skin and bleeding also signified her self punishment for being a Nazi in doing so.

Her agony in letting go of her murdered family also reflected her extremely arduous struggle to separate from her living nuclear family (see also LO's case described in Danieli, 1989). She used to be severely bulimic. She overcame her bulimia in therapy a year prior to this outbreak. This allowed her, for the first time in the history of her relationship with men, to choose an available one. A subsequent pilgrimage to her family's country of origin coincided with her struggle to choose between two men: An American Jew (not a child of survivors) who represents her identification with her present and future country, versus a Jewish child of survivors from her family's original country whom she fell in love with when he visited the United States. She chose to "confront the past and its lessons" in her artistic career, and to marry her American husband, with whom she happily has a boy and a girl.

The emergence of the leitmotif of the family tree in a "resurrection dream" of a daughter of survivors began the most meaningful change in her life. She dreamt that she was sitting on the edge of a grave, from which many hands were reaching out to her. Her associations led to her murdered relatives, and to imagining her parents' lives before the war. In particular, she pictured, with great longing, Friday evening dinner in a religious home, with lit candles, and prayers and songs, and the smell of the challah, and intimate family closeness and warmth. As she described her fantasies in great detail, she found herself jealous of her parents' prewar life, which was in sharp contrast to the fragmented and lonely life they had now, with their children, including LB, who was suffering from severe depressions, utter forlorness, and alcohol abuse. An artist, she began to draw the dream and related imagery, and decided to explore symbolic links to her family's prewar life. Beyond her art, her search led her to find new roots in Hasidism. She married a man with kindred aspirations and is in the process of building a large family in an Orthodox Jewish community of which she feels an integral part. Her change inspired the rest of her siblings to follow suit and to create a semblance of extended family for her parents as well.

Most children of survivors were named after murdered relatives. Some were namesakes of murdered half-siblings. Frequently, the idealized stories and fantasies of their namesakes determined the way their parents viewed and treated them and shaped parts of their identities. When they have to choose names for their own children, they have to decide whether to name them after a family member, as a first or second (mute) name. Is it the name their child is going to live by proudly and publicly or is it a secret, mute, private name, that others know only by initial (code)?

GP, a daughter of survivors who first maintained the fantasy that her being overweight protected her from becoming a visible corpse, later associated it with having to "carry the weight of the family tree for [her] parents, and provide for everyone," a meaning that she found "grounding." Her separation difficulties from her mother had to do with her association that, "When my mother separated from her mother [in Auschwitz], her mother went to the left [to the gas chambers] and my mother went to the right. How could I possibly do anything like

that?" A profound sense of resignation permeated every aspect of her life. Despite clear evidence of competence in almost anything she chose to do, her first response to anything was, "I can't." Having been married for 5 years at the beginning of treatment, she also felt deeply ambivalent about having children since, "for me, to have children is to affirm life, my life. Children mean that life has value, that it ought to be perpetuated. I never allowed myself the right to live. I never valued my life. So having children would be affirming my own life, saying that I have the right to live fully and connect with the continuity of life. Somehow it had to stop with me. I have no conception of it continuing."

It was to the delight of everyone in the Project when she decided, during her sixth year of combined individual and group therapy, that she wanted to have children. When in the fifth month of her pregnancy, she tragically discovered that she had developed breast cancer and had to undergo a mastectomy. Reflecting her sense of resignation, she responded, "I can't create life without the presence of death." Experiencing her physician's assertion that she must choose between her life and the baby's as a "return to Auschwitz, to Mengele," she chose to change physicians and hospitals, to postpone chemotherapy, and to not use any pain medications after her mastectomy, in order to hold onto the baby and to not harm it in any way. When the time came to give the baby a name, she decided not to have him commemorate anyone who was murdered, but named him after the first Jew, Avraham (who lived long before the Holocaust happened).

The therapeutic journeys of participants in the Group Project for Holocaust Survivors and their Children described in this chapter reflect the paramount centrality of the family in the lives of survivors and their offspring and, indeed, illustrate the diagnostic and therapeutic benefit of viewing these individuals within the context of their multigenerational family tree regardless of the therapeutic modality used. This therapeutic perspective may apply to other victim/survivors as well.

References

Auerhahn, N. C. (1980). *Reality, fantasy, and repetition in the concentration camp survivor and his child.* Paper presented at the meeting of the American Psychological Association, Montreal.

Auerhahn, N. C., & Laub, D. (1984). Annihilation and restoration: Post-traumatic memory as pathway and obstacle to recovery. *International Review of Psycho-Analysis, 11,* 327–344.

Axelrod, S., Schnipper, O. L., & Rau, J. H. (1980). Hospitalized offspring of Holocaust survivors: Problems and dynamics. *Bulletin of the Menninger Clinic, 44,* 1–14.

Barocas, H. A., & Barocas, C. B. (1979). Wounds of the fathers: The next generation of Holocaust victims. *International Review of Psycho-Analysis, 6,* 1–10.

Bergman M. S., & Jucovy, M. E. (Eds.). (1982). *Generations of the Holocaust.* New York: Basic Books.

Bettleheim, B. (1984). Afterword to C. Vegh, *I didn't say goodbye* (R. Schwartz, Trans.). New York: E. P. Dutton.

Blau, D., & Kahana, J. (Eds.). (1981). The aging survivor of the Holocaust (Special issue). *Journal of Geriatric Psychiatry, 14*(2).

Braham, R. L. (Ed.). (1988). *The psychological perspectives of the Holocaust and of its aftermath.* New York: Columbia University Press.

Bychowski, G. (1968). Permanent character changes as an aftereffect of persecution. In H. Krystal (Ed.), *Massive psychic trauma.* New York: International Universities Press.

Cahn, A. (1987). *The capacity to acknowledge experience in Holocaust survivors and their children.* Unpublished doctoral dissertation, Adelphi University.

Carmelly, F. (1975). Guilt feelings in concentration camp survivors: Comments of a "survivor." *Journal of Jewish Communal Service, 2,* 139–144.

Chodoff, P. (1975). Psychiatric aspects of the Nazi persecution. In S. Arieti (Ed.), *American handbook of psychiatry* (Vol. 6, 2nd ed.). New York: Basic Books.

Chodoff, P. (1980). Psychotherapy of the survivor. In J. E. Dimsdale (Ed.), *Survivors, victims and perpetrators: Essays on the Nazi Holocaust.* New York: Hemisphere.

Chodoff, P. (1981). Survivors of the Nazi Holocaust. *Children Today, 10*(5), 2–5.

Danieli, Y. (1980). Countertransference in the treatment and study of Nazi Holocaust survivors and their children. *Victimology: An International Journal. 5*(2–4), 355–367.

Danieli, Y. (1981a). Differing adaptational styles in families of survivors of the Nazi Holocaust: Some implications for treatment. *Children Today, 10*(5), 6–10, 34–35.

Danieli, Y. (1981b). Exploring the factors in Jewish identity formation (in children of survivors). In *Consultation on the psychodynamics of Jewish identity: Summary of proceedings* (pp. 22–25). American Jewish Committee and the Central Conference of American Rabbis, March 15–16, 1981.

Danieli, Y. (1981c). Families of survivors of the Nazi Holocaust: Some short- and long-term effects. In C. D. Speilberger, I. G. Sarason, & N. Milgram (Eds.), *Stress and anxiety* (Vol. 8). New York: McGraw-Hill/Hemisphere.

Danieli, Y. (1981d). Matching interventions to different adaptational styles of survivors. In *Massuah: A yearbook on the Holocaust and heroism* (Vol. 9). Tel-Aviv: M. Stern Press. (In Hebrew)

Danieli, Y. (1981e). On the achievement of integration in aging survivors of the Nazi Holocaust. *Journal of Geriatric Psychiatry, 14*(2), 191–210.

Danieli, Y. (1982a). Therapists' difficulties in treating survivors of the Nazi Holocaust and their children. (Doctoral dissertation, New York University, 1981.) *University Microfilms International,* No. 949–904.

Danieli, Y. (1982b). *Group project for Holocaust survivors and their children.* Prepared for National Institute of Mental Health, Mental Health Services Branch. Contract #092424762. Washington, DC.

Danieli, Y. (1984). Psychotherapists' participation in the conspiracy of silence about the Holocaust. *Psychoanalytic Psychology, 1*(1), 23–42.

Danieli, Y. (1985a). Separation and loss in families of survivors of the Nazi Holocaust. *Academy Forum, 29*(2), 7–10.

Danieli, Y. (1985b). The treatment and prevention of long-term effects and intergenerational transmission of victimization: A lesson from Holocaust survivors and their children. In C. R. Figley (Ed.), *Trauma and its wake* (pp. 295–313). New York: Brunner/Mazel.

Danieli, Y. (1988a). Confronting the unimaginable: Psychotherapists' reactions to victims of the Nazi Holocaust. In J. P. Wilson, Z. Harel, & B. Kahana (Eds.), *Human adaptation to extreme stress: From the Holocaust to Vietnam* (pp. 219–238). New York: Plenum Press.

Danieli, Y. (1988b). The heterogeneity of postwar adaptation in families of Holocaust survivors. In R. L. Braham (Ed.), *The psychological perspectives of the Holocaust and of its aftermath* (pp. 109–128). New York: Columbia University Press.

Danieli, Y. (1988c). Treating survivors and children of survivors of the Nazi Holocaust. In F. M. Ochberg (Ed.), *Post-traumatic therapy and victims of violence* (pp. 278–294). New York: Brunner/Mazel.

Danieli, Y. (1988d). The use of mutual support approaches in the treatment of victims. In E. Chigier (Ed.), *Grief and bereavement in contemporary society: Vol. 3. Support systems* (pp. 116–123). London: Freund Publishing House.

Danieli, Y. (1989). Mourning in survivors and children of survivors of the Nazi Holocaust: The role of group and community modalities. In D. R. Dietrich, & P. C. Shabad (Eds.), *The problem of loss and mourning: Psychoanalytic perspectives* (pp. 427–460). Madison, CT: International Universities Press.

Danieli, Y., & Krystal, J. H. (1989). *The initial report of the Presidential Task Force on Curriculum, Education and Training of the Society for Traumatic Stress Studies.* Chicago: The Society for Traumatic Stress Studies.

Dasberg, H. (1987). Psychological distress of Holocaust survivors and offspring in Israel, forty years later: A review. *Israel Journal of Psychiatry and Related Sciences, 23*(4), 243–256.

Davidson, S. (1984). Human reciprocity among the Jewish prisoners in the Nazi concentration camps. In Y. Gutman & A. Sat (Eds.), *Nazi concentration: Proceedings of the Fourth Yad Vashem International Historical Conference* (pp. 555–572). Jerusalem: Yad Vashem.

Des Pres, T. (1976). *The survivor: An anatomy of life in the death camps.* New York: Oxford University Press.

de Wind, E. (1972). Persecution, aggression and therapy. *International Journal of Psycho-Analysis, 53,* 173–177.

Dimsdale, J. E. (Ed.). (1980). *Survivors, victims and perpetrators: Essays on the Nazi Holocaust.* New York: Hemisphere.

Dor-Shav, K. N. (1978). On the long-range effects of concentration camp internment on Nazi victims: 25 years later. *Journal of Consulting and Clinical Psychology, 46,* 1–11.

Eitinger, L. (1980). The concentration camp syndrome and its late sequelae. In J. E. Dimsdale (Ed.), *Survivors, victims, and perpetrators: Essays on the Nazi Holocaust.* New York: Hemisphere.

Eitinger, L., & Krell, R. (Eds.). (1985). *The psychological and medical effects of concentration camps and related persecutions on survivors of the Holocaust: A research bibliography.* Vancouver: University of British Columbia Press.

Eitinger, L. (1972). *Concentration camp survivors in Norway and Israel.* The Hague: Martinus Nijhoff.

Frankle, H. (1978). The survivors as parent. *Journal of Jewish Communal Service, 54*(3), 241–246.

Freyberg, J. T. (1989). The emerging self in the survivor family. In P. Marcus & A. Rosenberg (Eds.), *Healing their wounds: Psychotherapy with Holocaust survivors and their families* (pp. 85–104). New York: Praeger.

Goodman, J. S. (1978). The transmission of parental trauma: Second generation effects of Nazi concentration camp survival. (Doctoral dissertation, California School of Professional Psychology, 1978.) *University Microfilms International,* No. 7901805.

Guerin, P. J., Jr., & Pendagast, E. G. (1976). Evaluation of family system and genogram. In P. J. Geurin, Jr. (Ed.), *Family therapy: Theory and practice* (pp. 450–464). New York: Gardner Press.

Kahana, B., Harel, Z., & Kahana, E. (1989). Clinical and gerontological issues facing survivors of the Nazi Holocaust. In P.

Marcus & A. Rosenberg (Eds.), *Healing their wounds: Psychotherapy with Holocaust survivors and their families* (pp. 197–211). New York: Praeger.

Kestenberg, J. (1989a). Transposition revisited: Clinical, therapeutic, and developmental considerations. In P. Marcus and A. Rosenberg (Eds.), *Healing their wounds: Psychotherapy with Holocaust survivors and their families* (pp. 67–82). New York: Praeger.

Kestenberg, J. S. (1989b). Coping with losses and survival. In D. R. Dietrich & P. C. Shabad (Eds.), *The problem of loss and mourning: Psychoanalytic perspectives* (pp. 381–404). Madison, CT: International Universities Press.

Klein, H. (1968). Problems in the psychotherapeutic treatment of Israeli survivors of the Holocaust. In H. Krystal (Ed.), *Massive psychic trauma*. New York: International Universities Press.

Klein-Parker, F. (1988). Dominant attitudes of adult children of Holocaust survivors toward their parents. In J. P. Wilson, Z. Harel, & B. Kahana (Eds.), *Human adaptation to extreme stress: From the Holocaust to Vietnam* (pp. 193–218). New York: Plenum Press.

Kleinplatz, M. M. (1980). *Contribution of support to the adaptation of survivors' children in two cultures*. Paper presented at the annual meeting of the American Psychological Association, Montreal.

Krystal H. (1968). *Massive psychic trauma*. New York: International Universities Press.

Krystal, H. (1975). Affect tolerance. *Annual of Psychoanalysis, 3*, 179–219.

Krystal, H. (1978). Trauma and affect. *Psychoanalytic Study of the Child, 33*, 81–116.

Krystal, H. (1981). Integration and self-healing in posttraumatic states. *Journal of Geriatric Psychiatry, 14*(2), 165–189.

Krystal, H. (1988). *Integration and self-healing*. Hillsdale, NJ: Analytic Press.

Krystal H., & Niederland, W. G. (1968). Clinical observations on the survivor syndrome. In H. Krystal (Ed.), *Massive psychic trauma*. New York: International Universities Press.

Krystal, H. & Niederland, W. G. (Eds.). (1971). *Psychic traumatization: Aftereffects in individuals and communities*. Boston: Little, Brown.

Leitner, I. (1985). *Saving the fragments*. New York: New American Library.

Lifton, R. J. (1973). The sense of immorality: On death and the continuity of life. *American Journal of Psychoanalysis, 33*, 3–15.

Lifton, R. J. (1979). *The broken connection*. New York: Simon & Schuster.

Lomranz, J., & Shmotkin, D. (1985). Time orientation in Nazi concentration camp survivors: Forty years after. *American Journal of Orthopsychiatry, 55*(2), 230–236.

Luchterhand, E. (1967). Prisoner behavior and social system in the Nazi concentration camps. *International Journal of Psychoanalysis, 13*(4), 245–264.

Luchterhand, E. (1971). Sociological approaches to massive stress in natural and man-made disasters. In H. Krystal & W. G. Niederland (Eds.), *Psychic traumatization: Aftereffects in individuals and communities*. New York: Little, Brown.

Marcus, P., & Rosenberg, A. (1989). The religious life of Holocaust survivors and its significance for psychotherapy. In P. Marcus & A. Rosenberg (Eds.), *Healing their wounds* (pp. 227–256). New York: Praeger.

Matussek, P. (1975). *Internment in concentration camps and its consequences* (D. Jordan & I. Jordan, Trans.). New York: Springer Verlag. (Original work published 1971)

Meerlo, J. A. M. (1963). Delayed mourning in victims of extermination camps. *Journal of Hillside Hospital, 12*(2), 96–98.

Moskovitz, S. (1983). *Love despite hope*. New York: Schoken.

Niederland, W. G. (1961). The problem of the survivor: Some remarks on the psychiatric evaluation of emotional disorders in survivors of the Nazi persecution. *Journal of the Hillside Hospital, 10*(3–4), 233–247.

Niederland, W. G. (1964). Psychiatric disorders among persecution victims: A contribution to the understanding of concentration camp pathology and its aftereffects. *Journal of Nervous and Mental Diseases, 139*, 458–474.

Phillips, R. D. (1978). Impact of Nazi Holocaust on children of survivors. *American Journal of Psychotherapy, 32*, 370–378.

Rakoff, V. A. (1966). A long-term effect of the concentration camp experience. *Viewpoints, 1*, 17–22.

Rich, M. S. (1982). *Children of Holocaust survivors: A concurrent validity study of a survivor family typology*. Unpublished doctoral dissertation, California School of Professional Psychology, Berkeley.

Rijswijk, Z. H. (Ed.). (1979). *Israel-Netherlands symposium on the impact of persecution* (Jerusalem, October, 1977). The Netherlands: Ministry of Cultural Affairs, Recreation and Social Weifare.

Rosenthal, P. A., & Rosenthal, S. (1980). Holocaust effect in the third generation: Child of another time. *American Journal of Psychotherapy, 34*(4), 572–580.

Roskies, D. G. (1984). *Against the Apocalypse: Responses to catastrophe in modern Jewish culture*. Cambridge: Harvard University Press.

Rubenstein, I. (1989, October). *Psychic trauma as a result of the Holocaust in three generations*. Paper presented at the Fifth Annual Meeting of the Society for Traumatic Stress Studies, San Francisco

Shafir, A., Hirsch, M., & Shepps, S. (1975). *The delayed mental influence of the Holocaust experience as projected in a psychodiagnostic battery*. Unpublished manuscript, Tel-Aviv University Medical School, Mental Health Clinic, Kupat Holim, Tel-Aviv.

Sigal J. J. (1971). Second-generation effects of massive psychic trauma. In H. Krystal & W. G. Niederland (Eds.), *Psychic traumatization: Aftereffects in individuals and communities* (pp. 67–92). Boston: Little, Brown.

Sigal, J. J., & Weinfeld, M. (1989). *Trauma and rebirth: Intergenerational effects of the Holocaust*. New York: Praeger.

Solomon, Z., Kotler, M., & Milkulincer, M. (1988). Combat-related post-traumatic stress disorders among second generation Holocaust survivors: Preliminary findings. *American Journal of Psychiatry, 145*, 865–868.

Spiegelman, A. (1986). *Maus*. New York: Pantheon Books.

Steinberg, A. (1989). Holocaust survivors and their children: A review of the clinical literature. In P. Marcus & A. Rosenberg (Eds.), *Healing their wounds: Psychotherapy with Holocaust survivors and their families* (pp. 23–48). New York: Praeger.

Terry, J. (1984). The damaging effects of the "survivor syndrome." In S. A. Luel & P. Marcus (Eds.), *Psychoanalytic reflections on the Holocaust: Selected essays* (pp. 135–148). New York: Holocaust Awareness Institute Center for Judaic Studies, University of Denver, and Ktav Publishing House.

Trautman, E. C. (1971). Violence and victims in Nazi concentration camps and the psychopathology of the survivors. In H. Krystal & W. G. Niederland (Eds.), *Psychic traumatization: Aftereffects in individuals and communities*. New York: Little, Brown.

Wachtel, E. F., & Wachtel, P. L. (1986). *Family dynamics in individual psychotherapy: A guide to clinical strategies*. New York: Guilford Press.

Wiesel, E. (1972). The watch. In E. Wiesel, *One generation after* (pp. 79–86). New York: Avon Books.

Wiesel, E. (1979). *Wind of Auschwitz*. Unpublished manuscript (poetry).

Wilson, A. (1985). On silence and the Holocaust: A contribution to clinical theory. *Psychoanalytical Inquiry*, 5(1), 63–84.

Winnicott, D. W. (1965). *The maturational processes and the facilitating environment*. London: Hogarth Press.

Organization, Social Policy Issues, and Critical Stress Incident Debriefing in Response to Victims of Trauma

Part VIII contains nine chapters concerned with social policy, organizational responsiveness to victims, and critical stress incident debriefing. Although it appears that the bulk of research from 1980 to the present was concerned with understanding the nature, dynamics, and vicissitudes of PTSD, far less attraction has been paid to social policy issues for the victim or in establishing organizational responsiveness to intervene and assist those adversely affected.

In Chapter 76, Jeffrey T. Mitchell and Atle Dyregrov discuss traumatic stress reactions in disaster workers and emergency medical service (EMS) personnel. By definition and the nature of their occupations, disaster workers and EMS personnel are exposed to highly stressful situations in which there is almost always an acute need for intervention to aid victims whose lives are often endangered. Clearly, such work carries with it the potential risk to develop stress reactions which, under certain conditions, could develop into PTSD.

The authors review the stress-related symptoms common to emergency work and organize their discussion into symptom clusters: cognitive, physical, emotional, behavioral, interpersonal, and delayed effects. Since it is inevitable that a range of stress reactions to emergency work will occur at some point in time for the EMS worker, the question that must be addressed is the issue of how to prevent or attenuate post-traumatic stress syndromes.

The authors discuss various approaches and techniques in order to maintain the optimal level of functioning for the employee. These include stress-mitigation programs, educational literature, postevent stress debriefing, individual counseling, and the training of management and supervisory personnel so that they can respond at the organizational level to the individual needs of EMS or disaster workers.

In Chapter 77, Arthur S. Blank, Jr., presents an overview and discussion of the Veterans Administration readjustment counseling program for Vietnam veterans. This program, which is also known colloquially as the Vet Centers, was established in 1979 in response to a growing concern about the emotional well-being of Vietnam veterans. Presently, there are 196 Vet Centers throughout the United States which have seen over 900,000 clients since the doors first opened. The initial concept of the program was to provide community-based centers, staffed by fellow veterans, and located in the veterans' neighborhoods so that peer support could be utilized in the form of individual counseling and support groups.

During the decade of its existence, the Vet Center program grew, expanded, and became more sophisticated in offering mental health services. Today, a broad range of services are offered and include individual counseling, crisis intervention, aftercare for substance abuse related to PTSD, referrals for employment assistance, and more. As Blank details in the chapter, the program was not only innovative and successful beyond expectations, but also cost-efficient and a model of a social movement in the mental health field whose impact has now been documented by conventional measures of organizational effectiveness.

In Chapter 78, Tom Williams discusses trauma in the workplace. The focus of his chapter is on stressful events that occur to ordinary workers who become victims of trauma.

To begin, Williams presents a prevention model that has three interrelated components. Primary prevention refers to attempts to reduce stressors on the job site by security protocols or similar procedures to guard against harmful exposure. Secondary prevention characterizes attempts to minimize the deleterious effects of exposure to a trauma. This phase includes critical stress incident debriefing. The third level of prevention concerns the provision of resources to facilitate individual or group counseling. Implicit in each phase of prevention, however, is knowledge of stress-response syndromes, about which the author recommends that employees become educated in detail. Toward this end, Williams presents a framework for understanding stress-response reactions and explains the acute and chronic symptoms that affect employees in the workplace. Furthermore, he notes that when PTSD develops following a trauma, the employee may be at risk for substance abuse, particularly if he or she experiences episodes of intrusive imagery alternating with denial processes. This observation is consistent with the psychobiology of trauma and alcohol addiction that was discussed by Matthew Friedman in Chapter 66. Similarly, Williams recommends that treatment must focus simultaneously on PTSD and alcohol abuse for successful amelioration.

In Chapter 79, Giovanni de Girolamo presents an international perspective in the treatment of PTSD. The author, an associate professional officer at the World Health Organization (WHO), provides an interesting framework by which to examine natural disasters and those of human origin, and to explain how social policies have been created at WHO, the United Nations, and other international organizations to address the care of victims. For example, he indicates that

> UN General Assembly Resolution 42/169, adopted on December 11, 1987, designated the 1990s as a decade for *natural disaster reduction*; it stated that natural disasters . . . have killed about 3 million people worldwide over the past two decades, adversely affected the lives of at least 800 million more, and resulted in immediate economic damage exceeding $23 billion.

These figures, and many more cited in the chapter, present a stark and disturbing image of how much global traumata exist as a consequence of different types of disasters. Thus, there exists a very strong need to create programs of prevention and treatment of traumatic stress reactions.

The author casts a perspective by which to discern the coordinated efforts of international agencies:

> The role of WHO has gradually shifted from relief to disaster preparedness and response, including involvement in training, in assessment of health situations and needs, and in coordination of large-scale disaster operations. WHO's target for the Eighth General Programme of

> Work, covering the years 1990–1995, is that by 1995, "70% of all countries will have developed
> master plans appropriate to their particular circumstances to deal with the health aspects of
> emergency and disaster situations."

An analysis of intervention programs is then presented in terms of how they attempt to address the psychiatric needs of the victims. At the end of this densely referenced chapter is the identification of seven areas needing future research, such as a broader search base on non-English populations as to the prevalence of PTSD and comorbidity.

In Chapter 80, Susan E. Salasin and Robert F. Rich discuss mental health policy for victims of violence with special emphasis on women as victims of discrimination in public policy. They state that

> it will be demonstrated that a woman who is a crime victim is a victim of "double-jeopardy":
> in jeopardy first from the "social envelope" of shame and social isolation engendered by her
> community of support; and in jeopardy second from the "policy envelope" of "woman as pro-
> vocateur," "woman as property," and "woman as liar," roles that the system assigns to her.

The authors argue that there are gender differences in reactions to assault, with women being more likely to internalize their anger than men and to have fewer socially acceptable outlets for their anger, hostility, and emotional distress. Furthermore, Salasin and Rich make the case that women are at risk as victims of violent crime since 10 million individuals are victimized yearly by domestic violence, rape, assault, and child physical and sexual abuse. As a consequence of these types of traumata, and "with devastating force, this event violates fundamental human assumptions about the integrity and control of one's body and one's self. Self-esteem is shattered, and the world no longer appears to be safe, just, and orderly." As has been noted throughout the chapters of this *Handbook*, PTSD is a common and expectable development following violent attack. Yet the authors point out that at state governmental levels throughout the United States and other countries as well, public policy and programs "are not oriented toward meeting the emotional and psychological needs of women as victims. Instead, the laws, taken as a whole, demonstrate contempt for these victims." After discussing the historical, political, and social bases of discrimination against women, a set of policy recommendations is presented which would serve to meet the needs of those women who are injured by acts of violence.

In Chapter 81, Liisa Eränen and Karmela Liebkind discuss the helping behavior of communities and individuals in coping with disaster. The authors create a social-psychological analysis of disasters, their dimensions and characteristics, before examining community reactions to the catastrophic event. They note, for example:

> The order of priorities and the consensus born in connection with a disaster are collectively
> called the *state of emergency consensus*. Under normal conditions, people identify with different
> social groups of which the most important is the family. Usually, when in a state of danger,
> people attempt to strengthen the primary group bonds and in disasters they take care first of
> those closest to them.

Thus, a disaster may cause temporary changes in values, attitudes toward subgroups in society, and the disposition of individuals to engage in prosocial behavior (voluntary helping). Four forms of voluntary helping are discussed by the authors who also make the point that a disaster provides the opportunity to bolster the self-esteem of the helper, since common group membership may create prosocial norms in the wake of the disaster.

However, for the disaster victim to receive help from volunteers, a psychosocial process of equalization of status within the emergent social structure created by the disaster itself may be necessary to ward off the effects of a lack of reciprocity between giving and receiving aid. The special value of a sociological perspective of disaster impacts is to examine changes at the macro level of community organization to determine precisely how the structural elements are altered by a disaster which, in turn, sets in motion temporary changes in groups and organizations that seek to provide assistance to the victim.

In Chapter 82, Renate Grønvold Bugge continues a discussion of creating temporary organizational structures for crisis intervention when a disaster strikes a community. Based on her experience with a major crisis in Norway in 1986, the Hotel Caledonian fire, which killed 14 persons and injured 67 others, the author had the responsibility of setting up emergency psychological services for the victims and their families.

To explain the processes that confront disaster workers in situations of crisis intervention, the author employs organization systems theory in order to identify clearly the roles, tasks, and responsibilities that have to be created (or changed within existing institutions—e.g., a hospital) in order to effectively meet the needs of the victims. In this regard, Bugge's chapter parallels the disaster work reported in Chapters 37, 38, 39, and 40 on the Kings Cross Fire, the North Sea oil rig disasters, and the Zeebrugge ferry disaster. Moreover, this chapter is especially important since it provides a generic model that indicates, in a step-by-step fashion, the sequence of tasks to be dealt with by the rescue workers and the specialist teams alike. For example:

> In an acute situation, such as a disaster, priorities can change quickly. It is therefore important to reexamine the situation continuously in deciding which tasks are primary and which are secondary. The goals of the permanent organization may have to be put aside during the acute phase to give priority to tasks that are dictated by the disaster. . . . When the support work started [in the hotel fire], the goals were quite unclear beyond providing phone service, comfort for the families who came to the hospital, and information for the clinical work. The goals had to be redefined within 48 hours.

It is the case, of course, that a disaster requires the existence of a unique organizational structure for crisis intervention and, in the chapter, Bugge categorizes and discusses each component and function of such a health care system. Among the issues included are: (1) establishing a time frame for operation and setting limits on responsibilities; (2) recruitment of volunteers and skilled persons to assist in the operation; (3) physical location and resource allocation; (4) leadership roles and the delegation of authority; (5) group process factors and stress debriefing of rescue workers; (6) lines of decision-making and communication among the staff of the temporary organization; and (7) evaluation of the crisis-intervention operation and the performances of the temporary organization staff and volunteers.

In Chapter 83, Linda Ann Stevenson presents a capsulized discussion of the role of voluntary organizations in the United Kingdom for disabled war veterans suffering from PTSD. The author's central point in the chapter is that PTSD affects a small but significant proportion of ex-servicemen and many do not receive adequate pensions or compensations for their service-connected disability. Thus, it is for this reason that voluntary organizations are established to aid war veterans in obtaining benefits that allow a reasonable standard of living. Stevenson discusses the work of the voluntary agencies and concludes that "the proper role of the voluntary organizations should be to provide social support and extend the amount and choices of care provided by the state."

In Chapter 84, the last chapter in Part VIII, Akbar Zargar, Bahman Najarian, and Derek Roger discuss settlement reconstruction and psychological recovery in Iran following the Iran–Iraq War. This chapter is unique because it details the attempt to integrate at the community level, an architectural reconstruction process of destroyed villages and towns to meet the psychological needs of the war victims. The ideas detailed in this chapter also parallel those presented in Chapters 20, 21, and 22 on World War II veterans from the United States, France, and Holland, for whom the issue of a supportive social network was a determinant of mental health in the aging process. The authors discuss how a cohesive and supportive social network, which affords the opportunity to develop a meaningful sense of connectedness to others, can reduce the severity of PTSD, in particular, and aid in the stress recovery process. Furthermore, they note that where the fabric of the community social structure has been damaged or eliminated entirely by the ravages of warfare, the systematic attempt to reconstruct communities so as to optimize patterns of behavior that have a salutary effect on coping with stress reactions can lead to positive mental health outcomes and stave off tendencies toward psychological isolation, anomie, alienation, and forms of emotional and interpersonal detachment.

All the chapters contained in Part VIII help to identify many areas for future research, education, training, and social policy work. These include (1) establishing Stage 1 forms of disaster intervention preparedness, (2) the proper training of voluntary and professional staff to deal with crisis situations, (3) the development of creative and highly effective forms of counseling to deal with the acute and prolonged effects of trauma, (4) longitudinal and cross-sectional studies of survivors and victims, (5) planning for the mental health needs of helpers, and (6) national and international coordination and program development in terms of social policies for the mental health of victims of trauma.

CHAPTER 76

Traumatic Stress in Disaster Workers and Emergency Personnel

Prevention and Intervention

Jeffrey T. Mitchell and Atle Dyregrov

Introduction

It has long been known that victims of disasters and other smaller, but still painful, life events suffer significant short- and/or long-term psychological sequelae. The focus of most psychosocial interventions and follow-up services or research during the last three or four decades has been on the actual victims and survivors of the distressing events. Those who came to help others (e.g., emergency medical service personnel) were thought to be trained not to react to human carnage and destruction or to the pain of the survivors. They were considered exempt from the psychological sequelae which befell the victims and survivors. However, recent research and experience with emergency personnel, such as firefighters, paramedics, police officers, and disaster workers, clearly indicates that these helpers are subjected to stressors which can produce an array of psychological, social, and physical reactions that may be extremely stressful.

This chapter has been designed to provide a framework to develop an understanding of emergency workers, their jobs, and their personalities. Such an understanding can assist mental health professionals in providing appropriate prevention-oriented strategies to mitigate the impact of traumatic events on emergency

personnel. In it, we will present a specially designed set of intervention strategies which can be utilized to assist emergency workers in recovering from or coping with the effects of traumatic stress.

Background

The paucity of literature related to emergency personnel and disaster workers before 1978 is noteworthy. It is as if researchers and clinicians failed to consider the potential deleterious impact that emergency work was having on the participants. Besides mentioning that firefighters in World War II in London had significant stress reactions after being exposed to continuous bombings, Glass (1959), in one of the early studies, offered little to complete an understanding of emergency services stress or its mitigation.

A document entitled *First Aid for Psychological Reactions in Disasters* was prepared in 1954 (American Psychiatric Association [APA], 1964). In it, emergency workers are cautioned, "You will naturally extend yourself to the limits of capacities. Do not push yourself beyond those limits, lest you become as ill as those who need your help" (p. 20). The document goes on to state, "Your training should prepare you to handle your own emotional problems first—and promptly . . . the training you received as a disaster worker will in itself protect you somewhat in time of stress" (pp. 20–21). Such statements, while admirable, lack an understanding of the *normality of stress responses* for the majority of emergency personnel and further contribute to the faulty concept that training alone is sufficient to eliminate significant

Jeffrey T. Mitchell • Emergency Health Services Department, University of Maryland, Baltimore County Campus, Catonsville, Maryland 21228.   **Atle Dyregrov** • Center for Crisis Psychology, Fabrikkgt 5, 5037 Solheimsvik, Norway.

International Handbook of Traumatic Stress Syndromes, edited by John P. Wilson and Beverley Raphael. Plenum Press, New York, 1993.

stress reactions in those who are exposed to horrible sights and sounds as they work with human pain.

Stressed Emergency Personnel

Fortunately, experienced clinicians like Duffy (1979; Staff, 1979) were later able to point out that no amount or type of training could eliminate stress reactions in those who walked among maimed bodies, disfigured body parts, and the array of human miseries which are present in disasters. Freeman (1979) reported that police officers who worked at a disaster site were requesting counseling and other psychological support for as long as a year after the incident. Kliman (1975) was convinced that rescue workers in the 1972 Corning, New York, flood were in need of psychological support. Other researchers point out that disaster relief workers are among those individuals who are most in need of psychological support (Cohen & Ahearn, 1980; Dunning & Silva, 1980; Hartsough, 1983; Mitchell, 1982, 1983; Peuler, 1984; Solomon, 1985). The effects of responding to and working at a disaster were compared to the effects of combat stress and found to be quite similar (Figley, 1981).

Disaster workers are not alone in their reactions to stressful work conditions. Rayner (1958) described over-intellectualization, emotional suppression, rigid thinking, and limited decision-making in emergency care nurses. Lippert and Ferrara (1981) reported that police officers who take a human life in the performance of their duties experience strong feelings of guilt, anger, immobilization, and denial. Direct work with people in need of help is, in and of itself, emotionally stressful and may produce feelings of fear, anger, embarrassment, frustration, and despair (Adams, 1980; Cherniss, 1980; Kahn, 1978; Maslach, 1978; Maslach & Jackson, 1979). The more closely one is involved with patients in the line of disaster relief work, the more vulnerable one becomes to losing one's objectivity and becoming abused (Shubin, 1979; Yager & Hubert, 1979).

Paramedics routinely list infant deaths, child abuse, mass casualties, disaster, and high-rise fires as the most stressful calls that they handle (McGlown, 1981). Furthermore, in questionnaires designed to measure job-related psychological stress, paramedics showed scores higher than firefighters whose scores were already elevated above the general population (Dutton, Smolensky, Lorimar, Hsi, & Leach, 1978). Emergency workers who do not have direct on-site involvement with the chaos and destruction or the victims themselves, may experience significant stress as a result of their work in support of more directly involved personnel. Police, fire, and emergency medical dispatchers, for example, are described in the literature as significantly stressed by their dispatch work (Doerner, 1987; Holt, 1980; Sewell & Crew, 1984; Weaver, 1987).

Those who are pressed into service during times of crisis but who normally would not perform emergency services are often seriously affected by their emergency work; perhaps even more than their emergency service counterparts who regularly perform various types of emergency work. Dyregrov (1988) found considerable stress among military personnel who were suddenly pressed into action in an attempt to find and rescue or recover victims of an avalanche in Norway. It should also be remembered, of course, that emergency work has effects which reach beyond the workers themselves and affects their families and friends as well. There are numerous descriptions in the literature of stress effects on family members of police officers and others in emergency services (Maslach & Jackson, 1979; Nordlicht, 1979).

Cognitive Effects of Emergency Work: Stress-Related Symptoms

Laube (1973) pointed out that trained emergency workers in a disaster are able to cope with their anxiety without impairment to their professional roles. However, individuals differ in their reactions, and notable signals of cognitive distress have been observed in disaster workers. High levels of anxiety and psychological stress are usually associated with poor cognitive performance (Eysenck, 1989). The more complex the cognitive task, the greater is the deficit in performance under stress. The performance on easy tasks does not seem to be seriously affected by stress (Mayer, 1977). Mental confusion is among the most frequently reported cognitive stress-response symptoms (Wilkinson & Vera, 1985). Memory problems, concentration difficulties, and poor attention span have also been observed as common signs of cognitive dysfunction as a result of stress (DSM-III-R) (APA, 1987). Constricted thought, denial, excessive use of fantasy, and selective inattention have been noted as defenses against distressing thoughts after disastrous events (Wilkinson & Vera, 1985). Furthermore, routine emergency work can also produce serious cognitive dysfunction. Among stressed subjects in general, Sedgwick (1975) noted an inability to think clearly, increased distractibility, and a reduced ability to master cognitive or eye-hand skill tasks. Lazarus (1969) reported cognitive rigidity and inflexibility and mental disorganization in stressed people. The study by Holsti in 1971 pointed to the fact that stressed people tend to display deteriorated verbal performance, diminished tolerance for ambiguity, reduced ability to concentrate, limited attention span, diminished perceptual activity, and reduced ability to discriminate the dangerous from the trivial stimuli.

Physical Effects of Emergency Work

Emergency work is filled with unanticipated and novel situations and is complicated by disturbed rest periods, long working hours, and limitations in staffing levels. All these factors tend to affect most workers negatively (Holsti, 1971; Staff, 1980). Among 2,300 police officers who were studied, Blackmore (1978) found 36% who stated that they were experiencing stress-related health problems. Numerous authors (Pelletier, 1977; Sarason, Johnson, Berberich, & Siegel, 1979; Stanley & Saxon, 1980) noted a variety of physical stress-related symptoms as a result of exposure to stressful events. Some physical effects of stress are immediate and manifest themselves in increased injury rates among emergency personnel. In his study, Keena (1981) pointed out that the injury rate among emergency medical technicians jumped from 22% in routine calls to 50% when the stress on the scene increased because of the severity of the patient's injuries was greater.

Byl and Sykes (1978) reported finding considerable physical fatigue and dizziness among stressed workers and Ilinitch and Titus (1977) described extensive physical symptoms of distress in emergency workers in the Big Thompson Dam flood in Colorado. Fatigue and psychomotor dysfunction were common in those rescue workers. Sleep disturbance, nausea, lowered sexual and eating appetites, and fatigue were present in emergency personnel 8 weeks after the 1982 Air Florida Flight 90 air crash in Washington, D.C. (Mitchell, 1982). Some physical effects of emergency work have been known to last for considerably longer periods of time (Appelbaum, 1981).

Emotional Effects of Emergency Work

The emotional effects of emergency work, as is the case with the cognitive and physical aspects of stress, are many and varied. Most people experiencing stress often reduce their capacity for pleasure as well as their ability to interact with others (Sargent, 1980). Health care workers who deal with crisis events in patients often react with anxiety and defensiveness when the clients complain or ask questions (Cherniss, 1980; Johnston, 1979).

Emergency workers readily admit that small mistakes in their work can have catastrophic consequences. This sets the foundation for considerable anxiety about their work (Graham, 1981). Routine and extraordinary emergency work stressors have equal potential to cause stress reactions in the workers. Ilinitch and Titus (1977) described anxiety, anger, and guilt in rescue workers. Cohen and Ahearn (1980) reported similar reactions in many of the emergency workers they contacted after work in stressful conditions. Anxiety, guilt, grief, depression, self-doubt, anger, irritability, victim concern, denial, and a need for emotional reassurance were found in air crash rescue workers (Mitchell, 1982). Emotional numbing and denial are also common reactions to emergency work (Duston, 1979).

Long-term emotional disability is not uncommon after extraordinary stressors. Henderson and Bostock (1977) found that five of seven shipwrecked survivors developed formal psychiatric disorders after the ordeal although none had a history of psychiatric disturbance before the event. The same psychiatric disorders can be found in emergency workers as a result of their work. Posttraumatic stress disorder (PTSD) (APA, 1980, 1987) has been recently noted in emergency workers (Mitchell, 1983; Mitchell & Bray, 1989) and medical professionals (Shovar, 1987).

Behavioral and Psychosocial Effects of Emergency Work

When cognitive, physical, and emotional factors are affected by stress, it is a virtual impossibility also not to affect a person's behavior. Hartsough (1985), Myers (1989), Butcher and Dunn (1989), and Gist and Lubin (1989) found a variety of behavioral manifestations of stress in disaster workers, including suppression of conversation, withdrawal from others, excessive talking, and under- or overeating. Glass (1959) reported that stressed emergency workers often become docile and suggestible and have decreased activity levels. They may grow apathetic and exhibit almost motionless behavior.

The behavioral manifestations of stress in emergency workers often affect their homelife. The study by Blackmore (1978) of 2,300 police officers supported that assertion. Approximately 37% of the officers reported serious marital problems which were linked to their work. Twenty-three percent of the sample reported drinking problems and another 10% said they abused other drugs. Mitchell (1982) reported that emergency personnel experienced lowered sexual appetites after highly stressful events.

Job turnover may also be negatively impacted by the stress associated with emergency work. Razen (1974) found a 70% turnover rate in special care units as compared with a 28% turnover for other units in the hospital. In addition, intensive care unit nurses left their jobs at a younger age than did nurses in units which provided more routine nursing care. Storlie (1979) stated that critical care personnel are more prone to experience job burnout than other nonemergency oriented personnel. Absenteeism, increased sick visits, decreased job satisfaction, the formation of antagonistic work factions, and mistakes in job performance appear to be prominent byproducts of stress in emergency workers and most other persons (Hall, Gardner, Perl, Stickney, & Pfefferbaum, 1979).

Delayed Effects of Emergency Work

Emergency personnel are very good at suppressing their reactions to a stressful event. Under field conditions, the ability to suppress immediate reactions is very important. It prevents them from being incapacitated by their reaction while still attempting to save the lives of others, treat their wounds, or limit property destruction.

When immediate reactions are successfully suppressed they are generally encountered later. Frederick (1981) stated that these symptoms and many others can occur much later; "emotional breakdowns can occur long after the crash site has been cleared and the physical injuries have been treated" (p. 17). The most common forms of expression for suppressed reactions tend to be nightmares and other intrusive images, such as flashbacks and obsessive thoughts about the incident, humor, physical activity, and at times, emotional outbursts (Forstenyer, 1980). Wilkinson (1983) found symptoms of distress in some people six or more months after an incident. Taylor and Frazer (1981) found 20% of recovery personnel, who worked on the Mount Erebus air crash, still experienced symptoms of distress 20 months after the tragic incident. Other researchers confirm the Taylor and Frazer (1981) study with similar results (Raphael, Singh, Bradbury, & Lambert, 1983–1984; Titchener & Lindy, 1980). Cox (1980) indicated that

it is not rare for there to be a latency period of a few months, or occasionally a few years, before the psychological reaction became apparent. This presents a major problem for the diagnosis of PTSD and the management of the post-trauma situation. (p. 621)

Prevention of Posttraumatic Stress Syndromes in Emergency Personnel

S. M. Miller and Birnbaum (1988) pointed out that individuals who lack the cognitive and social coping skills to deal with certain stressful events experience more physical and psychological stress and poor outcomes. The greater the disparity between the requirements of the situation and the cognitive and social skills of the person, the greater the disruption of the person (Bandura, 1977, 1981, 1985).

It seems apparent then that preincident stress education programs can play a vital role in reducing stress reactions in emergency personnel and disaster workers. Meichenbaum (1974) suggested that people could be taught stress control and that there was considerable promise in stress education programs. As early as 1959, N. E. Miller (1959) found that effective education was a key in learning behaviors which could reduce the fear of danger. N. E. Miller (1980) concluded that learning can affect visceral responses. Furthermore, Cox (1980) supported this conclusion and stated that the "ability to cope with stress can change with a number of positive factors, such as education and training" (p. 116).

Claus (1980) echoed Cox's premise and stated:

Training professionals how to manage stress in the environment is largely cognitively oriented. People can be taught to become aware of those stimuli which trigger defensive reactions and to develop coping strategies. (p. 11)

Other authors suggested that stress training and education programs play a role in stress prevention and mitigation. Simpson (1980) emphasized the prevention aspects of stress education and training. Everly and Girdano (1980) and Appelbaum (1981) reiterated the prevention role and also stated that stress management training can be instrumental in problem-solving and in the alleviation of existing stress.

Ellison and Geny (1978) in their work with police officers urged that training for the prevention and minimization of stress should begin at the recruitment level before police officers are exposed to the significant stressors associated with police work. Jaremko, Hadfield, and Walker (1980) agreed and emphasized that education is a potent part of stress prevention of "stress inoculation."

The use of preincident stress training and or stress education programs has shown considerable success. Hemenway (1981) reported that a large life insurance company realized an estimated return of five dollars on every dollar that was spent on stress-management training because of the decrease in absenteeism and other stress-related health problems. Executives in the Kennecott Copper Company attributed a 75% drop in sickness and accident costs to stress-management programs aimed at stress prevention and mitigation. Several clinicians and stress researchers have noted encouraging results of educational programs for emergency personnel. After 12 hours of training in relaxation and cognitive techniques, stress-trained police officers were rated as "significantly superior" to their untrained fellow officers in almost all aspects of case management in simulated exercises (Sarason et al., 1979). Novaco (1977) found similar success in teaching police officers anger control techniques. Graham (1981) and Claus (1980) pointed out positive effects of training nurses in stress management.

Likewise with paramedic populations, considerable success has been found in preventing or eliminating stress reactions by means of stress education programs (Mannon, 1981; McGlown, 1981; Schwettman, 1980; Staff, 1981). One of the authors of this chapter found a decrease in measured stress among paramedics 3 months after stress-management training (Mitchell, 1983).

Not all researchers agree that stress education is effective in reducing stress-response syndromes. Seligman (1975), Janis (1971), Zuckerman and Spielberger (1976), and N. E. Miller (1980) noted that stress education or training programs had little to no effect on stress produced by situations which were chronic, broad spectrum, or too complex. Sarason et al. (1979) further pointed out that evidence of long-term positive effects of stress-management training is minimal and further research will be necessary before conclusions can be drawn.

In spite of these objections, the positive evidence which does exist has encouraged us to proceed with the development and dissemination of stress education programs with the goal of mitigating the impact of emergency services job-related stress reactions. Obviously, the effectiveness of these programs must still be evaluated by further research. However, the consistently positive course evaluations and anecdotal records obtained may suggest both the value and utility of such training efforts.

Stress-Mitigation Education for Emergency Workers

Our own experience has demonstrated that stress education programs for emergency personnel have enhanced their sense of self-confidence in their ability to cope successfully with distressing events. These programs have partially desensitized emergency personnel to the sights, sounds and experience of the emergency scene so that they are less distressed by those stimuli. It has been our experience that stress-trained emergency workers recognize more readily stress reactions in themselves and others and are more prone to request help earlier. Stress-educated and trained emergency workers also face their stress reactions with a greater sense of control and a feeling that they are not abnormal or unique but expectable aspects of the work itself.

Stress-Mitigation Programs

The following factors are included in stress-mitigation programs for emergency personnel: (1) Emergency workers are given general information about the nature of stress-response syndromes and their causes and their effects on the average person. (2) Course material discusses and reviews *critical incident stress* or emergency stress reactions. (3) Significant differences are shown between the routine stress of everyday work (i.e., hassles) and the acute stress of emergency or disaster work. (4) Personnel are then presented with information on the typical signs and symptoms which are likely to appear during or shortly after an emergency team's participation in tragic events. Lists of cognitive, physical, emotional, and behavioral signs and symptoms of distress are presented in detail. Delayed stress reactions are also discussed. Additionally, the compounded negative effects of acute stress reactions which are mixed with underlying chronic stress conditions are also discussed. (5) Material is presented to emergency workers which describes stress survival strategies during the actual on-scene operations. For example, personnel are advised to take breaks frequently; limit their exposure to disturbing sights or sounds; limit the time frames in which they work to 1½ to 2 hours maximum before a break, and to take in sufficient amounts of food and fluid to maintain themselves in a condition of maximal efficiency. They are also advised to render support to one another during the mission and upon their return to routine duties. (6) Another prevention-oriented strategy is to provide stress-related information to spouses and significant others in stress workshops. In this way the significant others can be informed in order to be available to assist emergency workers in identifying and responding appropriately to the distress that is being experienced by the worker in the aftermath of a tragic event. The significant others can urge their loved ones to seek out more quickly the kind of help that can assist them in mitigating and reducing their stress reactions (Mitchell & Bray, 1989).

Additional Prevention-Oriented Stress Strategies

Howarth and Dussuyer (1988) identified four major factors which enhance a person's ability to resist the harmful effects of stress and to maintain physical and emotional balance as they face stressful events: (1) physical health, (2) self-esteem and personality, (3) social support, and (4) a sense of control over one's life.

It has long been assumed that good physical health can enhance a person's resistance to stress. At least one study (Shephard, 1983) supported this view. Since emergency personnel and disaster workers are frequently involved in situations which are quite disruptive to their routines and their family life, they are more prone to suffer the harmful consequences of stress. They are therefore urged to stay in a state of physical health which can withstand the rigors of their work. Regular exercise programs and a healthy diet are major factors in reducing the risks of severe stress reactions. One group of firefighters was studied to see if there are measurable benefits of physical fitness programs. It was found that firefighters who were physically fit experienced less injuries overall, and less serious injuries, when they were injured on the job than were firefighters who were less fit. Those who exercised regularly and ate balanced diets also felt better mentally and appeared to have less severe

reactions to traumatically stressful events (Mitchell & Bray, 1989). Moreover, Howarth and Dussuyer (1988) and Kobasa (1982) pointed out that "hardy" personalities appear to resist stress better than individuals without the core characteristics of the hardy police officer. Training programs for emergency personnel which emphasize assertiveness training, decision-making, conflict resolution, wellness, human communications skills in crisis intervention, and the other "human elements" are helpful in enhancing the skills which are associated with effective coping. Many who have been through such programs have reported positive benefits. Howarth and Dussuyer (1988) pointed out that numerous studies and articles have appeared in the literature which indicate that people who do feel in control of the harmful factors in their environment experience considerably less stress. Training which enhances a person's ability to cope effectively in a distressing environment is considered to be prevention-oriented and should be encouraged for emergency personnel. Additionally, other applied techniques can be utilized to prevent or limit stress reactions in emergency workers. For example, under highly stressful circumstances, small teams or task forces can be assigned to perform tasks which would normally be performed by one or two persons. Spreading the exposure effects across the team may effectively limit the more powerful exposures which might be encountered by an individual. Furthermore, whenever possible, predeployment briefings should be utilized to warn emergency personnel of the stressors associated with the event. The predeployment briefings should clearly state the type and nature of the event and any particular circumstances which accompany that event. These preparatory measures aid in creating realistic expectations as to what will be encountered in the line of duty. Based on our own experiences, command staff should meet during prolonged incidents and should exchange information and assure that all appropriate personnel throughout the ranks are informed of pertinent information regarding the incident and the operations which are underway.

As noted above, emergency and disaster workers should be limited to 1½- to 2-hour segments of time before obtaining a rest break. Appropriate rest breaks, of course, depend heavily on the type of event, the bioecological conditions, the numbers of staff, and other factors. Experience has demonstrated that a maximum of 12 hours at a scene prevents the adverse psychological sequelae associated with more extensive exposures. A minimum time of 6 hours away from the scene should be required before work crews are redeployed at the same event. Finally, other helpful techniques include resting work crews away from the immediate scene, breaks and meals taken together in groups, and short walks during breaks away from the site (Myers, 1989).

Intervention Strategies for Emergency Personnel

Prevention efforts, no matter how well organized, may not always be able to ameliorate the impact of disasters and other forms of crisis work on emergency personnel. In light of that fact, response agencies should preplan a variety of stress-reduction or stress-intervention strategies which can be employed when their workers have been adversely affected by their work. Some strategies will be useful in most situations; others will be useful only when the magnitude of an event is great enough to demand special strategies. Mental health support programs for emergency workers should be preset and developed in conjunction with emergency services response plans. They should begin operations on a small scale and escalate as the needs arise.

The *sine qua non* of mental health involvement in emergency services support programs is that the professionals chosen to work with emergency service personnel must be well versed in issues of stress, posttraumatic stress disorder (PTSD), psychotrauma, crisis intervention, and the nature and functions of emergency services work. Mental health professionals who are unknown to the emergency service personnel begin their work with a serious handicap. The lack of familiarity with the emergency workers causes a significant gap in credibility. The immediate response from provider groups will likely be mistrust, resistance, and anger (see Chapter 38, in this volume, for a discussion). Not all mental health professionals are suited by personality or training to provide services in the field of psychotrauma. In fact, the experience in the field clearly indicates that the wrong type of help provided by the wrong mental health professionals at the wrong time or under the wrong circumstances can be more damaging than no help at all.

Posttrauma Interventions for Emergency Personnel

Posttrauma interventions for emergency personnel can be summarized under two broad categories. The first includes support services provided *on site* or directly associated with the scene. The second group of support services includes activities which are provided immediately *after* an event or in the weeks or months which follow. These services include such items as psychological debriefing, individual counseling, assessments, referrals for additional services, spouse support programs, and debriefings (Mitchell & Bray, 1989).

On-site support services may be performed by specially trained peer support personnel, such as police officers, firefighters, or paramedics. They may also be provided by mental health professionals or by combined teams of peer support personnel and mental health professionals. The services at the scene can be categorized into three distinct areas of involvement. Support services may be provided to individuals who are showing obvious signs of distress at the scene. The obvious signs of distress include emotional lability, angry outbursts, severe withdrawal, psychomotor dysfunction, psychogenic shock, mental confusion, and dissociative reactions. Group intervention and counseling are not provided under field conditions since personnel are at various stages of distress and are often unprepared to manage their feelings in the context of a group setting. Individual contacts are therefore indicated when psychological first aid is presented under field conditions (Mitchell & Bray, 1989).

The second area of involvement for support services personnel is that of providing advice and counsel to command staff who are in charge of the personnel who are involved in the incident. When advice and counsel is given, it is typically limited to advice about appropriate rest schedules in the context of the event. However, little or no advice is given by support staff to the commanders regarding operational elements of the incident since that is outside of the area of responsibility and competence of the mental health professional.

Since many actual victims of an incident are often left to care for themselves while emergency services personnel are involved in the operations, the third task of support services personnel is to provide assistance to actual victims of the event and their families. This role, however, is usually delegated to other appropriate mental health agencies should they arrive at the scene. However, since mobilization of such resources is rather rare, it is more likely that emergency-oriented support services will provide for the needs of the victims, the survivors, and their families (see also Chapter 81, in this volume).

Postincident Intervention Strategies

Traumatic events, by definition, are capable of causing distress among emergency providers. A rapid deployment of psychological support services may be instrumental in limiting the impact of the event and in decreasing the potential for the development of PTSD.

There are many helpful stress-reduction and recovery-enhancement techniques which may be employed by well-trained mental health professionals or peer-support personnel who work under their supervision. Each technique requires appropriate familiarization to avoid producing harm where help was intended.

Decompression and defusing sessions are small group meetings provided by peers in proximity to the event. They are not provided at the scene itself but instead at a facility appropriate for such a group meeting. The defusing session has three basic parts: (1) an *introduction*, in which confidentiality is assured and the basic ground rules are described; (2) the *fact phase*, in which the participants describe what happened and how they are reacting; and (3) an *information phase*, in which the participants are given useful information which will help them to reduce their stress. The objectives of decompression are either to eliminate the need to provide a full debriefing or to enhance a full debriefing if one is indicated (Mitchell & Bray, 1989).

Deescalation and Demobilization

After large-scale incidents, such as disasters, another form of intervention is frequently utilized. It is called a "deescalation" or "demobilization" and is designed to reduce the distress associated with moving from a traumatic event into the routine of daily operational duties or home life. The deescalation procedure is a group meeting held away from the scene of the event; usually taking place immediately after personnel are released from operations and dispatched away from the scene. Personnel are brought to a large room and are divided into core working groups or homogeneous teams. A mental health professional then gives them a brief (e.g., 10-minute) talk on the stress symptoms which are most common after disasters and the types of techniques which can mitigate the stress. Personnel do not have to speak but they are afforded an opportunity to ask questions if they so choose. Once the 10-minute talk is concluded, emergency workers are given food and fluids and a rest period which lasts about 20 minutes. Then their commanders enter the room and give them instructions on returning to duty or going home. Before leaving the deescalation center, personnel are given traumatic stress handout material and advised that a debriefing is being planned for sometime within 10 days. Personnel are encouraged (or ordered if their commanders so desire) to attend the debriefing when it is conducted.

A Seven-Phase Debriefing Process

Debriefings are formal group meetings which generally last 2½ to 3 hours and are led by a team of mental health professionals and peer-support personnel. Debriefings follow a prescribed *seven-phase structure*. All personnel involved in the event are invited to come to the debriefing. Typically, four critical incident stress-debriefing team members lead the debriefing. Usually, the stress team leader is a mental health professional.

1. The debriefing begins with an introduction in which the *ground rules* of the process are described. Confidentiality is emphasized, and the participants are informed that the debriefing is not psychotherapy but a discussion with psychological and educational elements. Participants are urged to talk but they are advised that they do not have to speak if they choose not to.

2. The second phase of the debriefing process is the *fact of what happened* phase. In this phase, the participants are asked to describe what happened during the incident from their *own perspective*.

3. In the third phase of the debriefing, personnel are asked to personalize the experience of the event by describing their *own thoughts about it*. In this way, the attendees are able to move from a point in which they only relate to the facts of the situation to a point in which they develop a personal perspective of the event.

4. The fourth phase in the process is to have the participants move into a *discussion of the emotions* associated with the event. The typical question which begins this phase is, "What was the worst part about this event for you personally?" The participants may speak as openly and freely about the worst aspects of the situation as they wish.

5. The fifth phase of the debriefing is a *review of the signs and symptoms of distress* associated with the event. Stress symptoms are reviewed as they arose in personnel *at the scene*, afterward, and what symptoms remain at the time of the debriefing. In this manner, the critical incident stress team can obtain three "snapshot" pictures of distress in the personnel and determine if the symptoms are worsening or lessening. Symptoms which appear in any one of the four major symptom groups are considered important; that is, cognitive, physical, emotional, and behavioral symptoms are important to be reviewed.

6. The sixth phase of a debriefing is the *teaching phase*. In this phase, personnel are given information regarding stress reactions, the normal nature of the stress symptoms the personnel are experiencing, and specific techniques which may help to reduce the acute stress symptoms which were described in the previous phase. The teaching phase is adapted to the needs of the group and the issues which were discussed throughout the debriefing process.

7. The seventh and final phase of the debriefing is the *reentry phase*. This is a period of time in which the debriefing participants may ask questions, present new issues, or discuss issues already brought out in the debriefing but which may need additional review. The critical incident stress team will then make summary statements, and the debriefing draws to a close.

The critical incident stress team remains available after the debriefing to continue discussions with individuals who may need personal assistance in dealing with their reactions to the event itself or to the debriefing. Referrals are made when necessary.

After "defusings," deescalations, and debriefings, the critical incident stress team always follows up by means of visits, phone calls, and individual counseling sessions. Follow-up meetings which are not as formal and structured as the debriefing are frequently held after a debriefing as a way to check on an entire group. Usually, these meetings are held a week to 10 days after the debriefing. They are much shorter, and the typical questions which are asked are: "How are things since the debriefing?" "Is anyone stuck on any particular part of the incident?" "How have things been on your own (or off-duty) time?" "What else do you feel you might need to get you past this particularly bad event?"

The debriefing process has been utilized in a number of situations in which emergency personnel are not in need of assistance but others are. In our experience, school groups, companies and corporations, community groups, and others have benefitted from the process.

Many emergency personnel need individual consultations from critical incident stress team members. Both peer and professional short-term counseling services are available. If it is determined that long-term counseling is indicated, the emergency worker is referred for therapy.

When events are stressful enough to affect the workers negatively, their families, spouses, and significant others are subsequently invited to attend special debriefings which have been specifically designed for them. They are not included in the debriefings for emergency personnel since the issues are quite different between the groups of emergency workers and significant others.

Conclusion

Disaster and emergency personnel are not exempt from the devastating impact of tragic events on their emotions, their health, their careers, their families, or their lives. In fact, they may be more seriously affected because they suppress their reactions in order to maintain their ability to function during the crisis and later because they fear debilitation from their own emotions within their family systems or other aspects of their personal lives. However, the impact on emergency personnel is often hidden from the view of the general public. Specialized preventions and intervention programs, such as those described within this chapter, will be necessary to assist emergency personnel in maintaining physical and emotional health in the line of duty as well as a balanced life.

References

Adams, J. D. (1980). *Understanding and managing stress: A book of readings*. San Diego, CA: University Associates.

American Psychiatric Association. (1964). *First aid for psychological reactions in disasters*. Washington, DC: Author.

American Psychiatric Association. (1980). *Diagnostic and statistical manual of mental disorders* (3rd ed.). Washington, DC: Author.

American Psychiatric Association (1987). *Diagnostic and statistical manual of mental disorders* (3rd ed., rev.). Washington, DC: Author.

Appelbaum, S. H. (1981). *Stress management for health care professionals*. Rockville, MD: Aspen Systems.

Bandura, A. (1977). Self-efficacy: Toward a unifying theory of behavior change. *Psychological Review, 84*, 191–215.

Bandura, A. (1981). Self-referent thought: A developmental analysis of self-efficacy. In J. H. Flavell & L. D. Ross (Eds.), *Social cognitive development: Frontiers and possible futures* (pp. 200–239). London: Cambridge University Press.

Bandura, A. (1985). *Social foundations of thought and action: A social cognitive theory*. Englewood Cliffs, NJ: Prentice-Hall.

Blackmore, J. (1978). Are police allowed to have problems of their own? *Police Magazine, 1*(3), 47–55.

Butcher, J. N., & Dunn, L. A. (1989). Human responses and treatment needs in airline disasters. In R. Gist & B. Lubin (Eds.), *Psychosocial aspects of disaster*. New York: Wiley.

Byl, N., & Sykes, B. (1978). Work and health problems: An approach to managements for the professional and the community. *Community Health, 9*(3), 149–158.

Cherniss, C. (1980). *Professional burnout in human service organizations*. New York: Praeger.

Claus, K. E. (1980). The nature of stress. In K. E. Claus & J. T. Bailey (Eds.), *Living with stress and promoting well-being: A handbook for nurses*. St. Louis, MO: C. V. Mosby.

Cohen, R. E., & Ahearn, F. L. (1980). *Handbook for mental health care of disaster victims*. Baltimore, MD: The Johns Hopkins University Press.

Cox, J. D. (1980). *Occupational stress and individual strain: A social-psychological study of emergency medical personnel*. Unpublished doctoral dissertation, University of Utah, Salt Lake City.

Doerner, W. G. (1987). Police dispatcher stress. *Journal of Police Science and Administration, 15*(4), 257–261.

Duffy, J. (1979). The role of CMHCs in airport disasters. *Technical Assistance Center Report, 2*(1), 7–9.

Dunning, C., & Silva, M. (1980). Disaster induced trauma in rescue workers. *Victimology, 5*(2–4), 287–297.

Duston, H. (1979). The consequences of stress. In *Clinical roundtables*. Bloomfield, NJ: Roche Laboratories, Health Learning Systems.

Dutton, L. M., Smolensky, M. H., Lorimar, R., Hsi, B., & Leach, C. S. (1978, September/October). Psychological stress levels in paramedics. *Emergency Medical Services, 88*, 90–94.

Dyregrov, A. (1988, October). *The effects of children's trauma on the helping professional*. Paper presented at the Fourth Annual Meeting of the Society for Traumatic Stress Studies. Dallas, Texas.

Ellison, K. W., & Geny, J. L. (1978). Police officer as burned out samaritan. *FBI Law Enforcement Bulletin, 47*(3), 1–7

Everly, G., & Girdano, D. (1980, November). *Stress mess solution: The causes and cures of stress on the job*. Bowie, MD: Robert J. Brady.

Eysenck, M. W. (1989). Trait anxiety and stress. In S. Fisher & J. Reason (Eds.), *Handbook of life stress cognition and health*. New York: Wiley.

Figley, C. (1981, March). Working on a theory of what it takes to survive. *APA Monitor*, 9.

Forstenyer, A. (1980, July). Stress, the psychological scarring of air crash rescue personnel. *Firehouse*, pp. 50–52, 62.

Frederick, C. J. (Ed.). (1981). *Aircraft accidents: Emergency mental health problems*. Washington, DC: National Institute of Mental Health, U.S. Department of Health and Human Services.

Freeman, K. (1979). CMHC responses to the Chicago and San Diego airplane disasters. *Technical Assistance Center Report, 2*(1), 10–12.

Gist, R., & Lubin, B. (Eds.). (1989). *Psychosocial aspects of disaster*. New York: Wiley.

Glass, A. J. (1959). Psychological aspects of disaster. *Journal of the American Medical Association, 171*(2), 222–225.

Graham, N. K. (1981). Done in, fed up, burned out: Too much attrition in EMS. *Journal of Emergency Medical Services, 6*(1), 24–29.

Hall, R. C., Gardner, E. R., Perl, M., Stickney, S. K., & Pfefferbaum, B. (1979). The professional burnout syndrome. *Psychiatric Opinion, 16*(4), 12–13, 16–17.

Hartsough, D. (1983). *Mitigating the emotional consequences of disaster work: A guide for training and debriefing*. Unpublished manuscript, Purdue University.

Hartsough, D. M. (1985). Stress and Mental Health Interventions in three major disasters. In D. M. Hartsough & D. G. Myers (Eds.), *Disaster work and mental health: Prevention and control of stress among workers*. Washington, DC: Center for Mental Health and Human Services, National Institute of Mental Health.

Hemenway, P. T. M. (1981, November). Burnout update. . . . *The Philadelphia Bulletin*, pp. E2, E4.

Henderson, S., & Bostock, T. (1977). Coping behavior after shipwreck. *British Journal of Psychiatry, 131*, 15–20.

Holsti, O. R. (1971). Crisis, stress and decision making. *International Social Science Journal, 23*, 53–67.

Holt, F. X. (1980, November). The dispatcher and stress. *Firehouse*, pp. 18, 21.

Howarth, I., & Dussuyer, I. D. (1988). Helping people cope with the long-term effects of stress. In S. Fisher & J. Reason (Eds.), *Handbook of life stress, cognition and health* New York: Wiley.

Ilinitch, R. C., & Titus, M. P. (1977). Caretakers as victims: The Big Thompson flood, 1976. *Smith College Studies in Social Work, 48*(1), 67–68.

Janis, J. L. (1971). *Stress and frustration*. New York: Harcourt Brace Jovanovich.

Jaremko, M. E., Hadfield, R., & Walker, W. E. (1980). Contribution of an educational phase of stress inoculation of speech anxiety. *Perceptual and Motor Skills, 50*(2), 495–501.

Johnston, D. H. (1979). Crisis intervention. *Critical Care Update, 6*(4), 5–20.

Kahn, R. (1978). Job burnout prevention and remedies. *Public Welfare, 36*(2), 61.

Keena, B. (1981, Spring). What we've learned about firefighter safety and health. *Emergency Management, 33.*

Kliman, A. S. (1975). The Corning flood project: Psychological first-aid following a natural disaster. In H. J. Parad, H. L. P. Resnik, & L. G. Parad (Eds.), *Emergency and disaster management: A mental health sourcebook.* Bowie, MD: Charles Press.

Kobasa, S. C. (1982). The hardy personality: Toward a social psychology of stress and health. In G. S. Sanders & J. Suls (Eds.), *Social psychology of health and illness.* Hillsdale, NJ: Lawrence Erlbaum.

Laube, F. (1973). Psychological reactions in disaster. *Nursing Research, 22,* 343–347.

Lazarus, R. S. (1969). *Patterns of adjustment and human effectiveness.* New York: McGraw-Hill.

Lippert, W., & Ferrara, E. R. (1981, December). The cost of "coming out on top": Emotional responses to surviving the deadly battle. *FBI Law Enforcement Bulletin 50*(12), 6–10.

Mannon, J. M. (1981). Aiming for detached concern—How EMTs and paramedics cope. *Emergency Medical Services, 10*(3), 6–23.

Maslach, C. (1978). Job burnout: How people cope. *Public Welfare, 36*(2), 56–58.

Maslach, C., & Jackson, S. (1979, May). Burned out cops and their families. *Psychology Today,* p. 59.

Mayer, R. E. (1977). Problem solving performance with task overload: Effects of self-pacing and trait anxiety. *Bulletin of Psychonomic Society, 9,* 282–286.

Meichenbaum, D. (1974). *Cognitive behavior modification.* Morristown, NJ: General Learning Press.

McGlown, K. J. (1981). *Attrition in the fire service: A report.* Washington, DC: Federal Emergency Management Agency, U.S. Fire Administration.

Miller, N. E. (1959). Liberalization of basic S-R Concepts. Extensions to conflict behavior, motivation, and social learning. In S. Koch (Ed.), *Psychology: A study of science* (Vol. 2). New York: McGraw-Hill.

Miller, N. E. (1980). Effects of learning on physical symptoms produced by psychological stress. In H. Selye (Ed.), *Selye's guide to stress research.* New York: Van Nostrand Reinhold Co.

Miller, S. M., & Birnbaum, A. (1988). Putting the life back into "Life Events": Toward a cognitive social learning analysis of the coping process. In S. Fisher & J. Reason (Eds.), *Handbook of life stress, cognition, and health.* New York: Wiley.

Mitchell, J. T. (1982, October). The psychological impact of the Air Florida 90 disaster on fire-rescue, paramedic, and police officer personnel. In R. A. Cowley (Ed.), *Mass casualties: A lesson learned approach, accidents, civil disorders, natural disasters, terrorism* (DOT HS806302). Washington, DC: Department of Transportation.

Mitchell, J. T. (1983, February). Emergency medical stress. *APCO Bulletin, Journal of Association of Public Safety Communications Officers,* pp. 14–16.

Mitchell, J. T., & Bray, G. P. (1989). *Emergency services stress.* Englewood Cliffs, NJ: Prentice-Hall.

Myers, D. G. (1989). Mental health and disaster, preventive approaches to intervention. In R. Gist & B. Lubin (Eds.), *Psychological aspects of disaster.* New York: Wiley.

Nordlicht, S. (1979). Effects of stress on the police officer and family. *New York State Journal of Medicine, 79*(3), 400–401.

Novaco, R. W. (1977). A stress inoculation approach to anger management in the training of law enforcement officers. *American Journal of Community Psychology, 5*(3), 237–346.

Pelletier, K. (1977). *Mind as healer, mind as slayer.* New York: Delta Books.

Peuler, J. (1984). *Innovations in family and community outreach in times of disaster.* Paper presented at the National Institute of Mental Health Symposium on Innovations in Mental Health Care of Victims, Washington, DC.

Raphael, B., Singh, B., Bradbury, L., & Lambert, F. (1983–1984). Who helps the helper? The effects of disaster on the rescue worker. *Omega, 14*(1), 9–20.

Rayner, J. F. (1958). How do nurses behave in disaster? *Nursing Outlook, 6,* 572–576.

Razen, J. (1974). Nursing turnover in special care units. *Abstracts of Hospital Management Studies, 10,* 335.

Sarason, I. G., Johnson, J. H., Berberich, J. P., & Siegel, J. M. (1979). Helping police officers to cope with stress: A cognitive-behavioral approach. *American Journal of Community Psychiatry, 7*(6), 593–603.

Sargent, A. G. (1980). Androgyny as a stress management strategy. In J. D. Adams (Ed.), *Understanding and managing stress.* San Diego, CA: University Associates.

Schwettman, J. L. (1980). Proceedings: NAEMT hassle management seminar-EMT/paramedic burnout. *Emergency Medical Services, 9*(6), 137–143.

Sedgwick, R. (1975, September/October). Psychological response to stress. *Journal of Psychiatric Nursing and Mental Health Services, 74,* 12–17.

Seligman, M. E. P. (1975). *Helplessness: On depression, development, and death.* San Francisco: W. H. Freeman.

Sewell, J. D., & Crew, L. (1984, March). The forgotten victim: Stress and the police dispatcher. *FBI Law Enforcement Bulletin, 53*(3), 7–11.

Shephard, R. J. (1983). Employee health and fitness: The state of the art. *Preventative Medicine, 12,* 644–653.

Shovar, G. P. (1987). Medical professionals and PTSD. In T. Williams (Ed.), *Post-traumatic stress disorders: A handbook for clinicians.* Cincinnati, OH: Disabled American Veterans.

Shubin, S. (1979, January). Rx for stress—Your stress. *Nursing,* pp. 53–55.

Simpson, M. E. (1980). Societal support and educating. In I. L. Kutas & L. B. Schlesinger (Eds.), *Handbook on stress and anxiety: Contemporary knowledge, theory and treatment.* San Francisco: Jossey-Bass.

Solomon, S. (1985). Enhancing social support for disaster victims. In B. Sowder (Ed.), *Disasters and mental health: Selected contemporary perspectives* (DHHS Publications No. 14–8521, pp. 107–121). Washington, DC: U.S. Government Printing Office.

Staff (1979, January 8). Crash trauma, nightmares plague rescuers. *Time,* p. 61.

Staff (1980, November). Hotline: A year in review, common problems, uncommon solutions. *Firehouse,* pp. 78–82.

Staff (1981, September/October). Time management: A survival guide for EMS managers. *Emergency Medical Services* (pp. 68, 70–72).

Stanley, S. R., & Saxon, J. P. (1980). Occupational stress: Implications for vocational rehabilitation counselling. *Journal of Rehabilitation, 46*(2), 56–59.

Storlie, F. J. (1979, December). Burnout: The elaboration of a concept. *American Journal of Nursing,* pp. 2108–2111.

Taylor, A. J. W., & Frazer, A. G. (1981). Psychological sequelae of Operation Overdue following the DC-10 aircrash in Antarctica (Victoria University of Wellington Publications in Psychology No. 27). Wellington, New Zealand: Victoria University.

Titchener, J. L., & Lindy, J. D. (1980). *Affect defense and insight: Psychoanalytic observations of bereaved families and clinicians at a major disaster.* Unpublished manuscript, University of Cincinnati.

Weaver, W. C. (1987). Stress and the EMS dispatcher. *Emergency Medical Services, 16*(7), 18, 21, 23, 25–26.

Wilkinson, C. B. (1983). Aftermath of a disaster: The collapse of the Hyatt Regency Hotel skywalk. *American Journal of Psychiatry, 140,* 1134–1139.

Wilkinson, C. B., & Vera, E. (1985). The management and treatment of disaster victims. *Psychiatric Annals, 15*(3), 174–184.

Yager, J., & Hubert, D. (1979). Stress and coping in psychiatric residents. *Psychiatric Opinion, 16*(4), 21–24.

Zuckerman, M., & Spielberger, C. D. (Eds.). (1976). *Emotions and anxiety.* New York: Wiley.

CHAPTER 77

Vet Centers

A New Paradigm in Delivery of Services for Victims and Survivors of Traumatic Stress

Arthur S. Blank, Jr.

night. a wounded marine crawls, inches at a time, across a bridge. his blood flows from his body and down into the river of perfumes.[1] all through the night the people cry as the flames consume their homes and their city and at daybreak the refugees gather near the river of perfumes and watch the flow of a river of blood and the river flows raging into the ocean. . . .

the waters of the china sea become the waters of the pacific, and each wave . . . rolls through the timeless blue of the ocean and touches the lonely sands of america. my companions on this night are two drifters I have met on a beach in oregon. . . . I study their faces and suddenly know, yes, they have been there too, and have seen it all and are like me and have to keep moving because there seems to be nothing anymore that one can hold on to. for tonight, we have chosen this beach. and tomorrow?

—Quentin Mueller, Vietnam veteran (1976)

After years of wandering and problems with stress and depression I found help from the Vet Center. . . . With counseling and guidance I was able to find a job. . . . The Vet Center has lit a light of hope in what would otherwise have been a dim future.

—Veteran of the Vietnam War (1989)

Introduction

In 1979, during the sorrowful and fractious wake of the Vietnam War, the United States government established a nationwide system of outreach and counseling centers

(Vet Centers) to help veterans and their friends and family members with the psychological wounds and readjustment struggles arising from the Vietnam experience. At the time, the Congress and the President conceived of Vet Centers as a temporary expedient to overcome the mutual alienation of Vietnam veterans and the Veterans Administration (now the Department of Veterans Affairs [DVA]) health-care system. Twelve years and over

Arthur S. Blank, Jr. • Readjustment Counseling Service (10B/RC), Department of Veterans Affairs, Washington, DC 20420.

International Handbook of Traumatic Stress Syndromes, edited by John P. Wilson and Beverley Raphael. Plenum Press, New York, 1993.

[1]The River of Perfumes runs through the old imperial capital of Hue in Vietnam. The reference is to the battle of Hue during the Tet Offensive of 1968.

1,000,000 clients later, the 197 Vet Centers throughout the 50 states, Puerto Rico, the Virgin Islands, and Guam have discovered and refined a new paradigm in delivery of services for victims and survivors of traumatic stress. A uniquely constructed mix of services, a treatment model emphasizing the growth-enhancing potential of traumatic events, staffs which include both peers and professionals, a specialized organizational structure within a governmental department, and strong community and political support have all combined to produce a highly successful program.

In this chapter, I will analyze the development and features of the U.S. Vet Centers for those who wish to use this model in creating similar systems for veterans in other nations. My purpose also is to facilitate the translation of Vet Centers' effective qualities into service structures for survivors of traumatic encounters other than war.

Historical Background

Although American military personnel had been exposed to combat in Vietnam since the 1950s, veterans first began returning home from this war in large numbers in 1966. Reports from military psychiatrists serving in Vietnam early in the war (Johnson, Bowman, Byrdy, & Blank, 1967; *New York Times*, 1967) conveyed the finding that the war was producing little by way of acute or lasting traumatic stress reactions. However, by 1969, veterans themselves and a few civilian mental health professionals began to note classical symptoms of traumatic neurosis among returnees from the Vietnam War, complicated from the outset by the unusual social role of veterans resulting from the intense controversy in the United States about the war. In 1969, Senator Alan Cranston of California (later to become Chairman of the U.S. Senate Committee on Veterans Affairs) held Senate hearings in Washington, DC, on the psychological and readjustment difficulties of returning Vietnam veterans, and shortly thereafter introduced legislation to establish a special counseling program within the DVA. This began a 10-year legislative and political process, marked by recurrent hearings and offered legislation, and by persistent opposition to the creation of a service delivery system for Vietnam veterans.

This opposition was mirrored in the mental health arena by profound denial by professionals of the existence of traumatic stress effects in war veterans and in most other survivors. In 1968, the American Psychiatric Association (APA) had removed from its *Diagnostic and Statistical Manual of Mental Disorders* (DSM-II) (APA, 1968) any diagnosis which would have corresponded to posttraumatic stress disorder (PTSD). Throughout the 1970s, most Vietnam veterans with PTSD, along with victims and survivors of other traumata, if seen at all in a mental health context, were misdiagnosed as having other psychiatric disorders, and were provided treatment which did not take sufficient account of the unique psychological impact of trauma.

However, concurrently during the 1970s, two other developments occurred. A self-help movement arose among veterans, and by 1976 there were at least a few hundred organized self-help groups nationwide, some at churches or colleges and universities, and others in the form of community centers established by the veterans themselves. Also, a small number of professionals who were accurately diagnosing PTSD and providing psychotherapeutic treatment for veterans, established the Vietnam Veterans Working Group in 1976 (Shatan, Smith, & Haley, 1977). This group collected hundreds of case reports and began a process which ultimately led to the codification of the condition, formerly known as traumatic neurosis, as posttraumatic stress disorder in the third edition of the *Diagnostic and Statistical Manual of Mental Disorders* (DSM-III) (APA, 1980).

These developments, combined with continuing legislative leadership from Senator Cranston, were added to in the late 1970s by impetus provided by Max Clelland, the first Vietnam veteran chief of the DVA. The result was enactment of Public Law 96–22 in 1979, authorizing the DVA to provide a new category of services, to be known as *readjustment counseling*. The DVA and the Congress agreed that this service would be provided in community-based counseling centers. In its report on the readjustment counseling legislation, the Senate Veterans Affairs Committee specified it as most important that veterans understand "that seeking readjustment counseling does not imply or result in a diagnosis of mental illness" (U.S. Senate, 1979). The then Chief Medical Director of the DVA, Dr. James Crutcher, stated that

> We did not recognize . . . that Vietnam veterans had specific psychological readjustment problems . . . those patients came to us because of . . . difficulty in work, anxiety, and insomnia. We in the medical profession in the [DVA] admitted these patients . . . with diagnoses of situational maladjustment, free-floating anxiety, and some with depressive reactions. During the evaluation period it was possible to determine that the real problem was not a mental illness, but was an adjustment back to society. (U.S. Senate, 1979)

The Committee reported that DVA psychiatrists postulated that veterans were reluctant to seek help because of the stigma of mental illness.

Dr. Crutcher stated that the new legislation would provide that veterans with readjustment problems would be treated

> in the appropriate manner and not within the confines of psychiatric facilities, [and this will allow for] easy access to care and remove the stigma and maybe the reluctance of an individual suffering these problems to go through the route of a mental hygiene clinic or psychiatric admission.

The Senate Veterans Committee further specified that the DVA would hire paraprofessionals and utilize volunteers in furnishing readjustment counseling services, would mount an extensive outreach program, and that the centers for services would be located "in local communities with easy access . . . they can operate from independent store fronts, college campuses, offices within community mental health centers and offices within other sympathetic organizations."

Growth and Development of the Outreach Counseling Program

The first Vet Center began seeing clients on October 1, 1979. From that point through March, 1990, the Vet Center system has grown to encompass 197 Centers, 826 employees, an associated program for reimbursement of therapists in the private sector who treat Vietnam Era veterans, and an annual budget of $57 million. Along with extensive staff time devoted to education, consultation, and outreach, the Vet Centers accomplish approximately 640,000 visits by veterans and family members per year. Over 800,000 veterans and 300,000 family members have been seen during the past 12 years.

Services Offered

By design the Vet Centers provide a broad range of services, including psychotherapy and counseling for posttraumatic stress disorder, referral and aftercare for substance abuse related to PTSD, employment counseling, educational counseling, assistance with upgrade of military discharge, crisis intervention for acute PTSD symptoms, outreach, consultation, education of community professionals and the public, plus intensive networking and referral interactions with other community agencies. As implied by this array of services, Vet Center staff can confront and help with the full array of postwar readjustment difficulties in veterans: PTSD, employment and education career impairments, alienation and disconnection from community resources, and the like.

Basic Design Considerations

The definition, by the Congress and the Department of Veterans Affairs, of readjustment counseling and the system of community-based Vet Centers formulated to provide the services, reflect certain design considerations or basic concepts. This is a system formulated to serve a specific target population, such as might be set up for crime victims, disaster survivors, or former prisoners of war. The system was newly organized around the needs of that population, rather than around preexisting professional disciplines, institutions, or treatment methodologies. The pattern of advantages and disadvantages of a system newly designed from the ground up to serve a specific population, as compared to a preexisting system adapting itself to function in a new way, is of course complex. In the instance of the U.S. Vietnam Vet Centers, there has been an unusual degree of success, which will be analyzed in the remainder of this chapter.

Indicators of Success

The Vet Center system is an innovative experiment on the part of the federal government in establishing a nationwide organization for treatment of traumatic stress effects. After 12 years of experience, it is now possible to analyze systematically this experiment from the perspectives of organization, therapy, historical context, and the consumer. The factors which indicate that the system is highly successful will be looked at, followed by a further analysis of the probable reasons for the success.

The indicators or markers of success are the following:

1. *Positively regarded by consumers.* As of 1990, with over one million persons having been seen for services, only 45 letters of complaint about services have been received in the DVA headquarters in Washington, DC. Most referrals to Vet Centers are by word of mouth from other clients, a standard indicator of consumer satisfaction. Frequently local veterans organizations provide formal recognition of Vet Center services (see the Vet Center *Voice*, 1980–1990).

2. *Honored and valued community institution.* In communities throughout the nation, the Vietnam Vet Center has earned a place of respect and honor among community service agencies. This is indicated by the consistently favorable print and broadcast media coverage (DVA, 1990). In fact, to the best of my knowledge, during 12 years of operations, there have been no or almost no unfavorable investigative media reports on Vet Center services. In addition, a 2-year study carried out by the General Accounting Office (GAO) found that Vet Centers are highly regarded in communities (GAO, 1987).

3. *Volunteers.* Community support and success are persistently reflected in significant numbers of volunteers, both lay and professional, available to assist in the Vet Centers. The most frequent problem regarding volunteers is to find sufficient space for their work at the centers.

4. *Ability to recruit.* Vet Center staff are drawn from a highly specialized and relatively small male and female power pool nationwide, consisting of Vietnam theater or Vietnam era veterans,[2] who in addition to the personal military service background possess the required professional or paraprofessional counseling or mental health training or experience, as well as outreach skills. Also, in recent years, federal government pay scales for mental health professionals have lagged behind the private sector, requiring at some locations, considerable effort to overcome the unfavorable pay gradient. Nonetheless, Vet Centers continue to attract needed staff and are able to fill positions.

5. *Moderate staff burnout and turnover.* Notwithstanding the sometimes intense emotional stress of providing multiple services including counseling and psychotherapy to survivors of war, the annual staff turnover rate for Vet Centers is stable at 12%, which is approximately the same as for the 190,000 employees of the DVA medical branch, the Veterans Health Administration (VHA), of which the Vet Centers are a part.

6. *Productivity.* As measured in hours applied to

---

[2]Vietnam-theater veterans are those who served during the war in Vietnam, Laos, or Cambodia, or in the adjacent waters or airspace. Vietnam-era veterans are those who served in the military during the war, but not in the Vietnam theater.

outreach, consultation, and education, time spent with clients including travel time, and client visits per staff member, productivity consistently compares favorably with any mental health or counseling system. The resultant cost per visit and cost per staff services hour are such as to render the Vet Centers a good economic investment in an age of shrinking fiscal resources (DVA, 1980–1992).

7. *Low return rate.* Following the opening phase of Vet Center services in 1980–1981, the proportion of new clients seen each year, out of all veterans seen, has averaged 63.5%, with relatively low variance. The past two years (1988–1989) have shown the highest proportion of new clients since the opening phase (DVA, 1989). The lack of accumulation of chronic cases (in a clinical area where secondary gain and treatment dependency are sometimes feared, but do not occur in the presence of effective treatment), accompanied by indicators of positive consumer feedback, is a critical sign of program success. The actual observed proportion of long-term or return cases is appropriate, considering both the frequently cyclic character of recovery from PTSD, and the deep chronicity and complexity of many cases resulting from over a decade of nondiagnosis and nontreatment.

8. *Confirmation by formal oversight and evaluations.* Multiple oversight hearings by the Senate and House of Representatives Committees on Veterans Affairs, an evaluation study by the General Accounting Office, and internal evaluations within the DVA have confirmed the basic effectiveness of Vet Centers (Department of Veterans Affairs, 1981, 1986, 1987; U.S. House of Representatives, 1981, 1982; U.S. Senate, 1988).

9. *Congressional and Departmental support.* During the past decade, the Congress has four times passed, and the President signed, laws continuing Vet Centers, and in 1988, the Congress and the President removed any delimiting date for the centers. In addition, the Department of Veterans Affairs, in response to actual experience over time, has provided increasingly committed organizational, fiscal, and other types of support needed for effective services.

10. *Impact on larger system.* The Vet Centers have stimulated major changes and improvements with the large (172 hospitals and clinics, annual budget of approximately $16 billion) DVA medical system, in the diagnosis and treatment of PTSD. Directly or indirectly, Vet Centers, along with other influences, have contributed to the establishment in the DVA of (a) a high-level special committee of experts which advises the Chief Medical Director on PTSD, (b) a Departmental-level Advisory Committee on the Readjustment of Vietnam Veterans, (c) far-reaching new efforts to train mental health professionals within DVA medical facilities on PTSD, and (d) multiple new specialized PTSD services units in medical facilities.

11. *Survival.* This unique and highly innovative direct services program for war trauma and postwar readjustment has survived and flourished within the federal government over a 12-year period of intense downward pressure on fiscal resources throughout the government.

To summarize, Vet Centers are positively regarded by their clients, honored and valued as community institutions, attract significant numbers of professional and paraprofessional volunteers, are able to recruit highly specialized staff from a short-supply pool, experience comparatively low levels of burnout and turnover, show high productivity and low cost per visit, have a modest client return rate, are favorably evaluated by multiple governmental entities, attract continuing Congressional and Department of Veterans Affairs support, have a major impact on the large DVA medical system diagnosis and treatment of PTSD, and show good survival potential. In the interest of defining, for the benefit of those concerned with service delivery systems, the strengths which have caused this successful history, I will examine in the following sections the underlying reasons for success.

Organizational Features Promoting Success

At the management consulting firm of McKinsey & Co. (San Francisco, CA), Thomas J. Peters and Robert H. Waterman, Jr., in researching successful American companies, developed a framework for understanding organizations, which consists of seven variables: structure, staff, strategy, style, systems, skills, and shared values, which is known as the *McKinsey Seven S's* (Peters & Waterman, 1982). *Structure* refers to the design of the organization, how the pieces fit together. *Staff* covers the people who make up the organization. *Strategy* concerns the plans or long-term approaches. *Style* refers to the so-called soft features, the feelings and soul of the organization and its functioning. *Systems* addresses the functioning of the organization—for example, how communication takes place, how data are transmitted, stored, and analyzed, and how performance is evaluated. *Skills* refers to the abilities of people in the organization, including how those abilities are obtained, maintained, and improved. Finally, *shared values* refers to the underlying values of the organization, which endure over time and determine activities and decision-making. The advantage of such a deceptively simple scheme as the Seven S's is that it encourages the focusing of attention comprehensively over the full range of an organization's features, and the avoiding of too narrow preoccupation with only a few features. Thus, my analysis of the reasons for success of the Vet Centers flows according to these seven categories.

Structure

History and Sociopolitical Context

I consider here the developmental history of the centers and their place in the larger national community as part of the structure of the organization. Vet Centers came about as a result of strong public support expressed through elected representatives (the Congress). Probably, this support derived from a national need to reaffirm positive commitments to those who had served in the military as well as to make reparation to those who had thereby suffered emotional and life-development wounds. This public support, encouraged of course by Vietnam veteran advocates, found further expression in particular legislators, who were characterized by political prominence and vigor, and/or Vietnam veteran status, or some personal connection to the Vietnam War experience. The same type of commitment has been present in many Department of Veterans Affairs officials. The result of this political process was that the main features of Vet Centers were codified in law or in congressional reports which accompanied various statutes and hearings (e.g., U.S. Senate, 1979). A further important aspect of the strong support from the legislative and executive branches of government is that it has been persistent and enduring over time.

Organization and Management

Within the nationwide medical system of the DVA, the Vet Centers are organizationally discrete. Although reporting to the office of the Chief Medical Director in the Washington headquarters of the DVA, Vet Centers management, operational policy control, supervision, and fiscal authority are within the special office, the Readjustment Counseling Service, which operates the Vet Centers. From the Vet Centers' headquarters staff, line authority is carried out through Readjustment Counseling Service management staffs in each of several regions to the Vet Centers. All funds budgeted for Vet Centers must be used for that purpose and are tracked as such. This special line of authority within the larger organization is not unprecedented and is utilized for other highly specialized functions, including General Counsel (legal), public affairs, and medical educational centers. The specialized organizational setup is analogous to that of the Special Forces within the U.S. Department of the Army, and reflects several requirements of the mission. The discrete line of authority makes it possible for the top leadership of the Vet Center system to consist of Vietnam veterans (95% of the national and major regional management officials) and, in turn, makes it possible for a high level of Vietnam veteran staffing to be maintained among Vet Center service-providing staff nationwide (60% in addition to approximately 25% Vietnam-era veterans). Although both the management and the service-delivery staffs maintain these high levels of Vietnam veteran staffing, the special organizational framework also makes possible, as in the case of the Special Forces, a steady focus over time on the various components of a complex specialized mission.

Recruitment of Vietnam veterans who are also social workers, psychologists, psychiatric nurses, or professional or paraprofessional counselors draws from a very small pool of qualified persons. Therefore, recruitment can be effective only if coordinated on a national and regional basis, with extensive networking across the country in order to find new staff.

At the local level, the key structural features are the following: Each Vet Center is small, with a staff team averaging four persons. The centers are community-based, located in storefronts, former residential houses, shopping centers, or on the sidewalk level in small office buildings. With few exceptions, they are not physically associated with any hospital or medical clinic.

A critical structural feature at the local level is that each Vet Center is administratively supported by the nearest DVA medical center or clinic for supplies, personnel, fiscal processing, and other logistical services. Additionally, although each Vet Center is professionally and organizationally supervised by the regional and national management levels of the Readjustment Counseling Service, the service delivery program is closely coordinated with that of the nearest DVA medical center or clinic, with which the Vet Center works as part of a professional team.

Staff

Staff members of Vet Centers consist of a mix of professional and paraprofessional counselors, social workers, psychologists, and psychiatric nurses, plus office managers. Since staff are either themselves veterans or have some direct personal connection to the war, forceful personal commitment to work with war veterans and prior experience with PTSD are two important staff qualities.

The fact that a majority of staff members share with clients the experience of having served in Southeast Asia during the war gives unique and unprecedented qualities and potency to system operations and services. Many staff members were themselves traumatized or experienced postwar readjustment hurdles, and have successfully traveled the path along which they help their clients. Their work is a survivor mission, which makes for an intrepid personal commitment to excellence.

Also, such persons tend to show courage in confronting the traumatic experiences of their clients, they are not anxious in listening to painful and horrible events, and they are comfortable with the intense emotions which need to come forth in counseling and psychotherapy.

Staff must be comfortable with a small and interdisciplinary team and must be able to help each other in dealing with the stress of their work. Cross-training is a critical element. As will be described below, Vet Centers provide a broad mix of services, and since each team staff team is small, it needs persons with at least the potential for cross-training. For example, a psychologist who can perform outreach, networking, and public education as well as psychotherapy will contribute more than one who can do only the latter.

Staff is tailored to local needs, and service patterns vary according to the needs of the specific clientele. For example, one Vet Center may have a greater emphasis on psychological counseling and psychotherapy, another more on employment and educational counseling and direct mobilization of community resources for the client.

Finally, management at all levels for 13 years has seen to it that emphasis is placed on hiring staff from diverse ethnic backgrounds and also has promoted the hiring of female staff members. The ethnic and gender mix is therefore favorable for meeting various clinical needs.

Strategy

Strategy can be the linchpin of success for a group, clinic, or other service-delivery organization. Strategic decisions, made at various points in time, have contributed to the success of Vet Centers. Also, some aspects of strategy have emerged out of operations without conscious deliberations, but eventually could be discerned and codified.

A legislative-political process over ten years was required to establish Vet Centers. Therefore, many dialogues and hearings were tapped in order to define the mission. Thus, the mission was defined early, in-depth, and in a well-documented fashion. Currently, in the United States, any service-delivery element which is part of a large medical care delivery system is subject to significant pressures to make changes in its mission. A deliberate effort has been made to resist such casual or unofficial pressures.

A key element is the high priority given to outreach. Vet Centers emphasize outreach activities right up to the point of saturation of service-delivery capacity.

Another strategic priority is a commitment to serve as advocates and ombudspersons for veteran clients, within the limits imposed by sound psychotherapeutic principles. Decisions are made on a case-by-case basis. Sometimes it is most helpful to support clients in conducting their own interactions with employers, other service agencies, and the like. At other times, it is most useful to make calls for or accompany a client. The level of advocacy which is clinically indicated in the individual case is what is provided. For example, a Vet Center received a distress call from a veteran whose house was about to be foreclosed by the sheriff for nonpayment of the mortgage, and his eviction loomed. The veteran threatened to respond with violence. The Vet Center negotiated a delay with the sheriff, mobilized volunteers from the community to get the veteran's finances straightened away, looked after his children, helped him make improvements on the house, and then began provision of psychological help for the PTSD which lay behind his various difficulties.

The broad mix of readjustment counseling services, all organized at one site, is another key element of strategy. In addition to outreach and advocacy, services include (1) psychotherapy and psychological counseling (group, individual, and family), (2) networking and brokering of other community resources, (3) crisis intervention, (4) consulting with and educational activities for fellow professionals and the public concerning Vietnam veterans and their postwar readjustment, (5) employment counseling, (6) educational counseling, (7) prerelease counseling and technical services for incarcerated veterans, and (8) emergency food and shelter assistance.

Staff balance the advocacy-ombudsperson role with neutrality about political issues. For example, staff at all levels adhere to a nonpolitical stance about the Vietnam War out of respect for the widely differing values or attitudes about the war among the population which the Vet Centers are committed to serve and in order to be receptive to clients of all shades of opinion.

As a small service-delivery subsystem within a much larger government medical-care system, management takes special care to coordinate and harmonize the mission with the mission of the larger organization. This has turned out to be not difficult, because the mission of the Vet Centers is in fact central to the mission of the Department of Veterans Affairs. Sometimes, however, this fact must be clarified; management may have to seek opportunities to help both the subsystem and the larger organization retain awareness of the correspondence of mission.

Over time, it has become clear that as a new paradigm for service delivery, the community-based Vet Centers provide an organizational improvement for the larger organization, which is currently moving from a heavy reliance on hospital-based services into more frequent use of community-based medical care. In other words, there has been a serendipity factor. The strategic point for a traumatic stress service delivery system is that it may flourish to the extent that it can contribute to the strategies of the larger organization of which it is part, while maintaining its own specialized mission.

Certain design or operational decisions have been made in accordance with the special clinical characteristics of the client population. For example, Vietnam veterans with PTSD are often sensitive about controversial aspects of their war experiences and mistrustful of federal government elements for a variety of reasons. Therefore, the DVA decided at the outset that all Vet Center counseling records would be kept under the control of the client, except for the legal requirements of subpoena or duty to warn.

Style

As a place, the Vet Center is not altogether (1) a clinic, (2) a club, or (3) a community center, but in fact partakes of each of these and, in addition, it has qualities of (4) a refuge, (5) a resource base—through its links to other community agencies—and (6) a symbolic psychological holding environment pertaining to the Vietnam experience. The latter quality is symbolized by display of some Vietnam War military paraphernalia donated by clients.

The Center promotes an informal, noninstitutional, nonclinical, and nonmedical atmosphere or image. Room is provided for informal relaxing and socializing. Nonauthoritarian placement of furniture is emphasized; paperwork for clients is deemphasized. Clients may be seen without appointment whenever needed. As much as possible, the needs of the client determine administrative routines.

The Vet Center serves as a community focal point concerning the Vietnam experience, a place where students can call for leads on school research on Vietnam veterans, where community groups can provide ceremonies for honoring veterans, where holidays can be marked, and even sometimes where weddings are held. As these usages imply, the Vet Center role conveys a sense of ownership by the consumer, which is mediated by the staff who are stewards of the service functions. The emotional or holding environment or psychological container function derives not only from availability of counseling but also from the various social and community functions.

As implied by much of the foregoing material, an esprit or sense of heart or commitment is manifested in the style of the organization. This has many sources. One activity which is both a source and a manifestation is the work of Vet Center staff members in crisis intervention. As part of the outreach function, counselors call on veterans needing help, often going the extra mile to help a frightened or despairing person to form a therapeutic connection. Sometimes staff members are called on by police to help talk down and talk in a veteran who has created a hostage or barricade situation, usually directly resulting from overwhelming PTSD symptoms. Staff thereby help to save lives or to avert injury. Public response to this kind of outreach has fostered the Vet Center image of concern and caring which in turn has provided other veterans with the courage to ask for help directly.

The outreach and community roles of the centers, combined with direct counseling services, specifically address in a rational and deliberate fashion the isolation, aloneness, loneliness, and effects of rejection, distancing, and abandonment that is experienced sometimes for many years by many veterans with PTSD and other readjustment difficulties. Thus, the centers develop (similarly to self-help groups) an extended community of recovered survivors who can utilize supportive comradeship as part of their path to recovery.

Systems

Systems are the processes or the ways things work in an organization, including but not limited to the flow of information. Several essential systems for Vet Centers are (1) management information (teleconferences, meetings, minutes), (2) a nationwide staff newsletter distributed not only in-house but to persons and groups which interact with the counseling system, (3) automated hardware and software (computers, electronic mail, FAX, etc.), (4) supervisory systems in the form of regular site visits utilizing systematic protocols, (5) inservice training conferences, and (6) a formal quality assurance program including records review, assessment standards, systematic review of difficult cases, and the like.

Skills

The personal experience of the large majority of Vet Center service providers as Vietnam-theater or Vietnam-era veterans implies a set of personal skills based on both training and experience: adapting to traumatic and hardship situations, comprehension of the meaning of public service, a sense of humor in the face of adversity, working as a team member, knowing how to function in a large hierarchical organization, patience in dealing with uncertainty and disappointment, commitment to a mission under difficult and trying circumstances, awareness of cultural differences, and personal psychological coping skills for recovering from traumatic stress.

These personal skills form a foundation for professional skills. The professional skills required for readjustment counseling for war veterans in Vet Centers are an amalgam of traditional knowledge and skills drawn directly from the fields of counseling, clinical social work, clinical and counseling psychology, and psychiatric nursing, and, indirectly, from psychiatry.

Skills from a number of subdivisions within the counseling field are relevant. These skills are combined in a multidisciplinary fashion, encouraging cross-training among staff. The needs of the clientele at each individual center vary along a spectrum with diagnostic-level PTSD and the need for psychological counseling or psychotherapy at one end, and, at the other end, primarily social and employment adjustment difficulties requiring employment counseling and direct community interventions or skills training. Different staff members focus on particular parts of this spectrum according to their training and experience.

A unique quality of Vet Center staff is the inclusion of skills for networking with other community agencies, outreach activities, and for educational exercises for professionals and the public about the target population, all combined with direct client services. Thus, most staff members must possess or develop the skills required to play a multifaceted community role, in addition to the specific counseling services which they offer to individual clients.

From a discipline standpoint, the services provided are not a subspecialty of any particular mental health field, although it is interesting that some persons in each of the fields of social work, psychology, and psychiatry are inclined to claim readjustment counseling as a subspecialty. Rather, veterans readjustment counseling is an innovative combination of clinical skills from diverse sources, personal experience qualifications, and an array of community activist skills. The resulting combination is significantly different from the traditional mental health disciplines.

Shared or Superordinate Values

The last of the categories for organizational analysis is shared or superordinate values. These are the values which hold an organization together, keep it focused on its mission, and give individuals a sense of community with colleagues in their work. A coherent and consensually accepted set of values also provides staff with an edge of clarity and integrity in their work.

Therapeutic Model

The most important underlying value of the Vet Center system is its basic therapeutic philosophy concerning the nature of, and recovery from, posttraumatic stress disorder, and various functional impairments resulting from postwar readjustment experiences. Some key elements of the therapeutic model will now be reviewed.

A necessary (though not always sufficient) condition for recovery of most clients with PTSD, in the long run, is a degree of *revisiting* and *revivification* of the traumatic events, along with some amount of psychological working-through of their reactions. Thus, the treatment model is an uncovering and working-through model. Some would argue that this model is required for recovery from PTSD due to any type of trauma. However that may be, it is particularly relevant in the case of American Vietnam veterans, because there was very strong pressure from family, community, and society in the decade after the war to forget, to not talk about, and to suppress experiences in Vietnam. Because this pressure was so pervasive and often intense, the clinical assumption has to be made that any client may need some amount of revivification of memories and associated affects and conflicts.

Of course, the degree and duration of revivification and working-through varies widely between cases, from a few counseling visits, or a visit to the Vietnam Veterans Memorial, or joining a veterans organization, to medium- or long-term psychotherapy. Although this treatment model is central, it is not exclusive, and clinical services also include stress reduction and desensitizing techniques, along with social services which address real-life issues to the fullest extent necessary.

A second core aspect of the therapeutic model is that wartime traumatic events and difficulties in postwar readjustment, while having resulted in wounds which need healing, also contain challenges and opportunities for growth and development. Counseling emphasizes the impact, recovery, and growth-potential aspects of traumatic stress, rather than the disease aspects. On interpersonal or community levels, staff members search for the skills which the client learned in military training and in the war zone, and how those skills can be utilized productively throughout life. Second, staff members focus on the deeper understanding of human life—and death—which results from having been traumatized by war. Third, counselors attempt to find the sources of pride and strength which veterans possess from having survived, to help the veterans find forgiveness and reparation for any regrettable actions, and to help them to understand the admirable qualities of their performance and conduct in the military.

Thus, clients are not seen just as victims, but as survivors, who have the potential to use traumatic experiences to good effects for themselves and others.

Peer Staffing

Peer staffing is a fundamental superordinate value. A *sine qua non* for the success of this organization is maintaining minimum levels of service providers who were directly in the war zone, or who have been in the military during the Vietnam War and were proximate to the clients' historical experiences.

A Psychosocial Interpretation

It is understood by Vet Center staff that it is inevitable and appropriate for the life of a service-delivery system, which is directed at a particular type of trauma, to be permeated with reverberations, sometimes unconscious, of the particular traumatic experiences which are taken up in treatment. This can be understood as a transference phenomenon, where the past, channeled into current organizational life from the memories of clients and of staff, is reenacted. For example, we expect that both staff and clients will be mistrustful of authority, because in the Vietnam War a fundamental element of experience was that troops were let down by authority. Relations with others are colored at times by memories

of experiences with comrades in Vietnam. Such reenactments, accepted as a normal part of organizational life, can then be watched for, recognized, and, if necessary, defused or productively utilized.

A Psychohistorical Interpretation

Finally, another shared or superordinate value is the understanding that the Vietnam War experience was quite powerful and is sometimes still unresolved for many people other than veteran clients and staff. For example, a veteran client's difficulties with an employer may be contributed to by the employer's having gone to great lengths to avoid service in the war, or perhaps by the fact that a family member of the employer was killed in the war. Many citizens with whom veteran clients interact have unresolved feelings about the war, and they may have their own needs for understanding and working-through—needs which the client and the staff member may be able to address. Consequently, Vet Center staff members regularly function as consultants to the community about the Vietnam experience.

Summary

This chapter has considered a highly successful nationwide system of outreach and counseling services in the United States for veterans of the Vietnam War, their family, and their friends. The system is notable for its high valuation by its clients, and I have provided a summary of the qualities and forces which shape its success in the hope that this will be of benefit to those who work in or would design organizations for similar purposes. A closing note: It is my own experience that clinicians and program administrators who would help persons with the effects of traumatic stress sometimes must serve not only by providing good treatment, but also by advocating and defending their system in the other realms which may determine its fate—whether government, corporations, or the public. Understandably, many clinicians would wish to treat their clients or patients and to leave the fighting of battles on behalf of the treatment system to someone else. However, one thing I have learned in the Vet Center journey is that to maintain and improve services requires that those who know the victim and survivors well—their therapists—now and again stand up for them in the larger world.

Epilogue

In 1991, immediately after the conclusion of the Persian Gulf War, the U.S. Congress took account of the developments described in the foregoing chapter and opened the Department of Veterans Affairs Vet Centers to those who served in the Persian Gulf and also to those who served earlier in conflict zones in Lebanon, Grenada, and Panama. By the summer of 1992, Vet Centers had seen over 25,000 veterans of the Persian Gulf War, and over 2,000 veterans of Lebanon, Grenada, and Panama. This prompt legislative and VA response was in sharp contrast to the long delay in provision of assistance for Vietnam veterans and represents a lesson learned concerning the importance of early intervention for readjustment difficulties, acute stress reaction, and acute PTSD in war veterans.

References

American Psychiatric Association. (1968). *Diagnostic and statistical manual of mental disorders* (2nd ed.). Washington, DC: Author.

American Psychiatric Association. (1980). *Diagnostic and statistical manual of mental disorders* (3rd ed.). Washington, DC: Author.

Department of Veterans Affairs. (1986). *Report of the Vet Center Planning Committee*. Washington, DC: Author.

Department of Veterans Affairs, Office of Program Planning and Evaluation. (1981). *Readjustment counseling program for veterans of the Vietnam era: Program evaluation, formative phase*. Washington, DC: Author.

Department of Veterans Affairs, Office of Program Planning and Evaluation. (1987). *An evaluation of the Veterans Administration's readjustment counseling program for veterans of the Vietnam era*. Washington, DC: Author.

Department of Veterans Affairs, Readjustment Counseling Service (115). (1980–1992). *Workload and fiscal reports*. Washington, DC: Author.

Department of Veterans Affairs, Readjustment Counseling Service (115). (1992). *National workload summary*. Washington, DC: Author.

Department of Veterans Affairs, Readjustment Counseling Service (115). (1990). *Executive summary: News articles—Tenth anniversary Vietnam veterans outreach centers*. Washington, DC: Author.

General Accounting Office. (1987). *Vietnam veterans: A profile of VA's Readjustment Counseling Program* (GAO/HRD-87-63). Washington, DC: U. S. Government Printing Office.

G.I. Mood hailed by psychiatrist: Problems in Vietnam found low despite strain. (1967, January 4). *New York Times*, p. 30.

Johnson, A. W., Bowman, J. A., Byrdy, H. S., & Blank, A. S. (1967). Army psychiatry in Vietnam. In *Proceedings: Social and preventive psychiatry course* (pp. 41–76). Washington, DC: Walter Reed Army Institute of Research, Walter Reed Army Medical Center.

Mueller, Q. (1976). A song from the River of Perfumes. In J. Barry & W. D. Ehrhardt (Eds.), *Demilitarized zones: Veterans after Vietnam*. Perkasie, PA: East River Anthology.

Peters, T. J., & Waterman, R. H., Jr. (1982). *In search of excellence*. New York: Harper & Row.

Readjustment Counseling Service Vet Center. (1980–1990). *Voice* (Vet Center newsletter). Fargo, ND: Department of Veterans Affairs.

Shatan, C. F., Smith, J. R., & Haley, S. (1977). Johnny comes marching home: DSM-III and combat stress. In *130th Annual Meeting, American Psychiatric Association, Scientific Proceedings* (pp. 234–235). Toronto, Canada: American Psychiatric Association.

U. S. House of Representatives. (1981, April 8). *Hearing: Readjustment Counseling, Committee on Veterans Affairs, Subcommittee on Hospitals and Health Care* (Serial No. 97–20). Washington, DC: U. S. Government Printing Office.

U. S. House of Representatives. (1982, August 26). *Committee on Veterans Affairs, Subcommittee on Hospitals and Health Care, Hearing on Adequacy of Alcohol Treatment Program* (Serial No. 97–76). Washington, DC: U. S. Government Printing Office.

U. S. Senate. (1979, April 27). *Committee on Veterans Affairs Report to Accompany S.7* (Report No. 96–100). Washington, DC: U. S. Government Printing Office.

U. S. Senate. (1988, July 14). *Committee on Veterans Affairs, Hearing on Post-Traumatic Stress Disorder* (Senate Hearing 100–900). Washington, DC: U. S. Government Printing Office.

CHAPTER 78

Trauma in the Workplace

Tom Williams

Introduction

The inclusion of posttraumatic stress disorder (PTSD) in the DSM-III (American Psychiatric Association [APA], 1980) and its succeeding volume, the DSM-III-R (APA, 1987) has had profound effects on the mental health and the business communities. As perceived from a mental health standpoint, PTSD describes emotional distress, typically based on a discernible environmental event, which is the primary determinant of the symptom cluster. The kinds of stressors that cause PTSD are being well documented, researched, and treated clinically as evidenced by the various chapters of this *Handbook*. Although there is a known course for the emotional distress in PTSD, its mileposts are extremely variable from both the standpoint of the nature of the trauma and from that of the individual differences among the persons involved. Within the industrial-business sphere of economic enterprise, there is now legitimacy in the recognition of employment-related traumata as shown by disability pensions, workers' compensation, and veterans disability benefits. The U.S. Government, whose disability system for mental disorders is based on the current DSM-III-R, finds itself forced to address the issue of PTSD for federal employees. Workers' compensation laws in some states in the United States, as well as those European communities, often include emotional distress for events that occurred in the workplace. Many other states, by case law and precedent, hold the employer responsible for employment-related stressful events that harm or injure employees.

In Chapter 76, in this volume, the authors discussed the responsibility of employers not only to identify the potential stressors within the work environment, but also to develop strategies to prevent or reduce duty-related stressors or diminish the emotional aftermath of them (see also Wilson, 1989, for a review).

In this chapter, I will address the expected set of emotional responses to traumatic events in the workplace and make specific suggestions for diminishing the potential deleterious effects to well being. Further specific measures will be discussed for the amelioration and prevention of the onset of posttraumatic stress disorder.

Prevention Model

Primary Prevention

The primary prevention of PTSD in the workplace requires that the stressor itself be eliminated or substantially attenuated whenever possible. Clearly, this is the primary role of occupational safety and includes policies and procedures to prevent on-the-job injuries. Examples include such things as careful maintenance to reduce mechanical failures on equipment or theft-proof retail outlets or financial institutions, and well-defined sets of security procedures via protocols to reduce dangers or risks. However, primary prevention is difficult, if not impossible, in many high-risk occupations, such as law enforcement, firefighting, active-duty military forces, and in nonpredictable traumatic events and disasters. Pretrauma training and the development of a crisis-management plan are both useful and pragmatic procedures.

Secondary Prevention

Secondary prevention includes those measures that are employed to prevent the development of permanent emotional injuries by provision of direct services after a trauma and prior to the development of symptoms of emotional distress. This is the basis of *critical incident debriefing* (see Chapter 76, in this volume, for a discussion). Furthermore, although some employers may be able to provide trained internal resource personnel in

Tom Williams • Post Trauma Treatment Center, 31933 Miwok Trail, Evergreen, Colorado 80439.

International Handbook of Traumatic Stress Syndromes, edited by John P. Wilson and Beverley Raphael. Plenum Press, New York, 1993.

the event of a trauma, others most likely will have to seek out assistance beyond the responsibility of the employer.

Tertiary Prevention: Posttrauma Counseling and Assistance

Tertiary prevention consists mainly in providing resources to an individual or group after the emergence of symptoms or ongoing personal counseling associated with the trauma. These services are designed to treat symptom concerns and attempt to prevent recurrence of psychic dysfunction. They are also oriented toward PTSD-specific outpatient or inpatient occupational trauma programs. These programs have the specified focus of addressing posttrauma problems among employees who suffer stress-response syndromes.

Continuum of Trauma Risk in Occupations

It is clear that some occupations have predictable and repetitive traumata. Active military duty, especially in combat-related activity or paramilitary responsibilities, is one of many such conditions. For example, the utilization of military (e.g., Coast Guard) or paramilitary Drug Enforcement Agency (DEA) antidrug operations are examples within the United States. The more obvious and the common employment categories at risk for stress reactions are law enforcement, firefighting, and emergency medical technicians. Often neglected in servicing professions from this group are "command" personnel and support personnel, such as radio and telephone dispatchers.

Other groups subject to potential trauma include a rather broad spectrum of workers in industry as well as in transportation, construction, or similar occupations that expose employees to potentially dangerous situations which may be of low probability for occurrence such as hotel fires and natural and man-made disasters.

It is a truism, too, that the kinds of employees who are exposed to trauma form a cross-section of the normal population. Others, however, may be drawn toward high-risk occupations that are risky, dangerous, or "action-oriented." Their personality characteristics, as well as the demanding nature of their work, often lead them to band together socially. This affiliative cohesion often means that they draw their emotional support from co-workers and may begin to develop an "us/them" attitude toward people who are not in their line of work. Their friends and spouses tend to originate from the immediate work group or closely related fields. Frequently, a spirit of family and camaraderie exists within their industry. One consequence of this pattern of affiliation is that a major trauma or disaster will have systemic effects. The importance of an internal system for provision of crisis services is magnified within these occupations that have an us/them attitude. Outside resources and personnel, that may be pulled into play, must have prior experience or connection within that particular industrial group to be most effective. Internal resources and personnel, such as employee assistance programs (E.A.P.), find themselves overburdened with their normal duties when a disaster strikes their company or similar companies within the industry (Raphael, 1986). Experts in traumatic stress and PTSD as well as in debriefings may be required to facilitate processes to restore organizational and individual employee equilibrium associated with mental health and productivity.

Framework of Stress-Response Reactions

Acute Trauma Response

The *emotional response* to a traumatic event consists of several interacting factors (Figure 78.1). In severe traumata, PTSD may be a major factor. If death or permanent separation exists, *grief* is very likely another, with some common overlap of symptoms. *Individual variables*, which include personality styles, coping skills, and support systems, affect other aspects of emotional response. *Trauma-specific* elements, separate from the other factors, need to be understood and addressed. Responding to a fatal traffic accident is different than seeing a co-worker crushed by a piece of heavy equipment, although some individual emotional responses may be identical. *Duty-related* trauma programs need to address the entire spectrum of the affective responses of employees (see Green, Wilson, & Lindy, 1985; Wilson, 1989).

The emotional response to the trauma of individuals, work groups, and companies is depicted in Figure 78.2. Stressor experiences, as explained in the DSM-III-R, are events outside the normal range of human experience and that would cause *symptoms of distress* in most persons. If employees are well trained and somewhat inoculated to trauma (Meichenbaum, 1985), they tend to bypass the shock phase depicted in Figure 78.2, or they may have some of the psychological and physiological elements of the shock phase (e.g., numbing, denial). If

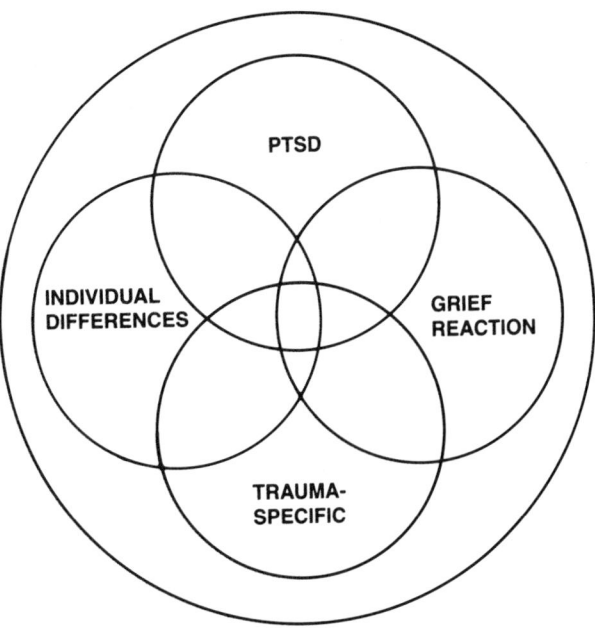

Figure 78.1. Factors affecting emotional responses.

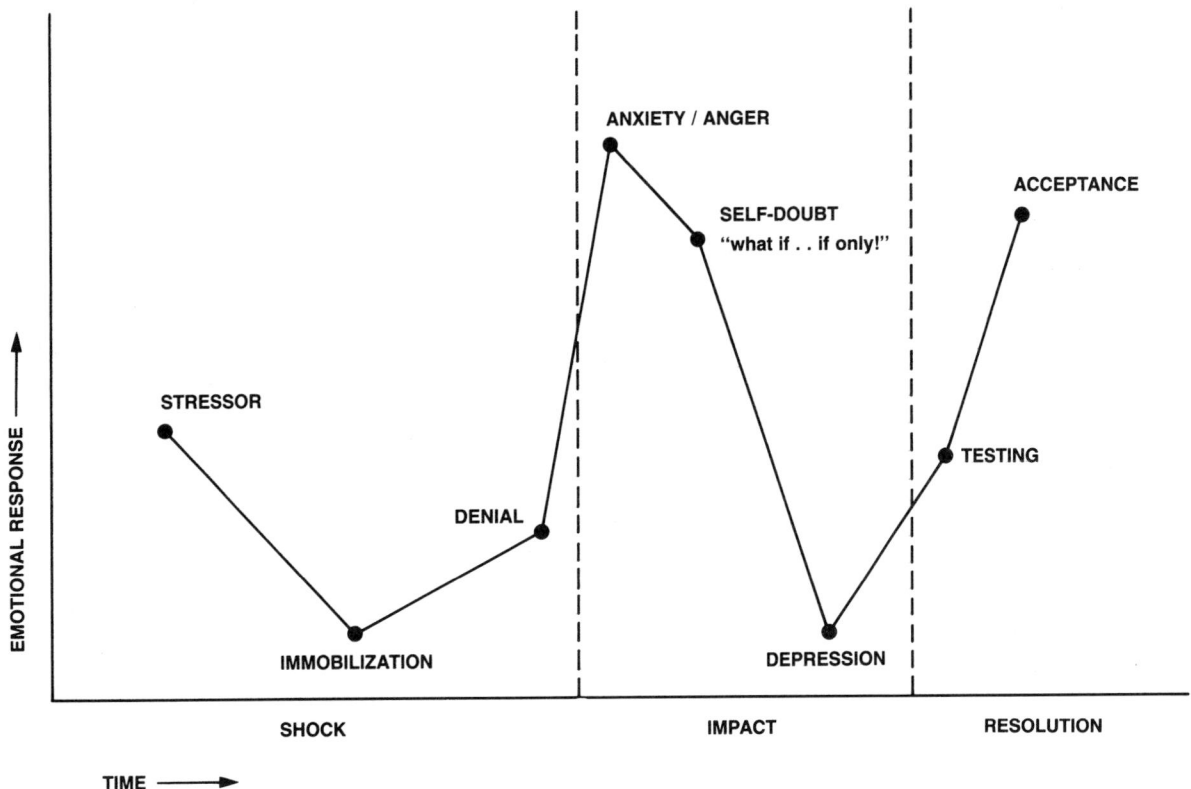

Figure 78.2. Phases of posttraumatic stress disorder.

the trauma is outside of their training and preparation or has special significance to them, they may react with signs and symptoms of stress or PTSD. Some of the special aspects of the traumatic stressor include the death of a co-worker, multiple deaths, mass destruction, or deaths of children. An individual employee may be more susceptible to a specific set of stressors. The previous trauma history of the employee may reduce or magnify the impact of this specific stressor on his or her subsequent patterns of adaptation.

Shock Phase

Essentially, the shock phase consists of physiological and psychological shock. Perceptual changes that often accompany this phase are time expansion, tunnel vision, and various dissociative states of consciousness (see also Chapter 32, in this volume). The body's "fight, flight, or freeze" response has alerted and prepared the individual for action. Usually, there is an intense focus on the trauma situation similar to "freeze framing" every millisecond of the trauma. The freeze framing may be associated with a perceptual distortion in the form of *time expansion*, whereas in others it may be associated with a sense of *time acceleration*. Although certain perceptual mechanisms may be adaptive in the traumatic situation, they may be difficult later when the survivor has a subjective belief of having had more time to be able to react or problem solve than was actually available during the event. This extreme focus on the trauma can leave the survivor with a psychological and physiological

sense of tunnel vision that may later become associated with survivor guilt. Clearly, there is a range of dissociative-like perceptual changes during a trauma which include forms of derealization often seen in survivors of sexual assault and observers of carnage. In some cases, these perceptual alterations may be related to the subsequent onset of flashbacks and possible complications of the development of long-term personality alterations, such as borderline or multiple-personality disorders.

Impact Phase

Although the shock phase is generally avoided for the well-trained workers, the impact phase generally produces emotional distress. The high state of emotional arousal, anger, anxiety, fear, rage, or tension is often accompanied with signs of hyperarousal and hypervigilance. Traditionally, people have a difficult time with sleep initiation, exaggerated startle response, memory impairment, trouble concentrating, nightmares, and flashbacks. The nightmares are related to the trauma and tend to follow general and specific elements of the traumatic event. It has been my experience that about 80% of the victims have "miniflashbacks," where the persons think or feel as though they are reliving the event for a very short period of time (seconds or microseconds). They report a *dual reality* of being oriented to reality and seeing the trauma situation again. Full-blown flashback episodes are possible and can be frequent in survivors of plane crashes and armed robbery.

The self-doubt step of the impact phase is of special importance to understanding duty-related trauma. This is characterized with the self-questioning of "Did I do the right thing?" "Should I have done something differently?" It also has an element of avoidance by asking such questions as "If only I hadn't worked that day or, if only I had not traded shifts then the outcome would have been better." Of course, a certain amount of the self-questioning is important and useful. It is vital to review carefully the elements of the traumatic situation with the employee to determine what they did and did not do in the situation. With a sensitive reappraisal of what happened, the employee will likely continue to progress through the natural stress recovery process without hindrance. Without examining step-by-step their role in the event, the employees may not be able to successfully reappraise their actions. Failure to do so, despite evidence to the contrary, may then be associated with assuming too much responsibility for the outcome of a particular aspect of the stressful event. This illogical assumption is often aided and reinforced by the perceptual changes that occurred in the traumatic event itself. The failure to process adequately the nature of the individual's role in the trauma may lead to continuing symptoms of anxiety and depression.

Survivor Guilt

Where there is death involved in the trauma, survivor guilt is likely to develop. I consider the survivor guilt, as discussed by Cobb and Lindemann (1943), as a form of *existential guilt*. The survivor often asks, "How come I lived and other people didn't?" Therapeutically, individuals may come to the realization that there were many factors that impinged on their behavior and that the responsibility for what occurred is spread across individuals, a fact which aids the process of positive reappraisal.

Another form of survivor guilt I term *content guilt* (Williams, 1988). Here the person feels guilty about behaviors he or she *failed to enact* during the traumatic situation (see Chapter 1, in this volume, for a discussion). In dealing with this step, the focus is to review the event step-by-step. The *perceptual alterations* that may have occurred during the event give the survivors the false impression that there was more they could have done to change the possible consequences. If workers emerge from this phase with the feeling that they applied all their resources appropriately to the situation, they will continue to recover. By the term *resources*, we refer to the time to respond, equipment, knowledge, training, backup support available, and previous experience.

There is a range of traumatic components in traumatic events and suffered by disaster workers (see Chapter 6, in this volume). Among the more troubling is the level of *responsibility trauma*, which include the various perceptions of responsibility and perceived consequence in relation to the outcome. Clearly, some work roles are inherently more likely to evoke guilt related to such responsibilities, and these role aspects will need to be understood and discussed. These issues are indeed further complicated where actual responsibility exists— particularly for the death or deaths of others, or where "scapegoating" or inquiry allocates blame. Detailed as-

sessment and working-through of such complex psychological issues are required. The final step in the impact phase is often some form of *depression*. The survivor feels tired much of the time, tends to oversleep and have a poor quality of sleep (i.e., sleep disturbance), has weight loss or weight gain, withdraws from family and friends, and reduces activities to a basic pattern of working, eating, and resting. In this phase, some people tend to be lethargic and irritable. With employees who change work shifts, it may be difficult to determine if this lethargy is a product of a stressor or simply shiftwork changes in behavior.

Recovery Phase

In the recovery phase, individuals often go through a testing period where they attempt to lead a normal life. They make decisions to "face" the trauma, for instance, to drive by the scene of the shooting. They may decide to assume greater control of their lives. The *acceptance step* of the recovery phase is when workers realize that the trauma is part of their life employment and continue their stream of adaptation. This concept of acceptance is often hampered by well-meaning employers, coworkers, and family members who continue to say, "Forget it, put it behind you, get back to normal." The survivors can get back to normal as long as they understand that it may be a "different" sense of normal for them than the pretrauma normal.

In Figure 78.2, the acceptance step is designated at a higher state of emotional response than when the stressor hit. If the person is subject to another traumatic event, he or she reenters the recovery process at a higher level of physiological and psychological tension. As discussed by the authors in Chapter 2 in this volume, survivors can be more susceptible to psychological and physiological stressors than persons without such experiences. Figure 78.3 depicts multiply traumatized people. The first portion of Figure 78.3 is identical to Figure 78.2. With the onset of additional stressors, individuals may bypass the immobilization phase, have some elements of denial, and then move into the impact phase. In this state of responsiveness, the individual has an even higher level of susceptibility to trauma. Persons who have not successfully resolved previous trauma often "stair-step" to more pathological and distressing emotional reactions to the new event. This is likened to the straw that broke the camel's back. The workers feel as though they are defective and may respond to what supervisors tell them: "If you can't tolerate the situation, then leave it." When a person leaves a stressful occupation, either through disability or normal retirement, that in itself can be a major stressor that can lead to symptoms of a stress disorder. This loss of life structure may precipitate an additional personal crisis. Examples of workers at risk for stair-stepping effects of stress exposure include emergency medical service personnel and police officers.

Phases of PTSD and Substance Abuse

The model of chronic PTSD (see Chapter 4, in this volume, for a discussion) has been modified on the basis

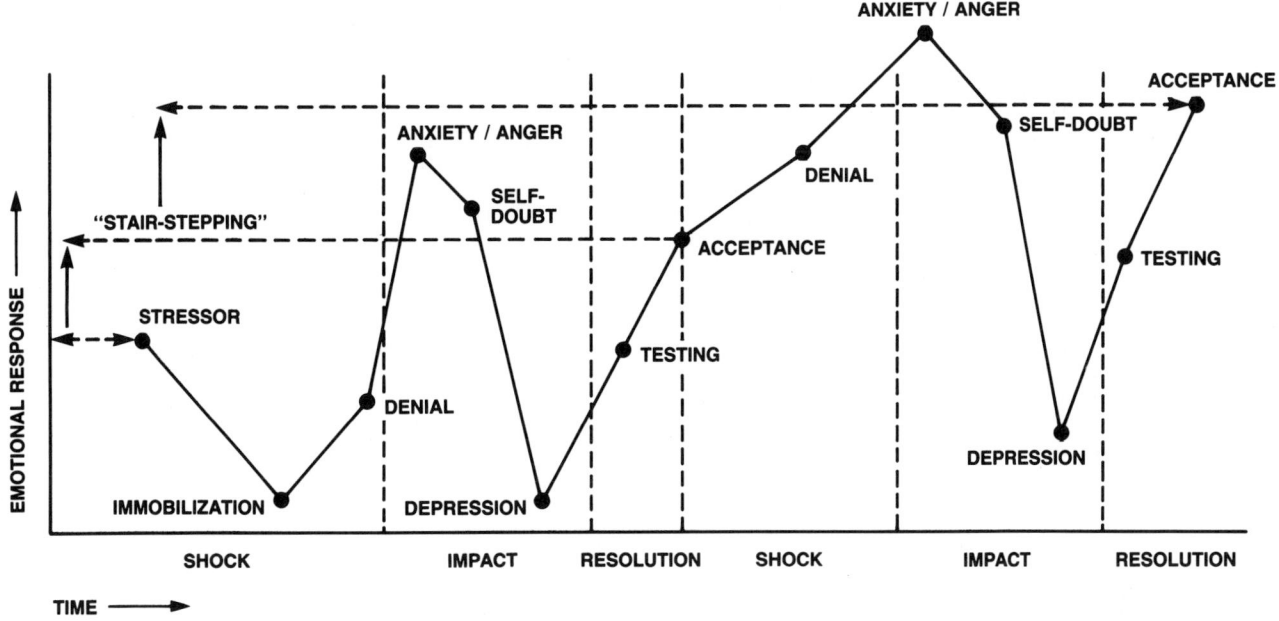

Figure 78.3. "Stair-stepping": Cumulative stressor effects.

of our clinical work. As noted in Figure 78.4, there are three main phases to chronic PTSD. The DSM-III-R organizes the symptom clusters in a similar manner of intrusion and hyperarousal versus avoidance, denial, and depressive symptoms. As indicated, there may be a symptom-free phase during which a person functions well. However, if one were to look closely, there may be problems of intimacy and substance abuse. When an-

other trauma occurs, there is a strong reminder of the original trauma, such as an anniversary date, and it may become fully symptomatic again. Upon exposure to a confluence of everyday stressors, they also may have their symptoms intensified. Persons with inadequate stress-coping techniques may find themselves symptomatic even after a minor stress. Similarly, when trauma occurs in the workplace, simply returning to that location may cause the person to experience intensification upon reexposure. An example would be a flight attendant being assigned to duty on the same type of aircraft as during an incident.

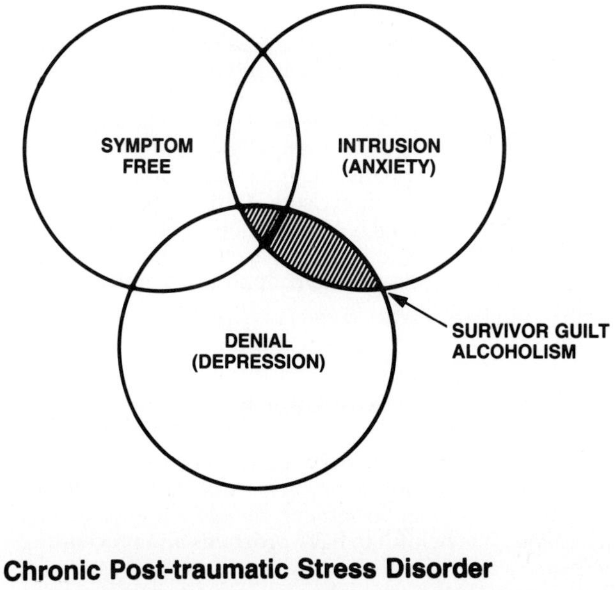

The intrusion phase, which may remain dormant for months or years, is characterized by psychologically reexperiencing the event. Typically, this is a very distressing phase, and people develop a variety of mechanisms to attempt to cope with this stage. Adaptive mechanisms include attempts at active mastery, exercise, relaxation techniques, increase of leisure time activities, and perhaps entry or reentry into counseling. Maladaptive techniques in this phase are generally related to reliance on alcohol or other chemicals to reduce the high levels of tension and anxiety, and fits of rage.

The denial/avoidance phase is often accompanied by depression. Generally, people avoid things that remind them of the trauma, an almost impossible task when their employment is related to the trauma. As a consequence, there is often observed an increase in sick leave, the quest for job change, irritability and dissatisfaction at work. Many people in this phase seek out high-risk activities which are helpful in warding off depression. They may choose skydiving, sports parachuting, scuba diving, race car driving, or mountain climbing, or seek numerous sexual encounters to block depression symptoms (Wilson, 1989).

Chronic Post-traumatic Stress Disorder

Figure 78.4. Overlapping symptoms in PTSD.

In the stress recovery process and with proper treatment, most individuals are able to return to the symptom-free phase. However, high levels of current stress may prevent the restoration of homeostasis. If the person has personality or emotional difficulties separate from PTSD, the effect may be that symptoms are magnified and the person fixates in a cyclical alternation between the intrusion and denial phases, as depicted by the overlap of the circles in Figure 78.4. Since employees in unusually stressful jobs have had more extensive pre-employment evaluations than the general work force, they are less likely to have premorbid psychopathology. With employment-related trauma, the most common reason is the inability to resolve satisfactorily the survivor guilt or development of substance abuse disorders in the attempt to self-medicate. Many treatment failures in traditional chemical dependency in-patient programs are due to the inability of the treatment program to address an underlying stress disorder.

In recent years, various approaches to the treatment of employment-related traumatic stresses have begun to emerge. First, employers must identify the type, amount, and location of stressors to which their employees may be exposed. Some events can be anticipated and some may actually be avoided by procedural changes, increased security, or increased maintenance. The ability to respond to traumatic events should be evaluated in the light of training, normal work loads that will increase in times of crisis, appropriateness, and the expected frequency of utilization. Organizations with a high potential for trauma need a strong response capability for employee assistance. In particular, peer-support programs have been found to be effective. Many peer-support programs have been an outgrowth of critical incident stress-debriefing programs. Alternatively, there are times when the extent or the nature of the trauma, such as the death of a fellow employee, can be so devastating that intraorganizational programs will lose their ability to function effectively. Nonetheless, internal resources such as an employee assistance program and a specially trained group of volunteers, supported by outside experts, can reduce the overall impact of a disaster. In times of disaster, the lack of a crisis-management plan perpetuates the disaster for decision makers and the company.

Training in emotional response to trauma for all employees in high-risk occupations is becoming a way of doing business in climates of increasing technology and crime rates. Appendix A contains a trauma response specialist training outline used by our center in the United States. It is only one of many such programs that are available to organizations.

Stress Debriefing

Talking with affected employees or customers after a traumatic event is often called *stress debriefing*. Debriefings can be technical when they review job performance during a crisis situation or they may be purely emotional, dealing with the affective consequences of tragedy. In debriefing survivors of airplane crashes, for example, it is important to review the flight attendants' and pilots' role-related behaviors during the tragedy and the emotional aftermath. Usually, passengers who may have no role other than attendance require only an emotional debriefing (see Chapter 76, in this volume, for a discussion).

Debriefings are conducted as soon as possible after the traumatic event. During periods of prolonged stress, such as rescue operations and body identifications, periodic debriefings are required. These are done on or close to the disaster site by highly experienced professionals.

The meetings are conducted in a secure area that is safe and is secluded from interruptions and the press. Debriefings are best done with the "cloak of confidentiality" from the treating professional and may or may not be time limited (see also Chapter 38, in this volume, for a discussion). The group's size should be manageable, 10 to 12 persons, but situations may dictate either individual debriefings or larger group sessions. The format includes what happened in a step-by-step sequential basis and what were the emotional responses at each step of the way. After the group has discussed the tragedy and their role in it, an educational portion of the debriefing is conducted. This consists of a discussion of the material contained in Figure 78.2. A handout, similar to the one in Appendix B, is provided at the end of the session so that the employees can share the information with co-workers, family, and friends. The debriefing should be conducted in proximity to the traumatic event. It is also true that the debriefers themselves may need to be debriefed by someone who is not associated with the stressful event.

In large transportation disasters, for example, employees are assigned liaison duties with survivors and next-of-kin families. Other employees are often assigned phone bank duties to answer queries from the families and friends of the passengers. Experience has shown that employees from both these groups can become dysfunctional during and after their utilization in these special cases. Preselection and pretraining of such employees, along with supervisory personnel and other incident-management persons, are mandatory. Once trained, these individuals will be more effective in dealing in their special roles and the possibility of they themselves becoming casualties is significantly reduced (see Chapter 82, in this volume, for a discussion). Supervisors also need to be aware of the possible long-term effects of trauma on their employees and of possible referral services. Appendix C is a sample of information for law-enforcement supervisors. Trauma specialists can be located through such organizations as the Society of Traumatic Stress Studies in the United States and Europe. Early identification and appropriate referral can reduce future claims.

Conclusion

Organizations have the responsibility to help identify and eliminate stress problems that are predictable within their work environment. Should a trauma be unavoidable, it is helpful to have programs and procedures in place to deal with the immediate effects of the trauma. This is often done through peer support, employee assistance programs, and outside resources. As reviewed in this chapter, posttraumatic intervention by the employers or outside professional experts can facilitate the normal stress recovery process and restabilization of the organization that is affected by the unexpected traumatic event or disaster.

Appendix A

Training Program

A company's response to a traumatic incident in the workplace can seriously affect operations, personnel, and the company's financial future. Immediate response to a catastrophic event through the use of company-trained "Trauma Response Specialists" will minimize personal trauma, the interruption of corporate operations, and corporate liability. The addition of a company trauma response team eliminates valuable time spent locating and hiring competent disaster response specialists from within each city, and provides the company with a group of trained specialists as a critical adjunct to an existing corporate disaster plan.

PROGRAM AGENDA

DAY ONE   A.M.
Introduction
- Program structure, philosophy, and history
- Preincident evaluation and preparedness
- Emotional response to trauma

P.M.
- Managing traumatic stress reactions in employees
- Long-term effects of trauma
- Posttraumatic stress disorder: When to seek help

DAY TWO   A.M.
Stress Debriefings
- Conducting a critical incident debriefing
- Conducting a death notification

P.M.
Counseling Techniques for Survivors: Victims, Families, and Next-of-Kin
- Organization
- Telling the story
- The consequences of surviving
- Steps toward recovery
- Closing and evaluation

DAY THREE   A.M.
Pretrauma Training
- Trauma coping tools
- Crisis techniques

P.M.
- Stress assessment techniques
- Stress management techniques
- Team building

DAY FOUR   A.M.
On-Site Management Skills
- Crisis management

- Development of local resources
- Press relations

P.M.
Communication Skills
- Individual and group communication
- Debriefing company employees: On-site/others
- Aftercare/reintegration to the workplace: Pathological bonding

DAY FIVE   A.M.
- Tracking
- Coordinating "Trauma Response Specialists"
- Communications
- After-action report

P.M.

- Legal aspects
- Trauma review

Appendix B

Sample Handout: Emotional Responses to Trauma

There are several predictable phases that persons who suffer a trauma tend to go through. The phases usually occur in the following order, but the phases may appear in any sequence.

Shock can last from a few hours to one week. This includes a feeling of immobilization, where you can't remember simple things like your own telephone number, where your keys are kept, what time it is, etc. This is followed by denial where you don't really believe what is happening or has happened. Often times you deny the fact that you were frightened and/or anxious.

Impact starts sometime after the incident and can last for up to two weeks. This is characterized by anger, sometimes directed toward your employer, fellow employees, police, or just society in general. This is usually dependent on what happened. In this phase you question yourself on how well you handled the situation with such self questions as, "Did I do the right thing?" This is the "what if" time when you think about what could have happened, or how you might have reacted differently. These self doubts are common and expected. Another frequent occurrence in this impact phase is the onset of depression. You can give in to feelings of hopelessness and impotence, unable to think of positive outcomes, see yourself as a helpless victim, and blame yourself for poor judgment and bad decisions.

Resolution may go on for up to two months. The first step is realizing that you probably did a good job with the "incident." The last step is one of acceptance, where you really understand what has happened, that fear is human, and stop second guessing yourself or blaming yourself or others.

If you have had a medical problem such as gastrointestinal disorder, hypertension, diabetes, seizure disorders, etc., be particularly aware of any changes in these medical conditions and seek medical evaluation immediately. A certain amount of emotional distress is common after trauma. If the anxiety, fear at work, depression or sleep disorders continue for more than a few days, you should seek professional assistance to help you with these difficulties. Do not be alone immediately following the incident. Avoid alcohol or other drugs that are not prescribed.

Dreaming about the incident is common, but should go away in a couple of weeks. There may be times where you think or feel that the incident is reoccurring, something like a "miniflashback."

You should talk about the experience with family and friends, and if possible with people who were there. The more you are able to talk about what happened with people who understand, the sooner the difficulties will pass and the associated problems will diminish.

Appendix C

The Management of Traumatic Stress Reactions in Police Officers

There are certain events which are so shocking or life-threatening that they cause symptoms of psychological distress in most people, even if they escape physical injury. The situation is aggravated for police officers in two ways:

1. Police officers are expected to deal with the trauma of others in a calm and professional manner.
2. The possibility of serious injury or death is part of the everyday work environment. Events which can be particularly damaging include: (a) violent confrontation in which injury occurs or is imminent, (b) automobile accidents, (c) hostage situations, (d) police-related shootings, (e) assaults on officers, (f) rescue operations, and (g) investigations into extraordinary criminal acts (i.e., homicides involving children, etc.).

Traumatized officers may or may not show overt signs of emotional distress following such incidents. Most of them, however, will go through the predictable phases of emotional response to trauma:

Shock occurs as an initial response lasting a few hours to a week during which the officer may appear dazed or preoccupied, have difficulty with remembering simple things, and act out of character (e.g., have outbursts of temper over inconsequential things).

Impact starts sometime after the initial crisis is over. Anger directed at management, other officers, or anyone "responsible" for the traumatic event is common. Self-blame is also common. Periods of depression nearly

always occur as the person allows the full impact of what happened to sink in.

Resolution may go on for up to two months. Depressive episodes become less frequent. The person begins to accept that he or she, co-workers, and management did the best they could to deal with the traumatic incident and prevent such things from happening in the future. Finally, the individual comes to accept that such events, as regrettable as they are, do happen.

There are certain steps which can be taken to facilitate the *normal recovery process* from psychological trauma:

1. *Debrief.* A Trauma Team conducts an initial debriefing, on site, for all officers involved in a traumatic incident. The debriefing is designed to allow the officers to process their emotional reactions to the incident. An effective debriefing is supportive and nonjudgmental, helping to regain their shaken sense of security and self-esteem. An on-site follow-up meeting with the Trauma Team normally takes place a week after the incident. This allows assessment of longer-term reactions and aids in further processing of the trauma.

2. *Encourage working-through.* The primary purpose of the debriefing is to encourage the officers to begin dealing with their responses to the traumatic event. The single most effective method for the *resolution* of traumatic stress is talking about the trauma with others who went through it. You should encourage your officers to talk about the trauma and meet periodically as a support group to monitor their progress.

3. *Manage the stress.* Keep in mind the traumatic stress reactions discussed above, and take steps to deal with them. These include dealing in a sensitive manner with periodic stress reactions during the *impact* phase and being alert to any symptoms which might indicate an officers is not successfully resolving their traumatic stress. In such cases, a referral to the Center should be made. Our experience has been that the support of co-workers during the weeks following the trauma is vital to *resolution.* Thus, you should encourage your officers to maintain their regular work schedules as much as possible following traumatic incidents.

Given a supportive work environment, most persons will successfully resolve their traumatic stress. Be alert, however, for signs of problems in resolution, which may appear early on or not surface until weeks after the trauma. These signs should become a matter of concern if they become habitual. A referral should be made if you observe:

• significant personality changes, such as isolation, irritability, or increased alcohol use
• deterioration in work habits or attitudes
• chronic lateness, absenteeism, or excessive use of sick leave.

Finally, investigations or court appearances related to the traumatic incident can be particularly stressful. "Replaying" an incident can cause symptoms to surface. Should this occur, we have staff members specially trained to assist in the process.

References

American Psychiatric Association. (1980). *Diagnostic and statistical manual of mental disorders* (3rd ed.). Washington, DC: Author.

American Psychiatric Association. (1987). *Diagnostic and statistical manual of mental disorders* (3rd ed., rev.). Washington, DC: Author.

Cobb, S., & Lindemann, E. (1943). Neuropsychiatric observation after the Coconut Grove fire. *Annals of Surgery, 117,* 814–824.

Green, B. L., Wilson, J. P., & Lindy, J. D. (1985). Conceptualizing post-traumatic stress disorder: A psychosocial framework. In C. R. Figley (Ed.), *Trauma and its wake: The study and treatment of posttraumatic stress disorder* (pp. 53–69). New York: Brunner/Mazel.

Meichenbaum, D. (1985). *Stress inoculation training.* New York: Pergamon Press.

Raphael, B. (1986). *When disaster strikes.* New York: Basic Books.

Williams, T. (1988). Diagnosis and treatment of survivor guilt: The bad penny syndrome. In J. P. Wilson, Z. Harel, & B. Kahana (Eds.), *Human adaptation to extreme stress: From the Holocaust to Vietnam* (pp. 319–336). New York: Plenum Press.

Wilson, J. P. (1989). *Trauma, transformation, and healing: An integrative approach to theory, research, and posttraumatic therapy.* New York: Brunner/Mazel.

CHAPTER 79

International Perspectives on the Treatment and Prevention of Posttraumatic Stress Disorder

Giovanni de Girolamo

Introduction

In the 10th revision of the *International Classification of Diseases*, Chapter 5, one may read that posttraumatic stress disorder (PTSD)

> arises as a delayed and/or protracted response to a stressful event or situation of an exceptionally threatening or catastrophic nature, which is likely to cause pervasive distress in almost anyone (e.g., natural or man-made disaster, combat, serious accident, witnessing the violent death of others, being the victim of torture, terrorism, rape or other crime). (World Health Organization [WHO], 1992a)

The identification of this new diagnostic category can be seen in the context of a more general trend in the psychological and psychiatric fields, by which, as noted by Figley (1988), "a number of concepts have merged which are associated with emotional reactions to environmental stimuli." Greater attention, then, has begun to be paid to the psychological aspects of human reactions to natural and man-made disasters, to violence, to war, and to severe accidents; the increasing amount of research focusing on stressful life events and their relationship with various indicators of psychological and somatic ill-health is related in part to this trend. New specialties have appeared in the scientific field, such as victimology, which studies the victims of criminal violence and their relationships to their violators (Helsinki Institute for Crime Prevention and Control, 1989; Sparr,

1989), while old specialties have substantially expanded their traditional areas of concern. Occupational medicine, for example, now includes the study of job-induced traumatic stress (Schottenfeld & Cullen, 1986), or the investigation of possible interventions for workers who are exposed to highly stressful events in the line of duty.

Although other chapters in this book are devoted to theoretical, clinical, and management-related issues of PTSD, in this chapter I will discuss some problems related to PTSD at an international level. Disasters and violence, as two of the major sources of PTSD, will be the main focus, with particular emphasis on these problems as reflected in developing countries. This choice is justified by the following points:

1. Both disasters and violence represent major public health problems, and are areas of major concern for such international organizations as WHO.
2. The numbers of people affected are large, and the impact on whole societies can be devastating, especially in developing countries, where the available coping resources are limited.
3. To deal effectively with disasters and violence, international effort and coordination are essential. Logical vehicles for such coordination are the international agencies of the United Nations (UN) system, such as WHO, the United Nations Disaster Relief Coordinator (UNDRO), the United Nations Development Programme, and others. The main activities and programs of these agencies in this area will be mentioned accordingly.

In this perspective, it will sometimes be conceptually and operationally coherent to consider PTSD within the broader field of psychosocial consequences of disasters and violence.

Therefore, in this chapter, I will first address some

Giovanni de Girolamo • Division of Mental Health, World Health Organization, 1211 Geneva 27, Switzerland.

International Handbook of Traumatic Stress Syndromes, edited by John P. Wilson and Beverley Raphael. Plenum Press, New York, 1993.

conceptual and epidemiological issues of disasters and subsequently will discuss the epidemiology of PTSD and other psychological disorders following a natural disaster. Problems of prevention and treatment of PTSD consequent to disasters will then be considered. In the second half of the chapter, problems of PTSD and man-made violence will be examined, focusing on implications for prevention and treatment.

Disasters: Conceptual Issues

As stated in the ICD-10 definition, disasters of any kind are one of the most common and most relevant causes of PTSD. Taylor (1987) proposed a taxonomy of disasters which classifies them according to the primary causes (natural, industrial, and humanistic) and the primary elements (earth, air, fire, water, and people); the traditional classification differentiates only between man-made (including both industrial and humanistic) and natural disasters. However, a clear distinction between what is man-made and what is natural is sometimes impossible, because of the increasing effects of man's actions on the overall ecological balance and the occurrence of "anthropogenic" natural disasters (Beinin, 1985).

Despite the apparent self-evidence of what is meant by "disaster," it is not easy to give a satisfactory definition of the term, and so this issue remains controversial. Korver (1987) found almost 40 different definitions of disaster in the literature. This conceptual difficulty is related to the fact that, as stressed by the same author, while "upwards a disaster is unlimited, downward, one has to draw a line somewhere." If we consider some of the most widely known definitions of disasters, however, it is possible to draw some unified conclusions:[1]

1. A disaster creates a discontinuity in the social structure, and the social aspects of the disaster situation should be considered as more important than the physical event and its components, as emphasized by Quarantelli (1980).

2. The magnitude of the disaster or the altered ecological balance is not to be considered as the key element of a disaster; rather, it is essential to consider the adjustment capacity of the victims and the relationship of the disaster to the resources that are available. This way of

conceptualizing a disaster has important implications when we evaluate psychological reactions to it, and is well reflected in the ongoing discussion concerning the relative importance to be attributed to the stressor itself or to individual vulnerability in the occurrence of PTSD.

3. The concept of disaster changes over time and among different cultures. Among some populations, especially in developing countries, a lengthy first-hand experience of coping with natural disasters has produced the creation of specific "disaster subcultures," which are likely to deeply affect their pattern of psychological reactions to the disaster situation, and should be considered carefully in evaluating PTSD from a cross-cultural perspective.

Epidemiology of Natural Disasters

A UN General Assembly Resolution 42/169, adopted on December 11, 1987, designated the 1990s as a decade for *natural disaster reduction*; it stated that natural disasters, such as those caused by earthquakes, windstorms, tsunamis, floods, landslides, volcanic eruptions, wildfires, and other calamities, have killed about 3 million people worldwide over the past two decades, adversely affected the lives of at least 800 million more, and resulted in immediate economic damage exceeding $23 billion. Africa's recent drought alone threatened the lives of more than 20 million people and uprooted millions of others. Other epidemiological estimates, obtained on the basis of the data collected by the U.S. Office of Foreign Disaster Assistance (Agency for International Development, 1989) concerning the major disasters which occurred worldwide from 1900 up to 1988, indicate that, in these 9 decades, about 339 million people have been affected by floods, with a total of 36 million rendered homeless; 26 million have been affected by earthquakes, with similar numbers affected by typhoons and cyclones, giving a total of almost 10 million homeless people; finally, 3.5 million have been affected by hurricanes, resulting in 1,300,000 people without homes. From 1970 to 1981, floods were the most frequent disaster, comprising more than one third of all disasters occurring in that decade. Windstorms were the next most frequent disaster (one fourth of the total number), whereas earthquakes caused the greatest number of deaths and monetary loss.

The geographic distribution of disasters between developed and developing countries deserves special attention, because there seems to be a special relationship between the location of a disaster on the one hand, and the severity of its consequences on the other. Out of the 109 worst natural disasters which occurred between 1960 and 1987, as selected and studied by Berz (1989), 41 occurred in developing countries; however, the number of deaths caused among the affected populations was far greater in the developing countries (758,850 deaths in developing countries as compared to only 11,441 in developed countries). In general, the number of deaths and injuries and the amount of damage is closely related to the prevailing level of economic development: As stated in the UNDRO manual on *Disaster Prevention and Mitigation* (1986), "The smallest and poorest countries

---

[1]According to the World Health Organization (1989g), "disasters are situations where there are unforeseen, serious and immediate threats to public health." The United Nations Disaster Relief Co-ordinator (1986) has adopted a definition originally proposed by Dynes, which states that "Sociologically, a disaster is an event, located in time and space, that produces the conditions whereby the continuity of the structure and processes of social units becomes problematic." The American College of Emergency Medicine (1976) has defined "a disaster as a sudden massive disproportion between hostile elements of any kind and the survival resources that are available to counterbalance these in the shortest period of time." Finally, Lechat (1979) suggested that "Natural disasters can be defined as ecological disruptions exceeding the adjustment capacity of the affected community."

are affected most severely by natural disasters, and the poorest and most disadvantaged members of a disaster affected community are likely to experience the most serious consequences." The UNDRO manual also shows a list of indicators of vulnerable and disaster-prone countries for the period 1960–1981, based on various sources of data; in this list, the disasters resulting in the greatest numbers of people killed all occurred in countries characterized by a low-income economy: Bangladesh (633,000 deaths), China (247,000 deaths), Nicaragua (106,000 deaths), and Ethiopia (103,000 deaths).

The extent of risk among many populations, especially in developing countries, has increased over the last few decades owing to increasing population size, greater population density in vulnerable areas, and the strong tendency of large populations toward urbanization. There has also been a concurrent increase in the magnitude of certain types of man-made disaster. One such man-made disaster can now affect several countries or even continents; some authors have proposed the term *planetary disasters* for these large-scale events (Manri & Magalini, 1989). We know very little about the stress-related disorders caused by such events, which represent an important area in need of investigation, particularly when new types of elements are involved (e.g., nuclear energy) (Alexandrowsky, 1989; Baum, Gatchel, & Schaeffer, 1983; de Girolamo, 1991; Dew, Bromet, Schulberg, Dunn, & Parkinson, 1987; Poumadere, 1990). We know only in very general terms that, as originally suggested by Barton (1969), forewarning, duration, and scope of impact of a disaster represent some of the main variables mediating its social, psychological, and physical consequences.

From all these considerations, it is possible to draw the following conclusions: (1) Despite remarkable differences in the available estimates, it is evident that natural (and man-made) disasters represent a phenomenon deeply affecting the lives of millions of people, and sometimes producing devastating effects on whole societies; for many developing countries they have represented and still represent a public health priority, and should be considered also as a mental health priority. (2) The effects of these disasters are unevenly distributed among different countries (mainly developed vs. developing countries) as well as within countries. (3) The change in magnitude of some disasters and the occurrence of new kinds of disasters, such as nuclear accidents, raise new problems regarding their psychological short- and long-term consequences. These new problems require investigation.

Epidemiology of PTSD and Other Psychological Disorders Following a Natural Disaster

As stated by Perry and Lindell (1978) and by the UNDRO (1986), different views have been expressed by various authors about the extent of psychological disorders following a disaster. Some hold the position that disasters represent catastrophic events producing adverse psychological reactions among most victims,

whereas others suggest that the extent of the problem has been overestimated, and that psychological problems that are due to the stressful events appear only among people with a preexisting vulnerability.

For instance, according to Frederick (1981), some 25% of people after a catastrophic event will become especially active and helpful, whereas another 25% will display some degree of psychological or behavioral disturbance, including PTSD. On the other hand, Duffy (1988) stated that a "disaster syndrome" is present in up to 75% of victims during the impact phase. Such contrasting findings can be explained in terms of differences in sampling methods, methodologies, diagnostic categories, and types of disasters under study, as well as differences in interpretations of the same data. Furthermore, since only in the last few years have operational diagnostic criteria for PTSD been defined, it is difficult to make reliable inferences as regards incidence and prevalence of this disorder from studies carried out in the past, which employed different criteria and concepts.

Some of the epidemiological research recently carried out in developed countries has found a high prevalence of psychological morbidity among people who were exposed to a natural disaster (McFarlane, 1987; Maj *et al.*, 1989; Shore, Tatum, & Vollmer, 1986). However, the two former studies did not assess specific types of disorders, such as PTSD, but employed the General Health Questionnaire and surveyed only the existence of nonspecific minor psychological morbidity among victims. The third study, which used the Diagnostic Interview Schedule (DIS), found a substantial prevalence of PTSD. A specific study focusing on PTSD was carried out in the United States after a tornado, among 116 disaster victims; 59% of them met DSM-III criteria for PTSD (Madakasira & O'Brien, 1987).

Unfortunately, the amount of epidemiological research carried out in developing countries and focusing on psychological morbidity related to natural disasters, and in, particular, on PTSD, is extremely limited. As stated by UNDRO (1986):

> In the field of mental health, with the exception of some recent work in the United States and Australia, almost nothing is known of the incidence of psychological traumas and related disturbances following disasters.

Because of the often devastating physical impact which natural disasters have on populations living in developing countries and because of the scarcity of resources there, interventions have generally been confined to rescue and to the provision of basic medical care, with a corresponding neglect of psychological needs and related epidemiological research and intervention. This limitation seems particularly significant in light of the fact that, as mentioned above, the largest numbers of affected populations are from developing countries. Furthermore, as mentioned above, the existence of some clear disaster subcultures among populations with lengthy experience in coping with natural disasters, especially in developing countries, makes it difficult to apply findings from research carried out among populations only exceptionally affected by a disaster: The different culture patterns, social structures, and coping behaviors may reasonably modify the incidence, the severity, and the outcome of a disorder such as PTSD (Boehnlein, 1987; Wilson, 1989). Among the limited research conducted in developing countries, there was one study carried out on the occasion of the Armero eruption and one after the Ecuador earthquake; in both, the administration of a screening questionnaire (the Self-Report Questionnaire) to primary care facility attenders showed a high rate of people in emotional distress (Lima, Pai, Santacruz, & Lozano, 1987; Lima, Chavez, et al., 1989). Again, the methodology of these studies, which assessed only the existence of psychological distress among samples of the affected populations attending health services, does not allow any conclusion regarding the prevalence of PTSD among general victim populations.

The type of diagnostic categories used to determine the presence of psychological disorders among populations or groups affected by a disaster can also deeply influence the rate of disorders found. For example, using a broader definition of PTSD, the percentage of people found to be suffering from psychological disorders because of a major natural disaster increased substantially (Shore, Vollmer, & Tatum, 1989). The importance of "victim variables," such as personal vulnerability, prior psychopathological status, presence of social support, and the like, and of "disaster variables," such as severity, duration, scope of impact, and the like, also need to be clarified (Breslau & Davis, 1987; Lindy, Green, & Grace, 1987; Silverman, 1986; Ursano, 1987).

One of the most in-depth investigations into mental health problems and intervention needs related to the occurrence of a major natural disaster is represented by the study carried out by Ross and Quarantelli (1976) on the occasion of the Xenia tornado, which occurred in Ohio in 1973. Their conclusions were the following:

1. A significant proportion of the population affected exhibited mental health needs related to general psychological distress following the tornado; however, the authors did not assess specifically the prevalence of PTSD among disaster victims.

2. The actual demand for mental health services seemed to be clearly below the existing needs, with the effect that the existing and the emergent mental health systems failed to reach all those who had mental health problems as a consequence of the disaster.

3. There was no increase in the number of people showing a severe psychopathology, but rather a decrease as shown by some indicators, such as hospitalization rates and psychoactive drug prescriptions.

4. Many problems with daily living emerged, and such needs were scarcely met by the health services. The relevance of living and social problems to the mental health status of the population affected has been demonstrated in other situations (Maj et al., 1989) and has been stressed by UNDRO (1986).

Finally, it should be mentioned that two recent studies, carried out on the occasion of two large-scale man-made disasters, namely the toxic oil syndrome catastrophe which occurred in Spain in 1981 and the gas disaster which occurred in Bhopal (India) in 1985, found a substantial rate of victims who were suffering from disaster-related psychological disorders (Lopez-Ibor, Soria, Canas, & Rodriguez-Gamazo, 1985; Sethi, Shar-

ma, Trivedi, & Singh, 1987). In the latter study, among 855 attenders of primary care clinics, 22.6% were identified by the administration of a structured interview (the Present State Examination), as suffering from a definite psychiatric disorder; 35% from this group were showing some sort of adjustment reaction. However, in neither study was an assessment of specifically defined PTSD carried out.

Although the above estimates, however varying, relate to populations specifically affected by a disaster, very few epidemiological estimates exist regarding the overall prevalence of PTSD (due to any cause) in the general population. One of the few studies in which this problem has been investigated is the ECA survey, where a lifetime PTSD rate of 0.5% among men and 1.3% among women was found; however, the number of those who experienced some symptoms after a trauma was substantially higher (15% among men and 16% among women), with an average of 2.4 symptoms (Helzer, Robins, & McEvoy, 1987). In half of those with symptoms, the symptoms lasted less than 6 months. These findings, however, have been criticized from a methodological point of view (Haber-Schaim, Solomon, Bleich, & Kottler, 1988; Keane & Penk, 1988). In a study carried out in two rural American communities, a PTSD lifetime rate of approximately 3% for both men and women was found (Shore et al., 1989).

To summarize, it can be safely said that a substantial proportion of the people affected by a natural (or man-made) disaster will show some degree of psychological distress; however, only a small minority of the people affected will feel incapacitated or panicky, with the majority soon assuming an active role, seeking safety, organizing rescue activities, and taking care of the most cogent needs, as emphasized by UNDRO (1986) and by other authors active in the field (Lechat, 1984). Little is known about the prevalence of true PTSD among victims of a natural disaster, and even less is known as regards the magnitude of the problem among populations from developing countries, who are more frequently and severely affected. Very limited information is also available as regards the number of people suffering from PTSD as a consequence of their exposition to *several* disasters, which is not an uncommon situation in developing countries.

Prevention and Treatment of PTSD Consequent to Natural Disasters

In the field of emergencies related to the occurrence of disasters, the role of WHO has gradually shifted from relief to disaster preparedness and response, including involvement in training, in assessment of health situations and needs, and in coordination of large-scale disaster operations. WHO's target for the Eighth General Programme of Work, covering the years 1990–1995, is that by 1995, "70% of all countries will have developed master plans appropriate to their particular circumstances to deal with the health aspects of emergency and disaster situations" (WHO, 1987). These master plans should include a mental health component because, as previously shown, in some countries disasters, because of their frequency and severity, represent a mental health priority (Lima, Pai, Santacruz, Lozano, Chavez, & Samaniego, 1989; WHO, 1992b).

In general, the key activities for coping with disasters and disaster risks are essentially *preparedness*, which involves all actions designed to minimize loss of life and damage, and to organize and facilitate timely and effective rescue, relief, and rehabilitation in case of disaster; *prevention*, which may be described as measures designed to prevent phenomena from causing or resulting in disasters or other related emergency situations; and finally *mitigation*, which means reducing the actual or probable effects of an extreme hazard on the people and their environment once it has occurred. The importance of preventive measures and preparedness, the integration of emergency response within regular WHO programs, and the linkage with development have been emphasized in the resolutions adopted by WHO in 1981 and 1985 (WHO, 1988, 1989a,b,c,e,f).

The importance of preventive measures for reducing the number and severity of natural (and man-made) disasters is self-evident; but such measures also play an essential role in preventing and minimizing the psychological consequences of disasters, especially the occurrence of PTSD.

From the psychological point of view, the primary prevention of disasters must deal with a common psychological reaction to be found among populations exposed to a threat (i.e., denial) (Kinston & Rosser, 1974). The negation of an imminent threat can make forewarning useless and can expose populations to risks otherwise avoidable by producing a delay in the adoption of essential preparedness measures. Health workers, therefore, may have an important role in definitely alerting the public and thus making timely and effective prevention possible.

In terms of intervention programs aimed at preventing and treating psychological stress-related disorders, as seen before, the main needs following natural disasters exist in developing countries and among socioeconomically deprived individuals. Because in developing countries the resources devoted to mental health are often inadequate to meet even the routine needs, the primary health care system is the first and often the only health network available in case of a disaster. Moreover, for socioeconomically deprived individuals, primary care is the only means of extending effective health and mental health services. There are other considerations which underscore the importance of integrating mental health services within the framework of the existing health system, and especially the primary-care system:

1. Many potential users do *not* come to a facility which is openly labeled as a mental health service, because they do not see themselves as people needing specialized help but consider themselves only as victims of extreme adversity. Moreover, the majority of people in developing countries tend to express psychological distress in somatic terms (Goldberg & Bridges, 1988), and, therefore, the primary health care worker represents the crucial locus for the intervention.

2. It is well known that the large majority of cases of psychological distress among attenders of health centers

go unrecognized, do not receive proper care, and represent an important burden for the health services. Better and prompt recognition and management of these disorders, including PTSD, can improve their outcome and reduce the burden on the health services.

3. The primary health care network, thanks to its central position in the community, can guarantee proper follow-up of victims and their families for as long as they need.

Therefore, the training of primary health care workers to give appropriate treatment to people attending health centers and showing emotional distress due to a very stressful event deserves maximum priority (Lima, 1986). Such training represents one of the main preparedness activities. The training of health workers should include knowledge of disaster behavior and of psychological reactions to disasters; basic knowledge of stress-related disorders to be found among populations affected by a disaster; understanding and knowledge of how to deal with the main psychosocial needs of affected populations; and dissemination of simple and effective skills to be used for the recognition and treatment of psychologically distressed victims (interviewing skills, counseling, brief and simple psychotherapeutic methods, targeted pharmacotherapy, group therapy, and the like).

The training of health workers in mental health seems to be effective and long-lasting. In the context of a WHO collaborative study in six developing countries, general health workers were assessed 18 months after their training which was aimed at improving their knowledge, attitudes, skills, and capacity of management in mental health care. It was shown that the improvement was still visible and was of equal magnitude in all countries (Ignacio *et al.*, 1989).

In this framework, the role of the specialized mental health team should essentially be one of supervision and training, and only especially difficult cases should be referred for direct treatment. Specific tasks of mental health teams intervening for disaster victims in various developed countries have been described in detail by Cohen (1982).

Attention should also be paid to the mental health needs of the caregivers themselves, who are faced with heavy demands during disasters and who are themselves exposed to a substantial risk of stress-related disorders.

As for service planning, it must be remembered that services should be provided on the basis of the actual needs rather than on the basis of the demand: This applies both to the timing and magnitude of the interventions (Ross & Quarantelli, 1976).

A major boon for the overall field of disaster prevention, preparedness, and mitigation should come from the UN General Assembly Resolution 42/169, mentioned above, designating the 1990s as the International Decade for Natural Disaster Reduction (IDNDR) (Lechat, 1990; WHO, 1989d,g). The objective of this decade would be to reduce the loss of life, property damage and social and economic disruption caused by natural disasters, particularly in developing countries. In the context of the IDNDR, WHO will play a major technical role in the health sector, including in the specific area of mental health.

PTSD and Man-Made Violence

One of the most common sources of PTSD is man-made violence, either individual, small-group, or large-scale violence. Man-made violence can be defined as the "interhuman infliction of significant and avoidable pain and suffering" (Harding, 1981). There are a number of specific emotional patterns of reaction and adaptation among victims of man-made violence which are different from those raised by violence related to natural events. As suggested by Frederick (1981), perhaps the most remarkable difference has to do with "the means by which events are precipitated. Natural disasters occur because of something entirely beyond the control of victims," while in the case of human-induced acts of violence it is common to believe that somehow the act of violence is precipitated by the victim. This belief can result in feelings of guilt in the victim, the importance of which in the genesis of PTSD has been underscored by Sonnenberg (1988), who has suggested that in psychodynamic terms, PTSD can be described just as a disease of guilt. Identification with the aggressor is another important psychological phenomenon totally lacking among victims of natural disasters.

Among the situations characterized by the infliction of man-made violence, war stands as the most ancient and the most important in terms of the magnitude of its effects. The potential stressful significance which war and the exposure to combat can have, both for soldiers and for civilian populations, is very well known, and has been the object of a great deal of literature (Kentsmith, 1986; Weil, 1985a,b,c). Moreover, long-term psychological sequelae of war involvement, mostly in terms of PTSD related to the experience of being a prisoner of war, have also been demonstrated (de Loos, 1988; Kluznik, Speed, Van Valkenburg, & Magraw, 1986; Miller, Martin, & Spiro, 1989). Many clinical descriptions under various labels can be found in texts of military psychiatry which would now be identified as PTSD (Ettedgui & Bridges, 1985; Peebles, 1989); however, it was the Vietnam War and its aftermath which stimulated a renewed and deeper attention to the psychological problems related to war stress and war involvement, and enhanced the overall field of research and investigation into what is now known as PTSD. The most comprehensive of the studies carried out among Vietnam veterans—the Vietnam Experience study—investigated 2,490 Vietnam veterans and 1,972 non-Vietnam veterans and found a substantial percentage (15%) of ex-soldiers from the first group who suffered from combat-related PTSD at some time during or after service (Centers for Disease Control Vietnam Experience Study, 1988). Moreover, 2.2% of the Vietnam veterans were still suffering from the disorder during the month prior to the interview. The rate of psychiatric co-morbidity among the veterans suffering from PTSD was also high.

Other studies have confirmed high psychological morbidity among Vietnam veterans (Faustman & White, 1989; Kolb, 1989; Palinkas & Coben, 1987). Recently, a study which evaluated the influence of military service during the Vietnam era on the occurrence of PTSD, using a sample of over 2,000 male-male monozygotic veteran twin pairs, found a prevalence of PTSD of almost 17% in twins who served in Southeast Asia compared with 5% in co-twins who did not serve in Southeast Asia (Goldberg, True, Eisen, & Henderson, 1990).

In general, a high prevalence of posttraumatic stress disorders and general psychological morbidity has been found among soldiers exposed to combat stress situations (Solomon, Weisenberg, Schwarzwald, & Mikulincer, 1987). In terms of long-term consequences, combat stress reactions and PTSD have been found to be associated with a decline in postwar social functioning (Solomon & Mikulincer, 1987). A few studies have also tried to clarify the relationship between life events, coping responses, and PTSD (Mikulincer & Solomon, 1988; Solomon, Mikulincer, & Flum, 1988, 1989).

However, despite these studies, no generalizable epidemiological estimates exist as regards the percentage of soldiers and civilians exposed to war situations who suffer from PTSD. The lack of data is again particularly striking in the case of developing countries, which have been, over the last few decades, the main theater in the world of various forms of military and political violence (Zwi & Ugalde, 1989). Still more limited in number are the studies carried out in situations characterized by long-lasting political violence other than conventional war. In some of these studies, a high rate of PTSD among samples of victims has been found (Bell, Kee, Loughrey, Roddy, & Curran, 1988; Curran, Bell, Murray, Loughrey, Roddy, & Rocke, 1990). However, on the basis of specific investigations, some authors have suggested that the effects of widespread violence because of political reasons might not be widely damaging for the mental health of the general population (Curran, 1988); some forms of denial seem to be, in these situations, the main form of coping behavior (Cairns & Wilson, 1989).

War and political violence not only cause direct psychosocial health problems in populations, but also result in the creation of refugees (World Health Organization, 1987). The experience of being a refugee is often associated with a substantial degree of psychological suffering, notably PTSD (League of Red Cross and Crescent Society, 1988). The problem of refugees has been markedly increasing around the world over the last few years: According to official United Nations High Commissioner for Refugee Programs (UNHCR) estimates, twenty years ago the refugee population stood at just under 2.5 million; by 1980 it had risen to 8.2 million (Editorial, 1990). At the end of 1991, the number of refugees cared for by UNHCR was approaching 17 million, plus two million Palestinians assisted by the United Nations Relief and Works Agency (UNRWA). The large majority of refugees live in developing countries. Yet, despite the magnitude of the problem, we do not know much about the percentage of such refugees suffering from specific psychological disorders such as PTSD. The few existing studies have been carried out among refugees living in resettlement countries (Beiser & Fleming, 1986; Kroll et al., 1989; Mollica, Wyshak, & Lavelle, 1987), and their findings are hardly generalizable to refugees living in crowded camps, often in staggeringly poor conditions. Nor do we know about the natural history and outcome of these disorders when they are untreated, and how the cultural norms and beliefs of the refugee populations could have a moderating effect on them. WHO has been expanding its activities in the field of psychosocial and mental health needs of refugees and displaced populations, and a number of projects have been initiated for Khmer displaced populations living in border encampments on the Thai-Kampuchean border (de Girolamo, Diekstra, & Williams, 1989), for Afghan refugees and displaced populations (El Fawal, 1990), for Namibian refugees (Aboo-Baker & Chikara, 1990), and Joz Yugoslav displaced people (WHO, 1992).

Another form of violence closely related to war and political violence is torture: Its physical and psychological sequelae, essentially in terms of PTSD, have been well documented (Goldfield, Mollica, Pesavento, & Faraone, 1988). The United Nations has made many efforts to eliminate the practice of torture; the UN General Assembly, in 1981, decided to set up a Voluntary Fund for Victims of Torture, and in 1984 adopted the International Convention against Torture and Cruel, Inhuman or Degrading Treatment and Punishment (Danielus, 1986). However, despite these efforts to ban torture from the world, it remains widespread for political or ideological reasons and still stands as a significant cause of post-traumatic psychological morbidity (Basoglu & Marks, 1988; Goldfield et al., 1988).

Many other situations characterized by the infliction of violence can be at the origin of PTSD, and are to be found in civilian life; the most important are related to crime and criminal behavior. Recently, a large survey has provided important data about the magnitude of this problem, although it includes only developed countries (van Dijk, Mayhew, & Killias, 1990). An average of 2,000 people have been interviewed in each of the 14 countries surveyed. The overall victimization rate for 5 years (1983–1988) was high, accounting in many countries for more than half of the population surveyed (in the United States 57.6%, in Australia 57.2%, in Canada 53%, in France 52%, in Spain and West Germany for more than 51%). The victimization rate for all crimes in 1988 was highest in the United States (28.8%), but high rates were also found in Canada (28.1%) and in Australia (27.8%). For most types of crimes the young tended to be more at risk than the elderly, men more than women, and city dwellers more than inhabitants of rural areas or of small towns. Rates for women tended to be substantially higher (similar to those of men) in the countries where female employment levels were more equal, such in the United States. Countries with the lowest crime rates were those with a low level of urbanization. Many crimes, especially robbery, assault, and sexual offenses, were underreported to the police. Among women, sexual incidents were reported most frequently again in Australia (7.3%), in the United States (4.5%) and in Canada (4.0%); the highest rates for sexual assaults were 2.3% (United States), 1.7% (Canada), and 1.6% (Australia). The authors of the survey note that they found higher rates of crime than expected. On average, only 3.8% of people said they had received any form of help or emotional support from the police. This rate was higher in the United States (10.0%), Belgium (6.4%), Canada (5.5%), England (4.0%), and Finland (4.4%). In general, many more would have appreciated assistance than actually got it. On the whole, 35% of victims said that the services of a support agency would have been useful for them, especially for victims of sexual assaults and violence. Again, however, we do not have from this survey any reliable estimates of the incidence of PTSD among victims of crime.

The relationship of violence to various psychiatric disorders is also demonstrated by the finding that among adult psychiatric patients, a high proportion of them (often half or more) suffered sexual abuse, other physical abuse, or both when children (Lindberg & Distad, 1985; Taylor, 1988). In particular, two studies (Harter, Alexander, & Neimeyer, 1988; Mullen, Romans-Clarksons, Walton, & Herbison, 1988) have clearly demonstrated the long-term psychological sequelae of physical and sexual abuse, and especially of a direct link between abuse in childhood and adult psychological disorders. Furthermore, children who are sexually abused are at great risk of displaying a variety of antisocial behaviors, especially personal violence, later on (Poythress, 1988).

Some groups are especially vulnerable to violence, such as the elderly (Hayes & Burke, 1987), children (Jones, 1989), youths (Krisberg, 1987), and women (Mehta & Dandrea, 1988). Both some agencies of the United Nations system and national health authorities have addressed these problems, producing detailed analysis of the phenomena and recommendations for dealing effectively with them (CIOMS/WHO, 1985; United Nations, 1989; U.S. Department of Health and Human Services, 1985). And violence can be disruptive for the psychological well-being of the whole family (Solomon, 1988). Specifically, PTSD consequent to violence can influence the overall family balance through the psychological suffering shown by children and relatives of victims, which has been called "secondary victimization" (Hueting, 1981).

It should be emphasized that violence, like any other behavior, is strongly shaped by cultural norms and values. For instance, it is likely that violence against women, or within the context of the family, is more common in those societies in which women's status is low compared to that of men, or in which violence against women is more "acceptable" than against other population groups. Gender, therefore, can deeply affect the overall range of exposure to violence. Similar considerations apply to violence perpetrated against minority groups, or groups having particular racial, ethnic, religious, or ideological backgrounds. Psychological expectations and cultural assumptions also apply to violence related to alcohol abuse: The expectation of behavioral changes subsequent to drinking may have more to do with such changes, and, therefore, more impact, than the alcohol itself; and the same phenomenon of abuse in different cultures can assume very different forms (World Health Organization, Regional Office for Europe, 1989).

Prevention and Treatment of PTSD Related to Man-Made Violence

As described above, violence represents a public health priority. Therefore, interventions aimed at reducing violent behaviors can deeply affect the overall health status of a population or of a group, especially of high-risk groups. Many of the observations raised above as regards prevention and treatment of PTSD related to disasters apply also in the case of PTSD related to man-made violence (WHO, 1992b). This is particularly true with regard to the need for effective strategies of prevention and treatment of victims of man-made violence in developing countries, which are characterized by the highest rate of large-scale violence. In these countries, political conflicts, dramatic socioeconomic changes, and demographic pressures are often associated with a substantial increase in man-made violence, while resources to cope with it are generally limited. Primary health care workers represent again the frontline intervention in these countries and need to be trained in dealing with psychological problems associated with man-made violence, especially PTSD.

A crucial place for meeting the early needs of victims of violence is the emergency room, which is usually the first place where victims of violence arrive and have their first contact with health services. It is important that assessment be carried out by personnel who are acceptable to victims (in terms of language, religion, ethnicity, and sex). Adequate training in medical ethics for all health personnel is important. Also, proper training for health workers is necessary because it is well known that dealing with victims of extremely distressing experiences, such as those involved in the onset of PTSD, is a painful experience even for a skilled therapist.

Victims often need practical help in terms of financial support, jobs, and housing, and nonmedical needs should receive proper attention. Adequate financial compensation may play an important role in helping victims of violence to recover from PTSD, but it should be remembered that a high number of offenders and perpetrators of severe violent acts remain undetected, and a substantial proportion of those who are arrested are subsequently acquitted (Hamilton, 1981), thus depriving the victim of legal compensation. Finally, self-help or peer groups should be encouraged.

Although an adequate intervention for victims of violence is important, it should be borne in mind the danger of labelling all victims as ill for the possible induction of a sick role (Harding, 1981) and the "creation of a stigmatizing 'victim status'" (World Health Organization, 1986).

Specific preventive programs should address specific problems: For instance, in the field of child abuse, a family planning policy must be encouraged as a starting point for prevention, and education for parenthood should be widely promoted (World Health Organization, 1988).

Prevention can also be fostered through the training of local health personnel in refugee settlements: Here, the training of local health workers in dealing with psychosocial problems related to the condition of being a refugee must be mandatory for sociocultural reasons, and can also be an important tool in fostering autonomy and self-reliance (Simmonds, Cutts, & Dick, 1985).

Areas Needing Further Research

Many issues remain to be tackled by researchers and clinicians and have been the object of detailed proposals (Boehnlein, 1989). The following issues seem to deserve priority and need international collaboration:

1. Much of the research into PTSD has been done with men and among Western populations; this is reflected in the very limited number of contributions on this topic from authors from non-English-speaking countries (Mendelson, 1987). It is therefore imperative to carry out extensive research with populations from developing countries, which are most affected by natural and man-made disasters of large and small scale. This research will allow the study of cross-cultural variations in frequency, symptomatology, temporal patterns, and outcome of PTSD and related disorders and will clarify the moderating effect of culture on this disorder. WHO multicentric studies, which have found significant variations between developed and developing countries in the course and outcome of a severe mental disorder such as schizophrenia (World Health Organization, 1979; Sartorius et al., 1986), clearly show the importance of the setting in shaping the course and the outcome of a psychiatric disorder. This research, to be practically and ethically feasible, needs to follow strict guidelines (Lima, Pai, et al., 1989; McFarlane, Wallace, & Cook, 1985).

2. Although there is agreement that social support and intense kin relationships are highly supportive and facilitate postdisaster recovery among victims (Cormie & Howell, 1988; Perry & Lindell, 1978; UNDRO, 1986), little empirical evidence is available in this regard. However, in some studies lack of social support was not associated with a greater psychological impairment (McFarlane, 1988). Therefore, the specific role of these variables in modifying the overall frequency, severity, and course of PTSD needs to be further explored, as do the importance of personal vulnerability and prior psychopathology in the occurrence of PTSD.

3. Investigations into physiological determinants and correlates of PTSD, so far primarily laboratory-based, should be strengthened, and should be mainly clinically based. Moreover, it is important to find some reliable, valid, and feasible physiological measures of stress to be used as diagnostic tools. For instance, in a recent study saliva cortisol appeared to be the best psychophysiological measure of stress (Rahe, Karson, Howard, Rubin, & Poland, 1990).

4. It has been argued that many of the defense styles related to PTSD can be interpreted as defense against trauma-related imagery (Brett & Ostroff, 1985). Therefore, the role of certain primary symptoms, such as imagery and sleep disorders, in the overall determinism of PTSD should be further explored. Diagnostic specificity of PTSD symptoms also needs to be further explored, as does the natural history of the disorder (Green, Lindy, & Grace, 1985).

5. An important area for research is co-morbidity, which has been frequently found in persons suffering from PTSD: For instance, substance abuse, frequently associated with PTSD, has been interpreted as a long-term attempt to numb oneself against intrusive images and nightmares, thus representing a secondary response to primary PTSD symptoms (Green et al., 1985).

6. The experience of facing a trauma as an individual versus the effect of trauma when experienced with others needs to be investigated.

7. Finally, treatment of PTSD is an important area in need of research. As regards pharmacotherapy, at the moment no effective drug treatment is available for PTSD, and only temporary symptom relief can be provided (Davidson & Nemeroff, 1989; Friedman, 1988). Some interesting brief psychotherapeutic methods have been suggested (Horowitz, 1986); these deserve detailed consideration and need to be adequately tested and verified for cross-cultural applicability as well as for general effectiveness.

ACKNOWLEDGMENTS

Many thanks are due to Drs. N. Sartorius and J. Orley for their helpful comments. J. Halpern contributed her invaluable editorial assistance and suggestions during the preparation of the manuscript for this chapter.

References

Aboo-Baker, F., & Chikara, F. (1990). *Report of a mission on mental health services in Namibia*. Geneva: World Health Organization.

Agency for International Development. (1989). Disaster history: Significant data on major disasters worldwide, 1900-present. Washington, DC: Office of U.S. Foreign Disaster Assistance, Agency for International Development.

Alexandrowsky, Y. A. (1989). Psychoneurotic disorders associated with the Chernobyl accident. In *Medical aspects of the Chernobyl accident* (pp. 283–902). Vienna: International Atomic Energy Agency.

American College of Emergency Medicine. (1976). The role of the emergency physician in mass casualty/disaster management. *JACEP, 5,* 901–902.

Barton, A. (1969). *Communities in disasters*. New York: Basic Books.

Basoglu, M., & Marks, I. (1988). Torture. *British Medical Journal, 297,* 1423–1424.

Baum, A., Gatchel, R. J. & Schaeffer, M. A. (1983). Emotional, behavioral and physiological effects of chronic stress at Three Mile Island. *Journal of Consulting and Clinical Psychology, 51,* 565–572.

Beinin, L. (1985). *Medical consequences of disasters*. Berlin: Springer.

Beiser, M., & Fleming, J. A. E. (1986). Measuring psychiatric disorder among Southeast Asian refugees. *Psychological Medicine, 16,* 627–639.

Bell, P., Kee, M., Loughrey, G. C., Roddy, R. J., & Curran, P. S. (1988). Posttraumatic stress in Northern Ireland. *Acta Psychiatrica Scandinavica, 77,* 166–169.

Berz, G. (1989). List of major natural disasters, 1960–1987. *Earthquakes & Volcanoes, 20,* 226–228.

Boehnlein, J. K. (1987). Culture and society in posttraumatic stress disorder: Implications for psychotherapy. *American Journal of Psychotherapy, 41,* 519–530.

Boehnlein, J. K. (1989). The process of research in posttraumatic stress disorder. *Perspectives in Biology and Medicine, 32,* 455–465.

Breslau, N., & Davis, G. C. (1987). Posttraumatic stress disorder: The stressor criterion. *Journal of Nervous and Mental Disease, 175,* 255–265.

Brett, E. A., & Ostroff, R. (1985). Imagery and posttraumatic stress disorder: An overview. *American Journal of Psychiatry, 142,* 417–424.

Cairns, E., & Wilson, R. (1989). Coping with political violence in Northern Ireland. *Social Science and Medicine, 28,* 621–624.

Centers for Disease Control Vietnam Experience Study. (1988). Health status of Vietnam veterans: I. Psychosocial characteristics. *Journal of the American Medical Association, 259*(18), 2701–2707.

Council for International Organizations of Medical Sciences/World Health Organization. (1985). *Battered children and child abuse*. Geneva: Author.

Cohen, R. E. (1982). Intervening with disaster victims. In M. Killilea & H. C. Schulberg (Eds.), *The modern practice of community mental health*. San Francisco: Jossey-Bass.

Cormie, K., & Howell, J. M. (1988). A mental health component in the public health response to disasters. *Canadian Journal of Public Health, 79,* 97–100.

Curran, P. S. (1988). Psychiatric aspects of terrorist violence: Northern Ireland 1969–1987. *British Journal of Psychiatry, 153,* 470–475.

Curran, P. S., Bell, P., Murray, A., Loughrey, G. C., Roddy, R. J., & Rocke, L. G. (1990). Psychological consequences of the Enniskillen bombing. *British Journal of Psychiatry, 156,* 479–482.

Danielus, H. (1986). The United Nations Fund for Torture Victims: The first years of activity. *Human Rights Quarterly, 8,* 294–305.

Davidson, J. R. T., & Nemeroff, C. B. (1989). Pharmacotherapy in posttraumatic stress disorder: Historical and clinical considerations and future directions. *Psychopharmacology Bulletin, 25,* 422–425.

de Girolamo, G. (1991). Psychosocial aspects of nuclear accidents: The role of the World Health Organization. *Disaster Management, 3,* 149–154.

de Girolamo, G., Diekstra, R., & Williams, C. (1989). *Report of a visit to border encampments on the Kampuchea-Thailand border* (MNH/PSF/90.1.). Geneva: World Health Organization.

de Loos, W. S. (1988). *Psychosomatic approach to war stress survivors and late somatic sequelae*. Paper presented to the First European Conference on Traumatic Stress Research, Lincoln, England.

Dew, M. A., Bromet, E. J., Schulberg, H. C., Dunn, L. O., & Parkinson, D. K. (1987). Mental health effects of the Three Mile Island nuclear reactor restart. *American Journal of Psychiatry, 144,* 1074–1077.

Duffy, J. C. (1988). Common psychological themes in societies' reaction to terrorism and disasters. *Military Medicine, 153,* 387–390.

Editorial. (1990). *Refugees, 73,* 5.

El Fawal, K. (1990). *Mental health programme for Afghanistan and for Afghan refugees in Pakistan*. Report of a mission. Geneva: World Health Organization.

Ettedgui, E., & Bridges, M. (1985). Posttraumatic stress disorder. *Psychiatric Clinics of North America, 8,* 89–103.

Faustman, W. O., & White, P. A. (1989). Diagnostic and psychopharmacological treatment characteristics of 536 inpatients with posttraumatic stress disorder. *Journal of Nervous and Mental Disease, 177,* 154–159.

Figley, C. R. (1988). Toward a field of traumatic stress. *Journal of Traumatic Stress, 1,* 3–16.

Frederick, C. J. (1981). Violence and disasters: Immediate and long-term consequences. In *Helping victims of violence* (pp. 32–46). Proceedings of a WHO Working Group on the Psychosocial Consequences of Violence, The Hague.

Friedman, M. J. (1988). Toward rational pharmacotherapy for posttraumatic stress disorder: An interim report. *American Journal of Psychiatry, 145,* 281–285.

Goldberg, D., & Bridges, K. (1988). Somatic presentation of psychiatric illness in primary care settings. *Journal of Psychosomatic Research, 32,* 137–144.

Goldberg, J., True, W. R., Eisen, S. A., & Henderson, W. G. (1990). A twin study of the effects of the Vietnam war on posttraumatic stress disorder. *Journal of the American Medical Association, 263,* 1227–1232.

Goldfield, A. E., Mollica, R. F., Pesavento, B. H., & Faraone, S. V. (1988). The physical and psychological sequelae of torture: Symptomatology and diagnosis. *Journal of the American Medical Association, 259,* 2725–2729.

Green, B. L., Lindy, J. D., & Grace, M. C. (1985). Posttraumatic stress disorder: Toward DSM-IV. *Journal of Nervous and Mental Disease, 173,* 406–411.

Haber-Schaim, N., Solomon, Z., Bleich, A., & Kottler, M. (1988). Letter to the Editor. *New England Journal of Medicine, 318,* 1691.

Hamilton, J. R. (1981). Identification of high risk groups. In *Helping victims of violence* (pp. 116–129). Proceedings of a WHO Working Group on the Psychosocial Consequences of Violence, The Hague.

Harding, T. (1981). Summary and recommendations. In *Helping victims of violence* (pp. 160–170). Proceedings of a WHO Working Group on the Psychosocial Consequences of Violence, The Hague.

Harter, S., Alexander, P. C., & Neimeyer, R. A. (1988). Long-term effects of incestuous child abuse in college women: Social adjustment, social cognition, and family characteristics. *Journal of Consulting and Clinical Psychology, 56,* 5–8.

Hayes, R. L., & Burke, M. J. (1987). Community-based prevention for elderly victims of crime and violence. *Journal of Mental Health Counseling, 9,* 210–219.

Helsinki Institute for Crime Prevention and Control. (1989). *Changing victims policy: The United Nations Victim Declaration and recent developments in Europe.* Report on the meeting of an ad hoc Expert Group Meeting, Helsinki, November, 1988, 17–20.

Helzer, J. E., Robins, L. N., & McEvoy, L. (1987). Posttraumatic stress disorder in the general population: Findings of the Epidemiological Catchment Area Survey. *New England Journal of Medicine, 317,* 1630–1634.

Horowitz, M. J. (1986). Stress-response syndromes: A review of posttraumatic and adjustment disorders. *Hospital and Community Psychiatry, 37,* 241–249.

Hueting, J. (1981). Psychosocial mechanisms of short-term and long-term reactions to violence. In *Helping victims of violence* (pp. 13–19). Proceedings of a WHO Working Group on the Psychosocial Consequences of Violence, The Hague.

Ignacio, L. L., De Arango, M. V., Baltazar, J., D'Arrigo Busnello, E., Climent, C. E., Elkahim, A., Giel, R., Harding, T. W., Ten Horn, G. H. M. M., Ibrahim, H. H. A., Srinivasa Murthy, R., & Wig, N. N. (1989). Knowledge and attitudes of primary health care personnel concerning mental health problems in developing countries: A follow-up study. *International Journal of Epidemiology, 18,* 669–673.

Jones, D. P. H. (1989). Child abuse. *Current Opinion in Psychiatry, 2,* 497–503.

Keane, T. M., & Penk, W. E. (1988). Letter to the Editor. *New England Journal of Medicine, 318,* 1690–1691.

Kentsmith, D. K. (1986). Principles of battlefield psychiatry. *Military Medicine, 151*(2), 89–96.

Kinston, W., & Rosser, R. (1974). Disaster: Effects on mental and physical state. *Journal of Psychosomatic Research, 18,* 437–456.

Kluznik, J. C., Speed, N., Van Valkenburg, C., & Magraw, R. (1986). Forty-year follow-up of United States prisoners of war. *American Journal of Psychiatry, 143,* 1443–1446.

Kolb, L. C. (1989). Chronic posttraumatic stress disorder: Implications of recent epidemiological and neuropsychological studies. *Psychological Medicine, 19,* 821–824.

Korver, A. J. H. (1987). What is a disaster? *Prehospital and Disaster Medicine, 2,* 152–153.

Krisberg, B. (1987). Preventing and controlling violent youth crime: The state of the art. In *Violent juvenile crime: What do we know about it and what can we do about it?* University of Minnesota: Center for the Study of Youth Policy.

Kroll, J., Habenicht, M., Mackenzie, T., Yang, M., Chan, S., Nguyen, T., Ly, M., Phommasouvanh, B., Nguyen, H., Vang, Y., Souvannasoth, L., & Cabugao, R. (1989). Depression and posttraumatic stress disorders in Southeast Asian refugees. *American Journal of Psychiatry, 146,* 1592–1597.

League of the Red Cross and Crescent Society. (1988). *Refugees: The trauma of exile.* Geneva: Author.

Lechat, M. (1990). The public health dimensions of disasters. *International Journal of Mental Health, 19,* 70–79.

Lechat, M. F. (1979). Disasters and public health. *Bulletin of the World Health Organization, 57*(1), 11–17.

Lechat, M. F. (1984). Natural and man-made disasters. In W. W. Holland & G. Knox (Eds.), *Oxford textbook of public health* (pp. 119–132). Oxford: Oxford University Press.

Lima, B. R. (1986). Primary mental health care for disaster victims in developing countries. *Disasters, 10,* 203–204.

Lima, B. R., Chavez, H., Samaniego, N., Pompei, M. S., Pai, S., Santacruz, H., & Lozano, J. (1989). Disaster severity and emotional disturbance: Implications for primary mental health care in developing countries. *Acta Psychiatrica Scandinavica, 79,* 74–82.

Lima, B. R., Pai, S., Santacruz, H., & Lozano, J. (1987). Screening for psychological consequences of a major disaster in a developing country: Armero, Colombia. *Acta Psychiatrica Scandinavica, 76,* 561–567.

Lima, B. R., Pai, S., Santacruz, H., Lozano, J., Chavez, H., & Samaniego, N. (1989). Conducting research on disaster mental health in developing countries: A proposed model. *Disasters, 13,* 177–184.

Lindberg, F. H., & Distad, L. J. (1985). Posttraumatic stress disorders in women who experienced childhood incest. *Child Abuse and Neglect, 9,* 329–334.

Lindy, J. D., Green, B. L., & Grace, M. C. (1987). The stressor criterion and posttraumatic stress disorder. *Journal of Nervous and Mental Disease, 175,* 269–272.

Lopez-Ibor, J. J., Soria, J., Canas, F., & Rodriguez-Gamazo, M. (1985). Psychopathological aspects of the toxic oil syndrome catastrophe. *British Journal of Psychiatry, 147,* 352–365.

Madakasira, S., & O'Brien, K. F. (1987). Acute posttraumatic stress disorder in victims of a natural disaster. *Journal of Nervous and Mental Disease, 175*(5), 286–290.

Maj, M., Starace, F., Crepet, P., Lobrace, S., Veltro, F., De Marco, F., & Kemali, D. (1989). Prevalence of psychiatric disorders among subjects exposed to natural disaster. *Acta Psychiatrica Scandinavica, 79,* 544–549.

Manni, C., & Magalini, S. (1989). Disaster medicine: A new discipline or a new approach? *Prehospital and Disaster Medicine, 4,* 167–170.

McFarlane, A. C. (1987). Life events and psychiatric disorder:

The role of a natural disaster. *British Journal of Psychiatry, 151,* 362–367.

McFarlane, A. C. (1988). The aetiology of posttraumatic stress disorders following a natural disaster. *British Journal of Psychiatry, 152,* 116–121.

McFarlane, A. C., Wallace, M., & Cook, P. (1985). Australian research into the psychological aspects of disasters. *Disasters, 9,* 32–34.

Mehta, P., & Dandrea, L. A. (1988). The battered woman. *American Family Physician, 37,* 193–199.

Mendelson, G. (1987). The concept of posttraumatic stress disorder: A review. *International Journal of Law and Psychiatry, 10,* 45–62.

Mikulincer, M., & Solomon, Z. (1988). Attributional style and combat-related posttraumatic stress disorder. *Journal of Abnormal Psychology, 97*(3), 308–313.

Miller, T. W., Martin, W., & Spiro, K. (1989). Traumatic stress disorder: Diagnostic and clinical issues in former prisoners of war. *Comprehensive Psychiatry, 30*(2), 139–148.

Mollica, R. F., Wyshak, G., & Lavelle, J. (1987). The psychosocial impact of war trauma and torture on Southeast Asian refugees. *American Journal of Psychiatry, 144,* 1567–1572.

Mullen, P. E., Romans-Clarsons, S. E., Walton, V. A., & Herbison, G. P. (1988). Impact of sexual and physical abuse on women's mental health. *Lancet, 1,* 842–845.

Palinkas, L. A., & Coben, P. (1987). Psychiatric disorders among United States Marines wounded in action in Vietnam. *Journal of Nervous and Mental Disease, 175*(5), 291–296.

Peebles, M. J. (1989). Posttraumatic stress disorder: A historical perspective on diagnosis and treatment. *Bulletin of the Menninger Clinic, 53,* 274–286.

Perry, R. W., & Lindell, M. K. (1978). The psychological consequences of natural disaster: A review of research on American communities. *Mass Emergencies, 3,* 105–115.

Poumadere, M. (1990). The credibility crisis. In B. Segerstahl & G. Kromer (Eds.), *Chernobyl and Europe: A policy response study.* Berlin: Springer.

Poythress, N. (1988). Violence and dangerousness. *Current Opinion in Psychiatry, 1,* 682–687.

Quarantelli, E. L. (1980, November). *Sociology and social pathology of disasters: Implications for Third World and developing countries.* Disaster Research Center, Ohio State University. Paper presented at the 9th World Civil Defense Conference in Rabat, Morocco.

Rahe, R. H., Karson, S., Howard, N. S., Rubin, R. T., & Poland, R. E. (1990). Psychological and physiological assessments on American hostages freed from captivity in Iran. *Psychosomatic Medicine, 52,* 1–16.

Ross, G. A., & Quarantelli, E. L. (1976). *Delivery of mental health services in disasters: The Xenia tornado and some implications.* Ohio State University: The Disaster Research Center Book and Monograph Series.

Sartorius, N., Jablensky, A., Korten, A., Ernberg, G., Anker, M., Cooper, J. E., & Day, R. (1986). Early manifestations and first-contact incidence of schizophrenia in different cultures. *Psychological Medicine, 16,* 909–928.

Sethi, B. B., Sharma, M., Trivedi, J. K., & Singh, H. (1987). Psychiatric morbidity in patients attending clinics in gas affected areas in Bhopal. *Indian Journal of Medical Research, 86*(Suppl.), 45–50.

Shore, J. H., Tatum, E. L., & Vollmer, W. M. (1986). Psychiatric reactions to disaster: The Mount St. Helens experience. *American Journal of Psychiatry, 143,* 590–595.

Shore, J. H., Vollmer, W. M., & Tatum, E. L. (1989). Community patterns of posttraumatic stress disorders. *Journal of Nervous and Mental Disease, 177,* 681–685.

Schottenfeld, R. S., & Cullen, M. R. (1986). Recognition of occupation-induced posttraumatic stress disorders. *Journal of Occupational Medicine, 28,* 365–369.

Silverman, J. J. (1986). Posttraumatic stress disorder. *Advances in Psychosomatic Medicine, 16,* 115–140.

Simmonds, S., Cutts, F., & Dick, B. (1985). Training refugees as primary health care workers: Past imperfect, future conditional. *Disasters, 9,* 61–68.

Solomon, Z. (1988). The effect of combat-related posttraumatic stress disorder on the family. *Psychiatry, 51,* 323–329.

Solomon, Z., & Mikulincer, M. (1987). Combat stress reactions, posttraumatic stress disorder, and social adjustment. *Journal of Nervous and Mental Disease, 175,* 277–285.

Solomon, Z., Mikulincer, M., & Flum, H. (1988). Negative life events, coping responses, and combat-related psychopathology: A prospective study. *Journal of Abnormal Psychology, 97,* 302–307.

Solomon, Z., Mikulincer, M., & Flum, H. (1989). The implications of life events and social integration in the course of combat-related posttraumatic stress disorder. *Social Psychiatry, 24,* 41–48.

Solomon, Z., Weisenberg, M., Schwarzwald, J., & Mikulincer, M. (1987). Posttraumatic stress disorder among frontline soldiers with combat stress reaction: The 1982 Israeli experience. *American Journal of Psychiatry, 144,* 448–454.

Sonnenberg, S. M. (1988). Victims of violence and posttraumatic stress disorder. *Psychiatric Clinics of North America, 11,* 581–590.

Sparr, L. F. (1989). Victims and survivors. *Current Opinion in Psychiatry, 2,* 757–763.

Taylor, A. J. (1987). A taxonomy of disasters and their victims. *Journal of Psychosomatic Research, 31,* 535–544.

Taylor, P. J. (1988). Victims and survivors. *Current Opinion in Psychiatry, 1,* 675–681.

United Nations. (1989). *Violence against women in the family.* New York: Author.

United Nations Disaster Relief Co-ordinator (UNDRO). (1986). *Disaster prevention and mitigation: Vols. 11 & 12. Preparedness and social aspects.* New York: United Nations.

Ursano, R. J. (1987). Posttraumatic stress disorder: The stressor criterion. *Journal of Nervous and Mental Disease, 175,* 273–275.

U.S. Department of Health and Human Services. (1985). *Surgeon general's workshop on violence and public health, report.* Leesburg, VA: U.S. Department of Health and Human Services.

van Dijk, J. J. M., Mayheew, P., & Killias, M. (1990). *Experiences of crime across the world.* Amsterdam: Unpublished report from the 1989 International Crime Survey.

Weil, F. (1985a). Treatment teams under war stress. *Psychiatric Journal of the University of Ottawa, 10*(1), 45–47.

Weil, F. (1985b). Soldiers under war stress. *Psychiatric Journal of the University of Ottawa, 10*(1), 48–52.

Weil, F. (1985c). Civilians under war stress. *Psychiatric Journal of the University of Ottawa, 10*(1), 53–55.

Wilson, J. P. (1989). *Trauma, transformation, and healing.* New York: Brunner/Mazel.

World Health Organization. (1979). *Schizophrenia: An international follow-up study.* Chichester: Wiley.

World Health Organization. (1986). *The health hazards of organized violence.* Report on a WHO meeting, Veldhoven, April 22–25 1986. Geneva: Author.

World Health Organization. (1987). *Eighth General Programme of Work, covering the period 1990–1995.* Geneva: Author.

World Health Organization. (1988). *Prevention of mental, neurological and psychosocial disorders* (WHO/MNH/EVA/88.1.). Geneva: Author.

World Health Organization. (1989a). *Emergency preparedness and response: Annual report 1988* (PCO/EPR/89.3). Geneva: Author.

World Health Organization. (1989b). *Emergency preparedness and response: Programme 1989–1991* (PCO/EPR/89.5). Geneva: Author.

World Health Organization. (1989c). *Emergency preparedness and response: Consultative meetings for programme development 1986–1989* (PCO/EPR/89.7). Geneva: Author.

World Health Organization. (1989d). *International decade for natural disaster reduction 1990–2000 (IDNDR)* (PCO/EPR/89.1). Geneva: Author.

World Health Organization. (1989e). *Report of the second interregional meeting on health emergency preparedness and response, Alexandria, June 11–13, 1989* (ERO/EPR/89.11). Geneva: Author.

World Health Organization. (1989f). *WHO action in emergencies and disasters: WHO Manual revision* (PCO/EPR/89.6). Geneva: Author.

World Health Organization. (1989g). *Resolution on the international decade for natural disaster reduction* (A/44/832/Add.1). Geneva: Author.

World Health Organization. (1992a). *The ICD-10 Classification of Mental and Behavioral Disorders: Clinical descriptions and diagnostic guidelines.* Geneva: Author.

World Health Organization. (1992b). *Psychosocial consequences of disasters: Prevention and management* (WHO/MNH/PSF/91.3). Geneva: Author.

World Health Organization. (1992c). *United Nations programme of humanitarian assistance in Yugoslavia: WHO mission on the mental health needs of refugees, displaced persons and others affected by the conflict.* (MNH 92.1, MNH 92.4). Geneva: Author.

World Health Organization Regional Office for Europe. (1989). *Different forms of social violence, with special reference to the influence of alcohol and other drugs.* Report on a WHO consultation, Leuven, September 25–28, 1988 (EUR/ICP/ADA/018). Copenhagen: Author.

Zwi, A., & Ugalde, A. (1989). Toward an epidemiology of political violence in the Third World. *Social Science and Medicine, 28,* 633–642.

CHAPTER 80

Mental Health Policy for Victims of Violence

The Case against Women

Susan E. Salasin and Robert F. Rich

Introduction

Public policy-making, as it is reflected in legislation and laws, represents a reactive process, a formalization with the force of law, of the values, norms, attitudes, and beliefs of society which are prevalent at a given period of time. The women's movement has focused our attention on this process. Discrimination against women in many areas of their social functioning has existed and we feel that it is now time to examine how this bias operates against women who are victims of crime and violence. The aftermath of such experiences often leads to the development of traumatic stress syndromes.

Although there is a substantial gap between the emotional and psychological needs of victims of crime and violence and the public policies which have been designed and implemented for crime victims at all levels of government in the United States, evidence will be provided and reasons advanced that this gap is a "yawning" gap when it comes to females. Indeed, it will be demonstrated that a woman who is a crime victim is a victim of "double jeopardy": in jeopardy first from the "social envelope" of shame and social isolation engendered by her community of support; and in jeopardy second from the "policy envelope" of "woman as provocateur," "woman as property," and "woman as liar"

roles that the system assigns to her. The following questions will serve as the focus of this chapter:

1. What are the emotional and psychological needs of victims of crime, and of women in particular?
2. What public policies have been designed and implemented to respond to the needs of these victims?
3. What is the gap between needs and programs that are available to respond to these needs?
4. What kinds of policies should we expect government to develop to be responsive; in particular, what is the role of government in responding to the emotional and psychological needs of women?

"Victims of crime and violence" is the topic of this chapter; therefore, we will organize our discussion around a definition which includes individuals who have been subject to a sudden, unanticipated (even though it may have been feared) assault on their person (physical and emotional), for which they have no ready recourse. As Bard and Sangrey (1979) have pointed out, the severity of this assault is proportional to the degree it is experienced as an assault on the "self." On a spectrum, burglary is a lesser assault, while rape constitutes the ultimate violation of the self.

Violence as a Stressor: Different Gender Responses

The evolution of the women's movement has brought us to a point in time where we can spotlight and systematically examine the "case" against women who are victims of crime and violence. Knowledge about what happens in the aftermath of personal violence has been derived from a body of research and clinical reports

Susan E. Salasin • Center for Mental Health Services, Department of Health and Human Services, 5600 Fishers Lane, Rockville, Maryland 20857. Robert F. Rich • Institute of Government and Public Affairs, University of Illinois, Urbana, Illinois 61801. The views presented here only reflect those of the authors and not their institutions of employment.

International Handbook of Traumatic Stress Syndromes, edited by John P. Wilson and Beverley Raphael. Plenum Press, New York, 1993.

gathered over the past 10 to 15 years. In the earlier phases of this initiative, these findings were produced in a "gender-blind" manner, and it was assumed that what was being learned was equally true for men and women.

Feminists started the focus on women as victims by asking: Who gets victimized? By whom? In what manner? Whose interests are served by these victimization patterns? Why are women stigmatized as having "caused it," and men absolved of responsibility? This feminist perspective was dramatically illustrated some time ago in Israel. The Israeli Parliament, alarmed by the rapidly rising rate of rape, voted to place a curfew on women to keep them in their homes from early evening until early morning. The rationale was that most of the rapes occurred during that time period. Prime Minister Golda Meir was so outraged at this that she proposed that the curfew be placed on men, since they were the ones doing the raping! (Bart & O'Brien, 1985).

This questioning by the feminist movement, with its forceful emphasis on the destructive and destabilizing impacts of crimes such as rape and domestic violence, brought a new focus on gender and impact. Many research and data-gathering efforts were mounted to examine women's responses to crimes of personal violence, or to compare sex differences in response to violence (Kelly, 1988). The investigators discovered that women get victimized in some special ways related to their sexuality. They also discovered that they get victimized in ways that serve to reinforce their powerless status in the family and society.

The picture that began emerging from gender-based studies was that men, for the most part, are victimized by other men. Women, for the most part, are victimized not by other women, but by men. Men tend to initiate or to be drawn into violence with other men in an effort to prove who is "more equal," or to defend self. Women are the subjects of violence as a function of their dependency and sexuality by a man who displays some combination of physical, economic, or social dominance. For both men and women, the attack of violence and its subsequent feeling of powerlessness puts their social and sexual identity on the line.

Men who are victimized typically respond to this threat to their macho image with anger and with physical and/or sexual aggression that confirms their male identity (Carmen & Rieker, 1989). Women who are victimized typically respond to this threat to their image of being "protected and taken care of" with anger also. An important difference, however, is that women feel that this anger cannot be expressed or experienced safely without rejection and/or retribution from those on whom they depend. Thus, because their anger cannot be expressed toward others, it is directed against the self (Carmen & Rieker, 1989). This, the statistics tell us, is the path taken by most women.

Female Crime Victims: At Risk

Over 6 million violent crimes are reported each year (assault, rape, robbery); close to half of these, an estimated 3 million, are committed against females (National Crime Survey, 1988). Furthermore, it is estimated that up to 50% of actual violent crimes are never reported. These victims are also female. This is yet another 3 million women per year who are victims of violence from men (Hamilton, 1989).

In addition, there are also crimes that are not "counted" as crimes (domestic violence, child physical and sexual abuse) (Hamilton, 1989). These crimes occur in greater proportion, an estimated 4 million per year, to the other crimes against women. The victims of all of these crimes are females. Thus, it is estimated that 10 million women are victims of violence from men each year.

Violence against women by men is so legion that some researchers have characterized it as a "normative developmental crisis" (Hamilton, 1989). That is to say, it is a crisis to be anticipated in the normal course of development in a woman's life. And no woman is immune from this potential crisis, for it occurs within every ethnic and racial group, and at every social class level.

And this violence is on the uptake. In preliminary Department of Justice crime figures for 1988, reported rape has increased 13% over 1987 (National Crime Survey, 1988). These "violence statistics" about women's lives dwarf those for breast cancer, other cancers, high blood pressure, and other public health issues. Society in the United States is the most violent in the developed world, and this violence is gender-driven.

In 1985, Surgeon General C. Everett Koop responded to the pervasive threat of violence in our society by mounting a public health initiative "Violence and Its Effects" (Koop, 1985). This was a sustained effort, during his tenure in office, to educate the public about the potentially hazardous aftermath of violence for the health and mental health of an individual. He did not, however, single out the particular jeopardy in which women live. But in 1986, an expert panel was convened by the National Institute of Mental Health, entitled "Women's Mental Health." This panel recommended that violence against women be one of the five priority areas for research in the prevention and treatment of the mental health problems of women (Eichler & Parron, 1987).

The trauma of violence is extremely difficult for women to integrate into their lives. With devastating force, this event violates fundamental human assumptions about the integrity and control of one's body and one's self. Self-esteem is shattered, and the world no longer appears to be safe, just, and orderly. This is a trauma very difficult for women to resolve with ordinary coping styles. As we will demonstrate in this chapter, this has very important mental health and public policy implications.

Historically, public policy for women as victims of crime has been particularly problematic for government. Police, prosecutors, and legislators have tended to view women's issues as ones which are tied to the family and to the marriage; consequently, government has felt that its intervention should be quite limited in this area. The limits of this intervention may well have served to exacerbate emotional and psychological problems for women as victims and as survivors.

In a competitive society, such as we are familiar with through most of our history, it is fashionable to stress "winning" over "losing" and to assign cultural contempt for victims or losers. This contempt is only mildly tempered by humanitarian concern and man's compassion for the less fortunate. People in trouble have to overcome many problems: their problem, whatever it is; the reluctance of society to accept someone as being needy; and the indifference of the systems that are supposed to help. Historically, society in the United States has been very reluctant to accept responsibility for victims (Rich, 1981; Rich & Stenzel, 1980).

As a society, we struggle with developing criteria that will help us decide when it is appropriate for the state to intervene, when the marketplace should be relied upon, and when we should enforce a conscious decision to let people act on their own and not be interfered with by big government. In the case of victims, we have never been quite certain what responsibilities to assign to the states, what responsibilities to assign the individual who is the offender, what responsibilities to assign to the victim, and what responsibilities the state has, if any, for the victim.

In essence, we are dealing with some very fundamental questions: In what areas should government intervene? What instruments of intervention are most appropriate?

A Framework for Understanding Public Policy

It is important to examine public policy in any given area because it represents the codification of core, societal values with respect to a particular issue or subject. Public policy-making institutions and processes attempt to identify a "majority view" on a subject which allows the State to reach closure and take some set of appropriate actions.

Public policy-making, as it is reflected in laws (legislation) represents a reactive process; it formalizes with the force of law, the values, norms, attitudes, and beliefs of society which are prevalent at a given moment in time. Public policy reflects societal beliefs; it does not tend to be instrumental in shaping and forming societal perspectives. In cases where there are tensions in society between competing values or in cases where there is no majority view, government tends to postpone action or it takes a symbolic action which delays any formal initiative to a point in time when mainstream beliefs can be clarified.

Within this framework, it is clear that public policy may change over time as different attitudes and beliefs emerge. The majority view in a given area may, indeed, change even in a relatively short period of time. Health care, mental health care, and civil rights each present cases where major changes in values and in corresponding public policy can be documented.

The rights and needs of victims present special problems for public policy as it relates to the criminal justice system in the United States. Historically, the criminal justice system is considered to be central to what government should be doing. It is one of the few areas where there is a general societal consensus on the need for government to intervene. American society is legendary for the importance it attaches to protecting private property and the rights of individuals. However, the right of an individual to exercise his or her free will ends at the point at which his or her fist hits another individual's chin. Each individual has a right to look to government to protect person and property.

Consequently, from the very first days of United States history, the criminal justice system has been seen as one of the central functions of governments. This system is designed to apprehend, try, and punish individuals who have violated another individual's rights—personal and property rights. Thus, the focus of the criminal justice system is on what the responsibilities of government are in protecting individual rights. At the same time, the system is also sensitive to protecting the rights of the accused: One is innocent until proven guilty.

Can we conceive of society possessing certain values which are passed on to citizens—either by consent or by coercion? At the most basic level, almost every social theorist and citizen can agree that the government exists to help protect citizens; therefore, a criminal justice system is an integral part of whatever—broad or limited—conception one has of government. The critical issue becomes: What are the limits to this criminal justice system?

- Simple laws to protect citizens?
- Enforcement of these laws?
- Punishment of citizens who do not obey the laws?
- Provision of some compensation to citizens who have been harmed by a convicted criminal?

We probably can all agree that government needs to formulate laws and enforce them—including providing some punishment to those who disobey; however, it is not at all clear as to whether the state has any responsibility to compensate those who have been harmed, other than compensation that comes from knowing that those who violated the social contract have been punished.

Alternatively, the state could recognize the right of families and individuals to seek retribution on their own. These fundamental questions are behind many of the debates about what constitutes appropriate victim services in American society and others. Does the state formally have a responsibility to victims and their families; and, if so, what is the breadth and scope of this responsibility?

Victims are therefore placed in a special predicament with respect to the criminal justice system on the one hand, and with respect to core societal values on the other. Historically, the system has not assigned the victim status within the system, other than the expectation that the victim will be fully cooperative with government in prosecuting a particular case. Within the context of the criminal justice system, the government does not see that it has special responsibilities to the victim; the system represents the victim through the process of prosecution.

Society also feels that victims are problematic from a public policy perspective. Victim status challenges strongly held social views:

- We should reward winners and not losers; victims are losers.
- We should only be willing to help those who are, in

---

turn, willing to cooperate in the formal criminal justice process.

- We should be willing and ready to pull ourselves up by our bootstraps and have the capacity to overcome adversity in the long run.
- If we do not overcome adversity, in the long run, we only have ourselves to blame.
- People are first-class citizens in society when they have a job and are able to hold a job.

These represent core American values which date back to the pioneering days of this country.

When victims are female and have children, victim status is even more problematic from a public policy perspective. Domestic violence is often considered to be a family matter and an issue which government should not interfere with. Family quarrels should be left to the family. Attempted rape, rape, domestic violence, and incest represent violent crimes which stigmatize women as "soiled" or "spoiled"; public policy has tended to be unresponsive to the needs of these victims.

Moreover, to the extent that public policy has recognized the needs of these victims, special mental health needs have been largely ignored. In part, this has been due to the fact that men are traditionally the breadwinner and must be able to function in the workplace. Women, however, did not carry this responsibility so their mental health problems could be ignored.

In addition, there are powerful reasons why the victim contributes to the maintenance of this state of ignorance. First, if one admits that he or she has emotional and psychological needs, this admission is seen as a sign of weakness and a sign that a person cannot overcome adversity as someone should be expected to. Second, if one is identified as having special mental health needs, there is the strong chance that one will be stigmatized. Third, if one exhibits long-term or delayed problems, it is often assumed that the person must have a history of mental illness or instability. It would be fair to conclude that public policy for female victims of violence who exhibit mental health needs is very unresponsive to the needs which exist.

The Social Envelope for Female Victims

In the immediate aftermath of victimization, a period usually persisting 3 to 6 months, a host of mental health needs and problems wrap themselves around the victim like a social envelope that is particularly corrosive for women. In addition to the victim trauma response—that quartet of fear, shame, guilt, and anger—the woman's psyche is further betrayed by the impact of the "second injury" (Symonds, 1980). This is a term coined to denote the victim's feelings of hurt and abandonment at the hands of police officers, nurses, and doctors who have first contact with the victim.

These professionals often assume an aloof or businesslike attitude to protect themselves emotionally and function effectively in a crisis. Victims interpret this emotional insulation as a personal rejection. Often, women feel that the rejection and lack of support from those in the helping roles are more devastating than the original attack. This is particularly true with their interactions with the criminal justice system.

Close upon the heels of the second injury, interacting with and reinforcing it, comes the sense of shame, of guilt, and stigmatization. This is especially true for women, who are likely to feel the brunt of the social mythology that claims that they "asked for it." Shame brings about a desire to conceal that the event happened, not to talk about it, which blocks off one of the most important routes to recovery.

Guilt and self-blame are very explosive issues in the immediate aftermath. Guilt, according to Robert Jay Lifton, comes when one feels responsible—either through action or inaction—for the precipitation of the trauma (see Chapter 1, in this volume, for a discussion). Women are very vulnerable to these feelings through the attempts of others to "blame the victim." Such self-blame also inhibits treatment-seeking behavior.

Women's reluctance to seek treatment in the immediate aftermath has been documented empirically. Rape victims rarely utilize formal assistance in the immediate or near aftermath of the trauma. In one study, only 5% of rape victims who were college students responded with efforts to gain assistance from a rape crisis center or professional psychotherapist (Koss & Burkhart, 1989).

Another study found that less than half of a sample of adult rape victims, judged three months later to be in need of psychotherapy, agreed to accept it. In a third study, only a quarter of the victims who entered an immediate postrape treatment program completed a 14-hour course of therapy (Koss & Burkhart, 1989).

Impact of the Trauma over Time

The bulk of improvement following victimization appears to take place, with good support and/or intervention, in about 1 to 3 months after the trauma. Evidence, however, from longer-term follow-up studies indicates that the majority of female crime victims do not experience rapid recovery.

In a typical follow-up study of rape victims 1 year after the event, evidence was given of 5 divorces immediately following the rape (in two cases the man left immediately). Jobs were lost by 13 more because of the severity of their reactions, and 12 had discussed it with no one (Ellis, Attkeson, & Calhoun, 1981). Other researchers have concluded that only 25% of rape victims were free of significant symptoms 1 year past the assault. Among samples of women raped 1 to 16 years previously, 48% stated that they eventually sought therapy (Koss & Burkhart, 1989).

Other figures recently made available on the effects of crime on women reveal some highly disturbing outcomes. Women who had been the victim of a violent rape were compared to women who had not been victims of rape. It was found that 19% of the rape victims had attempted suicide. Only 2% of the women who had not been victims of rape had attempted suicide (Berglas, 1985).

The psychosocial impacts on women who are victims of domestic violence are equally as sobering. Compared to nonbattered women, abused women are 5 times more likely to attempt suicide, 15 times more likely to abuse alcohol, 6 times more likely to report child abuse, and 3 times more likely to be diagnosed as depressed or psychotic. In absolute numbers, 19% of all battered women attempt suicide at least once, and 38% are diagnosed as depressed. And almost a third of psychiatric in- and outpatients are battered (Stark & Flitcraft, 1988).

Incest victims, in particular, do not fare well in their sexual and intimate relationships (see Chapter 50, in this volume). They are significantly more likely to report early pregnancy, marital separation and divorce, and repeated sexual victimization. These women are at extremely high risk for marriage to an abusive spouse. One study reported that a follow-up of incest victims some 20 years later revealed that fully 80% had attempted suicide at least once (Silver, Boon, & Stones, 1983).

For the woman, assimilation and resolution of the trauma depends, in part, on developing an interpretation of why and how it happened and its meaning for her as a woman. If this interpretation is not a positive one, then degradation and helplessness are integrated into her self-concept, beliefs, and behavior. This may mean leading a fear-dominated, constricted, and withdrawn life, or it may mean acting out a sense of powerlessness and unworthiness through a series of involvements in abusive relationships (Carmen & Rieker, 1989).

If the interpretation is a positive one, however, the victim comes to feel a sense of maturation, a strengthened belief in herself, an increased ability to think for herself and reject stereotypes (Burt & Katz, 1987). This may foster a sense of mission regarding the need to contribute in some meaningful way to the life of the family, community, or to society that had not been present previously.

In the first case, there is a disconfirmation of the self. In the latter case, there is a confirmation of self. In both cases, there has been a transformation of the self, but toward radically different ends. It will become evident as we examine the policy-making process that the net impact of existing public policies contributes to a disconfirmation of the self.

The Policy Envelope

Historical Background

Having examined the special mental health needs of female victims, it is appropriate to ask: What are the historical roots of public policy for victims in general, and for women in particular?

The criminal–victim relationship is probably as old as mankind. The victim–criminal relationship may be thought of as part of the individual's struggle to exist. In many societies, the victim responded to attacks with immediate revenge in the form of punishment. The victim and criminal both participated in a power struggle whose final goal was survival.

The notion of systematic retaliation developed as the first primitive social groupings, based on familial relationships, were formed. Some variety of kindred groups provided great support in obtaining redress of wrongs. Revenge acquired broad implications because an attack on a member of one's family weakened the entire kindred group relative to other families. It became

the duty of a family to respond to an offense, usually through aggressive retaliation. In a sense, legal protection and social order—concepts as we know them today—were defined by family ties. The fear of vendetta acted as a deterrent to disruption of social order, and, conversely, an individual without the support of a family had no legal protection and was left essentially defenseless.

Later, in some tribes, settlement took on a relatively civilized state characterized by the custom of paying goods to the victim as restitution for an offense. Accumulation of economic goods, which indicates a higher level of social development, leads to the correlation of physical or mental hurt with material items. Steven Schafer (1968) noted that among less sophisticated and less cohesive social groupings of gatherers and lower hunters, 12% allowed restitution in place of blood feud, among higher hunters 33% offered restitution as an alternative, and among the more highly developed societies of horticulturists, 45% allowed or required restitution for offenses. Restitution, in other words, became an integral part of a settled, stable community (Irish, 1981; Schafer, 1968).

The concept of restitution appeared in the Mosaic dispensation established among the Hebrews and in ancient Greece in the writings of Homer. Specifically, in the *Iliad*, Ajax reprimands Achilles for refusing reparation from Agamemnon, making reference to the practice of paying blood fines to appease a brother's death (Reiff, 1979, p. 133). The notoriously harsh Babylonian Code of Hammurabi, dating back more than 4,000 years, listed restitution and an-eye-for-an-eye punishment as remedies for a detailed series of crimes. Usually, punishment was administered by a member of the victim's family, and monetary reparation to the victim was generally made by the offender (Hobhouse, 1975, p. 8). The severity of the punishment or amount of the restitution were assessed according to the seriousness of the crime and the age and sex of both the victim and the offender. The high price of restitution required by the Code of Hammurabi and the Law of Moses suggests that responding to the needs of the victim was less a motive than ensuring severe punishment for the criminal.

It is probably worth noting that the penal law of ancient communities was a law of torts rather than a law of crimes. It was the victim, not the state, who was wronged. Restitution was aimed at satisfying the victim's desire for revenge. Although today theft, assault, robbery, and trespass are considered crimes against the state, under Roman law they were torts—a wrong committed by one person against another—remedied by monetary payments to the victim. Anglo-Saxon law also set a sum for compensation for every injury against one's person or honor (Meiners, 1978, p. 7).

Over time, the state wanted to be compensated in part for helping to arrange for compensation—and even more over time wrongs against victims were considered to be wrongs against the state and not the individual. Hence, civilization is marked by remedies by the state—ruling out remedies by families and kindred groups.

Modern societies consider theft, assault, and robbery to be crimes against the state. Even in the area of torts, the government provides the forum (i.e., the formal legal system) in which to adjudicate a particular case. In turn, the government provides for specific procedures for punishing the offender who has been found guilty of a specific crime. The criminal justice system is seen as an integral part of modern government. The state has a responsibility to (1) promulgate laws which are designed to protect citizens from property crimes and from crimes against the individual, (2) enforce the laws, and (3) punish citizens who do not obey the laws.

However, there is much less agreement as to what the role of the government should be, if any, in providing for monetary compensation and services for those who have been harmed other than the compensation which comes from knowing that a convicted criminal has been punished. Moreover, the state specifically forbids families and individuals from seeking retribution on their own.

There have been many explanations put forward as to why the society is so reluctant to provide services to victims. Most of these explanations have to do with the tendency to blame the victim for his or her problems or to feel that the victim was somehow predisposed to the problems he or she is experiencing (Rich, 1981; Rich & Stenzel, 1980; Ryan, 1971).

Public Policy as a Response to the Needs of Victims

As one examines more recent trends in public policy for victims, it is important to focus on a key question: Is current policy focusing on the needs of victims and their families?

It is our belief that one of the functions of our legal system is to codify through laws society's normative values and then to reinforce these cultural norms. Indeed, it is the primary responsibility of our legal system to preserve and uphold our cultural beliefs, our society's *raison d'être*. Nowhere are these underlying societal values more apparent than in the laws that have been developed in the victims' area.

Social Policies Concerned with Victims of Trauma

In a society which places a tremendous emphasis on a competitive ethos in which winning is everything, victims are viewed as losers who have somehow precipitated their own downfall. Social psychologists have suggested that this tendency to attribute blame to victims stems from a need to view the world as rationally ordered and therefore under our control (Coates *et al.*, 1979; Lerner & Simmons, 1966). If we can exercise control over our lives, it logically follows that those who are victimized have somehow done something to precipitate the unfortunate event. To admit that the victim was innocent would throw this strongly held belief in a just world into complete disarray.

Over the past 20 years, public policymakers have paid increased attention to victims (Sales, Rich, & Reich, 1987). The following types of programs/policies have been adopted as a response to the victims' movement:

1. *Victim compensation laws.* These laws have been adopted in over 40 states. They are modeled after work-

men's compensation laws, and they are designed to provide compensation for medical expenses, some losses of property, and loss of earnings from jobs. In almost all states, there is an upper limit which is placed on the awards that are given. Moreover, there are important exceptions/exclusions which are written into the law (Irish, 1981). Victims cannot be given financial awards if the crime was committed by a family member, if the victim somehow brought on the crime, and if they have significant financial means of their own. Only recently, has there been some minimal recognition of mental health needs. These programs will also not cover long-term expenses.

2. *Victim restitution laws.* These laws which are also popular in many states, stipulate that offenders must make some kind of financial restitution to the victims and/or their families. Moreover, they stipulate that earnings by an offender which are accrued while in prison must be used for purposes of restitution.

3. *Victim assistance programs.* These programs grew out of the LEAA experience in the 1970s. The programs are designed to facilitate cooperation of the victim with the criminal justice system. In addition, these programs also provide for short-term counseling, assistance in replacing locks or some other needs of this type, and protection from intimidation in the courtroom through such programs as separate waiting rooms.

4. *Victim impact statements.* These laws, which exist in a few states, provide victims with the opportunity to provide input to the judge on the impact of the crime on their lives. This information can be used by the judge in setting bail and in sentencing. The information may also be used in parole hearings.

5. *Victim's bills of rights.* In a small number of states, the legislature has adopted an overall "victim's bill of rights." This law is designed to recognize the special status of victims and to provide the victim with special status in the criminal justice system along with the state and the accused.

6. *Provision of services.* States have also designed a variety of service programs to meet the needs of victims. These services include shelters and crisis-intervention counseling (Rich, 1981; Rich & Cohen, 1982; Sales, Rich, & Reich, 1987).

These laws are important because they attempt to respond to some victim needs; however, each of these policies also contains critical *exclusionary clauses.* These clauses reflect core societal values; in other words, victims cannot receive benefits if:

- The crime is committed by a family member or even by someone in a common-law marriage
- The person did not provide proper resistance
- There are long-term needs

Indeed, in the context of these laws, one might argue that public policy has served to revictimize the victim. This is particularly true for women. Our investment in believing that people get what they deserve (i.e., that "good outcomes go to good people and bad things befall bad people") has become ingrained in our culture's attitude and treatment of victims. Nowhere is this pernicious myth of contributory negligence more apparent than in societal attitudes toward crime victims (in particular, victims of rape and domestic violence). Americans take a far more lenient view of victims of "acts of fate" because it is evident that the victim had no role in producing his or her condition. However, because crime victims suffer from a human-induced victimization, it is easy to believe that the victim's behavior could have precipitated the act; for example, the burglary victim should have taken better security precautions, the rape victim should not have worn such a short dress, or the battered wife should not have taunted her husband. This difference in society's perception of victimization is clearly expressed by Frederick (1980) in an article on human versus natural-induced disasters:

> The victims of a major disaster are accepted by other persons, and sympathy is quickly developed for them. Victims of human-induced violence often are rejected by other persons because there is a feeling of guilt by association or contamination, and because victims are thought to be particularly blameworthy. (p. 74)

This tendency to express more sympathy toward victims of natural disasters is reflected in the degree of federal assistance that has been allocated for different categories of victims. Victims of such natural disasters as the Johnstown flood, the Three Mile Island nuclear disaster, and the contamination of the Love Canal were the recipients of immediate federal assistance. In contrast, the federal government has, in the past, rejected several proposals (e.g., H.R. 4257—Victims of Crime Act, 1979) whereby by providing a 25% federal match states would be encouraged to establish victim compensation programs. This resistance was only overcome in 1984 with the passage of the Victims of Crime Act (VOCA) under President Ronald Reagan.

At present, victims who sustain physical injuries are entitled to compensation for medical expenses not reimbursed by other sources, for loss of earnings stemming from the injury, for a limited amount of mental health counseling, for the loss of the services of an injured family member, and for funeral and burial expenses (Irish, 1981). These provisions represent a step in the right direction, but systematically exclude significant sectors of the population, such as the elderly and others on fixed incomes. More significantly, most compensation statutes have built-in stipulations which further restrict the number of victims who are eligible for compensation. It is our contention that these restrictions are based on more than cost-effectiveness criteria, and reflect systematic societal biases against those who have been victimized.

Policymaking vis-à-vis Female Victims

The most blatant example of a systematic societal bias is when compensation is denied in cases where the victim has contributed (either by direct participation in an illegal activity or deliberate provocation of the offender) to his or her victimization. What more explicit evidence of society's proclivity to blame the victim do we need?

Another significant limitation on eligibility for victim compensation is the "familial exclusion role" which has been incorporated into the statutes of most of the states (Irish, 1981). According to this rule, victims are deemed ineligible for compensation if the offender is a member of his or her family. Family is defined quite broadly to include "individuals who share a common residence, maintain a common-law or sexual relationship, or who are related within the third degree of consanguinity or affinity" (U.S. Department of Justice, *Crime Victim Compensation*, cited in Irish, 1981, p. 62).

Taken together, these two provisions reflect society's tendency to blame all victims of one-to-one violent crimes, but particularly those crimes involving victims and offenders with blood ties. In practice, this burden most frequently falls on the woman who has either been raped or physically abused by a husband or lover.

Woman as Property

Rape victims and battered women are considered uniquely undeserving of public sympathy and assistance. This is expressed by two writers in an article on rape laws:

> there is still a widespread belief in our culture that women "ask for it," either individually or as a group. Curiously, society does not censure the robbery victim for walking around with $10, or the burglary victim for keeping all of those nice things in his house, or the car theft victim for showing off his flashy new machine. When a mugging victim is questioned, it is unlikely that he will be asked, "How often in the past have you given money voluntarily to drug addicts?" (Schwartz & Cleary, 1980, p. 133)

This bias against physical/sexual crimes against women represents two fundamental cultural beliefs: First, as the fundamental social unit of society, the nuclear family must at all costs be preserved. Second, that the inferior female—especially a married one—is the "property" of her male mate and as such he is given free rein to treat her as he sees fit. As one writer expresses it: "By marriage, the husband and wife are one person in law. The very being or legal existence of the woman is suspended during marriage, or at least is incorporated and consolidated into that of the husband" (Moore, 1979, p. 42). As the above discussion suggests, existing victim compensation laws systematically discriminate against rape victims and battered women. A closer examination of the laws and criminal justice practices that have been developed for dealing with cases of rape provides additional support for this contention.

Examination of some of the fundamental provisions of rape statutes makes it becomes readily apparent that this category of victims is afforded different treatment than victims of nonsexual criminal assaults. Because these laws are based on traditional attitudes about social roles and sexual mores, rape laws have tended to reinforce the belief that women are the sole property of men. This concept of women belonging to men, coupled with a strongly held belief in the sanctity of the nuclear family, has acted to prevent women from bringing criminal charges of rape against their husbands until recently. In all but a handful of states, husbands are exempt from prosecution on rape charges (Hui, 1981; Sales *et al.*, 1987). In fact, rape is the only felony charge in which marriage is considered a legal defense. In an article on rape reform legislation, the attitudes underlying this position are clearly articulated:

> Although there is a societal interest in protecting the marital relationship, there is an equal interest in safeguarding the individual from acts of violence. Both interests must be considered in the determination of legislative policy. Under present law, the integrity of the individual is subjugated to societal interest in protecting marital privacy. (Sasko, H. & Sesek, D., 1975, cited in Hui, 1981)

Woman as Liar

Another provision in rape laws which disproportionately discriminates against women victims is the material corroboration requirement whereby a case can only be successfully prosecuted if "external evidence" such as an eyewitness to the assault, medical evidence proving vaginal penetration, or physical injuries suffered by the victim, is provided. Until 1974, courts in New York State would not hear a rape victim's case without material corroboration after charges. Such a precondition is still emphasized in many jurisdictions and remains unique to rape trials; a mugging victim is not required to produce eyewitnesses to his attack in order to convince the judge and jury of his claims of truthfulness (Hui, 1981).

As Susan Sontag has noted when writing about AIDS, the metaphorical trappings that stigmatize crime victims, or victims of rape in particular, have real life consequences. One of these trappings is the theme of "woman as liar," so well expressed by Hilberman (1976):

> The theme of woman as liar pervades our constructs about rape victims and underlies the assumption that women often make false charges of rape against men, even men they do not know. While law enforcement personnel are aware that false charges of crime occur, it is only in rape cases that it is assumed that the usual safeguards in the system cannot protect the innocent from a lying witness. In robbery, for example, it is understood that property was taken from the victim without his/her consent, and there is no need to prove that fear of death or grave bodily harm was at issue. The law, then, grants more protection to property than to person, especially if the person is female.

Woman as Provocateur

Perhaps the most blatant example of society's tendency to place an inordinate amount of blame on victims is the "resistance requirement." This requirement forces the victim to demonstrate that she resisted the attack to the utmost even to the point of sustaining severe physical injuries. Without this demonstration of resistance, the chances of obtaining a conviction are greatly diminished (Hui, 1981). In other cases of assault and robbery, the individual is not expected to risk serious injury or death to protect himself and/or his property. In her analysis of the consent standard in rape laws, Harris (1976) pointed out:

> In robbery cases, the court set a low standard of force to prove victim fear and hence non-consent, applying a rea-

sonable man test. . . . The law does not expect the person to risk serious injury or death in defense of self or property. . . . only the law of rape makes unjustified adverse assumptions about the general sincerity of the alleged victims, which lead to requirements of much higher levels of proof of force and resistance. Such requirements leave the physical safety of women correspondingly less protected in cases of rape than in cases of robbery or simple assault. (p. 624)

The imposition of this requirement in rape cases reflects a societal skepticism toward the legitimacy of women's allegations of rape. This skepticism is buttressed by the admissibility of evidence regarding the woman's prior sexual history. The rationale being that if it can be demonstrated that a woman consented, or was "unchaste" in the past, she most likely consented in the current rape. As Harris (1976) rightly suggests:

> once a woman has voluntarily engaged in intercourse, the law grants less protection to her right to refuse intercourse in the future, without consideration of whether her past decision expresses anything about the likelihood of her having exercised her choice in the present case. (p. 624)

Research conducted by social psychologists has also demonstrated that individuals are more likely to infer guilt in rape cases in which the victim was a prostitute than when the victim was a college sophomore (Coates et al., 1979).

These explicit statutory provisions and their implicit assumptions refute basic legal principles, such as "innocent until proven guilty," and serve to deny rape victims equal protection under the law. Instead, the law appears to blame these victims for precipitating their own misfortune, and hence denies them the fair and equitable treatment provided to other crime victims.

Public Policy: Playing Catch-Up

Fortunately, there seems to be a shift in societal attitudes toward rape victims. In large part stimulated by the women's movement in the late 1960s and 1970s, there is a growing recognition that rape constitutes a serious offense and that the treatment of offenders should be similar to that of other offenses of comparable magnitude. Rape is now included in the FBI Crime Index, which represents a measure of serious offenses in which better reporting and more active prosecution has been encouraged.

The growing concern over the plight of rape victims and the concomitant belief that society should do something to help these victims has resulted in the passage in some states of laws and legislation mandating equitable treatment of victims of rape as for victims of other crimes. Examples of some of the changes in rape laws include:

- The marital rape exemption has been completely eliminated in some states.
- The requirement of material corroboration for a successful conviction has been abolished in a few states.
- The admissibility of prior sexual conduct and reputation of the victim, making it more difficult for the

defense counsel to defame the victim's testimony on the grounds of "unchastity," has been restricted in some states.

- Rape victims are now eligible for victim compensation funds in some states (Hui, 1981, p. 113).

These new statutes provide greater legal protection to rape victims and reduce some of the inequities suffered by rape victims in their dealings with the criminal justice system. These laws challenge the traditional societal values that have consistently plagued rape victims: the myth that as property, husbands are entitled to rape their wives; the belief that women cry rape too easily and secretly are asking for it to happen; and the myth that an unchaste woman freely gives her consent to any man at any time. Although more legislation is needed, particularly in clarifying the legal definition of force, consent, and how much resistance indicates nonconsent, the new statutes enacted in such states as Iowa, Wisconsin, Oregon, and Washington reflect the beginnings of a societal acceptance of rape victims as legitimate victims, deserving of equal protection and treatment under the law.

Although the clinical evidence points to a predictable potential response to the victimization experience (which appears to cut across various types of victimization), public policymakers, responsible for guiding and funding public agencies that provide services to victims, do not appear to have placed a high priority of a long-termed and delayed emotional reaction of the victims and their families. There is a gap between recognizing a need and translating that recognition into an effective public policy.

Conclusion

In his unpublished paper entitled *Diminished Man*, Paul Weiss (1980) analyzes the societal mechanisms which are employed to strengthen an individual or which may be used to "diminish" him or her. It is clear that societies develop norms/standards for what is considered to be accepted behavior and for what is considered to be deviant. These standards are then translated into public programs, legislation, and policy at the federal and state levels.

As we have pointed out in this chapter, the programs and policies which currently exist (mostly at the state level in the United States) are not oriented toward meeting the emotional and psychological needs of women as victims. Instead, the laws, taken as a whole, demonstrate contempt for these victims.

The policies reflect mainstream societal values which have not internalized the process of transforming a woman from victim to survivor. New laws and programs have been reactive to political and social pressures and have met some minimal needs, including the needs to recognize (1) that sexual assault can occur within the family; (2) that women do not need to be subject to interrogation concerning their previous sexual history (this is not admissible evidence in court); (3) that government should provide protection and assistance to victims of domestic violence; and (4) that police and law enforcement officers need professional training in how to work effectively and sensitively with these victims.

However, even with this progress, there are a series of tensions/conflicts over competing societal values which have not been addressed:

1. Should government provide long term assistance to women as victims?
2. Does the need for long-term emotional and psychological assistance imply that a victim had a previous "history of mental illness?"
3. Which, if any, of the "exclusionary clauses" have been written into law are appropriate?
4. Should governmental programs recognize the possibility of "delayed stress" related to the victimization experience?

Up to this point in time, society has not been willing to recognize long-term needs or the delayed-stress phenomena as direct by-products of the victimization experience.

It is also clear that public policy in this area, as in many other areas, has not adopted a proactive stance; instead, it has reacted to mainstream values on the one hand and to political pressure on the other. If we are to make progress in overcoming the case against women outlined in this chapter, government will need to adopt a proactive stance and to educate the public about the need to work with women in becoming survivors and working with society in fundamentally changing its attitudes so that they are not facilitating the victimization process.

References

Bard, M., & Sangrey, D. (1979). *The crime victim's book* (pp. 10–28). New York: Basic Books.

Bart, P. B., & O'Brien, P. H. (Eds.). (1985). *Stopping rape: Successful survival strategies* (pp. 1–10). New York: Pergamon Press.

Berglas, S. (1985, February). Why did this happen to me? *Psychology Today*, pp. 44–48.

Burt, M. R., & Katz, B. L. (1987). Dimensions of recovery from rape: Focus on growth outcomes. *Journal of Interpersonal Violence*, 2, pp. 55–82.

Carmen, E. H., & Rieker, P. (1989). A psychosocial model of the victim-to-patient process. *Psychiatric Clinics of North America*, 12(2), 431–443.

Coates, D., Wortman, C., & Abbey, A. (1979). Reacting to victims. In I. H. Frieze, D. Bar-Tal & J. S. Caroll (Eds.), *New approaches to social problems*. San Francisco: Jossey-Bass.

Eichler, A., & Parron, D. (1987). *Women's mental health: Agenda for research* (DHHS Publication No. ADM 87–1542). Washington, DC: U.S. Government Printing Office.

Ellis, E., Attkeson, B., & Calhoun, K. (1981). An assessment of long-term reactions to rape. *Journal of Abnormal Psychology*, 90(3), 363–366.

Frederick, C. J. (1980). Effects of natural vs. human induced violence upon victims. In *Evaluation and change: Special issue* (pp. 71–75). Minneapolis: Minneapolis Medical Research Foundation.

Hamilton, J. (1989). Emotional consequences of victimization and discrimination in special populations of women. *Psychiatric Clinics of North America*, 12(1), 35–51.

Harris, L. R. (1976). Toward a consent standard in the law of rape. *University of Chicago Law Review*, 43(3), 613–645.

Hilberman, E. (1976). Rape: The ultimate violation of self. *American Journal of Psychiatry*, 133(4), 436–437.

Hobhouse, L. T. (1975). Law and justice. In J. Hudson & B. Galaway (Eds.), *Considering the victim: Readings in restitution*. Springfield, IL: Charles C Thomas.

Hui, A. (1981). *Responding to victims of rape and spouse abuse: The criminal justice system and the law as mirrors of societal attitudes and prejudices*. Unpublished undergraduate thesis, Princeton University.

Irish, L. W. (1981). *On the imbalance of justice: State compensation to crime victims*. Unpublished undergraduate thesis, Princeton University.

Kelly, L. (1988). *Surviving sexual violence* (pp. 43–73). Minneapolis: University of Minnesota Press.

Koop, E. (1985). *Proceedings of the Surgeon General's Workshop on Violence and Public Health*, DHHS, PHS.

Koss, M. P., & Burkhart, B. R. (1989). A conceptual analysis of rape victimization. *Psychology of Women Quarterly, 13*, 27–40.

Lerner, M. J., & Simmons, C. (1966). Observer's reaction to the innocent victim. *Journal of Personality and Social Psychology, 4*, 203–210.

Lifton, R. J. (1976). *Death in life* (pp. 31–56). New York: Touchstone Books.

Meiners, R. E. (1978). *Victim compensation: Economic, legal, and political aspects*. Lexington, MA: Lexington Books.

Moore, D. (Ed.). (1979). *Battered women*. Beverly Hills, CA: Sage Publications.

National Crime Survey. (Preliminary, 1988). Washington, DC: Department of Justice.

Reiff, R. (1979). *The invisible victim: The criminal justice system's forgotten responsibility*. New York: Basic Books.

Rich, R. F. (1981). Evaluating mental health services for victims: Perspectives on policies and services in the United States. In S. E. Salasin (Ed.), *Evaluating victim services* (pp. 128–142). Beverly Hills: Sage Publications.

Rich, R. F., & Cohen, D. (1982). Victims of crime: Public policy perspectives and models for services. Unpublished manuscript prepared for the World Federation for Mental Health.

Rich, R. F., & Stenzel, S. (1980). Mental health services for victims: policy paradigms. In *Evaluation and change: Special issue* (pp. 47–54). Minneapolis: Minneapolis Medical Research Foundation.

Ryan, W. (1971). *Blaming the victim*. New York: Vintage Books.

Sales, B., Rich, R. F., & Reich, J. (1987). Victimization policy research. *Professional Psychology: Research and Practice, 18*(4), 326–337.

Sasko, H., & Sesek, D. (1975). Rape reform legislation: Is it the solution? *Cleveland State Law Review, 24*(3), 463–503.

Schafer, S. (1968). *The victim and his criminal: A study in functional responsibility*. New York: Random House.

Schwartz, M. D., & Cleary, T. (1980). Toward a new law on rape. *Crime and Delinquency, 26*(2), 129–151.

Silver, R. L., Boon, C., & Stones, M. H. (1983). The search for meaning in misfortune: Making sense of incest. *Journal of Social Issues, 39*(2), 81–102.

Stark, E., & Flitcraft, A. (1988). Personal power and institutional victimization: Treating the dual trauma of woman battering. In F. Ochberg (Ed.), *Post-traumatic therapy and victims of violence* (pp. 115–151). New York: Brunner/Mazel.

Symonds, M. (1980). The second injury to victims. *Evaluation and change: Special issue* (pp. 36–38). Minneapolis: Minneapolis Medical Research Foundation.

Weiss, P. (1980). *Diminished man*. Unpublished manuscript for the Smithsonian Woodrow Wilson International Center for Scholars, Washington, DC.

CHAPTER 81

Coping with Disaster

The Helping Behavior of Communities and Individuals

Liisa Eränen and Karmela Liebkind

Introduction

Disaster research in the behavioral sciences is a relatively new area. With the exception of the major pioneering studies, research concerned with disasters began systematically in the United States in the 1950s and in Europe and Japan in the following decades (Dynes, 1987a; Hultaker, 1983; Raphael, 1986; United Nations, 1986). Early disaster research was by nature documentary and descriptive and lacking in well-specified conceptual and methodological approaches. As descriptive research studies accumulated, however, they made possible more sophisticated analytical studies of the effects of disaster. Methodologically and ethically, researchers can study disasters only *post hoc*, of course, and this presents many problems concerned with psychosocial outcomes (see Chapter 10, in this volume). Among the persistent problems is that of delineating the interactive effects of individual differences variables and pervasive situational and environmental effects common to all disaster situations (Hultaker, 1983; Wilson, 1989).

Presently, there are different conceptions as to what differentiates natural disasters from direct or indirect man-made disasters (Perry, 1985, p. 14). The conceptual boundary between the two types of events is flexible to some extent since humankind, through their own actions, could provoke a natural disaster (e.g., excessive harvesting of timberlands causing a flood) (B. A. Turner, 1978, p. 2). As is now generally believed, the consequences may produce very different effects on mental

Liisa Eränen and Karmela Liebkind • Department of Social Psychology, University of Helsinki, SF-00100 Helsinki, Finland.
International Handbook of Traumatic Stress Syndromes, edited by John P. Wilson and Beverley Raphael. Plenum Press, New York, 1993.

health outcome (Frederick, 1980; Lifton & Olson, 1976). One fundamental difference is that *natural* disasters are often beyond our control and occur rapidly and often without warning. In this regard, they may lead to a distressing sense of loss of control (Baum, Fleming, & Singer, 1983). However, because human beings believe in their power to control technology, a man-made disaster might induce a greater sense of loss of control than natural disasters, which are not expected to be in our control.

There is no simple definition of the concept of disaster and, indeed, the literature is marked by a number of varying concepts and definitions (Quarantelli, 1985a). Moreover, the definition of disaster has developed and changed considerably over the years. From one perspective, a disaster was defined as a physical event or on the basis of an assessment of the *physical impact* of an event. In research in the social and behavioral sciences, however, disasters are not studied primarily as a physical event but as a social psychological phenomenon (Quarantelli, 1980). Early definitions assumed that the greater the physical destruction of a disaster, the greater would be the social disruption. Nevertheless, there is not necessarily a direct or isomorphic connection between physical impact and psychosocial functioning or mental health outcome. What may be more crucial is not the existence of a physical disaster impact, but the psychological belief that important personal, social, and environmental resources are in danger (Quarantelli, 1985a, pp. 41–46). Thus, if a situation is construed psychologically as threatening, dangerous, or associated with a loss of control, then this becomes the important phenomenological reality (W. I. Thomas & D. S. Thomas, 1928).

In the most recent definitions of disaster, the aim has been to treat disaster as a social phenomenon and to emphasize the social and psychological aspects of the situation instead of the physical events. According to Quarantelli (1980), a *social-consensus* type of crisis situation is one in which there is little internal conflict within the society regarding what has happened in the disaster. Quarantelli defined a disaster as a social-consensus type crisis in which there is an *imbalance* in the *demand-capability ratio*. In such a situation, the emphasis is on the *collective efforts* being made to terminate a particular crisis by restoring capabilities to the level of demands. This definition thus reflects the unpredictable and uncontrollable nature of many disaster situations. The utility of this definition is that it is applicable whether it is a question of an actual disaster or only the *threat of disaster* and is not dependent on the special or unique characteristics of a particular disaster. Also, the definition is applicable on the level of individual and societal levels of analysis.

In most Western countries, the attitudes toward disaster are reflected in culture-specific ways in terms of attempts to prevent, limit, and control disaster effects. Related importantly to cultural mechanisms of coping with disasters is the issue of cognitive attribution in terms of expectation for locus of control. Fatalistic, externalized belief attributions (e.g., it is God's punishment) may result in learned helplessness and the failure to learn alternative ways to cope with the aftermath of a disaster (Caporale, 1987). On the other hand, where the culture emphasizes a belief in an internal locus of causation and effective coping, disaster impacts might be less pathological and lead to more adaptive forms of postdisaster learning and future preparation.

Dimensions of Disaster

The distinction between a disaster and an accident is one of degree, and not all studies make a clear distinction between *individual* and *collective* disasters (see Erikson, 1976, for a discussion). For example, in studies of posttraumatic stress disorder (PTSD), individual and collective stress situations are sometimes considered to be of a comparable magnitude. From the social-psychological perspective, research emphasizes the *community* nature of disasters. The essential characteristic here is that the disaster affects the structure and functioning of the community itself. Thus, among the crucial differences between a disaster and an accident is that in a disaster the social structure and processes are affected to the extent that the disaster threatens the very existence and functioning of the community. This difference, then, places disasters among the relatively rare human experiences in the course of the life cycle (Britton, 1987, pp. 50–52; Erikson, 1976; Quarantelli, 1985a). In studying individual reactions, a difference can be made between *agent-generated* and *response-generated* reactions (Wilson, Smith, & Johnson, 1985). This distinction separates the effects and demands created by the disaster agent from others that take place when responding to the disaster situation. Thus, the community is regarded as forming a *recovery environment* which may either prevent and ameliorate the worst of the damage caused by the disaster or intensify its effects depending on how the rescue and disaster aid are implemented (Quarantelli, 1985b, pp. 200–201; Perry & Lindell, 1978).

In the definition of disaster, the attempt is made to emphasize those general characteristics which apply to all disasters as well as to the unique characteristics related to particular disasters (e.g., a nuclear meltdown). Clearly, these different dimensions affect how the disaster is appraised and processed psychologically. Moreover, as noted by Wilson (1989) and Wilson et al. (1985), traumatically stressful events such as a disaster contain many types of stressors that contribute differentially to postdisaster adaptation (Wilson et al., 1985). Similar analyses of the role of the disaster impacts have been discussed by Quarantelli (1985a), Barton (1969), and Raphael (1986, p. 103).

Community Reactions to Disaster

Changes in Values and Functions

Disasters are typically conceptualized in terms of the loss and destruction they produce (Quarantelli & Dynes, 1985, p. 160). The effects of a disaster on a community are, however, paradoxical since they can lead to massive disorganization and patterns of prosocial cooperation and integration. Above all, the integrating factors are the consensus-generated norms which support altruistic behavior (Dynes, 1970, p. 204).

From a functional perspective, a community is a social organization which provides people with the indispensable functions they need for everyday life (Quarantelli & Dynes, 1985, p. 158). In all communities, of course, there is the potential for conflict since the members of the community may have conflicting goals. Sometimes disasters alter this situation in positive, prosocial ways. In the face of an external objective threat, the values of the community may be placed in a new hierarchical order of importance; one which places the welfare of others and the need to rebuild the infrastructure as humanistic, first-order goals. For the moment, conflicts lose their customary significance. In the wake of a disaster, most activity is strongly concentrated in the present moment, primarily in caring for the victims. The predisaster forms of production, distribution, and consumption are often radically altered or redirected. In a disaster situation, only absolutely necessary production continues: Normal trade may cease and production will be distributed and consumed according to need. In some emergencies, violations of the rules are overlooked and social participation is channeled at an unofficial level and directed at tasks created by the disaster. When destabilization of the infrastructure occurs, old regulations and norms may not be operative, and individuals have the autonomy to decide when and how things should be done, as long as their actions are in line with the goals the community has given first priority at that moment (Dynes, 1970, pp. 84–97, 102–108).

The order of priorities and the consensus born in connection with a disaster are collectively called the *state of emergency consensus*. Under normal conditions, people identify with different social groups of which the most important is the family. Usually, when in a state of danger, people attempt to strengthen the primary group bonds and in disasters they take care first of those closest to them. According to R. H. Turner (1967), in a disaster the community returns to a "mechanical solidarity." Mechanical solidarity is based on the concept of homogenization and a reduction in role differentiation and status rankings. When the disaster is widespread, mechanical solidarity permeates the various social groups and increases identification among victims, and previous class, race, ethnic, and social class barriers temporarily disappear (Barton, 1969, pp. 230–233; Dynes, 1970, pp. 84–87; R. H. Turner, 1967). In a disaster situation, mechanical solidarity is based on shared fate, similar affective reactions, and a sense of likeness among those caught in the disaster (Dynes, 1970, pp. 102–108; Edberg & Lustig, 1983, pp. 27–33; R. H. Turner, 1967). At these times, the community is served by different utilization of resources (personal, social, economic, and environmental) than under normal conditions since social status no longer has an exchange value in a crisis situation. Thus, the earlier power structure of the community changes and the individual's identification with the community is therefore strengthened, because of the disaster impacts (Wenger, 1978, p. 37).

The common identification among the victims and the desire to help are crucially affected by the extent of the destruction and suffering. In most disasters, the degree of prosocial behavior has been significant, but there are exceptions. In an "ordinary" disaster, the relative deprivation mechanism alleviates feelings of suffering: The knowledge that you are only one among many sufferers decreases one's own feelings of loss. Nonetheless, those who have suffered severe losses are worried only about their own difficulties. Usually, the helpers are those whose own average losses are slight, so that they have more actual or personal resources and motivation to help others. The greater the proportion of those who feel they have suffered severe losses, the smaller is the proportion of the population whose losses seem slight and who have the empathic reserves toward other victims. When the destruction is widespread, the level of needs clearly exceeds the available resources (Barton, 1969, pp. 25–27; Dynes & Quarantelli, 1980, pp. 339–354; Fritz, 1961, pp. 684–687; Wolfenstein, 1957, pp. 189–198).

When group membership is particularly salient to a person, his or her perceived similarity and/or identification to the group and conformity to its norms will increase. After a disaster, communities often exhibit internal solidarity and a tendency to define their in-groups in terms of shared feelings and experiences. The emotional experience of the disaster becomes the criterion attribute necessary for admittance to their group. The cognitive result of this social identification is the appearance of stereotypical perception which guides behavior. This implies a tendency for people to observe themselves and others in the light of a stereotype. The characteristics belonging to exemplar individuals in the in-group are assigned to oneself and other members of the group. The stereotypical in-group attributes include emotional experiences, needs, goals, attitudes, and behavioral norms. Thus, social identification can directly increase group cohesion. Altruism and cooperation are mediated by the perception of common group membership, that is, social identification. The most important condition of this membership is the perception of "we-group ties" between individuals. Thus, in this situation, altruism represents behavior based on the cognitive extension of the self (J. C. Turner, 1982, pp. 30–31).

Helping as a Social-Organizational Phenomenon

After a disaster, a community has been described as a therapeutic and altruistic society. What, then, is meant by altruism? Altruism is one form of helping. Helping can also be divided into those activities which are ways of achieving another goal, that is, which have an egoistic motive, and altruistic helping, which is a goal in itself. It is difficult to find a general theory of altruism because different prosocial activities motivate people for different reasons (see Aronoff & Wilson, 1985, for a review). From the point of view of the beneficiary, it is, of course, not always important whether the motive was selfish or not. In research studies, altruism is indeed often defined as the effect of an attitude or behavior and not on the basis of motive (Kemper, 1980, pp. 307–338). However, there are important personality characteristics and motives that are associated with altruism (see Aronoff & Wilson, 1985; Staub, 1978).

Dynes and Quarantelli (1980) have studied helping as a social-organizational phenomenon. Norms regulate the behavior which takes place within a given framework of social relationships. According to Dynes and Quarantelli, disasters do not change the factors affecting behavior but create new tasks for the group. Following a disaster, the reaction of a community can then be seen as a system of helping behavior born entirely from the situation so that separating helping behavior from other activities is difficult (Dynes & Quarantelli, 1980; Kemper, 1980).

The most important resources for the society in coping with the problems caused by a disaster are its social organizations. Evidently, help channeled through these organizations is more efficient than uncoordinated individual activity. A community has at least four possibilities in trying to cope with the new tasks: (1) It can intensify the activities of established organizations carrying out their regular activities (e.g., hospitals). (2) Those organized activities which do not directly relate to problems created by the disaster (e.g., construction) can be redirected by the community. (3) The community can make use of individuals who ordinarily might not offer emergency help. (4) The community can create new roles to cope with tasks lacking predisaster equivalence. Voluntary help could be used in handling these tasks (Dynes & Quarantelli, 1980).

Although organizations are an important resource in coping with disaster, in the actions that are taken following a disaster, cooperation between organizations is often a central and difficult problem. A disaster situation requires cooperation between several different organizations, and often each organization has its own disaster plan, but there may not be a coordinated community plan. Problems may be created by unclear responsibility and authority relationships and insufficient communication between organizations. When cooperation is deficient, workers may be unsure of their tasks and positions (Drabek, 1985, 1986; Green, 1985). Disagreements between organizations have been known to lead to open conflict and a quarrel over "whose disaster and whose victims are really in question" (Raphael, 1986, p. 240; Berah, Jones, & Valent, 1984).

Helping in Mental Health Organizations

In the mental health sector, there are two different models of the organization of services during and after a disaster. The traditional clinical approach, which is based on the so-called disease model, emphasizes the diagnosis and cure of disorders. The community-oriented, psychosocial model emphasizes prevention and work within the social environment. The clinical model is still predominant; but in disaster situations the established mental health system has often proved to be inadequate to deal with the problems caused by the disaster (Taylor, Ross, & Quarantelli, 1976, pp. 82–85).

When there is no experience with disaster, mental health organizations are generally not taken into account in planning for required services (Baisden & Quarantelli, 1981). In most cases, planning and organizing of mental health services are begun only after the disaster has already occurred. How they are organized depends to a great extent on what types of problems the disaster is believed to have caused (Taylor *et al.*, 1976). According to Baisden and Quarantelli (1981), the mental health sector usually has a strong ideology which says that something "must be done" for disaster victims. Physicians, psychologists, and social workers have varying concepts of what types of problems are to be expected. Common to all is that they are prepared for "something" which is coming, if not immediately, then at least later, and it is to be expected that there will be many people in need of help (Taylor *et al.*, 1976, pp. 66–77).

Experience suggests that mental health organizations are generally reluctant to change their methods, even if there is no demand for their services. At first, traditional medical models tend to dominate but as the crisis situation continues, other services exceed clinical wisdom and knowledge, and, consequently, methods change, usually to include more social services and legal activities (e.g., hearing of complaints, distribution of material, aid in filling out forms, etc.) (Baisden & Quarantelli, 1981).

Voluntary Helping

Volunteer aid in disasters can be channeled in many different ways. Dynes and Quarantelli (1980) distinguished four forms of voluntary helping: (1) People may be members of organizations that have emergency responsibility written into their charters. These people work within the framework of ordinary social relationships and roles that form part of a previously prepared plan. Such organizations (e.g., the Red Cross) have a latent structure that is activated when emergencies occur. (2) An individual may be a member of an organization which has no specific, emergency-related purposes (group volunteer) but which extends its activities during a disaster. The volunteering is not done on the part of the individual but of the organization to which he or she belongs. (3) Individuals may expand their normal professional roles and carry out tasks which are similar but not identical to those they usually perform. For example, a physician who normally sees only private patients may work in the emergency ward of the clinic of a hospital. (4) Part of helping behavior may be interpreted as an expansion of the more abstract role of a community

member to include a certain "civic duty." Normative constraints are already present, at least in a latent form, in existing role obligations. Dynes interpreted this as an expansion of the role of a citizen but does not explain the underlying psychological processes (Dynes, 1970; Dynes & Quarantelli, 1980).

Because the organizations are not able, at least immediately, to cope with all the tasks and problems created by the disaster, people spontaneously form groups to fill the gaps (Dynes, 1987b, p. 98; Forrest, 1974, pp. 38–40; 1978, pp. 114–117). For example, the failure of institutionalized mental health organizations to supply needed services gives rise to voluntary groups which organize themselves as they go along. The emergent system may include, for example, religious groups which already have better connections with other organizations than do the mental health organizations (Taylor *et al.*, 1976, p. 135).

Primary Victims of Disaster

People act according to certain basic assumptions about themselves and the world. Most people share a basic assumption as to a belief in their own invulnerability and a vision of the world as a predictable place in which events do not occur at random. Individuals also need a certain degree of autonomy and attempt to control the events in their environment. By its very nature, a disaster is an uncontrollable situation so that these basic cognitive beliefs may be undermined. It is common for a person's sense of invulnerability to be changed. Hence, if individuals find it difficult to believe in random chance, it becomes difficult for them to understand a disaster. As noted by many observers of massive psychic trauma, a disasterlike event can profoundly affect ideological, belief, religious, and attributional systems.

It is possible for a feeling of invulnerability to change at the time of a disaster into an *illusion of centrality*; for example, that only one's own house has met with disaster or is, at the very least, at the center of the disaster. The central experiences of disaster are feelings of helplessness and abandonment. Individuals may have experienced a shocking loss of control of their environment, and loss of emotional control is usually viewed as a further threat. The reaction that sets in after a disaster can be seen as an attempt to understand what has happened and to find a satisfactory explanation for it. On the other hand, there is also the attempt to regain lost autonomy and the feeling of control of the environment. This requires a reevaluation of one's own beliefs. The change from victim to survivor requires that one be able to accept the undeniable fact that "bad" things can happen in the world and to oneself while also realizing that the world is not necessarily a bad place and one is not uniquely vulnerable (Bains, 1983, pp. 126–132; Janoff-Bulman, 1985, pp. 17–23; Lohman, 1969; Lifton, 1967; Raphael, 1986, pp. 55–60; Wolfenstein, 1957).

One way of reevaluating and reappraising a disaster experience is to ruminate about it obsessively or disclose pursuant feelings to others. The need to repeat an event in imagination may be related to the amount of anticipatory preparation and the strength of the experienced loss of control involved. If there were no anticipatory fantasies due to the suddenness of the event or the refusal to admit the existence of danger, the experienced loss of control will have been stronger and reestablishing control more difficult. Telling the experience to others provides a possibility to become gradually desensitized to the experience.

Self-disclosure also changes an individual from a passive to an active mode of processing and coping. A sudden disaster causes a strong need for action but may not provide opportunity for it. In the same way as inhibited emotional reactions, the actions not taken (i.e., failed enactments; Wilson, 1989) form part of reliving the event afterward. Reliving an event by talking about it may also be a defense against one's own helplessness. To avoid pain, the individual tries to apportion the experience according to his or her ability to tolerate it. Some details may be more difficult than others and, for this reason, the narratives of others may be a threat since they may activate material which the individual may not be ready to work-through (Figley, 1985, p. 404; Raphael, 1986, p. 94; Wolfenstein, 1957, pp. 135–143).

For those who have experienced a disaster, the ordinary reaction is a fear of the event reoccurring. The feeling of invulnerability of a victim of disaster has been altered; the world has changed from a safe place into one in which disasters happen. The fear of repetition may be associated with a delayed emotional reaction and a tendency to relive the disaster experience. A state of tension and the alertness created by the disaster may develop into vigilance or hypervigilance. Central to speculations as to the potential for reoccurrence are such concerns as: Can I prepare for it this time? Will I be overwhelmed again? Who will be injured? Thus, depending on the personality dynamics of the victim, vigilance or hypervigilance may lead to states of preparedness or maladaptive avoidance.

Emergency Worker as a Secondary Victim

Those persons who work with disaster, such as police, fire, and medical personnel, are trained and experienced in working with crisis situations and with the dead and the wounded. It has been believed, and in many quarters is still believed, that this protects them from psychological damage. By definition, disasters are exceptional situations, so that it is very probable that in each disaster the majority of the emergency workers will have no previous experience of death and suffering on such a wide scale. Emergency workers have begun to be thought of as *secondary victims* of a disaster. Although they do not personally experience the physical effects of the disaster, they do see the destruction it has produced and experience secondhand the losses of others (Bolin, 1985, p. 6).

In a disaster, the demand–capability ratio is out of balance and in many cases the demands exceed resources. Qualitative loading of an emergency or of disaster work refers to the difficulty and complexity of the task (Aronoff & Wilson, 1985). In a disaster, work may be loaded both *quantitatively* and *qualitatively*. For example, work is often done under pressure, in haste with many competing demands. There are time limits involved in getting the wounded to proper medical treatment. If these limits are exceeded, the chances of the wounded for survival decrease. The incessant and urgent demands inherent in disasters often demand and require that those who are engaged in helping try to establish control, aid, and care in the face of the disaster (Raphael, 1986, pp. 230–232). Moreover, disaster workers often set high expectations for themselves at this task; consequently, failure or inability in helping to reduce the trauma of the situation may lead to feelings of personal failure (Hartsough & Myers, 1985).

On the other hand, working in a disaster is also rewarding in many respects. One of the inspiring sides of disaster work is the satisfaction that saving human life brings. The atmosphere is typically very intense, and sharing experiences creates a feeling of closeness and common purpose. Often, workers feel that they are doing something much more important, valuable, and meaningful than mundane jobs. The relationship between the workers and the victims is often much closer emotionally than in normal working life. The victims of disaster are chosen by fate. Identification with the victim may be strong, which is one of the principal reasons why the worker feels the grief and suffering of the victim so strongly. Identification with the victim may also strengthen the helpers' own feelings of vulnerability and make them more reflective on the meaning of life and death.

As Wilson (1989) and others have noted, working with victims of trauma and disaster can lead to powerful countertransference reactions, which must be fully recognized to aid in the successful process of rendering help and assistance (see Berah *et al.*, 1984; Raphael, 1986, pp. 232–238).

Mitigating the Psychological Effects of Disaster: Group-Based Self-Esteem

It is a truism that individuals have a need for positive self-esteem. When a social group affects the definition of the self, the need for self-esteem motivates a desire to evaluate that group more positively. Tajfel and Turner (1979) referred to this as the need for positive social identity. In a disaster, the victims and those helpers who are involved initially begin to form an in-group. One's own group is often evaluated in comparison to other groups with respect to central values. Moreover, social categories are evaluated through social comparisons with other categories as to relevant value dimensions (Festinger, 1954). The need for positive social identity motivates individuals to look for and reinforce the positive aspects of their group in relation to other groups, that is, to prefer their own group in social perception. The mere division into in- and out-groups is often sufficient for the creation of intergroup discrimination even in situations of disaster (J. C. Turner, 1982, pp. 33–34).

Common group membership has the potential to motivate altruistic behavior. In a disaster, helping may become a group norm in which the victims cooperate to aid less fortunate others. Social identification with the changed social order then explains the expansion of the citizen's civic role described by Dynes (1970) and the creation of new norms. One's own group is then evaluated positively. Many victims emphasize the positive effect of the experience on the community and how well it, in turn, has coped with the disaster.

Organizations external to the trauma, which were not on the scene from the beginning, may very well become an out-group, because they do not share the victims' emotional experiences and common social identity. When a disaster is exceptionally destructive, the resources limited, and help is lacking, unavailable, or ineffective, it may become difficult for an individual to find positive characteristics in the group which would increase self-esteem. When there are no positive differentiating features in the group, individuals are motivated to dissociate themselves from the group. Such cognitive operations may result in not helping others, since the feeling of being a member of a group (which, in turn, forms the basis for altruism in disasters) is lacking.

The creation of norms which support prosocial behavior aids the recovery process but may set limits on posttraumatic reactions. Norms may be created in the community which, for example, regulate the way in which grief at a loss is expressed. Such norms may then complicate the individual recovery process.

Helping as a Means to Positive Identity

In the area of altruism and prosocial behavior, motives for helping have been studied, but little attention has been paid to the effects on the recipient (Aronoff & Wilson, 1985). According to attribution theory, receiving help and seeking help may be interpreted as negative or unfavorable information about one's own abilities. When receiving help becomes a norm, however, this normativeness can directly affect attribution processes. Thus, if the persons receiving help believe that everyone in a similar situation would need help, they would not necessarily doubt their own abilities or suffer a loss of self-esteem. We believe that personal reasons for seeking aid which is based on need causes more negative attributions than external normative factors which, in turn, are reflected in the attitudes of both the persons seeking help and those of others (Gross, Wallston, & Piliavin, 1980).

According to the theory of reciprocity, a feeling of independence requires reciprocal give and take. An inability to "pay back" makes reciprocity difficult and may lead to feelings of dislike toward the helpers, especially if they expect gratitude or recognition for their actions. From a social-psychological perspective, reciprocity is easier to maintain within relationships of friendship and family ties, and it is toward them the victims of a disaster try to get help. Reciprocity theory suggests that victims may strengthen their feelings of independence by accepting less help than is being offered or actually refusing certain types of help. In this way, they are able to decrease the power of the helpers over them.

The conceptions of the need for help held by some mental health workers and by disaster victims may conflict. Most disaster victims do not regard themselves as suffering from mental health problems in the immediate aftermath of a catastrophe and therefore do not believe that they need help. The disinclination of disaster victims to use mental health services is sometimes interpreted as reflecting a desire to avoid accepting the role of victim. The victim's role is often situationally determined, and mental health professionals have been criticized because they may enhance or enable the survivors to become locked into roles of passivity and dependence (Dynes, 1987b, pp. 88–89). Some guidelines for emergency workers presumptuously state that even if someone appears to be physically in good shape and capable of functioning, they could be severely affected nonetheless. Even the most capable-appearing disaster victim should, according to these guidelines, be expected to need psychiatric help (Mitchell, 1981).

Psychosocial Support

When mental health plans for intervention are revised, Hartsough (1982) suggested that it is possible to change either the helper, the services, the place, or the target group. In *planning* mental health programs for disasters, the things most ordinarily changed are the *target group* and the *place* where services will be offered. The aim is to bring the most effective services to the victims as soon as possible (Hartsough, 1982; Taylor *et al.*, 1976).

To recover psychologically from a disaster requires the return of feelings of autonomy and control so that feelings of helplessness decrease as well as other negative emotions. It also requires understanding of the event and what happened to the individual as well their attempts to integrate the experience. Usually, the victims of disaster have a need to change passivity into activity through talking and working-through the stressful and overwhelming aspects of the trauma they have undergone, and their specific role in the event. This represents the kind of emotional support that is most beneficial to restoring the normal stress recovery process (Horowitz, 1986; Raphael, 1986; Wilson, 1989).

Although disaster workers have the responsibility to provide the victims with emotional support as well, it is not always possible for several reasons indigenous to this type of work. First, carrying out certain tasks may require the suppression of feelings. The suppression or numbing of feelings may diminish empathic responding and effective problem-solving. Second, the sheer magnitude of a disaster may become a traumatic stressor for the disaster relief worker and lead to acute symptoms of PTSD. Third, the demands to help the victims may lead to a denial of personal feelings that only emerge at a later time.

Research results concerned with the factors which increase the risk of long-term or strong stress reactions are conflicting to some extent. The greatest agreement is found in risk factors which concern the *severity* of the disaster experience (Drabek, 1986, pp. 205–207). Intervention arranged for risk groups also succeed better when services are organized in connection with other help offered during the disaster, at least in the early stages (Raphael, 1986, pp. 269, 276). Also, early intervention has the advantage of creating an atmosphere in which the disaster relief workers are viewed as part of the total group and thus are more readily accepted (Peuler, 1985, pp. 19–20). Furthermore, mental health workers who take part in the work done immediately after the disaster are more empathetic and better able to understand the experiences of the victims (Raphael, 1986).

From the point of view of the prevention of psychological damage and the most effective crisis intervention, it is essential that there be cooperation with the organizations involved in the emergency work proper. Because the relationship between the mental health organization and the disaster organizations is often weak, it is important to create such liaison. Interagency cooperation and the careful orchestration of their different strengths, resources, and abilities can be mobilized to render maximum assistance to the disaster victims (Cohen & Ahearn, 1980, pp. 63–65; Raphael, 1986, pp. 251–252). For other perspectives on factors that mitigate stress reactions, see Chapters 65, 66, and 67 in this volume.

Conclusion

From our psychosocial perspective, one of the central issues in disasters is to a great extent a problem of perceived or actual control. It is also reflected in the myths that emerge and surround disasters and their effects. Such myths contain themes of destruction, panic, and chaos. These themes suggest a situation in which control has been lost.

The effects of a disaster and the problems created by it can be addressed on different levels. On the *societal level*, the problem is the maintaining of social order. On the *community level*, the problem is how to act efficiently and stabilize the chaotic situation created by the disaster. In estimating and evaluating the work of organizations, the expectations of control contained in the culture may be at odds with the situation, especially if the disaster is massive and not easily remedied.

Working in a disaster has been found to place stressful and often overwhelming demands on emergency workers. As noted by other authors in this *Handbook*, a disaster is often a traumatic experience for emergency workers. However, where disaster relief organizations adequately prepare, train, and debrief (i.e., facilitate the stress recovery process) the emotional reactions can be diminished and effectively dealt with.

Moreover, adequate training and preparation can, in turn, facilitate the effectiveness of the worker in the disaster. The workers should be made aware of the process leading to the development of prosocial, altruistic norms within the victimized population. Such developmental prosocial norms alter the existing social structure temporarily because the previous status roles in power structure function in nonoperative ways. Thus, the self-esteem of the worker and the victim can be enhanced with prosocial activity. However, reciprocity theory specifies that some victims of a disaster may not be able to accept help from workers who expect gratitude since it leads to a diminished sense of self-worth. Through the equalization of status with the emergent social structure of a disaster situation, prosocial behavior may lead to positive group identification and enhance the stress recovery process itself.

References

Aronoff, J., & Wilson, J. P. (1985). *Personality in the social process.* Hillsdale, NJ: Lawrence Erlbaum.

Bains, G. (1983). Explanations and the need for control. In M. Hewstone (Ed.), *Attribution theory: Social and functional extensions.* Oxford, England: Basil Blackwell.

Baisden, B., & Quarantelli, E. L. (1981). The delivery of mental health services in community disasters: An outline of research findings. *Journal of Community Psychology, 9,* 195–203.

Barton, A. (1969). *Communities in disasters: A sociological analysis of collective stress situations.* New York: Raven Press.

Baum, A., Fleming, R., & Singer, J. (1983). Coping with victimization by technological disaster. *Journal of Social Issues, 2,* 117–138.

Berah, E. F., Jones, H. J. & Valent, P. (1984). The experience of a mental health team involved in the early phase of a disaster. *Australian and New Zealand Journal of Psychiatry, 18,* 354–358.

Bolin, R. (1985). Disaster characteristics and psychosocial impacts. In B. J. Sowder (Ed.), *Disasters and mental health: Selected contemporary perspectives.* Rockville, MD: National Institute of Mental Health.

Britton, N. R. (1987). Toward a reconceptualization of disaster for the enhancement of social preparation. In R. R. Dynes, B. De Marchi, & C. Pelanda (Eds.), *Sociology of disasters.* Milan, Italy: Franco Angeli.

Caporale, R. (Speaker). (1987). *Differential vulnerability of social systems to natural disasters.* (Lecture). Helsinki: University of Helsinki.

Cohen, R. E. & Ahearn, F. L. (1980). *Handbook for mental health care of disaster victims.* Baltimore: Johns Hopkins University Press.

Drabek, T. E. (1985). Institutional and political contexts. In *Proceedings from a 1984 workshop sponsored by the National Institute of Mental Health and the Federal Emergency Management Agency.* Rockville, MD: National Institute of Mental Health.

Drabek, T. E. (1986). *Human system responses to disaster. An inventory of sociological findings.* New York: Springer-Verlag.

Dynes, R. R. (1970). *Organized behavior in disasters.* Lexington, MA: Heath Lexington Books.

Dynes, R. R. (1987a). Introduction. In R. R. Dynes, B. De Marchi, & C. Pelanda (Eds.), *Sociology of disasters. Contribution of sociology to disaster research.* Milan, Italy: Franco Angeli.

Dynes, R. R. (1987b). The concept of role in disaster research. In R. R. Dynes, B. De Marchi, & C. Pelanda (Eds.), *Sociology of disasters. Contribution of sociology to disaster research.* Milan, Italy: Franco Angeli.

Dynes, R. R., & Quarantelli, E. L. (1980). Helping behavior in large-scale disasters. In D. H. Smith, J. Macalay, & Associates (Eds.), *Participation in social and political activities.* San Francisco: Jossey-Bass.

Edberg, A. K., & Lustig, B. I. (1983). *Solidaritet och konflikt.* [Disaster Studies 14]. Uppsala, Sweden: University of Uppsala.

Erikson, K. (1976). *Everything in its path.* New York: Simon & Schuster.

Festinger, L. (1954). A theory of social comparison processes. *Human Relations, 7,* 117–140.

Figley, C. R. (1985). From victim to survivor: Social responsibility in the wake of catastrophe. In C. R. Figley (Ed.), *Trauma and its wake: The study and treatment of post-traumatic stress disorder.* New York: Brunner/Mazel.

Forrest, T. R. (1974). *Structural differentiation in emergent groups*

(Disaster Research Center Report Series No. 15). Columbus: Ohio State University Press.

Forrest, T. R. (1978). Group emergence in disasters. In E. L. Quarantelli (Ed.), *Disasters: Theory and research*. Beverly Hills: Sage Publications.

Frederick, C. J. (1980). Effects of natural vs. human-induced violence upon victims [Special Issue]. *Evaluation and Change*, 71–75.

Fritz, C. (1961). Disaster. In R. K. Merton & R. A. Nisbet (Eds.), *Contemporary social problems*. New York: Harcourt, Brace & World.

Green, B. L. (1985). Overview and research recommendations. In *Role stressors and supports for emergency workers. Proceedings from a 1984 Workshop Sponsored by the National Institute of Mental Health and the Federal Emergency Management Agency*. Rockville, MD: National Institute of Mental Health.

Gross, A. E., Wallston, B. S., & Piliavin, I. M. (1980). The help recipient's perspective. In D. H. Smith, J. Macalay, & Associates (Eds.), *Participation in social and political activities*. San Francisco: Jossey-Bass.

Hartsough, D. M. (1982). Planning for disaster: A new community outreach program for mental health centers. *Journal of Community Psychology, 10*, 255–264.

Hartsough, D. M., & Myers, D. G. (1985). *Disaster work and mental health: Prevention and control of stress among workers*. Rockville, MD: National Institute of Mental Health.

Hultaker, O. (1983). Family and disaster. *International Journal of Mass Emergencies and Disasters, 1*, 7–19.

Janoff-Bulman, R. (1985). The aftermath of victimization: Rebuilding shattered assumptions. In C. R. Figley (Ed.), *Trauma and its wake: The study and treatment of post-traumatic stress disorder* (pp. 15–35). New York: Brunner/Mazel.

Kemper, T. D. (1980). Altruism and voluntary action. In D. H. Smith, J. Macalay, & Associates (Eds.), *Participation in social and political activities*. San Francisco: Jossey-Bass.

Lifton, R. J. (1967). *Death in life: Survivors of Hiroshima*. New York: Simon & Schuster.

Lifton, R. J., & Olson, E. (1976). The human meaning of total disaster: The Buffalo Creek experience. *Psychiatry, 39*, 1–18.

Lohman, H. (1969). *Leva under hot. Om mánniskors beteende i katastrofsituationer* (Living under threat: On human behavior in disasters) (Aldusserien 273). Stockholm: Bokförlaget Aldus/Bonniers.

Mitchell, J. T. (1981). Multi-casualty situations. In J. T. Mitchell & H. L. P. Resnik (Eds.), *Emergency response to crisis: A crisis intervention guidebook for emergency service personnel*. London: Prentice-Hall International.

Perry, R. W. (1985). *Comprehensive emergency management: Evacuating threatened populations*. Greenwich, CT: JAI Press.

Perry, R. W., & Lindell, M. K. (1978). The psychological consequences of natural disaster: A review of research on American communities. *Mass Emergencies, 3*, 105–115.

Peuler, J. (1985). Family and community outreach in times of disaster: The Santa Cruz experience. In M. Lystad (Ed.), *Innovations in mental health services to disaster victims*. Rockville, MD: National Institute of Mental Health.

Quarantelli, E. L. (1980). *Sociology and social psychology of disasters: Implications for third world and developing countries*. Department of Sociology, Disaster Research Center, Ohio State University, Columbus.

Quarantelli, E. L. (1985a). What is disaster: The need for clarification in definition and conceptualization in research. In B. J. Sowder (Ed.), *Disasters and mental health: Selected contemporary perspectives*. Rockville, MD: National Institute of Mental Health.

Quarantelli, E. L. (1985b). An assessment of conflicting views on mental health: The consequences of traumatic events. In C. R. Figley (Ed.), *Trauma and its wake: The study and treatment of post-traumatic stress disorder* (pp. 173–215). New York: Brunner/Mazel.

Quarantelli, E. L., & Dynes, R. R. (1985). Community responses to disasters. In B. Sowder (Ed.), *Disasters and mental health: Selected contemporary perspectives*. Rockville, MD: National Institute of Mental Health.

Raphael, B. (1986). *When disaster strikes: How individuals and communities cope with catastrophe*. New York: Basic Books.

Staub, E. (1978). *Positive social behavior and morality*. New York: Academic Press.

Tajfel, H., & Turner, J. C. (1979). An integrative theory of intergroup conflict. In W. G. Austin & S. Worchel (Eds.), *The social psychology of intergroup relations*. Monterey, CA: Brooks/Cole.

Taylor, V., Ross, G. A., & Quarantelli, E. L. (1976). *Delivery of mental health services in disasters: The Xenia tornado and some implications* (Disaster Research Center, Book and Monograph Series No. 11). Columbus: Ohio State University Press.

Thomas, W. I., & Thomas, D. S. (1928). *The child in America: Behavior problems and programs*. New York: Knopf.

Turner, B. A. (1978). *Man-made disasters*. London: Wykenham Publications.

Turner, J. C. (1982). Towards a cognitive redefinition of the social group. In H. Tajfel (Ed.), *Social identity and intergroup relations*. Cambridge: Cambridge University Press.

Turner, R. H. (1967). Types of solidarity in the reconstituting of groups. *Pacific Sociological Review, 10*, 60–68.

United Nations. (1986). *Disaster prevention and mitigation*. New York: Author.

Wenger, D. E. (1978). Community response to disaster: Functional and structural alterations. In E. L. Quarantelli (Ed.), *Disasters: Theory and research*. Beverly Hills: Sage Publications.

Wilson, J. P., Smith, W. K., & Johnson, S. (1985). A comparative analysis of PTSD among various survivor groups. In C. J. Figley (Ed.), *Trauma and its wake: The study and treatment of post-traumatic stress disorder* (pp. 142–172). New York: Brunner/Mazel.

Wilson, J. P. (1989). *Trauma, transformation, and healing: An integrative approach to theory, research, and post-traumatic therapy*. New York: Brunner/Mazel.

Wolfenstein, M. (1957). *Disaster: A psychological essay*. London: Routledge & Kegan Paul.

CHAPTER 82

Temporary Organization for Crisis Intervention

When Disaster—A Hotel Fire—Strikes a Community

Renate Grønvold Bugge

Introduction

When disaster strikes a community, confusion often results. Usually, the implementation of contingency plans requires the cooperation of different organizations, groups, and individuals. Frequently, such units are poorly coordinated, at least initially. In addition, there will always be volunteers who want to help.

Often, in the acute circumstances of a disaster, there will be a lack of well-defined goals beyond the immediate goal of saving lives, and there will be a lack of clear priorities among the measures to be taken, which may lead to conflict and overreaction. Personnel who are involved in rescue work and crisis intervention tend to focus on their own specific areas of responsibility and action; they may fail to assess correctly the overall situation. As a result, there may be contradictory information regarding the extent of damage, the numbers of injured and dead, and precisely who is involved. This state of confusion will affect all participants from organizations down to individuals.

My personal point of view, nonetheless, is that temporary organizations will be formed during disaster situations, whether planned or not, either as totally new constellations of individuals or as a direct outgrowth of existing permanent organizations.

Temporary organizations exist only to carry out specific tasks and, when the task is finished, are disbanded.

Renate Grønvold Bugge • Vest-Agder Sentralsykehus, 4600 Kristiansand South, Norway.

International Handbook of Traumatic Stress Syndromes, edited by John P. Wilson and Beverley Raphael. Plenum Press, New York, 1993.

It will always be a challenge to make temporary organizations function adequately in the face of a disaster. Every critical situation brings with it unforeseen difficulties, making flexibility an important characteristic. Nevertheless, proper planning in the various permanent organizations will improve the effectiveness of temporary organizations as the need for them arises.

In this context, ordinary community agencies, such as the police, rescue agencies, and hospitals, should plan coordinated actions to cover acute rescue work and psychosocial crisis intervention. Also, it is of the utmost importance that transportation agencies, schools, and other enterprises develop contingency plans for disaster. When planning ahead, it will be helpful to focus on problems of organization, taking into account the experience gained from earlier crises (Turner, Thompson, & Rosser, 1989). In this chapter, I will cite the experience that was obtained during a specific disaster—a hotel fire in Norway.

Disaster Situation

The Caledonian Hotel, which was built in 1969, was the newest hotel in Southern Norway. It was generally believed to be very safe because it was built in full compliance with Norway's relatively strict building codes. The maximum capacity of the hotel's 230 rooms was approximately 400 guests. On the night of the fire, 113 were guests registered.

Several conferences had ended the night before the fire. Most of the participants had departed for England, Sweden, or various destinations in Norway. Some stayed, however, and woke up to a disaster in the early morning hours on September 5, 1986.

Four hours after the rescue work started the following facts were known: (1) 14 hotel guests had lost their lives, not by fire but by asphyxiation—the rescuers had arrived too late for them; (2) 54 hotel guests had been treated by the hospital staff, and (3) 13 of those who received treatment were hospitalized because of injuries with 2 being seriously injured. The next day, however, all of them were released either to go home or for transfer to other hospitals in their home communities. Colleagues, family members, the townspeople of Kristiansand, and the whole country were overwhelmed with emotion at the news of the disaster.

It seemed unreal to hear news of a catastrophic fire in our town. At that hour no one could yet say what the dimensions of the disaster were.

In the acute phase, immediately after the rescue operations, the guests were brought to a military camp nearby where several agencies took care of them. Teams from two psychiatric hospitals were sent to the main evacuation site.

Rescue Operations in the Hotel Fire Disaster

The rescue operations and assistance offered in connection with the fire can be summarized roughly as follows:

1. *Acute/emergency assistance*: The medical and physical treatment lasted from 4:40 a.m. to about 9:00 a.m.
2. *Preventive psychiatric assistance*: (a) Psychiatric teams were in operation from 9:30 a.m. to 2:00 p.m.; (b) an office for bereaved families was opened at 1:00 p.m. and remained open throughout the day; and (c) psychological assistance started at 7:10 p.m.

The following day, debriefing groups were started and information and letters were dispatched to involved groups. Debriefing groups and psychological support work continued throughout the following 9 days. We concentrated our efforts on these groups: (1) bereaved families; (2) hotel guests (both hospitalized and released); (3) relatives, colleagues, and friends; (4) rescue and medical personnel; and (5) observers.

We found that we had to cope with different emotional reactions, depending upon affected person's involvement with the fire. We dealt mainly with the following reactions: (1) anxiety, (2) loss/grief, (3) shock, and (4) reactivation (Weisæth, 1986).

At the time of the hotel disaster, I was in charge of the children's psychiatric department at the main hospital. I received authority from the catastrophe leader, who was the head of the medical department at the hospital, to organize the psychological support work. His decision to delegate the responsibility for organizing the psychological support work was made at a meeting where a representative from the Norwegian Director of Health was present together with professionals from the state level who had special experience from previous catastro-

phes. In my position as organizer of psychological assistance and debriefing, I reported to the catastrophe leader at the hospital. Different lines of cooperation and report seemed to be necessary, however, because the support work involved several local, regional, national, and international institutions.

When a disaster strikes (Raphael, 1986) there will always be several organizations and professions involved. Each organization will have plans for crisis intervention. In Norway, the chief of the local police department is in charge of coordinating rescue operations.

The hospital is a permanent institution with its structures of organization that are meant to fulfil certain goals. When disaster strikes, a *temporary organization* has to be created. Often it is created out of the basic elements of a permanent organization. In an emergency situation, new forms of cooperation among several organizations must emerge. Furthermore, in a crisis, subgroups from several professions work together under new leadership. Rescue personnel from different organizations are scattered on different teams. Medical personnel from different organizations will cooperate in the acute situation.

In this chapter, I will deal with some of the experiences from my position in the temporary organization that was created in September, 1986, when the Caledonian Hotel in Kristiansand, Norway, burned. As a starting point, I will explain the Tavistock model of group relations as it pertains to the development of temporary organizations following disasters.

In a catastrophe situation special plans are put into action. This situation can be compared to a temporary organization with several subgroups. The hospital's temporary organization includes all responsibility in the work that has to be carried out in the acute medical phase. In addition, psychological support work was brought into function on this particular occasion.

Theoretical Background: The Tavistock Model

The analysis of these experiences will be based on the theoretical frame of reference known as the *Tavistock model*. The Tavistock model was developed at the Tavistock Institute of Human Relations and is now used in Group Relations Training Programs in several countries. The Tavistock aspiration and goal was to develop an integrated science of human behavior. These theoretical concepts will be used in explaining social policy issues in disaster intervention. "We try to develop a theory of organization that reconciles tasks, human activities, and organization within one general framework" (Miller & Rice, 1967).

The term "Tavistock model" refers to a heuristic framework for identifying and understanding what conscious and unconscious processes take place within and between groups of people. The usage of the word "model" implies a tradition with identifiable, experiential, and intellectual roots that is being reinterpreted and reworked by representatives of different organizations (Lawrence, 1979).

Bion (1961) elaborates the working hypotheses and methodology on which the Tavistock model is founded.

Bion was able to see that in any group there are simultaneously present two groups: the *work group* and the *basic assumption group*. The work group supports the skills of its members and recognizes their differences in a realistic way. This kind of group is not fixed to roles or to a structure, to a past history, or to an exclusive future organization. Such a group can change according to the changing circumstances of the environment.

Parallel with the work group, some groups operate on certain unspoken assumptions. Bion (1961) identifies three basic assumption groups:

1. The basic assumption *dependency* group (BaD). This group is dependent on one leader who is experienced as omnipotent in contrast to other participants as helpless.
2. The basic assumption *pairing* group (BaP). This group has a model of expectancy and hopefulness, longing for a savior.
3. The basic assumption *fight/flight* group (BaF/F). This group is one of action. The role of the leader is to mobilize fight or flight processes in order to preserve the group. Feelings of paranoia are typically projected out of the group.

Bion's hypotheses essentially address the myths on which groups of people operate. There is always, in any group, a conflict between the individual and the group. If we think conceptually about individuals and groups as open systems, this conflict can become a positive way of testing realities in a changing environment. In reality it is more often likely that both the individual and the group are looked upon as closed systems. When this occurs, the individual faces the risk of being "lost in the group."

Subdivisions by Content Area

My role at the main hospital in Kristiansand, in the southern part of Norway, gave me some perspectives on how a temporary organization can work. This means a temporary organization on different levels, whether national, regional, local, or in a single organization. I will emphasize the temporary organization within the frame of the hospital, although I have to take into account the cooperation with organizations on the other levels (see Figure 82.1).

In Figure 82.2, I present some of the reactions that occurred when other organizations were involved, either through representatives in the local organization or by delegation of tasks.

I next focus specifically on the groups responsible for psychological assistance. These groups may be regarded as comprising an organization on their own, though they are only part of the whole crisis unit at the hospital.

Finally, on a microlevel, I will analyze some of the reactions that occurred within the involved groups and individuals and discuss the connection between reactions and roles in the organization. This discussion will include roles from different systems/organizations such as rescue personnel, hotel staff, medical personnel, expert teams, survivors, and bereaved families (see Figure 82.3).

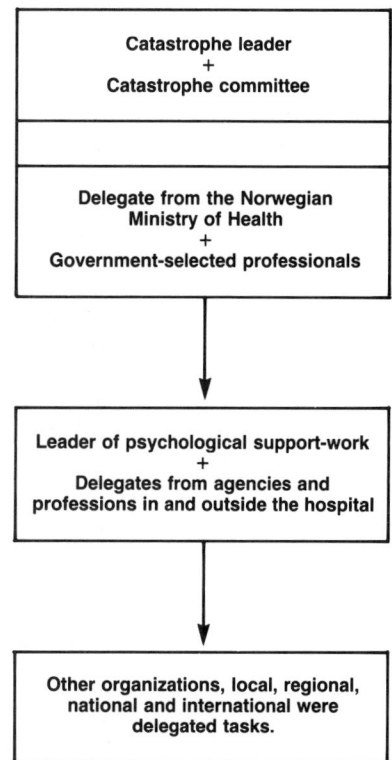

Figure 82.1. Lines of delegation.

There was no precedence, either at the hospital or in the community, for giving assistance after the rescue operation or the emergency medical treatment. When the psychological assistance started, the medical and physical treatment had been terminated several hours earlier. The crisis manager returned to his position as hospital chief-of-staff, without realizing that our work was part of the emergency situation and required more time than the medical emergency phase.

We realized that we needed his leadership for the duration of the whole task. This was an important realization and it made clear to us how much confusion can arise during a crisis because the staff either leave their positions or others take on more work than they are supposed to, or external experts fail to properly transfer the tasks they have been involved to others who would assume their responsibilities.

When the crisis manager at the hospital delegated the organizational work to me, neither of us had any hypotheses about what the work would consist of. It was urgent to recruit professionals for the work ahead. Since this was a disaster that effected the whole region, we called professionals from several agencies. These included: (1) doctors from the national health service; (2) school psychologists; (3) medical nurses from the national health service; (4) social workers; (5) psychiatric nurses; (6) members of the clergy; and (7) psychiatrists.

It was a clear policy to recruit assistance from the local health and social services to underline that immediate crisis intervention can be offered at the local level. It

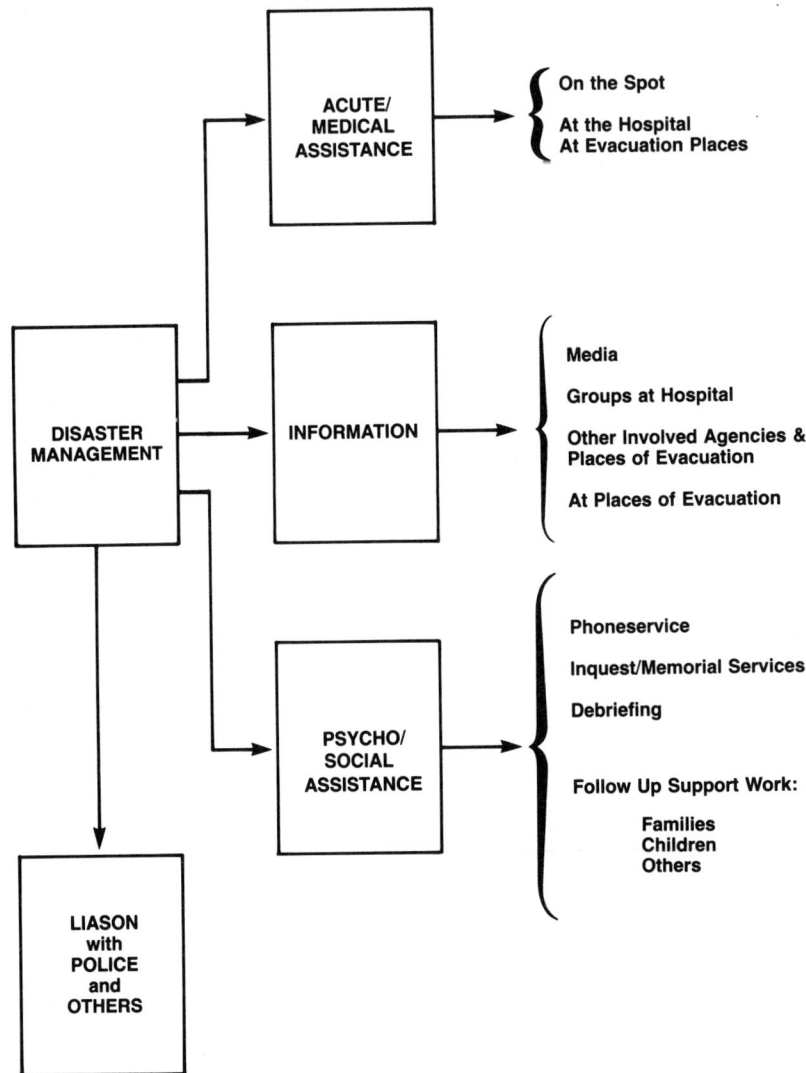

Figure 82.2. Temporary organization for crisis intervention.

is not necessary to think of crisis intervention as a new field of expertise offered by just a few. Everyone who was recruited joined the team of psychological support workers and accepted the leadership that was provided by the hospital. In organizational terms, this meant that each was a representative from a different permanent organization. These organizations granted leaves of absence to their professionals who joined the disaster team. The professionals were contacted by telephone and told when they were expected at the hospital. There was already a list of those who were willing to volunteer for this kind of service.

In these circumstances, negotiation and goal definition are important in creating cooperation between different groups. Furthermore, it is important to be clear about different levels of representation and what kind of authority is connected with representation. It is often the case that failure to formally delegate responsibility to representatives destroys the possibilities for cooperation between groups.

The clear delegation of authority, with direct lines up to the Director of Health, made it possible for us to give assistance throughout Norway and foreign countries, too. There was a group from Scandinavian Airlines System (SAS) at the hotel. Their home base was Stockholm, Sweden. The SAS personnel cooperated with our support team at the hospital. Several of them came back to Kristiansand within a few days to face the reality of their survival. SAS also asked for advice on how to prevent posttraumatic stress disorders (PTSD). This meant, for instance, establishing a training program to make the survivors able to continue to travel and stay in hotels, to prevent phobic reactions that might otherwise make invalids of their employees (see Chapter 78, in this volume, for a discussion of employee assistance programs for PTSD).

There were also other foreign visitors involved; it was important to establish contact with official channels of information and to create possibilities for those involved or families of the bereaved to come to Norway.

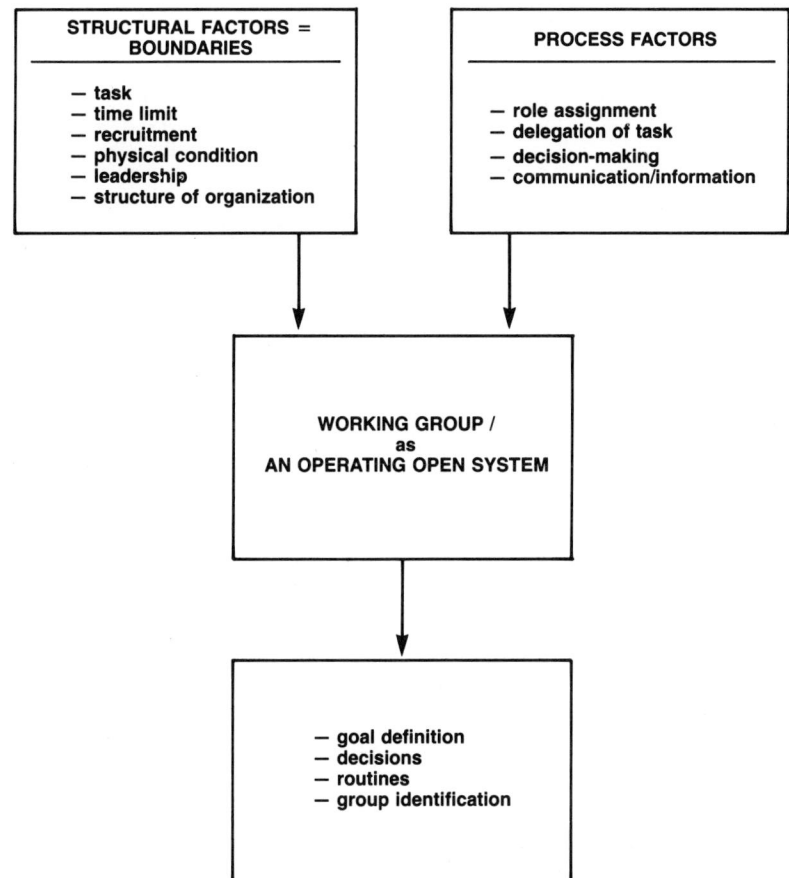

Figure 82.3. Model for evaluating an organization as a working group (i.e., an open operating system).

Domestically we were unable to offer all the victims crisis assistance directly. In several cases, we asked for assistance from the local communities where those involved were living. For instance, we phoned mental health personnel in different regions during the follow-up. We contacted key persons in the actual areas for the necessary aid to high-risk victims. We were sometimes met by bureaucratic boundaries but could put force behind our requests for assistance because our authority was given directly by the Director of Health. We also asked the police for assistance in delivering messages to families. We had to establish cooperation with the police to prepare for the following inquest. Sometimes this came into conflict with identification procedures.

These are examples of the importance of clear leadership. Formal leadership, delegated from above and supported and accepted by co-workers and other agencies, provides authority. This kind of authority enabled us to make decisions and use resources commensurate with the situation. The more complicated a task is, and the more agencies, professionals, and regions involved, the more important it is that the responsible leader has clearly delegated authority and that this authority is accepted by co-workers (see Figures 82.1 and 82.2). This psychological support work was carried out by what developed into an autonomous organization, but it is important to emphasize that it was conducted within the larger crisis-management organization at the hospital.

We ran into some problems in coordinating our efforts. Frustration developed between our workers and the switchboard operators, for example. It turned out that the switchboard had received no prior information about our work. We then established regular communication on every shift, exchanging information on what could be expected, the names of those on duty, and which phones and offices were in use.

The hospital had established an office for the survivors and bereaved families as part of the ordinary plan for disaster and crisis management. It was necessary to establish an exchange of information to prevent duplication of effort and avoid contradictory information.

On paper, there was a plan to coordinate the release of information to newspapers, radio, and television. But, in fact, reporters came directly to the support team because it was a new aspect in the management of a local civilian disaster. There was also a lack of communication between the different teams of helpers. We found that it was quite important to keep in touch with the catastrophe organization as a whole. However, this was often complicated due to the following problems: (1) psychological assistance was not part of the ordinary plan for crisis/disasters, and (2) there was too little awareness of the fact that psychological assistance would take time.

The fire broke out on a Friday morning. The work through the weekend could go on without interfering with ordinary work at the hospital. When the ordinary hospital service started again on Monday a conflict arose. Resources such as telephones, offices, and personnel that had been recruited by crisis management were called for when the ordinary hospital service started again. We had to negotiate and ended up with compromises so that both the permanent organization and the temporary organization could meet their primary tasks.

For both organizations, meeting tasks required keeping focus on clientele. For the permanent organization, this meant patients with appointments and scheduled examinations. For the temporary organization, this meant family members and survivors who were in the middle of an emergency. When the rescue and medical-emergency phase was concluded, an evaluation was done. At this time the psychological work was still at its peak; it was a very tense situation. One part of the temporary organization had ended its work and the other part still was in the middle of it. It seemed like a collision of two different cultures with different traditions and different modes of thought. Ordinarily, medical-emergency work is finished when there are no more lives to be saved. *But it is at that time that psychosocial reactions begin reaching the surface.*

We found that it was necessary to use the media to provide information about preventive intervention in schools and nurseries after we became aware that children were affected. Several youngsters had been at the hotel site without permission, a number of parents had been there as onlookers, and children of rescue workers had posttraumatic reactions connected with their awareness of the danger. It proved useful to supply information and instructions through the media.

These interventions were offered at a time when it was a conviction in the medical community that the need for such assistance was exaggerated. This again illustrates that we have to be aware of *potentially conflicting communities* within the health services. And we must emphasize again that it is not a question of being right or wrong, but of combining professional knowledge and resources for the benefit of those who are involved when disaster strikes a community. These experiences certainly carry consequences for the future integration of medical-emergency assistance with psychological crisis intervention.

Psychological Support Work as a Part of Temporary Crisis Organization

Application of Concepts from the Tavistock Group Relation Model

During the hotel fire, a temporary organization was created from scratch. Experience from group-relations conference work was used to build the organization and to put it into operation. It was important to focus attention on some of the major concepts from the model, such as the primary task and the differing roles and functions in a temporary organization, in order to clarify the importance of authority and delegation.

Definition of Goals and Methods

The primary task all this time was crisis intervention, debriefing and optimizing the benefits for those affected. An important part of this was always to take care of phone calls and the people affected by the disaster. The door to the office was always open and the team leader was always responsible for the phone.

In this kind of intensive and personally stressful work, it is very important to get a sense of the psychological condition of the support workers as well. If someone had personal problems, he or she would have to leave for a while and be debriefed. Such problems could only be worked out within the team if there were quiet periods. This can be compared to the processes occurring in groups when conflict develops between a basic assumption group and a work group. There were always desires to work out personal reactions. These differed between the groups on duty.

Guidelines in the Temporary Organization

In creating a working organization, it is necessary to establish guidelines that have to be followed by everyone joining the organization. In the case of the actual support work, this meant guidelines for *establishing contact*. In handling telephone calls this meant:

1. *Presenting oneself* by name and saying that one worked with the psychological support team. This made contact with the same worker possible in case of follow-up calls.

2. Immediately asking for the *caller's name, phone number, and address* to make it possible to call back in case of interruption, which had to be expected under chaotic circumstances and with a shortage of telephone lines.

3. Ascertaining the caller's *role in the disaster*. The roles included (a) directly involved in the present disaster as survivors, involved family members, bereaved family members, or rescue workers; or (b) indirectly involved when earlier traumatic situations get reactivated by the present disaster.

4. Making a *clinical evaluation* of the caller by listening to his or her tone of voice, choice of words, and level of coherence. This was important in judging the caller's psychological state to establish whether depression, anxiety, anger, or guilt were expressed. It was important to be aware of the danger of suicide as a posttraumatic reaction.

5. Making sure to ask about the caller's *present social situation*. Was the person alone or with family or friends. If the caller was alone, we encouraged the individual to contact neighbors and/or friends, even at night. If the caller was isolated, we made sure he or she made contact with professionals in the local network.

6. *Following up* to make sure that arrangements were carried through. We were aware that promises that are not kept increase anxiety and discomfort.

7. Keeping everyone connected with the support work *up to date on information*. This helped prevent rumors and frustration, keeping the different groups together in the crisis organization. Where there is a lack of up-to-date information, working groups are known to

split into basic assumption groups, in which the climate of dependency, pairing, and fight/flight flourishes. It is well known that in situations of stress, conflict and co-operation tend to grow, mirroring these group processes.

Structure and Organization of the Temporary Agency of Crisis Intervention

Because of my experience as a staff member in group relation conferences, I was able to apply this model to the structure of the subsystem to attempt to make it function adequately.

Specifically, this meant designing an organization in which:

1. It was known at all times who was the leader in authority.
2. The 55 volunteers from different agencies in the region were organized into teams working on 8-hour shifts each day for the first 5 days. Then, the next 4 days, they did phone-calling.
3. All teams received a brief introduction from the subsystem leader to the procedures associated with their different tasks expected. All information was passed on formally to prevent rumors and wrong decisions.
4. A team leader was assigned.
5. All team leaders had to report to the subsystem leader. This leader met each team leader either before the worker went on duty or early in the morning at the end of the shift.
6. Each team member was to fulfill his or her job and report to the team leader. The team leader was responsible for collecting all the material on what had been done during the last shift.

Individual Roles in the Disaster Work

In what follows I focus on the individual roles of team workers in the organization of psychological support work.

As mentioned above, the team members were recruited from different agencies and professions. They had to clarify their involvement on their own with their employment authorities. Their positions in their home agencies did not determine their positions in the temporary organization. In the organization, positions were assigned on the basis of professional competence, experience, and personal ability. This meant, for instance, that a psychiatric nurse was preferred as administrative team leader because of specific abilities and prior experience in administration. Team members comprised members of the clergy, doctors, and psychologists.

It was also important to look for special professional competence in working with bereaved children. Psychologists from child and youth psychiatric clinics were asked to take this task. Split families also needed special professional attention. Empathy and an elementary knowledge of crisis intervention were not sufficient.

Before the temporary organization for psychological support work disbanded, we had a staff meeting which all 55 volunteers were asked to attend, along with the

crisis manager. He gave a review of the whole crisis organization with its different elements. In the course of psychological debriefing, each member talked about his role in the temporary organization. For example:

1. I was told several times by Renate to stay on duty, in case I was needed. I kept close to the telephone, but did not get one single call. I feel very frustrated about not being used in spite of being told to stay ready.

2. I wonder why I was used in almost every role, as administrator and as professional in different complicated situations. I was exhausted and quite frustrated at hearing that others were not called upon at all.

These two examples illustrate what seemed to be obvious in other groups within the medical system: (1) Frustration is created when helpers are prepared to work without getting the chance. (2) Stress results when team members are overwhelmed by responsibility. The concept of roles is also useful in analyzing different individuals and groups at risk. Crisis produces stress for many kinds of groups. In general, those whose workplace is endangered, along with rescue personnel, hospital staff, and family members face a great risk of stress overload.

Role Stress in the Crisis Intervention Worker

The role played by the involved person might have a great impact on his reactions. Let me give some examples.

Workplace

Elected union leaders have to carry the burden of anxiety for their colleagues. Will they lose their jobs? What will the future bring? Substitute leaders are also put under pressure. They must suddenly carry out responsibilities in an acute situation, which they may not be prepared for. Employees must evaluate dangerous situations or work under hazardous conditions.

The wife of a hotel staff member telephoned. She was very upset about her husband. He had crawled into bed and stayed there drinking all the time. She described totally regressive behavior. At last it was possible to make him come to the telephone. Our team worker motivated him to come and see us. He could not understand his own reactions. He felt afraid, scared, and he did not want to meet his colleagues although he knew that they cared about him. He told us that he was the vice president of the local union for hotel staff members. The president was on vacation and therefore he suddenly had to face all the anxiety of his colleagues. He carried the burden of the questions: Will we lose our jobs? Will we be fired? He also knew that he would be called for military service within a few days. He simply could not cope with the idea of leaving home to face such a situation. It was a relief to him to become aware of his position in the hotel organization. Because of his place in the organization, he had to carry a lot of projections from his colleagues. In this case, his role in the organization, anxiety, and life situation together led to the extreme reaction of regression.

One of the chambermaids phoned. She did not like her reactions because they did not go along with her image of herself as a strong person. In this first session it turned out that several earlier traumatic experiences had been reactivated. Her anxiety about becoming insane did not improve at the second session. She was the leader of the chambermaids. At that time, it was decided that this group should start going through the rooms in the hotel to remove personal belongings left by the guests. In her staff many developed quite strong phobic reactions to this task. Some of them had personal grief too, because they had known some of the deceased guests quite well. She wanted to protect her staff from the pain. On the other hand, she was put under pressure because her staff was expected to do this work. Her staff was an invisible group in the hotel organization. This group had no way to make its grief and reactions visible, in contrast to some of the other staff groups who were quite central. When she began to realize that she, because of her role at the hotel, had a real burden to carry, she became relieved of her personal concern about her own insanity.

Family Members

Ex-family members are put under special pressure. Ex-wives have no official status as bereaved widows, but may still have close ties to their deceased spouse. Bereaved teenagers are often overlooked, and are confused about how to relate to a dead or injured parent if he or she has established a new family. Smaller children are often excluded from crisis intervention activities such as inquests and memorial ceremonies. Even when they are involved, the assistance they receive is often insufficient.

A father and his two minor sons started to work with their grief. Wife and mother, who was dead, would not come back any more. It was important to talk through how it would be meaningful to say a formal good-bye to her. I asked the children, "What would you have liked to tell her if she were still here? Perhaps you could write her a letter and put it in her coffin? What did you like to play with her? Perhaps you could take the little matchbox car when you take leave with her? You could express what you feel by drawing her a picture." I helped the boy and put the drawing into the coffin in front of his mother's face. Afterwards I asked the boys what they were going to remember from these hours in the church at their mother's coffin. The smaller one said: "I didn't expect mother to be lying as she did." I kept thinking about this and finally realized that his angle of view as a little boy was very different. None of us adults had lifted him up so that he could see his mother from a natural position.

Rescue and Medical Personnel

Those who have just started in a new job such as nurses and doctors in training, part-time workers, who often lack the feeling of identity and support from their colleagues in working through the trauma, and rescue personnel who have been mobilized but not used might also experience psychological difficulty. This is true especially if these workers wait for hours without knowing if they are to be used and without knowing when the operation has been terminated.

Others

This group includes all the spectators who watch the catastrophe unfold either on the spot or through the media. It is especially important to consider children's reactions. Children who have been at the disaster site without their parents' knowledge, for example, do not know how to unload their reactions and impressions.

Discussion and Conclusion

In a disaster, conflicts will arise between permanent organizations and the temporary organization that is set up to deal with the situation. The temporary organization is usually planned on paper. Leadership, areas of responsibility, and delegative authority seem clear in organizations such as the police, fire department, and hospital. Still, evaluation reports often reveal chaos and confusion in plans of action, lines of communication, acts of delegation, and the integration of different subgroups.

In connection with the hotel fire, the hospital's disaster plan was invoked and several wards were alerted, but several of the emergency wards failed to get the message that their services were *not* needed. The personnel were under pressure for many hours and then had the experience of not even being noticed.

In an acute situation, different groups or individuals often start with the same kind of work. In the ordinary disaster plan at the hospital, there is a routine for establishing an information office for involved and bereaved families. When psychological assistance began there were no lines of communication between this service and the established office. There was also a lack of communication between these offices and the police. This led to confusion during the identification of the victims.

These are examples of what can happen in a small community. In large communities, it is well known that chaos can arise when several agencies or organizations offer psychosocial assistance independently of the other providers. However, in both small and large scale disasters, it is necessary to share a coordinating leader who can define and delegate responsibility both in the acute phase—lasting up to two weeks after a disaster—and in the follow-up work for at least a year after the disaster. The primary task of rescue operations, medical aid, and psychological assistance is management focused on survivors, bereaved families, and helpers. The crucial question will be: How does one organize for the problems that have to be solved?

Different views of what is necessary stem from the different roles found in permanent organizations. A medical doctor will concentrate on his primary task: to save life, even in a crisis. A social worker, psychiatrist, or psychologist will focus on psychosocial aspects both in the acute phase and in follow-up. These are not contradictory aims: The focus is on crisis management. But each role affects perception. The challenge in every crisis is to integrate the acute rescue/medical work with the psychosocial crisis management. Both should be recognized and integrated in a temporary organization. Survivors and helpers may become "secondary victims" of a rivalry between different experts or psychosocial assistants. This will occur if there is a lack of integration between traditional crisis-management organizations on national, regional, and local levels.

Over time, permanent organizations develop special means to provide for their own survival. Survival of the organization will be seen as more important than will a continuous redefinition of its tasks. A temporary organization which is designed on paper to manage crises will also tend to have the characteristics of a permanent organization.

In a hospital, the responsible leader will typically be a doctor, supported by the head doctors of other departments. This does not mean that the responsible crisis manager will have any particular knowledge of crisis management. He will judge the situation from his ordinary position and knowledge. It will be necessary, therefore, to bring in other professionals in different roles. The existence of a temporary role assumes perception of different sectors that may complete the actions of assistance; this assumption does not discredit other roles in the permanent system.

Lessons Learned from the Disaster: Effective Intervention upon Recurrence

In June, 1989, there was a large NATO exercise in Norway. Kristiansand was the site of a large rescue operation which involved the central rescue headquarters for southern Norway, the Kristiansand Police Department, and the hospital; the exercise included an actual plane crash. It proved useful to take advantage of the experience gained from the hotel fire in 1986, thus showing how a temporary organization designed for disasters can adjust to the primary task at hand.

In 1986, it was not clear that psychosocial assistance should be included in disaster plans. In 1989, psychosocial personnel were alerted immediately along with medical personnel. In 1986, there was no organized communication between the police, the crisis manager, and the head of the psychosocial assistance group. In 1989, a representative from this subsystem was sent to the police to coordinate all necessary information. This improved the work done with survivors and involved/bereaved families. In 1989, we used the experience gained in 1986 to provide within the first hour two teams of psychiatric personnel at the sites where victims were expected to be sent.

In 1986, there was no organized care for those who were sent to the hospital. Those who were not hurt had to leave again without special attention. In 1989, we organized personnel who were not involved in the emergency medical care to join groups of families and survivors. This made it possible to provide them with information and reduce confusion and anxiety. At the main evaluation and debriefing meetings, it became obvious that the police officer in charge did not know that the psychosocial assistance team had been alerted, too. He openly expressed approval, however, for the fact that the hospital had included this form of assistance in their crisis-management plan. It is hoped that an information coordinator between the hospital and the police

will be called into action the next time disaster strikes, whether in reality or in an exercise.

Summary

When a disaster strikes, many different organizations become involved. Family and personal tragedies can often be resolved in a satisfactory way if rescue and psychological assistance are organized according to the need.

In this presentation, I have illustrated how concepts and methods taken from group-relations conferences in that Tavistock tradition may be useful in creating a temporary organization to meet an extraordinary situation. The presentation also emphasizes how important it is to define responsibility and leadership clearly.

An individual's role in the organization (both formal and informal), that person's life circumstances, and the anxiety the participant feels in the emergency situation are the three main factors contributing to an emergency worker's reaction. Strong leadership and good communication are necessary in the temporary organization during the acute phase if problems in further cooperation are to be avoided afterward.

Areas of responsibility have to be maintained clearly throughout a crisis; a crisis itself will ordinarily engender chaos. It is important that everyone knows who is in charge and when and to whom responsibility is transferred.

Resource people (e.g., professionals from diverse fields) have to cooperate with local leaders, following supervision and/or temporary leadership. It is important to acknowledge the authority of the local leaders during the acute phase because they have to continue working after the acute phase.

The design of the work conference in the Tavistock tradition reflects conflicts between the basic assumption group and the work group. These conflicts are also seen in temporary organizations set up to deal with crisis.

The work conference also reflects the complexity of organizations where there is often tension between the individual and the group, between subgroups within the organization, and between management and members. In crises, tension between outside experts and local professionals can also arise, especially if the delegation of responsibility is unclear.

Concepts taken from group-relations conferences can be applied usefully both in creating temporary organizations and in evaluating their performance. In the future, it would be useful for persons working in critical incident stress debriefing and disaster intervention to jointly share the collected knowledge to further advance our knowledge of how to create temporary organizations to meet the various needs of disaster victims in order to promote psychological well-being.

References

Bion, W. R. (1961). *Experiences in groups*. London: Tavistock Publications.

Lawrence, W. G. (Ed.). (1979). Introductory essay: Exploring boundaries. In *Exploring individual and organizational boundaries: A Tavistock open systems approach* (pp. 1–20). New York: Wiley.

Miller, E. J., & Rice, A. K. (1967). *Systems of organization*. London: Tavistock Publications.

Raphael, B. (1986). *When disaster strikes*. New York: Basic Books.

Turner, S. W., Thompson, J. A., & Rosser, R. M. (1989). The Kings Cross Fire: Planning a "Phase Two" psychosocial response. *Disaster Management*, 2, 31–37.

Weisæth, L. (1986). Post-traumatic stress disorder after an industrial disaster. In P. Pichot, P. Berner, P. Wolf, & K. Thau (Eds.), *Psychiatry—The state of the art* (pp. 299–307). New York: Plenum Press.

CHAPTER 83

Role of Voluntary Organizations in the United Kingdom for Disabled Veterans Suffering from War Trauma and Posttraumatic Stress Disorder

Linda Ann Stevenson

Introduction

All wars leave legacies, and many of those who are scarred by combat live quietly with deep emotional pain and memories that never fade from the horrors of war. Many ex-servicemen in the United Kingdom who are suffering from the long-term effects of posttraumatic stress disorder (PTSD) have been unable to qualify for war pensions, despite the fact that their mental injury has had a disabling effect upon their lives.

In this chapter, I will examine the role of voluntary organizations in the United Kingdom in providing care for disabled veterans. It is also believed that many of the policy issues apply to other countries as well. For many veterans, their emotional problems have not been accurately diagnosed or treated, and they have been left to cope and adapt without the help and support of the statutory services. Clearly many ex-servicemen since World War II have been reliant upon different voluntary groups.

> Surveys of disabled ex-servicemen have shown that serious and persistent psychological damage remains the most frequent sequela of the traumatic deprivations of captivity or of severe battle stress. Mental injury is man-

ifest in many forms, in depressions, anxiety states, all manner of irrational fears, chronic tension states with restlessness, pathological instability or sensitivity leading to social withdrawal and inability to relate to others. (Murphy, 1987, p. 6)

Experience has shown that some ex-servicemen will never fully recover from their damaging war experiences and will need help and support from others for the rest of their lives. These findings by Brigadier Murphy (1987) are consistent with a 20-year follow-up study of war veterans in the United States (Archibald & Tuddenham, 1965) where it was reported that many veterans retained their original symptoms of such gross stress reactions as startle reaction, recurrent nightmares, irritability, and headaches, which remain largely unchanged after a decade and a half. More recently, the Falklands War (see Chapter 25, in this volume) has renewed attention on traumata brought on by combat exposure. However, despite the efforts by some to highlight the needs of those who are psychologically damaged by warfare, little is being done by the statutory agencies to provide specialist care for the victims.

In 1988, the First European Conference on Traumatic Stress Studies, which took place in Lincoln, England, brought together delegates from throughout the world who were working with trauma victims. In Britain, statutory care has been mobilized to help survivors of such civilian disasters as the Zeebrugee Ferry disaster (see Chapter 40, in this volume) where survivors have been awarded compensation for PTSD; this has not happened for survivors of the Falklands War, yet their needs are similar—to be able to come to terms with what has been

Linda Ann Stevenson • 104 Moore Road, Mapperley, Nottingham NG3 6EJ, England.
International Handbook of Traumatic Stress Syndromes, edited by John P. Wilson and Beverley Raphael. Plenum Press, New York, 1993.

for them a traumatizing experience. After interviewing survivors from the Falklands War, Carr (1984) concluded that "the Government which had sent them to war did little about the welfare of the 777 injured servicemen, leaving it instead to the armed forces and public charities" (p. 155).

For the first time, however, a psychiatrist accompanied the Task Force to the Falklands to assess the psychological effects of warfare. Although he is continuing to work with active duty personnel, many are left to readjust to civilian life without debriefing. In many cases, the psychological trauma of war has taken years to emerge. It is these men, and others like them, who have perhaps left the services over 40 years ago following World War II who may require the assistance of voluntary organizations.

It has long been recognized that men who enlist in the military have to undergo a readjustment of many of their previously held standards of socialization, morality, and conduct and need to formulate new rules by which to live. In times of war, failure to adjust to these new rules has been shown to lead to neurosis (Kardiner, 1943). Among the major causes of traumatic neuroses in this situation are fear, apprehension, and intensely terrifying anxiety (see Chapter 1, in this volume, for a review of these points).

The continuation of these morbid fears, following the cessation of hostilities and upon the return to normal life situations, has been classified by the American Psychiatric Association (APA) as PTSD and has been recognized in the *Diagnostic and Statistical Manual of Mental Disorders* (DSM-III-R) (APA, 1987) as a potentially chronic mental disorder. In the United States, work with Vietnam War veterans has shown that the syndrome is widespread. Wilson (1978, 1980) and Levenberg (1983) estimated that between 500,000 and 700,000 of the approximately 1.2 million Vietnam combat veterans suffer from PTSD. Wilson (1980, 1988a,b) and Wilson and Krauss (1985) have empirically investigated the factors that are predictive of PTSD and reviewed their causal link to the nature and dynamics of the syndrome. Noteworthy is his finding that *psychological isolation* upon homecoming was highly associated with the severity of the disorder.

The research data from the studies of American Vietnam veterans may have implications for the treatment of war veterans in the United Kingdom. Adequate psychological support and counseling may help to prevent prolonged stress reactions. Even though the problem is by no means on the same scale as the American Vietnam experience, the onus of responsibility rests with the government and the statutory services to provide whatever long- or short-term care that is necessary. In the United States, the federal government has funded over 185 readjustment counseling centers, which are staffed by Vietnam veterans and professionals who are able to give this much needed support (see Chapter 77, in this volume, for a review). A similar service has been created in Australia for their Vietnam veterans. For many, PTSD is not a transient experience and symptoms may persist for years. Yet, with support, most of the veterans can be reintegrated into society and lead more productive lives.

Current Provisions for War Pensions in the United Kingdom

Currently, there are over 290,000 disabled ex-servicemen and their dependents in receipt of war pensions in the United Kingdom, the vast majority of whom served and were disabled in the World War II. Pensions, once awarded, are generally adequate, and the welfare services are accessible for all pensioners. However, for some, the pensions do not cover the basic necessities of life and they find themselves turning to the voluntary organizations for additional help. Others, although qualified for pensions, may not have applied. Thus, the voluntary groups function in helping them claim their proper entitlements. In the United States, many veterans organizations perform a similar service (e.g., Disabled American Veterans, American Legion, Vietnam Veterans of America, etc.).

In the United Kingdom, the voluntary sector is very active in giving support and advice to disabled ex-servicemen and women. In 1972, following a representation from the National Federation of the Far Eastern Prisoners of War Clubs and Associations to the Department of Social Security (DSS), a special unit was set up to deal with claims made by former prisoners of war in the Far East. This action has resulted in a full accounts being taken of the special difficulties that arise in the consideration of their cases. Diseases and afflictions such as beriberi, malaria, hepatitis, eye problems, and nervous disorders may lead to eligibility for war pensions. The Far Eastern Prisoners of War Association has encouraged ex-servicemen to come forward so that they can help them claim retrospective pensions. In some cases, the causal connection between the disease and war service is easy to prove, as it is unlikely that certain diseases such, as malaria, could have been contracted elsewhere, but other claims, such as PTSD, are much more difficult to prove. The expertise of the association has proved it to be an effective special interest group, in that it has successfully lobbied the British Government to provide the needed services for its members.

It is estimated that there are about 120,000 surviving former prisoners of war (POWs), many of whom need help for problems originating from deprivations they suffered during wartime (see Chapters 19, 21, and 24, in this volume). As a result of their cases being highlighted, and pressure being brought to bear on the government by the voluntary organizations, many veterans are now presenting themselves for medical examinations, and problems that have been neglected or that have lingered for years are now being treated.

Historical Perspective of the Development of War Pensions

Compensation by the state was first introduced in England by King Charles II who, having realized that voluntary subscription was inadequate, came to the conclusion that state intervention was inevitable. Today, the government continues to provide pensions for those who become disabled while in the armed forces. The Department of Social Security set up a War Pensions

Welfare Service whose task it is to help pensioners meet and overcome difficulties and stresses that are caused by their disabilities. Nationally, there are 30 Welfare Service Offices where the staff are able to maintain a regular visiting list of around 20,000 pensioners. Despite their workload, they aim to contact all pensioners who have a 100% disability assessment. And the voluntary sector is able to extend and supplement many of the services provided by the state. Through the respective service organizations, they are able to improve the quality of the services and extend the choices that are available. However, it would appear that there is a place for voluntary organizations in the United Kingdom in terms of health care benefits and support to ex-servicemen.

In 1978, the Wolfenden Report looked at the future role of voluntary organizations and pointed out that they are in a unique position to alleviate many social needs in British society. They concluded: "In our view, the informal and statutory systems, taken together, constitute the principal means of meeting social needs in our society" (Wolfenden Committee, 1978).

Recent figures for the number of pension awards show a sharp decline when compared with the numbers of casualties following World War I and World War II. Many ex-servicemen from World War II are now reaching old age and are at a time of life when their personal needs are more pressing. The Ministry of Defence has reported that they envisage the number of elderly pensions will have reached a peak in 1990. Voluntary organizations have been approached and have indicated their willingness to share the additional work load necessitated by the number of pensioners. Such groups as the Ex-Services Mental Welfare Society have already begun to recruit additional volunteers to cope with this increased work load. As the Welfare Officers from the DSS are only able to regularly visit a small percentage of the present pensioners, the voluntary groups provide a valuable back-up service by providing support. For some veterans, a regular friendly visit from a caring individual may be all they need; others are in need of specialist help. The voluntary workers can help to identify their problems and present them to the professional staff. This is especially relevant where psychological disturbances that may have remained dormant for years begin to surface in later life.

Following World War II, 27,000 pensions were awarded for neurosis and other nervous disorders, but many other veterans had *delayed effects* that were never attributed to their war experiences. In the past, it has proved difficult for those with PTSD to claim pensions. If more emphasis were to be made about possible, and actual, psychological problems arising from war experiences, perhaps the government would be more willing to establish criteria to properly compensate veterans with service-connected PTSD, as has been done by the Department of Veterans Affairs in the United States (see Chapter 77, in this volume, for a discussion of these issues).

War Pensions

The burden of proof has always been upon the ex-servicemen to claim pensions and seek help for service-connected disabilities. It is possible to claim a pension for mental injury. A successful claim can be made for acute hysteria or neurosis provided it is proved to have been caused, or aggravated, by service in the armed forces. Alternatively, if an anxiety state is brought on by worry over a disease, in respect of which a pension is already being paid, the claimant can apply for an increase in the assessment for the first disease, rather than make a fresh claim. The case of *Freeman* v. *the Ministry of Pensions* (1966) concerned an ex-serviceman who took his own life because the pain and anxiety suffered as a result of a disability which itself had been due to his war service had become unbearable. The man's dependents were awarded a pension and, when summing up the case, the judge emphasized that each claim for a pension must be carefully considered. The level of awards for disabled ex-servicemen and women has always been based upon entitlement and compare favorably with industrial injury benefits in Britain.

The force of popular sentiment cannot be overlooked because many of the servicemen injured during the two World Wars were conscripts, and it has always been felt that they should be treated generously. This does not mean, however, that an injured soldier, or the family of a serviceman who has been killed, is assured of a pension. Article 4 of the Service Pensions Order, 1978, sets out the basic conditions of entitlement to a pension, on a claim in respect of the disablement brought on within 7 years of the end of the member's service, or when the death of a member occurs within that period. There must always be some causal connection between the service and the injury or death; it is not enough that it occurred during service. Disablement that is entirely unrelated to service is expected to be covered by the general social security provisions.

The principle of assessing the basic award is almost identical to those adopted by the industrial sector. The degree of disability is determined by comparing the disabled person with

> the condition of a normal healthy person of the same age and sex, without taking into account the earning capacity of the member in his disabled condition in his own or any other specific trade or occupation, and without taking into account the effect of any individual factors or extraneous circumstances. (Service Pensions Order, 1978)

In addition, widows are only awarded pensions if it can be established that the husband's death was caused or aggravated by injuries received as a result of his service to the Crown. Once the Crown is satisfied that a disabled ex-serviceman's injuries can be properly attributed to his service, a pension is granted. However, for servicemen who suffer psychological disturbances, proving their case is not always easy, and some may not be emotionally strong enough to fight for their statutory rights and as a result fail to get their proper entitlement.

Work of Voluntary Organizations

Over the years, the voluntary organizations have taken an active part in caring for ex-servicemen and their dependents. In the United Kingdom, one of the oldest and most highly respected of these organizations is the Soldiers, Sailors, and Airmen's Families Association (SSAFA). Originally, the SSAFA was founded in 1885 for the purpose of looking after the wives and dependents of soldiers who were serving overseas. Soon the organization established a visiting service to the homes of soldiers' families and took a keen interest in their welfare. Voluntary representatives were recruited, and by the beginning of the South African War, there were over 3,000 members in the association. Following the formation of the Royal Air Force in 1921, the scope and work of the association was extended to include airmen and their families.

During the early years of the organization, they worked closely with the government of the day. Service pay was poor and there was widespread distress among service families; as a result, thousands of them had to turn to the organization for help. The association made strong representations to the government to call for widows and orphans of servicemen to be given pensions as a statutory right independent of charity or the rates. This, then, was the beginning of their unending campaign to improve conditions. By 1915, the government accepted for the first time the state's liability for war pension's when the Ministry of Pensions was set up in 1917. This action was a tremendous achievement for the organization. Over the years, the volume of work for the SSAFA has declined steadily to a peacetime level. Even so, they continue to provide a valuable service by looking after the welfare of the families of service and ex-servicemen and women. The volunteers act as friendly advisers to these families, whatever their problems or difficulties, however personal and varied. They also help them with financial problems and will represent the cause of any of these families to the appropriate government departments where there is reason to do so.

Today, the organization has a total of 4,500 voluntary workers throughout the United Kingdom, and 12,000 throughout the world. They work alongside the services and supplement the welfare and financial provisions of the state. Other voluntary organizations (e.g., Far Eastern P.O.W. Club) provide similar services to ex-servicemen in the United Kingdom.

Role of the Voluntary Organization

Voluntary organizations can be said to extend the absolute amount of resources available to the social services by attracting people, ideas and material resources, that would not have been attracted by the statutory organizations. (Wolfenden Committee, 1978, p. 27)

As noted above, voluntary organizations have always been willing to provide support and assistance to disabled ex-servicemen. Clearly, the proper role of the voluntary organizations should be to provide social support and extend the amount and choices of care provided by the state.

Summary

My review of the role of voluntary organizations in the health care of veterans in the United Kingdom has

shown that long-term care is needed for those who have been psychologically affected by their war experiences. Active combat service in wartime is a stressful time for nearly all servicemen, and there is no way of knowing who is likely to suffer PTSD. In fact, "the majority of trauma experts believe that given sufficient emotional stress, neurotic symptoms may appear in anyone" (Gillespie, 1942). Not only is it difficult to foresee who will be adversely affected, the prognosis for some chronic cases may not be good, and they may need help for many years. In chronic cases, "war neurosis proper has, by association of current with older conflicts, passed over into a peace neurosis and become consolidated as such" (Jones, 1924). The veteran may need long term care which may prove to be expensive and beyond the resources of the voluntary sector. Many veterans who have suffered battle trauma have had no previous psychological problems but were merely reacting logically to illogical situations. That such reactions persist calls for the need of private, voluntary groups to aid those who suffer from PTSD and other forms of traumatic stress reactions.

References

American Psychiatric Association. (1987). *Diagnostic and statistical manual of mental disorders* (3rd ed., rev.). Washington, DC: Author.

Archibald, H. C., & Tuddenham, R. D. (1965). Persistent stress reactions following combat: A 20-year follow-up. *Archives of General Psychiatry*, 12, 475–481.

Carr, J. (1984). *Another story*. London: Hamish Hamilton.

Gillespie, R. D. (1942). *Psychological effects of war on citizen and soldier*. New York: W. W. Norton.

Jones, E. (1924). *Psychoanalysis and war neurosis*. New York: W. W. Norton.

Kardiner, A. (1943). *The traumatic neuroses of war*. New York: Paul B. Hoeber.

Levenberg, S. (1983). Vietnam combat veterans from perpetrator to victim. *Family and Community Health*, 5, 69–76.

Murphy, J. F. D. (Brigadier). (1987). Tyger, tyger, burning bright. *Menews*, 10, 6.

Service Pensions Order. (1978). Article 9(2)(a), (SI 1978/1525). London: Her Majesty's Stationery Office.

Wilson, J. P. (1978). *Identity, ideology, and crisis: The Vietnam veteran in transition* (Vol. 2). Washington, DC: Disabled American Veterans.

Wilson, J. P. (1980). Conflict, stress and growth: The effects of war on psychosocial development among Vietnam veterans. In C. R. Figley & S. Leventman (Eds.), *Strangers at home: Vietnam veterans since the war*. New York: Praeger.

Wilson, J. P. (1988a). Understanding the Vietnam veteran. In F. Ochberg (Ed.), *Post-traumatic therapy and victims of violence* (pp. 227–253). New York: Brunner/Mazel.

Wilson, J. P. (1988b). Treating the Vietnam veteran. In F. Ochberg (Ed.), *Post-traumatic therapy of victims of violence* (pp. 254–277). New York: Brunner/Mazel.

Wilson, J. P., & Krauss, G. E. (1985). Predicting post-traumatic stress syndromes among Vietnam veterans. In W. Kelly (Ed.), *Post-traumatic stress disorder and the war veteran patient*. New York: Brunner/Mazel.

Wolfenden Committee. (1978). *Report on the future of voluntary organizations*. London: Her Majesty's Stationery Office.

CHAPTER 84

Settlement Reconstruction and Psychological Recovery in Iran

Akbar Zargar, Bahman Najarian, and Derek Roger

Introduction

The effects of disasters may be either tangible or latent (Raphael, 1986). Unlike material losses, social and psychological consequences tend to fall into the latter category, and are often overlooked during reconstruction and rehabilitation following disasters. A survey of the current literature shows clearly the emphasis on material aspects of disasters. For example, in a recent publication which summarized all disasters which took place during 1987 (UNDRO, 1988), the main criteria for the declaration of a disaster were property damages in excess of $1 million (United States dollars) and the loss of 10 lives. One might well ask why so relative a measure as a given amount of property damage should feature as prominently as it does. One problem is that the psychological consequences of disasters, unlike material losses, are difficult to quantify. Disasters differ widely in the way people perceive their intensity and even the degree of physical damage which they bring about (Barton, 1962, 1969; Fritz, 1961). However, the psychological aspects of disasters can be documented and understood, and posttraumatic stress disorder (PTSD) is now formally acknowledged by the American Psychiatric Association (1980, 1987) as a recognizable syndrome of psychopathology.

In this chapter, we will focus on the association between psychological aspects of disasters and the process of reconstructing both dwellings and the community infrastructure, and will take account of the existing litera-

ture on the subject as well as the results of survey data obtained by the first author from resettled rural survivors of the Iraq–Iran conflict. The chapter is divided into three sections. First, we will consider the *psychological aspects* of disasters and will conclude with some discussion of two theoretical models which are particularly relevant to disasters: life-events and learned helplessness. Second, we will review the factors affecting the implementation of *reconstruction policies*, focusing on the provision of emergency and temporary shelter and on such issues as site selection and house design during reconstruction. Third, we will examine factors which govern the *timing of the return of the survivors* to the new site, including conditions in the emergency shelters and potential future threats. In this section, we will conclude with a brief consideration of the role of the survivors themselves during the reconstruction process, in relation to decision-making and to physical rebuilding. It is hoped that the integration of prior theoretical and empirical work, together with recent first-hand evidence, will contribute toward a more comprehensive understanding of the complex interactive effects of psychological responses and physical reconstruction.

Overview of the Psychological Aspects of Disasters

The prolonged effects experienced by the victims of large-scale disasters have only recently received serious academic and scientific attention (Drabek, 1986). For example, the psychological aftereffects on the survivors of Hiroshima and Nagasaki were first investigated 17 years after the event (Kinston & Rosser, 1974; Lifton, 1967). Kinston and Rosser argued that the lack of adequate assessment may be due partly to a failure to take full account of the many elements which must be considered when investigating postdisaster psychological adjustment. These include features of the disaster itself, such

Akbar Zargar • Department of Architecture, University of Shahid Beheshti, Tehran, Iran. **Bahman Najarian** • Department of Psychology, University of Shahid Chamran, Ahwaz, Iran. **Derek Roger** • Department of Psychology, University of York, Heslington, York 5DD, England.

International Handbook of Traumatic Stress Syndromes, edited by John P. Wilson and Beverley Raphael. Plenum Press, New York, 1993.

as the number of homeless people and nonfatal casualties, the number of survivors in public shelters, the number of families in which a fatality has occurred, or the number of visible casualties seen by survivors (see Janis, 1974). In turn, these will be mediated by such factors as the degree of social support and the effects of attempts to overcome the trauma by means of cognitive control, temporary denial defense techniques, and a persistent sense of hope for better times to come (Drabek, 1986; Raphael, 1977, 1986).

An added complication is that the psychological consequences of disasters are not limited to the victims and survivors alone, but may also extend to the rescue staff and workers involved in the relief operations (Raphael, 1986). Reactions to disasters may also vary according to whether they are man-made or natural (Warheit, 1976). Perhaps the major difference between them lies in the anger which survivors feel and express towards those who they feel are responsible for such man-made disasters as wars, coupled with their feelings of meaninglessness and dehumanization (see I. G. Sarason & B. R. Sarason, 1987). War is a catastrophic event but an aspect of society (Fantino & Reynolds, 1975), and must be taken into account in any study of the effects of disasters. Over one half of all nations have taken part in at least one war since the turn of the century (Lefrancois, 1980). Kidron and Smith (1983) estimated that there have been about 300 wars since 1945; indeed, there has been no single day free of war since that time.

The most obvious consequences of war are the human and property losses suffered by the victims. Although the negative impacts are much worse for those who lose members of their family than for those who lose only materials or land (Drabek, 1986), all survivors are potentially at risk for lifelong adverse psychological and somatic consequences (see Lefrancois, 1980; I. G. Sarason & B. R. Sarason, 1987). For example, it is reliably estimated that half a million American Vietnam veterans still suffer from postdisaster symptoms (Wilson, 1978, 1980; Wilson, Harel, & Kahana, 1988). A number of case studies have shown that these may continue to affect individuals many years after the event (see Amen, 1985).

In fact, whatever the causal agents might be, disasters have consistently been shown to result in a variety of psychological symptoms, and the more severe the disaster the more serious and complex the psychological reactions of the survivors (I.G. Sarason & B.R. Sarason, 1987; Schwarzwald, Solomon, Weisenberg, & Mikulincer, 1987; Wilson, Smith, & Johnson, 1985). Although a range of positive responses to disasters has been reported, including altruism and enthusiastic participation in repair (UNDRO, 1982), as many as 75% of survivors may show overt symptoms of PTSD. These include apathy, passivity, aimless pottering around, and extreme suggestibility, and 12% to 25% may suffer serious psychological reactions, including clinical cases requiring formal diagnosis and hospitalization (Kinston & Rosser, 1974; Mileti, Drabek, & Haas, 1975; Thompson, 1985; Wilson, 1988).

There are many theoretical models which could be used to account for the relationship between disasters and subsequent psychological distress, but it is beyond the scope of this chapter to consider them all in detail. However, there are two approaches which present particularly promising avenues for research: *life events* and *learned helplessness*. Work on life events stems from pioneering studies by Holmes and Rahe (1967) and their colleagues, who developed a series of scales in which a range of life experiences is listed. Subjects are asked to endorse those items which have occurred over a retrospective period (typically 3 to 6 months previously), and a number of studies have reported low but significant correlations between life-event frequency and the incidence of mental and physical illness.

The life-events approach is beset by many methodological problems, but the relationship between event frequencies and illness is preserved when attempts are made to partial these out (B. S. Dohrenwend & B. P. Dohrenwend, 1978; Tausig, 1982). The general model of progressive exhaustion and concomitant lowering of resistance upon which the approach is based thus appears to be fundamentally sound, and the work on life events has important implications for the present discussion. One of these is that disasters are, by definition, stressful events in themselves, and the findings from research on the effects of other events will apply to them as well. More importantly, the survivors' capacity to cope with disaster will depend upon preceding events. This will be particularly true of protracted disasters, such as war, where the continuing demand for coping may undermine the efforts of even the most resilient individuals.

Particular life events may also act as triggers for posttraumatic stress responses. Amen (1985), for example, showed how a series of negative life experiences served to precipitate a delayed traumatic response to the stresses of service in Vietnam. Five years after a flood in the United States, 30% of the survivors still showed symptoms of postdisaster syndrome, many of which were phobic reactions toward cues related to the flood (see Popovic & Petrovic, 1964). Again, Ploeger (1974) indicated that 10 years after the occurrence of a disaster in Germany, its victims still manifested some symptoms of the postdisaster syndrome which were aggravated by exposure to even mild provocations, such as talking about the event or the season of the disaster.

As has been pointed out, one of the consequences of disaster is that victims may become apathetic and incapable of any further response. In the psychological literature this behavior is sometimes referred to as *learned helplessness*, a construct which arose from laboratory experiments showing that continued exposure to unpredictable stressors resulted in a suppression of normal coping responses (Seligman, 1974). Helplessness following trauma is regarded as a response to the trauma itself because it is uncharacteristic; that is, individuals who were previously capable of responding appropriately are reduced to seeming apathy by the experience of helplessness (Wilson et al., 1985). In an account of the psychological consequences of man-made disasters, this state of resignation is described by Bastiaans (1985) as *exhaustion*, evidenced, for example, in delayed recovery following trauma among war veterans and concentration camp victims. A similar point has been made in relation to the survivors of Hiroshima and Nagasaki, who were described in 1991 by the authors of a Committee Report on the Effects of Nuclear Attack as suffering from almost inconsolable feelings of hopelessness following the bombings.

Although the long-term psychological effects of disasters are less clear-cut than the immediate and short-term ones (see Drabek, 1986), there is no doubt that they may persist over many years following the events. It is also clear that the outcomes depend not only on the features of the disasters themselves but also on the psychological makeup of the survivors and the incidence of prior and subsequent events. These findings are important because effective reconstruction depends in part upon the responses of the survivors themselves, and the lack of motivation which characterizes helplessness may have a significant effect on their capacity to adapt during the recovery phase following disasters.

Factors Relating to Policy Decisions on Physical Reconstruction

The Four Phases of Recovery

Reconstruction following disasters is concerned with more than simply rebuilding houses. As it has already been pointed out, social *and* psychological rehabilitation are equally important. As far as physical recovery is concerned, four phases have been identified (UNDRO, 1982). The first is referred to as Phase zero and includes any predisaster planning strategies for mitigating the effects of future hazards, based upon a study of permanent housing prior to the disaster. Phase 1, the period of emergency shelter, typically lasts for up to 5 days, and is followed by Phase 2, temporary accommodation, which may last for up to 5 or 6 months. The final phases occur with the reconstruction of new permanent housing.

For our purposes in this section, Phases 1 and 2 will be discussed together and will be described as *emergency shelter* and *temporary accommodation*. The process of reconstruction itself will then be discussed under the following headings: site selection, site organization and house design, reintegration into communities, and materials and technology used for reconstruction. Each category will be discussed in turn and will include general considerations derived from earlier work as well as reference to some of the observations and findings of a recent study conducted by the first author. This study involved the administration of a structured interview to 132 survivors of the Iraq–Iran War after they had been resettled in newly built houses. The participants came from 11 villages in southern Iran in the province of Khusestan. All were selected by a stratified random-sampling procedure, and the interviews took place in the villages (the interested reader is referred to Zargar, 1988, for a more detailed account of the procedure).

Phase 1

1. *Emergency shelter and temporary accommodation.* The period immediately following a disaster is characterized by confusion and uncertainty. Orner (1988) succinctly describes this situation as "living in utter limbo," and the provision of temporary accommodation for the survivors forms a crucial period in the reconstruction

process. Maslow (1970) described human growth and adjustment as a progression up a hierarchy of needs, from basic physical and safety needs as primary to self-esteem and self-actualization as well as later developmental processes. According to Maslow, refugees may have safety needs activated as prepotent as a result of the abrupt and intense change in their lives. The adverse conditions encountered in temporary shelters such as overcrowding and unemployment (Loizos, 1977) may add to their existing distress, and these additional adverse life events may be sufficient to precipitate complete demoralization and breakdown (Rossi, Wright, Weber-Burdin, & Pereira, 1983).

Kinston and Rosser (1974) described a particular frame of mind which they call "camp mentality," which includes such characteristics as selfishness, lack of compassion, and egotistical behavior. This description will apply to most disaster-related temporary shelters, since the negative consequences of living in these circumstances have been shown to develop even in the most sophisticated and advanced camps (Kinston & Rosser, 1974; Orner, 1988). Clearly, postdisaster policies should be directed toward making this temporary settlement period as short as possible. Indeed, one useful measure of the success of settlement reconstruction plans and policies may be the brevity of emergency shelter provision (Davis, 1978). In this context, it should be borne in mind that survivors may be quite capable of building emergency shelters for themselves using indigenous techniques and salvaged materials from the ruins (Geiple, 1982; Nehnevajsa & Wong, 1977). In principle, refugees ought to be given an opportunity to establish a form of community as similar as possible to their own experience, avoiding in particular military-style camp layout (MacAdam, 1987; Davis, 1978; United Nations High Commissioner for Refugees Program, 1982), although the dangers to them must of course be borne in mind.

Phase 2

2. *Site selection.* The construction of permanent housing is one of the main priorities for the survivors of a disaster. Indeed, in the survey of survivors of the Iraq–Iran war, 45% of those interviewed placed housing as their first priority, followed by land restoration (38%), and such public services as schools and drinking water (16%). Survivors may resort to a variety of sources to assist in the problems of homelessness (Bolin & Trainer, 1978), but the main issue revolves around whether or not they should return to their original position. Thus, selection of a suitable location is a complex and delicate process (see Davis, 1975, 1987), and must be made with respect to the cultural, ethnic, personal and social needs and interests of the survivors (Perry & Muskkatel, 1984).

When survivors have been given an opportunity to decide about the site of their new homes, usually they prefer the original site and even the same spots, and may show considerable resistance to moving (Quarantelli, 1982). Survivors have been known to refuse to sell their lands to the government even when there was a potential threat on these lands. When they have been forcibly relocated, they may ignore official warnings and move back to their original land (Mitchell, 1977), and there have been cases where the whole community has evacuated their reconstructed homes at a new site and moved back to the original one (Aysan, 1987).

Perhaps this is not surprising since relocation changes not only the geographical site of their homes but also important aspects of their social and familial lives. Shelters built by survivors from salvaged materials may well be more efficient and comfortable for victims than the commonly used tents, and a degree of self-help may, in fact, serve to reduce feelings of helplessness. The preference of survivors to remain near the ruins of their demolished houses was clearly supported by the survey of victims of the Iraq–Iran war, which was carried out by the first author, an attitude which was apparently unrelated to the circumstances in which they were living. In fact, evidence from Turkish studies shows clearly that survivors prefer to remain where they are rather than being evacuated (UNDRO, 1977a).

The preference among survivors to return to their old locations, their strong resistance to any sort of change and their insistence upon sameness in various aspects of their lives after the disaster no doubt reflect the anxiety which accompanies uncertainty. Consequently, returning to their origins may well be beneficial to their psychological well-being. Indeed, Bolin (1976) argued that "residential dislocation" can give rise to additional adverse postdisaster effects (see also Raphael, 1986), and Thompson (1985) pointed out that the "overlearned familiar routines" of the old environment may be an effective way of alleviating distress. These views are consistent with the work, discussed earlier, on the adverse effects of life events. Returning victims to their original homes may thus be considered less "transitional" than relocation, and since victims usually assess and compare their losses relative to those of other victims (Barton, 1969), authorities must be consistent in their policies if they are to avoid incurring further distress among survivors.

There are many factors which influence site preferences amongst survivors, including age, sex and occupation (Boileau, Cattarinussi, Zotti, Pelanda, Strassoldo, & Tellia, 1978). Thus, older victims are more adaptable to new locations, and generally show better adjustment to relocations and postdisaster effects than younger victims (Schiff, 1977). Suitability of the land itself is obviously important, especially since unsuitable sites may in themselves contribute to the occurrence of some disasters. In many major cities in the developing countries, such as Mexico City, squatter settlements are vulnerable to mud slides, fire, and earthquakes. Also, many villages located on flat, fertile plains to facilitate the reestablishment of agricultural production might be at risk of flooding (Davis, 1987). This dilemma was born out in the survey of survivors of the Iraq–Iran conflict: 87% of resettled villagers expressed their satisfaction with the sites, but in fact 60% of them are subject to flooding. If there is a continuing probability of future threats to an old site, it may be more appropriate to disregard the survivors' preferences in determining relocation sites (Boileau *et al.*, 1978; Oliver-Smith, 1977), and the probability of a disaster recurring should be taken into account when considering the site for selection (Goldsteen & Schorr, 1982; R. K. Leik, S. A. Leik, Ekker, & Gilfford,

1982). Furthermore, reminders of the catastrophic event may trigger the "original trauma" in some victims when they return to the place of the event (Amen, 1985).

These and other factors may necessitate relocating survivors to land where the risk of future disasters is low, but this change may seriously disrupt the social organization of the community (Davis, 1981, 1987; UNDRO, 1977b). In fact, complete relocation of survivors to other sites rarely occurs in practice (Drabek, 1986), but in planning the location of even temporary sites authorities should bear in mind that the great the number of postdisaster residential moves, the less chance the survivors may have of successfully coping with the consequences of the disaster (Bolin, 1982). As has been discussed earlier, life changes of any description may provoke distress, even under normal conditions.

An equally important issue in deciding upon resettlement policies is consultation with the survivors themselves. If they are given the opportunity to contribute to the decision, the chance of successful resettlement may be significantly enhanced, in part, because the sense of helplessness is mitigated by active participation. Relating this to our own work with the survivors of the Iraq–Iran war, the 87% who expressed satisfaction with the sites did so partly because 79% of them claimed that their representatives had been consulted about site designation. Local institutions had also been give a chance to express their opinions, and there can be little doubt that these opportunities contributed to the success of the site locations.

3. Population integration. The importance of maintaining community structure as far as possible cannot be overemphasized, and the study among the survivors of the Iraq–Iran war showed a clear preference for preserving the predisaster population configuration for each village. Nearly all the survivors preferred the original community and resented having to live with strangers in reconstructed villages. For example, in response to the question of whether or not they preferred to be living with other villagers in the new settlement, 82% of the participants expressed their dissatisfaction with the idea of integration with other communities in their reconstructed villages. Again, these findings support the view that change should be minimized during the postdisaster period; survivors do not want the additional demand of having to form new social and community relationships. Having old friends, kin, and neighbors helps to maintain continuity in the struggle to return to normality after the disaster.

Undoubtedly, cultural factors played a role in reconstruction in the Iran study, since the majority of the resettled communities were Arabs with particular tribal backgrounds who strongly guarded their own traditions. In fact, authorities did decide in some situations to build clusters of villages, where each cluster consisted of a few small villages built close to one another in a particular area. The residents of these close-by villages are apparently doing their best to maintain their "territorial privacy," by avoiding routine and frequent interactions and communications with nearby villages, again supporting the view that psychological recovery is enhanced where survivors are able to live with those whom they know and can relate to (see also Demerath &

Anthony, 1957; Golek, 1983; Warrick *et al.*, 1981). There are cases reported in the literature where simple events, such as finding an "incompatible" neighbor, have forced the victims to abandon their homes and resort to a more familiar and "friendly site" (Ciborowiski, 1967; Hogg, 1980), and similar instances were found in some of the rural areas of Khusestan.

4. *Site organization and house design.* It would appear that the more similar the organization of the site and the design of the new houses to that of the original dwellings, the less disturbance and stress there may be for the survivors. However, owing to the vulnerability of the old houses, the implementation of new designs sometimes may be inevitable. When new designs are to be introduced, the policy should be directed toward appropriateness, something not too different from the original. Failing to select a proper design may result in a variety of problems including those of maintaining the new house properly. Whenever changes are to be implemented, designers and builders should try to produce plans which are consistent with the traditional aspects of the user's life (Aysan & Oliver, 1987; Davis, 1975); the greater the similarity between the pre- and postdisaster social and physical aspects, the fewer the adaptations required (Mileti *et al.*, 1975).

One advantage of keeping house designs the same (or very similar) is that it gives the victims a sense of control over their houses, in terms of understanding and being able to manipulate their design and structure if necessary. As we have seen, the perception of control over the environment may be a key factor in facilitating postdisaster adaptation and may explain why people are so resistant to change and become disoriented when change occurs (Morris, 1974). The outcome of our survey of the survivors of the Iraq–Iran war certainly favors the idea that victims should not be deprived of their original housing designs. Alterations in the design of some buildings meant in some cases that survivors were no longer able to live with all members of their family or kin, as they had been accustomed to doing. In fact, where a significantly different design from the original was imposed, the occupants frequently altered the building, and the same thing has been observed with the layout of the villages themselves. The results of the survey showed that 86% of those who were given the opportunity to participate in the design and building of their houses were satisfied with them, whereas only 69% of a group who were given little or no opportunity to contribute expressed satisfaction.

5. *Policies on materials and technology.* Materials and technology used in reconstruction may represent the final result of the interrelationships among a number of factors, including stability of the site, the local building patterns, aesthetic improvements to the buildings, and changes aimed at lowering the liability of the buildings to future disasters (Bates, Timothy, & Glittenberg, 1979; Tonkinson, 1979). Many authorities believe that postdisaster conditions are good opportunities for introducing substantial improvements in social systems anyway (Fritz, 1961). Snarr and Brown (1978) argue that victims, in general, receive a more or less improved quality of housing after disasters.

However, not all these changes in design and structure will be based upon the pattern and plans (Bates,

Fogleman, Pareton, Pittman, & Tracy, 1963; see also Lessa, 1964; Oliver-Smith, 1979; Prince, 1920), and it is well documented that people will do all they can to alter those aspects of their reconstructed villages which they do not find consistent with their needs and tastes. This tendency to modify their new homes diminishes only when victims feel secure and in a "balanced place" (Baron, Byrne, & Griffitt, 1979; Spielberger & Sarason, 1985). Furthermore, some technological improvements in construction may increase survivors' vulnerability by producing dependence on less reliable artifacts (Davis, 1981; Perrow, 1984). Orr (1979) pointed out that technological changes may bring about extensive adverse side-effects and even social disruption (also Lewis, O'Keefe, & Westgate, 1977; Long, 1978), and using new designs and new materials may impose additional psychological stress by virtue of the fact that some people may not know how to use and repair them.

This was borne out in the Khusestan survey, where the significant change which occurred in the survivors' habits, attitudes, and acceptances of new building materials was not necessarily for the better; indeed, 77% of the respondents felt that they had learned nothing about the new building methods during the reconstruction period. The new houses were constructed from burned brick and cement, whereas the original dwellings were made from rammed earth and mud. In the survey, 96% said that they would prefer to use the new materials for expanding or modifying their rebuilt homes, and about 80% would like to use cement blocks for new stables. No such attitudes and tastes had ever been expressed (let alone practiced) prior to the war. The use of these new materials in such circumstances has changed the survivors' opinions about their indigenous building materials, which are more readily available and perhaps much cheaper (if not free) than the new ones.

Another change was that nearly all of those interviewed said that they would like to extend their new houses in order "to complete them." No doubt this preference arose from the fact that about 50% of houses contained more than one family after resettlement, and many of these families comprised more than five members. However, favoring improvements in this way was interesting because the new houses had no fewer rooms than the original ones, indicating a significant change in the expectations of the villagers after resettlement. Perhaps the most conspicuous change in the expectations of the villagers is reflected in the preference for air conditioning in the new houses. More than 61% of the households installed some form of air conditioning (mainly fans and coolers), compared with only 17% prior to the disaster. However, this might simply be a function of the changes in financial circumstances, since 82% of those who were interviewed reported that they were better off than they had been before the war.

Factors Affecting the Return of Survivors to the New Site

Bearing in mind the deleterious effects of living in even the most well-organized temporary shelters, the importance for survivors of returning to permanent housing is paramount. Survivors have been known to become so frustrated and aggressive as a result of long periods of living in temporary shelters and waiting to return home that they became hostile toward the very people and agencies who are endeavoring to help them (Krell, 1978; Lacey, 1972; Mileti *et al.*, 1975). The timing of the return to permanent homes may be mediated by four main factors: completion of the buildings, the conditions in the emergency shelter, potential threats, and progress toward psychological recovery by the victims.

Phase 3

1. *Completion of the buildings.* Survivors can only return to their permanent homes when building work is completed. Consequently, the process of rebuilding damaged homes should be kept as simple and short as possible. In fact, it has been found that survivors prefer to return home even before the completion of their homes rather than remain in temporary shelters (Drabek, 1986). Our findings with the victims of the Iraq–Iran conflict are in complete agreement with the latter claim. Indeed, most subjects who were interviewed indicated their unequivocal preference for returning to the ruins of their houses rather than living in the confined environment of emergency shelters. One important qualification to this principle is that urban survivors generally lack construction skills with indigenous materials, and are therefore more dependent on external aid than rural people who generally possess these skills.

2. *Conditions of the emergency shelter.* Survivors of disasters general appreciate that the process of rebuilding and returning home may take considerable time (Drabek, 1986). However, as mentioned earlier, the period of having to live in temporary shelter should be kept as short as possible (Birnbaum, Coplon, & Drabek, 1973). In fact, Erikson's "two-disaster theory" (i.e., collective and individual traumata) refers to the side-effects of temporary shelter as the second disaster, and the slower the process of reconstruction and the longer the emergency period, the greater the long-term effects on the victims are likely to be (Erikson, 1976). One of these effects is learned helplessness, discussed in the previous section, which gradually erodes the survivors' optimism and hopes for betterment as the emergency shelter period is prolonged (Birnbaum *et al.*, 1973). Another consequence of remaining for prolonged periods in temporary accommodation is that survivors may become so alienated from the communities in which they lived prior to the disaster that they are reluctant to return when the time comes (Milne, 1979).

3. *Potential threats.* The likelihood of further disasters recurring in the future remains a potential problem with those who remain at the original site, and will also color the victims' perception of postdisaster life. The probability of such events must always be considered before advising victims to return home, a fact which can be appreciated by bearing in mind the primary reasons for the evacuation's taking place (Hultaker, 1977). Some steps can be taken to predict the likelihood of natural disasters recurring, but risk assessment is much more difficult in the case of man-made disasters (UNDRO, 1980). During wars, for example, the front lines may change drastically overnight. In Iran, the situation five months after the commencement of a cease fire was that many areas still could not be settled because of the risk of renewed hostilities.

4. *Psychological recovery of victims.* Timing the return home will also be influenced by the degree to which survivors have been affected psychologically. Many survivors show a remarkable capacity to adapt to adversity. Often, their main concern is to have the problems of reconstruction sorted out as quickly as possible so that they can return home (Drabek, 1986). Indeed, there have been cases where survivors of earthquakes have returned to their damaged homes within minutes following the impact (Takuma, 1972). However, even though serious symptoms may not be commonplace, most survivors are likely to be affected to some degree in the period following the disaster.

Among the general changes in behavior which have been noted is a gradual decrease in the altruism which characterizes efforts to rebuild communities immediately following the disaster; this seems to revert to predisaster levels within six months (Barton, 1962, 1969; Fritz, 1961). It has also been reported that survivors become particularly cautious some months after the disaster, arranging all kinds of protective insurance against a possible recurrence of the disaster in the future (Drabek, 1986; Drabek & Key, 1984). Informal observation suggests a similar phenomenon in Iran, where building insurance increased dramatically following the heavy missile attacks which occurred in 1988.

The rate of recovery from the trauma of disaster varies from one community to another, and is related to the type and scale of the impact (Drabek, 1986) as well as various social characteristics of the community; for example, having family friends in the same temporary shelter appears to increase the victims' chances of coping successfully with their stressors (Drabek, 1986). As a consequence of these differences, estimates of the appropriate time to return survivors to their reconstructed villages vary widely. Thompson (1985), for example, argued that a year may pass before victims can integrate in the social system effectively, and that this period may be significantly prolonged for those who have lost some members of their family. Wallace (1956), on the other hand, reported that the postdisaster syndrome may only last for a few weeks. These variations clearly pose a major problem for the authorities in deciding on the appropriate timing for the return.

Another important factor affecting the time of the return is that particular periods in the year may have become associated with emotional upset over the disaster. This was discussed earlier with regard to the role of subsequent life events in triggering a recurrence of symptoms. I. G. Sarason and B. R. Sarason (1987) described an "anniversary syndrome" in which depression, anxiety, and other psychological problems occur on the anniversary date of the catastrophe. Finally, decision-making about time of the return should take into account the season and circumstances prevailing on the original site, in terms of the provision of shelter and other facilities.

Phase 4

5. *Participation in the reconstruction.* Although survivors need time to recover from the aftereffects of disasters, they are nonetheless the best source of help and

guidance throughout the reconstruction period. In practice, participation could occur at many levels, but participation by survivors can best be considered in relation to two aspects: *policy and decision-making* and actual *physical reconstruction.*

Although a lack of trust in aid officials will not occur following all disasters (Rossi *et al.,* 1983), authorities working with survivors should be prepared for distrust or even hostility being directed toward them (Schorr, Goldsteen, & Cortes, 1982). Thus, Horige and Oura (1979) reported a significant rise in the negative attitudes of survivors, revolving mainly around "blame assignation" to authorities.

One obvious way to deal with these negative attitudes is to avoid impersonal and excessively bureaucratic approaches, and to attempt to resolve the problems as promptly as possible (Bolin, 1982; Taylor, Ross, & Quarantelli, 1976). A more important strategy, however, is to give survivors themselves a chance to take part in decision-making. Providing such opportunities facilitates the transfer of control over survivors' lives into their own hands, and may contribute significantly toward alleviating conflict between themselves and the authorities.

Allowing survivors to participate in decision-making also increases the probability that they will like the new settlements (Perry & Muskkatel, 1984). Indeed, Drabek (1986) argued that the best way of assessing the quality of settlement reconstruction programs should be the degree to which victims are satisfied with their homes.

The results of the survey of survivors of the Iraq–Iran war showed that 86% of those who were fully consulted about the design of the new houses reported complete satisfaction with them; in the worst case, where no consultation took place, only 14% reported satisfaction. The authors therefore favor strongly the principle of consulting and informing survivors about the process of reconstruction. Quite apart from ensuring satisfaction with the finished product, continuous consultation during the reconstruction process minimizes the potentially harmful effects of rumors which arise in response to uncertainty (Thompson, 1985).

One question which naturally arises is how soon survivors could be expected to participate, given the intensity of the trauma which could follow disasters. Drabek (1986) suggested that survivors usually come to terms with their circumstances within 2 weeks, but there is no clear-cut criterion which could be used. Mawson, Mark, Ramm, and Stern (1981) proposed procedures for encouraging adaptation by survivors, including visiting places associated with the disaster to allow the free expression of emotion. According to these authors, a gradual and selective approach to the "avoidance cues" is psychologically beneficial to the victims, even though grief symptoms may temporarily increase when they are first exposed (I. G. Sarason & B. R. Sarason, 1987).

The long period of temporary settlement may be substantially eased if the victims are given a chance to take part in some sort of training which could help them cope with their existing distress and their future responsibilities (Leslie, 1986). Even under normal conditions, mastery over the environment is an important factor in psychological well-being, and Cox (1978) showed that training and educating people who are under stress is extremely beneficial to them.

The particular skills which could most usefully be taught will depend upon the circumstances (I. G. Sarason & B. R. Sarason, 1987), but the existing skills of the survivors should be exploited as far as possible to facilitate their contribution to the recovery effort (Hewitt & Burton, 1971; McComb, 1980; Syren, 1981). Giving survivors the opportunity to function normally as employed and working people, or even to take the main responsibility and share in the reconstruction of their settlement contributes directly to the reduction of feelings of helplessness. Promoting the establishment of social and personal bonds through employment also helps to divert the constant preoccupation with the past which frequently hampers recovery (I. G. Sarason & B. R. Sarason, 1987).

Active participation by survivors also helps to change attitudes about control and dependency in relation to possible future disasters. For example, in our own study, 39% of the survivors reported that they expected the full intervention of the state to rebuild their houses in the event of a recurrence, whereas 58% said that they would be prepared to cooperate with the government and take part in the reconstruction. In the past, these villagers have been found to be quite capable of rebuilding their own houses without external help, and we would like to argue that a far smaller percentage would have indicated an unwillingness to take part in the physical work of reconstruction had they done so on this occasion.

Conclusions

The main conclusions of the foregoing review may be summarized as follows:

1. The psychological and physical aspects of reconstruction following disasters are closely related to one another, and both can contribute to facilitating or hindering the process of recovery. For this reason, reconstruction strategies should be coordinated with continued monitoring of psychological recovery. There are many factors which might be considered in relation to survivors' coping skills, but two which were presented as particularly important in the context of the present chapter are *learned helplessness,* which is associated with the uncertainty and lack of perceived control following catastrophes, and the *role of life events,* partly in sensitizing individuals to distress but more importantly in precipitating or triggering posttraumatic stress disorders.

2. In view of the strong desire on the part of survivors to return to their homes, the emergency shelter period should be kept as short as possible; the shorter the period of postdisaster temporary settlement, the faster and more successful the survivors' recovery is likely to be. Indeed, in many cases, temporary settlement on the original site is better than a distant refugee camp, although the probability of a recurrence of the disaster would have to be taken into consideration here.

3. The settlement site layout, housing design, technology, and use of materials policies should be as similar to the old ones as possible, and where changes are inevitable, alterations should be consistent with the victims' needs and interests. Such an approach should ensure that victims will be content with their rebuilt homes and

not feel the need to undertake major alterations to them, or even to abandon them after a short while. The introduction of new technology should be approached with great caution, since it is crucial that the survivors be able to repair and maintain the new houses themselves.

4. Survivors should be given every opportunity to take part in the decision-making processes concerning their current life in the emergency shelter and their future life in their prospective homes. This should include decisions over policy as well as direct participation in the work of rebuilding which is contrary to the claim that presenting survivors with a ready-made building will facilitate recovery. Rather, taking part in the actual process of physical reconstruction appears to be psychologically helpful to survivors as well as economically beneficial to the authorities. However, to achieve this objective, the agencies involved should implement training and employment policies that aimed at creating new skills as well as exploiting existing ones.

References

Amen, D. G. (1985). Post-Vietnam stress disorder: A metaphor for current and past life events. *American Journal of Psychotherapy, 41,* 580–586.

American Psychological Association. (1980). *Diagnostic and statistical manual of mental disorders* (3rd ed.). Washington, DC: Author.

American Psychiatric Association. (1987). *Diagnostic and statistical manual of mental disorders* (3rd ed., rev.). Washington, DC: Author.

Aysan, Y. (1987). Homeless in 42m2. *Open House International, 12(3),* 21–26.

Aysan, Y., & Oliver, P. (1987). *Housing and culture after earthquakes: A guide for future policy making on housing in seismic areas.* Oxford, England: Oxford Polytechnic Press.

Baron, R. A., Byrne, D., & Griffitt, W. (1979). *Social psychology: Understanding human interaction.* Boston: Allyn & Bacon.

Barton, A. H. (1962). The emergency social system. In G. W. Baker & D. W. Chapman (Eds.), *Man and society in disaster* (pp. 222–267). New York: Basic Books.

Barton, A. H. (1969). *Communities in disaster: A sociological analysis of collective stress situations.* Garden City: Doubleday.

Bastiaans, J. (1985). The psychosomatic consequences of manmade disasters. In C. D. Spielberger & I. G. Sarason (Eds.), *Stress and anxiety* (pp. 111–118). New York: McGraw-Hill.

Bates, F. L., Fogleman, C. W., Pareton, V. J., Pittman, R. H., & Tracy, G. S. (1963). *The social and psychological consequences of a natural disaster.* National Research Council Disaster Study 18. Washington, DC: National Academy of Sciences.

Bates, F. L., Timothy, F., & Glittenberg, J. K. (1979). Some changes in housing characteristics in Guatemala following the February 1976 earthquake and their implications for future earthquake vulnerability. *Mass Emergencies, 4,* 121–133.

Birnbaum, F., Coplon, J., & Drabek, S. (1973). Crisis intervention after a natural disaster. *Social Casework, 54,* 545–551.

Boileau, A. M., Cattarinussi, B., Zotti, G. D., Pelanda, C., Strassoldo, R. & Tellia, B. (1978). *Friuli: La Prova del Terremoto* [need English trans.]. Milan, Italy: Franco Angeli.

Bolin, R. C. (1976). Family recovery from natural disaster: A preliminary model. *Mass Emergencies, 1,* 267–277.

Bolin, R. C. (1982). *Long-term family recovery from disaster.* Boul-

der, Colorado: Institute of Behavioral Science, University of Colorado.

Bolin, R. C., & Trainer, P. C. (1978). Modes of family recovery following disaster: A cross-national study. In E. L. Quarantelli (Ed.), *Disasters: Theory and research* (pp. 233–247). Beverly Hills: Sage Publications.

Ciborowski, A. (1967). Some aspects of town reconstruction (Warsaw and Skopje). *Impact, 17,* 31–48.

Cox, T. (1978). *Stress.* Hong Kong: Macmillan.

Davis, I. (1975, January). Disaster housing: A case study of Managua. *Architectural Design,* 42–47.

Davis, I. (1978). *Shelter after disaster.* Oxford, England: Oxford Polytechnic Press.

Davis, I. (1981). Disasters and settlement—Towards an understanding of the key issues. In I. Davis (Ed.), *Disasters and the small dwellings.* Oxford, England: Pergamon Press.

Davis, I. (1987). Safe shelter within unsafe cities: Disaster vulnerability and rapid urbanization. *Open House International, 12(3),* 5–15.

Demerath, N. J., & Anthony, F. C. W. (1957). Human adaptation to disaster. *Human Organization, 16,* 1–2.

Dohrenwend, B. S., & Dohrenwend, B. P. (1978). *Some issues in research on stressful life events.* New York: Wiley.

Drabek, T. E. (1986). *Human system responses to disaster: An inventory of sociological findings.* New York: Springer-Verlag.

Drabek, T. E., & Key W. H. (1984). *Conquering disaster: Family recovery and long-term consequences.* New York: Irvington Publishers.

Erikson, K. T. (1976). Loss of community at Buffalo Creek. *American Journal of Psychiatry, 133,* 302–305.

Fantino, E., & Reynolds, G. S. (1975). *Introduction to contemporary psychology.* San Francisco: W. H. Freeman.

Fritz, C. E. (1961). Disasters. In R. K. Merton & R. A. Nisbet (Eds.), *Contemporary social problems* (pp. 651–694). New York: Harcourt.

Geiple, R. (1982). *Disasters and reconstruction: The Friuli (Italy) Earthquakes of 1979.* London: George Allen & Unwin.

Goldsteen, R., & Schorr, J. L. (1982). The long-term impact of a man-made disaster: An examination of a small town in the aftermath of the Three Mile Island nuclear reactor accident. *Disasters, 6(1),* 50–59.

Golec, J. A. (1983). A contextual approach to the social psychological study of disaster recovery. *International Journal of Mass Emergencies and Disasters, 1,* 255–276.

Hewitt, K., & Burton, I. (1971). The hazardousness of a place. *Department of Geography Research Publication, 6.* Toronto: University of Toronto.

Hogg, S. J. (1980). Reconstruction following seismic disaster in Venzone, Friuli. *Disasters, 4(2),* 173–185.

Holmes, T. H., & Rahe, R. H. (1967). The social adjustment rating scale. *Journal of Psychosomatic Research, 11,* 213–218.

Horige, K., & Oura, H. (1979). The cognition of the damages caused by the 1978 Miyagiken Oki earthquake, and its corresponding behaviors. *Study of Sociology (Shakaigaku Kenkyu), 38,* 9–67.

Hultaker, O. (1977). Evakueringar i stobritannien under valdskriget [Evacuation in Great Britain during World War II]. *Disaster Studies 4.* Uppsala, Sweden: University of Uppsala.

Janis, I. L. (1974). *Psychological stress: Psychoanalytic and behavioral studies of surgical patients.* New York: Academic Press.

Kinston, W., & Rosser, R. (1974). Disaster: Effects on mental and physical state. *Journal of Psychosomatic Research, 18,* 437–456.

Kidron, M., & Smith, D. (1983). *The war atlas: Armed conflict-armed peace.* London: Pan Books.

Krell, G. I. (1978). Managing the psychological factor in disaster programs. *Health and Social Work, 3,* 139–154.

Lacey G. N. (1972). Observations on Abervan. *Journal of Psychosomatic Research, 16,* 257.

Lefrancois, G. R. (1980). *Psychology.* Belmont, CA: Wadsworth Publishing.

Leik, R. K., Leik, S. A., Ekker, K., & Gilfford G. A. (1982). *Under the threat of Mount St. Helens: A study of chronic family stress.* Minneapolis: Family Study Center, University of Minnesota.

Leslie, J. (1986). A building education program in North Yemen. *Disasters, 10*(3), 163–171.

Lessa, W. A. (1964). The social effects of Typhoon Ophelia (1960) on Ulitha. *Micronesia, 1*(1–2), 1–47.

Lewis, J., O'Keefe, P., & Westgate, K. N. (1977). A philosophy of precautionary planning. *Mass Emergencies, 2,* 95–104.

Loizos, P. (1977). A struggle for meaning: Reaction to disaster amongst Cypriot refugees. *Disasters, 1*(3), 231–239.

Long, F. (1978). The impact of natural disasters on Third World agriculture: An exploratory survey of the need for some new dimensions in development planning. *American Journal of Economics and Sociology, 37,* 149–163.

MacAdam, R. (1987). REDR—Engineering's humanitarian response. *Structural Engineer, 65A*(8), 297–302.

Maslow, A. H. (1970). *Motivation and personality* (2nd ed.). New York: Harper & Row.

Mawson, D., Mark, I. M., Ramm, L., & Stern, R. S. (1981). Guided mourning for morbid grief: A controlled study. *British Journal of Psychiatry, 138,* 185–193.

McComb, D. (1980). *Bit Thompson: Profile of a natural disaster.* Boulder, CO: Pruett Publishing.

Mileti, D. S., Drabek, E. M., & Haas J. E. (1975). *Human systems in extreme environments.* Boulder, CO: Institute of Behavioral Science, University of Colorado.

Milne, G. (1979). Cyclone Tracy: Psychological and social consequences. In J. I. Reid (Ed.), *Planning for people in natural disasters* (pp. 116–123). Townsville, Queensland, Australia: James Cook University of North Queensland.

Mitchell, W. A. (1977). Partial recovery and reconstruction after disaster: The Lice case. *Mass Emergencies, 2,* 233–247.

Morris, J. (1974). *Conundrum.* Harcourt, Brace & Jovanovich.

Nehnevajsa, J., & Wong, H. (1977). *Flood preparedness 1977: A Pittsburgh area study.* Pittsburgh: University of Pittsburgh, University Center for Urban Research.

Oliver-Smith, A. (1977). Traditional agriculture, central places, and postdisaster urban relocation in Peru. *American Ethnologist, 4*(1), 102–116.

Oliver-Smith, A. (1979). The Yungay avalanche of 1970: Anthropological perspectives on disaster and social change. *Disasters, 3*(1), 95–101.

Orner, R. (1988). *The human element in post war settlement reconstruction: Tragedy.* Paper presented at the Post War Settlement Reconstruction Workshop, Institute of Advanced Architectural Studies, University of York, England.

Orr, D. W. (1979). Catastrophe and social order. *Human Ecology, 7,* 41–52.

Perrow, C. (1984). *Normal accidents: Living with high risk technologies.* New York: Basic Books.

Perry, R. W., & Muskkatel, A. H. (1984). *Disaster management: Warning response and community relocation.* London: Quorum Books.

Ploeger, A. (1974). Lengede-Zehn Jahre danach: Medizinisch-Psychologische Katamnese einer extremen Belastungssituatuion [Lengede—Ten years later: Ten-year follow-up of miners trapped for two weeks in 1963]. *Psychotherapie und Medizinsche Psychologie, 24,* 137–143.

Popovic, M., & Petrovic, D. (1964). After the earthquake. *Lancet, 2,* 1169.

Prince, S. H. (1920). *Catastrophe and social change, based upon a sociological study of the Halifax disaster.* Unpublished Ph.D. thesis, New York: Columbia University Department of Political Science.

Quarantelli, E. L. (1982). *Sheltering and housing after major community disasters: Case studies and general conclusions.* Columbus, Ohio: Disaster Research Center, Ohio State University.

Raphael, B. (1977). The Granville train disaster—Psychological needs and their management. *Medical Journal of Australia, 1,* 303–305.

Raphael, B. (1986). *When disaster strikes: A handbook for the caring professions.* London: Hutchinson.

Rossi, P. H., Wright, J. D., Weber-Burdin, E., & Pereira, J. (1983). *Victims of the environment: Loss from natural hazards in the United States, 1970–1980.* New York: Plenum Press.

Rubin, C. B., & Barbee, D. G. (1985). Disaster recovery and hazard mitigation: Bridging the intergovernmental gap. *Public Administration Review, 45,* 57–63.

Sarason, I. G., & Sarason, B. R. (1987). *Abnormal psychology: The problem of maladaptive behavior* (5th ed.). Englewood Cliffs, NJ: Prentice Hall.

Schiff, M. (1977). Hazard adjustment, locus of control, and sensation seeking: Some null findings. *Environment and Behavior, 9,* 233–254.

Schorr, J. K., Goldsteen, R., & Cortes, C. H. (1982, August). *The long-term impact of man-made disaster: A sociological examination of a small town in the aftermath of the Three Mile Island nuclear reactor accident.* Paper presented at the Tenth World Congress of Sociology, Mexico City, Mexico.

Schwarzwald, J., Solomon, Z., Weisenberg, M., & Mikulincer, M. (1987). Validation of Impact of Event Scale for psychological sequelae of combat. *Journal of Consulting and Clinical Psychology, 55,* 251–256.

Seligman, M. W. P. (1974). Depression and learned helplessness. In R. J. Friedman & M. M. Kalz (Eds.), *The psychology of depression: Contemporary theory and research* (pp. 83–125). Washington, DC: V. H. Winston.

Snarr, D. N., & Brown, L. E. (1978). Post-disaster housing in Honduras after Hurricane Fifi: An assessment of some objectives. *Mass Emergencies, 3,* 239–250.

Spielberger, C. D., & Sarason, I.G. (1985). (Eds.). *Stress and anxiety.* New York: McGraw-Hill.

Syren, S. (1981). Organiserad aktivitet efter Tuveskredet [The Tuve land-slide organized activities]. *Disaster Studies, 10.* Uppsala, Sweden: Uppsala University.

Takuma, T. (1972). Immediate responses at disaster sites. *Proceedings of the Japan-United States Disaster Research Seminar: Organizational and community responses to disasters* (pp. 184–195). Columbus, OH: Disaster Research Center, Ohio State University.

Tausig, M. (1982). Measuring life events. *Journal of Health and Social Behavior, 23,* 52–64.

Taylor, V., Ross, G. A. & Quarantelli, E. L. (1976). *Delivery of mental health services in disasters: The Xenia tornado and some implications.* Disaster Research Center, Ohio State University.

Thompson, J. A. (1985). *Psychological aspects of nuclear war.* New York: Wiley.

Tonkinson, R. (1979). The paradox of permanency in a resettled New Hebridean community. *Mass Emergencies, 4,* 105–116.

UNDRO. (1977a). *Case report: Earthquake* (24th November, 1976). Turkey: Van Province.

UNDRO. (1977b). *Emergency shelter study, phase 1, volume 1, the provision of emergency shelter: Issues and perspectives.* New York: Office of the United Nations Disaster Relief Co-ordinator (submitted in 1977).

UNDRO. (1980). *Natural disasters and vulnerability analysis*, Report of Expert Group Meeting. Geneva: United Nations.

UNDRO. (1982). *Shelter after disaster: Guidelines for assistance.* New York: United Nations.

UNDRO. (1988). *Disaster news in brief* (7th January—31st December, 1987). New York: United Nations.

United Nations High Commissioner for Refugees Program (UNHCR). (1982). *Handbook for emergencies.* Geneva: United Nations.

Warheit, G. J. (1976). A note on natural disasters and civil disturbances: Similarities and differences. *Mass Emergencies, 1,* 131–137.

Warrick, R. A., Anderson, J., Dowing, T., Lyons, J., Ressler, J., Warrick, M., & Warrick, T. (1981). *Four communities under ash after Mount St. Helens.* Boulder, CO: Institute of Behavioral Science, University of Colorado.

Wilson, J. P. (1978). *The forgotten warrior.* Washington, DC: Disabled American Veterans.

Wilson, J. P. (1980). Conflict, stress and growth: The effects of war on psychosocial development of Vietnam veterans. In C. R. Figley (Ed.), *Strangers at home: Vietnam since the war.* New York: Praeger

Wilson, J. P. (1988). Understanding the Vietnam veteran. In F. Ochberg (Ed.), *Post-traumatic therapy and victims of violence* (pp. 227–254). New York: Brunner/Mazel.

Wilson, J. P., Harel, Z., & Kahana, B. (Eds.). (1988). *Human adaptation to extreme stress: From the Holocaust to Vietnam.* New York: Plenum Press.

Wilson, J. P., Smith, W. K., & Johnson, S. (1985). A comparative analysis of PTSD among various survivor groups. In C. R. Figley (Ed.), *Trauma and its wake.* New York: Brunner/Mazel.

Zargar, A. (1988). Reconstruction and development. *Open House International, 13*(2), 22–36.

Index